Grainger & Allison's Diagnostic Radiology

A Textbook of Medical Imaging

FIFTH EDITION

VOLUME TWO

Edited by

Andy Adam
MBBS (Hons), FRCP, FRCS, FRCR, FFRRCSI (Hon)
Professor of Interventional Radiology
Department of Radiology
St Thomas' Hospital
King's College London
London, UK

Adrian K. Dixon
MD, FRCR, FRCP, FRCS, FMedSci, FFRRCSI (Hon), FRANZCR (Hon)
Professor of Radiology
Department of Radiology
Addenbrooke's Hospital
University of Cambridge
Cambridge, UK

Consulting Editors

Ronald G. Grainger
MB ChB(Hons), MD, FRCP, DMRD, FRCR, FACR(Hon), FRACR(Hon)
Professor of Diagnostic Radiology (Emeritus)
University of Sheffield
Honorary Consultant Radiologist,
Royal Hallamshire Hospital and Northern General Hospital
Sheffield, UK

David J. Allison
BSc, MD, MRCS, LRCP, MBBS, DMRD, FRCR, FRCP
Emeritus Professor of Imaging
Imperial College
London, UK

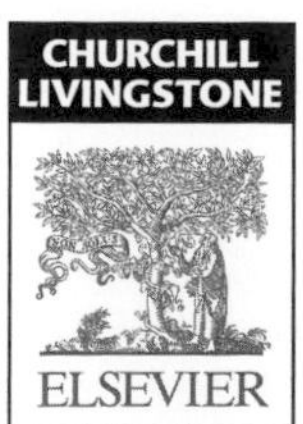

ELSEVIER
CHURCHILL
LIVINGSTONE

An imprint of Elsevier Limited

Fifth edition published 2008

ISBN 978-0-443-10163-2

British Library Cataloguing in Publication Data
A catalogue record for this book is available from the British Library.

Library of Congress Cataloging in Publication Data
A catalog record for this book is available from the Library of Congress.

Notice
Medical knowledge is constantly changing. Standard safety precautions must be followed, but as new research and clinical experience broaden our knowledge, changes in treatment and drug therapy may become necessary or appropriate. Readers are advised to check the most current product information provided by the manufacturer of each drug to be administered to verify the recommended dose, the method and duration of administration, and contraindications. It is the responsibility of the practitioner, relying on experience and knowledge of the patient, to determine dosages and the best treatment for each individual patient. Neither the publisher nor the editors and authors assume any liability for any injury and/or damage to persons or property arising from this publication.

The Publisher

The publisher's policy is to use **paper manufactured from sustainable forests**

Printed in China
Last digit is the print number: 9 8 7 6 5 4 3 2 1

T021520

Not to be
taken from
the Library

Grainger & Allison's

Diagnostic Radiology

A Textbook of Medical Imaging

This work is dedicated
with our love
to

our dear wives

Ruth *Deirdre*

Jane *Anne*

and
our children and their families

R.G.G. **D.J.A.**

A.A. **A.K.D.**

Commissioning Editor: *Michael Houston*
Development Editor: *Gavin Smith*
Editorial Assistant: *Elizabeth MacSween*
Project Manager: *Naughton Project Management/Anne Dickie*
Illustration Manager: *Gillian Richards*
Illustrators: *David Graham, Paul Banville*
Text Design: *Jayne Jones*
Cover Design: *Stewart Larking*
Marketing Managers: *Ria Timmerman (UK), Matt Latuchie (USA)*

Contents

SECTION EIGHT
Paediatric imaging

SECTION NINE
Miscellaneous disorders

Contributors

† : deceased

Andy Adam MBBS (Hons), FRCP, FRCS, FRCR, FFRRCSI (Hon)
Professor of Interventional Radiology
Department of Radiology
St Thomas' Hospital
King's College London
London, UK

E. Jane Adam MBBS, MRCP, FRCR
Consultant Radiologist
Department of Radiology
St George's Hospital
London, UK

Judith E. Adams MBBS, FRCR, FRCP
Chair, Diagnostic Radiology
Imaging Science and Biomedical Engineering
University of Manchester
Honorary Consultant Radiologist
Royal Infirmary
Manchester, UK

David J. Allison BSc, MD, MRCS, LRCP, MBBS, DMRD, FRCR, FRCP
Emeritus Professor of Imaging
Imperial College
London, UK

Sandra Allison MD
Assistant Professor of Radiology
Director, Radiology Residency Program
Director, Ultrasound
Georgetown University Hospital
Washington DC, USA

Philip Anslow FRCR
Consultant Neuroradiologist
Department of Radiology
Radcliffe Infirmary
Oxford, UK

Susan M. Ascher MD
Georgetown University Medical Center
Washington DC, USA

Zelena A. Aziz MD, MRCP, FRCR
Consultant Radiologist
Department of Radiology
London Chest Hospital
London, UK

Clive I. Bartram FRCS, FRCP, FRCR
Emeritus Consultant, St Mark's Hospital and Honorary Professor of Gastrointestinal Radiology
Faculty of Medicine
Imperial College
London, UK

Philip P. W. Bearcroft FRCP, FRCR
Consultant Radiologist
Department of Radiology
Cambridge University Hospitals NHS Foundation Trust
Addenbrooke's Hospital
Cambridge, UK

Anna-Maria Belli DMRD, FRCR
Consultant Vascular Radiologist and Reader in Radiology
Department of Radiology
St George's Hospital
London, UK

Anthony R. Berendt BM, BCh, FRCP
Consultant Physician-in-Charge
Bone Infection Unit
Nuffield Orthopaedic Centre
Oxford, UK

Lol Berman FRCP, FRCR
University Department of Radiology
Addenbrooke's Hospital
Cambridge, UK

Martin J. K. Blomley†

Carol A. Boles MD
Associate Professor of Radiology
Associate, Surgical Sciences
Orthopedic Surgery
Wake Forest University
North Carolina, USA

Jamshed B. Bomanji MBBS, MSc, PhD
Consultant in Nuclear Medicine
UCLH Trust
Middlesex Hospital
London, UK

Gisele Brasil Caseiras PhD
Research Fellow
Insitute of Neurology
University College London
London, UK

Jackie E. Brown BDS, MSc, FDSRCP, DDRRCR
Consultant Oral and Maxillofacial Radiologist
Kings College London Dental Institute
Guy's Dental Hospital
London, UK

Dina F. Caroline MD, PhD
Professor Emerita
Department of Radiology
Temple University Hospital
Philadelphia
Pennsylvania, USA

Silvia D. Chang MD, FRCP(C)
Assistant Professor
University of British Columbia
Department of Radiology
Vancouver General Hospital
Vancouver, Canada

W. K. 'Kling' Chong BMedSci, MD, MRCP, FRCR
Consultant Neuroradiologist
Department of Radiology
Great Ormond Street Hospital for Children NHS Trust
London, UK

Bairbre Connolly MBBCh, BAO, FRCSI, MCH, FFRRCSI, FRCP(C)
Medical Director and Division Head of Image Guided Therapy
Pediatric Interventional Radiologist
Assistant Professor, University of Toronto
Department of Diagnostic Imaging
The Hospital for Sick Children
Toronto, Canada

Susan J. Copley MBBS, MD, MRCP, FRCR
Consultant Radiologist and Honorary Senior Lecturer
Radiology Department
Hammersmith Hospital
London, UK

David O. Cosgrove MA, MSc, FRCP, FRCR
Emeritus Professor
Imaging Sciences Department
Faculty of Medicine
Imperial College
Hammersmith Hospital
London, UK

Nigel Cowan PGDipLATHE, FRCP
Oxford, UK

Justin J. Cross MRCP, FRCR
Consultant Neuroradiologist
Department of Radiology
Addenbrooke's Hospital
Cambridge, UK

Paras Dalal BSc, MRCP, FRCR
Research Fellow in Thoracic Imaging
Department of Radiology
Royal Brompton Hospital
London, UK

Maria Daskalogiannaki MD
Registrar in Radiology
Department of Radiology
University Hospital of Heraklion
Crete, Greece

A. Mark Davies FRCR
Consultant Radiologist
Royal Orthopaedic Hospital
Birmingham, UK

Adrian K. Dixon MD, FRCR, FRCP, FRCS, FMedSci, FFRRCSI (Hon), FRANZCR (Hon)
Professor of Radiology
Department of Radiology
Addenbrooke's Hospital
University of Cambridge
Cambridge, UK

Rose de Bruyn DMRD, FRCR
Consultant Radiologist
Department of Radiology
Great Ormond Street Hospital for Sick Children NHS Trust
London, UK

Claudio Defilippi MD
Consultant Radiologist
Department of Radiology
OIRM - S. Anna Hospital
Turin, Italy

Sujal R. Desai MD, MRCP, FRCR
Consultant Radiologist
Department of Radiology
King's College Hospital
London, UK

Robert J. Eckersley PhD
Research Associate
Imaging Sciences Department
Faculty of Medicine
Imperial College
Hammersmith Hospital
London, UK

Andrew J. Evans MRCP, FRCR
Consultant Radiologist
Nottingham Breast Institute
Nottingham City Hospital
Nottingham, UK

Jane Evanson BSc, MBBS, MRCP, FRCR
Consultant Neuroradiologist, Barts & The London Hospital NHS Trust
The Royal London Hospital
London, UK

Laura Fender BMedSci, BMBS, MRCP, FRCR
Consultant Radiologist
Nottingham University Hospital
Nottingham, UK

Alan H. Freeman MBBS, FRCR
Consultant Radiologist
Department of Radiology
Addenbrooke's Hospital
Cambridge, UK

Julia Gates MD
Assistant Professor of Radiology
Department of Radiology
Tufts University School of Medicine
Springfield
Massachusetts, USA

Robert N. Gibson MBBS, MD, FRANZCR, DDU
Professor of Radiology
Department of Radiology
University of Melbourne
Royal Melbourne Hospital
Victoria, Australia

Raymond J. Godwin MA, MB, Bchir, FRCP, FRCR
Consultant Radiologist
Department of Radiology
West Suffolk Hospital
Suffolk, UK

Karen Goldstone BSc, MSc, Csci, FIPEM
Radiation Protection Advisor
Acting Head of Department of Medical Physics and Clinical Engineering
East Anglian Regional Radiation Protection Service (EARRPS)
Addenbrooke's Hospital
Cambridge, UK

Philip C. Goodman MD
Professor of Radiology
Chief, Thoracic Imaging Division
Department of Radiology
Duke University Medical Center
Durham
North Carolina, USA

Isky Gordon FRCR, FRCP
Professor of Paediatric Imaging
Institute of Child Health
London, UK

Nicholas Gourtsoyiannis FRCR (Hon)
Professor of Radiology
University of Crete
Faculty of Medicine
Heraklion, Crete
Greece

Andrew J. Grainger BM, BS, MRCP, FRCR
Consultant Radiologist
Chapel Allerton Orthopaedic Centre
Leeds Teaching Hospitals
Leeds, UK

Ronald G. Grainger MB ChB(Hons), MD, FRCP, DMRD, FRCR, FACR(Hon), FRACR(Hon)
Professor of Diagnostic Radiology (Emeritus)
University of Sheffield
Honorary Consultant Radiologist
Royal Hallamshire Hospital and Northern General Hospital
Sheffield, UK

Philippe Grenier FRCR (Hon)
Professor of Radiology
Service de Radiologie Polyvalente Diagnostique et Interventionnelle
Hôpital Pitié-Salpêtrière
Paris, France

Roxana S. Gunny BS, BSc, MRCP, FRCR
Consulant Neuroradiologist
Department of Radiology
Great Ormond Street Hospital for Children NHS Trust
London, UK

Christine M. Hall MBBS, DMRD, FRCR MD
Professor of Paediatric Radiology
Great Ormond Street Hospital for Children NHS Trust
London, UK

David M. Hansell MD, FRCP, FRCR, LRSM
Professor of Thoracic Imaging
Department of Radiology
Royal Brompton Hospital
London, UK

George G. Hartnell FRCR, FRCP
Director of Cardiovascular and Interventional Radiology
Department of Radiology
Baystate Medical Center
Springfield
Professor of Radiology
Tufts University Medical School
Boston
Massachusetts, USA

Hedvig Hricak MD, Dr. Med, SC, Dr. h.c, FRCR (Hon)
Chairman, Department of Radiology
Carroll and Milton Petrie Chair
Professor of Radiology, Weill Medical College of Cornell University
Memorial Sloan-Kettering Cancer Center
New York, USA

James E. Jackson MRCP, FRCR
Consultant Radiologist
Department of Imaging
Hammersmith Hospital
London, UK

H. Rolf Jäger FRCR, MD
Reader in Neuroradiology
Institute of Neurology
University College London
Honorary Consultant Neuroradiologist
The National Hospital for Neurology and Neurosurgery and University College Hospital
London, UK

Jonathan J. James BMBS, FRCR
Consultant Radiologist
Nottingham Breast Institute
Nottingham City Hospital
Nottingham, UK

Renee M. Kendzierski DO
Assistant Professor of Radiology
Department of Radiology
Temple University Hospital
Philadelphia
Pennsylvania, USA

Dow-Mu Koh MRCP, FRCP
Senior Lecturer and Honorary Consultant
Department of Radiology
Royal Marsden Hospital
Sutton, UK

Isla Lang MBChB, MRCP, FRCR
Consultant Paediatric Radiologist
Sheffield Children's Hospital
Sheffield, UK

Adrian K. P. Lim MD, FRCR
Consultant Radiologist and Senior Lecturer
Imaging Sciences Department
Faculty of Medicine Imperial College
Hammersmith Hospital
London, UK

David J. Lomas MA, MB, BChir, FRCR, FRCP
Professor of Clinical Magnetic Resonance Imaging
Department of Radiology
Addenbrooke's Hospital
Cambridge, UK

Sharyn L. S. MacDonald MBChB, FRANZCR
Consultant Radiologist
Department of Radiology
Christchurch Hospital
Christchurch, New Zealand

David MacVicar MA, MRCP, FRCP, FRCR
Consultant Radiologist
Department of Diagnostic Radiology
Royal Marsden Hospital
Sutton, UK

Adrian Manhire BSc, MBBS, FRCP, FRCR
Consultant Radiologist
Nottingham City Hospital
Nottingham, UK

Tarik F. Massoud MA, MD, PhD, FRCR
University Lecturer and Honorary Consultant in Neuroradiology
University Department of Radiology
University of Cambridge School of Clinical Medicine
Addenbrooke's Hospital
Cambridge, UK

Kieran McHugh FRCPI, DCH, FRCR
Department of Radiology
Great Ormond Street Hospital for Sick Children NHS Trust
London, UK

James Meaney FRCR, FFRRCSI
Director of MRI
St James's Hospital
Dublin, Ireland

Hylton B. Meire FRCR, DRCOG, DMRD
Consultant Radiologist (Retired)
King's College Hospital
London, UK

Kenneth A. Miles MD, FRCR, MSc, FRCP
Clinical Imaging Sciences Centre
Brighton and Sussex Medical School
University of Sussex
Falmar, Brighton, UK

Stuart E. Mirvis MD, FACR
Professor of Radiology
Department of Radiology
University of Maryland School of Medicine
Baltimore
Maryland, USA

Sameh K. Morcos FRCS, FFRRCSI, FRCR
Professor of Diagnostic Imaging
University of Sheffield
Consultant Radiologist
Department of Diagnostic Imaging
Northern General Hospital
Sheffield, UK

Robert A. Morgan MBChB, MRCP, FRCR
Consultant Radiologist
Department of Radiology
St George's Hospital
London, UK

Iain Morrison MBBS, MRCP, FRCR
Consultant Radiologist
Radiology Department
Kent and Canterbury Hospital
Canterbury, UK

Nestor L. Müller MD, PhD, FRCPC
Professor and Chairman
Department of Radiology
University of British Columbia
Head and Medical Director
Department of Radiology
Vancouver General Hospital
Vancouver, Canada

Graham Munneke MRCP, FRCR
Consultant in Interventional Radiology
Department of Radiology
St. George's Hospital
London, UK

Alison D. Murray MB ChB (Hons), FRCR, FRCP
Senior Lecturer in Radiology
Department of Radiology
University of Aberdeen
Aberdeen, UK

Richard A. Nakielny FRCR
Honorary Clinical Lecturer
Directorate of Medical Imaging & Medical Physics
Royal Hallamshire Hospital
Sheffield, UK

Hrudaya Nath MD
Professor of Radiology
Department of Radiology
University of Alabama Hospitals
Birmingham
Alabama, USA

Tony Nicholson MSc, FRCR
Consultant Vascular Radiologist
Department of Clinical Radiology
Leeds Teaching Hospitals
Leeds, UK

Amaka C. Offiah BSc, MBBS, MRCP, FRCR, PhD
Consultant Radiologist (Academic)
Great Ormond Street Hospital for Children NHS Trust
London, UK

Simon Padley BSc, MBBS, FRCP, FRCR
Consultant Radiologist
Department of Radiology
Chelsea and Westminster Hospital
London, UK

Martyn N. J. Paley PhD, FInstP
Professor of MR Physics
Academic Radiology
University of Sheffield
Sheffield, UK

Nickolas Papanikolaou PhD
Biomedical Engineer
Department of Radiology
University Hospital of Heraklion
Crete, Greece

Jai Patel MBChB, MRCP, FRCR
Consultant Vascular Radiologist
Department of Clinical Radiology
St James's University Hospital
Leeds, UK

Anne Paterson MBBS, MRCP, FRCR, FFR RCSI
Consultant Paediatric Radiologist
Radiology Department
Royal Belfast Hospital for Sick Children
Belfast, UK

Praveen Peddu MRCS, FRCR
Specialist Registrar in Radiology
Department of Radiology
King's College Hospital
London, UK

A. Michael Peters BSc, MD, MSc, MRCP, MRCPath, FRCR
Professor of Nuclear Medicine
Brighton and Sussex Medical School
University of Sussex
Brighton, UK

William H. Ramsden BM, FRCR
Consultant Paediatric Radiologist
Department of Clinical Radiology
St James's University Hospital
Leeds, UK

Sheila Rankin FRCR
Consultant Radiologist
Department of Radiology
Guy's and St. Thomas' Foundation Trust
London, UK

Padma Rao MBBS, BSc, MRCP, FRCR, FRANZCR
Consultant Paediatric Radiologist
Royal Children's Hospital
Parkville
Melbourne
Victoria, Australia

Christine Reek BSc, FRCR
Consultant Radiologist
Department of Radiology
Greenfield Hospital
Leicester, UK

John H. Reynolds DMRD, FRCR, MMedSci
Consultant Radiologist
Birmingham Heartlands Hospital
Birmingham, UK

Rodney H. Reznek FRANZCR (Hon), FRCP, FRCR
Professor of Diagnostic Imaging
The Centre for Cancer Imaging
St Bartholomew's Hospital and The London Queen Mary's School of Medicine and Dentistry
London, UK

Philip M. Rich BSc, FRCS, FRCR
Consultant Neuroradiologist
Department of Neuroradiology
Atkinson Morley Wing
St George's Hospital
London, UK

Andrea Rockall MD, BS, BSc, MRCP, FRCP
Department of Radiology
St Bartholomew's Hospital
London, UK

Giles Roditi FRCP, FRCR
Consultant Radiologist
Department of Radiology
Glasgow Royal Infirmary
Glasgow, UK

Lee F. Rogers MD
Clinical Professor of Radiology
Department of Radiology
University of Arizona Health Services
Tucson
Arizona, USA

Giles Rottenberg FRCR
Consultant Radiologist
Department of Radiology
Guy's and St. Thomas' Foundation Trust
London, UK

John Rout BDS, FDSRCS, MDentSc, DDRRCR, FRCR
Consultant Oral and Maxillofacial Radiologist
Birmingham Dental Hospital
Birmingham, UK

Michael B. Rubens MB, DMRD, FRCR
Consultant Radiologist
Department of Radiology
Royal Brompton Hospital
London, UK

Asif Saifuddin BSc (Hons), MBChB, MRCP, FRCR
Consultant Radiologist
Department of Radiology
Royal National Orthopaedic Hospital NHS Trust
Stanmore, UK

Evis Sala MD, PhD, FRCR
University Lecturer in Oncology Imaging
University Department of Radiology
Addenbrooke's Hospital
Cambridge, UK

Caron Sandhu FRCR
Consultant Radiologist
Department of Radiology
Guy's and St. Thomas' Hospital
London, UK

Dawn Saunders MD, MRCP, FRCR
Consultant Neuroradiologist
Department of Radiology
Great Ormond Street Hospital for Children NHS Trust
London, UK

Daniel J. Scoffings MRCP, FRCR
Specialist Registrar in Neuroradiology
Addenbrooke's Hospital
Cambridge, UK

Djilda Segerman MA, MSc, MIPEM
Head of Nuclear Medicine Physics
Department of Medical Physics
Brighton and Sussex University Hospitals NHS Trust
Brighton, UK

Kathirkama Shanmuganathan MD
Associate Professor of Radiology
Department of Radiology
University of Maryland School of Medicine
Baltimore
Maryland, USA

Ashley S. Shaw MRCP, FRCR
Consultant Radiologist
Department of Radiology
Addenbrooke's Hospital
Cambridge, UK

Satinder P. Singh MD, FCCP
Associate Professor of Radiology
Director Cardiac CT
Director, Combined Cardiopulmonary and Abdominal Fellowship
Chief of Cardiopulmonary Radiology
Department of Radiology
University of Alabama Hospitals
Birmingham
Alabama, USA

S. Aslam A. Sohaib MRCP, FRCR
Radiology Department
Royal Marsden Hospital
London, UK

Alan Sprigg MBChB, DCH, DRCOG, DMRD, FRCR, FRCPCH
Consultant Paediatric Radiologist
Sheffield Children's Hospital
Sheffield, UK

John M. Stevens MBBS, DRACR, FRCR
Lyshom Department of Neuroradiology
Radiology Department
The National Hospital for Neurology and Neurosurgery
London, UK

Dennis J. Stoker MB, FRCP, FRCS, FRCR
Emeritus Consultant Radiologist
Henley-on-Thames, UK

Nicola H. Strickland BM BCh, MA (Hons), (Oxon), FRCP, FRCR
Consultant Radiologist
Imaging Department
Hammersmith Hospitals NHS Trust
Honorary Senior Lecturer
Imperial College
London, UK

Louise E. Sweeney MBBCH, BAO, DCH, DMRD, FRCR, FFR, RCSI
Consultant Paediatric Radiologist
Radiology Department
Royal Belfast Hospital for Sick Children
Belfast, UK

Mihra S. Taljanovic MD, MA
Associate Professor of Clinical Radiology and Clinical Orthopedic Surgery
Head - Musculoskeletal Imaging Section
Department of Radiology
Tucson
Arizona, USA

Andrew M. Taylor BA (Hons), BM BCh, MRCP FRCR
Consultant Radiologist
Department of Clinical Radiology
Great Ormond Street Hospital for Children NHS Trust
London, UK

Stuart Taylor BSc, MD, MRCP, FRCR
Consultant Radiologist
Department of Intestinal Imaging
St Marks Hospital
Northwick Park
Harrow, UK

Henrik S. Thomsen MD
Professor and Chairman
Department of Diagnostic Radiology
Copenhagen University Hospital
Herlev, Denmark

Paolo Toma MD
Radiologist-in-Chief
Radiology Department
G. Gaslini Institute
Genoa, Italy

Peter Twining FRCR, BSc, BS MB
Consultant Radiologist
Nottingham University Hospital
Nottingham, UK

John A. Verschakelen MD, PhD
Professor of Chest Radiology
Department of Radiology
University Hospitals Gasthuisberg
Leuven, Belgium

Sarah J. Vinnicombe BSc, MRCP, FRCR
Consultant Radiologist
Department of Radiology
St Bartholomew's Hospital
London, UK

Gustav K. von Schulthess MD, PhD
Professor and Director
Department of Radiology
University Hospital
Zurich, Switzerland

Iain D. Wilkinson BSc, MSc, PhD, CSci, ARCP, FIPEM
Reader in Magnetic Resonance & Consultant Clinical Scientist
Academic Radiology
University of Sheffield and Sheffield Teaching Hospitals NHS Foundation Trust
Sheffield, UK

A. Robin M. Wilson FRCR, FRCP(E)
Consultant Radiologist
King's College Hospital and Guy's and St Thomas' Foundation Trusts
London, UK

David J. Wilson MBBS, BSc, FRCP, FRCR
Consultant Musculoskeletal Radiologist
Nuffield Orthopaedic Centre and University of Oxford
Oxford, UK

Stuart J. Yates MSci, MSc, CSci, MIPEM
Principal Physicist
Department of Medical Physics & Clinical Engineering
Cambridge University Hospitals NHS Foundation Trust
Cambridge, UK

Preface

We hope that this 5th edition of *Diagnostic Radiology* will continue to build on the original vision of Professors Grainger and Allison who, back in the early 1980s, saw the need for a 'bible' for doctors studying for postgraduate examinations in radiology, and to provide a bench book for reporting and reference. The success of the first four editions, which were extremely well received by an increasingly international readership, speaks for the realisation of their dream. Few could have predicted at that stage the extraordinary growth of radiology, or its increasing importance within all aspects of modern medicine. The unprecedented expansion in the imaging repertoire, together with the trend for increasing subspecialisation, have led to changes in training and in the methods used for teaching and learning. This book has had to evolve to reflect these changes, adapting to the perceived needs of those facing postgraduate examinations and also to all radiologists who wish to have an up-to-date basic general textbook for ready reference and illustration.

An attempt to cover every subject in detail would have resulted in a huge book that would have been very difficult to use. We have chosen to concentrate on those subjects that most radiologists need to know well, and to pay special attention to the needs of trainee radiologists preparing for examinations. Because training throughout Europe is moving towards a three year basic course followed by two years of training in selected subspecialties, the factual examination in the UK has moved to an earlier stage in training with less emphasis on some of the diagnostic rarities so beloved by examiners of old. The curriculum is now somewhat less comprehensive and the reduction in size of this 5th Edition reflects that – down from three volumes to two. In this electronic age there are many databases of images available on the internet, with accompanying text. Nevertheless, we believe that well structured textbooks remain an essential part of medical education and practice as they present information in a format that facilitates learning, guiding the reader through an unfamiliar field. We are convinced that *Diagnostic Radiology* will remain a valuable resource for many years to come.

We are again extremely grateful to the distinguished international cast of authors who have all worked hard to deliver fresh and up-to-date material. We are also most grateful to Michael Houston, Gavin Smith and Nora Naughton for their professional skills and publishing expertise and to Jeremy Rabouhans for invaluable help with proof reading. We could never have done it without them!

Andy Adam
Adrian Dixon

Acknowledgements

This edition could not have occured without the large amount of work done by all the contributing authors and their colleagues. However, the vision and overall planning of Michael Houston at Elsevier have been fundamental in bringing the book to fruition. So, too, has the meticulous gathering and editing of material by Gavin Smith. Finally, the skilful copy-editing, and other tasks provided by Nora Naughton, and her remarkable team, must not be forgotten; without them the Editors simply could not have managed. All of these colleagues remained remarkably cheerful throughout and kept strong heads even when chapters were late, images missing, and all the other hiccups that can hinder progress in a project of this kind. At a local level, all the Editors would like to thank their various secretaries, technicians and colleagues who have helped proofread, collect material and made various other invaluable contributions.

The Editors

SECTION 5

The Musculoskeletal System

CHAPTER

45 Techniques and Imaging of Soft Tissues

A. Mark Davies and Andrew J. Grainger

The imaging evaluation of the soft tissues has undergone a rapid evolution with the application of computed tomography (CT), magnetic resonance imaging (MRI), and recently high resolution ultrasound (US). Consideration must be given to the financial costs and invasiveness of each technique balanced against the diagnostic reward. No examination should be reported in isolation without knowledge of relevant clinical details and results of previous investigations.

IMAGING TECHNIQUES

Radiography

The relative lack of soft tissue contrast resolution is a well-recognized limitation of radiography. Only those structures exhibiting a radiodensity sufficiently different to that of water can be distinguished from other soft tissues. Thus fat and gas yield a discernible radiodensity less than that of muscle (Fig. 45.1). Increased radiodensity may be seen in soft tissues with haemosiderin deposition, mineralization, be it calcification or ossification, and certain foreign bodies. A low kilovoltage technique will accentuate the density differences between fat and muscle. Density differences can also be maximized with digital radiography where the broad exposure range means that it is difficult to make an inadequate exposure. A free choice of data processing allows control of the grey scales, contrast, etc., which can be optimized to highlight soft tissue disease. When evaluating a radiograph it is important to remember that numerous extraneous factors may mimic soft tissue abnormalities. These include skin folds, clothing, hair artefacts and companion shadows. Also, iatrogenic conditions may pose diagnostic problems to the unwary such as the sites of old bismuth injections in the buttocks and tantalum gauze previously used in hernia repairs.

Ultrasound

Diagnostic ultrasound has been applied to the musculoskeletal system since B-mode techniques became available. There have been rapid developments in ultrasound technology over recent years and these, along with the widespread availability of ultrasound and relatively low cost, have resulted in a vast expansion in the evaluation of the soft tissues. Ultrasound has an important role in the assessment of soft tissue masses, being able to reliably distinguish solid from cystic (Fig. 45.2) and abnormal tissue from normal variants such as accessory muscles. The advent of high frequency (>10 MHz) transducers with their improved spatial resolution, along with other developments such as multifrequency transducers, compound imaging and

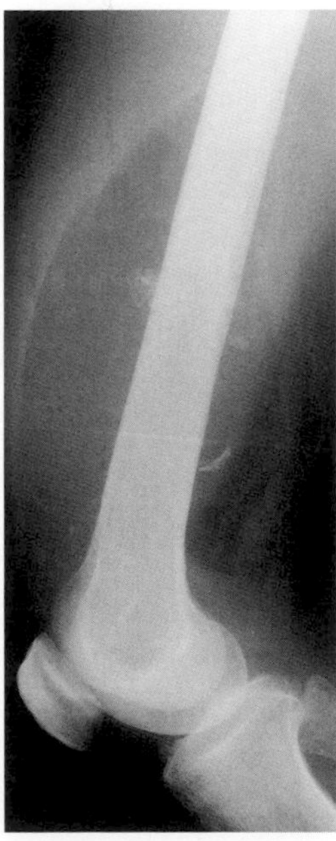

Figure 45.1 Lipoma. Lateral radiograph of the thigh showing a hypodense lipoma containing foci of calcification and ossification.

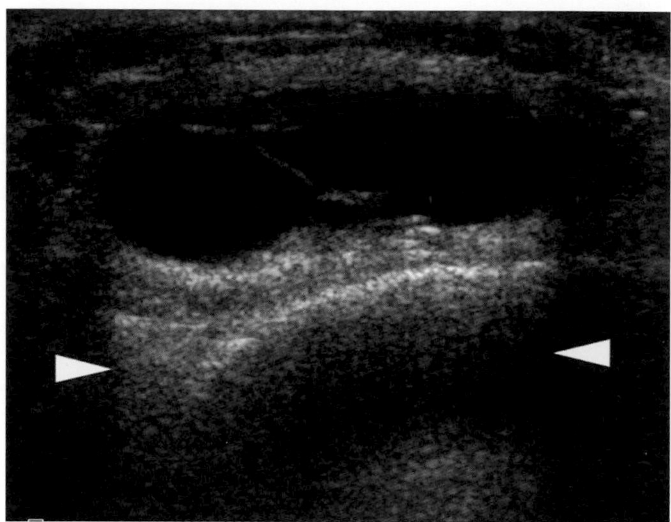

Figure 45.2 Ganglion cyst. Transverse US. Septa are seen within the otherwise anechoic cyst lying on the dorsum of the foot and found to be arising from the talonavicular joint. Its cystic nature is also indicated by the posterior enhancement in reflectivity due to increased transmission of sound waves through the cyst (arrowheads).

beam steering, has meant that further applications for musculoskeletal ultrasound continue to be introduced. Tendons, ligaments, nerves and muscle are now readily shown with ultrasound. The physics of ultrasound means there will always be a trade-off between image resolution and depth of penetration. Nevertheless the majority of musculoskeletal soft tissue structures lie superficially and are readily amenable to high resolution ultrasound assessment. Indeed images obtained on modern equipment can surpass MRI in resolution and detail of information obtained. Other advantages of ultrasound over MRI include its real-time ability to assess structures dynamically, its capability, using Doppler technology, to assess vascular flow and to guide interventional procedures such as joint aspirations and soft tissue biopsies. The trade-off between resolution and penetration means that some deeper structures, such as the deep musculature about the adult hip, remain difficult to assess with ultrasound, particularly in larger patients. Furthermore ultrasound is unable to see behind or into bone. This means that structures in the acoustic shadow of bone are not demonstrated and the bones themselves cannot be examined beyond an assessment of the cortical surface. Other disadvantages of ultrasound over MRI include its relatively limited field of view, marked operator dependency and poor demonstration of findings on hard copy images; although extended field of view imaging, now available on many machines, has gone some way to resolve this last issue (Fig. 45.3A).

Computed tomography

The introduction of computed tomography (CT) proved a revolution in the detection of soft tissue masses and the preoperative staging of soft tissue tumours. Although these functions have now largely been superseded by US and MRI, it remains an adequate alternative where access to these techniques is limited. CT, by virtue of its ability to assign a numerical value (Hounsfield number) to X-ray attenuation, produces good qualitative and quantitative assessment of soft tissues, offering an opportunity to distinguish the nature of a mass whether it is muscle, fat, fluid or tumour, and not solely on morphology (Fig. 45.4). The high spatial resolution of CT, of the order of 1 mm, allows for masses as small as 1 cm to be detected, depending on differential attenuation between the lesion and the surrounding soft tissues. The contrast sensitivity and cross-sectional ability of CT will reveal soft tissue masses and calcifications that are not visible on conventional radiography. Conversely, the demonstration of normal anatomy will exclude all but the smallest lesions. Lesion conspicuity can be increased with intravenous (IV) iodinated contrast medium. The window

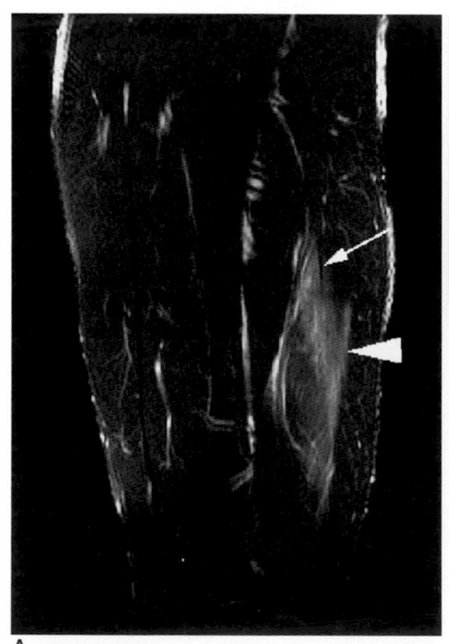

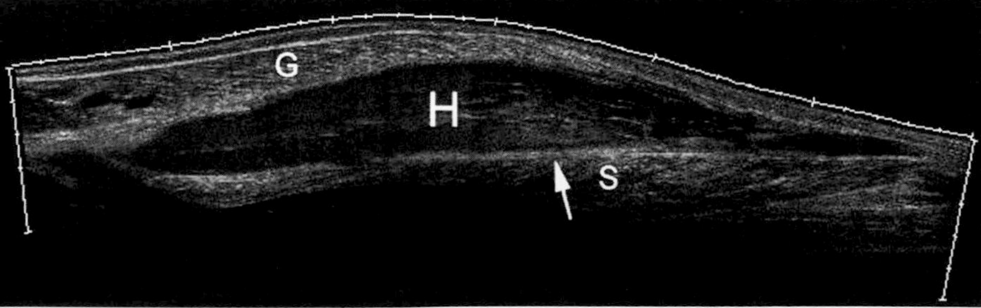

Figure 45.3 Muscle tears. (A) T2-weighted sagittal MRI showing a grade 1 muscle tear of biceps femoris. This is seen as high signal feathery oedematous change within the muscle (arrowhead). The tear has occurred at the myotendinous junction and the tendon is shown (arrow).
(B) Longitudinal extended field of view US demonstrates a grade 2 muscle tear of the medial head of gastrocnemius in a different patient. The retracted medial head of gastrocnemius muscle (G) is seen separated from the underlying tendon aponeurosis (arrow) and soleus muscle (S) by haematoma (H).

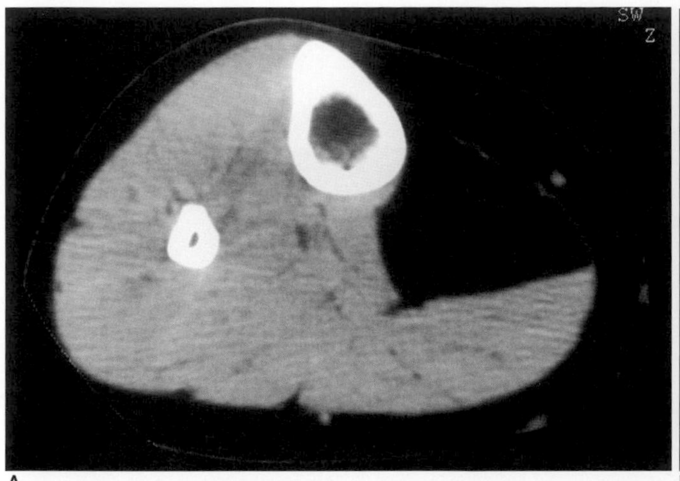

A

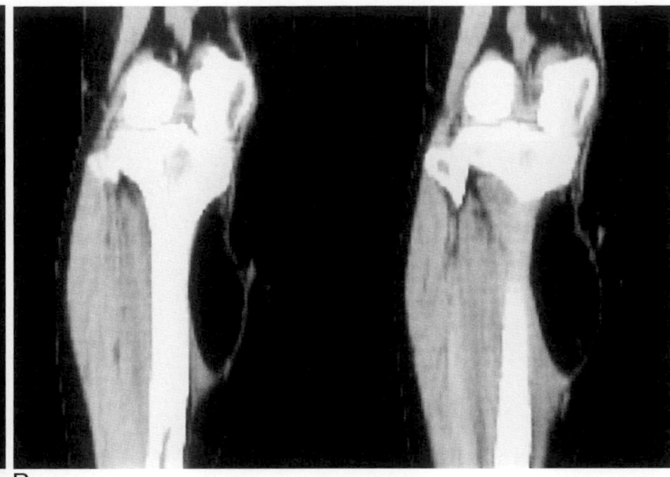

B

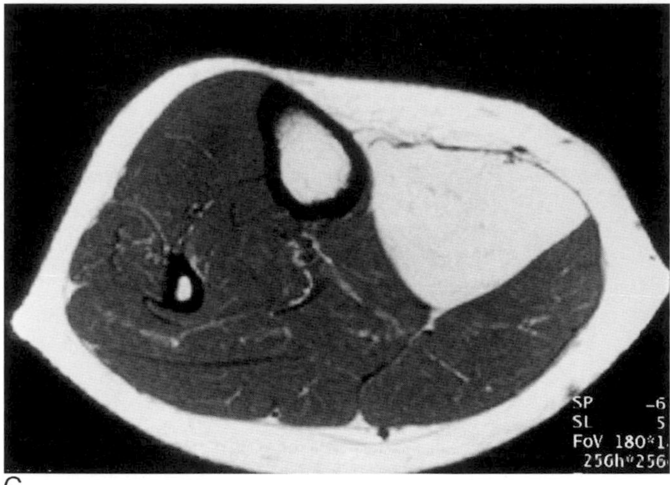

C

Figure 45.4 Lipoma. (A) Axial CT of the calf showing the low attenuation lipoma. (B) Coronal CT reconstructions. (C) Axial T1-weighted MRI showing the lesion to be hyperintense.

levels utilized to review the images will depend on personal preference but narrow window settings are required for small density differences. The full extent of a lesion can be displayed by performing multiplanar reconstructions (Fig. 45.4B).

Magnetic resonance imaging

Like ultrasound, MRI has the distinct advantage of not using ionizing radiation. Its superior soft tissue contrast resolution and multiplanar capability means that it has superseded CT in the imaging of most soft tissue problems. Soft tissue lesions can be categorized by MRI according to site, morphological changes and signal characteristics. To maximize the potential diagnostic yield, protocols should include sequences in at least two orthogonal planes and with differing weighting to illustrate both the T1- and T2-weighted characteristics of the lesion. Although there are continuing major advances in MR technology, spin-echo (SE) sequences will suffice in the evaluation of most soft tissue lesions. Reduced data acquisition times with increased image sharpness are an advantage of fast spin-echo (FSE) techniques, also called turbo spin-echo. A drawback of FSE is the paucity of contrast on the T2-weighted images between fat and fluid thereby reducing the conspicuity of many lesions. This problem can be overcome by the use of fat suppression either as part of the spin-echo sequence or utilizing a short TI inversion recovery (STIR) sequence (Fig. 45.5A). Both T2-weighted fat-suppressed and STIR sequences are particularly sensitive to small variations in the fluid content of lesions and they are ideally suited for the detection of subtle soft tissue abnormalities. Many soft tissue lesions will appear isointense with surrounding musculature on T1-weighted images (Fig. 45.5B).

Gradient echo (GE) techniques were originally introduced to reduce data acquisition times. Occasionally GE images can be helpful by exploiting the increased susceptibility effects that can be found with blood breakdown products (haemosiderin), fine calcifications and small loculi of gas. GE techniques are also useful when performing a dynamic contrast-enhanced sequence (see below).

Contrast enhancement following the IV injection of a gadolinium chelate will result in a decrease in the T1 relaxation time and show up soft tissue lesions due to their different vascularization and perfusion (Fig. 45.5B,C). Enhancement can be most clearly identified on fat-suppressed T1-weighted images but enhancement is rarely necessary in the detection of soft tissue abnormalities where fat-suppressed T2-weighted or STIR sequences will suffice without the additional expense of the contrast medium. Similarly, many soft tissue abnormalities

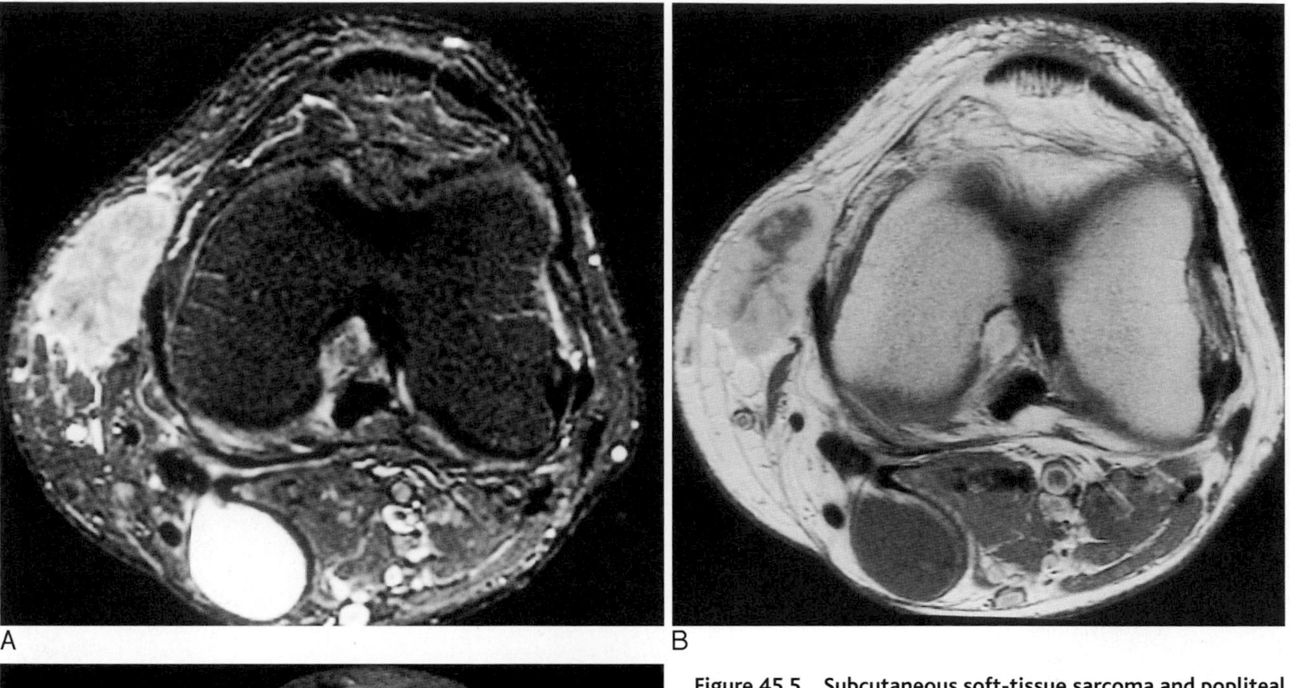

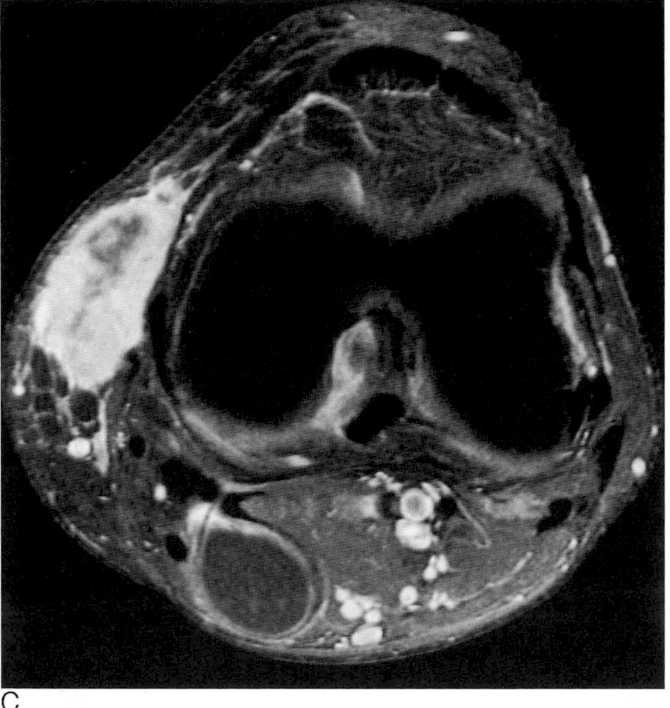

Figure 45.5 Subcutaneous soft-tissue sarcoma and popliteal (Baker's) cyst. (A) Axial T2-weighted fat-suppressed fast spin-echo MRI showing the sarcoma to be hyperintense but heterogeneous, whereas the fluid-filled popliteal 'cyst' (gastrocnemius-semimembranosus bursa) is hyperintense and homogeneous. (B) Axial T1-weighted spin-echo post gadolinium shows enhancement of the sarcoma with central non-enhancement indicating necrosis. Only rim enhancement is evident in the popliteal cyst. (C) Axial T1-weighted fat-suppressed spin-echo post gadolinium showing increased conspicuity of the enhancement as compared to Figure 45.5B.

can be adequately categorized on MRI without contrast medium, e.g. ganglion, lipoma, haemangioma, etc. In equivocal cases, contrast agents can be of value in helping to distinguish cystic from solid lesions and thereby identifying the most appropriate portion of a lesion to biopsy (Fig. 45.5B,C). MRI is the best technique for staging soft tissue tumours and for follow-up. With the increasing use of adjuvant chemotherapy for soft tissue sarcomas, dynamic contrast-enhanced techniques will be increasingly used to assess angiogenesis and response.

Radionuclide imaging

Numerous soft tissue lesions concentrate bone-seeking radiopharmaceuticals[1]. When presented with increased activity in the soft tissues, correlation with a radiograph of the affected area is mandatory. Any soft tissue abnormality with the propensity to develop mineralization can show ectopic activity on skeletal scintigraphy. These include congenital abnormalities such as fibrodysplasia ossificans progressiva (Fig. 45.6), collagen vascular disorders such as dermatomyositis, trauma as in myositis ossificans and neoplasia as in extraskeletal osteosarcoma and synovial sarcoma. Skeletal scintigraphy may be helpful in assessing the maturity of ectopic ossification as can be seen with spinal cord injuries. In this situation surgical resection is best deferred until the ossification becomes stable to minimize the risk of recurrence. Scintigraphy is not routinely indicated in the surgical staging of soft tissue sarcomas.

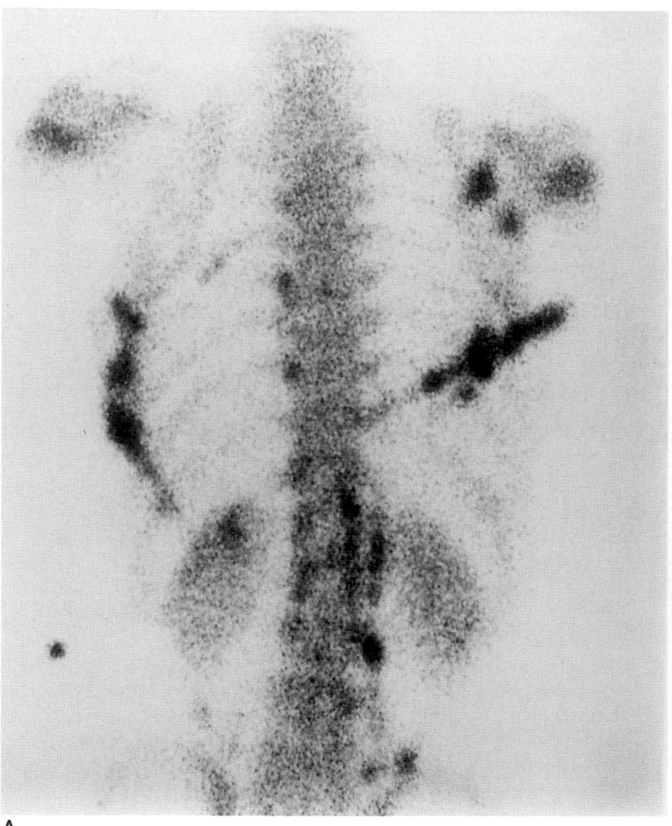
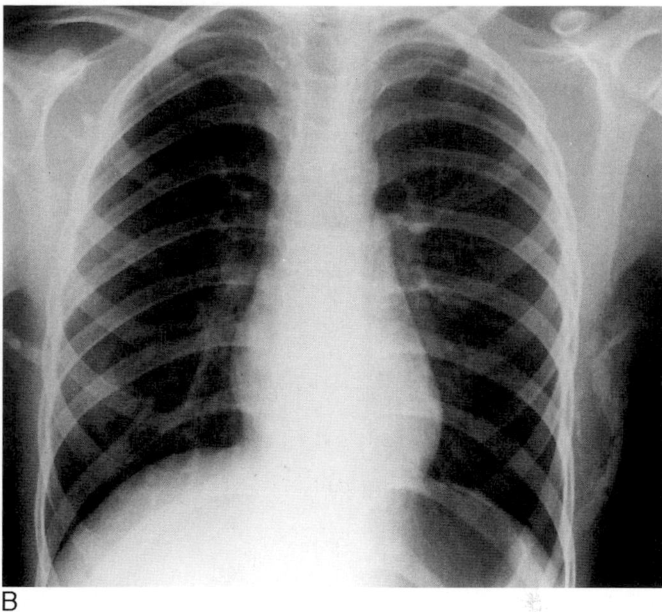

A B

Figure 45.6 Fibrodysplasia ossificans progressiva. (A) Posterior 3-h skeletal scintigram of the trunk showing linear foci of increased activity corresponding to the soft tissue ossification. (B) Chest radiograph showing bilateral chest wall ossification.

Local osseous extension is uncommon and is best demonstrated by MRI. Bone metastases from soft tissue sarcomas are rare in the absence of disseminated disease elsewhere, notably the lungs, but can be seen in alveolar soft part sarcoma and rhabdomyosarcoma. Positron emission tomography (PET) with [F-18] fluorodeoxyglucose has not yet been widely studied for soft tissue lesions; it can be used to assess soft tissue tumour metabolism in order to grade tumours[2] and to assess relapse. It may also be helpful in assessing malignant transformation of peripheral nerve sheath tumours in neurofibromatosis.

RADIOGRAPHIC OBSERVATIONS

CALCIFICATION AND OSSIFICATION

The deposition of amorphous calcium salts within the soft tissues is variously called mineralization or calcification. Two forms of calcium salts may be found in the soft tissues: calcium pyrophosphate dihydrate and calcium hydroxyapatite. If bony trabeculae are discernible within the mineralized focus the term 'ossification' is used, sometimes prefixed with the terms ectopic or heterotopic. There is a wide differential diagnosis, which can be divided into generalized calcification, localized calcification and ossification (Table 45.1).

CALCIFICATION—GENERALIZED

Metabolic disorders

Prolonged elevation of the serum calcium or, more importantly, the serum phosphate, irrespective of the cause, will result in the deposition of calcium salts in the soft tissues. In primary hyperparathyroidism this is typically seen in arteries, cartilage (chondrocalcinosis) and the periarticular tissues. This is uncommon today as primary hyperparathyroidism is usually detected by identification of serum biochemical abnormalities before the more florid radiographic abnormalities have the opportunity to develop. In secondary hyperparathyroidism, typically associated with renal failure, arterial and soft tissue calcification are frequent findings (Fig. 45.7). Periarticular calcification is a prominent feature, particularly in those on long-term renal dialysis (Fig. 45.7B). Conversely, chondrocalcinosis is an infrequent finding in secondary hyperparathyroidism.

Soft tissue calcification has also been described in hypoparathyroidism, pseudohypoparathyroidism and pseudopseudohypoparathyroidism. In hypoparathyroidism there is a deficiency in parathormone (PTH), usually secondary to excision or surgical trauma but rarely idiopathic. Subcutaneous calcification, basal ganglia calcification, osteosclerosis and premature closure of epiphyses are typical of the primary disease. Occasionally, band-like paraspinal calcification may be seen mimicking diffuse idiopathic skeletal hyperostosis. Pseudohypoparathyroidism, a rare inherited X-linked dominant disease in which there is end-organ resistance to PTH, exhibits similar features to hypoparathyroidism. Features that distinguish it from

Table 45.1 CONDITIONS SHOWING SOFT TISSUE CALCIFICATION AND/OR OSSIFICATION

Generalized conditions

1. Metabolic disorders
With hypercalcaemia
Hyperparathyroidism
Hypervitaminosis D
Idiopathic hypercalcaemia
Milk-alkali syndrome
Without hypercalcaemia
Chronic renal disease with secondary hyperparathyroidism
Hypoparathyroidism
Pseudo- and pseudopseudohypoparathyroidism
Gout
Ochronosis (alkaptonuria)

2. Vascular disorders
Arterial and venous
Connective tissue associated with oedema

3. Infection
Bacterial
Miliary tuberculosis
Leprosy (nerves)
Parasitic
Cysticercosis
Guinea worm (dracunculosis)
Loa-loa
Armillifer armillatus

4. Connective tissue disorders
Congenital
Fibrodysplasia ossificans progressiva
Ehlers–Danlos syndrome
Pseudoxanthoma elasticum
Werner's syndrome
Acquired
Calcium pyrophosphate deposition disease (CPPD)
Hydroxyapatite deposition disease (HADD)
Dermatomyositis
Progressive systemic sclerosis (scleroderma)
CREST syndrome (calcification, Raynaud's phenomenon, oesophageal dysmotility, scleroderma, telangiectasia)

5. Miscellaneous
Tumoral calcinosis
Renal osteodystrophy
Idiopathic calcinosis universalis
Sarcoidosis with hypercalcaemia

Localized conditions

1. Soft tissue necrosis
Injection sites
Thermal injuries (burns and frost-bite)

2. Trauma
Haematoma/subperiosteal
Haematoma/cephalhaematoma
Myositis ossificans
Neurogenic heterotopic ossification

3. Tumours
Benign
Haemangioma (phleboliths)
Lipoma
Soft tissue chondroma
Soft tissue aneurysmal bone cyst
Malignant
Synovial sarcoma
Soft tissue osteosarcoma
Soft tissue chondrosarcoma

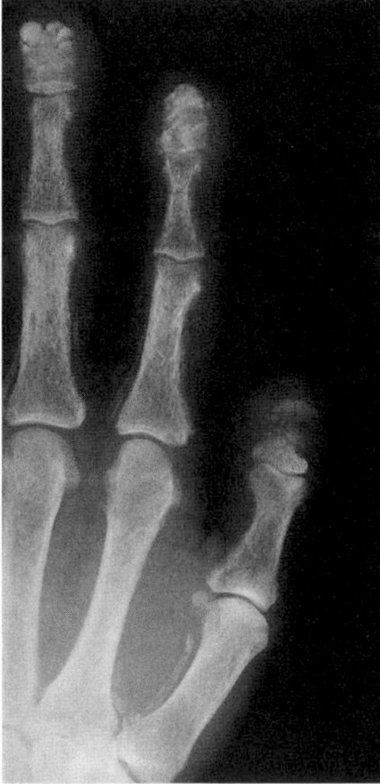

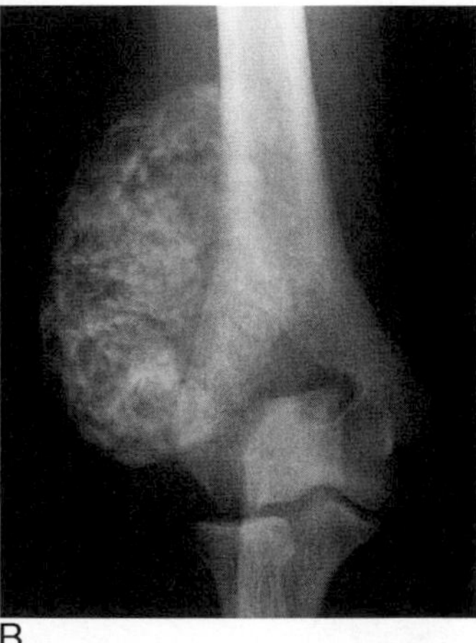

Figure 45.7 Chronic renal failure (two different cases). (A) PA hand radiograph showing the florid features of secondary hyperparathyroidism including terminal phalangeal resorption, soft tissue calcification, subperiosteal resorption, vascular calcification and osteopenia. (B) Tumoral calcinosis with heavy periarticular calcification.

hypoparathyroidism are growth deformities, with broad bones and cone epiphyses, brachydactyly with short metacarpals and metatarsals, especially the first, fourth and fifth, and small exostoses projected at right angles from the bone. In pseudopseudohypoparathyroidism, in which the serum calcium and phosphate levels are normal, the radiographic abnormalities are identical to those of pseudohypoparathyroidism.

Hypervitaminosis D usually occurs due to the administration of excessive levels of the vitamin in the treatment of rickets and osteomalacia but can also be found in granulomatous diseases, Paget's disease and rheumatological conditions such as rheumatoid arthritis and gout. Smooth, lobulated amorphous masses of calcium, usually calcium hydroxyapatite, occur in the periarticular regions, bursae, tendons sheaths, and both within the capsule and cavity of joints. The bony manifestations of vitamin D intoxication depend on the age of the patient, with dense metaphyseal bands and cortical thickening with or without generalized osteosclerosis seen in infants and children. Adults merely show varying degrees of osteoporosis.

A generalized increase in bone density is a feature of idiopathic infantile hypercalcaemia where there are associated clinical manifestations of hypotonia and mental and physical retardation. The condition is thought to be due to inappropriate sensitivity to vitamin D.

Milk-alkali syndrome is reported in patients with chronic peptic ulcer disease and renal impairment in whom the excessive ingestion of alkali, usually calcium carbonate, and milk leads to diffuse calcifications in the soft tissues, kidneys and eyes.

Reversibility depends on the chronicity of the disorder. The soft tissue calcifications are typically periarticular, amorphous and vary in size from small nodules to large masses. Similar deposits may be seen in renal osteodystrophy, collagen vascular disorders, hypervitaminosis D and idiopathic tumoral calcinosis.

Deposits of monosodium urate in gout, so-called 'tophi', are not radio-opaque. However, calcification within the tophi can occur as a secondary phenomenon. The incidence of chronic tophaceous gout has decreased considerably with the introduction of effective anti-uricaemic drugs.

Vascular disorders

Arterial calcification

Some degree of arterial disease is an almost inevitable part of the ageing process in the developed world so that atheromatous calcification is considered a normal variant on most radiographs in middle-aged and elderly patients. The spectrum of calcification ranges from irregular plaques to extensive tram-line calcification predominantly affecting the aorta and pelvic and lower limb arteries. Finer 'pipe-stem' calcification is seen in medial degeneration (Mönckeberg's arteriosclerosis) which also shows a similar propensity for the lower limbs, as does the calcification associated with diabetes mellitus (Fig. 45.8). A finer more generalized pattern of arterial calcification is seen in renal failure and hyperparathyroidism (Fig. 45.7A). Rounded, curvilinear or crescentic calcification is a typical feature of aneurysms on radiographs irrespective of site.

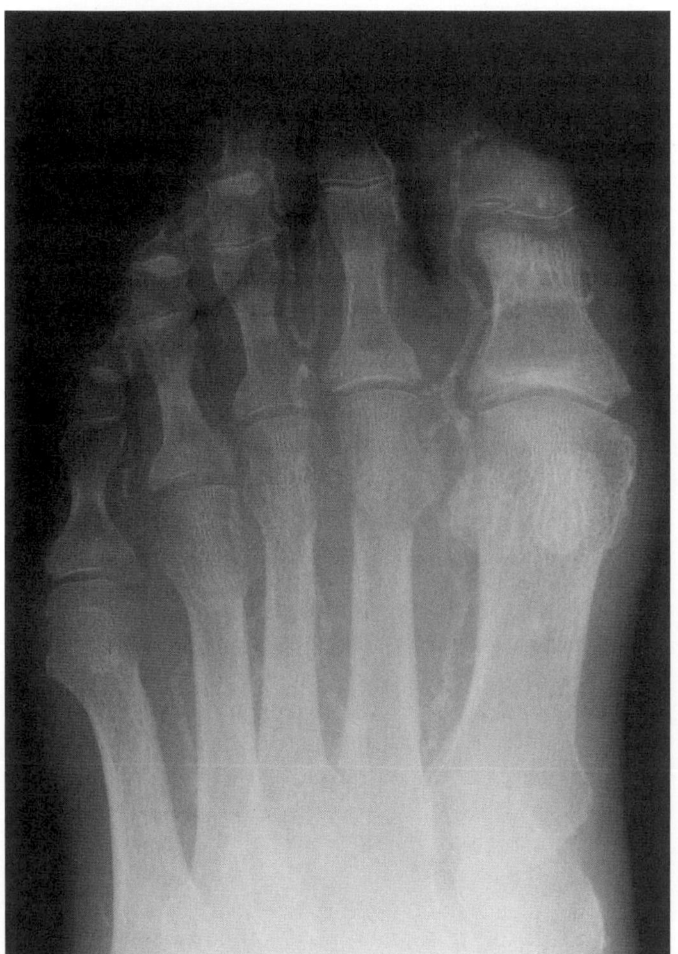

Figure 45.8 Arterial calcification. Heavy vascular calcification in a diabetic patient. Resorption of the first and second terminal phalanges due to repeated infection.

Venous calcification

Venous mural calcification is rare, whereas small circular calcified densities, phleboliths, are common, especially in the pelvic veins. They are also seen in chronic varicosities and haemangiomas, most frequently cavernous (Fig. 45.9A). Phleboliths may be the only radiographic soft tissue abnormality indicative of haemangiomas in patients with Maffucci's syndrome, which is the combination of multiple enchondromas (Ollier's disease) and haemangiomas (Fig. 45.9B). Subcutaneous calcification and organized periosteal new bone formation may occur in chronic oedema associated with venous incompetence.

Infection

Bacterial

Diffuse calcification is extremely rare in bacterial infection. Dystrophic calcification may occur in resolving abscesses, particularly in tuberculosis of the spine (Fig. 45.10). Extensive calcified lymphadenitis is highly suggestive of an old tuberculous infection and, in endemic areas, the fungal infections histoplasmosis and coccidioidomycosis. Leprosy is a rare cause of nerve calcification.

Parasitic

Most of the parasitic infestations that result in calcifications on radiographs are rare in the developed world but crop up from time to time in visitors or immigrants from endemic regions. These infections are produced by worms (helminths). Two of the commoner worm infestations, echinococcosis (hydatid disease) and schistosomiasis, are renowned for calcifications in the liver and urinary tract, respectively, rather than the peripheral soft tissues. Intramuscular or subcutaneous calcification is a feature of the following infections. Cysticercosis infection

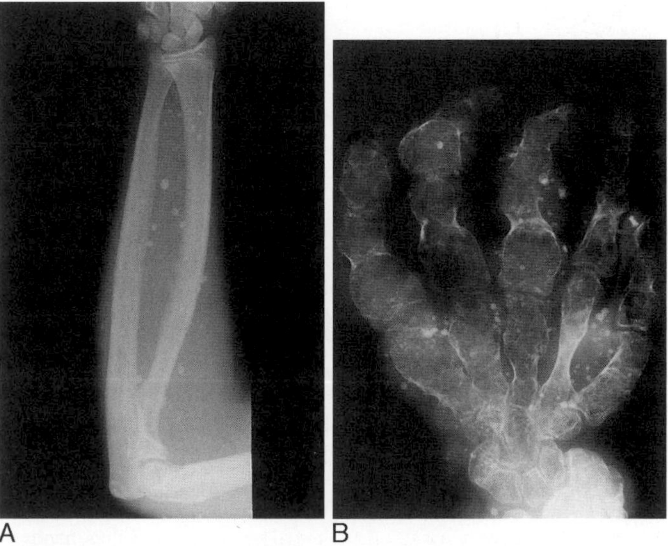

Figure 45.9 Haemangiomas (two different cases). (A) Extensive cavernous haemangioma of the forearm indicated by the numerous phleboliths. (B) Maffucci's syndrome with multiple enchondromas and soft tissue haemangiomas.

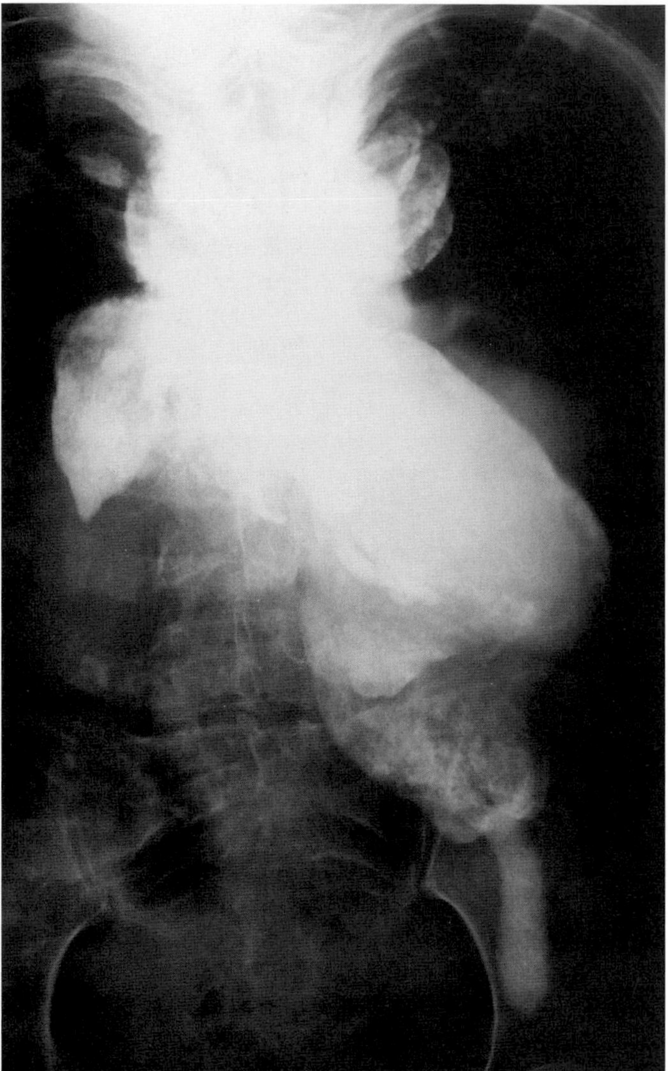

Figure 45.10 Old tuberculosis (Pott's disease) of the spine. The resultant spinal deformity is obscured by the massive calcified paravertebral abscesses.

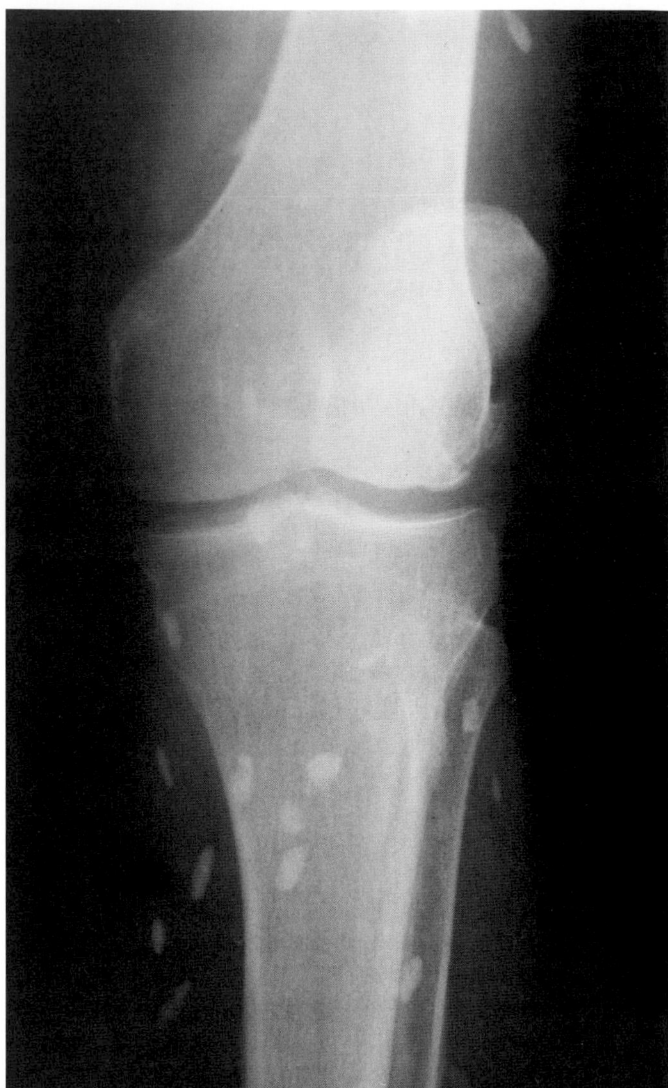

Figure 45.11 Cysticercosis. AP radiograph of the knee showing multiple calcified oval cysts aligned along muscle planes.

remains prevalent in Central and South America, Africa, Asia and parts of Eastern Europe. Cysticercosis is due to the pork tapeworm *Taenia solium*. Humans may be the intermediate host of the larval stage or the definitive host of the adult tapeworm. Deposits of the larval form show a predilection for muscle, subcutaneous tissues and brain where they encyst (*Cysticercus cellulosae*). The calcified dead cysts are typically oval with a lucent centre, up to 1 cm in length, and orientated in the direction of the muscle fibres (Fig. 45.11). Infestation with the guinea worm (*Dracunculus medinensis*) is found in tropical Africa, the Middle East, India, Far East and northern South America. The larvae are ingested in contaminated drinking water and penetrate the intestinal wall to mature in the subcutaneous tissues. When the female guinea worms die, they produce long coiled or curled calcifications which in time can break up due to the action of adjacent muscles. Infection with the filaria *Loa loa* (loiasis) is prevalent in West and Central Africa. Infection is by a fly bite with the larvae developing into the mature worm in the subcutaneous tissues. The dead worm may calcify to produce a fine linear or coiled thread-like appearance. This may occur at any site in the body but is best visualized in the hands and feet.

Connective tissue disorders

Congenital

Fibrodysplasia ossificans progressiva Previously known by the synonym myositis ossificans progressiva this is an inherited autosomal disorder with variable penetrance. It causes progressive swelling and ossification of the fascia, aponeuroses, ligaments, tendons and connective tissue of skeletal muscle, and is entirely unrelated to myositis ossificans. The initial manifestation is swelling of the muscular fascial planes, usually affecting the neck and shoulder girdle first, before the onset of multifocal calcification progressing to ossification. Early changes can be detected by CT, MRI and skeletal scintigraphy (Fig. 45.6). The progressive ossification produces large masses that can bridge between bones, which in the thorax can result in respiratory compromise. The disorder can be suspected before the development of soft tissue swellings by identification of associated skeletal abnormalities. These are short first metacarpals and metatarsals and small cervical vertebral bodies with relative prominence of the pedicles.

Acquired

Crystal deposition diseases Crystal deposition in a joint will stimulate a synovitis due to one of the following crystalline arthropathies:

1 gout
2 calcium pyrophosphate dihydrate deposition disease (CPPD)
3 calcium hydroxyapatite deposition disease (HADD)
4 mixed crystal deposition disease.

CPPD is the general term for the deposition of calcium pyrophosphate dihydrate crystals in and around joints, and in the annulus of the intervertebral disc. The latter is a useful distinguishing feature from ochronosis which involves the nucleus pulposus. There are three manifestations of CPPD, which can occur in isolation or combination. These are: acute intermittent synovitis (pseudogout), chronic pyrophosphate arthropathy and chondrocalcinosis (Fig. 45.12). Pyrophosphate arthropathy has many similar radiographic appearances to osteoarthritis. It is for this reason that many cases will pass through orthopaedic clinics simply labelled as osteoarthritis. Features suggestive of pyrophosphate arthropathy include unusual distribution (e.g. patellofemoral, radiocarpal and elbow joints), prominent subchondral cyst formation and relative paucity of osteophytes. Chondrocalcinosis affects both fibrocartilage (menisci, triangular fibrocartilage, symphysis pubis and annulus fibrosus) and hyaline cartilage of the knee, wrist, elbow and hip (Fig. 45.12). CPPD is associated with many conditions, such as hyperparathyroidism, haemochromatosis, gout, Wilson's disease and diabetes mellitus.

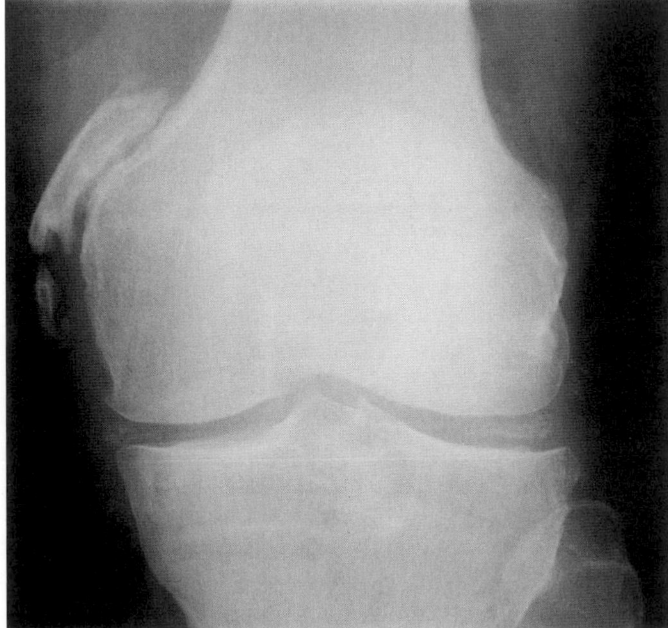

Figure 45.12 Chondrocalcinosis of the menisci. Ossification adjacent to the medial femoral condyle indicates old medial collateral ligament injury (Pellegrini–Stieda lesion).

HADD typically has a monoarticular presentation in the middle-aged and elderly. It is characterized by homogeneous cloud-like periarticular calcification, most commonly affecting the shoulder in and around the supraspinatus tendon (Fig. 45.13). Aetiology is thought to be related to repetitive minor trauma with a cycle of necrosis and inflammation leading to dystrophic calcification. Pain, which can be severe, is related to the release of crystals into the surrounding tissues, most notably joints and bursae. Over time, dependent on the clinical course, the calcifications may increase in size, remain unchanged or regress.

Dermatomyositis This is a condition of unknown aetiology that produces inflammation and muscle degeneration. It is more common in women than men, typically of middle age, but a severe form can be seen in children. It is frequently associated with nonspecific subcutaneous calcification with less common, albeit characteristic, sheet-like calcification along fascial and muscle planes, particularly involving the proximal large muscles. The major differential diagnoses for such calcification are idiopathic calcinosis universalis and hyperparathyroidism. The childhood form may be associated with hypogammaglobulinaemia or leukaemia. In older patients it may be associated with malignancy; the most common associations are with carcinoma of the bronchus, breast, stomach and ovary.

Progressive systemic sclerosis (scleroderma) This condition, with unknown aetiology, causes small vessel disease and fibrosis in several organs. Scleroderma is the cutaneous manifestation of the disease. It often presents with Raynaud's phenomenon and skin changes. Typical features in the hands are terminal phalangeal resorption (acro-osteolysis) due to pressure atrophy, discrete dense plaques of calcification (calcinosis circumscripta) and occasional intra-articular calcification (Fig. 45.14). Erosive changes can occur which may be due to concurrent rheumatoid arthritis or some form of overlapping condition. The related CREST syndrome is due to the combination of calcinosis,

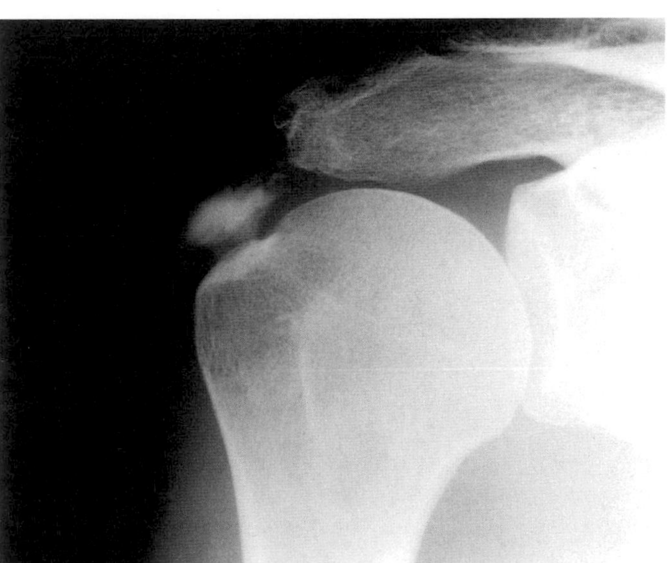

Figure 45.13 Calcium hydroxyapatite deposition disease (HADD). Heavy calcification in the distal supraspinatus tendon.

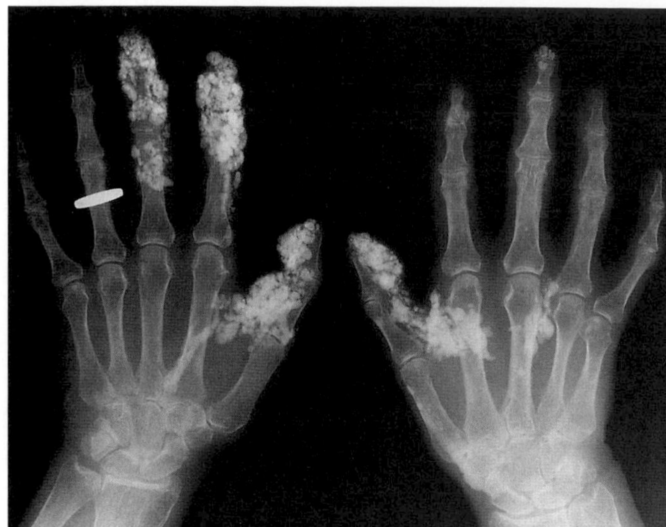

Figure 45.14 Scleroderma. Widespread digital calcification (calcinosis circumscripta).

Raynaud's phenomenon, oesophageal dysmotility, scleroderma and telangiectasia. The only radiographic difference from that described above is that the calcification may also involve the tendon sheaths.

Miscellaneous

Tumoral calcinosis

This is an autosomal dominant condition with variable clinical expression, due to a biochemical defect of phosphorus metabolism. To make the diagnosis it is important that there is a normal serum calcium level and that renal, metabolic and collagen vascular disorders have been excluded. It leads to large multilocular juxta-articular cystic lesions filled with calcific fluid (calcium hydroxyapatite) with or without fluid–fluid levels. By virtue of their site and size, these masses can lead to restricted joint motion, bone erosion and superficial ulceration and secondary infection. Treatment relies on phosphate depletion. Surgery is frequently associated with recurrence of the mass. This condition should not be mistaken for the similarly termed and appearing 'tumoral calcinosis', otherwise known as 'metastatic calcification', secondary to renal failure (Fig. 45.7B).

CALCIFICATION—LOCALIZED

The first radiographic sign of soft tissue mineralization will be faint calcification. In time this may become more extensive and therefore more conspicuous. Alternatively, in certain conditions the mineralization can develop into woven bone. Therefore, localized calcification may be the precursor of conditions typically associated with ossification described below.

Trauma

Any condition that results in focal soft tissue necrosis may predispose to calcification. These include injection sites, radiation damage to the soft tissues and thermal injuries, both burns and frost-bite. Blunt trauma may cause fat necrosis within the subcutaneous tissues with areas of dystrophic calcification. Calcification of atrophic muscles may be seen 1–2 months after severe crush injury (calcific myonecrosis). The appearance may simulate localized tumoral calcinosis with occasional liquefaction[3]. Any haematoma, particularly if in a subperiosteal location, may calcify. This includes the subperiosteal (pericranial) haematoma seen in the skull of babies, usually as a result of birth trauma.

Tumours

Widespread soft tissue calcification is a rare manifestation of disseminated malignancies (e.g. metastases, leukaemia and myeloma) where there is hypercalcaemia associated with extensive bone destruction. Localized intratumoral calcification may occur within any soft tissue tumour due to haemorrhage and/or necrosis. Benign soft tissue tumours with the propensity to mineralize include soft tissue chondromas (punctate or 'ring-and-arc' calcification), lipomas, particularly if in a parosteal location (ossification), haemangiomas (phleboliths) and soft tissue aneurysmal bone cyst. The typical malignant soft tissue tumours that calcify are extraskeletal osteosarcoma, extraskeletal chondrosarcoma and synovial sarcoma (Fig. 45.15). In the latter entity calcification occurs in approximately 30% of patients with a central rather than a peripheral distribution[4]. A rare benign tumour that can mimic myositis ossificans with peripheral calcification is the ossifying fibromyxoid tumour of soft parts.

OSSIFICATION

Many calcifying lesions may proceed to ossification with the production of woven bone. The radiological distinction may not be straightforward. The deposits of calcium salts tend to be more densely sclerotic than comparable amounts of bone. If there is doubt, CT can readily distinguish the amorphous quality of calcium salts from the trabecular pattern of ossification. Heterotopic ossification is a common complication of many conditions (see Table 45.1) and is thought to be due to inappropriate differentiation of fibroblasts into osteoblasts in response to a local inflammatory process. Developmental causes include fibrodysplasia ossificans progressiva, melorheostosis and progressive osseous heteroplasia (Fig. 45.6). The majority of other causes of heterotopic ossification are traumatic in origin.

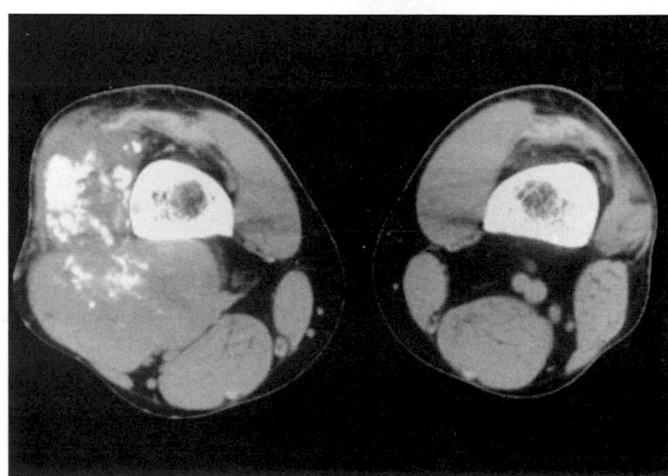

Figure 45.15 Synovial sarcoma. Axial CT demonstrating a soft tissue mass lateral and posterior to the femur containing calcifications.

Soft tissue ossification as a result of surgery is well recognized, particularly after total hip arthroplasty. In most cases the ossification is of little clinical significance, but in a few, pain and restricted motion requires surgical intervention. Post-traumatic or post-surgical ossification is common in tendons and ligaments. Examples include the Achilles tendon and the medial collateral ligament of the knee (Pellegrini–Stieda lesion; Fig. 45.12). Ossification may occur in patients with severe thermal and electrical burns.

Acute detachment or repeated trauma to a tendino-osseous junction can lead to soft tissue ossification with underlying cortical irregularity. In the skeletally immature, an avulsed ossification centre may continue to grow, presenting at a later stage with a large ossified mass in the soft tissues. These types of avulsion injury classically affect the pelvis, particularly the origin of the hamstrings (Fig. 45.16).

Trauma can also be an indirect cause of soft tissue ossification when associated with injuries to the central nervous system, be it prolonged unconsciousness or spinal trauma. In this situation it is known as neurogenic heterotopic ossification. It typically exhibits a periarticular distribution with the hips most commonly affected. The shoulders and elbows are usually only involved with head or higher spinal injuries. Surgical excision is frequently associated with recurrence.

Heterotopic bone formation in muscles, tendons and fascia following trauma is known as myositis ossificans. A very similar condition (radiographically and pathologically) occurring in the absence of trauma is the pseudomalignant osseous tumour of soft tissues; this is also known as pseudomalignant myositis ossificans. Initially there is interstitial haemorrhage with subsequent mineralization. The mineralization is seen first in the periphery; there is a gradual reduction in size of the mass (Fig. 45.17). Both are helpful distinguishing features from a mineralizing soft tissue sarcoma. The lesions will appear hypervascular on angiography and show increased activity on bone scintigraphy. Where possible, early biopsy should be avoided as the immature lesion can pathologically resemble a soft tissue osteosarcoma. The MRI features of the early lesion can also be confusing showing florid perilesional oedema involving the whole affected muscle compartment on T2-weighted or STIR images[5].

GAS IN SOFT TISSUES

Gas/air may be introduced into the soft tissues from within and without the body. It may also be formed directly within the soft tissues. Gas in the soft tissue can be recognized radiographically by increased radiolucency outlining the soft tissue planes. Care should be taken not to confuse ectopic viscera with soft tissue gas. A prime example would be bowel gas within an inguinal hernia which can overlie the soft tissues of the groin or scrotum.

Gas arising within the body

Air may enter the soft tissues whenever there is a breach in the integrity of the lining of either the respiratory or gastrointestinal tract. In the chest and retroperitoneum this is known as surgical emphysema. Common causes in the chest include blunt trauma with a fractured rib puncturing the lung, penetrating lung trauma and following chest surgery. It can also be a complication of interventional procedures such as the insertion of central lines and biopsy and drainage procedures.

Gas formed within the soft tissues is a manifestation of infection (Fig. 45.18). The classic example is gas gangrene which is a bacterial infection caused by several clostridial species. The condition is characterized by a severe toxic state, extensive oedema and necrosis with gas production. The infection usually follows open, contaminated wounds with concomitant vascular compromise. Another form of clostridial infection is

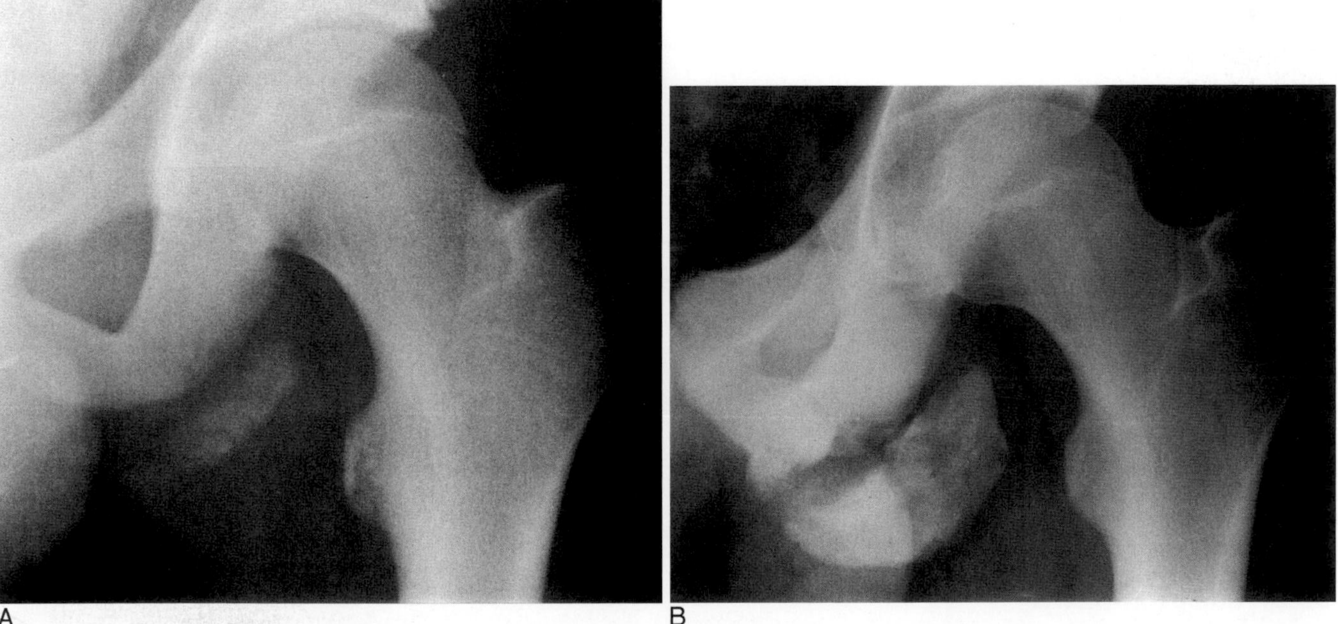

Figure 45.16 Ischial avulsion. (A) Radiograph at presentation shows the avulsed ischial apophysis lying in the soft tissues. (B) Three years later the apophysis has continued to grow to form a large ossified mass.

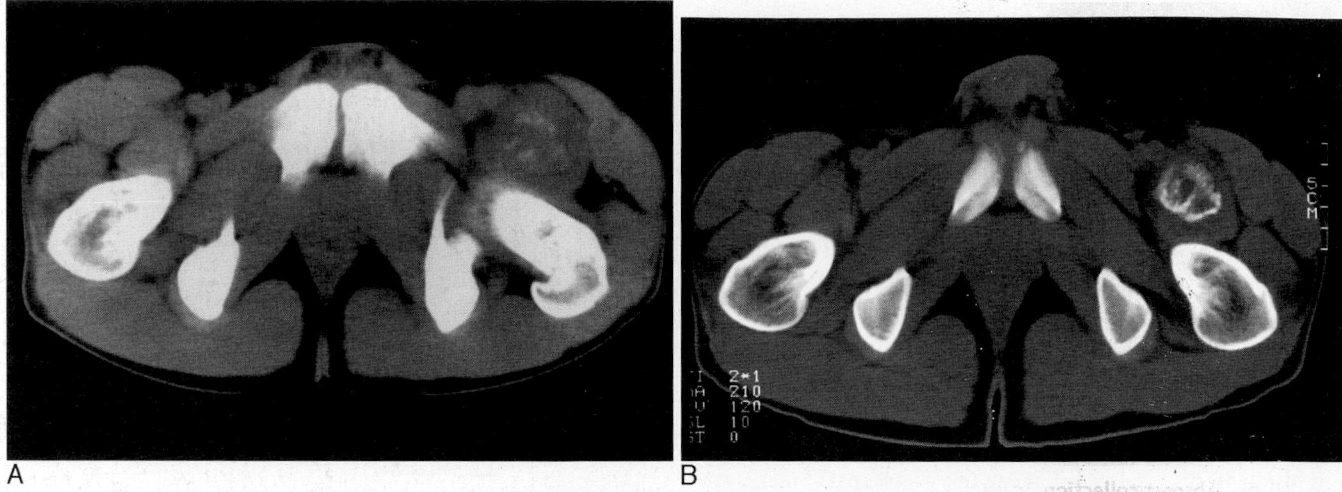

Figure 45.17 Myositis ossificans. (A) Axial CT at presentation showing early peripheral mineralization. (B) Six weeks later there has been maturation with well-organized peripheral ossification.

anaerobic cellulitis where the gas is confined to the subcutaneous and superficial fascial layers. Other anaerobic infections may also produce gas. These include coliforms, anaerobic *Streptococcus*, *Bacteroides* and *Aerobacter aerogenes*. These tend to be less severe than clostridial infections with more localized collections of gas.

Gas introduced from without

Air may be introduced into the soft tissues as a result of penetrating injuries or compound fractures. This can be distinguished from infection in that it is present on the initial radiograph, whereas the gas associated with infection usually takes several days to develop. Dead wood contains considerable air, and thus small wooden foreign bodies within the soft tissues can appear on CT to be comprised entirely of air with no apparent 'solid' component. In time the wood will absorb water from the surrounding tissues and be rendered isodense with muscle. Frequently, air can be identified within joints and soft tissues following therapeutic injections and surgical procedures.

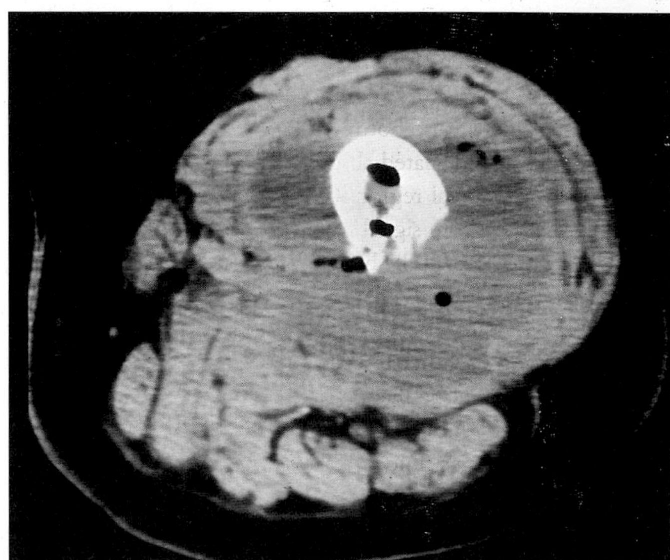

Figure 45.18 Clostridial osteomyelitis. The axial CT shows the relatively hypodense abscess collection surrounding the abnormal femur containing multiple loculi of gas.

SOFT TISSUE INFECTION

Infections in the soft tissues are common and may require percutaneous or surgical intervention. Gas may be seen in the soft tissues in association with infection; this has been discussed in the preceding section, as has the appearance of soft tissue calcification seen with parasitic infections, healing abscesses and tuberculosis. With the exception of soft tissue swelling and blurring of normal fat planes, most soft tissue infections do not give rise to radiographic changes and cross-sectional imaging techniques are required.

Abscess and pyomyositis

Abscesses may develop in the soft tissues either from extrinsic sources, for instance following a puncture wound, or from an intrinsic source either via haematogenous spread or direct spread from a nearby source such as a bowel fistula or infected joint. Unless very deeply placed, abscesses are readily identified on US and appear as predominantly cystic structures, often of a complex multiloculated nature. Posterior acoustic enhancement will be seen. The cyst contents can vary considerably in echogenicity depending on the nature of the collection and on the amount of soft tissue debris present, and may be shown to swirl around with gentle probe pressure. Although the collection itself will not show any Doppler signal, the tissues surrounding the collection may appear markedly hypervascular (Fig. 45.19)[6].

In cases where the infection has resulted from the introduction of a foreign body, this may be still present. Although

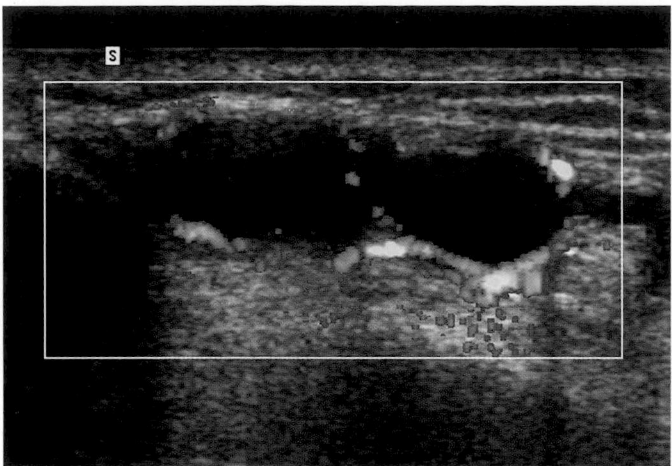

Figure 45.19 Abscess collection. Transverse US with power Doppler. A largely anechoic collection lying in the thigh of this diabetic patient was found to contain pus. Note the marked vascularity of the soft tissues surrounding the collection shown.

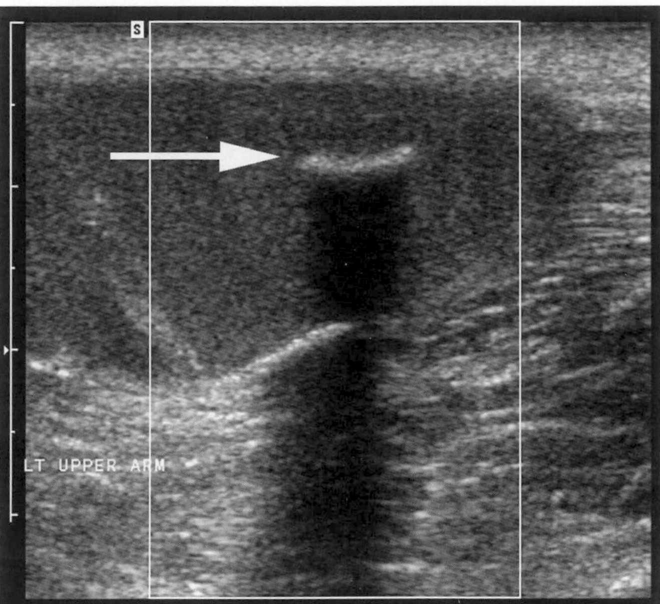

Figure 45.20 Wooden foreign body. Transverse US. A piece of bamboo cane seen here in transverse section (arrow) is located in an abscess collection in the subcutaneous tissues of the upper arm. Note the acoustic shadowing behind the foreign body.

radio-opaque matter may be seen on conventional radiographs, ultrasound is excellent for looking for non-radio-opaque foreign bodies (Fig. 45.20).

MRI and CT will also both show abscess collections and may be required for deep-seated abscesses such as those in the psoas muscle or deep gluteal region. On MRI the collection will be of low to intermediate signal on T1 weighting and high signal on T2 weighting and will show peripheral enhancement with gadolinium. Oedematous change in the surrounding tissues will usually be present and seen as less well defined increased T2 signal, often with a rather feathery appearance. CT will usually show abscesses as a nonenhancing area of lower attenuation than the surrounding tissues, although the presence of haemorrhage or very proteinaceous fluid may result in increased attenuation. The surrounding tissues may enhance following intravenous contrast medium. US or CT is ideally suited for guiding aspiration and drainage of soft tissue abscess collections.

In the western world pyomyositis is most frequently seen in immunocompromised individuals. MRI best shows the generalized change seen throughout the affected muscle in pyomyositis in the form of heterogeneous increased signal on T2-weighted imaging, although ultrasound will also show generalized alteration in echogenicity[7]. As the disease progresses, small pockets of fluid form within the muscle with similar imaging characteristics to abscesses. MRI is the most sensitive investigation in pyomyositis[8].

Cellulitis

Cellulitis represents a superficial infection involving the subcutaneous tissues. Clinically the tissues appear erythematous and swollen. Imaging reveals thickening of the skin and subcutaneous tissues. Fluid is seen tracking between the lobules of subcutaneous fat. On ultrasound these appear as low reflective septa, while on T2-weighted MRI these thickened septa yield increased signal. Increased signal is also seen in the skin itself and underlying fascia. Since these changes are nonspecific and will be seen with noninfective causes of soft tissue oedema, clinical correlation is essential. Imaging remains useful to demonstrate any associated abscess formation and may be required to exclude involvement of other local structures such as bone or joint.

NEUROMUSCULAR DISORDERS

A wide-ranging and diverse group of conditions can be considered under the broad heading of neuromuscular disorders. These include the congenital and acquired myopathies and neuropathies, all of which bring about muscle changes as their end point. Conditions include those affecting the nerve supply to muscles, such as the congenital and acquired spinal muscle atrophies and peripheral neuropathies, and those affecting the muscles themselves such as the congenital, inflammatory and metabolic dystrophies and myopathies. Despite the rather complex range and classification of congenital and acquired neuromuscular disorders, the response that skeletal muscle makes to these conditions and insults is fairly narrow. This means that the changes that can be demonstrated in muscle using conventional imaging techniques are also limited. The key changes seen in muscle pathology are hypertrophy and atrophy, oedema-like change and fat infiltration and calcification. The term 'oedema-like' change is preferred to oedematous, as muscles showing this change on MRI are not actually oedematous when examined histologically[9].

Conventional radiographs have a limited role to play in the diagnosis of these conditions. Fat atrophy may be apparent on plain radiography while calcification within skeletal muscle can be seen both following trauma (as in myositis ossificans) and in inflammatory conditions such as dermatomyositis. These situations are further discussed elsewhere in this chapter.

Hypertrophy and atrophy may be detected using US, although when these changes are generalized they can be difficult to appreciate. Fat infiltration is easier to recognize on US as the normal striated architecture of the muscle is lost and the affected muscles show an increase in reflectivity. The main disadvantage of US is its small field of view, which makes it a difficult tool for examining generalized muscle conditions. US can be useful when nerve compression is suspected as many of the peripheral nerves can be easily followed and causes of nerve entrapment may be identified. US also has a role in guiding muscle biopsies. Atrophy, hypertrophy and fat infiltration are easier to identify on CT and certainly larger areas of muscle can be screened effectively.

Considerable interest exists in the use of MRI in neuromuscular disorders. Normal muscle shows intermediate signal on both T1- and T2-weighted imaging. Indeed, when MRI changes are reported as showing high or low signal, this is usually assessed relative to skeletal muscle. Fat appears bright on T1-weighted imaging and its signal can be suppressed using standard techniques such as inversion recovery and spectral fat suppression. Consequently fat infiltration of muscle is easy to recognize on MRI. Oedema-like change in muscle will appear as increased signal on T2-weighted imaging, and this is most clearly shown on fat-suppressed T2 and STIR imaging.

T1 and fat-suppressed T2 (or STIR) sequences are fundamental to the diagnosis of neuromuscular disorders[10]. While coronal and sagittal imaging may be useful in assessing the longitudinal extent of muscle involvement, it is axial imaging that provides the best demonstration of the muscle compartments for identifying patterns of muscle involvement and the individual muscles or muscle groups involved. Axial imaging also allows the contralateral side to be included in the same field of view, making comparisons easy in asymmetrical disease.

As can be seen, the signal changes seen on MRI in neuromuscular pathology are nonspecific and are generally not helpful in distinguishing between different types of disease. It has been said that more diffuse muscle atrophy is seen in spinal muscle atrophy when compared with the muscular dystrophies, but others have commented that the difference is not as clear-cut as that[10]. The pattern of signal intensity does give some useful information about the chronicity of a muscle disorder. Fat infiltration represents a long-standing irreversible process, while oedema-like signal change represents acute or subacute and potentially reversible muscle damage.

Occasionally, when a muscle undergoes significant fat replacement the fat has the effect of causing pseudohypertrophy of the muscle, although this is a relatively rare finding.

Muscle denervation

MRI is not very sensitive to early changes in muscle following denervation. The earliest reliable changes are seen after around 1 month with the affected muscle or muscles yielding increased signal on T2-weighted and STIR imaging[11]. About a year after denervation fatty infiltration becomes apparent.

SOFT TISSUE INJURY

The advent of MRI and high resolution US has revolutionized our ability to image soft tissue injury. Soft tissue injuries can be grouped into acute injuries or more chronic injuries which generally occur as a result of sustained or repetitive trauma. A brief overview of the role of imaging in tendon and muscle injury is given here since these topics, along with ligament injuries, are presented in more detail elsewhere in this text.

Tendon injury

On US, tendons are visualized as linear structures comprising multiple parallel echogenic bands representing the interfaces between collagen bundles (Fig. 45.21A). Vascular flow is not shown in the normal tendon. Using MRI the normal tendon is visualized as a nonenhancing low signal structure on all conventional sequences.

Tendons are comprised of highly organized linear bundles of collagen microfibrils with an extremely regular and ordered structure. The regular structure results in an alteration in the imaging characteristics of tendons on US and MR depending on the tendon alignment relative to the ultrasound beam or static magnetic field (B_0). This property is known as anisotropy. To see the normal echogenic fibrillar pattern in tendons on US the tendon must be aligned perpendicular to the ultrasound beam. Any significant angulation of the incident ultrasound beam to the tendon will result in echoes generated by the tendon being reflected back at an angle and not returned to the transducer. This leads to the tendon appearing hypo- or even anechoic (Fig. 45.21B). Since one indication of tendon pathology is a loss of the normal bright fibrillar reflections, a careful technique is needed to ensure optimal visualization of the tendon. The anisotropy of tendons on MRI is the result of the so-called 'magic angle phenomenon'. This can result in artefactual increased signal from tendons on short TE imaging sequences. Normally tendons have an extremely short T2 relaxation time, giving them the signal void seen with conventional MRI techniques. However, when the alignment of the tendon (and therefore the collagen bundles within it) approaches 55 degrees to the static magnetic field (B_0), known as the magic angle, the T2 relaxation lengthens and signal is seen from within the tendon. This effect is only seen on short TE imaging sequences (T1 and proton density) and is important because tendon abnormalities usually yield increased signal from within the tendon on short TE imaging. Lesions can be distinguished from the magic angle effect by the persistence of abnormal signal on long TE sequences. The magic angle effect is not exclusive to tendons and may also be seen in ligaments, menisci and articular cartilage.

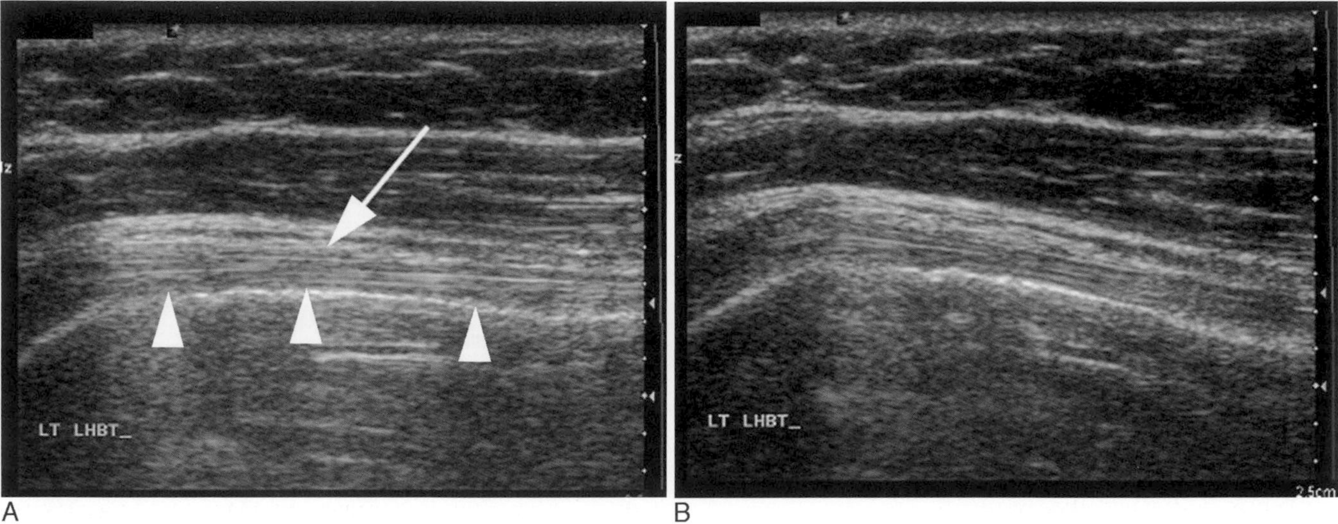

Figure 45.21 Long head of biceps tendon shown on ultrasound. (A) Longitudinal US of the normal long head of biceps tendon shows the tendon (arrow) as parallel brightly reflective bands running along the cortical surface of the humerus (arrowheads). (B) Longitudinal US. The probe face has been angled so it no longer lies parallel to the tendon, which now loses some of its echogenicity due to the effect of anisotropy.

Chronic tendon injury

Chronic or repetitive trauma to a tendon results in degenerative change within the tendon which has become known as tendinopathy or tendinosis. These terms have replaced the older term of tendonitis, which implies an inflammatory component to the disease process; inflammation is not seen to exist histologically. Changes seen within the tendon include degeneration and disorganization of the collagen bundles along with vascular ingrowth. Calcific deposits may form within the tendon and these can be demonstrated on conventional radiographs. Some tendons, such as the extensors and flexors of the hand and foot, have a synovial tendon sheath; where this becomes involved in the process the condition is known as tenosynovitis. Many tendons do not have a tendon sheath (for instance the Achilles and patellar tendons) and are instead surrounded by loose connective tissue known as the paratenon. This may also become involved, a condition known as paratenonitis.

A common feature seen on both MRI and US in tendinopathic tendons is thickening of the affected tendon. Using US, areas of low reflectivity will be seen within the tendon with loss of the normal fibrillar architecture (Fig. 45.22A). Neovascularization may also be seen with Doppler techniques demonstrating blood flow within the normally avascular tendon (Fig. 45.22B). On MRI increased signal will be seen within the tendon on both short and long TE sequences (Fig. 45.22C). If tenosynovitis is present this will be seen on US and MRI as synovial thickening and fluid surrounding the tendon. Paratenonitis is seen on US as a low reflective 'halo' surrounding the tendon and on MRI as a thin high signal rim on T2 imaging which enhances with gadolinium on T1 imaging.

Calcium deposition in affected tendons is readily shown on US as bright reflective foci. As expected, calcium will yield low signal on MRI although there may be increased signal in the surrounding tissues due to inflammatory response. Tendon calcification can cause susceptibility artefact. In acute calcium deposition the calcific material is liquid or semiliquid and may show fluid–fluid levels on MRI.

Tendon tears

Tendon tears are unusual in an otherwise normal tendon. When a tendon undergoes tendinopathic change it becomes weaker and at this point tears may occur. A tendon tear may either be full or partial thickness. Full thickness tears are generally easily recognized at US and MRI. Retraction of the torn ends will be seen and, depending on how acute the tear is, haematoma or fluid will be seen filling the gap. Both techniques are able to give an indication of the tendon gap, and assessment of the tendon dynamically with US helps confirm the full thickness nature of the tear. Disruption of a tendon without tendinopathic change is usually the result of avulsion of the tendon from the bone. In this case the avulsed bone fragment may be seen on conventional radiographs, but its tendon attachment can be confirmed at US or MRI.

Partial thickness tears are also visualized at MRI or US. The distinction between a partial thickness tear and tendinopathy may be difficult at US and MRI. Tears will appear as well-defined low reflective areas or clefts extending into the substance of the tendon on US, and the presence of high signal on T2-weighted MRI extending to a tendon surface is also indicative of a partial thickness tear. Using US, Doppler will help distinguish a tear from vessels formed in an area of tendinopathy.

In general, studies would suggest that in many cases there is little to choose between MRI and US when diagnosing tendon abnormalities[12].

Muscle injury

Acute muscle injury

Muscle injuries are common, especially in those undertaking athletic activities. Movement in muscle is transmitted to the skeleton through the kinetic chain comprising muscle

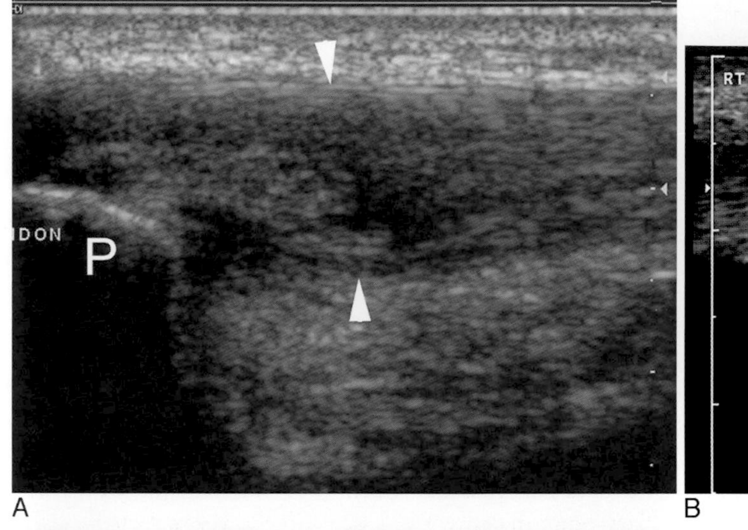

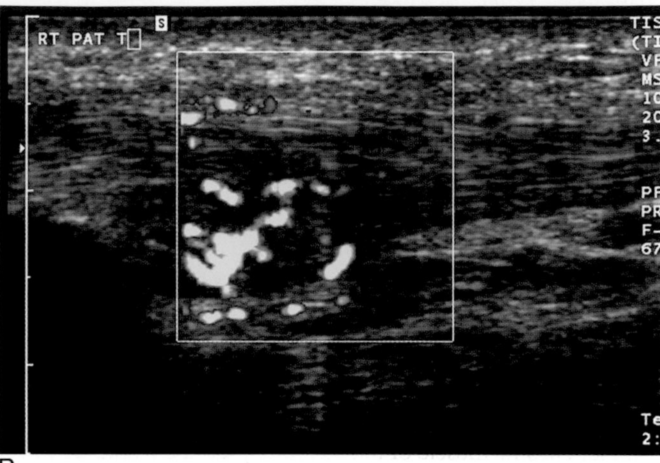

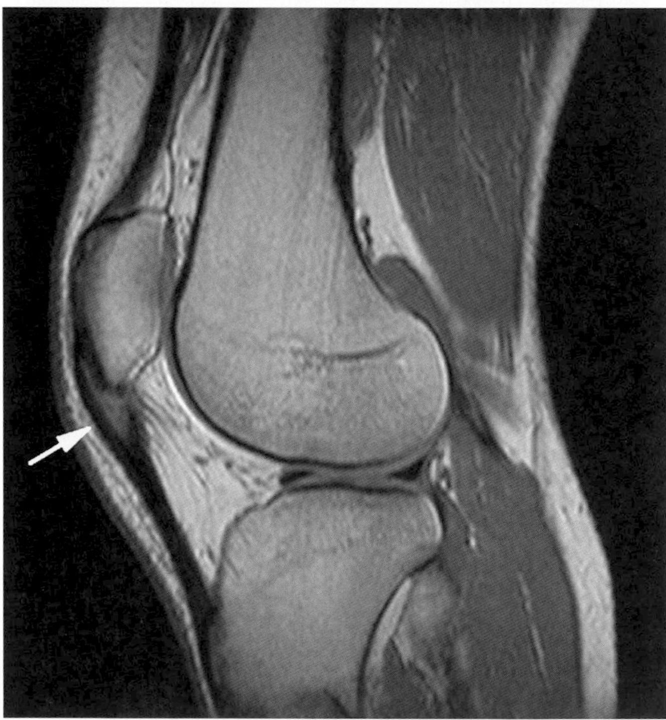

Figure 45.22 Patellar tendinopathy. (A) Longitudinal US shows the thickened patellar tendon (between the arrowheads) at its insertion into the patella (P). Note the low reflective change within its substance. (B) A similar section, this time with power Doppler, shows the intense neovascularization seen within the tendinopathic tendon. Normal tendon is avascular. (C) Sagittal proton density MR image of the patellar tendon shows thickening and increased intrasubstance signal at its proximal insertion (arrow).

connecting to tendon connecting to bone. The majority of 'muscle' tears in fact represent tears at the myotendinous junction where the tendon arises from the muscle, a relatively weak point in the kinetic chain. The diagnosis of muscle tears is normally a clinical one. In some situations imaging can be helpful, particularly when dealing with athletes where an indication of the degree of severity of the muscle injury can be helpful in predicting the likely time before the athlete can return to competition.

Acute muscle injuries range from strains to complete rupture and are graded 1 to 3.

A grade 1 tear or strain represents microscopic tearing of muscle fibres, usually without loss of muscle strength. No macroscopic tear in the muscle fibres is seen, but oedema and haemorrhage may occur within the muscle. Appearances are usually normal on US although occasionally a mild increase in reflectivity can be seen[13]. On MRI the appearances will depend on the relative amount and age of haemorrhage and oedema. The majority of acute muscle strains appear as intermediate signal on T1 and increased signal on T2-weighted imaging (Fig. 45.3B). There is usually a poor relationship between the severity of the patient's symptoms and the MRI findings; the latter may persist for some time after the patient has made a full recovery[14].

Grade 3 tears represent a full thickness tear of the muscle with complete separation of the torn ends of the muscle, or more commonly the muscle from the tendon. Grade 2 tears represent partial tears where there is macroscopic but incomplete separation of muscle or muscle and tendon. In these more severe muscle injuries the muscle belly will be retracted at the site of the tear, opening a gap which will be filled with haematoma or fluid[15]. This is readily seen with US (Fig. 45.3A) and MRI. Depending on the age of the tear the haematoma may appear anechoic or more complex. The demonstration of muscle retraction may be helped by examining the area dynamically while the patient tenses the affected muscle against resistance. Both US and MRI may show fluid tracking around the muscle adjacent to the covering fascia.

Blunt trauma to a muscle will result in haemorrhage into the muscle (often with some swelling). Where muscles overlie each other, two or more muscles (or even muscle groups) may be involved. The diagnosis is normally clear from the history, but imaging will show haemorrhage and oedema within the muscle. This is often subtle on US and the characteristic finding is increased reflectivity and some focal swelling of the muscle.

Chronic muscle injuries

Disuse atrophy of muscle may be seen from a variety of causes including chronic muscle or tendon injury and denervation. The loss of muscle bulk may be obvious on cross-sectional imaging. In addition the muscle undergoes a process of fatty infiltration seen as increased signal on T1-weighted MRI, as increased echogenicity on US, and as areas of fat attenuation on CT. This has been discussed further in Section 4.

Delayed onset muscle soreness (DOMS)

DOMS is a well-recognized phenomenon where muscular pain develops hours or days after muscle activity. It remains poorly understood but is manifest on MRI as oedematous change (increased signal on T2 weighting and STIR imaging) in the affected muscles. The appearances are therefore similar to those of a muscle strain, but the clinical picture differs in that the symptoms come on some time after the exercise. As with muscle strains, the MRI findings take longer to resolve than the muscular pain.

Myositis ossificans

Myositis ossificans may develop following muscle trauma. In this condition ossification occurs in the muscle and may be visible on plain radiography and CT (Fig. 45.17). Ultrasound will show the area of ossification as a dense reflection from within the muscle with posterior acoustic shadowing. MRI initially shows oedema-type change in the muscle. This gradually organizes, becoming better defined. Cortical bone developing around the edges of the lesion is of low signal intensity on all sequences. In the mature lesions the centre of the area becomes filled with bone trabeculae surrounded by fatty bone marrow. The latter will show signal characteristics of fat.

Muscle hernias

Muscle hernias usually present as a lump which the patient may notice becomes more prominent when the muscle is tensed. They represent muscle fibres herniating out through a tear or weakness in the muscular fascia. Such weaknesses are often associated with perforating veins in the lower limb. Ultrasound during muscle contraction is readily able to show muscle hernias and provide reassurance that the palpable mass is composed of normal muscle tissue.

SOFT TISSUE TUMOURS

Soft tissue tumours, taken in the literal sense to mean a mass or swelling, can be classified as neoplastic and non-neoplastic or as benign and malignant. The role of imaging is first to detect or exclude the presence of a mass and then, where possible, to characterize the lesion. After preliminary radiography, which may reveal useful diagnostic information, US is the quickest and most cost-effective means of confirming the presence or absence of a mass. At this stage the prevalence and distribution of diagnoses of soft tissue masses by age, sex and location should be considered. In this way it is possible to reduce the differential diagnosis on the basis of probability. For example, in one series of 18 677 benign soft tissue tumours, giant cell tumour of tendon sheath made up only 4% of the cases; however the prevalence of this particular tumour rises to 20–23% when looking at benign tumours of the hand and wrist in adults[16]. Similarly, in a series of 12 370 malignant soft tissue tumours, synovial sarcoma made up only 5.4% of the cases, whereas the proportion of synovial sarcoma in the lower extremity rises to 22–33% of 6- to 35-year-olds[17]. When considering the published figures, the referral bias of the reader's unit needs to be borne in mind. The prevalence of malignancy in soft tissue masses presenting to a district general hospital varies between one in 20 and one in 100 cases. This increases to between one in two and one in three patients seen at a tertiary referral centre. A useful adage is that all deep-seated lesions greater than 5 cm in diameter should be clinically considered malignant until imaging, with or without subsequent biopsy, proves otherwise. Because of its high intrinsic contrast resolution, MRI has some potential for the classification of soft tissue tumours. Depending on the case mix, the correct histological diagnosis reached on the basis of imaging studies varies between 25 and 44%[16,18]. The majority of the cases diagnosed with confidence on MRI in the 44% of 225 soft tissue tumours were benign lesions such as lipomas, haemangiomas, arteriovenous malformations, benign neural tumours, periarticular cysts, haematomas, pigmented villonodular synovitis (PVNS) and giant cell tumours of tendon sheath[18]. The more common conditions and those with relatively specific imaging appearances are briefly described below.

Synovial cysts, bursae and ganglia

Synovial 'cysts' are benign uni- or multilocular soft tissue masses found in the periarticular tissues. They represent a continuation or herniation of synovial tissue through the joint capsule and are therefore fluid-filled and lined with synovium. They may be due to a distended bursa as frequently seen with the classic popliteal (semimembranosus-gastrocnemius bursa or Baker's) cyst (Fig. 45.5). Bursae are open or closed synovium-lined sacs usually found over bony prominences or between muscles and tendons. They occur at numerous sites but the most frequently encountered and imaged include the subacromial/subdeltoid, olecranon, iliopsoas, pre-patellar and semimembranosus-gastrocnemius bursae. Ganglia, the commonest cause of a mass in the hand and wrist, are also cystic but filled with a myxoid matrix and differ from synovial cysts and bursae in that they are not lined with synovium. A variant form of ganglion cyst with joint communication is the meniscal cyst of the knee where most are associated with myxoid degeneration and horizontal cleavage tears of the underlying meniscus. It is largely a semantic argument to differentiate the precise nature of synovial cysts, bursae or ganglia as the imaging characteristics are so similar and the surgical management, if required, is simple excision. The exception is the meniscal cyst: here surgery of the meniscus is also usually required. All these lesions tend to show a well-defined homogeneous mass that is hypoechoic on US with posterior acoustic enhancement (Fig. 45.2), slightly hypodense with respect to muscle on CT and hyperintense on T2-weighted and STIR sequences on MRI (Fig. 45.5A). Only the periphery of the main cystic mass will show enhancement with iodinated contrast medium on CT or paramagnetic contrast medium on MRI (Fig. 45.5B,C). Occasionally a more heterogeneous mass may be seen if there has been previous haemorrhage within. Also, if there is a high protein content within the cyst resulting in T1 shortening, the mass may appear isointense or even slightly hyperintense to muscle on T1-weighted images.

Synovial proliferative disorders

In the patient presenting with a monoarticular mass, several benign proliferative disorders of the synovium should be considered. These include synovial chondromatosis, PVNS and lipoma arborescens. These are considered metaplastic rather than neoplastic conditions. True benign neoplasms of synovium such as synovial haemangioma and synovial chondroma are rare.

Synovial chondromatosis can be classified as primary or secondary. The more common secondary form classically appears as multiple intra-articular osteochondral loose bodies against a background of degenerative joint disease. The primary form presents with a synovial mass which frequently contains fine 'ring-and-arc' calcification indicating the cartilage nature of the lesion (Fig. 45.23). In the absence of this calcification the lesion may be distinguishable from the intra-articular variant of synovial sarcoma. In time the synovial masses will recede with the development of intra-articular chondral bodies. In the early stages the treatment involves synovectomy but recurrence is common. There is rare association between synovial chondromatosis and synovial chondrosarcoma although the histological distinction between these two conditions can be difficult. MRI is ideally suited to demonstrate the synovial masses with small signal voids corresponding to the foci of mineralization.

Pigmented villonodular synovitis and lipoma arborescens

Pigmented villonodular synovitis (PVNS) may arise from the synovium of joints, less commonly bursae and from tendon sheaths when it is known as giant cell tumour of tendon sheath. The articular variety may be focal or more commonly generalized within the one joint. The typical clinical picture is that of an insidious onset of a monoarticular arthropathy in a young adult. The pathology consists of hyperplastic synovium with lipid-laden foam cells, histiocytes, giant cells and haemosiderin deposition. Radiographs may show a soft tissue mass which can be relatively radiodense due to the haemosiderin.

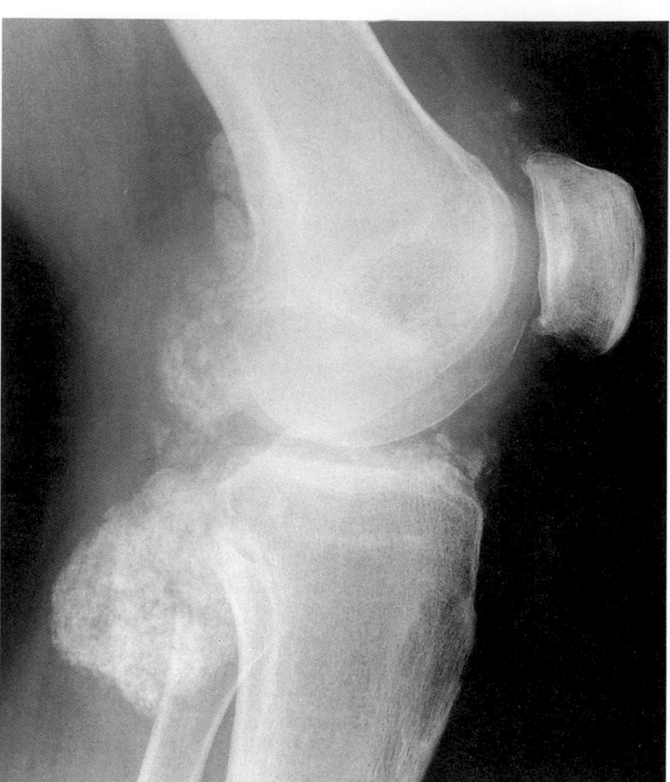

Figure 45.23 Synovial osteochondromatosis. Lateral radiograph showing the fine cartilage calcifications of primary synovial osteochondromatosis.

Relatively well defined erosions and subchondral cysts affect both sides of the joint. The MRI appearances are typical with low signal intensity synovial masses on all sequences due to the haemosiderin (Fig. 45.24). This so-called 'black synovium' may also be seen with amyloid deposition or in any condition associated with recurrent intra-articular bleeding such as haemophiliac arthropathy. Where PVNS arises from tendon sheaths, US readily identifies the solid mass and its association with the tendon sheath.

A rare synovial metaplastic condition readily diagnosed on MRI is lipoma arborescens. In this benign condition, delicate branching fronds of fat, high signal intensity on T1-weighted images, can be identified within synovial hypertrophy.

Lipomatous tumours

Lipomatous tumours may be benign or malignant. A number of cases will exhibit imaging features sufficiently distinctive for a specific diagnosis to be made. The benign lipoma is the most common of all mesenchymal tumours and can be superficially or deeply located. It comprises a well-defined mass of mature fat (adipocytes) and will appear as radiolucent on radiographs, low attenuation on CT (−65 to −120 HU) and hyperintense on T1-weighted MRI (Fig. 45.4). Fine septations can be seen on both CT and MRI. Subcutaneous lipomata are well seen with US and their precise appearance is variable ranging from a focus of increased reflectivity in the fat to a lesion with the same echo characteristics as the surrounding fat. Calcification or ossification can occur in long-standing lesions (Fig. 45.1). Larger lesions may cause pressure erosion of underlying cortical bone. High-grade liposarcomas will show features indistin-

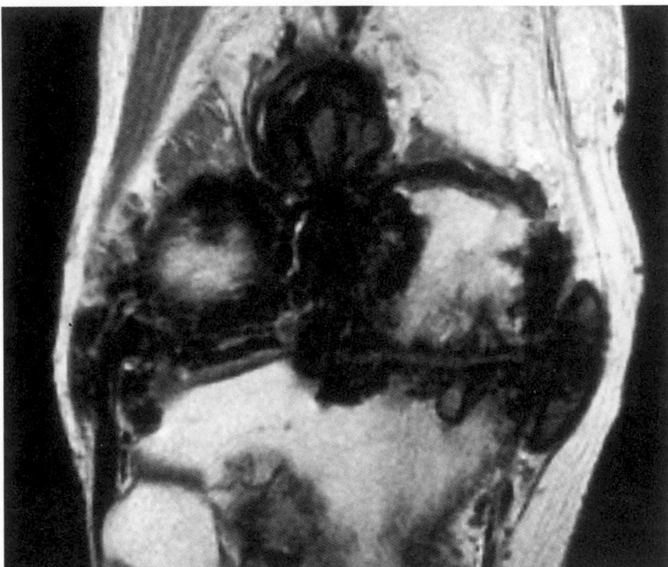

Figure 45.24 Pigmented villonodular synovitis (PVNS). Coronal T1-weighted MR image showing dark synovial masses due to haemosiderin deposition against a background of degenerative joint disease.

guishable from other soft tissue sarcomas (see below). There is another intermediate category, the low-grade or well-differentiated liposarcoma, also known as an atypical lipoma. These show a propensity for local recurrence but do not tend to metastasize. This entity should be suspected if the fat-suppression images on MRI do not appear homogeneous. Occasionally lipomatous tumours will appear biphasic comprising areas of simple lipoma with intermediate-to high-grade sarcoma (Fig. 45.25). MRI is valuable in distinguishing the various components and indicating the most appropriate site for biopsy.

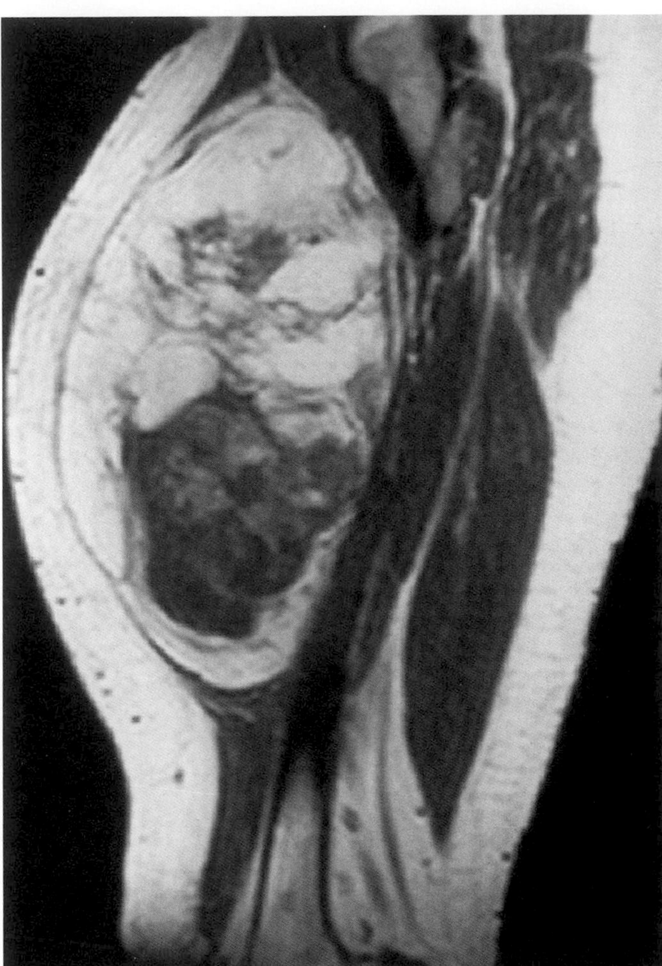

Figure 45.25 Low-grade liposarcoma. Sagittal T1-weighted MR image of the thigh showing a heterogeneous mass. The cephalic portion is hyperintense, typical of simple lipoma, whereas the caudal component is isointense with muscle, much more suggestive of sarcoma.

Vascular tumours

The commonest vascular 'tumour' of soft tissues is a haematoma. The typical appearance of a subacute haematoma on T1-weighted MRI is that of a mass with a thin dark rim of haemosiderin surrounding a hyperintense layer representing methaemoglobin and an isointense centre of liquefaction. There remains some debate as to whether real vascular tumours are developmental malformations or true tumours. There are various different categories of haemangioma including capillary, cavernous and venous. Haemangiomas and vascular malformations may be found in association with a number of congenital syndromes including Kasabach–Merritt, Maffucci, Osler–Weber–Rendu, Klippel–Trenaunay–Weber, Gorham and Proteus syndromes. On radiographs the presence of phleboliths is a specific sign (Fig. 45.9). Angiography is rarely used these days to diagnose a haemangioma but can be useful for preoperative planning or as a prelude to embolization therapy. US can be helpful in demonstrating a mass and identifying phleboliths as echogenic foci with acoustic shadowing. Doppler studies give further information regarding the type and rate of blood flow within the lesion. MRI frequently shows distinctive serpiginous vessels against a high signal background due to a combination of fat and pooled blood. Fluid–fluid levels and the so-called 'bunch of grapes' appearance are said to be typical but can also be seen with haemorrhagic necrotic sarcomas, particularly synovial sarcoma. The flow rate within a haemangioma can be determined with dynamic contrast-enhanced MRI. High-flow lesions tend to have signal voids on all sequences.

Neurogenic tumours

Benign nerve sheath tumours are subdivided into schwannoma and neurofibroma. Malignant nerve sheath tumours are known by a confusing number of different names, usually including the terms either malignant or sarcoma. On MRI, schwannomas typically present as a small fusiform mass with tapering margins. Schwannomas tend to arise eccentrically from the underlying nerve, whereas neurofibromas are centrally sited. The target appearance on T2-weighted MRI is said to be distinctive of a neurofibroma; it can be seen with schwannomas but not usually with malignant peripheral nerve sheath tumours. A variant of neurofibroma is the plexiform neurofibroma in which there is diffuse enlargement and distortion of a major nerve trunk. The diagnostic criteria for neurofibromatosis type 1 (von Recklinghausen's disease) include café-au-lait spots, one plexiform neurofibroma, or more than one neurofibroma. The target sign can sometimes be recognized on US.

As with MRI, US will often demonstrate the associated nerve entering or leaving the lesion (Fig. 45.26).

Morton's neuroma is a misnomer in that it is due to perineural fibrosis of the plantar digital nerve and not a tumour originating from Schwann cells. It typically occurs level with the metatarsal heads, most frequently between the third and fourth metatarsals. Both US and MRI may be used to confirm these lesions, which are usually obvious on clinical grounds. Because of their fibrous nature the lesions are most conspicuous on T1-weighted images, particularly fat-suppressed contrast-enhanced[19]. Morton's neuroma can be associated with a distended intermetatarsal bursa which will be revealed on T2-weighted or STIR images. US shows the lesion as a low reflective intermetatarsal mass. Applying compression during the examination helps distinguish the neuroma from any associated compressible bursa.

Fibrous tumours

There are numerous tumours of fibrous origin. Many occur in infancy and childhood, such as fibromatosis colli, which presents in the first few weeks of life with a torticollis due to a benign fibroblastic lesion of the sternocleidomastoid muscle. Imaging will show a diffuse swelling of the affected muscle. In itself this is not specific but the age and site are so characteristic that the diagnosis is not usually in doubt.

One benign fibrous tumour which is locally invasive is aggressive fibromatosis (extra-abdominal desmoid). Radiography is usually normal although bone erosion may occur in up to a third of chronic cases. The tumours are made up of elongated spindle cells (fibroblasts) with varying amounts of collagen. It is because of the latter that these tumours frequently appear relatively hypointense on MRI unlike many other soft tissue tumours (Fig. 45.27). Indeed it may be difficult to see the lesion at all on a fat-suppressed T2-weighted image and enhancement can be limited due to the relatively hypovascular nature of the tumour. Arguably, intermediate weighting images (proton density) best demonstrate the lesion. Nevertheless MRI frequently underestimates the full extent of fibromatosis. Although the mainstay of treatment is surgery, local recurrence is common. Fortunately, fibromatosis may remain relatively dormant for many years. In cases where surgical options have been exhausted, both radiotherapy and chemotherapy have been used with varying success.

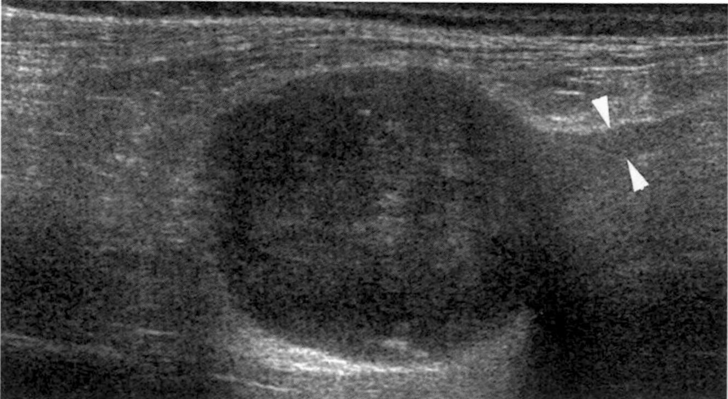

Figure 45.26 Schwannoma. A longitudinal US image of the antecubital fossa demonstrates a solid soft tissue mass arising from the median nerve. The mass is predominantly of low reflectivity, but note that the centre of the lesion is more reflective than the periphery (target sign). The clue to the diagnosis lies in the fact that the lesion arises from the median nerve which can be seen extending distally from the mass, arising from the lesion like a rat's tail (arrows).

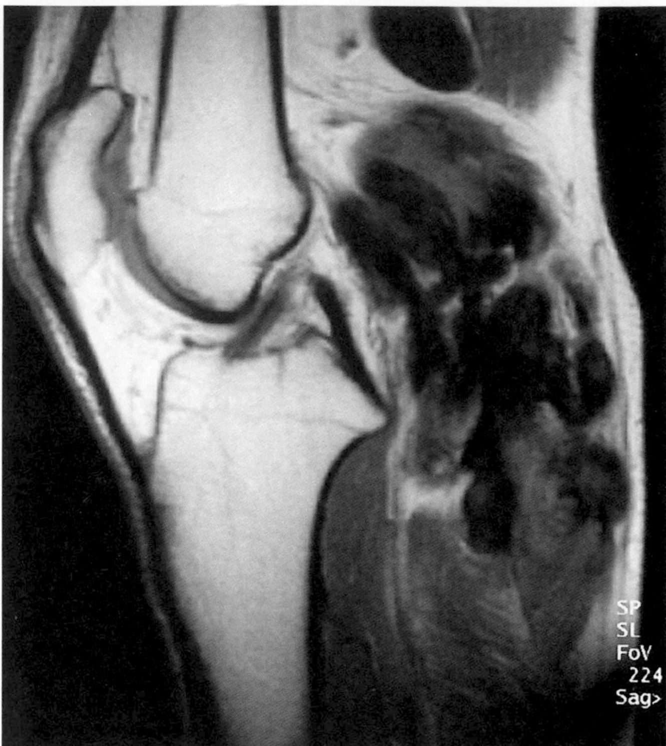

Figure 45.27 Aggressive fibromatosis (extra-abdominal desmoid). Sagittal T1-weighted MR image showing an extensive low signal intensity mass behind the knee. The low signal intensity is due to the hypocellular nature of the lesion with fibrous tissue and hyalinized collagen.

Soft tissue sarcoma

The vast majority of soft tissue sarcomas, irrespective of the precise tissue of origin, will exhibit a similar spectrum of imaging findings. Calcification on radiography will suggest synovial sarcoma, extraskeletal osteosarcoma and soft tissue chondrosarcoma but can be seen rarely with other malignancies (Fig. 45.15). US is generally unhelpful in further evaluating these lesions, but it does have an important role to play in guiding percutaneous biopsy. Many studies using MRI have attempted to differentiate benign from malignant soft tissue masses by looking at differing parameters[20,21]. However, an ill-defined margin is of no value in predicting malignancy[22]. Most soft tissue malignancies are well defined, due to the presence of a pseudocapsule around the tumour (Fig. 45.5). Ill-defined lesions are in fact frequently benign, such as inflammatory processes including infections, aggressive fibromatosis and post-traumatic[5,23]. Homogeneous lesions on T1- and T2-weighted images tend to be benign, whereas malignant lesions are usually heterogeneous, particularly on T2-weighted images (Fig. 45.5). By combining the MRI parameters it is possible to predict malignancy with a sensitivity and specificity of approximately 80% respectively[24]. While this is of academic interest, the accuracy is not sufficient for individual patient management. Unless the imaging features, particularly on MRI, are reasonably specific, a soft tissue mass should be considered as a possible malignancy and plans should be made for biopsy after appropriate staging studies.

Tumour staging

Staging of a suspected soft tissue malignancy is a mandatory part of the preoperative evaluation. The purpose of staging is twofold: first, to accurately delineate the tumour for planning surgery, second, to establish a standard nomenclature by which the extent of a tumour can be categorized. This is of limited value to the individual patient but is important when the efficacy of different treatments is being assessed. A number of staging systems have been advocated. These include the American Joint Commission on Cancer system, the Musculoskeletal Tumor Society system, the Hajdu staging system and the Memorial Sloan-Kettering system. Arguably, the most straightforward is the Musculoskeletal Society system which has the added advantage of being equally applicable to bone sarcomas[25]. With this system the tumour is classified by histological grade, local extent and presence or absence of metastatic disease. Staging of the primary tumour is best performed with MRI. The local extent of the tumour should be accurately documented noting intra- and extracompartmental spread. The relationship of the tumour to adjacent structures, bones, joints and neurovascular bundle should be noted (Fig. 45.28). The initial imaging staging also requires a chest radiograph and a chest CT to exclude occult pulmonary metastases. Occasionally, soft tissue sarcomas such as epithelioid sarcoma can metastasize to lymph nodes. Again, MRI is useful and the examination should be extended proximal to a tumour if there is any suggestion of local lymphadenopathy. Where possible, the staging studies should be performed before biopsy as the trauma of the procedure may exaggerate the apparent extent of the tumour, and the imaging may suggest the most appropriate site for the biopsy. The mainstay

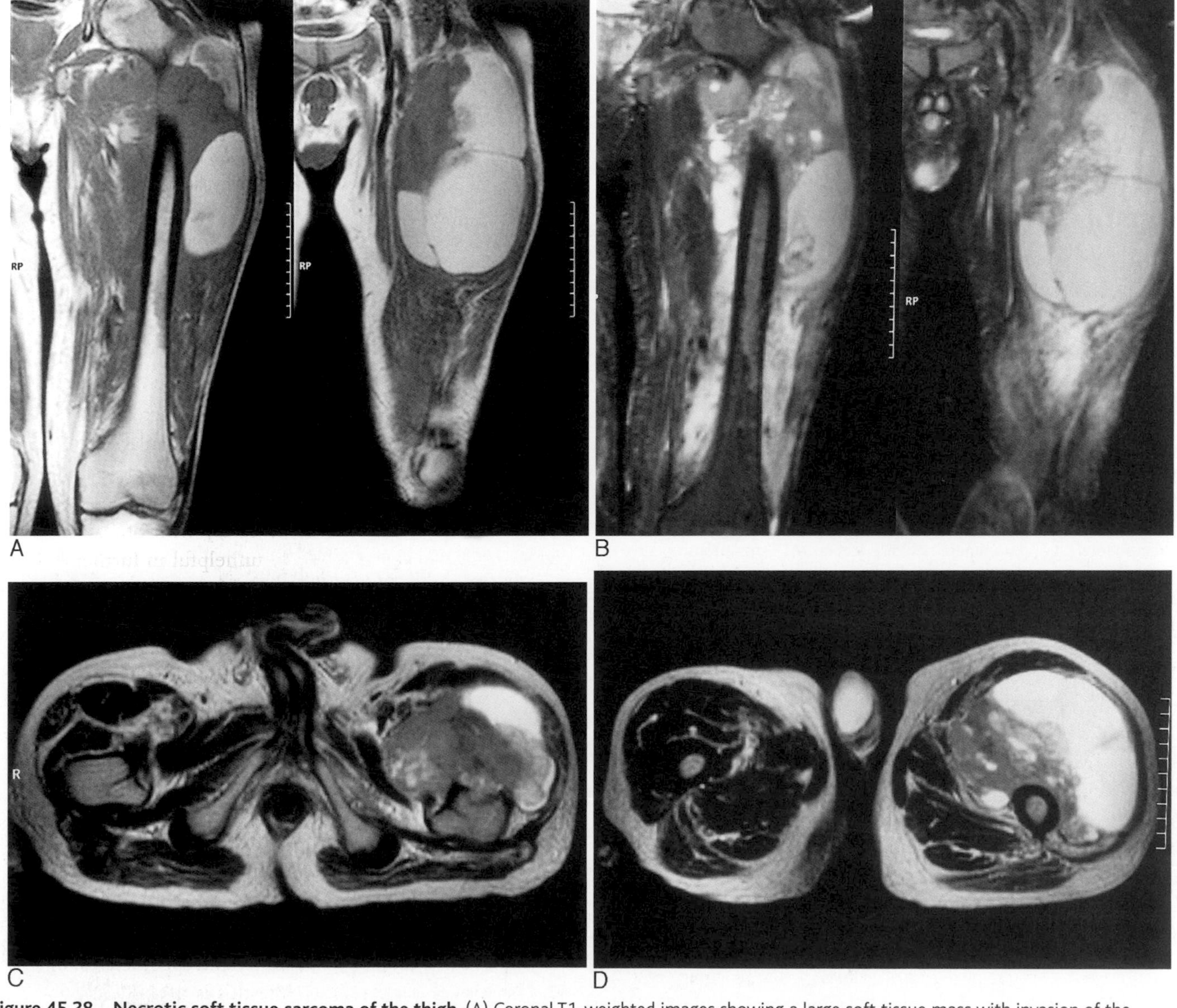

Figure 45.28 Necrotic soft tissue sarcoma of the thigh. (A) Coronal T1-weighted images showing a large soft tissue mass with invasion of the proximal femoral diaphysis. The mass shows hyperintense areas either due to subacute haemorrhage or fat. (B) Coronal STIR images. The hyperintense areas in Figure 45.28A do not fat suppress, indicating that this represents haemorrhage and not a lipomatous tumour. (C, D) Two axial T2-weighted fast spin-echo images showing the solid and cystic/necrotic components of the tumour as well as the invasion of the anterior femur.

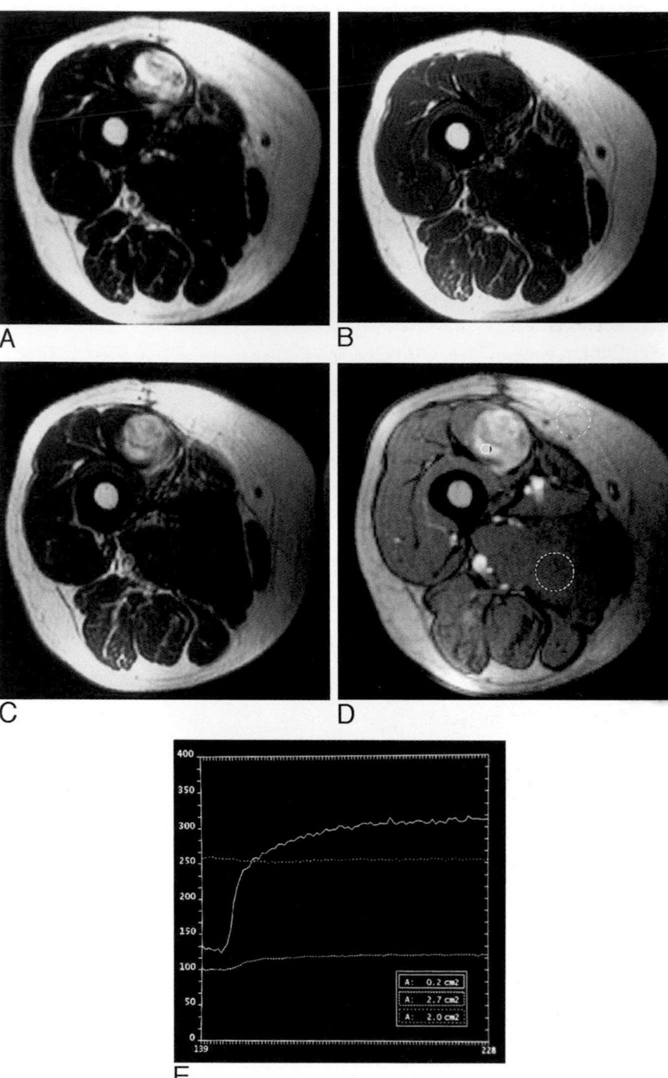

Figure 45.29 Recurrent soft tissue sarcoma. (A) Axial T2-weighted MR image of the thigh shows a hyperintense mass lesion in the rectus femoris muscle. (B) Axial T1-weighted image. The mass is isointense with muscle. (C) Axial T1-weighted image post gadolinium. The mass shows diffuse enhancement. (D) Three-second gradient-echo image obtained as part of a dynamic sequence. Regions of interest (ROI) were drawn on the tumour, subcutaneous fat and unaffected muscle (circle). (E) Time-intensity curve plotted from the dynamic sequence showing rapid enhancement from the tumour, minimal enhancement of the muscle, and absent enhancement of the subcutaneous fat.

of treatment of soft tissue sarcomas is surgery. The value of neoadjuvant chemotherapy remains controversial. Where it is employed, however, repeat staging with MRI of the primary tumour and CT of the chest is required before definitive surgery to assess the response to the chemotherapy and to ensure the planned surgery remains appropriate. Both dynamic contrast-enhanced MRI and colour flow power Doppler US can be used to assess tumour response to chemotherapy[26]. Accurate assessment requires the comparison of standardized examinations performed before and after the chemotherapy.

Tumour follow-up

Following surgery, be it limb salvage or amputation, patients are closely monitored at increasing intervals for evidence of local recurrence and metastatic disease. Local recurrence is a major potential problem with soft tissue sarcomas, particularly when they are high grade. It is almost inevitable if the original surgical resection was intralesional or marginal. At the first suggestion of recurrence some form of cross-sectional imaging is required—CT, MRI or US[27]. MRI and CT have a similar sensitivity in the detection of local recurrent disease when the mass is 15 cm^3 or more[28]. MRI is the technique of choice in the detection of early recurrence when local control may still be surgically achievable. While US does have some financial attractions, MRI will still be required for preoperative planning if a recurrence is identified. On MRI, a T2-weighted or STIR sequence is most useful in demonstrating recurrence as a high signal intensity mass (Fig. 45.29)[29]. In the absence of a high signal intensity mass the likelihood of recurrence is remote. Diffuse high signal intensity is frequently seen shortly after surgery or can be prolonged after radiation therapy[30]. The use of gadolinium-DTPA will help differentiate between enhancing recurrent tumour and nonenhancing non-neoplastic complications such as seromas and haematomas (Fig. 45.29C). Dynamic contrast-enhanced MRI can be helpful in equivocal cases (Fig. 45.29C,D)[31].

Follow-up imaging studies for possible metastatic disease are targeted at the commonest site for distant spread, the lungs. In the author's unit, chest radiographs are obtained after surgery every 3 months for 2 years, every 6 months for a further 2 years and then annually. Routine follow-up with serial chest CT is of doubtful value, but CT is indicated if at any stage the chest radiograph is suspicious of metastatic disease.

REFERENCES

1. Peller P J, Ho V B, Kransdorf M J 1993 Extraosseous Tc-99m MDP uptake: a pathophysiologic approach. RadioGraphics 13: 715–734
2. Eary J F, Conrad E U 1999 Positron emission tomography in grading soft tissue sarcomas. Semin Musculoskelet Radiol 3: 135–138
3. Dhillon M, Davies A M, Benham J, Evans N, Mangham D C, Grimer R J 2004 Calcific myonecrosis: a report of 10 new cases with an emphasis on MR imaging. Eur Radiol 14: 1974–1979
4. Sanchez Reyes J M, Alcaraz M M, Quinones T D, Aramburu J A 1997 Extensively calcified synovial sarcoma. Skeletal Radiol 26: 671–673
5. Shirkhoda A, Armin A R, Bis K G, Makris J, Irwin R B, Shetty A N 1995 MR imaging of myositis ossificans: variable patterns at different stages. J Magn Reson Imaging 5: 287–292
6. Chau C L, Griffith J F 2005 Musculoskeletal infections: ultrasound appearances. Clin Radiol 60: 149–159
7. Belli L, Reggiori A, Cocozza E, Riboldi L 1992 Ultrasound in tropical pyomyositis. Skeletal Radiol 21: 107–109
8. Trusen A, Beissert M, Schultz G, Chittka B, Darge K 2003 Ultrasound and MRI features of pyomyositis in children. Eur Radiol 13: 1050–1055
9. Polak J F, Jolesz F A, Adams D F 1988 Magnetic resonance imaging of skeletal muscle. Prolongation of T1 and T2 subsequent to denervation. Invest Radiol 23: 365–369
10. Fleckenstein J L 2000 MRI of neuromuscular disease: The basics. Semin Musculoskelet Radiol 4: 393–419
11. Fleckenstein J L, Watumull D, Conner K E et al 1993 Denervated human skeletal muscle: MR imaging evaluation. Radiology 187: 213–218
12. Campbell R S, Grainger A J 2001 Current concepts in imaging of tendinopathy. Clin Radiol 56: 253–267
13. Takebayashi S, Takasawa H, Banzai Y et al 1995 Sonographic findings in muscle strain injury: clinical and MR imaging correlation. J Ultrasound Med 14: 899–905

14. Fleckenstein J L, Weatherall P T, Parkey R W, Payne J A, Peshock R M 1989 Sports-related muscle injuries: evaluation with MR imaging. Radiology 172: 793–798
15. De Smet A A 1993 Magnetic resonance findings in skeletal muscle tears. Skeletal Radiol 22: 479–484
16. Kransdorf M J 1995 Benign soft-tissue tumors in a large referral population: distribution of diagnoses by age, sex and location. Am J Roentgenol 164: 395–402
17. Kransdorf M J 1995 Malignant soft-tissue tumors in a large referral population: distribution of diagnoses by age, sex and location. Am J Roentgenol 164: 129–134
18. Moulton J, Blebea J, Dunco D, Braley S, Bisset G, Emery K 1995 MR imaging of soft tissue masses: diagnostic efficacy and value of distinguishing between benign and malignant lesions. Am J Roentgenol 164: 1191–1199
19. Terk M R, Kwong P K, Suthar M et al 1993 Morton neuroma: evaluation with MR imaging performed with contrast enhancement and fat suppression. Radiology 189: 239–241
20. Berquist T, Ehman R, King B, Hodgman C, Ilstrup D 1990 Value of MR imaging in differentiating benign from malignant soft tissue masses: study of 95 lesions. Am J Roentgenol 155: 1251–1255
21. Crim J, Seeger L, Yao L, Chadnani V, Eckardt J 1992 Diagnosis of soft tissue masses with MR imaging: can benign masses be differentiated from malignant ones? Radiology 185: 581–587
22. Ma L, Frassica F, Scott E, Fishman E, Zerhouni E 1995 Differentiation of benign and malignant musculoskeletal tumors: potential pitfalls with MR imaging. RadioGraphics 15: 349–366
23. Sánchez-Márquez A, Gil-Garcia M, Valls C et al 1999 Sports-related muscle injuries of the lower extremity: MR imaging appearances. Eur Radiol 9: 1088–1093
24. De Schepper A, Ramon D, Degryse H 1992 Statistical analysis of MRI parameters predicting malignancy in 14122 soft tissue masses. Fortschr Röntgenstr 156: 587–591
25. Enneking W F, Spanier S S, Goodman M A 1980 A system for the surgical staging of musculoskeletal sarcoma. Clin Orthop 153: 106–120
26. van der Woude H J, Bloem J L, van Oostayen J A et al 1995 Treatment of high grade sarcomas with neoadjuvant chemotherapy: the utility of colour Doppler sonography in predicting histopathologic response. Am J Roentgenol 165: 125–133
27. Choi H, Varma D G K, Fornage B D, Kim E E, Johnston D A 1991 Soft tissue sarcoma: MR imaging vs sonography for detection of local recurrence after surgery. Radiology 157: 353–358
28. Reuther G, Mutschler W 1990 Detection of local recurrent disease in musculoskeletal tumours: MR imaging versus CT. Skeletal Radiol 19: 85–90
29. Vanel D, Lacombe M J, Couanet D, Kalifa C, Spielmann M, Genin J 1994 Musculoskeletal tumor: follow-up with MR imaging after treatment with surgery and radiation therapy. Radiology 164: 243–245
30. Richardson M L, Zink-Brody G C, Patten R M, Koh W J, Conrad E U 1996 MR characterization of post-radiation soft tissue edema. Skeletal Radiol 25: 537–543
31. Vanel D, Shapeero L G, Tardivon A, Western A, Guinebretiere J M 1998 Dynamic contrast-enhanced MRI with subtraction of aggressive soft tissue tumors after resection. Skeletal Radiol 27: 505–510

CHAPTER 46

Skeletal Trauma

Lee F. Rogers, Mihra S. Taljanovic and Carol A. Boles

Even when the presence and severity of a fracture is apparent clinically, radiological examination is important to document the nature and extent of the injury and identify any additional bony injuries. The evaluation of the acutely injured patient has long depended on conventional radiographs. More recently, advanced imaging techniques have assumed an important role. This section presents general considerations in the imaging of skeletal trauma in adolescents and adults with identification and description of certain 'classic' lesions, which deserve special mention due to their frequency and/or clinical importance. Paediatric skeletal trauma is covered in Chapter 68 of this book.

IMAGING TECHNIQUES

Radiography (X-rays) is the mainstay in trauma imaging as most traumatic lesions of the skeleton can be documented on standard radiographs. Two orthogonal views (at right angles to one another) are required to characterize most lesions. The location and nature of a fracture are usually readily demonstrated on radiographs; however the adjacent soft tissues are usually difficult, if not impossible, to assess.

Skeletal scintigraphy (radionuclide radiology) is a very sensitive method of detection for stress fractures or non-displaced hip fractures that are often not visible on conventional radiographs. Uptake of the radiopharmaceutical (usually a phosphate analogue) is related to osteoblastic activity; the radioactive tracer, attached to the phosphate compound, is incorporated into new bone as it is built. Thus fractures with a high rate of bone turnover demonstrate increased radioactivity.

Computed tomography (CT) is more sensitive and specific than conventional radiography in the detection and full depiction of fractures involving regions of complex anatomy such as the face, spine and pelvis. Reconstructed CT images in the sagittal and coronal planes are particularly helpful. A disadvantage of CT is that fractures may not be detected due to volume averaging. For this reason, radiographs or preliminary digital images must always be reviewed when interpreting CT examinations of skeletal trauma to avoid overlooking fractures lying in the axial plane.

Magnetic resonance imaging (MRI) is unique in its ability to demonstrate the nature and extent of injuries involving the soft tissues: ligaments, tendons, cartilage and muscles. MRI is also exquisitely sensitive to changes in bone marrow. Imaging can be accomplished in any plane without moving the patient, and a variety of pulse sequences can be used to characterize tissue in great detail. In general, fat will appear as high signal (bright) on T1-weighted sequences and will become progressively darker on T2-weighted images. Water (and oedema) will have low signal (i.e. will appear dark) on T1-weighted images and will become very bright on T2-weighted sequences. Fat suppression, accomplished by a variety of methods, can make intramedullary abnormalities within the bone and soft tissues more conspicuous.

Ultrasound (US) evaluation of musculoskeletal injuries is more commonly utilized to detect soft tissue injuries. Higher resolution, near-field, linear-array electronic transducers provide good images of superficial structures. Tendon injuries are the most frequently evaluated, but muscle and ligament injuries and some fractures can be seen. Tendons are usually imaged in the longitudinal and transverse axes, with the transducer parallel or perpendicular to the tendon. Side-to-side US comparison with the unaffected side will aid in the evaluation.

GENERAL CONSIDERATIONS

A fracture is identified on a radiograph as a linear lucency within bone and a disruption or break in the adjacent cortex accompanied by varying degrees of displacement of the fracture fragments. Impaction and overlap of fracture fragments results in an increased density of bone: sharply defined and linear with overlap, and band-like and less well defined where impacted. Soft tissue swelling is usually present adjacent to an acute fracture.

Displacement or obliteration of normal fat pads can be a clue to acute fracture haematoma or joint distension. Specific examples of how this clue may be used are described with the associated injury, below. The presence of a lipohaemarthrosis (fat and blood within a joint space) is prima facie evidence of an intra-articular fracture and is best assessed with a cross-table radiograph (i.e. horizontal X-ray beam) (Fig. 46.1). This is of particular importance in knee trauma.

Fractures may occur under a variety of clinical circumstances. Most commonly, a fracture is the result of a large force acting acutely on an otherwise normal bone and disrupting the normal bony architecture. If the affected bone is already weakened, however, substantially less force may be required to cause a fracture. Such injuries are referred to as *pathological fractures*. Metastatic disease is the most common underlying process, but pathological fractures through benign tumours such as enchondroma or solitary bone cyst are not unusual and are often the initial presentation of a previously unsuspected lesion. Bone weakening due to Paget's disease, renal osteodystrophy or osteogenesis imperfecta may result in pathological fractures. A key feature of pathological fractures is that they tend to be oriented transversely in long bones ('banana fracture'; Fig. 46.2).

Stress fractures (fatigue fractures) occur due to chronic repetitive trauma, ultimately resulting in structural failure of the bone. Such injuries may be difficult to diagnose at initial presentation; subtle periosteal reaction or a transverse band of linear sclerosis may develop 1–2 weeks after the onset of symptoms. A similar event can occur in abnormal bone secondary to normal activity; such an injury is termed an *insufficiency fracture* and is often seen in osteopenic bone in the elderly.

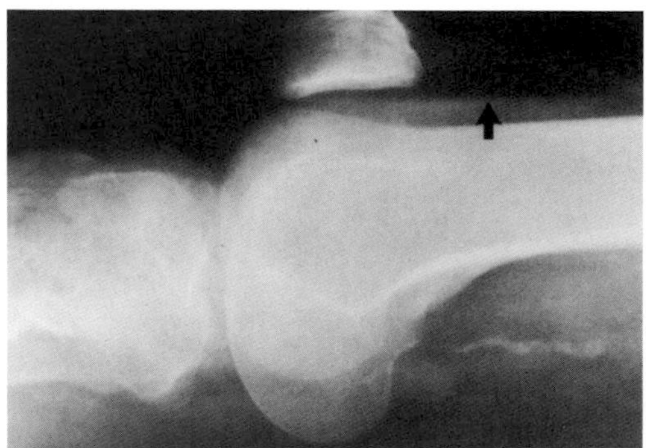

Figure 46.1 Lipohaemarthrosis in the knee is seen as a fat–fluid level (arrow) in the suprapatellar recess on a horizontal beam lateral view. This finding is pathognomonic for an acute intra-articular fracture, usually in the tibial plateau.

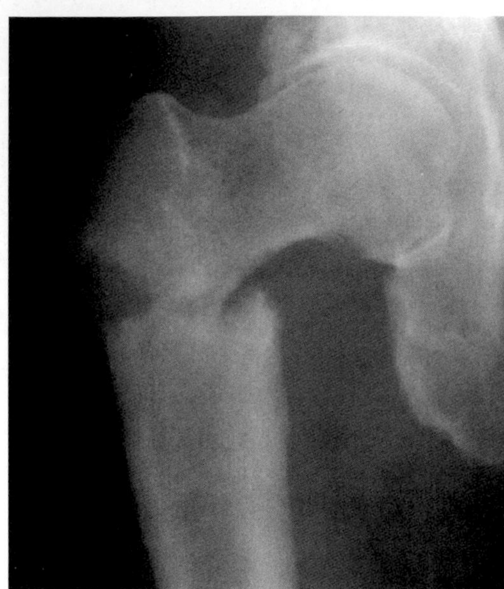

Figure 46.2 Pathological 'banana fracture'. A transverse subtrochanteric fracture of the right femur with varus angulation is demonstrated. A transverse fracture in a long bone, particularly in the subtrochanteric region of the femur, is almost always due to an underlying abnormality. In this case, there is a metastatic lesion in the lateral cortex which led to the fracture.

The fracture line is often never identified. Skeletal scintigraphy and MRI[1] are very sensitive methods of detection for this type of injury and may be positive in the face of a normal radiographic examination. Common locations for stress fractures include the metatarsal shafts (first described in military recruits and thus termed 'march fractures', see Fig. 46.99), the pubic rami, the femoral neck, the tibial (Fig. 46.3) and fibular shafts and the tuberosity of the calcaneus.

Neuropathic injury or Charcot joints refers to fractures and/or dislocations occurring in relatively denervated areas. The classic example is the diabetic foot. Typical radiographic findings include the 'five Ds': destruction, dislocation, disorganization, density (heterotopic new bone and sclerosis) and debris (Fig. 46.4).

Soft tissue injury

Soft tissue injury involving the ligaments, tendons, muscles and cartilage is not usually evident on radiographs. These are best studied with MRI, which relies on changes in signal and morphology to detect injury to tendons and ligaments. Normal tendons and ligaments are devoid of signal on all routine pulse sequences, due to their lack of mobile protons in a tightly organized matrix. Intrasubstance injury (sprain, partial tear, oedema) increases the water content in and around these structures, which is manifested by increased signal in these locations, particularly on long TR sequences. Fat-suppressed sequences increase the conspicuity of the increased signal.

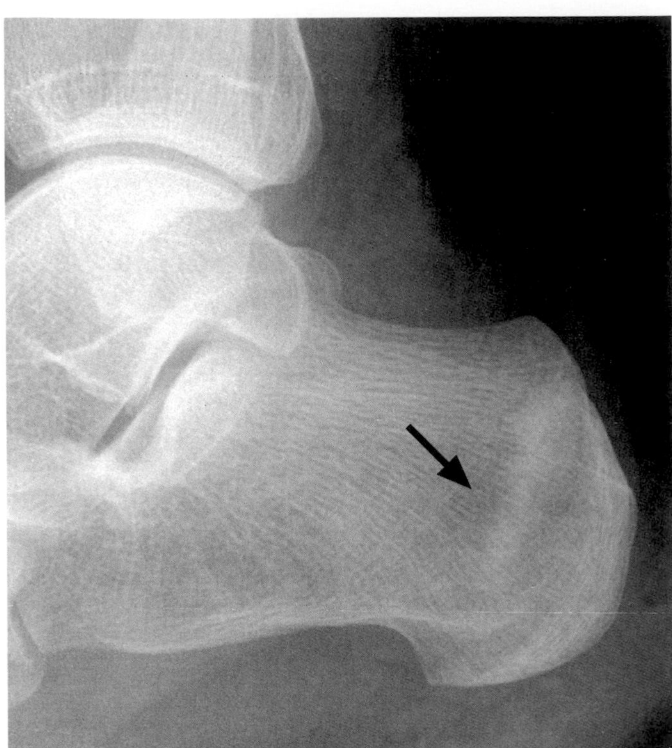

Figure 46.3 Calcaneal stress fracture. A lateral view of the calcaneus in a young male runner who complained of heel pain for one month. Note linear sclerosis in tuberosity (arrow) of a stress fracture.

Tendons may become inflamed due to acute injury or chronic overuse (tendinitis); findings usually include enlargement of the tendon and increased intratendinous MR signal (Fig. 46.5). A partial tear may be seen as an irregularity in the shape of the tendon (i.e. a defect in the border of the tendon) with associated high signal on T2-weighted sequences. A complete tear is diagnosed when the tendon is discontinuous, absent, or unrecognizable (Fig. 46.6).

The MRI assessment of ligamentous injury is similar. A basic grading system includes three levels of injury, corresponding roughly to steps of clinical severity. Grade I injury, or mild sprain, is described as abnormal increased signal around an otherwise normal-appearing ligament. Grade II injury is consistent with a severe sprain and demonstrates abnormal thickening and/or abnormal signal within the ligament. Grade III injury represents a complete disruption of the ligament.

On ultrasound, normal tendons appear as hyperechoic parallel lines in the longitudinal plane (see Fig. 46.89B). Artefactual areas of hypoechogenicity may result from incorrect transducer placement. Tears are demonstrated as a hypoechoic gap in the tendon, often with fluid in the tendon sheath. Tendinitis is seen as increased thickness of the tendon with altered echogenicity, either focally or diffusely. The tendons of the rotator cuff have been the most evaluated. In the shoulder, *four groups* have been described based on US appearance: *non-visualization* of the cuff, *localized absence* or *focal non-visualization*, *discontinuity* and *focal abnormal echogenicity*.

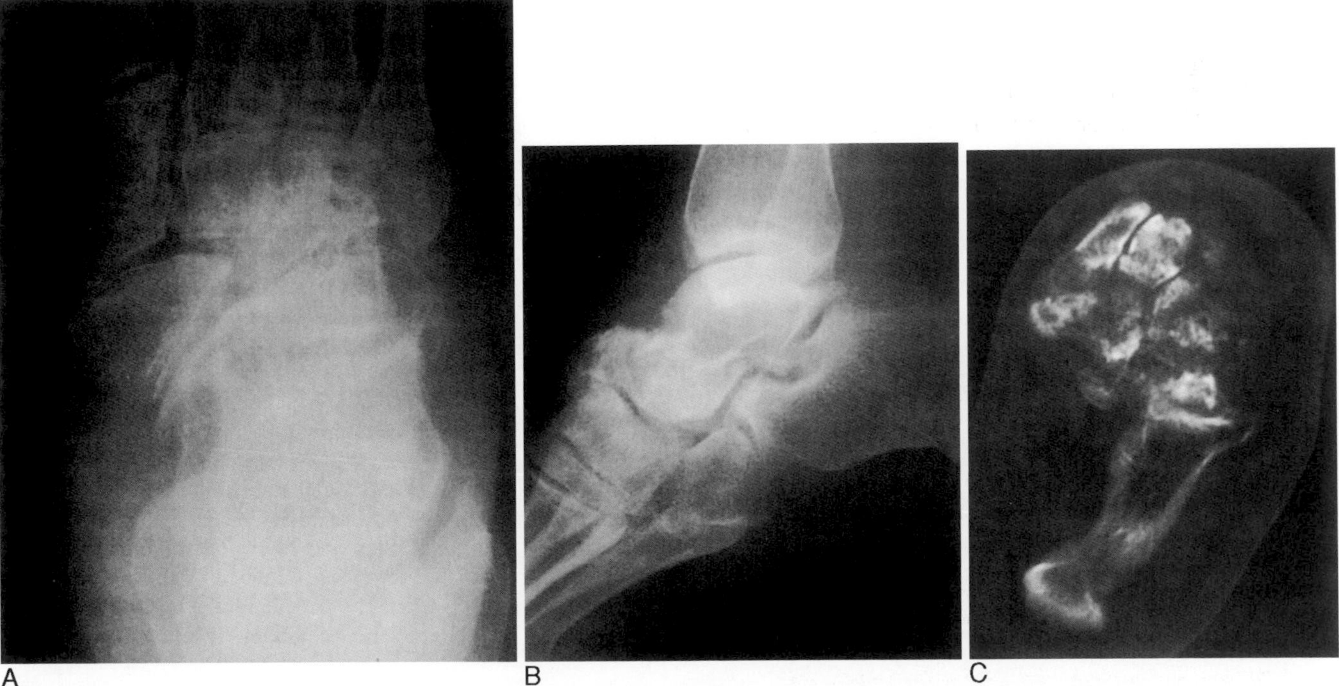

Figure 46.4 Neuropathic changes in the foot and ankle. AP (A) and lateral (B) views of the foot in a diabetic demonstrate destructive changes in the midfoot, with multiple fracture fragments. Note the sclerosis and deformity of the navicular, cuboid and lateral cuneiform. The more distal foot demonstrates normal mineralization; because of the lack of sensation, disuse osteopenia is not usually seen. Axial CT in the same patient (C) demonstrates these findings.

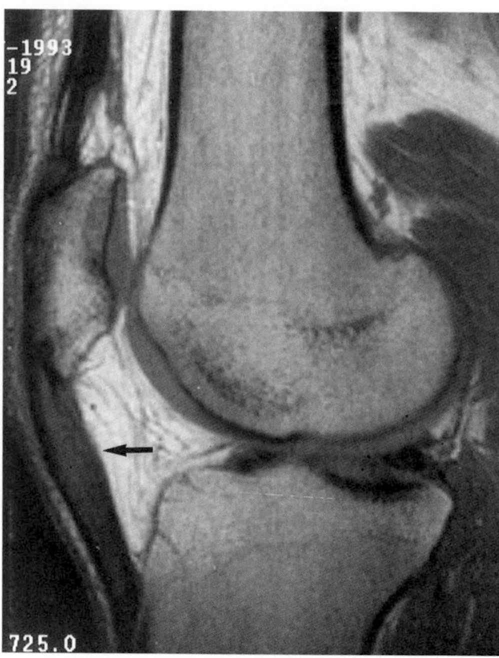

Figure 46.5 MRI appearance of tendinitis. Sagittal T1-weighted image of the knee in a professional basketball player demonstrates abnormal signal and increased size in the patellar tendon, consistent with severe tendinitis (arrow). The tendon is normally devoid of signal.

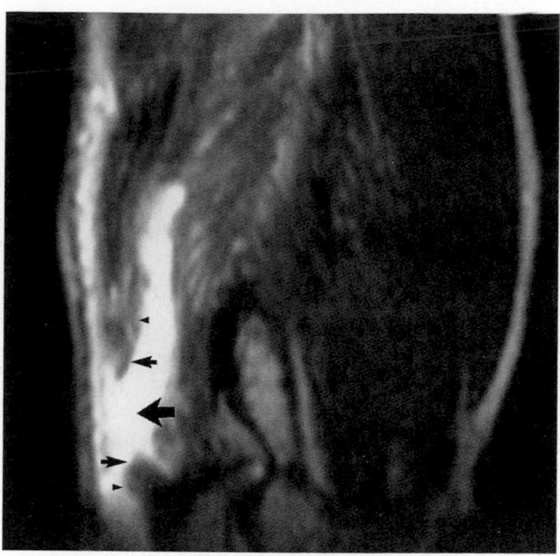

Figure 46.6 MRI appearance of a tendon disruption. Sagittal T2-weighted MRI in a patient who suffered complete rupture of the distal triceps brachii tendon after a fall. Note the large area of high signal (large arrow), indicating oedema and haemorrhage, and discontinuity of the tendon ends (smaller arrows and arrowheads). The tendon has low signal and is dark on the illustration.

THE PELVIS

The routine radiographic assessment of the pelvis always begins with a standard anteroposterior (AP) view and can be augmented with a variety of oblique views. Inlet and outlet views, obtained by angling the tube caudally and cranially respectively, can help in visualizing the obturator rings and assessing the integrity of the pelvic ring (Fig. 46.7). Judet views, obtained by rolling the patient to one obliquity or the other, can be valuable in assessing the anterior or posterior walls of the acetabula. CT[2] is a more precise method of evaluating the acutely injured pelvis, allowing detection and characterization of subtle fractures and fragments in areas of complex anatomy (Fig. 46.8). In addition, it provides detailed information about the soft tissues in and around the pelvis, such as haematomas. With post-processing techniques, three-dimensional reconstructions of the traumatized pelvis can be created and manipulated to provide the orthopaedic surgeon with information useful in planning treatment (Fig. 46.9).

To understand the mechanics of fractures of the pelvis, it is best to think of the pelvis as a ring; any disruption of one part of the ring necessitates a matching disruption elsewhere in the ring. Smaller rings exist around the obturator foramina, to which the same rule generally applies.

The injury patterns seen in the pelvis are generally related to certain specific force patterns, and are divided into *stable* and *unstable injuries*. Unstable injuries involve fractures or dislocations in the anterior and posterior aspects of the pelvic ring; these may be due to lateral compression, AP compression, or vertical shearing forces.

Lateral compressive forces usually result in bilateral fractures of the superior and inferior pubic bones associated with a unilateral fracture of the sacral alae. Displacement is uncommon in such injuries.

AP compression causes disruption of the sacroiliac joints and pubic symphysis. When all three of these are disrupted, the pelvis is widened and flattened in an 'open book' appearance (Fig. 46.10). There may be no associated fracture.

Vertical shear forces often result in a particular pattern of injury (Malgaigne complex, Fig. 46.11) in which a fracture of the medial ilium or sacrum is seen in conjunction with fractures of the superior and inferior rami on the ipsilateral side with superior displacement of the affected hemipelvis.

Stable pelvic fractures may be due to direct blows or avulsions, or may be stress injuries. Direct blows to the pelvis can result in localized fractures to the iliac wings (Fig. 46.12). A straddle injury (caused by landing on a hard object in a straddle position, as is seen in bicycle accidents) causes fractures of the ischial and pubic rami, often bilaterally, with superior displacement of the medial fragments (Fig. 46.13). Urethral injury is very commonly associated with such an

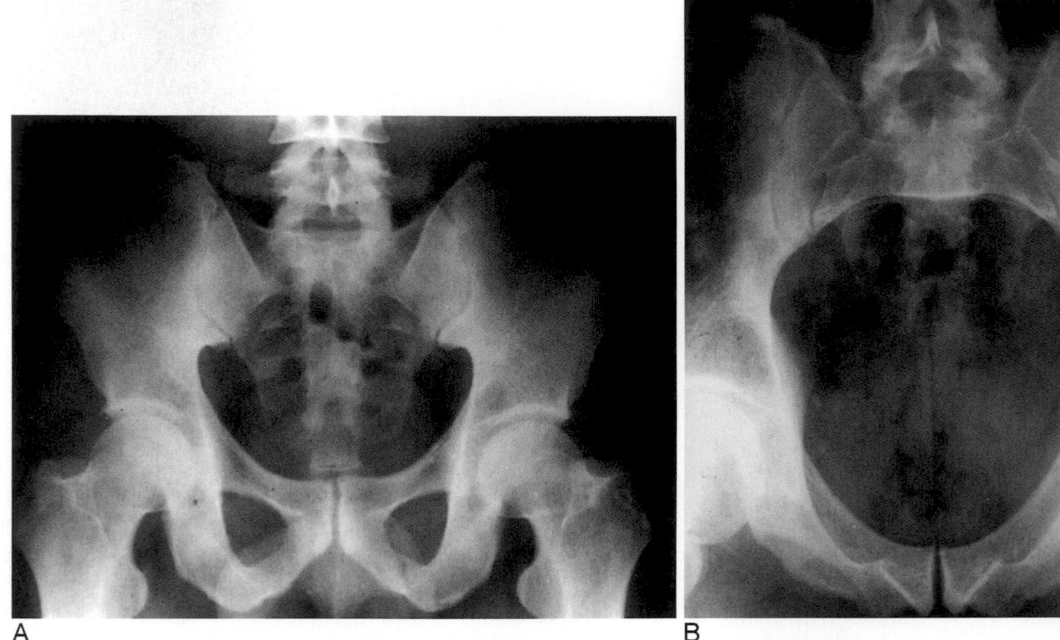

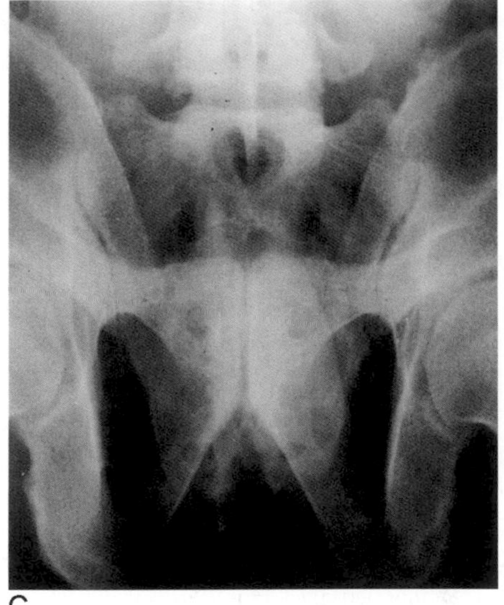

Figure 46.7 Normal views of the pelvis. AP (A), outlet (B) and inlet (C) views of the pelvis are easily obtained without manipulating the acutely injured patient.

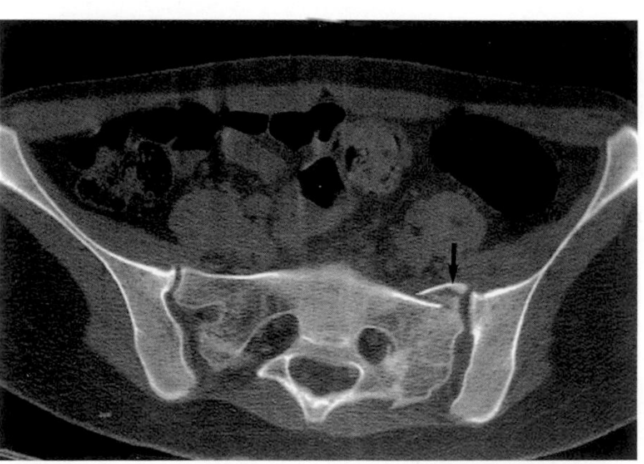

Figure 46.8 CT of a pelvic fracture. Note the fracture fragment arising from the anterior sacrum adjacent to the left sacroiliac joint (arrow). Such fractures can be very difficult to identify and characterize on routine radiographs.

injury, and a retrograde cystourethrogram should always be considered in such an instance. Transverse fractures of the lower sacrum or coccyx are usually the result of a fall on the buttocks and are best diagnosed on the lateral film.

Avulsion injuries occur at certain characteristic locations and are due to the action of the associated muscles. Such injuries are more common in children and adolescents, particularly in athletes. Avulsion of the anterior superior iliac spine is related to sartorius injury; a similar injury in the anterior inferior iliac spine reflects avulsion of the rectus femoris (Fig. 46.14). Hamstring avulsion affects the ischial tuberosity (Fig. 46.15), adductor avulsion affects the inferior ischial ramus and iliopsoas avulsion is seen off the lesser femoral trochanter.

In the elderly, insufficiency fractures of the pelvis are common in the sacral alae. They are difficult to identify on

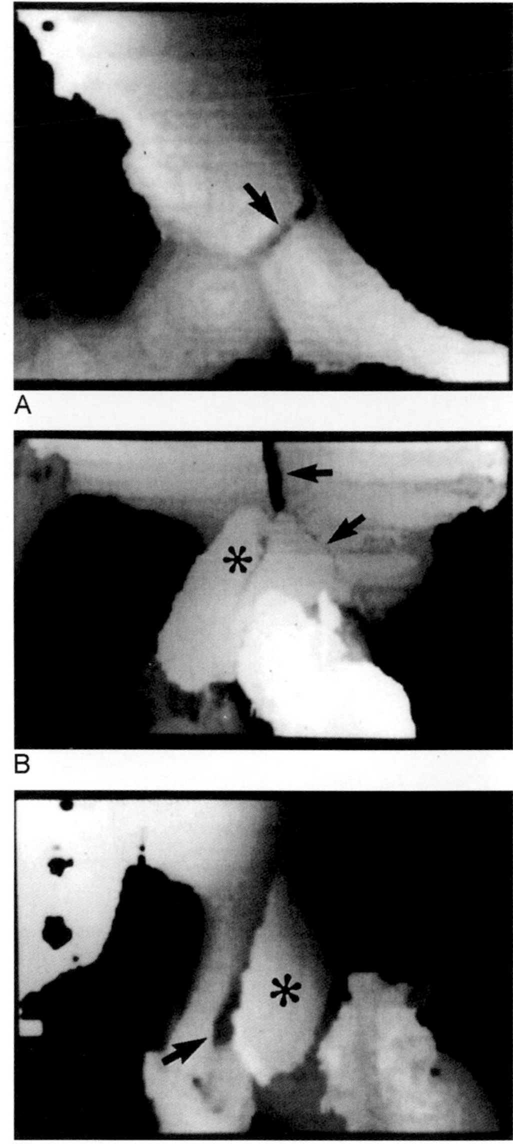

Figure 46.9 **3D reconstruction of CT images of an acetabular fracture**. Frontal (A), lateral (B) and posterior (C) projections demonstrate the fracture (arrows) with a large separated fragment (*).

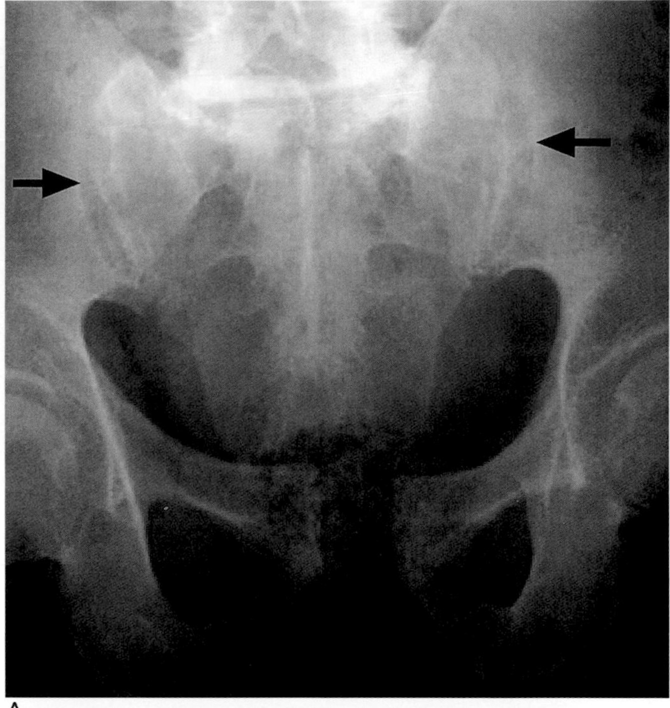

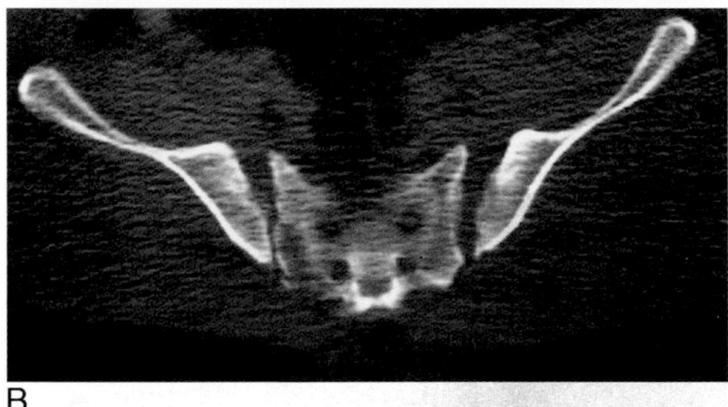

Figure 46.10 **Open book injury of the pelvis**. An AP radiograph of the pelvis (A) demonstrates widening of the sacroiliac joints (arrows) and diastasis of the symphysis pubis. CT of a different patient (B) shows the widening of the sacroiliac joints and the external angulation of the iliac wings.

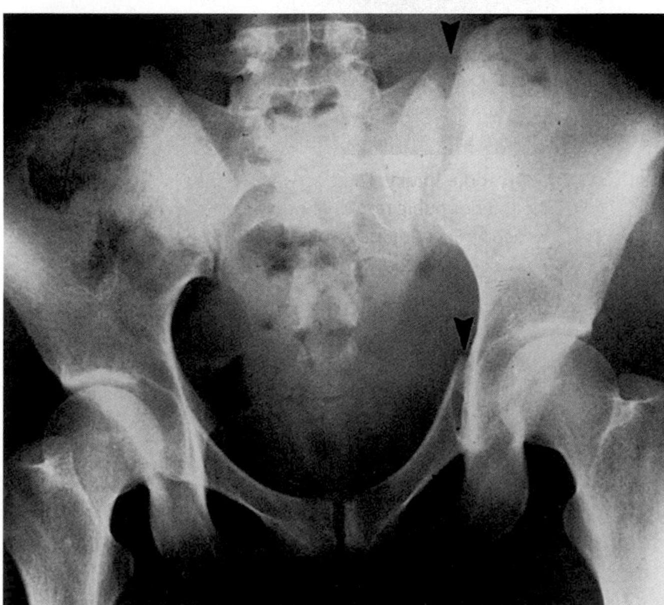

Figure 46.11 **A Malgaigne fracture**. Note fractures in the left superior and inferior pubic rami and in the posterior portion of the left iliac wing adjacent to the sacroiliac joint (arrowheads). There is superior displacement of the left hemipelvis, including the hip.

radiographs because of complex anatomy and overlying bowel, but are easily recognized on skeletal scintigraphy or MRI[3,4] as an area of increased activity in the shape of a capital letter 'H' (this is referred to as the 'Honda sign'; Fig. 46.16). Sacral insufficiency fractures are usually accompanied by insufficiency fractures of the body of the pubis.

Acetabular fractures are generally described in terms of involvement of the anterior or posterior columns, or may be centrally located. They are often associated with dislocation of the hip (Fig. 46.17). Acetabular fractures are discussed below in the section 'The Hip'.

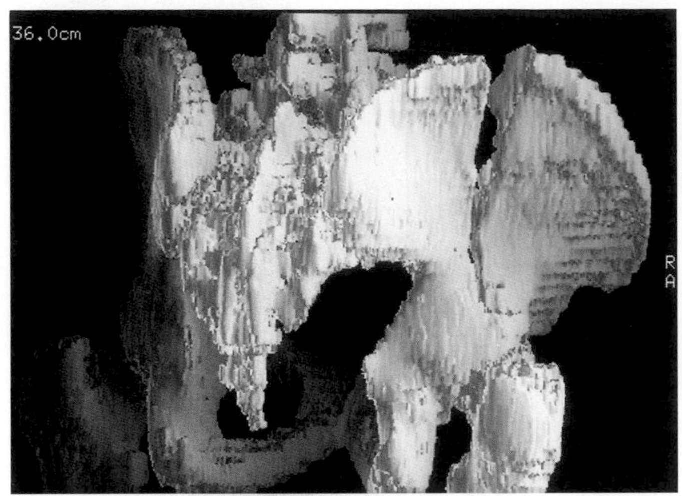

Figure 46.12 Fracture of the right iliac wing. Such fractures are associated with lateral compressive forces, as in this patient involved in a motor vehicle accident. This oblique posterior view from a 3D-reconstructed CT image demonstrates the lesion, but does not replace the radiographs and axial CT. Extension into the acetabulum is not seen on this 3D reconstruction.

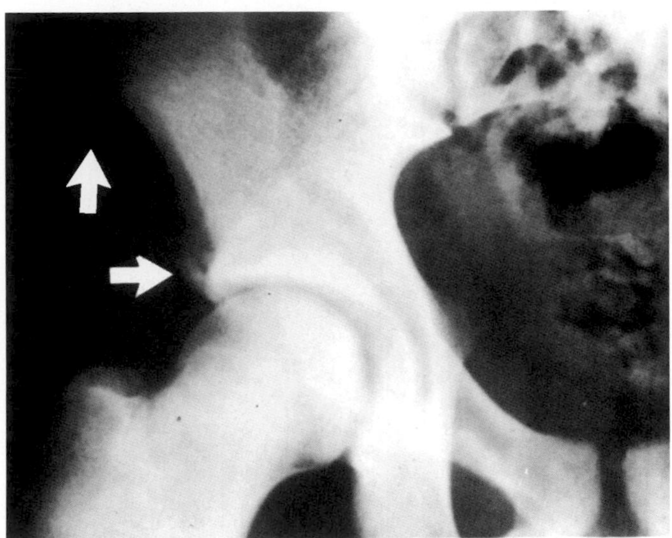

Figure 46.14 Acute traumatic avulsion of the right superior (vertical arrow) and inferior (horizontal arrow) iliac spine apophyses, due to traction on the sartorius and rectus femoris, respectively.

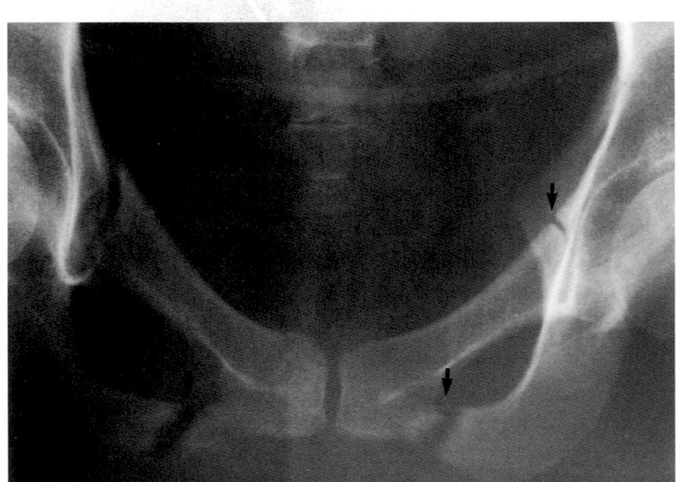

Figure 46.13 Straddle injury. There are slightly displaced fractures of the superior and inferior pubic rami bilaterally (arrows), due to a direct blow to the perineum. Such injuries are frequently associated with trauma to the urinary bladder or urethra.

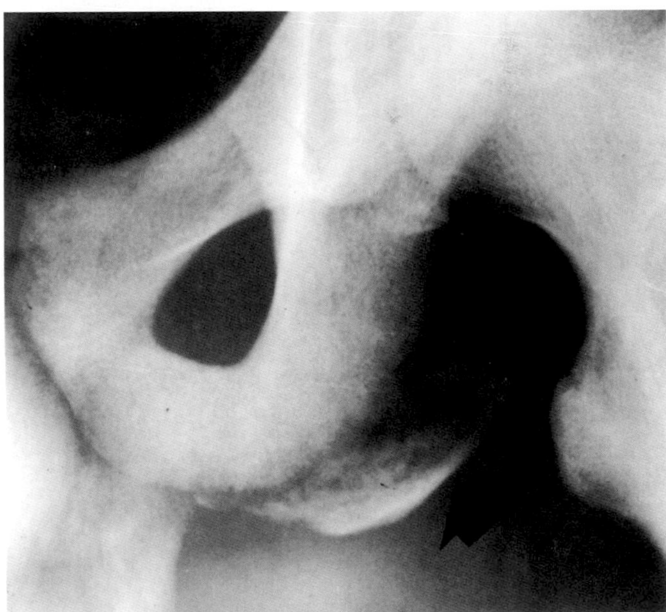

Figure 46.15 Acute traumatic avulsion of the ischial tuberosity apophysis due to traction of the hamstrings (arrow).

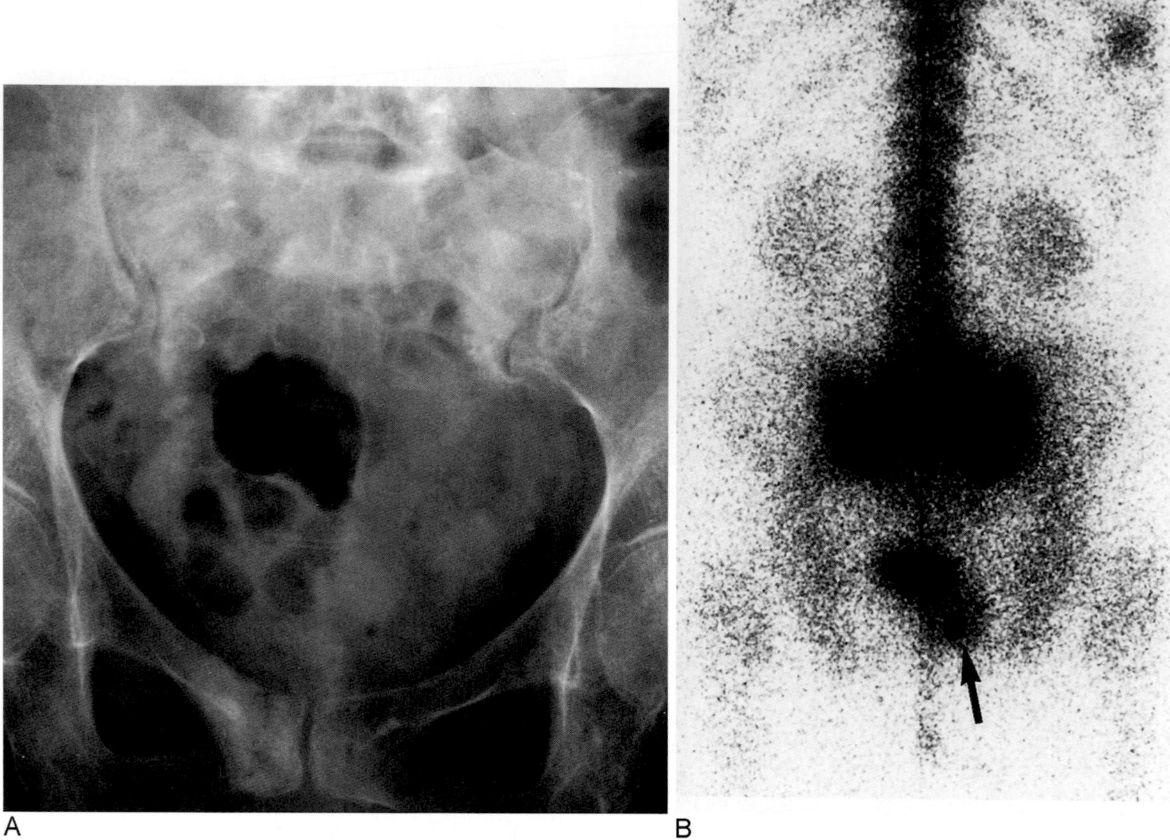

Figure 46.16 Insufficiency fracture of the sacrum. An AP radiograph (A) demonstrates sclerosis in the sacral ala paralleling the sacroiliac joints bilaterally. No distinct fracture line is evident. There was also a focus of sclerosis in the right pubis. Spot image from a bone scintigram (B) demonstrates the classic 'H' pattern of increased tracer uptake in the sacrum seen in insufficiency fracture. A fracture of the right pubis is also noted (arrow).

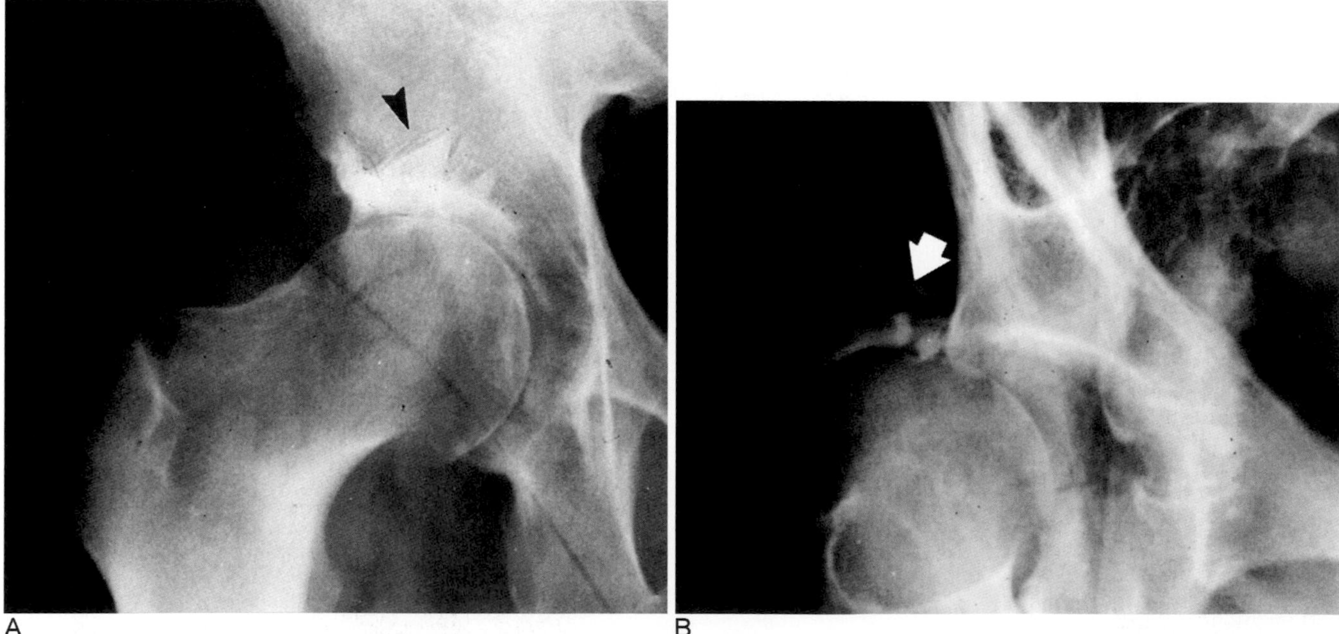

Figure 46.17 Fracture-dislocation of the right hip. An AP radiograph (A) demonstrates a curvilinear density superior to the acetabulum (arrowhead), suggesting a fracture. In an oblique (Judet) projection (B), the displaced posterosuperior fragment is well demonstrated (arrow). Note posterior subluxation of the hip.

APPENDICULAR SKELETON

Fracture description

Fractures involving the long bones in adults are described by certain universally accepted descriptive terms to make it easier to communicate with the referring clinician.

The location of the fracture should be described in precise terms. In general, the location of fractures involving the shaft of a long bone can be described by dividing the shaft into thirds (proximal, middle and distal), and placing the injury by reference to this division (e.g. 'junction of the proximal and middle third of the shaft', 'midshaft').

Perhaps the most important feature of a fracture is the distinction between *open fractures* (in which the overlying skin is disrupted and the fracture is connected with the outside environment) and *closed fractures* (in which the overlying skin is intact). This distinction is usually best made on clinical grounds, although subtle radiological clues, such as gas in the adjacent soft tissues, may suggest previous transient exposure of the bone to air in the absence of obvious clinical evidence.

Fractures extending across the full width of a bone (i.e. involving 'both cortices' radiographically) are called *complete fractures*. Fractures that do not extend all the way across the bone are referred to as *incomplete*. Incomplete fractures, such as greenstick fractures, are more common in children. *Complete fractures* should be further characterized according to their orientation. *Transverse fractures* are those that run at right angles to the long axis of the affected bone (Fig. 46.2). Oblique fractures cross the shaft at an angle (Fig. 46.18). If the inciting injury involved significant torsion, a *spiral fracture* may occur; the fragments created by a spiral fracture are often very sharp and pointed (Fig. 46.19). Any fracture that divides the bone into more than two separate fragments is said to be *comminuted*; the degree of comminution is often directly related to the force of the injury. A *segmental* fracture refers to an injury that results from two separate complete (usually transverse) fractures, and divides the bones into three large fragments (Fig. 46.20). A *butterfly fragment* is a large triangular fragment, usually oriented along the long axis of the bone (Fig. 46.21).

The relationship of the fracture fragments to each other is another important descriptive element of the trauma report. In general, the proximal fragment, *regardless of its relative size, is considered the point of reference* when describing fragment

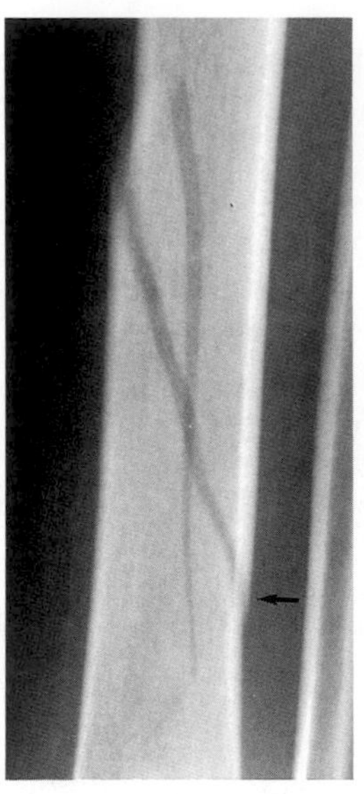

Figure 46.19 Spiral fracture. AP projection of the leg demonstrates a spiral fracture of the tibia. Note the sharp ends of the fracture fragments (arrows), which may cause significant soft tissue injury.

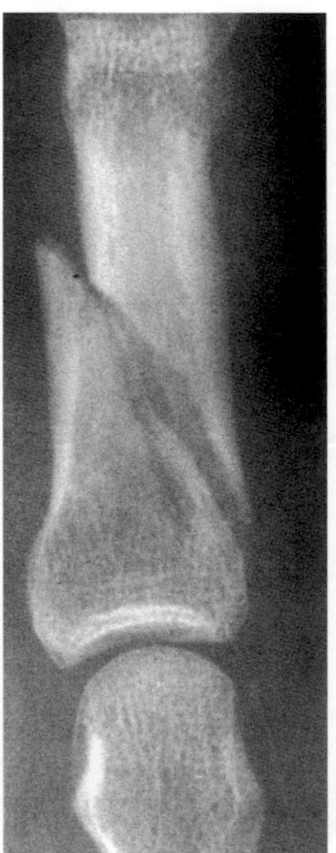

Figure 46.18 An oblique fracture of the proximal phalanx of the fourth digit. There is minimal override of the fracture fragments.

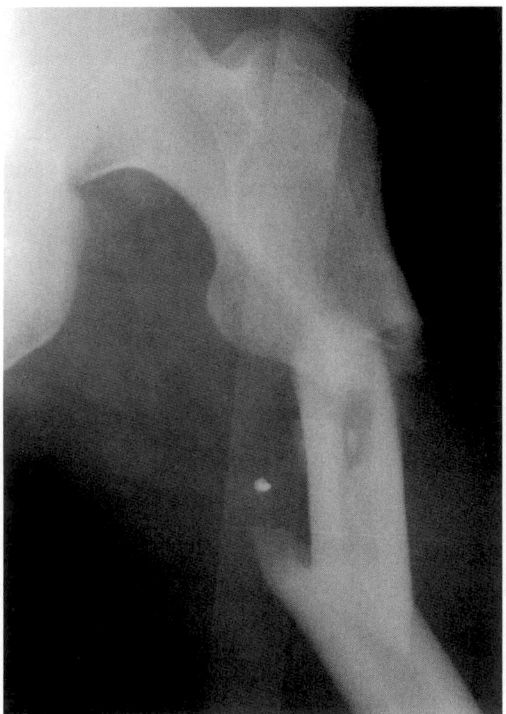

Figure 46.20 Segmental fracture. AP view of the left hip demonstrates a three-part fracture of the proximal femoral shaft, due to massive trauma in a motor vehicle accident.

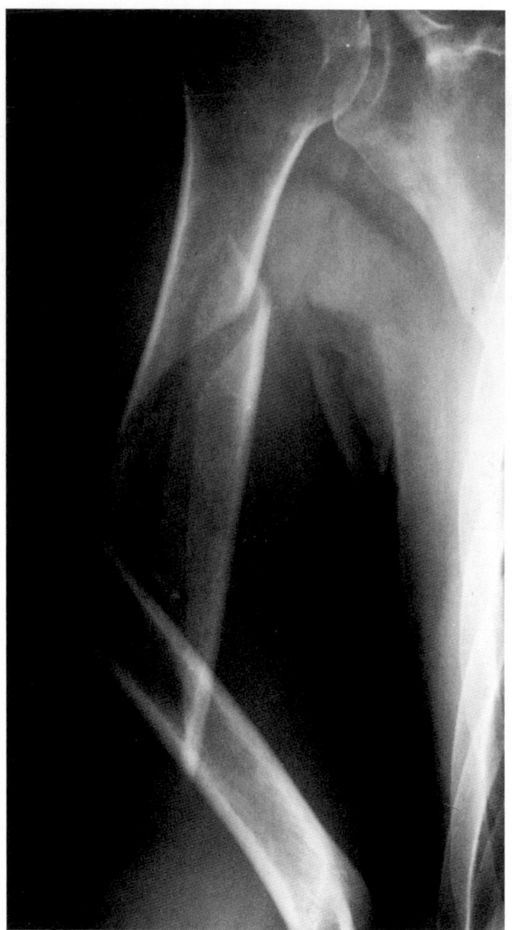

Figure 46.21 A comminuted fracture of the midshaft of the right humerus demonstrates a large medial butterfly fragment (large arrow). There is marked lateral angulation at the fracture line between the major fracture fragments.

displacement. Displacement refers to the linear translation of the distal fragment(s) relative to the proximal fragment. Displacement should be described in two planes (e.g. anterior/posterior and medial/lateral), so it is imperative to obtain orthogonal views of all long bone fractures (Fig. 46.22). While measurement of the displacement may be given precisely (e.g. in mm), such measurements may be inaccurate due to the magnification inherent in the image. A better approximation can be achieved by expressing displacement in terms of the cortical width or shaft width of the affected bone (e.g. 'one shaft width medial displacement').

Angulation refers to the shifted direction of the long axis of the *distal fragment* relative to that of the proximal fragment. The most commonly used method of description refers to the *angle made* by the *major fracture fragments at the site of the fracture*; if the fragments form an arrow pointing laterally, we say '*there is lateral angulation at the fracture line*' (Fig. 46.23). Alternatively, this same fracture could be described in terms of the motion of the distal fragment relative to the proximal one: '*there is medial angulation of the distal fracture fragment*'. Notice that although these two descriptions of the injury sound like opposites, they are really saying the same thing. Alternatively, some would call this a fracture with *varus angulation*. Any joint or fracture in which the *distal fragment is angulated medially* is termed *varus*; if the distal bone or fragment is angulated away from the midline, it is termed *valgus*.

It is imperative that the joints above and below a fracture be included in the radiograph so that the degree of angulation can be evaluated properly.

Distraction and impaction refer to the separation or pressing together, respectively, of fracture fragments along the long axis

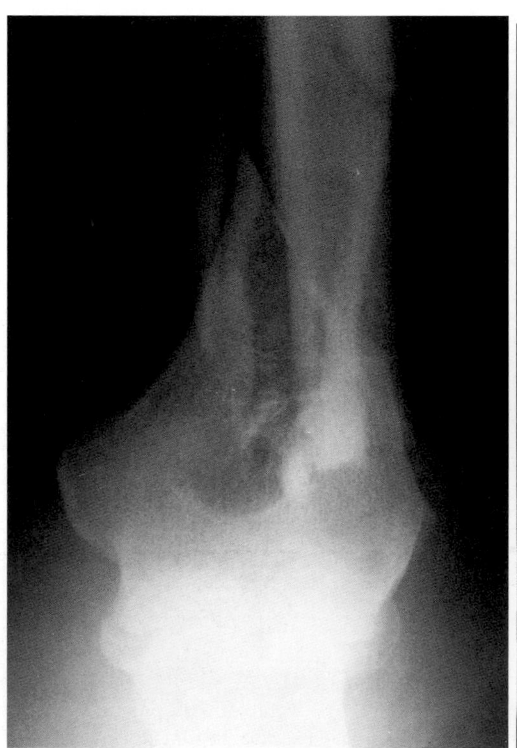

A

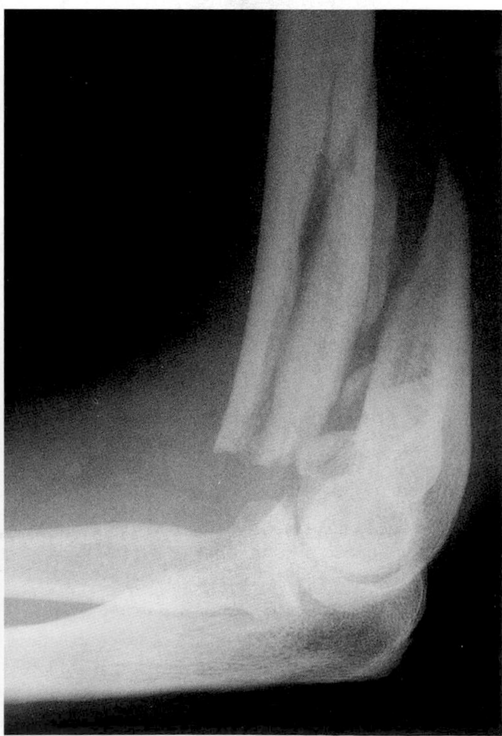

B

Figure 46.22 Fragment displacement. AP (A) and lateral (B) views of an acute comminuted fracture of the supracondylar humerus demonstrate one-half shaft width medial displacement (seen on the AP view), and posterior displacement by more than one complete shaft width (on the lateral view) of the major distal fracture fragment. There is no significant angulation.

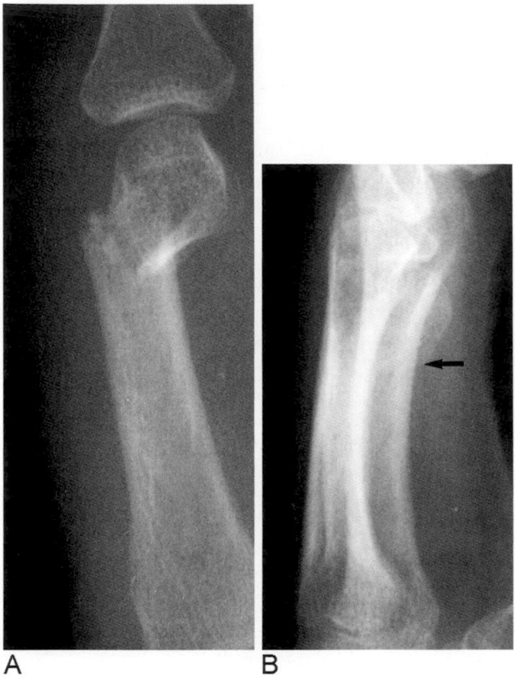

Figure 46.23 Angulation of fracture fragments. AP (A) and lateral (B) views of a 'boxer's fracture' of the distal fifth metacarpal demonstrates typical radial and volar angulation of the distal fragment (arrow).

of the bone (Fig. 46.24). If the fragments overlap one another without impaction, they are said to be overriding or bayoneting. As with displacement, it is probably better to relate the degree of distraction or compression to a reproducible entity such as the cortical width of the bone.

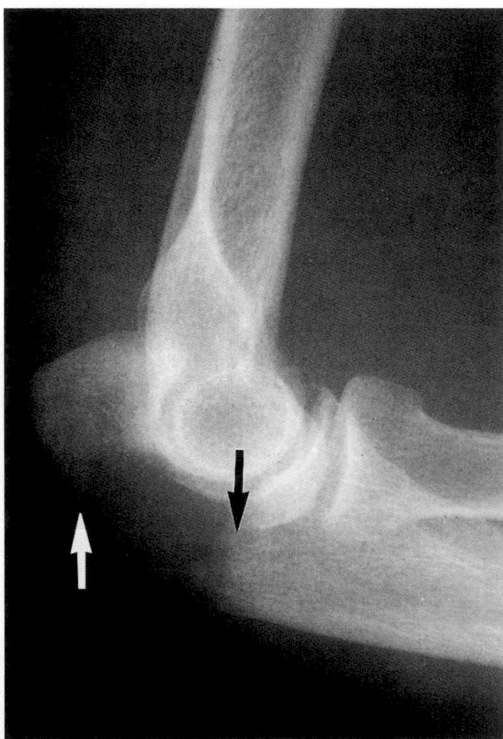

Figure 46.24 Distracted fracture of the olecranon. Lateral view of the elbow in a patient who was struck by a bus, causing fracture of the olecranon process of the ulna (arrows). Note the wide distraction of the fragments, caused by retraction of the triceps brachii inserting on the proximal fragment.

Displacements involving the components of a joint are described with two additional terms: dislocation refers to the condition in which the articular surfaces normally in contact are completely separated, while subluxation occurs when the surfaces make only partial contact (Fig. 46.25).

Avulsion fracture refers to the separation of a (usually small) bone fragment at the attachment site of a ligament or a tendon. Avulsion injuries are common about the ankle and in the fingers. Occasionally, the avulsed bone fragment may be quite large; the fracture line is almost always transverse (Fig. 46.26). Because the avulsion fracture is functionally equivalent to disruption of the attached soft tissue structure, the importance of this type of injury depends on the nature and importance of that structure. If the tendon or ligament is disrupted from the bony attachment site, there is often no associated finding on routine radiographs except soft tissue swelling. MRI can directly visualize tendon or ligament injuries. US may also demonstrate tendon disruption.

An osteochondral fracture is a disruption of articular cartilage and the underlying subchondral bone, usually seen as a curvilinear zone of abnormality at the articular end of a bone (Fig. 46.27). The fragment may become completely detached and separate from the native bone, leaving a defect in the joint surface; the fragment may enter the joint space as a loose body. Common sites of this type of injury include the femoral condyles, patella and the talar dome. MRI can identify injuries of the joint surface (Fig. 46.28).

The term occult fracture is used to describe an injury to bone that is clinically suspected, but cannot be identified on initial radiographs. Subsequent hyperaemia and local deossification around the fracture site may render the fracture more visible later; a repeat radiograph in 7–10 days may reveal a fracture line. A *bone bruise* or *contusion* is defined as an area of acute bone marrow oedema secondary to trauma without a definable fracture line and is the result of microtrabecular disruption with associated haemorrhage and oedema. While undetectable with conventional radiography or CT, bone

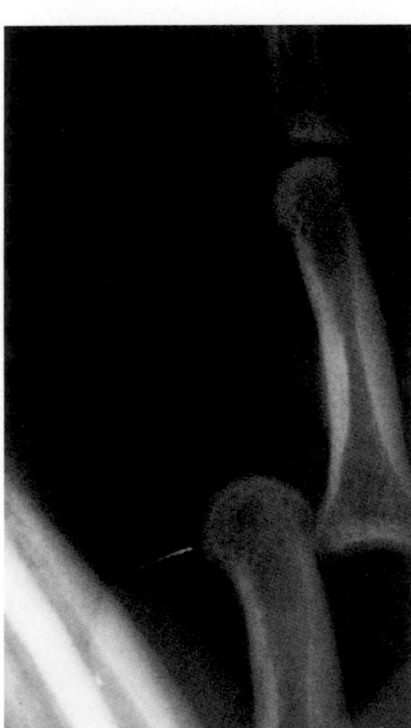

Figure 46.25 Dislocation at the proximal interphalangeal joint of the fourth finger. There is complete separation of the articular surfaces of the bones (arrows).

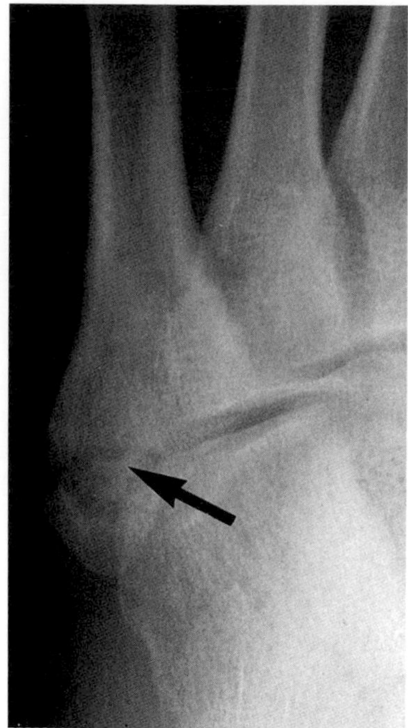

Figure 46.26 Avulsion fracture. AP views of the foot demonstrate a horizontal lucency at the base of the fifth metatarsal (arrow), representing an avulsion injury at the insertion site of the peroneus brevis tendon.

bruises and contusions are readily diagnosed with MRI (Fig. 46.29).

SPECIFIC INJURIES

The shoulder

The routine radiographic evaluation of the shoulder should include AP views with both internal and external humeral rotation (with the arm at the side). These can be augmented with: a true tangential view of the glenohumeral joint (Grashey view), which is obtained by rotating the patient towards the affected side; an axillary view, which requires abduction of the arm and can be difficult for patients in pain; and the transscapular ('Y') view, which projects along the long axis of the scapula (approximately 20 degrees off true lateral) (Fig. 46.30).

The shoulder is a very mobile joint, and dislocation of the shoulder is a common injury. The vast majority (about 90%) of shoulder dislocations involve *anterior dislocation of the humeral head* relative to the glenoid fossa. Usually there is medial and inferior displacement, so that the humeral head ends up

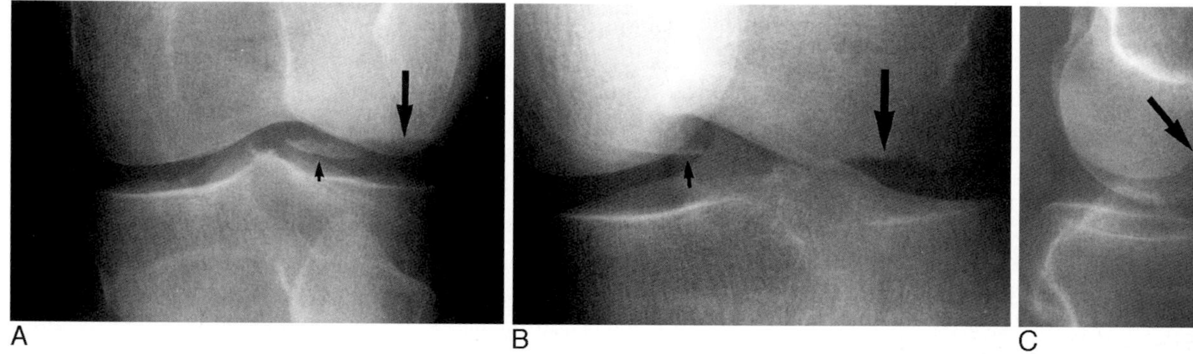

Figure 46.27 Osteochondral fracture. AP (A) oblique (B) and lateral (C) views of the knee demonstrate a curvilinear defect in the lateral femoral condyle (arrow) representing an osteochondral injury and the displaced fragment (small arrow) located in the knee joint. Such injuries involve subchondral bone and the overlying cartilage, and are often the result of impaction forces.

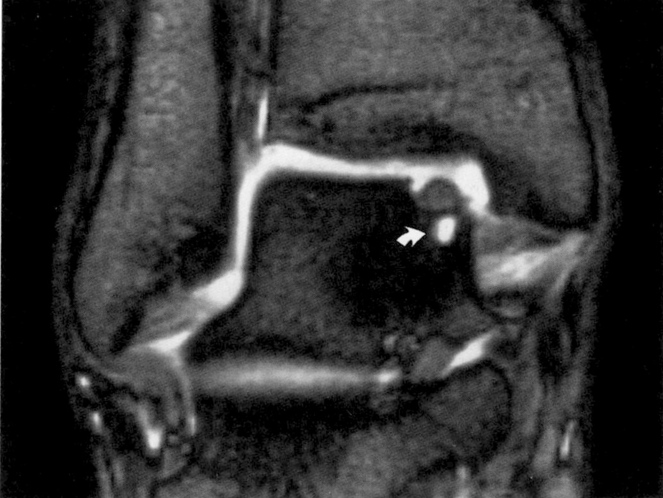

Figure 46.28 MRI of an osteochondral fracture. Coronal T2-weighted image of an ankle demonstrates high signal fluid between a fracture fragment in the talar dome and the native talus (arrow). Fluid can track between the fragment and the talus only if the overlying cartilage is disrupted.

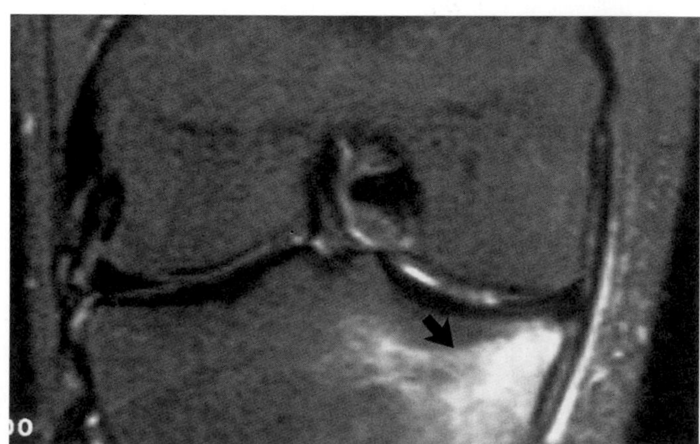

Figure 46.29 Bone contusion demonstrated with MRI. Coronal STIR (fat-suppressed T2-weighted) image of the knee demonstrates an area of high signal oedema in the medial proximal tibia (arrow) without gross disruption of the cortex. This is a bone contusion due to a direct blow to the tibia.

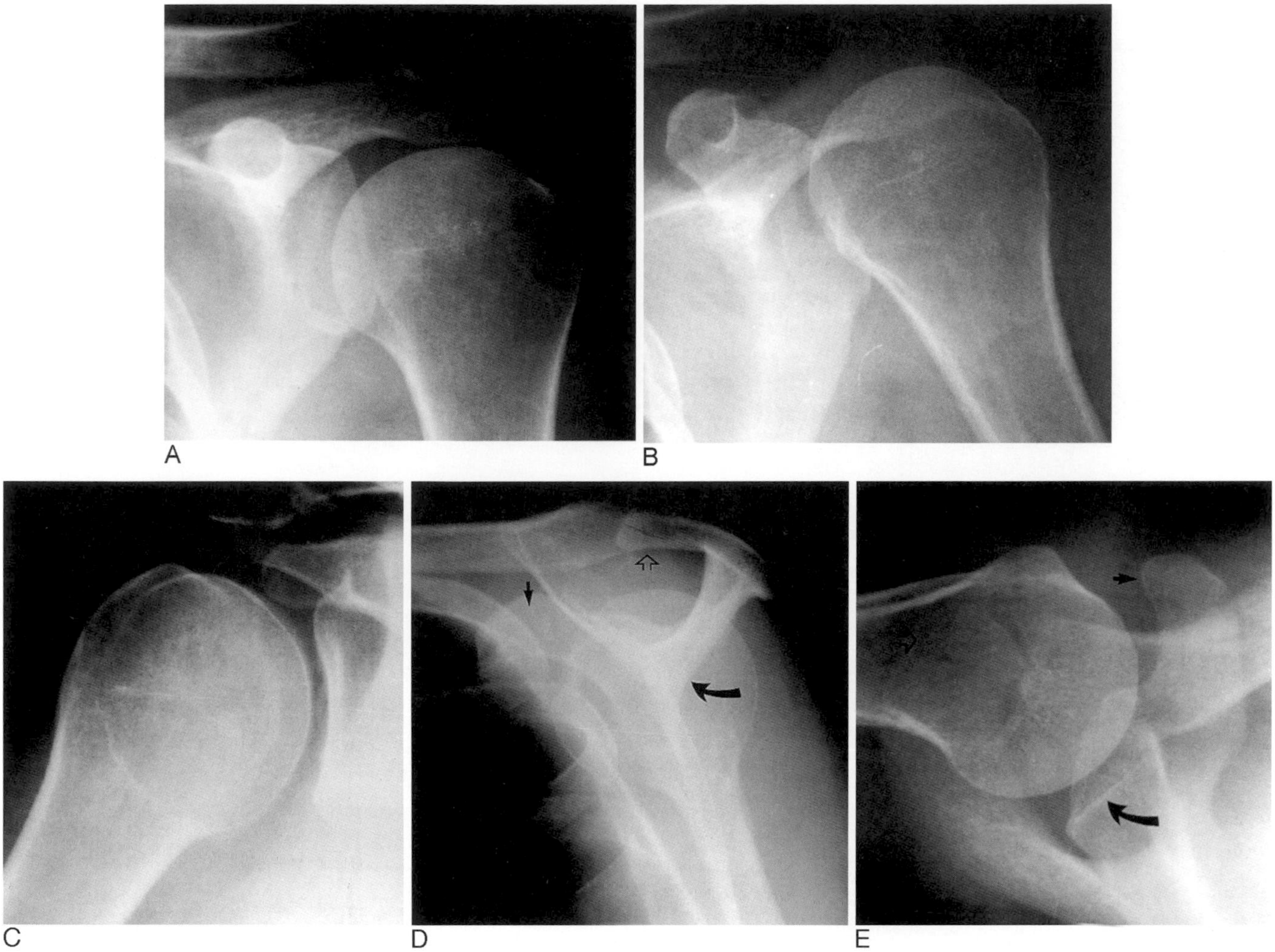

Figure 46.30 Normal shoulder. AP projections with the humerus in external (A) and internal (B) rotation demonstrate the glenohumeral joint in obliquity. The greater humeral tuberosity is profiled in external rotation, but is superimposed over the humeral head in internal rotation. The Grashey view (C) is an oblique AP designed to demonstrate the glenohumeral joint in tangent; it is obtained by rotating the patient about 40 degrees towards the side being imaged. Trans-scapular (D) and axillary (E) views demonstrate the acromion (open arrow), coracoid (small arrow) and glenoid fossa (curved arrow).

beneath the coracoid process; this is referred to as a subcoracoid dislocation (Fig. 46.31). The humerus is in external rotation with anterior dislocation. Avulsion fractures of the greater tuberosity are commonly associated with an anterior dislocation. About 20% of anterior shoulder dislocations result in an impaction fracture of the posterior superior humeral head where the head strikes the inferior glenoid after coming to rest in a subcoracoid dislocation. This indentation defect is termed a Hill–Sachs fracture and is best seen on internal rotation (Fig. 46.32) or axillary views. A fracture of the antero-inferior glenoid rim, referred to as a Bankart lesion (Fig. 46.33), may also occur. The presence of one or both of these lesions increases the chance of recurrent dislocations.

Posterior shoulder dislocations account for about 5% of shoulder dislocations. Approximately half of these are related to seizures or electrocutions; simultaneous and bilateral injuries may occur in this circumstance. A direct blow to the anterior humeral head can also cause a posterior shoulder dislocation. Diagnosis of a posterior shoulder dislocation on the routine anteroposterior shoulder radiograph is often difficult. Typically, the humerus is in fixed *internal rotation*, causing

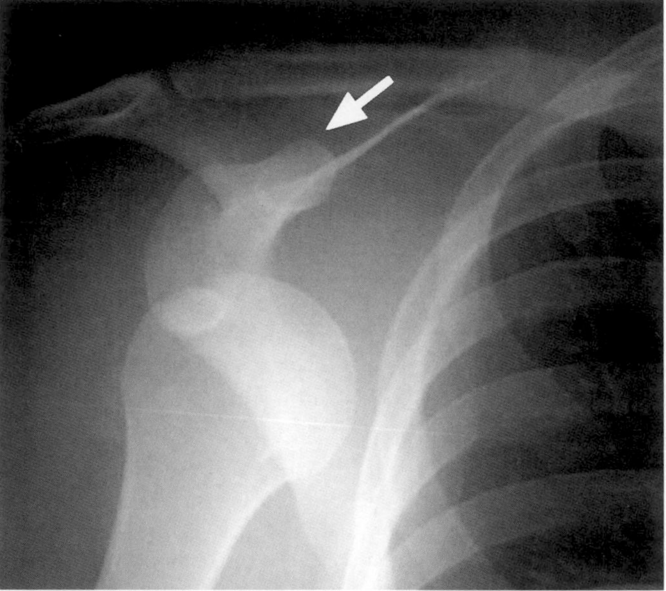

Figure 46.31 Anterior (subcoracoid) shoulder dislocation. AP radiograph demonstrates the humeral head located inferomedial to the glenoid, beneath the coracoid process (arrow). This appearance is pathognomonic of anterior dislocation.

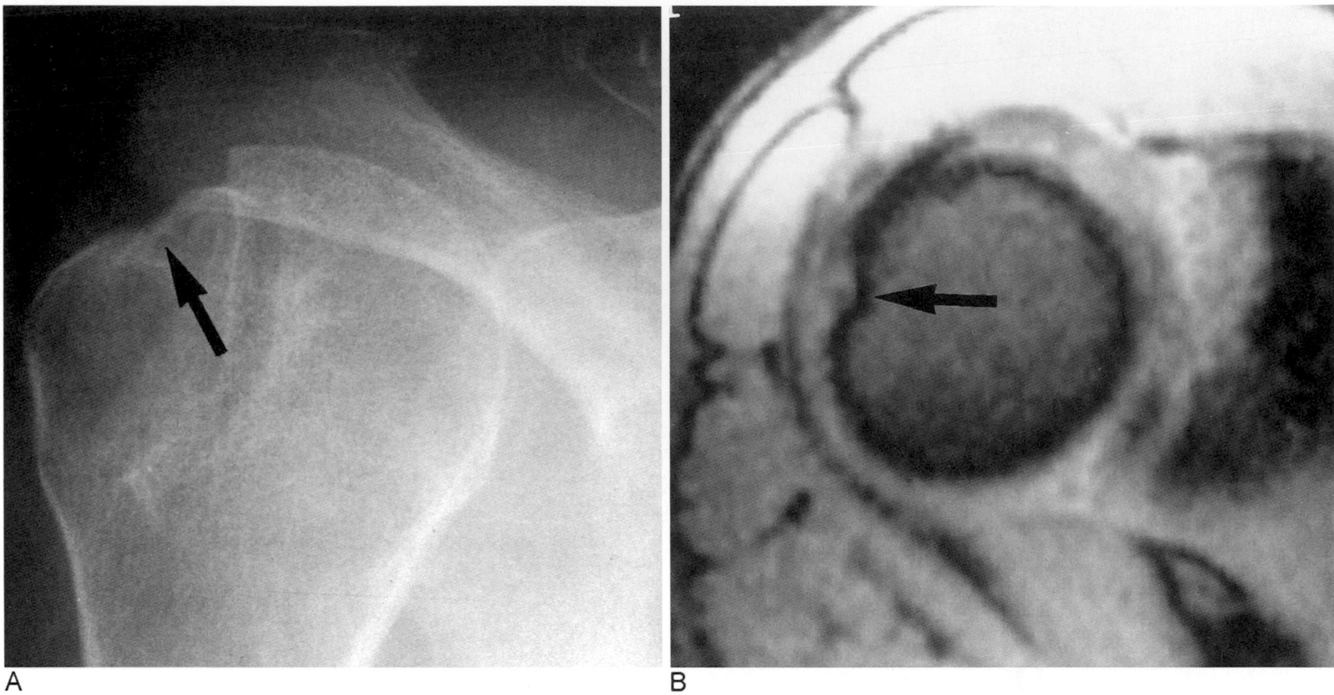

Figure 46.32 Hill–Sachs deformity of the humerus. Internal rotation view of the shoulder (A) shows a notch in the posterolateral aspect of the humeral head (arrow). (B) Axial T2-weighted MRI from another patient who previously suffered an anterior shoulder dislocation demonstrates a Hill–Sachs defect (arrow). The Hill–Sachs defect is seen as a notch in the posterolateral humeral head above or at the level of the coracoid process.

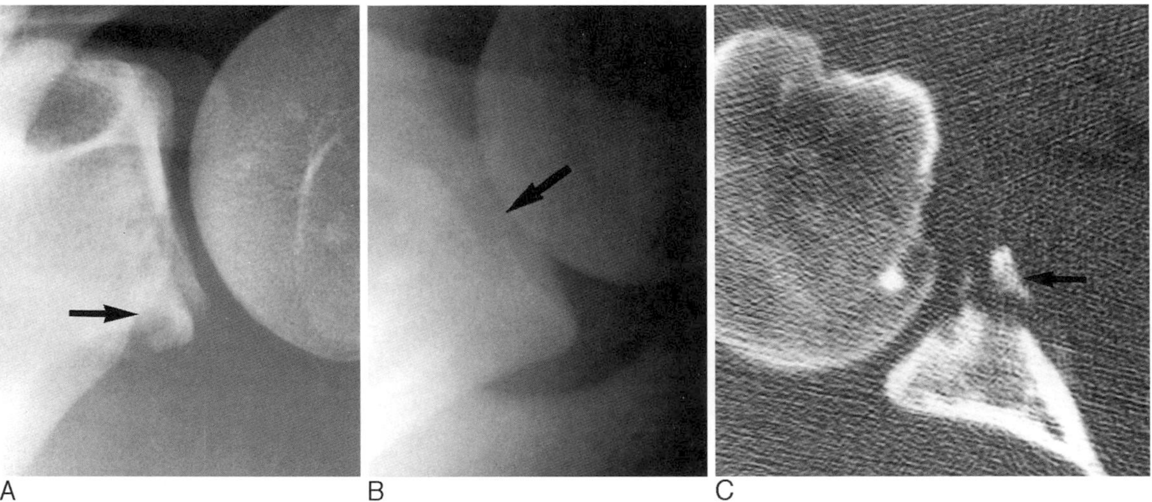

Figure 46.33 Bankhart injury of the inferior glenoid rim. AP (A) and axillary (B) radiographs in a patient who suffered an anterior shoulder dislocation show an irregularity in the inferior bony glenoid, consistent with a Bankhart fracture (arrow). The shoulder has been reduced. Axial CT (C) from the same patient shows the relationship of the fragment (arrow) to the glenoid.

the head and neck of the humerus to appear like an electric light bulb—the *'light bulb sign'*. The craniocaudal relationship of the humerus and the bony glenoid is not usually disturbed, but subtle *widening of the joint* (greater than 6 mm) may be detected. Alternatively, the joint may be diminished, or the bones may actually overlap on the Grashey view. A Y view or axillary view may confirm. The corresponding fracture involves the medial humeral head and appears as a vertical line of sclerotic density paralleling the medial cortex; this impaction fracture is referred to as the *trough sign* (Fig. 46.34).

CT of the shoulder can exclude or identify entrapped fragments and evaluate the integrity of the bony glenoid. The cartilaginous glenoid labrum, however, is best studied with MRI or postarthrogram MRI or CT (Fig. 46.35).

The term 'pseudo-dislocation of the shoulder' has been used to describe the inferolateral displacement of the humeral head relative to the glenoid, secondary to a large haemarthrosis following comminuted intra-articular humeral fractures (Fig. 46.36). While there is obvious incongruity of the joint in this setting, the joint alignment returns to normal after aspiration or resorption of the intra-articular fluid.

Tears of the rotator cuff may result from an acute trauma, particularly in younger patients. As bony evidence of this injury is usually absent, evaluation with MRI is required to identify the

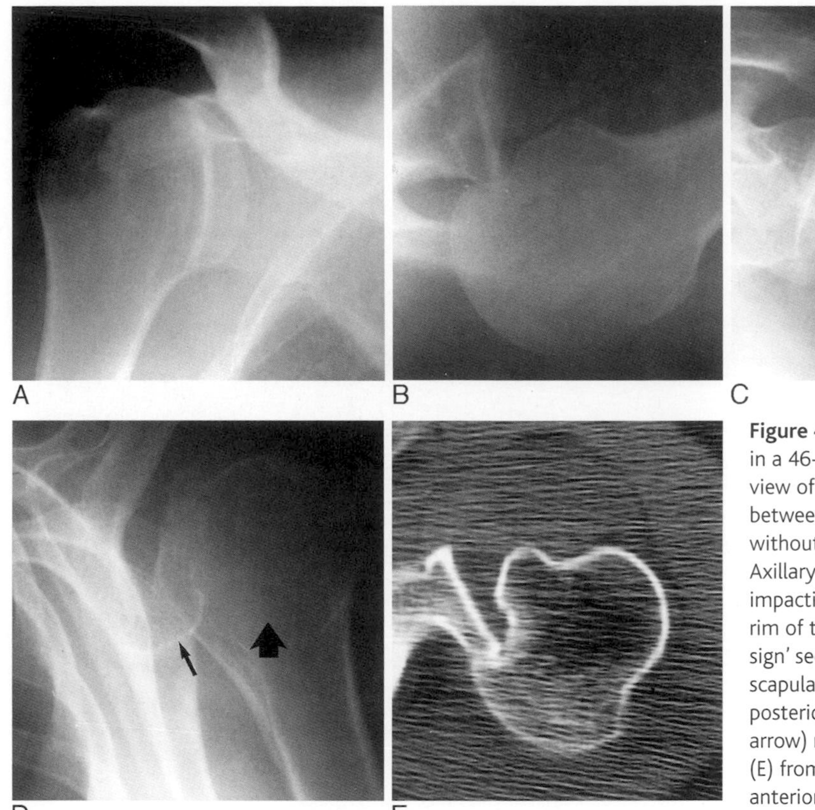

Figure 46.34 Posterior shoulder dislocation in a 46-year-old man who was assaulted. Grashey view of the right shoulder demonstrates overlap between the humeral head and the glenoid fossa without significant craniocaudal displacement. Axillary view from a different patient (B) shows impaction of the humeral head on the posterior rim of the glenoid; this leads to (C) the 'trough sign' seen on an AP radiograph (arrow). Trans-scapular radiograph from a third patient shows posterior dislocation of the humeral head (large arrow) relative to the glenoid (small arrow). CT (E) from the patient in (D) shows impaction of the anterior humeral head on the posterior glenoid.

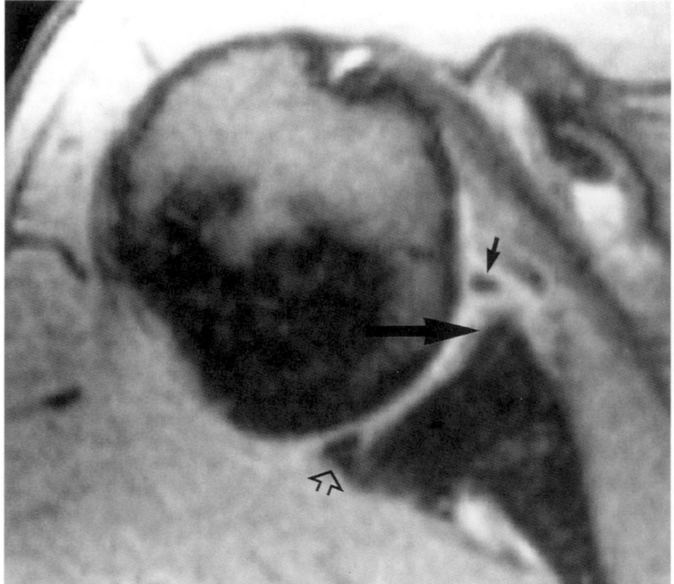

Figure 46.35 Tear of the glenoid labrum. Axial T2-weighted image in a patient who previously suffered an anterior shoulder dislocation demonstrates separation of the anterior glenoid labrum (arrow) from the bony glenoid (large arrow). The posterior labrum (open arrow) remains intact.

tear. The supraspinatus is the most commonly injured of the cuff musculature; tears generally occur within 2 cm of the attachment to the greater tuberosity and appear as areas of high signal and discontinuity within the normal tendinous signal void on T2-weighted images (Fig. 46.37). Increased signal on gradient echo, T1- and proton density-weighted sequences may be the result

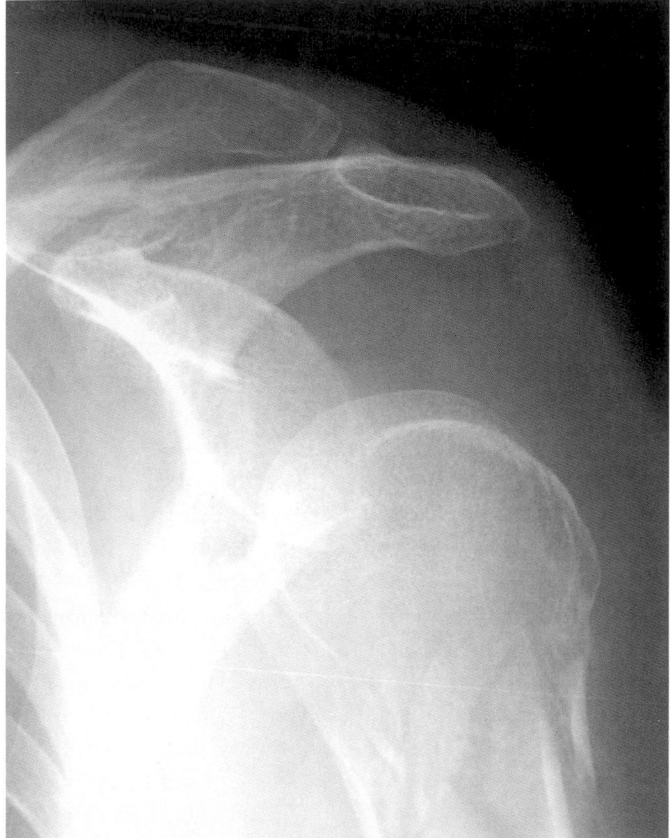

Figure 46.36 Pseudodislocation of the shoulder. AP radiograph demonstrates a comminuted fracture of the surgical neck of the left humerus. There is inferior pseudosubluxation of the humerus relative to the glenoid due to large haemarthrosis.

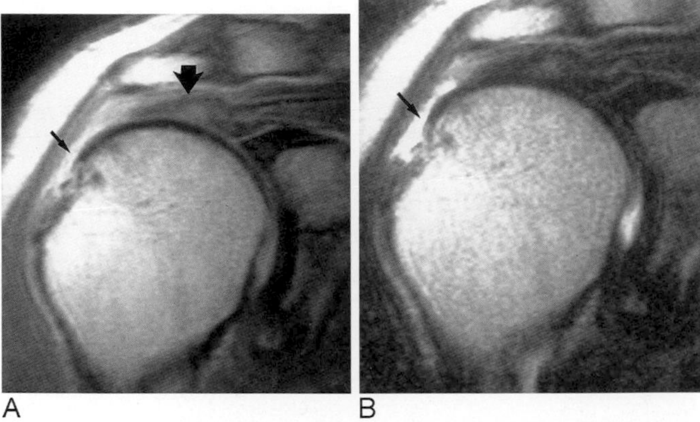

Figure 46.37 Rotator cuff tear. Coronal oblique proton density (A) and T2-weighted images demonstrate abnormal high signal in the expected region of the distal supraspinatus tendon (small arrow), consistent with a complete tear. The supraspinatus tendon is retracted (large arrow).

of an artefact due to 'magic angle'. These sequences should not be used without correlation to the T2-weighted sequences in the diagnosis of rotator cuff disease. A mechanically equivalent injury is avulsion of the greater humeral tuberosity.

Scapula

Fractures of the scapula are most often due to falls or a crushing injury. They are usually located in the scapular neck or body. Ipsilateral upper rib and clavicle fractures, pulmonary contusion and pleural effusion are often seen in association with scapular fracture.

Clavicle

Evaluation of the clavicle requires a straight and a cranially angled AP view. Fractures of the mid-third of the shaft (Fig. 46.38A) are most common. Fractures involving the distal aspect of the clavicle may disrupt the coraco-clavicular ligaments and/or enter the acromio-clavicular joint.

Acromio-clavicular joint injury

Subluxation or dislocation of the acromio-clavicular (AC) joint involves various degrees of disruption of the AC and coraco-clavicular ligaments. Often referred to as a 'shoulder separation', they most often result from a direct blow as occurs in a fall or frontal impact with a large stationary object (e.g. hitting a tree while skiing). Normal alignment of the joint is present on an AP view when the AC joint measures less than 5 mm wide and the undersurfaces of the acromion and the distal clavicle form an uninterrupted arc. The evaluation of the AC joint following trauma is easily accomplished with an AP view of both sides performed with the patient holding 6–9 kg (15–20 lb) weights in each hand (stress view) in order to emphasize ligamentous laxity or disruption. AC joint separations (Fig. 46.38 B, C) are classified according to the degree of displacement of normal structures. Grade I injuries represent incomplete disruption of the acromio-clavicular ligaments, and are manifested by widening of the AC joint (particularly on stress views). Grade II injuries represent complete disruption of the AC ligaments and partial disruption of the coraco-

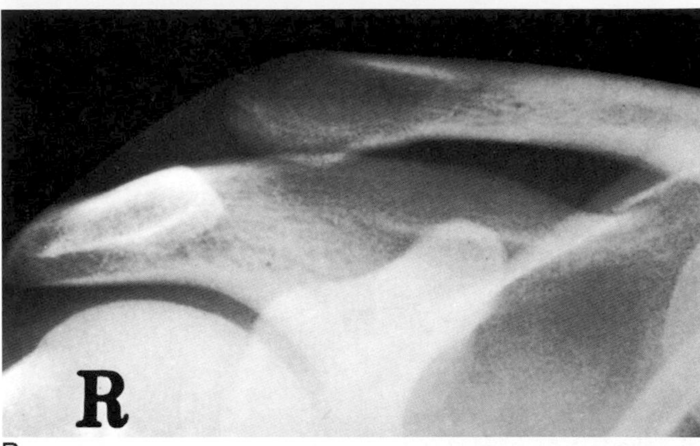

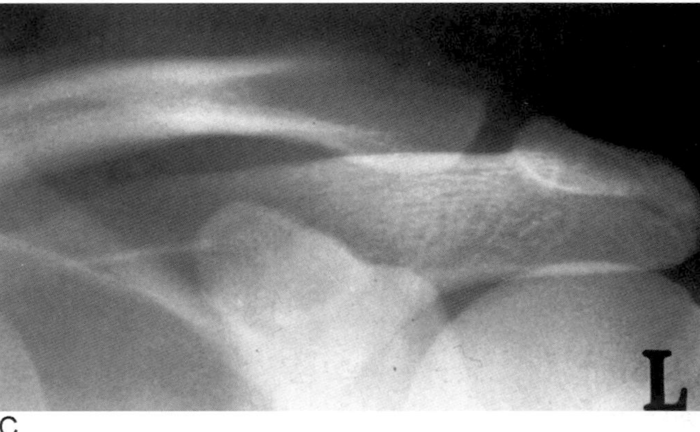

Figure 46.38 Clavicular injuries. The middle third of the clavicle (A) is the most common location for clavicle fractures. (B) First degree separation of the right acromio-clavicular joint on weight bearing (10–20 lb held in the hands). Normal left acromio-clavicular joint (C) for comparison.

clavicular ligaments; they are manifested by elevation of the clavicle less than a complete shaft width above the acromion. Grade III injuries are the most severe, and involve complete disruption of the AC and coraco-clavicular ligaments with elevation of the clavicle as determined by an increased distance between the superior surface of the coracoid process and undersurface of the clavicle. The normal coraco-clavicular distance is 1.1–1.2 cm. Stress views are unnecessary to diagnose Grade III AC separation evident on the initial radiographs.

Sternoclavicular dislocation

This uncommon injury is difficult to diagnose with routine radiographs. While an AP radiograph may demonstrate widening of the joint or overlap of the medial clavicle and the manubrium, CT is the preferred method for evaluating this injury. Anterior dislocation of the clavicle is the more common injury and results in superior displacement of the clavicle relative to the normal side. The less common posterior displacement is, however, more dangerous, because there could be an injury to the great vessels at the thoracic inlet. The veins are more frequently compromised than the arteries, but the trachea may also be compressed (Fig. 46.39).

Humerus

Fractures of the proximal humerus most commonly occur in the elderly; the surgical neck of the humerus is the most typical location. These fractures are often associated with separation of the greater tuberosity (Fig. 46.40).

Fractures of the humeral shaft tend to be angulated and overriding, due to muscular contraction on the individual fragments. Fractures of the distal humeral shaft are frequently spiral fractures.

Elbow

The routine evaluation of the elbow should include AP, flexed lateral and external oblique views (Fig. 46.41). Falls on an outstretched hand in an adult may result in a radial head fracture, which is usually oriented vertically, or may cause a radial neck fracture, which tends to be impacted and slightly angulated (Fig. 46.42). Radial head fractures are commonly difficult to identify on AP and lateral views of the elbow, and may then be only obvious on the oblique projection. In some cases, even these additional efforts will not reveal a subtle fracture, and so secondary signs of fracture become important in recognizing the severity of the injury. The most important of these signs is the *fat pad sign*.

There are normal focal accumulations of fat adjacent to the elbow joint synovium: on a lateral view of the normal elbow, the posterior fat pad is not visible between the humeral condyles. The anterior fat pad is usually seen as a fusiform fat collection along the anterior distal humeral cortex (Fig. 46.41). If the elbow joint becomes distended by fluid for any reason, the expansion of the synovial margins displaces these fat pads away from the humerus, resulting in visualization of the posterior fat pad and displacement of the anterior fat pad superiorly (the

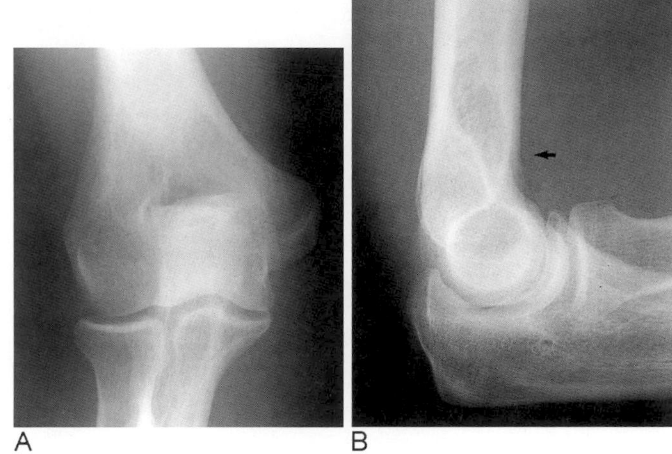

Figure 46.41 Normal elbow. AP (A) and lateral (B) views of a normal elbow demonstrate the normal bony alignment. Note the smooth rounded anterior fat pad (arrow) on the lateral view. A posterior fat pad is not seen in the normal elbow.

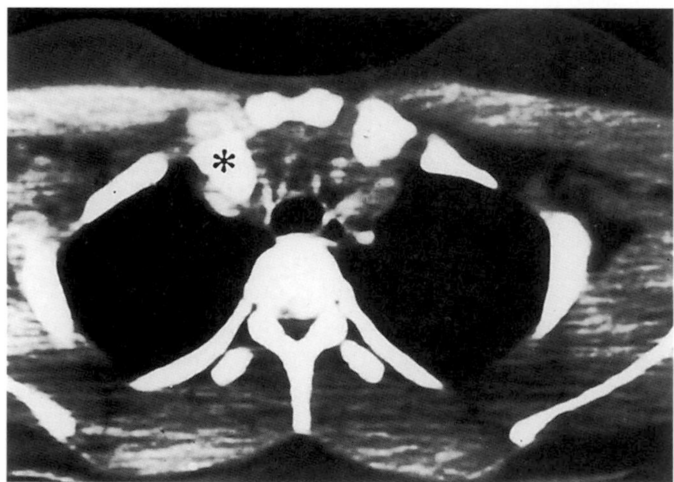

Figure 46.39 Posterior sternoclavicular joint dislocation. CT image demonstrates posterior displacement of the medial right clavicle (*) relative to the manubrium.

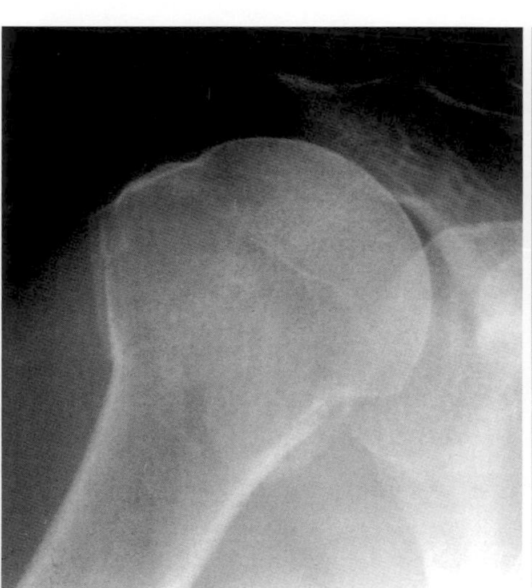

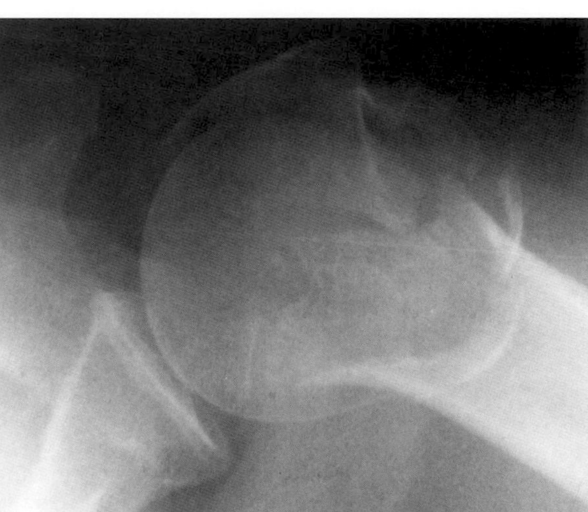

Figure 46.40 Fracture of the humeral neck. AP (A) and axillary (B) views of the left shoulder demonstrate an acute comminuted fracture of the surgical neck of the humerus. Note the separation of the greater and lesser tuberosities.

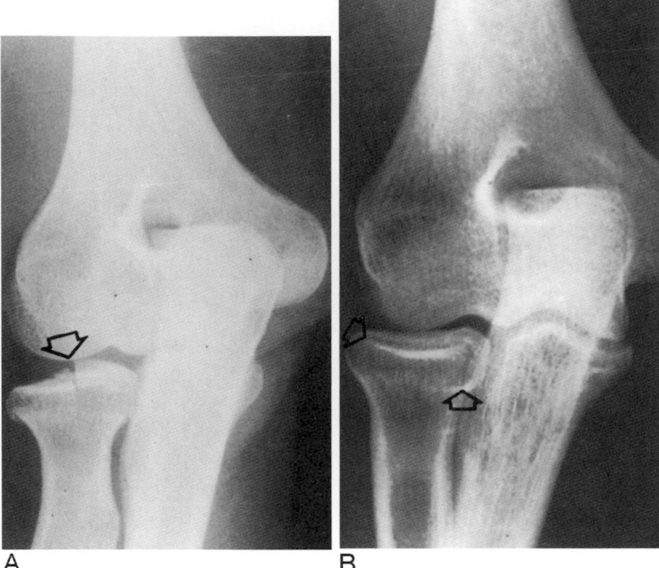

Figure 46.42 Fracture of the radial head. Oblique (A) radiograph of the elbow demonstrates a fracture of the radial head (arrow). The AP projection (B) demonstrates a curvilinear density indicating impaction of the radial head cortex and a faint vertical lucency in the ulnar aspect of the radial head, representing the fracture (arrow).

'sail sign') (Fig. 46.43). The appearance of a positive fat pad sign is a non-specific marker for an elbow joint effusion; however, in the setting of acute elbow trauma it strongly suggests the presence of a haemarthrosis secondary to an intra-articular fracture, usually a radial head fracture.

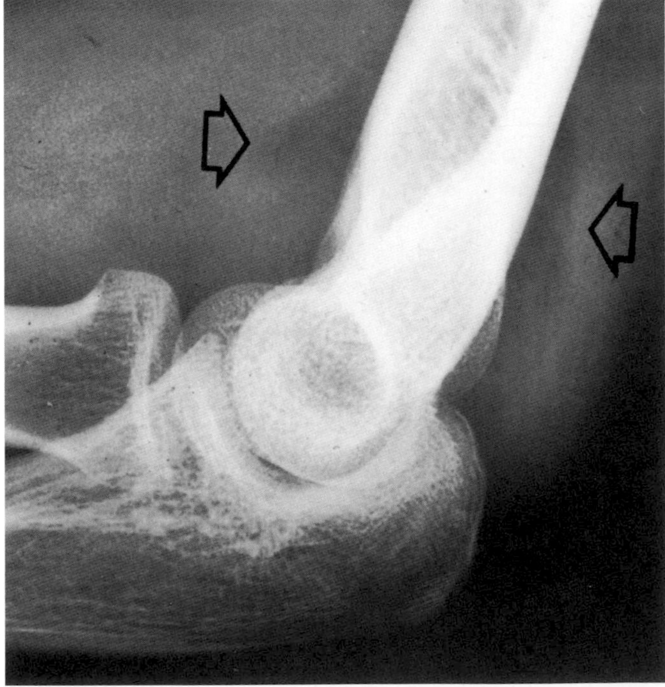

Figure 46.43 Elevation of the periarticular fat pads due to haemarthrosis of the elbow. Note the lucencies anterior and posterior to the distal humeral shaft, representing elevation of the periarticular fat pads of the elbow (arrows). The normal anterior fat pad is rounded; the posterior fat pad is not normally visualized.

Fractures of the capitellum usually result from valgus impaction forces. They may be linear, but are most often osteochondral injuries and as such may be quite difficult to diagnose on plain radiographs. MRI is very sensitive to such lesions.

Olecranon fractures may result from a direct blow to the elbow, or may be due to an avulsion injury related to contraction of the triceps muscle. The fracture fragments are often distracted due to muscular contraction (Fig. 46.24).

Dislocations of the elbow almost invariably involve posterior and lateral dislocation of the radius and ulna in relation to the humerus (Fig. 46.44). A fracture of the ulnar coronoid process is frequently present. Isolated dislocations of the radial head are extremely rare in adults; a thorough search for a fracture of the ulna should be made.

Traumatic avulsion of the medial (ulnar) collateral ligament is often seen in association with impaction injuries to the radiocapitellar joint due to valgus forces, and is best assessed with MRI. The normal ligament runs from the medial epicondyle to the proximal ulna, and is best seen on coronal images. On T2-weighted images, disruption is manifested by discontinuity of the normal, low-signal ligamentous fibres in association with high signal from surrounding oedema (Fig. 46.45).

Forearm

In general, fractures in the forearm either involve both bones, or a fracture of one is associated with a dislocation of the other. Occasionally, only one bone (usually the ulna) will fracture with no resulting displacement; the classic example is the nightstick injury, which represents a distal ulnar fracture due to a direct blow from an unforgiving object (e.g. policeman's baton).

As in the leg, when two bones (i.e. the radius and ulna) are fixed along their length by an interosseous membrane, a displaced fracture of one bone necessitates fracture or displacement of the other. Although both are rare, the two classic examples of forearm fracture-dislocation complexes are the Monteggia injury, which is characterized by an anteriorly angulated fracture of the proximal ulna associated with anterior dislocation of the radial head (Fig. 46.46) and the Galeazzi

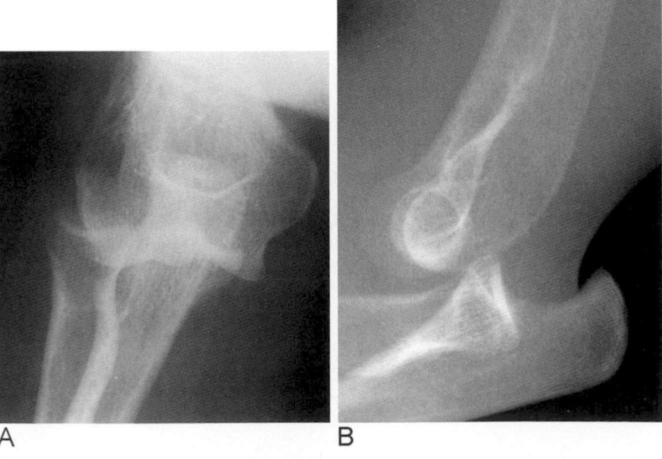

Figure 46.44 Complete dislocation of the elbow. AP (A) and lateral (B) radiographs demonstrate posterior dislocation of the radius and ulna relative to the humerus. Ulnar coronoid process fractures are often associated with this injury.

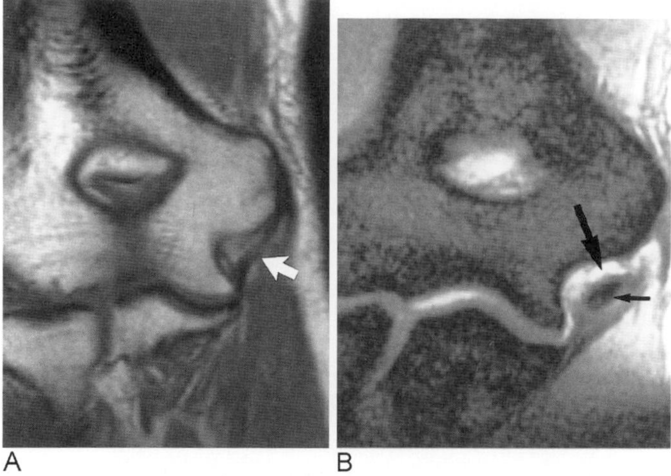

Figure 46.45 Tear of the medial (ulnar) collateral ligament (MCL) of the elbow. Coronal T1-weighted image (A) of a normal elbow demonstrates an intact MCL as a linear low signal structure extending from the medial humeral epicondyle to the proximal ulna (arrow). Coronal T2-weighted image (B) from a different patient demonstrates disruption of the ulnar collateral, with high signal seen at the expected site of humeral attachment (arrow). A small focus of low signal is noted at the proximal end of the ligament, which may represent an avulsion fragment (small arrow). The patient was a professional baseball pitcher; such athletes are prone to MCL tears due to marked valgus stress during pitching.

injury, in which a dorsally angulated distal radial fracture is seen in conjunction with a disruption of the distal radioulnar joint (Fig. 46.47). Both classically occur when the patient falls onto a flexed arm. Although uncommon in clinical practice, these injuries have a mysterious way of appearing on radiological board or College examinations.

Wrist

Radiological evaluation of the acutely injured wrist should include PA and lateral radiographs (Fig. 46.48), to be supplemented according to the specific situation as described below. In general, when an injury to the carpus is suspected, multiple views are necessary.

Injuries to the wrist typically occur as a result of a fall on an outstretched hand. Fracture patterns generally correspond to the age of the patient. In children and in adults over 40, fractures of the distal radius predominate. In young adults, fractures of the scaphoid are most common. Carpal fractures are very uncommon before age 12 and after 45 years.

The term Colles' fracture is often (inappropriately) used to refer to any fracture of the distal radius resulting from a fall on an outstretched hand, yet Colles specifically described an

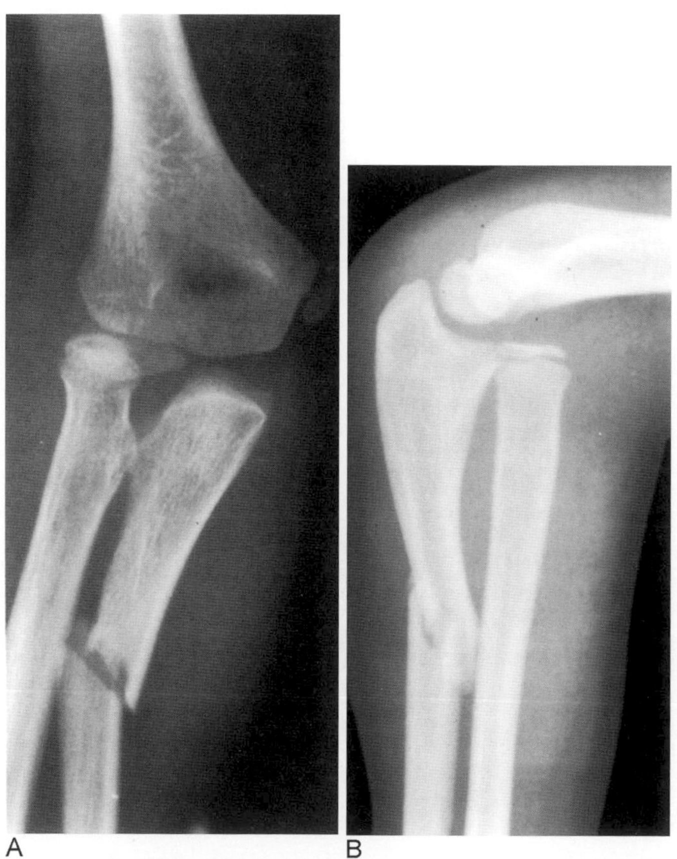

Figure 46.46 Monteggia fracture-dislocation of the proximal forearm. AP (A) and lateral (B) views demonstrate an anteriorly angulated fracture of the proximal ulna and anterior dislocation of the radius relative to the capitellum.

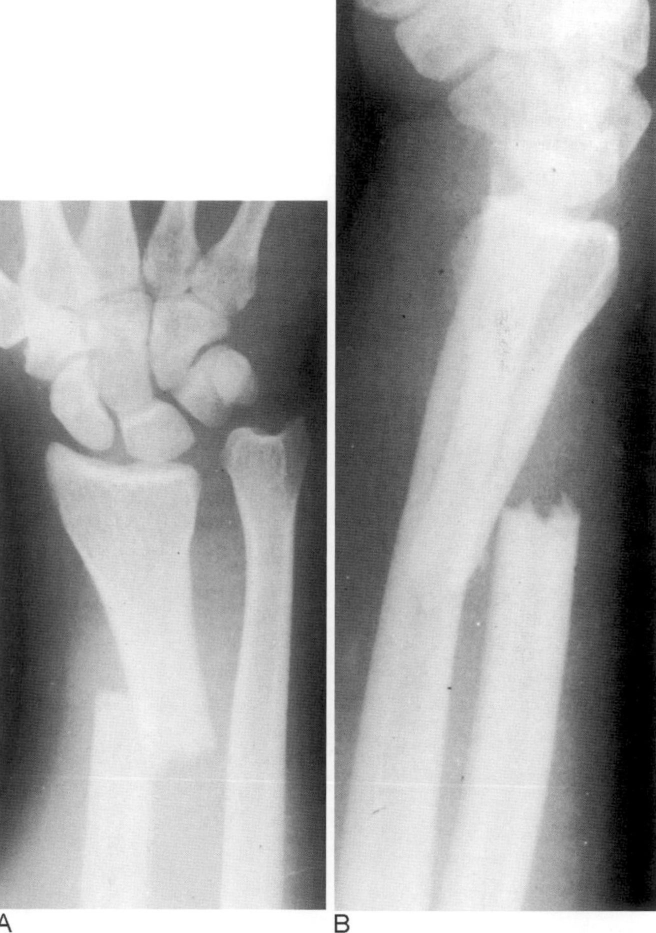

Figure 46.47 Galeazzi fracture-dislocation of the distal forearm. AP (A) and lateral (B) views of the distal arm demonstrate a displaced fracture of the radius and diastasis of the distal radioulnar joint, with ulnar dislocation.

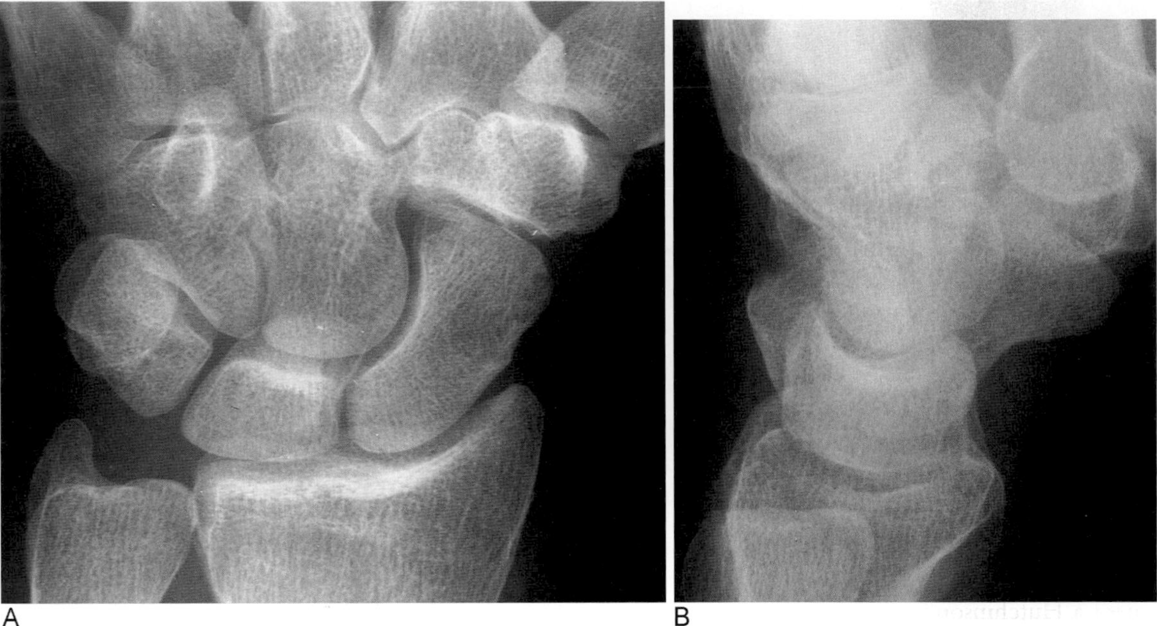

Figure 46.48 Normal wrist. PA (A) and lateral (B) views.

impacted fracture of the distal radius with dorsal displacement of the distal fracture fragment. Although not in the original description, this fracture is often associated with an avulsion of the ulnar styloid. Neutralization or reversal of the normal slight (10 degrees) volar tilt of the distal radial articular surface is abnormal and connotes an impacted fracture (Fig. 46.49).

Other eponyms have been attached to different distal radial fractures; the student is urged not to use these names but to use basic fracture description terms in order to make sure the radiology report is as accurate as possible and to avoid potential confusion. A distal radial fracture with a volarly displaced distal fragment is referred to as a Smith's fracture (or a reverse Colles' fracture); a displaced fracture of the volar lip of the distal radius without involvement of the dorsal lip is a Barton's fracture (Fig. 46.50) and the opposite condition (fracture of the dorsal lip) is termed a reverse Barton's fracture. An isolated

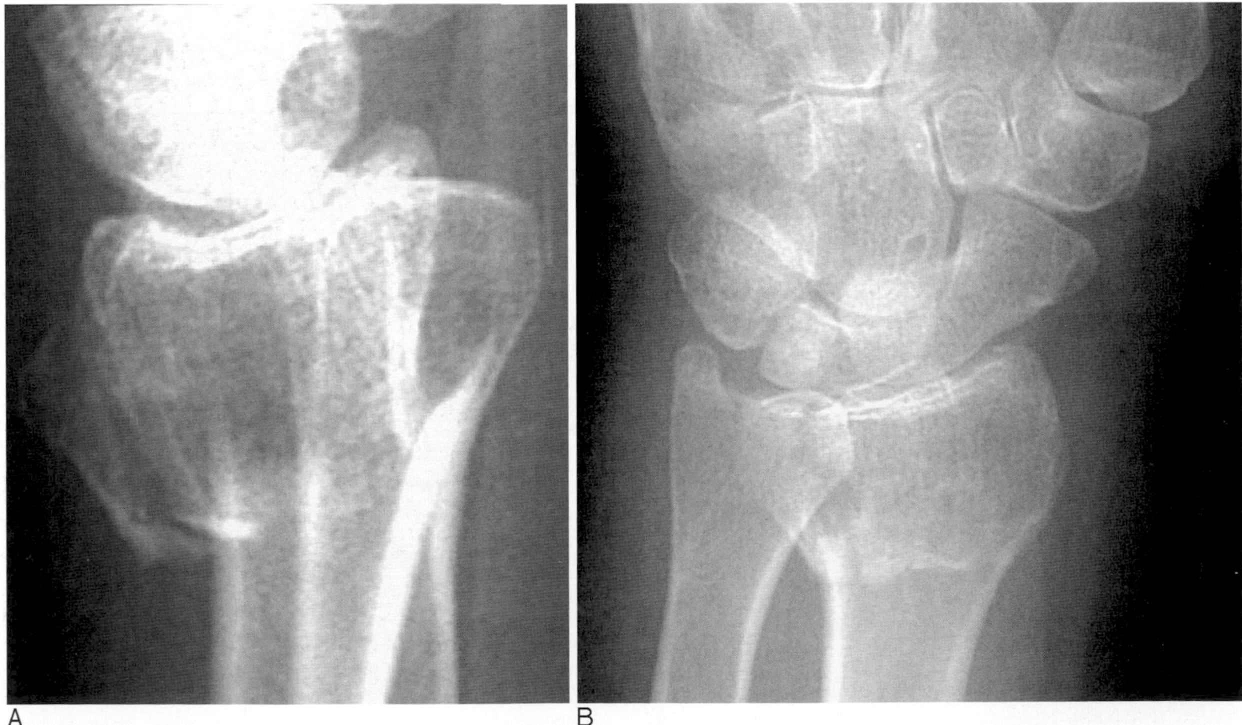

Figure 46.49 Colles' fracture of the distal radius. Lateral (A) and PA (B) views demonstrate an impacted fracture of the distal radius with dorsal angulation of the distal fracture fragment. The ulnar styloid process is intact. (Case courtesy of Tim B. Hunter, M.D., Tucson, Arizona)

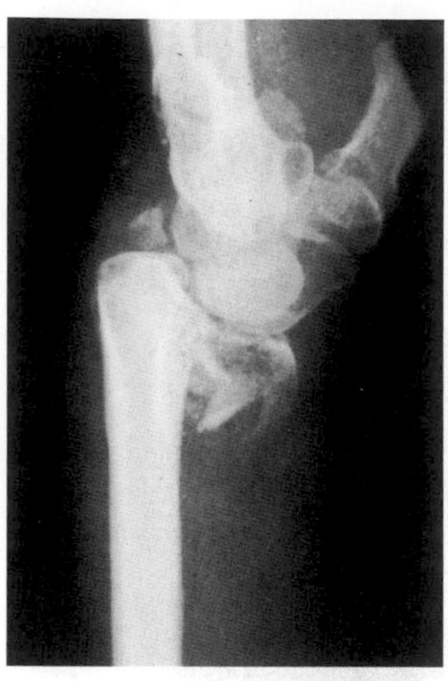

Figure 46.50 Barton's fracture. Lateral view of a comminuted fracture of the volar rim of the distal radius.

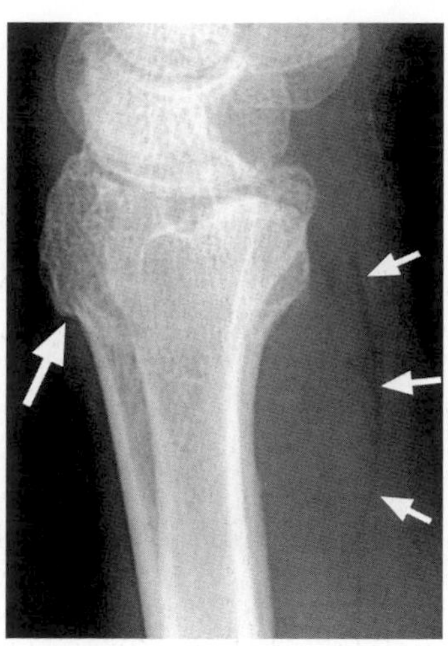

Figure 46.52 Elevation of the pronator quadratus fat plane (small arrows) in a patient who suffered a subtle fracture of the distal radius (large arrow).

fracture of the radial styloid process (usually due to a direct blow) is termed a Hutchinson's (or chauffeur's crank handle) fracture (Fig. 46.51).

An indirect sign of an acute distal forearm fracture is displacement or obliteration of the pronator quadratus fat plane. This line of fat is seen on the lateral radiograph of the wrist; normally it lies in close approximation to the anterior surface of the distal radius. When a distal forearm fracture causes swelling, the fat plane is displaced away from the bones, or may be obliterated by the blood and oedema (Fig. 46.52).

The most common carpal bone fractured is the *scaphoid*, which accounts for about 75% of carpal fractures. Evaluation of the scaphoid usually requires several views in addition to the routine PA and lateral: a PA view in maximum ulnar deviation tends to display the scaphoid in profile to its best advantage and is most likely to identify otherwise subtle or inapparent fractures of the scaphoid.

Fractures of the scaphoid typically present with pain in the anatomical 'snuff box'. Most are non-displaced transverse fractures through the middle, or 'waist', of the scaphoid (Fig. 46.53). These fractures may be invisible even with a magnifying glass on the immediately post-traumatic film. If there is any clinical or radiological doubt, MRI can be performed at outset or a series of scintigraphy or scaphoid radiographic views must be taken 7–10 days after the original trauma, by which time osteoclasis will have widened the fracture line. Occasionally, fractures may occur in the proximal or distal pole. Because the blood supply to the scaphoid is via artery entering the bone at its waist, nonunion of the fracture fragments interrupts the blood supply to the proximal fragment, leading to osteonecrosis of that fragment. Early osteonecrosis can be suggested with MRI or scintigraphy; on CT or radiographs the condition is evident only late in its course. Typically, the necrotic fragment will appear dense compared to the surrounding bones on radiographs or CT. This is due to a combination of disuse osteoporosis of the surrounding normal bone and fat necrosis in the avascular segment causing sclerosis (Fig. 46.54). Relative

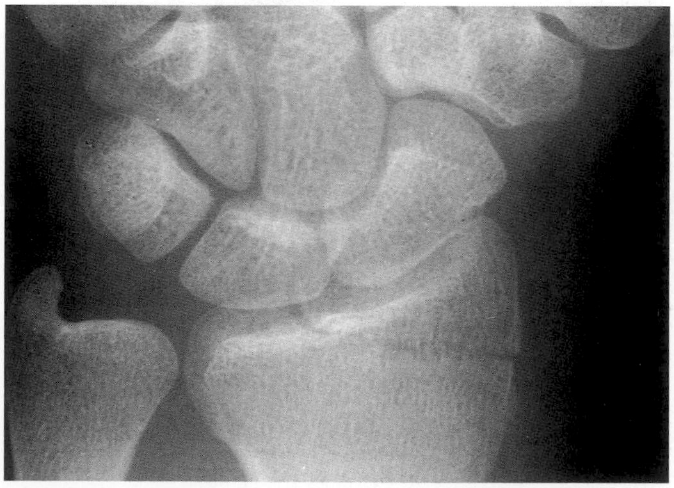

Figure 46.51 Hutchinson's fracture of the radial styloid, usually due to a direct blow.

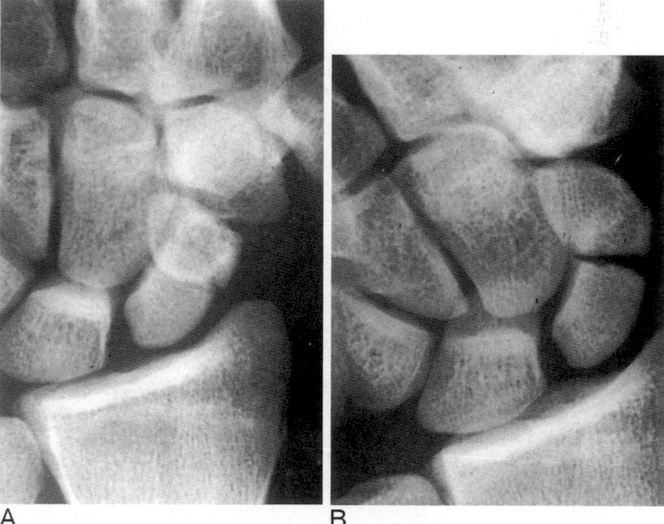

Figure 46.53 Fracture of the scaphoid. In the PA projection (A), the scaphoid is somewhat rotated, and a fracture is difficult to see. The navicular view with the wrist in ulnar deviation (B) demonstrates a lucent band traversing the waist of the scaphoid, representing a fracture. Such fractures can be difficult to detect in the acute setting; occasionally, re-imaging the patient 7–10 days after injury may demonstrate the fracture due to hyperaemia of the surrounding bone.

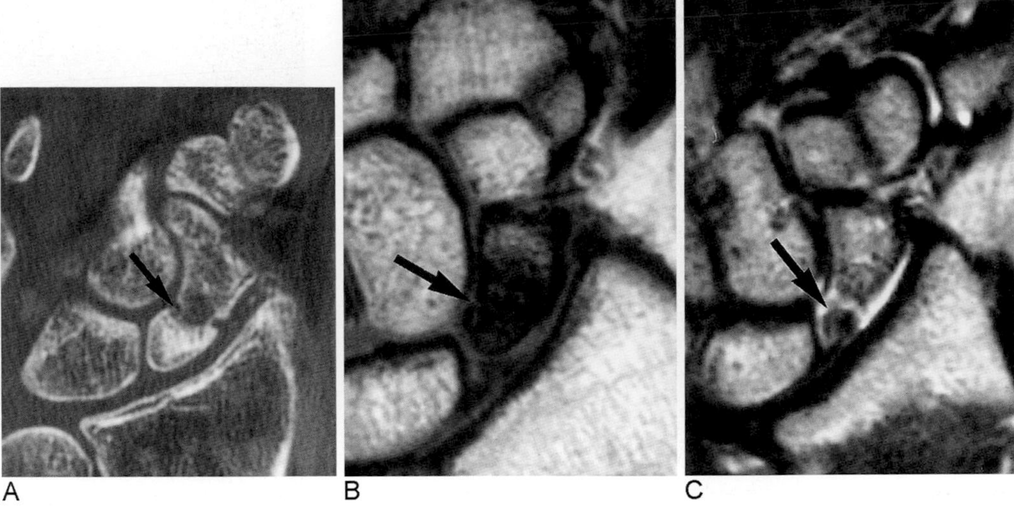

Figure 46.54 Osteonecrosis of the proximal pole of the scaphoid. Direct coronal CT. (A) demonstrates the unhealed fracture through the waist of the scaphoid (arrow). The proximal pole is dense, indicating ischaemia or osteonecrosis. Coronal T1-weighted (B) and T2-weighted (C) images demonstrate abnormal low signal in the proximal fragment (arrow).

ischaemia from disruption of part of the blood supply of the proximal pole may also result in increased density of the proximal pole. This may return to normal as the fracture heals.

Fractures of the triquetrum are the second most common carpal fractures, accounting for about 15%. The most common pattern of injury is a small avulsion fragment on the dorsal surface of the bone at the attachment site of the dorsal radiocarpal ligament, seen best on the lateral radiograph (Fig. 46.55). Fractures of the hamate may involve the hook (not uncommonly seen in golfers or baseball players) (Fig. 46.56), or may involve the dorsal surface. Trapezium fractures occur secondary to abduction and hyperextension of the thumb, and manifest as vertical fractures in the lateral aspect of the bone. All other carpal fractures are relatively rare.

Important soft tissue injuries to the wrist include tears of the scapho-lunate and luno-triquetral ligaments, and of the triangular fibrocartilage complex on the ulnar aspect of the wrist. Imaging of such tears was traditionally performed using arthrography, often involving injections of three separate joint compartments (Fig. 46.57). It has been shown that MRI can accurately assess the integrity of these structures[5] (Fig. 46.58).

Carpal dislocations

Dislocations of the carpus are generally the result of ligamentous disruption. The ligaments surrounding the lunate provide much of the intrinsic stability of the carpus, so it should not be surprising that disruption of these structures results in dislocations and instabilities of varying severity.

In *scapho-lunate dissociation* (the simplest and most common of these injuries) the scapho-lunate ligament is disrupted, widening the scapho-lunate space on the PA radiograph. Normal intercarpal distance is about 2 mm; a space wider than 4 mm is clearly abnormal (Fig. 46.59). Such a finding has been termed the '*Terry Thomas sign*' after the famous English comedian who had a prominent gap between his two upper incisors; younger American readers may prefer the 'David Letterman sign' or the 'Lauren Hutton sign'! This separation is best demonstrated on ulnarly deviated anterior views. Because of the disruption of the scapho-lunate ligament, the scaphoid may rotate on its axis so that its distal pole moves volarly. The resultant angle between the short axis of the lunate and the long axis of the scaphoid, as seen on the lateral view, will exceed 60 degrees (normal is 30–34 degrees) (Fig. 46.60). This rotation of the scaphoid, or

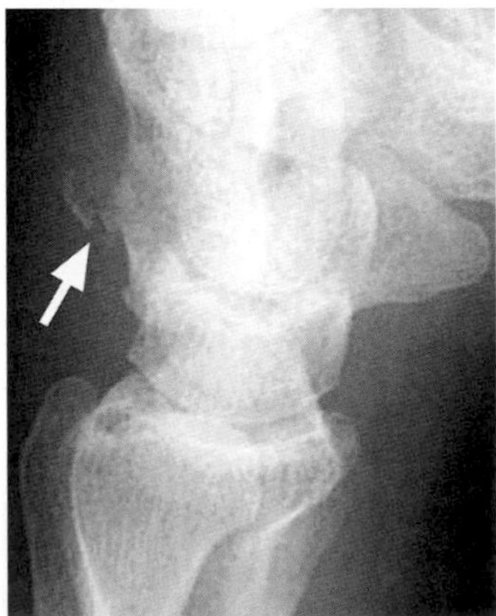

Figure 46.55 Dorsal chip fracture of the triquetrum (arrow). This common injury is usually seen only in the lateral projection.

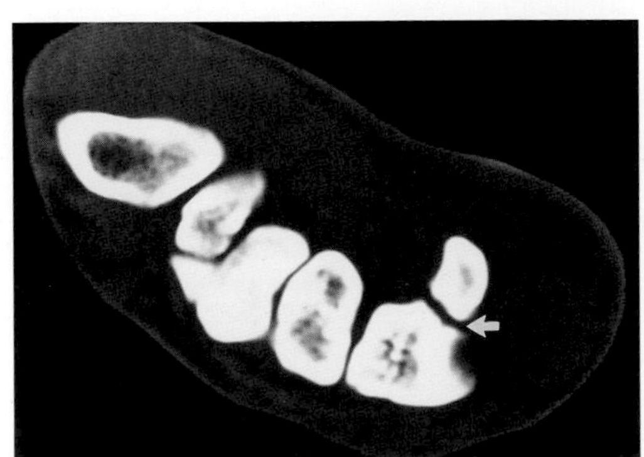

Figure 46.56 Fracture of the hook of the hamate. Axial CT demonstrates separation of the hook of the hamate (arrow), indicating an acute fracture.

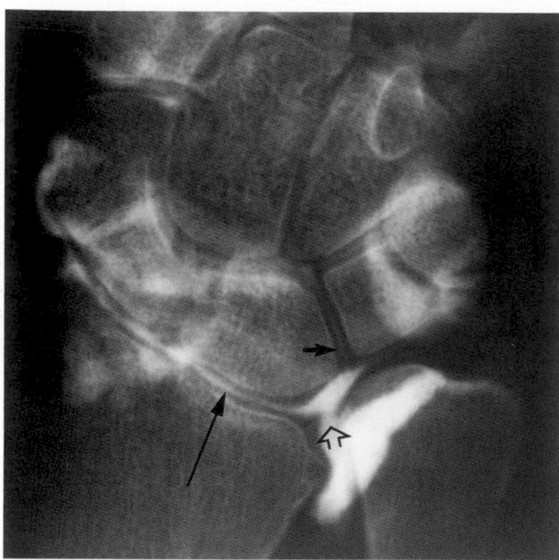

Figure 46.57 Arthrography: evaluation of the intrinsic ligaments of the wrist. An AP radiograph after injection of contrast medium into the radiocarpal joint (long arrow) shows spread into the midcarpal space through the lunotriquetral ligament (small arrow) and into the distal radioulnar joint through a tear in the triangular fibrocartilage (open arrow).

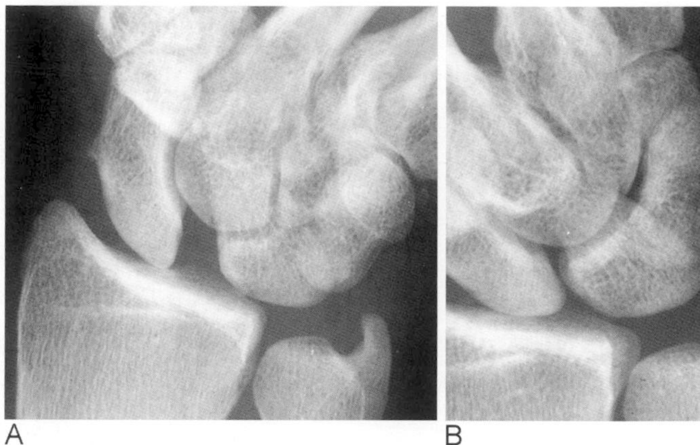

Figure 46.59 Scapholunate dissociation. PA view of the wrist in ulnar deviation (A) shows abnormal widening of the scapholunate distance (greater than 4 mm), consistent with disruption of the scapholunate ligament. View in radial deviation (B) demonstrates no significant abnormality; the widening is not apparent.

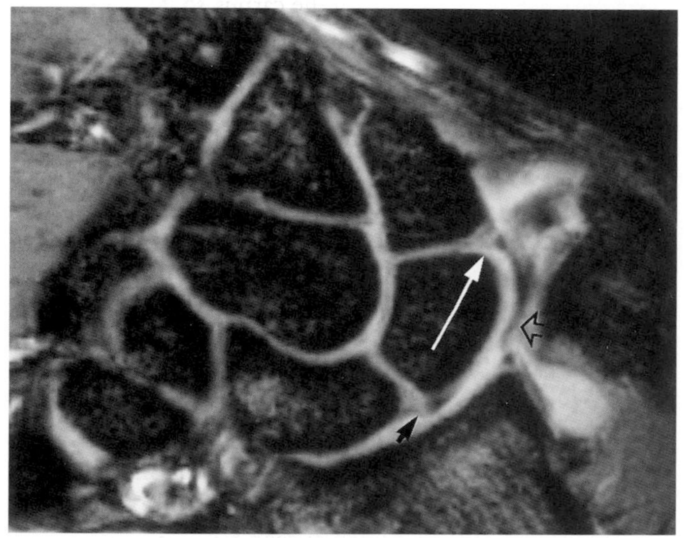

Figure 46.58 MRI of the wrist. Coronal T2-weighted MRI demonstrates an intact scapholunate ligament (black arrow) and the normal triangular fibrocartilage (open arrow). The lunotriquetral ligament is often not visualized, and absence of this structure on MRI is not an accurate predictor of ligamentous injury (long arrow).

rotatory subluxation, can result in apparent foreshortening of the scaphoid on the PA view with projection of the cortex of the distal pole over the waist (the 'signet ring' sign).

In the normal wrist, the radius, lunate and capitate line up together in the sagittal plane, forming a series of parallel arcs on the lateral radiograph (Fig. 46.48). A *perilunate dislocation* occurs due to disruption of the scapho-lunate, luno-capitate and luno-triquetral ligaments. The result is that the lunate maintains its normal relationship to the radius, while the remainder of the carpus and hand shift dorsally. On the anterior view, the lunate loses its normal trapezoidal configuration and takes on the appearance of a triangular wedge of pie. Fractures of the scaphoid or, less commonly, capitate are associated with dorsal perilunate dislocations (Fig. 46.61).

If disruption of the volar radiocarpal ligaments occurs in addition to the ligamentous disruptions described in a perilunate dislocation, the result is a *lunate dislocation*. Typically, the lunate dislocates anteriorly (volarly) and tilts so that its distal articular surface faces the palm. The remaining carpal bones maintain their normal relationships with each other and with the radius. The appearance of a lunate and a perilunate dislocation on a PA radiograph can be identical (Fig. 46.62).

Dislocations may occur at the fourth and fifth carpometacarpal joints commonly associated with fractures of the base of the metacarpals. The proximal metacarpals usually move dorsally and towards the ulnar aspect.

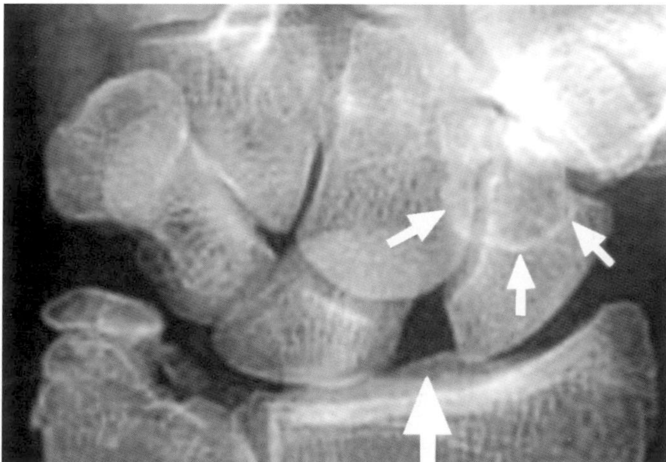

Figure 46.60 Scapholunate dissociation. The PA view shows rotation of the scaphoid, so that the distal pole is seen on end (the 'signet ring' sign) (small arrows). The scapholunate space is abnormally wide (large arrow). Note also old ununited fracture of the ulnar styloid and ossification in triangular fibrocartilage from previous injury.

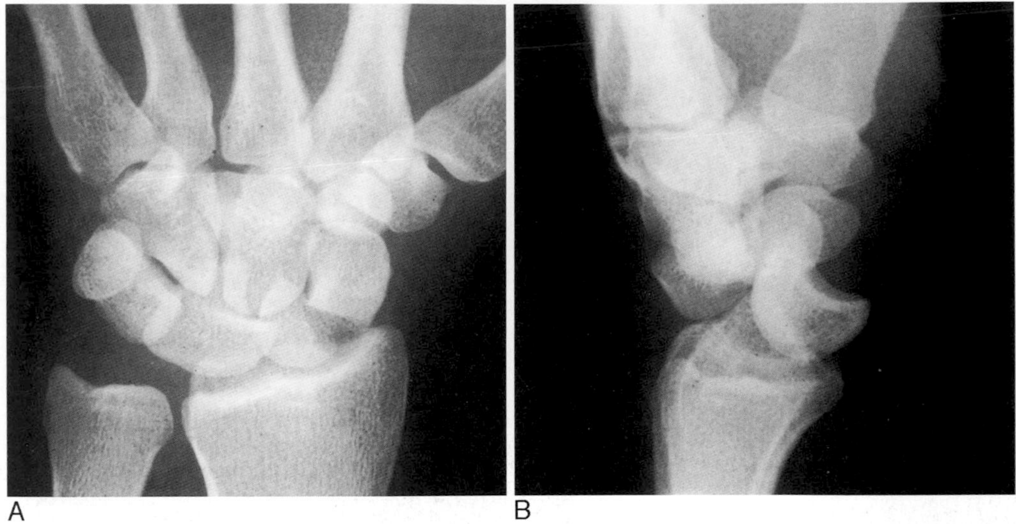

Figure 46.61 Posterior trans-scaphoid perilunate fracture-dislocation. The PA view (A) demonstrates overlap of the lunate and capitate, with a 'wedge of pie' appearance of the lunate. There is a fracture of the scaphoid. The lateral view (B) demonstrates slight volar tilt of the lunate, with the remainder of the carpus and hand posteriorly dislocated.

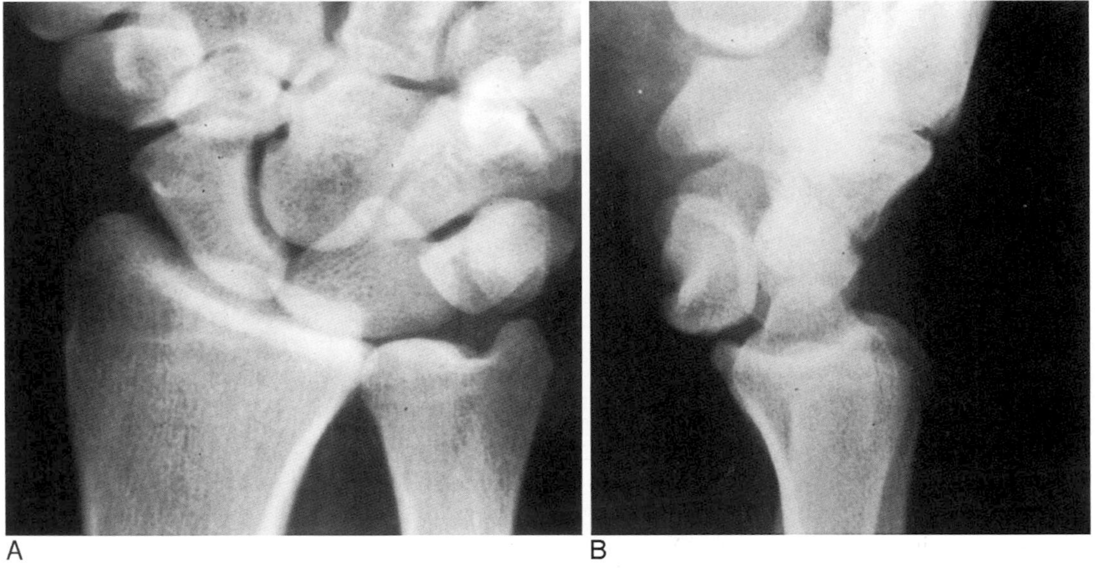

Figure 46.62 Anterior lunate dislocation. PA view (A) can be indistinguishable from a perilunate dislocation. The lateral view (B) shows volar displacement, dislocation and tilt of the lunate. The remainder of the carpus is normally aligned with the radius.

The hand

Fractures of the fourth and fifth metacarpals are common and are usually the result of punching a hard object (boxer's fracture). The fracture may involve the midshaft or distal end of the bone, and the distal fragment is usually volarly angulated (Fig. 46.23).

An oblique fracture at the base of the first metacarpal that involves the first carpometacarpal joint space is termed a Bennett's fracture. Such a fracture is often unstable, as the distal fragment is distracted by the unopposed abductor pollicis longus muscle, and may require surgical intervention (Fig. 46.63). A similar fracture with comminution of the metacarpal is referred to as Rolando's fracture. This injury is actually less prone to displacement of the distal fragment due to the comminution of the thumb base (Fig. 46.64).

Forced abduction of the thumb can result in disruption of the ulnar collateral ligament of the metacarpophalangeal joint (MCP) of the thumb, a major stabilizer of the thumb. Traditionally termed 'gamekeeper's thumb' because it so often resulted from breaking the necks of rabbits, it has lately earned the additional name of 'skier's thumb', being frequently found when a skier falls onto an outstretched hand before releasing the ski pole. This lesion is frequently radiographically occult unless associated with a small avulsion fragment arising from the base of the proximal phalanx (Fig. 46.65). Views with the thumb radially stressed will demonstrate radial deviation at the MCP. The treatment of this lesion depends on the degree of displacement of the disrupted ligament, and on the presence or absence of entrapment of its severed end by surrounding structures. US and MRI may demonstrate the

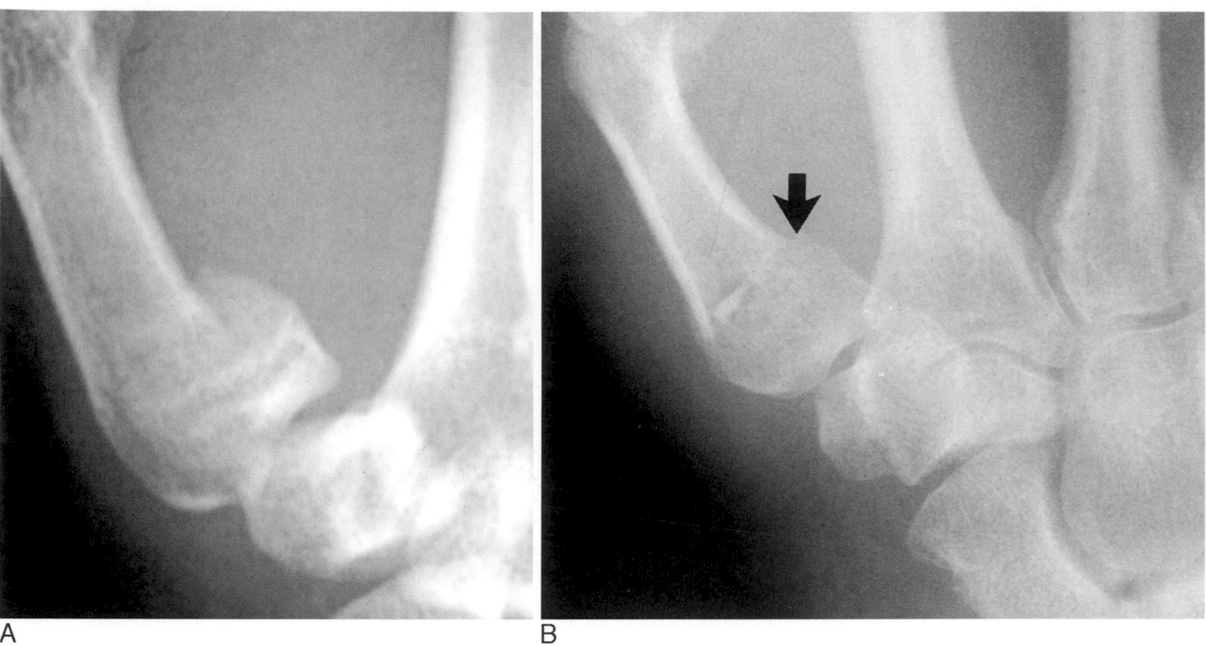

Figure 46.63 (A) **Bennett's fracture-dislocation of the base of the thumb.** Note that the oblique fracture extends into the joint. Note also the radial and proximal displacement of the metacarpal shaft, due to contraction of the abductor pollicis longus. (Case courtesy of Dr. Tim B. Hunter, Tucson, Arizona). Extra-articular fracture (arrow, B) generally does not require surgical fixation.

torn ligament and potential entrapment, which is termed the 'Stener lesion'.

Fractures and dislocations in the phalanges are quite common. Specific mention should be made of two specific injury patterns. The first of these occurs at either the proximal or distal interphalangeal joint (PIP, DIP) as a result of forced hyperextension, with or without dislocation. Lateral radiographs may reveal a subtle flake of bone arising, but separate, from the volar aspect of the base of the more distal phalanx involved (Fig. 46.66). This bony fragment represents an avulsion of the volar plate, the palmar ligamentous stabilizer of the interphalangeal joint.

The second is a similar injury occurring at the DIP due to a direct blow to the fingertip causing hyperflexion of the DIP with disruption of the deep component of the extensor tendon. An avulsion fragment may be seen adjacent to the dorsal aspect of the base of the distal phalanx (Fig. 46.67). This injury, known as baseball, mallet, or drop finger, can result in a flexion deformity. Avulsion of the extensor tendon may occur without an associated fracture. The lateral radiograph will then show the joint held in flexion which is sufficient to make the diagnosis of disruption of the extensor tendon.

The hip

The standard radiographic evaluation of the hip includes an AP view with the hip in internal rotation (thus demonstrating the greater and lesser trochanters in profile, and the femoral neck along its long axis), and a frog-leg lateral, which

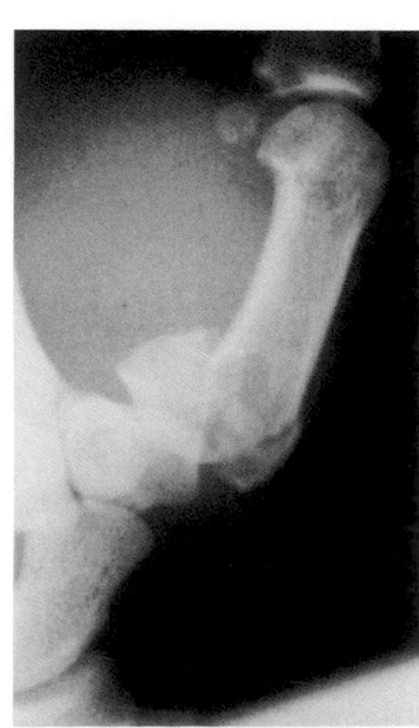

Figure 46.64 Rolando's fracture of the thumb. Comminution of this intra-articular fracture prevents abduction and retraction of the metacarpal shaft, and is less likely to require surgical fixation than is a Bennett's fracture.

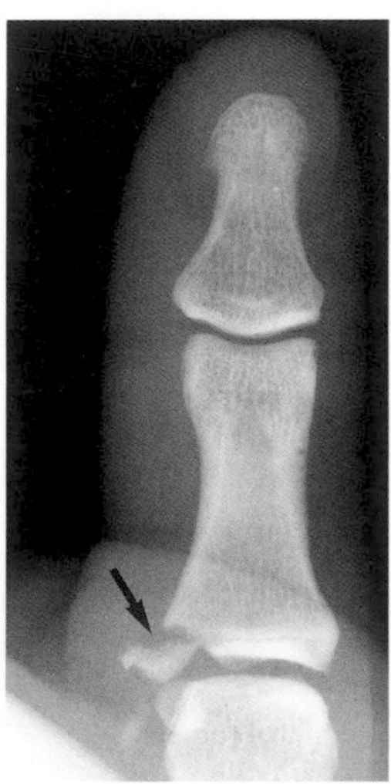

Figure 46.65 Gamekeeper's, or ski pole, fracture. An AP view of the thumb demonstrates a bony fragment adjacent to the medial aspect of the base of the proximal phalanx of the thumb (arrow); this represents avulsion of the ulnar collateral ligament of the MCP joint, and leads to significant instability of the thumb.

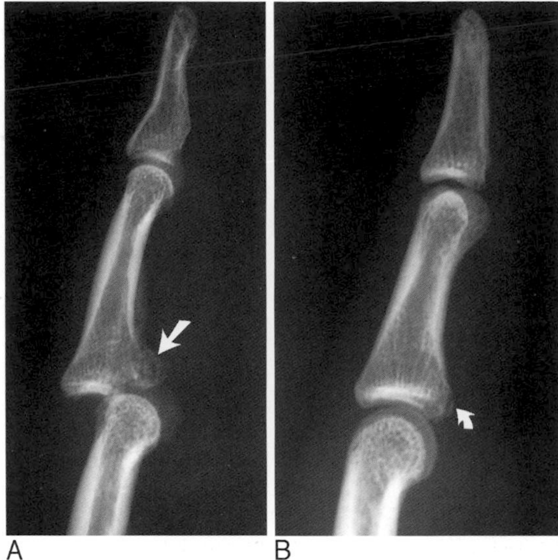

Figure 46.66 Volar plate avulsion. The patient in (A) demonstrates dorsal subluxation of the middle phalanx, with a volarly displaced fracture fragment (arrow) representing an avulsion of the volar plate. In a different patient (B), there is no displacement; the fracture fragment is very subtle (arrow).

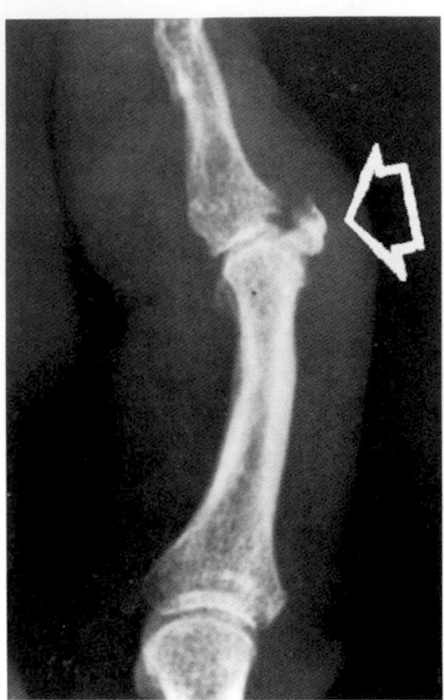

Figure 46.67 Baseball finger. There is a fracture fragment dorsal to the base of the distal phalanx, indicating avulsion of the extensor tendon. The fixed flexion deformity at the DIP is due to the unopposed action of the flexor tendon.

is essentially an AP view of the hip with the hip externally rotated and abducted (Fig. 46.68). Patients with acute injury to the hip will often not be able to cooperate with the position necessary to obtain a frog-leg lateral view; a groin lateral view requires no motion of the injured hip and demonstrates the anterior and posterior cortices of the femoral neck. Displaced fractures of the femoral neck usually result in external rotation of the femoral neck and shaft relative to the femoral head.

Hip fractures in the elderly are a major cause of morbidity and mortality in western society. While hip fractures in younger adults are frequently due to severe trauma such as motor vehicle accidents or falls from a great height, hip fractures in the elderly often occur as a result of a simple fall. Osteoporosis makes bones more susceptible to fracture following relatively mild trauma and superimposed medical conditions may increase the likelihood of a fall. While radiography can detect many, if not most, acute hip fractures, it

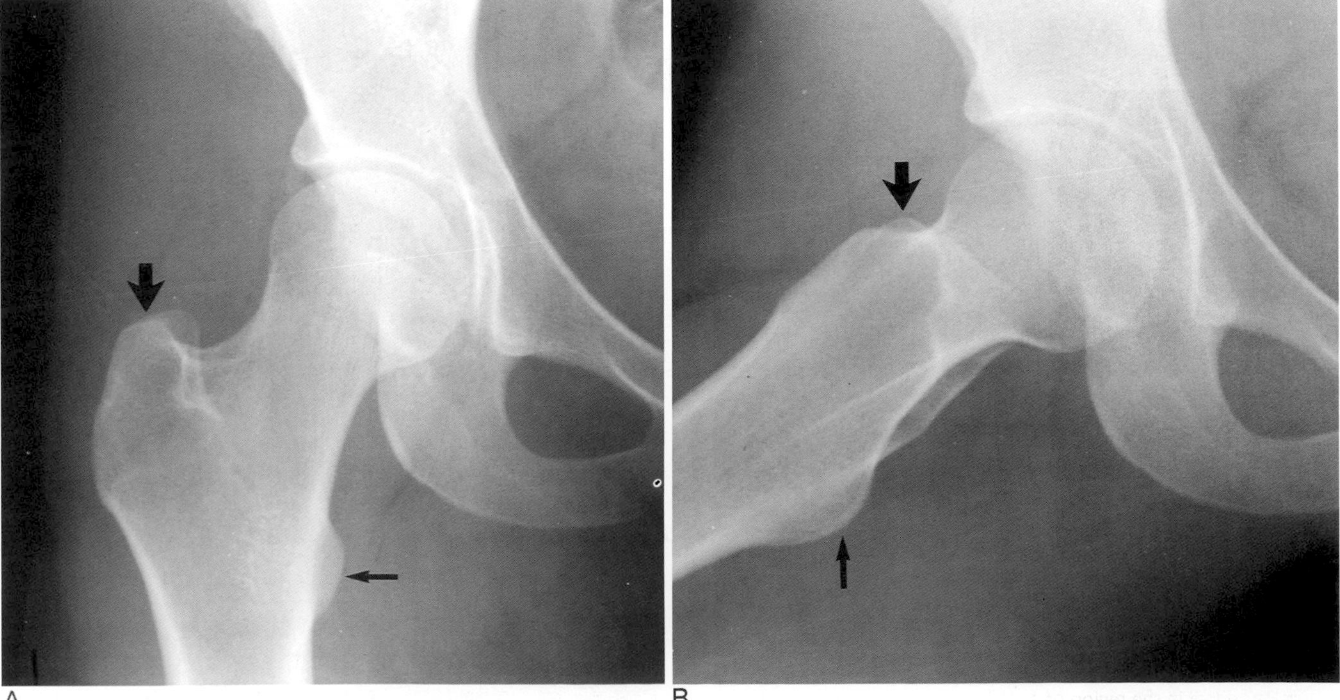

Figure 46.68 Normal hip. AP (A) and frog-leg (B) views of the hip demonstrate the normal alignment of the hip joint, as well as the positions of the greater (arrow) and lesser (thin arrow) trochanters.

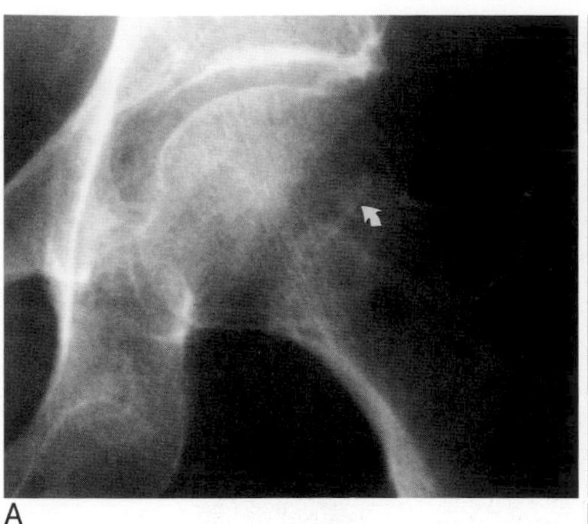
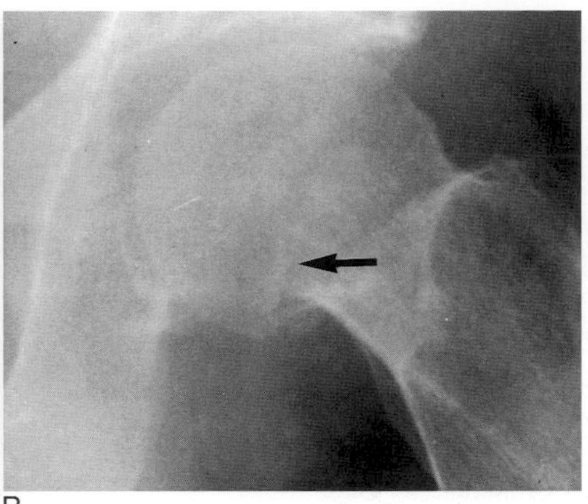

Figure 46.69 Non-displaced fracture of the femoral neck. AP radiograph (A) demonstrates subtle sclerosis in the subcapital region of the femoral neck, consistent with a fracture (arrow). Frog-leg view (B) confirms the fracture (arrow) and demonstrates cortical disruption. Such non-displaced fractures often progress to displaced fractures if the patient continues to bear weight on the hip.

should be borne in mind that subtle nondisplaced fractures may go undiagnosed initially, only to present at a later time after displacement has occurred.

A non-displaced impacted femoral neck fracture may only be represented by a band of sclerosis traversing the femoral neck, or by subtle disruption of the normal trabecular pattern of the femoral neck/head junction with valgus angulation of the primary compressive trabeculae (Fig. 46.69). Displacement of the femoral fracture fragments can drastically increase the rate of complications such as poor union, arthritis and avascular necrosis.

Because the blood supply to the adult femoral head is principally via recurrent arteries entering the hip from the lateral aspect of the femoral neck, fractures proximal to this site may disrupt blood flow to the femoral head and result in avascular necrosis (AVN) (Fig. 46.70). The risk of AVN is directly related to the proximity of the femoral neck fracture; unfortunately, most femoral neck fractures in the elderly are subcapital (at the head/neck junction), putting such patients at very high risk for AVN. If the fracture is impacted, the risk is somewhat diminished. In fact, while impacted valgus fractures of the femoral neck are usually stabilized with compression screws and allowed to heal, the risk of AVN in displaced complete fractures is so great that the femoral head is often resected preemptively and a prosthesis implanted.

Intertrochanteric fractures do not disrupt the blood supply to the femoral head, and thus do not impose a significant risk of AVN. Fractures in this location are often comminuted, involving separation of the greater and/or lesser trochanter (Fig. 46.71). A compression screw and plate combination designed to allow impaction of the fragments on weight bearing stabilizes intertrochanteric fractures.

Isolated fractures of the greater trochanter are common, resulting from falls in the elderly. Isolated fractures of the lesser trochanter are uncommon in the elderly; if present, they are often pathological and an underlying condition such as a

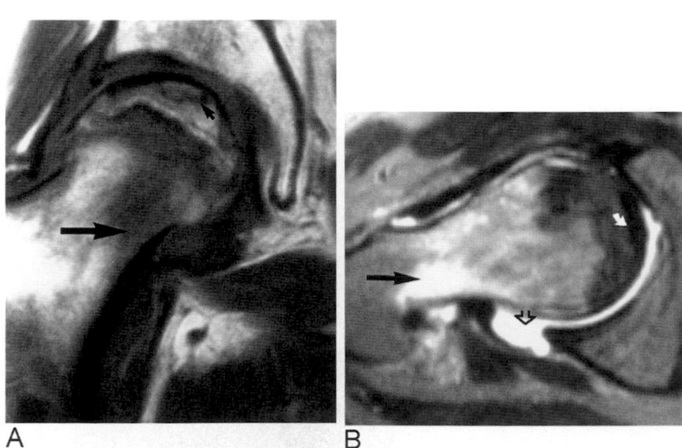

Figure 46.70 Coronal T1-weighted MRI (A) in a patient with Cushing's syndrome demonstrates a well-defined lesion in the subcortical bone demarcated by a line of low signal, consistent with avascular necrosis of the femoral head (small arrow). An ill-defined zone of decreased signal in the medial femoral neck (arrow) represents a subcapital fracture. An oblique axial STIR image oriented along the long axis of the femoral neck (B) shows low signal in the region of AVN (small arrow) and high signal in the posterior femoral neck fracture (arrow). There is a small joint effusion (open arrow).

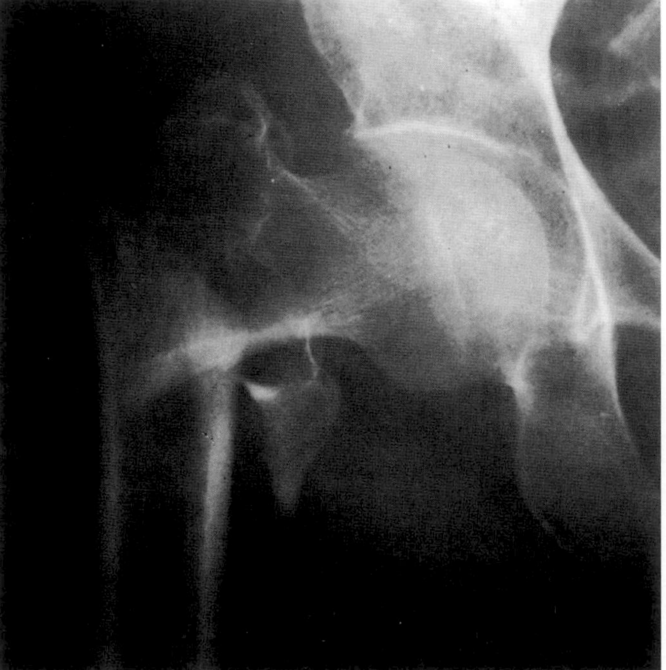

Figure 46.71 Intertrochanteric fracture. There is varus deformity and separation of the trochanters.

metastasis should be excluded (Fig. 46.72). Subtrochanteric fractures (Fig. 46.2) are also frequently pathological and are usually transversely orientated. They are seen in the setting of metastatic disease, myeloma and Paget's disease.

The accurate and timely detection and characterization of these injuries may have a major impact on the patient's functional level. Skeletal scintigraphy and MRI have been shown to be highly sensitive for undisplaced fractures, and should be considered if a suspected hip fracture cannot be demonstrated on routine radiography[6–8]. Scintigraphy may have a lag time (during which it will yield a false-negative result) of between 24 and 72 h following trauma to the hip, while MRI should demonstrate positive findings immediately and is thus preferred (Fig. 46.73).

Dislocations of the hip are usually related to motor vehicle accidents, and result from the femur being driven posteriorly by the dashboard; thus, most hip dislocations involve posterior displacement of the femur relative to the acetabulum. Often there will also be a fracture of the posterior wall of the acetabulum, which may not be detected initially. CT is frequently able to demonstrate small fragments inside and outside the joint after relocation, or may clarify the cause of a difficult relocation (Fig. 46.74). Anterior dislocations are uncommon, and tend to result in displacement of the femoral head into the obturator foramen.

Femoral shaft

The femur is the strongest bone in the body, and fractures involving the femoral shaft in a healthy person require extreme force. Unfortunately, accidents involving high-speed motor vehicle collisions provide such forces, and associated trauma to the hip or knee is common, particularly femoral neck fractures and dislocations of the hip. It is, therefore, imperative that the entire length of the femur, including the joints above and below the injury, be included in the initial radiographic assessment.

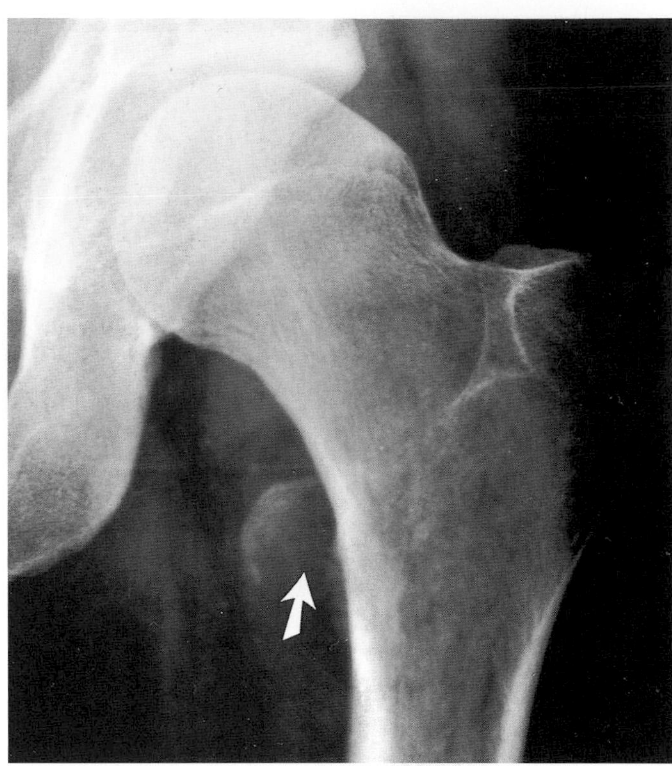

Figure 46.72 Avulsion fracture of the lesser trochanter. Note the separation of the lesser trochanter (arrow) in an area of permeative bone destruction. Such fractures are almost always pathological when seen in adults; this patient had multiple myeloma.

The knee

Trauma to the knee is very common in athletically active people. The standard radiographic series for evaluation of the knee should include an AP and lateral view, and should be supplemented by oblique views to increase sensitivity of fracture detection. Special views for visualization of the patellofemoral joint (e.g. the sunrise view) may also be obtained. In the setting of acute severe trauma, special care should be taken

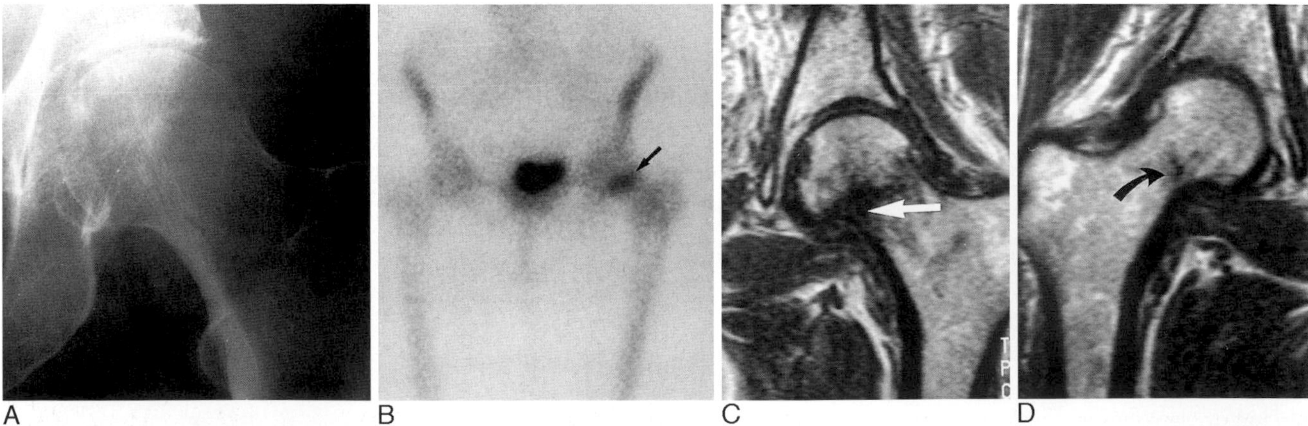

Figure 46.73 Imaging of occult hip fracture. AP radiograph of the **left** hip (A) demonstrates no evidence of fracture. Bone scintigram (B) demonstrates increased radionuclide activity in the **left** subcapital region, consistent with a fracture (arrow); the right hip was read as normal. Coronal T1-weighted MRI the next day (C) clearly shows a well-demarcated line of decreased signal in the subcapital region of the **left** femoral neck consistent with a non-displaced fracture (arrow). MRI of the **right** hip (D) shows a subtle medial femoral neck fracture (curved arrow) not demonstrated on the skeletal scintigram or on the conventional radiograph.

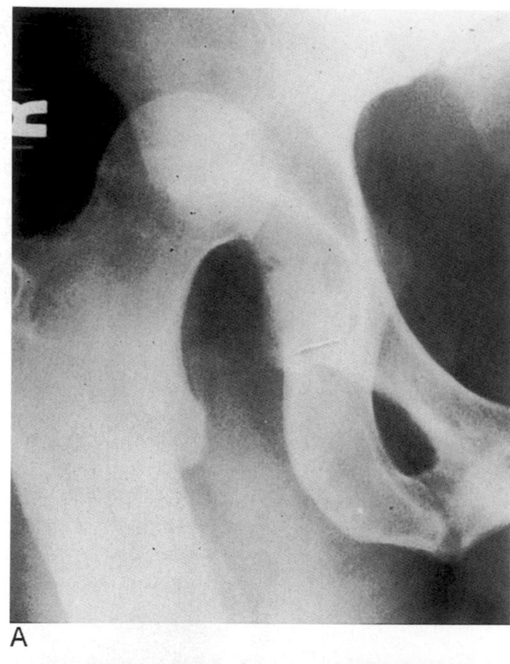

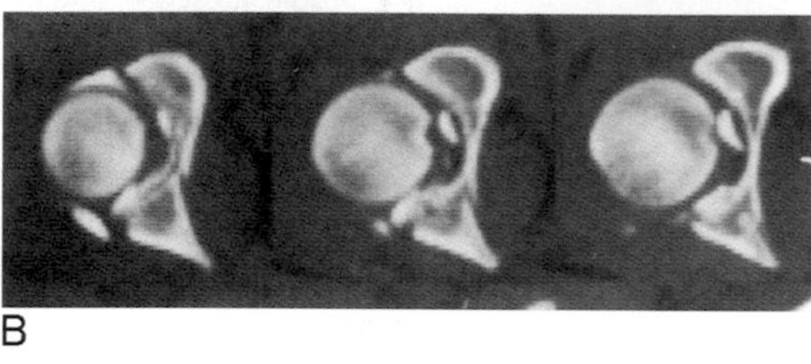

Figure 46.74 Fracture-dislocation of the right hip. AP radiograph (A) before relocation shows the femur dislocated posterosuperiorly. No bony fragments are seen. CT images (B) after relocation. Multiple fragments are seen, including a large intra-articular fragment. There is a fracture of the posterior acetabular wall.

to include a cross-table lateral view, as explained below. While some (usually more severe) injuries are detectable with radiographs, most involve soft tissue structures better demonstrated with MRI.

Fractures involving the distal femur are usually supracondylar (i.e. above the condyles), but often have a vertical extension between the condyles and extend into the knee joint.

The most common fractures about the knee detected on radiographs are those involving the tibial plateau. Lateral plateau fractures are more common than those of the medial plateau, and are generally due to valgus impaction injuries (Fig. 46.75). The presence and degree of impaction of articular surface fragments will largely determine the type of treatment indicated; fragments depressed more than 8–10 mm are usually surgically lifted. The presence of a non-displaced tibial plateau fracture can be difficult to detect; these are often best seen on oblique views.

Ancillary imaging methods are also useful in the evaluation of tibial plateau fractures; MRI and CT (with reconstructions in the long axis) can define the position and size of comminuted fragments and display the surrounding soft tissues (Fig. 46.76).

Avulsion fractures involving the lateral margin of the tibial plateau represent avulsions of the ilotibial band and herald an accompanying disruption of the anterior cruciate ligament (ACL). This complex is referred to as a Segond fracture (Fig. 46.77).

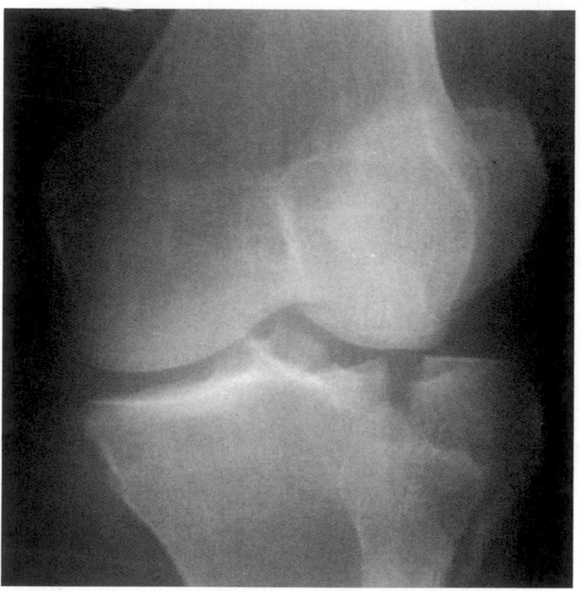

Figure 46.75 Lateral tibial plateau fracture without significant depression.

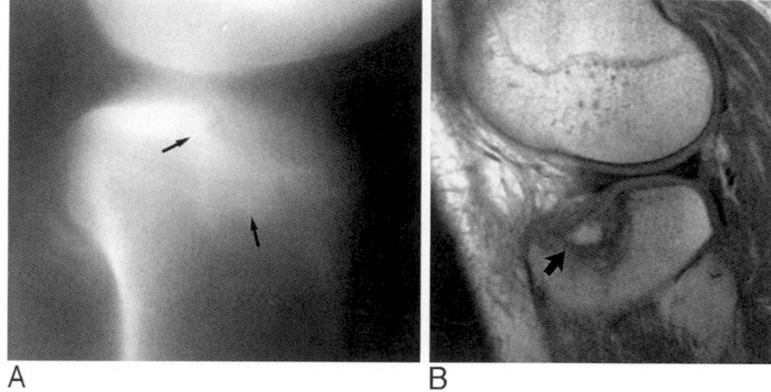

Figure 46.76 A subtle lateral tibial plateau fracture was very difficult to detect on the AP radiographs, but is much better demonstrated on the lateral view (arrows). Sagittal MRI (B) illustrates very clearly the depression of the fragment (arrow).

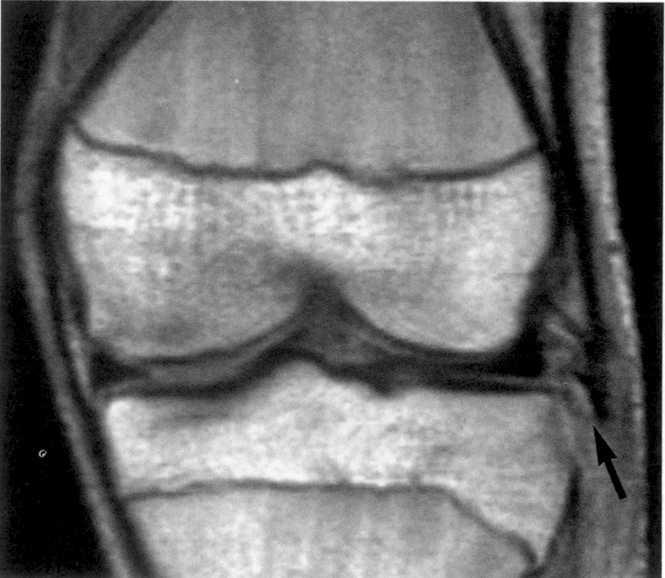

Figure 46.77 Segond fracture of the knee. Coronal proton density-weighted MRI demonstrates avulsion of the bony insertion of the iliotibial band (arrow). Avulsions of the lateral collateral ligament complex have a close association with ACL injury.

Fractures of the patella may be due to a direct blow or due to forced contraction of the quadriceps mechanism with the knee fixed in flexion. The latter mechanism usually results in a transverse fracture and retraction of the quadriceps; the former may result in linear fractures, or stellate patterns if greater forces are involved. It is generally not difficult to distinguish an acute patellar fracture from a bipartite patella (a normal variant consisting of a separate ossification centre in the superolateral aspect of the patella): the bipartite fragment will have a smooth, well-corticated edge, unlike the acute fracture fragment (Fig. 46.78). Bipartite patellae are bilateral in about 80% of cases.

Osteochondral fractures in the knee usually occur in the articular surfaces of the patella or femoral condyles. MRI can demonstrate the size and location of the lesion, and help to determine the integrity of the overlying cartilage. If the cartilage is disrupted, fluid from the joint can track into the space between the fragment and the remainder of the bone; a T2-weighted image will demonstrate this as high signal extending between the two areas of bone (Fig. 46.27).

Acute intra-articular fractures with extension into the marrow cavity allow blood and marrow fat to extrude into the joint space; the resulting lipohaemarthrosis can be demonstrated on a radiograph using a cross-table X-ray beam as described above. Thus, the horizontal cross-table lateral view of the knee may be very helpful in determining the presence of an occult intra-articular fracture: if a lipohaemarthrosis is present, a fat–fluid level will be visible in the suprapatellar recess of the knee joint (Fig. 46.1).

True dislocation of the knee (i.e. at the tibiofemoral joint) is an unusual injury that is due to a strong force. The tibia may dislocate anteriorly or posteriorly. Because there is a close association with intimal injury or disruption of the popliteal artery, angiography is generally performed when a knee dislocation is documented and there is a decrease in or absence of the dorsal pedal pulse suggesting such an injury.

The most common dislocation involving the knee is a *patellofemoral dislocation*. This relatively common injury is clinically undiagnosed at initial presentation in the majority of cases[9] and is difficult to detect on routine radiographs. Valgus stress with internal rotation, often combined with a medial blow to the patella, causes lateral dislocation of the patella relative to the trochlear groove of the femur. This usually results in disruption of the medial patellar retinaculum and matching osteochondral fractures or contusions in the medial aspect of the patella and the lateral femoral condyle (Fig. 46.79). A large joint effusion is frequently present. Patients usually relocate the patella spontaneously or purposely before presenting for medical evaluation; MRI[9] illustrates the residual injuries to best advantage (Fig. 46.80).

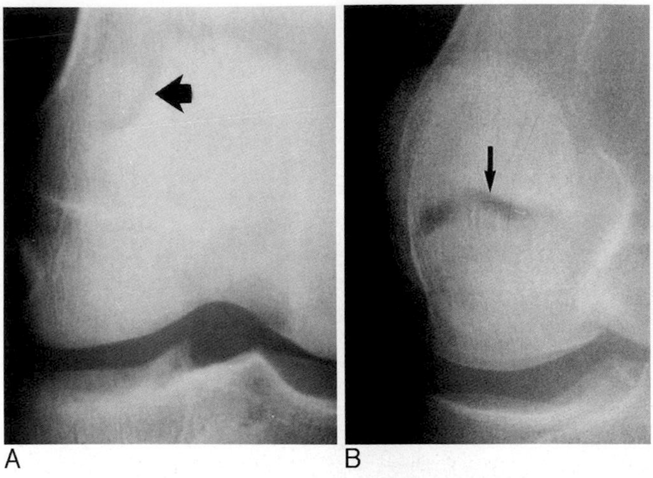

Figure 46.78 Bipartite patella (A) is usually superolateral in location; the fragment is often smaller than the 'defect' in the patella. The edges are smooth and sclerotic (arrow). In comparison, an acute fracture of the patella (B) demonstrates fragments that fit together like puzzle pieces; the edges are indistinct (arrow).

Internal derangement of the knee

MR imaging has made possible the evaluation of the internal structures of the acutely injured knee and has proven to be accurate in the evaluation of injury to the ligamentous and cartilaginous structures.

Injury to the *anterior cruciate ligament* (ACL) can be easily documented with MRI. The normal ACL is represented on oblique sagittal images (along the course of the ligament) by an elongated ovoid signal void that extends from the medial

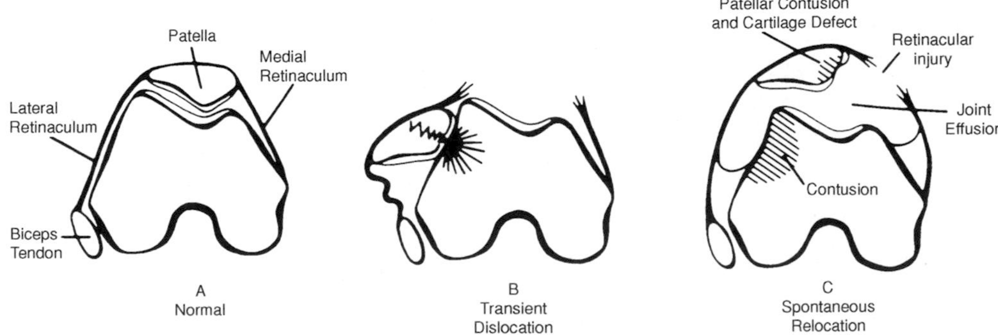

Figure 46.79 Transient patellar dislocation. (A) Normal relationship of the patella and retinacula in extension. (B) Transient lateral patellar dislocation results in disruption of the medial retinaculum. Contractile force of the vastus medialis causes the medial facet of the patella to strike the lateral femoral condyle. The patella usually reduces back into the intercondylar notch spontaneously with knee extension. (C) The resultant MR findings are delineated: disruption of the medial patellar retinaculum, patellar and femoral contusions and joint effusion. (Reprinted with permission from Kirsch et al 1993 Am J Roentgenol[9].)

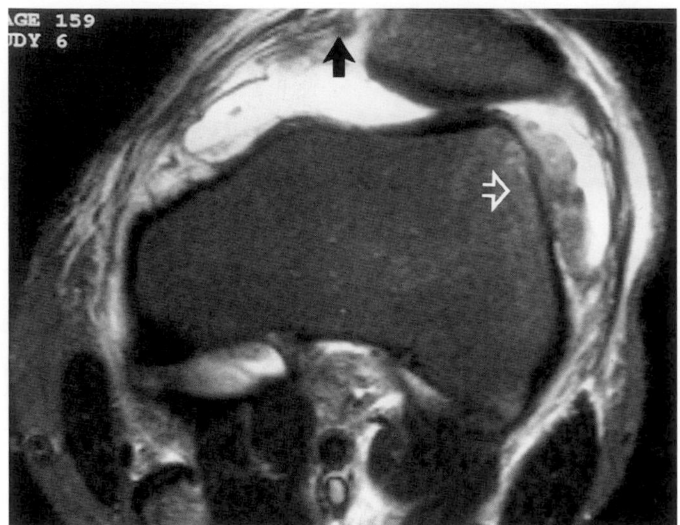

Figure 46.80 MRI appearance of transient patello-femoral dislocation. Axial STIR image of the knee in a patient who had experienced transient patellar dislocation demonstrates disruption of, and abnormal high signal surrounding the medial patellar retinaculum (solid arrow). Oedema in the medial patella and lateral femoral condyle (open arrow) represents contusions. There is a moderate joint effusion. The patella remains subluxed.

aspect of the lateral femoral condyle to the anterior tibial spine. Disruption of the ACL is manifested by replacement of the normal ligamentous signal void with amorphous intermediate signal representing oedema and haemorrhage (Fig. 46.81). If the ACL is not visualized and no oedematous tissue is seen in its expected location, a chronic ACL injury can be inferred. Interpretation of the status of the ACL based solely on the sagittal images can be misleading; confirmation in the coronal and axial planes may significantly increase diagnostic accuracy[10,11]. An important ancillary finding in acute ACL injury is the presence of bone contusions in the posterolateral aspect of the tibia, and in the articular surface of the lateral femoral condyle (Fig. 46.81). This pattern is essentially pathognomonic for ACL injury[10–12]. Rarely, the tibial insertion site of the ACL may be the point of disruption; in this case, an avulsion fragment will be seen arising from the anterior aspect of the tibial spine.

The *posterior cruciate ligament* (PCL) is less commonly injured than the ACL. The normal PCL is represented on sagittal images as a thick, curved signal void extending from the medial femoral condyle to a bony shelf just below the midportion of the posterior tibial plateau. Abnormal internal signal, thickening or disruption are signs of PCL injury[13,14]. The most common mechanisms of PCL injury are posterior translation of the tibia in a flexed knee (dashboard injury) and hyperextension (often associated with ACL tear).

The *medial and lateral collateral ligament complexes* (MCL and LCL) are seen on coronal images as thin bands of signal void extending from the distal femur to the tibia and fibula. As in the cruciate ligaments, abnormal signal surrounding, or within, the ligaments or complete disruption of the structures are signs of acute injury to the collateral ligaments. In general, MCL disruption is seen in association with valgus stress and LCL injury occurs with varus stress (although frequently the injury patterns are more complex and involve other structures). As mentioned above, an avulsion of the lateral tibial rim insertion of the LCL (Segond fracture) heralds the presence of an associated ACL injury.

MRI may document meniscal tears with a high degree of sensitivity and specificity. Normally depicted as a triangular area of signal void, a torn meniscus will demonstrate a linear or globular collection of abnormal intermediate or high signal within its substance, extending to either the superior or inferior articular surface. Extension to the capsular surface of the meniscus does not represent a tear; such signal is frequently seen in normal menisci and represents mucoid degeneration (Fig. 46.82). Tears may also manifest as changes in shape or size of the meniscus;

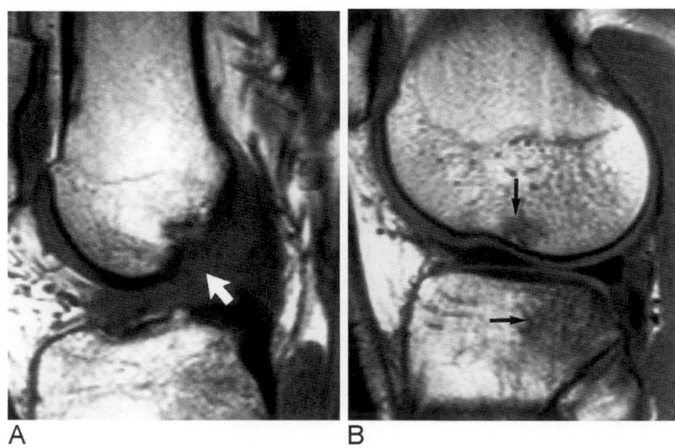

Figure 46.81 MRI appearance of acute rupture of the ACL. Sagittal T1-weighted MRI of the knee (A) demonstrates a mass of intermediate amorphous signal in the expected location of the anterior cruciate ligament (arrow), consistent with a complete tear of the ACL. Further laterally (B), low signal in the posterior tibia and lateral femoral condyle represents typical contusions seen in association with ACL injury (small arrows).

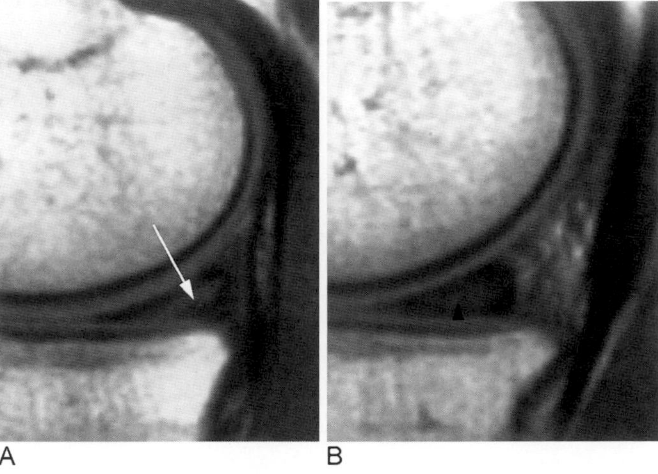

Figure 46.82 MRI appearance of meniscal injury. Sagittal T1-weighted MRI of the knee (A) demonstrates linear high signal in the posterior horn of the medial meniscus extending to the inferior articular surface, consistent with a tear (arrow). In a different patient (B), high signal (arrowhead) that does not extend to the articular surface probably represents mucoid degeneration.

comparison with other meniscal segments should reveal that the posterior horn of the medial meniscus is at least as large as any other quadrant. Bucket-handle tears, which involve displacement of the free edge of the meniscus into the intercondylar notch, can be best documented in the coronal plane (Fig. 46.83).

Injury to the *extensor mechanism* of the knee comprises trauma to the quadriceps muscle group, the patella and the patellar tendon. As in assessment of the cruciate and collateral ligaments, abnormal signal or size of the musculotendinous unit (MTU) suggests intrasubstance injury or partial tear, while complete disruption is usually manifested as discontinuity of the normal black tendon fibres. Complete disruptions are usually associated with retraction of the associated muscle groups and redundancy of the severed tendon margin (Fig. 46.84).

The lower leg

Fractures of the leg most commonly involve the distal ends of the tibia and fibula, which will be discussed in the ankle section. Direct blows to the leg may cause fracture of one or both bones. The classic injuries are the tibial fracture, either due to a direct blow or related to chronic stress (seen in runners), and the 'bumper fracture', a fracture of the proximal fibula (often occurring in a pedestrian struck by an automobile bumper). Because the peroneal nerve is anatomically close, it may be damaged in bumper fractures.

Stress injuries, as elsewhere in the body, may manifest only as slight thickening of the cortex or subtle periosteal reaction, or the radiograph may be normal (Fig. 46.3). Scintigraphy, or MRI, may be necessary to make the correct diagnosis.

The ankle

The standard radiographic evaluation of the ankle includes AP, lateral and an internally rotated oblique view (mortise view). The mortise view is designed to demonstrate the true ankle joint; the space around the talar dome should be approximately 4 mm in all directions (Fig. 46.85). Stress views with the ankle forced into inversion (supination) or eversion (pronation) can be performed to assess laxity or disruption of ankle ligaments, manifested by widening or narrowing of this space.

Ankle injuries are one of the most common causes for emergency room visits. The mechanics of ankle trauma are best explained in terms of inversion or eversion of the foot relative to the leg, with resulting distraction/avulsion injury on one side of the ankle and corresponding impaction injury on the other side. For example, the most common ankle injury is due to external rotation of the foot relative to the leg (although in reality, the leg is internally rotated relative to the planted foot). The result is a spiral or oblique fracture of the lateral malleolus (due to impaction) and avulsion of the deltoid ligament medially (with or without an associated avulsion fracture fragment arising from the medial malleolus) (Fig. 46.86). In the case of an inversion injury, the opposite applies: a transverse fracture of the lateral malleolus from distraction of the lateral ankle and an oblique fracture of the medial malleolus from impaction forces would be expected.

It is important to realize that distraction of the ankle medially or laterally can result in stretching or disruption of the supporting ligaments on that side (i.e. a sprain). If the ligament ruptures in its midportion, there will be no radiographic evidence other than soft tissue swelling in the region. When the ligament ruptures at its insertion onto one of the bones, it may cause an avulsion fracture; these injuries usually occur at the proximal aspect of the ligament (i.e. at the malleoli) and can be seen on routine radiographs. The fracture fragments are generally very small and are located just distal to the tip of the malleolus. Occasionally, the avulsion fragment may be quite large; in this setting, a transverse fracture of the malleolus is identified. Although not usually necessary for diagnosis, the integrity of the ankle ligaments can be assessed with MRI, either at the time of injury or in the setting of chronic instability.

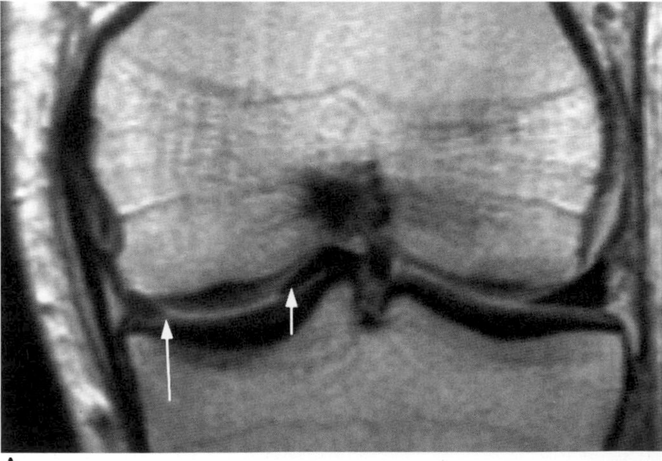

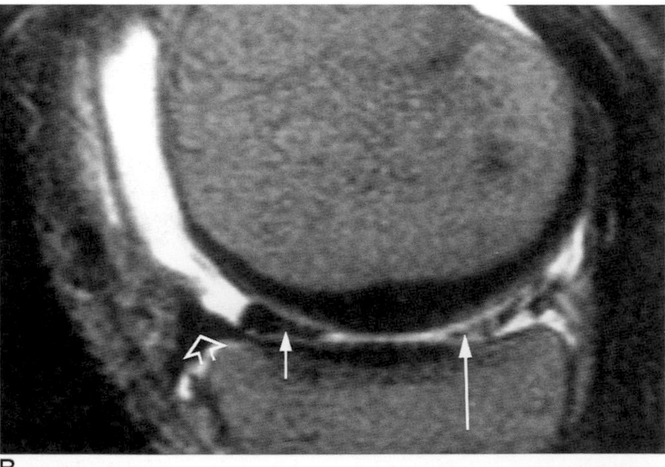

Figure 46.83 Bucket-handle tear of the medial meniscus. Coronal proton density-weighted image (A) shows decreased size of the medial meniscus (long arrow) and a meniscal fragment displaced medially into the intercondylar notch (small arrow). Sagittal T2-weighted MRI of the knee (B) shows irregular shape and small size of the posterior horn of the medial meniscus (long arrow). The posterior horn of the meniscus should be at least as large as any other meniscal quadrant. There is a large area of signal void in the anterior joint (small arrow), separate from the anterior horn of the meniscus (open arrow), that represents a fragment of the meniscus that has separated and migrated anteriorly.

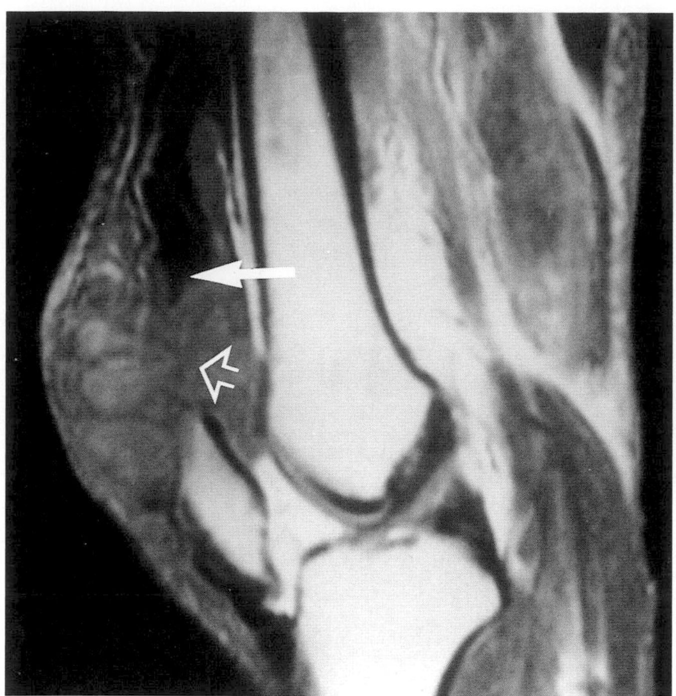

Figure 46.84 Complete rupture of the quadriceps tendon in a dialysis patient. Sagittal T1-weighted MRI of the knee demonstrates disruption of the quadriceps tendon with a large amorphous area of haemorrhage (open arrow) just above the inferiorly retracted patella. Note the retraction of the quadriceps tendon (long arrow).

Often a well-corticated bony fragment will be seen adjacent to one or both malleoli; the aetiology of these ossicles is debatable. Many sources believe these to be normal accessory ossification centres (they occur at predictable sites), but others feel that at least some of these ossicles represent the sequelae of previous traumatic avulsion injuries. Regardless of their aetiology, it is important to distinguish such ossicles from acute avulsion fragments. Typical features of chronic ossicles are round shape, well-defined cortical margins and a uniform space between the ossicle and the malleolus. The reader is referred to *Keats' Atlas of Normal Radiographic Variants* for more detailed descriptions and examples.

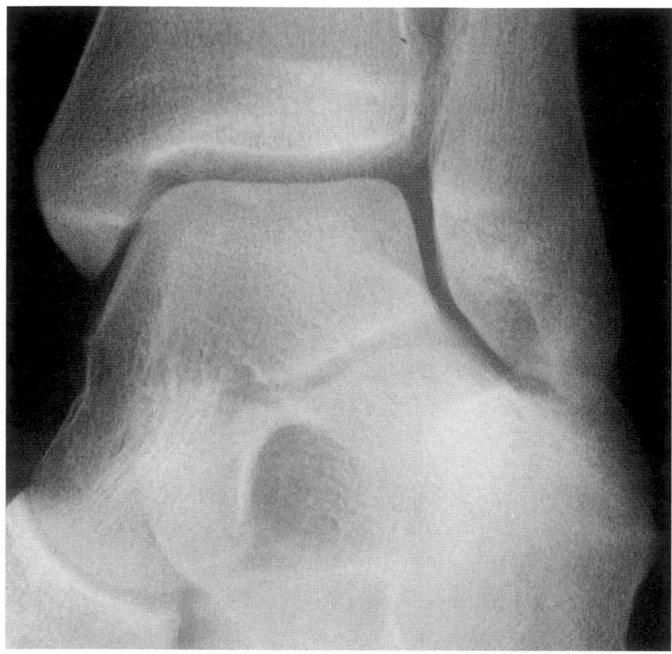

Figure 46.85 Oblique (mortise) view of the normal ankle demonstrates a uniform 3–4 mm space around the talus.

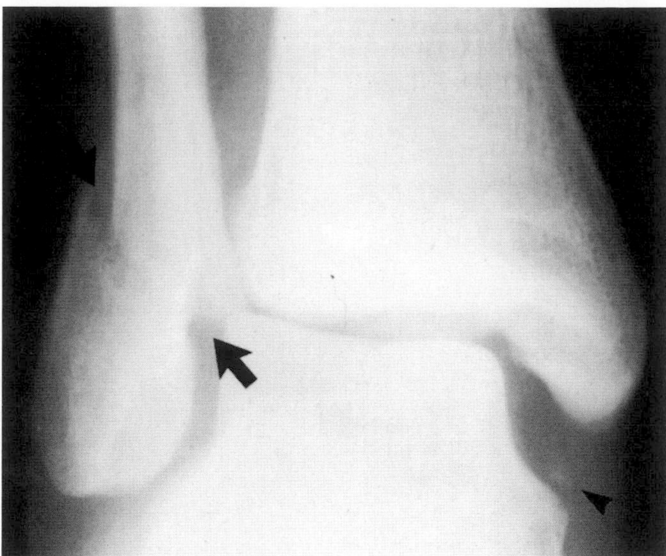

Figure 46.86 An eversion injury of the ankle involving an oblique impaction fracture of the lateral malleolus (arrow), lateral subluxation of the talus, and a small avulsion fracture of the medial malleolus (arrowhead).

An important stabilizing influence in the ankle is the distal tibiofibular syndesmosis. If a fibular fracture extends superiorly to the level of the syndesmosis or above it, the syndesmosis is considered disrupted. Rarely, an eversion injury may result in an avulsion of the medial malleolus without a visible lateral malleolar fracture; the force may be dissipated superiorly, causing disruption of the interosseous ligament joining the shafts of the fibula and tibia, with fracture of the proximal fibula. Such a complex is referred to as a Maisonneuve fracture (Fig. 46.87).

The posterior lip of the distal tibia may be fractured either in combination with the medial and lateral malleoli due to massive force (trimalleolar fracture), or due to vertical compressive force in a dorsiflexed foot. Impaction of the dome of the talus against the plafond creates comminuted fractures of the distal tibial joint surface known as pilon fractures.

Soft tissue injury about the ankle

Rupture of the Achilles tendon may occur due to athletic trauma (jumping), or can be seen following normal activity in patients with underlying systemic diseases. Patients with diabetes mellitus, chronic renal failure, hyperparathyroidism, gout and connective tissue disorders are particularly susceptible to tendon tears. When the Achilles tendon is disrupted, the injury usually occurs within 2–3 cm of the distal insertion point on the calcaneal tuberosity, in a relatively avascular zone. While swelling of the tendon and obliteration of the pre-Achilles fat pad may be clues to the diagnosis on a lateral radiograph, MRI is a very sensitive and specific method of

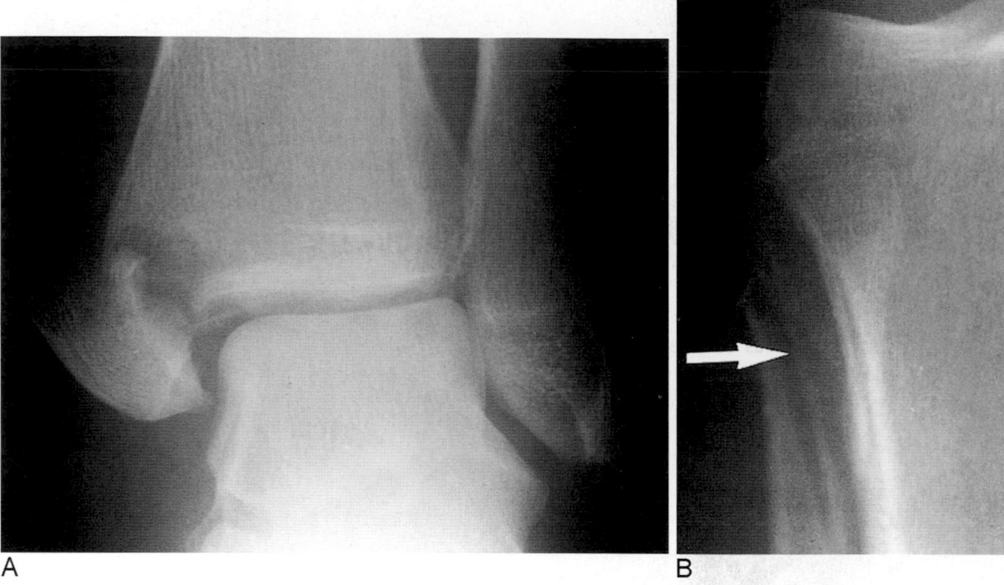

Figure 46.87 Maisonneuve fracture. AP radiograph of the ankle (A) demonstrates a transverse fracture of the medial malleolus. More cranially (B) there is a fracture of the proximal fibula (arrow), indicating extension of the injury plane along the interosseous membrane.

evaluating this structure. As elsewhere, the normal tendon will demonstrate signal void on all sequences. Sagittal and axial images are most useful in the evaluation of the Achilles tendon; on axial images the tendon should be semilunar in shape. A complete disruption will demonstrate discontinuity of the tendon fibres on sagittal T2-weighted images, with high signal fluid and oedema between and surrounding the redundant tendon ends. There is often some degree of retraction of the proximal portion of the tendon (Fig. 46.88).

Similarly, US may demonstrate tendon disruption or tendinitis. Real-time US allows determination of distance between ruptured tendon portions in maximal plantar flexion. Tendinitis is seen as thickening of the tendon with areas of altered echogenicity (Fig. 46.89). Comparison with the unaffected side may be useful.

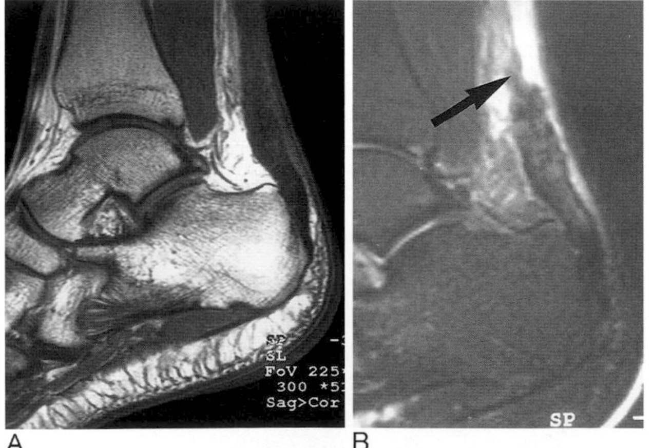

Figure 46.88 Achilles tendon rupture. Sagittal T1-weighted (A) and STIR (B) MRI demonstrate discontinuity of the Achilles tendon, with abnormal signal (arrow, B) representing haemorrhage and oedema. Note how poorly the T1-weighted image demonstrates the disruption; this is because oedematous tendon and fluid may look identical with such sequences.

Injury to the posterior tibialis tendon (PTT) is the next most common tendon injury in the ankle region. The normal PTT should be approximately twice as large as the adjacent flexor digitorum longus tendon on an axial MRI. Increased signal or enlargement of the tendon indicates tendon injury (Fig. 46.90). Inversion injury can cause partial or complete rupture of the peroneus longus and brevis tendons in the lateral aspect of the ankle. Familiarity with the normal anatomy and an appreciation of a change in morphology and signal are necessary to diagnose such injuries with MRI. US may also demonstrate the transverse and longitudinal tears, altered echogenicity and fluid in the tendon sheath.

The hindfoot

The talus has no muscular or tendinous attachments. It is attached to the adjacent bones by ligaments and the ankle joint capsule. In severe trauma, these attachments may be disrupted and the talus may be dislocated, usually anteriorly. Because the talar blood supply is through the capsular attachments, such an injury is almost invariably associated with osteonecrosis of the talus. Most of the blood supply to the talar dome enters through the more distal talus; fracture of the talar neck can result in *osteonecrosis of the dome* (Fig. 46.91). Avulsion fractures of the dorsal surface of the head and neck of the talus are not unusual. Osteochondral fractures of the talar dome can occur due to impaction injuries; these are very difficult to diagnose with routine radiographs, and MRI is often necessary to elucidate the cause of ongoing pain after an ankle injury (Fig. 46.92).

Fractures of the calcaneus are usually due to compressive forces, as in a fall from a height. Comminuted impaction occurs in the body of the calcaneus, with flattening of the subtalar portion of the bone. Boehler's angle is formed by the intersection of lines drawn on a lateral view from the anterior superior and posterior superior edges of the calcaneus to the highest point of the articular surface (Fig. 46.93). A normal Boehler's angle should be between 20 and 40 degrees. An impacted fracture of the calcaneus will reduce or even

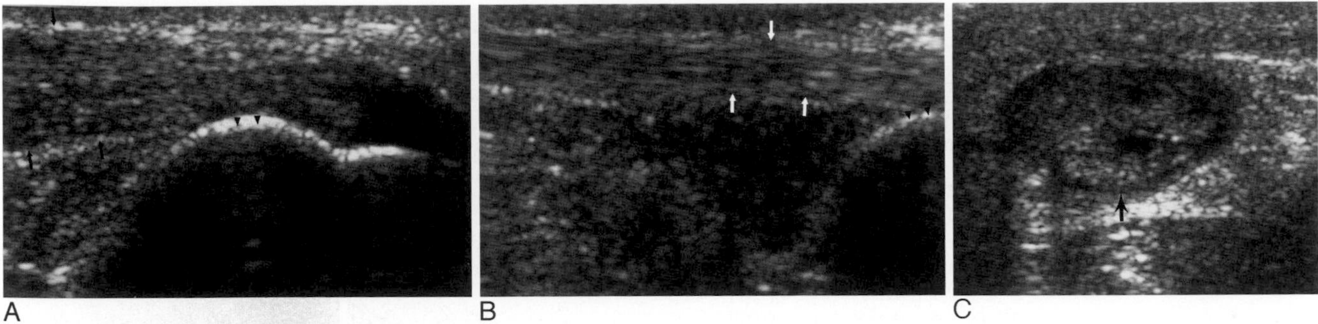

Figure 46.89 Partial tear/strain of the Achilles tendon. A 21-year-old man injured his ankle while playing rugby. He had soreness in the region of the right distal gastrocnemius muscles, but no weakness. Longitudinal US (A) demonstrates thickening of the tendon (arrows) proximal to its calcaneal attachment. The left side (B) demonstrates his normal Achilles tendon (arrows). There is shadowing by the calcaneus (arrowheads) in (A) and (B). Axial US in the midsubstance of the abnormal right tendon (C) reveals a rounded anterior margin (arrow) and focal areas of decreased echogenicity.

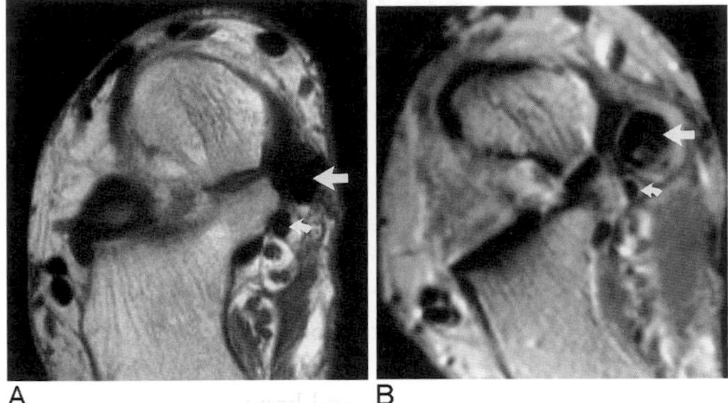

Figure 46.90 Partial tear of the posterior tibialis tendon. Oblique axial T1-weighted MRI of a normal ankle (A) demonstrates the normal 2:1 size ratio of the posterior tibialis (arrow) and flexor digitorum longus (small arrow) tendons. Axial proton density image from a patient who experienced ankle trauma (B) shows enlargement of, and abnormal signal within, the posterior tibialis tendon, consistent with a partial tear of that structure (arrow). The flexor digitorum longus tendon is normal (small arrow).

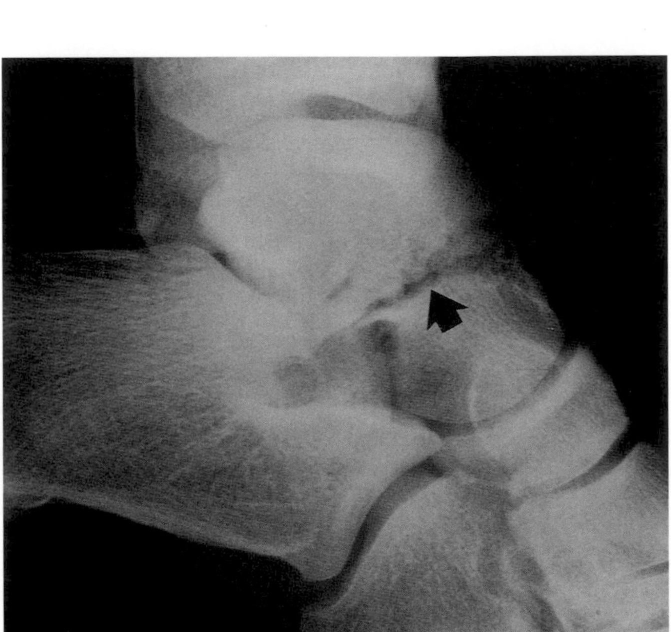

Figure 46.91 Fracture of the neck of the talus (arrow). This injury has a high incidence of subsequent AVN of the talar dome, particularly with associated subtalar dislocation.

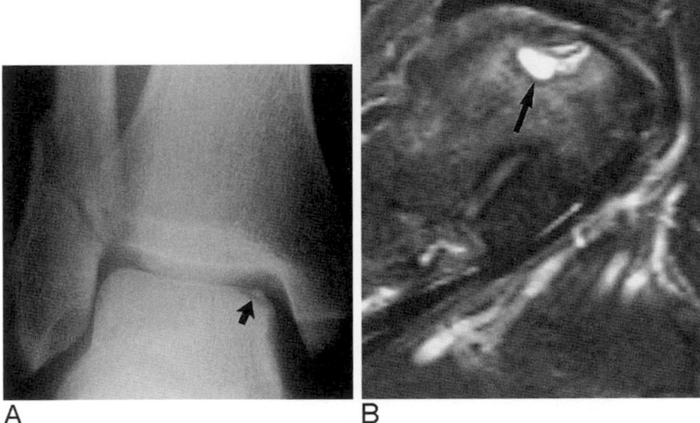

Figure 46.92 Osteochondral fracture of the medial talar dome. Oblique view of the ankle (A) demonstrates a lucency separating a small bony fragment from the remainder of the talar dome, consistent with an osteochondral fracture (arrow). There is also a fracture of the lateral malleolus. Sagittal STIR MR image from another patient (B) demonstrates an osteochondral fragment of the talar dome separated from the remainder of the talus by high signal fluid (arrow).

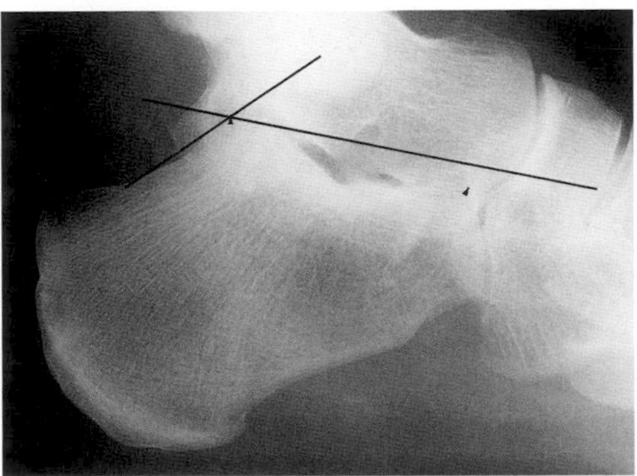

Figure 46.93 Lateral view of the calcaneus demonstrating the proper measurement of Boehler's angle, which is normally 20–40 degrees.

reverse Boehler's angle. Most calcaneal fractures are evident enough to make it unnecessary to measure Boehler's angle (Fig. 46.94). Such fractures are also well seen in axial views of the heel (Harris view); however, complex calcaneal fractures are studied to best advantage with CT (Fig. 46.95). The extension of impacted calcaneal fractures into the subtalar joints, particularly the posterior, is well evaluated with direct coronal CT. It should be remembered that impacted calcaneal fractures are commonly associated with compression fractures in the lumbar spine. Fractures without change in Boehler's angle may occur in the anterior process, the posterior tuberosity, or the lateral margin of the bone (Fig. 46.96). Stress fractures are common in the tuberosity (see Fig. 46.3).

The mid- and forefoot

Fractures of the remaining tarsal bones are unusual. The most common is an avulsion injury on the dorsal surface of the navicular. Fracture-dislocations may occur at the common tarsometatarsal joint (Lisfranc's joint). These injuries are often the result of severe shear forces due to forced plantar flexion, as in motor vehicle or parachuting accidents. They are frequently seen as neuropathic fracture-dislocations in the diabetic foot. Lisfranc injuries are classified as homolateral (in which all the metatarsals are shifted laterally) (Fig. 46.97) or divergent (in which the first metatarsal shifts medially and the remainder of the forefoot shifts laterally) (Fig. 46.98). Normal alignment must be understood in order to recognize a subtle dislocation at this joint; the first metatarsal is aligned with the medial cuneiform, the second metatarsal with the middle cuneiform, the third metatarsal with the lateral cuneiform and the fourth and fifth metatarsals with the cuboid. These are best seen on oblique views. In addition, there is usually a fracture in the recessed base of the second metatarsal, and other smaller fractures along the margins of the tarsometatarsal joints.

Stress fractures of the metatarsals are common following various kinds of overuse; the classic is the *march fracture* seen in military recruits and runners, usually manifested as periosteal new bone formation along the shafts of the second, third, or fourth metatarsals (Fig. 46.99).

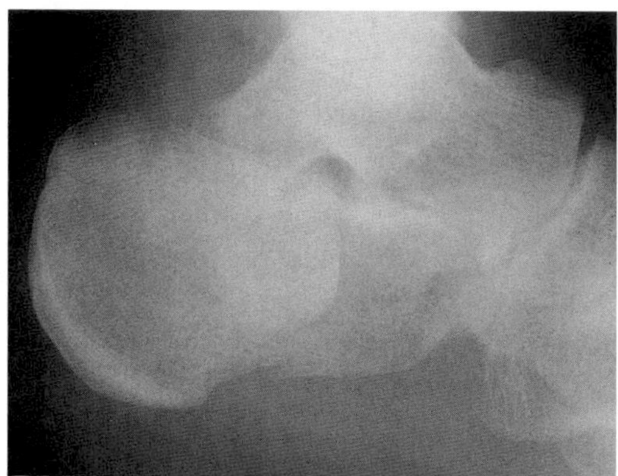

Figure 46.94 Fracture of the calcaneus causing flattening of Boehler's angle.

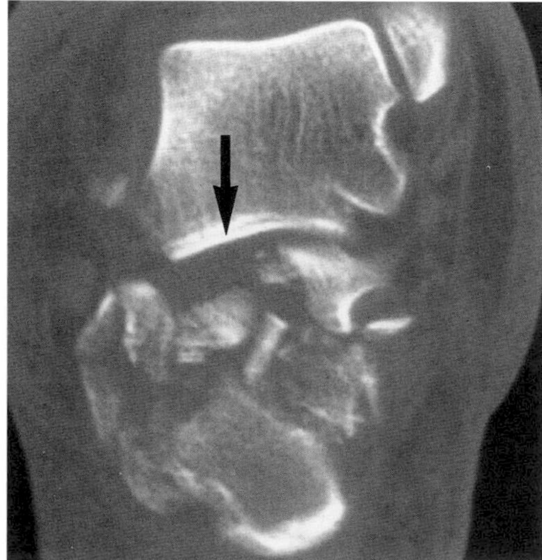

Figure 46.95 CT of a comminuted fracture of the calcaneus demonstrates complete disruption of the posterior subtalar joint (arrow). Such fractures are very difficult to characterize with plain radiographs.

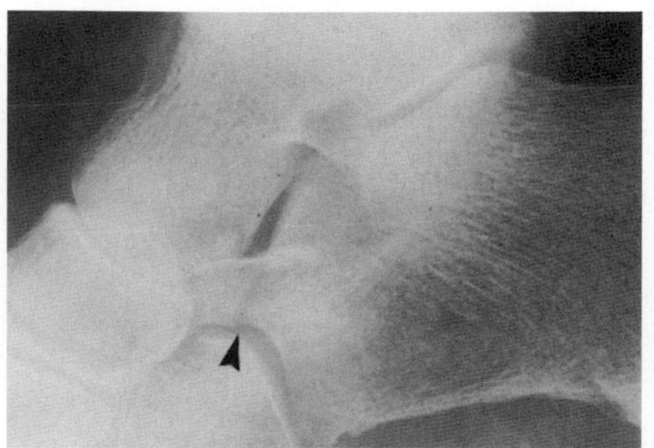

Figure 46.96 Fracture of the anterior process of the calcaneus (arrowhead).

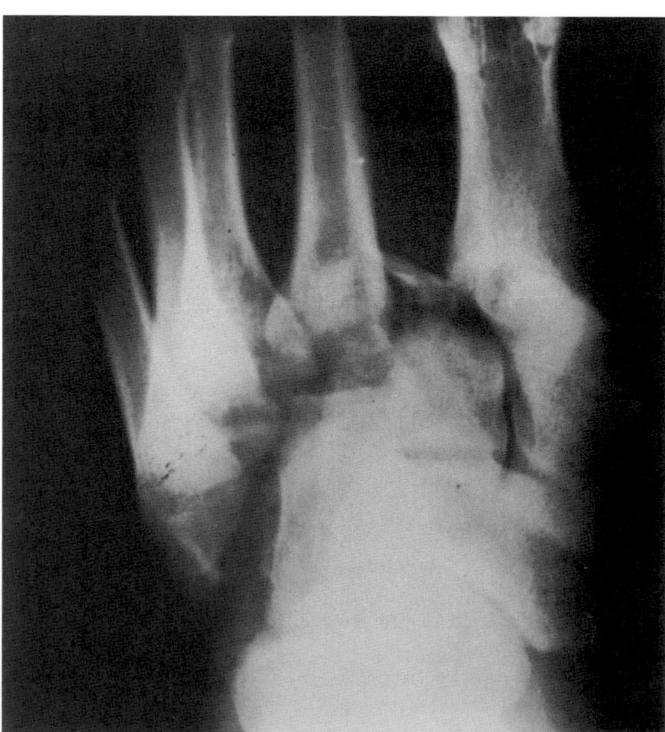

Figure 46.97 Homolateral Lisfranc fracture-dislocation. All five metatarsals are displaced laterally.

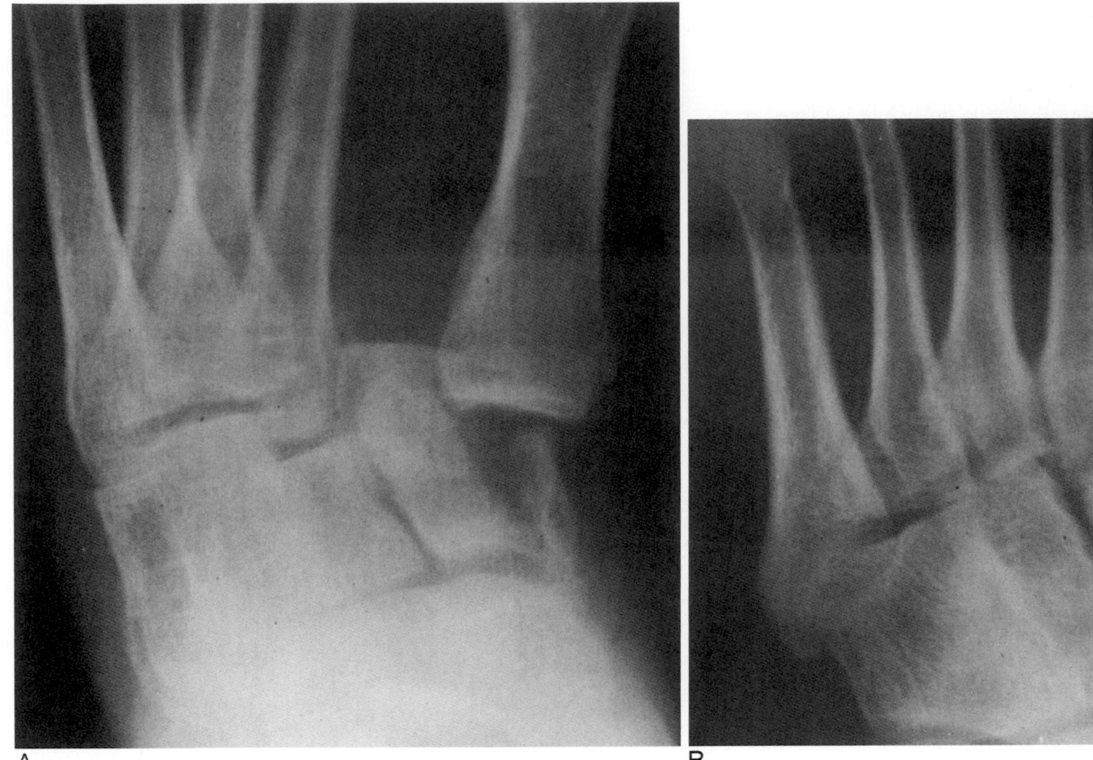

Figure 46.98 Oblique (A) and AP (B) projections of a divergent Lisfranc fracture-dislocation, which includes medial displacement of the first metatarsal (seen on A) and lateral displacement of the second to fifth metatarsals (seen on B). There is also a fracture of the medial cuneiform.

Forced inversion of the foot may result in an important avulsion fracture at the base of the fifth metatarsal. Rupture of the attachment site of the peroneus brevis may cause an avulsion of a small to moderate bony fragment from this site. The fracture line will invariably be *transverse*; this is an important point because this injury must be distinguished from a normal accessory ossification centre at the base of the fifth metatarsal. This accessory centre appears as a longitudinal lucency in the lateral aspect of the base of the fifth metatarsal. The Jones' fracture is an

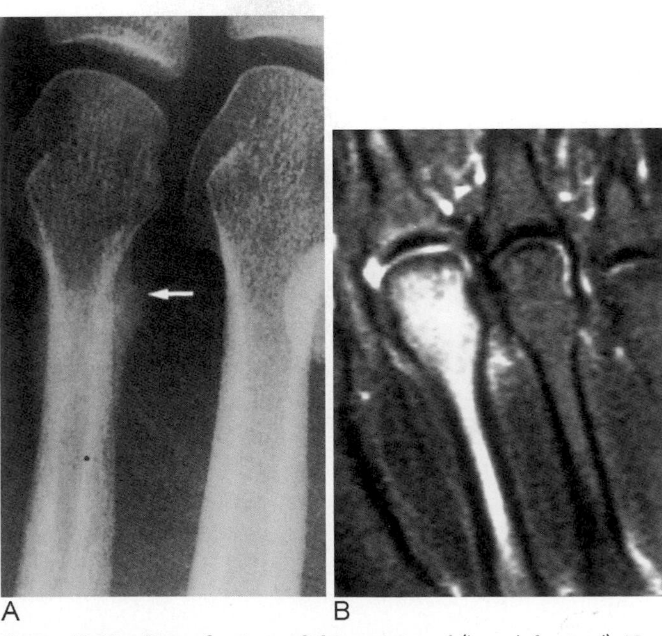

Figure 46.99 **Stress fracture of the metatarsal** ('march fracture'). AP radiograph (A) demonstrates fluffy periosteal new bone along the distal shaft of the third metatarsal (arrow); the patient had foot pain for 16 days. In another patient, coronal STIR MRI (B) demonstrates increased signal in the distal second metatarsal diffusely, consistent with stress injury.

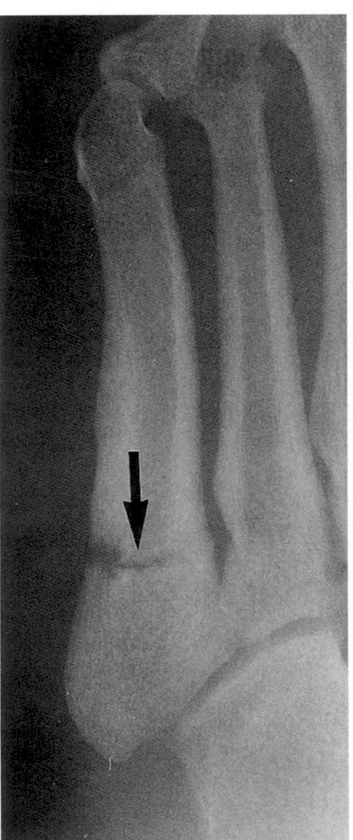

Figure 46.100 **Fracture of the proximal shaft of the fifth metatarsal** ('true Jones fracture') (arrow). Jones originally described a fracture in this location, which he himself suffered while dancing.

extra-articular fracture of the proximal aspect of the fifth metatarsal (Fig. 46.100).

Fractures of the phalanges of the toes are common and relatively insignificant. The only exception is a fracture of the distal phalanx of the great toe with extension into the nail bed, which increases the risk of infection and frequently requires debridement.

THE SPINE

The purpose of the radiographic examination of the potentially injured spine is to identify or exclude the presence of fractures and dislocations and to determine the extent of injury, once identified. Injuries to the spinal cord may occur without associated fracture or dislocation of the spine but these are uncommon and found under certain predictable circumstances. Care is needed in handling patients with suspected spinal injuries so as not to create a cord injury where none existed before, or to cause more extensive cord injury than may already be present. Movement of the injured patient's head and neck should be restricted until spinal fracture and dislocations have been excluded. Because physical examination of the spine is difficult, this exclusion is usually accomplished by radiographic examination, but the correct views must be obtained. AP and lateral projections of the area of the spine in question obtained with the patient in the recumbent position are the minimum (Fig. 46.101). Oblique radiographs of the cervical and lumbar spines might be considered in less severely injured patients. Oblique views are of limited value in the thoracic spine and can be safely omitted.

CT[15,16] is utilized to clarify doubtful findings, to identify obscure injuries (particularly in the posterior elements) and for further evaluation of obvious fractures and dislocations (Fig. 46.101D). Volume averaging limits the demonstration of fractures in the axial plane, but displacement and malalignment is displayed by image reconstruction. CT, with image reconstruction in the sagittal and coronal planes, has become the accepted means of 'clearing' the cervical spine in patients who have sustained significant trauma[15,16].

MRI provides valuable and unique information about the status of ligaments, intervertebral discs and spinal cord[17,18] (Fig. 46.101E). There is a direct correlation between the MR signal characteristics and the histopathology of cord trauma.

Fractures and dislocations are most common in the lower cervical spine (C4–C7), at the thoracolumbar junction (T10–L2) and at the craniovertebral junction (C1–C2). Fractures usually involve the vertebral body and may be accompanied by fractures of the posterior elements. The important radiographic observations are to determine:

1 whether or not the height of the vertebral bodies is maintained
2 whether the alignment of the spine is normal
3 if the distances between the vertebrae at the intervertebral disc spaces, facet joints and spinous processes remain normal
4 if the contiguous surfaces of the joints and vertebral end-plates remain parallel.

Fractures and dislocations are manifested by a loss of vertebral body height, disruption of the cortical margins, malalignment of the spine and a loss of the parallel apposing cortical surfaces of bone at the facet joints or intervertebral disc spaces.

Fractures limited to the vertebral body or posterior elements are considered *stable*; those involving both the vertebral body and posterior elements are considered *unstable*. Paraspinal haematomas may point to an otherwise obscure fracture or dislocation in the cervical or thoracic spine. The haematomas present as retropharyngeal masses in the cervical spine and as paraspinal masses on the frontal projection in the dorsal spine but are difficult to identify in the lumbar spine because they are of the same density as the paraspinal muscles.

Fractures of the spine

Compression fractures

A compression fracture is manifested by an anterior wedged deformity of the vertebral body or a depression limited to the vertebral end-plate, usually the superior end-plate (Fig. 46.102). The fracture is commonly caused by flexion of the spine. A faint band of sclerosis may be identified just beneath the deformed end-plate, indicating a zone of bony impaction. Rarely the injury is limited to the inferior end-plate of the vertebral body.

With severe compression injuries, a portion of the vertebral body may be displaced into the spinal canal, compromising the spinal cord or nerve roots. This is most commonly encountered in the form of a teardrop fracture in the cervical spine and in burst fractures at the thoracolumbar junction. Whenever a compression fracture is encountered, retropulsion of a fragment of the vertebral body must be considered.

Fracture-dislocations

Fracture-dislocations occur most commonly in the lower cervical spine (Fig. 46.103) and at the thoracolumbar junction. Usually the upper vertebral body is displaced anteriorly relative to the lower vertebral body. There is often an anterior wedged compression fracture of the lower vertebral body and fractures involving the laminae, facets, or spinous processes.

Alternatively, there may be disruption of the joint capsule of the facet joints and interspinous ligament without associated fractures. At times there may be no significant fracture associated with a dislocation, since the injury is limited to the intervertebral disc, facet joint capsules and intervening ligaments. This more commonly occurs in the cervical spine. The degree of dislocation is variable. If minimal, it is often referred to as a 'subluxation', whereas 'dislocation' is used to indicate a more extensive or complete displacement of one vertebra relative to the other.

Fractures of the posterior elements

Fractures of the posterior elements do not commonly occur without accompanying fractures of the vertebral bodies, except

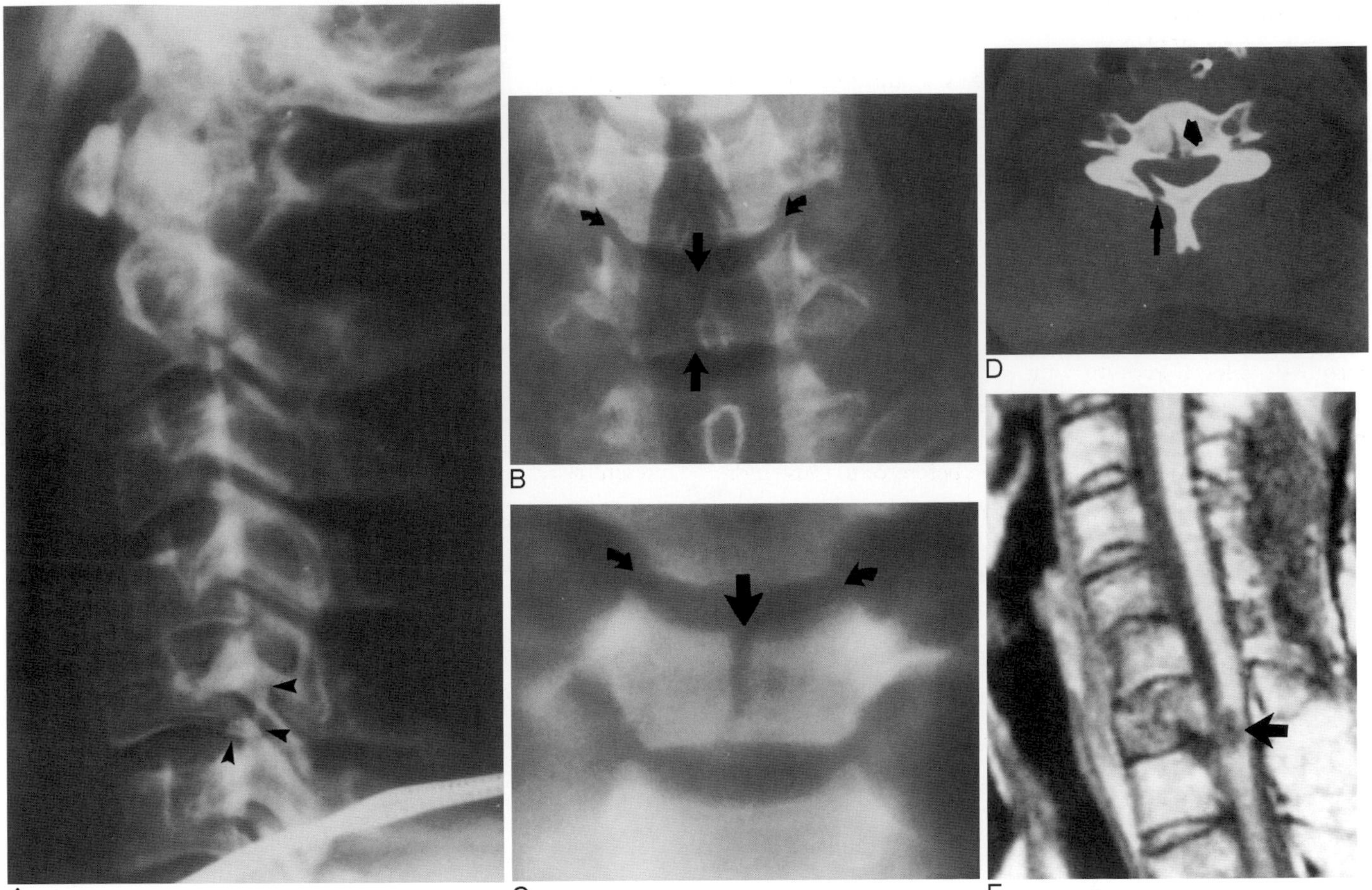

Figure 46.101 Teardrop (bursting, dispersion) fracture of C5. In lateral projection (A), the body of C5 is severely comminuted, with posterior fragments (arrowheads) retropulsed into the spinal canal. In the frontal projection (B,C), a vertical fracture line is present in the vertebral body (arrows) and the Luschka joints at the C4–5 level are diastatic (curved arrows) secondary to dispersion of the body fragments. The CT image (D) demonstrates the linear body fracture (broad arrow) as well as the characteristic laminar component (long-stemmed arrow) of the burst fracture. (E) MRI of another teardrop fracture in another patient, which demonstrates retropulsion of the posterior fragment with myelomalacia within the adjacent spinal cord (arrow).

for fractures of the transverse processes of the lumbar spine, the neural arches of the first and second cervical vertebrae and the spinous processes at the cervicothoracic junction. Isolated fractures of the vertebra at other locations are often difficult to diagnose and require CT to establish with certainty.

Classification of injuries

Acute traumatic injuries of the spine are often pragmatically classified on the basis of mechanism of injury: pure, dominant, or combined forces (Fig. 46.104). Injuries may be grouped into those caused by hyperflexion, flexion-rotation, extension-rotation, vertical compression (axial-loading), hyperextension, lateral flexion and the unclassifiable ones, in which the mechanism of injury is either diverse or imprecisely understood.

Cervical spine

The X-ray examination of the cervical spine depends upon the patient's clinical condition. In severely injured patients

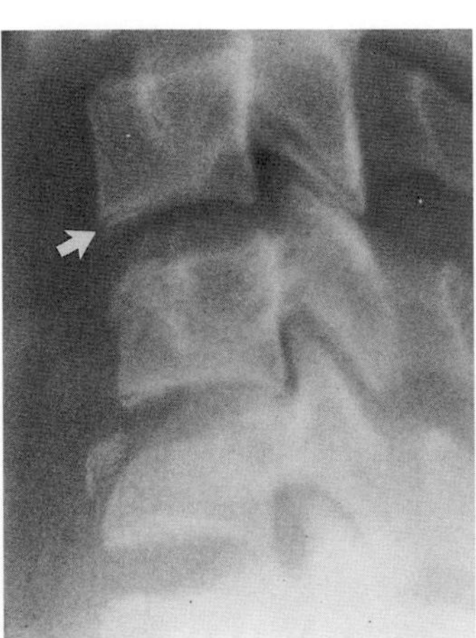

Figure 46.102 Simple wedge compression fracture of C7. Anterior wedging of the vertebral body involving the superior end-plate, with a separate fragment arising from the anterior superior margin of the body. The posterior elements are intact and the height of the posterior margin of the vertebral body is maintained. Note the normal vertebral apophyseal rings on the adjacent vertebrae (arrows) in this 13-year-old boy.

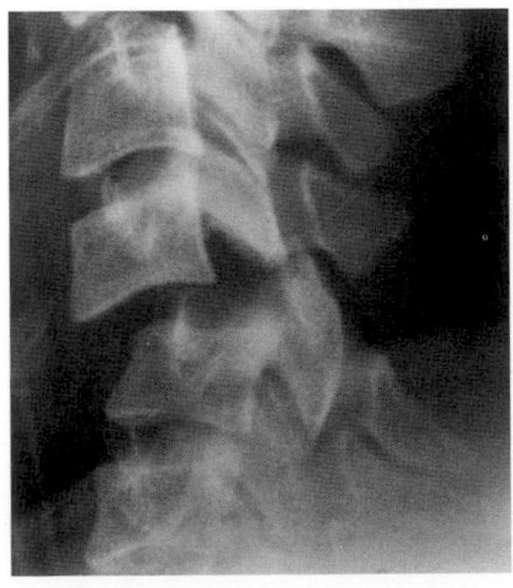

Figure 46.103 Fracture-dislocation at C4–5. There is a disruption of the facet joints and the intervertebral disc with the characteristic anterior displacement of the vertebra above the level of the dislocation. The interspinous ligaments are also disrupted, as evidenced by the separation of the spinous processes. The facets above are locked anterior to the facets below. This therefore represents a bilateral locked facet.

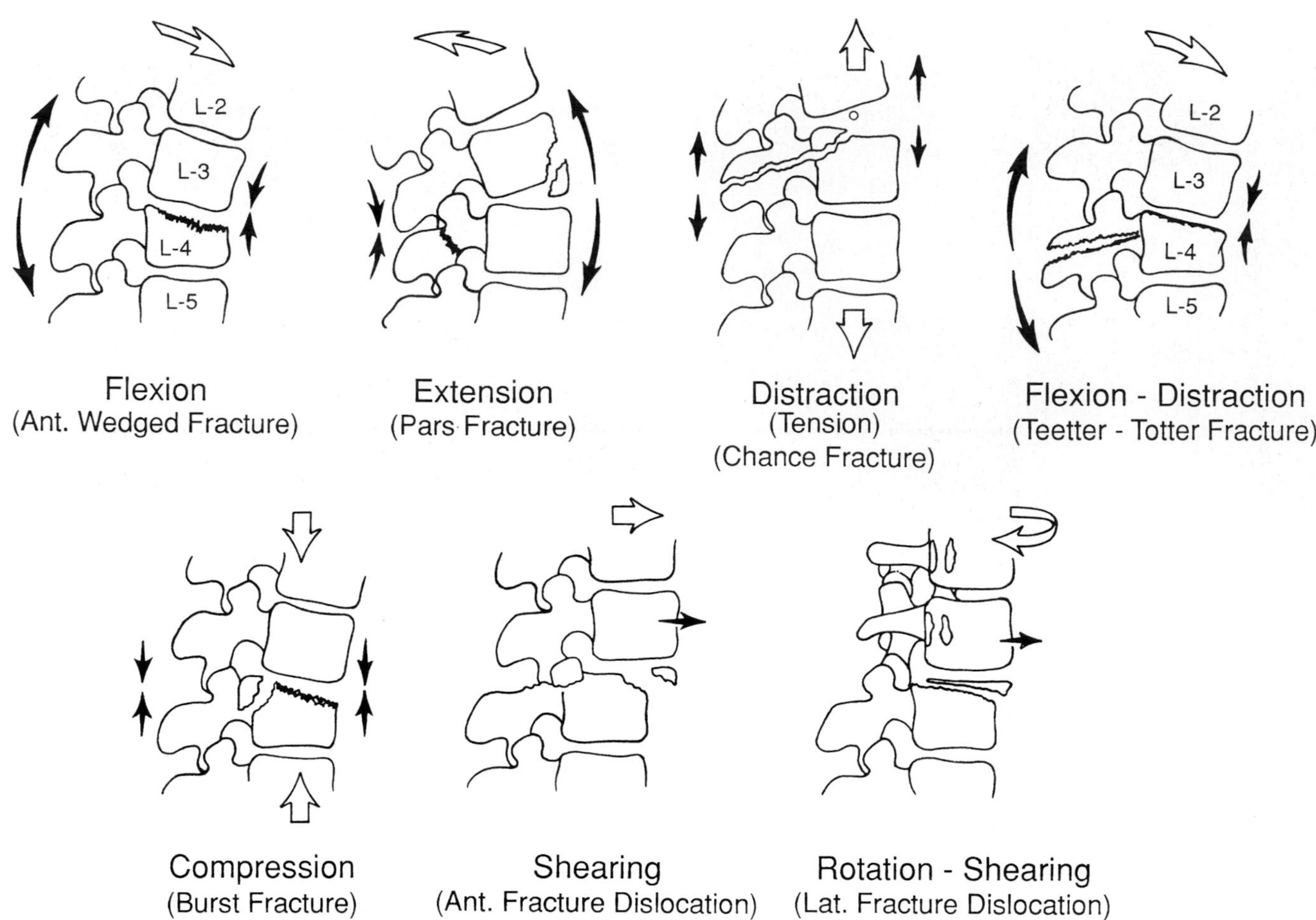

Figure 46.104 Pathomechanics of spinal injury. Each force produces a characteristic injury as visualized on the lateral radiograph. **Flexion** creates an anterior wedged deformity of the vertebral body. **Extension** results in a small triangular fragment separated from the anterior inferior margin of the vertebral body. **Distraction** creates horizontal fractures in the posterior element and little or no wedging of the vertebral body. **Flexion-distraction** creates a horizontal fracture of the posterior elements and anterior wedging of the vertebral body. **Axial compression** is characterized by anterior wedging of the vertebral body and retropulsion of the posterior superior margin of the vertebral body as in burst fractures. **Shearing** results in fracture–dislocations manifested by anterior displacement of the vertebra above the level of dislocation carrying with it a triangular avulsed fragment from the anterior superior margin of the vertebral body below. Fractures of the laminae and superior facets are commonly encountered. **Rotational** forces are combined with shearing to produce an anterior lateral dislocation of the spine.

(unconscious, major head or neck trauma, spinal cord or root signs, multiple organ system injuries, or multiple fractures), the *single most important radiographic examination is the horizontal beam lateral of the cervical spine.* Care must be taken to ensure that all seven cervical vertebrae are included. If not, a repeat examination should be obtained while pulling down on the patient's arms (Fig. 46.105). *Failure to visualize the seventh cervical vertebra and the C7/thoracic junction* is the most common error made in the radiographic assessment of cervical spine injury[19,20]. Two additional views are obtained: an AP radiograph of the lower cervical spine and AP open-mouth projection of the atlanto-axial articulation. CT with image reconstruction in both the coronal and sagittal planes is performed for patients who have sustained severe trauma, as in motor vehicle accidents.

Retropharyngeal haematomas point to underlying fractures or dislocations of the cervical spine. In adults, the soft tissues anterior to the arch of C1 measure approximately 10 mm; anterior to C4, 3–7 mm and anterior to C6, 16–20 mm. Measurements of soft tissue in excess of these amounts should suggest the possibility of underlying fracture or dislocation. Measurements anterior to the mid-cervical spine on films obtained in the emergency department are quite variable, and in fact measurements up to 7 mm are common. If the measurement is much greater than 7 mm, a fracture is likely and the neck should be immobilized until a fracture is identified or the situation clarified. Under these circumstances, the injury is often ultimately found at either extreme—the craniovertebral or cervicothoracic junction.

The atlas—C1

Fractures of the first cervical vertebra or atlas are relatively uncommon. The most common is an isolated fracture of the posterior or neural arch of the atlas (Fig. 46.106). This results from compression of the arch between the occiput and the spinous process of C2 during hyperextension. These fractures are commonly non-displaced and bilateral. Care must be taken to differentiate these fractures from gaps in the neural arch that occur as normal variations. This injury is neurologically benign and mechanically stable, and should not be misinterpreted as a Jefferson fracture.

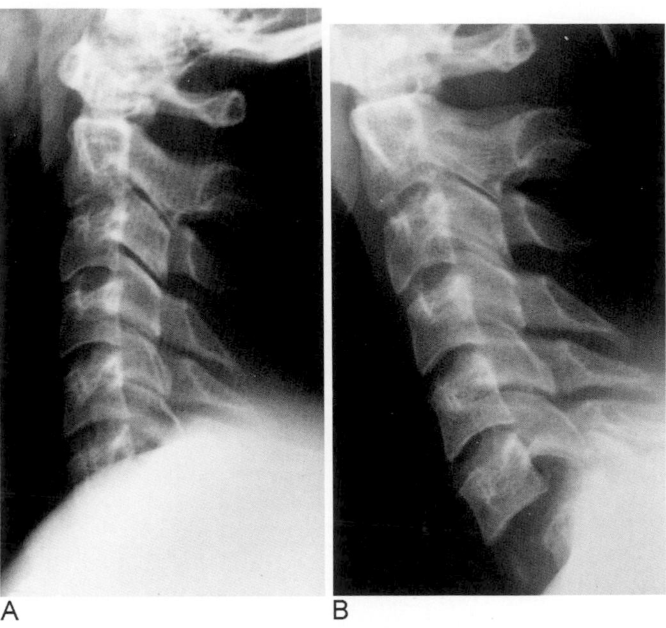

Figure 46.105 We must demonstrate all seven cervical vertebrae. (A) Initial cross-table lateral radiographic examination of the spine reveals only six cervical vertebrae. (B) A repeat examination was obtained while pulling down on the shoulder which demonstrates a fracture-dislocation at C6–7 not apparent on the initial radiograph.

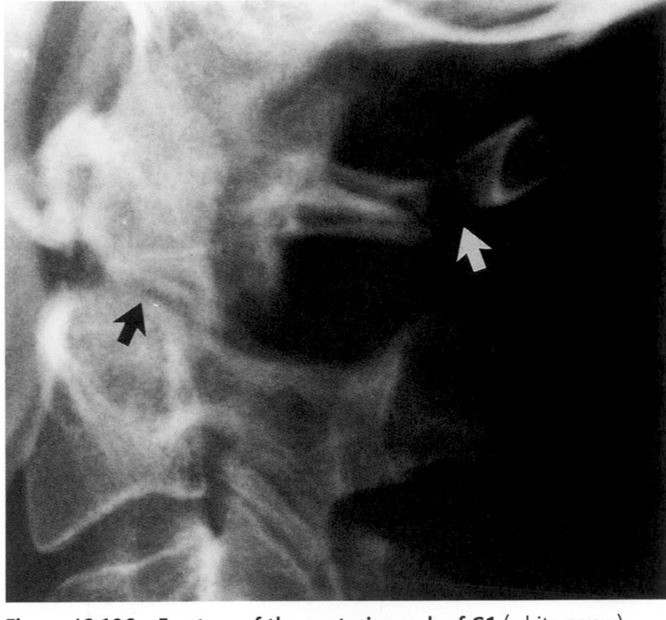

Figure 46.106 Fracture of the posterior arch of C1 (white arrow) combined with fracture at the base of the dens. Note the posterior dislocation (black arrow). This is a Type 3 fracture as it includes the superior articular facet of C2.

Jefferson fracture is an uncommon injury characterized by disruption of the anterior and posterior arches of the atlas (Fig. 46.107). Jefferson described bilateral anterior and posterior atlantal arch fractures. CT has demonstrated that only a single disruption of each arch can result in a Jefferson fracture.

The Jefferson fracture results from a force delivered to the top of the skull. The force is transmitted to the occipital condyles and thence to the superior articulating surfaces of the lateral masses of the atlas. The latter, which are oblique and superiorly concave to articulate with the occipital condyles, may be driven downward and laterally, with the force dissipated through disruptions of the anterior and posterior arch fractures.

In lateral projection, the Jefferson fracture may be *impossible to distinguish from the isolated fracture of the posterior arch of the atlas* caused by hyperextension (Figs 46.106, 46.107A). However, in many cases no fracture is evident on the lateral projection and the diagnosis depends on findings in the AP projection. Characteristically, a Jefferson fracture is identified by a bilateral offset of the lateral masses of C1 relative to C2 on the frontal projection (Fig. 46.107B). Tilting or rotation of the head may cause a unilateral offset, but this should be associated with a corresponding inset of the lateral masses on the contralateral side. Whenever there is a bilateral offset, a Jefferson fracture is suggested. Often the fractures of the AP arch cannot be identified on the plain radiographs. CT will visualize the fracture sites (Fig. 46.107C,D).

The axis—C2

Fractures of the axis are quite common and at times are radiographically obscure. Therefore C2 should be scrutinized for evidence of injury in *every* case of suspected neck injury.

Hangman's fracture (traumatic spondylolysis of the axis) represents fractures of the neural arch of C2 that are produced by a hyperextension force such as that commonly experienced when the head or face hits the windshield or steering wheel in a motor vehicle accident. This may result in bilateral fractures of the neural arch anterior to the inferior facets. (This is the same fracture as caused by judicial hanging and it is therefore often referred to as a *hangman's fracture*.)

The fracture lines are usually oblique (Fig. 46.108) and tend to be relatively symmetrical and often associated with dislocation of C2 on C3 (Figs 46.109, 46.110). There may be an avulsion fracture of the anteroinferior margin of C2 (Fig. 46.110). Neurological consequences of the hangman's fracture are often less severe than might be anticipated, for two reasons. First, the normal cervical cord occupies only approximately one-third to one-half of the AP diameter of the normal spinal canal at this level. Second, the bilateral isthmus fracture produces a decompression of the canal. These combine to spare the upper cervical cord.

Fractures of the odontoid are also quite common. They are usually transversely oriented and situated at the base of the odontoid (Figs 46.106, 46.111). There may be anterior or posterior displacement, depending upon the nature of the injuring force. Dens fractures are usually radiographically subtle. The most reliable, though non-specific, marker of a dens fracture is soft tissue swelling anterior to the atlanto-axial articulation.

Dens fractures have been classified into Types 1, 2 and 3. Type 1 is an avulsion fracture of the superolateral portion of the tip of the dens by the intact alar ligament. Type 2 is a transverse fracture at the base of the dens (Fig. 46.111). Type 3 is a fracture, not of the dens, but of the superior portion of the axis body with extension through one or both of its superior articular

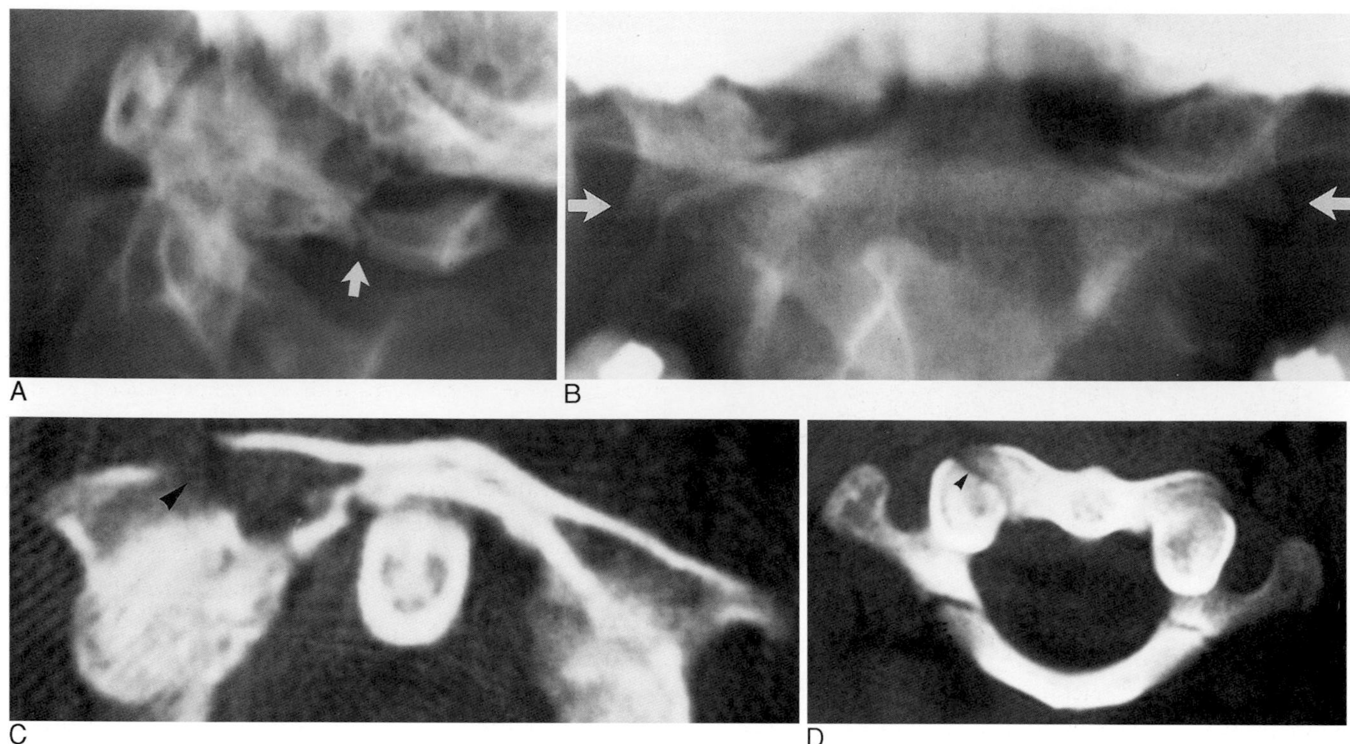

Figure 46.107 Jefferson fracture of C1. (A) Lateral radiograph demonstrates fracture of the posterior arch of atlas indistinguishable from the isolated fracture seen in Figure 46.106. (B) The open-mouth view demonstrates bilateral displacement of the lateral masses relative to the lateral border of C1 and relative to the lateral margin of the vertebral body of C2 (arrows). Note also the widening of the space between the dens and medial border of the lateral masses of C1. These findings are characteristic of a Jefferson fracture. (C,D) CT demonstrates a single fracture in the right portion of the anterior arch (arrowhead) and bilateral fractures of the posterior arch.

facets (Fig. 46.112). Types 1 and 2 are also known as 'high' and Type 3 as 'low' dens fractures. The diagnosis is often difficult because the fractures are minimally displaced and therefore obscure. CT with image reconstruction is most helpful.

In the frontal view, the Mach effect caused by the inferior cortical margin of the posterior arch of the atlas crossing the base of the dens may simulate a dens fracture. Simply repeating the open-mouth projection with slightly different angulation will establish the aetiology of this transverse lucency. Type 3, or low fractures, may not be evident on the frontal projection except by noting that the dens is tilted 7 degrees or more off the vertical axis of the body of C2. Such a fracture is identified on the lateral view by noting disruption of the 'ring' of C2 (Fig. 46.112B). Plain film tomography may be superior to CT in the

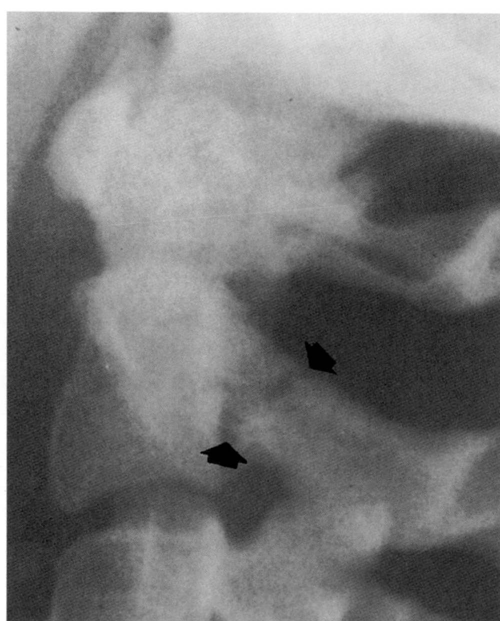

Figure 46.108 Undisplaced hangman's fracture. The arrow indicates the fracture of the pars interarticularis.

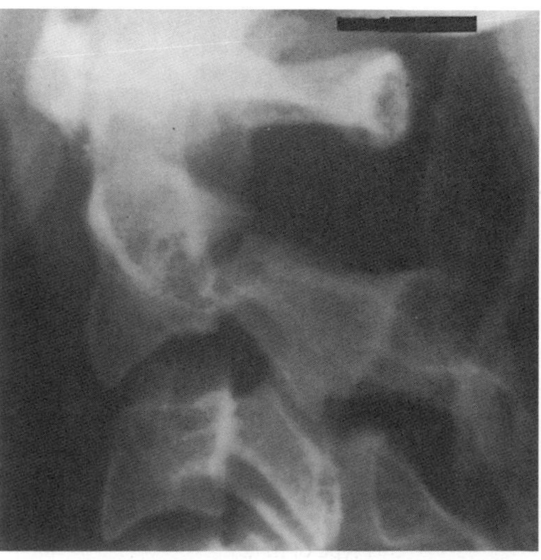

Figure 46.109 This is a hangman's fracture with subluxation of C2 upon C3 and widely displaced fracture in the neural arch.

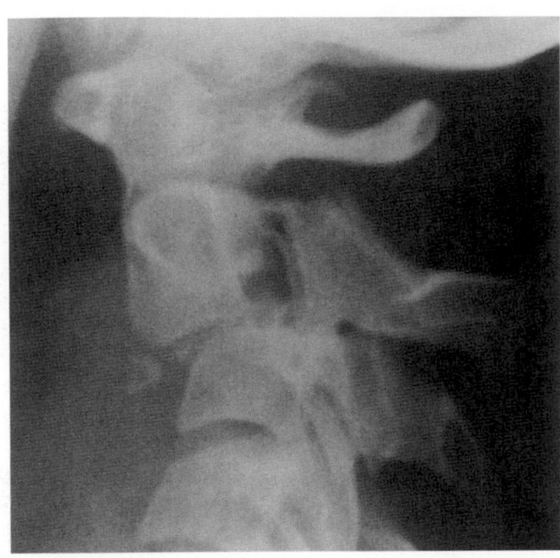

Figure 46.110 Hangman's fracture with wide separation of the fracture fragments and locking of the C2 facets anterior to C3. There is also a small fragment arising from the anterior margin of the vertebral body of C2.

detection of subtle dens fractures (Fig. 46.112C) because the fracture line may lie precisely in the plane of a CT image and be obscured by volume averaging and therefore not recorded.

Extension teardrop fracture is a fracture of the anteroinferior corner of the body of C2 avulsed by the intact anterior longitudinal ligament (Fig. 46.113). The vertical height of the extension teardrop fragment equals or exceeds its horizontal width. It is not associated with neurological deficit. This fracture may occur in isolation or be associated with a hangman's fracture (see Fig. 46.110). Before accepting it as an isolated injury, the possibility of a hangman's fracture should be excluded. The identical fractures avulsed by fibres of the anterior longitudinal ligament may occasionally involve lower cervical vertebral bodies.

The lower cervical spine—C3–C7

Injuries of the lower cervical spine consist of various fractures of the vertebral body with or without associated dislocation or subluxation, with or without significant fractures of the vertebral body and fractures limited to the posterior elements without associated dislocation. The most common error is failure to recognize that all seven cervical vertebrae are not included on the lateral radiograph (Fig. 46.114). This leads to the oversight of fractures or dislocations of the lower cervical vertebrae or cervicothoracic junction. *Make certain all seven cervical vertebrae are visualized!*

A simple wedge compression fracture results from compression of a vertebral body between adjacent bodies during flexion; the vertical height of the affected vertebral body is decreased anteriorly ('wedged') (see Fig. 46.102). The posterior height of the vertebral body is maintained. The posterior elements are commonly intact.

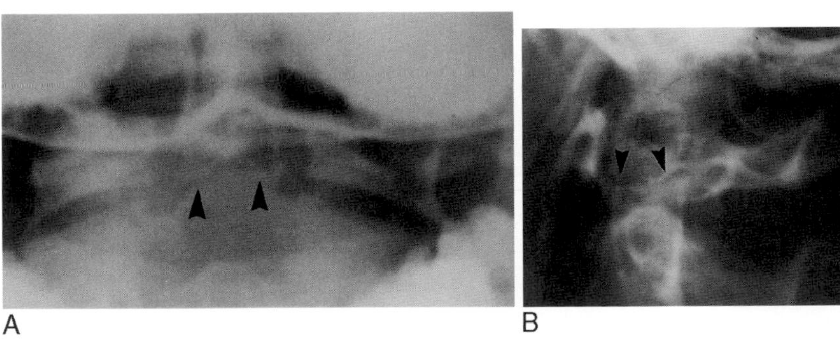

Figure 46.111 High (Type II) dens fracture in frontal (A) and lateral (B) projections. The fracture lines (arrowheads) are confined entirely to the base of the dens.

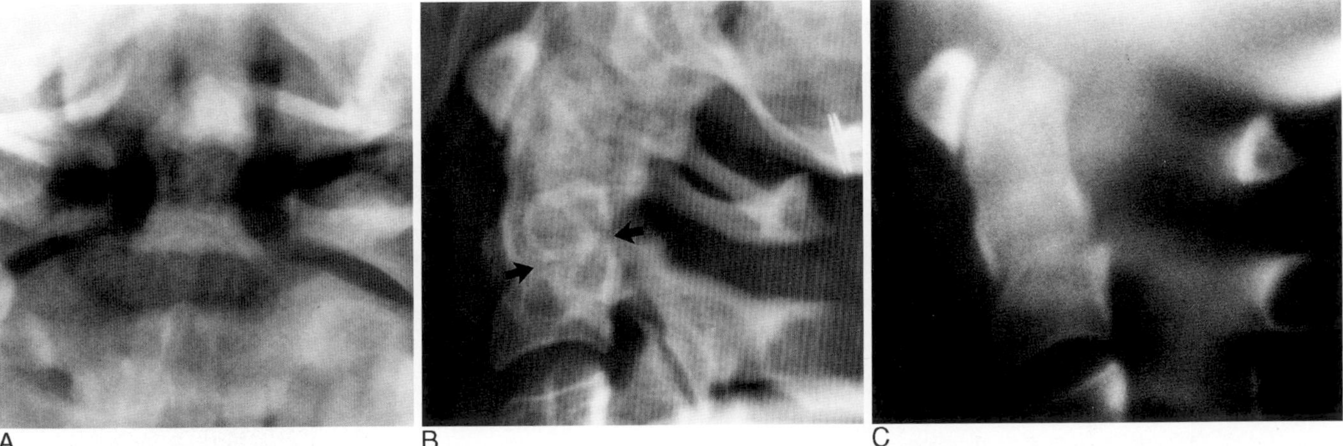

Figure 46.112 Low (Type III) dens fracture. (A) AP open-mouth view demonstrates lateral tilting of the dens. No fracture line is apparent. This is frequently the case in this type of fracture. (B) Lateral view demonstrates disruption of the ring of C2 (arrows). There is slight anterior tilting of the long axis of the dens. The dens is usually either in neutral or posterior angulation relative to the body of C2 in lateral projection. (C) A lateral tomogram clearly demonstrates the fracture line and the tilting of the dens.

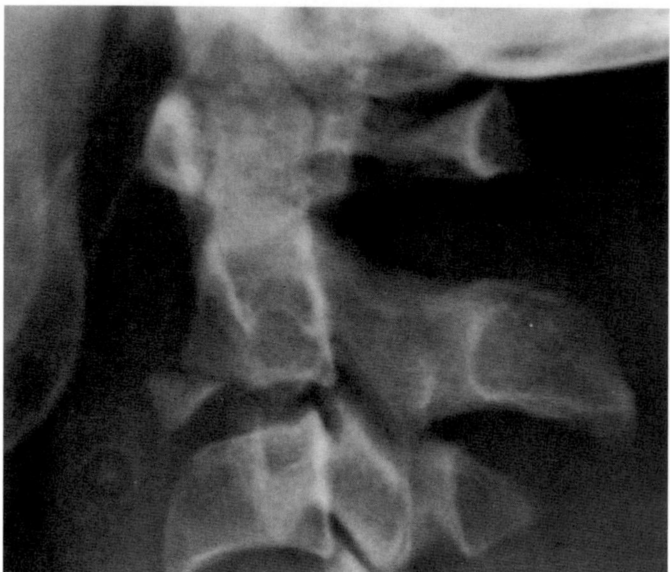

Figure 46.113 Extension teardrop fracture of C2. Note the triangular fragment arising from the anterior inferior margin of the vertebral body and the marked swelling in the retropharyngeal tissue representing a haematoma. The circular lucency within the soft tissues projected within the retropharyngeal soft tissues represents a snap on the cervical collar. There is slight posterior subluxation of C2 upon C3 in keeping with the hyperextension mechanism and disruption of the intervertebral disc.

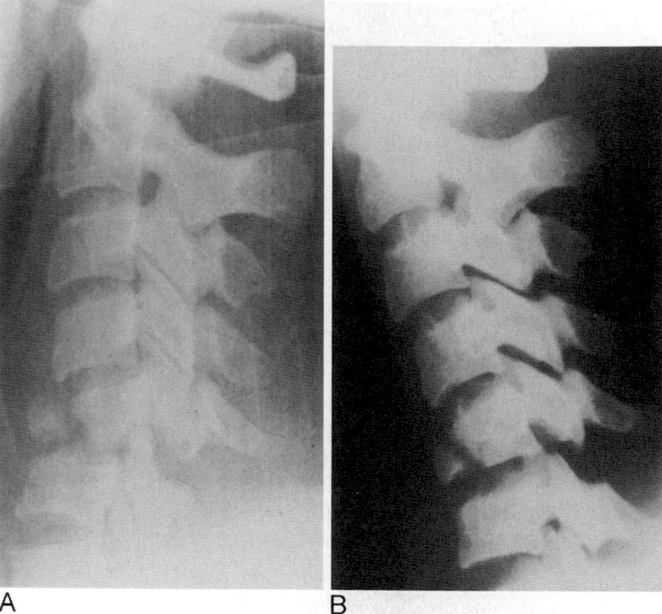

Figure 46.115 Flexion teardrop fracture. (A) In the lateral radiograph of the cervical spine obtained immediately after the injury, the cervical spine is in the flexed attitude. A single large fragment consisting of the anteroinferior corner of the body of C5 is present. The fifth vertebral body is posteriorly displaced and, in addition, widening of the interfacetal and interspinous spaces between C5 and C6 indicates complete disruption of the posterior ligament complex and bilateral interfacetal dislocation. (B) In the lateral examination carried out 2 weeks after the injury, the characteristic teardrop-shaped fragment is seen. In addition, the subjacent intervertebral disc space is abnormally widened, as are the interfacetal and interspinous spaces, indicating complete soft tissue disruption at the involved level.

The teardrop fracture is a fracture-dislocation due to flexion and axial compression. These are usually associated with spinal cord injury. A teardrop fracture is characterized by a distinct triangular fragment of the anteroinferior aspect of the vertebral body involved and is said to resemble a teardrop (Fig. 46.115). The anterior height of the vertebral body is reduced. Diffuse prevertebral soft tissue swelling is common. The posterior displacement of the fractured vertebra and diastasis of the interfacetal joints indicate disruption of the longitudinal ligaments, intervertebral disc and posterior ligament complex. These fractures are caused by motor vehicle accidents and diving into shallow water.

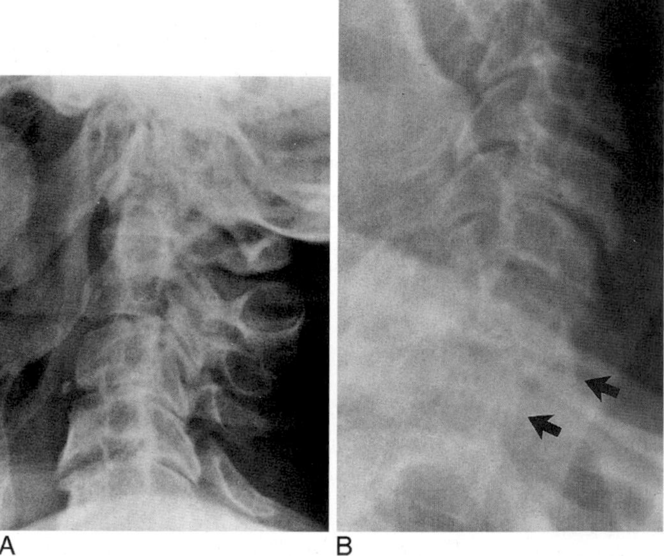

Figure 46.114 Value of swimmer's projection in demonstration of the cervicothoracic junction. Initial lateral radiograph includes only the first five cervical vertebrae. There is a small fracture from the anterior inferior margin of C3. (B) A swimmer's projection clearly demonstrates dislocation at C7–T1 (arrows).

Bilateral locked facets or bilateral interfacetal dislocation (BID) may occur at any level of the lower cervical spine and is usually associated with some degree of neurological deficit. Both facet joints at the level of injury are dislocated and all the interosseous ligaments, including the intervertebral disc, are disrupted, thereby permitting marked forward displacement of the involved vertebrae. The characteristic radiographic features are anterior displacement of the involved vertebrae for a distance of at least one-half the sagittal diameter of a vertebral body and complete dislocation of the articular masses of the involved vertebrae (Fig. 46.116). The articular masses of the vertebra above lie completely anterior to the articular masses of the vertebra below, thus 'locking' the facets. This is often accompanied by bilateral laminar fractures of the vertebra above, the laminae and spinous process remaining aligned with the opposing elements of the vertebra below.

Unilateral locked facets, or unilateral interfacetal dislocation (UID), is caused by simultaneous flexion and rotation. With flexion and rotation, the involved vertebra moves anteriorly and rotates on its vertical axis, causing dislocation of the

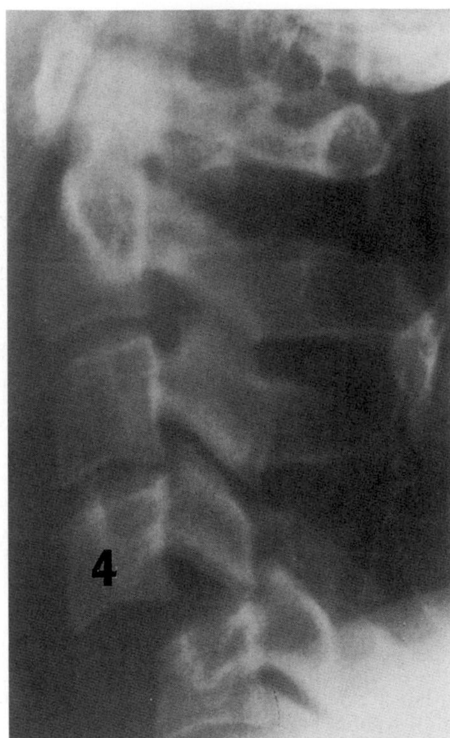

Figure 46.116 Bilateral locked facets at C4–5 (interfacetal dislocation). Note that the lateral mass of the inferior facet of C4 is locked anteriorly to the superior facet of C5.

interfacetal joint on the side opposite the direction of rotation. The dislocated facet comes to rest anterior to the subjacent facet and is thus 'locked'.

In the frontal radiograph (Fig. 46.117A) the spinous processes from the level of the dislocation cephalad are rotated off the midline in the direction opposite that of rotation and therefore point to the side of dislocation. In the lateral projection (Fig. 46.117B), the dislocated vertebra is anteriorly displaced 25% of the sagittal diameter of a cervical vertebral body. The articular masses and interfacetal joints are no longer superimposed from the level of the dislocation upward. The spine above the level of dislocation is obliquely oriented, with the spine below in direct lateral orientation. The oblique orientation gives rise to a '*bow tie*' or '*butterfly*' appearance of the rotated articular masses (Fig. 46.118). The distance between the posterior surface of the articular mass and the spinolaminar junction line of the vertebrae below the dislocation is greater than that of the vertebrae above with an abrupt change in this distance at the level of the dislocation.

Associated fracture of either the dislocated or contiguous articular mass is common. The anterior displacement of the cephalad vertebra may decrease as a result of the fracture. CT best demonstrates the abnormalities (Figs 46.119, 46.120).

Hyperflexion sprain (Fig. 46.121) is a pure soft tissue and ligamentous injury caused by acute flexion without axial compression. The principal radiographic sign is localized kyphotic angulation. This must be differentiated from a reversal of cervical lordosis due to muscle spasm. Signs of hyperflexion strain on the lateral view include widening of the interspinous or interlaminar space ('fanning'), subluxation of the interfacetal joints and posterior widening and anterior narrowing of the intervertebral disc with or without 1–3 mm of anterior displacement of the vertebra. The findings may be accentuated by carrying out a lateral view in flexion and diminished

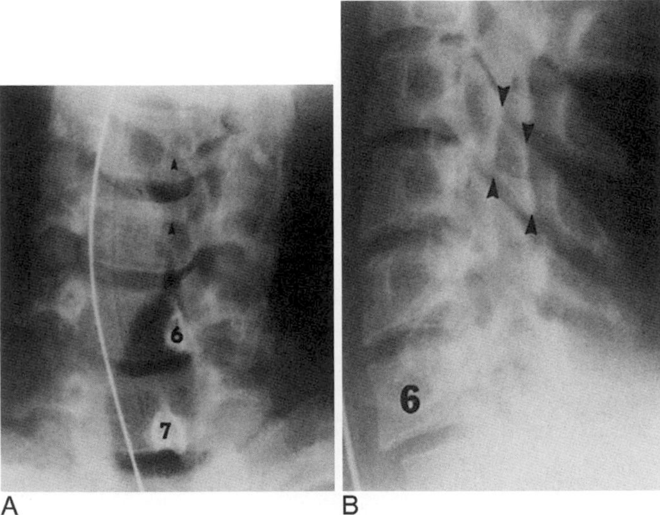

Figure 46.117 Unilateral locked facets. In the frontal projection (A), the spinous processes from C6 and above (arrowheads) are rotated off the midline. In the lateral projection (B), the sixth cervical vertebra is displaced slightly anteriorly on C7 by a distance less than half the anteroposterior diameter of a cervical vertebral body. Additionally, from the level of C6 upwards, the posterior cortical margins of the articular masses (arrowheads) are not superimposed, reflecting the rotational components of this injury.

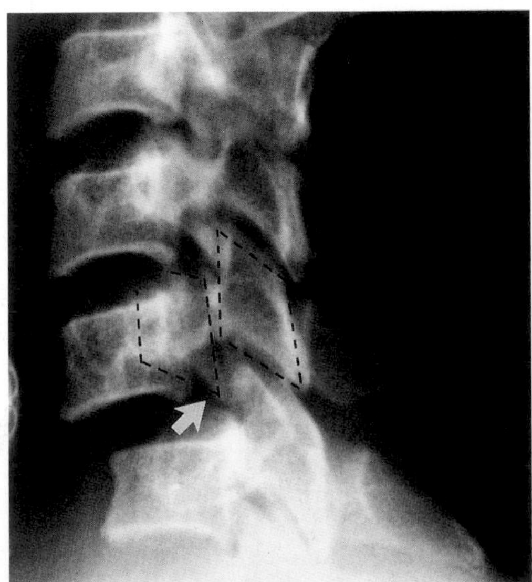

Figure 46.118 Unilateral locked facets at C5–6. In this case the 'bow tie' or 'butterfly' configuration of the facet is characteristic of this lesion and is clearly depicted by the dashed lines. Note that at the level of dislocation, the vertebrae above are in the oblique projection and those below are in the lateral projection. The distance between the posterior surface of the facets and the spinolaminar line above the level of dislocation is obliterated, whereas the space is preserved below the level of dislocation. This is a very sensitive indicator that the vertebrae above are rotated and those below are in the lateral projection. One can see that the inferior facet of one side (arrow) lies anterior to the vertebra below.

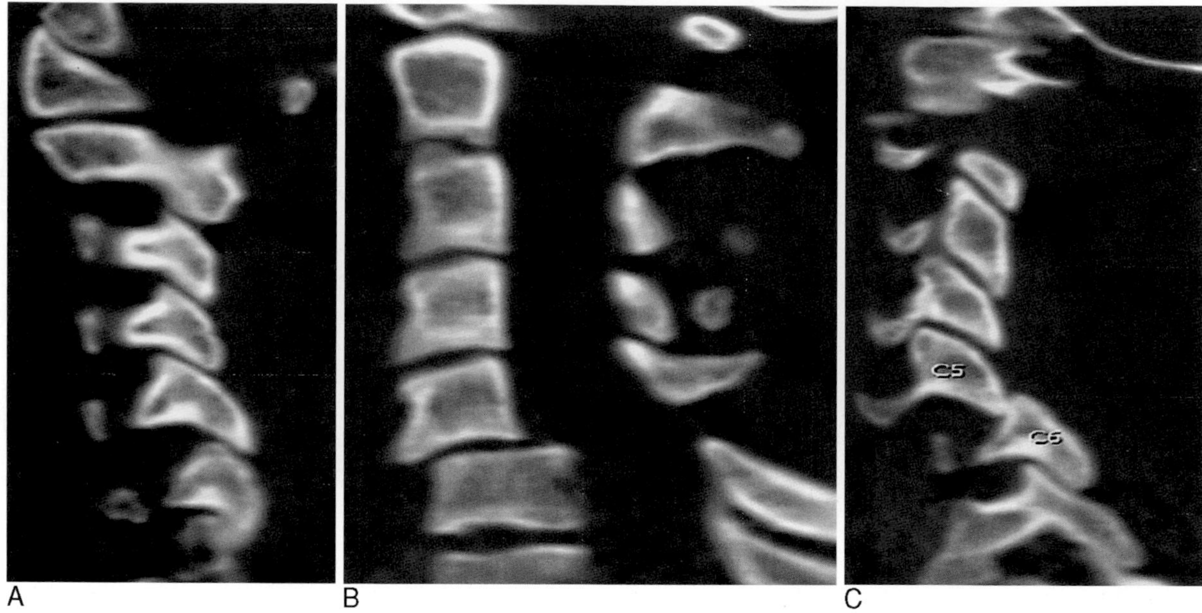

Figure 46.119 Unilateral locked facets of C6 on the left. CT images. The facet joints at C5/C6 are subluxed on the right side (A). The midline images (B) show that C5 is subluxed anteriorly upon C6 approximately 25% of the width of vertebral body. The C5 facet is locked anterior to C6 facet on the left side (C). (Case courtesy of Dr. Raymond F. Carmody, Tucson, Arizona).

by doing a similar view in extension. When performing lateral flexion and extension views, the radiologist must personally control the positioning of the patient's head and preclude forced flexion and extension, which might precipitate or aggravate cervical cord or root injury.

Hyperflexion sprain is associated with 30–50% incidence of delayed instability due to failure of ligamentous healing. A posterior fusion is often required to prevent subsequent anterior subluxation or dislocation.

Hyperextension injury in spondylosis Older patients with spondylosis of the cervical spine may sustain a spinal cord injury as a result of a simple fall (Fig. 46.122). Hyperextension of the head upon the neck causes the cord to be pinched

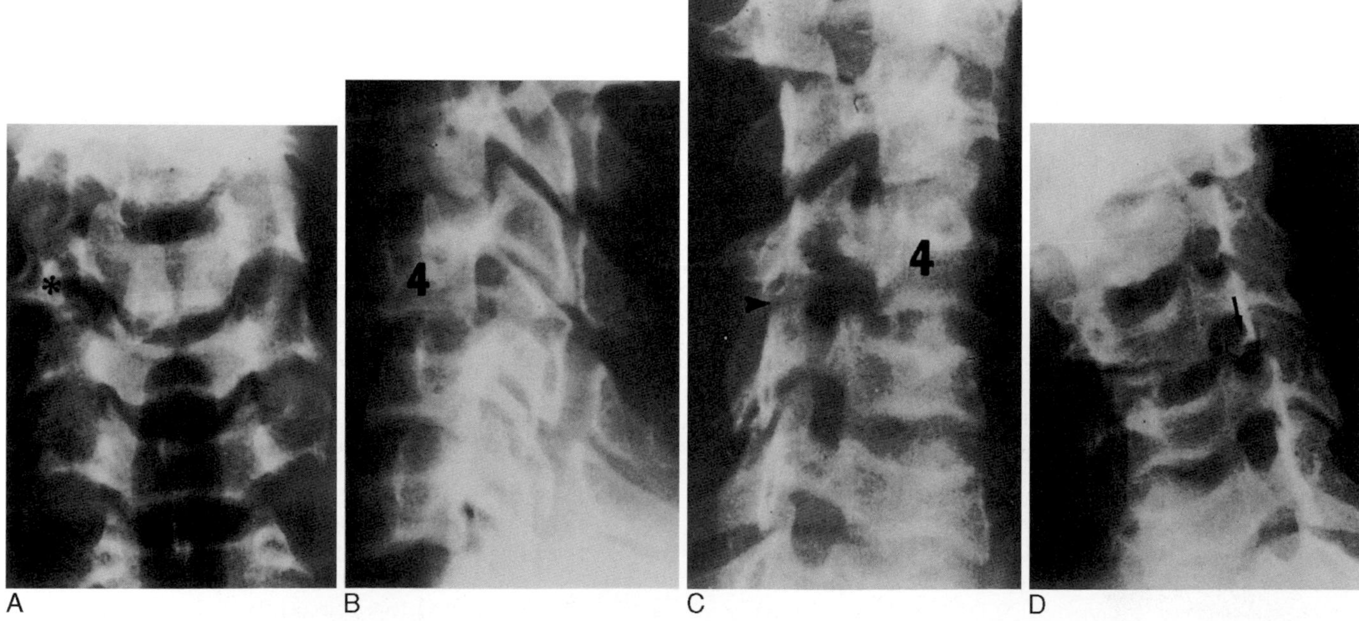

Figure 46.120 Hyperextension fracture-dislocation of C4. The frontal projection (A) shows a comminuted fracture of the articular mass of C4 on the right (*). The lateral projection (B) shows that the body of C4 is anteriorly displaced. The anatomy of the posterior elements at the C4–5 level is completely disorganized. In the right anterior oblique projection (C) the articular mass of C4 is shown to be severely comminuted. The inferior articulating facet of C4 has been completely destroyed ('flattened facet' sign). In addition, there is a transverse fracture through the superior articulating facet of C5 (arrowhead). In the left anterior oblique projection (D) there is an interfacetal dislocation of C4 with respect to C5 (stemmed arrow).

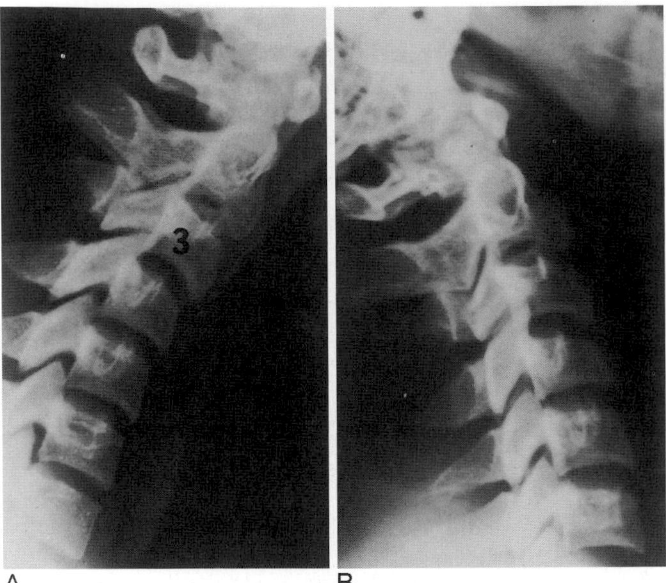

Figure 46.121 Anterior subluxation of C3 on C4. In the flexed position (A), C3 is anteriorly displaced with respect to C4 by a distance of 2–3 mm. In addition C3 has pivoted upon the anteroinferior corner of its vertebral body, and this, coupled with the anterior translation, has caused a hyperkyphotic angulation at the C2–3 level. The interfacetal joint space is widened posteriorly and the interspinous space is widened ('fanning'). In the same patient, in the hyperextended position (B) the spine appears normal.

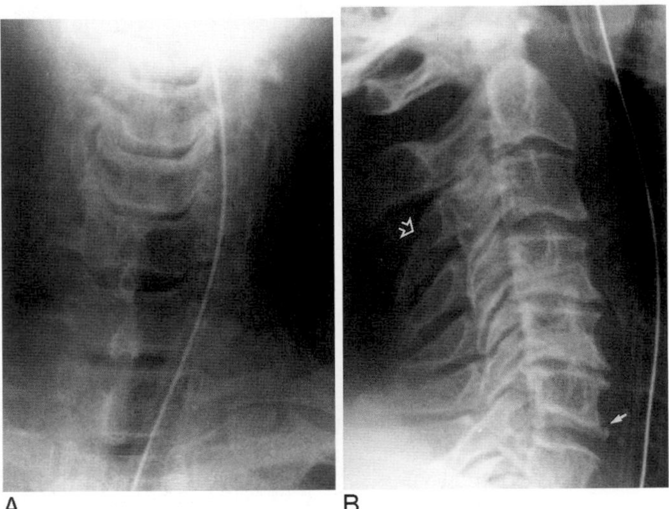

Figure 46.122 Spondylosis with quadriplegia following minor trauma (A). The AP and lateral projections demonstrate changes of degenerative arthritis. The lateral projection (B) shows retropharyngeal soft tissue swelling and a small fracture from the anterior inferior margin of C6 (arrow) and a fracture of the spinous process of C3 (open arrow). These two fractures attest to the hyperextension mechanism of injury.

between posterior vertebral osteophytes and the thickened ligamentum flavum, resulting in a spinal cord injury. This is often associated with a retropharyngeal haematoma secondary to a disruption of the anterior longitudinal ligament. Occasionally, a small fracture of the anteroinferior surface of the vertebra results from an avulsion fracture at the site of the tear in the anterior longitudinal ligament. Despite the profound neurological deficit, there is often no evidence of fracture or dislocation. This injury results in the central cervical cord syndrome, characterized by flaccid paralysis from the level of dislocation and sensory changes that are greater in the upper extremity than in the lower. The extent and nature (oedema or haemorrhage) of the cord injury determine whether the neurological changes are minimal and transitory or severe and permanent.

Isolated fractures of the posterior elements are rare and difficult to visualize on plain radiographs. The only exception is the 'clay shoveller's fracture' (Fig. 46.123A), an avulsion of the spinous process of C6, C7 or T1 caused either by rotation of the upper trunk when the cervical spine is relatively fixed or, less commonly, as the result of a direct blow. CT may demonstrate other fractures of the posterior elements (Fig. 46.123B). Thus CT should be obtained on patients with initial negative plain radiographs who experience continued pain following trauma.

Whiplash injury The so-called 'whiplash injury of the cervical spine' is of considerable importance because of its legal implications. The injury is caused by a sudden deceleration of the body, as occurs when an automobile is stopped suddenly by collision or when a stationary automobile is struck from behind by a moving vehicle. The head is thus snapped back and forth—'whiplashed'. There is considerable difference

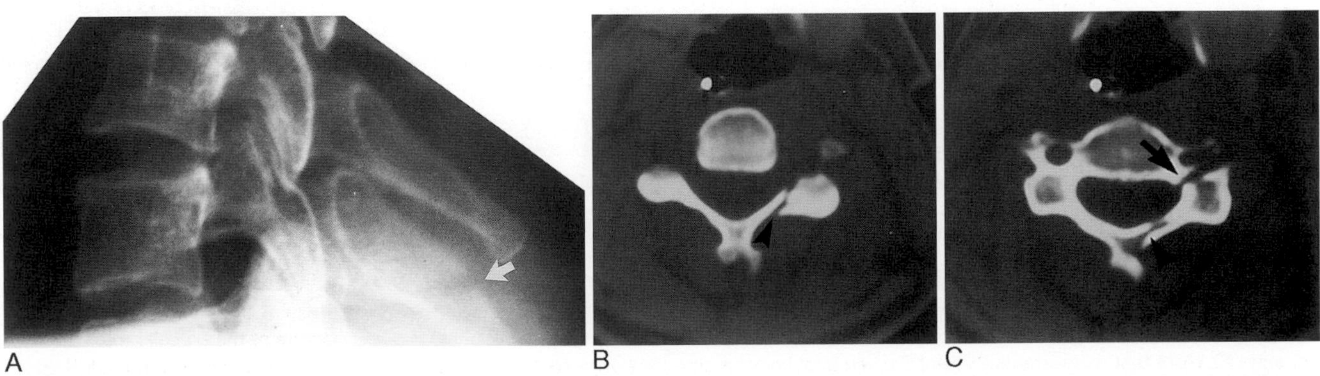

Figure 46.123 Fractures of the posterior elements. (A) Clay shoveller's fracture (arrow) of the spinous process of C6–7. (B,C) **Left pediculolaminar fracture.** The plain radiographs were unremarkable. The arrow indicates the fracture of the pedicle and transverse process. The laminar fracture is identified by arrowheads.

of opinion about the importance of the whiplash injury as a cause of clinical complaints and disability.

Minor degrees of reversal of the cervical curve, as well as minimal offset of one cervical vertebra on another, may be produced by voluntary muscle contraction and therefore presumably can be produced by muscle spasm secondary to pain, without any actual ligamentous injury of the cervical spine. This adds to the difficulty in assessing the significance of minor variations in the cervical spine. Care should be taken not to overemphasize these variations.

Thoracic spine

The routine radiographic examination of the thoracic spine includes AP and lateral projections. In the lateral projection, the upper three or four thoracic vertebrae are not usually visible because of the superimposed shoulders. To demonstrate this area, the 'swimmer's' (Fletcher) projection is obtained (see Fig. 46.114). This is a steeply oblique view obtained by turning the shoulders.

Compression, impaction and shearing forces cause the majority of thoracic spine fractures. Compressive forces dissipated through the longitudinal axis of the thoracic spine result in simple wedge (compression) fracture. Impaction forces, such as occur on landing on the back from a fall, usually cause fractures of the posterior elements and injuries of the costovertebral joints as well as vertebral body fractures. Shearing forces cause fracture-dislocations.

Simple wedge (compression) fractures

Most fractures of the thoracic and lumbar vertebrae tend to be anterior compressions, which are usually readily observed in the lateral projections (Fig. 46.124) and may be evident on the frontal projection because of loss of height or obliteration of the superior end-plate of the involved vertebra. The involved vertebral body is characteristically wedged anteriorly. Disruption of the superior end-plate is frequently, but not always, visible. The anterior cortical margin of the involved vertebra may be disrupted, angulated, or impacted (Fig. 46.124). The posterior cortex remains intact. In the AP radiograph, these changes are usually subtle. Localized lateral bulging of the mediastinal stripe secondary to a paraspinous haematoma is a reliable marker of an acute fracture (Fig. 46.125). The usually smooth concave lateral cortex of the vertebral body may be disrupted, angulated, convex (Fig. 46.125) or impacted, and it may even be possible to detect a decrease in height of the involved vertebral body.

Lesions that might be confused with acute compression fractures of the thoracic spine include non-united vertebral ring epiphyses (see Fig. 46.102), Schmorl's nodes, limbus vertebrae and old healed compression fractures. Ring epiphyses appear from 6–8 years in girls and 7–9 years in boys, become partially fused at age 14–15 and are usually completely fused by age 20 in both sexes. Schmorl's nodes are usually multiple, typically located in the end-plates and characterized by irregular sclerotic margins surrounding an irregular lucent defect (Fig. 46.126A). A limbus vertebra is a distant separate ossicle, well marginated by cortical bone (Fig. 46.126B), found on the anterior superior margin of the vertebral body. It represents a developmental abnormality of the ring apophysis. The age or acuity of compression fractures in older patients with osteoporosis frequently cannot be established radiographically and must be determined on the basis of clinical findings.

Fracture-dislocation

Fracture-dislocation commonly occurs in the lower thoracic and upper lumbar spine, the thoracolumbar junction. It is the

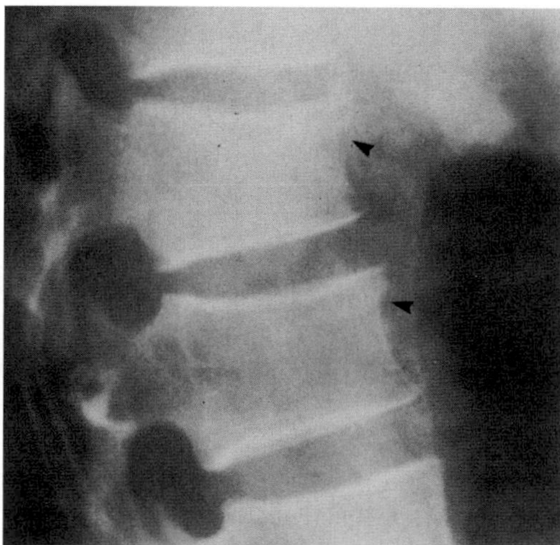

Figure 46.124 Simple wedge (compression) fracture of the bodies of T11 and T12. Note that the posterior walls of the vertebral bodies are maintained and the posterior elements are intact without evidence of dislocation. Fractures of contiguous vertebrae are common in the thoracic spine.

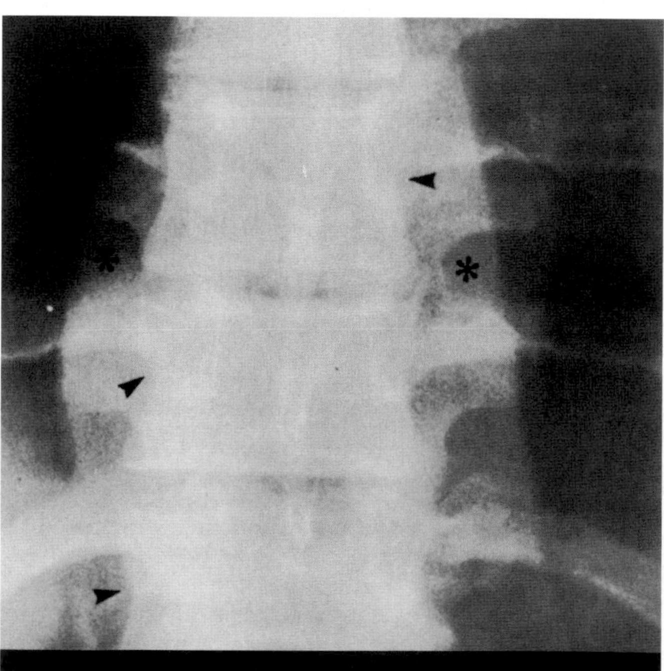

Figure 46.125 Compression fractures of T9, T10 and T11. Bilateral paraspinous haematomas are indicated by asterisks. Disruption, angulation and impaction of the lateral cortical margins of the involved vertebral bodies are indicated by arrowheads.

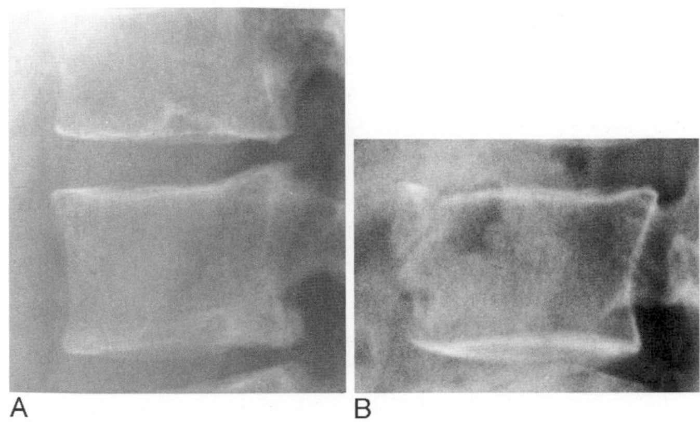

Figure 46.126 Schmorl's nodes and limbus vertebra. Note the sharply defined dome-like-densities arising from the end-plate in these two adjacent vertebrae (A). (B) **Limbus vertebra.** There is a well-marginated ossicle at the anterior superior margin of the vertebral body. Note that the underlying vertebral body margin is also well defined. This represents a developmental defect, presumably of the ring apophysis.

result of combined shearing rotation and flexion forces which disrupt the lamina and facet joints and displace the vertebra above the level anteriorly, while creating an anteriorly wedged compression fracture of the vertebra below (Fig. 46.127). The anteriorly displaced vertebral body above is usually accompanied by a triangular bony fragment avulsed from the anterior superior surface of the vertebral body below. CT is required to fully visualize such injuries.

Lumbar spine

The most common fracture is a *simple wedge (compression) fracture* without distraction of the posterior elements (Fig. 46.128). The absence of a fracture of the posterior wall of the vertebral body distinguishes this type of fracture from the less common but more severe burst fracture described below. The fracture is usually limited to the superior end-plate and subjacent portion of the vertebral body, sparing the inferior end-plate. Occasionally the opposite occurs. In the elderly, one should look closely for evidence of bone destruction in the pedicles and cortical margins of the vertebral bodies to identify a pathological fracture due to metastatic disease.

Burst fractures are common at the thoracolumbar junction. These are due to axial compression forces. In this injury, a fragment from the superoposterior margin of the vertebral body is displaced into the spinal canal (Fig. 46.129) and may cause a neurological injury of the spinal cord, conus medullaris, or nerve roots. Every compression fracture should be closely examined for evidence of a retropulsed fragment, to distinguish between a simple wedged compression and a burst fracture. The posterior cortex of the vertebral body should be identified in every wedged vertebral body. If intact, it is a simple, wedged compression fracture; if it is disrupted and a fragment is displaced into the spinal canal, it is a burst fracture.

CT is an excellent means of visualizing such fragments (Fig. 46.130). The characteristic findings are: a retropulsed fragment from the posterosuperior margin of the vertebra lying between the pedicles; a sagittal fracture of the inferior half of

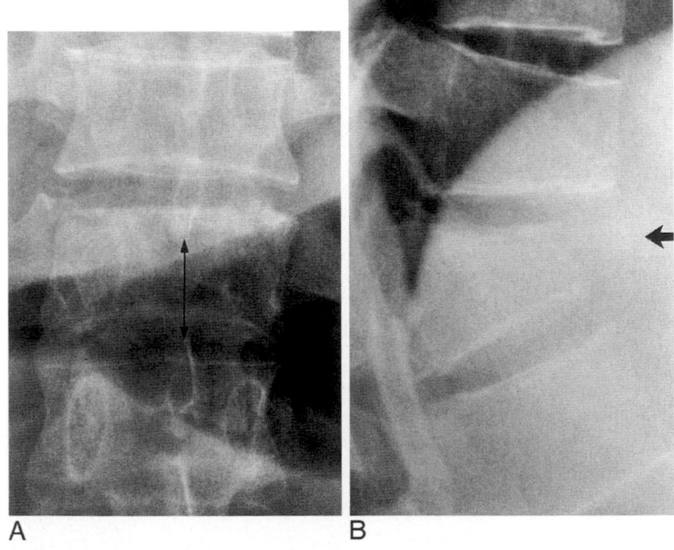

Figure 46.127 Fracture-dislocation of T11–12. The AP projection (A) shows very few findings. Closer examination reveals a wide separation of the spinous processes of T11–12 (arrows) and obliteration of the T12–L1 vertebral disc space. There is also a fracture from the anterior superior margin of the 12th vertebral body on the right. (B) A dislocation is demonstrated, with displacement of a small fragment of bone from the anterior superior margin of the vertebra below the level of dislocation (arrow). The fractures of the posterior elements are not well visualized due to overlying ribs. There is characteristic wedging of the vertebral body below the level of dislocation.

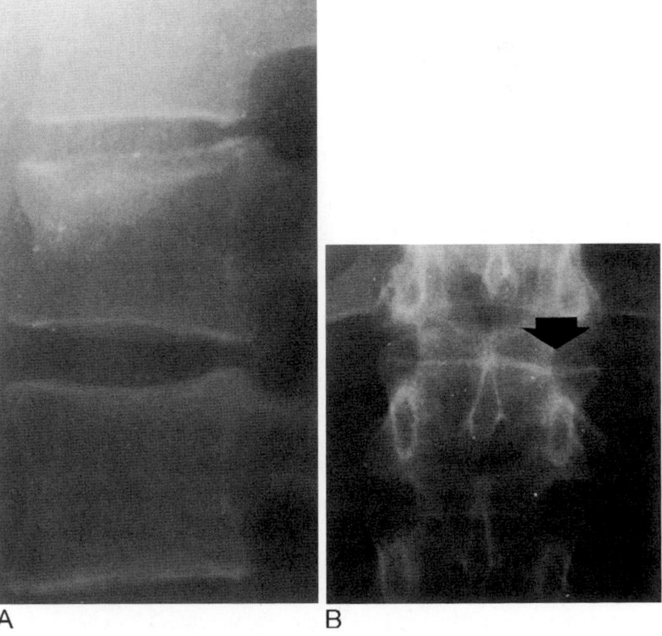

Figure 46.128 Simple wedge compression fracture of L1. In lateral projection (A), the fracture is evidenced by disruption, impaction and anterior sloping of the superior end-plate and by disruption of the superior aspect of the anterior cortex of the vertebral body. In frontal projection (B), the left half of the superior end-plate is depressed (arrow).

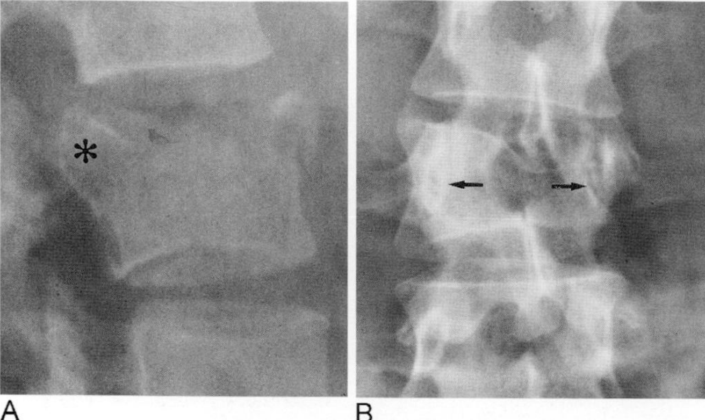

Figure 46.129 Burst fracture of L3. (A) Lateral projection demonstrates slight anterior wedging with obvious compression of the vertebra. Note the retropulsion of the fragment rising from the superior margin of the vertebra (*). This fragment is displaced into the spinal canal and may result in neurological injury. (B) AP projection demonstrates compression of the vertebra. Note the widening of the interpediculate distance (arrows), indicating presence of a sagittal fracture in the vertebra and posterior elements, allowing lateral displacement. These findings are characteristic of a burst fracture.

the vertebral body; and a fracture of the lamina, often at the junction of the lamina and spinous process.

The severity of neurological deficit depends on the degree of posterior displacement of the posterior body fragments into the neural canal.

The Chance fracture is a horizontal fracture with little or no compression of the vertebral body. This is also known as a seatbelt fracture, since it is commonly associated with the wearing of lap-type seatbelts. At times, a horizontal fracture of the posterior elements may be associated with a horizontal fracture through the vertebral body (Fig. 46.131), or alternatively there may be a disruption of the ligaments and intervertebral discs without fractures (Fig. 46.132).

The cause of these injuries is a flexion of the trunk over an object, such as a seatbelt, that serves as a fulcrum. The fulcrum of the flexion forces is displaced forward to the object over which the body is flexed, and therefore no significant compression fracture results from such injuries.

The Chance fracture is characterized in the AP projection by a transverse fracture of the spinous process and, frequently, the pedicles (Fig. 46.131), and widening of the interspinous space is common due to separation and angulation of the vertebrae at the affected interspace. In the lateral radiograph, the Chance fracture is characterized by horizontal fracture involving the spinous process and/or the laminae and the articular masses in addition to a horizontal or obliquely horizontal fracture of the vertebral body. The vertebral body is tilted with little or no anterior wedging. Lap seatbelt injuries differ from flexion injuries of the lumbar spine by virtue of their frequent association with intra-abdominal soft tissue injury and neurological injury when angulated or displaced.

Isolated fractures of the posterior elements are unusual with the exception of those involving the transverse process. Fractures of transverse processes may occur in association with severe injury anywhere in the spine, but in the lumbar area there may be an isolated injury due to local trauma, the result of either muscle pull or direct local injury. Beware that radiolucent lines simulating fracture of transverse processes may be produced by the psoas shadow, intra-abdominal gas, or un-united ossification centre.

ACKNOWLEDGEMENTS

The chapter on Skeletal Trauma in the first edition of this book was superbly written by Dr John H Harris Jr of Houston, Texas. The chapter in the second edition was written by Dr J H Harris Jr in association with his son Dr R D Harris of Hanover, New Hampshire.

Figure 46.130 Burst fracture of L3. In the lateral projection (A), anterior wedging of the involved vertebral bodies suggests a simple wedge fracture, but note that the entire vertebral body is posteriorly displaced and is comminuted. These findings are not characteristic of a simple wedge fracture. Computed tomography (B) reveals the severe comminution of the vertebral body and a fracture at the junction of the lamina and spinous process on the right. Note the posterior displacement of the posterior fragments into the neural canal.

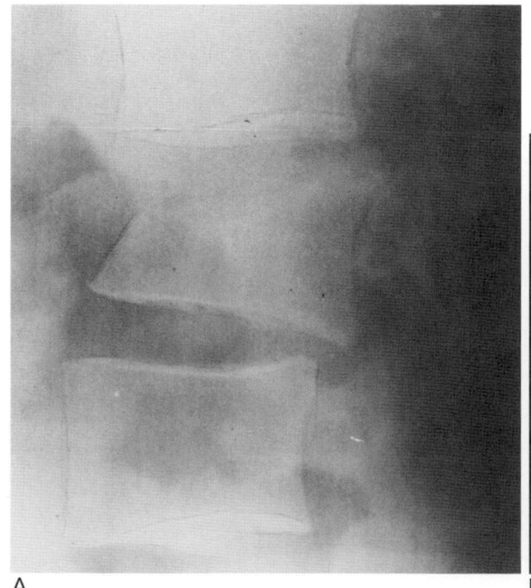

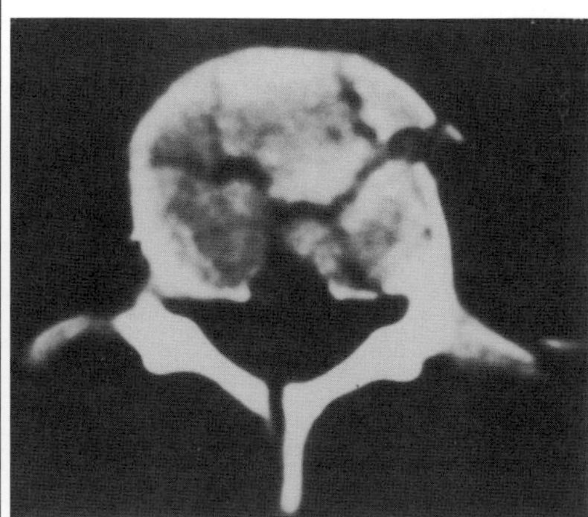

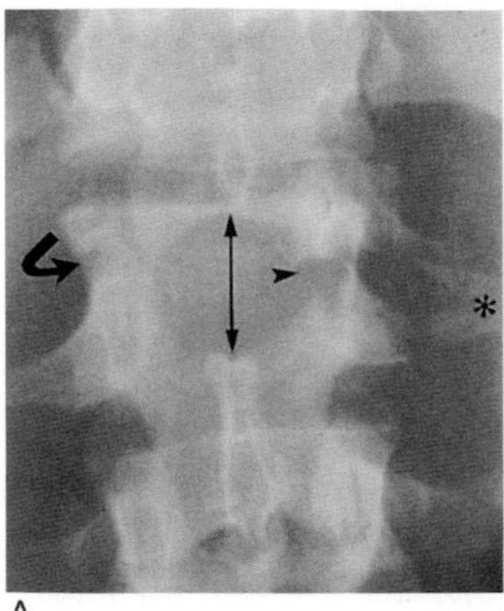
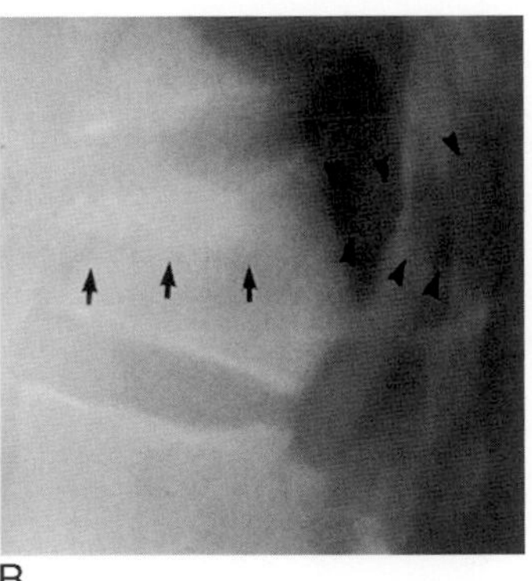

A B

Figure 46.131 Chance fracture of L1. The frontal projection (A) shows a comminuted fracture of the left transverse process (*), transverse fracture of the left pedicle (arrowhead), separation of the T12 and L1 laminae and spinous processes (double arrow) and a fracture of the right superolateral cortex of L1 (curved arrow). In the lateral projection (B) the arrowheads indicate a distracted transverse fracture of the spinous process and laminae and the arrows indicate the horizontal fracture of the body with anterior wedging.

The chapter on Skeletal Trauma for the third edition was completely rewritten by Dr Andrew H Sonin and Dr Lee F Rogers of Chicago. Drs J H Harris Jr and R D Harris most graciously offered them full use of all their many excellent illustrations from the previous two editions. The fourth edition was updated by Dr Carol A Boles and Dr Lee F Rogers of Winston-Salem, North Carolina.

REFERENCES

1. Ahovuo J A, Kiuru M J, Kinnunen J J et al 2002 MR imaging of fatigue stress injuries to bones: intra- and interobserver agreement. Magn Reson Imaging 20: 401–406
2. Falchi M, Rollandi G A 2004 CT of pelvic fractures. Eur J Radiol 50: 96–105
3. Kanberoglu K, Kantarci F, Cebi D et al 2005 Magnetic resonance imaging in osteomalacic insufficiency fractures of the pelvis. Clin Radiol 60: 105–111
4. Blake S P, Connors A M 2004 Sacral insufficiency fracture. Br J Radiol 77: 891–896
5. Zanetti M, Hodler J, Gilula L A 1998 Assessment of dorsal or ventral intercalated segmental instability configurations of the wrist: reliability of sagittal MR images. Radiology 206: 339–345
6. Oka M, Monu J U 2004 Prevalence and patterns of occult hip fractures and mimics revealed by MRI. AJR Am J Roentgenol 182: 283–288
7. Pandev R, McNally E, Ali A et al 1998 The role of MRI in the diagnosis of occult hip fractures. Injury 29: 61–63
8. Verbeeten K M, Hermann K L, Hasselqvist M et al 2005 The advantages of MRI in the detection of occult hip fractures. Eur Radiol 15: 165–169. Epub 2004 Jul 27
9. Kirsch M D, Fitzgerald S W, Friedman H, Rogers L F 1993 Transient lateral patellar dislocation: Diagnosis with MR imaging. Am J Roentgenol 161: 109–113
10. Remer E M, Fitzgerald S W, Friedman H et al 1992 Anterior cruciate ligament injury: MR imaging diagnosis and patterns of injury. RadioGraphics 12: 901–915
11. Fitzgerald S W, Remer E M, Friedman H et al 1993 MR evaluation of the anterior cruciate ligament: Value of supplementing sagittal images with coronal and axial images. Am J Roentgenol 160: 1233–1237
12. Sonin A H, Fitzgerald S W, Friedman H et al 1994 Posterior cruciate ligament injury: MR diagnosis and patterns of injury. Radiology 190: 455–458
13. Sonin A H, Fitzgerald S W, Hoff F L et al 1995 MR imaging of the posterior cruciate ligament: normal, abnormal, and associated injury patterns. Radiographics 15: 551–561
14. Sonin A H 1994 Magnetic resonance imaging of the extensor mechanism. In: Fitzgerald S W (ed) The knee. MRI Clin North Am 2: 401–411
15. Van Goethem J W, Maes M, Ozsarlak O et al 2005 Imaging in spinal trauma. Eur Radiol 15: 582–590. Epub 2005 Feb 5
16. Richards P J 2005 Cervical spine clearance: a review. Injury 36: 248–269; discussion 270
17. Tewari M K, Gifti D S, Singh P et al 2005 Diagnosis and prognostication of adult spinal cord injury without radiographic abnormality using magnetic resonance imaging: analysis of 40 patients. Surg Neurol 63: 204–209; discussion 209
18. Hall A J, Wagle V G, Raycroft J et al 1993 Magnetic resonance imaging in cervical spine trauma. J Trauma 34: 21–26
19. Daffner R H 1992 Evaluation of cervical vertebral injuries. Semin Roentgenol 27: 239–253
20. Davis J W, Phreaner D L, Hoyt D B, Mackersie R C 1993 The etiology of missed cervical spine injuries. J Trauma 34: 342–346

FURTHER READING

Fornage B D 1995 Musculoskeletal ultrasound. Churchill Livingstone, New York.

A basic introduction to musculoskeletal ultrasound

Keats T E, Anderson M W 2005 Atlas of normal roentgen variants that may simulate disease, 6th edn. Mosby, St Louis.

The most complete collection of unusual variants that often masquerade as fractures. No Accident and Emergency Department should be without it

Rockwood C A Jr, Green D P, Bucholz R W 2002 Fractures in adults, 5th edn. Lippincott Williams & Wilkins, Philadelphia.

The complete work used by orthopaedic trauma surgeons

Rogers L F 2002 Radiology of skeletal trauma, 3rd edn. Churchill Livingstone, New York.

The definitive work for the radiology of skeletal trauma

Schmidt H, Freyschmidt J (eds) 1993 Koehler and Zimmer: Borderlands of normal and early pathologic findings in skeletal radiography, 4th edn. Thieme, New York.

A classic guide to the sometimes murky territory between what may be normal and what is abnormal in the skeletal system

CHAPTER 47

Bone Tumours (1): General Characteristics and Benign Lesions

Dennis J. Stoker and Asif Saifuddin

GENERAL CHARACTERISTICS OF BONE TUMOURS

Bone 'tumours' may be benign or malignant. Benign tumours include both true neoplasms and tumour-like lesions, which will be discussed since their mode of presentation and management is similar. All malignant bone tumours are neoplastic, either primary or secondary. The pre-biopsy diagnosis of a bone tumour depends upon several features, including age of the patient, site of the lesion within the skeleton and the individual bone and finally the radiological characteristics. The last will allow an assessment of the rate of growth (indicative of likely benignity or malignancy) and underlying histological subtype (Table 47.1).

Age at presentation

The majority of bone tumours show a peak incidence confined to one or more decades and a range of common incidence beyond which their occurrence is rare. Metastases are the commonest malignant bone tumours in patients over 45 years of age. An atypical metastasis is more common in this age group than a classical primary malignant tumour, so that a lesion with spiculated periosteal new bone formation and soft tissue mass in a man of 70 years is far more likely to be a prostatic metastasis than a primary osteosarcoma.

Primary malignant bone tumours are rare before 5 years of age, while the first decade is the most common for disseminated bone lesions of leukaemia and neuroblastoma. In the second decade, osteosarcoma and Ewing's sarcoma are prevalent.

RADIOLOGICAL ASSESSMENT OF BONE TUMOURS[1]

Location

The location of the lesion within the skeleton (appendicular, axial) and within the individual bone (epiphysis, metaphysis, diaphysis; intramedullary, intracortical, surface) must be considered in detail when discussing individual tumours.

Rate of growth

When considering rate of growth, the most important feature is the nature of the margin. In benign and low-grade malignant neoplasms, this margin is sharp (geographical, Lodwick pattern I) with a zone of transition extending over only a few millimetres (Fig. 47.1A). The degree of marginal sclerosis is variable. The most actively growing lesions, such as giant cell tumour, have a non-sclerotic margin. Conversely, the least aggressive lesions show a sclerotic rim of varying thickness.

The next most aggressive pattern (moth-eaten, Lodwick pattern II) is characterized by a zone of destruction made up of multiple lucent areas measuring 2–5 mm in diameter. Each lucent area is ill defined and tends to coalesce with adjoining lesions. As purely medullary lesions of this size are not visible radiographically, a moth-eaten pattern generally implies widespread cortical involvement. Moth-eaten destruction is observed in a variety of malignant neoplasms (Fig. 47.1B).

Table 47.1 HISTOLOGICAL TYPING OF PRIMARY BONE TUMOUR-LIKE LESIONS (MODIFIED FROM WHO CLASSIFICATION)		
	Benign	**Malignant**
I. Bone-forming tumours	Osteoma	Osteosarcoma
	Osteoid osteoma	Parosteal osteosarcoma
	Osteoblastoma	Periosteal osteosarcoma
		Telangiectatic osteosarcoma and many other types
II. Cartilage-forming tumours	Chondroma	Chondrosarcoma
	Osteochondroma (cartilage-capped exostosis)	Mesenchymal chondrosarcoma
	Chondroblastoma	Clear-cell chondrosarcoma
	Chondromyxoid fibroma	
III. Giant cell tumour		Malignant giant cell tumour
IV. Marrow tumours		
a. Round cell tumours		Ewing's sarcoma
		Atypical Ewing's sarcoma
		Primitive neuroectodermal tumours
b. Lymphoma		Hodgkin's disease
		Non-Hodgkin's lymphoma
c. Plasma cell tumours		Solitary myeloma (plasmacytoma)
d. Leukaemia		Granulocytic sarcoma (chloroma)
V. Vascular tumours	Haemangioma	Haemangioendothelioma
	Lymphangioma	
	Glomus tumour	
	Intermediate	
	Haemangiopericytoma	
	Massive osteolysis	
VI. Other connective tissue tumours	Non-ossifying fibroma	Fibrosarcoma
	Benign fibrous histiocytoma	Malignant fibrous histiocytoma
	Desmoplastic fibroma	
	Lipoma	Liposarcoma
	Fibromatoses	Malignant mesenchymoma
VII. Other miscellaneous tumours	Neurilemmoma	Neurosarcoma
	Neurofibroma	Chordoma
		Adamantinoma of long bones
VIII. Unclassified tumours		Undifferentiated primary sarcoma
IX. Tumour-like lesions	Solitary bone cyst	
	Aneurysmal bone cyst	
	Langerhans cell histiocytosis (eosinophilic granuloma)	
	Fibrous dysplasia	
	Osteofibrous dysplasia	
	Implantation epidermoid	
	Reparative giant cell granuloma	

The most malignant pattern (permeative, Lodwick pattern III) is composed of multiple coalescing small ill-defined lesions 1 mm or less in diameter with a zone of transition of several centimetres (Fig. 47.1C). Plain radiography inevitably underestimates the extent of involvement in such cases, as even in areas where no destruction is visible, neoplastic cells have probably infiltrated the marrow spaces and their presence is more clearly shown on MRI. Regions with apparently intact cortex may show extracortical tumour masses. This phenomenon often leads, in highly malignant tumours such as Ewing's sarcoma, to saucerization of the outer cortical margin as the tumour, temporarily restrained by the periosteum, erodes back through the cortical bone. A permeative pattern is observed particularly in malignant round cell tumours, osteosarcoma and most metastases. The pattern may occur at certain stages of osteomyelitis or other non-neoplastic conditions such as Langerhans cell histiocytosis (LCH).

Benign or low-grade malignant neoplasms tend to remain within the intramedullary cavity until late in their development. Typically, the cortex is not destroyed, but slow erosion

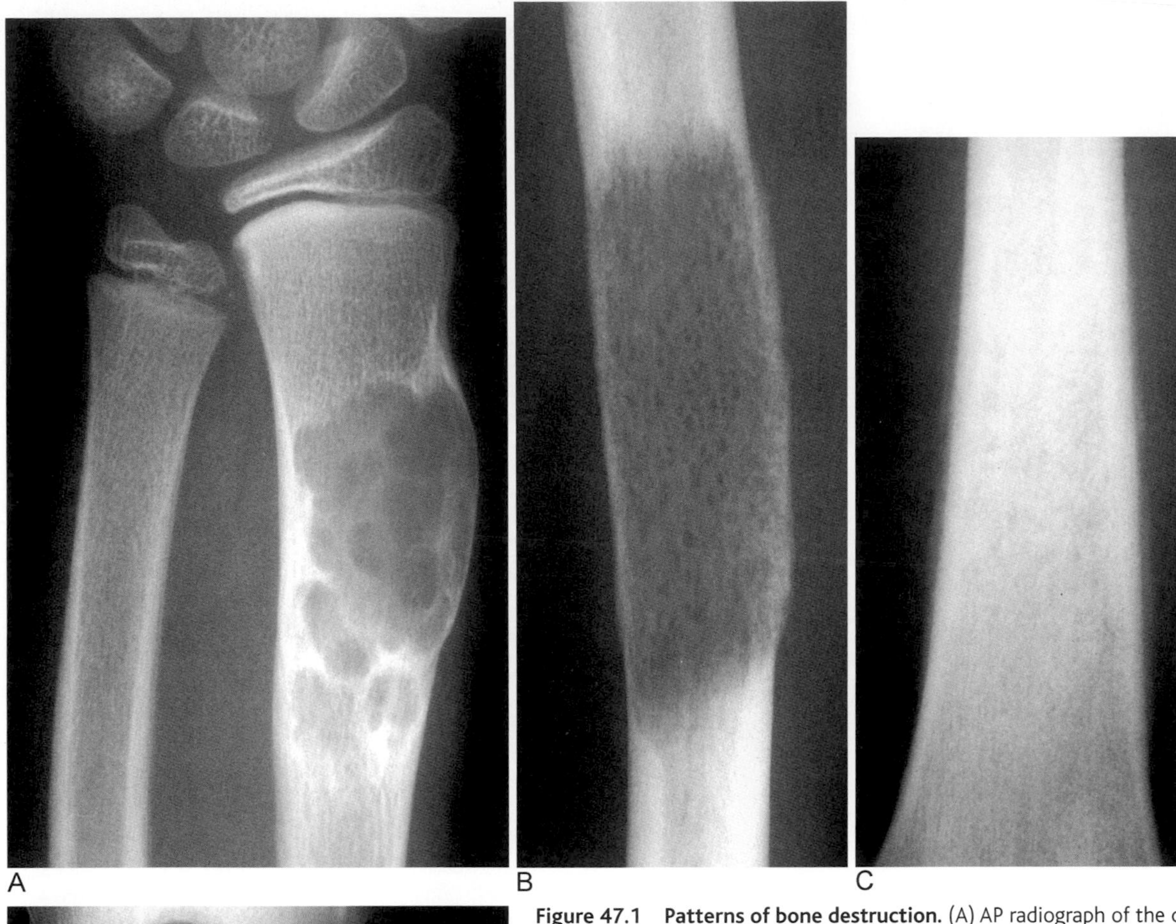

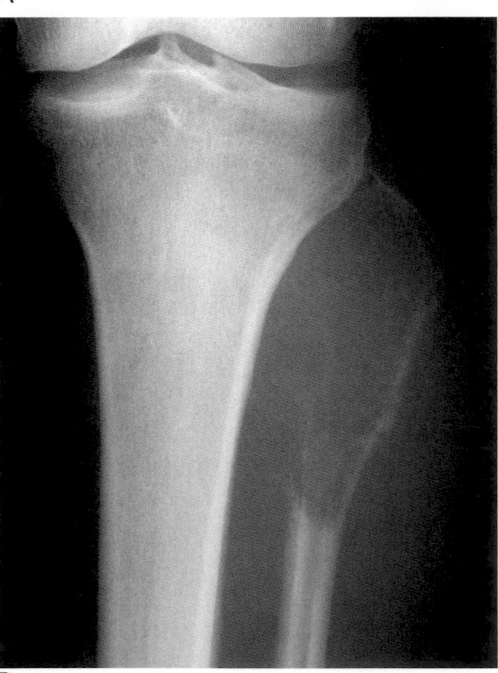

Figure 47.1 Patterns of bone destruction. (A) AP radiograph of the distal radius in a patient with non-ossifying fibroma (NOF), demonstrating the sharp, 'geographic' margin indicating slow growth. Endosteal scalloping and bone expansion with an intact overlying cortex are additional features of slow growth. (B) AP radiograph of the humerus showing a 'moth-eaten' appearance caused by the coalescence of multiple small lytic areas in a patient with renal carcinoma metastasis. (C) AP radiograph of the distal femur showing a 'permeative' pattern of bone destruction in a patient with primary bone lymphoma. (D) AP radiograph of the fibula showing a lytic lesion with expansion and destruction of the cortex indicating an aggressive growth pattern.

of its endosteal surface (endosteal scalloping) together with periosteal new bone formation results in expansion of bone (Fig. 47.1A). Conversely, high-grade malignant tumours commonly extend through the cortex by the time of presentation, resulting in cortical destruction and an adjacent extraosseous mass (Fig. 47.1D).

Periosteal reaction[2]

Periosteal reaction may be of various types with none being pathognomonic of any particular tumour. Rather, the type helps to indicate the aggressiveness of the lesion. A thick, well-formed (solid) periosteal reaction (Fig. 47.2A) indicates a slow rate of growth but not necessarily a benign tumour since it

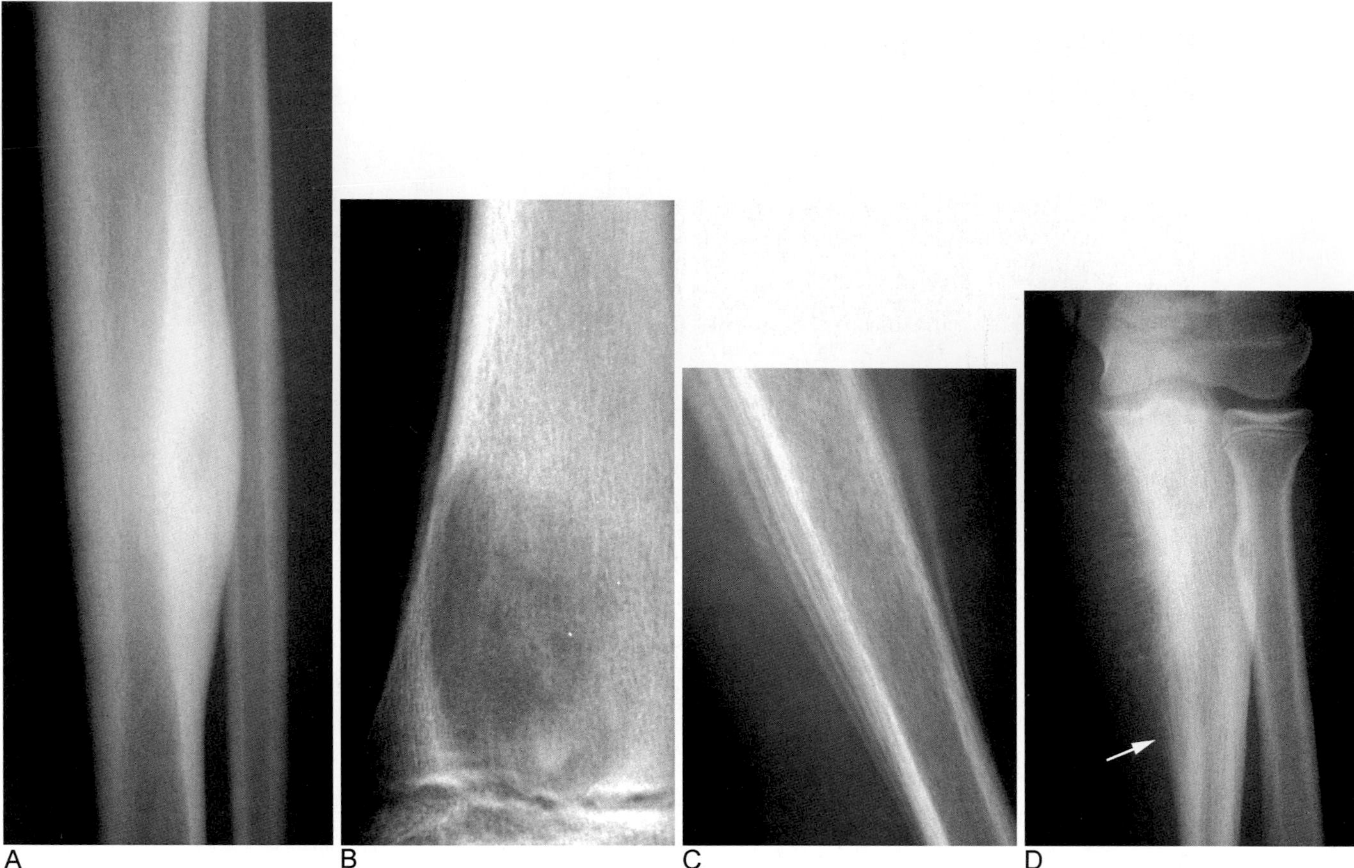

Figure 47.2 Patterns of periosteal reaction. (A) Lateral radiograph of the tibia showing a solid periosteal reaction due to osteoid osteoma. (B) AP radiograph of the distal tibia showing a single, laminated periosteal reaction associated with a Brodie's abscess. (C) AP radiograph of the humerus showing a multilaminated periosteal reaction associated with Ewing's sarcoma. (D) AP radiograph of the proximal ulna showing a 'hair-on-end' type vertical periosteal reaction associated with Ewing's sarcoma. Note also the Codman's triangle (arrow).

may be seen with low-grade chondrosarcoma. Laminated periosteal reaction (Fig. 47.2B) indicates subperiosteal extension of tumour, infection or haematoma. Lesions demonstrating periodic growth, such as Ewing's sarcoma, may show a multilaminated pattern (Fig. 47.2C). A Codman's triangle indicates the limit of subperiosteal tumour in a longitudinal direction. Spiculated, vertical or 'hair-on-end' types of periosteal reaction (Fig. 47.2D) are seen with the most aggressive tumours such as osteosarcoma and Ewing's sarcoma. However, the most rapidly growing lesions may not be associated with any radiographically visible periosteal reaction, since mineralization of the deep layer of periosteum can take two weeks.

Matrix mineralization

The matrix of a tumour represents the extracellular material produced by the tumour cells within which the tumour cells lie. Certain tumours produce characteristic radiographically visible matrix mineralization, which allows the histological cell type to be predicted. Chondral calcifications (Fig. 47.3A) are typically linear, curvilinear, ring-like, punctate or nodular. Osseous mineralization (Fig. 47.3B) is cloud-like and poorly defined whereas diffuse matrix mineralization in benign fibrous tumours produces the characteristic 'ground-glass' appearance (Fig. 47.3C) seen most commonly in fibrous dysplasia. Some neoplasms, such as adenocarcinoma metastases, can provoke reactive mineralization, whereas calcifications within an intraosseous lipoma are due to associated fat necrosis. Also, some tumours such as malignant fibrous histiocytoma may develop on underlying calcified bone infarcts (Fig. 47.3D).

CT and MRI in diagnosis and staging

CT is excellent for demonstrating the presence of radiographically occult matrix mineralization (Fig. 47.4A) and the persistence of a thin cortical shell indicating that the tumour still lies deep to the periosteum. CT also plays a major role in the investigation of cortical thickening, allowing the demonstration of the cause, such as the nidus of an osteoid osteoma (Fig. 47.4B) or a stress fracture.

The major role of MRI is in local staging, particularly for high-grade malignant tumours such as osteosarcoma, where the intraosseous extent (Fig. 47.5A), identification of 'skip' lesions (Fig.47.5B) and involvement of the neurovascular bundle (Fig. 47.5C) and adjacent joint (Fig. 47.5D) can all be assessed with great accuracy[3]. Such information is vital for planning surgical management, be it limb salvage or amputation. Dynamic contrast enhanced MRI has been advocated for determining chemotherapeutic response[4].

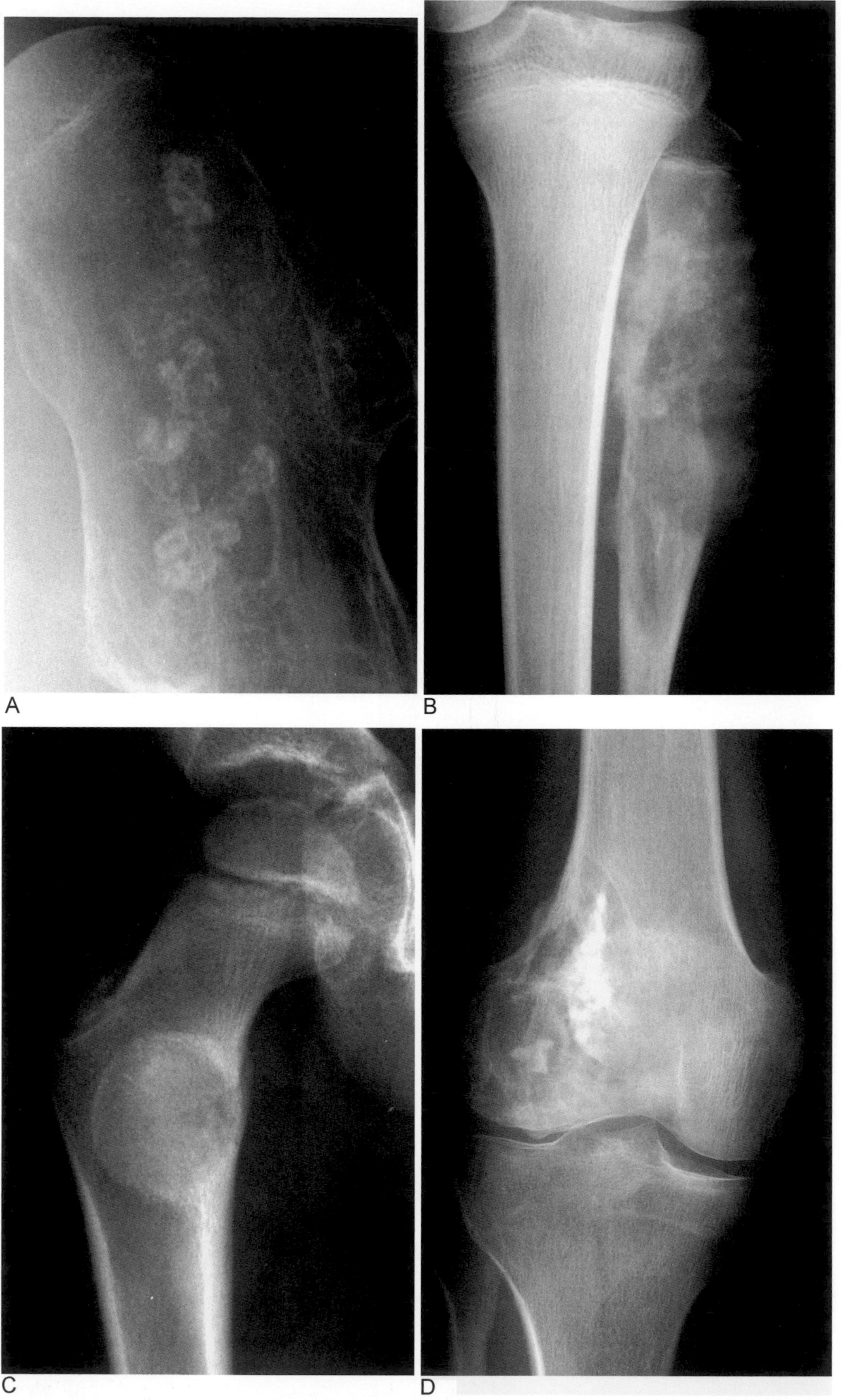

Figure 47.3 Patterns of matrix mineralization. (A) AP radiograph of the proximal humerus in a patient with metachondromatosis, showing typical chondroid calcification. (B) AP radiograph of the proximal fibula in a patient with osteosarcoma showing typical osseous mineralization. (C) AP radiograph of the proximal femur in a patient with fibrous dysplasia showing typical ground-glass mineralization. (D) AP radiograph of the distal femur in a patient with malignant fibrous histiocytoma complicating a heavily calcified medullary bone infarct.

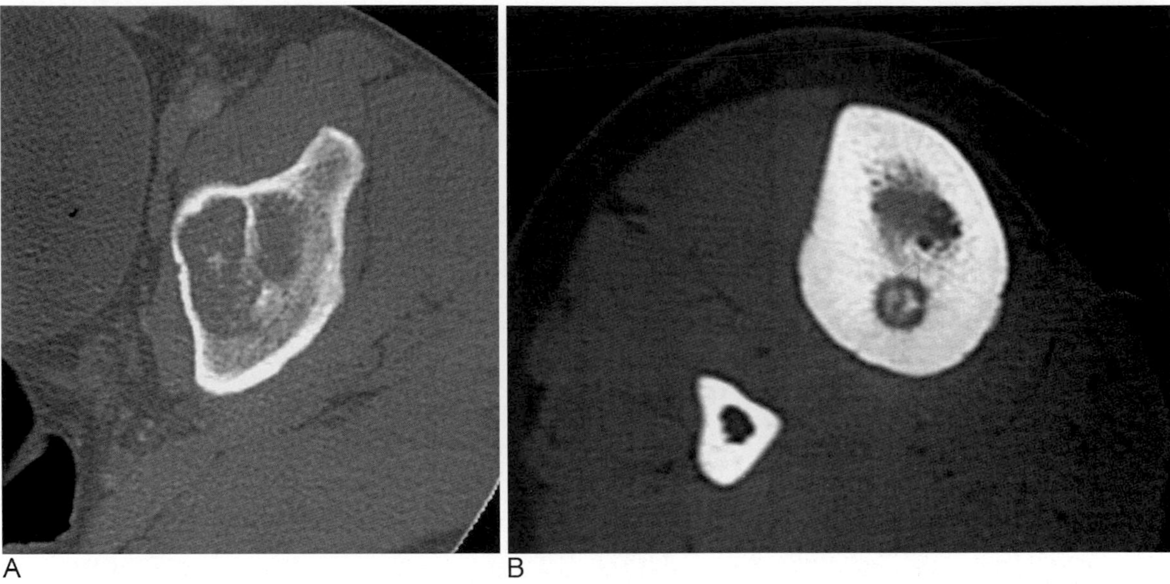

Figure 47.4 Role of CT in lesion characterization. (A) CT through the left acetabulum showing radiographically occult chondroid matrix mineralization in a patient with grade 1 chondrosarcoma. (B) CT through the tibia showing the nidus of an osteoid osteoma (same patient as in Fig. 47.2A).

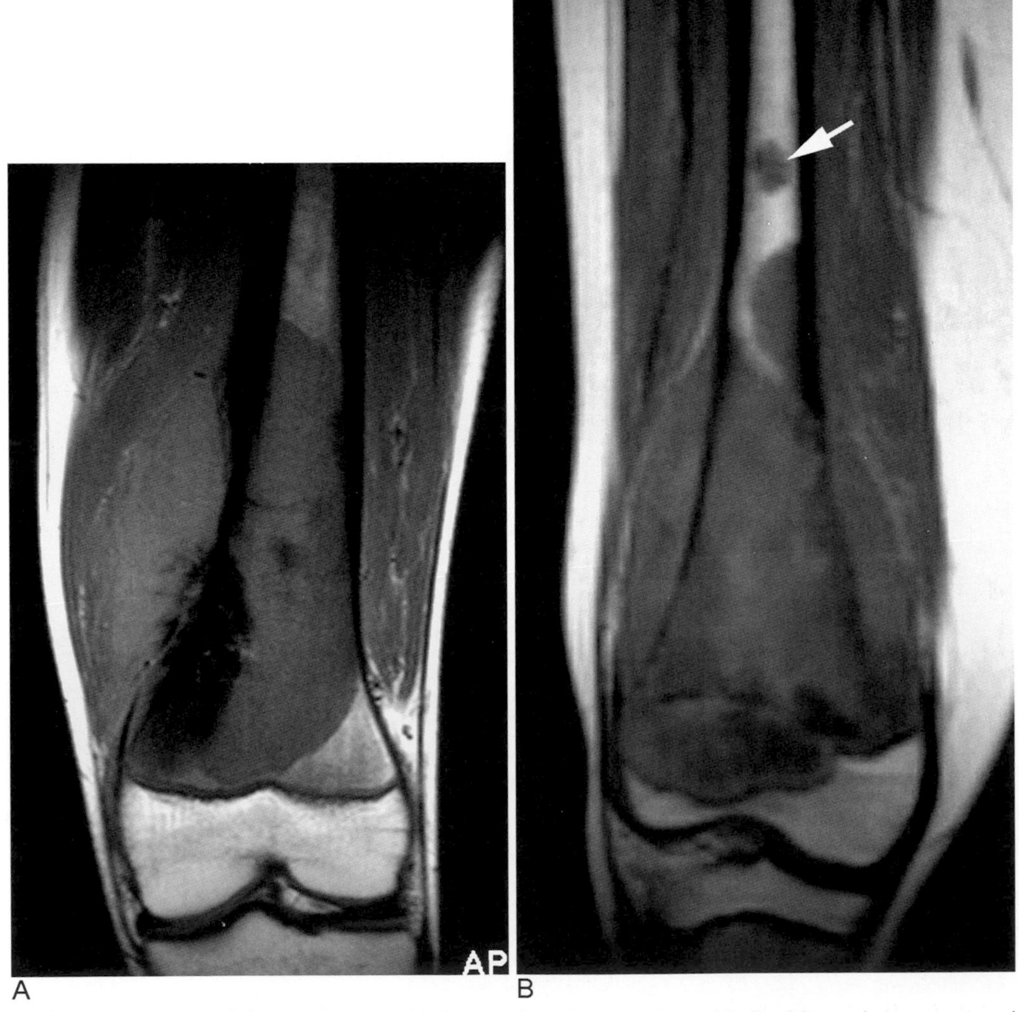

Figure 47.5 Role of MRI in local staging. (A) Coronal T1-weighted spin-echo MRI in a patient with distal femoral osteosarcoma showing the intraosseous tumour extent represented by intermediate signal intensity (SI) contrasting against the hyperintense fatty marrow. (B) Coronal T1-weighted spin-echo MRI in a patient with distal femoral osteosarcoma showing a 'skip' metastasis (arrow).

Continued

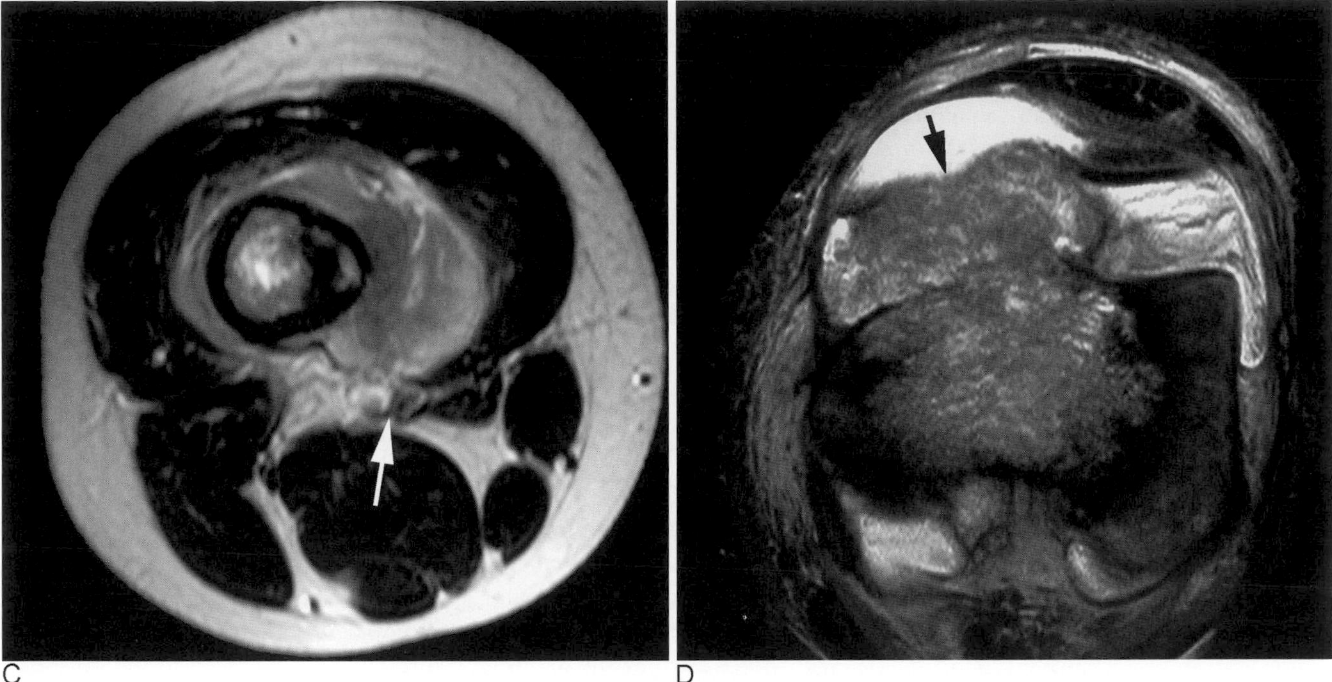

Figure 47.5 Cont'd (C) Axial T2-weighted fast spin-echo MRI in a patient with distal femoral osteosarcoma showing extraosseous tumour abutting the neurovascular bundle (arrow). (D) Axial fat suppressed T2-weighted fast spin-echo MRI through the distal femur in a patient with osteosarcoma showing joint involvement (arrow).

In the presence of a purely lytic lesion, several MRI features may help in lesion characterization. The presence of low signal intensity (SI) on T2-weighted images indicates chronic haemorrhage and may be seen with giant cell tumour. MRI is very sensitive to the presence of fluid levels and the degree of fluid level change is related to the histological diagnosis[5]. Lesions that are completely filled with fluid levels are almost always aneurysmal bone cysts. MRI can also demonstrate a fatty matrix as seen with haemangioma and intraosseous lipoma. The vascular nature of renal metastases has been demonstrated by the presence of the 'flow-void' sign[6]. MRI is very sensitive to reactive medullary and soft-tissue oedema, which characterizes certain lesions such as osteoid osteoma, osteoblastoma, chondroblastoma and Brodie's abscess[7].

Bone scintigraphy plays little role in the diagnostic work-up of a suspected primary bone tumour, with the possible exception of osteoid osteoma or osteoblastoma, particularly in the spine. However, scintigraphy is still useful for the identification of skeletal metastases, although this role has recently been challenged by whole body MRI[8]. The position of techniques such as MR spectroscopy[9], positron emission tomography (PET) and CT-PET[10] in the management of suspected bone tumours is as yet unclear.

Finally, the use of ultrasound[11] and CT[12] for image-guided needle biopsy is well established although the likely future route of approach and surgical options should be considered in an appropriate clinical setting.

BENIGN TUMOURS

CHONDROID ORIGIN[13]

Benign tumours apparently derived from cartilage comprise:

1 **Chondroma**. This is commonly central in its situation in the bone (then referred to as enchondroma), but may be eccentric, e.g. in a subperiosteal location (periosteal chondroma). Multiple enchondromas are found in enchondromatosis (Ollier's disease), Maffucci's syndrome (multiple enchondromas with soft-tissue haemangiomas) and metachondromatosis (combination of multiple enchondromas and osteochondromas).

2 **Osteochondroma** (cartilage-capped exostosis). This peripherally situated benign tumour is usually solitary. When multiple, the term 'diaphyseal aclasis' (multiple hereditary exostoses—MHE) is employed.

3 **Chondroblastoma**.

4 **Chondromyxoid fibroma**.

(En)Chondroma

Enchondroma represents a benign intramedullary neoplasm made up of lobules of hyaline cartilage. Solitary enchondroma is the second commonest benign chondral lesion after osteochondroma and accounts for 3–17% of all primary bone tumours in large biopsy series. Enchondromas affect the tubular bones of the hands and feet in 40–65% of cases and present either when they become symptomatic, due to size or pathological fracture (in 60% of cases), or as incidental findings. The majority arise in the proximal phalanges (40–50%) followed by the metacarpals (15–30%) and middle phalanges (20–30%). The small bones of the feet are involved in 7% of cases. Approximately 25% are found in the femur, tibia and humerus. Other sites are very rare.

The age range is 10–80 years, with most presenting in the second to fourth decades. The sex incidence is equal. Any chondroma that becomes painful in the absence of fracture, or shows recent increase in size, should be regarded as potentially malignant and biopsied.

Radiological features

Most enchondromas arise centrally in the phalanges and metacarpals. Lesions are typically metaphyseal or diaphyseal with epiphyseal location accounting for only 2–5%. Enchondromas are often eccentric and mostly (75%) solitary. They are typically well-circumscribed, lobulated or oval lytic lesions, which may expand the cortex (Fig. 47.6). Size at presentation ranges from 10 to 30 mm. Chondral-type calcification may be identified within the matrix. Lesions involving slender bones such as rib or fibula may show eccentric expansion, when the term enchondroma protuberans has been used.

Outside the hands and feet, the ratio of chondrosarcoma to chondroma is 5:1[14]. Features most consistent with a benign lesion in these bones include:

1 age under 20 years; chondrosarcoma is rare under this age
2 a purely medullary lesion consisting of well-formed circular, curvilinear or nodular calcific densities ('popcorn' calcification) without focal lytic areas
3 a well-defined round or elliptical margin
4 no cortical destruction, periosteal new bone formation or soft tissue mass
5 slow growth.

In comparison, features indicative of chondrosarcoma include deep endosteal scalloping, cortical destruction with soft tissue mass and periosteal reaction[15].

On scintigraphy, chondromas tend to show activity that is equal to or less than that of the iliac crest. Chondroid tumours have characteristic features on MRI, appearing of intermediate SI on T1-weighted images and as hyperintense, lobulated lesions on T2-weighted images. Matrix mineralization manifests as punctate areas of signal void (Fig. 47.7). A hypointense rim and septations may be seen, the latter showing enhancement following IV gadolinium[16].

Less common varieties of chondroma

Periosteal chondroma[17] These are rare lesions affecting children and young adults and located in the metaphyses of tubular bones, most commonly the proximal humerus followed by the femur and tibia. They are also seen in the small bones of the hands and feet. Radiologically, each appears as a well-defined area of cortical erosion typically measuring 1–3 cm with mature periosteal reaction and sometimes a thin external shell of bone. Cartilaginous matrix mineralization is observed in half the cases (Fig. 47.8A). MRI shows the features of a chondral lesion with a lobulated hyperintense mass on T2-weighted images adjacent to but not infiltrating the underlying cortex (Fig. 47.8B). The differential diagnosis includes periosteal chondrosarcoma and periosteal osteosarcoma. Malignant transformation has not been reported.

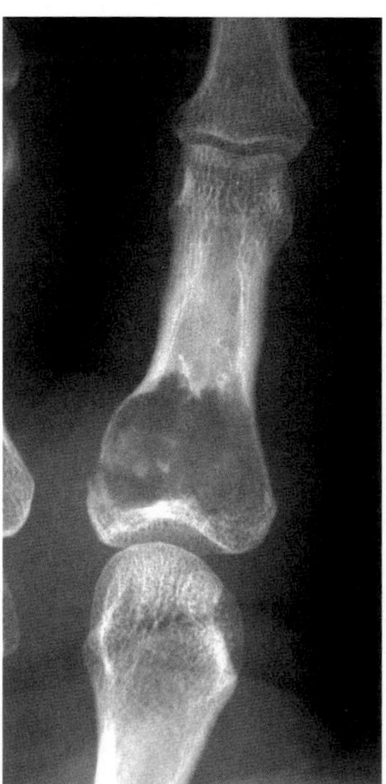

Figure 47.6 Proximal phalangeal enchondroma. AP radiograph of the index finger showing a pathological fracture.

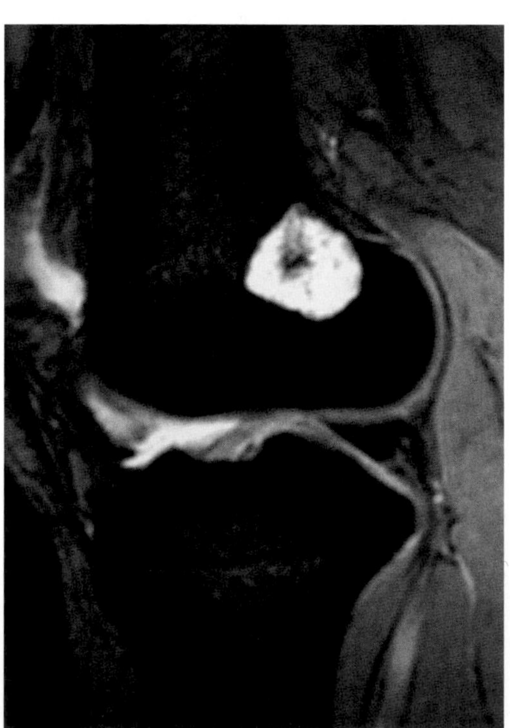

Figure 47.7 Distal femoral chondroma. Sagittal T2*-weighted gradient-echo MR image showing classical appearances of a chondroma. Calcification is manifest as focal areas of signal void.

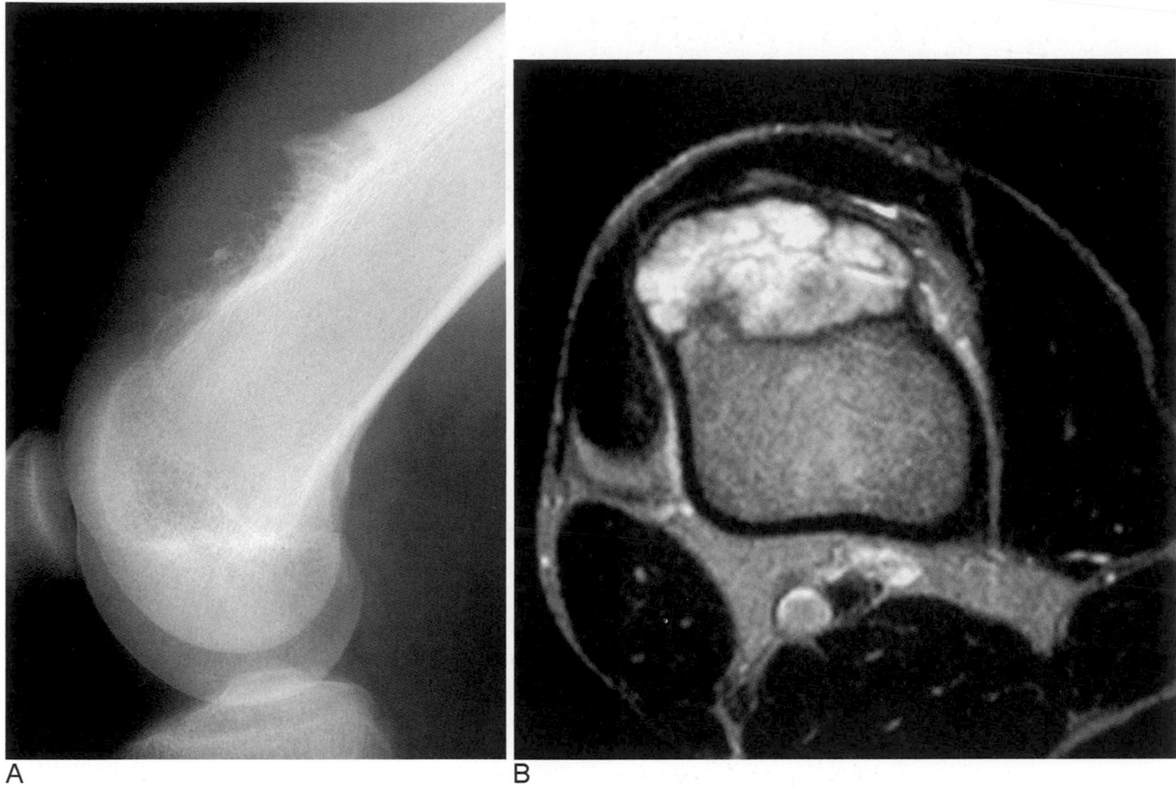

Figure 47.8 Periosteal chondroma. (A) Lateral radiograph of the distal femur showing a calcified surface lesion. (B) Axial fat-suppressed T2-weighted fast spin-echo MRI showing a hyperintense lobulated lesion, without medullary infiltration.

Multiple chondromas (enchondromatosis, Ollier's disease) This disorder is sporadic, *not* genetically inherited and is typically unilateral. In addition to multiple enchondromas, flame-like rests of cartilage in the metaphyses impede bone growth and may result in bowing or angulation (Fig. 47.9).

Malignant change is reported in 5–30% of cases. These patients are also at risk of developing gliomas and pancreatic or ovarian carcinoma.

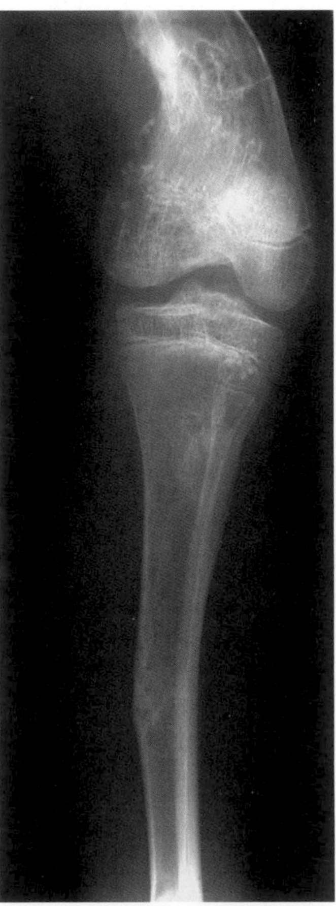

Figure 47.9 Enchondromatosis. AP radiograph of the distal femur and tibia showing multiple enchondromas and distal femoral deformity consistent with Ollier's disease.

Enchondromatosis with haemangiomas (Maffucci's syndrome) This rare disorder combines multiple enchondromas and soft tissue haemangiomas (occasionally lymphangiomas). The condition is unilateral in 50% of cases. The presence of soft tissue haemangiomas with phleboliths differentiates the disorder from Ollier's disease. The true incidence of chondrosarcomatous change is uncertain because of the rarity of the disease, but is reported in approximately 20% of cases, usually in patients over the age of 40 years.

Osteochondroma (cartilage-capped exostosis)[18]

This tumour is classified with chondroid tumours as it has a cartilage cap that is actively growing. It is generally accepted to be a developmental anomaly, but may arise following radiotherapy. It accounts for approximately 35% of benign bone tumours and nearly 10% of all bone tumours. Osteochondromas may present at any age from 2 to 60 years, but the highest incidence is in the second decade. The male to female ratio is 1.8:1.

Long bones are commonly affected, especially around the knee (35% of cases). The commonest locations are the distal femur, proximal humerus, proximal tibia and proximal femur. The commonest flat bones affected are the ilium and scapula. The solitary or multiple lesions are initially metaphyseal but migrate to the diaphysis with time, leading to the classical 'coat-hanger' variety of osteochondroma, pointing *away from* the adjacent joint. Both pedunculated and sessile forms are recognized. Multiple osteochondromas (diaphyseal aclasis) constitute an uncommon autosomal dominant disorder. The exostoses may be larger than the solitary variety and may lead to shortening or deformity of the affected limbs. The metaphyses in this condition are also typically widened and dysplastic (Fig. 47.10).

Osteochondromas present with mechanical problems such as an enlarging mass, pressure on adjoining structures or rarely fracture of the bony stem. Mechanical irritation of overlying soft tissues may result in bursa formation, which can mimic sarcomatous degeneration. MRI is highly accurate in the assessment of symptomatic osteochondromas[19]. The incidence of chondrosarcomatous change in the cartilage cap is very small in a solitary osteochondroma (probably less than 1%). Malignant degeneration in diaphyseal aclasis is approximated at 3–5%.

Radiological features

The lesion appears as an outgrowth from the normal cortex, with which it is continuous. Pedunculated lesions have a long slim neck (Fig. 47.11A) whereas sessile lesions have a broad base with the bone of origin (Fig. 47.11B). As the lesion grows, the marrow cavity extends into the exostosis (Fig. 47.12A).

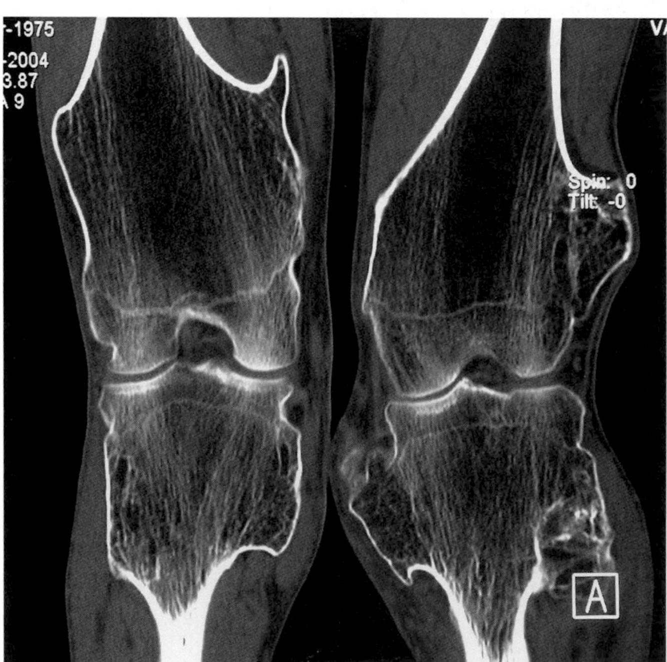

Figure 47.10 Diaphyseal aclasis. Coronal multiplanar reconstruction from a multislice CT study of the knees showing classical features of diaphyseal aclasis with multiple osteochondromas and metaphyseal expansion.

The actively growing cartilage cap is not visible radiologically, but can be shown by ultrasound or CT. It is shown particularly well with T2-weighted MRI when the hyperintense cartilage contrasts well against adjacent hypointense muscle (Fig. 47.12B). With age, however, the cap becomes increasingly calcified in a punctate or nodular fashion. Differential diagnosis of a sessile lesion includes periosteal chondroma or parosteal osteosarcoma. Scintigraphy shows variable activity and is of no value in identifying malignant change.

Bizarre parosteal osteochondromatous proliferation (BPOP)[20]

This rare lesion is a tumour-like disorder, which is included here for reasons of differential diagnosis. It arises adjacent to the cortex of the small tubular bones of the hands or feet and may resemble an osteochondroma. However, continuity between the lesion and underlying bone is not found (Fig. 47.13).

Differential diagnosis includes soft tissue chondroma and florid reactive periostitis, which some suggest is a precursor to BPOP.

Chondroblastoma[21]

Chondroblastoma accounts for approximately 1% of all bone neoplasms with 80–90% occurring between the ages of 5 and 25 years (mean age 18 years). The tumour is rare after the age of 30 years, when flat bones are mostly affected. The male to female ratio is almost 2:1. Chondroblastoma has rarely been associated with metastases (especially to the lung) and a rare variant termed 'aggressive' (atypical) chondroblastoma, associated with cortical destruction and soft tissue extension, has been described.

Chondroblastoma usually presents with joint pain, since it is typically located in the epiphysis of a long bone and may promote a synovial reaction. Forty per cent arise around the knee, while the proximal femur is the commonest single location, accounting for 33% of all cases. Chondroblastoma is usually located eccentrically in the epiphysis (40%), but with partial closure of the growth plate it usually extends to involve the metaphysis (55%). Epiphyseal equivalents such as the apophyses and sesamoid bones can also be involved, accounting for locations such as the greater trochanter of the femur, the greater tuberosity of the humerus and the acromion. Less than 4% are located purely within the metaphysis. In the feet, the calcaneus and talus are most commonly involved, while chondroblastoma is the commonest tumour of the patella.

Radiological features

The lesion is usually spherical or lobular with a fine sclerotic margin (Fig. 47.14). Matrix mineralization is demonstrated in only 10% radiographically, although it is much more commonly seen at CT. Linear periosteal reaction is present in 30–50% of cases, usually distant to the epiphyseal tumour. MRI shows variable SI on T2-weighted images (Fig. 47.15), including hypointensity and fluid levels due to secondary aneurysmal bone cyst (ABC) change in 15% of cases. Associated marrow and soft tissue oedema and reactive joint effusion are almost invariable.

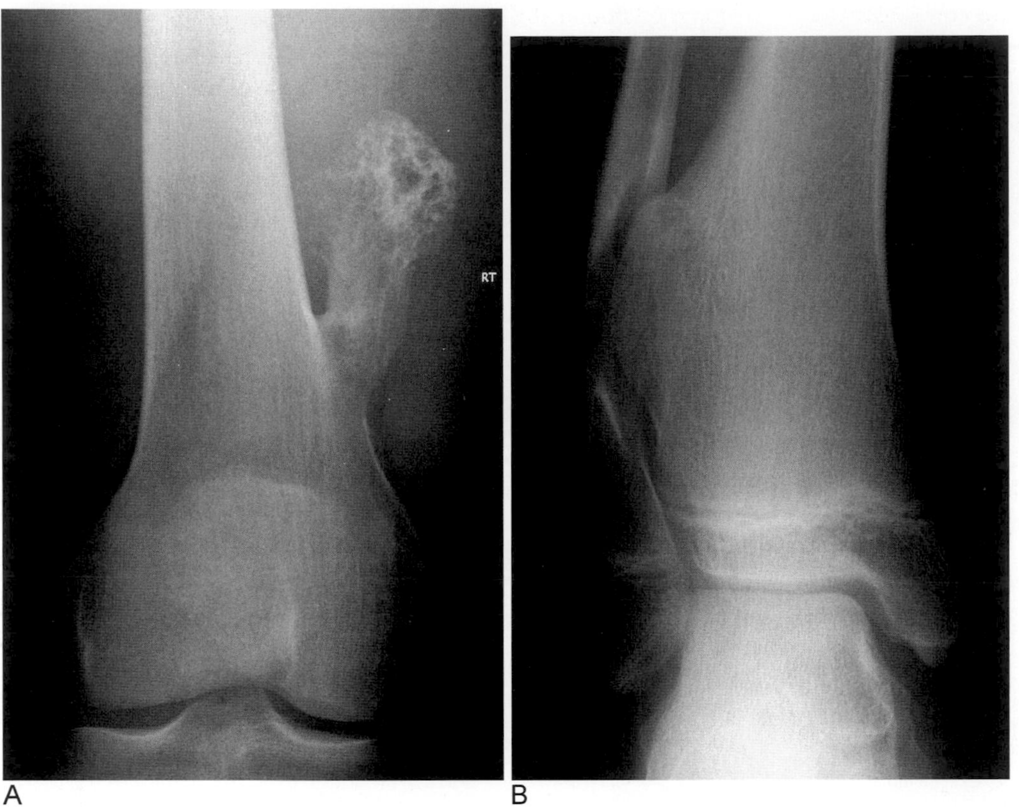

Figure 47.11 Osteochondroma. (A) AP radiograph showing a typical pedunculated osteochondroma of the distal femur. (B) AP radiograph of the distal tibia showing a sessile osteochondroma with associated modelling deformity of the adjacent fibula.

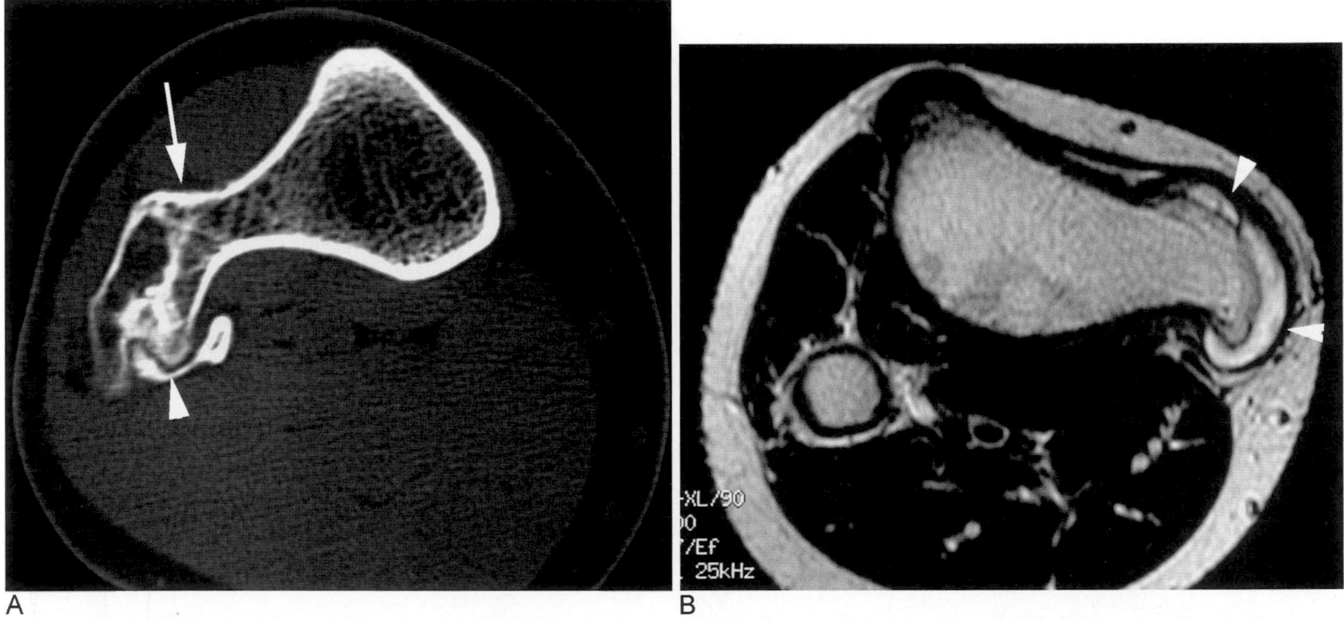

Figure 47.12 Osteochondroma. CT and MRI features. (A) CT through the proximal tibia showing a tibial osteochondroma (arrow) causing marked thinning of the adjacent fibula (arrowhead). (B) Axial T2-weighted MRI showing a uniformly thin, hyperintense cartilage cap (arrowheads).

The differential diagnosis of lytic epiphyseal lesions in children includes Brodie's abscess. In adults, subchondral cysts and clear cell chondrosarcoma need to be considered.

Chondromyxoid fibroma[22]

Chondromyxoid fibroma accounts for less than 0.5% of biopsied primary bone tumours with 75% of cases occurring between 10 and 30 years of age (mean age 23 years). Most lesions are metaphyseal and eccentric within the medulla resulting in thinning and expansion of the cortex. The long bones account for 60% of cases with 40% arising in the flat bones (ilium 10%) or small tubular bones of the hands and feet (17%). The upper third of the tibia accounts for approximately 25% of chondromyxoid fibromas. Juxtacortical lesions have also been reported.

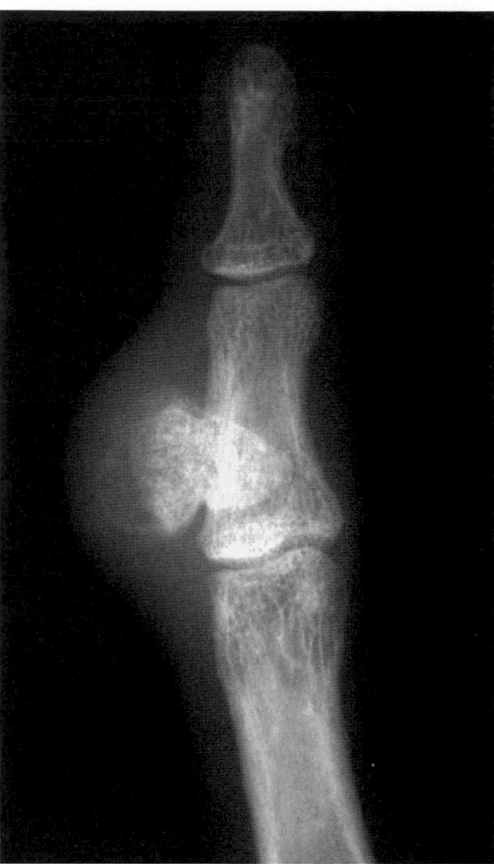

Figure 47.13 BPOP. AP radiograph of the little finger showing a bizarre parosteal osteochondromatous proliferation adjacent to the middle phalanx.

Radiological features

In the proximal tibial shaft, chondromyxoid fibroma appears as an eccentric, lobulated lesion with a sclerotic margin (Fig. 47.16). Periosteal reaction and soft tissue extension are uncommon and matrix calcification is seen in only 12.5% of lesions[23]. MRI shows no particular diagnostic features. Outside its classical location, it has no characteristic appearances.

OSTEOID ORIGIN[24]

Enostosis (bone island)[25]

An enostosis or bone island represents a focus of cortical bone located within the medulla and is congenital or developmental in origin. Bone islands are usually incidental findings, being most commonly seen in the pelvis, femur and other long bones. Multiple lesions are seen in osteopoikilosis and osteopathia striata. These are both autosomal dominant conditions in which multiple bone islands are present in a periarticular distribution, appearing either round (osteopoikilosis) or elongated (osteopathia striata).

Radiological features

Classical radiological features consist of a dense sclerotic focus with a characteristic spiculated margin that blends with the trabeculae of the host bone (Fig. 47.17). On MRI, the lesion has very low SI on all pulse sequences, being equal to that of cortical bone. Bone islands typically show no uptake on skeletal scintigraphy, allowing differentiation from osteoblastic metastases. However, approximately 25% of 'giant' bone islands show increased activity on scintigraphy.

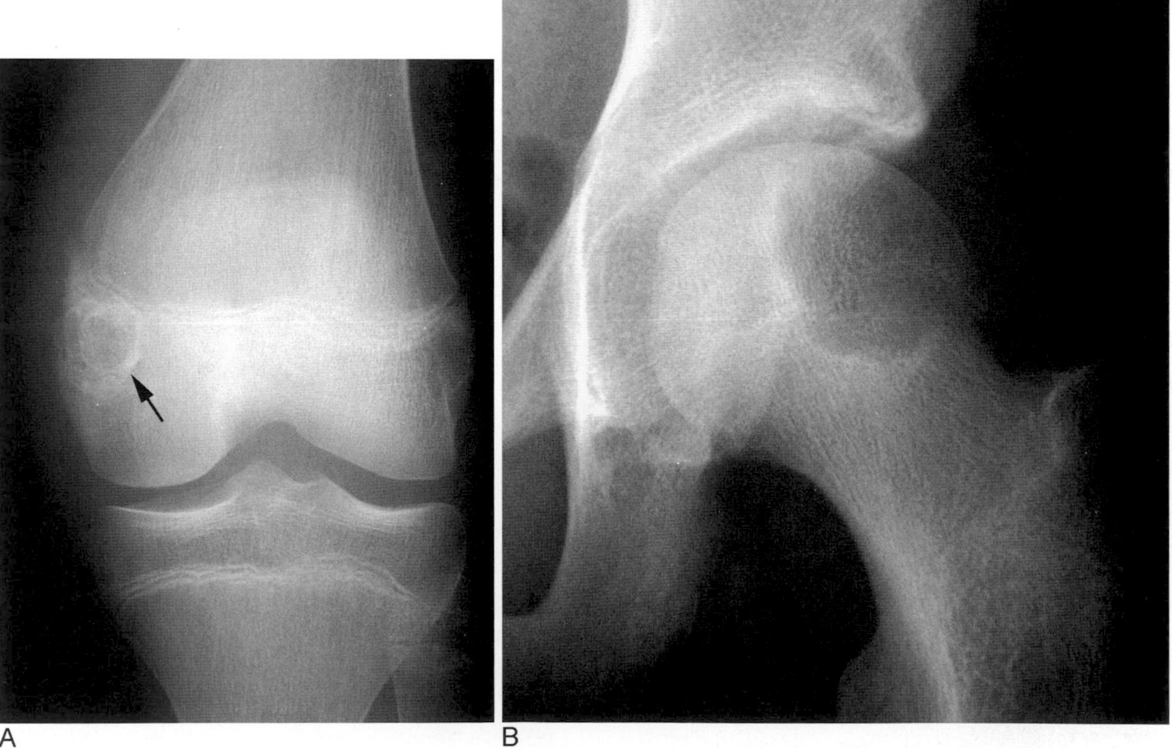

Figure 47.14 Chondroblastoma in the immature and mature skeleton. (A) AP radiograph of the knee showing a lobulated, lytic lesion (arrow) adjacent to the open growth plate and limited to the epiphysis. (B) AP radiograph of the hip showing extension of the lesion across the fused growth plate.

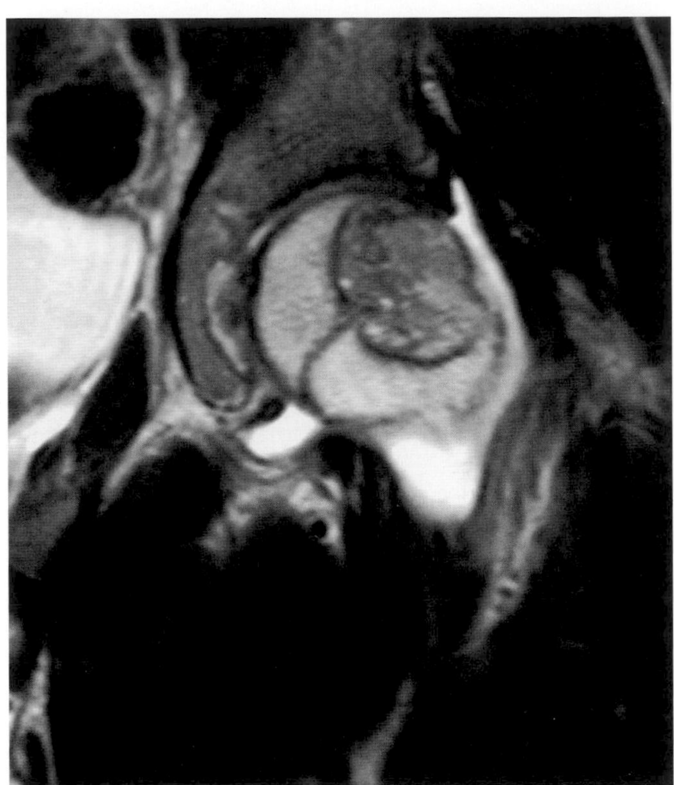

Figure 47.15 Chondroblastoma of the left femoral head. Coronal fat-suppressed T2-weighted fast spin-echo MRI showing the hypointense lesion with surrounding marrow oedema and reactive joint effusion.

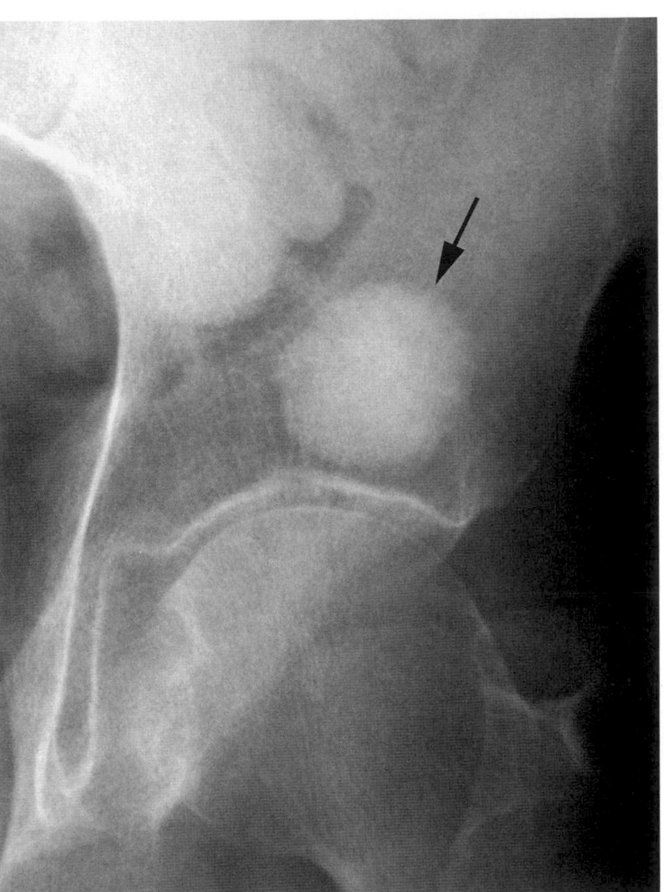

Figure 47.17 Giant bone island. AP radiograph of the left hip showing a uniformly sclerotic bone island (arrow) in the supra-acetabular region of the ilium.

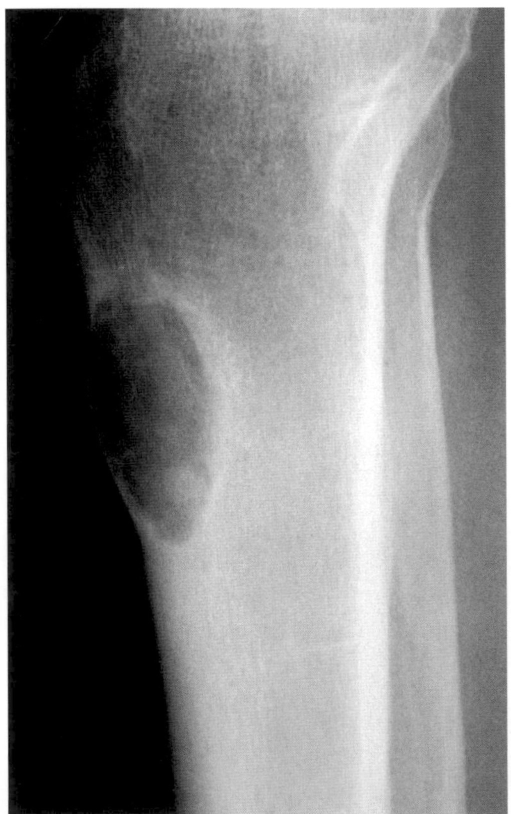

Figure 47.16 Chondromyxoid fibroma. Lateral radiograph of the proximal tibia showing expansion of the anterior cortex.

Osteoma

These tumours may consist of predominantly cortical or cancellous bone. Cortical (ivory) osteomas commonly affect the paranasal sinuses and are slowly growing, dense lesions usually showing a well-defined spherical or hemispherical margin. They are usually incidental findings and rarely exceed 2–3 cm in diameter. However, they may interfere with drainage of the sinuses or result in cerebrospinal fluid (CSF) rhinorrhoea, pneumocephalus or even meningitis.

Outside the paranasal sinuses, osteomas are rare and, if multiple, occur in Gardner's syndrome. Solitary osteomas may involve the long bones and spine[26], where they present with dull aching pain. Radiologically, they are homogeneously dense lesions with smooth or lobulated margins. Cancellous osteomas are less common but may also be found in the paranasal sinuses. Isolated parosteal osteomas are also described[27].

Osteoid osteoma

This small benign tumour is essentially a hamartoma and is often associated with a characteristic clinical picture of night pain relieved by aspirin. It accounts for approximately 10% of all biopsied benign tumours. Most patients present in the second and third decades of life and the male to female ratio is 2–3:1. The paucity of early plain radiographic changes often results in diagnosis being delayed for between 6 months and several years. Pain and disuse may result in osteoporosis, muscle wasting and even altered tendon reflexes, suggesting a neurological lesion. Approximately 13% of cases are intra-articular, cause synovitis and present as a monoarthropathy[28]. Spinal lesions commonly manifest as painful scoliosis[29].

Almost no skeletal site is exempt, with the lesion affecting the medullary cavity, cortex or subperiosteal region. Osteoid osteoma is most common in the appendicular skeleton, with over 50% occurring in the diaphysis or metaphysis of the tibia or femur. In the spine, more than 90% of lesions are located in the neural arch.

Radiological features

The characteristic feature of the lesion is the nidus, which may appear lucent, sclerotic or of mixed density depending upon the degree of mineralization. By arbitrary definition, the nidus of an osteoid osteoma measures no more than 10–15 mm in diameter and most do not exceed 5 mm (Fig. 47.18). The nidus is surrounded by a region of reactive medullary sclerosis and periosteal reaction, the degree of which depends upon the age of the patient and the location within the bone (subperiosteal lesions and those in younger patients being more reactive than medullary or intra-articular lesions). Dense bony reactive changes may obscure the nidus on plain radiographs. Rarely, a multifocal nidus is found.

Bone scintigraphy is almost invariably abnormal, showing the characteristic 'double density sign' with an area of focal intense activity corresponding to the nidus, and a surrounding area of slightly lesser intensity produced by the reactive sclerosis (Fig. 47.19). Increased activity is also seen on the vascular and blood pool phases.

CT may fail to identify a small lesion unless 2–3 mm slices are used (Fig. 47.20). Periosteal reaction is absent with intra-articular lesions (Fig. 47.21), lesions in the terminal phalanges and those deep in medullary bone or at tendinous or ligamentous insertions. Sometimes periosteal reaction and soft tissue oedema will be observed distant from the affected region.

Although MRI can demonstrate osteoid osteoma (Fig. 47.22), it is rarely required for diagnosis and may be very misleading due to the associated reactive bone oedema, soft tissue oedema and soft tissue mass[30]. Another difficulty with MRI is the inability to demonstrate a very small nidus.

The natural history of osteoid osteoma is one of spontaneous resolution, and symptomatic treatment with nonsteroidal anti-inflammatory drugs is possible. However, the current treatment of choice is CT-guided radiofrequency ablation (Fig. 47.23), which is minimally invasive and has a high success rate[31].

Osteoblastoma

Osteoblastoma possesses histological similarities to osteoid osteoma and is differentiated primarily by its size, being typically greater than 1.5–2 cm in diameter. It is a rare tumour accounting for less than 1% of all primary bone neoplasms. Over 80% of patients are under the age of 30 years and the male to female ratio is 2–3:1. The presentation differs from osteoid osteoma in that pain is not usually acute or severe and is rarely relieved by aspirin.

The spine, including the sacrum, is the commonest location for osteoblastoma, accounting for 40–50% of cases. Over 90% involve the neural arch eccentrically and typically lead to painful scoliosis[29]. The other major sites are the diaphyses or metaphyses of long bones, most commonly the femur.

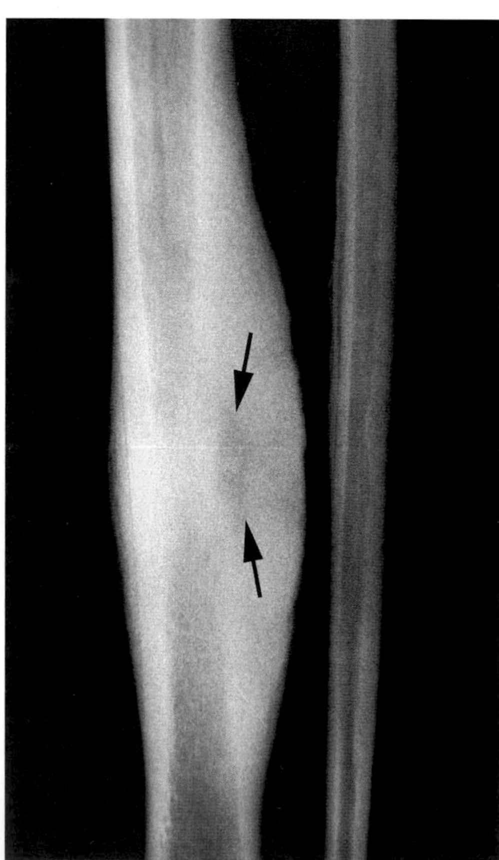

Figure 47.18 Osteoid osteoma. AP radiograph of the tibia shows solid thickening of the anterolateral tibial cortex containing a small nidus (arrows).

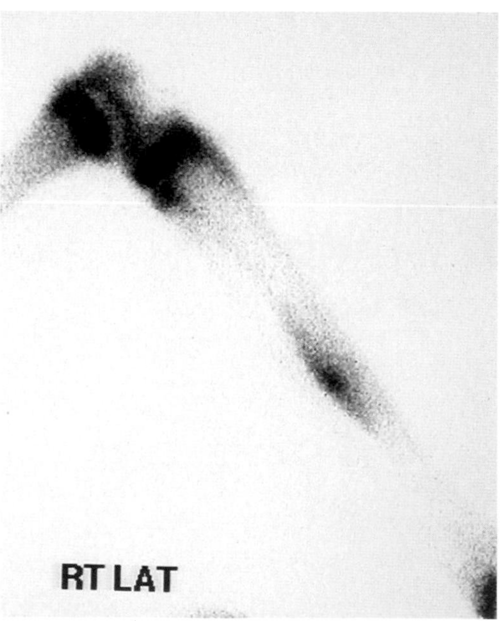

Figure 47.19 Osteoid osteoma. Lateral ^{99m}Tc-MDP scintigram showing the 'double-density' sign.

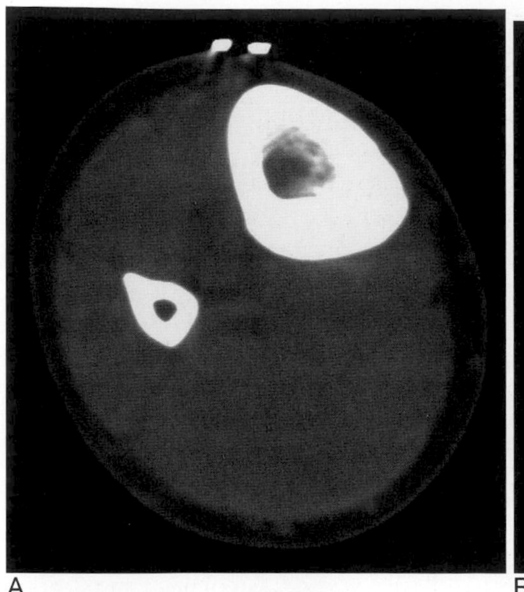

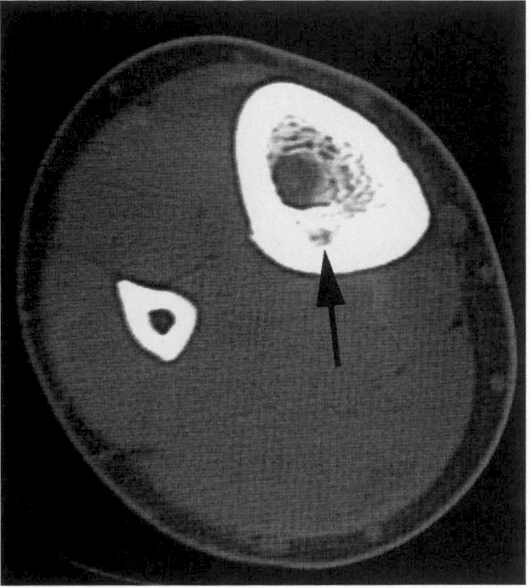

Figure 47.20 Osteoid osteoma. (A) 5 mm axial CT through the tibia showing only a thickened posterior tibial cortex. (B) Repeat 2 mm CT slice demonstrates the nidus (arrow).

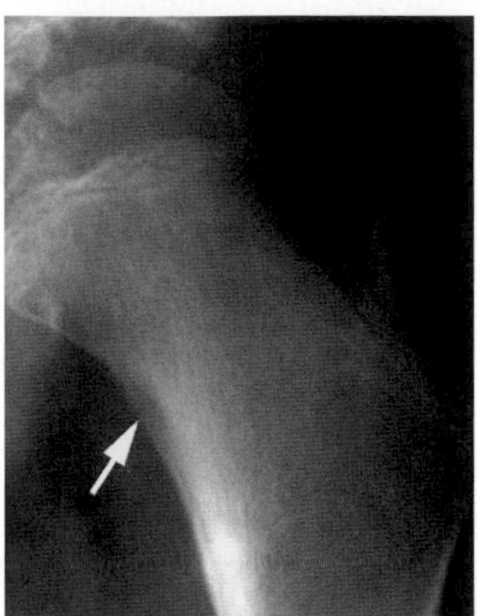

Figure 47.21 Osteoid osteoma. AP radiograph of the hip showing an intra-articular osteoid osteoma involving the medial femoral neck (arrow).

A variant of osteoblastoma termed 'aggressive osteoblastoma' is most commonly reported in the sacrum. It is locally aggressive, more likely to recur and is capable of metastasizing.

Radiological features[32]

The lesion is predominantly lytic, measuring 10–100 mm in diameter, with larger lesions showing a greater degree of matrix mineralization (Fig. 47.24). Spinal lesions result in scoliosis with the tumour located at the apex of the concavity of the curve, where expansion or absence of the pedicle may be seen. CT often reveals occult calcification, which can be punctate, nodular or generalized. Larger lesions may result in bony expansion with or without a surrounding shell of reactive bone.

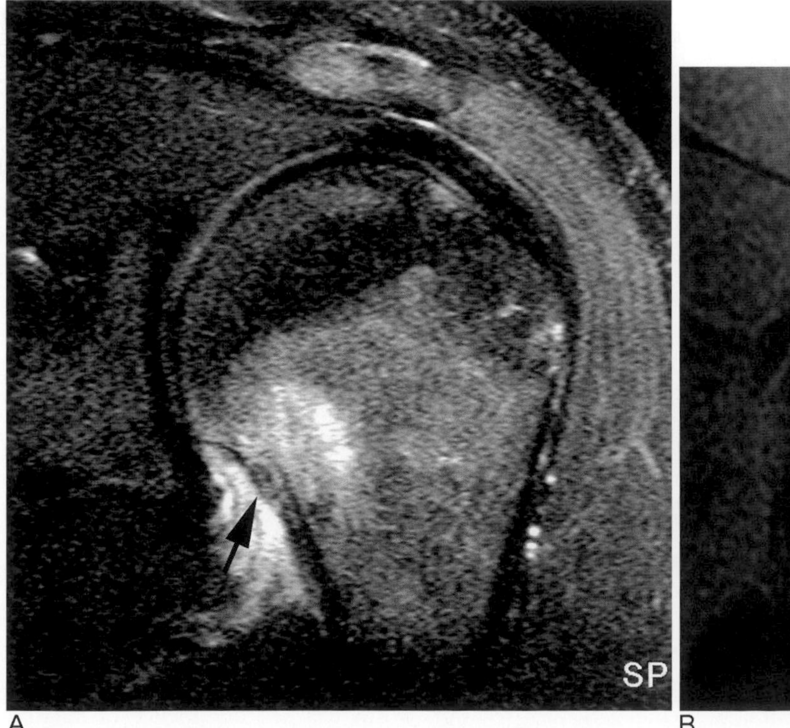

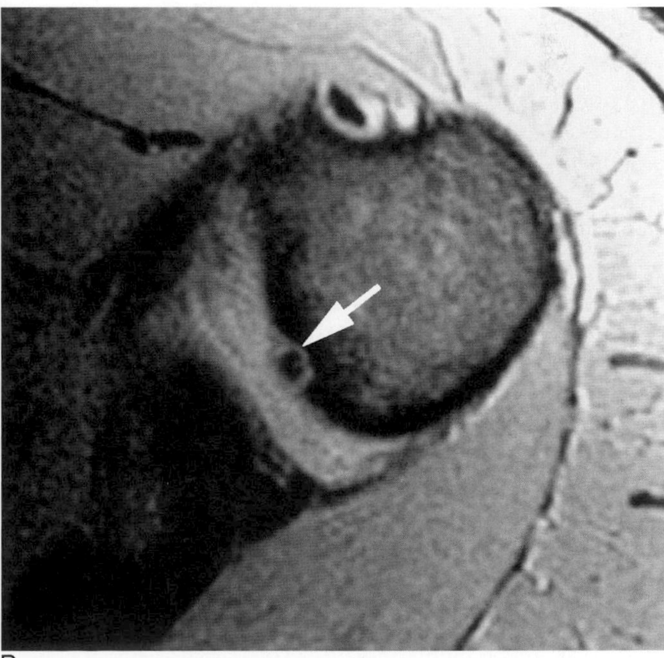

Figure 47.22 Osteoid osteoma of the proximal humerus. MRI features. (A) Coronal fat-suppressed T2-weighted fast spin-echo MRI shows a hypointense nidus (arrow) with adjacent reactive soft tissue and medullary oedema. (B) Axial T2*-weighted gradient-echo MRI shows the nidus in a medial subperiosteal location (arrow).

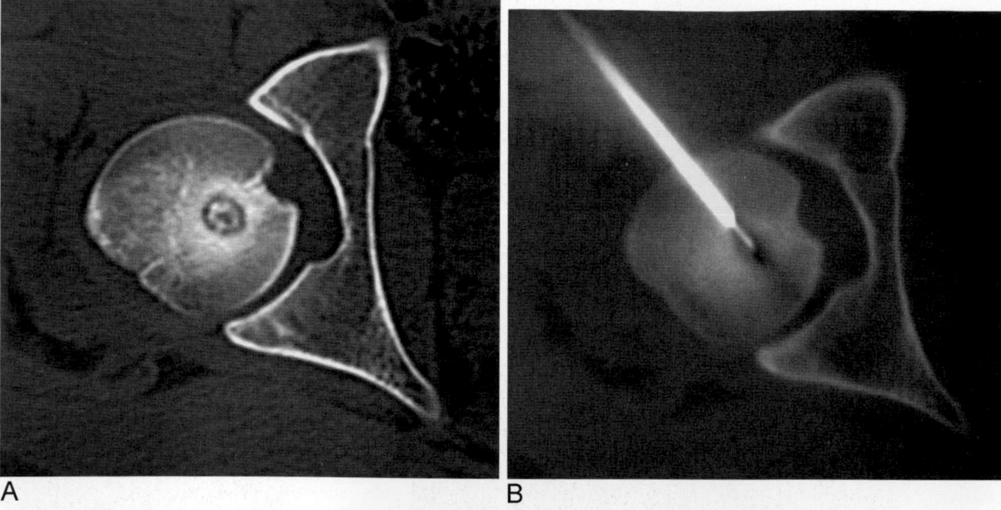

Figure 47.23 Radiofrequency ablation for osteoid osteoma of the femoral head. (A) Axial CT shows typical appearances of a calcified nidus. (B) CT showing radiofrequency ablation of the lesion.

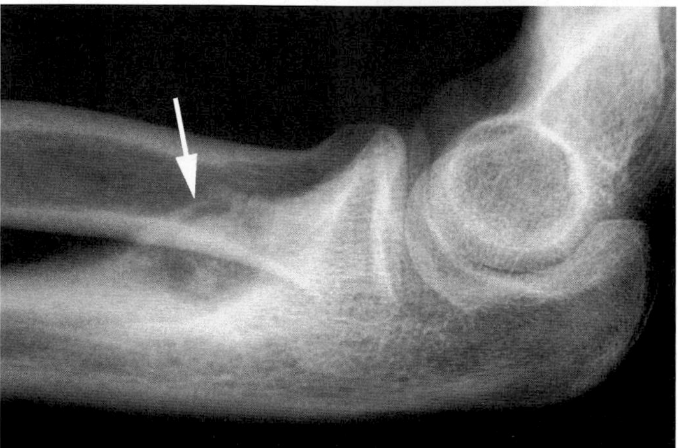

Figure 47.24 Osteoblastoma of the proximal ulna. Lateral radiograph shows a calcified, expanded lytic lesion (arrow) with surrounding reactive medullary sclerosis.

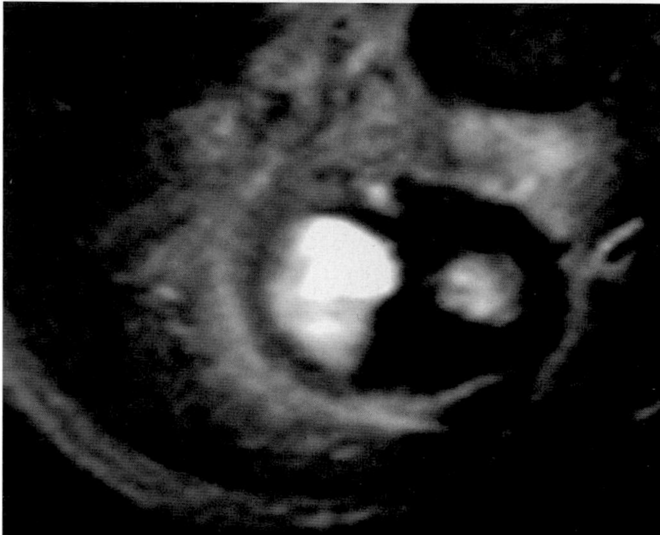

Figure 47.25 Osteoblastoma of the proximal ulna. Axial STIR MRI showing fluid levels indicative of secondary aneurysmal bone cyst change. Note also extensive reactive soft tissue oedema.

Osteoblastoma can also produce an extracortical mass, which may be reactive or due to tumour extension and may result in spinal cord compression. As with osteoid osteoma, scintigraphy is always positive and the MRI features are dominated by the reactive marrow and soft tissue changes, which may extend across several vertebral levels[33]. MRI may also demonstrate secondary ABC change (Fig. 47.25).

In long bones, the differential diagnosis includes Brodie's abscess, chondromyxoid fibroma and LCH.

CYSTIC LESIONS OF BONE[34]

Simple bone cyst[35]

Simple bone cyst (SBC—unicameral bone cyst) is a lesion of unknown aetiology and is not considered truly neoplastic. By definition, these cysts are solitary, but not always unilocular. Most occur between the ages of 5 and 15 years with less than 15% reported over the age of 20 years. The male to female ratio is 2.5:1 and presentation with pathological fracture is classical, especially with humeral lesions.

The proximal humerus is by far the commonest site (over 60% of cases), followed by the proximal femur (approximately 30% of cases). Other reported sites, which tend to affect adults, include the distal calcaneus and the ilium adjacent to the sacroiliac joint.

Radiological features

Initially, SBC is located in the proximal metaphysis of the humerus or femur and progresses into the diaphysis with skeletal growth (Fig. 47.26). Eventually, they may reach the junction of the middle and distal thirds of the shaft, by which time they are usually healed. Occasionally, the cyst adheres to the growth plate and extension into the epiphysis/apophysis is reported in 2% of lesions. SBC usually lies centrally in the shaft, expanding the bone symmetrically and thinning the cortex. The lesion is typically 6–8 cm in size. Apparent trabeculation is common, but periosteal reaction is not seen in the absence of fracture. Fracture may result in a fragment of cortex penetrating the cyst lining, resulting in the 'falling fragment' sign, in which movement of the bone fragment in response to gravity definitively

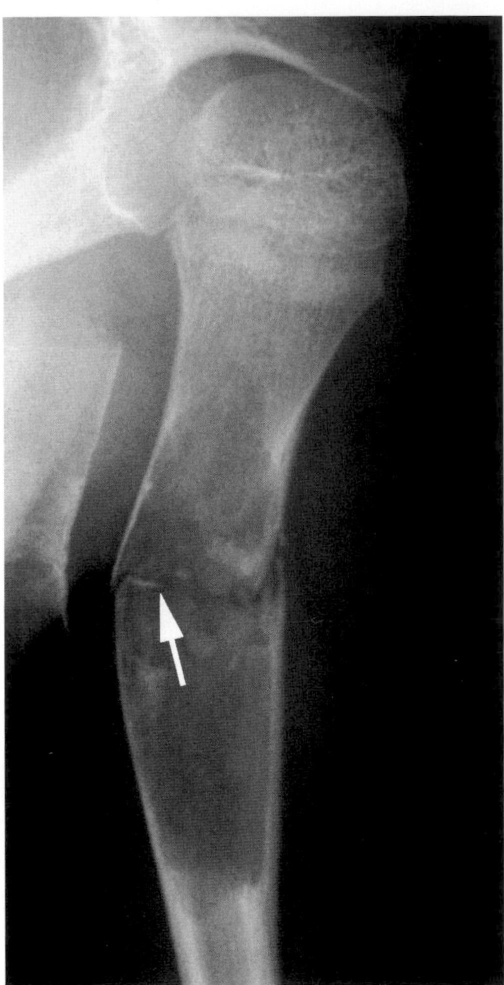

Figure 47.26 **Simple bone cyst.** AP radiograph of the left arm showing a fractured proximal humeral simple bone cyst with a 'fallen fragment' (arrow).

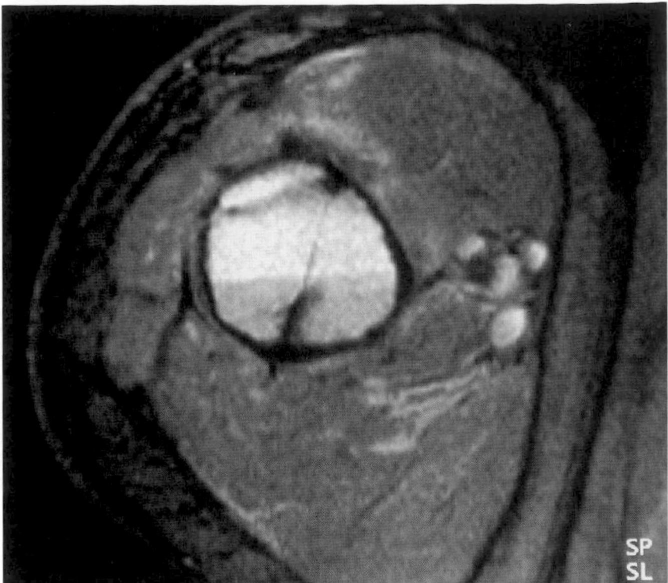

Figure 47.27 **Simple bone cyst of the proximal humerus.** Axial T2-weighted fast spin-echo MRI shows fluid levels indicative of previous fracture.

establishes the diagnosis of a cystic lesion. However, this sign is reported in only 5% of cases.

MRI demonstrates the fluid content of the lesion, homogeneous low to intermediate SI on T1-weighted images (although mild hyperintensity due to a high protein content may be seen) and marked hyperintensity on T2-weighted or STIR images. These appearances are altered by the presence of fracture, in which case haemorrhage may result in the presence of fluid–fluid levels (Fig. 47.27) and pericystic oedema[36].

The major differential diagnosis includes ABC and fibrous dysplasia.

Aneurysmal bone cyst[37]

Recent cytogenetic studies indicate that primary aneurysmal bone cyst (ABC) represents a true neoplasm, rather than a benign reactive lesion. Secondary ABC change can develop in a variety of preceding benign or malignant lesions, including nonossifying fibroma, chondroblastoma, giant cell tumour, fibrous dysplasia, osteoblastoma and osteosarcoma.

Primary ABC accounts for 1–2% of all primary bone lesions and usually presents in the second decade, with 70–80% occurring between 5 and 20 years of age. The male to female ratio is equal. ABC can involve many sites, but the long bones (over 50% of cases) and spine (20% of cases) are most common. Involvement of flat bones is most common in the pelvis. Vertebral lesions may result in structural scoliosis or neurological symptoms including paraparesis.

Radiological features[38]

The classical lesion (accounting for 75–80% of cases) is a purely lytic, expanding intramedullary lesion in the metaphysis of a long bone extending to the growth plate (Fig. 47.28).

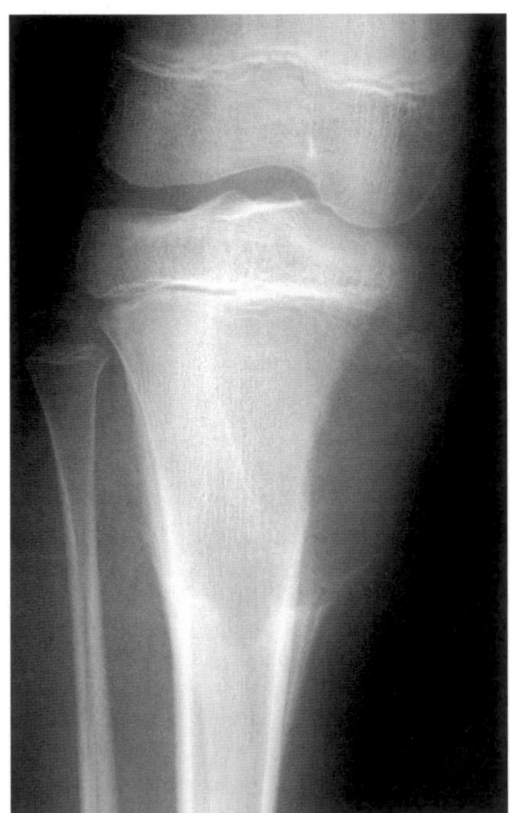

Figure 47.28 AP radiograph showing an aneurysmal bone cyst of the proximal tibial metaphysis.

The lesion may be central or, more commonly, eccentric. Twenty per cent of long bone ABCs involve the diaphysis. A thin 'egg-shell' covering of expanded cortex is often identified, particularly with CT, which may also demonstrate fine septal ossification (Fig. 47.29). Apparent trabeculation due to ridging of the endosteal cortex is also a feature, as is marginal periosteal reaction. Intracortical or subperiosteal ABC is also observed (Fig. 47.30)[39]. In the spine, ABCs usually arise in the neural arch, commonly with extension into the vertebral body, when unilateral collapse can result in structural scoliosis.

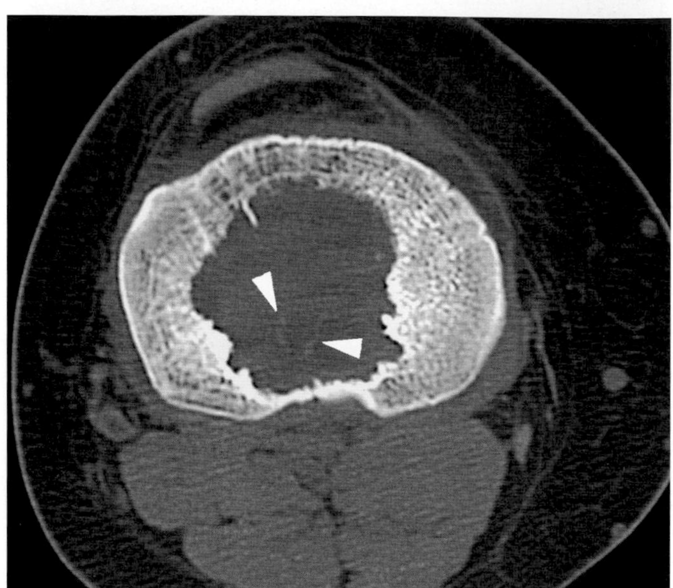

Figure 47.29 CT showing a proximal tibial aneurysmal bone cyst with evidence of faint septal ossification (arrowheads).

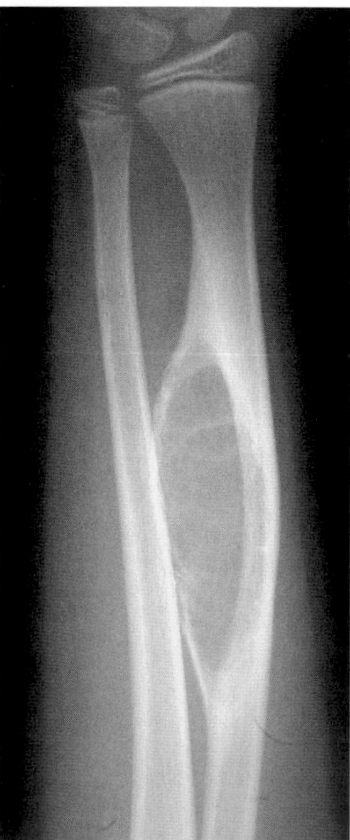

Figure 47.30 AP radiograph of the forearm showing a subperiosteal aneurysmal bone cyst of the radius.

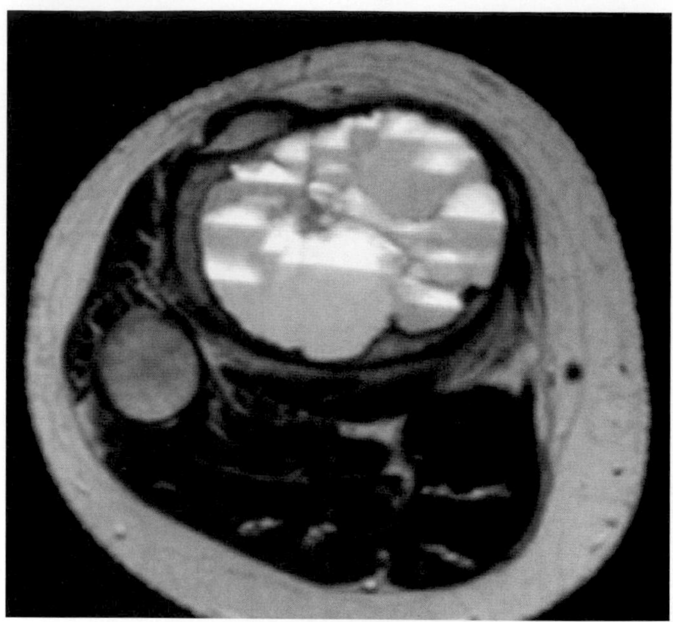

Figure 47.31 Axial T2-weighted fast spin-echo MRI showing multiple fluid levels in a proximal tibial aneurysmal bone cyst.

With CT and particularly T2-weighted MRI, fluid–fluid levels may be identified (Fig. 47.31). The lesion commonly shows a thin rim and internal septa, which may enhance following gadolinium. Reactive medullary oedema is also a frequent feature. The absence of fluid levels may indicate a 'solid' variant of ABC, which is most commonly reported in the long bones[40].

The most important differential diagnosis of ABC is telangiectatic osteosarcoma.

Giant cell tumour[41]

Giant cell tumour (GCT) is an aggressive benign neoplasm accounting for approximately 5% of primary bone tumours and 20% of benign neoplasms. However, malignant change in GCT is recognized, being either primary or secondary[42], and benign lesions may rarely metastasize to the lungs[43]. Multifocal, metachronous GCT has also been reported[44], in which case hyperparathyroidism must be excluded. GCT can also complicate Paget's disease of bone. Approximately 80% occur between 18 and 45 years of age with the male to female ratio being 2:3. The tumour nearly always occurs in a subarticular or subcortical region (adjacent to a fused apophysis) of a long bone, with the knee (distal femur and proximal tibia—55%), distal radius (10%) and proximal humerus (6%) being the commonest sites. The sacrum (7% of cases) is the most frequently affected site in the spine. Unlike most benign spinal tumours, GCT primarily involves the vertebral body rather than the neural arch.

Radiological features

GCT is classically a subarticular, eccentric, lytic lesion with a geographic, non-sclerotic margin. However, a poorly defined margin indicative of a more aggressive lesion may be identified in 10–15% of cases. Involvement of the subchondral or apophyseal bone is seen in 95–99% of GCTs at presentation, although lesions arising in the immature skeleton involve the metaphysis adjacent to the growth plate. The tumour usually measures 5–7 cm in size at presentation. Apparent trabeculation and cortical expansion are common features (Fig. 47.32) but periosteal reaction is seen in 10–15% of cases, indicating healing of a pathological fracture. Cortical destruction with extra-osseous extension may occur in up to 50% of cases. Sacral lesions typically present as lytic destructive lesions extending to the margin of the sacroiliac joint (Fig. 47.33).

On MRI, the tumour is iso- or hypointense on T1-weighted images and shows heterogeneous hyperintensity on STIR images. Areas of hyperintensity on T1 weighting indicate the presence of haemorrhage. Profound hypointensity on T2-weighted images in solid areas of the tumour is seen in the majority of cases, being due to the deposition of haemosiderin from chronic recurrent haemorrhage (Fig. 47.34). Marrow

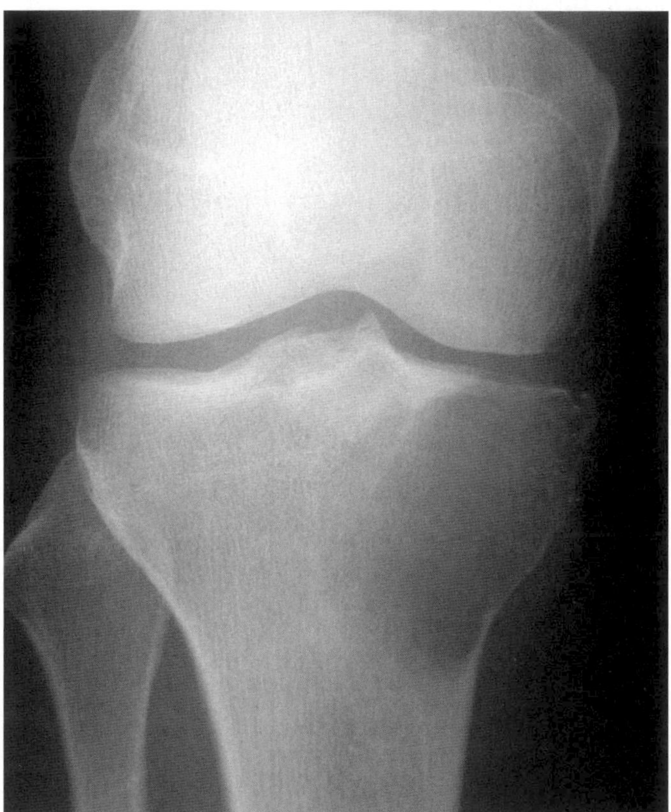

Figure 47.32 AP radiograph of the knee showing a proximal tibial giant cell tumour. Note the eccentric subarticular location.

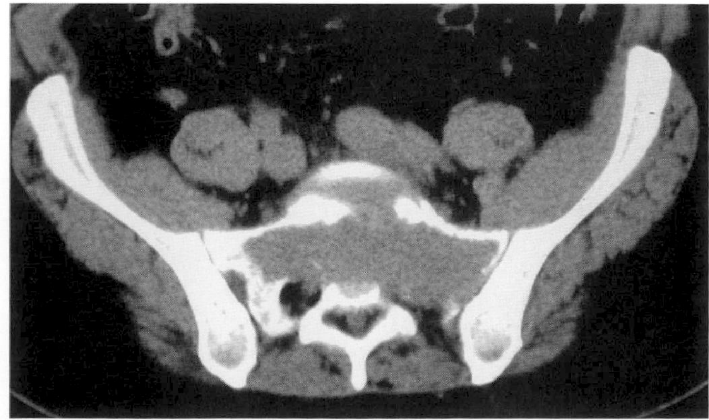

Figure 47.33 CT of the sacrum showing a giant cell tumour. Note the extension to the left sacroiliac joint.

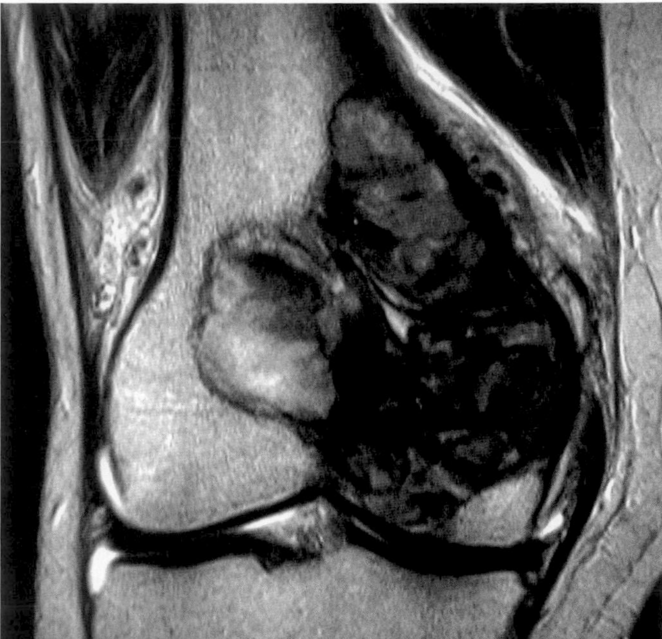

Figure 47.34 Coronal T2-weighted fast spin-echo MRI showing a distal femoral giant cell tumour with predominantly low SI due to haemosiderin deposition from chronic haemorrhage.

oedema is also demonstrated, while fluid–fluid levels indicate the presence of secondary ABC change, which is reported in approximately 15% of cases. Malignant GCT has no characteristic distinguishing features.

The most important differential diagnostic considerations are lytic osteosarcoma and, in older patients, malignant fibrous histiocytoma or lytic metastasis, particularly from a primary renal tumour.

FIBROUS ORIGIN[45]

Fibrous cortical defect

Fibrous cortical defect (FCD) is common in childhood and can almost be regarded as a normal variant, possibly due to a growth disturbance related to subclinical injury at a tendon insertion. FCD is most commonly identified in the distal femoral and proximal tibial metaphyses as an incidental finding. It has the same appearance, location and histology as a nonossifying fibroma, the lesions differing only in their size, with FCD usually 1–1.5 cm in maximal dimensions (Fig. 47.35). FCD typically disappears with time.

Nonossifying fibroma

Nonossifying fibroma (NOF—fibroxanthoma) is considered a benign neoplasm, with symptoms typically arising when it is large enough to cause pathological fracture. Most patients present in the second decade of life, but some NOFs have been reported presenting as late as the fifth decade. A slight male preponderance is recorded and the majority (90%) involve the lower limbs, particularly the tibia and distal end of the femur.

Multiple lesions are found and occasionally a familial incidence is reported. An association with neurofibromatosis (5%) may be present in such cases[46]. The Jaffe–Campanacci

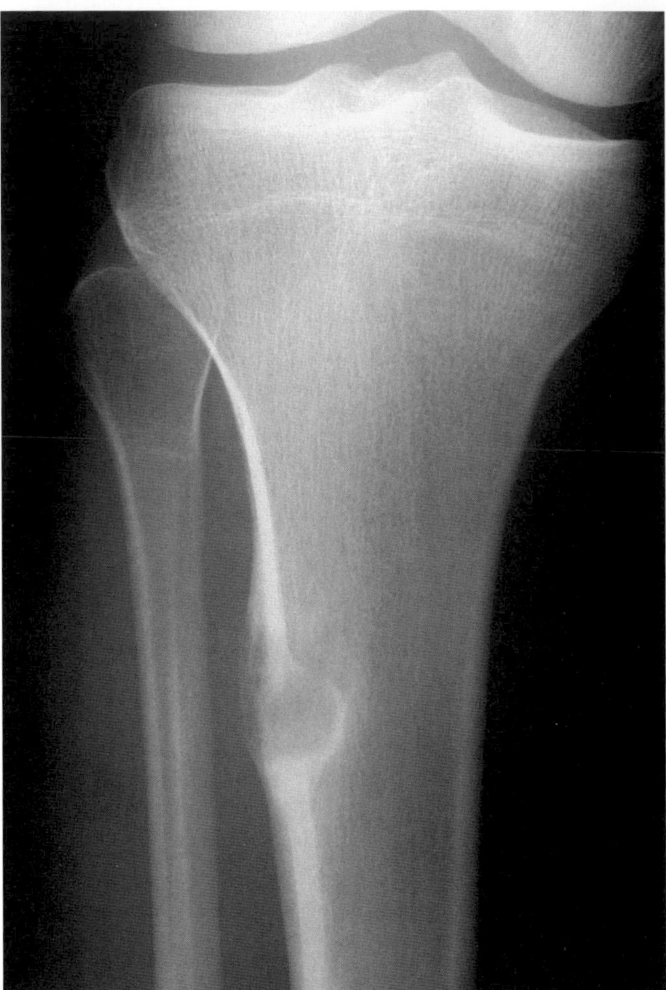

Figure 47.35 AP radiograph of the proximal tibia showing a diaphyseal fibrous cortical defect. Note the ground-glass appearance of the matrix.

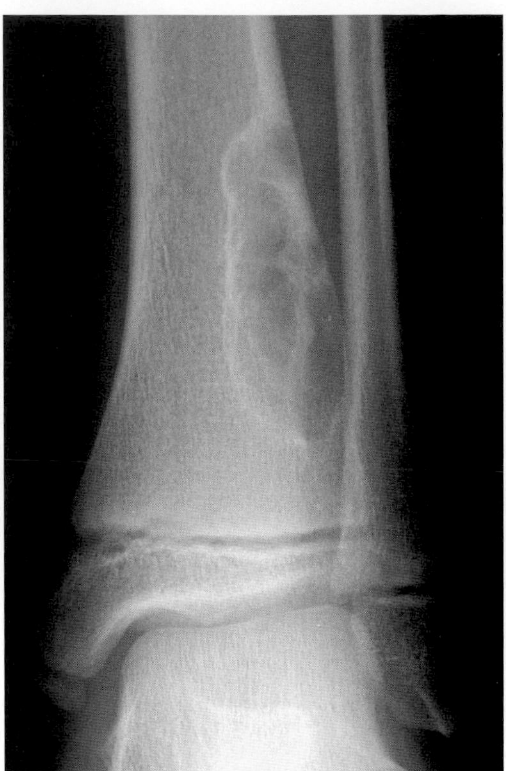

Figure 47.36 AP radiograph of the ankle showing a classical distal tibial nonossifying fibroma.

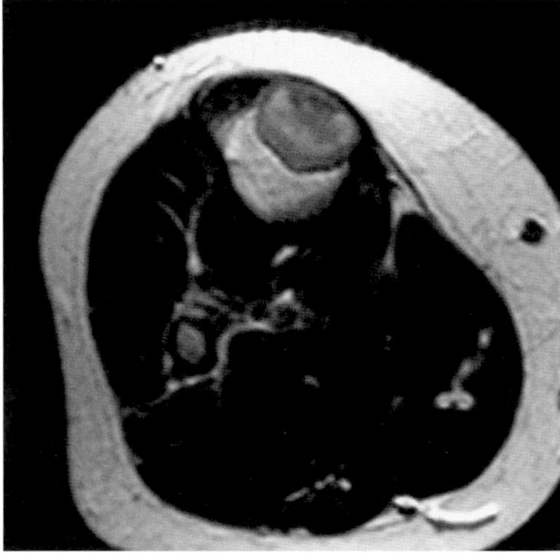

Figure 47.37 Axial T2-weighted MRI showing a proximal tibial nonossifying fibroma with relatively low SI due to its fibrous nature.

syndrome consists of multiple (usually unilateral) NOFs with café-au-lait spots but no other stigmata of neurofibromatosis. NOF can usually be diagnosed radiologically, in which case biopsy is unnecessary.

Radiological features

The lesions are metaphyseal or diametaphyseal and essentially intracortical. A lobulated 'soap bubble' appearance is classical, with the lesion usually enlarging into the medullary cavity. The tumour is oval with its long axis in the line of the bone (Fig. 47.36). When NOF arises in a slim bone such as the fibula, it crosses the shaft readily and its characteristic intracortical origin is less obvious. It may then resemble other entities, such as ABC. Periosteal reaction is typically seen only after fracture.

On MRI, NOF shows intermediate SI on T1-weighted images and enhances following intravenous gadolinium. On T2-weighted images (Fig. 47.37), approximately 80% are hypointense, but with marginal or septal hyperintensity, and the remainder are hyperintense. Marginal sclerosis appears as a hypointense rim[47].

Benign fibrous histiocytoma[48]

Benign fibrous histiocytoma (BFH) is an uncommon lesion having the same histology as that of a NOF, but occurring in an older age group and in a different location. BFH presents between 20 and 50 years, with a mean age in the third decade. The male to female ratio is equal.

Radiological features

Most frequently the lesion resembles a giant cell tumour, occurring in an eccentric subarticular location, but with a well-defined sclerotic margin, indicating slower growth (Fig. 47.38). About one-third occur on either side of the knee. The MRI features are also similar to GCT.

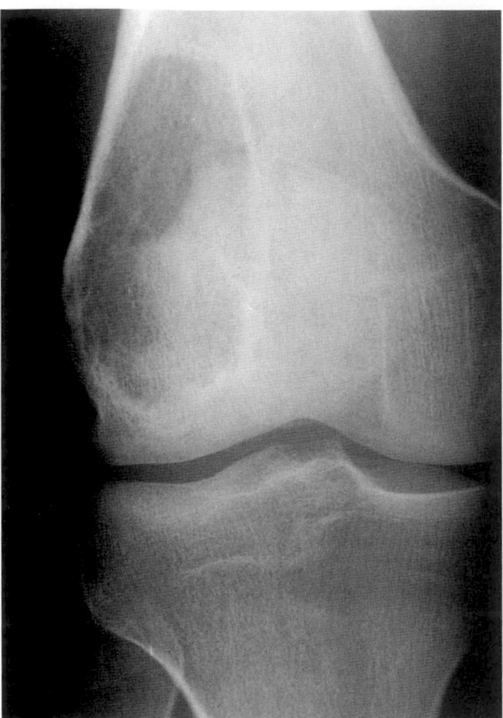

Figure 47.38 AP radiograph of the distal femur showing a benign fibrous histiocytoma.

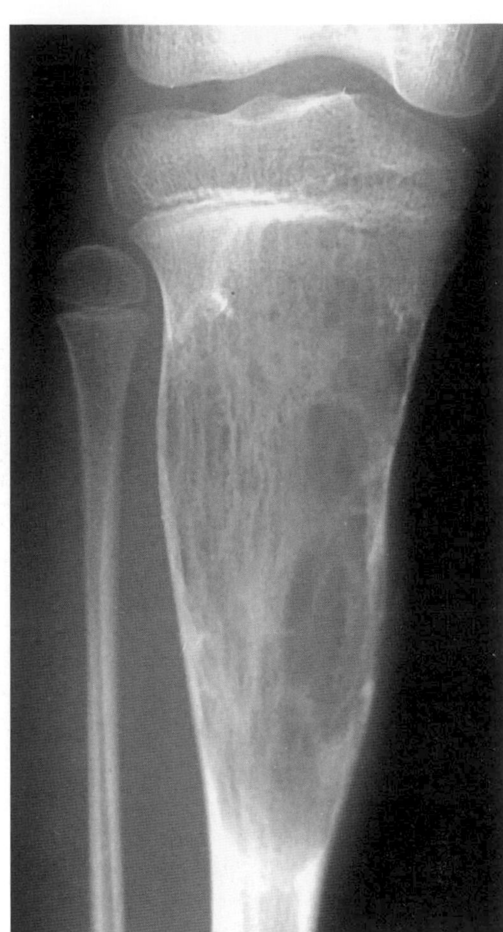

Figure 47.39 AP radiograph of the proximal tibia showing a desmoplastic fibroma.

Desmoplastic fibroma (desmoid tumour)[49]

Desmoplastic fibroma is a rare, locally aggressive benign neoplasm with similar histological features to soft tissue fibromatosis. It accounts for 0.06% of all bone tumours and 0.3% of benign bone neoplasms. Seventy per cent of cases present between 10 and 30 years of age (mean age 21 years) with no particular difference between men and women. Desmoplastic fibroma usually arises in the metaphyseal regions of long bones (femur, humerus, tibia and radius constitute 56% of cases), the mandible (26%) and ilium (14%). It is rarely associated with fibrous dysplasia.

Radiological features

Most lesions are diametaphyseal and arise as either subperiosteal or intraosseous tumours. Many are large at presentation (over 50 mm in diameter) and two patterns are seen, an ill-defined moth-eaten or permeative lesion and an expanding, trabeculated lesion (Fig. 47.39). The MRI features are non-specific, showing heterogeneous intermediate SI on T1-weighted and hyperintensity on T2-weighted images with irregular enhancement following gadolinium[50]. When the soft tissues are invaded, it may be difficult to distinguish from bony invasion by soft tissue fibromatosis. Although desmoplastic fibroma is considered a benign lesion, metastasis has been reported following local recurrence.

Post-traumatic cortical desmoid (avulsive cortical irregularity, Bufkin lesion)

Described by Bufkin in 1971[51], this benign lesion probably results from chronic avulsive stress at the femoral origin of the medial head of gastrocnemius. The lesion is usually an incidental finding, but may cause mild pain in children, usually in the 10–15-year age group. It is twice as common in the left femur; one-third are bilateral. Similar lesions are described in the humerus at the insertions of the pectoralis major and deltoid muscles.

The characteristic site is the posterior aspect of the supracondylar ridge of the medial femoral condyle (Fig. 47.40A). Periosteal reaction is seen, but there is no soft tissue extension. On MRI (Fig. 47.40B), lesions may appear concave or convex and MRI may demonstrate radiologically occult lesions[52]. The lesion heals without treatment and can be regarded as a normal variant.

VASCULAR TUMOURS[53,54]

Haemangioma and lymphangioma

Both single and multiple haemangiomas and lymphangiomas occur in bone and may be regarded as congenital vascular malformations. However, many present as isolated bone lesions and are therefore included in the differential diagnosis of a bone tumour. Haemangiomas are classified histologically as capillary, cavernous, arteriovenous or venous. Osseous capillary haemangiomas most commonly affect the vertebral body, whereas osseous cavernous haemangiomas affect the skull vault.

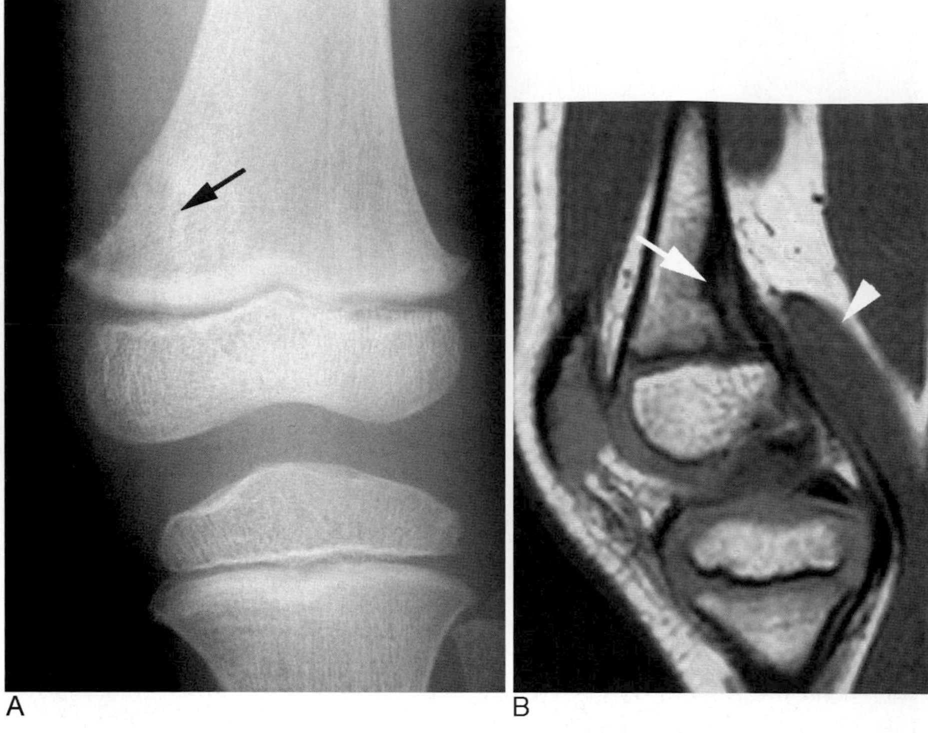

Figure 47.40 Cortical desmoid (Bufkin lesion). (A) AP radiograph of the knee showing a distal femoral metaphyseal cortical desmoid (arrow) appearing as a poorly defined lytic lesion. (B) Sagittal T1-weighted MRI showing the lesion (arrow) at the site of origin of the medial head of gastrocnemius (arrowhead).

Haemangiomas of the spine are reported in 11% of cases in large autopsy series and constitute 28% of all skeletal haemangiomas. They are multifocal in 25–30% of cases. The second commonest site is the calvaria. Vertebral and calvarial haemangiomas are commonly asymptomatic lesions. However, vertebral collapse can occur and extraosseous extension, indicating a diagnosis of aggressive haemangioma, may cause neurological complications.

Radiological features

In vertebral lesions, fine or coarse vertical trabeculation is typically seen, due to hypertrophy of the primary trabeculae and erosion of the secondary trabeculae. This appearance is mainly found in the vertebral body, but may extend into the neural arch (Fig. 47.41A). Similar striated lesions are found in the epiphyses and metaphyses of long bones with the direction of the linear striations running along the axis of the bone. Occasionally, well-defined vascular channels may be evident (Fig. 47.41B). CT shows the thickened trabeculation as dense 'dots' within a fatty matrix (Fig. 47.42A). On MRI, vertebral haemangiomas typically show increased SI on T1- and T2-weighted images because of their increased fat content (Fig. 47.42B, C). However, vascular haemangiomas may have reduced SI on T1 weighting, in which case CT is valuable

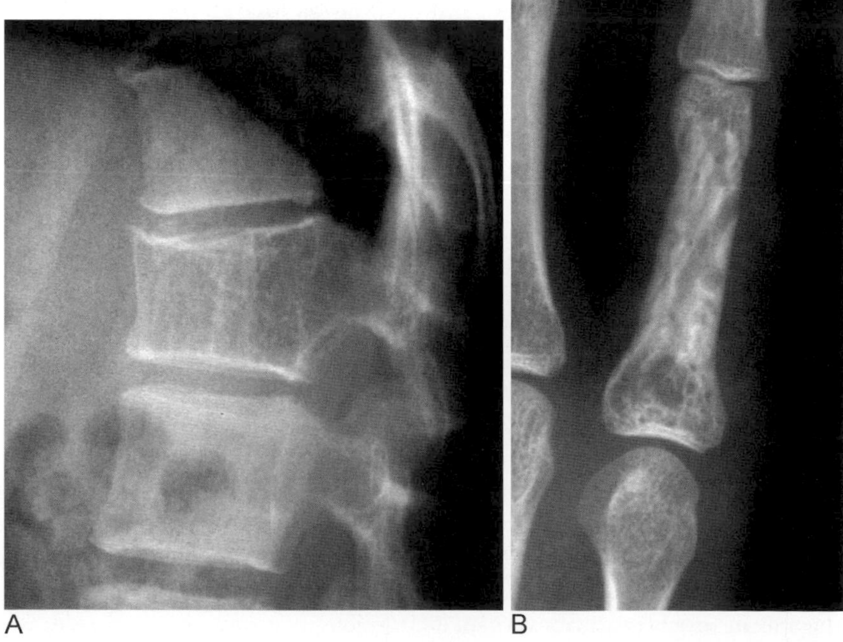

Figure 47.41 Haemangioma of bone. (A) Coned lateral radiograph of the thoraco-lumbar junction showing a diffuse haemangioma of the T12 vertebral body. (B) AP radiograph of the little finger metacarpal showing a haemangioma with multiple intraosseous vascular channels.

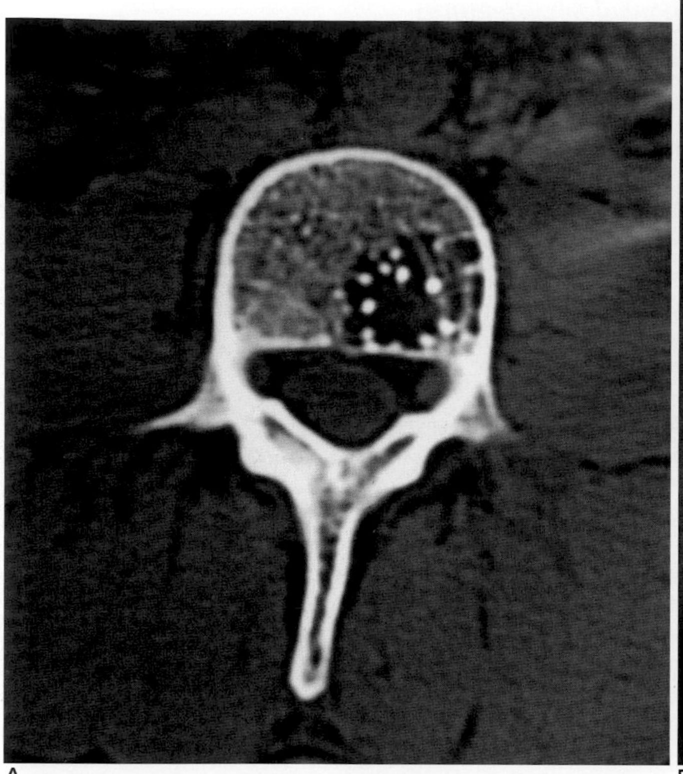

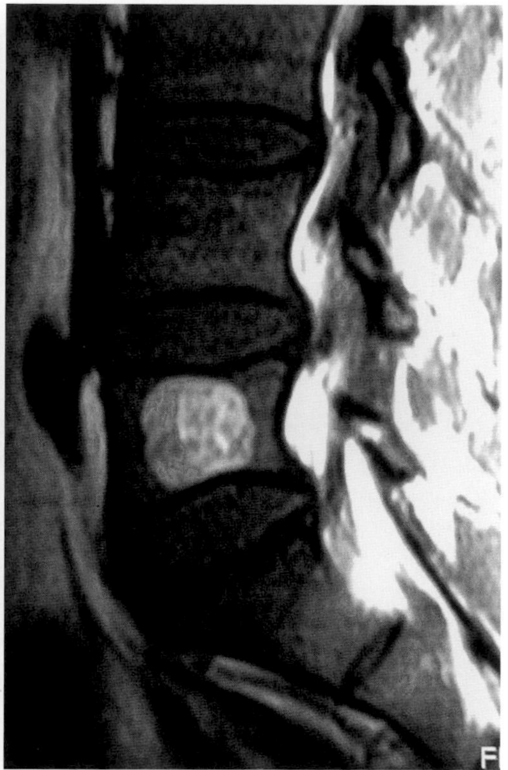

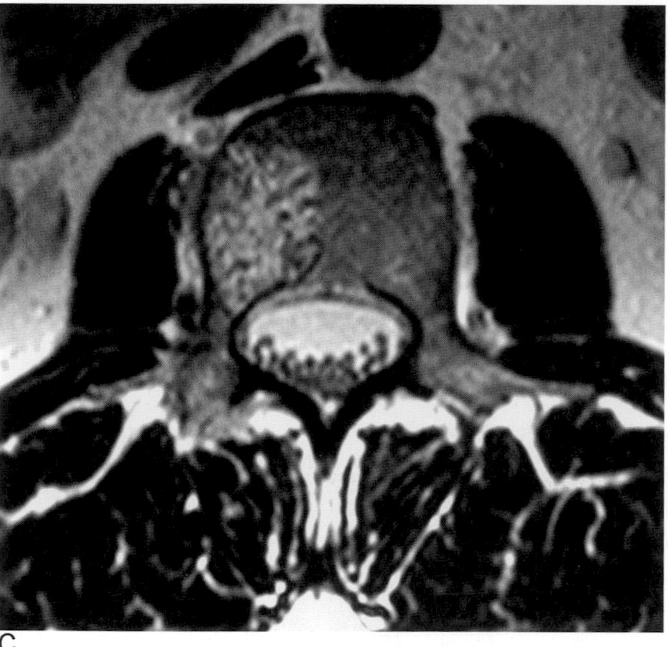

Figure 47.42 Haemangioma of bone. (A) Axial CT through the L3 vertebra showing a haemangioma with fatty matrix and thickened primary trabeculae. (B) Sagittal T1-weighted MRI of the lumbar spine showing a haemangioma of L5 with high SI due to fat. (C) Axial T2-weighted fast spin-echo MRI showing typical features of a vertebral haemangioma in the right side of L2.

in characterization by demonstrating the typical thickened trabeculae. With aggressive haemangioma, the extraosseous component shows intermediate T1-weighted SI.

In flat bones, multiple, well-defined lytic lesions produce a soap-bubble effect, while in the skull radiating mature spiculation can produce a 'sunburst' appearance (Fig. 47.43).

Cystic angiomatosis[55]

Cystic angiomatosis is a multifocal condition of either blood or lymphatic vessels. The age at presentation is variable, although 50% are diagnosed before the age of 20 years. Most patients present in adolescence due to pain and swelling as a result of enlargement of viscera, especially the spleen. Skeletal lesions are usually discovered incidentally unless pathological fracture occurs. Diffuse skeletal angiomatosis embraces these cases but covers a wider spectrum of angiomatous lesions.

Radiological features

Numerous lytic lesions are present, especially in the ribs (Fig. 47.44) and pelvis. The disease is centripetal in its distribution, with few lesions occurring distal to the elbow or knee. Individual lesions are round or oval with a fine sclerotic rim, although mainly sclerotic lesions have been reported. The prognosis of the disease is unrelated to the bone lesions and is worse with

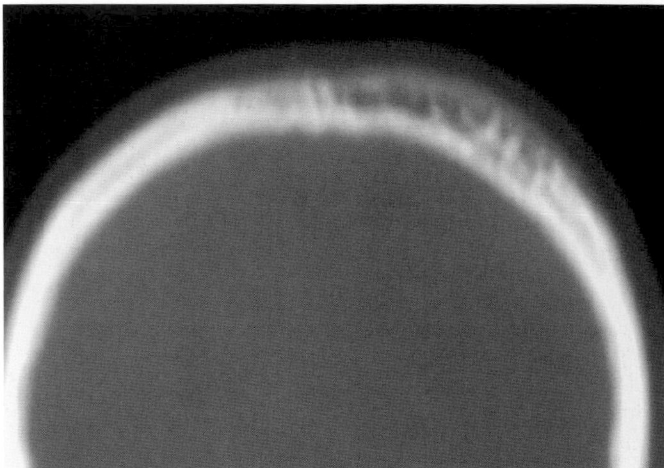

Figure 47.43 Coronal CT multiplanar reconstruction showing a haemangioma of the skull vault.

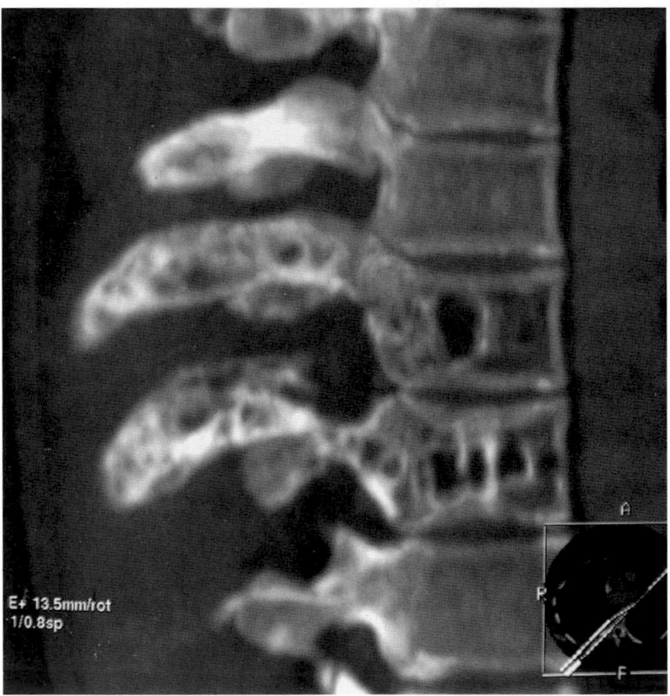

Figure 47.44 Coronal oblique CT multiplanar reconstruction showing angiomatosis affecting the vertebrae and adjacent ribs.

visceral involvement. In a proportion of patients with cystic lymphangiomatosis, chylous pleural effusions may develop.

Massive osteolysis (Gorham's disease, vanishing bone disease)

This rare, non-inheritable disorder has also been called 'haemangiomatosis'. It predominates in children and young adults and is characterized by a non-malignant proliferation of vascular or lymphatic structures of bone, which results in progressive bony destruction, often with extension into surrounding soft tissues. Commonly affected sites include the shoulder region, mandible and pelvis. Progressive resorption of a single bone occurs, but paired bones, several contiguous ribs and segments of the spine have also been affected. Spontaneous arrest is rarely reported.

Radiological features

Purely lytic destruction of the metaphysis or diaphysis of a long bone with associated cortical erosion is seen (Fig. 47.45). Subsequent pathological fracture produces little or no callus and no attempt at healing. Further resorption produces tapering of the bone ends. When the spine or thorax is involved, life may be threatened by the relentless bone destruction. Only complete excision of the affected bone can halt the progress of the disease. CT and MRI[56] are useful in delineating the local extent of the lesion but do not show any characteristic appearances except for the absence of a major soft tissue mass.

Other vascular tumours

The rare, related entities of haemangiopericytoma and glomus tumour usually arise in soft tissue and involve bone secondarily. Occasionally, a primary bony focus occurs.

MISCELLANEOUS LESIONS

Tumours of neural tissue

Both schwannoma and neurofibroma may cause pressure erosion when arising in close proximity to bone and this is particularly so with intraspinal lesions. Intraosseous benign nerve

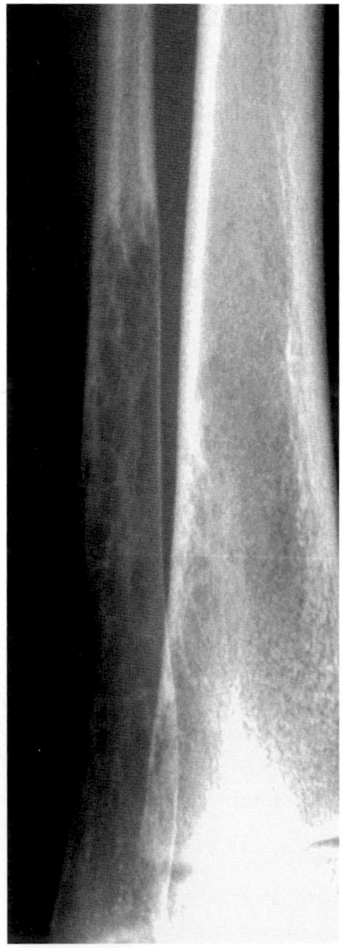

Figure 47.45 Gorham's disease of the fibula. AP radiograph showing extensive lytic destruction of the fibular metaphysis and diaphysis.

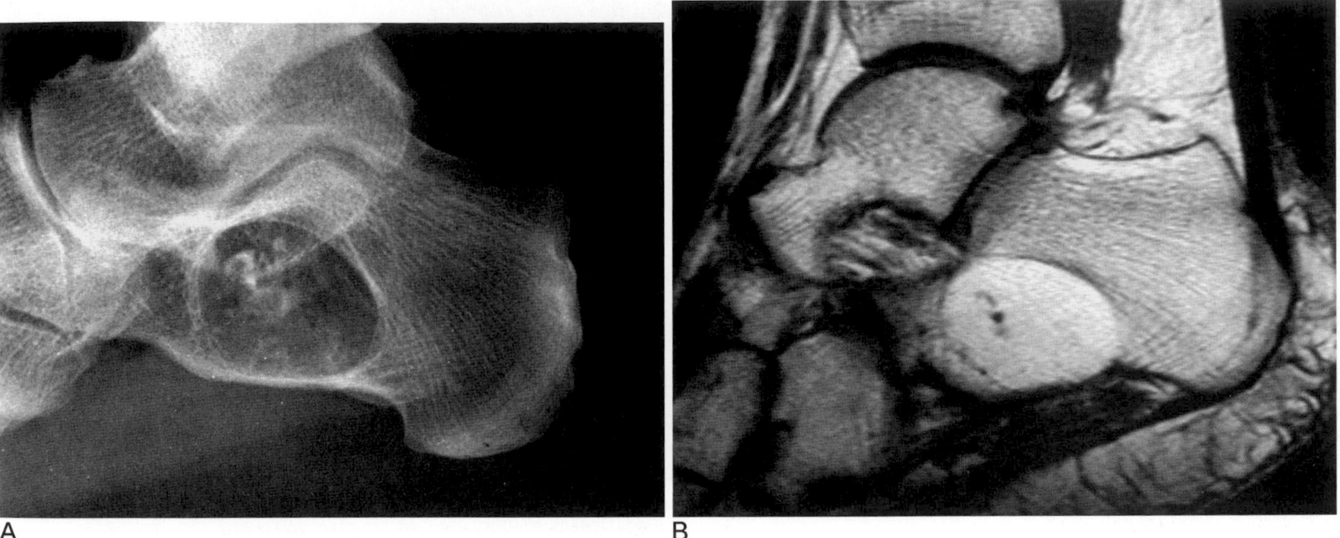

Figure 47.46 Intraosseous lipoma of the calcaneus. (A) Lateral radiograph showing a geographic, calcified lytic lesion. (B) Sagittal T1-weighted spin-echo MRI showing the hyperintense fatty nature of the lesion.

sheath tumours are very rare and most commonly involve the jaw. Lesions arising in the appendicular skeleton are extremely rare and show no diagnostic radiological features[57].

It should be noted that in neurofibromatosis, skeletal lesions such as the classical pseudarthrosis of the tibia or spinal deformity[58] are rarely due to intraosseous neural tissue, but are related to the overall mesenchymal disturbance.

Lipomatous lesions of bone

Two types of this rare benign lesion of bone occur:

1 True intraosseous lipoma[59] arises in the medulla and produces expansion, sometimes with endosteal scalloping and trabeculation, resembling a cyst or even fibrous dysplasia. Calcification is also seen. Most affect the lower limb, with a predilection for the calcaneus (Fig. 47.46A). CT and MRI aid in diagnosis by demonstrating the fatty nature of the matrix (Fig. 47.46B).

2 Parosteal lipoma[60], which may cause benign pressure erosion of the bone and the formation of circumferential periosteal new bone (Fig. 47.47). The combination of such peripheral ossification with a tumour of otherwise fatty matrix establishes the radiological diagnosis.

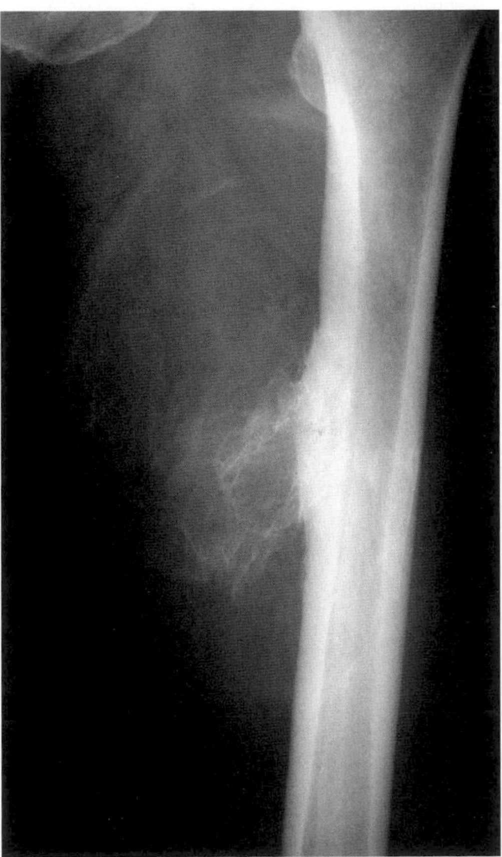

Figure 47.47 AP radiograph of the proximal thigh showing a parosteal lipoma of the femur.

TUMOUR-LIKE DISORDERS

Implantation epidermoid

This lesion is a cyst lined by epidermis and containing exfoliated squames. It is almost always confined to a terminal phalanx in the hand and sometimes associated with a previous history of a penetrating injury to the digit[61].

Radiologically, usually a slightly expanded terminal phalanx contains a well-defined round lytic lesion; however, the lesion can sometimes occur elsewhere in the skeleton (Fig. 47.48). The cortex is not always intact on both sides and pathological fracture may occur. The differential diagnosis includes

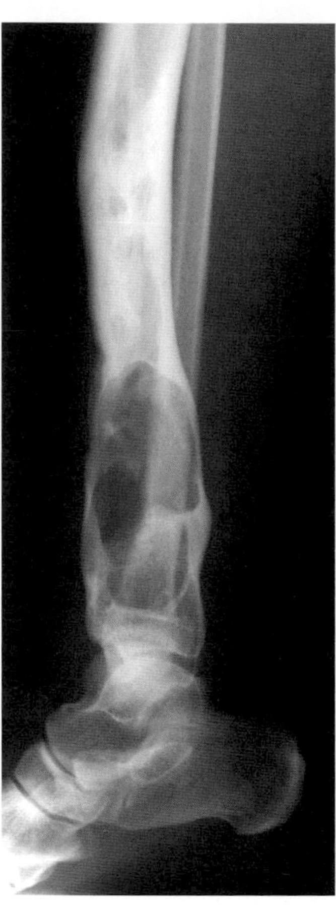

Figure 47.48 Lateral radiograph of the distal tibia showing a large implantation epidermoid.

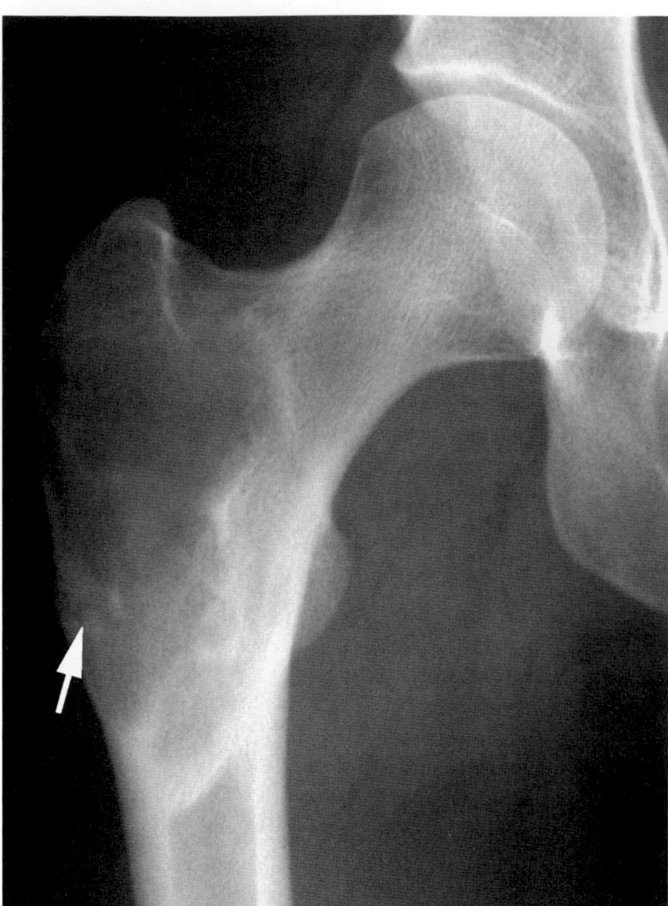

Figure 47.49 Fibrous dysplasia. AP radiograph of the proximal femur showing a well-defined expanded lesion with typical ground-glass matrix mineralization and a thick, sclerotic margin (rind sign). A stress fracture is present in the lateral cortex (arrow).

enchondroma, which, however, rarely presents in the terminal phalanx.

Fibrous dysplasia[62]

Fibrous dysplasia (FD) is a developmental disorder of bone accounting for 7% of benign bone tumours and may be either monostotic (70–85%) or polyostotic. Unlike many bone tumours, however, FD is usually painless unless a fracture has occurred. Seventy-five per cent of cases present before the age of 30 years and there is no sex predilection. The commonest sites of monostotic FD are the ribs (28%), proximal femur (23%) and craniofacial bones (20%). Polyostotic FD may range from the involvement of two bones to more than 75% of the skeleton.

Approximately 30–50% of patients with polyostotic disease have café-au-lait spots. FD may be associated with a variety of syndromes. McCune–Albright syndrome consists of polyostotic FD (typically unilateral), ipsilateral café-au-lait spots and endocrine disturbance, most commonly precocious puberty in girls. Mazabraud's syndrome consists of FD (most commonly polyostotic) and soft tissue myxomata.

Radiological features

Radiologically, FD presents as a geographic lesion that may cause bone expansion and deformity with diffuse ground-glass matrix mineralization. A thick sclerotic margin ('rind' sign) is characteristic (Fig. 47.49). The metadiaphyseal region is typically affected in long bones. Periosteal reaction is not a feature in the absence of fracture. Varus deformity of the proximal femur (shepherd's crook deformity) is a characteristic late finding.

Scintigraphy is the best technique for identifying polyostotic disease (Fig. 47.50). On MRI[63], lesions are hypointense on T1W and either hypointense or hyperintense on T2W. Mild hyperintensity on T1W may be due to haemorrhage. Internal septations and cystic change with fluid levels may all be seen. Following intravenous contrast medium, either uniform or septal enhancement is described.

The identification of associated chondroid calcification (Fig. 47.51) indicates a diagnosis of fibrocartilaginous dysplasia[64]. Malignant change in fibrous dysplasia is rare, being reported in 0.5% of cases. It is more common in polyostotic disease and may follow prior radiotherapy.

Osteofibrous dysplasia[65]

Osteofibrous dysplasia[66] (OFD, ossifying fibroma of Kempson) is a rare lesion that histologically resembles fibrous dysplasia and the stroma of adamantinoma. However, it has a specific clinical and radiological picture. Presentation is from birth to 40 years, with almost 50% occurring under the age of 10 years. The male to female ratio is equal. The tibia is affected

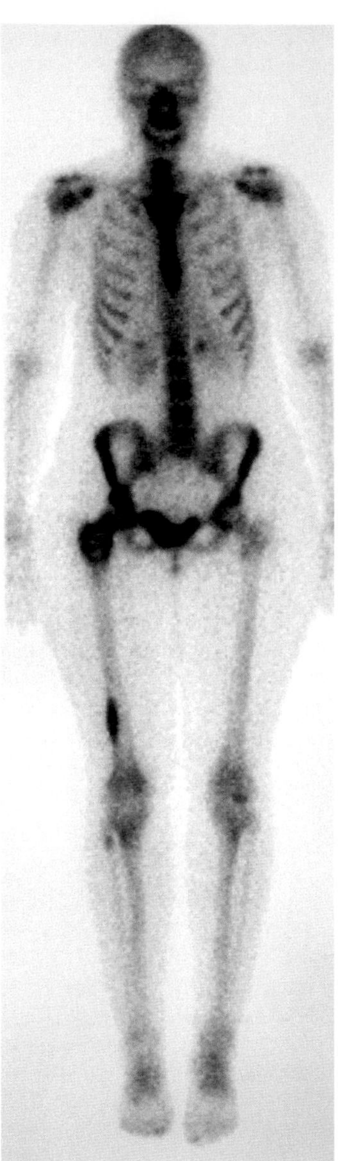

Figure 47.50 Polyostotic fibrous dysplasia. Whole body ^{99m}Tc-MDP bone scan showing multiple lesions in the right ilium, acetabulum and femur.

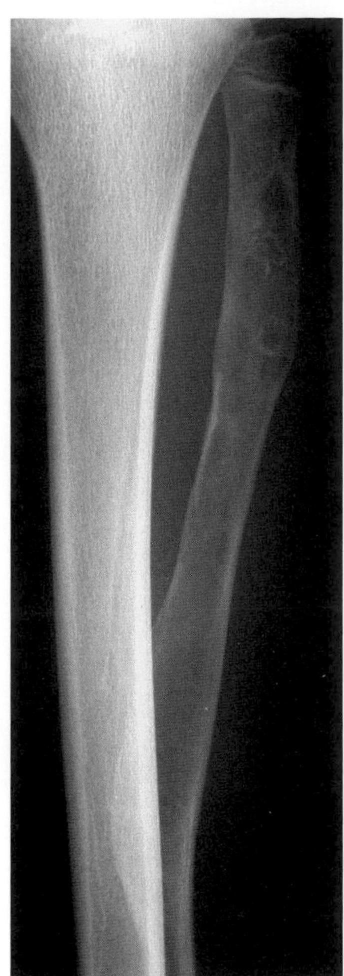

Figure 47.51 Fibrocartilaginous dysplasia. AP radiograph of the left lower limb showing changes consistent with fibrous dysplasia in the fibula, but with associated cartilaginous matrix mineralization.

in over 90% of cases and in two-thirds of these the anterior mid-diaphyseal cortex is involved. Multiple lesions may occur in the same bone, but the ipsilateral fibula is affected in 20% of cases. Bilateral involvement may be seen.

Radiological features

In early infancy the lesion expands and bows the tibia with a sclerotic rim. After 3 months of age, the lesion is eccentric, multilocular and may show a ground-glass matrix mineralization similar to FD (Fig. 47.52). Cross-sectional imaging confirms its intracortical origin, but otherwise it shows no characteristic features. The lesion is typically active on scintigraphy. If surgery can be withheld in early infancy, spontaneous healing can occur. It seems very possible that in some patients OFD is a precursor of, or at least associated with, adamantinoma.

Brown tumours of hyperparathyoidism

So-called because of their brownish appearance at surgery, due to haemorrhage and altered blood, brown tumours of hyperparathyoidism (HPT) may be single or multiple well-defined lytic lesions, comprised of fibrous tissue containing giant cells. Other features of the disease (primary or secondary HPT) are usually evident and a brown tumour is rarely the cause of presentation. Histologically, they mimic giant cell tumours and the diagnosis is established biochemically.

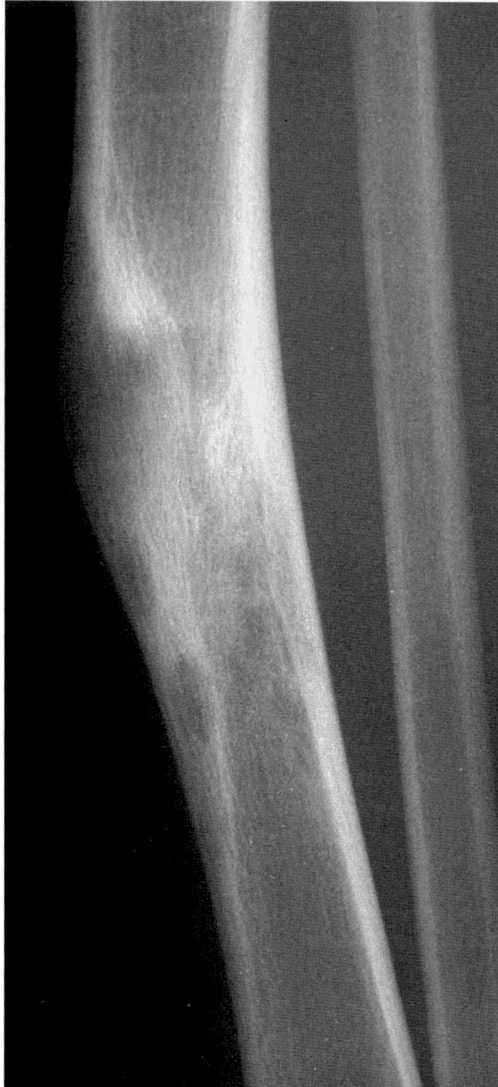

Figure 47.52 Osteofibrous dysplasia. Lateral radiograph of the tibia showing anterior cortical expansion and ground-glass mineralization.

REFERENCES

1. Lodwick G S, Wilson A J, Farrell C et al 1980 Determining bone growth rates of focal lesions of bone from radiographs. Radiology 134: 577–583.
2. Wenaden A E, Szyszko T A, Saifuddin A 2005 Imaging of periosteal reactions associated with focal lesions of bone. Clin Radiol 60: 439–456.
3. Saifuddin A 2002 The accuracy of imaging in the local staging of appendicular osteosarcoma. Skeletal Radiol 31: 191–201.
4. van der Woude H J, Bloem J L, Hogendoorn P C 1998 Preoperative evaluation and monitoring chemotherapy in patients with high-grade osteogenic and Ewing's sarcoma: review of current imaging modalities. Skeletal Radiol 27: 57–71.
5. O'Donnell P, Saifuddin A 2004 The prevalence and diagnostic significance of fluid–fluid levels in focal lesions of bone. Skeletal Radiol 33: 330–336.
6. Choi JA, Lee KH, Jun WS et al 2003 Osseous metastasis from renal cell carcinoma: "flow-void" sign at MR imaging. Radiology 228: 629–634.
7. Azouz EM 2002 Magnetic resonance imaging of benign bone lesions: cysts and tumors. Top Magn Reson Imaging 13: 219–229.
8. Daldrup-Link H E, Franzius C, Link T M et al 2001 Whole-body MR imaging for detection of bone metastases in children and young adults: comparison with skeletal scintigraphy and FDG PET. AJR Am J Roentgenol 177: 229–236.
9. Wang C K, Li C W, Hsieh T J et al 2004 Characterization of bone and soft-tissue tumors with in vivo 1H MR spectroscopy: initial results. Radiology 232: 599–605.
10. Even-Sapir E, Metser U, Flusser G et al 2004 Assessment of malignant skeletal disease: initial experience with 18F-fluoride PET/CT and comparison between 18F-fluoride PET and 18F-fluoride PET/CT. J Nucl Med 45: 272–278.
11. Saifuddin A, Mitchell R, Burnett S J, Sandison A, Pringle J A 2000 Ultrasound-guided needle biopsy of primary bone tumours. J Bone Joint Surg Br 82: 50–54.
12. Jelinek J S, Murphey M D, Welker J A 2002 Diagnosis of primary bone tumors with image-guided percutaneous biopsy: experience with 110 tumors. Radiology 223: 731–737.
13. Robbin M R, Murphey M D 2000 Benign chondroid neoplasms of bone. Semin Musculoskelet Radiol 4: 45–58.
14. Unni K K 1996 Dahlin's Bone tumors, 5th edn. Lippincott-Raven, Philadelphia.
15. Murphey M D, Flemming D J, Boyea SR, Bojescul J A, Sweet D E, Temple H T 1998 Enchondroma versus chondrosarcoma in the appendicular skeleton: differentiating features. Radiographics 18: 1213–1237.
16. De Beuckeler L H, De Schepper A M, Ramon F, Somville J 1995 Magnetic resonance imaging of cartilaginous tumors: a retrospective study of 79 patients. Eur J Radiol 21: 34–40.
17. Robinson P, White L M, Sundaram M et al 2001 Periosteal chondroid tumors: radiological evaluation with pathologic correlation. AJR Am J Roentgenol 177: 1183–1188.
18. Murphey M D, Choi J J, Kransdorf M J, Flemming D J, Gannon F H 2000 Imaging of osteochondroma: variants and complications with radiologic-pathologic correlation. Radiographics 20: 1407–1434.
19. Lee K C, Davies A M, Cassar-Pullicino V N 2002 Imaging the complications of osteochondromas. Clin Radiol 57: 18–28.
20. Tannenbaum D A, Biermann J S 1997 Bizarre parosteal osteochondromatous proliferation of bone. Orthopedics 20: 1186–1188.
21. Kaim A H, Hugli R, Bonel H M, Jundt G 2002 Chondroblastoma and clear cell chondrosarcoma: radiological and MRI characteristics with histopathological correlation. Skeletal Radiol 31: 88–95.
22. Wu C T, Inwards C Y, O'Laughlin S, Rock M G, Beabout J W, Unni K K 1998 Chondromyxoid fibroma of bone: a clinicopathologic review of 278 cases. Hum Pathol 29: 438–446.
23. Yamaguchi T, Dorfman H D 1998 Radiographic and histologic patterns of calcification in chondromyxoid fibroma. Skeletal Radiol 27: 559–564.
24. White L M, Kandel R 2000 Osteoid-producing tumors of bone. Semin Musculoskelet Radiol 4: 25–43.
25. Greenspan A 1995 Bone island (enostosis): current concept—a review. Skeletal Radiol 24: 111–115.
26. Peyser A B, Makley J T, Callewart C C, Brackett B, Carter J R, Abdul-Karim F W 1996 Osteoma of the long bones and the spine. A study of eleven patients and a review of the literature. J Bone Joint Surg Am 78: 1172–1180.
27. Bertoni F, Unni K K, Beabout J W, Sim F H 1995 Parosteal osteoma of bones other than of the skull and face. Cancer 75: 2466–2473.
28. Allen S D, Saifuddin A 2003 Imaging of intra-articular osteoid osteoma. Clin Radiol 58: 845–852.
29. Saifuddin A, White J, Sherazi Z, Shaikh M I, Natali C, Ransford A O 1998 Osteoid osteoma and osteoblastoma of the spine. Factors associated with the presence of scoliosis. Spine 23: 47–53.
30. Davies M, Cassar-Pullicino V N, Davies A M, McCall I W, Tyrrell P N 2002 The diagnostic accuracy of MR imaging in osteoid osteoma. Skeletal Radiol 31: 559–569.
31. Cioni R, Armillotta N, Bargellini I et al 2004 CT-guided radiofrequency ablation of osteoid osteoma: long-term results. Eur Radiol 14: 1203–1208.
32. Kroon H M, Schurmans J 1990 Osteoblastoma: clinical and radiologic findings in 98 new cases. Radiology 175: 783–790.
33. Shaikh M I, Saifuddin A, Pringle J, Natali C, Sherazi Z 1999 Spinal osteoblastoma: CT and MR imaging with pathological correlation. Skeletal Radiol 28: 33–40.
34. Parman LM, Murphey MD 2000 Alphabet soup: cystic lesions of bone. Semin Musculoskelet Radiol 4: 89–101.

35. Wilkins R M 2000 Unicameral bone cysts. J Am Acad Orthop Surg 8: 217–224.
36. Margau R, Babyn P, Cole W et al 2000 MR imaging of simple bone cysts in children: not so simple. Pediatr Radiol 30: 551–557.
37. Kransdorf M J, Sweet D E 1995 Aneurysmal bone cyst: concept, controversy, clinical presentation, and imaging. AJR Am J Roentgenol 164: 573–580.
38. Mahnken A H, Nolte-Ernsting C C, Wildberger J E et al 2003 Aneurysmal bone cyst: value of MR imaging and conventional radiography. Eur Radiol 13: 1118–1124.
39. Maiya S, Davies M, Evans N, Grimer J 2002 Surface aneurysmal bone cysts: a pictorial review. Eur Radiol 12: 99–108.
40. Ilaslan H, Sundaram M, Unni K K 2003 Solid variant of aneurysmal bone cysts in long tubular bones: giant cell reparative granuloma. AJR Am J Roentgenol 180: 1681–1687.
41. Murphy M D, Nomikos G C, Flemming D J et al 2001 From the archives of AFIP. Imaging of giant cell tumor and giant cell reparative granuloma of bone: radiologic-pathologic correlation. Radiographics 21: 1283–1309.
42. Bertoni F, Bacchini P, Staals E L 2003 Malignancy in giant cell tumor of bone. Cancer 97: 2520–2529.
43. Siebenrock K A, Unni K K, Rock M G 1998 Giant-cell tumour of bone metastasizing to the lungs. A long-term follow-up. J Bone Joint Surg Br 80: 43–47.
44. Dumford K, Moore T E, Walker C W, Jaksha J 2003 Multifocal, metachronous, giant cell tumor of the lower limb. Skeletal Radiol 32: 147–150.
45. Smith S E, Kransdorf M J 2000 Primary musculoskeletal tumors of fibrous origin. Semin Musculoskelet Radiol 4: 73–88.
46. Gross M L, Soberman N, Dorfman H D et al 1989 Case report 556: Multiple non-ossifying fibromas of long bones in a patient with neurofibromatosis. Skeletal Radiol 5: 389–391.
47. Jee W H, Choe B Y, Kang H S et al 1998 Non-ossifying fibroma: characteristics at MR imaging with pathologic correlation. Radiology 209: 197–202.
48. Hamada T, Ito H, Araki Y et al 1996 Benign fibrous histiocytoma of the femur: review of three cases. Skeletal Radiol 25: 25–29.
49. Taconis W K, Schutte H E, Heul R O 1994 Desmoplastic fibroma of bone: a report of 18 cases. Skeletal Radiol 23: 283–288.
50. Mahnken A H, Nolte-Ernsting C C, Wildberger J E et al 2001 Cross-sectional imaging patterns of desmoplastic fibroma. Eur Radiol 11: 1105–1110.
51. Bufkin W J 1971 The avulsive cortical irregularity. AJR Am J Roentgenol 112: 487–492.
52. Suh J S, Cho J H, Shin K H et al 1996 MR appearance of distal femoral cortical irregularity (cortical desmoid). J Comput Assist Tomogr 20: 328–332.
53. Wenger D E, Wold L E 2000 Benign vascular lesions of bone: radiologic and pathologic features. Skeletal Radiol 29: 63–74.
54. Vilanova J C, Barcelo J, Smirniotopoulos J G et al 2004 Hemangioma from head to toe: MR imaging with pathologic correlation. Radiographics 24: 367–385.
55. Levey D S, MacCormack L M, Sartoris D J et al 1996 Cystic angiomatosis: case report and review of the literature. Skeletal Radiol 25: 287–293.
56. Yoo S Y, Hong S H, Chung H W et al 2002 MRI of Gorham's disease: findings in two cases. Skeletal Radiol 31: 301–306.
57. Mutema G K, Sorger J 2002 Intraosseous schwannoma of the humerus. Skeletal Radiol 31: 419–421.
58. Tsirikos A I, Ramachandran M, Lee J, Saifuddin A 2004 Assessment of vertebral scalloping in neurofibromatosis type 1 with plain radiography and MRI. Clin Radiol 59: 1009–1017.
59. Campbell R S, Grainger A J, Mangham D C, Beggs I, Teh J, Davies A M 2003 Intraosseous lipoma: report of 35 new cases and a review of the literature. Skeletal Radiol 32: 209–222.
60. Yu J S, Weis L, Becker W 2000 MR imaging of a parosteal lipoma. Clin Imaging 24: 15–18.
61. McGraw P, Bonvento B, Moholkar K 2004 Phalangeal intraosseous epidermoid cyst. Acta Orthop Belg 70: 365–367.
62. Parekh S G, Donthineni-Rao R, Ricchetti E, Lackman R D 2004 Fibrous dysplasia. J Am Acad Orthop Surg 12: 305–313.
63. Jee W H, Choi K H, Choe B Y, Park J M, Shinn K S 1996 Fibrous dysplasia: MR imaging characteristics with radiopathologic correlation. AJR Am J Roentgenol 167: 1523–1527.
64. Kyriakos M, McDonald D J, Sundaram M 2004 Fibrous dysplasia with cartilaginous differentiation ("fibrocartilaginous dysplasia"): a review, with an illustrative case followed for 18 years. Skeletal Radiol 33: 51–62.
65. McCaffrey M, Letts M, Carpenter B, Kabir A, Davidson D, Seip J 2003 Osteofibrous dysplasia: a review of the literature and presentation of an additional 3 cases. Am J Orthop 32: 479–486.

CHAPTER 48

Bone Tumours (2): Malignant Lesions

Dennis J. Stoker and Asif Saifuddin

- Bone metastases

Primary malignant neoplasms of bone

- Chondroid origin
- Osteoid origin
- Fibrous origin
- Marrow tumours
- Notochordal origin
- Miscellaneous lesions

BONE METASTASES

Bone metastases are common and often multiple. However, 9% of carcinoma bone metastases are solitary[1], making a solitary metastasis muchmore common than a primary neoplasm. At the time of presentation, a solitary lesion in a middle-aged or elderly patient is still more likely to be an atypical metastasis than the most typical of primary malignant bone tumours.

Evidence indicates that distant metastases result from venous tumour emboli[2], either from the primary tumour, from regional nodes or other metastases, e.g. in the lung. Venous embolization of neoplastic cells may be found in any soft tissue neoplasm, and is particularly related to vascularity of the primary tumour or access to a valveless venous plexus, e.g. Batson's vertebral plexus.

Bone metastasis is a relatively late occurrence because the lungs trap most tumour emboli. Appearance in bone without pulmonary involvement occurs with:

1 pulmonary lesions that are present but occult
2 transpulmonary passage of malignant cells[3]
3 paradoxical embolism (passage of emboli through a patent foramen ovale)
4 retrograde venous embolism with involvement of the vertebral column by intra-abdominal cancer.

The overall incidence of skeletal metastases in carcinoma during life is unclear. At autopsy[4], skeletal metastases have been found in 27% of all patients with carcinoma.

Bone metastasis is most common with carcinoma of the breast, bronchus, prostate, kidney and thyroid. The incidence of skeletal metastases is very high in carcinoma of the breast: 73% in autopsy cases[4], and 84% by scintigraphy in advanced mammary cancer in vivo[5]. A similar incidence is observed in prostatic cancer: 84% at autopsy[4] and 70% by scintigraphy. Carcinoma of the bronchus (especially small-cell) is the next most common, having an incidence of metastases at autopsy of 30–55%.

Thyroid carcinoma produces bone metastases in 50–60% of autopsy cases[4], but accounts for only 0.5% of all cancer deaths. Renal carcinoma (hypernephroma) characteristically metastasizes to bone. Therefore, in the case of a solitary lesion a renal ultrasound (US) is a reasonable next investigation. However, the type and origin of the metastasis may commonly be suggested by needle biopsy. Hypernephroma accounts for 2.5% of all cancer deaths, one-tenth the prevalence of gastric carcinoma. Therefore, bone metastases from carcinoma of stomach, bowel or pancreas are probably more common than those of hypernephroma.

Table 48.1 shows the incidence of skeletal metastases based on the literature and Table 48.2 provides a simplified list of common and less common sites of primary tumour.

Table 48.1 FREQUENCY OF SKELETAL METASTASES FROM DIFFERENT PRIMARY TUMOURS (DESCENDING ORDER OF FREQUENCY)

Johnston (1970)[1]	Lodwick (1975)	Schwinn (1981)
Autopsy	Radiology	Pathology
Bronchus	Breast	Bronchus
Breast	Prostate	Breast
Prostate	Bronchus	Prostate
Pancreas	Kidney	Kidney
Stomach	Uterus	Colon
	Thyroid	Melanoma
	Stomach	
	Colon	

Table 48.2 FREQUENCY OF PRIMARY CARCINOMA CAUSING SKELETAL METASTASES (INCIDENCE OF METASTASES RELATED TO INCIDENCE OF PRIMARY TUMOUR) AFTER ABRAMS ET AL[4]

Order of frequency	Whole population	Men	Women
1	Breast	Prostate	Breast
2	Prostate	Bronchus	Uterus
3	Bronchus	Bladder	Colon
4	Colon	Stomach	Stomach
5	Stomach	Rectum	Rectum
6	Bladder	Colon	Bladder
7	Uterus	Kidney	Thyroid
8	Rectum	Pancreas	Ovary
9	Thyroid	Thyroid	Bronchus
10	Kidney		Kidney
11	Ovary		

Distribution of skeletal metastases

The commonest sites of metastatic involvement are those containing red bone marrow, explaining why the axial skeleton is affected more commonly than the appendicular skeleton in adults[6]. Bone metastases, therefore, commonly involve the vertebrae, pelvis, proximal femora and humeri skull, and ribs (Fig. 48.1). Peripheral metastases are rare and 50% of these are from bronchus[7].

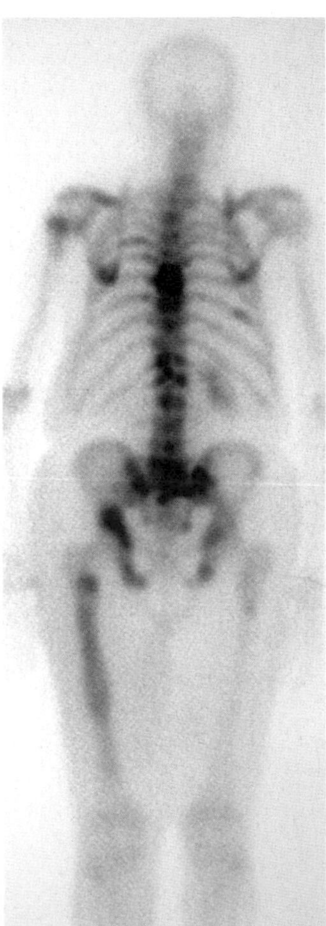

Figure 48.1 Whole body ^{99m}Tc-MDP (methylene diphosphonate) bone scintigram (posterior view) showing multiple regions of increased uptake due to prostatic carcinoma metastases. Involvement typically occurs in the spine, pelvis and ribs.

Spinal metastases occur most commonly in the thoracic vertebrae, but carcinomas arising within the pelvis, particularly prostatic carcinoma, show a predilection for the lumbosacral spine.

Diagnosis of bone metastases

Clinical

Unexplained back or limb pain in a patient with known carcinoma may indicate skeletal metastasis. A pathological fracture is suggested when the force applied is less than that required to fracture a normal bone. Imaging is necessary to reveal a pre-existing lesion.

Elevation of the serum alkaline phosphatase is a nonspecific finding and may not occur until multiple bone metastases have developed.

Radiological features[8,9]

Bone metastases are commonly lytic and multiple. Radiography is poor at defining medullary destruction and only a lesion of approximately 20 mm can usually be visualized. In osteoporosis, even larger metastases may not be revealed radiographically. As the destructive process extends to involve the cortex, a periosteal reaction or soft tissue mass may develop. Some carcinomas, such as hypernephroma, almost always produce lytic metastases. Some, such as prostate, are most commonly osteoblastic, while breast carcinoma metastases may show a mixed appearance. Osteoblastic change reflects a tissue response of the host bone rather than production of tumour bone, which is a characteristic feature of osteosarcoma.

The importance of identifying multiple lesions cannot be overemphasized as individual metastases may mimic primary malignant tumours of bone (Fig. 48.2). For this purpose, ^{99m}Tc-MDP bone scintigraphy remains the most cost-effective method[9], although it is known that whole body

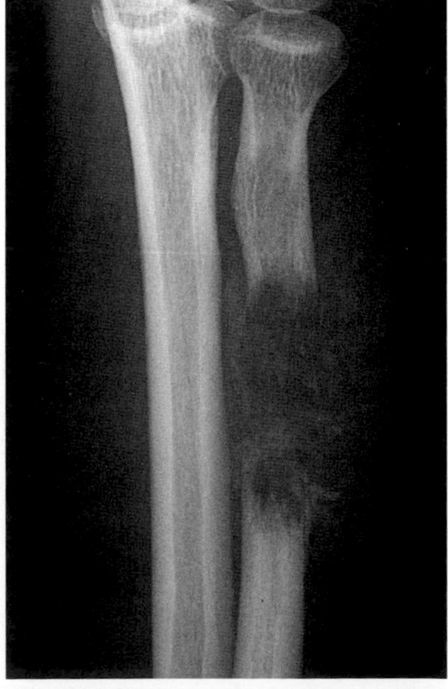

Figure 48.2 AP radiograph of the proximal forearm showing a mineralized squamous carcinoma metastasis to the radius.

MRI is a more sensitive technique[10]. A variety of scintigraphic abnormalities are seen, the most common being multiple sites of increased skeletal activity, typically in the axial skeleton (Fig. 48.1). Abnormal uptake on bone scintigraphy relies on intact local blood flow and increased osteoblastic activity. Therefore, lesions that infarct or stimulate no osteoblastic response may appear as photopenic areas or 'cold spots' (Fig. 48.3), most commonly seen with renal metastasis. Occasionally, a combination of 'hot' and 'cold' lesions occurs. Diffuse osteoblastic metastatic disease, typically from breast or prostate, may result in a 'superscan' appearance, which is suggested by the presence of generalized increase in skeletal activity with reduced or absent renal activity. Recently ^{18}F-fluoride PET/CT has proven both sensitive and specific for metastasis[11].

Sometimes, increased uptake on scintigraphy may be present at one or more sites and radiography shows a benign cause, such as a healing fracture, an appearance consistent with metastasis or normal appearances. Any region of unexplained abnormal uptake should be examined by MRI, which is more sensitive than radiography, and more specific than scintigraphy. Most metastases are located in the medulla and show reduced signal intensity (SI) on T1-weighted sequences, with increased SI on T2-weighted or fat-suppressed sequences. The identification of a hyperintense 'halo' around a lesion is a highly specific feature of metastasis on T2-weighted sequences[12] (Fig. 48.4).

Breast Breast cancer metastases are demonstrated by bone scintigraphy in 24% of early cases and 84% of advanced cases[2]. Most lesions are lytic but breast carcinoma is the commonest cause of osteoblastic metastases in women. About 10% of metastases are purely osteoblastic and 10% mixed. Lesions commonly involve the vertebrae, pelvis and ribs. Diffuse marrow infiltration may occur and only become evident radiographically when sclerosis follows therapy.

The differential diagnosis in a middle-aged or elderly woman includes vertebral collapse due to osteoporosis or myeloma. In neither of these conditions would widespread skeletal activity be expected on scintigraphy. In myeloma, the abnormal plasma electrophoresis may aid diagnosis.

Prostate Prostatic metastases are predominantly osteoblastic or mixed, with purely lytic lesions being very rare. Individual lesions may cause a florid 'sunburst' periosteal reaction (Fig. 48.5) mimicking osteosarcoma, which is rare at this age in the absence of Paget's disease or previous radiotherapy. Occasionally, diffuse or confluent osteosclerosis simulates other disorders such as myelofibrosis.

Lung Metastasis to bone is common, mostly to the axial skeleton. However, peripheral metastases to the hands and feet most commonly arise from bronchial carcinoma[7]. The majority of metastases are lytic, usually from squamous-cell and small-cell carcinomas. Adenocarcinoma and bronchial carcinoid, which metastasize to bone in approximately 10% of cases, normally produce focal or diffuse osteoblastic lesions.

Kidney Metastases from hypernephroma are almost always lytic, osteoblastic metastases being very rare. Expanded subarticular lesions resembling giant cell tumour (GCT) radiologically

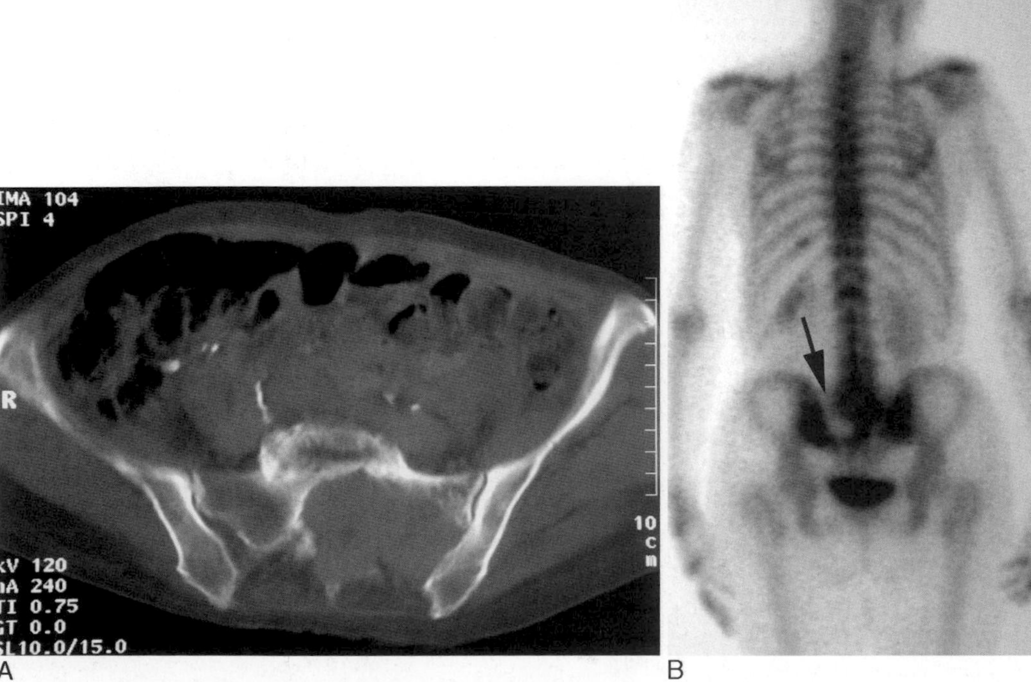

Figure 48.3 Cold metastasis due to hypernephroma metastasis to the sacrum. CT (A) shows a lytic destructive lesion of the left sacral ala manifest as a 'cold' spot on the bone scintigram (arrow) (B).

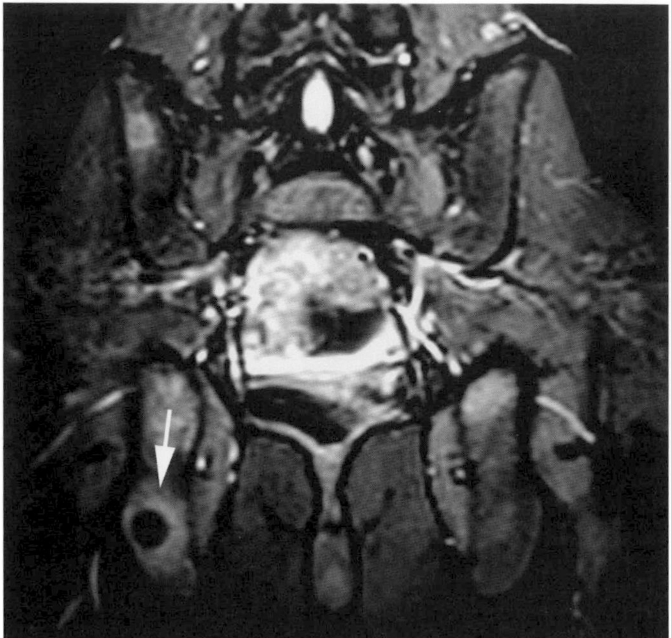

Figure 48.4 Osteosarcoma metastasis. Coronal STIR MR image through the posterior pelvis showing a sclerotic osteosarcoma metastasis of the right ischium with a hyperintense 'halo' (arrow) surrounding the lesion.

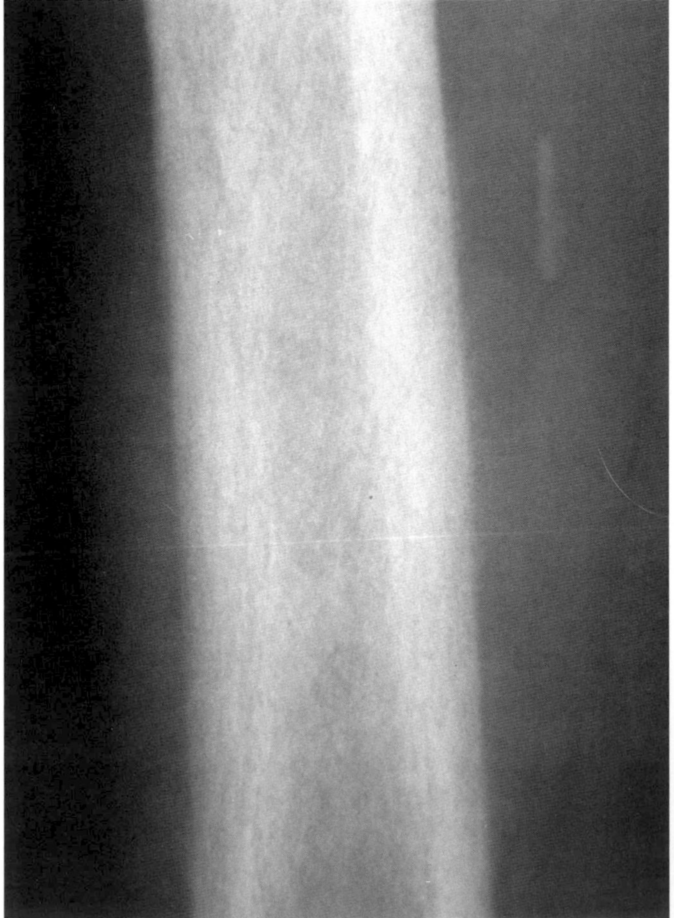

Figure 48.5 Sunburst periosteal reaction. AP radiograph of the femoral diaphysis showing a spiculated periosteal reaction mimicking osteosarcoma in a patient with prostatic metastasis.

are not uncommon (Fig. 48.6). Classical Wilms' tumours usually metastasize to the lungs and rarely involve bone.

Thyroid Metastases are usually lytic but, like those from hypernephroma, may expand the bone and present a trabeculated appearance. The combination of a lytic metastasis and diffuse neoplastic (sometimes miliary) lung involvement is suggestive of a thyroid origin.

Gastrointestinal tract Bone metastases occur in less than 7% of patients with colonic carcinoma and metastases confined to the skeleton occur in under 2%. The incidence in gastric carcinoma is similar. These cancers are, however, more common than those of kidney and thyroid. In Abrams' series[4], carcinoma of the colon and stomach respectively were the fourth and fifth commonest primary source of bone metastases (Table 48.2). Although usually lytic, like other adenocarcinomas, sclerotic metastases are also found. Calcification is also a feature.

Bladder Bone metastases are usually lytic, but occasionally osteoblastic, with exuberant periosteal new bone. An unusual predilection for the lower limbs may be shown. Adenocarcinomas arising in other pelvic organs share such a tendency.

Uterus Uterine cancer is of two types. The more common carcinoma of the cervix usually involves bone by direct spread to the bony pelvis. Blood-borne metastases are uncommon and usually lytic, but may rarely be osteoblastic or mixed. Carcinoma of the uterine body is an adenocarcinoma and, like that of the ovary, may produce osteoblastic metastases, particularly of the vertebrae.

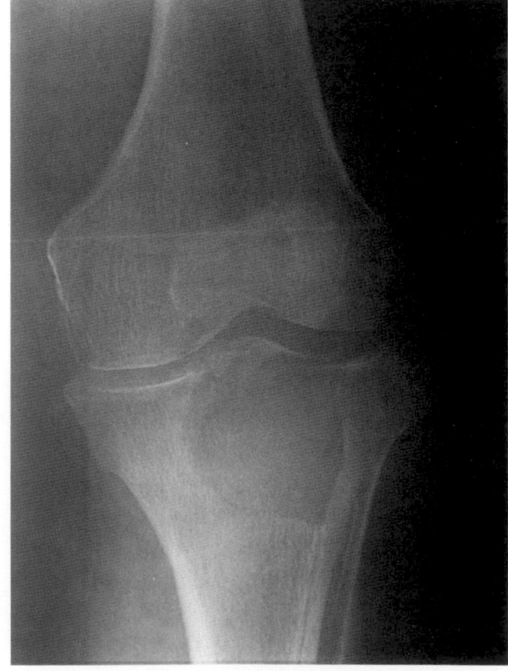

Figure 48.6 Renal carcinoma metastasis. AP radiograph of the knee showing a lytic, subarticular tibial lesion mimicking giant cell tumour.

Pancreas A relatively silent tumour when involving the body or tail, the incidence of bone metastasis is unknown, although a figure of 12% has been reported[1]. Although lytic lesions are usually described, osteoblastic vertebral metastases are probably more common than generally recognized.

Melanoma Spread to bone is rare and mainly to the axial skeleton, with an incidence of approximately 7%. The primary tumour may be insignificant or may have been removed years before. Metastases are usually lytic.

Table 48.3 RADIOGRAPHIC FEATURES FAVOURING DIAGNOSIS OF A METASTASIS RATHER THAN A PRIMARY MALIGNANCY OF BONE

Positive features	Features suggesting another diagnosis
Diaphyseal location in long bones	Absence of bone expansion
Vertebral body involved	Absence of florid periosteal reaction
Pedicles involved	Absence of tumour bone formation
	Absence of large soft tissue mass

Differential diagnosis of skeletal metastases

A solitary metastasis may resemble a primary malignant bone tumour, an aggressive primary benign tumour such as GCT, infection and miscellaneous disorders such as Paget's disease. Some helpful diagnostic indications are presented in Table 48.3. No single investigation, apart from biopsy, will provide a specific diagnosis of a metastasis or its site of origin.

The radiological investigation of metastatic disease

The presence of a primary malignant neoplasm may be known and the presence or absence of metastases must be established as part of the staging process. Radiography of symptomatic areas is useful. However, skeletal surveys are both ineffective and wasteful.

Skeletal scintigraphy (Fig. 48.1) is the primary investigation for assessing the whole skeleton. Whole body MRI correlates well with scintigraphy although some lesions are missed by one technique yet detected by the other[10]. Biopsy may not be indicated unless a solitary lesion has unexpected features. In these circumstances, biopsy could reveal a lesion of different histology and alter the staging of the cancer and its prognosis.

The second radiological presentation is with a solitary bone lesion, which could be a metastasis. The questions to consider are whether the lesion is solitary or multiple, and the source of the primary tumour.

The first consideration is resolved by skeletal scintigraphy, possibly followed by imaging of any area that shows increased uptake to confirm or exclude the presence of an additional metastasis. The second consideration may be answered by simple noninvasive investigations such as chest radiography and renal US. Further investigation, such as abdominal and pelvic CT, is not justified. In many cases, image-guided needle biopsy will suggest or exclude the likely site of origin. However, it should be recognized that the site of the primary carcinoma may remain unknown, even after full investigation, and that the prognosis may not be altered in, for example, metastatic adenocarcinoma, by merely identifying the site of the primary tumour.

In the setting of a solitary metastasis, local staging before surgical excision is achieved with MRI, as for any primary bone tumour.

Skeletal metastases in children

This is a less common occurrence than in adults. The commonest disseminated paediatric neoplasms affecting bone are neuroblastoma and leukaemia, which may have identical radiological appearances. Other soft tissue sarcomas, such as rhabdomyosarcoma, are less common. Primary retinoblastoma may involve bone by direct spread. Its blood-borne metastases may be lytic or osteoblastic. Osteosarcoma and Ewing's sarcoma may metastasize to bone with metastases from Ewing's sarcoma tending to resemble leukaemia or secondary neuroblastoma. The commonest intracranial neoplasm to metastasize to bones outside the skull is cerebellar medulloblastoma. Such metastases are rarely purely lytic. The vast majority occur after surgery has produced a neovascularity connecting the cerebral and extracerebral circulations, and few preoperative skeletal metastases have been reported.

PRIMARY MALIGNANT NEOPLASMS OF BONE

All primary malignant bone neoplasms are rare. Recent advances in chemotherapy and limb-salvage surgery have revolutionized the outcome, such that in specialist centres a patient with an appendicular osteosarcoma without metastases at presentation has a greater than 60% chance of 5-year survival.

The radiological investigation of a suspected malignant primary bone tumour includes characterization with radiography, local staging with MRI, and assessment of metastatic disease with chest CT and whole body skeletal scintigraphy.

Both dynamic enhanced MRI[13] and Doppler US[14] are accurate at determining response to chemotherapy, but the clinical utility of these techniques is as yet unproven. MRI has proved particularly valuable in demonstrating local recurrence following radiation therapy and surgery[15]. A 96% sensitivity was found for the exclusion of residual or recurrent tumour in patients with either osseous or soft tissue neoplasms where the T2-weighted sequences showed no increase in signal intensity. However, when high signal intensity was seen on the T2-weighted sequence, the sensitivity for disease activity was only 70%.

CHONDROID ORIGIN

Chondrosarcoma[16,17]

Chondrosarcoma is a malignant cartilage-producing tumour accounting for 8–17% of biopsied primary bone tumours and 25% of all biopsied malignant bone tumours. It is classified as primary or secondary and central (intramedullary) or peripheral. Secondary chondrosarcomas arise in a pre-existing bony lesion, usually an enchondroma (central) or an osteochondroma (peripheral—more frequently when these are familial and multiple), and only rarely in chondromyxoid fibroma, chondroblastoma or synovial chondromatosis.

Chondrosarcoma may also be classified according to its histological grade as low grade (grade 1; 45–50% of cases), myxoid (grade 2; 30–43% of cases), high grade (grade 3; 8–25% of cases) or dedifferentiated, which refers to the development of an adjacent high-grade nonchondroid neoplasm, typically osteosarcoma or malignant fibrous histiocytoma. Other distinct varieties include mesenchymal and clear-cell chondrosarcoma.

Clinical presentation

Although reported at most ages, chondrosarcoma is rare in children and should be differentiated from chondroblastic osteosarcoma. Over 50% of patients are more than 40 years old with a mean peak incidence of approximately 50 years. A male to female ratio of 1.5 to 1 is reported. Most patients complain of pain of insidious onset with a palpable mass reported in 28% of cases and pathological fracture in 27%. The tumour may be quite large at presentation, particularly when arising from the pelvis. The common sites of chondrosarcoma are the pelvis, proximal femur and proximal humerus. Chondrosarcomas in the hands and feet account for 1–4% of all cases.

A major consideration is the differentiation between chondroma and low-grade chondrosarcoma. It is reasonable to suggest that all central chondroid tumours in adults have a malignant potential. Thus, in the presence of pain or increased growth, lesions should be regarded as chondrosarcoma until proven otherwise by biopsy or their benign clinical progress.

Bone scintigraphy has demonstrated activity in many calcified medullary lesions in the middle-aged and elderly, indicating that chondroid growth has not ceased. Most such lesions, however, prove to be benign or of an extremely low grade of malignancy (grade 1 chondrosarcoma) and probably need observation only. Chondrosarcoma is suggested if the level of scintigraphic activity in the lesion is greater than that in the anterior iliac crest. It has been suggested that Gd-DTPA-enhanced MRI can aid in the diagnosis of low-grade chondrosarcomas.

Radiological features

A small low-grade chondrosarcoma may not be differentiated from a chondroma, appearing as a well-defined lytic lesion with chondroid matrix mineralization (Fig. 48.7). Calcification occurs in 75% of cases on radiography and 92% at CT. Slow growth allows reactive change to occur in the normal bone, so that as endosteal resorption takes place (Fig. 48.8) periosteal new bone is laid down and bone expansion occurs, particularly with more aggressive myxoid tumours (Fig. 48.9). Deep endosteal cortical scalloping (greater than two-thirds) is suggestive of chondrosarcoma as opposed to chondroma. The zone between normal and abnormal bone is narrow, although plain radiography may not accurately define medullary involvement. In the more malignant tumours, cortical destruction reveals the aggressive nature of the process. The presence of unusually aggressive radiological appearances should raise the suspicion of dedifferentiation to a more malignant neoplasm[18,19] (Fig. 48.10).

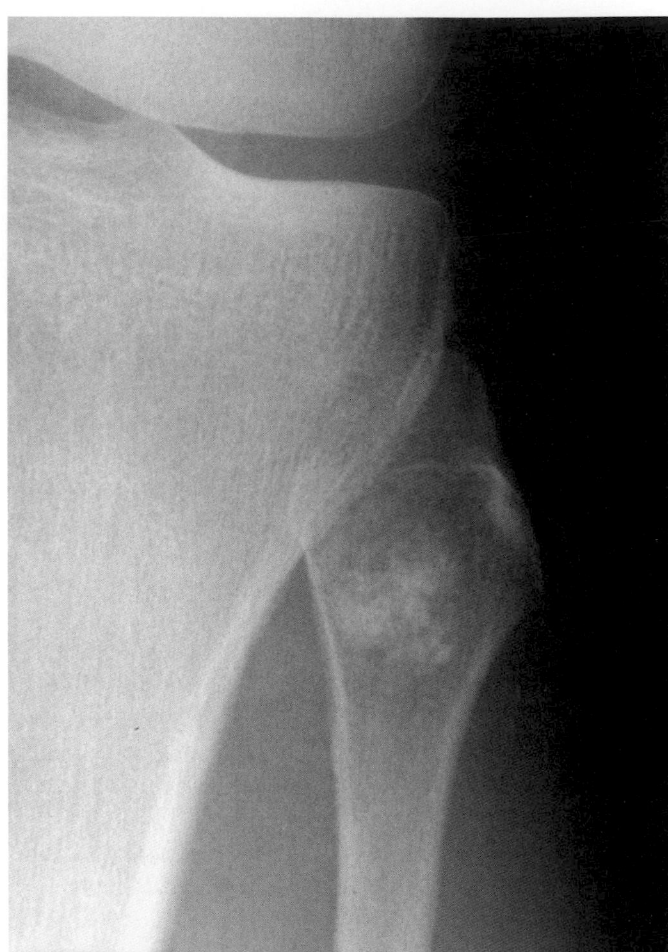

Figure 48.7 Chondrosarcoma. AP radiograph of the proximal tibiofibular joint showing a mineralized lesion of the fibula due to low-grade chondrosarcoma. The lesion cannot be radiologically differentiated from a chondroma.

Periosteal reaction is identifiable in up to half the patients. Despite the cortical scalloping, the laying down of appositional new bone by the periosteum usually means that the cortical thickness is increased.

A large extraosseous mass is very common with pelvic lesions but is often radiographically occult. CT and MRI will demonstrate such soft tissue extension with greater accuracy (Fig. 48.11). MRI has proven to be particularly valuable in local staging since malignant cartilage shows characteristic increased SI on T2-weighted images and a multilobulated appearance (Fig. 48.12). The lesion is slightly hypo-intense to muscle on T1-weighted images and may show focal areas of hyperintensity due to trapped areas of marrow. Matrix mineralization manifests as focal areas of signal void. Most chondrosarcomas are poorly vascularized and enhancement after intravenous contrast medium is minimal, typically showing a peripheral or septal pattern.

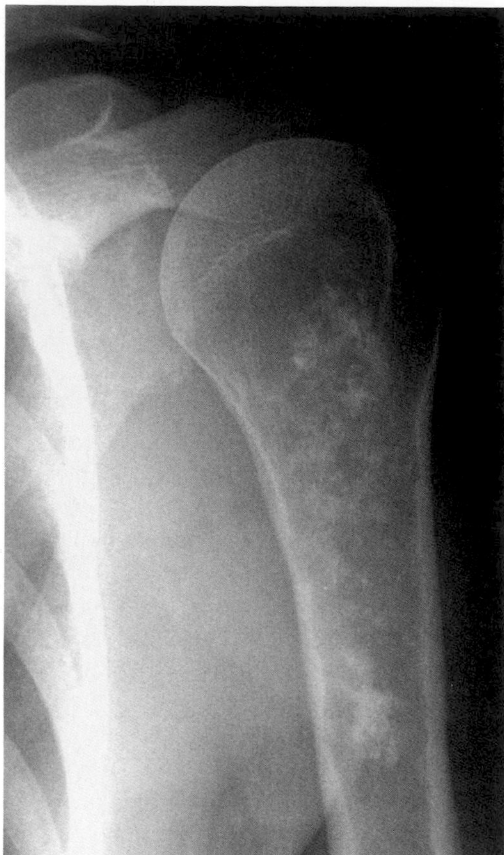

Figure 48.8 Chondrosarcoma. AP radiograph of the proximal humerus showing a typical low-grade chondrosarcoma with extensive chondral mineralization and endosteal scalloping.

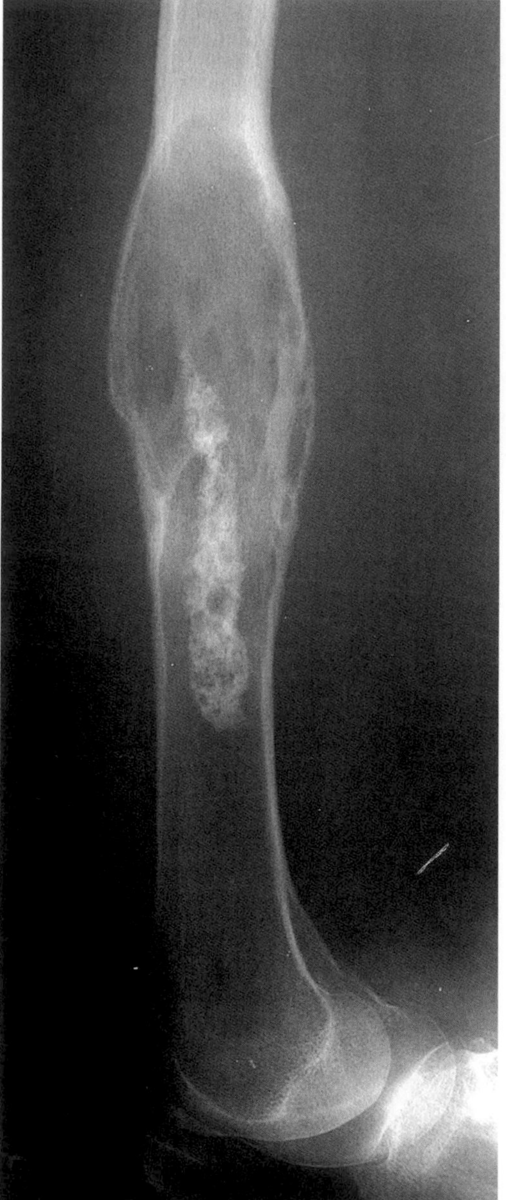

Figure 48.9 Myxoid chondrosarcoma. Lateral radiograph of the femur showing a grade 2 myxoid chondrosarcoma. Bone expansion indicates a more aggressive behaviour.

T2-weighted MRI has also proven valuable in the identification of dedifferentiation, in which case a region of intermediate SI adjacent to the typical hyperintense chondral tumour mass is seen[18]. Such areas should be targeted for image-guided needle biopsy[20].

Identification of secondary peripheral chondrosarcoma from an osteochondroma should be suspected clinically if pain develops or continued growth occurs after skeletal maturity. Radiological features of malignant change consist of destruction of part of the calcified cap or ossified stem of the osteochondroma. The thickness of the cartilage cap cannot usually be assessed radiographically but can be readily determined by US, CT or MRI. Most osteochondromas have cartilage caps no thicker than 5 mm and a cap in excess of 20 mm is likely to be malignant (Fig. 48.13). Pain and swelling over a cartilage cap may also be due to bursa formation.

Other varieties of chondrosarcoma

Periosteal chondrosarcoma[21] This rare form of chondrosarcoma typically involves the long bones, most commonly the distal femoral and proximal humeral metaphyses. It is more commonly seen in men, with a wide range of presentation. Radiologically, a calcified juxtacortical mass is identified, with associated cortical thickening and periosteal reaction. Involvement of the medulla is rare. The prognosis following adequate local resection is good.

Mesenchymal chondrosarcoma[22] Occurring at a rather younger age than conventional chondrosarcoma (third and fourth decade), this is a rare but specific entity containing cartilage but with a very much more cellular malignant matrix than a normal chondrosarcoma. Radiologically, it is indistinguishable from a central chondrosarcoma and often shows characteristic chondroid calcification. Involvement of many different bones is reported, with some predilection for the ribs and mandible. Local recurrence and disseminated metastases occur early and more frequently than with conventional chondrosarcoma.

Clear-cell chondrosarcoma[23] This histological variant, accounting for only 2% of all chondrosarcomas, is a low-grade chondrosarcoma with a long history and a better prognosis. Radiographically, it may resemble chondroblastoma or even

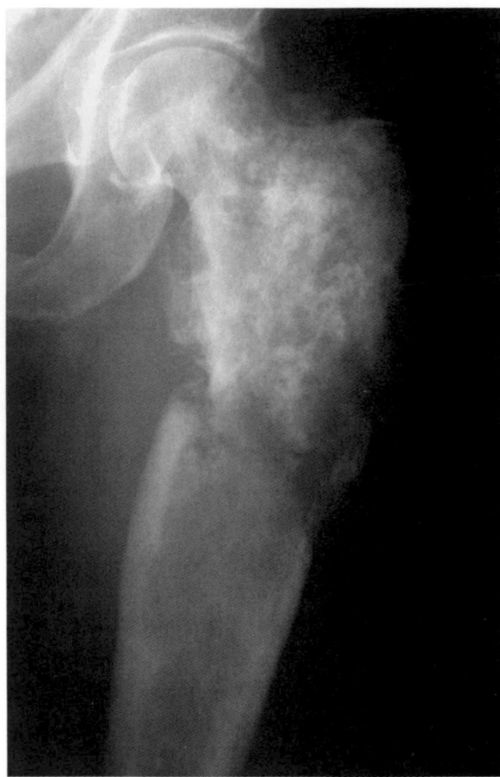

Figure 48.10 Dedifferentiated chondrosarcoma. AP radiograph of the left femur showing a proximal femoral chondrosarcoma with an adjacent area of lytic destruction and pathological fracture, due to associated dedifferentiation to malignant fibrous histiocytoma.

chondromyxoid fibroma, except that it almost always involves the ends of long bones (particularly the proximal ends of the femur or humerus) after closure of the growth plate. The lesion is usually lytic and may present a loculated or 'soap-bubble' appearance (Fig. 48.14).

OSTEOID ORIGIN

Osteosarcoma[24]

This primary malignant bone-forming neoplasm is rare, but is still the commonest primary malignant lesion of bone after myeloma. Primary osteosarcoma is classified according to site as central (conventional high-grade and low-grade), intracortical or surface (parosteal, periosteal or high-grade). Osteosarcoma may occasionally be multicentric (osteosarcomatosis) or arise in the soft tissues (extraskeletal).

Osteosarcoma may also occur secondary to Paget's disease (Paget's sarcoma), radiotherapy (post-radiation sarcoma) or as the dedifferentiated part of chondrosarcoma. Dedifferentiation into high-grade osteosarcoma can also occur from parosteal osteosarcoma. An association with several rare clinical syndromes is reported. These include Rothmund–Thompson syndrome, Li–Fraumeni syndrome and familial retinoblastoma.

Central osteosarcomas

Conventional central osteosarcoma

Clinical presentation This is the commonest form, accounting for 75% of all osteosarcomas. Approximately 80% of patients present before 30 years of age. The tumour is uncommon under the age of 10 years and very rare under the age of 5 years. The disease is therefore predominantly one of the second and third decades. In patients over the age of 40 years (10% of cases), osteosarcoma more commonly occurs in the flat bones or vertebrae and is usually secondary to a pre-existing disorder of bone, such as Paget's disease. However, this is not always the case as a minor peak of incidence may be observed in the fifth decade and later. Similarly, osteosarcoma of the jaws occurs in an older age group than that of the appendicular skeleton and carries a better prognosis. The male to female ratio is 2:1.

Presentation is typically with pain and a palpable mass, the swelling commonly being attributed to trauma. Osteosarcoma classically affects the metaphyseal region of the growing end of a long bone and about 50–75% are found in the distal femur or proximal tibia. Diaphyseal osteosarcoma accounts for 2–11% of cases. Other commonly affected sites include the proximal humerus and femur. Rarer sites include the ilium, ribs, vertebrae and jaw.

The tumour is generally greater than 6 cm in diameter at presentation and has usually extended outside the cortex but may remain deep to the periosteum. It is often highly vascular,

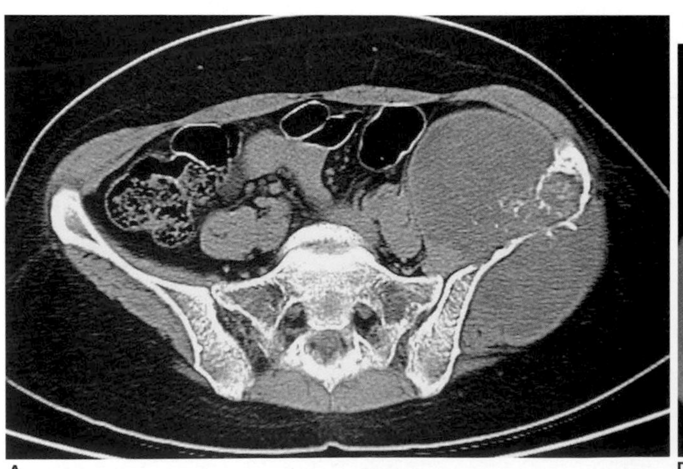

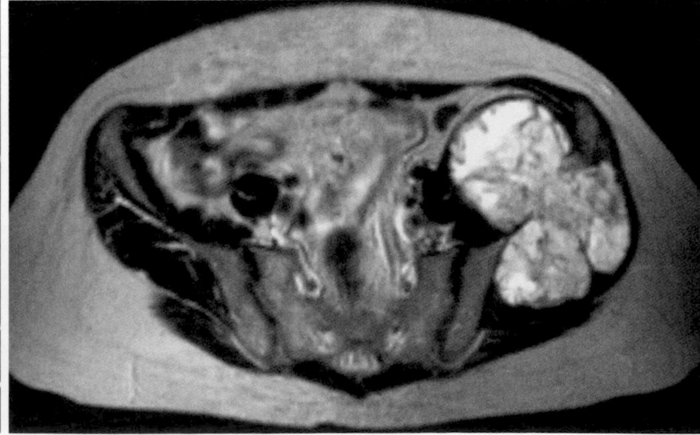

Figure 48.11 Chondrosarcoma of the left ilium. Axial CT (A) and T2-weighted MRI (B) show a large extraosseous mass.

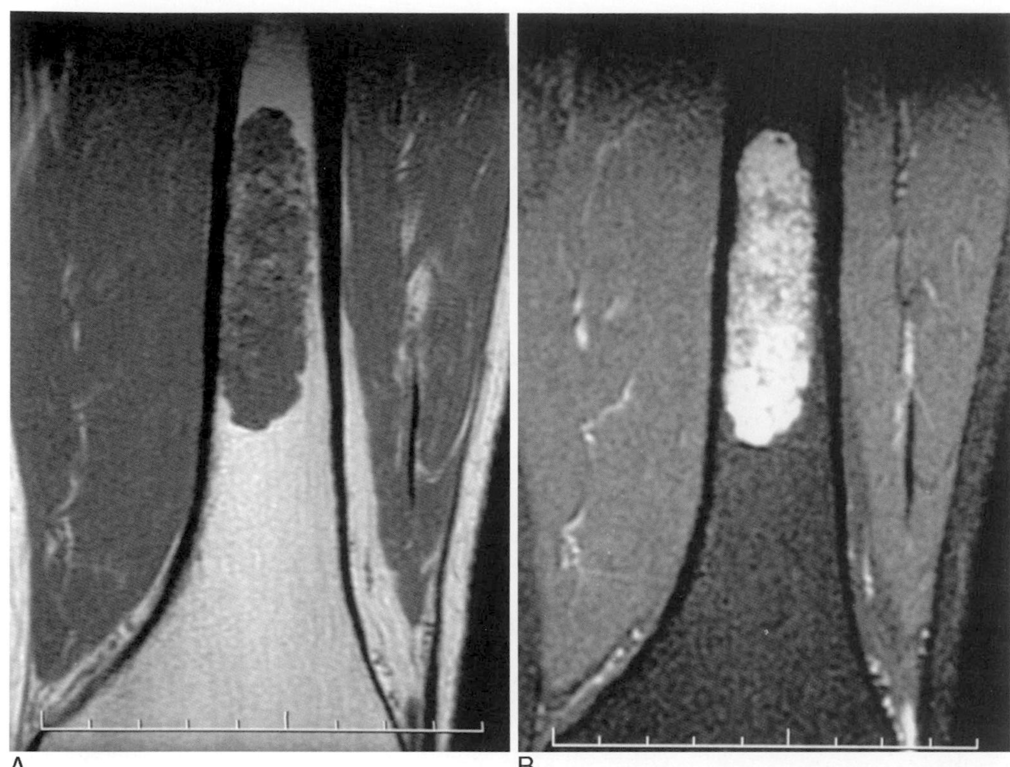

Figure 48.12 Chondrosarcoma of the femur. (A) Coronal T1-weighted spin-echo and (B) STIR MR images show a large lobulated intramedullary lesion, which is particularly hyperintense on STIR.

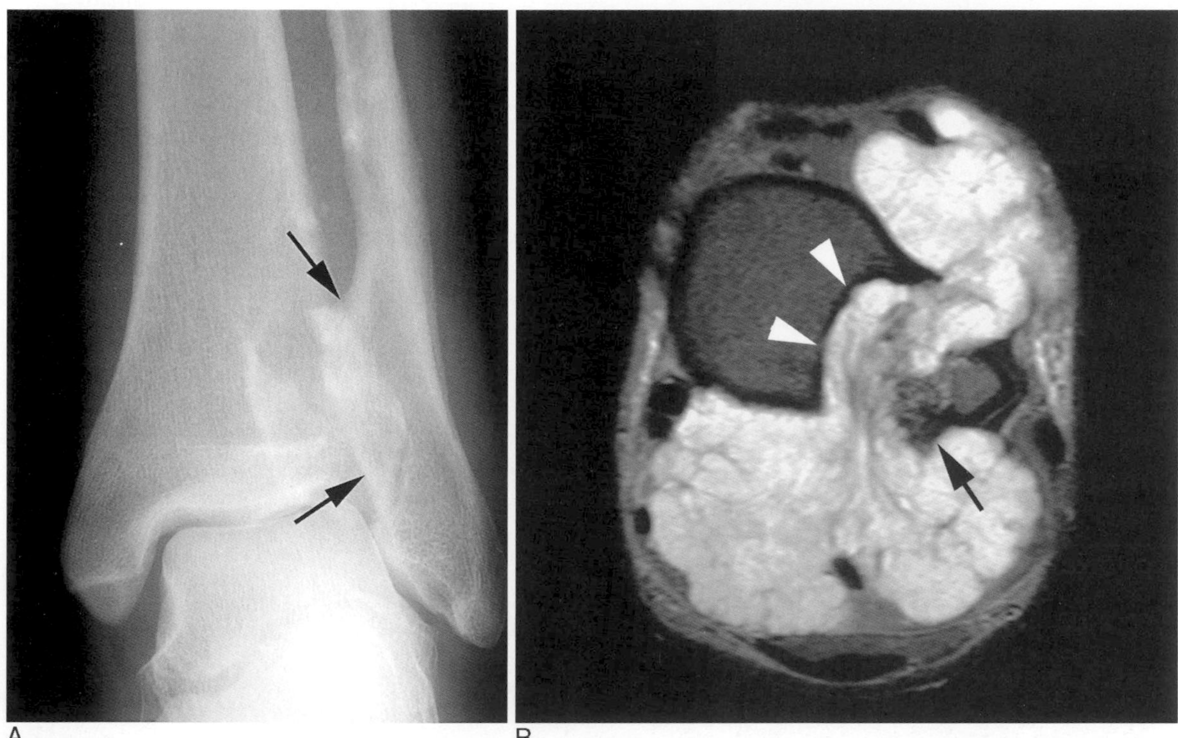

Figure 48.13 Peripheral chondrosarcoma. (A) AP radiograph of the ankle showing an osteochondroma of the distal fibula (arrows). (B) Axial fat-suppressed T2-weighted FSE MR image shows a large malignant cartilage cap surrounding the osteochondroma (arrow) and causing pressure erosion of the adjacent tibia (arrowheads).

accounting for the early haematogenous metastases to the lungs and less commonly the skeleton. A 'skip' metastasis refers to a metastasis occurring in the same bone as the primary lesion and is seen in approximately 5–8% of cases. Lymphatic metastases are occasionally identified in cases of osteoblastic osteosarcoma.

Radiological features Osteosarcoma typically presents as a metaphyseal lesion with a moth-eaten or permeative pattern of bone destruction. The medullary lesion is predominantly lytic but mineralization of the tumour osteoid leads to a characteristic associated medullary sclerosis (Fig. 48.15A). Occasionally the intramedullary component shows purely dense sclerosis

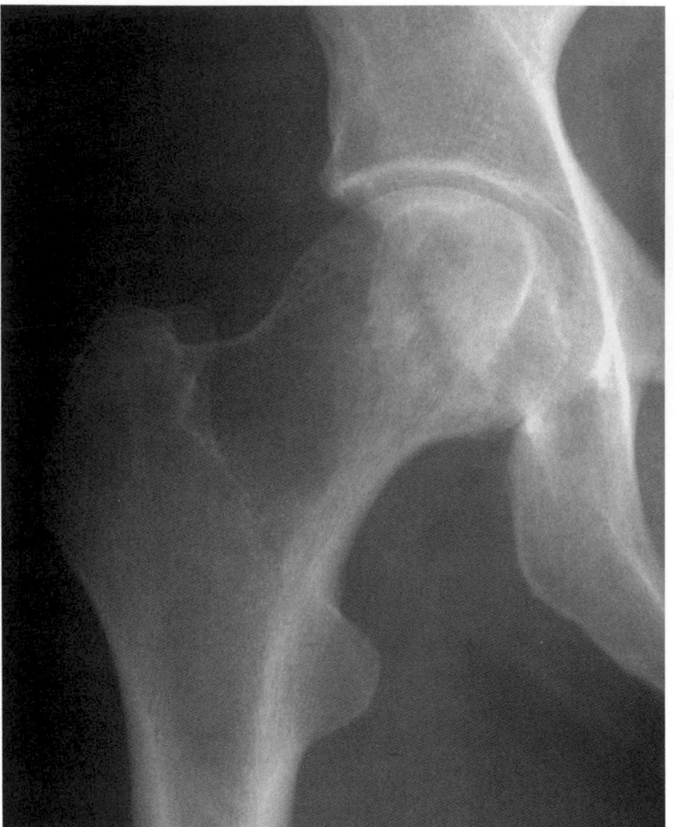

Figure 48.14 Clear-cell chondrosarcoma of the proximal femur appearing as a subarticular, lobulated lytic lesion.

(Fig. 48.15B). Cortical destruction is common, resulting in the development of an eccentric extraosseous mass, which commonly shows typical osseous 'cloud-like' matrix mineralization. The density of the extraosseous mass is increased by periosteal reaction, which is usually disorganized or perpendicular to the cortex or producing a 'sunburst' appearance. Reactive Codman's triangles may form at the margin of the lesion.

Variations of this classical appearance include entirely lytic osteosarcoma, accounting for approximately 13% of cases[25] (Fig. 48.16). A 'pseudocystic' form of osteosarcoma has also been recently described[26] (Fig. 48.17). Both of these types may mimic aneurysmal bone cyst.

Although MRI contributes little to the radiological diagnosis, it is invaluable for local staging by defining the extent of the tumour. Both intramedullary and extraosseous extension are accurately demonstrated, as is extension into the adjacent joint. MRI may also demonstrate extension of tumour across the open growth plate. Skip metastases, although rare, can be identified and it is essential to image the entire bone[27].

The natural history of osteosarcoma is for haematogenous spread with the production of pulmonary metastases. These contain osteoid and may be identified on bone scintigraphy or appear calcified on radiography and chest CT. Pulmonary metastases are typically sub-pleural and, rarely, may result in pneumothorax.

Other varieties of central osteosarcoma

***Telangiectatic osteosarcoma*[28]** This neoplasm is characterized by the formation of large septated blood-filled cavities and hence may be mistaken for an aneurysmal bone cyst. It accounts for 3.5–11% of all osteosarcomas and is twice as common in males with a mean age at presentation of 24 years. The femur, tibia and humerus are most commonly involved. Radiographs show a predominantly lytic lesion (Fig. 48.18). Subtle matrix mineralization may be demonstrated by CT, while both CT and MRI show extensive haemorrhage and

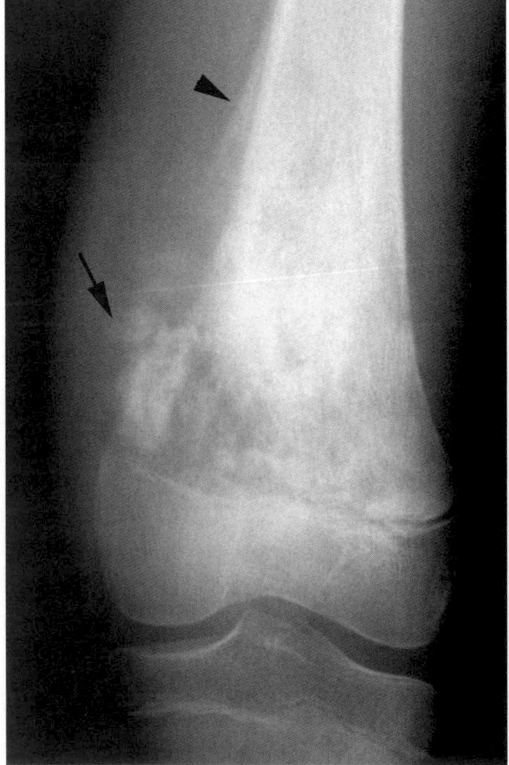

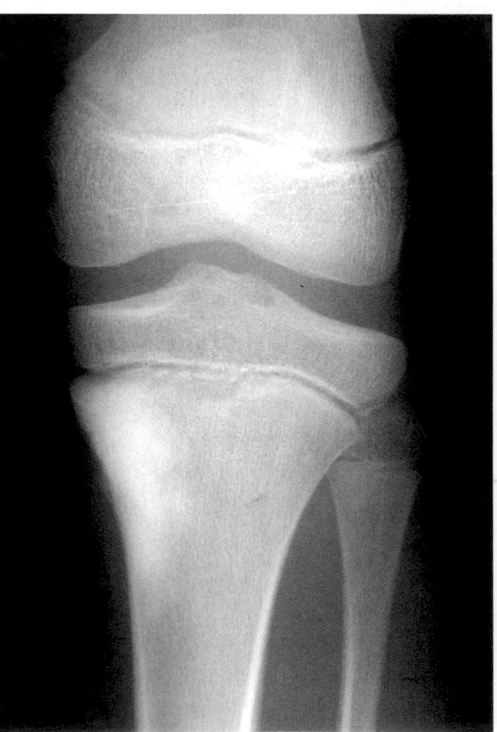

A B

Figure 48.15 Conventional central osteosarcoma. (A) AP radiograph of the distal femur showing a classical osteosarcoma with mixed lytic and sclerotic areas, tumour bone formation in the extraosseous mass (arrow), and a proximal Codman's triangle (arrowhead). (B) AP radiograph of the proximal tibia showing dense metaphyseal sclerosis due to an osteoblastic osteosarcoma.

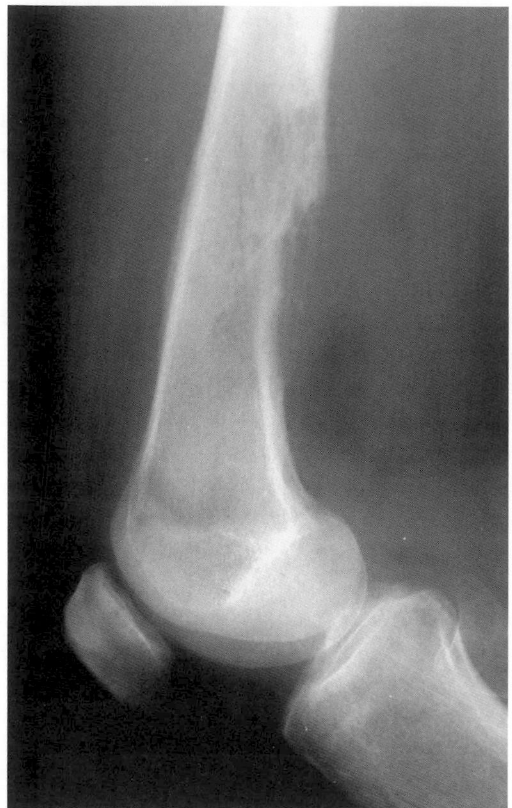

Figure 48.16 Lytic osteosarcoma. Lateral radiograph of the distal femur showing a lytic osteosarcoma.

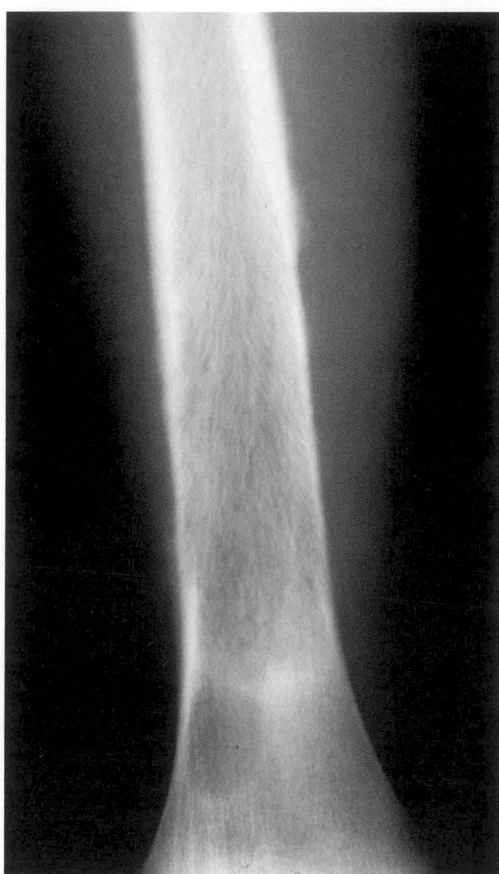

Figure 48.18 Telangiectatic osteosarcoma. AP radiograph of the distal femur showing the classical 'iron-filing' type destruction of the cortex.

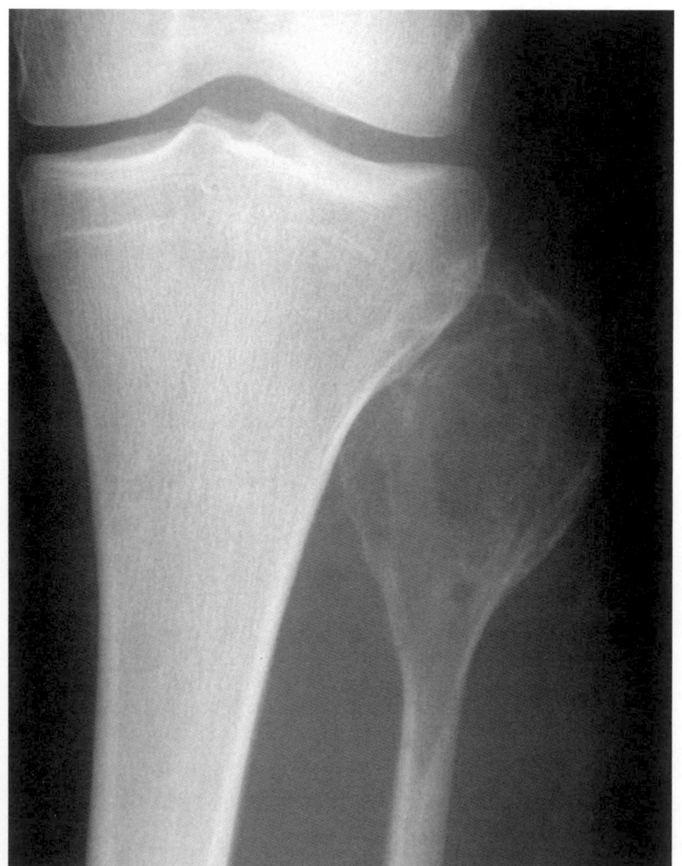

Figure 48.17 Pseudocystic osteosarcoma. AP radiograph of the proximal fibula showing an expanded, lytic lesion mimicking an aneurysmal bone cyst.

fluid levels, mimicking aneurysmal bone cyst. However, the demonstration of thick peripheral, septal and nodular enhancement of solid viable tissue on post-contrast studies is a consistent finding which helps to differentiate telangiectatic osteosarcoma from aneurysmal bone cyst. Extraosseous extension is also commonly demonstrated.

Small cell osteosarcoma The small cell variety accounts for 1% of cases. The age range, clinical presentation, sites of occurrence and radiological features are as for conventional central osteosarcoma.

Low-grade intramedullary osteosarcoma[29] This accounts for less than 1% of cases of osteosarcoma. It is a well-differentiated tumour presenting at a mean age of 34 years and with a slight female preponderance, affecting mainly the femur and tibia around the knee. Four radiological patterns have been described: lytic with varying degrees of coarse trabeculation (Fig. 48.19), lytic with little trabeculation, densely sclerotic and mixed lytic/sclerotic. Due to the relatively benign appearance, the tumour may be mistaken for fibrous dysplasia, osteoblastoma, or a low-grade chondroid tumour. However, CT or MRI commonly shows extraosseous extension, which should aid in differential diagnosis.

Intracortical osteosarcoma[30]

Intracortical osteosarcoma is the rarest form of osteosarcoma, accounting for less than 1% of cases. All reported cases have

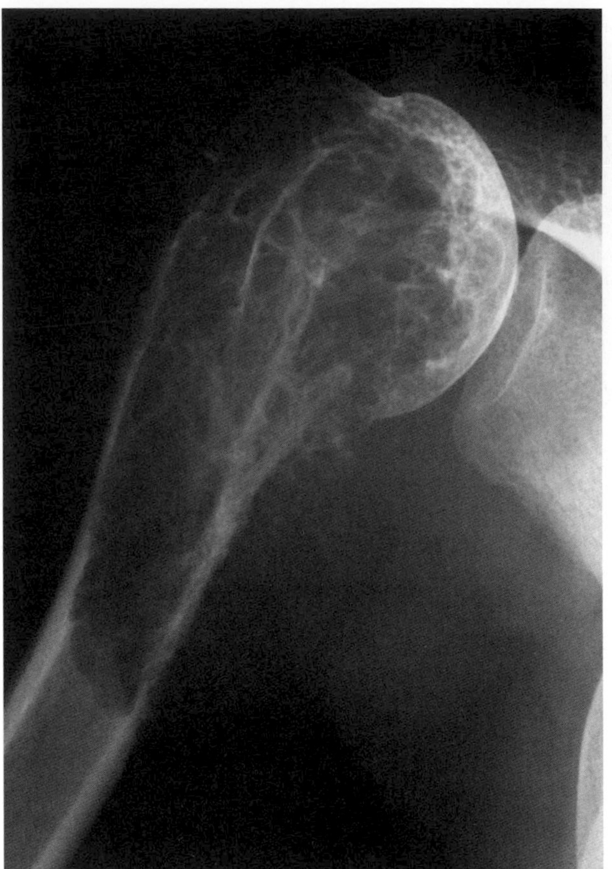

Figure 48.19 Low-grade central osteosarcoma. AP radiograph of the proximal humerus showing the lytic, trabeculated pattern.

arisen in the cortex of the femur or tibia. Patients present between the ages of 10 and 43 years (mean age in the second decade) and the tumour is twice as common in males. Radiologically, the tumour appears as a small lytic lesion surrounded by thickened cortex, resembling an osteoid osteoma or osteoblastoma. CT and MRI show absence of medullary involvement. However, in cases showing associated peritumoural and medullary oedema, microscopic medullary invasion has been reported. The lesion has a good prognosis compared to conventional intramedullary osteosarcoma.

Surface osteosarcoma[31]

This designation refers to a group of tumours that arise from the surface of the bone and includes parosteal, periosteal and high-grade lesions. Surface osteosarcomas account for 4–10% of cases.

Parosteal osteosarcoma[32] Parosteal osteosarcoma accounts for approximately 3–4% of all osteosarcomas. It affects both sexes equally in a wider, but generally older, age group. Although cases have been reported under 10 and over 50 years, most patients affected are in the third and fourth decades. Clinical symptoms are minimal. The natural history may extend to 5 years or longer before metastasis occurs. The prognosis following adequate surgical local resection is usually excellent. Dedifferentiation may occur in as many as one in six cases and particularly following local resection.

Most of the neoplasms involve the posterior aspect of the distal femur (60% of cases), proximal humerus or the tibia.

The characteristic feature is of a dense bony mass enveloping the distal femoral metaphysis (Fig. 48.20A). A well-defined, radiolucent line may separate the tumour from the normal cortex (Fig. 48.20B). Small satellite bony masses may appear in the soft tissues close to the main tumour, especially in the case of a recurrence. Medullary involvement is best appreciated with CT or MRI and is reported in 8–59% of cases. MRI typically shows a mass of low SI due to the sclerotic nature of the lesion. However, areas of intermediate T1-weighted SI or increased T2-weighted SI at the periphery of the lesion may indicate regions of higher grade or dedifferentiation (Fig. 48.20C)[33]. These areas should be targeted for needle biopsy.

The differential diagnosis includes a heavily mineralized osteochondroma and juxtacortical myositis ossificans, which is differentiated by its peripheral mineralization pattern.

Periosteal osteosarcoma[34] Periosteal osteosarcoma is an intermediate-grade chondroblastic osteosarcoma accounting for 1–2% of all osteosarcomas. It has a mean age of occurrence of 20 years and a slight male preponderance. It most commonly arises from the proximal tibial or distal femoral diaphyses.

Typical radiological features are of a small periosteal lesion with associated cortical thickening or erosion and perpendicular periosteal reaction (Fig. 48.21A). Occasionally, the tumour shows a thin peripheral 'cortex'. Rarely, nodular calcification is seen within the matrix. MRI classically shows hyperintensity on T2-weighted images due to the chondroblastic nature of the lesion (Fig. 48.21B). Reactive marrow SI changes may be present but true marrow invasion is extremely rare.

High-grade surface osteosarcoma[35] This very rare surface lesion accounts for 8–10% of surface lesions and less than 1% of all osteosarcomas. It has the same histological features as conventional central osteosarcoma and therefore a very much poorer prognosis than other surface tumours. The radiological features are similar to those of periosteal osteosarcoma but more aggressive in that the tumour is usually larger and there is a greater degree of cortical destruction (Fig. 48.22).

Secondary osteosarcoma

Approximately 5–7% of osteosarcomas are secondary, most commonly seen following Paget's disease (commonest) and radiotherapy. Rarely, osteosarcoma develops in association with osteonecrosis, fibrous dysplasia, osteogenesis imperfecta, metal prostheses and chronic osteomyelitis.

Paget's sarcoma[36] Many bone sarcomas arising after the age of 50 years are secondary to Paget's disease and at least 50% of these are osteosarcomas; fibrosarcoma or malignant fibrous histiocytoma account for 25% and the remainder are anaplastic sarcomas or occasionally giant cell tumours. Malignant change is reported in 3–14% of patients with Paget's disease.

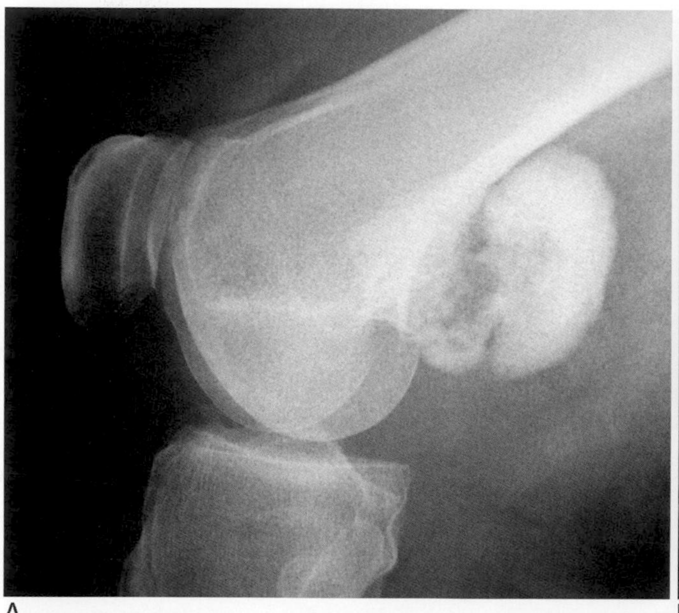

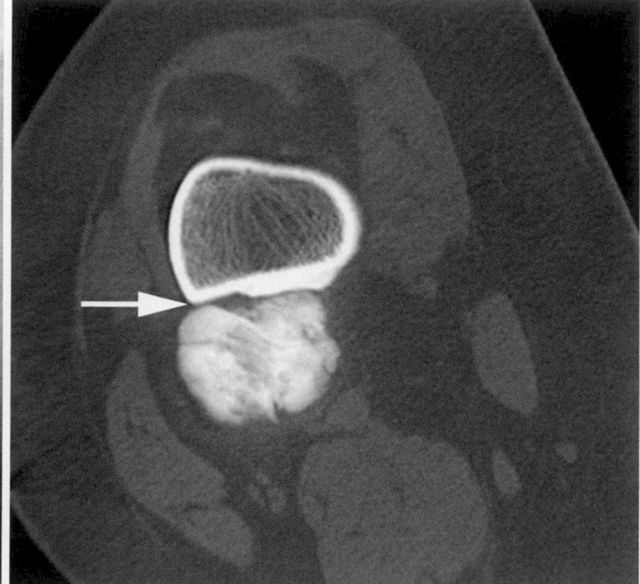

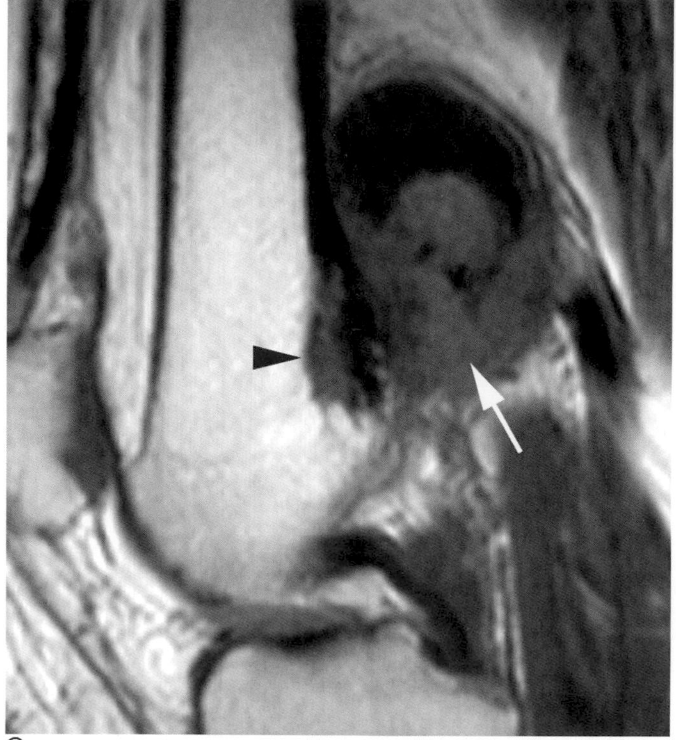

Figure 48.20 Parosteal osteosarcoma. (A) Lateral radiograph of the knee showing a dense, lobulated mass of bone arising from the posterior distal femur. (B) Axial CT shows a lucent line (arrow) separating the lesion from the underlying cortex. (C) Sagittal T1-weighted spin-echo MR image shows the low SI mass with central intermediate SI (arrow) indicating a region of dedifferentiation to high-grade tumour. Note also the intramedullary extension (arrowhead).

The overall prevalence is likely to be under 1%, with the incidence increasing to 5–10% in patients with widespread Paget's disease. However, sarcoma can occur in a patient with monostotic disease. Most patients are over the age of 45 years, with a mean age incidence of 55 in the USA and 67.6 years in England. The sex incidence of Paget's sarcoma is similar to that of the primary disease, with men affected twice as often as women. Malignant change is suggested clinically by a change in type or severity of bone pain and sometimes by an enlarging mass or a pathological fracture.

Radiologically, the commonest sites for Paget's disease, the pelvis and femur, are common locations for malignant change. The spine is typically spared. Usually a region of bone destruction is apparent with a wide zone of transition and evidence of a large soft tissue mass, best shown with CT and MRI (Fig. 48.23A). MRI is extremely valuable in identifying sarcomatous degeneration, based on the presence of marrow infiltration on a T1-weighted image (Fig. 48.23B)[37]. Scintigraphy is relatively insensitive to malignant transformation, which may be indicated by a focal region of reduced activity. In a few cases, the sarcomas are multifocal. The prognosis is extremely poor, with most patients succumbing within a year of diagnosis.

An important differential to consider is the rare pseudosarcoma, which may also present with an extraosseous mass[38]. Biopsy is therefore important in making a definitive diagnosis.

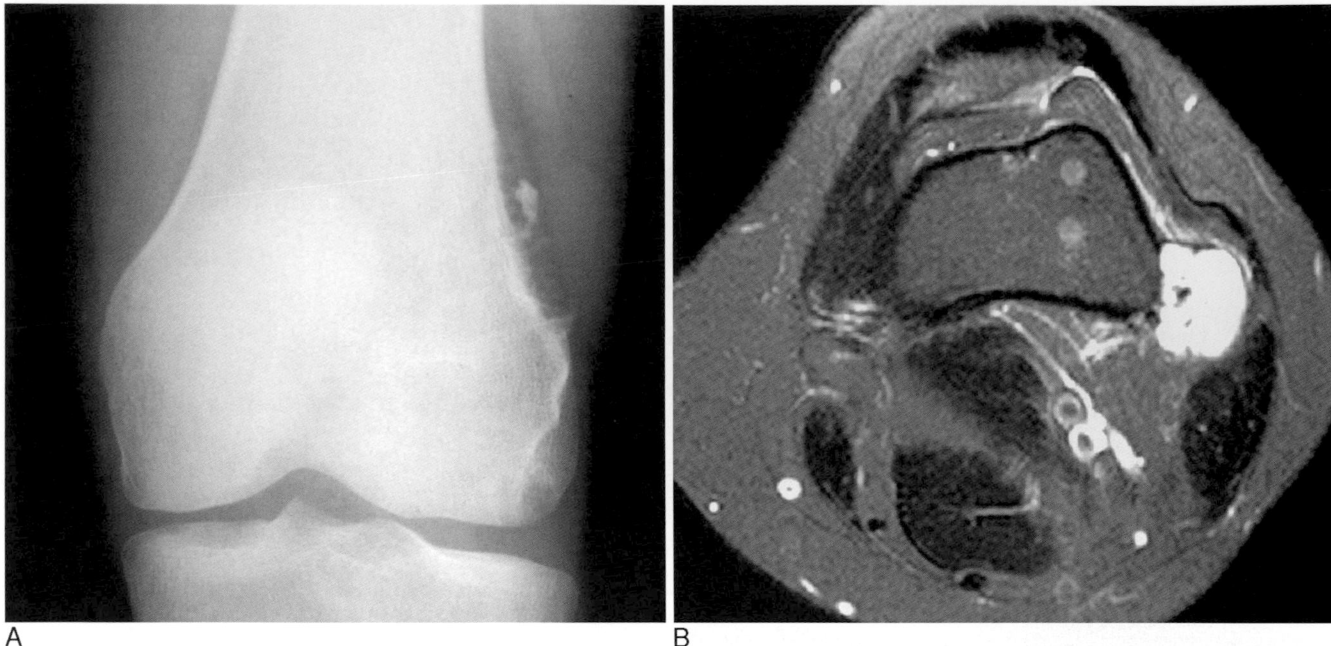

Figure 48.21 Periosteal osteosarcoma. (A) AP radiograph of the knee showing a spiculated periosteal reaction from the lateral femoral condyle and nodular matrix mineralization. (B) Axial fat-suppressed T2-weighted FSE MR image shows a lobular, hyperintense surface lesion consistent with a chondroblastic tumour.

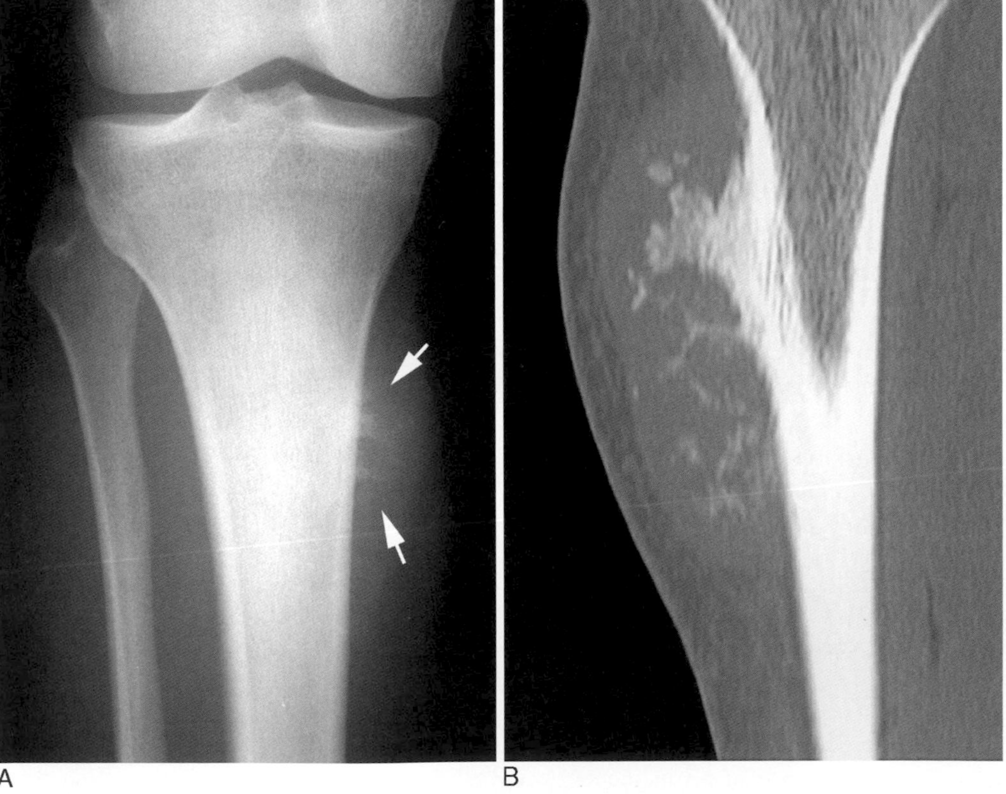

Figure 48.22 High-grade surface osteosarcoma of the proximal tibia. (A) AP radiograph shows a vertical periosteal reaction (arrows) arising from the medial metaphysis. (B) Sagittal CT multiplanar reconstruction shows the large associated soft tissue component. The features are similar to periosteal osteosarcoma, but more aggressive.

Post-radiation sarcoma[39] Post-radiation sarcoma (PRS) is now the preferred term (compared to radiation-induced sarcoma) for bone and soft tissue sarcoma that develops following previous radiotherapy. They account for 0.5–5.5% of all sarcomas. The criteria for diagnosis of a PRS include the following:

1 a history of radiation therapy
2 the development of a neoplasm in the radiation field
3 a latent period of several years (minimum 3–4 years)
4 histological proof of a sarcoma, which differs significantly from that initially treated.

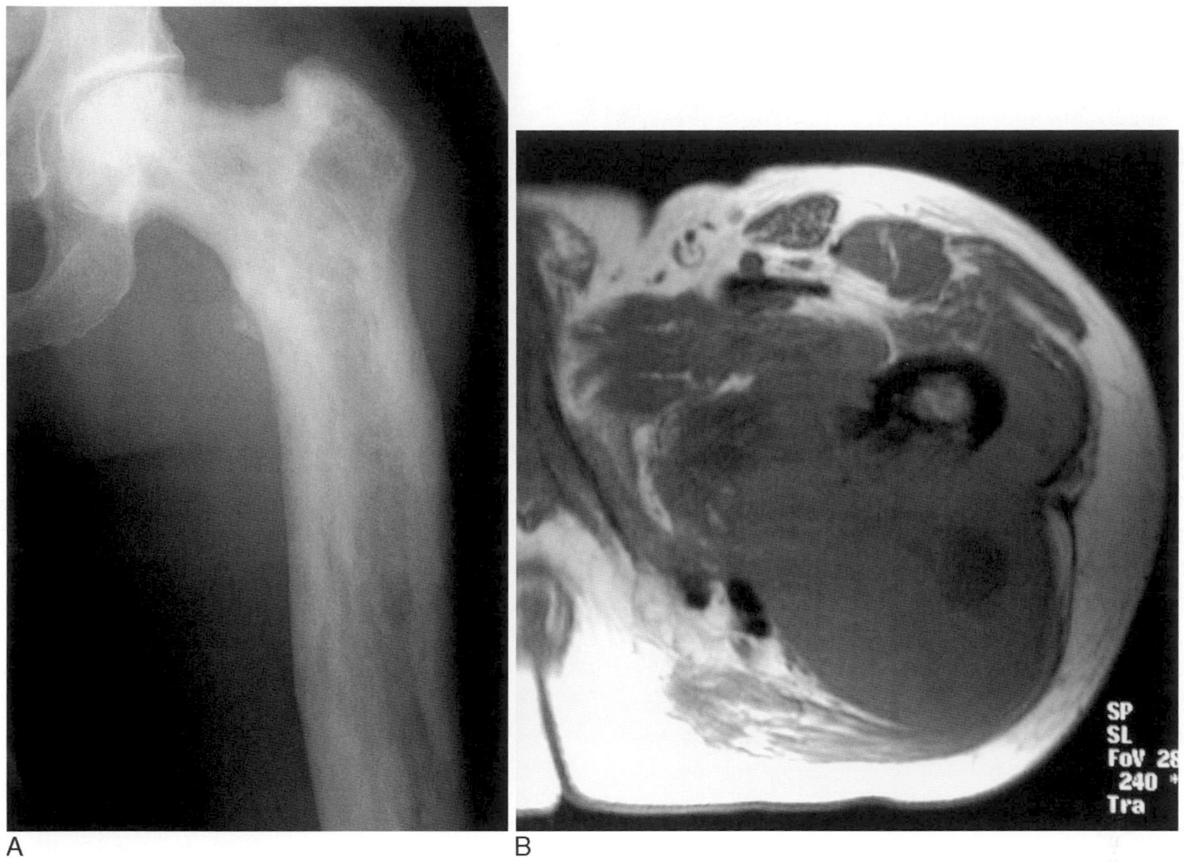

Figure 48.23 Paget's sarcoma. (A) AP radiograph of the proximal femur showing Paget's disease. (B) Axial T1-weighted spin-echo MR image shows an associated large soft tissue mass due to sarcomatous change.

The treated tumours mostly commonly resulting in the development of PRS are breast carcinoma, lymphoma, head and neck cancers and gynaecological malignancies. This accounts for the increased incidence in women. The mean age at presentation is in the sixth decade with a mean latency period before PRS development of approximately 15 years. It is considered that a minimal dose of 30 Gy is required to induce a PRS and it is also suggested that the concurrent use of chemotherapy increases the risk of sarcoma development.

The commonest PRS is osteosarcoma followed by malignant fibrous histiocytoma (MFH). The commonest sites are the pelvis and shoulder girdle. Typical radiological features include bone destruction (83% of cases), soft tissue mass (96% of cases), matrix mineralization and periosteal reaction (Fig. 48.24). There may also be evidence of radiation change in the underlying bone (radiation osteitis and marrow infarction) on both radiography and MRI, which may show fatty replacement of normal red marrow. The tumours have no specific signal characteristics, being of intermediate SI on T1 weighting and heterogeneous increased SI on T2 weighting. The prognosis is universally poor.

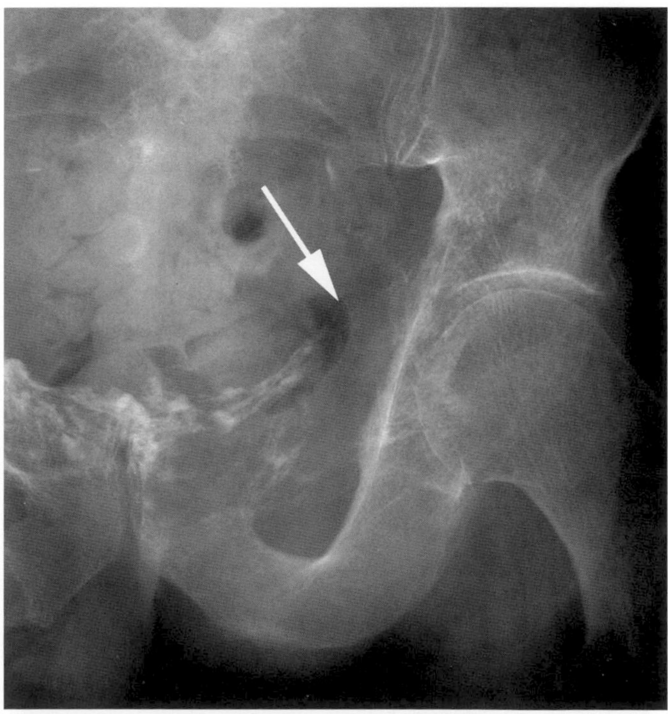

Figure 48.24 Radiation-induced sarcoma of the left superior pubic ramus manifest as a region of lytic bone destruction (arrow) with underlying radiation osteitis.

Primary multicentric osteosarcoma[40,41]

Multicentric osteosarcoma may be either synchronous or metachronous. The disorder is characterized by the presence of multiple foci of bony osteosarcoma without pulmonary metastases at presentation. The synchronous type typically consists of multiple metaphyseal lesions developing simultaneously, usually in children or adolescents. The lesions are usually osteoblastic (Fig. 48.25) and a poor prognosis with mean survival of 8 months has been reported. In the metachronous type, presentation is with a solitary lesion in a long or flat bone with the development of multiple lesions after a period of greater than 5 months. The lesions may be lytic or sclerotic. Patients are usually older and the condition is associated with a better prognosis.

FIBROUS ORIGIN

Malignant fibrous histiocytoma[42,43]

Malignant fibrous histiocytoma (MFH) is the most common primary malignant tumour of fibrous origin affecting bone. Together with fibrosarcoma, it accounts for 5% of primary malignant bone tumours. Approximately 25–30% of MFH arise in a pre-existing lesion, especially Paget's disease, post radiotherapy, bone infarction and in relation to dedifferentiated chondrosarcoma. Rarely, it is associated with fibrous dysplasia, nonossifying fibroma, chronic osteomyelitis and total hip replacement. Clinical features are nonspecific, usually presenting with pain and swelling of insidious onset, although pathological fracture is common, reported in 20% at presentation.

The metaphyses of long bones are predominantly involved (75% of cases), particularly around the knee. After the femur and the tibia, the humerus and pelvis are most commonly affected. The lesion involves the central metaphyseal region in 90% of cases. In 21% of cases, the pelvis, spine or ribs are involved, and multicentric MFH is also recognized.

The age range is from 6 to 80 years with the peak incidence in the fourth decade. The male to female ratio is 1.5:1.

Radiological features

Primary MFH is lytic and destructive, resembling a metastasis (Fig. 48.26). Central mineralization is rare, but central photon-poor regions are seen sometimes on scintigraphy, occasionally

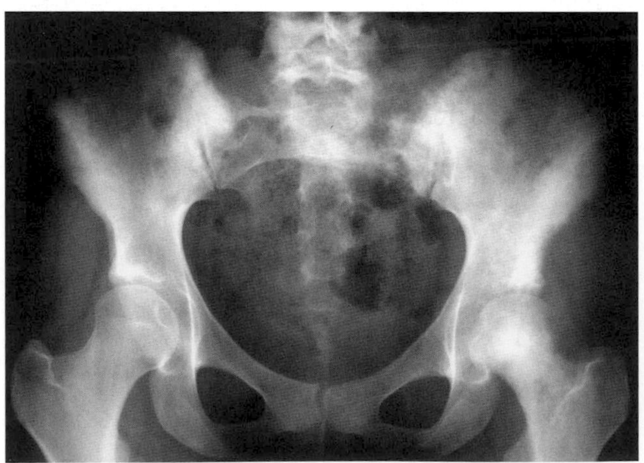

Figure 48.25 Osteosarcomatosis. AP radiograph of the pelvis shows multiple poorly defined osteoblastic lesions.

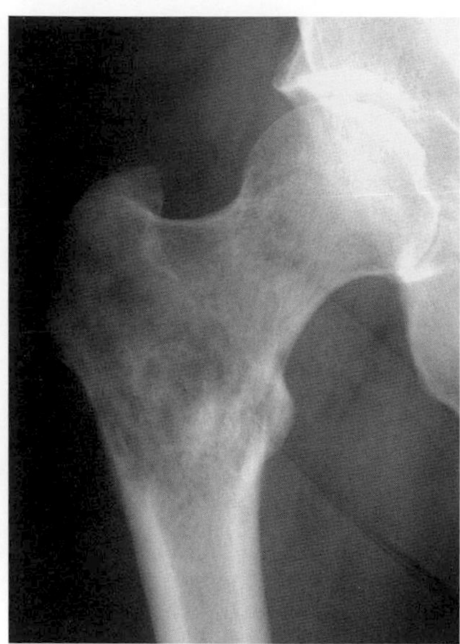

Figure 48.26 Malignant fibrous histiocytoma. AP radiograph of the proximal femur showing a moth-eaten destructive lesion with no characteristic features.

related to a pre-existing bone infarct. Periosteal reaction is uncommon but an extraosseous mass may be evident. The lesion may extend to the subarticular surface, mimicking giant cell tumour. No specific diagnostic features are found on MRI, although 'skip' metastases may be demonstrated.

Fibrosarcoma[44]

Fibrosarcoma is uncommon in children, with most patients presenting between 20 and 50 years of age. Sex incidence is equal. Patients usually present with pain and swelling of insidious onset. Pathological fractures are relatively common in the long bones. The lesion most commonly affects the long bones (70% of cases), with 50% arising in the lower limb, particularly around the knee (femur 40% and tibia 16%). Extension to the epiphysis is not uncommon while purely diaphyseal lesions are reported in 7% of cases. Less common sites include the pelvis (13%), humerus (10%) and jaw (8%). Most neoplasms arise in the medulla, although often eccentrically within the bone.

As with MFH, fibrosarcoma is reported as a secondary occurrence in Paget's disease, dedifferentiated chondrosarcoma, bone infarction following irradiation and in the chronic sinus tracts of osteomyelitis.

Radiological features

Fibrosarcoma shows 'moth-eaten' destruction of bone with a wide zone of transition in the more malignant tumours. Proximal intraosseous spread with 'skip' lesions may sometimes occur. Cortical destruction is common, with little periosteal reaction, and although a soft tissue mass is often demonstrated, this is usually small. Calcification, if it occurs within the soft tissue mass, tends to be punctate.

The differential diagnosis of fibrosarcoma includes other neoplasms such as a lytic osteosarcoma, chondrosarcoma and metastasis.

MARROW TUMOURS

Malignant round cell tumours of bone

The group of malignant small round cell tumours (MRCT) comprises Ewing's sarcoma, peripheral primitive neuroectodermal tumour (PNET), primary lymphoma of bone (formerly reticulum cell sarcoma), metastatic neuroblastoma and small cell osteosarcoma.

Ewing's sarcoma[45,46]

This rare, highly malignant primary bone neoplasm accounts for approximately 5% of biopsied primary tumours and, together with osteosarcoma, represents 90% of primary malignant bone tumours in children. Cytogenetic analysis shows a specific constant reciprocal translocation between chromosomes 11 and 22, which is shared with extraskeletal Ewing's sarcoma, PNET and Askin tumours.

Seventy-five per cent of patients are under the age of 20 years at presentation, most between 5 and 15 years, and 90% are under the age of 30 years. The male to female ratio is 2:1 and 95% occur in Caucasians. Characteristically, presentation is with localized pain and swelling. The presence of systemic symptoms, including pyrexia and elevation of the ESR, simulates infection and signifies disseminated disease, thus indicating a poor prognosis.

Usually a single bone is involved, but multiple lesions occur at presentation in 10% of cases and more commonly later in the disease, as Ewing's sarcoma is one of the few bone tumours that metastasizes readily to bone. In comparison to other sarcomas, most cases show extensive involvement of the diaphysis (35%) or the metadiaphyseal region (59%) of a long bone. Bones most commonly affected are the femur and humerus (together 31% of cases), the pelvic bones (21% of cases, most commonly the ilium) and ribs (6.5–8% of cases). The distal appendicular skeleton is involved in 27% of cases. The neoplasm is usually medullary in origin, but subperiosteal tumours may occur[47].

Radiological features The tumour produces a permeative pattern of predominantly lytic bone destruction with a wide zone of transition (Fig. 48.27A). The destructive process in bone may be radiographically occult in the most aggressive lesions. The tumour rapidly extends through the cortex producing a large extraosseous, sub-periosteal mass, which is sometimes disproportionate to the degree of medullary involvement. Soft tissue involvement is radiographically evident in 80%. The sub-periosteal tumour mass may cause erosion of the outer cortex, producing so-called 'saucerization' (Fig.48.27B). The classic multilaminar ('onion peel') periosteal reaction is uncommon, but confirms the periodic activity of the lesion. An incomplete laminar periosteal reaction is more common, with marginal Codman's triangles. A vertical 'hair-on-end' type of periosteal reaction is also classical of Ewing's sarcoma. Other reported features include cortical thickening and rarely pathological fracture or bone expansion.

Occasionally, Ewing's sarcoma shows a mixed or mainly sclerotic appearance, especially in the flat bones (Fig. 48.27C) and spine. These lesions may resemble osteosarcoma. Radiologically atypical Ewing's sarcoma has also been described, in which the lesion is predominantly eccentric with a very small intraosseous component[48].

CT and MRI typically show a large extraosseous component (Fig. 48.28). Intraosseous extent is accurately demonstrated and 'skip' metastases may be identified.

Differential diagnosis in the early stages includes osteomyelitis or trauma, particularly stress fracture. Each of these may

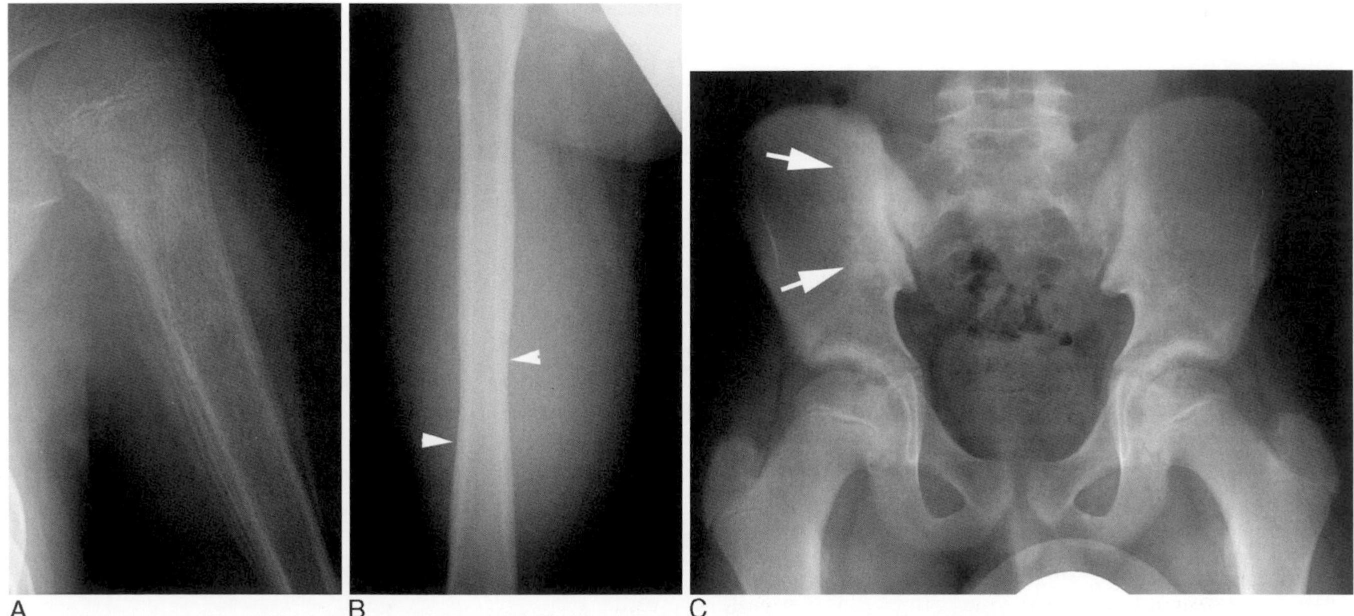

Figure 48.27 Ewing's sarcoma. (A) Typical appearance in the proximal humeral metadiaphysis with permeative marrow destruction, 'hair-on-end' and multilaminated periosteal reaction. (B) AP radiograph of the femur showing cortical 'saucerization' (arrowheads). (C) AP radiograph of the pelvis showing a sclerotic Ewing's sarcoma of the right ilium (arrows).

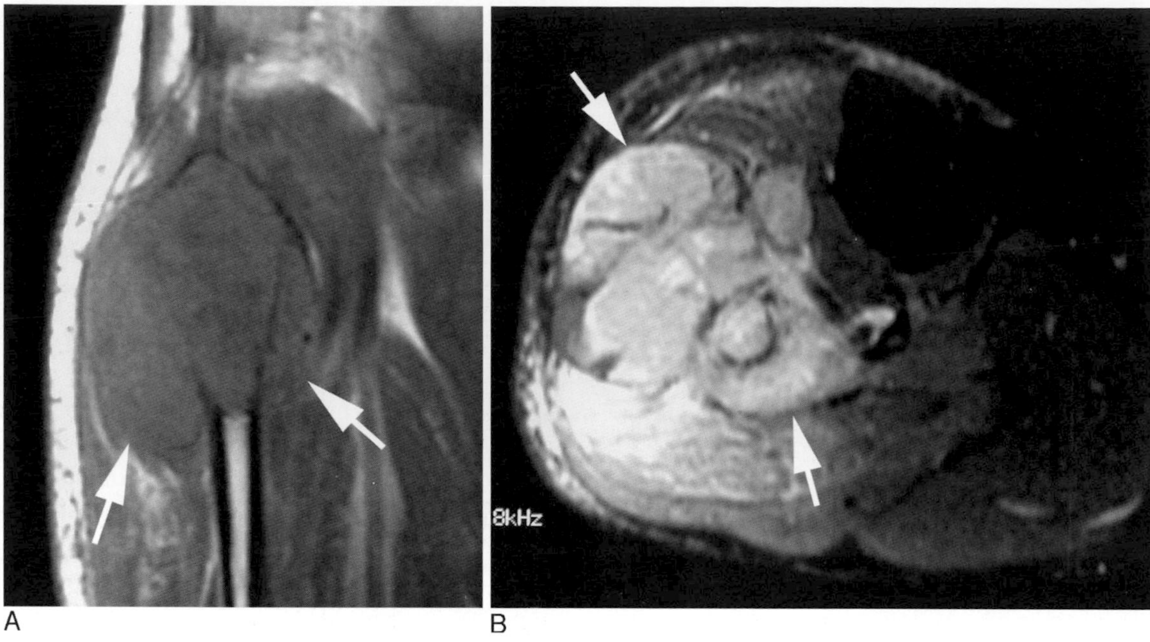

Figure 48.28 Ewing's sarcoma of the proximal fibula. (A) Coronal T1-weighted spin-echo and (B) axial STIR MR images show a large extraosseous mass (arrows).

produce a periosteal reaction with little bone destruction. A lytic osteosarcoma may be indistinguishable from Ewing's tumour. Primary lymphoma of bone should be suspected if the patient is over 30 years of age. Langerhans cell histiocytosis may occasionally mimic Ewing's sarcoma, especially when presenting at an early destructive stage and involving the pelvis.

Askin tumour[49]

This is a rare PNET of the chest wall occurring in children and young adults. Imaging typically demonstrates a lytic extrapleural mass with rib involvement in approximately 66% of cases. Invasion of the underlying lung is not a feature. The soft tissue mass tends to be slightly hyperintense to muscle on T1-weighted images.

Primitive neuroectodermal tumour of bone[50]

These rare tumours of bone resemble Ewing's tumours clinically except that they are more common in the female sex. Radiologically, they resemble Ewing's sarcoma in being destructive ill-defined neoplasms, which readily spread into the soft tissues. Involvement of the metaphyses and diaphyses of the lower limbs, humerus, pelvis and scapula, in that order of frequency, is found.

Primary bone lymphoma[51,52] (syn: lymphosarcoma of bone, reticulum cell sarcoma of bone)

The diagnosis of primary lymphoma of bone (PLB) depends on involvement of a single site in bone with no evidence of disease elsewhere in the body for at least 6 months after diagnosis, excluding regional lymph node disease. It is the rarest primary intraosseous malignancy, accounting for approximately 3% of malignant bone tumours, and is usually a non-Hodgkin's B-cell lymphoma. Primary Hodgkin's disease of bone is extremely rare[53] and accounts for 6% of PLB.

The age at presentation is wide, from the second to the eighth decades. The mean age is approximately 50 years but with a slightly biphasic distribution, showing peaks around 20 and 50 years. The male to female ratio is 1.6:1. Patients usually present with chronic pain and a palpable mass is present in one-third of cases.

The metadiaphyses of long bones are most commonly involved, particularly the femur, tibia and humerus. Pathological fractures are relatively common. Flat bones are also involved, especially the ilium and scapula. Spinal involvement has been reported in 25% of cases.

Radiological features The radiological features are similar to those described for Ewing's sarcoma, with a predominantly lytic permeative destructive lesion reported in 74% of cases (Fig. 48.29A) and associated soft tissue mass present in all cases imaged with MRI. Relative absence of cortical destruction is a characteristic feature. Periosteal reaction is demonstrated in 58% of cases. Nearly half the cases show some reactive sclerosis, while a predominantly sclerotic tumour is found in approximately 20% of cases and more commonly in Hodgkin's lymphoma. Additional characteristic features include the presence of sequestra in 11–16% of cases (Fig. 48.29B) and transarticular extension. Pathological fracture is reported in approximately 25% of cases.

MRI typically shows extensive involvement of the medullary canal with little cortical destruction but a large extraosseous mass (Fig. 48.29C).

NOTOCHORDAL ORIGIN

Chordoma[54,55]

Chordoma is a neoplasm originating from ectopic cellular remnants of the notochord and therefore arises from the

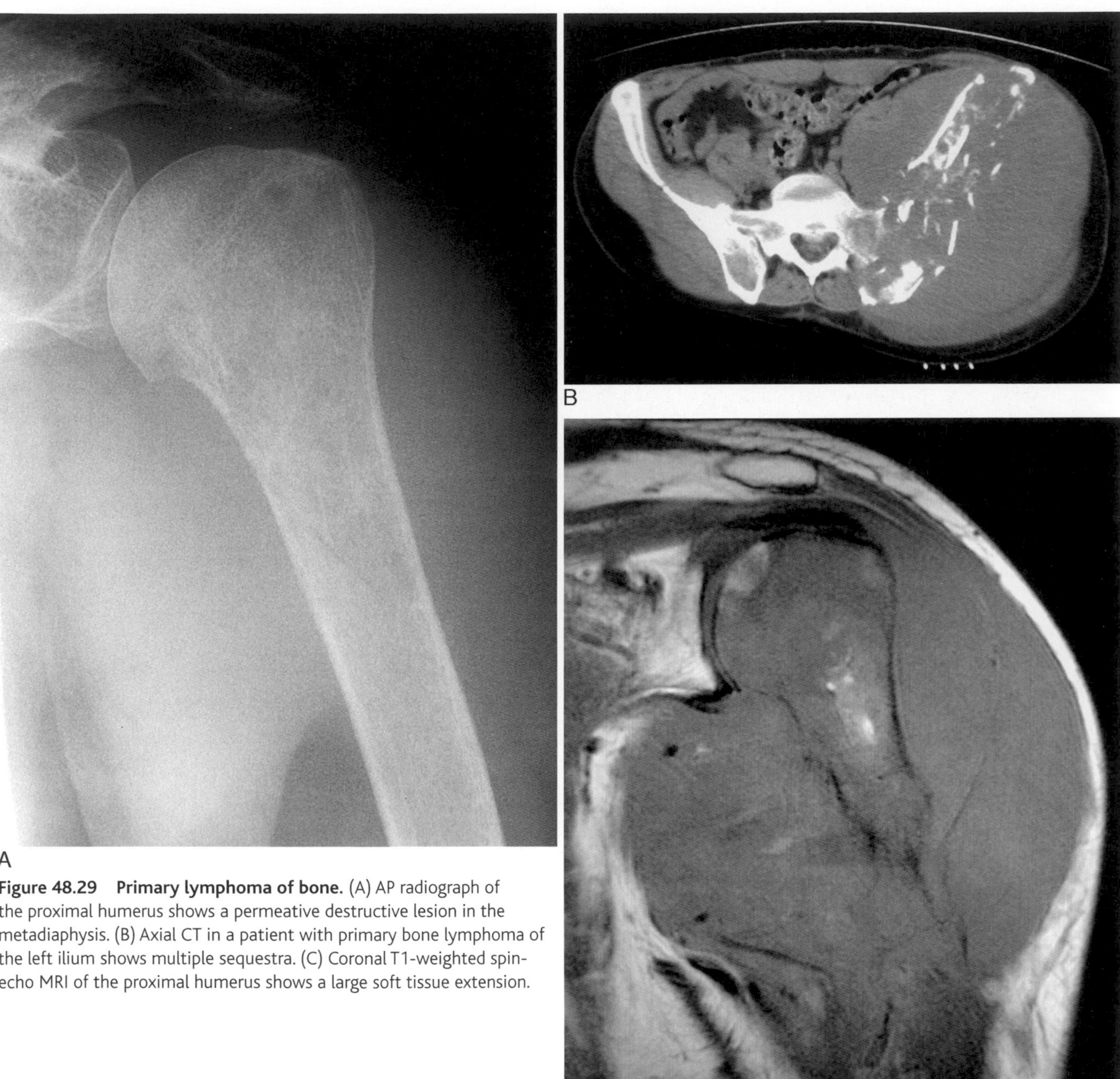

Figure 48.29 Primary lymphoma of bone. (A) AP radiograph of the proximal humerus shows a permeative destructive lesion in the metadiaphysis. (B) Axial CT in a patient with primary bone lymphoma of the left ilium shows multiple sequestra. (C) Coronal T1-weighted spin-echo MRI of the proximal humerus shows a large soft tissue extension.

midline of the axial skeleton. It accounts for 2–4% of all primary malignant bone tumours. Chordoma is the second commonest primary malignancy of the spine and accounts for over 50% of primary sacral tumours. The neoplasm has a predilection for the sacrococcygeal (50%) and clival (40%) regions, with other areas of the spine rarely involved. More than one vertebral body can be affected in half the cases. Chordomas most commonly present between 50 and 70 years of age. Sex incidence is equal below 40 years, but men are affected twice as often at older ages, particularly in the sacral region.

Symptoms are usually present for 1 year or longer before presentation. Pain is usual and additional symptoms relate to local pressure effects, including bladder dysfunction and constipation in the sacral region, or cranial nerve palsies in the clival region. The tumour grows slowly and is almost always associated with a large soft tissue mass by the time of presentation.

Dedifferentiation is rarely seen with chordoma and typically occurs in the setting of local recurrence or following radiotherapy.

Radiological features

Sacral lesions may be radiographically occult or show a large area of bone destruction with well-defined margins (Fig. 48.30). The size of any extraosseous mass is not appreciated radiographically. Amorphous calcification is present in a minority of cases, optimally demonstrated by CT (Fig. 48.31). In spheno-occipital chordoma, the dorsal aspect of the sella and clivus may be destroyed. A soft tissue mass frequently indents the nasopharynx.

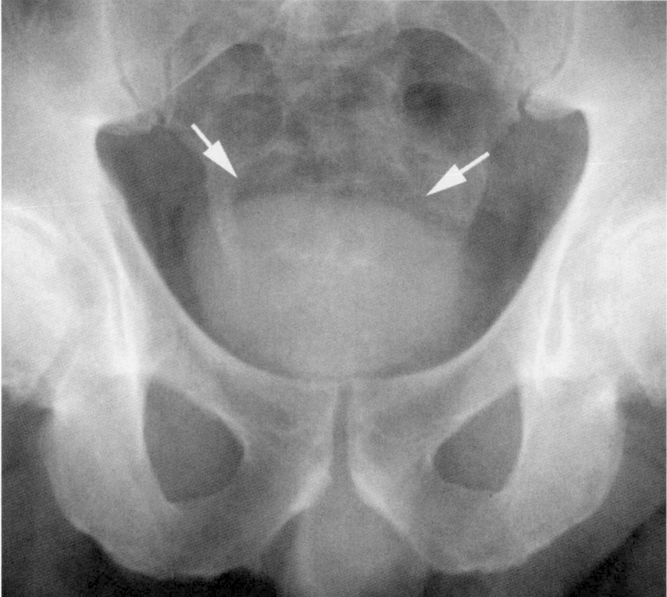

Figure 48.30 Sacral chordoma. AP radiograph of the sacrum shows a central, lytic destructive lesion (arrows).

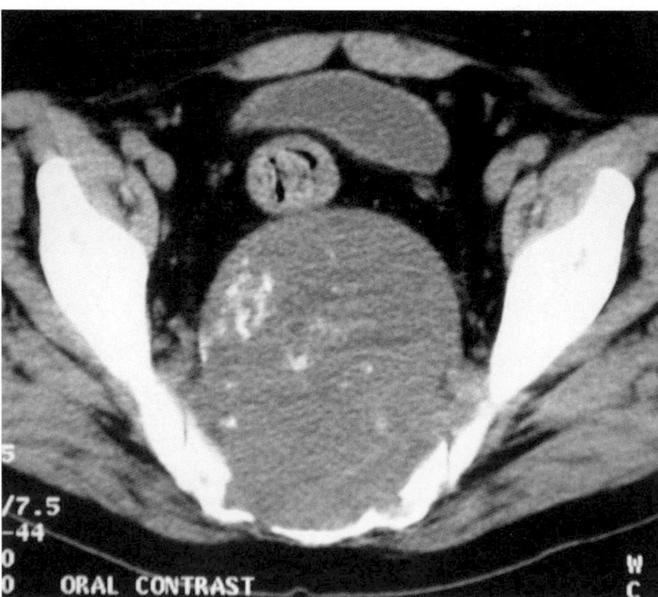

Figure 48.31 Sacral chordoma. CT shows a predominantly lytic mass with small foci of calcification.

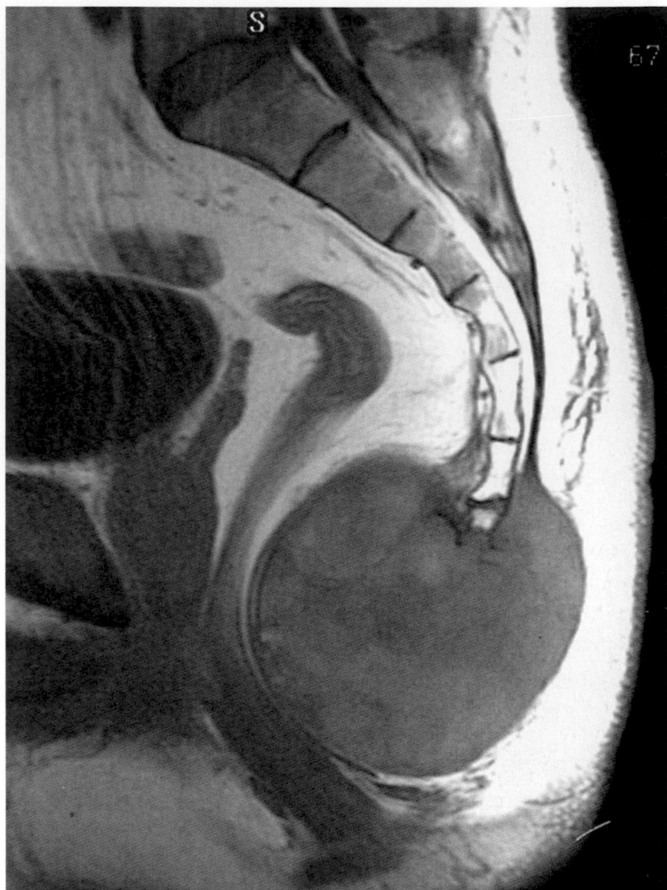

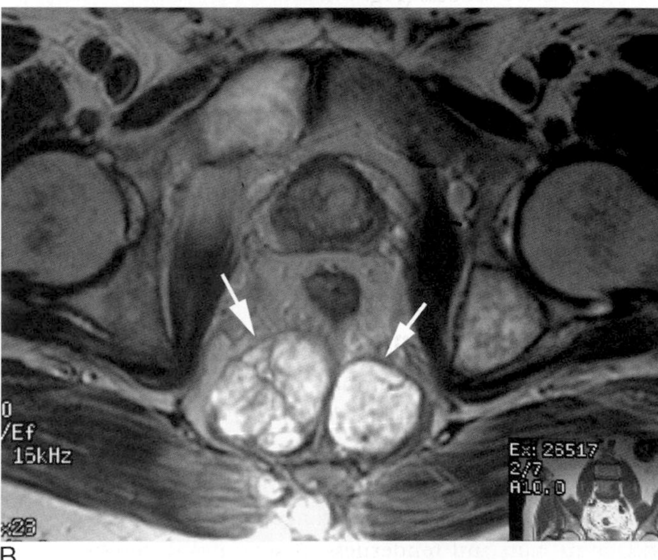

Figure 48.32 Sacrococcygeal chordoma. (A) Sagittal T1-weighted spin-echo MR image shows the intraosseous extent of the lesion and the relationship to the anterior pelvic viscera. (B) Axial T2-weighted FSE MR image shows the classical hyperintense, lobulated nature of the lesion (arrows).

MRI is essential for local staging before surgical excision. With regard to sacral lesions, sagittal T1-weighted images demonstrate the upper level of sacral involvement and also identify the relationship of anterior soft tissue extension to the recto-sigmoid (Fig. 48.32A). Involvement of the gluteal muscles and sacroiliac joints is also well demonstrated. SI on T1 weighting is variable, with areas of hyperintensity due to focal haemorrhage or high protein content being relatively common. T2-weighted images demonstrate a classical lobulated, hyperintense mass with internal septations and well-defined margins (Fig. 48.32B). Areas of low T2-weighted SI may be due to haemosiderin deposition. Heterogeneous or septal enhancement is typically seen following gadolinium.

MISCELLANEOUS LESIONS

Malignant vascular tumours[56]

Malignant vascular tumours of bone are rare and include haemangioendothelioma, epithelioid haemangioendothelioma and angiosarcoma.

Haemangioendothelioma

This is a low-grade malignant endothelial tumour, which affects a wide age group of patients and presents as a multifocal lesion in 25% of cases. The radiological features of individual lesions are nonspecific but the presence of multifocal disease, either within the same bone or in different bones, is a clue to the diagnosis. Multifocal lesions may affect a single limb or be randomly scattered throughout the skeleton. Each lesion is typically lytic although mixed lytic/sclerotic tumours can be seen. Periosteal reaction, cortical destruction and extraosseous extension are uncommon.

Epithelioid haemangioendothelioma is multifocal in approximately 40% of cases but has a propensity to be limited to a single anatomic region. Individual lesions are lytic with a small extraosseous mass identified in 40% of cases.

Angiosarcoma

Angiosarcoma represents a high-grade vascular neoplasm, which may also be unifocal or multifocal. The mean age of presentation is in the third to fourth decades of life. The radiological features are nonspecific, being those of an aggressive, lytic destructive process (Fig. 48.33). Sclerotic lesions are rarely encountered and periosteal reaction or pathological fractures are uncommon.

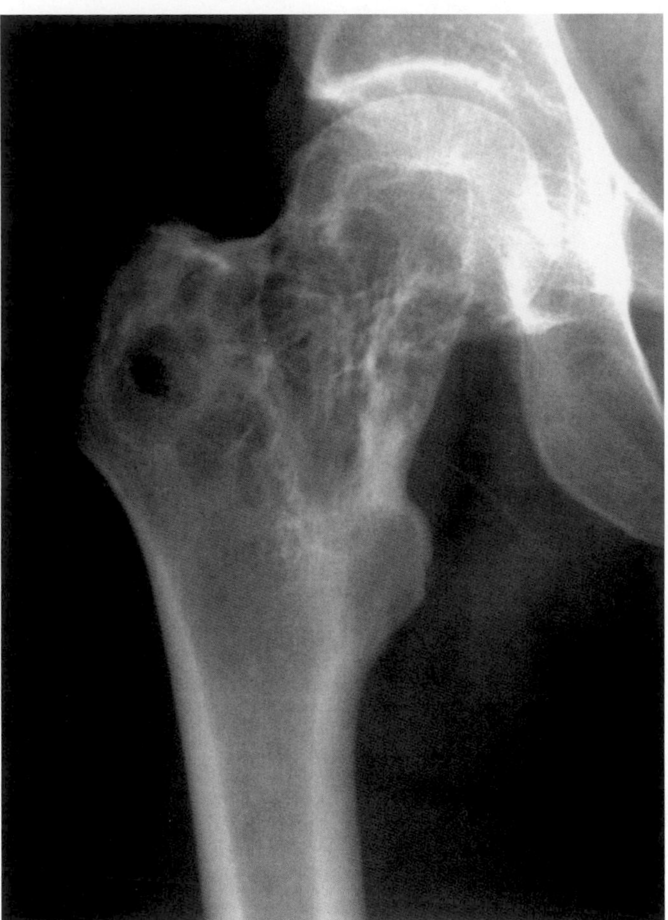

Figure 48.33 Angiosarcoma. AP radiograph of the proximal femur shows an aggressive, lytic destructive lesion with no specific features.

Anaplastic sarcoma

With some highly malignant tumours, the neoplastic cells are so immature that the tissue of origin cannot be determined pathologically. Most of these tumours are lytic, locally aggressive and exhibit no specific diagnostic radiological features.

Adamantinoma of long bones[57,58]

Adamantinoma is a rare tumour, accounting for 0.1–0.5% of all malignant bone tumours. Most cases occur between 10 and 50 years with an average age of 35 years. The male to female ratio is 5:4, but a higher female incidence is found at the younger end of the age range. Patients usually present with local pain and tenderness of several months to several years duration.

Approximately 85% occur in the tibia, mostly in the midshaft, but almost as commonly towards either metaphysis. Synchronous involvement of the tibia and fibula is reported in 10% of cases, with other bones rarely affected. Multifocal lesions in the same long bone are occasionally seen. Initially the tumours are eccentric but eventually they involve the whole depth of the shaft.

Histologically, differentiation is made between classical adamantinoma and osteofibrous dysplasia-like adamantinoma. This differentiation is of clinical importance since the former is more likely to metastasize.

Radiological features

Eccentric involvement of the diaphysis of the tibia is classical. The majority are predominantly intracortical, showing a geographic type of cortical destruction. The lesion is usually lytic with a sclerotic, lobulated margin and internal ossification or septations (Fig. 48.34). A multilocular appearance and satellite lesions, although rarely evident radiologically, are useful diagnostic features. In approximately 15% of cases, extracortical extension is seen. Rarer findings include anterior tibial bowing, moth-eaten destruction, ground-glass mineralization and bony expansion.

MRI is invaluable for local staging of adamantinoma, although differentiation between the two histological subtypes is not possible[58]. Features that may not be easily appreciated radiologically include extension into the marrow cavity in 60% of cases (Fig. 48.35), extraosseous extension and multifocal lesions in 27% of cases. A lobulated growth pattern is typical but there are no specific signal characteristics. Intense, uniform enhancement is seen following gadolinium.

Adamantinoma is locally aggressive and will readily recur if incompletely removed; metastases to lung have been reported in about 10% of cases. Early and complete resection is advisable.

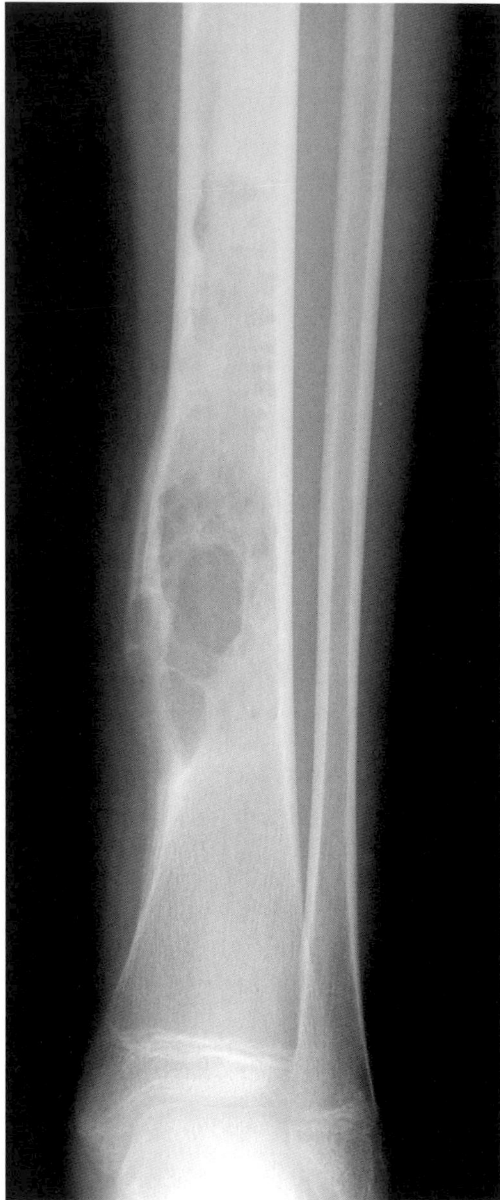

Figure 48.34 Adamantinoma. AP radiograph of the tibia showing a multiloculated, lytic lesion expanding the cortex.

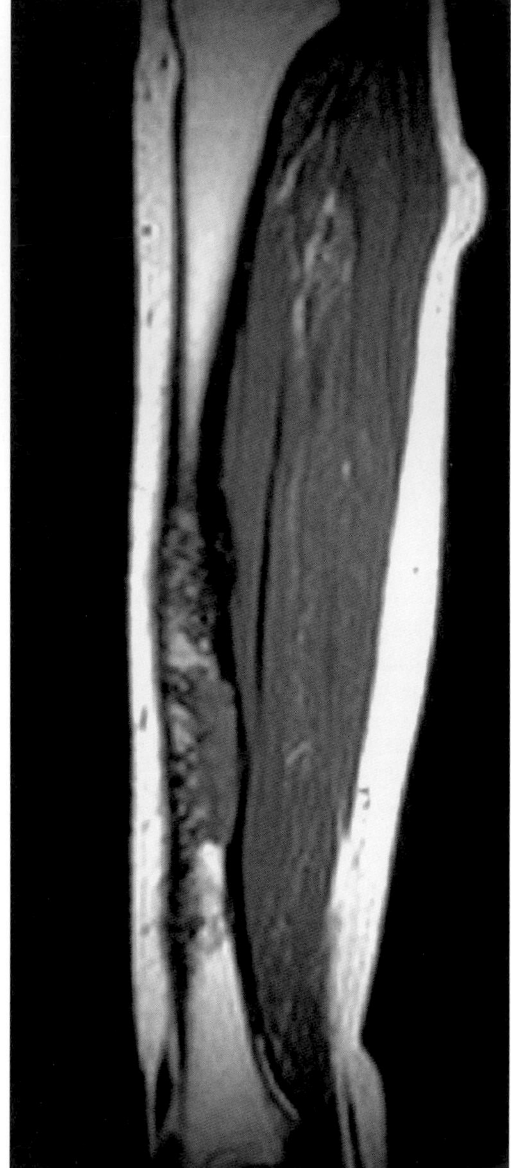

Figure 48.35 Adamantinoma. Sagittal T1-weighted MRI showing a lobulated diaphyseal lesion with extension into the medullary cavity.

REFERENCES

1. Johnston A D 1970 Pathology of metastatic tumor in bone. Clin Orthop 73: 8–32
2. Galasko C S B 1981 The anatomy and pathways of skeletal metastases. In: Weiss L, Gilbert H A (eds) Bone metastases. G K Hall, Boston, pp 49–63
3. Carter R L 1978 General pathology of the metastatic process. In: Baldwin RW (ed) Secondary spread of cancer. Academic Press, London
4. Abrams H L, Sprio R, Goldstein N 1950 Metastases in carcinoma. Analysis of 1000 autopsied cases. Cancer 3: 74–85
5. Galasko C S 1972 Skeletal metastases and mammary cancer. Ann R Coll Surg Engl 50: 3–28
6. Kricun M E 1985 Red-yellow marrow conversion: its effect on the location of some solitary bone lesions. Skeletal Radiol 14: 10–19
7. Libson E, Bloom R A, Husband J E, Stoker D J 1987 Metastatic tumours of bones of the hand and foot. Skeletal Radiol 16: 387–392
8. Soderlund V 1996 Radiological diagnosis of skeletal metastases. Eur Radiol 6: 587–595
9. Rosenthal D I 2001 Radiologic imaging for the diagnosis of bone metastases. Q J Nucl Med 45: 53–64
10. Lauenstein T C, Fredenberg L S, Goehde S C et al 2002 Whole-body MRI using a rolling table platform for the detection of bone metastases. Eur Radiol 12: 2091–2099
11. Even-Sapir E, Metser U, Flusser G et al 2004 Assessment of malignant skeletal disease: initial experience with 18F-fluoride PET/CT and comparison between 18F-fluoride PET and 18F-fluoride PET/CT. J Nucl Med 45: 272–278
12. Schweitzer M E, Levine C, Mitchell D G, Gannon F H, Gomella L G 1993 Bull's-eyes and halos: useful MR discriminators of osseous metastases. Radiology 188: 249–252
13. van der Woude H J, Bloem J L, Hogendoorn P C 1998 Preoperative evaluation and monitoring chemotherapy in patients with high-grade osteogenic and Ewing's sarcoma: review of current imaging modalities. Skeletal Radiol 27: 57–71
14. Bramer J A, Gubler F M, Maas M et al 2004 Colour Doppler ultrasound predicts chemotherapy response, but not survival in paediatric osteosarcoma. Pediatr Radiol 34: 614–619

15. Vanel D, Lacombe M J, Couanet D, Kalifa C, Spielmann M, Genin J 1987 Musculoskeletal tumors: follow-up with MR imaging after treatment with surgery and radiation therapy. Radiology 164: 243–245
16. Flemming D J, Murphey M D 2000 Enchondroma and chondrosarcoma. Semin Musculoskelet Radiol 4: 59–72
17. Murphey M D, Walker E A, Wilson A J, Kransdorf M J, Temple H T, Gannon F H 2003 From the archives of the AFIP: imaging of primary chondrosarcoma: radiologic-pathologic correlation. Radiographics 23: 1245–1278.
18. MacSweeney F, Darby A, Saifuddin A 2003 Differentiated chondrosarcoma of the appendicular skeleton: MRI-pathological correlation. Skeletal Radiol 32: 671–678
19. Littrell L A, Wenger D E, Wold L E et al 2004 Radiographic, CT, and MR imaging features of dedifferentiated chondrosarcomas: a retrospective review of 174 de novo cases. RadioGraphics 24: 1397–1409
20. Saifuddin A, Mann B S, Mahroof S, Pringle J A, Briggs T W, Cannon S R 2004 Dedifferentiated chondrosarcoma: use of MRI to guide needle biopsy. Clin Radiol 59: 268–272
21. Vanel D, De Paolis M, Monti C, Mercuri M, Picci P 2001 Radiological features of 24 periosteal chondrosarcomas. Skeletal Radiol 30: 208–212
22. Nakashima Y, Unni K K, Shives T C, Swee R G, Dahlin D C 1986 Mesenchymal chondrosarcoma of bone and soft tissue. A review of 111 cases. Cancer 57: 2444–2453
23. Collins M S, Koyama T, Swee R G, Inwards C Y 2003 Clear cell chondrosarcoma: radiographic, computed tomographic, and magnetic resonance findings in 34 patients with pathologic correlation. Skeletal Radiol 32: 687–694
24. White L M, Kandel R 2000 Osteoid-producing tumours of bone. Semin Musculoskelet Radiol 4: 25–43
25. deSantos L A, Edeiken B 1982 Purely lytic osteosarcoma. Skeletal Radiol 9: 1–7
26. Sundaram M, Totty W G, Kyriakos M, McDonald D J, Merkel K 2001 Imaging findings in pseudocystic osteosarcoma. Am J Roentgenol 176: 783–788
27. Saifuddin A 2002 The accuracy of imaging in the local staging of appendicular osteosarcoma. Skeletal Radiol 31: 191–201
28. Murphey M D, wan Jaovisidha S, Temple H T, Gannon F H, Jelinek J S, Malawer M M 2003 Telangiectatic osteosarcoma: radiologic-pathologic comparison. Radiology 229: 545–553
29. Andresen K J, Sundaram M, Unni K K, Sim F H 2004 Imaging features of low-grade central osteosarcoma of the long bones and pelvis. Skeletal Radiol 33: 373–379
30. Raymond A K 1991 Surface osteosarcoma. Clin Orthop 270: 140–148
31. Hermann G, Klein M J, Springfield D, Abdelwahab I F, Dan S J 2002 Intracortical osteosarcoma; two-year delay in diagnosis. Skeletal Radiol 31: 592–596
32. Okada K, Frassica F J, Sim F H, Beabout J W, Bond J R, Unni K K 1994 Parosteal osteosarcoma: a clinicopathologic study. J Bone Joint Surg 76(A): 366–378
33. Jelinek J S, Murphey M D, Kransdorf M J, Shmookler B M, Malawer M M, Hur R C 1996 Parosteal osteosarcoma: value of MR imaging and CT in the prediction of histologic grade. Radiology 201: 837–842
34. Murphy M D, Jelinek J S, Temple H T, Flemming D J, Gannon F H 2004 Imaging of periosteal osteosarcoma: radiologic-pathologic comparison. Radiology 233: 129–138
35. Okada K, Kubota H, Ebina T, Kobayashi T, Abe E, Sato K 1995 High-grade surface osteosarcoma of the humerus. Skeletal Radiol 24: 531–534
36. Smith S E, Murphey M D, Motamedi K, Mulligan ME, Resnik C S, Gannon F H 2002 From the archives of the AFIP. Radiologic spectrum of Paget disease of bone and its complications with pathologic correlation. Radiographics 22: 1191–1216
37. Whitten C R, Saifuddin A 2003 MRI of Paget's disease of bone. Clin Radiol 58: 763–769
38. Tins B J, Davies A M, Mangham D C 2001 MR imaging of pseudosarcoma in Paget's disease of bone: a report of two cases. Skeletal Radiol 30: 161–165
39. Sheppard D G, Libshitz H I 2001 Post-radiation sarcomas: a review of the clinical and imaging features in 63 cases. Clin Radiol 56: 22–29
40. Daffner R H, Kennedy S L, Fox K R, Crowley J J, Sauser D D, Cooperstein L A 1997 Synchronous multicentric osteosarcoma: the case for metastases. Skeletal Radiol 26: 569–578
41. Aizawa T, Okada K, Abe E, Tsuchida S, Shimada Y, Itoi E 2004 Multicentric osteosarcoma with long-term survival. Skeletal Radiol 33: 41–45
42. Link T M, Haeussler M D, Poppek S et al 1998 Malignant fibrous histiocytoma of bone: conventional X-ray and MR imaging features. Skeletal Radiol 27: 552–558
43. Smith S E, Kransdorf M J 2000 Primary musculoskeletal tumors of fibrous origin. Semin Musculoskelet Radiol 4: 73–88
44. Papagelopoulos P J, Galanis E C, Trantafyllidis P, Boscainos P J, Sim F H, Unni K K 2002 Clinicopathologic features, diagnosis, and treatment of fibrosarcoma of bone. Am J Orthop 31: 253–257
45. Zelazny A, Reinus W R, Wilson A J 1997 Quantitative analysis of the plain radiographic appearance of Ewing's sarcoma of bone. Invest Radiol 32: 59–65
46. Kransdorf M, Smith S E 2000 Lesions of unknown histogenesis: Langerhans cell histiocytosis and Ewing sarcoma. Semin Musculoskelet Radiol 4: 1123–1126
47. Shapeero L G, Vanel D, Sundaram M et al 1994 Periosteal Ewing sarcoma. Radiology 191: 825–831
48. Saifuddin A, Whelan J, Pringle J A, Cannon S R 2000 Malignant round cell tumours of bone: atypical clinical and imaging features. Skeletal Radiol 29: 646–651
49. Sallustio G, Pirronti T, Lasorella A, Natale L, Bray A, Marano P 1998 Diagnostic imaging of primitive neuroectodermal tumour of the chest wall (Askin tumour). Pediatr Radiol 28: 697–702
50. Rousselin B, Vanel D, Terrier-Lacombe M J, Istria B J, Spielman M, Masselot J 1989 Clinical and radiologic analysis of 13 cases of primary neuroectodermal tumors of bone. Skeletal Radiol 18: 115–120
51. Mulligan M E 2000 Myeloma and lymphoma. Semin Musculoskelet Radiol 4: 127–136
52. Krishan A, Shirkhoda A, Tehranzadeh J, Armin A R, Irwin R, Les K 2003 Primary bone lymphoma: radiographic-MR imaging correlation. Radiographics 23: 1371–1383
53. Gross S B, Robertson W W Jr, Lange B J, Bunin N J, Drummond D S 1992 Primary Hodgkin's disease of bone. A report of two cases in adolescents and review of the literature. Clin Orthop 283: 276–280
54. Papagelopoulos P J, Mavrogenis A F, Galanis E C et al 2004 Chordoma of the spine: clinicopathological features, diagnosis, and treatment. Orthopedics 27: 1256–1263
55. Sung M S, Lee G K, Kang H S et al 2005 Sacrococcygeal chordoma: MR imaging in 30 patients. Skeletal Radiol 34: 87–94
56. Wenger D E, Wold L E 2000 Malignant vascular lesions of bone: radiologic and pathologic features. Skeletal Radiol 29: 619–631
57. Kahn L B 2003 Adamantinoma, osteofibrous dysplasia and differentiated adamantinoma. Skeletal Radiol 32: 245–258
58. Van der Woude H J, Hazelbag H M, Bloem J L, Taminiau A H, Hogendoorn P C 2004 MRI of adamantinoma of long bones in correlation with histopathology. Am J Roentgenol 183: 1737–1744

CHAPTER 49

Metabolic and Endocrine Skeletal Disease

Judith E. Adams

Metabolic diseases of the skeleton affect bone as a tissue; all bones are involved, although radiological abnormalities are not always evident. Such disorders can be caused by genetic, endocrine, nutritional or biochemical factors. Knowledge of bone structure, development and physiology is essential to the understanding of the effects that metabolic bone disorders have on the skeleton and in interpreting the abnormalities which may be evident on radiographs and other imaging techniques1.

BONE STRUCTURE, GROWTH AND PHYSIOLOGY

Bone is a highly specialized rigid tissue that protects internal organs and has to withstand the load-bearing requirements of the skeleton without fracturing. It consists of crystals of hydroxyapatite embedded within organic matrix, principally triple helical fibres of Type I collagen. Bones are generally divided into flat and tubular bones. Tubular bones are designed for weight bearing. Bone is normally present in anatomical bones in two forms:

1 **compact (cortical) bone**, which forms the outer shell of bones
2 **trabecular (cancellous) bone**, which is found mainly in vertebral bodies, the pelvis and the metaphyseal regions of long bones.

All bones contain both types of bony tissue, although the relative amounts of each vary, and both contribute to bone strength. Despite its hardness, bone remains a *metabolically active tissue throughout life*, being constantly resorbed and laid down by bone cells, the activity of which can be modified by many factors[2]. As a consequence, bones remodel from birth to maturity, maintaining their basic shape, repairing following fracture, and responding to physical forces (i.e. mechanical stresses related to bone deformity) throughout life. The strength of bone is related not only to its hardness and other physical properties, but also to the architectural arrangement of the compact and trabecular bone. The skeleton contains 99% of the total body calcium and therefore plays a vital role in the maintenance of calcium homeostasis.

Bone cells

Osteoblasts are bone-forming cells which synthesize and secrete Type I collagen and mucopolysaccharides to form layers of bone matrix (osteoid) which subsequently becomes mineralized. Osteoblasts also synthesize collagenase, prostaglandin E_2 (PGE_2), and bone associated proteins, osteocalcin and osteonectin. Osteoblasts have receptors for parathyroid hormone, vitamin D, prostaglandin E_2 and glucocorticosteroids.

Osteocytes are derived from the osteoblast and are initially present on the surface of bone but subsequently become encased within bone. Each osteocyte lies within a lacuna and is interconnected to other osteocytes and osteoblasts by cytoplasmic extensions within canaliculi. The osteocyte has a role in maintenance of bone matrix which is facilitated by the transport of material and fluid via these canaliculi. At one time osteocytes were considered to be relatively inactive, but it has been shown that they respond to micro-strains to which bone is exposed (loading), calcitonin and parathyroid hormone, and so play an important role in maintaining constant levels of calcium within the body fluids.

Osteoclasts are multinuclear giant cells that resorb both calcified bone and cartilage and derive from the mononuclear phagocytic cell line of haemopoietic stem cells. Osteoclasts lie on the surface of bone causing active resorption and forming Howship's lacunae. Osteoclasts in contact with bone develop motile microvilli which cause the cell to adhere to the bone surface and result in a microenvironment between the osteoclast and the mineralized bone. This brush border of microvilli increases with activation by such factors as prostaglandin, vitamin D and parathyroid hormone. Osteoclasts secrete acid hydrolases and neutral proteases which degrade the bone matrix following its demineralization. As there are no receptors for 1,25-dihydroxy vitamin D (1,25(OH)D), on the surface of the osteoclast, it is probable that factors such as vitamin D and parathyroid hormone activate the osteoclasts through their effects on the osteoblast.

Bone formation and turnover

Bone formation (osteoblastic activity) and bone resorption (osteoclastic activity) constitutes bone turnover[3], a process which takes place on bone surfaces and continues throughout life. Bone formation and resorption are linked in a consistent sequence under normal circumstances. Precursor bone cells are activated at a particular skeletal site to form osteoclasts which erode a fairly constant amount of bone. After a period of time the resorption stops and osteoblasts are recruited to fill the eroded space with new bone (Fig. 49.1A). This coupling of osteoblastic and osteoclastic activity constitutes the basal multicellular unit (BMU) of bone. In healthy young adults the resorptive phase of the turnover cycle lasts about 30 days and the formation phase about 90 days. The length of the turnover cycle increases in later life and the rate of bone turnover is reduced. Uncoupling of the process (excessive osteoclastic resorption or defective osteoblastic function) results in a net loss of bone **(osteoporosis).** If there is both increased bone resorption and formation this constitutes increased bone turnover. Woven immature, instead of mature lamellar, bone is laid down, as in Paget's disease of bone (Fig. 49.2D). Increased activation frequency of resorption units also results in high turnover state (hyperparathyroidism, postmenopausal bone loss). Bisphosphonate therapy reduces the activation of resorption units by inhibiting osteoclasts, and reversal in the mineral deficit contributes to increase in bone mineral density (BMD).

Bones grow in length by endochondral ossification at the physis, and remodel by periosteal apposition of bone, endosteal resorption and osteoclastic resorption along the periosteal surface of the metaphysis (Fig. 49.1B). Defective osteoclastic function prevents this normal resorption of bone which is essential to maintain bone health by continual slow renewal throughout life. Defective osteoclastic function[4] in some diseases (i.e. osteopetrosis) can result in abnormal bone modelling and sclerosis on radiographs (Fig. 49.2C). Bone resorption by osteoclasts is a single-stage process in which collagen and mineral are removed together. Bone formation is a two-stage process: osteoblasts lay down osteoid, which subsequently becomes mineralized. Prerequisites for normal mineralization are vitamin D ($1,25[OH]_2D_3$), normal levels of phosphorus and alkaline phosphatase, adequate intake of calcium and a normal pH. Defects in the mineralization process will result in rickets or osteomalacia (Fig.49.2B).

Bone growth and development

Early in fetal development the framework of the skeleton is in place but without mineralization. At about 26 weeks of gestation the long bones assume their future shape and proportion. Bones grow in size and change in shape during childhood and adolescence, particularly during the pubertal growth spurt (Fig. 49.2C). Skeletal growth occurs primarily by endochondral ossification at the metaphyses and epiphyses. At birth about 25 g of calcium is present in the skeleton; the mineral required for the fetal skeleton is acquired from the mother. Bone develops by a process of either intramembranous or endochondral bone formation. In intramembranous formation, osteoblasts differentiate from mesenchymal cells and deposit osteoid which subsequently is mineralized. Bone is initially deposited as a network of immature woven trabeculae called the primary spongiosa. This is replaced by secondary, or mature, bone with the formation of bone marrow spaces, bone trabeculae and cortices. Bones which form by intramembranous ossification include the cranial vault, mandible, maxilla and middle portion of the clavicle.

Other bones, including the tubular bones, form and grow by endochondral ossification by which cartilaginous tissue which is derived from mesenchymal tissue is eventually replaced by bone. The primary centre of ossification in the tubular bones is in the centre of the cartilaginous template. The secondary, later developing, centres (epiphyses) are located at the ends of the developing bones (Fig. 49.1B). In endochondral ossification there is hypertrophy of cartilage cells and glycogen accumulation. Subsequently these cells undergo degeneration and become calcified (the provisional zone of calcification). The deeper perichondrial cells transform into osteoblasts through a process of intramembranous ossification. These osteoblasts, and vascular tissue, invade the cartilaginous matrix and lay down osteoid which becomes mineralized. Osteoblasts become trapped within the developing bone and transform into osteocytes.

Increase in bone length takes place at the metaphyses of long bones, which adjoin the cartilaginous growth plate. This cartilaginous growth plate remains between the ossification primary and secondary centres until growth ceases and skeletal maturity is reached. The distal remnant of the cartilage of the epiphyses is destined to become the articular surface of the adjacent joint. If endochondral ossification ceases for some reason (illness, nutritional deprivation) then the zone of pro-

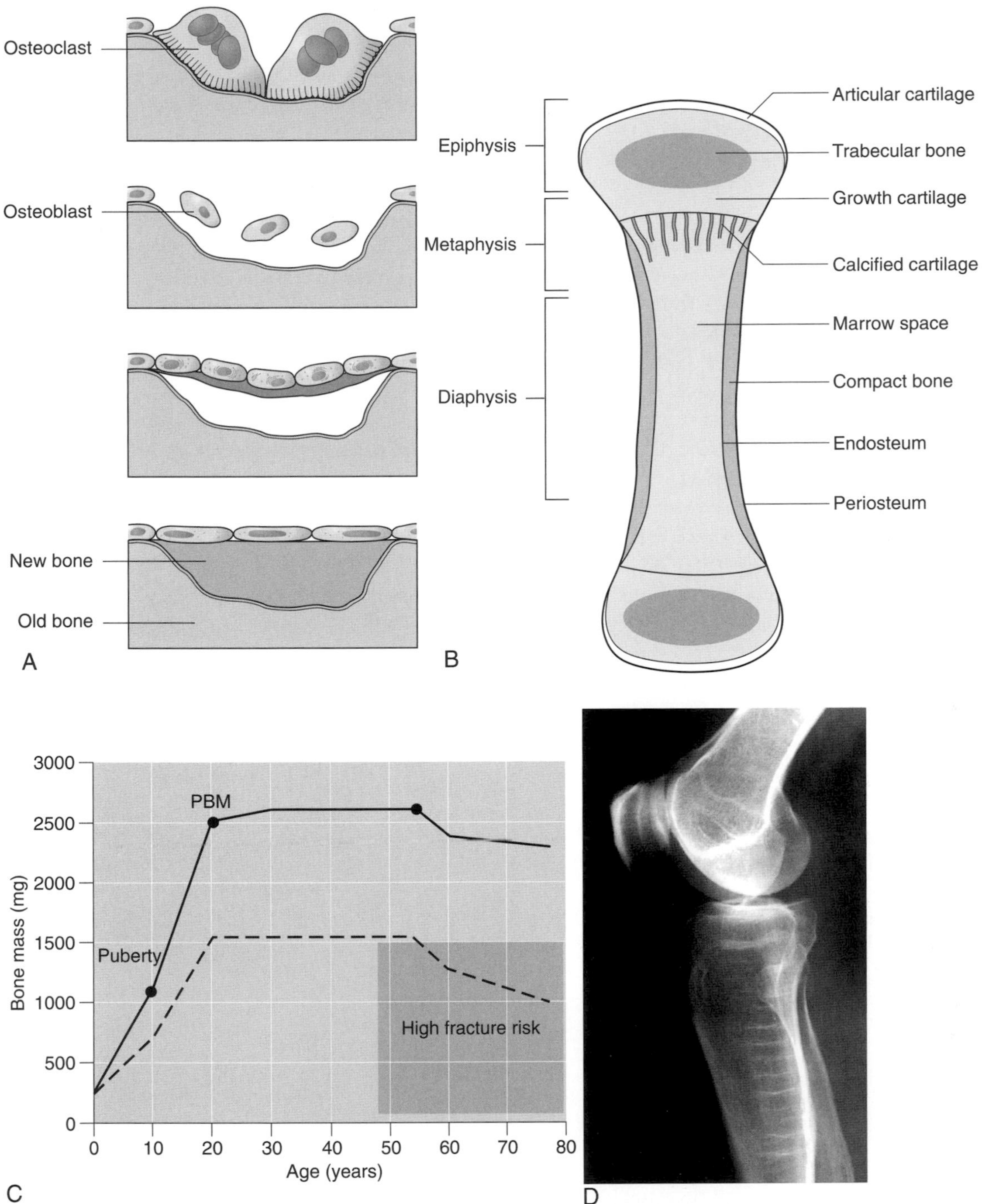

Figure 49.1 Bone growth, development and turnover. (A) The basal metabolic unit (BMU). Bone turnover continues throughout life so that old bone is replaced by stronger new bone; osteoclasts erode a pit of bone (top) and subsequently osteoblasts are recruited and fill the eroded pit with osteoid, which becomes mineralized. Normally this process is in balance and takes about 3–4 months to complete. If the process becomes uncoupled and erosion is excessive or the pit is incompletely filled with bone, there will be a net loss of bone over time (osteoporosis). Increase in both resorption and formation results in a high turnover state, e.g. Paget's disease. (B) Tubular bones consist of an outer shell of cortical bone with inner trabecular bone, particularly at the ends of the bones, and haemopoietic marrow. They grow in length by endochondral ossification which takes place at the physis (growth plate) between the distal epiphysis and the metaphysis. (C) Bone gain and loss during life: during childhood and adolescence there is accumulation of mineral in the bones which are growing in length and size, particularly at the time of puberty. Bones are larger and heavier in men than in women. Peak bone mass (PBM) is reached in the 20s and remains constant until about 35 years. At the time of the menopause, females lose bone due to oestrogen lack; both men and women lose bone with age. Maximizing PBM and minimizing bone loss by lifestyle factors such as regular exercise, good nutrition (adequate calcium and vitamin D) and avoiding risk factors (e.g. smoking, excess alcohol consumption) will prevent osteoporosis. (Adapted from Heaney et al 2000[175]). (D) Harris growth arrest lines (lateral radiograph knee). If endochondral ossification ceases for any reason (e.g. period of illness, hypothyroidism) the zone of provisional calcification is left as a thin, horizontal, dense white line when the bone is at that particular stage of development. There are several Harris lines in the proximal tibia. (With kind permission of Springer Science and Business Media.)

visional calcification present at that particular stage of skeletal development may remain as a thin white line (Harris growth arrest line) on radiographs (Fig. 49.1D).

Bones consist of an outer shell of compact (cortical) bone with a central cavity which contains the marrow space, and 'lace-like' trabecular bone which is prominent in the axial skeleton and at the ends of long bones. Compact cortical bone constitutes about 80% of skeletal mass. Cancellous (trabecular) bone constitutes 20% of total skeletal mass, but contributes importantly to skeletal strength. The bone trabeculae are arranged to resist tensile deforming stresses, either from weight bearing or muscular activity. The number, thickness and distribution of trabeculae are related to the forces to which they are subjected. Trabeculae provide a large surface area on which metabolic processes can take place and have a higher rate (× 8) of turnover and richer blood supply than compact bone. Around the cortex of the bone is a layer of periosteum and adjacent to the marrow cavity is its endosteal surface. Excessive osteoclastic activity (i.e. in hyperparathyroidism) causes resorption of cortical bone which may be visible radiologically (cortical 'tunnelling') and is indicative of increased bone turnover. Resorption and formation takes place not only within the cortex of bone, but also at the periosteal and endosteal surfaces.

At the endosteal surface, slightly more bone is removed than is replaced, resulting in a net loss of bone at this site. This causes the marrow cavity to enlarge and the bony trabeculae to become thinner—some may ultimately disappear. This expansion of the marrow cavity and loss of trabeculae is a normal phenomenon that occurs with age. At the periosteal surface, resorption takes place which is important in maintaining the normal shape of bones as they grow in length. There is a net gain of bone at the periosteal surface throughout life, so that tubular bones progressively increase in width as age advances[5].

The bones grow during the first two decades of life with a pubertal spurt during adolescence. Skeletal maturity is achieved at an earlier age in girls (16–18 years) than in boys (18–20 years). Some disorders (hypothyroidism, chronic ill health) may retard skeletal development. Skeletal maturation is assessed radiologically from a hand (non-dominant) radiograph (including wrists) which is then compared with an atlas of hand radiographs of normal American Caucasian boys and girls of different ages (Greulich and Pyle 1959)[6] or using the Tanner and Whitehouse bone score (TW2) method, which assesses changes in presence, size and shape of certain bones with age[7] (Fig. 49.2A). The latter method is more time consuming; both methods provide comparable results and reproducibility[8]. Auto-

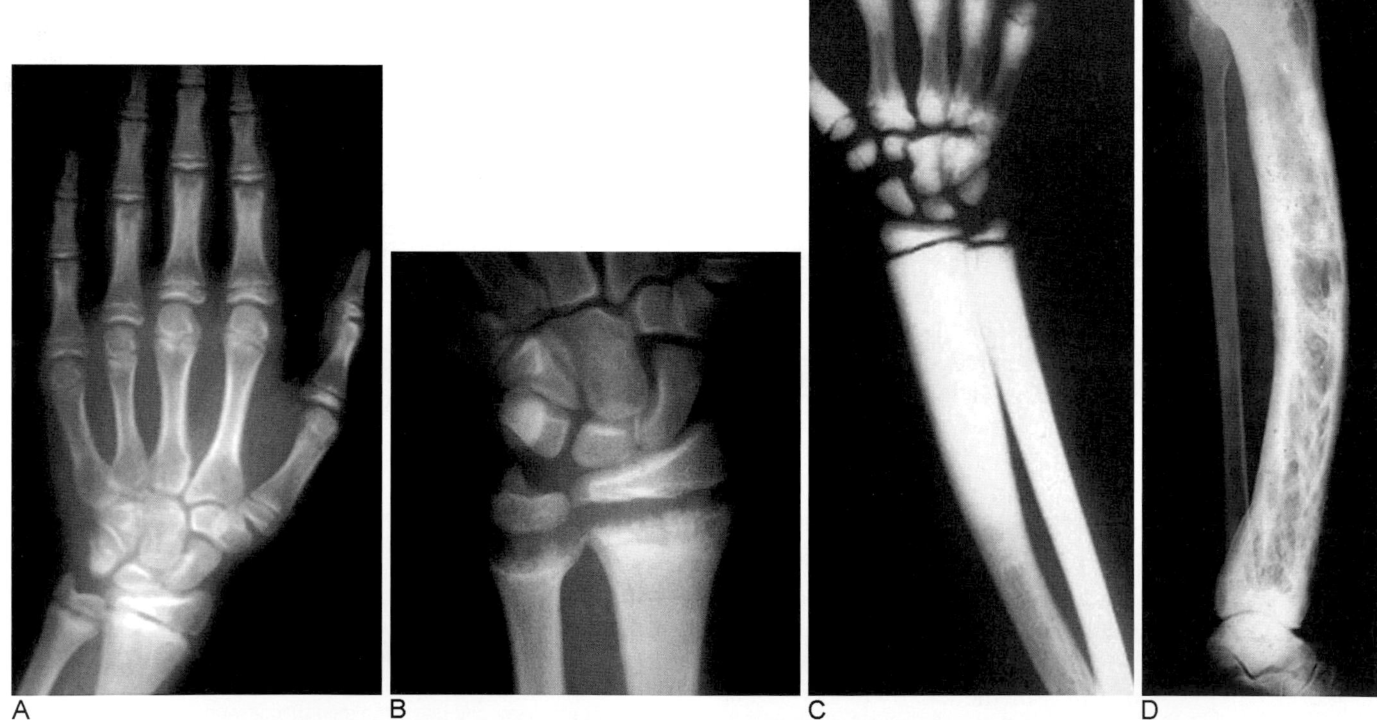

Figure 49.2 Radiographic evidence of normal and abnormal bone growth and development. (A) Normal hand radiograph in a child; this is used to assess skeletal maturity using either the Greulich and Pyle atlas or the Tanner and Whitehouse score (TW2 method). Both assess the change in size and shape of the epiphyses and carpal bones in the nondominant hand with age. (B) Rickets in the wrist of a child. There is increase in the width of the growth plate and cupping and splaying of the metaphysis, which is poorly mineralized. These radiographic features can occur as a result of vitamin D deficiency (lack of active metabolite 1,25$(OH)_2D_3$) from nutritional lack (dietary or lack of sunlight), malabsorption, liver disease or chronic renal failure, hypophosphataemia, hypophosphatasia, acidaemia and low calcium intake. (C) Defective osteoclastic function as evidenced by dense bones and abnormal bone modelling (lack of tubulation of the distal radius) in the forearm in a child with osteopetrosis. (D) Increase in both osteoclastic bone resorption and osteoblastic bone formation results in increased bone turnover, with immature woven bone being laid down instead of normal lamellar bone, as occurs in Paget's disease. In this radiograph of the tibia there are the characteristic features of Paget's disease with coarse and disordered trabecular pattern, cortical 'tunnelling', and expansion and deformity of bone, due to bone softening.

mated, computer-based techniques have potential to be applied to this quantitative assessment of the skeleton[9,10].

Following attainment of skeletal maturity there then follows a period of consolidation during which peak bone mass is achieved (Fig. 49.1C). For cortical bone this is reached at about 35 years of age, and a little earlier for trabecular bone. Although the long bones grow in length at the metaphyses, they are remodelled in shape during development by endosteal resorption and periosteal apposition.

The size and shape of the skeleton and its individual bones are determined by genetic factors, but are influenced by endocrine and local growth factors, nutrition and physical activity. Remodelling allows the skeleton to adjust to mechanical forces to which it is exposed. There is considerable variation in skeletal size and weight, both within and between races[11]. Black races have larger and heavier bones than whites, and Chinese have a small skeletal mass and size. Although genetic factors are important, they are modified by environmental differences such as diet and physical activity[12–14].

In mature healthy adults, bone turnover for the whole skeleton is about 2% per year, with maintenance of a constant bone mass. Bone formation is increased during periods of rapid growth and stimulated by physical activity, growth and thyroid hormones. Bone formation is decreased as a consequence of immobilization, undernutrition, deficiencies of thyroid and growth hormone and glucocorticoid excess[15]. After the attainment of peak bone mass, bone loss, particularly of trabecular bone, is believed to occur from the third decade of life[16–18]. Bone loss is a phenomenon which occurs in all races. Generally both men and women lose bone as they grow older, but women lose more than men. Women lose approximately 15–30% of their total bone mass between maturity and the seventh decade, whereas men lose only about half this amount. Relatively more trabecular bone is lost (40–50%) than compact bone (5%). After the age of 35, women lose bone at an annual rate of approximately 0.75–1.0% which increases to a rate of 2–3% in the postmenopausal period. This loss affects both cortical and trabecular bone, but the effect on trabecular bone predominates. In contrast, cortical bone is well preserved until the fifth decade of life when there is a linear loss in both sexes, such that men lose about 25% of their cortical bone whilst women lose about 30%. Low bone mineral density may be the result of either (A) low peak bone mass or (B) accelerated bone loss.

The amount of bone in the skeleton at any moment in time depends on peak bone mass and the balance between bone resorption and formation. The most common metabolic disorders of bone are: **osteoporosis**, in which there is a deficiency of bone mass leading to insufficiency (low-trauma) fractures; **rickets and osteomalacia**, in which there is a defective mineralization of bone osteoid (Fig. 49.2B) due to vitamin D deficiency, hypophosphataemia, lack of alkaline phosphatase or calcium, or severe acidaemia; and **hyperparathyroidism**, in which a tumour or hyperplasia of the parathyroid glands causes increase in parathyroid hormone production and stimulation of osteoclasts. Other metabolic bone disorders include osteogenesis imperfecta, hyperphosphatasia and osteopetrosis (Fig. 49.2C). Paget's disease is not strictly a metabolic bone disease, since it can be monostotic or polyostotic and does not involve the entire skeleton, but because it involves increased bone turnover (Fig. 49.2D) it is often included in this group of disease[19].

OSTEOPOROSIS

Osteoporosis is the most common metabolic bone disease and is claimed to affect 1 in 2 women and 1 in 5 men over the age of 50 years in their lifetime in the western world[20]. It is a quantitative abnormality of bone ('too little bone'); there is reduced bone mass and altered trabecular structure. Bones become brittle and fracture with little, or no, trauma (insufficiency fractures).

Osteoporosis is now defined as 'a systemic skeletal disease characterized by low bone mass and micro-architectural deterioration of bone tissue, with a consequent increase in bone fragility and susceptibility to fracture'[21]. Not only is the amount of bone tissue reduced, the structural integrity of bone is compromised by destruction of trabeculae resulting in loss of continuity and interconnectivity of these bone struts. With the introduction of noninvasive methods of bone densitometry, it is possible to define osteoporosis on the basis of bone mineral density (**BMD**) measured at the hip and spine by dual energy X-ray absorptiometry (**DXA**) as defined by the World Health Organization[22]:

Normal: BMD above −1 standard deviation (SD) of the young adult reference mean (peak bone mass)

Osteopenia: BMD between −1 and −2.5 SD below that of the young adult reference mean

Osteoporosis: BMD more than −2.5 SD below the young adult reference mean

Severe osteoporosis: BMD in the osteoporotic range with one or more low-trauma fractures.

This definition is now also applied to males, but importantly it is *not* appropriate in children or adolescents who have not yet reached peak bone mass[23]. In these patient groups, osteoporosis would appropriately be defined as a BMD which is more than 2 standard deviations below the mean BMD matched for age, gender and ethnicity. The WHO definition is *not applicable* to other bone densitometry techniques (quantitative computed tomography, QCT; quantitative ultrasound, QUS) or other anatomical sites (e.g. calcaneus).

Osteoporosis should not be considered as a single disease entity, but rather an end result of many disease processes[24] (Table 49.1). It may result from defective skeletal accretion during bone growth and development. Alternatively, it may result from disease processes in which bone resorption exceeds new bone formation, resulting in a net loss of bone mass and consequent compromise to skeletal strength.

Table 49.1 MAIN CAUSES OF OSTEOPOROSIS
Primary
Juvenile
Idiopathic of young adults
Postmenopausal
Senile
Secondary
Endocrine
Glucocorticoid excess
Oestrogen/testosterone deficiency
Hyperthyroidism
Hyperparathyroidism
Growth hormone deficiency (childhood onset)
Nutritional
Intestinal malabsorption
Chronic alcoholism
Chronic liver disease
Partial gastrectomy
Vitamin C deficiency (scurvy)
Hereditary
Osteogenesis imperfecta
Homocystinuria
Marfan's syndrome
Ehlers–Danlos syndrome
Haematological
Thalassaemia
Sickle-cell disease
Gaucher's disease
Other
Rheumatoid arthritis
Haemochromatosis

RADIOLOGICAL FEATURES

General

As there is less bone in osteoporotic bone than in normal bone, this will be evident radiographically by decreased radiodensity of bone. A useful descriptive term to use if fractures are not present is 'osteopenia'[25–27] (Fig. 49.3). Reduced bone density is often more prominent in areas of the skeleton rich in trabecular bone, particularly in the axial skeleton (vertebrae, pelvis, ribs and sternum). Eventually, changes may also be evident in the bones of the appendicular skeleton. Trabeculae become thin and may disappear completely; they may be sparse, but those that remain may become thickened due to stresses to which the skeleton is exposed. The cortex becomes reduced in width through endosteal bone resorption, and in states of increased bone turnover there will be intracortical tunnelling and porosity.

Osteoporotic bone is less able to withstand the stresses to which the skeleton is exposed than is normal bone, and this leads to the cardinal clinical feature of low-trauma fractures. Such fractures can occur at any skeletal site, but they are most common in sites of the skeleton rich in trabecular bone, particularly the vertebrae, the distal forearm and the proximal femur. These fractures may be associated with considerable pain and deformity. Femoral neck fractures carry significant morbidity (20%) and considerable socio-economic impact: a significant number (50%) of the elderly population affected by femoral neck fracture require subsequent nursing home care[28].

Spine

Perhaps related to biomechanical forces through the spine, as trabeculae are lost, the process of osteoporosis particularly involves the horizontally orientated secondary trabeculae. The vertical trabeculae actually become more prominent and thickened[27,29] (Fig. 49.4B). This results in a vertical 'striated' appearance to the vertebral body on lateral spinal radiographs. This feature is generally seen in several, or all, of the vertebrae when it is related to osteoporosis, which serves to distinguish a similar appearance in a single vertebral body when it is related to haemangioma.

Vertebral fractures are the most common of osteoporotic fractures (Fig. 49.4C). The anterior and central mid portion of the vertebrae withstand compression forces less well than the posterior and outer ring elements of the vertebrae, resulting in wedge or end-plate fractures or, less commonly, crush fractures[30,31]. Vertebral fractures can be graded as mild (grade 1), moderate (grade 2) and severe (grade 3)[32] (Fig. 49.4D). This semiquantitative grading method is the one currently most

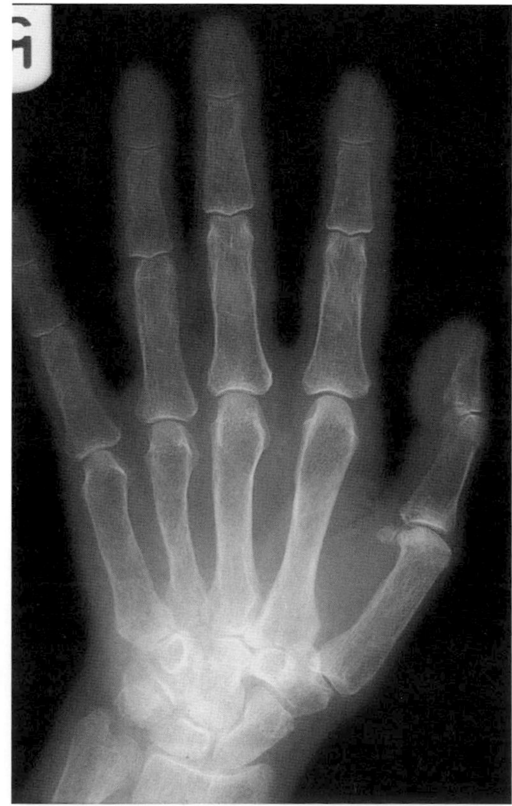

Figure 49.3 Osteoporosis. The hand of an elderly women shows reduced bone density, thinned cortex and reduced number of trabeculae, those which remain appearing more prominent.

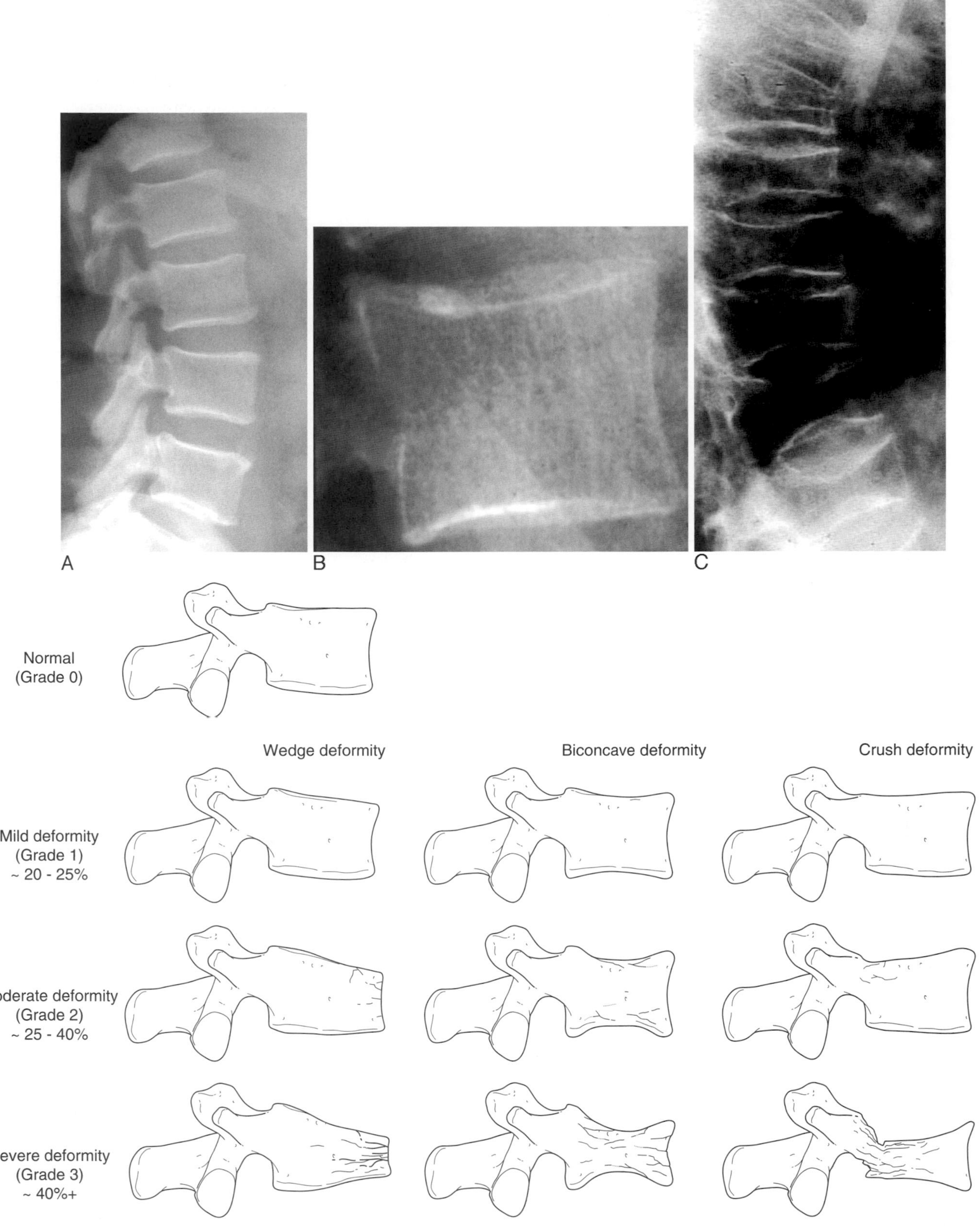

Figure 49.4 Osteoporosis—vertebral osteoporosis and fracture. (A) Lateral radiograph of normal vertebrae. (B) There is loss of the transverse trabeculae, resulting in prominence of the vertical trabeculae, giving a striated appearance. (C) Lateral thoracic radiograph with multiple wedge and end-plate osteoporotic vertebral fractures of varying grades. (D) The semiquantitative method of grading of Genant et al[32] which is widely used in epidemiology and pharmaceutical studies. Vertebral fractures are strong predictors of future fractures (×5 for vertebral fracture; ×2 for hip fracture) so it is important that they are accurately and clearly reported by radiologists. The higher the grade of vertebral fracture, the higher the risk of future fracture.

frequently applied to define the prevalence and incidence of vertebral fractures in epidemiology studies and pharmaceutical trials of the efficacy of new osteoporosis therapies.

The more severe the grade of vertebral fracture, the greater the risk of future fracture. Vertebral fractures are powerful predictors of future fracture (hip × 2; vertebral × 5). It is therefore extremely important that, if present, they are accurately and clearly reported by radiologists as fractures; other terms, such as 'deformities', must be avoided. There is evidence that vertebral fractures are being under-reported by radiologists, with the result that patients who should be receiving treatment to reduce their risk of future fractures are not being identified[33,34]. As a consequence there is currently a joint initiative between the International Osteoporosis Foundation (IOF) and the European Society of Skeletal Radiology (Osteoporosis Group) to improve the sensitivity and accuracy of reporting of vertebral fractures by radiologists, and an interactive teaching CD is available, or can be downloaded, from www.osteofound.org

Vertebral fracture may occur as an acute event related to minor trauma and be accompanied by pain, which generally resolves spontaneously over 6–8 weeks. This resolution of symptoms serves to distinguish osteoporotic vertebral fractures from similar events due to more sinister pathology, such as metastases, in which the symptoms are more protracted. However, 30% of vertebral fractures may be present in asymptomatic patients. Osteoporotic fractures occur most commonly in the thoracic and thoraco-lumbar regions and result in progressive loss of height in affected individuals. Osteoporotic fractures are uncommon above T7; if fractures are present above this anatomical region, metastases should be considered. Wedging of multiple vertebral bodies in the thoracic spine can lead to increased kyphosis (dowager hump) which, if severe, may result in the ribs abutting on the iliac crests and compromise of respiratory function.

Vertebroplasty

Vertebroplasty has selected application in patients with osteoporotic vertebral fractures that are persistently painful. Although it is performed by several medical specialists, radiologists are probably the most appropriate group to perform this image-guided interventional technique, particularly as imaging (radiographs, RNS, CT and MR) plays a role in selecting patients appropriate for the procedure[35].

Vertebroplasty is the injection of cement (methylmethacrylate) into a fractured vertebral body as a means of treating pain (Fig. 49.5). Injection is generally made by passing the introduction needle through the pedicles. Kyphoplasty is the injection of cement into the fractured vertebral body after a balloon has been used to decompress the fracture and correct some of the deformity[36,37]. Both techniques are intended to relieve pain in patients who have not responded to conservative measures and time.

There is no clear evidence as to how long to wait before treating with vertebroplasty, but the current consensus is that a minimum of 4 weeks should pass with adequate medical treatment; some clinicians will delay the procedure 6–8 weeks. Adequate medical treatment should include analgesia, and many consider there should be a trial of bisphosphonates. Patient selection is crucial to success. The pain should arise from vertebral fractures that are temporally related to the onset of symptoms. Magnetic resonance imaging with water-sensitive sequences and fat suppression (fast STIR) will show oedema and haemorrhage in a fracture of recent onset.

There are no randomised controlled trials that compare medical management with vertebroplasty, although some are in progress. The chance of successful pain relief by vertebroplasty for osteoporotic fracture is between 70% and 95%[38]. There are fewer data on the efficacy of kyphoplasty and none to show that this relatively complex procedure has an advantage in outcome when compared to vertebroplasty.

There are potential risks of vertebroplasty; these may be needle related (pedicle fracture, needle breakage, pneumothorax, haemorrhage, infection), cement related (root compression, cord compression, cement embolus), procedure related (fat embolus, rib or vertebral fracture), sedation related (respiratory arrest, airway injuries, cardiac arrest) or drug related (allergy). The overall complication rate from reports suggests that symptom-inducing or potentially serious complications occur in approximately 2% of patients treated for osteoporotic fracture[39,40].

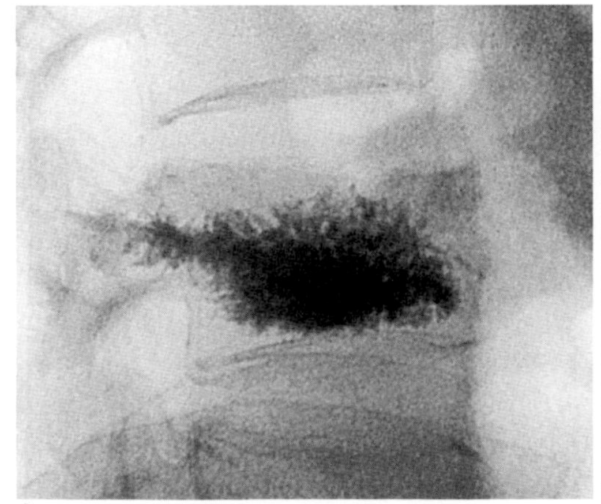
A

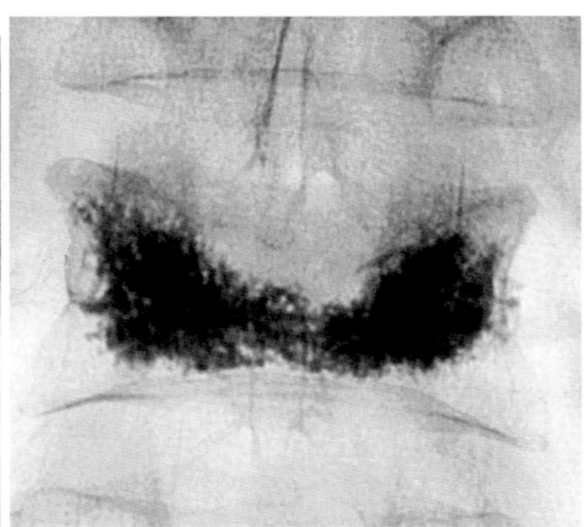
B

Figure 49.5 Osteoporosis—vertebroplasty. In selected cases, pain from osteoporotic vertebral fractures which has not responded to conservative and bisphosphonate therapy may be treated by injection of cement (methylmethacrylate) into the vertebral body. The cement is made radio-opaque so that it can be visualized during injection, and is seen in the lateral (A) and frontal (B) projection. Such vertebroplasty in the lumbar spine will cause false elevation on bone mineral density (BMD) as measured by DXA, and would have to be excluded from analysis. The introductory needle is generally passed through the pedicle.

Most cases are treated under conscious sedation with analgesia, but in some patients general anaesthesia is required. For needle placement, high quality fluoroscopy in either a biplane or C-arm configuration is recommended. Needles, injector sets and cements are now manufactured specifically for vertebroplasty. Care should be taken to ensure a sterile environment. All patients treated by vertebroplasty or kyphoplasty for osteoporotic compression fractures should be under the care of a clinician with special interest in osteoporosis management and on appropriate medical therapy to reduce future fracture risk.

Hands

The hands are often radiographed in metabolic bone disorders. In osteoporosis the trabeculae at the ends of the bones will be reduced in number and those that remain appear more prominent (Fig. 49.3). Normally, cortical bone appears as a solid white line on a radiograph with a smooth inner (endosteal) and outer (periosteal) surface. In osteoporosis, cortical bone is thinned by endosteal resorption, which causes it to become scalloped and irregular in outline. Within the cortical bone, Haversian systems and Volkmann's canals enlarge and become visible as longitudinal radiolucent striations within the cortex. Such features are better demonstrated if single-sided, non-screen fine grain film and a fine X-ray focal spot tube are used to optimize spatial resolution, and enhanced by magnification techniques which are possible in peripheral skeletal sites[41,42].

Other skeletal sites

Elsewhere in the skeleton similar changes occur, with reduction in trabecular number and cortical width. The trabecular pattern in the femoral neck has been quantified as an index of osteoporosis (Singh index)[43,44]. Fractures that occur in osteoporosis generally heal well with satisfactory callus formation. In some sites the presence of multiple micro-fractures and callus formation can cause osteosclerosis on a radiograph; this must be distinguished from other more sinister malignant pathologies. Such insufficiency fractures occur in particular anatomical sites, including the symphysis pubis, the sacrum, pubic rami and calcaneus. Other sites involved are the sternum, supra-acetabular area and elsewhere in the pelvis, femoral neck and proximal and distal tibia[45–48]. Some of these fractures may be accompanied by considerable osteolysis, particularly those involving the symphysis pubis, and may be erroneously diagnosed on radiographs as due to malignant tumour.

Other imaging techniques (radionuclide, CT and MR imaging) may help to differentiate insufficiency fractures from other pathologies. On radionuclide scans there is increased uptake in regions of acute insufficiency fractures.

When the sacrum is involved, there is often a characteristic H pattern (Honda sign) of radionuclide uptake[49]. CT is particularly helpful in defining the fracture lines of insufficiency fractures involving the sacrum (fractures usually occur parallel to the sacroiliac joint) and in the calcaneus. In these sites fractures may not be identified on radiographs because of complex anatomy and overlying structures. MR is helpful in differentiating vertebral fractures resulting from osteoporosis from those caused by other pathologies (myeloma, metastases)[50]. MR is particularly sensitive at identifying insufficiency fractures in the femoral neck before they are evident radiographically, as is skeletal scintigraphy[51].

AETIOLOGY

Osteoporosis can be classified as generalized, regional (involving a segment of the skeleton) or localized.

Regional osteoporosis

This can occur in disuse and reflex sympathetic dystrophy (RDS, Sudeck's atrophy) following fracture, or related to other pathologies (primary and secondary tumours)[27,52,53]. Chronic disuse is characterized by a uniform pattern of bone loss; acute immobilization causes more focal and irregular bone formation and resorption. This results in different patterns of bone loss which include diffuse osteopenia, linear translucent bands, speckled radiolucent areas and cortical bone resorption[54]. RDS is a clinical syndrome which can occur in children and adults and may be precipitated by a variety of processes[55,56]. There is overactivity of the sympathetic nervous system initially causing pain, soft tissue swelling and hyperaemia, with excessive bone resorption (probably stimulated by cytokines), which occurs particularly in a peri-articular distribution and may simulate malignant disease[57,58].

There are also conditions which cause focal or migratory and transient osteoporosis, usually in the region of large joints (hip, knee), the aetiology of which is uncertain. Transient osteoporosis of the hip occurs in youth and middle age, more frequently in men than women. There is sudden onset of pain without preceding trauma. Radiographically there is reduction in density of the proximal femur. There may be an underlying abnormality of perfusion of the marrow, which is oedematous. MR imaging is sensitive in demonstrating such changes in the marrow before any radiographic abnormality is present[59,60]. Focal bone loss can also occur with tumour, arthritis or infection.

Generalized osteoporosis

There are many causes of osteoporosis, falling into four categories:

1 factors which reduce peak adult bone mass
2 age-related bone loss
3 bone loss associated with the menopause or hypogonadal state
4 bone loss that is secondary to other medical conditions and drugs (Table 49.1).

Idiopathic juvenile osteoporosis (IJO)

This self-limiting form of osteoporosis occurs in pre-pubertal children and must be differentiated from osteogenesis imperfecta and other forms of juvenile osteoporosis. It is a rare disorder, first described by Dent and Friedman[61]. It occurs in children aged between 8 and 14 years who have previously been healthy. The disease runs an acute course over a period of 2–4 years, during which there is growth arrest and fractures. A wide spectrum of severity is seen, and both cortical and trabecular bone are affected. In the mild form, only one or two vertebral fractures may be present, but in more severe cases deformity involves all the vertebrae and the extremities, particularly the metaphyseal region of the distal tibia. A few affected patients may develop severe kyphoscoliosis, deformities of the extremities, and even die from respiratory failure due to thoracic deformity. The disease is reversible and remits spontaneously. Affected patients may be left with only a mild or moderate kyphosis, short stature and some bone deformity following fractures[61]. Investigations indicate uncoupling of the two components of bone turnover due to both increase in resorption and decrease in formation. The important differential diagnosis in children with vertebral fracture is hypercortisolism and leukaemia. Affected patients do not have the blue sclerae characteristic of osteogenesis imperfecta.

Osteoporosis of young adults

This heterogeneous condition occurs equally in young men and women[62]. The disease generally runs a mild course with multiple vertebral fractures occurring over a decade or more, with associated loss in height. Fractures of metatarsals and ribs are also common, and hip fractures may occur. The cause of the condition is uncertain and in some it may simply be that inadequate bone mass has been formed during skeletal growth. Some affected individuals may have a mild variant of osteogenesis imperfecta. Exceptionally, osteoporosis may present during pregnancy, but whether this is a causal or coincidental association is unknown.

Post-menopausal osteoporosis

At the time of the menopause, lack of oestrogen will result in some women losing trabecular bone at a rate three times greater than is usual (2–10% per annum). The condition, previously referred to as type I osteoporosis, characteristically becomes clinically evident in women 15–20 years after the menopause. Fractures occur in sites of the skeleton rich in trabecular bone, including the vertebral bodies and distal forearm (Colles' fracture).

Senile osteoporosis

This condition, previously referred to as type II involutional osteoporosis, occurs in both men and women of 75 years or older and is due to age-related bone loss. This occurs as a consequence of age-related impaired bone formation associated with secondary hyperparathyroidism caused by reduced intestinal calcium absorption due to decreased levels of $1,25(OH)_2D$ production in the elderly[63]. There is reduction in both cortical and trabecular bone. The syndrome manifests mainly as hip fractures and wedge fractures of the vertebrae, but fractures may also occur in the proximal tibia, proximal humerus and pelvis.

Secondary osteoporosis

A large number of conditions may lead to osteoporosis (Table 49.1). Radiologically these may be indistinguishable from age-related osteoporosis. However, some may have specific and diagnostic radiological features (i.e. subperiosteal erosions of the phalanges in primary hyperparathyroidism). In glucocorticoid excess (endogenous and exogenous)[64], there is reduced bone formation due to a direct effect on the osteoblast, and increased osteoclastic activity, probably mediated through secondary hyperparathyroidism, stimulated by reduced gastrointestinal absorption of calcium[65]. There is also evidence that glucocorticoids induce premature apoptosis of both osteoblasts and osteoclasts[66]. The effect is primarily on trabecular bone. Fractures occur particularly in the vertebral bodies and ribs; the latter may heal with profuse callus formation.

Peri-articular osteoporosis is a characteristic early feature of rheumatoid arthritis, but a generalized reduction in bone mass can occur, involving both compact and trabecular bone. There is generally increased bone resorption, with normal or reduced bone formation. The causes of these changes are complex. Immobilization and glucocorticoid therapy contribute to the osteoporosis.

OSTEOGENESIS IMPERFECTA

A number of inherited disorders of connective tissue may result in osteoporosis. Osteogenesis imperfecta (OI), or brittle bone syndrome, results from mutations affecting either the *COL1A1* or *COL1A2* gene of Type I collagen[67–71]. Although the disease is usually apparent at birth or in childhood, more mild forms of the disease may not become apparent until adulthood, when affected individuals may present with insufficiency fractures and osteopenia (Fig. 49.6). Radiographic features vary according to the type of disease and its severity and include osteopenia and fractures, which may heal with florid callus formation, mimicking osteosarcoma. Bones are thin and under-tubulated (gracile), normal in length or shortened, thickened and deformed by multiple fractures. Intra-sutural (Wormian) bones can be identified on skull radiographs[70]. In severe forms of osteogenesis imperfecta the diagnosis may be made before birth by detailed ultrasound in the second trimester. Diagnostic features include cranial enlargement, reduced echogenicity of bone and deformity and shortening of limb bones as a result of intrauterine fractures (Fig. 49.6A).

The classification of osteogenesis imperfecta is that devised by Sillence et al in 1979 and modified in 1986[67]. The important characteristics in this classification include blue sclerae, the severity of the disorder and the mode of inheritance (dominant, recessive, sporadic/new mutation), although accurate classification is difficult because of phenotypic overlap[68]. Affected subjects who do not have dental involvement are designated as group A. Subjects with dentinogenesis imperfecta are designated as group B.

Type I

This is the mildest and most prevalent form of the disease and may only become apparent in adulthood. There is a history of fractures, generally dating back to childhood. In children the fractures may become radiographically and clinically apparent as the child becomes more active (5+ years), and may take the form of overt fractures or micro-fractures involving the metaphyses. In infancy these features may resemble those found in non-accidental injury[72]. The differential diagnosis can usually be resolved by the presence of associated

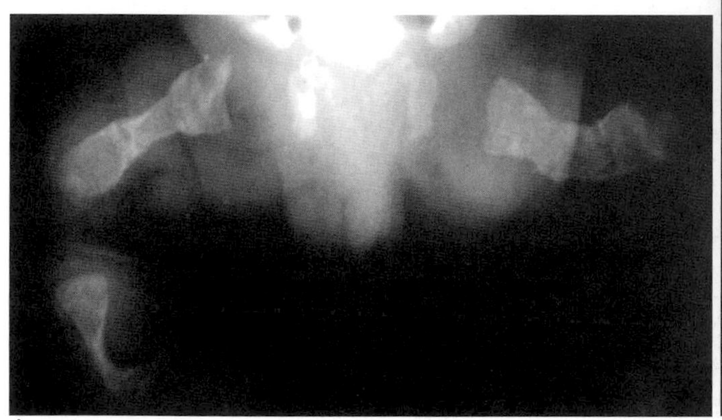

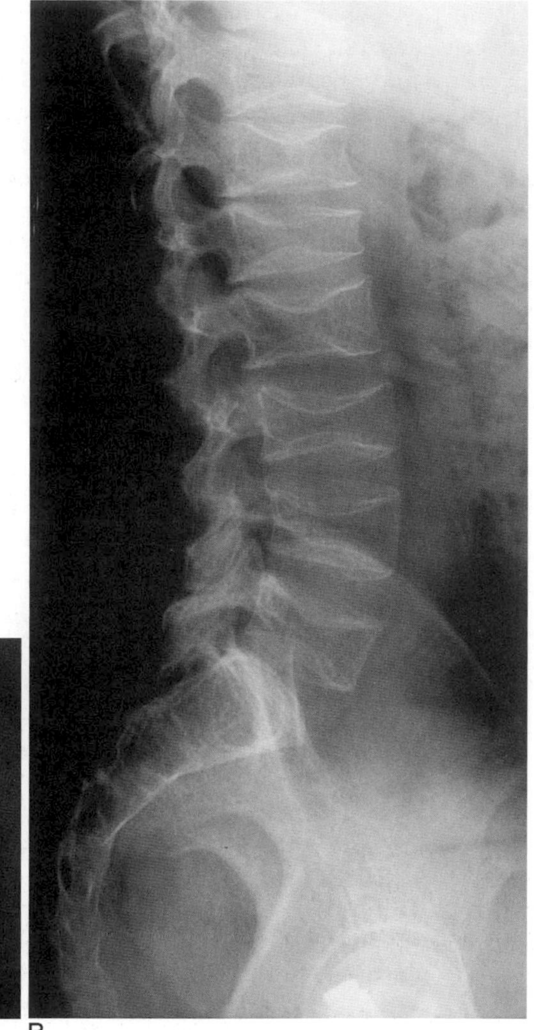

Figure 49.6 Osteogenesis imperfecta. This is a disorder which results from genetic mutations causing abnormalities in Type I collagen, and resulting in osteoporosis and low-trauma fractures (brittle bone disease). The different types vary in clinical presentation and severity. (A) Frontal view of the femora in an infant showing reduced bone density and marked deformity due to multiple fractures. (B) Lateral spinal radiograph in a 30-year-old man showing reduced bone density and end-plate fractures of all vertebrae. There is also evidence of a metallic pin in a previous hip fracture. Osteoporosis is much less common in men than in women, and more likely to be related to secondary causes, especially excess alcohol intake.

extraskeletal manifestations of osteogenesis imperfecta (blue sclerae, dentinogenesis imperfecta), or evidence of a family history of the condition, so that bone biopsy for diagnosis is infrequently required. Affected patients are short in stature, only 10% being of normal height, with joint laxity, blue sclerae and presenile hearing loss. Transmission is by autosomal dominant trait. Radiologically the bones are usually reduced in radiodensity, although some patients may have normal bone density. Bones may be thin and under-tubulated (gracile), or modelled normally. Vertebral fractures often occur in the fourth decade. When scoliosis is present, it is mild.

Type II (lethal perinatal)

Affected infants are small for dates with deep blue sclerae and shortened and deformed limbs due to multiple fractures. Fractures involve the ribs, and death is usually the result of pulmonary insufficiency. Survival is rare beyond the first three months of postnatal life. Other complications include brain and spinal cord injury. Radiologically, multiple fractures are present with a characteristic 'concertina' deformity of the lower limbs. The ribs may appear 'beaded' due to multiple rib fractures, which can occur in utero. The cranial vault is severely under-mineralized and may be distorted by moulding, with Wormian bones in the occipital and parietal region. Platyspondyly is present. Histology reveals defective endochondral ossification at the epiphyses, which appear disorganized with persistent islands of calcified cartilage and under-mineralized bone. There is defective transformation of woven bone to lamellar bone in both the cortical and trabecular skeletal components. Formation of membrane bone is also deficient, accounting for the marked calvarial thinning.

Type III (severe progressive)

This is inherited as an autosomal recessive trait. Fractures are usually present at birth and involve the long bones, clavicles, ribs and cranium, leading to deformity. Although size at birth is normal, growth retardation is evident in the first year of life and many affected patients only reach 0.9–1.2 m (3–4 ft) in height. As growth proceeds, increasing deformity of the calvaria occurs, with associated facial distortion, malocclusion and mild prognathism, basilar invagination, and progressive hearing loss. Sclerae are blue at birth, but this diminishes with age, and sclerae are white in adults. Vertebral fractures occur at an early age and contribute to the progressive and severe kyphoscoliosis which develops during childhood. Affected patients tend to be wheelchair bound because of the progressive deformities resulting from fractures. Complications include progressive pulmonary insufficiency through distortion of the thorax. Radiologically, the bones may be slender or broad due to recurrent fractures. Epiphyses are abnormal, with expansion and islands of calcified ('popcorn') cartilage[73]. As with other forms of osteogenesis imperfecta, the incidence of fracture declines following puberty.

Type IV (moderately severe)

This is inherited as an autosomal dominant trait and can vary in severity. It is sometimes confused with either type I or type III. There is generally more severe osteopenia and more extensive bone deformity than in type I. The sclerae are blue in children, and although this may persist into adulthood, they may also fade to white. Individuals are short in stature, with abnormal moulding of the calvaria and basilar invagination in a high proportion of patients. Bones in the axial and appendicular skeleton are osteoporotic and dysplastic, resulting in scoliosis and deformity, particularly of the pelvis. Joint laxity can result in dislocation, particularly of the ankle or knee.

METHODS OF QUANTITATIVE SKELETAL ASSESSMENT

MORPHOMETRY

For many years methods have been used to try and standardize measurement of cortical thickness (radiogrammetry), trabecular pattern (Singh index) and vertebral deformity (morphometry) from radiographs.

Radiogrammetry

Radiogrammetry involves the measurement on radiographs of cortical thickness in various long bones. The bone most frequently used is the second metacarpal of the nondominant hand, but the method has also been applied to other bones (clavicle, radius, humerus, femur and tibia). In the metacarpal the diameter of the bone in its mid portion (from each periosteal surface) and the medullary width (distance between endosteal surfaces) are measured using calipers[74,75]. A variety of indices have been described, including cortical thickness, metacarpal index and parameters of cortical area. The technique is simple to perform, uses a low radiation dose, and was widely applied. However, the reproducibility is limited (coefficient of variation [CV] up to 11%). This is because the endosteal surface becomes irregular and more difficult to identify with bone resorption. Consequently, longitudinal studies had to extend over a decade or more to assess change with time. Now modern computer vision methods (active shape models, ASM) have been applied and improve precision to better than 1% (digital X-ray radiogrammetry, DXR) (Fig. 49.7A).

Singh index

In the femoral neck there are two principal arches of trabeculae: the compressive group lie in the medial portion of the femoral neck and the tensile group in the lateral aspect. The number, thickness and arrangement of trabeculae in the femoral neck change with age, due to resorption and altered stresses. On radiographs this change in trabecular pattern can be graded as an index of osteopenia. Six grades were described by Singh et al (1970) ranging from grade 6 (normal) to grade 1 (severe osteoporosis)[44]. The subjectivity of the Singh grading scale limits its reproducibility. However, computer analysis has the potential to make the measurement more rapid and accurate[76].

Vertebral morphometry

Over the past decade efforts have been made to standardize the subjective visual assessment of vertebral fracture, and to quantitate alterations in vertebral height and shape[77]. These developments have been stimulated not only by the need for comparable methods to be used in epidemiological studies, but also by the fact that the prevalence and incidence of vertebral fractures are used as inclusion criteria and treatment outcome measures in therapeutic trials in which the efficacy of new drugs for the treatment of osteoporosis is being assessed.

The technique for spinal radiography should be standardized, with a fixed film focus distance (FFD), and the spine parallel to the radiographic table. Any scoliosis or tilting of the spine due to poor positioning will cause apparent, but false, biconcavity of the end-plates ('bean-can effect'). Centring is at T7 spinous process for the lateral thoracic spine and L3 spinous process for the lateral lumbar spine projections. Assessments for vertebral fractures are usually made from T4 to L4 on the lateral spinal projections. Vertebral fractures are defined as end-plate, wedge or crush. Changes in shape of the vertebrae (deforming events) are generally defined by the 6-point method, in which the anterior, mid and posterior points of the superior and inferior end-plates of the vertebral body are identified to measure anterior, mid and posterior heights (Fig. 49.7B). These points can be placed directly on a radiograph or, more usually, the radiograph is digitized and the points placed using a translucent cursor on a digitizing tablet. Vertebral deformity is defined by relating the anterior or mid vertical heights to the posterior height, expressed as a percentage (15% mild, 20% moderate or 25% severe deformity) or by specified standard deviations from normal reference data for vertebral size[78,79]. A vertebral fracture can be defined by grading from 0 (normal) to grade 3 (obvious fracture) in a semiquantitative scheme[32], which has now largely replaced 6-point morphometry.

The introduction of fan beam technology in dual energy X-ray absorptiometry (DXA) has enabled good quality (dual and single energy modes) images (postero-anterior and lateral projections) of the thoracic and lumbar spine from which instant vertebral assessment (IVA) and morphometric measurements can be made (MXA)[80,81]. It may be feasible for

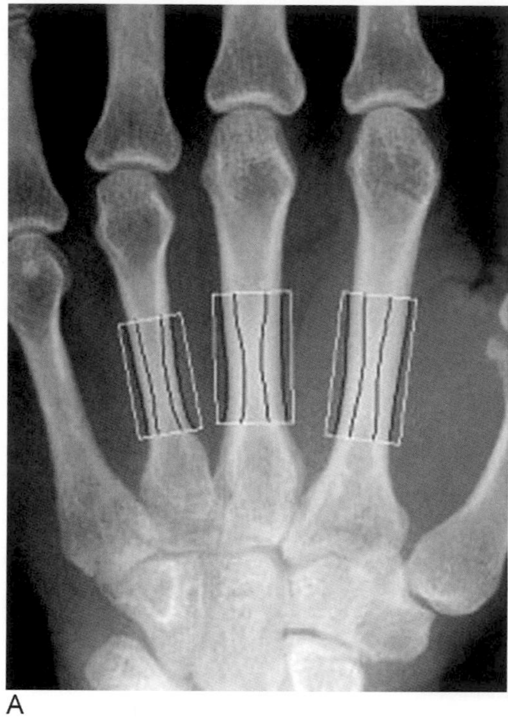

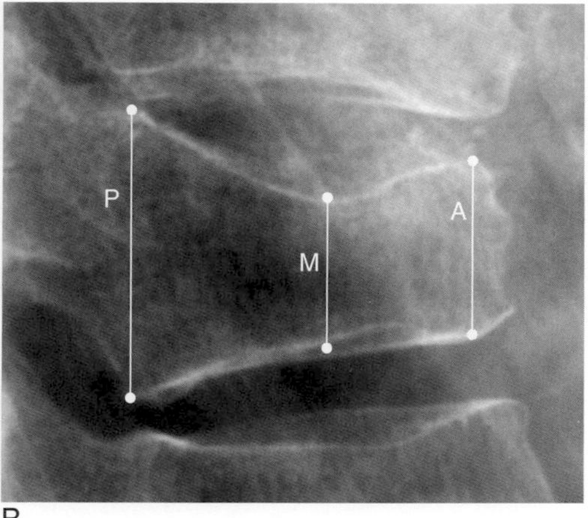

Figure 49.7 Quantitative assessment of the skeleton—radiogrammetry and morphometry. (A) Radiogrammetry. This is a long-established technique with measurement of the cortical thickness in the mid shaft of the second metacarpal of the nondominant hand (metacarpal index) using calipers. More recently there has been application of computer vision methods (active shape models, ASM) to automate this measurement to the 2nd–4th metacarpals, which improves precision (digital X-ray radiogrammetry, DXR). (B) Morphometry. Measurement of change in vertebral shape has been made by placing six points on the vertebra on a lateral spinal radiograph—on the top and bottom of the anterior A, middle M, and posterior P aspect of the vertebra as shown. From these are calculated the ratios of anterior to posterior heights (wedge), middle to posterior heights (end-plate) and posterior height of one vertebrae to that of its neighbouring vertebrae (crush) to define and grade fractures.

this process to be automated by computer techniques[82]. The advantages of MXA over conventional spinal radiography are a lower radiation dose (1/100th), less end-plate distortion since the X-ray beam is parallel to the end-plate at each vertebral level, and the entire spine is visualized on a single image (Fig. 49.8E).

BONE DENSITOMETRY

Treatment of established osteoporosis was, in the past, limited and unsatisfactory. However, over recent years, bisphosphonates, selective oestrogen receptor modulators (SERMs), teriparatide (parathyroid hormone) and strontium ranelate have been shown to increase bone mineral density and, more importantly, reduce future fracture[83]. Treatment strategies have generally favoured prevention of osteoporosis by maximizing peak bone mass, minimizing age-related and post-menopausal bone loss (hormone replacement therapy in premature menopause) and avoidance of risk factors (e.g. smoking) with adequate dietary intake of calcium and increased physical activity.

Whether a fracture occurs depends on a variety of factors, including the patient's propensity to fall and response to the fall. However, bone mineral density (BMD) is the single most important determinant of fracture, accounting for approximately 70% of bone strength. Reduced BMD is a useful predictor of increased fracture risk. The lower the peak bone density, the higher the risk of fracture in later life. Methods of measuring bone density are therefore relevant to the study of skeletal development, the detection of osteopenia, and assessment of efficacy of treatment of osteoporosis. Such methods for measuring BMD should be accurate, precise (reproducible), sensitive both to small changes with time and to differences in patient groups (i.e. fracture compared to non-fracture), inexpensive and involve minimal exposure to ionizing radiation. Some of the techniques now available come close to these ideal requirements[84,85].

Accuracy expresses how close the measurements made are to the actual bone mineral density measured by chemical analysis. All the quantitative methods available have some inaccuracies caused by variable fat content, either within the marrow of trabecular bone (single energy quantitative computed tomography, QCT) or by the fat content of extra-osseous soft tissue (other photon absorptiometric techniques, DXA). Changes in body composition or marrow fat may introduce errors in the measurement depending upon the technique and measurement site used.

Precision assesses the reproducibility of the measurement technique and is usually expressed as a percentage of coefficient of variation (CV%). A high precision (low CV% in the region of 1%) is essential in longitudinal studies to detect small changes over reasonable periods of time. Short-term precision reflects principally repositioning errors, whilst long-term precision using calibration phantoms reflects machine instability. Change in BMD is best evaluated by calculating the percentage change; the least significant change from two measures ($p = 0.05$) is given by 2.77 × precision error of the method[86].

Dual energy X-ray absorptiometry (DXA)[87,88]

DXA has now become the most widely available bone density technique after its introduction in 1987. X-ray beams of two peak energies are produced by a variety of techniques

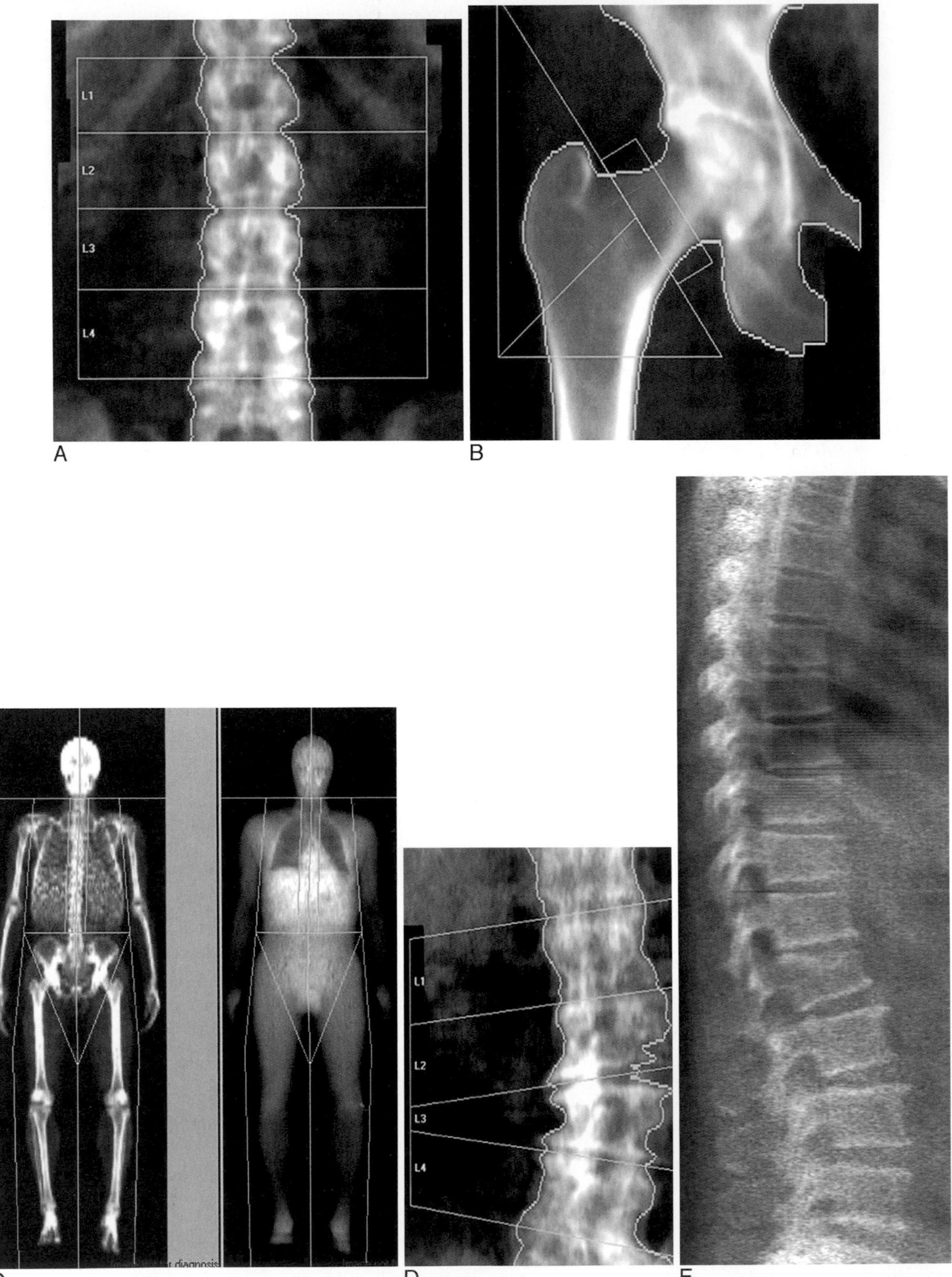

Figure 49.8 Quantitative assessment of the skeleton—DXA. Dual energy X-ray absorptiometry (DXA) provides 'areal' BMD (g cm^{-2}) and is currently the 'gold standard' method for diagnosis of osteoporosis by bone densitometry (WHO definition T score −2.5 or below) in (A) PA lumbar spine (L1–4) or (B) hip (femoral neck or total). (A) Osteophytes at L2/3 and L3/4 will cause false elevation of bone mineral density (BMD) in this anatomical site, especially in the elderly. DXA of the whole body can provide information on (C) total and regional BMD and (D) body composition (fat and muscle mass). (E) Vertebral assessment can be made from lateral images (single and dual energy; latter superior for imaging thoracic region) obtained on fan beam DXA systems at about 1/100th of the dose of conventional radiography (fractures present at L2).

(k-edged filtration, energy switching) by different scanner manufacturers. The energies used are selected to optimize the separation of the mineralized and soft tissue components of the areas scanned. Original machines had a pencil beam and coupled detector, and scanned in a rectilinear fashion. Modern machines have a fan beam X-ray source and banks of detectors. These allow rapid data acquisition with improved spatial resolution. The higher photon flux enables lateral imaging of the entire spine (single or dual energy) from which morphometric X-ray absorptiometry analysis (MXA) of vertebral fractures can be made[89]. In clinical diagnosis DXA is applied to the lumbar spine (L1–L4) and the proximal femur (regions of analysis include the femoral neck, trochanter, Ward's area and total hip); diagnosis is generally made on spine, femoral neck and total hip (Fig. 49.8A, B).

Whole body DXA with regional analysis gives information not only on bone density but also on body composition (lean muscle mass and fat mass) (Fig. 49.8C). DXA measures integral (trabecular + cortical) BMD. Different skeletal sites have variable cortical/trabecular ratios: 50/50 in the lumbar spine (PA), 10/90 in the lateral projection of the lumbar spine, 60/40 in the proximal femur and 80/20 in the whole body[84]. The accuracy of DXA is between 3% and 8%, with good precision (CV%) better than 1% in PA spine and total femur, and 1–2% in femoral neck. The advantages of DXA are the rapid scanning (less than 1 minute) and precise results if performed with meticulous care, and extremely low doses of radiation (1–6 μSv per site examined). There are, however, some limitations. Measurements are of integral bone and projected 'areal' (g cm^{-2}), rather than true volumetric (g cm^{-3}) density. DXA measurements are therefore size dependent, a particular problem in children in whom the bones are growing in size and changing in shape[23,90].

Additionally, all calcium within the path of the photon beam contributes to the BMD. Extraneous calcification (wall of aorta, and particularly degenerative and hyperostotic changes consequent to disc and apophyseal joint disease) will cause inaccuracies and overestimation of BMD (Fig. 49.8C). This limits the usefulness and sensitivity of spinal DXA in elderly patients in whom such degenerative changes are commonly present (60% in those aged 70 years or more). Other causes of falsely high BMD on DXA include vertebral wedge or crush fracture (same bone mineral content (BMC) in reduced area), Paget's disease of bone, sclerotic metastases, vertebral haemangioma, spinal metallic pinning or plating, calcified lymph nodes, residual Myodil and navel rings. Such artefacts require the results from affected individual vertebral bodies to be excluded from analysis; a minimum of two vertebrae must be available for analysis.

Treatment with strontium ranelate causes artefactual increase in BMD, approximately 50% of the increase being due to the high atomic number strontium in the bones. DXA body systems can now be used for examining peripheral sites (forearm), and to study regional bone density around a prosthesis following hip arthroplasty. Small, less expensive and more mobile DXA machines are manufactured for specific application to the forearm and the calcaneus (peripheral DXA, pDXA).

Quantitative computed tomography (QCT)[91,92]

QCT uniquely allows for the separate estimation of trabecular and cortical BMD and provides a true volumetric density in g l^{-1} (mg cm^{3}), rather than the 'areal' (mg cm^{-2}) of DXA. QCT is therefore not size dependent; it is of particular relevance in children and in diseases which result in small stature (Turner's syndrome, growth hormone deficiency, ill health). The technique is generally applied to the lumbar spine. A lateral projection radiograph is obtained, and for 2D QCT a plane is selected (10 mm slice) through the middle of each vertebra, generally T12–L3, parallel to the end-plates (Fig. 49.9A, B). If vertebral fractures are present, thinner (5 mm) sections may be required to avoid including the vertebral end-plate in the section, which will cause overestimation of BMD. A low dose technique (80 kV, 70 mA, 2 seconds) can be used to reduce patient radiation dose[93]. The entry of the basivertebral vein on the transverse axial section confirms the section to be in the mid plane of the vertebral body (Fig. 49.9D). An oval region of interest to include as much of the vertebral trabecular bone as possible, without including the cortical rim or basivertebral vein, is selected for analysis. QCT is performed with a calibration reference phantom to transform Hounsfield units into bone mineral equivalents (Fig. 49.9B). These phantoms were initially fluid (K_2HPO_4) but are now made of solid hydroxyapatite material. The results from different types of calibration phantoms are not interchangeable, unless a cross-calibration calculation can be made. In longitudinal studies it is preferable that the same reference phantom be used.

Original CT systems used rotate-translate technology which permitted only single 2D sections. The recent technical developments in CT of continuous spiral rotation of the X-ray tube and multiple rows of detectors enable rapid 3D volume data acquisition (Fig. 49.9C). As a consequence, precision has improved (better than CV 1%) and the method is applicable to measure bone size and density in the hip.

Although QCT is usually applied to the vertebral trabecular bone, more recently dedicated small CT machines (pQCT) have been developed which allow separate analysis of cortical and trabecular bone in the nondominant forearm (Fig. 49.9E, F) and in other sites of the skeleton, including the tibia. Measurement of cross-sectional bone and muscle area, and certain biomechanical parameters, can also be made[94].

Radiation dose

DXA entails extremely low radiation doses at between 1 and 6 μSv per site examined, equivalent to about 3 hours of background equivalent radiation (BER approximately 2400–7200 μSv, depending on geographic area). The radiation dose from QCT is higher but still compares favourably with conventional radiographic exposures. Using a low kV, the dose for QCT (including the initial scoutview) will be approximately 90 μSv[95].

Interpretation of results[96]

To interpret BMD results in an individual patient it is essential to have appropriate race- and sex-matched BMD

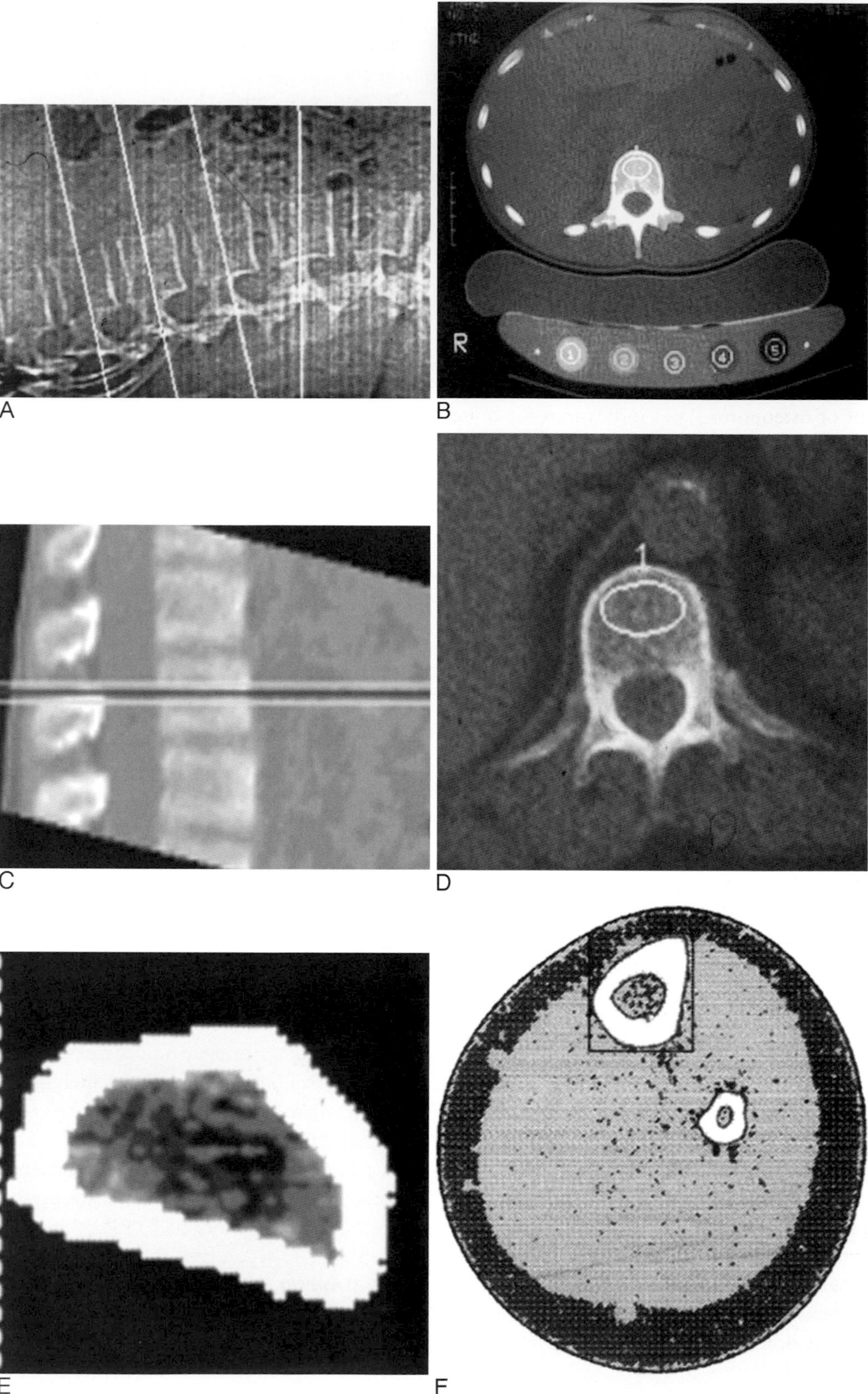

Figure 49.9 Quantitative assessment of the skeleton—quantitative computed tomography (CT). This method uniquely provides separate measures of cortical and trabecular BMD as true volumetric density (mg/cm^3) and is applied to the spine (A–D) and peripheral (pQCT) sites (forearm and tibia, E and F). For single-slice 2D QCT of the spine (A) a lateral projection radiograph is performed to identify the mid plane of four lumbar vertebrae (usually L1–4) and (B) the patient is examined lying on a bone mineral phantom (initially a fluid phantom K_2HPO_4 as in illustration, now solid hydroxyapatite phantoms are favoured) which enables Hounsfield numbers to be transformed into bone mineral equivalents. (C) With technical developments in CT (spiral, multi-slice), 3D volume imaging improves precision to CV 1%, and the appropriate section can be selected for analysis, and (D) the radiolucent area in the posterior aspect of the vertebral body confirms that the section is in the mid-plane. pQCT is generally performed in (E) the distal radius (4% site) to provide volumetric BMD of the cortical and trabecular bone and at (F) the mid shaft 50% site from which can be measured cortical thickness and density, endosteal and periosteal cross-sectional area, from which biomechanical parameters (moment of inertia and stress strain index) can be extracted, and cross-sectional muscle area.

reference ranges, since there are ethnic differences in BMD and fracture prevalence. The patient's results can then be expressed as a standard deviation (SD; Z score), percentage of expected or percentile of mean for age and sex, or as SD (T score), percentage of expected or percentile of sex-matched young normal individuals (peak bone mass)[97] (Fig. 49.1C). The Z and T score methods are currently most commonly applied. The World Health Organization has defined osteoporosis as a T score of below −2.5. Although there is consensus on this diagnostic definition from bone density, there is as yet no similar consensus on how these diagnostic definitions might most appropriately be applied consistently to therapeutic intervention. There are many and varied local and national guidelines published on the diagnosis, prevention and treatment of osteoporosis and indications for bone densitometry[98].

In longitudinal studies the absolute BMD is used to calculate change with time or treatment in an individual patient. The interval of time between measurements will depend on the site of measurement (axial or appendicular skeleton), the type of bone measured (trabecular, cortical or integral), the expected rate of change in BMD, the measuring technique used and its precision. The preferred measurement site for assessing change is the lumbar spine by DXA (high precision of better than 1%). In individual patients a minimum period of one, but preferably two, years should elapse between measurements to ensure change in BMD is significant (2.77 × precision error)[86].

Other research methods

Quantitative ultrasound (QUS) measures broadband ultrasound attenuation (BUA) and speed of sound (SOS)[99]. It is predominantly applied to the calcaneus, where it predicts fracture risk in elderly females. However, it cannot be used to diagnose osteoporosis as defined by the WHO, is temperature sensitive, is a poor monitoring tool, has been applied to numerous other skeletal sites (e.g. phalanges), and it is not clear how it should be used in clinical practice in other patient groups (men, young women and children). Quantitative magnetic resonance (QMR) has been applied in research to assess bone density and trabecular bone structure[100]. The diameter of bone trabeculae ranges from about 50 to 200 μm. Trabecular structure can be demonstrated on conventional radiographs, particularly in the appendicular skeleton (hands), where visualization can be enhanced by magnification techniques. More recently, there has been increased research application of high resolution computed tomography (HR-CT) and high resolution magnetic resonance imaging (HR-MRI) to examine trabecular structure in vivo. Micro CT systems with increased spatial resolution are under development, but these are generally only applicable to examine small tissue samples in vitro.

PARATHYROID DISORDERS

Most parathyroid tumours are functionally active and result in the clinical syndrome of primary hyperparathyroidism. This is the most common endocrine disorder after diabetes and thyroid disease, with an incidence within the population of about 1 in 1000 (0.1%). The incidence is higher in the elderly than those under 40, and is most common in women aged 60 or older. Over the past 50 years the diagnosed prevalence of the condition has increased some tenfold; this increase is due principally to the detection by chance of hypercalcaemia in patients, many of whom are asymptomatic, through routine use of multi-channel auto-analysis of serum samples since the 1970s.

HYPERPARATHYROIDISM

Primary hyperparathyroidism

The majority (80%) of patients with primary hyperparathyroidism have a single adenoma[101]. Multiple parathyroid adenomas may occur in 4% of cases. Chief cell hyperplasia of all glands occurs in 15–20% of patients; the histological diagnosis depends on the finding that more than one parathyroid gland is affected. Genetic factors are relevant in a proportion of these patients (familial hyperplasia, multiple endocrine neoplasia [MEN] syndromes). Carcinoma of the parathyroid is an infrequent cause of primary hyperparathyroidism (0.5%)[102]; the malignant tumour is slow growing but locally invasive. Cure may be obtained by adequate surgical excision and there is a 50% or greater 5-year survival rate. Recurrence is common (30%) and metastases to regional lymph nodes, lung, liver and bone occur late in 30% of cases. Biochemical remission may rarely occur spontaneously, presumably due to infarction of the tumour, but this is extremely rare since the parathyroid glands have a very rich blood supply from both the inferior and superior thyroid arteries. Metastases, when solitary, may be resected with benefit.

Secondary hyperparathyroidism

Secondary hyperparathyroidism is induced by any condition, or circumstance, which causes the serum calcium to fall. This occurs in vitamin D deficiency, intestinal malabsorption of calcium, chronic renal failure (through lack of the active metabolite of vitamin D, $1,25(OH)_2D$), and retention of phosphorus. If this secondary hyperparathyroidism is of sufficiently long standing, an autonomous adenoma may develop in the hyperplastic parathyroid glands, a condition referred to as tertiary hyperparathyroidism. This is usually associated with chronic renal disease but it has also been observed in patients with long-standing vitamin D deficiency and osteomalacia from other causes.

Clinical presentation

Most patients with primary hyperparathyroidism have mild disease and commonly have no symptoms, the diagnosis being made by the finding of asymptomatic hypercalcaemia. The most common clinical presentations, particularly in younger patients, are related to renal stones and nephrocalcinosis

(25–35%), high blood pressure (40–60%), acute arthropathy (pseudogout) caused by calcium pyrophosphate dihydrate deposition (chondrocalcinosis) (Fig. 49.10A, B), osteoporosis, peptic ulcer and acute pancreatitis, depression, confusional states, proximal muscle weakness and mild nonspecific symptoms such as lethargy, arthralgia and difficulties with mental concentration.

Treatment

Surgical removal of the overactive parathyroid tissue is generally recommended. In experienced hands surgical excision is successful in curing the condition in over 90% of patients[103]. The decision to operate, particularly in the elderly and those with asymptomatic disease, requires careful assessment[104]. Conservative treatment may be judged to be the management of choice with monitoring of the serum calcium, renal function, blood pressure and bone density at regular intervals[105,106].

Radiological findings

With the increased number of patients with primary hyperparathyroidism being diagnosed with asymptomatic hypercalcaemia, the majority (95%) of patients will have no radiological abnormalities.

Subperiosteal erosions

Subperiosteal erosion of cortical bone, particularly in the phalanges, is pathognomonic of hyperparathyroidism[101,107] (Fig. 49.10C). The most sensitive site in which to identify this early subperiosteal erosion is along the radial aspects of the middle phalanges of the index and middle fingers. Other sites may be involved including the distal phalanges (acro-osteolysis) (Fig. 49.10C), the outer ends of the clavicle, the symphysis pubis, the sacroiliac joints, the proximal medial cortex of the tibia, the proximal humeral shaft, ribs and femur. However, if no subperiosteal erosions are identified in the phalanges, they are unlikely to be identified radiographically elsewhere in the skeleton. Subperiosteal erosions in sites other than the phalanges indicate more severe and long-standing hyperparathyroidism, such as may be found secondary to chronic renal impairment.

Intracortical bone resorption

This results from increased osteoclastic activity in Haversian canals. Radiographically it causes linear translucencies within the cortex (cortical 'tunnelling') (Fig. 49.10D). This feature is not specific for hyperparathyroidism and may be found in other conditions in which bone turnover is increased (e.g. normal childhood, Paget's disease of bone).

Chondrocalcinosis

The deposition of calcium pyrophosphate dihydrate (CPPD) causes articular cartilage and fibrocartilage to become visible on radiographs[108] (Fig. 49.10A, B). This is most likely to be identified on radiographs of the hand (triangular ligament), the knees (articular cartilage and menisci) and symphysis pubis. Other joints less commonly involved are the shoulder and the hip. Clinically the patients may present with acute pain resembling gout, but on joint aspiration pyrophosphate crystals, rather than urate crystals, are found. Affected joints may however be asymptomatic, and chondrocalcinosis noted radiographically might bring the diagnosis of hyperparathyroidism to light in an asymptomatic patient. The combination of chondrocalcinosis in the symphysis pubis and nephrocalcinosis on an abdominal radiograph is diagnostic of hyperparathyroidism. Chondrocalcinosis is a feature of primary disease, rather than that secondary to chronic renal impairment.

Brown tumours (osteitis fibrosa cystica)

Brown tumours are cystic lesions within bone in which there has been excessive osteoclastic resorption (Fig. 49.10E). Histologically the cavities are filled with fibrous tissue and osteoclasts, with necrosis and haemorrhagic liquefaction. Radiographically, brown tumours appear as low density, multiloculated cysts that can occur in any skeletal site and may cause expansion of bones. They are now rarely seen.

Osteosclerosis

Osteosclerosis occurs uncommonly in primary hyperparathyroidism[109] but is a common feature of disease secondary to chronic renal impairment[110]. In primary disease with normal renal function it results from an exaggerated osteoblastic response following bone resorption. In secondary causes of hyperparathyroidism it results from excessive accumulation of poorly mineralized osteoid, which appears more dense radiographically than normal bone. The increase in bone density affects particularly the axial skeleton. In the vertebral bodies the end-plates are preferentially involved, giving bands of dense bones adjacent to the end-plates with a central band of lower normal bone density. These alternating bands of normal and sclerotic bone give a stripped pattern described as a 'rugger jersey' spine.

Osteoporosis

With excessive bone resorption the bones may appear reduced in radio-density in some patients. This may particularly occur in postmenopausal women and the elderly, in whom bone resorption exceeds new bone formation, with a net reduction in bone mass. This can be confirmed by bone densitometry, which is an integral component in the evaluation of hyperparathyroidism. In primary hyperparathyroidism there is a pattern of skeletal involvement that preferentially affects the cortical, as opposed to the trabecular, bone. Bone mineral density measurements made in sites in which cortical bone predominates, e.g. in the distal forearm, may show the most marked reduction[111]. Bone density increases after parathyroidectomy in primary hyperparathyroidism[112].

Metastatic calcification

Soft tissue calcification, other than in articular cartilage and fibrocartilage, does not occur in primary hyperparathyroidism unless there is associated reduced glomerular function resulting in phosphate retention. The latter results in an increase in the calcium × phosphate product, and as a consequence amorphous calcium phosphate is precipitated in organs, blood vessels and soft tissues[113] (Fig. 49.10C, F). If

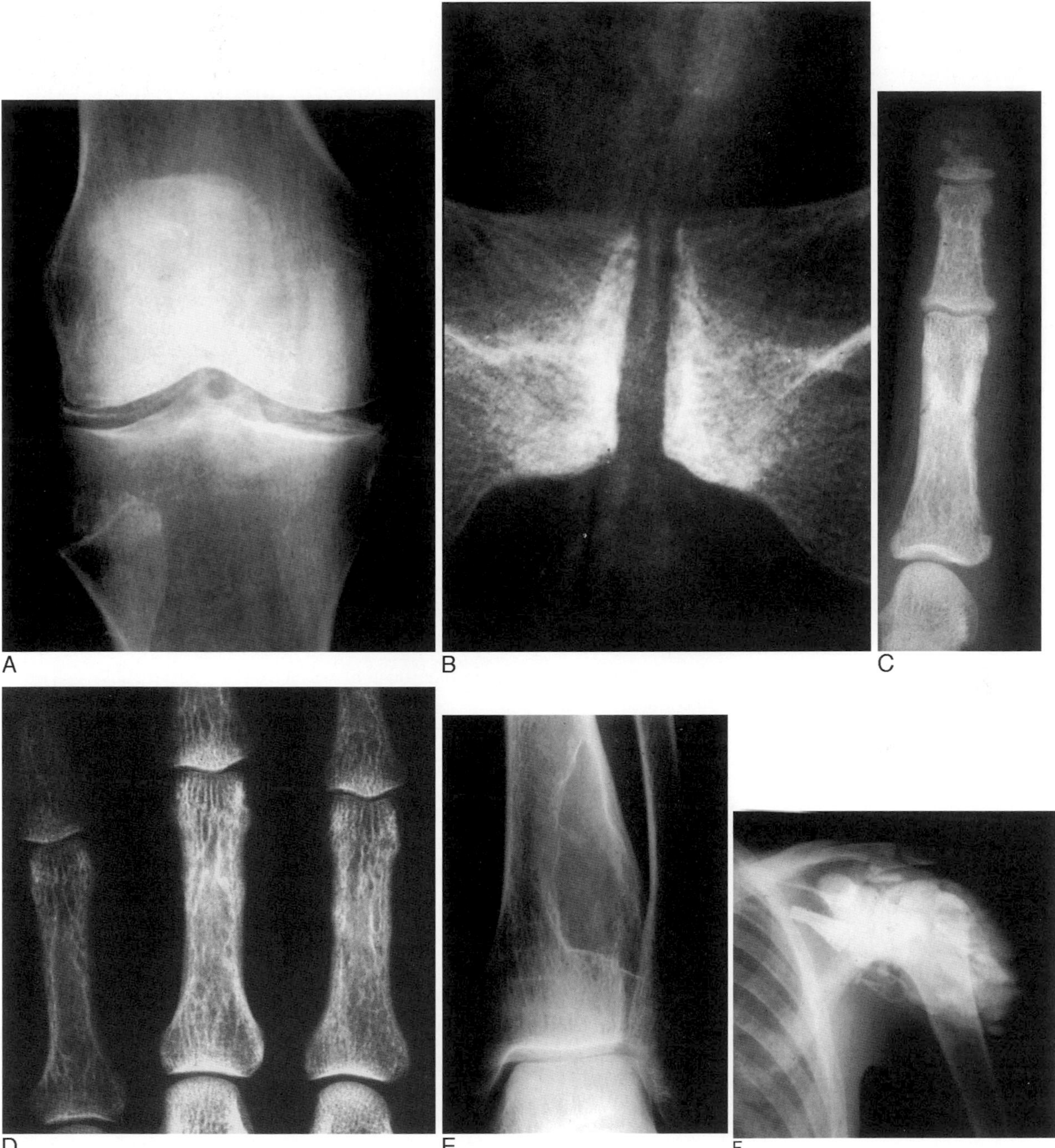

Figure 49.10 Hyperparathyroidism. In primary hyperparathyroidism there may be chondrocalcinosis (calcification of cartilage) as illustrated in (A) the knee and (B) the symphysis pubis. Other sites where this may be present are the triradiate ligament of the wrist and the large joints (hip and shoulder). Because of increased osteoclastic activity (C), subperiosteal erosions may be present and are most likely to be evident radiographically along the radial side of the middle phalanges of the 2nd and 3rd fingers. Acro-osteolysis is also present. As there is calcification of the digital artery (metastatic calcification), this is secondary hyperparathyroidism related to chronic renal failure (phosphate retention). Also related to increased osteoclastic resorption there can be (D) cortical 'tunnelling' (areas of resorption within the bone cortex) as in the proximal phalanges. (E) Bone cysts (brown tumours, osteitis fibrosa cystica) can occur in any site, seen here in the distal tibia. These cysts are less commonly seen now, as the diagnosis may come to attention in mild or asymptomatic patients who are found to have hypercalcaemia on routine blood testing. In hyperparathyroidism secondary to chronic renal disease there is phosphate retention, increase in the phosphate × calcium product and precipitation on amorphous calcium phosphate in the vessels and in soft tissues, usually around large joints, as seen (F) in the left shoulder.

there are features of hyperparathyroidism, i.e. subperiosteal erosions and additionally extensive vascular or soft tissue calcifications, e.g. around joints and in tendons, this implies impaired renal function in association with hyperparathyroidism.

HYPOPARATHYROIDISM

Aetiology

Hypoparathyroidism can result from reduced or absent parathyroid hormone production or from end organ (kidney, bone or both) resistance. This may be the result of the parathyroid glands failing to develop, the glands being damaged or removed, the function of the glands being reduced by altered regulation, or the action of parathyroid hormone (PTH) being impaired[114]. The biochemical abnormality which results is hypocalcaemia; this can clinically cause neuromuscular symptoms and signs such as tetany and fits. Acquired hypoparathyroidism results from either surgical removal of the parathyroid glands or from autoimmune disorders. Post-surgical hypoparathyroidism is more common and occurs in approximately 13% of patients following thyroid or parathyroid surgery. Idiopathic hypoparathyroidism usually presents during childhood, is more common in girls and is rare in black races. It may be associated with pernicious anaemia and Addison's disease. There may be antibodies to a number of endocrine glands as part of a generalized autoimmune disorder.

Radiological abnormalities

There may be localized (23%) or generalized (9%) osteosclerosis in affected patients[115]. This particularly affects the skull where the vault is thickened. At an early age of onset, the dentition is hypoplastic. Metastatic calcification may be present in the basal ganglia or in the subcutaneous tissue, particularly about the hips and shoulders (Fig. 49.11A). A rare but recognized complication of hypoparathyroidism is an enthesopathy with extraskeletal ossification in a paraspinal distribution and elsewhere. In the spine this skeletal hyperostosis resembles most closely that described by Forestier as 'senile' hyperostosis[116,117]. Differentiating features from ankylosing spondylitis are that there is no erosive arthropathy and the sacroiliac joints appear normal. Clinically the patients may have pain and stiffness in the back with limitation of movement. Extraskeletal ossification may be present around the pelvis, hip and in the interosseous membranes and tendinous insertions elsewhere.

Pseudohypoparathyroidism (PHP)

Pseudohypoparathyroidism describes a group of genetic disorders characterized by hypocalcaemia, hyperphosphataemia, raised PTH and target tissue unresponsiveness to PTH, first described by Albright et al in 1942[117–121]. Affected patients are short in stature, have reduced intellect, rounded faces and shortened metacarpals, particularly the fourth and fifth (Fig. 49.11B). Metastatic calcification, bowing of long bones and exostoses can occur. Clinical features include tetany, cataracts and nail dystrophy. Some of the clinical and radiological features of PHP may resemble those in other hereditary syndromes, including Turner's syndrome, acrodysostosis, Prader–Willi syndrome, fibrodysplasia ossificans progressiva and multiple hereditary exostosis. In PHP there is end organ unresponsiveness to PTH since the parathyroid glands are normal and produce PTH. This usually involves unresponsiveness of both bone and kidneys. However, there is a rare variation of PHP in which the kidneys are unresponsive to PTH but the osseous response to the hormone is normal[122]. The condition is referred to as pseudohypohyperparathyroidism, and the histological and radiological features resemble those of azotaemic osteodystrophy.

Radiographic abnormalities

Abnormalities may not be evident at birth but subsequently there develops premature epiphyseal fusion, calvarial thickening, bone exostoses and calcification in the basal ganglia and the soft tissue (Fig. 49.11A). Metacarpal shortening is present, particularly affecting the fourth and fifth digits (Fig. 49.11B). This may result in a positive metacarpal sign in which, if a line is drawn tangential to the heads of the fourth and fifth metacarpals, the

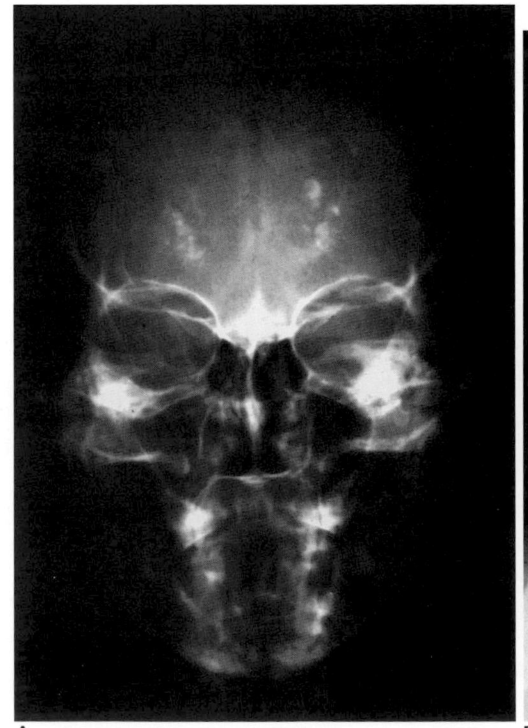

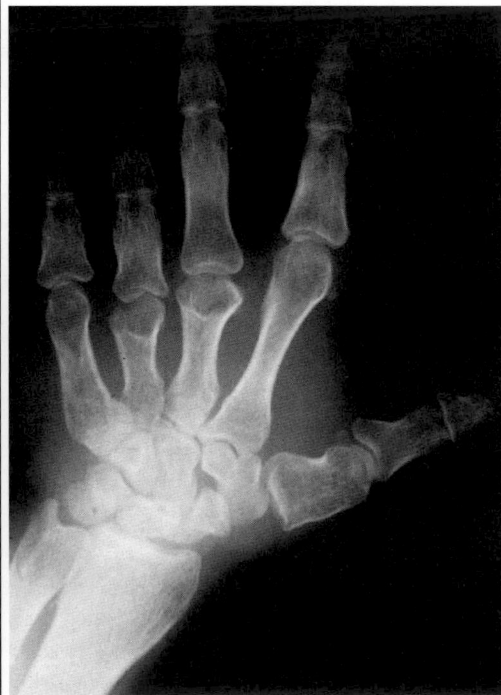

Figure 49.11 Hypoparathyroidism. (A) Soft tissue calcification may be present, seen here in the basal ganglia. (B) In pseudo-hypoparathyroidism (PHP of Albright) affected individuals are short in stature, and there are dysplastic features, including shortened metacarpals, particularly the fourth and fifth.

line should not normally intersect the third metacarpal, but does if there is shorting of the fourth metacarpal. This feature is not specific for PHP and can occur in other congenital (Beckwith–Wiedemann and basal cell naevus syndromes, multiple epiphyseal dysplasia) and acquired (juvenile chronic arthritis, sickle-cell disease with infarction) conditions. Soft tissue calcification occurs in a plaque-like distribution in the subcutaneous area. Rarely, soft tissue ossification can occur in a peri-articular distribution, usually involving the hands and feet.

Pseudo-pseudohypoparathyroidism (PPHP)

In these affected individuals the dysplastic and other features are the same as PHP, but there are no associated parathyroid or other biochemical abnormalities. The abnormalities include metacarpal and metatarsal shortening, calvarial thickening and exostoses; soft tissue calcification and ossification are best identified on radiographs. CT of the brain may be more sensitive at identifying basal ganglia calcification. Bone density may be normal, reduced or increased.

RICKETS AND OSTEOMALACIA

Mineralization of bone matrix depends on the presence of adequate supplies of 1,25-dihydroxy vitamin D (1,25(OH)$_2$D), calcium, phosphorus and alkaline phosphatase, and on a normal body pH. If there is a deficiency of any of these substances, or if there is severe systemic acidosis, the mineralization of bone will be defective. This results in a qualitative abnormality of bone, with a reduction in the mineral to osteoid ratio, resulting in rickets in children and osteomalacia in adults. Rickets and osteomalacia are therefore synonymous and represent the same disease process, but manifest in either the growing or the mature skeleton.

In the immature skeleton the radiographic abnormalities predominate at the growing ends of the bones where enchondral ossification is taking place, giving the classic appearance of rickets.

At skeletal maturity, when the process of enchondral ossification has ceased, the defective mineralization of osteoid is evident radiographically as Looser's zones (pseudofractures, Milkman's fracture), which are pathognomonic of osteomalacia[123,124]. Many different conditions can cause the same radiological abnormalities of rickets and osteomalacia. In the past there was much confusion between conditions that had similar clinical and radiological features, but with different patterns of progression and responses to therapies of the day. These causes of confusion have largely been clarified with the increased understanding during the late twentieth century of the structure and function of vitamin D and its metabolites.

The pro-hormone forms of vitamin D require two hydroxylation stages to form the active metabolite, through which the hormone exerts its physiological action. There are two pro-hormonal forms of 1,25-dihydroxy vitamin D in humans: vitamin D$_2$ and vitamin D$_3$. Vitamin D$_2$ is prepared by irradiation of ergosterol obtained from yeast or fungi, and is used for food supplementation and pharmaceutical preparations. Vitamin D$_3$ occurs naturally through the interaction of ultraviolet light on 7-dehydrocholesterol in the deep layers of the skin. Vitamin D$_2$ and D$_3$ are initially hydroxylated at the 25 position to form 25(OH)D$_2$ and 25(OH)D$_3$, the latter predominating and circulating bound to a specific protein. This hydroxylation occurs predominantly in the liver. A further hydroxylation in the 1 position in the kidney produces 1,25(OH)$_2$D, which is the active form of the hormone.

VITAMIN D DEFICIENCY

Deficiency may occur as a consequence of simple nutritional lack (diet, lack of sunlight), malabsorption states (vitamin D is fat soluble and absorbed in the small bowel), chronic liver disease (which affects hydroxylation at the 25 position) and chronic renal disease (in which the active metabolite 1,25-dihydroxy D is not produced). Consequently, a wide variety of diseases may result in vitamin D deficiency; the radiological features will be similar, being those of rickets or osteomalacia. This similarity of radiological features, but variation in response to treatment, contributed to some of the early confusion. Rickets due to nutritional deprivation was cured by ultraviolet light or physiological doses of vitamin D (400 IU per day), but that associated with chronic renal disease was not, except when very large pharmacological doses (up to 300 000 IU per day) were used. This led to the terms 'refractory rickets' and 'vitamin D resistant rickets' being used for these conditions. Within these terms were included the diseases that cause the clinical and radiological features of rickets, but were related to phosphate, not vitamin D, deficiency, such as X-linked hypophosphataemia, and genetic disorders involving defects in 1-alpha hydroxylase and the vitamin D receptor.

Genetic disorders of vitamin D metabolism

Prader et al in 1961 described the condition in which rickets occurred within the first year of life, was characterized by severe hypocalcaemia and dental enamel hypoplasia, and responded to large amounts of vitamin D. The term 'vitamin D dependency' was used for this syndrome. It is now recognized that this disease is due to an inborn error of metabolism in which there is defective hydroxylation of 25(OH)D in the kidney due to defective activity of the renal 25(OH)D 1-alpha hydroxylase. This results in insufficient synthesis of 1,25(OH)$_2$D. The preferred term for this condition is pseudo vitamin D deficiency rickets (PDDR) and it is inherited as an autosomal recessive trait[125].

Another inborn error of vitamin D metabolism was described in 1978[126]. Clinically it resembled pseudo vitamin D deficiency rickets but with high circulating concentrations of 1,25(OH)$_2$D. This condition results from a spectrum of mutations which affect the vitamin D receptor (VDR) in target tissues, causing resistance to the action of 1,25(OH)$_2$D (end organ resistance). Affected patients have complete alopecia.

Radiological appearances

Rickets

In the immature skeleton the effect of vitamin D deficiency and the consequent defective mineralization of osteoid is seen principally at the growing ends of bones[123,124,127]. In the early stage there is apparent widening of the growth plate which is the translucent 'unmineralized' gap between the mineralized metaphysis and epiphysis (Fig. 49.12). More severe change produces 'cupping' of the metaphysis, with irregular and poor mineralization (Fig. 49.2B). Some expansion in width of the metaphysis results in the swelling around the ends of the long bones affected. This expansion of the anterior ends of the ribs is referred to as a 'rachitic rosary'. There may be a thin 'ghost-like' rim of mineralization at the periphery of the metaphysis, as this mineralization occurs by membranous ossification at the periosteum. The margin of the epiphysis appears indistinct as enchondral ossification at this site is also defective. These changes predominate at the sites of bones which are growing most actively. These sites are around the knee (Fig. 49.12), the wrist (particularly the ulna) (Fig. 49.2B), the anterior ends of the middle ribs, the proximal femur and the distal tibia, and depend on the age of the child. If rickets is suspected, it is these anatomical sites which are most likely to show radiographic abnormality.

Rachitic bone is soft and bends, and this results in genu valgum or genu varum, deformity of the hips (coxa valga or more commonly coxa vara), in-drawing of the ribs at the insertion of the diaphragm (Harrison's sulcus) and protrusio acetabuli and triradiate deformity of the pelvis, which can cause problems with subsequent parturition. Involvement of the bones in the thorax and respiratory tract (larynx and trachea) rarely results in stridor and respiratory distress. In very severe rickets, when little skeletal growth is taking place (i.e. owing to nutritional deprivation or chronic ill health), paradoxically the radiological features of rickets may not be evident at the growth plate. In rickets of prematurity, little abnormality may be present at the metaphysis since no skeletal growth is taking place in the premature infant. However, the bones are osteopenic and prone to fractures. In mild vitamin D deficiency the radiographic features of rickets may only become apparent at puberty during the growth spurt, and the metaphyseal abnormalities predominate at the knee.

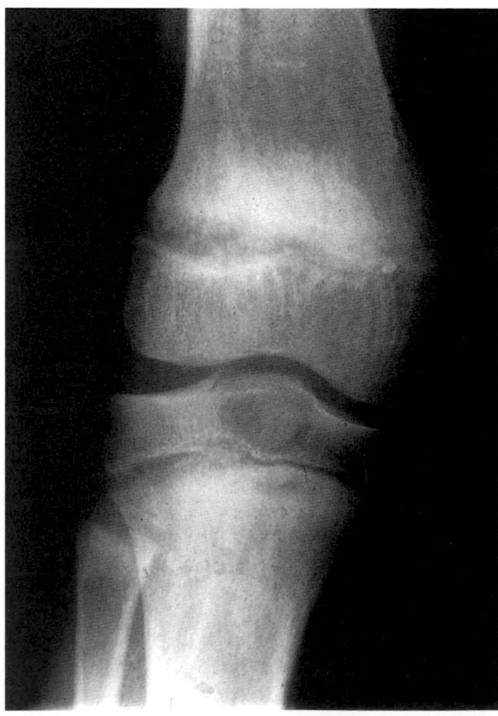

Figure 49.12 Rickets. In the immature skeleton, evidence of defective mineralization is evident in sites of endochondral ossification. The growth plate is widened; the metaphysis may be splayed and irregularly mineralized. The abnormalities will be most apparent in sites of the skeleton which are growing most rapidly (knee, as in the illustration; wrist; ankle) and which are therefore most likely to show the features on radiographs.

With appropriate treatment of vitamin D deficiency, the radiographic features of healing lag behind the improvement in biochemical parameters (2 weeks) and clinical symptoms. With treatment, the zone of provisional calcification will mineralize. This mineralized zone is initially separated by translucent osteoid from the shaft of the bone, and may be mistaken for a metaphyseal fracture of child abuse[128]. Reduced bone density and poor definition of epiphyses are helpful distinguishing features for rickets. The section of abnormal bone following healing of rickets may be visible for a period of time, and give some indication as to the age of onset and duration of the period of rickets. Eventually this zone will become indistinguishable from normal bone with remodelling over a period of 3–4 months. The zone of provisional calcification which was present at the onset of the disturbance to enchondral ossification may remain (Harris growth arrest line)[129] as a marker of the age of skeletal maturity at which the rickets occurred. However, this is not specific for rickets and may occur in any condition (e.g. period of ill health, lead poisoning) that inhibits normal enchondral ossification. There will be evidence of retarded growth and development in rickets, but in this author's experience, this tends to be more marked when the vitamin D deficiency is associated with chronic diseases that reduce calorie intake, general well-being and activity (i.e. malabsorption, chronic renal disease) than with simple nutritional vitamin D deficiency.

Vitamin D deficiency is associated with hypocalcaemia. In an attempt to maintain calcium homeostasis, the parathyroid glands are stimulated to secrete PTH. This results in another important feature of vitamin D deficiency rickets. Evidence of secondary hyperparathyroidism, with increased osteoclastic resorption, is always evident histologically, although not always radiographically.

Metaphyseal chondrodysplasias

In a variety of inherited bone dysplasias there are metaphyseal abnormalities which may range from mild (Schmit type) to severe (Jansen)[130]. Normal serum biochemistry serves to differentiate these dysplasias from other rachitic disorders which the radiographic abnormalities at the metaphyses may simulate.

Osteomalacia

At skeletal maturity the epiphysis fuses to the metaphysis with obliteration of the growth plate and cessation of longitudinal bone growth. However, bone turnover continues throughout life to maintain the tensile integrity of the skeleton. Vitamin D deficiency in the adult skeleton results in osteomalacia, the pathognomonic radiographic feature of which is the Looser's zone (1908)[131] (Fig. 49.13). Looser's zones (pseudo-fractures, Milkman's fractures)[132] are translucent areas in the bone that are composed of unmineralized osteoid. They are typically (but not always) bilateral and symmetrical. Radiographically they appear as radiolucent lines that are perpendicular to the bone cortex, do not usually extend across the entire bone shaft, and characteristically have a slightly sclerotic margin. Looser's zones can occur in any bone but most typically are found in the medial aspect of the femoral neck, the pubic rami, the lateral border of the scapula and the ribs. They may involve the first and second ribs, in which traumatic fractures are uncommon, being usually associated with severe trauma. Other less common sites for Looser's zones are the metatarsals and metacarpals, the base of the acromion and the ilium. They may not always be visible on radiographs; radionuclide bone scans are more sensitive in identifying radiographic occult Looser's zones[49].

Looser's zones must be differentiated from insufficiency fractures that may occur in osteoporotic bone, particularly in the pubic rami, sacrum and calcaneus. Such insufficiency fractures consist of multiple micro-fractures in brittle osteoporotic bone and often show florid callus formation, serving to differentiate them from Looser's zones[133,134]. Incremental fractures occur in Paget's disease of bone and resemble Looser's zones in appearance, but tend to occur on the convexity of the cortex of the bone involved[135,136], rather than medially on the concave side, as in osteomalacia. The other typical features of Paget's disease serve as distinguishing radiological features.

Complete fractures can occur through Looser's zones, but with no evidence of callus formation until the osteomalacia is treated with vitamin D. Then there will be quite florid callus formation around fractures with healing of the fractures and Looser's zones with little residual deformity. However, as in rickets, osteomalacic bone is soft and bends. This is evident

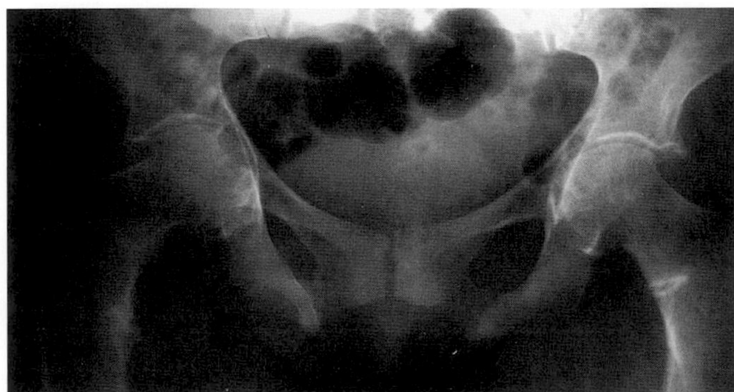

Figure 49.13 Osteomalacia. In the mature skeleton after fusion of the growth plate, the pathognomonic radiographic feature is the Looser's zone. These are radiolucent, unmineralized linear areas which are perpendicular to the cortex and which may have a sclerotic margin. They occur most frequently in the medial aspects of the femoral necks (as present in this case of a patient with coeliac disease), symphysis pubis, ribs and lateral borders of the scapulae. The malacic bones are soft and bend, and there is protrusio acetabulae bilaterally.

radiographically by protrusio acetabuli, in which the femoral head deforms the acetabular margin so that the normal 'teardrop' outline is lost. There may be bowing of the long bones of the legs and a triradiate deformity of the pelvis, particularly if the cause of the vitamin D deficiency has persisted since childhood and has been inadequately treated or untreated.

In osteomalacia, as in rickets, hypocalcaemia acts as stimulus to *secondary hyperparathyroidism*. This may be manifested radiographically as subperiosteal erosion, particularly in the phalanges but other sites (sacroiliac joints, symphysis pubis, proximal tibia, outer ends of the clavicle, skull vault—'pepperpot' skull) may be involved, depending on the intensity of the hyperparathyroidism and how long it has been present. There may also be cortical tunnelling and a hazy trabecular pattern. Generalized osteopenia may occur and vertebral bodies may have biconcave endplates, due to deformation of the malacic bone by the cartilaginous intervertebral disc ('cod fish' deformity)[137].

RENAL OSTEODYSTROPHY

The bone disease associated with chronic renal impairment is complex and multifactorial, and has changed over past decades[110,138]. Whereas originally features of vitamin D deficiency (rickets/osteomalacia) and secondary hyperparathyroidism (erosions, osteosclerosis, brown cysts) predominated, improvements in management and therapy have resulted in such radiographic features being present in only a minority of patients. Soft tissue and extensive vascular metastatic calcification (Fig. 49.10C, F) and 'adynamic' bone develop as a complication of disease (phosphate retention) and treatment (phosphate binders). New complications (amyloid deposition, noninfective spondyloarthropathy, osteonecrosis) are now seen in long-term haemodialysis and/or renal transplantation. Radiographs remain the most important imaging technique, but occasionally other imaging and quantitative techniques (CT, MRI, bone densitometry) are relevant to diagnosis and management.

In extreme cases of soft tissue calcification there may be ischaemic necrosis of the skin, muscle and subcutaneous tissue, referred to as 'calciphylaxis'. This condition can occur in patients with advanced renal disease, in those on regular dialysis, and also those with functioning renal allografts[139].

Renal tubular defects

Glucose, inorganic phosphate and amino acids are absorbed in the proximal renal tubule. Concentration and acidification of urine in exchange for a fixed base occur in the distal renal tubule. Renal tubular disorders may involve either the proximal or the distal tubule, or both. Such disorders result in a spectrum of biochemical disturbances that may result in loss of phosphate, glucose, or amino acids alone, or in combination, with additional defects in urine acidification and concentration. Such defects of tubular function may be inherited and present from birth (Toni–Fanconi syndrome, cystinosis, X-linked hypophosphataemia) or later in life (e.g. tubular function being compromised by deposition of copper in Wilson's disease, hereditary tyrosinaemia). Renal tubular dysfunction may also be acquired by tubular dysfunction being induced by the effects of toxins or therapies (paraquat,

Lysol burns, toluene 'glue sniffing' inhalation, ifosfamide, gentamicin, streptozotocin, valproic acid), deposition of heavy metals or other substances (multiple myeloma, cadmium, lead, mercury), related to immunological disorders (interstitial nephritis, renal transplantation), or with the production of a humoral substance in tumour-induced osteomalacia (TIO), also known as 'oncogenic rickets'[140,141]. In these renal tubular disorders, rickets or osteomalacia can be caused by multiple factors, including hyperphosphaturia, hypophosphataemia and reduced 1-alpha hydroxylation of 25(OH)D. Where the serum calcium is generally normal, secondary hyperparathyroidism does not occur.

X-linked hypophosphataemia (XLH)

This genetic disorder is transmitted as an X-linked dominant trait[142]. Sporadic cases also occur through spontaneous mutations. The incidence is approximately 1 in 25 000, and XLH is now the most common cause of genetically induced rickets. The disease is characterized by phosphaturia throughout life, hypophosphataemia, rickets and osteomalacia. Clinically affected individuals may be short in stature, principally due to defective growth in the legs, which are bowed; the trunk is usually normal[143]. Rickets becomes clinically evident at about 6–12 months of age or older. Treatment with phosphate supplements and large pharmacological doses of vitamin D (hence the term 'vitamin D-resistant rickets') can heal the radiological features of rickets and also increase longitudinal growth[144]. The radiological features of XLH are characteristic[145]. There is defective mineralization of the metaphysis and widening of the growth plate (rickets). The metaphyseal margin tends to be less indistinct than in nutritional rickets and the affected metaphysis is not as wide. Changes are most marked at the knee, wrist, ankle and proximal femur. Healing can be induced with appropriate treatment (phosphate supplements, $1,25(OH)_2D$)[144]. The growth plates fuse normally at skeletal maturation. The bones are often short and under-tubulated (shaft wide in relation to bone length) with bowing of the femur and tibia, which may be marked. Following skeletal maturation, Looser's zones appear and persist in patients with XLH (Fig. 49.14A). They tend to be in sites which are different from those which occur in nutritional osteomalacia, and often affect the outer cortex of the bowed femur, although they also occur along the medial cortex of the shaft. Looser's zones in the ribs and pelvis are rare. Although Looser's zones may heal with appropriate treatment, those that have been present for many years persist radiographically and are presumably filled with fibrous tissue.

Although there is defective mineralization of osteoid in XLH, the bones are commonly and characteristically increased in radio-density with a coarse and prominent trabecular pattern. This is a feature of the disease, and is not related to treatment with vitamin D and phosphate supplements, as it is present in those who have not received treatment. This bone sclerosis can involve the petrous bone and structures of the inner ear, and may be responsible for the hydropic cochlea pattern of deafness that these patients may develop in later life[146]. X-linked hypophosphataemia is characterized by an enthesopathy, in which there is inflammation in the junctional area between bone and tendon insertion that heals by ossification at affected sites[147] (Fig. 49.14B). As a result, ectopic bone forms around the pelvis and spine. This may result in complete ankylosis of the spine, resembling ankylosing spondylitis, and clinically limiting mobility. However, the

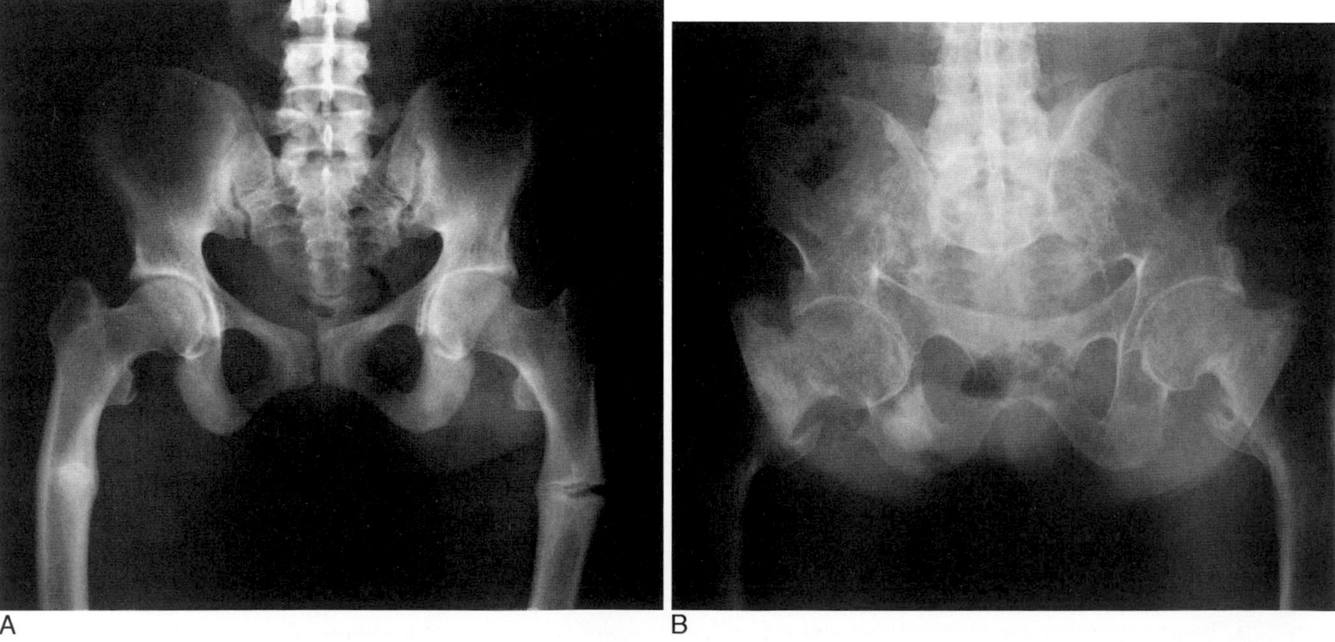

Figure 49.14 X-linked hypophosphataemic osteomalacia. This is the most common of the genetic causes of rickets and osteomalacia. There is a renal tubular abnormality which results in phosphaturia and hypophosphataemia. The bones may be radio-dense with a coarse trabecular pattern. In affected children there will be evidence of rickets. (A) In adults chronic Looser's zones may be present, as in the outer cortex of both femora. (B) There may be evidence of an enthesopathy in older patients with ossification of ligamentous insertion to bone, as present in the pelvis at the psoas insertion to the lesser trochanters. The paraspinal ossification resembles ankylosing spondylitis, but the sacroiliac joints are not eroded.

absence of inflammatory arthritis, with normal sacroiliac joints, serves to differentiate XLH from ankylosing spondylitis.

Ossification may occur in the interosseous membrane of the forearm and in the leg between the tibia and the fibula. Separate, small ossicles may occur around the joints of the hands and ossification of tendon insertions in the hands causes 'whiskering' of bone margins.

A rare, but recognized, important complication of XLH is spinal cord compression caused by a combination of ossification of the ligamentum flavum, thickening of the laminae and hyperostosis around the apophyseal joints[148]. Ossification of the ligamentum flavum causes the most significant narrowing of the spinal canal and occurs most commonly in the thoracic spine, generally involving two or three adjacent segments. Affected patients may be asymptomatic, even when there is severe spinal canal narrowing. Acute spinal cord compression can be precipitated by quite minor trauma. It is important to be aware of this rare complication of the disease since surgical decompression by laminectomy is curative and is best performed as an elective procedure by an experienced surgeon rather than as an emergency. The extent of intraspinal ossification cannot be predicted by the degree of paraspinal or extraskeletal ossification at other sites. CT is a useful imaging technique for demonstrating the extent of intraspinal ossification.

Extraskeletal ossification is uncommon in patients with XLH before the age of 40 years. The extent to which radiographic abnormalities of rickets and osteomalacia, osteosclerosis, abnormalities of bone modelling and extraskeletal ossification are present varies between affected individuals[149]. In some patients, all the features are present and so are diagnostic of the condition. In others, there may only be minor abnormalities and the diagnosis of X-linked hypophosphataemic rickets may be overlooked[150].

Tumour induced 'oncogenic' rickets/ osteomalacia (TIO)

'Oncogenic' rickets and osteomalacia was first reported in 1947[151]. The condition is characterized by phosphaturia and hypophosphataemia induced by a factor ('phosphatonin') produced by the tumour which has various effects (inhibiting production of 1,25$(OH)_2$D; direct effect on the renal tubule) and is associated with the clinical and radiographic features of rickets and osteomalacia. Such features may precede identification of the causative tumour by long periods (1–16 years). The tumours are usually small, benign and of vascular origin (haemangiopericytoma), but there is now known to be a wide spectrum of tumours, some of which may be malignant[152], that may result in this syndrome. The causative lesions may originate in the skeleton and occur in neurofibromatosis. The biochemical abnormalities will be cured, and the rickets and osteomalacia will heal, with surgical removal of the tumour[153]. Often the tumours are extremely small and elude detection for many years. It is important that the affected patient is vigilant about self examination and reports any small palpable lump or skin lesion. More sophisticated imaging (CT, MRI) may be helpful in localizing deep-seated lesions[152].

OTHER CAUSES OF RICKETS AND OSTEOMALACIA (Not related to vitamin D deficiency or hypophosphataemia)

Hypophosphatasia

This rare disorder was first described by Rathbun in 1948[154]. It is generally transmitted as an autosomal recessive trait, but autosomal dominant inheritance has also been reported. The disease is characterized by reduced levels of serum alkaline phosphatase (both bone and liver isoenzymes), with raised levels of phosphoethanolamine in both the blood and the urine. Serum calcium and phosphorus levels are not reduced; in perinatal and infantile disease there can be hypercalciuria and hypercalcaemia attributed to the imbalance between calcium absorption from the gut and defective growth and mineralization of the skeleton. The latter results in rickets in childhood and osteomalacia in adults. The severity of the condition varies greatly, being diagnosed either in the perinatal period, in infancy or childhood, but in some patients only becoming apparent in adult life[155]. The condition can wax and wane and tends to be more severe in children than when it becomes apparent in later life.

In severely affected neonates there is little, if any, evidence of mineralization of the skeleton; in extreme cases there may be such poor mineralization that only the skull base is visualized radiographically. Death ensues soon after birth since there is inadequate bony support for the thorax or brain. Less severely

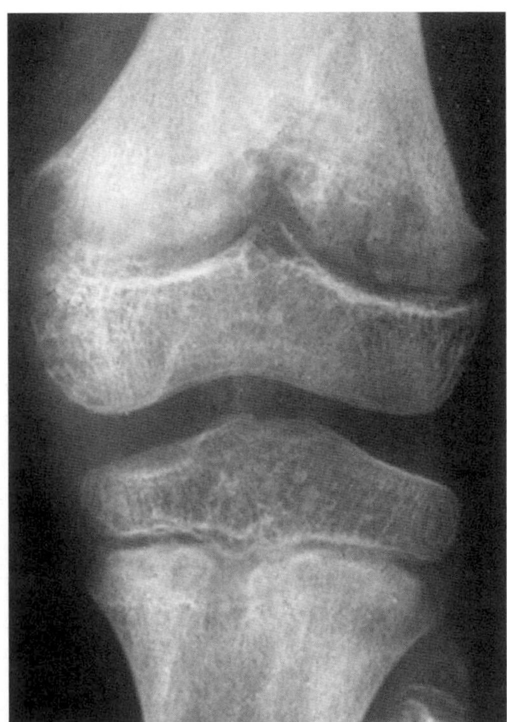

Figure 49.15 Hypophosphatasia. Affected patients may have rickets in childhood and osteomalacia in adulthood. The AP radiograph of the knee shows widened growth plates, particularly in the distal femur, and rather more patchy deficiency of calcification of the metaphysis that is characteristic of rickets due to vitamin D deficiency. There is no specific treatment for the condition.

affected children survive with rachitic metaphyseal changes appearing soon after birth as growth proceeds. The abnormalities at the growth plates resemble nutritional vitamin D deficiency rickets, but in hypophosphatasia larger, irregular lucent defects often extend into the metaphyses and diaphyses (Fig. 49.15). There may be generalized reduction in bone density with a coarse trabecular pattern. The long bones, particularly those in the lower limbs, become bowed; fractures may occur and be the presenting feature. Such fractures may or may not heal; when they do unite, it is through subperiosteal new bone formation.

In severe disease, multiple fractures may cause deformity and limb shortening. Initially the skull sutures are widened due to poor mineralization of the skull vault, but later premature fusion may lead to craniostenosis. This can result in raised intracranial pressure, bulging of the anterior fontanelle, proptosis and papilloedema. Wormian (intersutural) bones may be present.

In adult onset of the disease, the presenting clinical feature is usually a fracture occurring after relatively minor trauma, particularly in the metatarsals. Fracture healing is slow or absent with little callus formation, but will occur following intramedullary nailing[156]. The features of osteomalacia may be present with Looser's zones, a coarse trabecular pattern and bowing deformities of the limbs. Chondrocalcinosis and extraskeletal ossification of tendinous and ligamentous insertions to bone may occur[157]. The diagnosis is confirmed by the biochemical changes of reduced alkaline phosphatase and raised blood and urine phosphoethanolamine. As there is no effective treatment for hypophosphatasia, severely affected patients can prove a severe challenge to orthopaedic management[158].

OTHER METABOLIC BONE DISORDERS

A number of congenital and familial disorders can be associated with increased bone density (osteosclerosis) and abnormal bone modelling. These include osteopetrosis, pyknodysostosis, metaphyseal dysplasia (Pyle's disease), craniometaphyseal dysplasia, frontometaphyseal dysplasia, osteodysplasty (Melnick–Needles syndrome), progressive diaphyseal dysplasia (Camurati–Engelmann disease), hereditary multiple diaphyseal sclerosis (Ribbing's disease), craniodiaphyseal dysplasia, endosteal hyperostosis (Worth and Van Buchem types), dysosteosclerosis, tubular stenosis, and oculodento-osseous dysplasia[158]. All are rare and have different natural histories, genetic transmission, complications and radiographic features. Many are dysplasias rather than metabolic bone disorders.

OSTEOPETROSIS

In osteopetrosis there is defective osteoclastic resorption of the primary spongiosa of bone. Osteoclasts in affected bone are usually devoid of the ruffled borders by which osteoclasts adhere to the bone surface and through which their resorptive activity is expressed. In the presence of continued bone formation, there is generalized osteosclerosis and abnormalities of metaphyseal modelling[159] (Fig. 49.16). There have been reports of reversal of the osteosclerosis following successful bone marrow transplantation.

Osteopetrosis was first described by Albers-Schönberg in 1904, and is sometimes referred to as marble bone disease, osteosclerosis fragilis generalisata and osteopetrosis generalisata. There are two main clinical forms:

1 the lethal form of osteopetrosis with precocious manifestations and an autosomal recessive transmission
2 benign osteopetrosis with late manifestations, inherited by autosomal dominant transmission.

There is also a rarer autosomal recessive (intermediate) form which presents during childhood with the signs and symptoms of the lethal form but the outcome on life expectancy is not known. The syndrome previously described as osteopetrosis with renal tubular acidosis and cerebral calcification is now recognized as an inborn error of metabolism, carbonic anhydrase II deficiency. Neuronal storage disease with malignant osteopetrosis has been described, as has the rare lethal, transient infantile and postinfectious form of the disorder.

Autosomal recessive lethal type of osteoporosis

In affected individuals there is obliteration of the marrow cavity leading to anaemia, thrombocytopenia and recurrent infection. Clinically there is hepatosplenovmegaly, hydrocephalus and cranial nerve involvement resulting in

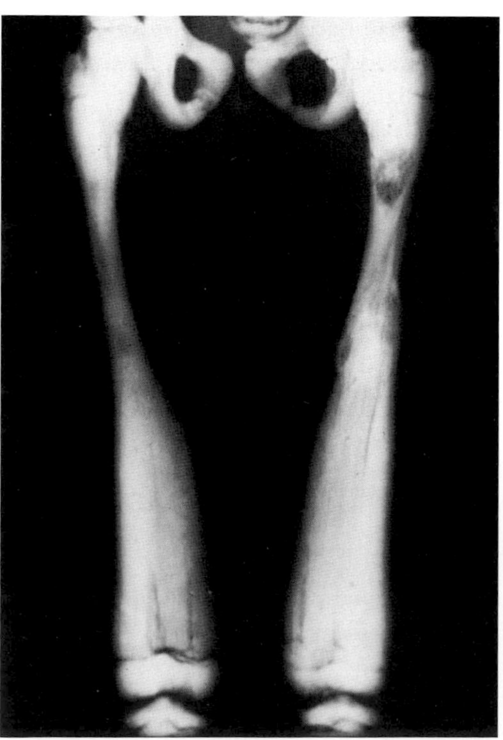

Figure 49.16 Osteopetrosis. Osteoclastic function is defective, resulting in dense sclerotic bones which are brittle and prone to fracture. There is evidence of abnormal modelling of the long bones, as in the distal femora, due to the failure of normal osteoclastic periosteal bone resorption which remodels the bones as they grow in length by endochondral ossification.

blindness and deafness. Radiographically all the bones are dense with lack of corticomedullary differentiation. Modelling of affected bones is abnormal with expansion of the metaphyseal region and under-tubulation of bone. This is most evident in the long bones, particularly the distal femur and proximal humerus. Although the bones are dense, they are brittle, and horizontal pathological fractures are common. The entire skull, particularly the base, is involved and the paranasal and mastoid air cells are poorly developed. Sclerosis of end-plates of the vertebral bodies produces a 'sandwich' appearance. MR imaging may assist in monitoring those with severe disease who undergo marrow transplantation, since success will be indicated by expansion of the marrow cavity. Findings on MR and CT of the brain have been described.

There is an intermediate recessive form of the disease which is milder than that seen in infants and distinct from the less severe autosomal dominant disease. Affected individuals suffer pathological fracture and anaemia and are of short stature, with hepatomegaly. The radiographic features include diffuse osteosclerosis with involvement of the skull base and facial bones, abnormal bone modelling and a 'bone within a bone' appearance.

Benign, autosomal dominant type of osteopetrosis (Albers-Schönberg disease)

This is often asymptomatic, and the diagnosis may come to light either incidentally or through the occurrence of a pathological fracture. Other presentations include anaemia and facial palsy or deafness from cranial nerve compression. Problems may occur after tooth extraction, and there is an increased incidence of osteomyelitis, particularly of the mandible. Radiographic features are similar to those of the autosomal recessive form of the disease, but are less severe. The bones are diffusely sclerotic, with thickened cortices and defective modelling. There may be alternating sclerotic and radiolucent bands at the ends of diaphyses, a 'bone within a bone' appearance and the vertebral end-plates appear sclerotic. In 1987, Andersen and Bollerslev classified this form of the disease into two distinct radiological types. In type I fractures are unusual, in contrast to type II in which fractures are common. Transverse bands in the metaphyses are more commonly a feature in type II disease, as is a raised serum acid phosphatase.

HYPERPHOSPHATASIA

Hyperphosphatasia is a rare genetic disorder resulting from mutations in osteoprotegerin (OPG), and is characterized by markedly elevated serum alkaline phosphatase levels[160]. Affected children have episodes of fever, bone pain and progressive enlargement of the skull, with bowing of the long bones and associated pathological fractures. Radiographically the features resemble Paget's disease of bone, and it is sometimes referred to as 'juvenile' Paget's disease, osteitis deformans in children or hyperostosis corticalis (Fig. 49.17). There is an increased rate of bone turnover, with woven bone failing to mature into lamellar bone.

Radiographically, this increased rate of bone turnover is evidenced by decreased bone radio-density with coarsening and disorganization of the trabecular pattern. In the skull the diploic space is widened and there is patchy sclerosis. The diaphyses of the long bones become expanded with cortical thickening along their concave aspects. The long bones may be bowed, resulting in coxa vara and protrusio acetabulae. The vertebral bodies are reduced in radio-density, reduced in height and biconcave. The bowing of the limbs causes affected individuals to be short in height. There is often premature loss of dentition due to resorption of dentine with replacement of the pulp by osteoid.

The radiographic features closely resemble those of Paget's disease but are diagnostic as they involve the whole skeleton and affect children from the age of 2 years. In contrast, Paget's disease is rare before the age of 40 years and skeletal involvement is either monostotic or asymmetrically polyostotic. On radionuclide scanning there is generalized increase in uptake giving a 'super scan' due to excessive osteoblastic activity with absence of evidence of renal uptake.

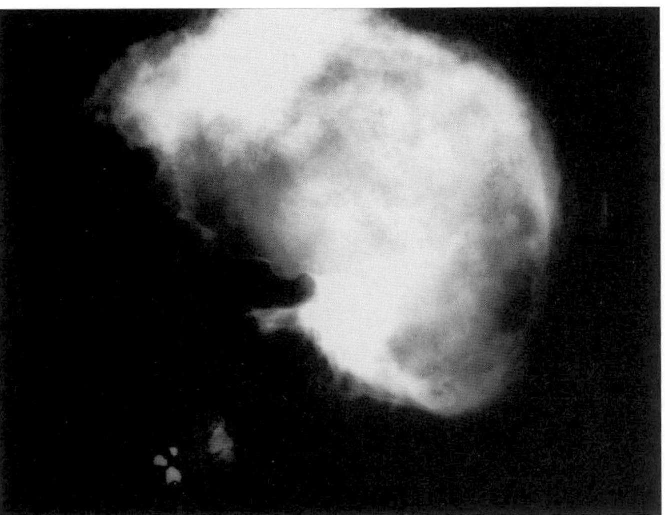

Figure 49.17 Hyperphosphatasia (juvenile Paget's disease). There is increased bone turnover resulting in immature woven bone being formed instead of mature lamellar bone. Bones are under-tubulated with a disorganized trabecular pattern, resembling the radiographic features of Paget's disease. In the lateral skull radiograph there is sclerosis, thickening of the skull vault and evidence of bone softening with basilar invagination. Platyspondyly may also be present.

MISCELLANEOUS

VITAMIN D INTOXICATION

In the past, vitamin D was advocated in the treatment of a variety of conditions including sarcoidosis, tuberculosis (especially lupus vulgaris), rheumatoid arthritis, hayfever, chilblains and asthma. The treatment had no beneficial effect in these conditions and its use was eventually abandoned. However, this was not before cases of vitamin D intoxication had been described. Vitamin D intoxication has become less common with the introduction of $1,25(OH)_2D$ and other active metabolites. However, the more recent use of vitamin D to treat cancer, psoriasis and immunological disease may result in a resurgence of interest in vitamin D intoxication. The clinical symptoms include fatigue, malaise, weakness, thirst and polyuria, anorexia, nausea and vomiting due to hypercalcaemia. The latter results in hypercalciuria, nephrocalcinosis, impaired renal function and hypertension. Radiographically, metastatic calcification may be present in tendons, ligaments, fascial planes and arteries, and in the periosteum, resembling periostitis and causing bone sclerosis[161–163].

HYPERVITAMINOSIS A

Hypervitaminosis A can occur in those who are receiving vitamin A or one of its synthetic derivatives (retinoic acids) for treatment of skin disorders (refractory cystic acne, keratinizing dermatoses, psoriasis)[140,164,165]. The skeletal manifestations include large bone outgrowths from the spine, particularly in the cervical region. In the peripheral skeleton there is evidence of a mild enthesopathy. In affected children there can occur cupping and splaying of the metaphyses, diaphyseal periostitis, particularly in the metatarsals and ulnae, and widening of the cranial sutures.

FLUOROSIS

Fluorosis results from the long-term ingestion of excessive amounts of fluoride. In some parts of the world fluorosis is endemic. The radiological features that result include osteosclerosis, particularly in the axial skeleton, and an enthesopathy with ossification of ligaments and large spinal osteophytes[166]. The paraspinal ossification may cause compression myelopathy[167].

OTHER ENDOCRINE DISEASES

Cushing's disease is caused by a basophil pituitary adenoma; Cushing's syndrome is caused by a tumour of the adrenal glands (adenoma, carcinoma), ectopic ACTH production by a tumour (e.g. bronchial carcinoma), or iatrogenically by treatment with glucocorticoids[168]. The cardinal skeletal manifestation is osteoporosis which affects sites rich in trabecular bone (axial skeleton). Low-trauma fractures can occur, and these may heal with exuberant callus formation. Avascular necrosis of the hip may also occur.

Thyroid disease There may be over- or under-activity of the gland (thyrotoxicosis and myxoedema respectively). Thyroid disease in adults may be a cause of osteoporosis. Congenital or childhood onset of hypothyroidism (cretinism) results in retarded skeletal maturation, fragmented epiphyses, 'slipper-shaped' vertebrae and Wormian bones in the skull[169]. Thyroid acropachy is the triad of pre-tibial myxoedema, thyroid eye disease (exophthalmos) and clubbing of the fingers. Radiologically there may be diaphyseal periostitis, predominantly involving the tubular bones of the hand[170–172]. Patients may be thyrotoxic, euthyroid or hypothyroid.

Acromegaly is the result of an eosinophilic adenoma of the pituitary gland; if it occurs in children gigantism results. There is overgrowth of all tissues and organs. The hypertrophied cartilage may initially cause widening of the joints, seen best in the hand radiograph in the metacarpal phalangeal (MCP) joints. However the hypertrophied cartilage is poor in tensile strength and liable to fissures. This results in premature osteoarthritis (acromegalic arthropathy)[173,174]. When the joints in the spine are involved, cord compression can occur. Acromegaly can also result in generalized osteoporosis.

REFERENCES

1. Adams J E 2005 Metabolic bone disease. In: von Schulthess G K, Zollikofer C L, Hodler J (eds) Musculoskeletal diseases: diagnostic imaging and interventional techniques. Springer-Verlag, Italia, pp 89–105
2. Mundy G R1999 Bone remodelling and its disorders, 2nd edn. Martin Dunitz, London, pp 1–82
3. Parfitt A M 1988 Bone remodelling: Relationship to the amount and structure of bone, and the pathogenesis and prevention of fracture. In: Riggs B L, Melton L J (eds) Osteoporosis—etiology, diagnosis and management. Raven Press, New York, pp 45–93
4. Mundy G R1999 Osteopetrosis. In: Bone remodelling and its disorders, 2nd edn. Martin Dunitz, London, pp 193–199
5. Adams P, Davies G T, Sweetnam P 1970 Osteoporosis and the effects of ageing on bone mass in elderly men and women. Q J Med 39: 601–615
6. Greulich W W, Pyle S I 1959 Radiographic atlas of skeletal development of the hand and wrist, 2nd edn. Stanford University Press, Stanford, California
7. Tanner J M, Whitehouse R H, Cameron N et al 1983 Assessment of skeletal maturity and prediction of adult height (TW2 method), 2nd edn. Academic Press, London
8. King D G, Steventon D M, O'Sullivan M P et al 1994 Reproducibility of bone ages when performed by radiology registrars: an audit of Tanner and Whitehouse II versus Greulich and Pyle methods. Br J Radiol 67: 848–851
9. Gross G W, Boone J M, Bishop D M 1995 Pediatric skeletal age: Determination with neural networks. Radiology 195: 689–695
10. Cao F, Huang H K, Pietka E, Gilsanz V 2000 Digital hand atlas and web-based bone age assessment: system design and implementation. Comput Med Imaging Graph 24: 297–307

11. Nelson D A, Kleerekoper M, Parfitt A M 1988 Bone mass, skin color and body size among black and white women. Bone Miner 4: 257–264
12. Jouanny P, Guillemin F, Kuntz C et al 1995 Environmental and genetic factors affecting bone mass. Similarity of bone density among members of healthy families. Arthritis Rheum 38: 61–67
13. Ralston S H 1997 The genetics of osteoporosis. Q J Med 90: 247–251
14. Krall E A, Dawson-Hughes B 1993 Heritable and life-style determinants of bone mineral density. J Bone Miner Res 8: 1–9
15. Sambrook P N 2005 How to prevent steroid induced osteoporosis. Ann Rheum Dis 64: 2176–2178
16. Melton L J, Riggs B L 1988 Clinical spectrum. In: Riggs B L, Melton L J (eds) Osteoporosis: Etiology, diagnosis and management. Raven Press, New York, pp 155–179
17. Newton-John H F, Morgan D B 1970 The loss of bone with age, osteoporosis and fractures. Clin Orthoped 71: 229–252
18. Mazess R B 1982 On ageing bone loss. Clin Orthoped 165: 239–252
19. Whitehouse R W 2002 Paget's disease of bone. Semin Musculoskelet Radiol 6: 313–322
20. van Staa T P, Dennison E M, Leufkens H G, Cooper C 2001 Epidemiology of fractures in England and Wales. Bone 29: 517–522
21. Consensus Development Conference: Prophylaxis and treatment of osteoporosis 1993 Am J Med 94: 646–650
22. WHO Study Group on assessment of fracture risk and its application to screening for postmenopausal osteoporosis 1994 Technical report 843. World Health Organization, Geneva, Switzerland, pp 5
23. A practical guide to bone densitometry in children 2004 National Osteoporosis Society, Camerton, Bath, BA2 0PJ, UK. www.nos.org.uk; email: info@nos.org.uk
24. Marcus R, Feldman D, Kelsey J (eds) 1996 Osteoporosis. Academic Press, San Diego, California
25. Mayo-Smith W, Rosenthal D I 1991 Radiographic appearances of osteopenia. Radiol Clin North Am 29: 37–47
26. Pitt M 1983 Osteopenic bone disease. Orthop Clin North Am 14: 65–80
27. Quek S T, Peh W C 2002 Radiology of osteoporosis. Semin Musculoskelet Radiol 6: 3197–3206
28. Grimley-Evans J 1990 The significance of osteoporosis. In: Smith R (ed) Osteoporosis. Royal College of Physicians, London, pp 1–8
29. Resnick D, Niwayama G 1995 Osteoporosis. In: Resnick D (ed) Diagnosis of bone and joint disorders, 3rd edn. W B Saunders, Philadelphia, pp 1783–1853
30. Jiang G, Eastell R, Barrington N A, Ferrar L 2004 Comparison of methods for the visualisation of prevalent vertebral fracture in osteoporosis. Osteoporos Int 15: 11887–11896
31. Ferrar L, Jiang G, Adams J, Eastell R 2005 Identification of vertebral fractures: an update. Osteoporos Int 16: 717–728
32. Genant H K, Wu C Y, van Kuijk C, Nevitt M C 1993 Vertebral fracture assessment using a semi-quantitative technique. J Bone Miner Res 8: 1137–1148
33. Gehlbach S H, Bigelow C, Heimisdottir M et al 2000 Recognition of vertebral fracture in a clinical setting. Osteoporos Int 11: 577–582
34. Delmas PD, van de Langerijt L, Watts N et al 2005 Underdiagnosis of vertebral fractures is a worldwide problem: the IMPACT study. J Bone Miner Res 20: 557–563
35. Peh W C, Gilula L A 2003 Percutaneous vertebroplasty: indications, contraindications, and technique. Br J Radiol 76: 69–75
36. Dixon R G, Mathis J M 2004 Vertebroplasty and kyphoplasty: rapid pain relief for vertebral compression fractures. Curr Osteoporos Rep 2: 369–375
37. Wong W H, Olan W J, Belkoff S M 2002 Balloon kyphoplasty. In: Mathis J M, Deramond H, Belkoff S M (eds) Percutaneous vertebroplasty. Springer-Verlag, New York, pp 109–124
38. McGraw J K, Lippert J A, Minkus K D et al 2002 Prospective evaluation of pain relief in 100 patients undergoing percutaneous vertebroplasty: results and follow-up. J Vasc Interv Radiol 13: 883–886
39. Deramond H, Mathis J M 2002 Vertebroplasty in osteoporosis. Semin Musculoskelet Radiol 6: 263–268
40. Gangi A, Guth S, Imbert J P et al 2003 Percutaneous vertebroplasty: indications, technique and results. Radiographics 23: e10
41. Buckland Wright J C, Bradshaw C R 1989 Clinical applications of high definition microfocal radiography. Br J Radiol 62: 209–217
42. Mall J C, Genant H K, Rossman K 1973 Improved optical magnification for fine-detail radiography. Radiology 108: 707–708
43. Garn S M, Poznanski A K, Nagy J M 1971 Bone measurement in the differential diagnosis of osteopenia and osteoporosis. Radiology 100: 509–518
44. Singh M, Nagrath A R, Maini P S 1970 Changes in trabecular pattern of the upper end of the femur as an index of osteoporosis. J Bone Joint Surg (Am) 52: 457–467
45. Peh W 1996 Imaging of pelvic insufficiency fracture. Radiographics 16: 335–348
46. De Smet A A, Neff J R 1985 Pubic and sacral insufficiency fractures: clinical course and radiologic findings. Am J Roentgenol 145: 601–606
47. Cooper K L, Beabout J W, McCleod R A 1985 Supra-acetabular insufficiency fractures. Radiology 157: 15–17
48. Manco L G, Schneider R, Pavlov H 1983 Insufficiency fractures of the tibial plateau. Am J Roentgenol 140: 1211–1215
49. Hain S F, Fogelman I 2002 Nuclear medicine studies in metabolic bone disease. Semin Musculoskelet Radiol 6: 323–329
50. Baur A, Stabler A, Bruning R et al 1998 Diffusion-weighted MR imaging of bone marrow: differentiation of benign versus pathologic compression fractures. Radiology 207: 349–356
51. Haramati N, Staron R B, Barax C, Feldman F 1994 Magnetic resonance imaging of occult fractures of the proximal femur. Skelet Radiol 23: 19–22
52. Schartzman R J, McLellan T L 1987 Reflex sympathetic dystrophy. A review. Arch Neurol 44: 555–561
53. Ameratunga R, Daly M, Caughey D E 1989 Metastatic malignancy associated with reflex sympathetic dystrophy. J Rheumatol 16: 406–407
54. Jones G 1969 Radiological appearance of disuse osteoporosis. Clin Radiol 20: 345–353
55. Kozin F 1986 Reflex sympathetic dystrophy syndrome. Bull Rheum Dis 36: 1–8
56. Wilder R T, Berde C B, Wolohan M et al 1992 Reflex sympathetic dystrophy in children. Clinical characteristics and follow-up of seventy patients. J Bone Joint Surg (Am) 69: 910–919
57. Doherty M, Watt I, Dieppe P 1980 Apparent bone erosions in painful regional osteoporosis. Rheumatol Rehabil 1: 95–96
58. Keats T E, Harrison R B 1978 A pattern of post-traumatic demineralization of bone simulating permeative neoplastic replacement: potential source of misinterpretation. Skelet Radiol 3: 113–114
59. Bloem J L 1988 Transient osteoporosis of the hip: MR imaging. Radiology 167: 753–755
60. Hayes C W, Conway W F, Daniel W W 1993 MR imaging of bone marrow edema pattern: transient osteoporosis, transient bone marrow edema syndrome, or osteonecrosis. Radiographics 13: 1001–1011
61. Dent C E, Friedman M 1965 Idiopathic juvenile osteoporosis. Q J Med 34: 177–210
62. Smith R 1980 Idiopathic osteoporosis in the young. J Bone Joint Surg Br 62: 417–427
63. Riggs B L, Melton L J 1986 Involutional osteoporosis. N Engl J Med 314: 1676–1686
64. van Staa T P, Leufkens H G, Cooper C 2002 The epidemiology of corticosteroid induced osteoporosis: a meta-analysis. Osteoporos Int 13: 777–787
65. Lukert B 1996 Glucocorticoid-induced osteoporosis. In: Marcus R, Feldman D, Kelsey J (eds) Osteoporosis. Academic Press, San Diego, California, pp 801–820
66. Manolagas S C, Weinstein R S 1999 New developments in the pathogenesis and treatment of steroid-induced osteoporosis. J Bone Miner Res 14: 1061–1066
67. Sillence D 1981 Osteogenesis imperfecta: an expanding panorama of variants. Clin Orthop Rel Res 59: 11–25
68. Rauch F, Glorieux F H 2004 Osteogenesis imperfecta. Lancet 363: 1377–1385
69. Tsipouras P 1993 Osteogenesis imperfecta. In: McKusick's Heritable disorders of connective tissue, 5th edn. Mosby, New York, pp 281–314

70. Cremin B, Goodman H, Prax M et al 1982 Wormian bones in osteogenesis imperfecta and other disorders. Skelet Radiol 8: 35–38
71. Beighton P, dePaepe A, Danks D, Finidori G et al 1986 International nosology of heritable disorders of connective tissue, Berlin 1986. Am J Med Gen 29: 581–594
72. Gahagan S, Rimsza M E 1991 Child abuse or osteogenesis imperfecta: how can we tell? Pediatrics 88: 987–992
73. Goldman A B, Davidson D, Pavlov H, Bullough P G 1980 Popcorn calcification: a prognostic sign in osteogenesis imperfecta. Radiology 136: 351–358
74. Barnett E, Nordin B E C 1960 The radiological diagnosis of osteoporosis: a new approach. Clin Radiol 11: 166–174
75. Horsman A, Simpson M 1975 The measurement of sequential changes in cortical bone geometry. Br J Radiol 48: 471–476
76. Smyth P P, Adams J E, Whitehouse R W, Taylor C J 1997 Application of computer texture analysis to the Singh Index. Br J Radiol 70: 242–247
77. Genant H K, Jergas M, van Kuijk C (eds) 1995 Vertebral fracture in osteoporosis. Osteoporosis Research Group, University of San Francisco, San Francisco, California
78. McCloskey E, Spector T, Eyres K et al 1993 The assessment of vertebral deformity: a method for use in population studies and clinical trials. Osteoporos Int 3: 138–147
79. Eastell R, Cedel S, Wahner H et al 1991 Classification of vertebral fractures. J Bone Miner Res 6: 207–215
80. Rea J A, Steiger P, Blake G M, Fogelman I 1998 Optimizing data acquisition and analysis of morphometric X-ray absorptiometry. Osteoporos Int 8: 177–183
81. Jiang G, Eastell R, Barrington N A, Ferrar L 2004 Comparison of methods for the visualisation of prevalent vertebral fracture in osteoporosis. Osteoporos Int 15: 887–896
82. Smyth P P, Taylor C J, Adams J E 1999 Vertebral shape: automatic measurement with active shape models. Radiology 211: 571–578
83. Eastell R 1998 Treatment of postmenopausal osteoporosis. N Engl J Med 338: 736–746
84. Faulkner K, Gluer C C, Majumdar S et al 1991 Noninvasive measurements of bone mass, structure, and strength: current methods and experimental techniques. Am J Roentgenol 157: 1229–1237
85. Kanis J A, Gluer C-C 2000 An update on the diagnosis and assessment of osteoporosis with densitometry. Osteoporosis Int 11: 192–202
86. Gluer CC 1999 Monitoring skeletal changes by radiological techniques. J Bone Miner Res 14: 1952–1962
87. Adams J E 1998 Single- and dual-energy: X-ray absorptiometry. In: Genant H K, Guglielmi G, Jergas M (eds) Bone densitometry and osteoporosis. Springer-Verlag, Berlin, pp 305–334
88. Blake G M, Wahner H W, Fogelman I 1999 The evaluation of osteoporosis: dual energy X-ray absorptiometry and ultrasound in clinical practice, 2nd edn. Marin Dunitz, London
89. Rea J A, Li J, Blake G M et al 2000 Visual assessment of vertebral deformity by X-ray absorptiometry: a highly predictive method to exclude vertebral deformity Osteoporos Int 11: 660–668
90. Adams J E 1989 Quantitative computed tomography. In: Galasko C B S, Isherwood I (eds) Imaging in orthopaedics. Springer-Verlag, London, pp 259–268
91. Mughal M, Ward K, Adams J 2004 Assessment of bone status in children by densitometric and quantitative ultrasound techniques. In: Carty H (ed) Imaging in children. Elsevier Science, Edinburgh, pp 477–486
92. Guglielmi G, Lang T F 2002 Quantitative computed tomography. Semin Musculoskelet Radiol 6: 219–227
93. Cann C 1981 Low dose CT scanning for quantitative spinal mineral analysis. Radiology 140: 813–815
94. Schneider P, Reiners C 1998 Peripheral quantitative computed tomography. In: Genant H K, Guglielmi G, Jergas M (eds) Bone densitometry and osteoporosis. Springer-Verlag, Berlin, pp 349–363
95. Kalender W A 1992 Effective dose values in bone mineral measurements by photon absorptiometry and computed tomography. Osteoporos Int 2: 82–87
96. Blake G M, Fogelman I 1997 Interpretation of bone densitometry studies. Semin Nucl Med 27: 248–260
97. Parfitt A M 1990 Interpretation of bone densitometry measurements: disadvantages of a percentage scale and a discussion of some alternatives. J Bone Miner Res 5: 537–540
98. Osteoporosis: clinical guidelines for prevention and treatment 1999 Royal College of Physicians, London
99. Njeh C F, Hans D, Fuerst T, Gluer C C, Genant H K (eds) 1999 Quantitative ultrasound: Assessment of osteoporosis and bone status. Martin Dunitz, London
100. Link T M, Bauer J S 2002 Imaging of trabecular bone structure. Semin Musculoskelet Radiol 6: 253–261
101. Hayes C W, Conway W F 1991 Hyperparathyroidism. Radiol Clin North Am 29: 85–96
102. Wynne A G, Van Heerden J, Carney J A, Fitzpatrick L A 1992 Parathyroid carcinoma: clinical and pathological features in 43 patients. Medicine 71: 197–205
103. Kaplan E L, Yoshiro Y, Salti G 1992 Primary hyperparathyroidism in the 1990s. Ann Surg 215: 300–315
104. NIH Conference: Diagnosis and management of asymptomatic primary hyperparathyroidism: Consensus Development Conference Statement 1990. Ann Intern Med 114: 593–597
105. Davies M 1992 Primary hyperparathyroidism: aggressive or conservative treatment? Clin Endocrinol 36: 325–332
106. Davies M, Fraser W D, Hosking D J 2002 The management of primary hyperparathyroidism. Clin Endocrinol 57: 145–155
107. Genant H K, Heck L L, Lanzl L H et al 1973 Primary hyperparathyroidism: A comprehensive study of clinical, biochemical, and radiographic manifestations. Radiology 109: 513–524
108. Dodds W J, Steinbach H L 1968 Hyperparathyroidism and articular cartilage calcification. Am J Roentgenol 104: 884–892
109. Genant H K, Baron J M, Strauss F H et al 1975 Osteosclerosis in primary hyperparathyroidism. Am J Med 59: 104–113
110. Sundaram M 1989 Renal osteodystrophy. Skelet Radiol 18: 415–426
111. Wishart J, Horowitz M, Need A, Nordin B E 1990 Relationship between forearm and vertebral mineral density in postmenopausal women with primary hyperparathyroidism. Arch Intern Med 150: 1329–1331
112. Silverberg S J, Gartenberg F, Jacobs T P et al 1995 Increased bone density after parathyroidectomy in primary hyperparathyroidism. J Clin Endocrinol Metab 80: 729–734
113. Parfitt A M 1969 Soft tissue calcification in uraemia. Arch Intern Med 124: 544–556
114. Dimich A, Bedrossian P B, Wallach S 1967 Hypoparathyroidism. Arch Intern Med 120: 449–458
115. Steinbach H, Waldron B R 1952 Idiopathic hypoparathyroidism: analysis of 52 cases, including report of new case. Medicine 31: 133–154
116. Salvesen H A, Boe J 1953 Idiopathic hypoparathyroidism. Acta Endocrinol 14: 214–226
117. Adams J E, Davies M 1977 Paravertebral and ligamentous ossification, an unusual association of hypoparathyroidism. Postgrad Med J 53: 167–172
118. Albright F, Burnett C H, Smith P H et al 1942 Pseudohypoparathyroidism—An example of Seabright-Bantam syndrome. Report of 3 cases. Endocrinol 30: 922–932
119. Steinbach H L, Young D A 1966 The Roentgen appearances of pseudohypoparathyroidism (PH) and pseudo-pseudohypoparathyroidism (PPH). Differentiation from other syndromes associated with short metacarpals, metatarsals and phalangeals. Am J Roentgenol 97: 49–66
120. Posnanski A K, Werden E A, Giedion A et al 1977 The pattern of shortening of the bones of the hands in PHP and PPHP—a comparison with brachydactyly E, Turner's syndrome, and acrodysostosis. Radiology 123: 707–718
121. Wilson L C, Hall C M 2002 Albright's osteodystrophy and pseudohypo parathyroidism. Semin Musculoskelet Radiol 6: 273–284
122. Kolb F O, Steinbach H L 1962 Pseudohypoparathyroidism with secondary hyperparathyroidism and osteitis fibrosa. J Clin Endocrinol 22: 59–70

123. Adams J E 2005 Radiology of rickets and osteomalacia. In: Feldman D, Glorieux F H, Pike J W (eds) Vitamin D, 2nd edn, vol 2. Elsevier, San Diego, pp 967–994

124. Pitt M J 1981 Rachitic and osteomalacic syndromes. Radiol Clin North Am 19: 582–598

125. Glorieux F H, St-Arnaud R 1997 Vitamin D pseudodeficiency. In: Feldman D, Glorieux F H, Pike J W (eds) Vitamin D. Academic Press, San Diego, pp 755–764

126. Brooks M H, Bell N H, Love L et al 1978 Vitamin D dependent rickets Type II, resistance of target organs to 1,25-dihydroxyvitamin D. N Engl J Med 293: 996–999

127. Pitt M J 1993 Rickets and osteomalacia are still around. Radiol Clin North Am 29: 97–118

128. Brill P W, Winchester P, Kleinman P K 1998 Differential diagnosis 1: diseases simulating abuse. In: Kleinman P K (ed) Diagnostic imaging of child abuse, 2nd edn. Mosby, St. Louis, pp 178–196

129. Harris H A 1933 Rickets. In: Bone growth in health and disease. Oxford Medical Publications, Oxford University Press, London, p 87

130. Taybi H, Lachman R 1996 Radiology of syndromes, metabolic disorders and skeletal dysplasias, 4th edn. Mosby Year Book, St. Louis

131. Looser E 1920 Uber spatrachitis und osteomalacie Klinishe ront-genologische und pathologischanatomische Untersuchungen. Drsch Z Chir 152: 210–357

132. Milkman LA 1930 Pseudofractures (hunger osteopathy, late rickets, osteomalacia). Am J Roentgenol 24: 29–37

133. DeSmet A A, Neff J R 1985 Pubic and sacral insufficiency fractures: clinical course and radiological findings. Am J Roentgenol 145: 601–606

134. McKenna M J, Kleerekoper M, Ellis B I et al 1987 Atypical insufficiency fractures confused with Looser zones of osteomalacia. Bone 8: 71–78

135. Milgram J W1977 Radiographical and pathological assessment of the activity of Paget's disease of bone. Clin Orthop 127: 63–69

136. Whitehouse R W 2002 Paget's disease of bone. Semin Musculoskelet Radiol 6: 313–322

137. Resnick D L 1982 Fish vertebrae. Arthritis Rheum 25: 1073–1077

138. Adams J E 2002 Dialysis bone disease. Semin Dial 15: 277–289

139. Gipstein R M, Coburn J W, Adams J A et al 1976 Calciphylaxis in man: A syndrome of tissue necrosis and vascular calcification in 11 patients with chronic renal failure. Arch Intern Med 136: 1273–1280

140. Lawson J 2002 Drug-induced metabolic bone disorders. Semin Musculoskelet Radiol 6: 285–297

141. Ryan E A, Reiss E 1984 Oncogenous osteomalacia: Review of the world literature of 42 cases. Am J Med 77: 501–512

142. Weisman Y, Hochberg Z 1994 Genetic rickets and osteomalacia. Curr Ther Endocrinol Metab 5: 492–495

143. Steendijk R, Hauspie R C 1992 The pattern of growth and growth retardation of patients with hypophosphataemic vitamin D-resistant rickets: longitudinal study. Eur J Pediatr 151: 422–427

144. Glorieux F H, Marie P J, Pettifor J M, Delvin E E 1980 Bone response to phosphate salts, ergocalciferol and calcitriol in hypophosphatemic vitamin D-resistant rickets. N Engl J Med 303: 1023–1031

145. Milgram J W, Compere C L 1981 Hypophosphatemic vitamin D refractory osteomalacia with bilateral pseudofractures. Clin Orthop 160: 78–85

146. O'Malley S P, Adams J E, Davies M, Ramsden R T 1988 The petrous temporal bone and deafness in X-linked hypophosphataemic osteomalacia. Clin Radiol 39: 528–530

147. Polisson R P, Martinez S, Khoury M et al 1985 Calcification of entheses associated with X-linked hypophosphatemic osteomalacia. N Engl J Med 313: 1–6

148. Adams J E, Davies M 1986 Intra-spinal new bone formation and spinal cord compression in familial hypophosphataemic vitamin D resistant osteomalacia. Q J Med 61: 1117–1129

149. Hardy D C, Murphy W A, Siegal B A et al 1989 X-linked hypophosphatemia in adults: prevalence of skeletal radiographic and scintigraphic features. Radiology 171: 403–414

150. Econs M J, Samsa G P, Monger M et al 1994 X -linked hypophosphatemic rickets: a disease often unknown to affected patients. Bone Miner 24: 17–24

151. McCance R A 1947 Osteomalacia with Looser's nodes (Milkman's syndrome) due to raised resistance to vitamin D acquired about the age of 15 years. Q J Med 16: 33–47

152. Edmister K A, Sundaram M 2002 Oncogenic osteomalacia. Semin Musculoskelet Radiol 6: 191–196

153. Linovitz R J, Resnick D, Keissling P et al 1976 Tumor-induced osteomalacia: a surgically curable syndrome, report of two cases. J Bone Joint Surg Am 58: 419–423

154. Rathbun J C, MacDonald J W, Robinson H M C, Wanklin J M 1961 Hypophosphatasia: a genetic study. Arch Dis Child 36: 540–542

155. Weinstein R S, Whyte M P 1981 Heterogeneity of adult hypophosphatasia: report of severe and mild cases. Arch Intern Med 141: 727–731

156. Anderton J M 1979 Orthopedic problems in adult hypophosphatasia: a report of two cases. J Bone Joint Surg Br 61: 82–84

157. Chuck A J, Pattrick M G, Hamilton E et al 1989 Crystal deposition in hypophosphatasia: a reappraisal. Ann Rheum Dis 48: 571–576

158. Greenspan A 1991 Sclerosing bone dysplasias. Skelet Radiol 20: 561–583

159. Stoker D J 2002 Osteopetrosis. Semin Musculoskelet Radiol 6: 299–305

160. Cundy T 2002 Idiopathic hyperphosphatasia. Semin Musculoskelet Radiol 6: 307–312

161. Holman C B 1952 Roentgenologic manifestations of vitamin D intoxication. Radiology 59: 805–815

162. DeWind L T 1961 Hypervitaminosis D with osteosclerosis. Arch Dis Child 36: 373–380

163. Davies M, Adams P H 1978 The continuing risk of vitamin D intoxification. Lancet ii: 621–623

164. Binkley N, Krueger D 2000 Hypervitaminosis A and bone. Nutr Rev 58: 138–144

165. Pierrotta S, Nobili B, Rossi F et al 2003 Vitamin A and infancy: biochemical, functional and clinical aspects. Vitam Horm 66: 457–591

166. Singh A, Jolly S S 1961 Endemic fluorosis. Q J Med 30: 357–372

167. Muthukumar N 2005 Ossification of the ligamentum flavum as a result of fluorosis causing myelopathy: report of two cases. Neurosurgery 56: E622; discussion E622

168. Sambrook P N 2005 How to prevent steroid induced osteoporosis. Ann Rheum Dis 64: 176–178

169. Mann D C 1996 Endocrine disorders and orthopedic problems in children. Curr Opin Pediatr 8: 68–70

170. Torres-Reyes E, Staple T W 1970 Roentgenographic appearance of thyroid acropachy. Clin Radiol 21: 95–100

171. Winkler A, Wilson D 1985 Thyroid acropachy. Case report and literature review. Mo Med 82: 756–761

172. Weetman A P 1993 Extrathyroidal complications of Graves disease. Q J Med 86: 473–477

173. Bluestone R, Bywaters E G, Hartog M et al 1971 Acromegalic arthropathy. Ann Rheum Dis 30: 243–258

174. Colao A, Pivonello R, Scarpa R et al 2005 The acromegalic arthropathy. J Endocrinol Invest 28(8 suppl): 24–31

175. Heaney R P, Abrams S, Dawson-Hughes B et al 2000 Peak bone mass. Osteoporos Int 11 (12): 985–1009

CHAPTER 50

Joint Disease

Philip P. W. Bearcroft

- Osteoarthritis and related conditions
- Inflammatory arthritis
- Crystal deposition and related arthropathies
- Polyarthritis associated with other diseases
- Synovial metaplasia and neoplasia
- Arthrography
- Differential diagnosis of joint disease based on the radiological features
- Joint diseases at specific sites

OSTEOARTHRITIS AND RELATED CONDITIONS

Osteoarthritis

Osteoarthritis (OA, osteoarthrosis) is the most common disorder that affects joints, affecting the majority of elderly patients. It is a dynamic phenomenon that reflects a balance between joint tissue destruction and repair. The clinical and radiological features in any affected joint are determined by the relative vigour of these opposing processes. It can involve the peripheral joints as well as the central skeleton, and the joints most at risk are the thumb base (carpometacarpal joint), distal interphalangeal (IP) joints, acromioclavicular joints, knees, hips, first metatarsophalangeal (MTP) joints and spinal apophyseal joints.

There is no universally accepted definition of OA, and our understanding of this common process is evolving. It is understood that alterations to the collagen and protein polysaccharide structure of cartilage lead to changes in the water content and ionic distribution and the resulting reduced turgor leads to joint space narrowing.

Osteoarthritis can be considered as primary or secondary: if no underlying cause is identified then it is designated primary. Secondary OA develops in joints damaged by previous disease (Table 50.1)

Radiological pathological correlation

Plain radiographs are the most useful technique to understand the radiological features of OA. OA is initiated within cartilage and bone at points of focal stress. This results in degeneration or fibrillation of the cartilage exposing the subarticular bone plate, with fragmentation of the subchondral trabeculae. This is accompanied by hypertrophic new bone production, osteophyte formation and bone remodelling (Table 50.2). The different radiological features produced in the stressed (destructive changes) and non-stressed (productive changes)

Table 50.1 CLASSIFICATION OF OSTEOARTHRITIS
Primary (idiopathic)
Peripheral joints
Spine
Apophyseal joints
Intervertebral joints
Secondary
Trauma
Acute
Chronic (occupational, sport)
Systemic, metabolic or endocrine disorders
Rheumatoid arthritis
Alkaptonuria (ochronosis)
Wilson's disease
Haemochromatosis
Kashin–Beck disease
Acromegaly
Hyperparathyroidism
Crystal disposition disease
Calcium pyrophosphate dihydrate (CPPD)
Basic calcium phosphate (hydroxyapatite)
Monosodium urate monohydrate (gout)
Neuropathic disorders
Tabes dorsalis
Diabetes mellitus
Hereditary (Type 2 collagen gene mutations)
Stickler's disease
Miscellaneous
Bone dysplasia

Table 50.2 PLAIN RADIOGRAPHIC FINDINGS IN PRIMARY OSTEOARTHRITIS AND CORRESPONDING UNDERLYING PATHOPHYSIOLOGICAL CAUSES

Radiological findings	Pathological cause
Localized joint space narrowing	Articular cartilage fibrillation, ulceration and erosion lead to changes in collagen and protein polysaccharide structure of cartilage. This results in reduced turgor
Subchondral bony sclerosis	Increased osteoblastic activity resulting in new bone formation and increased cellularity of the subchondral bone
Osteophyte formation (most commonly marginal)	Cartilage and bone proliferation and revascularization of remaining cartilage
Bone cysts and bone collapse	Subchondral micro-fractures and passage of synovial fluid under pressure through the damaged cartilage to excavate a subchondral cyst
Gross deformity with subluxation	Ligamentous laxity resulting from mechanical forces applied after the distortion of capsular structures
Loose bodies	Fragments of bone and cartilage become separated and, if not resorbed, become loose in the joint. They may reattach to the membrane, become vascularized and undergo endochondral ossification
Fibrocartilage or hyaline cartilage calcification	This is usually due to calcium pyrophosphate deposition disease (CPPD). The reparative response is usually quite florid

segments result in the characteristic bone changes which give OA its distinctive radiological findings (Fig. 50.1).

In hypertrophic OA, the repair phenomena and osteophyte growth predominate. This is the commonest presentation, and these changes help to distinguish OA from inflammatory 'atrophic' arthritis, such as rheumatoid and other inflammatory arthritides. In some cases, however, particularly in the elderly, there is little or no attempt at repair and the radiological changes resemble those of an erosive arthritis; the clinical and radiological deterioration of these individuals is often more rapid than usual.

In addition to these primary underlying processes, other issues that involve the joints can have an effect on both the radiological appearances and on the rate of progression of disease. These include: (1) recurrent synovial inflammation due to shedding of articular debris or the appearance of calcium-containing crystals in the joint; (2) ischaemic necrosis of the subchondral bone, particularly in the elderly; and (3) the development of the joint instability.

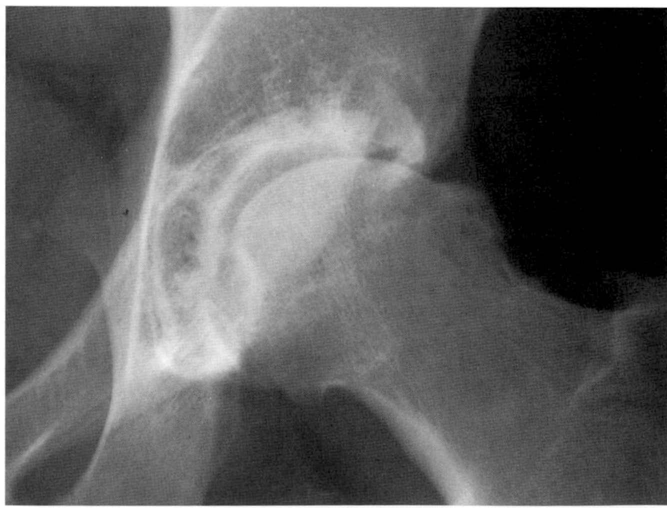

Figure 50.1 Osteoarthritis. There is an acetabular subchondral cyst, and subchondral sclerosis is maximal on the acetabular side of the joint in this individual. Marginal osteophytes are seen medially and laterally.

Aims of imaging

The noninvasive assessment of OA relies entirely on plain radiographs: other laboratory tests are not available. Imaging allows:

- Diagnosis of OA. Plain radiographs show the characteristic features of OA in the absence of evidence of inflammatory arthritis.
- Assessment of the structural severity.
- Identification of chondrocalcinosis.
- Identification of complications of OA (e.g. subchondral bone necrosis).
- Classification into primary or secondary (see Table 50.1).

Primary osteoarthritis

This form develops in the absence of any initiating factor. It occurs in the context of normal biomechanical forces which, due to some intrinsic abnormality within the cartilage, cause it to become degenerate. The condition is typically asymmetrical and it most commonly affects the hands, the spine and large weight-bearing joints.

Radiological appearances of primary and secondary osteoarthritis are similar. They are characterized by joint space narrowing, marginal osteophytes, subchondral cysts and subchondral sclerosis. Alterations of joint alignment such as subluxation are uncommon and bone mineralization is generally preserved, which helps to distinguish OA from other inflammatory causes of arthritis. Slow progression of the disease is the norm.

In the hand, the interphalangeal joints, the metacarpophalangeal (MCP) joint of the thumb and the scaphotriquetral joint are most commonly affected. Distal and proximal interphalangeal joint prominences are commonly encountered clinically and relate to underlying osteophytes. They are termed Heberden's and Bouchard's nodes respectively. When destructive changes outstrip the productive changes, the pattern can appear more 'erosive'. The resulting erosive osteoarthritis can be differentiated from psoriatic arthritis, which also affects the distal interphalangeal joints, by the presence of central erosions and osteophyte formation, in comparison to marginal erosions and no true osteophytes in psoriasis.

In the knee, joint space narrowing does not typically involve all three compartments (lateral and medial tibiofemoral and patellofemoral compartments) uniformly. The weight-bearing portion is subject to greater stress (usually the medial compartment) and shows the earliest and the greatest narrowing. Weight-bearing radiographs show this to advantage. Chondrocalcinosis is frequently associated with advanced disease and may involve articular hyaline cartilage or fibrocartilaginous menisci. When the patellofemoral joint is involved the lateral facet is most usually affected. Subarticular cysts and marginal osteophytes can become large. Chondromalacia patellae is a related condition occurring in younger patients, characterized by 'softening' of patellar cartilage. The condition is thought to be related to repetitive trauma and MRI can be useful to show the details of articular cartilage damage before bony changes are apparent on plain films (Fig. 50.2). Ossification of the medial collateral ligament (Pellegrini–Stieda disease) may be associated with degenerative change or may occur in isolation (Fig. 50.3).

In the foot and ankle, the most common site of involvement is the first metatarsophalangeal joint, often associated with hallux valgus. In the tarsus, the talonavicular joint is commonly involved, often with the formation of a bony spur dorsally. When this spur is florid, the possibility of an associated underlying congenital tarsal coalition should be considered. Called a 'talar beak', this is caused by overriding of the navicula on the talus.

The hip typically shows loss of joint space in the superior weight-bearing surface. This is followed by the typical marginal osteophyte formation and subarticular cyst formation and sclerosis (Fig. 50.1). Before these signs are seen, developing osteoarthritis may be suspected by the tendency of the femoral head to sublux laterally. This can be appreciated by comparing the width of the medial joint space to the opposite side. Medial migration may also occur, but this is uncommon unless there has been previous inflammatory disease.

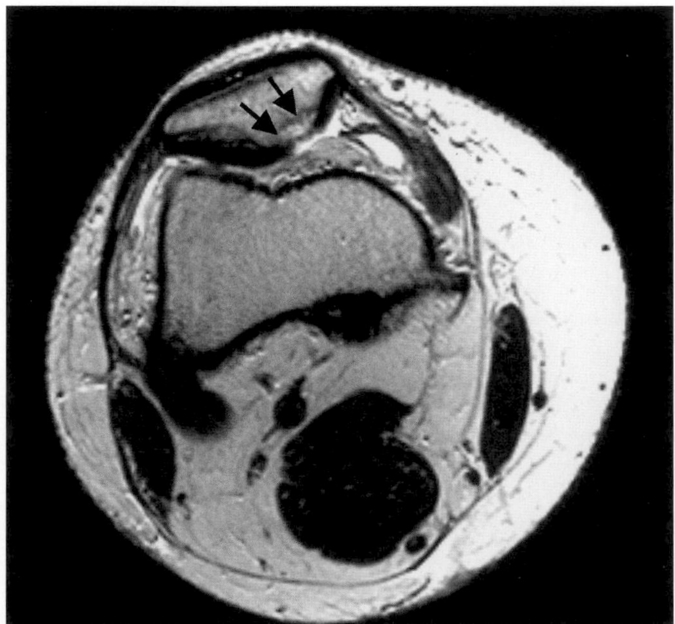

Figure 50.2 Chondromalacia patellae. FSE T2-weighted MR image demonstrates that the cartilage on the medial facet of the patella is denuded, with cystic change in the underlying bone (arrows). The appearances indicate advanced chondromalacia.

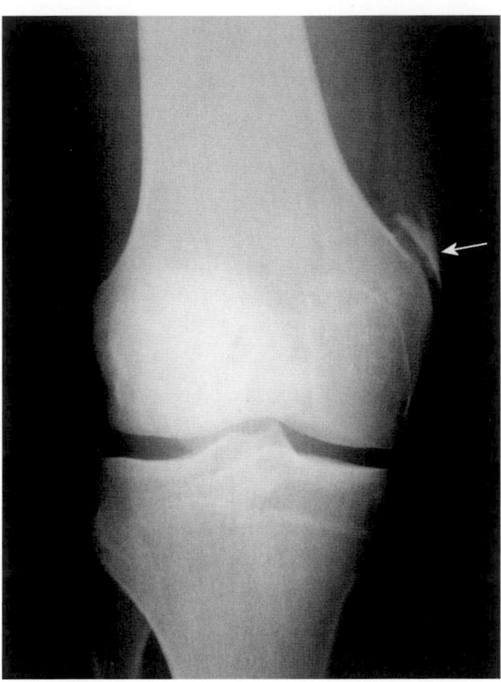

Figure 50.3 Pellegrini–Stieda lesion. Calcification/ossification is seen related to the superior portion of the medial femoral condyle (arrow).

Secondary osteoarthritis

This form most commonly results from previous inflammation or trauma, or secondary to abnormal biomechanical stresses (Table 50.1). The radiological pattern of osteoarthritis is identical to primary 'idiopathic' osteoarthritis and it is often not possible to identify the underlying cause.

Diffuse idiopathic skeletal hyperostosis

Diffuse idiopathic skeletal hyperostosis (DISH, hyperostotic spondylosis, Forestier's disease) is a common finding in elderly patients. It was originally described in 1950 by the French neurologist Jacques Forestier. It is a multifocal entity characterized by 'flowing' ligamentous ossification of the spine involving four or more contiguous vertebrae with preservation of underlying disc height (as opposed to degenerative disc disease), without apophyseal or sacroiliac joint fusion (as opposed to ankylosing spondylitis), and with hyperostosis of certain ligamentous attachments[1,2]. Ossification can also affect tendons and ligaments of the pelvis, as it may the superior third of the sacroiliac joints, the symphysis pubis, the calcaneus, tarsal bones, patella, olecranon, humerus or hands. It is considered to be a reaction to stress, and not an arthritis as such. Clinically, DISH may be asymptomatic or may present with variety of symptoms including back pain, stiffness, restricted movement, or symptoms of tendinosis, most commonly at the elbow or heel.

In the spine, the most commonly affected region is between T7 and T12, and at this level the process is typically right sided

(Fig. 50.4). It is thought that the pulsating aorta acts as an inhibitory factor that reduces the ossification on the left side of the vertebral bodies. In cases of a right-sided aorta and co-existent DISH the hyperostotic changes are reported to be more marked on the left-hand side. At the affected levels, the anterior longitudinal ligament is ossified and thickened from a few millimetres to 2 cm, and large pointed spurs develop that may fuse with corresponding spurs on adjacent levels. All segments of the spine may be involved. Cervical spine involvement may be accompanied by dysphagia due to anterior impingement on the oesophagus by the hypertrophic new bone, especially if only one segment remains mobile and exuberant osteophytes develop at that level as a consequence. Ossification of the posterior longitudinal ligament (PLL) may occur and may be extensive leading to spinal stenosis. Ossification of the PLL (OPLL) can occur as an isolated condition which is particularly prevalent in Japan. Retinoid intake is also associated with OPLL[3].

Extraspinal involvement with DISH occurs in the form of an enthesopathy. Heel and elbow spurs and a more whiskered appearance to the pelvis may all reflect this condition. The diagnosis, however, is made on the basis of the typical changes seen on radiographs of the spine.

Haemophilic arthropathy

Haemophilia is the general term for a group of disorders characterized by a deficiency of blood clotting factors. The two disorders most commonly associated with osseous and articular problems are classic haemophilia (haemophilia A, factor VIII deficiency) and Christmas disease (haemophilia B, factor IX deficiency). As X-linked recessive disorders, both are only expressed in males although both can be transmitted by female carriers. The blood dyscrasia leads to recurrent bleeding into joints, particularly the knee, elbow, ankle and shoulder. Small peripheral joints are only rarely involved. Involvement of the various joints is neither uniform nor symmetrical. Myositis ossificans is another recognized feature, especially in the pelvis and lower limb[4].

Early in the disease, joint effusion and oedema are the only findings and these are difficult to detect radiologically. Recurrent bleeds lead to increased radio-opacity of the periarticular soft tissues and synovium due to haemosiderin deposition. As a result of haemorrhage there is periarticular hyperaemia which leads to juxta-articular osteoporosis. If the condition affects the joint before closure of the epiphyseal plate, epiphyseal enlargement and overgrowth may also develop and accelerated maturation of the epiphysis is an expected finding if hyperaemia is

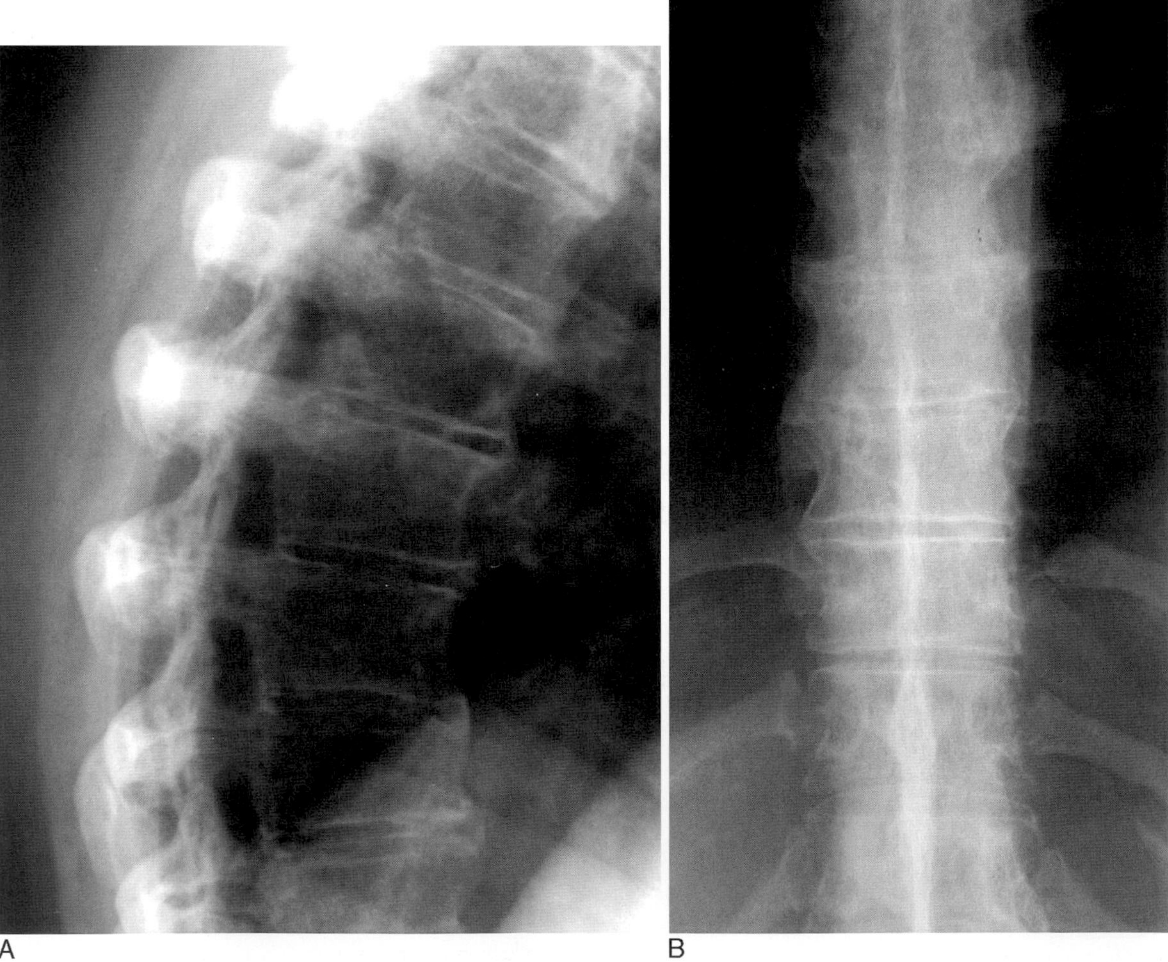

Figure 50.4 Diffuse idiopathic skeletal hyperostosis (DISH, Forestier's disease). (A) Lateral and (B) AP radiographs show bridging osteophytes at multiple levels, out of proportion to the degree of underlying degenerative change.

chronic. The thickened synovium can cause erosions on the articular surface, and cartilage destruction can lead to secondary OA. Subchondral cysts are common.

Intraosseous, subperiosteal and soft tissue pseudotumours may develop from the repeated bouts of haemorrhage, particularly in the femur and around the pelvis. An intraosseous pseudotumour is typically characterized by extensive bone destruction. MRI can be used to detect early synovial and cartilaginous changes that may not be evident on plain radiographs and to differentiate between acute and chronic bleeding in soft tissues[5]. The thickened irregular synovium with fibrosis and haemosiderin deposition shows low signal intensity foci on both T1- and T2-weighted spin-echo (SE) sequences with blooming on the gradient-echo (GE) sequences.

Ultrasound can also be useful in the assessment of soft tissue haematomas. Septic arthritis has been reported as a rare complication of haemophilia[6]. Arthropathy similar to that found in haemophilia has been described in the Klippel–Trenaunay and Kasabach–Merritt syndromes[7].

Neuropathic arthropathy (Charcot joint)

Neuropathic arthropathy refers to a destructive and productive articular abnormality occurring in association with a loss of pain sensation, proprioception, or both. The arthropathy occurs in a number of diseases that have neurological sequelae and the anatomical distribution depends on the underlying condition (Table 50.3). Intra-articular steroid injections may result in changes that resemble a neuropathic joint. Despite the underlying neuropathy, an involved joint may nevertheless be painful due to capsular distension and soft tissue trauma.

There are two forms of this arthropathy, atrophic and hypertrophic, although a combination may occur. Atrophic arthropathy is encountered early in the disease process, is more acute and is characterized by resorption of the ends of the affected bones resulting in sharp pointed ends. There is an absence of osteoporosis, sclerosis, fragmentation or soft tissue debris. The joint destruction often leads to dislocation.

The hypertrophic form begins with a joint effusion and progression is usually slow. The joint spaces are initially widened, then narrowed, and there is marked bony sclerosis. Osteoporosis is not seen with this condition. Pathological fractures and fragmentation of the articular surfaces result in bony debris, which may later fuse into a large dense well-organized corticated bony mass. This mass may fuse with the underlying bone, or bone fragments may break out of the periarticular space and dissect along muscle planes. Periosteal new bone formation may occur, and subluxation and dislocation proceed to destruction, and finally totally disorganization of the joint (Fig. 50.5). An important differential diagnosis is the pseudoneuropathic form of calcium pyrophosphate deposition disease (CPPD).

Table 50.3 CONDITIONS ASSOCIATED WITH NEUROPATHIC ARTHROPATHY

Condition	Prevalence of arthropathy	Joints most commonly affected
Congenital insensitivity to pain	100%	Ankle, tarsal, knee, hip
Syringomyelia	20–50%	Shoulder, elbow, wrist, cervical spine
Neurosyphilis	5–10%	Knee, hip
Diabetes mellitus	1%	Midfoot, forefoot
Alcohol related	Rare	Foot

Degenerative disease of the spine

Degenerative changes of the spine may affect (1) the nucleus pulposus leading to degenerative disc disease; (2) the annulus fibrosis leading to spondylosis deformans; (3) the apophyseal and costovertebral joints leading to osteoarthritis; or (4) in the cervical region, the uncovertebral joints of Luschka.

Degenerative disc disease is most common in the lower cervical and lower lumbar spine, although it can affect any segment. Classical features include disc space narrowing, small peripheral osteophytes, reactive subchondral sclerosis and internuclear gas (as a result of vacuum phenomenon). It is thought that degenerative disc disease results from biomechanical factors and is maximal at the junction between mobile and immobile segments (for example L5/S1).

Isolated spondylosis deformans is characterized by marginal osteophytes, but with preservation of the disc space. It is often, however, associated with degenerative disc disease (Fig. 50.6).

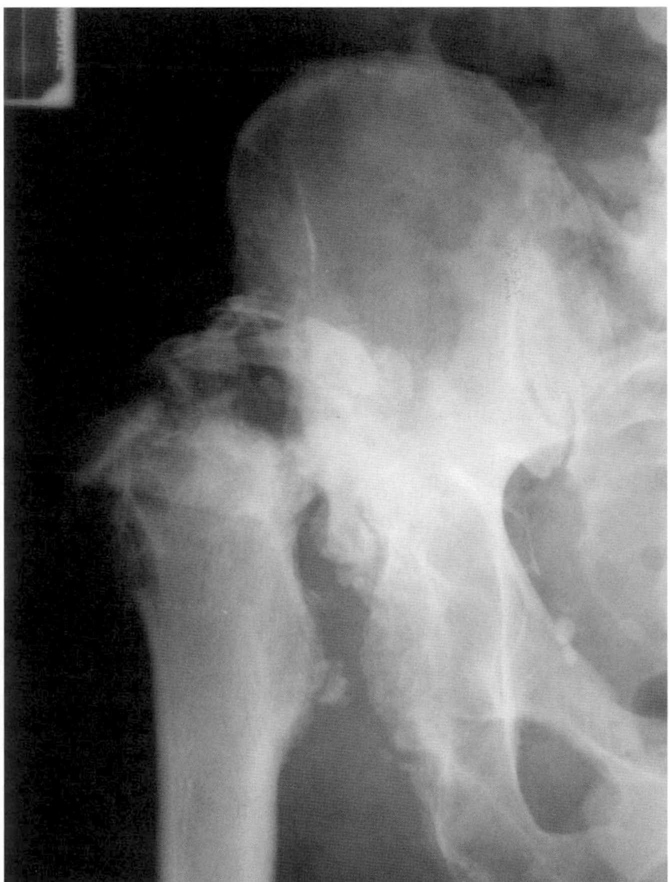

Figure 50.5 Neuropathic arthropathy of the right hip. There is destruction and fragmentation of the right femoral head leading to bony dislocation and disorganization of the joint. The underlying cause in this patient was syphilis.

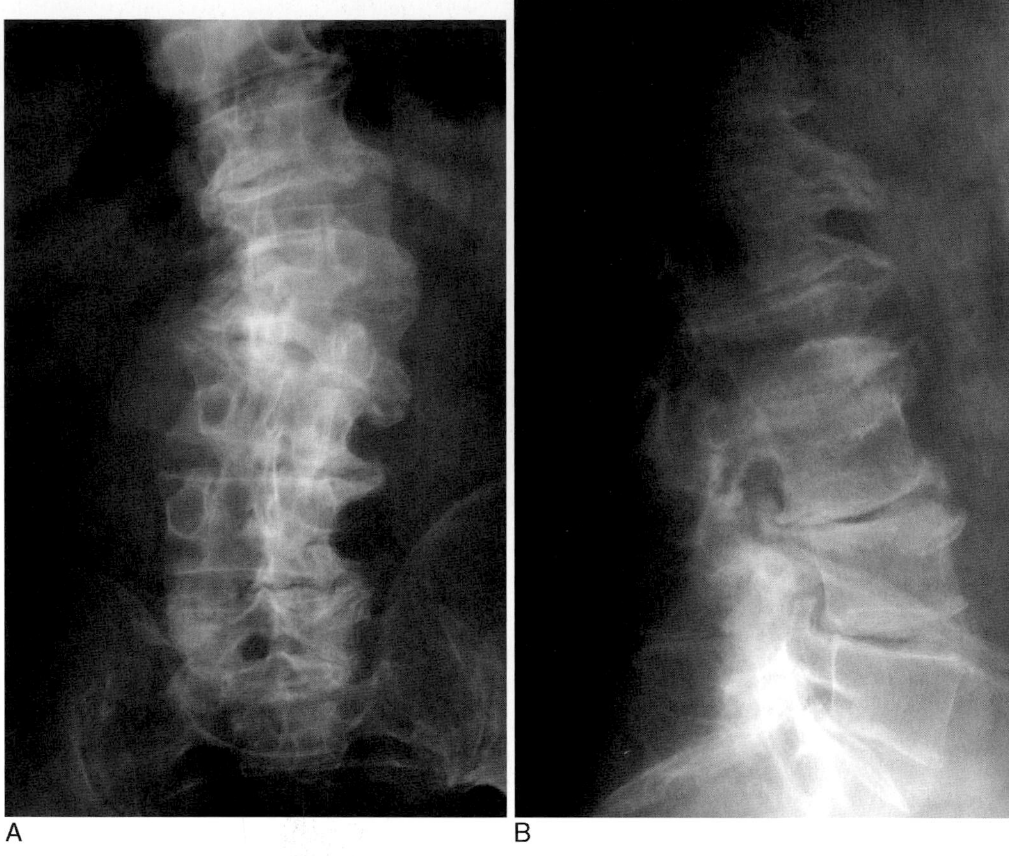

Figure 50.6 Spondylosis deformans. (A) AP and (B) lateral radiographs of the lumbar spine show degenerative change at multiple lumbar levels, with a scoliosis concave to the right, associated with pronounced marginal osteophyte formation.

Apophyseal joint osteoarthritis is characterized by joint space narrowing, sclerosis and hypertrophic bone formation of the apophyseal joints, which may contribute to neural encroachment and compression of the spinal nerve roots or spinal cord. In the cervical spine, uncovertebral joint degeneration leads to narrowing of the exiting foramina and compression of the nerve roots at that level (cervical spondylosis).

Spondylolisthesis refers to anterior displacement of a vertebral body with respect to the one below. True spondylolisthesis is associated with spondylolysis. Spondylolysis refers to a defect in the pars intraarticularis, best appreciated on oblique radiographs or CT, and commonly results in spondylolisthesis. It is most common at the L5 level and is seen in younger patients. Degenerative spondylolisthesis results from degenerative changes of the intervertebral disc facet joints, allowing loosening of the connecting ligaments. This form is more commonly seen in patients over 45 years old. A reverse spondylolisthesis or retrolisthesis due to degenerative changes results in a step-like interruption of the posterior vertebral contour. The intervertebral foramen is narrowed as a result.

INFLAMMATORY ARTHRITIS

Rheumatoid arthritis

Rheumatoid arthritis (RA) is an inflammatory arthritis of unknown aetiology. The currently accepted classification scheme for RA is the 1987 American College of Rheumatology (ACR) criteria set. The diagnostic criteria are dominated by signs and symptoms related to the locomotive system. This is despite the fact that RA is a multisystem disease. The major abnormalities appear in the synovial joints. If a patient meets four or more of the following seven criteria he or she may be given a diagnosis of RA (sensitivity 90%, specificity 90%):

1. morning stiffness for at least 1 hour
2. soft tissue swelling or effusion of three or more joints for more than 6 weeks (particularly the wrist, MCP, MTP and proximal IP joints)
3. arthritis of hand joints
4. symmetrical joint swelling
5. positive rheumatoid factor
6. the presence or one or more rheumatoid nodules
7. radiological changes (it must include erosions or unequivocal bony decalcification most marked adjacent to the involved joints).

The main radiological findings and the underlying pathophysiological causes are outlined in Table 50.4.

Clinical features

RA affects approximately 1% of population and is more common in women than men. The prevalence increases with age in both men and women[8]. Laboratory testing will usually show some sign of an acute phase reaction (thrombocytosis, raised ESR or CRP) although these do not correlate necessarily with disease activity. Rheumatoid factor is positive in the majority of patients with RA but is not independently specific for the disease.

Table 50.4 PLAIN RADIOGRAPHIC FINDINGS IN RHEUMATOID ARTHRITIS AND CORRESPONDING PATHOPHYSIOLOGICAL CAUSES

Radiological findings	Pathological cause
Periarticular osteoporosis	This reflects localized hyperaemia and is most pronounced in acute stages of the disease
Soft tissue swelling	This represents synovial hypertrophy, joint effusion and periarticular soft tissue oedema, and is typically symmetrical
Erosions	These are marginal in location caused by the inflammatory and erosive effect of the inflamed synovium on the 'bare area' of the joint (that part of the joint adjacent to the synovium which is not covered by cartilage)
Joint space narrowing	This results from cartilage loss. Early uniform cartilage loss results from interruption of the flow of synovial fluid nutrients by the pannus. Later the hypertrophied synovium causes direct destruction with undermining of the cartilage and destruction of the subchondral bone. There may be joint widening in the early stages or ankylosis in the end stages of the disease
Subchondral cysts	These result from destruction of the subchondral plate by pannus, which allows joint fluid to be forced into the subchondral bone under pressure
Joint subluxation and dislocation	These are due to damage or destruction to tendons and ligaments as a result of the inflammatory pannus. In the early stages the deformity may be reversible and therefore underestimated on plain films
Generalized regional osteoporosis	This results from pain-induced disuse and may be exacerbated by the effects of therapy (e.g. steroids)

Radiological features

RA is characterized by a symmetrical arthritis of the small joints, which is associated with soft tissue swelling in the initial stages. Large joints are moderately frequently involved. Conversely the spine is usually spared (apart from the cervical region).

Peripheral joints The conventional radiograph of the hand and wrist is used to determine the state and/or progression of disease and therefore high quality images must be produced with appropriate exposure and positioning. The earliest radiographic changes seen in the hands are juxta-articular osteopenia and symmetrical soft tissue swelling. Although these findings are nonspecific, they help to confirm the presence of underlying inflammation. Marginal erosions at the bare area (areas lacking articular cartilage) indicate a more aggressive arthropathy. These may be subtle. The early soft tissue changes occur most commonly at the metacarpophalangeal and interphalangeal joints, the ulnar styloid, the radial styloid, the mid portion of the scaphoid, and lateral portion of the hamate as it articulates with the fifth metacarpal. Erosions occur before joint space narrowing is evident, and indeed at this stage there may be slight apparent widening of the joint space due to the interposition of pannus between the articular surfaces. Tenosynovitis is commonly present at presentation and when it affects the flexor compartment or the wrist can lead to carpal tunnel syndrome due to pressure on the median nerve in the carpal tunnel.

Later changes in the fingers show joint space narrowing, with reduced soft tissue swelling. The juxta-articular osteoporosis progresses to diffuse osteoporosis and the marginal erosions increase in size and coalesce. Subluxation due to ligamentous laxity and damage is common, particularly in the form of swan neck or boutonnière lesions of the fingers, ulnar deviation and volar subluxation and dislocation of the phalanges at the MCP joint, rotatory subluxation of the scaphoid and drift of the entire carpus in an ulnar and/or volar direction (Fig. 50.7). Such malalignment can occur early, even before the advent of bony erosions. Tenosynovitis can lead to tendon rupture, particularly the extensor carpi ulnaris. Bony ankylosis is uncommon, but when seen occurs typically in the carpus (Fig. 50.7). End-stage disease is characterized by pancompartmental loss of the joint spaces, resorption of the carpal bones and 'arthritis mutilans'.

The foot is involved in 80–90% of RA patients. Some studies indicate that 10–20% of patients will have foot involvement before hand involvement but in these studies not all available radiographic views of the hands were performed. It is generally considered that changes in the feet accompany or lag somewhat behind the changes in the hands. Juxta-articular osteoporosis and soft tissue swelling is usually pronounced first at the MTP joints, with erosions occurring on the bare areas of the heads of the metatarsals. Later changes show progression of the marginal erosions to large subchondral erosions with loss of joint space. Lateral subluxation of the lateral phalanges with dorsiflexion deformities of the PIP joints is typical. Further

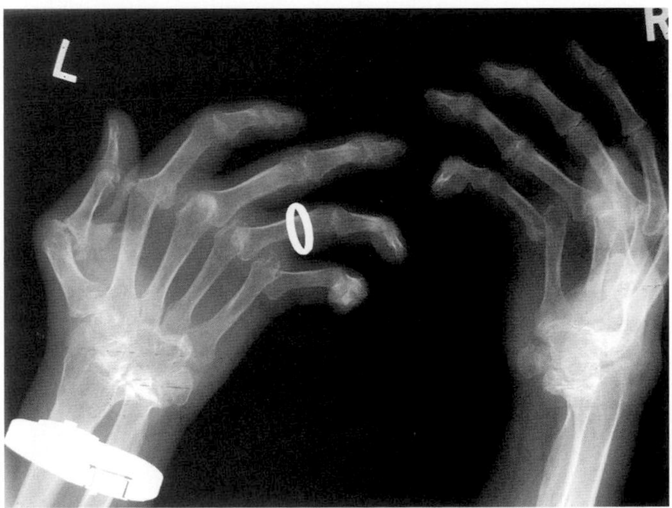

Figure 50.7 Rheumatoid arthritis. Involvement of the MCP joints with ligamentous damage or laxity has resulted in ulnar dislocation at all MCP joints, associated with underlying typical erosive changes. Bony ankylosis of the left wrist is pronounced involving the carpus.

progression may involve the tarsal bones symmetrically, and bony ankylosis is a feature of long-standing disease.

The knees, hips, shoulders and elbows are commonly involved, and involvement is typically symmetrical. Although marginal erosions may be present (Fig. 50.8), uniform loss of cartilage is the predominant feature and there is a propensity to develop intraosseous synovial cysts, which can grow to several centimetres in size. In these cases the synovium breaks through the cartilage and protrudes into the bone. A ball valve effect of the synovial fluid within the cyst causes enlargement. These should not be mistaken for a neoplastic lesion.

Spine and sacroiliac joints The cervical spine becomes involved in 70–80% of patients, whereas the thoracic and lumbar spine is uncommonly involved. Although the cervical spine may be involved anywhere from the occiput to T1, the most common finding is atlantoaxial subluxation due to damage or laxity of the cruciate ligament that holds the odontoid to the atlas. This can be associated with erosion of the odontoid due to involvement of the synovial joint between the odontoid peg and the cruciate ligament, or may result from bursal involvement of small bursae adjacent to the odontoid. Atlantoaxial subluxation is best demonstrated on a (controlled) flexed lateral radiograph of the cervical spine (Fig. 50.8), although CT and MRI can also be used to show neural compromise. Finally, due to erosions and/or osteopenia, the odontoid may fracture, or in the late stages of rheumatoid arthritis basilar invagination may occur. Such changes should be excluded before anaesthetic procedures.

The apophyseal joints or disc spaces are infrequently involved with RA. Sacroiliac joint involvement is recognized but the appearance is usually less aggressive than in other synovial joints and is typically symmetrical. Bony fusion is uncommon.

MRI and rheumatoid arthritis

MRI studies have shown a direct causal relationship between synovitis, bone marrow oedema and erosions, allowing a diagnosis of RA before the occurrence of radiographic erosions.

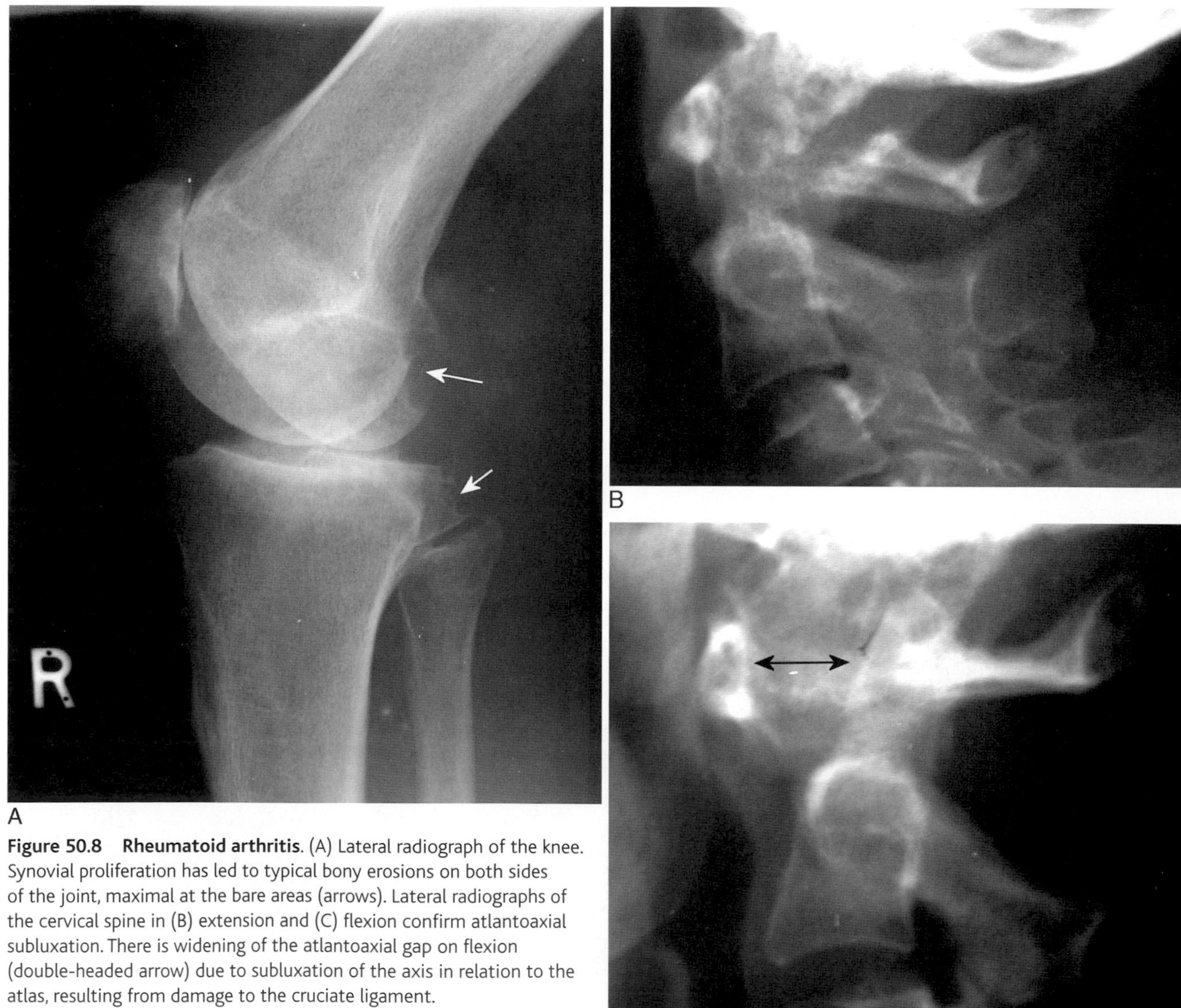

Figure 50.8 Rheumatoid arthritis. (A) Lateral radiograph of the knee. Synovial proliferation has led to typical bony erosions on both sides of the joint, maximal at the bare areas (arrows). Lateral radiographs of the cervical spine in (B) extension and (C) flexion confirm atlantoaxial subluxation. There is widening of the atlantoaxial gap on flexion (double-headed arrow) due to subluxation of the axis in relation to the atlas, resulting from damage to the cruciate ligament.

Indeed bone marrow oedema has been shown to appear at only 4 weeks after presentation. MRI is more sensitive than radiographs for erosion detection[9] due to its tomographic nature[10], shows erosions earlier than radiographs[11], and is also more sensitive for picking up erosions in larger joints[12]. However, it is not clear whether all erosions detected in MRI eventually become visible on plain radiographs.

Using MRI at the time of diagnosis of early RA may help to predict which patients will go on to erosive changes[13] and similarly MRI may offer a more sensitive approach to monitoring the effect of treatment than the plain films that are currently employed (Fig. 50.9).

Complications of rheumatoid arthritis

The main complications of RA are secondary infection, stress fracture and avascular necrosis due to steroid administration. Infection should be considered when there is rapid deterioration of the joint, particularly in the presence of an effusion. Fractures are also common complications and are of two types: insufficiency and stress fractures. Both of these develop in osteoporotic bone due to minor trauma or relatively normal activity respectively. The distal radius, the distal tibia and thoracolumbar vertebral bodies are most commonly affected. Avascular necrosis is most common in the hip and results from corticosteroid therapy in particular. *Baker's* cyst synovitis may lead to distension of the semimembranosus-gastrocnemius bursa posteromedial to the knee; rupture of this bursa can lead to painful swelling of the calf that mimics deep venous thrombosis.

Juvenile idiopathic arthritis

The term juvenile idiopathic arthritis (JIA) is used as a compromise between the American term, juvenile rheumatoid arthritis (JRA), and the European classification, juvenile chronic arthritis (JCA). There are several other synonyms, and up to seven subgroups. JIA is an inflammatory disorder of the connective tissues characterized by joint swelling and pain or tenderness that affects one or more joints for at least six weeks in patients under the age of 16. Rheumatoid factor is positive in only approximately 10% and the clinical onset may be extra-articular (20%). Articular presentation may be pauciarticular (four or fewer joints involved) or polyarticular (five or more joints involved) and each type is approximately equally common. Rarely, the disease can affect patients over the age of 16[14].

Radiological findings

Soft tissue swelling and synovitis predominate initially, when plain radiographs can be normal, although periarticular osteopenia is a feature. As a result of prolonged synovitis and hyperaemia, epiphyseal overgrowth occurs resulting in expansion of the epiphysis. Early closure of the epiphyseal plate is relatively common in severely affected patients, resulting in growth disturbances. Bone and cartilage changes occur late in the process and occasionally can lead to ankylosis.

Peripheral joints In the hand, any of the joints can be involved. The diaphyses are overtubulated and the epiphyses enlarged and osteoporotic with an increased internal trabecular pattern. Periosteal new bone formation and epiphyseal compression fractures may occur. One or more joints may be affected, and the pattern is frequently asymmetrical. Malalignment and subluxation are uncommon with JIA. Bony erosions are also uncommon, and joint space narrowing is a late feature. A useful discriminatory finding is the presence of periosteal new bone formation, which affects the phalangeal and metacarpal shafts and which may be florid. The foot shows similar changes. In the wrist, soft tissue swelling and osteoporosis are followed by the premature appearance of enlarged irregular and squared carpal bones, secondary to erosion and repair. The end result is often extensive ankylosis, most often in the carpometacarpal and mid-carpal joints with only one joint remaining open[15].

The shoulders, elbows, hips and knees are commonly also involved, with similar radiological changes seen to those in

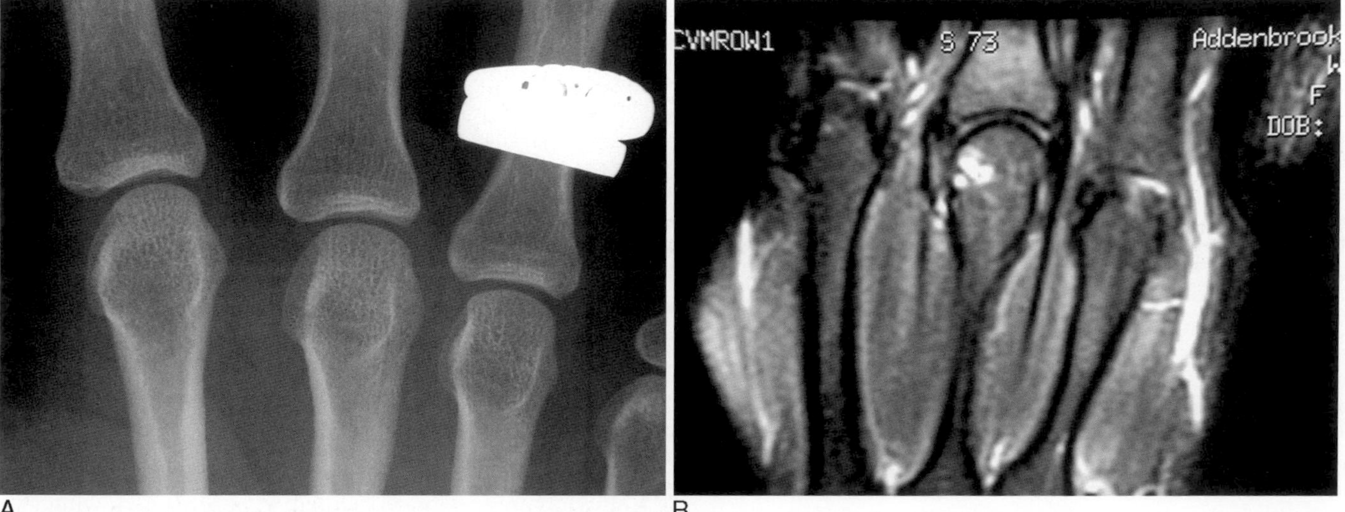

Figure 50.9 Early rheumatoid arthritis. (A) Plain radiographs are normal. (B) The corresponding MR shows oedema in the third metacarpal head, but the overlying cortex is intact. On subsequent radiographs, this eventually became an overt radiographic erosion.

the hands and feet. Early swelling, effusion, epiphyseal overgrowth, periarticular osteoporosis and preservation of cartilage are expected, with bone erosions, cartilage loss, ankylosis and deformity occurring as a late feature (Fig. 50.10).

Spine and sacroiliac joints In the spine, the cervical region is most commonly affected and involvement of the thoracolumbar spine and sacroiliac joints is uncommon. Atlantoaxial subluxation is common, particularly in seropositive patients. Underdevelopment of vertebral bodies and intervertebral discs occurs and may be associated with block fusion, resulting from ankylosis which affects both the disc and the apophyseal joints. The appearances can simulate Klippel–Feil syndrome, where block vertebrae and facet joint fusion are also seen. The spinous processes may be tapered, and compression fractures can be seen, possibly secondary to osteoporosis aggravated by steroid therapy. Scoliosis may occur in advanced disease[16].

Complications

The complications are related to the soft tissue swelling, synovitis and hyperaemia. These can result in leg length discrepancy resulting from growth plate disturbance, and chronic inflammation can lead to contractures.

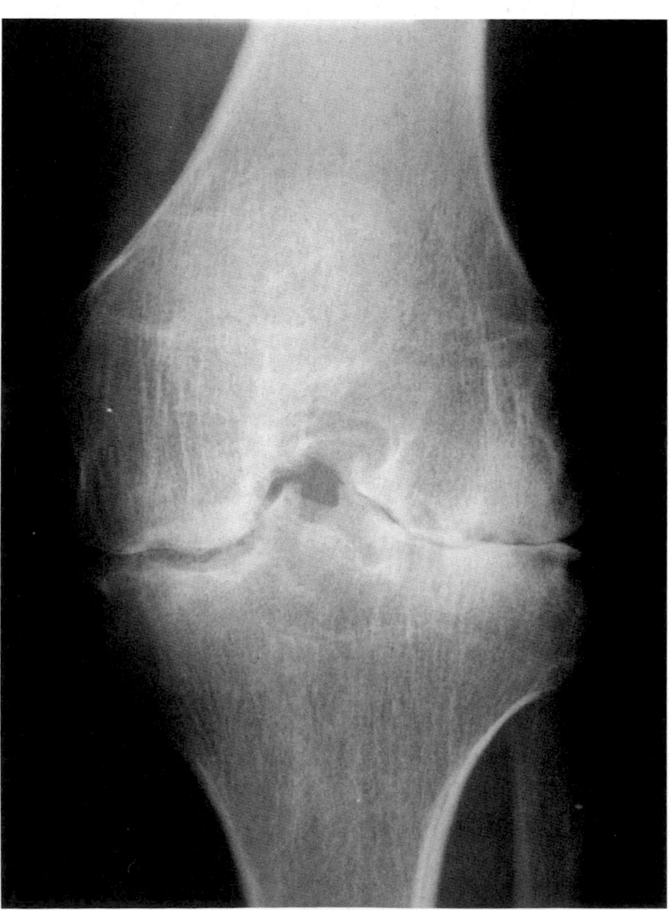

Figure 50.10 Juvenile inflammatory arthropathy of the knee. There is secondary degenerative change with loss of joint space and subchondral sclerosis associated with epiphyseal overgrowth and narrowing of the intercondylar notch. The epiphyseal overgrowth results from hyperaemia during the growth period in childhood.

Psoriatic arthropathy

Psoriatic arthritis represents a specific entity that affects up to 7% of patients with psoriasis, particularly between the ages of 30 and 50 years. Psoriasis affects approximately 1% of the population, and skin changes typically precede the arthropathy. Laboratory tests are nonspecific and the rheumatoid factor is absent. The finding of the psoriatic skin disease is critical in making the correct diagnosis.

Radiological features

The hands and feet, and the spine and sacroiliac joints are principally involved, and there are at least five patterns of clinical presentation[17]. The commonest form (70%) is an arthritis that affects one or possibly a few joints randomly. The second most common pattern is indistinguishable from rheumatoid arthritis (15%). In the third form, a destructive arthritis is seen affecting principally the distal interphalangeal joints (5%); nail pitting is strongly associated with this type. Rarely, the condition can present as an inflammatory arthritis of the spine with or without peripheral joint involvement, or with an aggressive arthritis mutilans, typically of the hands.

Peripheral skeleton In the hands and feet, the arthritis is usually bilateral but asymmetrical, is destructive in nature, affects predominantly the distal interphalangeal joints, and bony changes are preceded by soft tissue swelling. The joint space may be widened, and fluffy irregular or solid reactive marginal new bone formation or periosteal reaction along the diaphysis of the bone is observed (Fig. 50.11). Nail changes are obvious clinically and may even be detected on appropriate radiographs if they are severe. Advanced cases may proceed to tapering of the distal aspect of the head of the middle phalanx resulting in a 'pencil in cup' appearance. Bone mineral density is preserved until end-stage disease is present. The bony changes are often associated with soft tissue swelling of the entire finger (sausage digit) or underlying tenosynovitis. In addition to periosteal reactions or proliferative new bone formation, resorption of the distal phalangeal tufts is also typical. A minority of patients develop subluxation or cartilage loss, and spontaneous ankylosis of the IP joints is also characteristic of this form of arthritis. Extreme resorption and erosion of the metacarpals and phalanges with shortening of the digits and telescoping fingers is termed arthritis mutilans.

Wrist involvement is typically pancarpal, associated with erosions and bony destruction and proliferation, and this can lead to complete carpal fusion. The changes in the feet are similar to those in the hands. Symmetrical involvement of the distal interphalangeal joints is infrequent.

Involvement of the calcaneus will result in a picture similar to Reiter's disease with fluffy sclerosis and erosions at the insertion of the Achilles tendon. Involvement of the larger peripheral joints is usually asymmetrical or monoarticular, and soft tissue swelling or joint effusion are followed by marginal erosions with progression to uniform joint space narrowing in the context of preserved mineral content. New bone formation at the entheses or periosteal new bone formation may be seen.

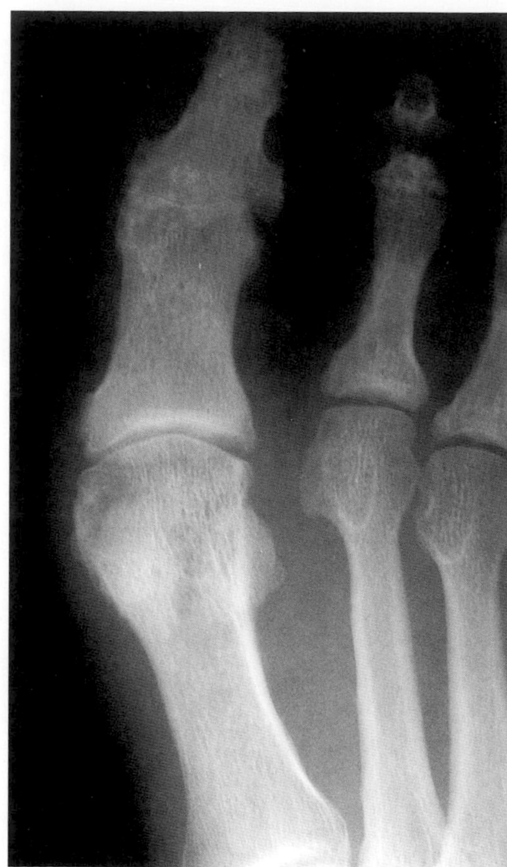

Figure 50.11 Psoriatic arthropathy. There is an inflammatory arthropathy of the IP joints of the great toe and second digit, associated with extra-articular erosions and fluffy irregular reactive margin new bone formation. The bone mineral density is preserved.

Spine and sacroiliac joints Up to 25% of patients with psoriatic arthritis have spine involvement. The characteristic findings are coarse asymmetrical non-marginal syndesmophytes that affect multiple levels with skip areas that are not affected. The syndesmophytes originate from the mid-vertebral body rather than the vertebral margins, and they are more superficially situated than in ankylosing spondylitis. They are less common in the cervical spine. Asymmetrical involvement is typical and occasionally the vertebral bodies may 'square' anteriorly as in ankylosing spondylitis.

Atlantoaxial subluxation is another recognized finding and this can be indistinguishable from rheumatoid arthritis. It is best demonstrated on a lateral radiograph of the spine in flexion. Sacroiliitis occurs in up to 25% of patients with psoriatic arthritis, and in the majority of patients the involvement is bilateral and symmetrical. Ankylosis is uncommon, but otherwise the appearances are indistinguishable from ankylosing spondylitis. Involvement of the iliac side of the joint first is typical, leading to blurring of the subchondral margins, erosions, narrowing of the joint space, and reactive sclerosis.

Differential diagnostic features

The following features in the hands would favour a diagnosis of psoriatic arthritis as opposed to rheumatoid arthritis: preservation of bone mineralization, proliferative marginal new bone formation or periosteal reaction, sausage digit, spontaneous bony ankylosis and enthesitis (see Table 50.7).

Reiter's syndrome

Classically, the Reiter's triad consists of conjunctivitis, urethritis and arthritis, but all three components are rarely seen at initial presentation. There is an association with the HLA-B27 antigen, and patients with the antigen have more acute disease, a higher prevalence of sacroiliitis and more frequent chronic back pain[18]. There is a clear association with infectious agents, particularly sexually transmitted disease (*Chlamydia*). The syndrome can also follow dysentery-like symptoms (*Salmonella, Shigella, Yersinia*, or *Campylobacter*). Of 600 men who developed *Shigella* dysentery, 10 developed post-dysentery Reiter's syndrome, and 6 were found to have persistent problems 10 years later[19].

Two additional consistent features are balanitis and a specific dermatitis (keratoderma blennorrhagicum). This characteristic lesion affects the palms of the hands and soles of the feet.

Radiological features

Although similar to psoriatic arthritis, the distribution is different. The disease characteristically affects the lower extremities, including the foot, knee and ankle, and the typical distribution is asymmetrical.

Peripheral skeleton Bone proliferation is prominent, and bone mineral density is preserved. Periosteal reactions and spontaneous joint effusions are common in the feet, and to a lesser extent the hands. In the acute inflammatory phase, periarticular osteoporosis is an expected feature. The calcaneus is involved in more than 50% of patients and may show erosions or a fluffy periosteal new bone formation and spurs, as well as increased density and size. The site of attachment of the Achilles tendon and the plantar surface are typically involved. Involvement of the small joints of the foot is random and asymmetrical, although the MTP joint of the hallux is most commonly involved. Uniform joint space narrowing and marginal erosions are seen, followed by destruction and dislocation. The knee may be involved unilaterally or bilaterally, and is characterized by joint effusion, local osteoporosis, and less commonly uniform joint space narrowing.

Spine and sacroiliac joints The most common involvement is that of the sacroiliac joints, although this site is less commonly involved than with psoriatic arthritis, and sacroiliitis is usually bilateral but asymmetrical. Changes are first seen on the iliac side of the joint, and complete fusion does not typically occur. The spine is less frequently involved than the sacroiliac joints resulting in asymmetric coarse non-marginal syndesmophytes with a discontinuous distribution (normal skip segments in between areas of abnormality).

Ankylosing spondylitis

Ankylosing spondylitis is a progressive chronic spondyloarthropathy and generally presents in young adults. It is characterized by involvement of the sacroiliac joints, the spinal apophyseal joints, the annulus fibrosus, and the deep layers of the anterior longitudinal ligament[20]. The disease is strongly linked to the HLA-B27 histocompatability antigen. The hallmark of the disease is joint ankylosis, and early diagnosis is important so that appropriate anti-inflammatory therapy can be initiated before fixed deformity is established. The male to female ratio is 10:1 and the peak age of onset is between 25 and 35 years. The histological features of proliferative chronic synovitis involving the diarthrodial joints are often indistinguishable from rheumatoid arthritis. There is a tendency towards capsular fibrosis and relatively rapid bony ankylosis.

Radiological features

The principal sites of involvement are the lower two-thirds of the sacroiliac joints and the spine. Other areas include the hips, shoulders, knees, ankles, costovertebral joints, manubriosternal joint, symphysis pubis and temporomandibular joints. Involvement of the small joints of the hands and feet is unusual.

Spine and sacroiliac joints In the spine, ankylosing spondylitis most commonly begins in the thoracolumbar region and progresses cranially. Spinal involvement generally precedes sacroiliitis and consists of early erosion and sclerosis of the anterior corners of the vertebral bodies resulting in vertebral body squaring, syndesmophyte formation, longitudinal ligamentous mineralization and eventually ankylosis of the apophyseal joints. Syndesmophytes represent ossification of the outer lamellae of the annulus fibrosus and the immediately adjacent anterior longitudinal ligament, which later blend with the periosteum. Vertebral body squaring results firstly from bone inflammation and erosion adjacent to the vertebral end plate (shiny or ivory corners) and secondly from mineralization of the anterior longitudinal ligament which fills in the normal anterior concavity of the vertical body (Fig. 50.12). With maturation the syndesmophytes produce the classic 'bamboo spine' (Fig. 50.13). The syndesmophytes can be differentiated from osteophytes by their vertical rather than horizontal origin, and can be differentiated from DISH by the lack of a radiolucent line between the calcified ligament and the anterior margin of the vertebral body. Degenerative change is secondary, and occurs between the fused segments. When the thoracic spine is involved, this is often characterized by marked kyphosis. Cervical spine involvement is late and uncommon. Eventually the entire spine becomes demineralized.

In the sacroiliac joints the process is most commonly bilateral and symmetrical, although asymmetry is encountered and in the early stages of the disease the process may appear to be unilateral. Radiologically, sacroiliitis involves the synovial component of the sacroiliac joint, and the initial finding is loss of definition of the joint margins. Then the joint space becomes widened or irregular, and focal erosions develop particularly on the iliac side of the joint, leading to sclerosis and ultimately ankylosis. In the ligamentous portion of the joint, both sacral and iliac cortices become indistinct due to 'whiskering' of the bone on either side of the joint, and finally this portion also undergoes ankylosis. MRI, CT or bone scintigraphy can help to detect the process before findings are apparent on plain radiographs.

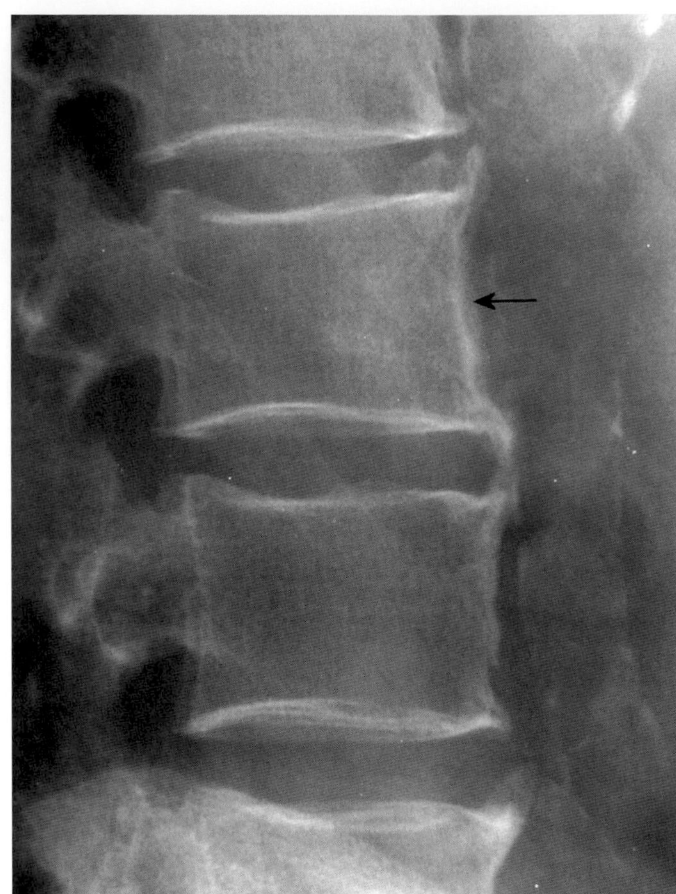

Figure 50.12 Ankylosing spondylitis of the spine. There is vertebral body squaring resulting from mineralization of the anterior longitudinal ligament which fills in the normal anterior concavity of the vertebral body (arrow).

Peripheral skeleton When large joints are involved, the hips, shoulders and knees are most commonly affected. When compared to rheumatoid arthritis, with which the disease is often mistaken, bony ankylosis predominates rather than erosions, and there is less demineralization and more reactive sclerosis. Arthritis mutilans does not occur with ankylosing spondylitis. The hands and feet are rarely involved clinically, and even more rarely involved radiologically.

Enthesitis The *enthesis* is a region of bone where a tendon, capsule or ligament attaches. *Enthesitis* refers to inflammation of this region, and is a typical feature of ankylosing spondylitis. It is also seen in psoriatic arthritis, enteropathic spondylitis and Reiter's syndrome. Enthesitis is seen as irregular new bone proliferation resulting in a 'whiskering' effect at the sites of muscle and tendon attachments, sometimes associated with reactive sclerosis. It is most common at the ischial tuberosity, iliac margins and the calcaneum. *Osteitis pubis*, is common particularly in women and is characterized by erosions, reactive sclerosis and later ankylosis of the symphysis pubis.

Complications

The rigid osteoporotic spine is prone to fractures, and these may lead to a pseudoarthrosis[21]. Such fractures are often not easily seen on conventional radiographs, prompting further

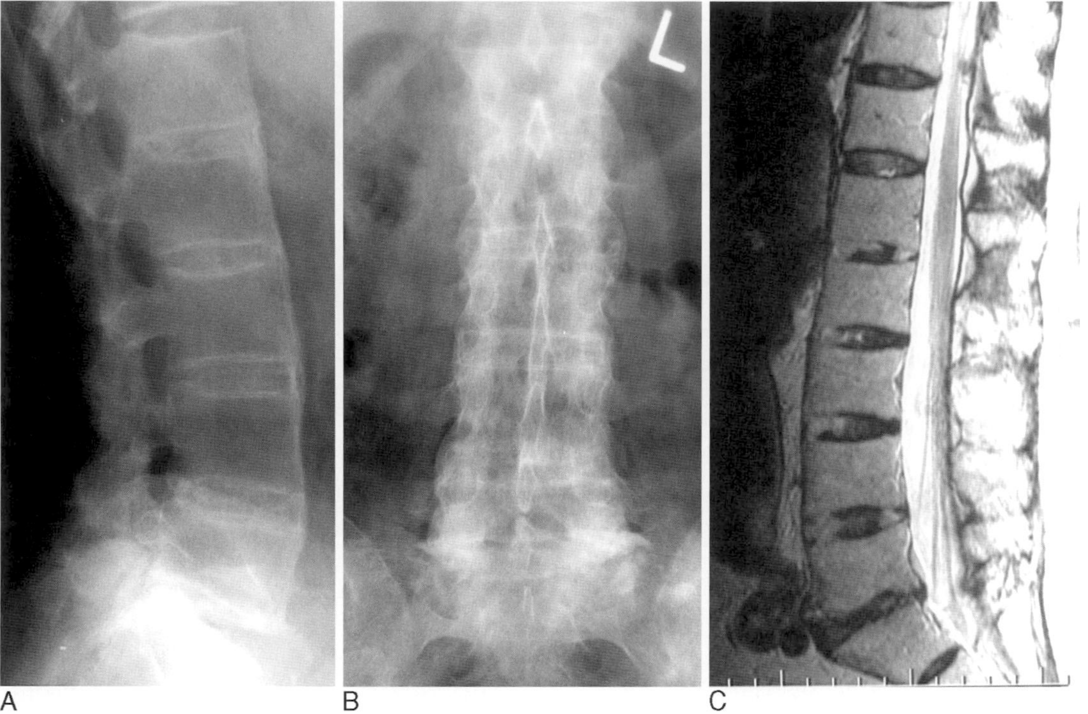

Figure 50.13 Advanced ankylosing spondylitis of the spine. (A) Lateral and (B) AP radiographs of the lumbar spine show that the syndesmophytes have matured to produce the classic 'bamboo spine'. (C) Corresponding MR shows the squaring of the vertebral bodies, calcification of the anterior longitudinal ligament, and increased signal in the anterior aspects of the discs.

assessment with bone scintigraphy, MRI or multidetector CT (MDCT). The multiplanar imaging ability of MRI makes it ideal in assessment of such injuries as the spinal cord can also be assessed together with complications such as epidural haematoma, spinal cord contusion or post-traumatic myelomalacia. Destructive lesions in the vertebral bodies can occur in an unfused segment between two longer ankylosed segments, and result from exaggerated spinal motion of this site. Such lesions simulate infection. Visceral complications of ankylosing spondylitis include aortic valve disease and upper zone pulmonary fibrosis.

CRYSTAL DEPOSITION AND RELATED ARTHROPATHIES

The major crystal deposition diseases are gout and pseudogout. Chondrocalcinosis refers to the deposition of calcium salts in fibrocartilage and hyaline cartilage (CPPD). When symptomatic, this condition is called pseudogout. Calcific deposits also occur in hydroxyapatite deposition disease (HADD), dialysis arthropathy and certain inborn errors of metabolism.

Gout

Gout (podagra) results from an inborn error of purine metabolism that causes hyperuricaemia and deposition of monosodium urate (MSU) crystals in joints and soft tissues resulting in recurrent episodes of acute arthritis. Under polarizing microscopy, MSU crystals are strongly negatively birefringent (Table 50.5). Primary gout is transmitted as an autosomal dominant condition with low penetrance in women. Only 5–10% of cases occur in women, in whom it usually occurs post-menopausally. Gout is less common in blacks than in whites. Symptomatically primary gout usually begins in the third decade of life, but can occur earlier[22]. Secondary hyperuricaemia may occur after a number of underlying conditions associated with either excessive breakdown of nuclear proteins (e.g. blood dyscrasias, leukaemia, lymphoma, myeloma, collagen storage diseases) or decreased renal excretion of uric acid (e.g. chronic renal disease, diuretics, low-dose salicylates).

The four stages in the evolution of gouty arthritis are: (1) asymptomatic hyperuricaemia; (2) acute gouty arthritis; (3) intercritical gout; (4) chronic tophaceous gout. Acute arthritis is the most common early clinical manifestation, typically affecting the first metatarsophalangeal joint. The first attack is usually monoarticular. The 'intercritical periods' are those between attacks. Early in the course of the disease, the patient is symptom-free during these intercritical periods, and the intercritical periods may last for many months. With recurring attacks the duration of the intercritical periods shortens and recovery between the attacks becomes incomplete. In chronic tophaceous gout, soft tissue lumps (tophi) occur containing deposits of monosodium urate crystals. On average they appear

Table 50.5 POLARIZING MICROSCOPE FINDINGS OF THE INTRA-ARTICULAR CRYSTALS FOUND IN CALCIUM PYROPHOSPHATE DIHYDRATE (CPPD, PSEUDOGOUT) AND MONOSODIUM URATE (MSU, GOUT) CRYSTAL DEPOSITION DISEASE

Crystal deposition	CPDD	MSU
Shape of crystals	Rhomboid	Needle shaped
Birefringence	Weak	Strong
Direction	Positive	Negative

approximately 10 years after the first episode of arthritis and, as a result of erosion of cartilage and subchondral bone caused by the chronic inflammatory reaction and crystal deposition, a deforming arthritis can develop.

Radiological features

During the early acute attacks, crystal shedding is associated with an intense inflammatory response and a joint effusion, but this pattern is not observed radiologically. Radiological findings occur only in chronic tophaceous gout, where typical erosions associated with eccentric soft tissue swellings are the hallmarks of the disease. The joints most often involved are the first metatarsophalangeal joints, the foot, hand, ankle, wrist, elbow and knee. Although destructive changes are seen in only approximately half of the patients, the degree of destruction can be severe.

Peripheral joints Involvement of the hand is asymmetric with random distribution of the lesions. Early acute changes relate to joint effusion and swelling localized to the affected joint. Periarticular osteoporosis is not a common feature. The joint space may be normal or uniformly narrowed. There may be periarticular, marginal or subchondral erosions, which are cyst-like or 'punched out' in that they have a sharp margin with a thin sclerotic rim, usually with little surrounding reactive sclerosis (Fig. 50.14). Typically they show sharp overhanging margins and are associated with adjacent eccentric soft tissue swelling. These destructive lesions are remote from the articular surface, which helps to differentiate this condition from rheumatoid arthritis where they are usually well demarcated and occur on the bare areas of the bone. Calcification within tophi may occur, as may bony ankylosis on occasion, but ulnar deviation does not occur.

Joint involvement in the hands is random and there may or may not be associated joint space narrowing. Severe deformities of the hand with telescoping of the digits may occur during treatment due to the rapid resorption of osseous tophi which are not replaced by bone matrix[23]. In the wrist, the carpometacarpal compartment is most commonly involved. Involvement of the shoulders, elbows or hips is uncommon. In the knees, tophi or an effusion may help to differentiate the condition, but more often the picture is that of osteoarthritis.

The hallmark location of gout is in the foot at the metatarsophalangeal joint of the great toe. In the acute stage it is exquisitely tender, and in the tophaceous stage the tophus is typically dorsally situated causing adjacent erosion. Hallux valgus is a common accompaniment and osteoporosis, absent in the early stages, becomes more prevalent as the disease progresses.

Spine and sacroiliac joints Spinal involvement is rare. Intervertebral disc narrowing is observed, as well as erosion of the odontoid peg process and atlantoaxial subluxation. Conversely, changes in the sacroiliac joints are not uncommon and include sclerosis, marginal irregularity, erosions and cyst-like changes with sclerotic margins.

Related conditions

Lesch–Nyhan syndrome is a rare syndrome of hyperuricaemia and mental retardation in children due to a metabolic enzyme deficiency. It is transmitted by a recessive gene on the X chromosome and thus occurs only in male children. Saturnine gout is a form of secondary gout caused by decreased renal urate clearance due to lead nephropathy. It affects patients with chronic lead toxicity and the radiological features are similar to those of primary gout.

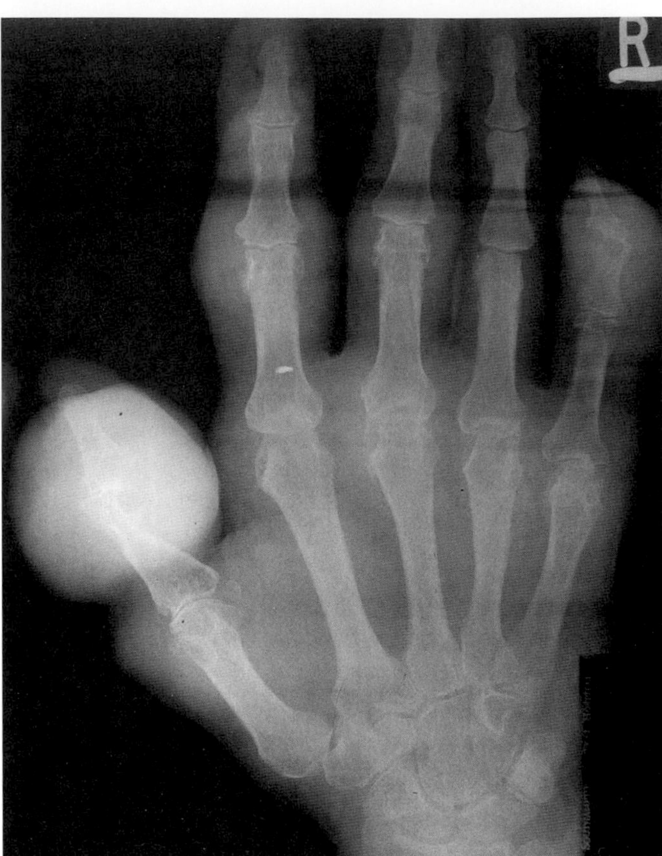

Figure 50.14 Chronic tophaceous gout. Large eccentric soft tissue lumps (tophi) occur asymmetrically resulting from monosodium urate crystal deposition. Underlying gouty erosions are seen at several sites, particularly the DIP joint of the right little finger and the CMC joint of the thumb.

Calcium pyrophosphate deposition disease

This results from the presence of calcium pyrophosphate dihydrate (CPPD) crystals in joints, bursae or tendon sheaths. In contrast to the MSU crystals seen in gout, CPPD crystals are weakly positively birefringent under polarizing light microscopy (Table 50.5). The condition may be symptomatic, in which case it is called pseudogout, or it may be asymptomatic, in which case the only radiological finding may be chondrocalcinosis. The term chondrocalcinosis relates to finding calcium salts in hyaline cartilage or fibrocartilage. These salts are most commonly CPPD, although hydroxyapatite or other calcium salt deposition would be indistinguishable radiologically, and chondrocalcinosis can also be seen in a number of other arthropathies such as gout, hyperparathyroidism, haemochromatosis, Wilson's disease and degenerative joint disease. Calcium pyrophosphate arthropathy refers to CPPD crystal deposition disease affecting joints and producing structural damage to the articular cartilage.

Radiological features

During acute attacks the resulting soft tissue oedema and joint effusions will not be appreciated well on plain radiographs although MRI or ultrasound might be used to demonstrate them. Chondrocalcinosis may or may not be present at this stage.

The chronic arthropathy, however, does have certain characteristic features. The most commonly affected joint is the knee, particularly the patellofemoral articulation. The radiocarpal, metacarpophalangeal and elbow joints are also commonly involved. Chondrocalcinosis is frequently but not invariably present. The arthropathy is characterized by uniform cartilage thinning, multiple subchondral cysts, osteophytes and a bilateral and symmetrical distribution. These appearances, and the lack of prominent subchondral sclerosis, help to differentiate the condition from OA. Giant cysts and structural collapse and fragmentation of the subchondral plate are recognized features. Periarticular calcific deposits, which may be large and can have an erosive pressure effect on adjacent bone, may occur and are termed tophaceous pseudogout. The crowned dens syndrome represents tophaceous pseudogout at the atlantoaxial joint with progressive cervical cord compression and it can mimic a number of unrelated conditions including polymyalgia rheumatica, giant cell arteritis, meningitis and spondylitis[24]. More commonly, cervical spine involvement is seen as intervertebral disc calcification and joint space narrowing. Lumbar and thoracic involvement is uncommon. The sacroiliac joints may show changes of osteoarthritis, and the symphysis pubis may show a thin vertical linear calcification.

Calcium hydroxyapatite and related crystal deposition disease

The crystals responsible for basic calcium phosphate (BCP) crystal deposition disease include hydroxyapatite (HA), octacalcium phosphate and tricalcium phosphate crystals. Several articular and periarticular syndromes have been described in association with BCP crystals (Table 50.6).

Hydroxyapatite deposition disease is known to occur both within a joint and in periarticular locations. Periarticular calcification is associated with the sudden onset of severe local pain, and is particularly common in the supraspinatus tendon (calcific tendinitis). Larger periarticular deposits may develop associated with metabolic diseases such as hyperparathyroidism, milk-alkali syndrome and tumoral calcinosis (Table 50.6).

Intra-articular deposition of HA crystals results in acute pain and swelling in the absence of chondrocalcinosis (unless there is additional CPPD). The picture ranges from monoarticular periarthritis to joint destruction. Radiologically, amorphous calcifications are seen around or within joints, tendons or bursae (Fig. 50.15). They vary in size from a few millimetres to several centimetres and may change in size over time. In articular disease, synovial and capsular calcification may occur. The joint space becomes narrowed followed by subchondral sclerosis and destructive changes. Osteophytes and subchondral cysts are absent unless there is associated secondary osteoarthritis. Occasionally periarticular calcifications have been reported following steroid injections[25].

Table 50.6 BASIC CALCIUM PHOSPHATE CRYSTAL JOINT AND ASSOCIATED SOFT TISSUE DISEASE
Calcific periarthritis
Unifocal, multifocal, linear
Calcific tendinitis/bursitis, intra-articular BCP
Acute gout-like attacks
Milwaukee shoulder syndrome
Erosive polyarticular disease
Mixed crystal deposition disease (CPPD and BCP)
Secondary BCP crystal deposition
Chronic renal failure
Collagen diseases (calcinosis)
Severe neurological injury sequelae
Post local steroid injection
Tumoral calcinosis
Hyperphosphataemic
Normophosphataemic

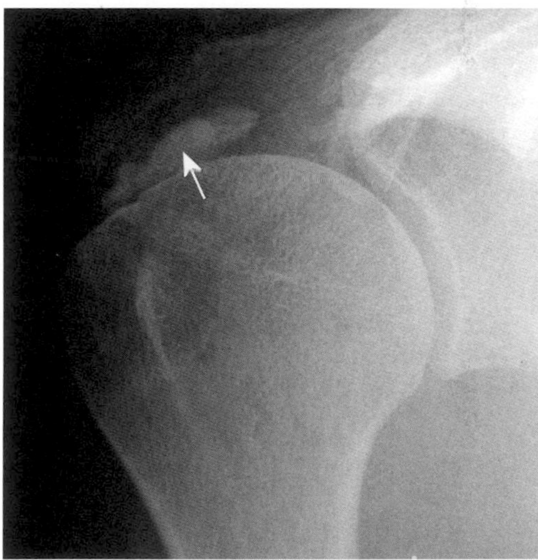
A

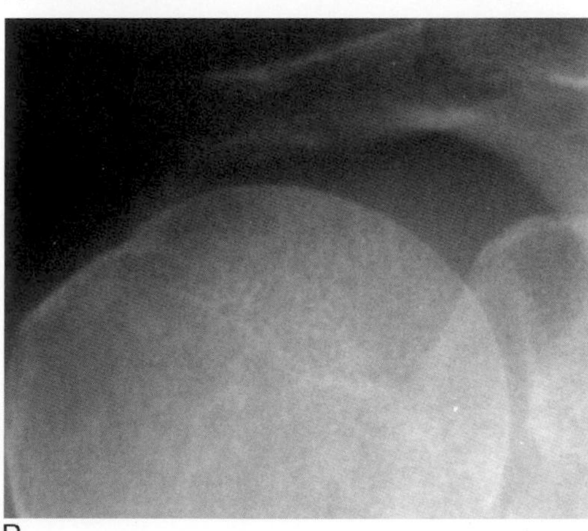
B

Figure 50.15 Calcific peritendonosis of the supraspinatus tendon. (A) At presentation there is a dense area of amorphous calcification (arrow) seen projected over the tendon. (B) Three weeks later, the calcification has largely been dispersed or been reabsorbed.

Haemochromatosis

Haemochromatosis is a chronic disease of iron overload in which excess iron is deposited in parenchymal tissues. It may be an acquired condition, or may be inherited secondary to a deficiency of hepatic xanthine oxidase. The male to female ratio is 10:1 and it usually occurs in the 40–60-year-old age group. The classic findings clinically are liver cirrhosis and 'bronze diabetes'. Radiologically, the findings are diffuse osteoporosis, chondrocalcinosis and a distinct arthropathy. The arthropathy occurs in the hands where symmetrical changes are seen at the index and middle finger metacarpophalangeal joints. The findings are joint space narrowing, well-defined 1–3 mm subarticular cysts and erosions, 'hook-like' osteophytes from the medial aspects of the heads of the metacarpals, sclerosis and irregularity of the articular surface, subluxation and flattening and widening of metacarpal heads (Fig. 50.16).

Ochronosis (alkaptonuria)

Alkaptonuria is a rare inborn error of metabolism which results from the congenital absence of the enzyme homogentisic acid oxidase; this results in an error in the tyrosine pathway, and the polymer homogentisic acid is excreted in the urine in excess. Homogentisic acid also accumulates in the soft tissues and the deposited material is coloured black (ochronosis). Affected articular cartilage becomes brittle leading to severe early degenerative change. The peak incidence of the arthropathy is in the 5th decade; men are twice as commonly affected as women. Spine involvement leading to spondylosis is more common than peripheral arthropathy and the lumbar region is often initially affected, followed by the thoracic and cervical spine. Intervertebral disc space narrowing occurs with dense calcification from associated calcium hydroxyapatite deposition. Diffuse osteoporosis results, and kyphosis and scoliosis may occur. The apophyseal joints are not involved. The shoulders, hips and knees are occasionally affected, in which case severe destruction can follow, but the other peripheral joints are rarely involved.

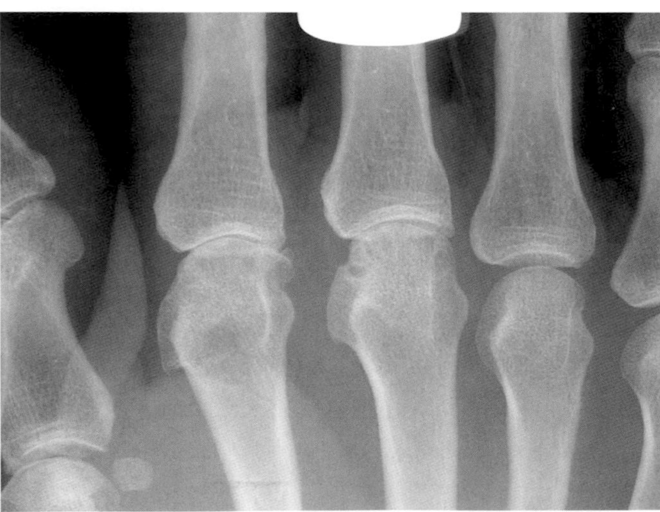

Figure 50.16 Haemochromatosis. Joint space narrowing is seen affecting specifically the MCP joints of the second and third digits with well-defined 1–3 mm subarticular cysts and erosions, hook-like osteophytes and articular surface irregularity.

Dialysis arthropathy

A wide variety of disorders can affect the musculoskeletal system in patients receiving long-term haemodialysis, either as a result of the treatment or as a result of the underlying condition. Septic arthritis and osteomyelitis, pseudogout, acute calcific polyarthritis, haemarthrosis and amyloid deposition have all been reported.

POLYARTHRITIS ASSOCIATED WITH OTHER DISEASES

Systemic lupus erythematosus

Systemic lupus erythematosus (SLE) is a systemic autoimmune disease characterized by production of antibodies directed against the cell nucleus and/or its components. The diagnosis is based on the presence of 4 out of 11 clinical or laboratory criteria[26]. Arthritis represents one of these criteria, and forms the basis of radiological diagnosis. The condition affects the hands, wrists and knees in a symmetrical fashion most commonly, and is characterized by an undulating course with exacerbations and remissions. Joint effusions are uncommon, and plain radiographs in these patients are frequently normal. The characteristic radiological findings are seen in the hands. Soft tissue atrophy is severe with concave rather than convex margins to the thenar and hypothenar borders and osteoporosis which may be periarticular or diffuse in distribution. Severe disease leads to subluxation and dislocation, in the absence of erosions. Indeed the hallmark sign is that of ulnar deviation at the MCP joint in the absence of erosions, with reversibility. This reversibility explains the observation that patients with ulnar deviation clinically may appear normal radiologically as the fingers are pushed back into their correct place at the time of radiographic exposure. Generalized osteopenia is more common and may be worsened by steroid therapy.

Scleroderma

Scleroderma or progressive systemic sclerosis is a systemic connective tissue disease characterized by excessive deposition of collagen in soft tissues that can result in fibrosis of the skin as well as of internal organs. Variations include the CREST syndrome, which is a combination of calcinosis, Raynaud's phenomenon, oesophageal dysmotility, sclerodactyly, and telangiectasia and Thibierge–Weissenbach syndrome, which is characterized by calcinosis and digital ischaemia. Scleroderma is also commonly accompanied by Raynaud's phenomenon in the absence of other features.

Radiologically, scleroderma is characterized in the hands by progressive soft tissue atrophy, terminal phalangeal resorption and soft tissue calcinosis (Fig. 50.17). These calcifications may be periarticular or may occur at the fingertips. Contractures and generalized osteopenia are frequently seen, and although bone erosions are uncommon, 'pencil-in-cup' deformities of the DIP joints have been described. Erosions at the distal ulna and radius may also be seen and occasionally subcutaneous, ligamentous, periarticular or intra-articular calcification may occur.

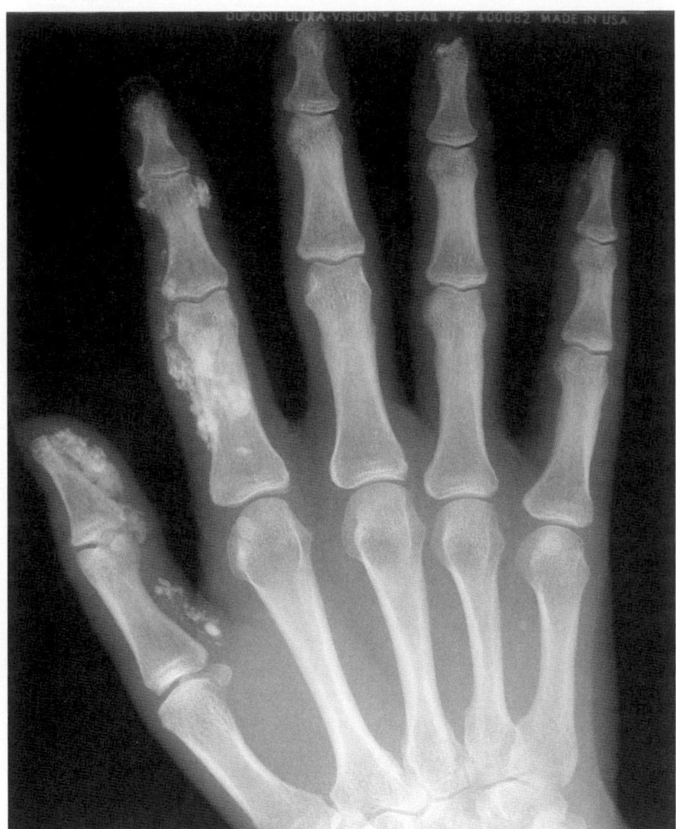

Figure 50.17 Scleroderma. There is soft tissue atrophy, particularly over the terminal tufts, with extensive soft tissue calcinosis, both along the shafts of several phalanges and also related to the terminal tuft of the fourth and fifth digits.

Mixed connective tissue disease

This is considered to be a specific syndrome combining features of scleroderma, polymyositis, rheumatoid arthritis and SLE. Patients with this 'overlap syndrome' possess an antinuclear antibody that reacts with ribonuclease-sensitive extractable nuclear antigen. Arthritis has been reported in over 75% of these patients although radiologically the features are variable. In the hands, osteoporosis, both periarticular and diffuse, soft tissue swelling and marginal erosions may be seen, together with flexion deformities, subluxation and marked ulnar deviation of the phalanges. Resorption of the terminal phalanges, soft tissue atrophy and calcification can simulate scleroderma. Large joint involvement is rare.

Jaccoud's arthritis

Jaccoud's arthritis uncommonly follows rheumatic fever and results in a severe nondestructive symmetrical polyarthropathy in the hands, associated with ulnar deviation that is reversible in the early stages. The bone is typically not involved, although erosions may follow in some cases. 'Hook-like' projections and pseudocysts at the radiopalmar aspects of the metacarpal heads may occur rarely, but only late in the disease, when contractures have also been found to occur.

Hypertrophic pulmonary osteoarthropathy

Hypertrophic pulmonary osteoarthropathy (HPOA) is a triad of periosteal new bone formation, painful clubbing of the fingers and synovitis. It was first recognized as an association with bronchogenic carcinoma, bronchiectasis and other chronic lung infections, pleural mesothelioma and cyanotic heart disease, but it has subsequently been seen in association with other conditions including ulcerative colitis, Crohn's disease and biliary cirrhosis.

Clubbing, periostitis and arthralgia may all be present or may occur in various combinations and in various order of appearance. Finger clubbing is the result of fibroelastic proliferation in the nail bed leading to thickening of the skin and subcutaneous tissues of the digits. When associated with bronchogenic carcinoma, the onset may be acute, and may be accompanied by hyperhydrosis. Synovitis occurs in over 30% of patients, and may be the presenting feature. The fingers are stiff, swollen and painful, and clinically the condition can resemble rheumatoid arthritis. Periosteal new bone formation and cortical thickening affects tubular bones and is evident in the diaphyses and metaphyses, with sparing of the epiphyses. In decreasing order of frequency, the following bones are most commonly affected: the radius and ulna, the tibia and fibula, the humerus and femur, metacarpals and metatarsals, proximal and middle phalanges. Long-standing periostitis results in cortical thickening.

Pachydermoperiostosis is generally regarded as the primary or idiopathic form of HPOA. It accounts for up to 5% of cases and has autosomal dominant transmission. It occurs predominantly in black men and is characterized by finger clubbing, generalized pachydermia including characteristic deep furrows of the face of the skin and scalp (cutis verticis gyrata) and excessive sweating. The coarse facies and enlargement of the extremities can produce a picture similar to acromegaly, but the growth hormone levels are normal and no pituitary tumour is present. Marrow failure due to endosteal cortical thickening resulting in reduced medullary haematopoiesis has been described[27].

Sarcoidosis

Sarcoidosis is a generalized systemic disease of unknown aetiology characterized by granulomatous changes in the skin, lungs, lymph nodes and viscera. Bone involvement occurs in approximately 10% of patients at some time during the course of the disease. The diagnosis is most commonly made on chest radiograph where lymphadenopathy and associated pulmonary fibrosis may be seen.

Radiologically, the bones most commonly affected are the distal and middle phalanges of the hands and feet; metacarpals and metatarsals are less commonly involved. Three patterns of bone involvement are described and they may co-exist (Fig. 50.18). (1) In diffuse sarcoidosis, the tubular bone is widened and there is a reticular or honeycomb appearance to the spongiosa, together with loss of definition between the cortex and medulla. (2) In circumscribed sarcoidosis, punched-out cyst-like lesions up to 5 mm in diameter are seen. (3) In mutilating sarcoidosis, the punched-out areas may coalesce forming larger areas of destruction. This is rare.

Multicentric reticulohistiocytosis

Multicentric reticulohistiocytosis (lipoid dermatoarthritis) is a rare disease of unknown aetiology in which cutaneous

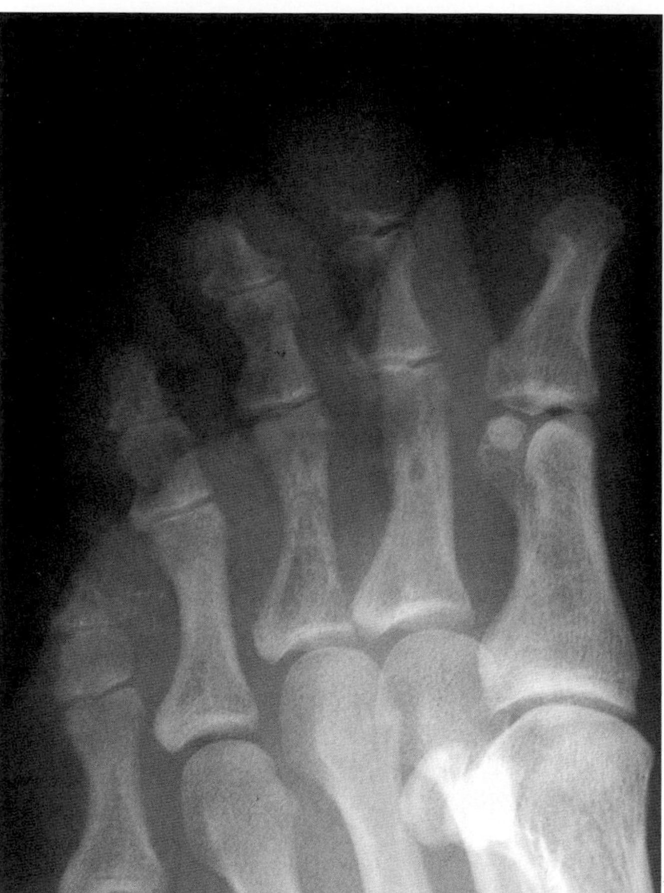

Figure 50.18 Sarcoidosis of bone. There is widening of the proximal phalanx of the second digit with a reticular or honeycomb appearance to the spongiosa of the proximal phalanges of the second and third digits, associated with areas of destruction particularly affecting the distal phalanx and the distal portions of the proximal and middle phalanges of the second digit. These are associated with soft tissue swelling.

xanthomas are associated with erosive arthritis leading to severe deformities. The disease is characterized by soft tissue infiltration by giant multinucleated vacuolated histiocytes. Articular disease is symmetrical and rapidly progressive, and usually predates the skin nodules. Radiologically, marginal erosions are seen with articular and subchondral bone destruction with little accompanying osteoporosis. The distal interphalangeal joints of the hands and feet show early involvement and the interphalangeal joints and carpal joints are usually involved before the metacarpophalangeal joints. Unremitting progression to arthritis mutilans is common. Other joints involved include the shoulder, elbow, wrist and hip, and in the cervical spine destruction and atlantoaxial subluxation is an expected feature.

Dermatomyositis/polymyositis

Polymyositis is an inflammatory condition of unknown aetiology that affects striated muscle. When it is accompanied by dermatological features, it is termed dermatomyositis. The age distribution is bimodal, with the condition occurring in children and the elderly. The disease is characterized by soft tissue oedema and atrophy in the acute stage, and subcutaneous or intermuscular fascial plane calcification developing during the healing phase. In chronic cases, flexion contractures present, and these can be severe. Steroid administration or limb disuse leads to osteopenia and fractures. Bone erosions are not a feature of these diseases.

Enteropathic arthropathies

Clinically, up to 10% of patients with ulcerative colitis and regional enteritis (Crohn's disease) have associated arthritis. Sacroiliitis and spondylitis identical to ankylosing spondylitis predominate and may precede the presentation of bowel disease, although usually the bowel disease precedes the arthropathy. Approximately 60% of patients are positive for the HLA-B27 antigen. Radiologically, the disease manifests as either a central or peripheral type. The two types co-exist in only a minority of patients. The central type mimics ankylosing spondylitis with syndesmophyte formation, which can be pronounced. In the peripheral form, the hands, wrists and feet may be involved with reduced periarticular osteopenia and joint space narrowing, and bouts of recurrent acute mild synovitis that coincide with exacerbations of bowel disease.

Peripheral arthritis tends to resolve after colectomy but central arthritis appears to be more independent of the underlying bowel disease. Whipple's disease may also be associated with arthritis occasionally, presenting as a migratory arthritis or arthralgia, sacroiliitis, erythema nodosum and uveitis in some patients.

Amyloid arthropathy

Radiological findings are periarticular osteoporosis and nodular soft tissue masses. Multiple erosions and subchondral intraosseous cysts are seen which may lead to pathological fracture. Joint space narrowing is not an expected feature and involvement is often bilateral and symmetrical. Large peripheral joints are most commonly involved.

Infectious arthritis

Infectious arthritis can result from bacterial, viral, fungal, parasitic and other infections and is considered in detail in Chapter 51. Infection, however, can co-exist with any one of the arthropathies mentioned in this chapter, and the presence of infection will make the diagnosis more difficult. A sudden worsening of symptoms or rapid joint or bony destruction should raise the possibility of a superadded infection and prompt an early diagnostic aspiration for culture. As infection is a differential diagnosis in any patient with monoarthritis, prompt aspiration for culture and microscopy is typically performed in any patient who presents with a monoarthropathy.

SYNOVIAL METAPLASIA AND NEOPLASIA

Pigmented villonodular synovitis

Pigmented villonodular synovitis (PVNS) is an uncommon disorder resulting from proliferation of the synovium of joints, bursae and tendons, most commonly affecting young adults. Patients present with intermittent pain and swelling of a joint, and typically the entire synovium is affected diffusely, although a localized form can also exist, particularly in the knee[28]. Erosion of bone occurs in approximately 50% of affected patients: cyst-like defects of varying sizes are present which show up sclerotic margins. In the hip, the erosions can lead to narrowing of the femoral neck (Fig. 50.19).

The disease may affect the synovium of a tendon sheath, in which case the condition is termed giant cell tumour of tendon sheath. Soft tissue calcification and osteophytes are not a feature of this condition. Repeated haemarthrosis is a common accompaniment and the resulting haemosiderin deposition accounts for the low signal intensity on T2/T2*-weighted images with MRI, particularly gradient-echo sequences, where the areas of haemosiderin deposition are seen to 'bloom'. Before the advent of MRI, it often took many years to make the diagnosis of PVNS, due to the nonspecific clinical presentation and slow progression of the condition.

Synovial (osteo-)chondromatosis

In this condition, metaplasia occurs in the subsynovial connective tissue in synovial joints and bursae, and rarely in tendon sheaths. The cartilage fragments that form become detached and float freely within the joint or bursal cavity (chondromatosis), where they are nourished by synovial fluid and grow.

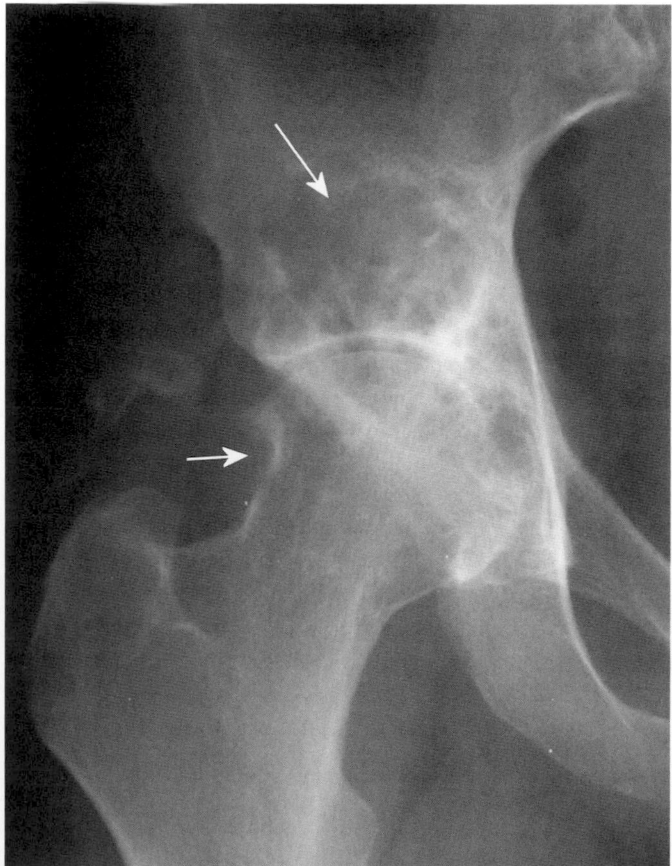

Figure 50.19 Pigmented villonodular synovitis (PVNS). In this advanced case, erosions are seen (arrows) on both sides of the joint, and are particularly large in the acetabulum. Along the femoral neck, erosion is maximal at the site of capsular insertion.

The cartilage eventually becomes calcified or ossified (osteochondromatosis). The condition is typically monoarticular, occurring in young or middle-aged adults; it is rare in children. The disease may be classified as primary, if no underlying cause is identified, or secondary to trauma, degenerative disease or inflammatory disease.

The most frequent sites of involvement are the knee, hip, elbow and shoulder. The characteristic finding is one of multiple small calcified loose bodies. In the early stages, before the nodules are calcified, plain radiographs will not detect the nodules themselves, but may show diffuse swelling.

Later, mineralization of the nodules produces multiple opacities with flecks of calcification and bony trabeculae. The presence of calcification can be confirmed on arthrography or ultrasound early in the condition but MRI and CT or CT arthrography are most commonly used to confirm the diagnosis. The presence of numerous similarly sized intra-articular ossicles in the absence of joint space narrowing helps to differentiate synovial osteochondromatosis from loose bodies associated with degenerative joint disease.

ARTHROGRAPHY

The use of diagnostic arthrography has reduced significantly wherever MRI is available. It remains a well-accepted special radiological procedure for evaluation of joint disease, and forms the basis of MR and CT arthrography. It is an effective safe technique for demonstrating the internal surfaces of diarthrodial joints and the technique can also be used to deliver steroid injections directly into the joint. It may prove to have a future benefit in the injection of viscosupplementation agents, such as hyaluronic acid, used in the management of patients with OA. Diagnostic shoulder arthrography still has a place in evaluation of patients with frozen shoulder where reduction in joint volume and lymphatic filling can be useful to demonstrate the tight joint (Fig. 50.20).

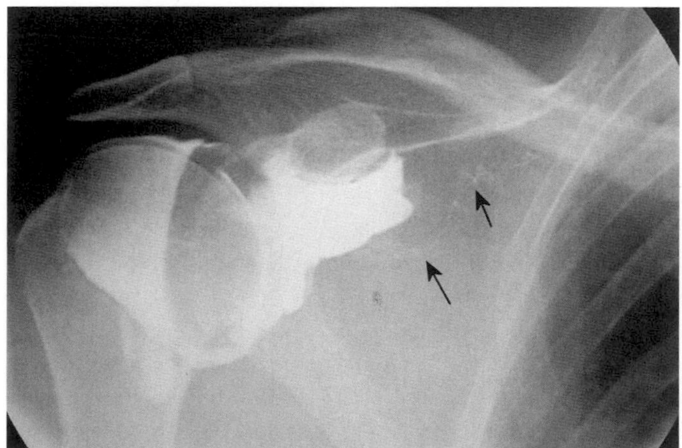

Figure 50.20 Capsulitis. At the time of shoulder arthrography, only 5 ml of contrast material could be injected into the joint before the patient found the injection uncomfortable, and the post-injection appearances confirm the presence of an obliterated axillary recess. Contrast has escaped into the lymphatics (arrows).

DIFFERENTIAL DIAGNOSIS OF JOINT DISEASE BASED ON THE RADIOLOGICAL FEATURES

Table 50.7 summarizes the clinical and radiological hallmarks of the more common degenerative and inflammatory joint diseases.

JOINT DISEASES AT SPECIFIC SITES

In addition to general arthritic conditions that may affect one of any number of different joints, there are certain conditions that have a predilection for a specific joint. In this section these conditions are explored together with the best imaging approach.

Hip

Avascular necrosis

Avascular necrosis (AVN) may affect any bone, but the commonest site of involvement is the femoral head. Many causes for this condition have been reported. In the elderly, the commonest cause relates to previous subcapital fracture of the femoral neck, but nontraumatic causes predominate in younger patients where the condition is commonly bilateral. The precise aetiology of atraumatic AVN is poorly understood. MRI has been demonstrated to be more sensitive than either CT or skeletal scintigraphy in the detection of early AVN[29]. Additional associated features can also be diagnosed on MRI (bone marrow oedema, articular cartilage damage and joint effusion). The conventional system for staging involves radiological and clinical aspects[30]. In the earliest stage (stage 0) the patient is asymptomatic and the condition is only diagnosed incidentally when the contralateral symptomatic avascular hip is being assessed. There are no plain radiographic changes at this stage, but bone marrow oedema within the femoral head can be demonstrated on MRI. It is the demonstration of asymptomatic contralateral avascular necrosis that necessitates the imaging of both hips when AVN is suspected.

In stage I disease, the trabeculae appear normal, and any osteoporosis is minor. More diffuse osteoporosis or subsequent sclerosis indicates stage II disease. By this stage, the infarct is distinguished from the normal bone by a shell of reactive tissue. In both these stages, the femoral head remains spherical. On MRI, the osteonecrotic lesion demonstrates varying signal characteristics depending on the severity and duration of avascularity[31]. In 80% of cases, a 'double line'[31] indicates the demarcation between normal and abnormal bone; this has been shown to be related to chemical shift effects. In stage III disease, the femoral head loses its spherical shape, although on plain radiographs this may only be visible on the lateral view. On MRI, a subchondral fracture is demonstrated as a low signal line paralleling the subarticular cortex and is of low signal intensity on all sequences. This precedes overt collapse of the femoral head. The joint space remains normal. The femoral head undergoes further collapse in stage IV disease which will lead to destruction of the cartilage and reduction in the joint space (Fig. 50.21).

Legg–Calvé–Perthes disease is a specific condition of unknown aetiology represented by AVN occurring without a recognized previous insult in children. Most common between 4 and 9 years, it must be a differential diagnosis in any child presenting with a painful limp and must be differentiated from an irritable hip or infective arthritis.

Transient osteoporosis of the hip

This is an uncommon condition that was initially thought to be found exclusively in women in their third trimester of pregnancy. It has now been described in men as well as in non-pregnant women. The cause remains unknown. The disease is self-limiting although it may take several months to resolve, and while the disease is active the patient complains of a hip pain. Plain radiographic findings are confined to regional osteoporosis and this is matched on MRI by a reduction in signal on T1 weighting within the femoral head, with a concomitant increase in signal on T2 weighting. The appearances are therefore of nonspecific bone marrow oedema, and the differential diagnosis includes early avascular necrosis, infiltration (e.g. malignancy), infection or trauma.

Iliopsoas bursitis

The commonest bursa around the hip to give rise to a soft tissue mass is the iliopsoas bursa, which communicates with the joint in 15% of individuals. It is interposed between the iliopsoas muscle and the anterior hip capsule, lateral to the femoral vessels. It is present as a collapsed structure in 98% of normal individuals but may become enlarged by any process that increases intra-articular fluid pressure such as osteoarthritis and rheumatoid arthritis. The clinical features are variable and include pain and swelling or femoral neuropathy due to pressure on the adjacent femoral nerve (Fig. 50.22). Other bursae in this region which can be symptomatic are those related to the ischial tuberosity and the greater trochanter.

Labral tears

Labral tears present with pain and clicking, often associated with a decreased range of motion. They are best evaluated with MRI. The normal labrum appears as a triangular structure seen best on coronal and sagittal images, returning low signal on both T1- and T2-weighted imaging sequences. Fat-saturated fast spin-echo (FSE) proton-density (PD) or T2* GE sequences with a small field of view (18 cm) and a surface coil can be useful to demonstrate tears within the labrum, although hip MR arthrography or even arthroscopy may be needed to achieve satisfactory results[32].

Slipped upper femoral epiphysis

Slipped upper femoral epiphysis (SUFE) can occur acutely or chronically in adolescent and young children. The slip is usually posterior, and therefore is best demonstrated on a frog leg lateral rather than an AP radiograph. Secondary avascular necrosis within the femoral head, which subsequently develops in 15% of individuals, can be detected by MRI at an early presymptomatic stage.

Knee

Meniscal degeneration and tears

The ability of the femur to rotate relative to a fixed tibia during flexion and extension puts the menisci at particular risk

Table 50.7 CLINICAL AND RADIOLOGICAL FINDINGS IN ARTHRITIS

Condition	Site of involvement	Discriminatory findings
Primary osteoarthritis (F>M, >45 years)	Hands	PIP/DIP involvement (Heberden's and Bouchard's nodes)
	Large joints, e.g. hip, knee	Joint space narrowing
		Subchondral sclerosis
		Subchondral cysts
		Marginal osteophytes
	Spine	Degenerative disc disease
		Spondylosis deformans
		Apophyseal joint involvement
		Spinal stenosis
		Foraminal stenosis
Erosive osteoarthritis (F; middle age)	Hands	PIP/DIP involvement
		Joint ankylosis
		Gull-wing deformities
		Heberden's nodes
Rheumatoid arthritis (F>M; Rh factor positive)	Hand and wrist	MCP/PIP involvement
		Periarticular osteoporosis
		Marginal erosions
		Subluxation: swan-neck and boutonnière deformity, hitchhiker's thumb
	Large joints, e.g. hip	Joint space narrowing
		Marginal erosions
		Synovial cysts
		Protrusio acetabulae
	Spine	Atlantoaxial subluxation
Juvenile idiopathic arthritis (M=F; children)	Hands	Joint ankylosis
		Periosteal reaction
	Large joints	Abnormalities of growth and maturation
	Cervical spine	Apophyseal joint fusion
		Atlantoaxial subluxation
Psoriatic arthritis (M>F; nail changes. HLA-B27 positive)	Hands and feet	Sausage digit
		DIPJ involvement
		Erosion of terminal tufts
		Pencil-in-cup deformities
		Joint ankylosis
		Periosteal reaction
		Preserved mineral density
	Sacroiliac joints	Asymmetric or unilateral sacroiliitis
	Spine	Coarse syndesmophytes
Reiter's syndrome (M, young adult)	Foot	Predominance of hallux involvement
		Erosions of calcaneum
	Spine	Coarse syndesmophytes
	Sacroiliac joints	Asymmetric or unilateral sacroiliitis
Ankylosing spondylitis (M>F; young adult. HLA-B27 positive in 95%)	Sacroiliac joints	Bilateral symmetrical sacroiliitis
		Ankylosis
	Spine	Anterior vertebral body squaring
		Syndesmophytes
		Paravertebral ossification
		Bamboo spine
	Pelvis	'Whiskering' of iliac crests and ischial tuberosity

Continued

Table 50.7 Cont'd CLINICAL AND RADIOLOGICAL FINDINGS IN ARTHRITIS

Condition	Site of involvement	Discriminatory findings
Enteropathic arthropathies	Sacroiliac joints	Symmetrical sacroiliitis
Gout (M>F)	Hands and feet, especially	Especially MTP joint of great toe
	great toe	Juxta-articular erosion, overhanging margin
		No periarticular osteoporosis
		Tophi
	Large joints	Erosion, overhanging margin
CPPD crystal deposition disease (M=F)	Any peripheral joint, predilection for the knee	Degenerative changes with chondrocalcinosis. Often bilateral
		Paucity of subchondral sclerosis
HA crystal deposition disease (F>M)	Predilection for shoulder	Periarticular calcification
	(supraspinatus tendon)	2nd and 3rd MCP involvement
Haemochromatosis (M>F)	Hands	Joint space narrowing
		Numerous subchondral cysts
		'Hook-like' osteophytes
Alkaptonuria (ochronosis) (M=F)	Intervertebral discs, sacroiliac	Disc calcification
	joints, large joints	Joint space narrowing
		Periarticular sclerosis
		Reversible MCP subluxation
Systemic lupus erythematosus (F>M, young adults)	Hands	IP joint arthritis
Scleroderma (F>M, adults)	Hands	Soft tissue calcifications
		Acro-osteolysis
Mixed connective tissue disease (overlap syndrome)	Hands	PIP, MCP, mid-carpal involvement
		Soft tissue swelling, calcifications or atrophy
Multicentric reticulohistiocytosis (F>M)	Hands and feet	IP joint involvement
		Soft tissue swelling
		Articular erosions
		Lack of osteoporosis
Polymyositis/dermatomyositis	Proximal extremities	Soft tissue calcification
	Hands	DIP joint erosions

of injury. Meniscal damage was traditionally evaluated with arthrography but MRI is now used almost exclusively. The intact meniscus demonstrates homogeneous low signal intensity on all pulse sequences, and degeneration or tears will result in increased signal within the meniscus, which is due to imbibed synovial fluid. The imbibed water molecules interact with large macromolecules within the meniscus, resulting in an alteration of both T1 and T2 values. Meniscal degeneration and tears are therefore apparent on T2, PD and T1 weighted sequences. In the earliest stages, such degeneration is represented on MR by focal or globular intrasubstance areas of increased signal intensity, which correlates histologically to foci of mucinous degeneration and chondrocyte-deficient or hypocellular lesions which have been termed interchangeably mucinous, myxoid or hyaline degeneration. In the past this change was erroneously called a 'grade I' tear of the meniscus, but it is clear that these changes can be observed in asymptomatic individuals, particularly athletes, and it is not considered a clinically significant finding.

Sometimes horizontal clefts of high signal are seen. These were originally termed 'grade II' tears. However, these extend to the capsular periphery of the meniscus not the articular surface. Although histologically these appearances correlate with a fissure within the substance of the meniscus, the 'tear' is not apparent arthroscopically as the meniscal surface is intact, and commonly these findings do not correlate with symptoms. However, it is considered that 'type II' changes predispose to subsequent meniscal tear, particularly when the posterior third of the medial meniscus is involved[33]. In the more advanced tears, the area of increased signal intensity, which is commonly linear, extends to one or more articular surfaces. Histologically, these appearances correlate with fibrocartilaginous separation or tears although, arthroscopically, approximately 5% of these 'grade III' meniscal tears correlate to what has been described in the orthopaedic literature as confined intrasubstance cleavage tears which require surgical probing during arthroscopy to diagnose, and which may be missed on conventional arthrography. Clinically the patient presents with pain, with or without knee locking.

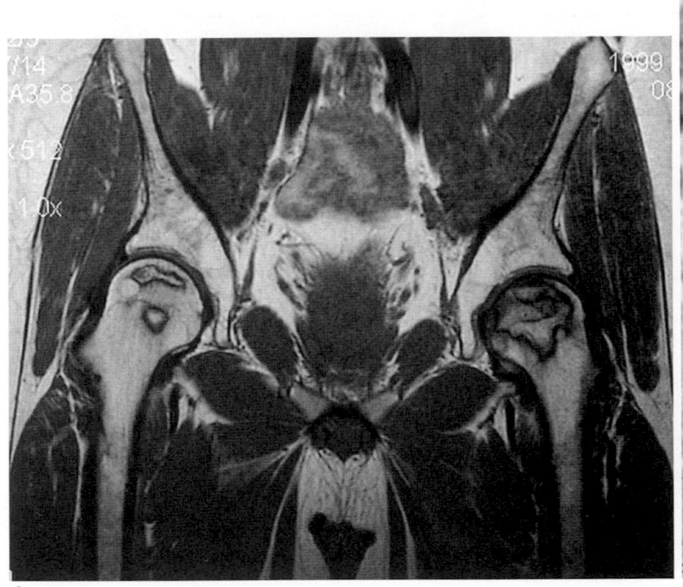

A

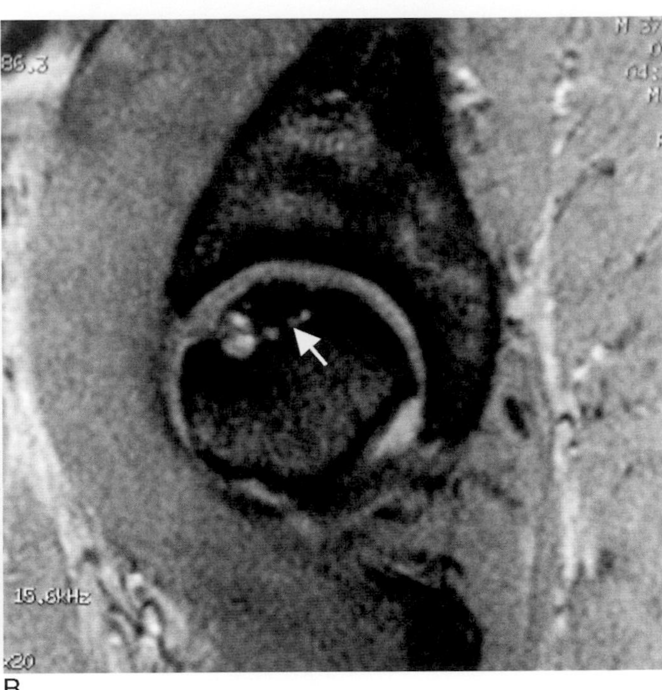

B

Figure 50.21 Avascular necrosis of the hip. (A) Coronal T1-weighted MR image through both hips confirms the presence of geographic areas of abnormality in both femoral heads which are well demarcated from the adjacent normal bone by a thin rim of low signal material. High signal within each abnormal area indicates viable fat. (B) Gradient-echo sagittal image demonstrates the osteochondral fragment, with fluid between the fragment and the parent bone (arrow) suggesting that the fragment itself is loose.

One particular type of tear is the bucket handle tear, which results when the free edge at the site of a vertical tear becomes dislodged and displaced within the joint. In the earliest stages, the torn free edge remains attached at either end of its length, but one or both of these attachments may become broken resulting in the fragment of fibrocartilage becoming loose within the joint. It commonly migrates to the intercondylar notch region (Fig. 50.23), but as with all loose bodies, it may appear anywhere within the joint. The medial meniscus is more often involved, and patients may present with a painful locked knee or lack the ability for full extension.

Figure 50.22 Iliopsoas bursa. A fluid-containing structure is seen to rise anterior to the left hip on a T2-weighted sequence in this patient with a hip effusion. The communication with the underlying joint via a neck lateral to the iliopsoas tendon is well demonstrated (arrows).

Meniscocapsular separations

Meniscocapsular separations or tears are more common in the medial meniscus, especially posteriorly, and result from damage to the meniscotibial or coronary ligaments. Even in the absence of 'type III' changes within the meniscus, such meniscocapsular separation can result in pain. Tears in excess of 1 cm commonly do not repair naturally, and require surgical intervention. On sagittal MR, the medial meniscus is displaced anteriorly resulting in excess of 5 mm of articular cartilage posteriorly being 'uncovered'. Unfortunately, however, the quantitative measurement of meniscal displacement may be unreliable. Furthermore, there is increasing interest in and recognition of the variability of the normal extent of meniscal movement. The diagnosis of a complete peripheral detachment of the posterior third is more reliable: it is seen as a free-floating meniscus, commonly associated with a medial collateral ligament tear.

Anterior cruciate ligament disruption

The anterior cruciate ligament (ACL) can be damaged by a variety of different mechanisms, and is particularly vulnerable after the collateral ligaments have been torn. Common to all forms of injury is rotation of the femur on the tibia at the time of injury, commonly associated with varus or valgus stress. For this reason, it is unusual for an ACL injury to exist in isolation and, in particular, meniscal tears are involved in up to 68% of acute injuries or in up to 91% of chronic ACL-deficient

Figure 50.23 Bucket handle tear. (A) Sagittal GE MR image shows an elongated structure of reduced signal within the intercondylar notch. (B) Corresponding coronal PD image shows the structure in cross section. The structure represents a large fragment of medial meniscus that has become detached and has moved into the intercondylar notch.

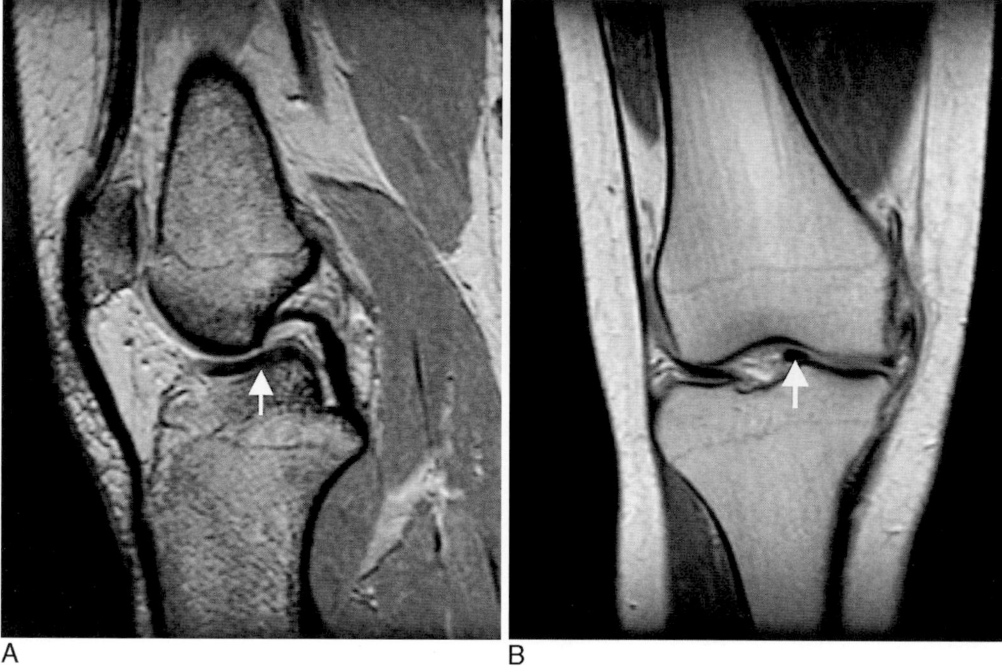

knees[34]. Collateral ligament injury is also a common accompanying finding, but may predate the ACL injury.

Acute ACL tears may be associated with an audible click at the time of injury[34] and the patient usually presents with a painful knee associated with acute haemarthrosis. A positive draw sign implies that the anteromedial band of the ACL must be disrupted, but commonly is also associated with disruption of the medial capsule. When the ACL tear is isolated, the classic anterior draw sign may be falsely negative.

The normal ACL is represented as one or more bands of low signal intensity, and the separate fibre bundles can be distinguished near the point of attachment, due to the interposition of fat between them. In a complete tear of the ACL, discontinuity in the low signal band is present (Fig. 50.24). Partial or incomplete disruptions may be associated with attenuation of some fascicles, which may appear indistinct due to adjacent oedema and haemorrhage. Secondary signs associated with ACL tear include a bunching up of

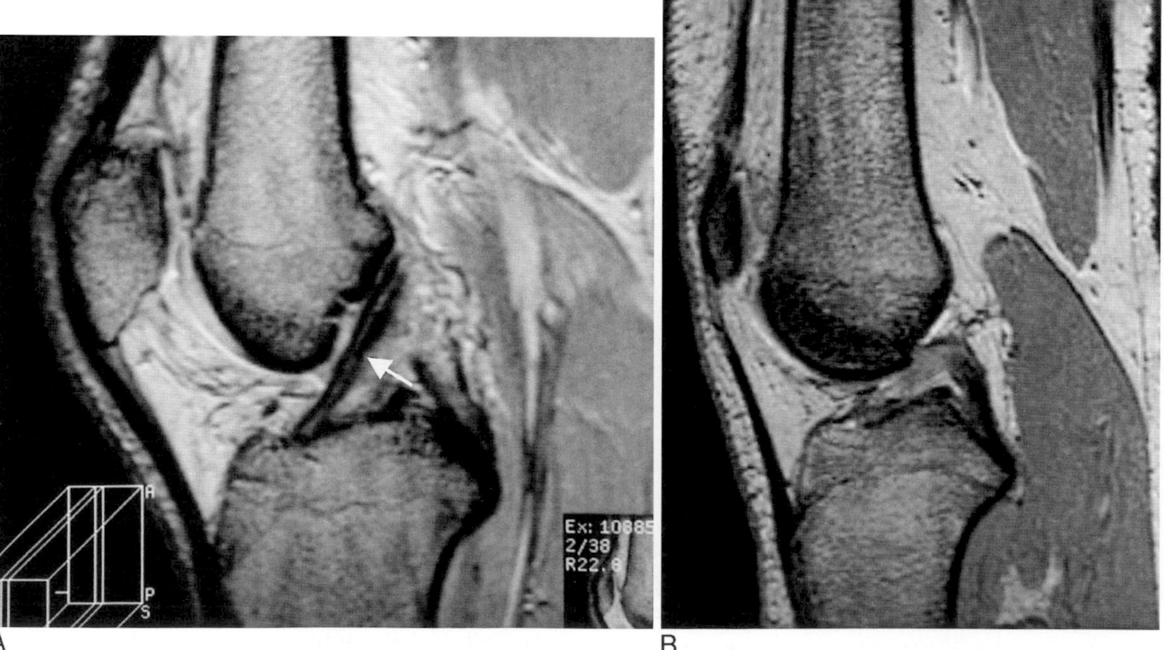

Figure 50.24 (A) Normal anterior cruciate ligament comprised of separate antero-medial and posterolateral bundles. (B) Sagittal GE image through the intercondylar region fails to demonstrate any normal anterior cruciate ligament indicating a chronic complete ACL rupture.

the posterior cruciate ligament, anterior translation of the femur on the tibial condyles and a wavy patellar ligament, although none of these signs in itself is specific. Absence of the ACL in both sagittal and coronal planes is diagnostic for ACL tear and the accuracy of MR in detecting ACL rupture is in excess of 95%. The anterior displacement of the tibia on the lateral sagittal images is a secondary sign but it is dependent on the degree of knee flexion. Another association of an acute ACL tear is the presence of a bony ligamentous avulsion of the meniscotibial portion of the middle third of the lateral capsule ligament. Additionally, fracture or bone bruising involving the posterolateral tibial plateau (Segond fracture) and lateral femoral condyle has been shown to be a relatively specific sign of an acute complete ACL tear[35], present in more than 90% of such injuries. This association of trabecular bone contusion is attributed to impingement of the lateral femoral condyle on the posterior tibia during either the initial rotatory subluxation or the subsequent lateral femoral condyle recoil.

The treatment of ACL injury is often conservative but may involve a primary repair or reconstruction. Repair is preferred when the tear is at either tibial or femoral attachment, and avulsion of an associated bony fragment is associated with a particularly good prognosis. Mid-substance interstitial tears are not good candidates for primary repair and ligamentous reconstruction is commonly preferred. A variety of surgical approaches have been described involving autogenous, allograft, xenograft and synthetic tissues. The radiologist is increasingly commonly asked to reassess the ACL postoperatively, and the images will need to be interpreted in the light of the surgical approach used. Sagittal oblique images parallel to the reconstructed ligament may allow visualization of the entire course of the reconstructed ACL, and recurrent tears of the ligament may be visualized directly (Fig. 50.25). More commonly, however, anterior translation of the tibia together with buckling of the PCL is a useful sign to indicate abnormal laxity of the reconstructed ACL, even in the absence of an interstitial tear. A further association exists between the slope of the intercondylar roof and the line of the tibial tunnel. If the tunnel lies anterior to the intercondylar notch then the tendon is at risk of impingement, which may be a cause of continuing symptoms.

Posterior cruciate ligament disruption

Rupture of the posterior cruciate ligament (PCL) may be caused either by excessive rotation or hyperextension or possibly by direct trauma when the knee is flexed. Isolated tears of the PCL are uncommon, and associated ACL meniscal or collateral ligament damage is usual. The patient presents with pain and locking, and a positive posterior draw sign may be present in only 60% of cases. As opposed to ACL tears, the mid-portion of the PCL is most commonly involved when torn (76%).

The PCL is seen on axial and sagittal images as a low signal intensity structure on all sequences, and the delineation of the PCL is not as sensitive to the position as that of the ACL. Increased signal within this structure focally on T1- or T2-weighted images should be interpreted as abnormal. Acute injuries may be associated with adjacent haemorrhage or oedema, which should result in an increase in signal of the adjacent tissues on T2-weighted images. A complete tear is represented as a discontinuity in the PCL, and is a straightforward MR diagnosis (Fig. 50.26). Partial tears and chronic tears where fibrous scarring is present can be more difficult to diagnose, particularly in the unusual situation where the PCL injury is isolated. Magic angle effect should be considered when signal change in the PCL is the only abnormality (see below).

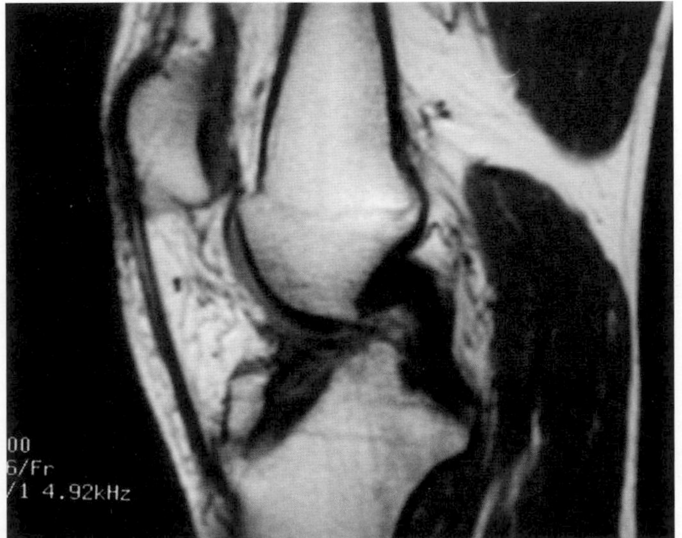

Figure 50.25 Torn reconstructed ACL. Sagittal T1-weighted MR image shows the tunnel for the reconstructed ACL. In the intercondylar notch, however, the reconstructed ligament is absent, and there is posterior translation of the femur on the tibia confirming that the ligament is completely torn.

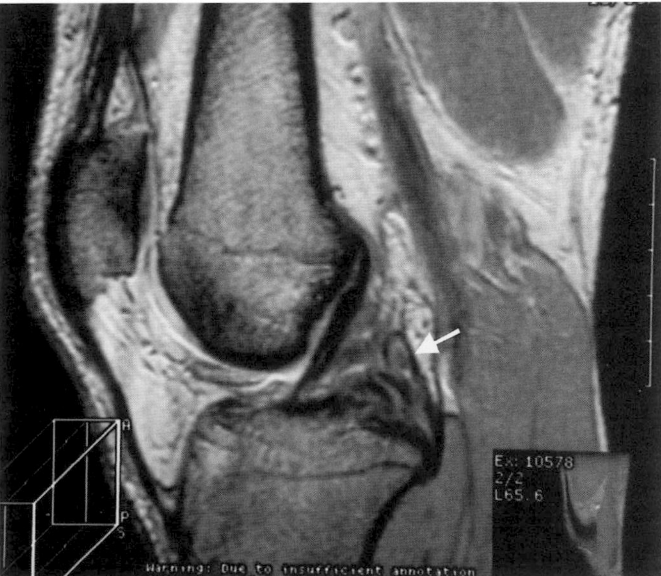

Figure 50.26 Torn PCL. The ACL in this individual is intact, but the PCL is torn from its proximal attachment (arrow).

Collateral ligaments

The medial collateral ligament (MCL) is injured with excess valgus force applied to a flexed knee. Sprains and partial ruptures involve the fibrous attachment of the ligament to the medial femoral condyle. Complete ruptures, however, are commonly associated with tears to the medial and posterior capsule, and if the force is sufficient, the ACL and medial meniscus may also be damaged (O'Donoghue's triad). MCL injuries are graded according to severity: grade I lesions are minimal tears in the absence of instability; grade II injuries are partial tears with minor instability; and grade III injuries are complete tears with gross instability. The degree of joint opening on stress views can be used to quantify the degree of instability. The patient with higher grade injuries presents with symptoms of pain and locking, but the symptoms are arising from the associated injuries more than from the collateral ligament damage itself. Acutely, oedema and haemorrhage are evident on T2-weighted sequences in relation to the MCL, but in grade I sprains, the MCL itself is of normal thickness, and appears closely applied to the underlying cortical bone. Displacement of ligamentous fibres away from cortical bone suggests a partial or grade II tear, and loss of continuity of the ligamentous fibres, with or without extension into the capsular layer, would indicate a full-thickness or grade III lesion. An associated joint effusion or haemarthrosis is typical of an acute injury and other associated findings would include a nondisplaced compression fracture or a bone contusion affecting the lateral tibial plateau. The MCL rupture heals with fibrosis and thickening, and occasionally with calcification. Accordingly, the MR appearances of a chronic tear show the MCL to be thickened, but the signal intensity is normal.

Isolated MCL tears and sprains are commonly treated nonsurgically. Even in isolated grade III MCL tears, there is no evidence that operative treatment is any more effective than inoperative rehabilitation. Combined MCL and ACL injuries are usually treated with surgical repair to the ACL.

The lateral collateral ligament (LCL) is seen on posterior coronal images as a low signal intensity band. Acute injuries are associated with oedema and haemorrhage in adjacent soft tissues, and the LCL itself appears thickened and returns increased signal intensity on T2-weighted images. In complete disruptions, the LCL may demonstrate a wavy contour and the discontinuity may be apparent on coronal images. Associated findings include medial tibial compression fractures and bone contusions, in keeping with the mechanism of injury involving forced varus strain on the knee. In severe injuries, the iliotibial band may also be disrupted, and this structure must be accurately visualized by including sufficiently anterior coronal images in the coronal series. Treatment is usually conservative but surgical repair of the LCL may be required when there are associated ACL injuries or when the knee is unstable (grade III tear).

Extensor mechanism abnormalities

Patellar tendinosis most commonly affects the superior or inferior insertion of the tendon. It is associated with overuse and sports involving jumping, hence its common name 'jumper's knee'. The patient presents with anterior knee pain, and focal tenderness over the site of injury is characteristic. Ultrasound demonstrates swelling of the affected tendon, with an area of reduced echogenicity and loss of the normal internal fibrillar pattern at the site of maximal tendon damage. Axial or sagittal MR images demonstrate a swollen oedematous tendon (with areas of increased signal on T2, and decreased signal on T1) and, uncommonly, a small bony fragment may be seen to be detached from the inferior pole of the patella.

Patella alta and baja On plain radiographs, the normal craniocaudal position of the patella is such that the length of the patellar tendon should be equal to the height of the patella, plus or minus 20%. Measurements on MRI allow a wider range for normality[36]. A high patella (patella alta) has been associated with the development of chondromalacia patellae, subluxation, cerebral palsy and quadriceps atrophy. A low patella (patella baja) is seen with polio, juvenile chronic arthritis and achondroplasia. However, patella alta and baja are often incidental findings.

Patellar bursae Inflammation of one of the two superficial bursae that overlie the patellar tendon results in bursitis. The resulting superficial infrapatellar bursitis or prepatellar bursitis results in lozenge-shaped structures with homogeneous low signal on T1 and high signal on T2 representing the contained fluid anterior to the proximal patella tendon or anterior to the patella respectively (Fig. 50.27). The fluid is often not contained within a discrete synovial structure, but instead is in the form of subcutaneous diffuse oedema, and therefore ultrasound is less reliable in diagnosis of this condition. Despite the colloquial name (housemaid's knee), the condition is not confined to individuals who spend significant time on their knees.

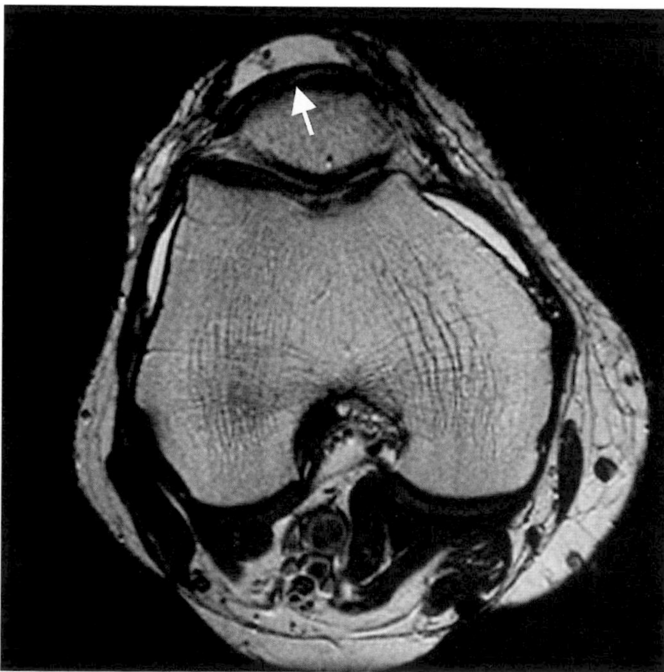

Figure 50.27 Prepatellar bursitis. An area of fluid signal is demonstrated anterior to the patella on this axial FSE T2-weighted image.

Cysts around the knee

The finding of a cystic structure in relation to the knee on MRI is a common occurrence, and three different pathological lesions must be recognized and distinguished: ganglion, meniscal cyst and bursa.

A ganglion cyst is filled with gelatinous viscous material. It does not usually communicate with a joint cavity or tendon sheath, and it is not lined by synovium. Although most commonly seen in relation to the wrist, they are a frequent finding on MRI examinations of the knee and can present with compressive nerve palsy, for example on the common peroneal nerve with a ganglion arising near the proximal tibiofibular joint. On MRI, they appear as well-marginated multiloculated structures, generally under 2 cm in size, returning typical characteristics of fluid (high T2, low T1). In some instances, a string of locules is seen extending towards the knee (Fig. 50.28). Treatment involves resection or rupture, although some clinicians advocate the injection of steroids into the structure. Recurrence is common.

A meniscal cyst is an accumulation of fluid in association with an adjacent meniscal tear extending from the joint surface of the meniscus to its outer border. Joint fluid is forced through the tear as the patient walks, and accumulates at the meniscocapsular margin. Thus it is a false cyst, and is not lined by synovium. It presents typically as a hard tense mass adjacent to the joint line. Lateral cysts are easier to diagnose clinically as they are palpable but these cysts are just as common on the medial side and they may be multiple. On ultrasound or MR, a complex cystic structure is demonstrated, but careful attention must be paid to the adjacent meniscus (Fig. 50.29). On MR, an increase in T2 within the cyst is expected, but T1 signal may be hypointense or isointense to normal muscle depending on the protein content of the fluid. Treatment involves addressing the underlying tear, in addition to removing the meniscal cyst.

A synovial cyst represents a herniation of fluid through a weakening of the joint capsule. The cyst is therefore lined by synovial membrane and filled with synovial fluid. The commonest such accumulation of fluid around the knee is within the semimembranosus-gastrocnemius bursa (Baker's cyst) which is a herniation from the posterior aspect of the knee through the gap between the medial head of gastrocnemius and the semimembranosus tendon. A corresponding cystic lesion is seen on ultrasound, and MRI gives the typical appearances of the fluid-containing structure, with high signal on T2 and low signal on T1. A definitive treatment has not been established, and generally the synovial cysts are treated conservatively unless they become symptomatic. Steroid injection or aspiration is advocated, but surgical removal is uncommon.

Ankle and foot

Transchondral fracture

The term 'transchondral fracture' is a preferred term encompassing the conditions talar dome fracture, osteochondritis dessecans and osteochondral fracture. All three conditions are thought to be related to previous trauma, commonly with an associated torsional component. The resulting talar dome defects occur medially or laterally with approximately equal incidence, and result from impingement of the talar dome with the posteromedial tibia or fibular styloid during injury respectively. Plain radiographs are notoriously unreliable in the early stages of this condition, and if the transchondral fracture has occurred in the absence of injury to the fibular collateral ligament, then the patient may be relatively asymptomatic. Nevertheless, a delay in diagnosis and treatment is associated with premature osteoarthrosis in up to 50% of patients in some

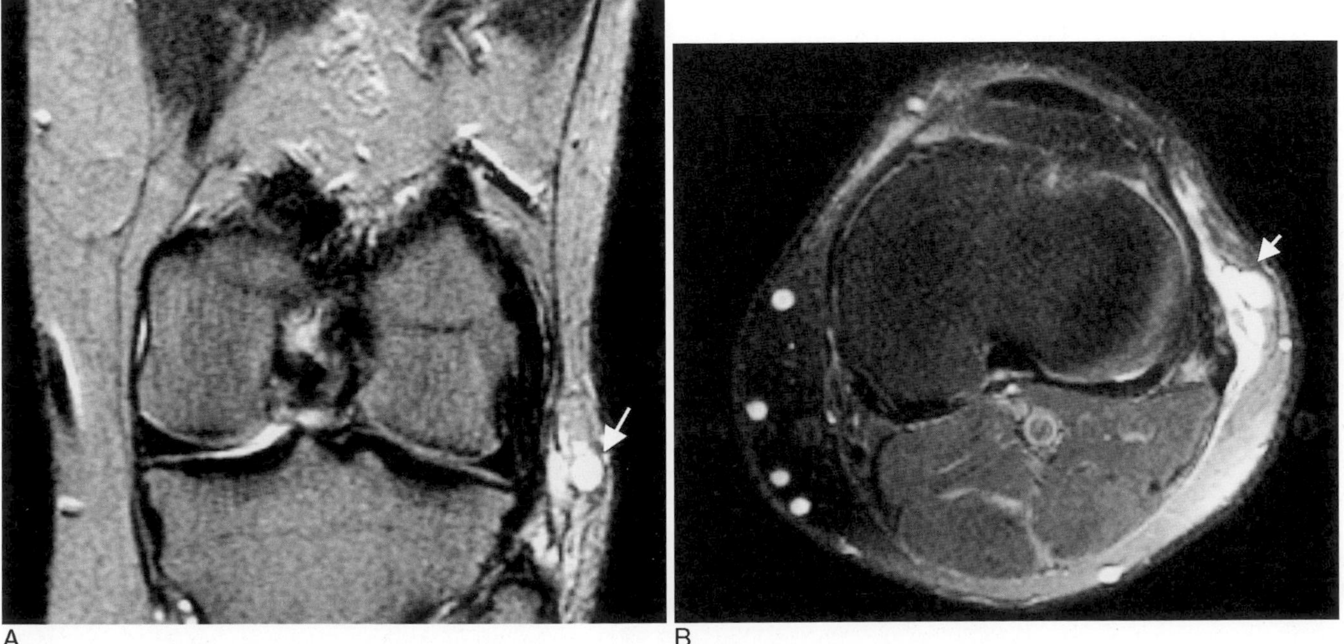

Figure 50.28 Ganglion. (A) A cystic structure is seen to arise lateral to the lateral meniscus (arrow) but the meniscus itself is normal. (B) Axial FSE T2-weighted MR image. There is no evidence of extension of the cystic lesion (arrow) deep to the lateral collateral ligament.

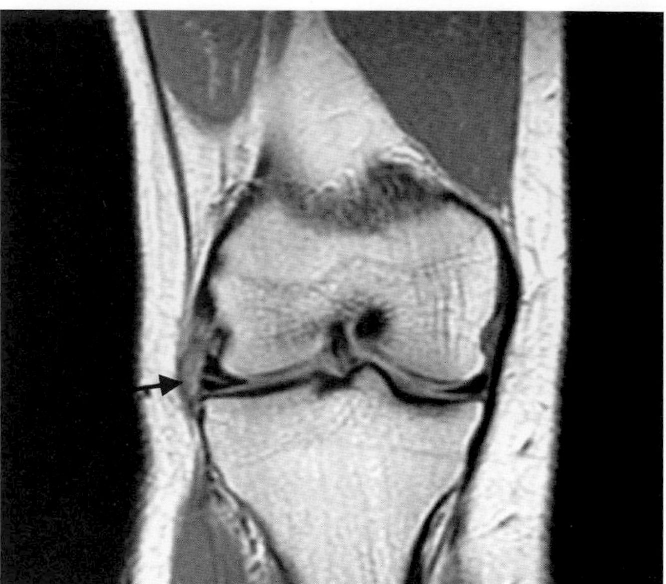

Figure 50.29 Meniscal cyst. A cystic structure is seen arising deep to the lateral collateral ligament (arrow), intimately related to the lateral meniscus. An oblique tear is seen through the meniscus confirming that this represents a meniscal cyst.

series, and MRI is indicated in individuals in whom pain persists for 2–3 months after an acute ankle injury. The staging of the condition with MR correlates well with the four-part staging system based on plain radiographs[37].

Stage I involves a compression fracture with normal plain radiographs. On MR, the only findings may relate to a focus of bone marrow oedema deep to the injured cartilage, but any flattening of the subarticular cortex will be minimal. Stage II lesions involve a partially detached osteochondral fragment, and fluid deep to the fragment and a discontinuity or fissure in the overlying cartilage indicates that the fragment is potentially at risk of becoming loose. A fat-saturated FSE T2-weighted or a STIR sequence in a coronal or sagittal plane will help assess whether a fragment is loose and will also optimally detect any adjacent bone marrow oedema. In stage III lesions, the osteochondral defect is detached and loose but remains within the underlying crater (Fig. 50.30) and in stage IV lesions the defect has become detached and has migrated. Although an effusion is a common accompanying finding, the absence of an effusion does not exclude the presence of an osteochondral defect.

The treatment in the early stages involves conservative management with immobilization, but stage II and III lesions are often treated surgically by curettage, drilling or pinning. A mobile osteochondral defect (stage IV) is typically excised to avoid excessive premature degenerative change. The objectives of imaging therefore are first to detect the condition and second to indicate whether the defect may be loose.

Tendon injuries

The most common tendon abnormalities in the ankle relate to injuries or chronic degeneration rather than inflammatory changes. The widely used term 'tendinitis' therefore is unfortunate, as evidence of inflammation within the tendon itself is absent histologically. Tendinosis is therefore a preferred term. Paratendonitis refers to inflammation in the soft tissues adjacent to a tendon, and may accompany tendinosis, and tenosynovitis relates to inflammation within a tendon sheath, often associated with fluid within the sheath. A normal tendon is represented by a well-defined linear structure of homogeneous low signal on all MR sequences and by an echogenic fibrillar structure on US. Acute ruptures of a normal tendon are unusual and are associated with high-impact injuries such as a road traffic accident. If a tendon ruptures under low-impact conditions it usually implies that the tendon was already abnormal and had undergone previous chronic degeneration. In its early stages, this is characterized by fusiform swelling of the tendon. On MR, low internal signal on all sequences

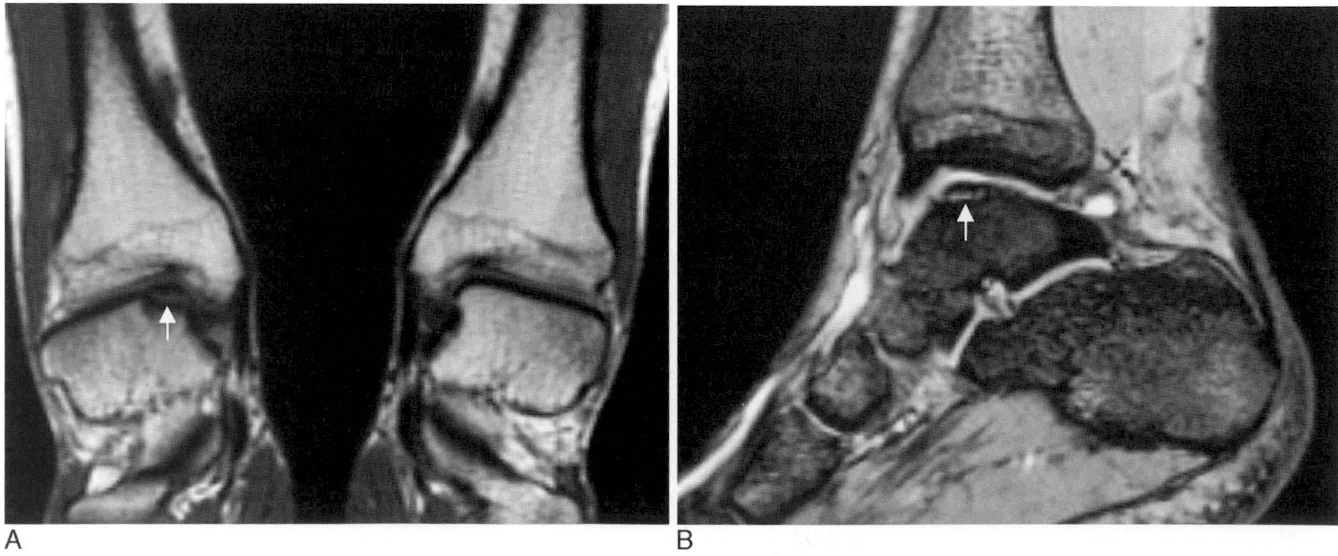

Figure 50.30 Transchondral fracture of the talar dome. (A) Six months after an acute injury, a focal abnormality is seen within the medial talar dome (arrow). (B) The osteochondral fragment is undermined by fluid (arrow) indicating that the fragment is loose.

within the tendon is preserved, and on ultrasound, there might be slight diffuse reduction in the fibrillar echogenicity. With further degeneration, focal areas of higher signal develop on MR, particularly on T2-, T2*-weighted or STIR sequences, which may be globular indicating cystic degeneration, or become linear indicating the development of a partial tear. On ultrasound, focal areas of reduced echogenicity indicate local intrasubstance damage, and partial tears will be seen as a discrete area of low echogenicity with no internal fibrillar pattern. Untreated, there is a tendency for the areas of partial tear and cystic change to coalesce, reducing the structural integrity of the tendon. Thinning of the tendon develops as bundles of fibres within it rupture, and this may eventually lead to a complete tear.

Achilles tendon

The normal Achilles tendon is the largest and strongest tendon in the human body and is formed by the common insertion of soleus, plantaris and gastrocnemius muscles. Injuries are most common in middle-aged men and are associated with sporting activity, although women may also be affected. Predisposing factors to degeneration include diabetes mellitus, gout, rheumatoid arthritis and other connective tissue disorders. Achilles tendinosis presents clinically with swelling of the tendon, most pronounced approximately 5 cm proximal to its insertion into the calcaneum. However, this stage is often missed, and the patient may present with an acutely ruptured tendon. It is not always possible to diagnose a tendon rupture by clinical diagnosis alone and the condition may be missed in up to 25% of cases, possibly due to the action of an intact plantaris.

MR findings of tendinosis include diffuse swelling or thickening, indicated in the early stages by increased signal on T2-weighted or STIR sequences. Sagittal images will demonstrate increased convexity anteriorly, and oedema, either diffusely within Kager's fat triangle or localized within the retrocalcaneal bursa, is typical. Linear focal regions of increased signal on T2-weighted images indicate progression to partial tear formation. The presence of a complete tear would be characterized by a disruption in the tendon morphology, associated with increased signal on T2-weighted images between the ends of the torn ligament (Fig. 50.31). In acute injuries, T1 signal can also be increased due to the presence of haemorrhage. Typically the tendon edges are frayed or corkscrewed, and the presence and degree of retraction of the proximal tendon is an important observation in those individuals in whom surgery is planned. US is often considered the preferred imaging technique for isolated Achilles abnormalities where facilities and operator experience are available, however, and the findings are indicated above.

Posterior tibial tendon

The posterior tibial tendon is a dynamic stabilizer of the medial arch of the foot, and rupture or damage to the tendon therefore is a common cause of acquired flat foot deformity. Chronic tendinosis can present with localized swelling of the tendon and pain, although this phase is commonly asymptomatic. Rupture most commonly occurs in women in their fifth and sixth decades, and a previous history of trauma is unusual. It is important when imaging the tendon to include its insertion on the navicular, as detachments are common at

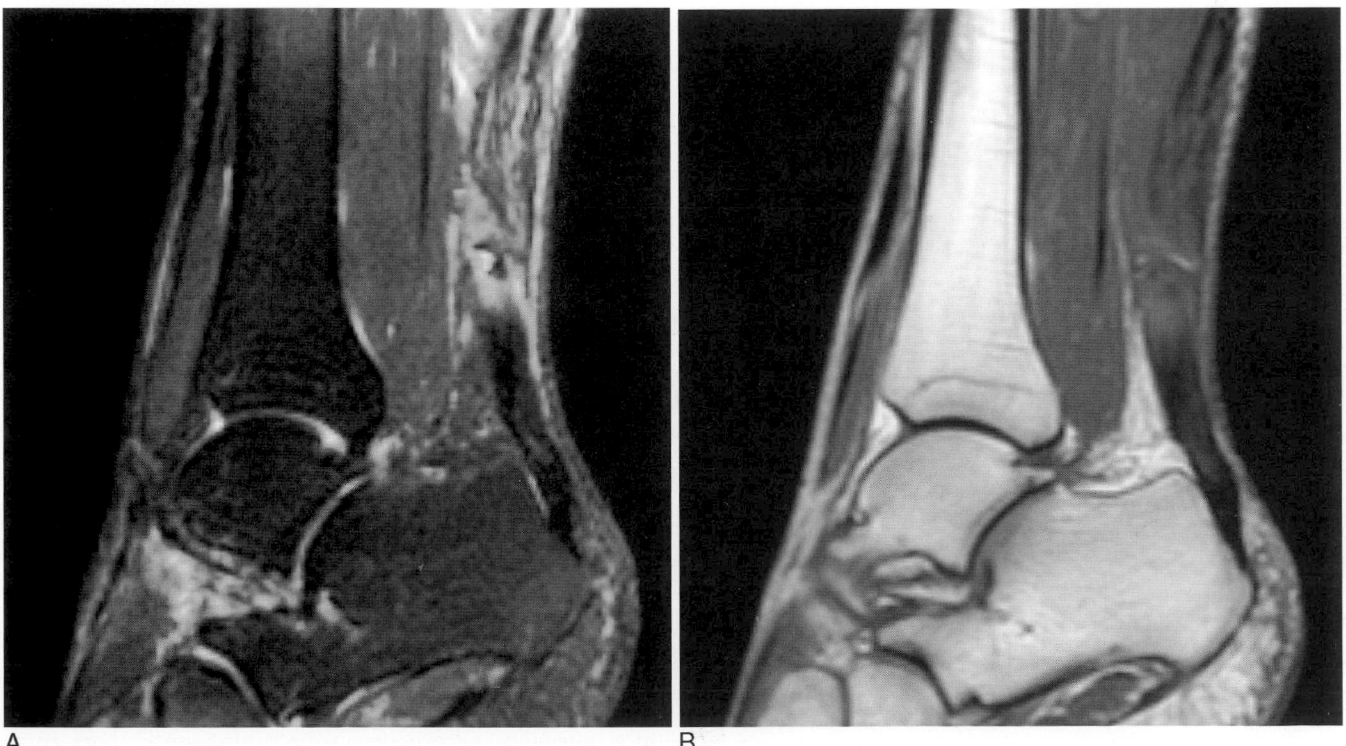

Figure 50.31 Complete rupture of the Achilles tendon. (A) T1- and (B) fat-saturated FSE T2-weighted MR images demonstrate swelling of the tendon, associated with haemorrhage (high signal on T1) and oedema (high signal on T2). The tear itself is well demonstrated on both sequences.

this site. Tears of the posterior tibial tendon are classified in one of three grades. Type I tears involve hypertrophy of the tendon, with reduced echogenicity on ultrasound and heterogeneous increased signal on T2-weighted or STIR images within the substance of the tendon (Fig. 50.32). Type II tears involve attenuated sections of the tendon which may or may not be associated with altered signal or echogenicity within. These two types of tear indicate a partial tear. In type III, a complete tear of the tendon is present, with a well-delineated tendinous gap between the ends of the tendons that appear frayed and irregular. Fluid within the tendon sheath is a common accompanying feature. The commonest part of the tendon to be involved is at the level of the medial malleolus, but partial or complete avulsion of the tendon from the navicular is more typical in younger patients, particularly those involved in high-impact sports.

Treatment involves support of the medial longitudinal arch with orthotics. If these fail, surgical intervention is considered, including re-siting of the insertion of the posterior tibial tendon, or arthrodesis.

Other tendon injuries

Any of the ankle tendons may become involved in injury. The peroneal tendons are most commonly injured in calcaneal fractures, where the tendons can become impacted between a laterally displaced calcaneal fragment and the distal tip of the fibula. The peroneal tendons can also become subluxed. Flexor hallucis longus injuries can be difficult to diagnose clinically, and are more common in ballet dancers due to the requirement to dance on tiptoes for prolonged periods. However, communication exists between the ankle joint and the flexor tendon sheaths in up to 20% of the normal population and therefore fluid within these sheaths may be a normal finding or may be secondary to problems within the ankle joint.

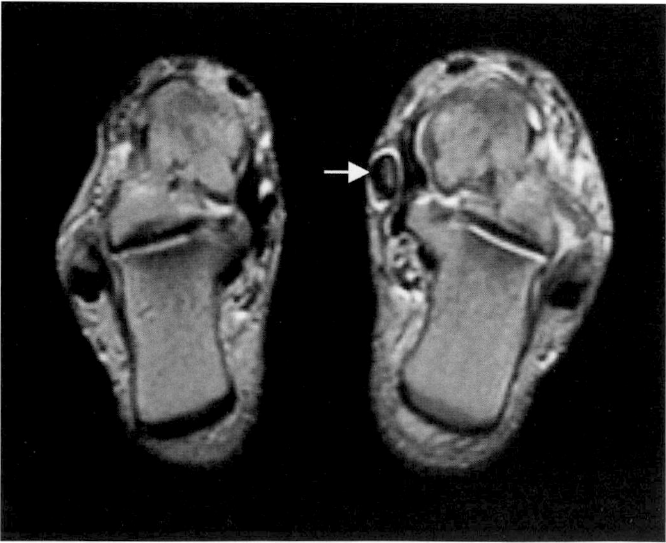

Figure 50.32 Posterior tibial tendon tendonosis. T2-weighted image shows that the posterior tibial tendon on the left (arrow) is swollen, and it contains increased signal indicative of tendonitis. The high signal surrounding the tendon indicates fluid within the tendon sheath (tenosynovitis).

Ligament injuries

Although ankle ligament injuries are common, they are not routinely evaluated with imaging. When performed, imaging is usually related to the evaluation of the lateral ligaments, where ankle sprains are divided clinically into three grades. The anterior talofibular ligament bundle is the weakest of the lateral ankle ligaments and is usually the first to be injured in forced inversion and plantar flexion. A grade I sprain involves stretching or tearing of this bundle. A grade II injury involves tearing the anterior talofibular ligament fibres and stretching the calcaneofibular ligament, and stage III results in an unstable ankle and involves disruption to both anterior and posterior talofibular ligaments together with the calcaneofibular ligament. Arthrography used to be the only technique to evaluate these injuries acutely, but now ultrasound or MRI is preferred.

Soft tissue masses

The commonest soft tissue masses to be found in the foot and ankle include ganglion cyst, haemangioma and giant cell tumour of the tendon sheath. When imaging a soft tissue mass in the foot it becomes particularly important to document the full anatomical extent of the lesion. In particular, lesions arising on the plantar aspect of the foot can, as they grow, extend between the metatarsals and present on the dorsal aspect of the foot. This is due to mechanical pressures on the lesion during walking, forcing the growth to be maximal superiorly. For this reason a careful analysis and description of the lesion is necessary to aid the surgeon to a complete excision.

Morton's neuroma This is a non-neoplastic swelling involving the interdigital nerve as it passes superficial to the deep intermetatarsal ligament.

Accessory muscles These normal variants can occur at any site. The commonest accessory muscle at the level of the ankle is an accessory soleus muscle, which represents persistence of the distal muscular portion of the soleus in the region of the pre-Achilles fat pad. It presents as a bulge on the posteromedial aspect of the ankle, associated with exercised-induced pain in an adolescent or young adult although it may represent an asymptomatic incidental finding on an MR examination of the ankle. The insertion of the accessory muscle is variable, but most commonly there is an accessory tubercle on the medial aspect of the calcaneum which receives the aberrant muscle. On MRI a rounded mass is seen within the pre-Achilles fat which returns a marbled signal identical to adjacent normal muscle (Fig. 50.33).

Shoulder

Shoulder impingement syndrome and rotator cuff tears

Neer clarified the concept of the shoulder impingement syndrome in 1972[38] and his insight has influenced a generation of orthopaedic surgeons. The basis of his concept is the presence of a restrictive space between the acromion, the coracoacromial arch and acromioclavicular joint (ACJ) superiorly and the humeral head and greater tuberosity inferiorly. Through

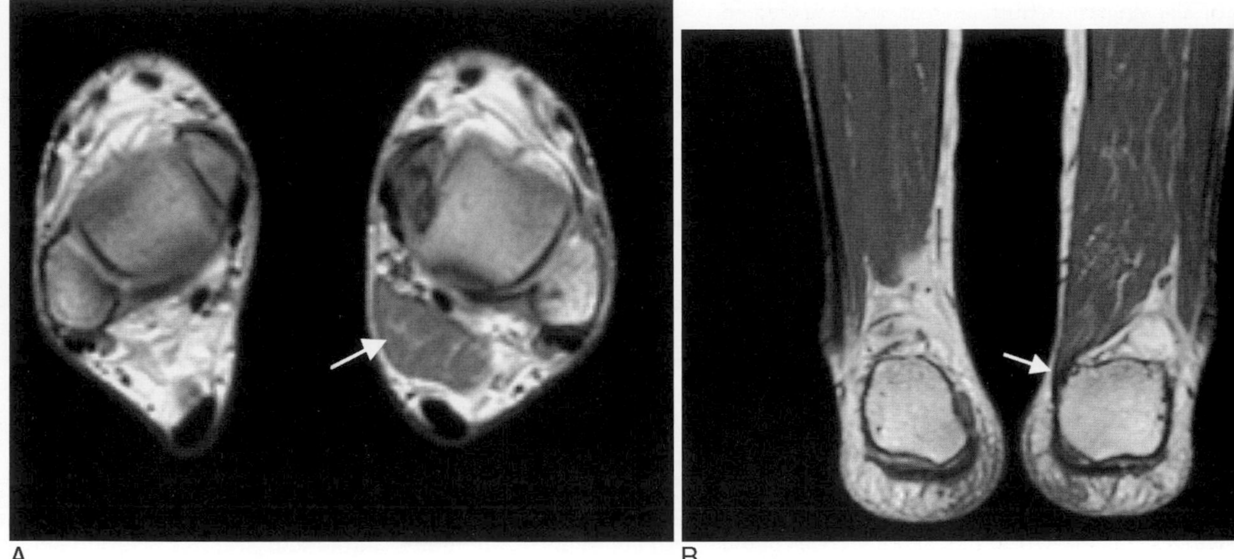

Figure 50.33 Accessory soleus muscle. (A) Axial proton-density weighted image confirms the presence of a soft tissue mass returning signal identical to muscle in the fat triangle anterior to the Achilles tendon on the left (arrow). (B) When compared to the contralateral side, the insertion of the accessory soleus onto a tubercle on the medial aspect of the calcaneus is demonstrated (arrow).

this space pass the tendons of the rotator cuff, particularly the supraspinatus and infraspinatus tendons, together with the subacromial-subdeltoid bursa, and a layer of fat. This anatomical configuration can lead to 'pinching' of the distal centimetre of supraspinatus tendon in particular, between the structures of the coracoacromial arch and the humeral head, especially on abduction and external rotation of the shoulder. Neer stressed that the tendon is particularly vulnerable at this site of pinching as it represents the watershed between two vascular territories (vessels travelling from the muscle belly and from the bone respectively); it is therefore relatively avascular and healing is suboptimal. In addition, anatomical variation in the shape of the acromion, particularly its inferior and anterior margin, and osteoarthritis can result in spurs and bony ridges that exacerbate the impingement. Neer classified the resulting changes within the damaged tendon into three stages. Stage 1 consists of reversible haemorrhage and oedema, typically seen in patients under 25. Stage II consists of tendinitis with fibrosis seen between the ages of 25 and 40. Stage III consists of partial and complete tendon rupture, in association with enthesophytes on the undersurface of the acromion which generally do not occur until the patient is over 40.

The advent of arthroscopy together with work from a variety of sources has built on Neer's original concept. Damage that occurs to the supraspinatus tendon is more normally considered in three stages of severity. Type I is where degeneration and tendinosis has occurred within the tendon but no surface defect is apparent. Type II damage is where partial thickness rotator cuff tears are present; these may be intrasubstance, or may open onto the superior or inferior surfaces. Type III tears involve a full thickness rotator cuff tear through the tendon, with communication between the subacromial-subdeltoid bursa and the shoulder joint. It was this latter condition which was the main focus of attention with shoulder arthrography, where contrast medium injected into the shoulder joint which extended into the subacromial-subdeltoid bursa was confirmatory evidence of the presence of a full thickness rotator cuff tear. Similarly, although Neer put great emphasis on the shape of the acromion, it is clear that subacromial spurs are seen in only a minority of patients referred to surgery for rotator cuff tendinosis, and in addition rotator cuff degeneration is observed in the absence of spurs.

MRI allows assessment of the rotator cuff tendons directly, together with evaluation of the acromion, the ACJ and subacromial-subdeltoid bursa. The normal rotator cuff tendon displays low signal intensity on all sequences. In cuff degeneration, areas of intermediate signal intensity develop on T1- and PD-weighted images, which display corresponding normal low or intermediate signal on heavily weighted T2 SE or FSE images. However, similar changes can be seen in normal volunteers and cadaveric studies in otherwise normal individuals where an area of intermediate signal or signal inhomogeneity can be seen on T1-weighted sequences within the distal supraspinatus tendon. These changes have also been attributed to the *magic angle* phenomenon at sites where the tendon orientation is at 55 degrees to the main magnetic field (B_0). At this angle the protons attached to water molecules are constrained in their direction of movement by the parallel cartilaginous macromolecule fibres. The resulting shortening of T1 relaxation results in an increase in the signal from the water molecules at this site, but the routine use of T2-weighted images, in which the phenomenon is not seen, should reduce the risk of misinterpretation. Nevertheless, it remains difficult to identify the earliest signs of cuff degeneration.

In the earliest stages of partial thickness tear of the supraspinatus or infraspinatus tendon, when the tear itself is not seen, differentiation between tendinosis and partial tear is difficult on MRI. However, once the partial tear has assumed a size where it is visible, its presence can often be detected. The presence of a full thickness cuff tear is characterized by increased signal on proton-density or T1-weighted sequences, matched by increased signal on T2-weighted sequences which can be seen to cross the full thickness of rotator cuff tendon (Fig. 50.34). Retraction of the tendon is seen as a gap that extends between the torn tendon ends, and the size of this gap can be measured accurately at MRI. Secondary signs associated with a full thickness rotator cuff tear include the presence of subacromial-subdeltoid bursal fluid, retraction of the supraspinatus musculotendinous junction, changes in the subacromial and subdeltoid peribursal fat, and fatty atrophy of the rotator cuff muscle. Although these features may provide useful secondary evidence, few of them are sufficiently reliable signs to diagnose rotator cuff tear in their own right.

In addition to visualizing the rotator cuff tendons directly, MRI provides valuable information about the osseous and articular structures adjacent to the tendons, which are often the primary cause for the impingement and which represent the focus of the surgeon's attention. In particular, degenerative change within the ACJ is a common accompaniment to rotator cuff degeneration and tear, and the extent of the inferior aspect of the degenerate joint is well visualized on MR (Fig. 50.34). Acromial and lateral clavicular spurs are also easily demonstrated on one of the multiple projections available during an MR examination. Degenerative cysts within the greater tuberosity of the humeral head are particularly common and are not a useful discriminator in determining the severity of impingement. The presence of an os acromiale is most easily seen on the axial sequence (Fig. 50.35), but cranial axial slices are needed to demonstrate the full extent of the acromion. The os acromiale, an unfused epiphysis, has been implicated in the development of ACJ degeneration and impingement, and must be recognized in advance of surgery to ensure that a stable acromion is not rendered unstable. The shape of the undersurface of the acromion can be well visualized on sagittal images, and has been variously classified[39]. The lateral down-sloping acromion, which narrows the acromiohumeral distance, is best appreciated on coronal oblique images.

The advent of high frequency linear array ultrasound probes has allowed accurate assessment of rotator cuff disease with ultrasound. As with tendons at other sites, a normal supraspinatus tendon is seen as an echogenic fibrillar structure and the earliest signs of tendinosis are when the structure is swollen when compared to the other side but otherwise appears normal. Thereafter the echogenicity is reduced, diffusely or focally, and a partial tear can be identified when a focal anechoic structure or fissure is seen within the degenerate tendon. The first sign of a full thickness tear is a flattening of the normally convex superficial surface of the supraspinatus tendon, leading to concavity as the underlying tendon loses substance. Thereafter the discrete tear can be seen traversing the full thickness of the tendon and its size can be measured both in terms of the cross-sectional area of the tendon involved and the degree of retraction longitudinally.

Rotator interval tears are often missed at MR examination unless MR arthrography is performed. They represent a tear in the thin elastic membranous tissue between tendons; the commonest site is between the supraspinatus and subscapularis tendons. T2-weighted images in a sagittal oblique plane may show the anterior extension of fluid across the rotator cuff interval, but the diagnosis is often only made at arthroscopy.

Subscapularis tendon tears occur almost exclusively in the presence of other rotator cuff tears, particularly of the supraspinatus tendon. Isolated tears to this tendon are seen in relation

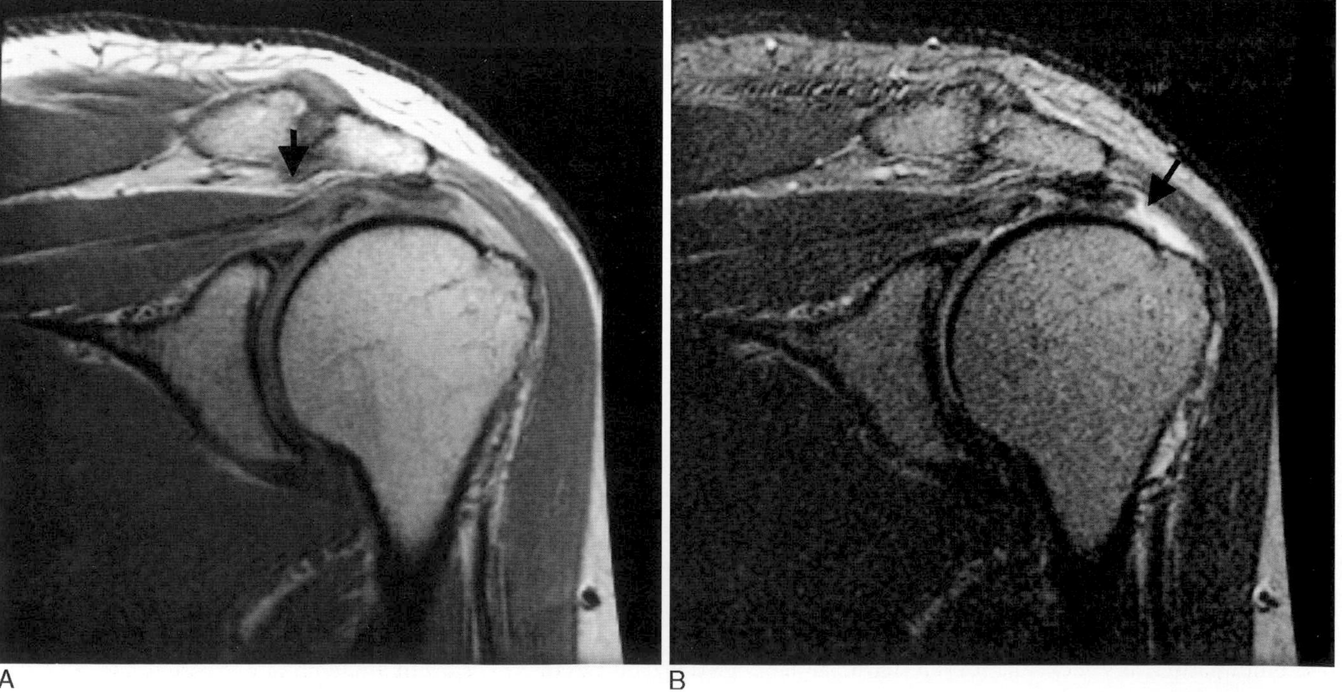

Figure 50.34 Supraspinatus tear. (A) Extensive degenerative change is present in the ACJ with fibrous tissue extending inferiorly to impinge upon the supraspinatus tendon (arrow). (B) The full thickness supraspinatus tear is indicated by termination of the tendon fibres abruptly with fluid within the empty space (arrow).

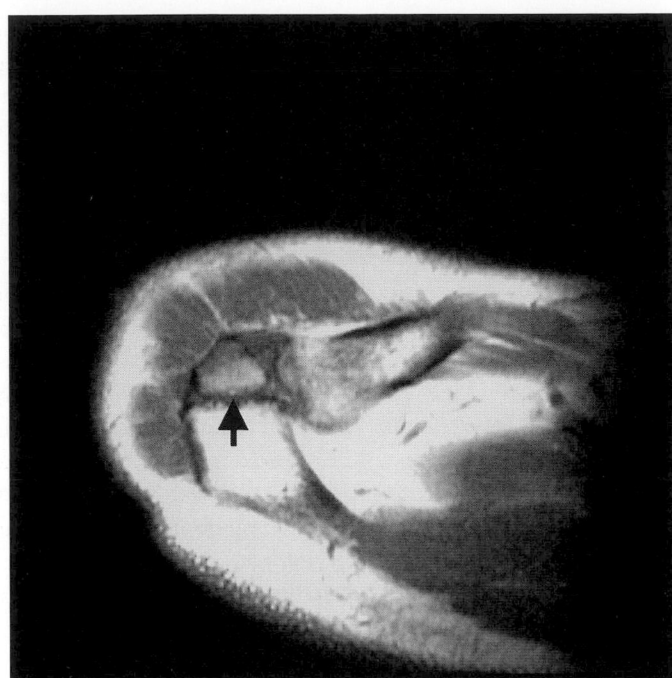

Figure 50.35 Os acromiale. Axial T1-weighted MR image. The os acromiale is well demonstrated on the cranial-most slice of the series.

to congenital lateral sloping of the coracoid process resulting in direct impingement between the coracoid process and the anterior aspect of the humeral head. Tears to *teres minor* tendon are uncommon, and are usually seen in association with global cuff tears. Both subscapularis and teres minor tendon tears are best visualized on axial images.

Evaluation of the shoulder in the postoperative patient can be challenging. The presence of susceptibility artefacts at the site of repair, probably associated with diathermy use, renders gradient-echo imaging difficult. Conventional spin-echo sequences minimize the artefact and can be useful in the demonstration of a retracted torn tendon.

Although the earlier stages of cuff degeneration are treated conservatively, the introduction of arthroscopy widely has revolutionized the management of shoulder impingement syndromes. Arthroscopic subacromial decompression has rapidly replaced open acromioplasty as the method of choice for the treatment of chronic subacromial outlet impingement. The coracoacromial ligament is detached from the anterior/inferior acromial surface, any frayed or inflamed cuff is debrided, and the undersurface of the acromion and the ACJ is flattened by use of a rotating burr under direct arthroscopic vision.

Glenohumeral joint instability

The bony contour of the glenohumeral joint is intrinsically unstable, and therefore the stability depends upon the muscular, tendinous and capsular structures that are related to the shoulder joint. The commonest form of instability is anterior instability, particularly seen in association with injuries to the labrum and the inferior glenohumeral ligament. Demonstration of associated abnormalities on MRI commonly requires MR or CT arthrography, as many of the findings are missed with a conventional MR technique. The commonest signs relate to avulsion of the anterior labrum, with or without a fracture involving the underlying inferior glenoid rim. Termed the Bankart lesion, the lesion is visualized best on axial sequences, where T1-weighted images will demonstrate changes in the subchondral bone, whereas T2*-weighted images will be more useful in evaluating the cartilaginous labrum. Changes in the humeral head in the form of posterolateral compression fracture (Hill–Sachs lesion) are seen in patients with a single and with recurrent episodes of anterior dislocation alike.

The posterior band of the inferior glenohumeral ligament is primarily responsible for posterior stability, augmented by the anterosuperior capsule. Posterior instability as an isolated finding represents less than 5% of patients with shoulder instability. The diagnosis is ultimately made during an examination under anaesthesia, when the posterior instability can be demonstrated dynamically. However, associated MR features include tear or fragmentation of the posterior labrum, possibly with a fracture in the underlying glenoid rim and a corresponding compression fracture involving the anterior surface of the humeral head (reverse Hill–Sachs deformity).

Multidirectional instability should be considered in young patients, particularly females, with generalized joint laxity with symptoms particularly referable to the shoulder. The underlying causative ligamentous laxity is atraumatic and often bilateral. Surgical intervention is often unhelpful, and treatment is most commonly in the form of physiotherapy and specific muscle rehabilitation. MRI is not normally required in the evaluation of these patients and will be normal.

Labral tears affecting the anterosuperior labrum with involvement of the biceps tendon are most commonly described in the high-performance throwing athlete, e.g. *SLAP* lesion (*s*uperior *l*abrum from *a*nterior to *p*osterior, in relation to the biceps tendon insertion). The importance of the differentiation of the types of SLAP lesion is discussed by Snyder and co-authors[40]. The clinical diagnosis of SLAP lesions is imperfect, as symptoms are often nonspecific. Treatment is surgical, and can usually be accomplished arthroscopically. The diagnosis of labral tears is unreliable on conventional MR, and can still be difficult on MR arthrography.

Adhesive capsulitis

This common condition, colloquially known as 'frozen shoulder', represents a clinical syndrome of pain associated with severely restricted shoulder joint movement. The diagnosis is commonly clinical, but arthrography has been useful to demonstrate the contraction of the joint capsule, with irregularity of the capsular insertion, reduction in joint volume, and early lymphatic filling. Despite the prevalence of capsulitis, neither ultrasound nor MRI has been shown to be useful in its determination.

Paralabral cyst

This is a cystic structure that is seen in relationship to a degenerate or torn labrum and commonly communicates with the joint. The paralabral cysts that attract most attention are those that extend into the spinoglenoid notch where they cause entrapment on the suprascapular nerve, resulting in atrophy of the infraspinatus and/or the supraspinatus muscles. Acutely, the affected muscles become inflated and therefore exhibit increased T2 and decreased T1 signal intensity. Chronic compression however leads to fatty atrophy, with corresponding increased signal on T1.

Elbow

Epicondylitis

Overuse syndromes are common. In the elbow, tearing of the extensor tendons attaching to the lateral epicondyle is known as *tennis elbow* and injuries to the common flexor/pronator muscle group attached to the medial epicondyle as golfer's elbow. In both cases, pain is elicited when the relevant muscle is contracted, and localized tenderness over the site of insertion is typical. The aetiology is thought to relate to chronic repetitive trauma, and despite their names, these conditions are not confined to sportsmen.

Plain radiographs are usually normal, and the diagnosis is usually clinical. If MR is performed, the earlier stages will be characterized by inflammatory changes within the tendinous attachment, which will be most evident on coronal T2-weighted images. Progression to tears will be indicated by a visible defect within the tendon, filled with fluid. Acute injuries may be associated with haemorrhage and haematoma formation. Careful analysis of the underlying ligaments must be made, as a ligamentous tear as an additional finding indicates a worse prognosis that may warrant surgical intervention. Ultrasound findings include swelling of the tendon, generalized reduced echogenicity, and focal hypoechoic areas that correspond to the presence of a tear. Treatment in the earlier stages of the disease is conservative consisting of rest and nonsteroidal anti-inflammatory drugs.

Biceps tendon rupture

The biceps tendon inserts distally onto the bicipital tuberosity of the radius and this is the commonest site of distal tears. Although the proximal tendon often retracts into the upper arm, the presence of a ligamentum lacerum may tether the proximal tendon distally and in those situations the patient will not exhibit the 'Popeye' appearance which is classically associated with biceps tendon rupture. The diagnosis of tendon rupture can be well demonstrated on MRI or ultrasound and the degree of any retraction can be estimated. On MRI, acute injuries associated with inflammation will be shown to advantage on STIR or fat-saturated T2-weighted sequences, and it is important that the axial images include slices distal to the proximal radioulnar joint, if they are not to miss the insertion of the tendon itself. Treatment involves primary repair of the ruptured tendon.

Cubital tunnel syndrome

The floor of the fibro-osseous cubital tunnel is formed by the medial capsule and the roof by the two heads of flexor carpi ulnaris. The walls are formed by two prominences projecting from the posteromedial aspect of the distal humerus. The tunnel transmits the ulnar nerve, and the space within the tunnel is diminished on flexion of the elbow. Compressive neuropathy may result in either motor or sensory defects, or both. Although ulnar nerve compression is an electrophysiological diagnosis, imaging can be useful to demonstrate the underlying compressive cause such as an osteophyte, a ganglion, or an accessory muscle. Changes within the ulnar nerve itself have been reported on MRI, resulting in increased signal on T2- or T2*-weighted images, but these cannot be relied upon to exclude a lesion within the nerve. Subluxation of the ulnar nerve is an associated condition, which will not be detected on static MRI. Ultrasound has the advantage in being able to evaluate the ulnar nerve dynamically and may also detect the cause of the nerve compression.

Wrist and hand

Ulnar variance

The concept of ulnar variance is central to the understanding of the development of triangular fibrocartilage (TFC) tears, ulnolunate impingement and Kienböck's disease. It refers to the relative levels of the distal articular surfaces of the ulna and radius with the forearm and carpus in neutral position. Negative ulnar variance indicates a relatively short ulna, and positive variance indicates a relatively long ulna. In the normal individual, the two distal surfaces should be within 2 mm of each other. The position of the wrist markedly affects the overall ulnar variance and for this reason it is important to ensure that the wrist and carpus are in a neutral position. Supination of the forearm results in relative ulnar shortening.

Triangular fibrocartilage complex tear

The triangular fibrocartilage complex (TFCC) remains under tension only while all of the suspensory attachments are intact. Arthroscopically, ballottement results in a 'trampoline' effect. This is lost when any one of the suspensory attachments is damaged, and this most commonly occurs at the radial or ulnar attachments. The central portion of the disc is thin and, when torn, can safely be excised surgically. The anterior and posterior limbs measure approximately 4 mm thick and they are particularly important mechanically. Poor results can be expected if these are resected surgically. Furthermore, the peripheral 15–20% of the articular disc is vascularized whereas the central portion is avascular. Central tears therefore are unlikely to heal spontaneously whereas peripheral tears may undergo a degree of spontaneous healing. In addition, peripheral ulnar avulsions can in some situations be treated by reimplantation.

Perforations can result from excessive loading, and are more common in patients with a positive ulnar variance (see below). Symptoms include pain localized to the ulnar side of the wrist with reduced mobility or clicking.

On MRI, the overall shape of the TFCC is visualized best on coronal images, and additionally the presence of ulnar variance can be assessed. In the axial plane, the disc is triangular in shape with its apex on the ulnar fovea. A thin layer of hyaline cartilage on the ulnar side of the distal radial articular surface represents the insertion of the annular disc and is represented as a high signal line on T2-weighted images, seemingly undermining the meniscus. This should not be misinterpreted as a tear. Central perforations are uncommon in the first three decades, but conversely, after the sixth decade, perforations occur frequently in asymptomatic individuals. This mirrors previous arthrographic findings that symptoms are not always associated with communication between the distal radioulnar joint and the radiocarpal compartment. Intrasubstance degeneration or tears of the anterior or posterior limbs of the TFC are best depicted on T2* images, and are represented as discontinuity or fragmentation, most commonly located adjacent to the radial attachment (Fig. 50.36). In more severe cases this leads to complete disruption of the articular cartilage with retraction.

Ulnolunate impingement syndrome

In neutral ulnar variance (normal), 80% of the axial loading from the carpus is transmitted to the radius, and 20% to the ulna. In positive ulnar variance, the ulna is subject to an increased proportion of this load and impinges on the medial aspect of the lunate. This painful compression leads to damage to the proximal articular surface of the lunate medially, and progressively this may lead to underlying bony changes within the lunate. Plain radiographs are initially normal with the exception of the presence of positive ulnar variance. Skeletal scintigraphy may show nonspecific uptake in the region of the lunate. On MRI, although the articular cartilage itself is not always visualized with enough spatial resolution to detect subtle abnormalities, the ulnar variance can be shown to advantage and early bone marrow oedema within the lunate or possibly within the impinging distal ulnar is characteristic. This will result in high signal on a T2-weighted or STIR sequence. This progresses to early sclerosis on plain radiographs with a corresponding reduction in signal returned from the proximal subarticular lunate on all sequences on MRI. Lunotriquetral ligament disruption and central TFC perforations are secondary associated signs.

Kienböck's disease

This eponymous disease refers to avascular necrosis of the lunate, a condition that is twice as common in men as women, which presents insidiously between the third and fifth decades, and which may be bilateral. Although the traditional staging of Kienböck's disease is based on plain film radiographs and clinical features, it should be noted that in the early stages the plain radiographs are normal. Traditionally, a three-phase technetium skeletal scintigram proved highly accurate in the assessment of patients with Kienböck's disease but MRI is now the preferred investigation as it allows accurate diagnosis and staging, and may also detect alternative diagnoses.

MR findings can be grouped into four stages[41]. In stage 1, the plain radiographs are usually normal, despite marrow necrosis being present pathologically, and MR shows bone oedema. The shape of the bone is preserved. In stage II disease, plain radiographs show lunate sclerosis which is matched by low signal on all MR sequences, although adjacent marrow may return increased signal on T2-weighted sequences due to the bone oedema. The bone morphology remains normal.

In stage III disease, the bone collapses craniocaudally, resulting in proximal migration of the capitate (Fig. 50.37). The presence of scapholunate ligament damage can result in rotatory subluxation of the scaphoid, allowing subdivision into two further subgroups, namely stage IIIA and IIIB, representing the absence and presence of rotatory subluxation respectively.

Stage IV disease represents the end-stage state, with sclerosis within the lunate radiographically, associated by widespread adjacent degenerative changes in the adjacent carpal bones and radius. Bone marrow oedema is not a feature of this advanced stage of disease, and lunate collapse is well defined in all three planes.

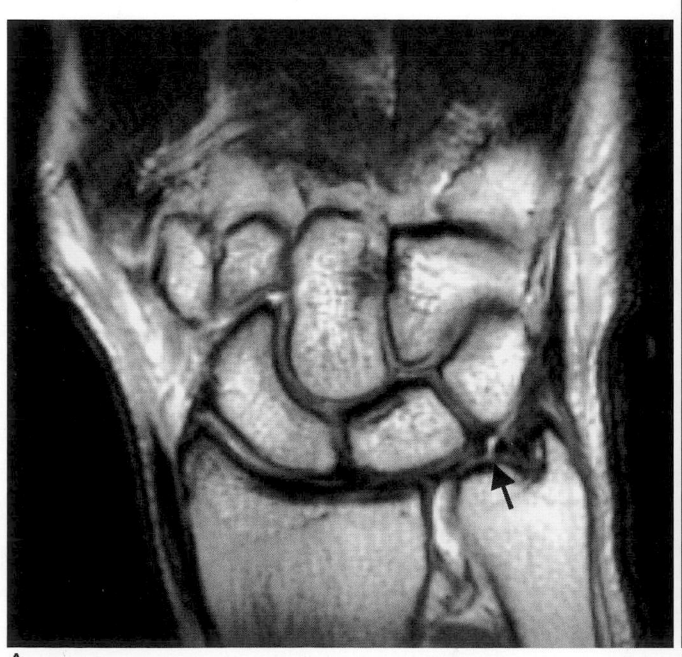

A

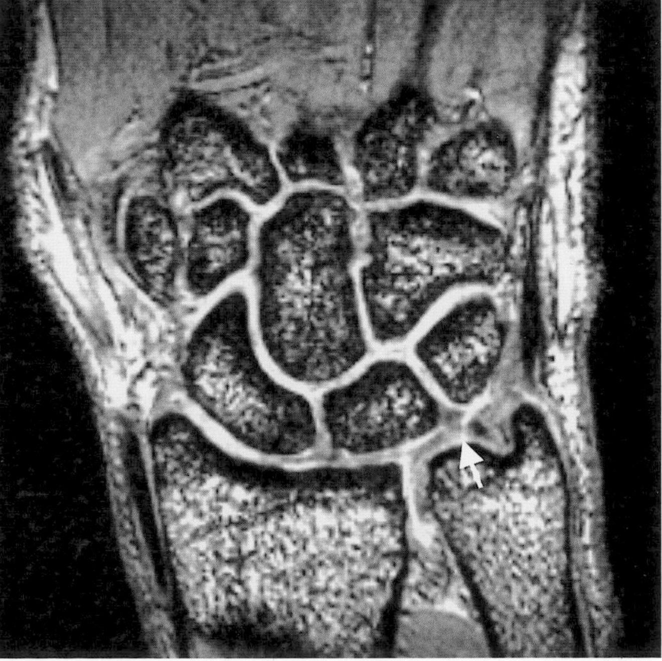

B

Figure 50.36 Torn TFCC. A focal tear is seen within the TFCC (arrow) on (A) coronal T1 and (B) GE images.

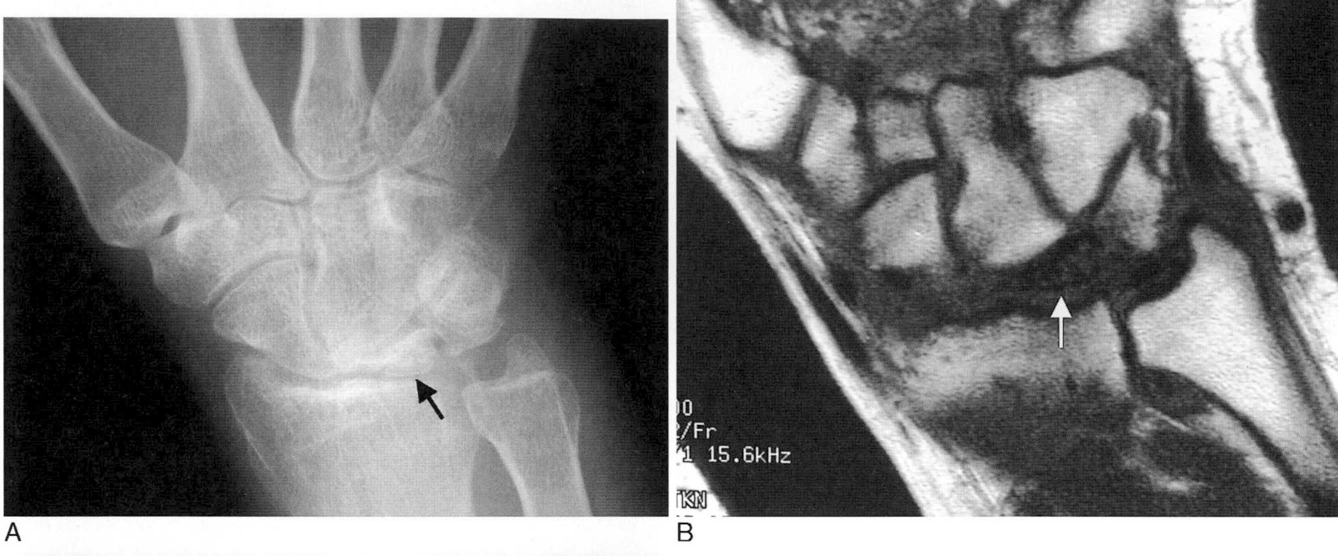

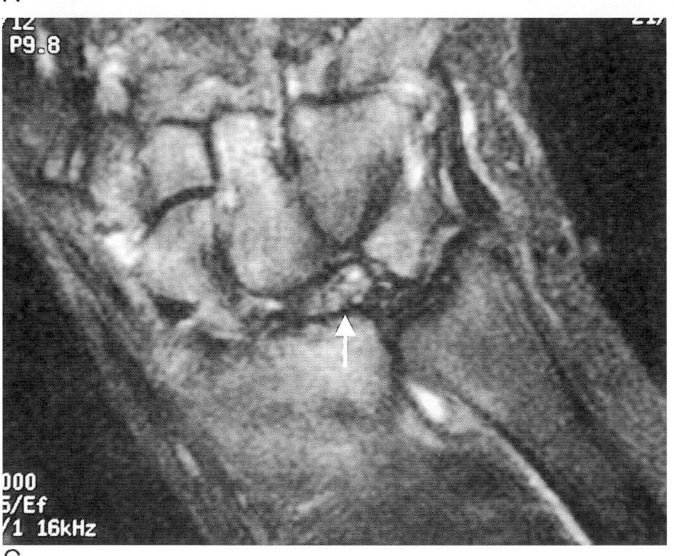

Figure 50.37 Kienböck's disease. (A) The lunate is collapsed and sclerotic indicating avascular necrosis (arrow). (B) T1-weighted MR image. The normal fatty marrow is replaced by low signal material indicating that the bone is avascular (arrow). (C) Fat-saturated FSE T2-weighted sequence shows a paucity of inflammatory change.

Avascular necrosis of the scaphoid

This condition is predominantly a post-traumatic event, secondary to fractures of the proximal pole or waist of the scaphoid which classically reduce the blood supply to the proximal pole. Plain radiographs demonstrate sclerosis, resorption and collapse in advanced disease, but MRI has the advantage in being able to demonstrate avascular necrosis at an earlier stage, when plain radiographs may be normal. Once again, early changes after the fracture are secondary to resulting bone marrow oedema, with high signal on T2-weighted or STIR images, commonly on both sides of the fracture line. Subsequently, the avascularity results in adipocyte death and as the acute bone marrow oedema subsides, an avascular proximal pole returns low signal on T1 and intermediate or low signal on T2-weighted sequences. MRI accurately demonstrates avascular necrosis when these two sequences are combined, but gradient-echo sequences cannot be relied upon to diagnose avascularity. Some authors suggest the additional use of intravenous gadolinium-DTPA to improve the accuracy by demonstrating lack of enhancement in the avascular pole, but its routine use is not recommended. However, the pattern of enhancement may enable an early accurate prediction of prognosis[42]. Early fixation of the proximal pole by the insertion of an intramedullary screw is indicated in the early stage of scaphoid fracture nonunion, before adipocyte death is complete, but a corticocancellous graft or prosthetic replacement of the proximal pole is required once avascularity is established.

Carpal tunnel syndrome

The fibroosseous carpal tunnel is made up of the convex volar aspect of the bones of the carpus and the flexor retinaculum. Through it pass the long flexor tendons to the fingers and the thumb, together with the median nerve. In certain positions, hypertrophied lumbricals enter the canal. Carpal tunnel syndrome results from crowding of structures within the cross-sectional area of the tunnel resulting in compression of the median nerve. It is bilateral in up to 50% of individuals and most common in women between their third and sixth decades. Causes include tenosynovitis of the flexor tendons, fracture to the distal radius or one or other carpal bones, carpometacarpal dislocation, inflammatory processes including RA or gout, or a soft tissue tumour (most commonly ganglion, lipoma or a haemangioma).

The diagnosis of carpal tunnel syndrome is electrophysiological, but MRI can determine an underlying cause when this is not clear from clinical examination. Changes in the median nerve may be present regardless of underlying aetiology: diffuse swelling or segmental enlargement, flattening, palmar bowing or increased signal intensity on T2-weighted images. However, none of these findings is sufficiently specific to replace electrophysiological diagnosis.

Treatment of the early stages is conservative involving splinting and nonsteroidal or steroidal drug therapy. Surgical decompression is reserved for those in whom sensory loss becomes progressive or muscle atrophy ensues. MRI in the postoperative wrist elegantly shows the inevitable fibrosis around the retinaculum and the immediately adjacent median nerve. However, it is often difficult to determine whether such fibrosis is responsible for continuing symptoms.

Soft tissue masses

The commonest lesions in the wrist include ganglion, tenosynovitis, haemangioma and giant cell tumour of the tendon sheath. Of these conditions, ganglion is by far the most prevalent (Fig. 50.38).

Tendon rupture

One of the commonest reasons for performing imaging of the finger relates to tendon injury. Both ultrasound and MRI can be used to identify the tendon involved, can delineate the site of the rupture, and can demonstrate the overall anatomy. Of particular importance, after rupture the proximal end can retract over several centimetres, and the use of imaging to demonstrate the position of this proximal fragment can help determine the extent of the surgical procedure.

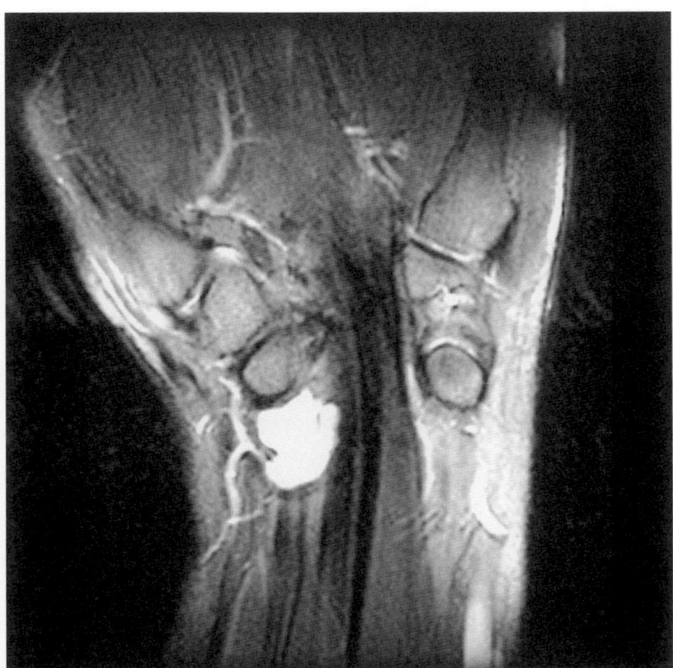

Figure 50.38 Ganglion. A 2 cm ganglion cyst has arisen proximal to the scaphoid on the volar aspect of the wrist. As expected from its fluid content, it returns increased signal on this fat-saturated T2-weighted sequence.

Guyon's canal lesions

Guyon's canal is a further fibroosseous tunnel made up of the pisiform and hamate bones, the transverse carpal ligament, and superficially the flexor carpi ulnaris insertion. The superficial and deep branches of the ulnar nerve pass through the tunnel, together with branches of the ulnar artery. The nerves supply sensation to the palmar skin of the fifth finger and the ulnar skin of the fourth finger and motor supply to the hypothenar muscles with exception of the adductor digiti minimi. A variety of causes of pressure on these nerves has been described, most commonly associated with trauma (particularly fracture to the hook of hamate), occupational or recreational compression (bicycle riding), or soft tissue mass including a ganglion, giant cell tumour of the tendon sheath, an aberrant muscle or ulnar artery aneurysm. Imaging is useful to detect mass encroachment on the nerves, aneurysmal dilatation of the ulnar artery or bone fragments within the canal. Although changes in the nerve can be demonstrated (predominantly oedema which is hyperintense on T2-weighted images or nerve swelling on MRI or ultrasound) these are not in themselves diagnostic.

REFERENCES

1. Resnick D, Niwayama G 1976 Radiographic and pathologic features of spinal involvement in diffuse idiopathic skeletal hyperostosis (DISH). Radiology 119: 559–568
2. Resnick D, Shaul S R, Robins J M 1975 Diffuse idiopathic skeletal hyperostosis (DISH): Forestier's disease with extraspinal manifestations. Radiology 115: 513–524
3. Pennes D R, Martel W, Ellis C N 1985 Retinoid-induced ossification of the posterior longitudinal ligament. Skeletal Radiol 14: 191–193
4. Vas W, Cockshott W P, Martin R F, Pai M K, Walker I 1981 Myositis ossificans in hemophilia. Skeletal Radiol 7: 27–31
5. Hermann G, Gilbert M S, Abdelwahab I F 1992 Hemophilia: evaluation of musculoskeletal involvement with CT, sonography, and MR imaging. Am J Roentgenol 158: 119–123
6. Wilkins R M, Wiedel J D 1983 Septic arthritis of the knee in a hemophiliac. A case report. J Bone Joint Surg Am 65: 267–268
7. Resnick D, Oliphant M 1975 Hemophilia-like arthropathy of the knee associated with cutaneous and synovial hemangiomas. Report of 3 cases and review of the literature. Radiology 114: 323–326
8. Hochberg M C 1981 Adult and juvenile rheumatoid arthritis: current epidemiologic concepts. Epidemiol Rev 3: 27–44
9. Peterfy C G 2001 Magnetic resonance imaging in rheumatoid arthritis: current status and future directions. J Rheumatol 28: 1134–1142
10. Ostergaard M, Hansen M, Stoltenberg M et al 1999 Magnetic resonance imaging-determined synovial membrane volume as a marker of disease activity and a predictor of progressive joint destruction in the wrists of patients with rheumatoid arthritis. Arthritis Rheum 42: 918–929
11. McQueen F M, Stewart N, Crabbe J et al 1999 Magnetic resonance imaging of the wrist in early rheumatoid arthritis reveals progression of erosions despite clinical improvement. Ann Rheum Dis 58: 156–163
12. Poleksic L, Zdravkovic D, Jablanovic D, Watt I, Bacic G 1993 Magnetic resonance imaging of bone destruction in rheumatoid arthritis: comparison with radiography. Skeletal Radiol 22: 577–580
13. Sugimoto H, Takeda A, Hyodoh K 2000 Early-stage rheumatoid arthritis: prospective study of the effectiveness of MR imaging for diagnosis. Radiology 216: 569–575
14. Fabricant M S, Chandor S B, Friou G J 1973 Still disease in adults. A cause of prolonged undiagnosed fever. JAMA 225: 273–276

15. Medsger T A Jr, Christy W C 1976 Carpal arthritis with ankylosis in late onset Still's disease. Arthritis Rheum 19: 232–242
16. Rombouts J J, Rombouts-Lindemans C 1974 Scoliosis in juvenile rheumatoid arthritis. J Bone Joint Surg Br 56B: 478–483
17. Moll J M, Wright V 1973 Psoriatic arthritis. Semin Arthritis Rheum 3: 55–78
18. Leirisalo M, Skylv G, Kousa M et al 1982 Followup study on patients with Reiter's disease and reactive arthritis, with special reference to HLA-B27. Arthritis Rheum 25: 249–259
19. Calin A, Fries J F 1976 An "experimental" epidemic of Reiter's syndrome revisited. Follow-up evidence on genetic and environmental factors. Ann Intern Med 84: 564–566
20. Berens D L 1971 Roentgen features of ankylosing spondylitis. Clin Orthop Relat Res 74: 20–33
21. Goldberg A L, Keaton N L, Rothfus W E, Daffner R H 1993 Ankylosing spondylitis complicated by trauma: MR findings correlated with plain radiographs and CT. Skeletal Radiol 22: 333–336
22. Resnick D, Reinke R T, Taketa R M 1975 Early-onset gouty arthritis. Radiology 114: 67–73
23. Gottlieb N L, Gray R G 1977 Allopurinol-associated hand and foot deformities in chronic tophaceous gout. JAMA 238: 1663–1664
24. Aouba A, Vuillemin-Bodaghi V, Mutschler C, De Bandt M 2004 Crowned dens syndrome misdiagnosed as polymyalgia rheumatica, giant cell arteritis, meningitis or spondylitis: an analysis of eight cases. Rheumatology (Oxford) 43: 1508–1512
25. Dalinka M K, Stewart V, Bomalaski J S, Halpern M, Kricun M E 1984 Periarticular calcifications in association with intra-articular corticosteroid injections. Radiology 153: 615–618
26. Arnett F C, Edworthy S M, Bloch D A et al 1988 The American Rheumatism Association 1987 revised criteria for the classification of rheumatoid arthritis. Arthritis Rheum 31: 315–324
27. Neiman H L, Gompels B M, Martel W 1974 Pachydermoperiostosis with bone marrow failure and gross extramedullary hematopoiesis. Report of a case. Radiology 110: 553–554
28. Goldman A B, DiCarlo E F 1988 Pigmented villonodular synovitis. Diagnosis and differential diagnosis. Radiol Clin North Am 26: 1327–1347
29. Glickstein M F, Burk D L Jr, Schiebler M L et al 1988 Avascular necrosis versus other diseases of the hip: sensitivity of MR imaging. Radiology 169: 213–215
30. Ehman R L, Berquist T H 1986 Magnetic resonance imaging of musculoskeletal trauma. Radiol Clin North Am 24: 291–319
31. Mitchell D G, Rao V M, Dalinka M K et al 1987 Femoral head avascular necrosis: correlation of MR imaging, radiographic staging, radionuclide imaging, and clinical findings. Radiology 162: 709–715
32. Edwards D J, Lomas D, Villar R N 1995 Diagnosis of the painful hip by magnetic resonance imaging and arthroscopy. J Bone Joint Surg Br 77: 374–376
33. Kornick J, Trefelner E, McCarthy S, Lange R, Lynch K, Jokl P 1990 Meniscal abnormalities in the asymptomatic population at MR imaging. Radiology 177: 463–465
34. Bessette G C, Hunter R E 1990 The anterior cruciate ligament. Orthopedics 13: 551–562
35. Murphy B J, Smith R L, Uribe J W, Janecki C J, Hechtman K S, Mangasarian R A 1992 Bone signal abnormalities in the posterolateral tibia and lateral femoral condyle in complete tears of the anterior cruciate ligament: a specific sign? Radiology 182: 221–224
36. Shabshin N, Schweitzer M E, Morrison W B, Parker L 2004 MRI criteria for patella alta and baja. Skeletal Radiol 33: 445–450
37. Berndt A L, Harty M 1959 Transchondral fractures (osteochondritis dissecans) of the talus. Am J Orthop 41-A: 988–1020
38. Neer C S 2005 Anterior acromioplasty for the chronic impingement syndrome in the shoulder. J Bone Joint Surg Am 87: 1399
39. Vanarthos W J, Monu J U Type 4 acromion: a new classification. Contemp Orthop 30: 227–229
40. Snyder S J, Karzel R P, Del Pizzo W, Ferkel R D, Friedman M J 1990 SLAP lesions of the shoulder. Arthroscopy 6: 274–279
41. Desser T S, McCarthy S, Trumble T 1990 Scaphoid fractures and Kienböck's disease of the lunate: MR imaging with histopathologic correlation. Magn Reson Imaging 8: 357–361
42. Kulkarni R W, Wollstein R, Tayar R, Citron N 1999 Patterns of healing of scaphoid fractures. The importance of vascularity. J Bone Joint Surg Br 81: 85–90

FURTHER READING

Resnick D 1997 Internal derangement of joints: Emphasis on MR imaging. W B Saunders, Philadelphia.

Vahlensieck M, Genant H K (eds), Winter P (trans) 2000 MRI of the musculoskeletal system. Thieme, Stuttgart.

Stoller D W 1997 Magnetic resonance imaging in orthopaedics and sports medicine, 2nd edn. Lippincott-Raven, Philadelphia.

Kransdorf M J, Murphy M D 1997 Imaging of soft tissue tumours. W B Saunders, Philadelphia.

Stoller D W 1999 MRI arthroscopic and surgical anatomy of the joints. Lippincott-Raven, Philadelphia.

Stoller D, Tirman P, Bredella M et al 2003 Diagnostic imaging: Orthopaedics. W B Saunders, Philadelphia.

Isenberg D A, Renton P 2003 Imaging in rheumatology. Oxford University Press, Oxford.

Greenfield G B, Arrington J A, Vasey F B 2001 Imaging in arthritis and related conditions. Lippincott-Raven, Philadelphia.

Resnick D 2002 Diagnosis of bone and joint disorders, 4th edn. W B Saunders, Philadelphia.

CHAPTER 51

Bone and Soft Tissue Infection

David J. Wilson and Anthony R. Berendt

INTRODUCTION

A range of microorganisms may infect any of the tissues of the musculoskeletal system where they usually cause symptom complexes of pain and loss of function, variably accompanied by fever and systemic illness. Joints and bone have a relatively poor blood supply compared to soft tissues and probably for this reason infections in these locations are more likely to become chronic and recurrent if they are not adequately treated in the early stages. On the other hand, infection of muscle and subcutaneous tissues, whilst potentially life threatening, tends to be limited to an acute and defined episode.

Even with antibiotic and surgical treatment, osteomyelitis is a difficult disease to treat and the infectious agent may be very difficult if not impossible to eradicate, while the symptomatic and structural problems that result can give rise to considerable morbidity and occasionally death. Early diagnosis and prompt appropriate treatment are therefore mandatory. The symptoms and signs of skeletal infection are varied and often nonspecific. Infection may mimic other conditions, most significantly degenerative disease, but also malignancy. Hence imaging has a crucial role in the detection, discrimination and diagnosis of infection of bone, joint and soft tissue and the radiologist is likely to play a pivotal role in management. Some presentations will require emergency investigation[1,2].

PATHOLOGICAL BASIS

Route of infection

Infection may be introduced via the bloodstream (haematogenous) or by direct inoculation, including by contiguous spread. Trauma, surgery and chronic ulceration are the most common causes of the latter. The type of organism that affects the bone or joint will to some extent depend on the route of infection. Pathogens causing haematogenous musculoskeletal infection are generally those associated with primary bacteraemias. Of these, *Staphylococcus aureus* is by far the most important, with *Haemophilus influenzae* (in the unimmunized), *Streptococcus pneumoniae*, the beta-haemolytic streptococci and the aerobic Gram-negative rods also playing a role. Where foreign bodies are present (prosthetic joints and other orthopaedic metal ware), pathogens include skin commensals of low virulence such as the coagulase-negative staphylococci. Implants may be infected haematogenously, but the majority of infections reflect contamination at the time of implantation. Fractures that were open at the time of injury are common sites for infection. The more complex the injury and the type of fracture, the greater is the risk. Early sepsis reflects direct implantation and causes include environmental organisms such as aerobic Gram-negative rods (e.g. *Pseudomonas*) and anaerobic Gram-positive rods (including *Clostridium* spp.) where debridement of contaminated or devitalized tissue has been inadequate, or involvement with skin pathogens and commensals after surgery and instrumentation (e.g. *Staphylococcus aureus*). It is unclear whether delayed onset infection is due to reactivation of a chronic and occult osteomyelitis or the result of blood-borne organisms settling in previously damaged, and hence compromised, tissue. It is probable that both these factors play a role.

Joint spaces are at particular risk of severe damage from infection. The articular cartilage is particularly susceptible to damage from infection and from the associated inflammatory response. Septic arthritis is a surgical emergency and treatment must be immediate and effective. Many surgeons would argue that prompt arthrotomy and lavage are mandatory; however, there is now increasing experience of conservative management of accessible joints with repeated aspiration. This is particularly appropriate in patients who are unwell for other reasons or unable to undergo anaesthesia and in small children. This strategy may also be the only way to manage septic arthritis with multiple joint involvement. The radiologist may be called upon to carry out image-guided drainage and catheter placement.

In the spine the disc spaces are the likeliest place for infection to arise. Osteochondrosis (degenerative disease of the disc) has a similar anatomical distribution and it is important to differentiate this condition from infection. Oedema and fluid in the disc are signs that make infection more likely than degeneration. Disease that is centred on the bone rather than the disc space is much less likely to be infection, and tumour and osteoporotic fracture should be considered. Circumstances that confuse these principles are when a tumour leads to a fracture and repair, when trauma accelerates degenerative change and when infection is low grade and indolent.

Immunocompromised patients are liable to rapid or occult infection. Advanced disease may present in bizarre fashion. The organisms may be unusual or rare and the rate of progress may be accelerated. Despite these factors the nature, appearance and pattern of infection is essentially the same and there is no need to alter the diagnostic principles outlined in this chapter.

Type of organisms

Bacteria, viruses and fungi can all infect bone, soft tissues and joints. The pattern of infection depends not only on the microorganism but also on the route of infection and the patient's resistance or immunity. In general, bacterial infections are more destructive and move rapidly. Fungi and atypical organisms such as *Actinomyces* tend to produce slow and chronic infections with an infiltrative pattern that may mimic malignancy. Tuberculosis and brucellosis exhibit a variety of patterns that range from aggressive to indolent and reparative. It is rare for imaging features to assist significantly in the identification of the type of microorganism. There is a large overlap in imaging appearances and a wide spectrum for each disease; guessing the type of infection will mislead more often than assist.

Bone reaction

There are limited ways in which bone can react to a disease process. These are lysis, sclerosis, fractures, heterotopic bone formation, bone expansion or remodelling and a periosteal reaction. Other diseases including tumour, trauma and degeneration can trigger many of these patterns. The hallmark of infection is that aggressive and rapidly changing features (lysis, cortical breach and fracture) are mixed with slower reactions (sclerosis, heterotopic bone and periosteal reaction).

If an abscess cavity forms in bone and breaks through to the soft tissues and skin the discharging sinus is a pathognomonic sign of infection. The hole in the bone develops a sclerotic margin and is called a cloaca. If a fragment of bone becomes avascular and separated mechanically it is called a sequestrum. A layer of living bone surrounding dead bone is called an involucrum, another classical sign of infection.

Periosteal reactions start as oedema immediately beneath the periosteum and may be seen on magnetic resonance imaging (MRI) or ultrasound (US)[3,4]. Then ossification occurs in the periosteum; this may be seen on radiography (Figs 51.1, 51.2, 51.3) but often not until two weeks after MR or US has demonstrated the abnormality. Untreated infection may produce a layered periosteal reaction—the 'onion skin' effect. This is not specific for infection and may be seen in neoplasia, typically in eosinophilic granulomas. Periosteal reaction may also be seen as a normal (physiological) finding in about half of all infants. It may be seen in other systemic disease including leukaemia,

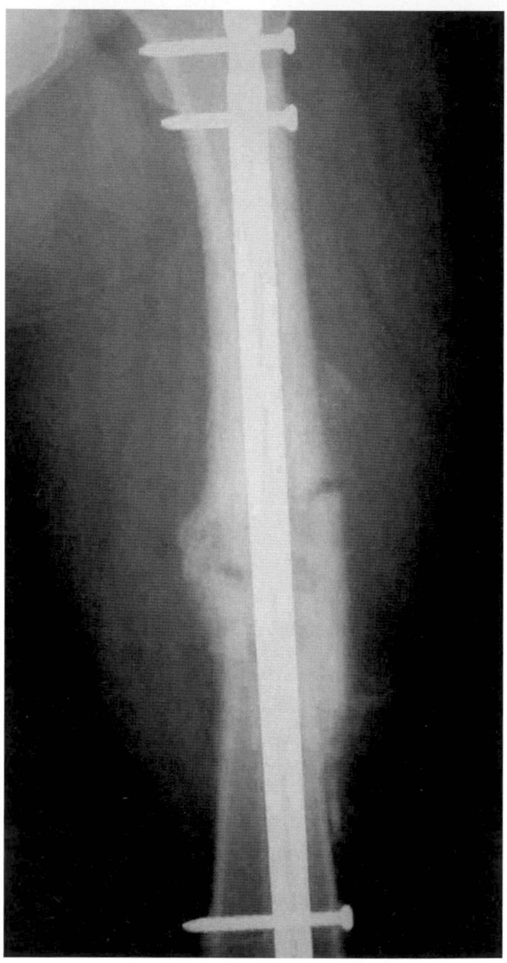

Figure 51.1 Infection at the fracture site has delayed union in the humerus. Note the extensive periosteal reaction.

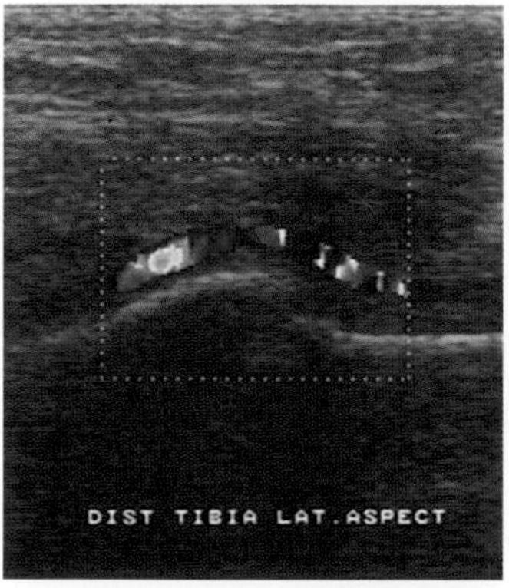

Figure 51. 2 An infected fracture of the tibia exhibits markedly increased flow on colour Doppler US. This may be judged by comparison with the normal side.

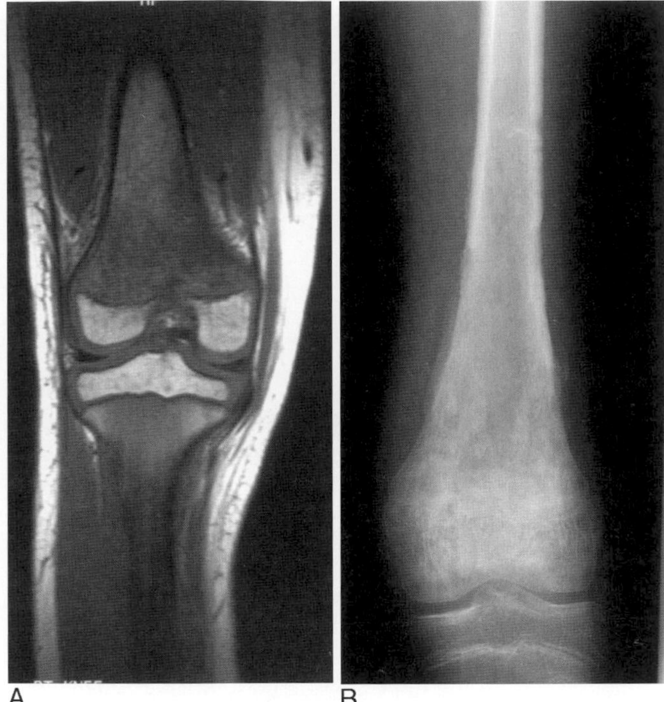

Figure 51.3 Osteomyelitis of the distal femur. The early MR (T1 SE) study (A) shows sparing of the epiphyses. The plain radiograph taken some months later (B) shows chronic osteomyelitis with sclerosis from the metaphyses and epiphysis. There are cortical defects and periosteal new bone.

neuroblastoma, and vitamin A poisoning. The latter is now most often seen in patients taking retinoid therapy (e.g. etretinate) for skin disease as these drugs are vitamin A analogues[5].

The progress of infection from onset to recovery or chronicity is characterized by normal looking bone (albeit infected) through periosteal reactions of increasing maturity, through lysis to mixed lytic and sclerotic lesions sometimes leading to sequestration and cloacae. The latter features are only seen in chronic infection.

Soft tissue reaction

Oedema and swelling are the principal response of soft tissues to infection. Cellulitis may progress with necrosis with cavitation, and sometimes haemorrhage may occur in the more fulminant disease process. As the organisms become established, collections of pus may develop in microabscesses. These may coalesce to create a macroscopic abscess. In due course an untreated abscess may point to the surface and discharge either onto the skin or into a viscus.

Potential cavities such as bursae or tendon sheaths may become infected although collections of fluid in these locations are more commonly the result of repetitive injury or inflammatory joint disease. Chronic soft tissue involvement may lead to indurated changes, especially in the case of the more indolent fungal infections. Calcification may occur in soft tissues secondary to local necrosis or in the wall of treated abscesses.

Joint reaction

A joint effusion is the nonspecific response to many irritants including infection. The effusion may be transparent and straw coloured but is more commonly hazy and turbid; haemorrhagic breakdown products and eventually frank pus are also encountered. By the time that pus is present in the joint there is a major risk of serious articular damage. The articular cartilage has a poor blood supply and is particularly sensitive to infection and inflammation. Cartilage oedema, thinning and focal destruction are the next stage. In animal models there is evidence that much of the joint destruction is due to the inflammatory response to the infection, with inflammatory tissue, effectively the same as pannus in rheumatoid disease, sweeping across and destroying the cartilage. The underlying bone will at first exhibit oedema and hyperaemia; then secondary direct infection may take place with all the features of conventional osteomyelitis. The more indolent infections may erode the margins of the joint, eating away at the cortex in the first instance. In children the growing epiphysis is at great risk and secondary growth arrest or disturbance is common. On the other hand, in chronic infection, hyperaemia of the adjacent bone may lead to overgrowth of the epiphysis with abnormally large metaphyses and epiphyses.

CLINICAL ENTITIES

Acute osteomyelitis

Typical acute osteomyelitis presents as an episode of local pain, reduced function and systemic ill health. The pain may be severe requiring opiate analgesics. Fever and toxicity are common but not universal. Oedema and redness of the soft tissues may occur but their absence does not exclude the diagnosis. Small children may not be able to explain that they have local pain and may present with irritability and reluctance to move the affected part or the entire limb served by the joint in question. Spinal infection in those too young to complain of back pain may manifest as a refusal to walk. If the symptoms are undiagnosed or unheeded then worsening pain and increasing general debility will ensue.

Chronic osteomyelitis

Symptoms vary from pain, swelling, general debility, chronic damage from a sinus and weight loss at one extreme to a complete absence of complaints at the other. The disability that ensues will depend on location and mechanical effects of the bony destruction. Chronic infection may lead to anaemia, cachexia, and on rare occasions to renal dysfunction secondary to amyloid deposition or the development of squamous metaplasia and, even, carcinoma in a chronic sinus. Flare-up of relatively acute symptoms and signs occurs at intervals often with years between. Dormant periods of over 40 years have been recorded.

Septic arthritis

Acute pain, effusion and limitation of movement are the commonest symptoms. It would be exceptionally rare for a joint to be infected but asymptomatic, but it is not uncommon to see presentations of chronic septic arthritis where the diagnosis was missed while acute. These cases present instead as rapidly progressive, destructive arthritis and the possibility of infection must be borne in mind to prevent joint replacement occurring without a concurrent strategy to manage the infection[6].

Cellulitis

Swelling, pain and heat are the hallmarks. Care must be taken to differentiate these features from those of vascular insufficiency (poor pulses) and deep venous thrombosis (sometimes very difficult to discriminate). All clinicians should be aware of the occasional presentation of necrotizing fasciitis, characterized by a degree of systemic illness and pain that is disproportionate to the physical signs, with the subsequent development of necrotic or blistering skin lesions. Imaging rarely adds to the diagnosis, which should be based on clinical signs. This is an acute problem which requires early management. MRI is a sensitive and specific tool to identify the extent of the disease and involvement of the fascia when there is soft tissue infection. It has a role in the staging of the extent and the planning of debridement and eventual soft tissue repair procedures.

Abscess

Pain, swelling and a prodromal illness are typical. A discharge is virtually pathognomonic. Abscess may be confused with a fast-growing soft tissue neoplasm. In some cases puncture and biopsy are the only means of discriminating between these entities. The cavity may contain debris and particulate matter. The surrounding tissues are oedematous and swollen, however imaging abnormalities do not necessarily indicate presence of the microorganism in the affected parts[7].

Pyomyositis

The signs and symptoms are very similar to those of cellulitis and abscess. In tropical countries where this condition is more common it will be considered early in the differential diagnosis but it is seen throughout the world. The symptoms may mimic musculoskeletal injury. *Staphylococcus aureus* is the commonest cause[8]. Imaging is important in the detection, staging and follow-up during treatment. Muscle enlargement and oedema with separate fluid collections in soft tissues are the principal features. Computed tomography (CT) and MR are the most useful techniques[9,10]. US will show abnormalities but is less valuable as a staging method. As percutaneous drainage may be part of the management[11] US and other guidance methods may be employed.

Necrotizing fasciitis

This life-threatening condition often commences with trauma although it may be minor in nature (cut or insect bite). Although group A *Streptococcus* is the most common bacterial isolate, a polymicrobial infection with a variety of Gram-positive, Gram-negative, aerobic and anaerobic bacteria is more common. Large areas of soft tissue and muscle are destroyed and devitalized. Gas formation in soft tissues may be present but its absence does not exclude the condition. Aggressive surgical debridement and a broad-spectrum antibiotic are essential to manage this potentially devastating disease[12–14].

Discitis

There may be a history of recent surgery or needle puncture (e.g. discography), but most cases arise spontaneously within degenerative discs. Increasing pain and limitation of movement are common. Some cases may resolve without treatment and milder forms are likely to be more common than has been recognized. Infection may ultimately produce paraspinal or iliopsoas abscesses, which give local symptoms and may discharge. It may also be complicated by spinal epidural abscess in which a pattern of progressively severe pain, accompanied by fever, is followed by neurological symptoms and subsequently signs[15,16].

RADIOLOGICAL APPEARANCES

Bone

Early

The earliest stage of osteomyelitis is not readily detected on any imaging technique. Most patients will undergo plain radiography and a normal study should not discourage further investigation. Skeletal scintigraphy should be positive at an early stage but this can occasionally be problematic in children as the growth plates are adjacent to the areas most often affected by bone infection. Ultrasound will show collections of fluid in the area immediately beneath the periosteum. They are seen as echo-free lines below the reflective line of the periosteum. Care must be taken to avoid confusion with muscle planes that are hypoechoic and with physiological cortical proliferation. Comparison with the opposite side is essential. It is likely that US evidence of periosteal oedema is one of the earliest imaging signs but unfortunately if it is not seen the diagnosis has not been fully excluded[4,17]. MR will show oedema on STIR or T2-weighted fat-suppressed images[18]. The affected area will enhance with intravenous Gd-DTPA[19]. However, most cases of osteomyelitis may be confidently diagnosed on MR without intravenous contrast medium. There are reports where MR failed to show any abnormality in early disease although some would argue that the lack of STIR images raises doubt regarding the MR techniques employed by the authors. The extent of the marrow oedema is likely to extend considerably beyond the limits of the truly infected bone. This difference will diminish as the infection takes hold. CT is perhaps the least useful technique in early disease as it does not show marrow oedema or subperiosteal collections adequately. CT may be of increased value in the later stages of the disease process.

It is important that the radiologist is aware that the diagnosis of acute osteomyelitis is, for management purposes, a clinical one. Antibiotic therapy in suspected acute osteomyelitis should generally not be delayed while waiting for imaging, as the immediate priority is to minimize the risk of bone death and resulting chronicity. Imaging can then be used in a confirmatory mode and for surgical planning if collections are found.

Intermediate

Those who have suffered from bone infection for several days will start to exhibit bone reaction and destruction. On plain radiographs a new periosteal reaction with a fluffy margin is typical. US will show increasing soft tissue oedema and subperiosteal fluid. MR is now probably the most sensitive technique as the marrow changes predominate. CT and US have limited roles. On MR a 'penumbra' sign has been described on T1 spin-echo images[20] (Fig. 51.4). This probably represents a layer of granulation tissue. The sign is more common than the double line observed at the margin of a lesion on T2-weighted

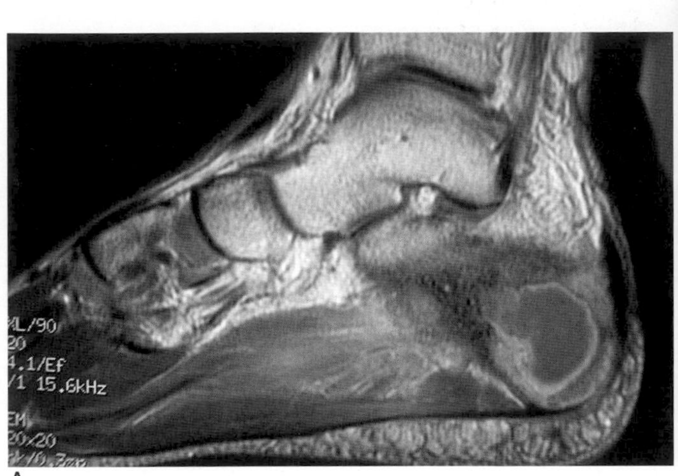

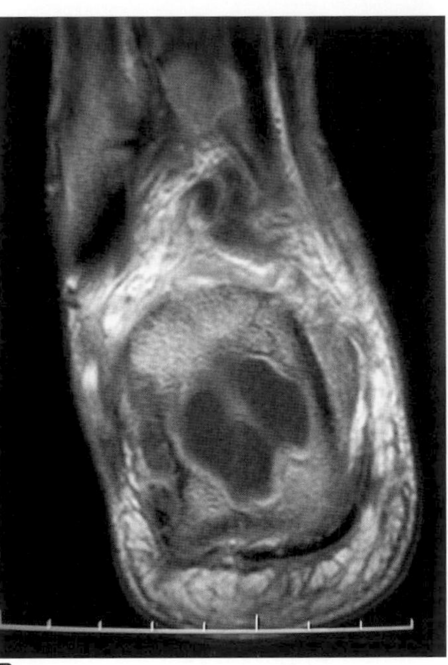

Figure 51.4 Penumbra sign. Sagittal (A) and coronal (B) MR images of the calcaneus show a circumscribed area of bone destruction with a halo or penumbra of granulation tissue and oedema.

and STIR images. It is strongly suggestive of osteomyelitis although it has been observed in cases of eosinophilic granuloma[21] and an unusual case of chondrosarcoma[22].

Late

Bone destruction followed by phases of healing and reaction leads to a mixed pattern that exhibits areas that seem to be aggressively changing and others that are indolent and repairing (Figs 51.5, 51.6). Hence the mixed pattern of destruction and bone remodelling that is almost diagnostic of chronic bone infection taken in isolation. The so-called 'sclerosing osteomyelitis of Garré' describes florid new bone formation and relatively dense bone, probably due to what we would now regard as classic untreated osteomyelitis[23]. This is fortunately rare in developed countries and the term is now used to describe a chronic osteomyelitis that shows a profound sclerotic reaction.

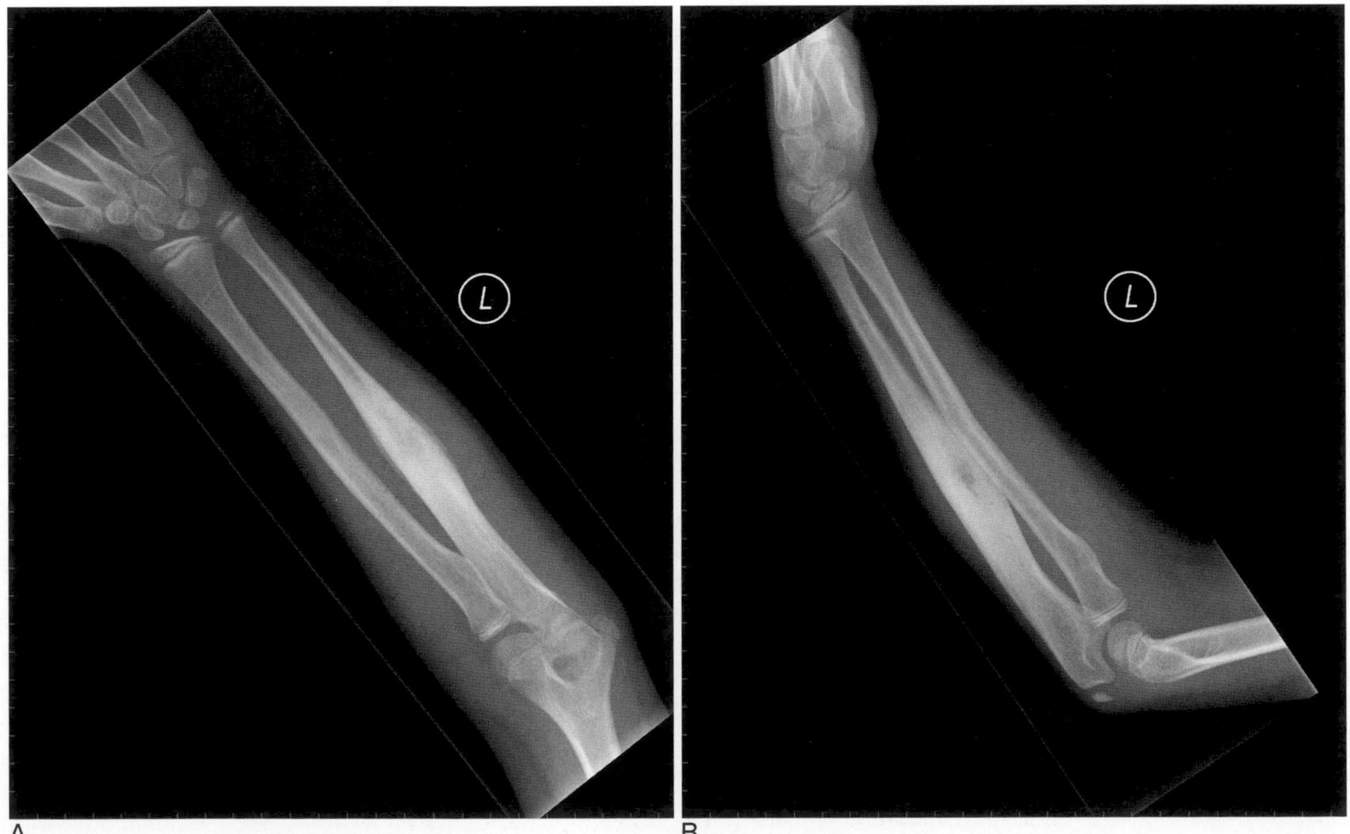

Figure 51.5 Chronic osteomyelitis of the ulna with plain radiographs (A, B),

Continued

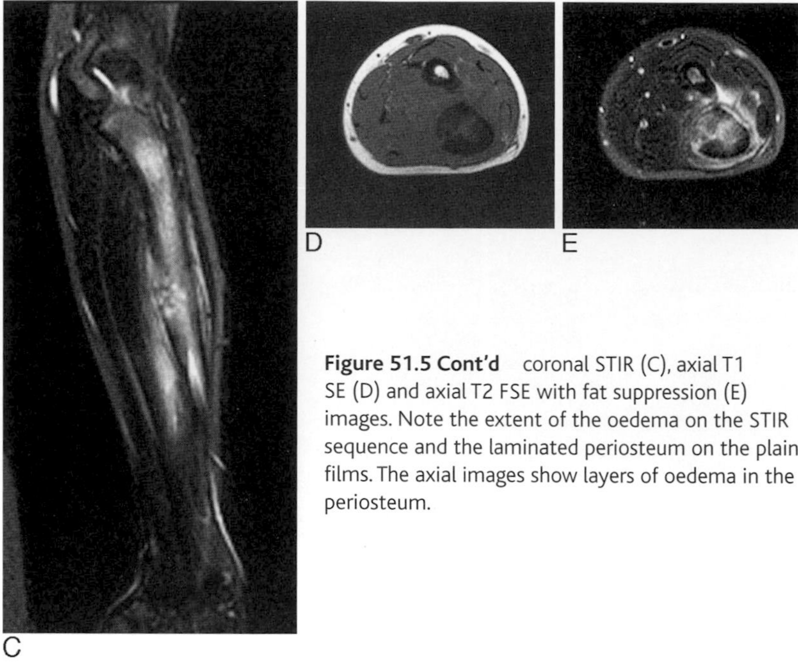

Figure 51.5 Cont'd coronal STIR (C), axial T1 SE (D) and axial T2 FSE with fat suppression (E) images. Note the extent of the oedema on the STIR sequence and the laminated periosteum on the plain films. The axial images show layers of oedema in the periosteum.

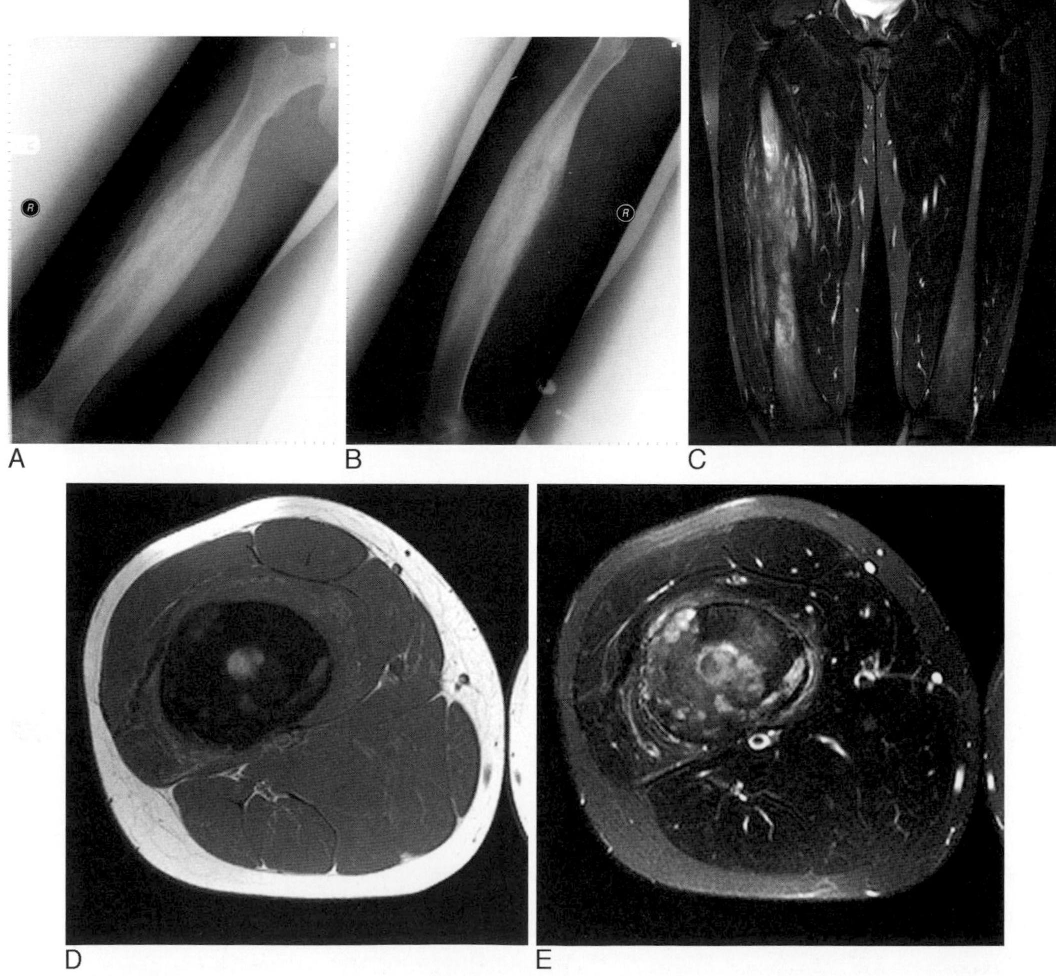

Figure 51.6 Chronic osteomyelitis of the femur with plain radiographs (A, B), coronal FSTIR (C), axial T1 SE (D) and axial T2 FSE (E) with fat suppression. This degree of periosteal new bone takes months if not years to develop.

Brodie's abscess is the description of an intraosseous abscess that has become somewhat 'walled off' and is seen much later in the progress of the infection. Signs are intense local sclerosis with relatively little to see on MR compared to the plain radiographic or CT appearances. This is one end of a spectrum of chronic or acute-on-chronic reactions and merges into other patterns. Sequestra are dead pieces of tissue, usually in the centre of the affected bone. They have lost their blood supply and are foci for the recurrence or flare-up of infection. Chronic discharge to the skin or a viscus may occur, the hole in the bone is known as a cloaca and the tract as a sinus. The route of the sinus may be tortuous.

Exceptionally rarely the bed of chronic infection may give rise to an aggressive sarcoma. These are very difficult to recognize early and carry a poor prognosis.

^{99m}Tc-MDP (monodiphosphonate) scintigraphy has high sensitivity but low specificity; ^{111}In-labelled white cell studies have high specificity but low sensitivity. This has led to suggestion by some authors that these tests should be combined[24]. However, many of the articles contain serious methodological flaws including the lack of defined standards for test assessment, lack of blinding, and in some cases, using the test result as part of the definition of infection! Notwithstanding these points, nuclear medicine has a useful screening role in identifying the location and extent of disease but it is not as valuable as MR. It may have a role in locating occult disease, especially using indium-labelled white cells or labelled autoantibodies. Gallium is now considered to be a less effective scintigraphy agent[25,26]. F-FDG PET and PET CT are likely to become increasingly used to detect musculoskeletal infection but there are few data to indicate superiority over MR[27–29].

Soft tissue

Early

Plain radiographs are insensitive to soft tissue infection. Oedema may be apparent but this should be obvious on clinical examination. The presence of gas in the soft tissue is ominous. Organisms of bowel origin or the causative agent of gas gangrene (*Clostridium*) may produce gas. Gas gangrene is an over-diagnosed condition; genuine cases are always severely ill with profound toxicity and there should be no doubt of the diagnosis when looking at the patient. US is not especially rewarding in early infections but is of value to exclude the later stages where abscesses start to form. Nuclear medicine studies are sometimes negative although the partial necrotic tissue in fulminant infection may take up bone-seeking agents. CT may show gas but has little useful role. MR is very helpful in defining the extent and nature of abnormal tissue (Figs 51.7, 51.8). It is especially valuable in excluding cavities and ruling out adjacent bone or joint involvement.

Intermediate

Abscesses cavitate and coalesce. US is useful in screening for and excluding this event; it also may be used to guide diagnostic puncture and therapeutic drainage[30–32]. In infection limited to soft tissues there have been successful treatment regimens that use only percutaneous drainage as opposed to conventional surgery. If these methods are used then careful review of the imaging is essential to exclude areas of necrosis, particularly in the obese patient or when bulky areas are scanned, e.g. the hip and buttock. Even with the best of imaging this diagnosis may still be overlooked; therefore if there is inadequate early improvement on drainage then early recourse to open surgery will be essential.

Late

Drainage and surgery are used to treat established abscesses. This is best planned using MR or CT. US is the best guidance method for percutaneous drainage. Associated deep venous thrombosis may be diagnosed by a combination of ultrasound compression, Doppler ultrasound and occasionally venography.

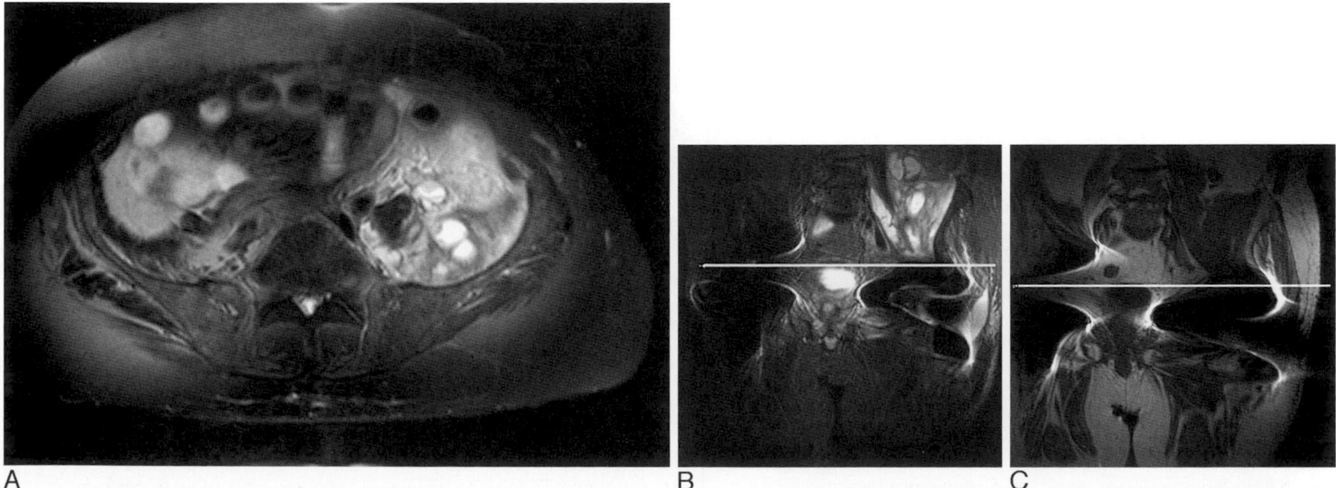

Figure 51.7 Iliopsoas abscess. (A–C) The abscess involves both psoas and iliacus muscles. There are cavities containing pus. The distortion on the coronal images is due to bilateral hip replacements. MR is often useful adjacent to metal but it should be remembered that the artefact masks areas and additional imaging (US/CT/NM) may be needed.

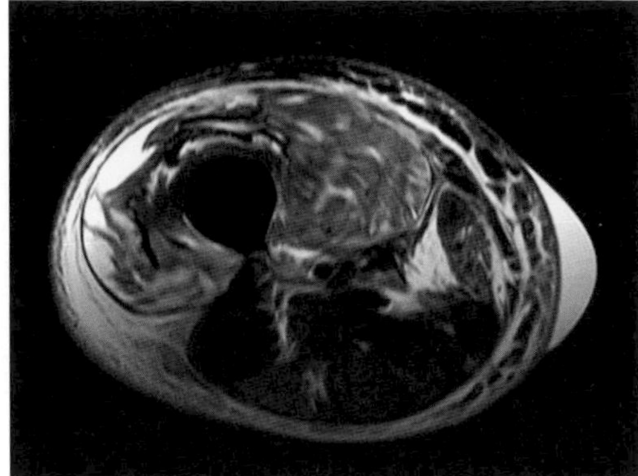

Figure 51.8 Necrotizing fasciitis. Axial T2-weighted MR shows extensive oedema and replacement of muscle by high signal material.

Joint

Early

Plain radiographs are usually normal in early joint infection but may show evidence of an effusion. This is relatively easy to detect in the knee and elbow but other joints are unlikely to show signs that are of any help. US is the best method of detecting or excluding joint fluid (Fig. 51.9). Note that the US appearances are nonspecific; it is not possible to accurately differentiate between pus, exudate, blood, or transudate[33]. Ultrasound can show synovial thickening but again this is not a specific sign for infection. The only reliable method of determining the nature of an effusion is to aspirate the joint. This is readily achieved with ultrasound control. Note that cases of genuine bacterial septic arthritis may have a normal body temperature, normal white cell counts and an unremarkable C-reactive protein (CRP). There is no reliable clinical method of deciding which case of monoarthropathy is due to infection. Skeletal scintigraphy, CT and MR are unlikely to be employed in early infection but will show less advanced changes of the type described below.

Intermediate

Osteopenia around the joint will become apparent on plain radiographs. CT will show effusion and loss of mineral. MR will demonstrate oedema in the adjacent bone as well as evidence of effusion and synovitis (Fig. 51.10). Early cartilage thinning will be apparent on all imaging and early cortical destruction in adjacent bones.

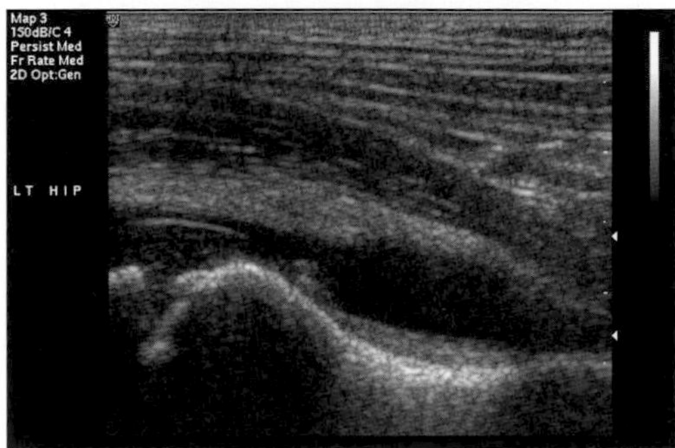

Figure 51.9 Ultrasound of the hip readily demonstrates an effusion but cannot determine whether it is due to transudate, pus or blood.

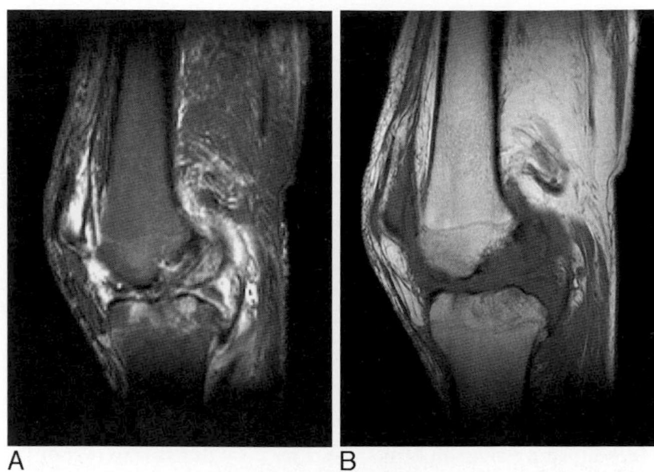

Figure 51.10 Septic arthritis. Sagittal T1 SE (A) and FSTIR (B) MR images show joint surface destruction and adjacent bone oedema. The synovium is irregular. These signs are nonspecific as they are also seen in advanced osteoarthritis and destructive arthropathies. Pus in the aspirate confirmed that this was an infected joint.

Late

Marginal destruction and bone erosion is clear on plain radiographs but more striking on CT (Fig. 51.11). MR will define the extent of bone and soft tissue involvement which is inevitably more dramatic than on any other imaging (Fig. 51.12). Sinus tracts may extend to the skin. The bone changes become identical to those of bone infection described above.

Muscle

Early

Plain radiographs are normal. US may show oedema by hypoechoic areas but as different muscle groups normally show varied patterns, great care must be taken to compare sides to avoid over-diagnosis. US will also allow differentiation of joint infection from muscle disease[34]. CT shows swelling but is far less useful than MR, which will demonstrate signal increase especially on STIR and fat-suppressed T2-weighted images. Skeletal scintigraphy may show increased tracer on the blood pool images.

Intermediate

The changes become more striking on all imaging. Cavitation and necrosis will be apparent on MR and US.

Late

Calcification in the margins of necrotic cavities is best seen on CT. The muscle may atrophy and be replaced by fat. Low attenuation on CT, hyperechogenicity on US, and increased fat signal on MR are observed.

Spine

Early

Infection in the spine almost always arises in the disc space and if it does not the organisms may well be unusual[35]. This is a relatively avascular area that is commonly the focus for mechanical degenerative changes (Fig. 51.13). It is probable that primary haematogenous osteomyelitis does arise, later affecting the vertebral

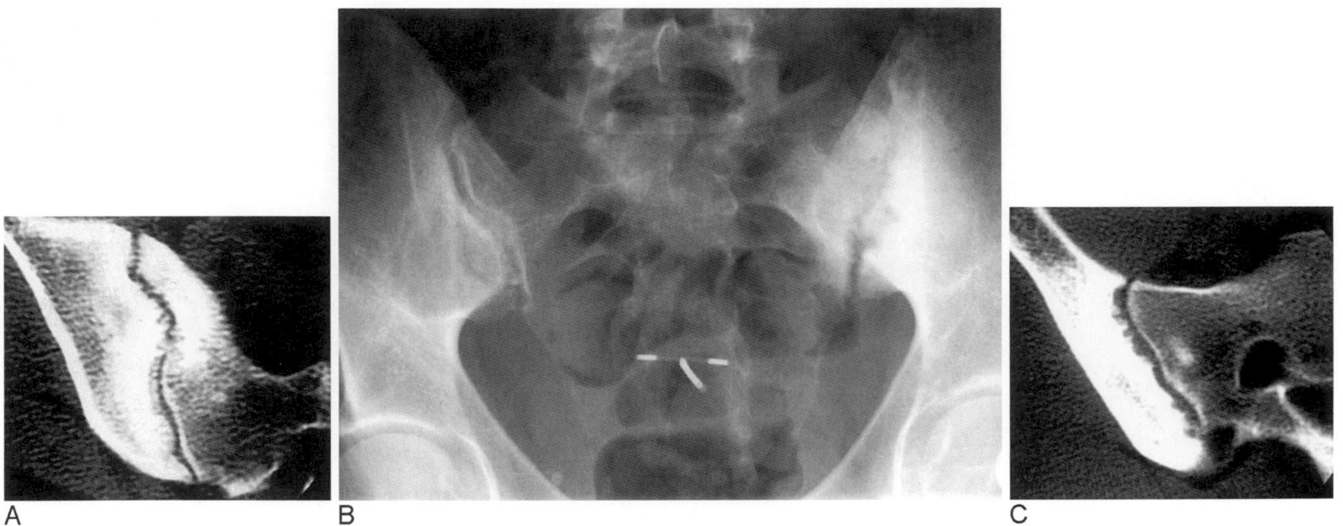

Figure 51.11 (A, B) CT cases of staphylococcal infective sacroiliitis shows irregularity of the joint surfaces and sclerosis either side of the joint. Compare this with (C), Reiter's syndrome, where the changes are confined to one side of the joint and erosions are prominent.

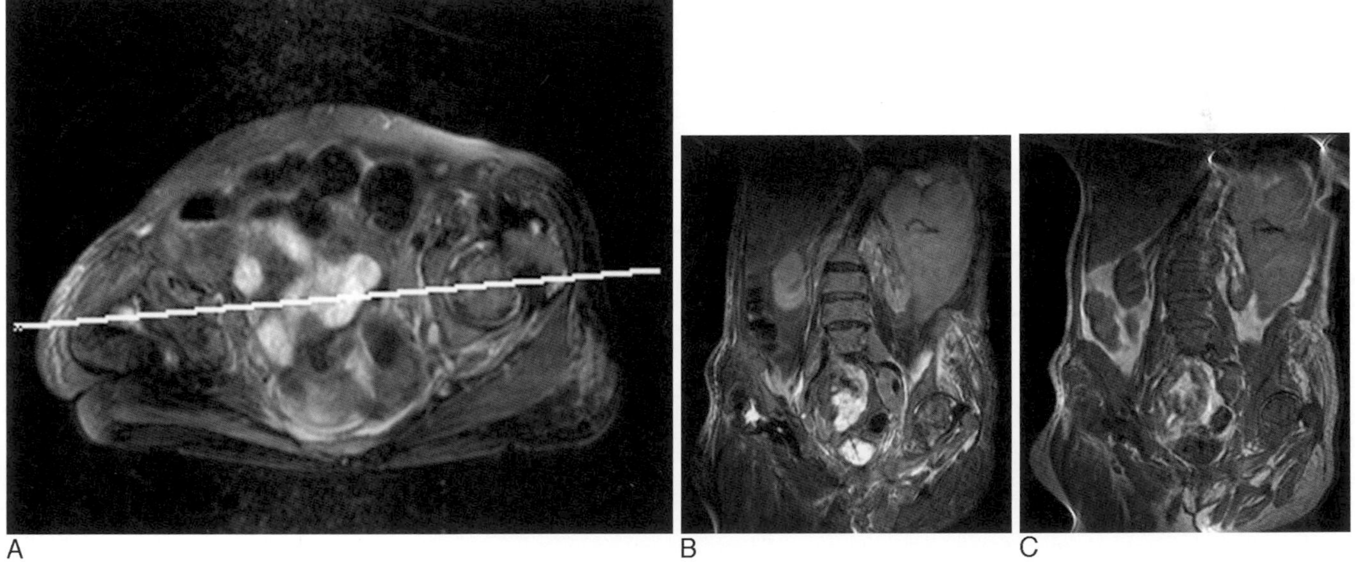

Figure 51.12 Excision arthroplasty for an infection. (A–C) On the left there is severe osteoarthritis and on the right a total hip replacement has been excised following infection leaving a cavity and pseudarthrosis. The left gluteal muscles are oedematous, raising the possibility of sepsis here as well. MR is useful in staging and following the extent of infection and response to treatment. Serial examinations will help judge the best time for formal replacement implant surgery but will also guide interventions such as debridement in the interim.

bodies. However, this would rapidly involve the disc space given the proximity to the trabecular bone, and disc involvement is a very early sign. The plain radiographic hallmarks are disc space narrowing, loss of clarity of the end-plates and paravertebral swelling (Figs 51.14, 51.15). Again the plain radiographs are often normal in the early stages. The area concerned is too deep for US; it is also surrounded by cortical bone that blocks sound. Nuclear medicine studies will be positive early although it might be necessary to resort to single photon emission computed tomography (SPECT) to identify detail of the abnormality.

Intermediate

Erosion of the bone occurs at the margins of the disc. In the more indolent infection, typically tuberculosis, the erosion and cortical destruction creeps along the vertebral margins under the anterior longitudinal ligament. The term 'tuberculous caries' has been employed. Plain radiographs readily demonstrate these changes as do CT and MR[36]. Scintigraphy will usually be positive but is nonspecific.

Late

As with all types of osteomyelitis, spine infections are associated with necrosis, cloacae, sequestra, and soft tissue and bone abscesses; the imaging of these is identical. In the spine, vertebral collapse may ensue, often leading to root and even cord compression. Epidural abscess may also occur, generally anterior to the cord/thecal sac, related to infected material in the disc space[37].

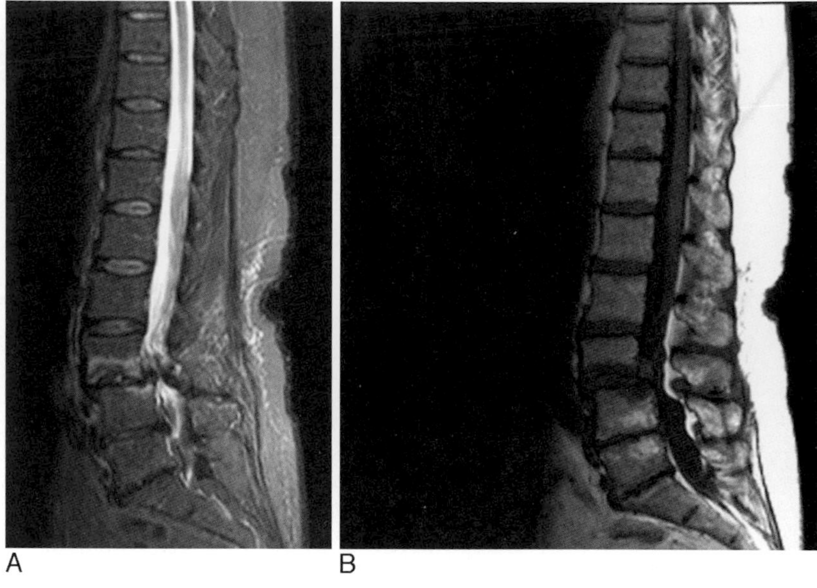

Figure 51.13 (A) Early infective discitis. T2W MR There is oedema in the L3/4 end-plates but this is the same sign as seen in degenerative stress change. The hallmark of infection is the high signal in the disc at a space that should be degenerate and therefore low signal. In this case there is also a degenerate slip of L3 on L4. Some believe that granulation tissue in the disc may be the cause of the high signal. There is a strong case for treating discitis as a degenerative condition with early follow-up and monitoring of systemic inflammatory markers. Early treatment with antibiotics is unlikely to help. (B) T1W MR shows chronic degenerative change (Modic Type 2) with fatty infiltration at L4/5.

Diabetic feet

In late diabetes the combination of a vasculitis and peripheral neuropathy often leads to chronic ulceration. Ulceration is due to the combination of loss of protective sensation, autonomic changes affecting skin pliability and altered architecture, with abnormal biomechanics due to motor neuropathy. Secondary infection is common. Here the imaging signs may be only of the features of bone infection that have been described above, but these are often superimposed on a destructive arthropathy with florid osteophytes and sclerosis due solely to neuropathy. In addition to this diabetic osteopathy, acute inflammation may occur in joints, commonly in the midfoot, due apparently to minor trauma, called an acute Charcot joint. This may be an aggressive process leading to major structural reorganization, most commonly a complete collapse and subsequent inversion of the plantar arch leading to the 'rocker bottom' deformity. The immediate clinical problem is how to differentiate active Charcot changes from infection that might require antibiotic therapy and surgery. In the longer term, Charcot rearrangements further affect the biomechanics of the foot and lead to ulceration that can be very difficult to treat.

Currently the best imaging methods are a combination of serial plain radiographs and MRI with contrast enhancement[38–42] although some authors question the need for contrast enhancement[43]. Nuclear medicine studies are very sensitive but also much less specific[44].

Rapid changes with bone destruction are possible in both neuropathic joints and infection but sepsis tends to be faster. Oedema in bone is also seen in both conditions but on balance infection is more likely to have an increased blood supply. Therefore, if an area of oedematous bone seen on a STIR image takes up contrast agent, it is more likely to be infected. Definitive discrimination is only possible with biopsy for histological analysis and culture. This can generally be performed under local anaesthetic using fluoroscopy and this is an important skill that the radiologist can bring to the multidisciplinary management of the diabetic foot. Imaging may render biopsy unnecessary and is essential for determining which piece of bone to sample[45–49].

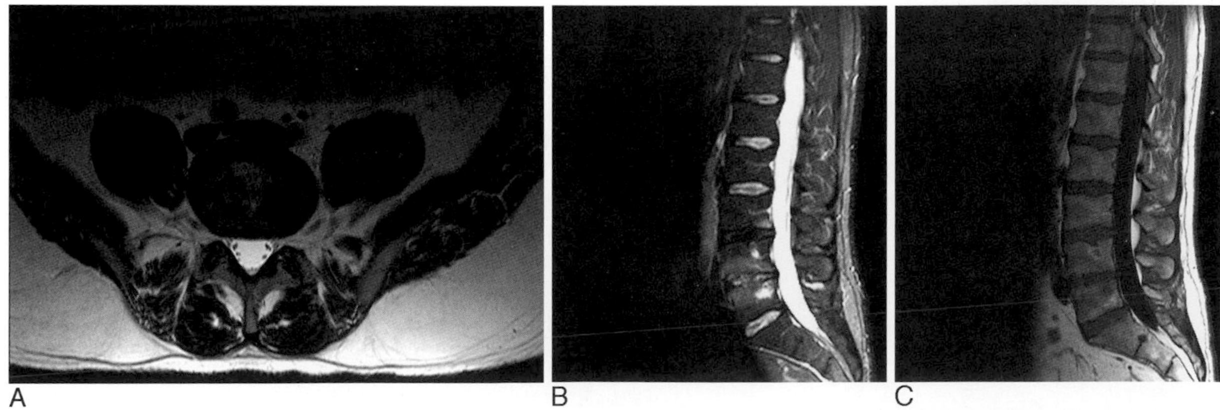

Figure 51.14 **Infective discitis at L4/5.** (A–C). A Axial T2W, B and C sagittal T2 and T1W MR images. Note the oedema on either side of the L4/5 disc. If this was a simple degenerative disc, it should be of low signal intensity on T2W. The fact that it yields high signal on T2W (B) indicates infection. Note how relatively normal the axial imae appears.

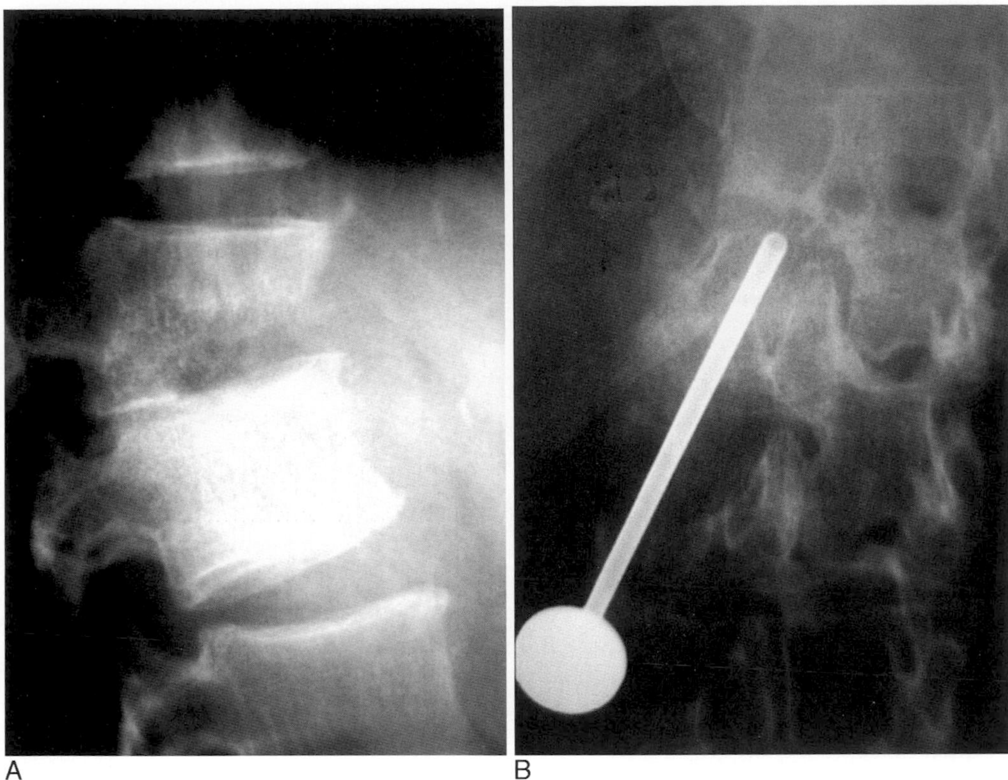

Figure 51.15 Infective discitis. (A) There is advanced end-plate destruction as well as sclerosis of the adjacent vertebrae. Biopsy will show abnormalities more reliably by histopathological examination. For this purpose, substantial core specimens assist the pathologist (B).

NAMED TYPES OF OSTEOMYELITIS

Some infections of bone have distinctive features. In reality there is a spectrum of response to infection and the following probably are best seen as ends of that range of response. The diagnoses of Brodie's abscess and of periostitis albuminosa have little impact on management.

Brodie's abscess

This is a description given to an intraosseous abscess that is surrounded by intense sclerosis (Fig. 51.16). It is probably one type of subacute infection. The plain radiographs may mimic osteoid osteoma but cross-sectional imaging will demonstrate a substantial cavity and biopsy will reveal infection[50].

Chronic multifocal osteomyelitis

In the 1970s it was noted that a number of children presented with a low-grade form of bone disease that behaved clinically like an acute osteomyelitis[51,52]. Typically it affected the long bones and went on to a sclerotic reaction. The first episode would settle and some months or even a few years later there would be recurrence at another site. No organisms are grown and the course of the disease becomes chronic and relapsing. The clinical importance is to avoid repeated biopsy once the relapsing nature of the condition has been recognized. Plain radiographs are essential to recognize the bone infection. Skeletal scintigraphy is a good method of screening for other lesions[53] whilst MRI is the best means of judging extent and activity.

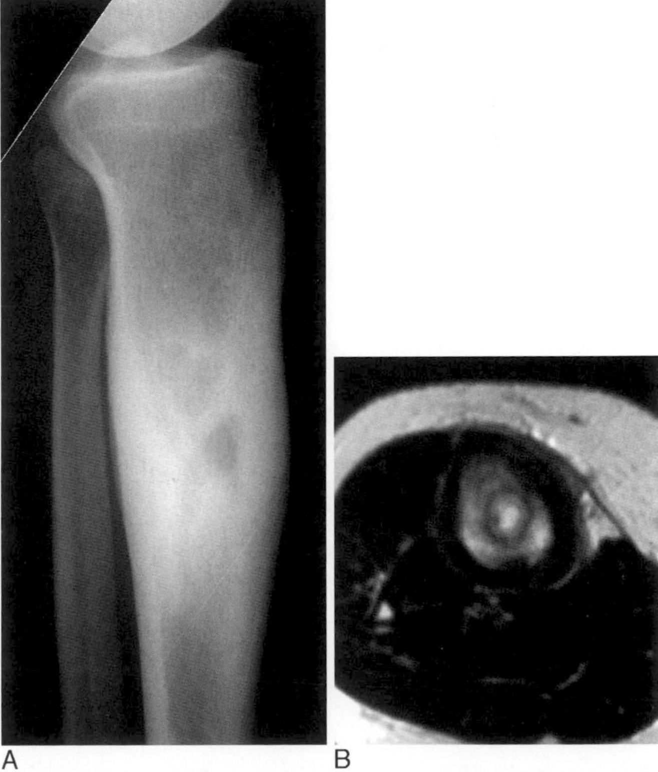

Figure 51.16 Brodie's abscess (A) with a penumbra sign on the axial MR image (B).

Sclerosing osteomyelitis of Garré

In the late 19th century Garré described four cases of children in their teens (aged 11–18) who suffered from osteomyelitis and had developed a collection of clear 'albumin containing' fluid adjacent to bone[23]. Each had presented acutely as pyogenic osteomyelitis. Pus was drained from the bone in two cases. As there was then no other treatment than surgery, all re-presented with recurrent symptoms. The interval varied from 10 months to 2 years. Aspirates at the second episode produced the 'albumin' containing fluid that in three of the four grew organisms (the types were not named in his paper). Garré was principally concerned that the bacteria were found despite the lack of frank pus. He termed the condition 'periostitis albuminosa'. He noted that Ollier had used the term much earlier in 1874.

Much later the term 'sclerosing osteomyelitis of Garré' was coined implying a separate disease entity. Reading the original work it is apparent that he was really describing the sequelae of osteomyelitis in the pre-antibiotic era. We now know that organisms persist for years despite a quiescent illness, in part due to Garré's observations.

From a practical point of view it is better to regard this as one type of reaction that may occur in chronic infection rather than a disease on its own[54].

Sickle-cell disease

Homozygous sickle-cell disease is associated with dactylitis and bone infarction. There is an increased risk of osteomyelitis and the problem is usually one of differentiating the direct effect of the disease from infection. MR seems the best solution although CT has also been advocated[55]. Abscess formation and cortical destruction are features that discriminate in favour of infection. The commonest infecting agents are the same as in those without haemoglobinopathy (*Staphylococcus aureus*, etc.); however, there is a higher incidence of *Salmonella* osteomyelitis than in the general population.

DIFFERENTIAL DIAGNOSIS

Tumour

Primary and secondary tumours of bone can also lead to lytic and sclerotic lesions and are part of the differential diagnosis of infection. Individual cases may be difficult to distinguish, especially when there are atypical features. The appearance of osteomyelitis may simulate almost the entire spectrum of bone tumours, and osteomyelitis should be considered the classic example of a 'bone tumour simulator'[22]. Often the issue is only resolved by biopsy but there are some general pointers that may assist.

Tumours tend to have a uniform and homogeneous appearance. In comparison, infection exhibits areas of rapid change alongside longer-standing features. Infection is more heterogeneous in pattern. Both may spread into the soft tissues but infection is more likely to produce soft tissue fluid-filled cavities. Secondary tumours are seen at multiple sites with each showing a fairly similar stage of development. The multifocal forms of osteomyelitis tend to show both new and established lesions. Infection may worsen and improve with time; without treatment tumours get worse.

Imaging is particularly useful in deciding which part of a mass to biopsy; the margins and areas of rapid change are more likely to show the definitive pathology.

Granulomatous disease

Eosinophilic granuloma and the more widespread lesions of Langerhans' histiocytosis can look very similar in appearance to infection[21,22]. Disseminated disease with lesions of the same age is less likely to be infection but here there will be difficulty in deciding whether it is metastatic tumour or widespread granulomas.

Degenerative disease

Aggressive forms of degeneration are commonly confused with infection. Rapidly progressive osteoarthritis seen in the shoulder (Milwaukee shoulder) and in the hip has a destructive pattern that may be indistinguishable from septic arthritis. Both destroy bone either side of the joint and both show large collections of fluid and debris in the joint. In the spine, advanced degenerative disc disease overlaps with disc space infection in the signs that it produces. High signal in the disc on T2-weighted MR or paraspinal abscesses are hallmarks of infection but do not always occur. It is probable that low-grade spinal infection does on occasion resolve spontaneously. When there are no symptoms or signs to suggest acute or subacute infection the best course of action is to wait and repeat the imaging (usually MR) in a few weeks. Active infection will progress whilst degeneration is unlikely to change over such a short interval. Early biopsy is indicated if there are clear signs of infection, systemic illness, or uncontrollable pain. It may be performed later in cases of doubt where time fails to resolve the diagnosis.

Irradiation

Areas of bone necrosis secondary to radiotherapy may look just like an aggressive infection. The destruction will traverse joints and be associated with osteopenia and soft tissue swelling. To confuse the diagnostician further, infection may occur in areas that have been irradiated[56].

SAPHO

The term SAPHO (Synovitis, Acne, Pustulosis, Hyperostosis, Osteomyelitis) has been coined for a series of similar conditions that link a bony sclerotic reaction that may mimic infection with sternoclavicular, spinal, pelvic and femoral hyperostosis, palmar-plantar pustulosis, acne, chronic relapsing multifocal osteomyelitis, unilateral sacroiliitis, psoriasis vulgaris and generalized pustular psoriasis[57].

SPECIFIC INFECTIONS

Brucellosis

Brucella behaves very much like tuberculosis of bone. Soft tissue ossification is perhaps more common. A history of farming contact or travel to endemic areas, including southern Europe, should be sought and specific antibodies tested in cases of undiagnosed infection, especially when the occupational or social history raises the possibility of exposure to *Brucella*. Gas is seen in the intervertebral disc although it is not fully understood why this occurs. The spine is most commonly affected. There are cases with focal involvement where the disc is preserved and the end-plates show changes. The more diffuse form involves the disc and may have some limited epidural extension. Many joints with scintigraphic detection of infection appear normal on plain radiographs[58]. If the radiologist sends samples for culture or histology in cases of suspected brucellosis or tuberculosis, it is essential to notify the laboratory of the risk of infection. Rarely, brucellosis can cause a culture-negative, presumed reactive arthritis or a chronic septic arthritis.

Fungi

A variety of fungi may affect bones and joints[59]. In general the infections tend to be slowly developing and difficult to eradicate; they may mimic tumours. There is an increased incidence in areas of the world where the organisms naturally reside[60]. Fungal infections in the musculoskeletal system are seen more often in immunosuppressed patients[41]. Fungi should be considered when the bacteriological findings do not fit the clinical presentation.

Actinomycosis

Seen most often in the USA, this mycosis commonly affects the lung and teeth. Direct invasion of ribs or mandible may result, giving a moth-eaten lytic destruction.

Blastomycosis

Occurring in the Americas and sometimes in Africa, a bone infection usually follows pulmonary or subcutaneous disease.

Candidiasis

Candida albicans may cause arthritis or osteomyelitis in immunosuppressed patients. Periarticular swelling and mild periosteal reactions are common.

Coccidioidomycosis

Seen in parts of the USA, pulmonary disease may disseminate to include bone involvement.

Histoplasmosis

Histoplasma capsulatum is found in the Mississippi valley and rarely affects bone. *Histoplasma duboisii* is confined to equatorial Africa and may affect bone with lytic lesions of the flat bones and spine. It mimics metastatic malignancy.

Streptomyces

Madura foot is a loose term used to describe direct chronic invasion of bone by mycotic organisms. The *Streptomyces* are the fungal infection often implicated. Seen largely in the Far East and India, the bone changes follow soft tissue infection and combine a chronic osteomyelitis with lytic expanded areas.

Haemophilus influenzae

Seen in primary osteomyelitis in children, this organism may also cause acute septic arthritis. It is especially liable to produce a haemorrhagic effusion within the affected joint. The availability of an effective vaccine has dramatically reduced the incidence of all invasive forms of infection with this pathogen in countries that can afford immunization.

HIV

Acquired immunodeficiency may be associated with osteomyelitis and joint infection from a wide range of organisms, many not normally seen in human infection, for example *Mycobacterium avium*[61,62] or bacillary angiomatosis[63]. Wide ranges of clinical and radiological features are seen but they are essentially exaggerations of the pattern of acute, subacute and chronic infection described above[62,64].

Hydatid

Multiloculated cysts are seen in the bone and adjacent soft tissue in bone and joint infection with this organism[60,65]. Sheep are the definitive host, the domestic dog being the intermediate host, and again occupational and travel history is important. Cystic degeneration in certain tumours may give very similar appearances. Serological studies are often positive in those from farming communities whether or not the bone is affected.

Infected prosthesis

Prosthetic joints and other orthopaedic implants are common sites of infection. The route is either by direct implantation at the time of the initial surgery or by haematogenous spread to sites that are relatively avascular and contain a foreign body (the implant). Infection may present as pain, swelling and systemic symptoms but more commonly it mimics aseptic loosening and takes a more chronic form (Fig. 51.17). The principal reason for making an early diagnosis in the more indolent infections is to allow proper planning of treatment.

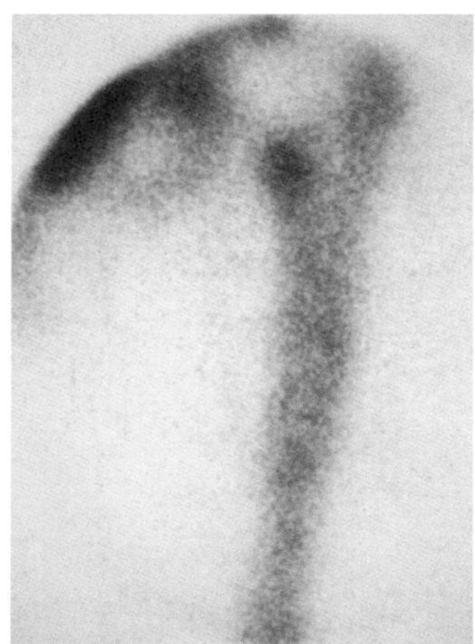

Figure 51.17 After a hip prosthesis has been in place for two years or more, a focal area of activity on skeletal scintigraphy (^{99m}Tc-MDP) is strongly suggestive of loosening or infection. The more diffuse uptake around the femoral component pushes the suspicions towards infection but these signs are not specific.

An infected prosthesis should be removed with antibiotic cover and continued antibiotic therapy. After an appropriate interval, repeat surgery with debridement of any dead tissue is followed by revision arthroplasty or sometimes a surgical fusion.

Plain radiographs will show osteopenia around the implant with progressive bony destruction. It is often impossible to differentiate these changes from aseptic mechanical loosening. The presence of focal bone destruction distant to the implant and a periosteal reaction favour infection but may also be seen in granulomatous reaction to the prosthesis. Some use scintigraphy to differentiate infection but even the more specific techniques (^{111}In white cell or ^{67}Ga citrate) have a significant false-positive rate and are rarely conclusive[26,66]. As it is essential to identify the organism, most units prefer to aspirate potentially infected joints for culture. There is a false-negative rate for this investigation and, in cases where there is doubt, a repeat aspiration with soft tissue biopsy may help. Finally, bone biopsy before or at the time of excision of the implant may be required.

Leprosy

Although progress has been made in the fight against leprosy (Hansen's disease—*Mycobacterium leprae*) the WHO estimates that there are about 1.15 million cases in the world compared to 10–12 million in the 1980s[67].

Articular manifestations with arthralgia and sacroiliitis are common[68].

The long-term effects of leprosy on bone are largely due to the anaesthesia produced in the periphery. The Charcot or neuropathic effects that ensue lead to the destruction of the ends of bone and heterotopic new bone formation. It is now possible to directly image thickening of nerves using US[69].

Lyme disease

Lyme disease is caused by *Borrelia burgdorferi*, a tick-borne spirochete that is found in North America and arboreal areas of Europe. It is the most common arthropod-borne infection in the USA and is found in most states. Typically it initially causes a skin rash (erythema chronicum migrans), which may later be complicated by involvement of the cardiac, nervous and musculoskeletal systems. In the skeleton, features are arthralgia, leading eventually to synovitis and arthritis. There may be destructive changes in the affected joints and the differential is with rheumatoid arthritis and seronegative arthropathy[70].

Melioidosis

Melioidosis is a tropical illness that causes pulmonary disease, abscess of skin and organs, meningitis, brain abscess and osteomyelitis[71]. The causative organism, *Burkholderia pseudomallei*, is found in the soil in the Far East, India and the Northern Territories of Australia[72,73]. Its musculoskeletal manifestations are identical to other infections[74]. Prompt recognition, antibiotic treatment and surgical drainage are necessary to optimize the chances of recovery.

Parasites

Infiltration of muscle by parasites can induce a variety of symptoms including arthritis, myositis and enthesitis. The imaging features are nonspecific in the early phase but calcification in and around the organism may be typical[75,76]. Infestations associated with musculoskeletal features include loiasis, echinococcosis and schistosomiasis.

Staphylococcus aureus

This is the commonest organism to affect bones and joints. Many asymptomatic people carry *Staphylococcus aureus*. There are resistant strains, including the difficult-to-manage type of methicillin-resistant bacteria (MRSA). The route of infection may be either blood-borne or due to direct inoculation. Presenting features include fever, toxicity and even frank septicaemia. At the other end of the spectrum some patients will have no symptoms and may have normal CRP and white cell counts. Common sites for infection are the metaphyses of long bones in children, the hip in children, joint replacements and the intervertebral discs.

Syphilis and yaws

Syphilis remains an epidemiological problem[77]. Skeletal presentations are varied and mimic many other diseases. Clinical presentation varies from arthralgia to osteomyelitis[78]. The manifestations may be exaggerated in HIV infection[79].

Congenital syphilis may cause a symmetric periostitis with lamination. Granulomas occurring in the metaphyses of long bones produce lytic areas known as Wimberger's sign. The growth plate may be abnormal with lytic bands in the adjacent bone. Although fortunately rare nowadays, occasional cases of tertiary syphilis present with osteitis and even frank osteomyelitis.

Yaws is caused by *Treponema pertenue* and still occurs in the tropics. It is associated with similar features to syphilis but chronic ulceration is more typical[80]. Late presentation of both yaws and syphilis may be as indolent chronic, sclerosing osteomyelitis.

Tuberculosis

As for other tuberculous infections, a myriad of presentations and appearances have been described[81] (Fig. 51.18). Perhaps the greatest problem is that tuberculosis is regarded as an 'old fashioned' infection and may be overlooked. Given that it is amenable to specific chemotherapy, errors of this sort are to be avoided. Bone infection is most typically slow growing and indolent. Tuberculous 'caries' is seen where the margin of the bone is scalloped and eaten away. Large 'cold' abscesses occur. This means that the patient is surprisingly well given the size of the collection. Patients with tuberculous infection may not be aware that their health and well-being is poor. The onset of the disease is insidious and the changes are so gradual that it may be unnoticed. Those who are treated and recover are often surprised at how much better they feel and may say that they did not know how ill they were. Tuberculosis should be considered in all cases of bone and soft tissue infection[81–83].

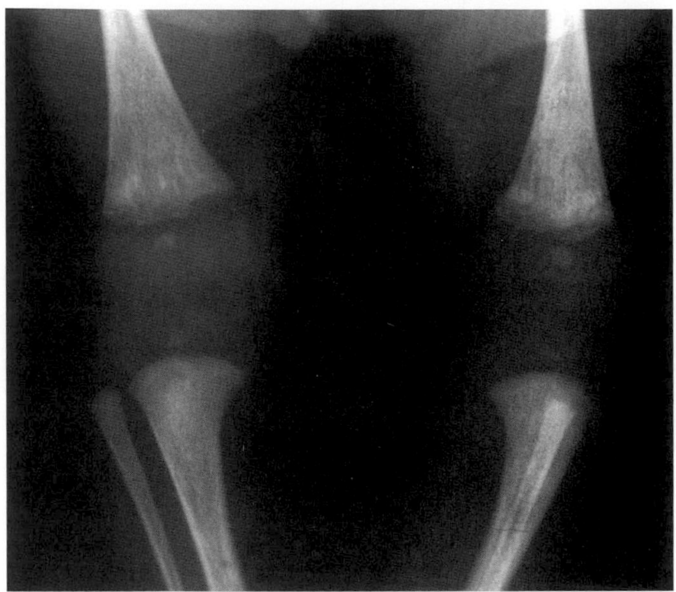

Figure 51.18 Tuberculosis may mimic many diseases. Here it produces a destructive synovitis.

Soft tissue infection with *Mycobacterium marinum* has been described in those who own and clean tropical fish tanks[84].

Viruses

Several viruses are known to affect bone. Before its virtual eradication, smallpox was known to cause joint effusions, dactylitis and periostitis. Focal lesions with epiphyseal lucencies have been reported. If the patient recovered these were associated with arthrodesis of the adjacent joint and focal growth arrest. Vaccinia and variola are both known to cause a hyperostosis and may cause joint effusions. Rubella may cause clinical arthritis and in the transplacental form may cause linear markings of sclerosis on the metaphyses of long bones described as 'celery stalk' (Fig. 51.19). Cytomegalic inclusion disease affects bone in a similar way to rubella. Lymphogranuloma venereum may cause focal lucencies in bone. Infantile cortical hyperostosis (Caffey's disease) and cat-scratch fever both exhibit periostitis and have an unproven link to viral disease[85].

MANAGEMENT

Role in diagnosis, relationship to biopsy

Imaging is crucial in several stages of the diagnostic process, in detecting the abnormality that leads to symptoms, in locating the source of symptoms and in determining that infection is a potential cause. CT and MR are very important in deciding which part to biopsy and by which route to approach. CT, US, fluoroscopy and MR can all be used to guide the biopsy, which is planned by the cross-sectional imaging appearances (Fig. 51.20). It is important to discuss the route of biopsy with the clinician who would perform the subsequent surgery if the lesion might be a tumour. It is wise also to consult the pathologist who will examine the specimen to agree on the type of tissue (soft tissue/bone) and the size and appropriateness of the specimen. There should be protocols for transfer and culture of the material. As the culture rate from chronic infection is low (variable but in the range < 30–60%), it is prudent always to send a sample for histopathology. Distinctive histological features include the presence of caseating granulomas in many cases of tuberculosis, visualizing fungal elements on special stains (and rarely bacteria) and the presence of polymorphs in periprosthetic tissues in cases of prosthetic joint infection.

Role in planning treatment

Surgical removal of dead or infected tissue is fundamental to the management of bone and soft tissue infection. This has in the past been performed by open exploration, cutting back to bleeding and 'live' bone. MR especially allows prediction of where the normal bone will be and so what excision will be necessary. Planning of this type helps reduce morbidity and complications and will allow more accurate informed consent by the patient, as well as guiding the subsequent reconstructive surgery necessary.

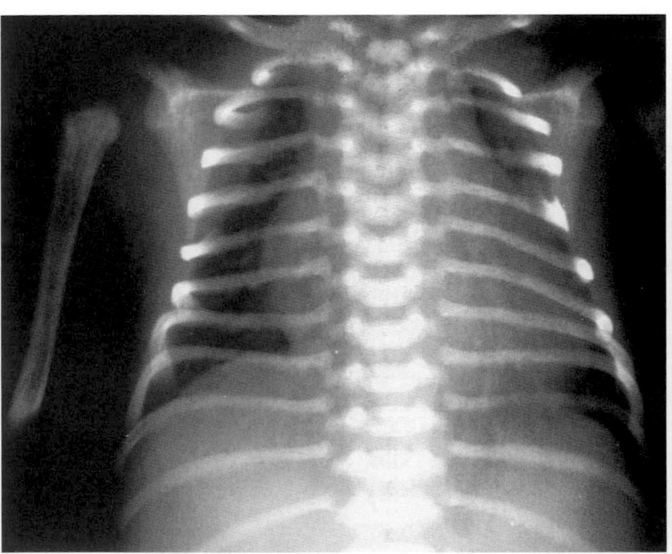

A

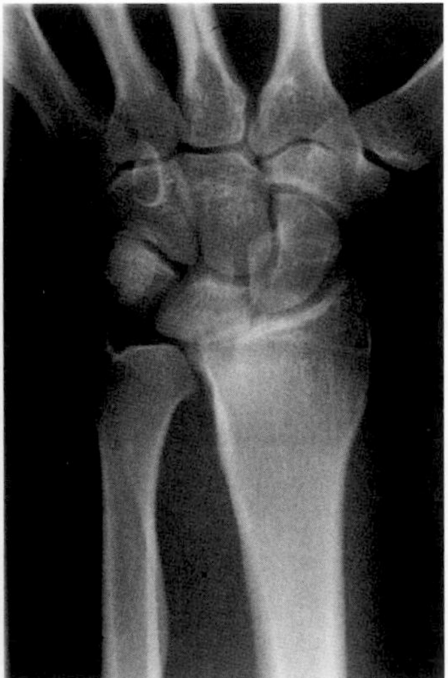

B

Figure 51.19 Congenital rubella produces a 'celery stick' striation in long bones (A) as well as a periosteal reaction (B). (Courtesy of Dr T. Chee, Tan Tock Seng Hospital, Singapore.)

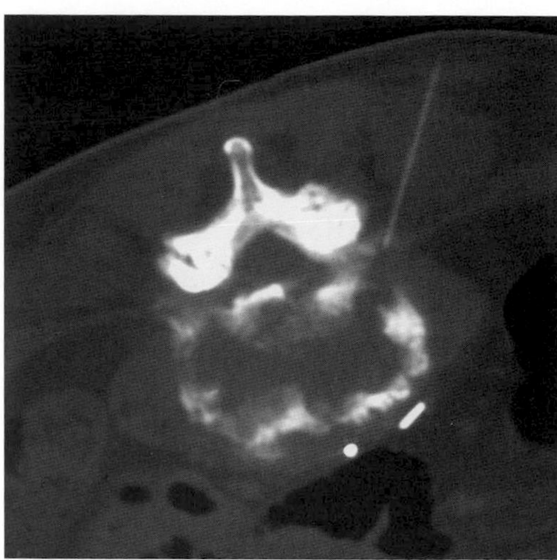

Figure 51.20 CT guidance for biopsy of infected discitis.

Radiological interventional techniques

Image-guided therapy includes the drainage of abscesses and placement of indwelling catheters. This is especially useful when the patient is not fit for more aggressive surgical procedures but it may also have a role in less severe cases. It is essential that the radiologist performing the procedure works closely with the surgeon and is aware of the need for careful monitoring of progress.

Cavities left after surgical debridement may cause mechanical instability, especially in the spine. Imaging may be used to assist the placement of implants or antibiotic-loaded cement in the cavity. In the spine this is a variation on the technique of vertebroplasty and it can be valuable in patients unfit for conventional spinal stabilization.

Role in monitoring treatment

Imaging is being used with increasing frequency in monitoring progress both after surgery and after antibiotic treatment. How often repeat studies should be performed depends on the case. It is rare to see significant change in under a week and it often takes much longer. The method that best demonstrates the lesion should be employed. It helps to use the same protocol and, whenever possible, the same machine and same radiologist. MR and CT are best suited to follow-up whilst US is less valuable as it is very observer dependent and so reproducible images are difficult to obtain. If US is used for follow-up it should be performed by the same radiologist, who should take detailed notes and diagrams to remember the extent of the disease. Difficulties with MR for follow-up include post-surgical artefact, metal artefact even from microscopic fragments after removal of orthopaedic metal ware and a long lag between clinical arrest of infection and complete resolution of MR changes.

ACKNOWLEDGEMENTS

Dr. Roland Werners for his assistance in translation of Garré's paper from the German.

REFERENCES

1. Boutin R D, Brossmann J, Sartoris D J, Reilly D, Resnick D 1998 Update on imaging of orthopedic infections. Orthop Clin North Am 29: 41–66.
2. Patton J T 1990 Manifestations of systemic disease and infections of the musculoskeletal system [published erratum appears in Curr Opin Radiol 1990; 2: 965]. Curr Opin Radiol 2: 678–683.
3. Abiri M M, Kirpekar M, Ablow R C 1989 Osteomyelitis: detection with US. Radiology 172: 509–511.
4. Nath A K, Sethu A U 1992 Use of ultrasound in osteomyelitis. Br J Radiol 65: 649–652.
5. Wilson D J, Kay V, Charig M, Hughes D G, Creasy T S 1988 Skeletal hyperostosis and extraosseous calcification in patients receiving long-term etretinate (Tigason). Br J Dermatol 119: 597–607.
6. Shirtliff M E, Mader J T 2002 Acute septic arthritis. Clin Microbiol Rev 15: 527–544.
7. Beltran J 1995 MR imaging of soft-tissue infection. Magn Reson Imaging Clin N Am 3: 743–751.
8. Hall R L, Callaghan J J, Moloney E, Martinez S, Harrelson J M 1990 Pyomyositis in a temperate climate. Presentation, diagnosis, and treatment. J Bone Joint Surg Am 72: 1240–1244.
9. Gordon B A, Martinez S, Collins A J 1995 Pyomyositis: characteristics at CT and MR imaging. Radiology 197: 279–286.
10. Garcia J 2000 MRI in inflammatory myopathies. Skeletal Radiol 29: 425–438.
11. Spiegel D A, Meyer J S, Dormans J P, Flynn J M, Drummond D S 1999 Pyomyositis in children and adolescents: report of 12 cases and review of the literature. J Pediatr Orthop 19: 143–150.
12. Urschel J D 1999 Necrotizing soft tissue infections. Postgrad Med J 75: 645–649.
13. Fontes R A, Ogilvie C M, Miclau T 2000 Necrotizing soft-tissue infections. J Am Acad Orthop Surg 8: 151–158.
14. Safran D B, Sullivan W G 2001 Necrotizing fasciitis of the chest wall. Ann Thorac Surg 72: 1362–1364.
15. Dagirmanjian A, Schils J, McHenry M C 1999 MR imaging of spinal infections. Magn Reson Imaging Clin N Am 7: 525–538.
16. Sadato N, Numaguchi Y, Rigamonti D, Kodama T, Nussbaum E, Sato S, Rothman M 1994 Spinal epidural abscess with gadolinium-enhanced MRI: serial follow-up studies and clinical correlations. Neuroradiology 36: 44–48.
17. Abiri M M, De Angelis G, Kirpekar M, Abou A N, Ablow R C 1992 Ultrasonic detection of osteomyelitis. Pathologic correlation in an animal model. Invest Radiol 27: 111–113.
18. Morrison W B, Schweitzer M E, Bock G W et al 1993 Diagnosis of osteomyelitis: utility of fat-suppressed contrast-enhanced MR imaging. Radiology 189: 251–257.
19. Hovi I, Lamminen A, Salonen O et al 1994 MR imaging of the lower spine. Differentiation between infectious and malignant disease. Acta Radiol 35: 532–540.
20. Grey A C, Davies A M, Mangham D C, Grimer R J, Ritchie D A 1998 The 'penumbra sign' on T1-weighted MR imaging in subacute osteomyelitis: frequency, cause and significance. Clin Radiol 53: 587–592.
21. Beltran J, Aparisi F, Bonmati L et al 1993 Eosinophilic granuloma: MRI manifestations. Skeletal Radiol 22: 157–161.
22. Fabiny R 1997 Bone tumour simulators. Problems and pitfalls in radiology. Acta Orthopaed Scand Suppl 273: 14–20.
23. Garré C 1893 Ueber besondere Formen und Fogelzustande der akuten infektiosen Osteomyelitis. Beitr Z Klin Chir 10: 241–298.
24. Hughes D K 2003 Nuclear medicine and infection detection: the relative effectiveness of imaging with 111In-oxine-, 99mTc-HMPAO-, and 99mTc-stannous fluoride colloid-labeled leukocytes and with 67Ga-citrate. J Nucl Med Technol 31: 196–201; quiz 203–204.
25. Seabold J E, Nepola J V, Marsh J L et al 1991 Postoperative bone marrow alterations: potential pitfalls in the diagnosis of osteomyelitis with In-111-labeled leukocyte scintigraphy. Radiology 180: 741–747.
26. Seabold J E, Nepola J V 1999 Imaging techniques for evaluation of postoperative orthopedic infections. Q J Nucl Med 43: 21–28.
27. El-Haddad G, Zhuang H, Gupta N, Alavi A 2004 Evolving role of positron emission tomography in the management of patients with inflammatory and other benign disorders. Semin Nucl Med 34: 313–329.

28. Crymes W B Jr, Demos H, Gordon L 2004 Detection of musculoskeletal infection with 18F-FDG PET: review of the current literature. J Nucl Med Technol 32: 12–15.
29. Zhuang H, Yu J Q, Alavi A 2005 Applications of fluorodeoxyglucose-PET imaging in the detection of infection and inflammation and other benign disorders. Radiol Clin North Am 43: 121–134.
30. Cardinal E, Bureau N, Aubin B, Chem R 2001 Role of ultrasound in musculoskeletal infections. Radiol Clin North Am 39: 191–201.
31. Kothari N A, Pelchovitz D J, Meyer J S 2001 Imaging of musculoskeletal infections. Radiol Clin North Am 39: 653–671.
32. Robben S G 2004 Ultrasonography of musculoskeletal infections in children. Eur Radiol 14 Suppl 4: L65–77.
33. Wilson D J, Green D J, MacLarnon J C 1984 Arthrosonography of the painful hip. Clin Radiol 35: 17–19.
34. Song J, Letts M, Monson R 2001 Differentiation of psoas muscle abscess from septic arthritis of the hip in children. Clin Orthop 391: 258–265.
35. Kayani I, Syed I, Saifuddin A 2004 Vertebral osteomyelitis without disc involvement. Clin Radiol 59: 881–891.
36. Teo H E, Peh W C 2004 Skeletal tuberculosis in children. Pediatr Radiol 34: 853–860.
37. Gasbarrini A L, Bandiera S, Barbanti Bròdano G et al 2005 Clinical features, diagnostic and therapeutic approaches to haematogenous vertebral osteomyelitis. Eur Rev Med Pharmacol Sci 9: 53–66.
38. Spaeth H J J, Dardani M 1994 Magnetic resonance imaging of the diabetic foot. Magn Reson Imaging Clin N Am 2: 123–130.
39. Yuh W T, Corson J D, Baraniewski H M et al 1989 Osteomyelitis of the foot in diabetic patients: evaluation with plain film, 99mTc-MDP bone scintigraphy, and MR imaging. AJR Am J Roentgenol 152: 795–800.
40. Morrison W B, Schweitzer M E, Batte W G et al 1998 Osteomyelitis of the foot: relative importance of primary and secondary MR imaging signs. Radiology 207: 625–632.
41. Aliabadi P, Nikpoor N, Alparslan L 2003 Imaging of neuropathic arthropathy. Semin Musculoskelet Radiol 7: 217–225.
42. Sella E J, Grosser D M 2003 Imaging modalities of the diabetic foot. Clin Podiatr Med Surg 20: 729–740.
43. Craig J G, Amin M B, Wu K et al 1997 Osteomyelitis of the diabetic foot: MR imaging-pathologic correlation. Radiology 203: 849–855.
44. Lipman B T, Collier B C, Carrera G F et al 1998 Detection of osteomyelitis in the neuropathic foot: nuclear medicine, MRI and conventional radiography. Clin Nucl Med 23: 77–82.
45. Sartoris D J 1994 Cross-sectional imaging of the diabetic foot. J Foot Ankle Surg 33: 531–545.
46. Loredo R, Metter D 1997 Imaging of the diabetic foot. Emphasis on nuclear medicine and magnetic resonance imaging. Clin Podiatr Med Surg 14: 235–264.
47. Marcus C D, Ladam-Marcus V J, Leone J et al 1996 MR imaging of osteomyelitis and neuropathic osteoarthropathy in the feet of diabetics. Radiographics 16: 1337–1348.
48. Vesco L, Boulahdour H, Hamissa S et al 1999 The value of combined radionuclide and magnetic resonance imaging in the diagnosis and conservative management of minimal or localized osteomyelitis of the foot in diabetic patients. Metabolism 48: 922–927.
49. Berendt A R, Lipsky B 2004 Is this bone infected or not? Differentiating neuro-osteoarthropathy from osteomyelitis in the diabetic foot. Curr Diab Rep 4: 424–429.
50. Lopes T D, Reinus W R, Wilson A J 1997 Quantitative analysis of the plain radiographic appearance of Brodie's abscess. Invest Radiol 32: 51–58.
51. Jurik A G, Egund N 1997 MRI in chronic recurrent multifocal osteomyelitis. Skeletal Radiol 26: 230–238.
52. Jurik A G 2004 Chronic recurrent multifocal osteomyelitis. Semin Musculoskelet Radiol 8: 243–253.
53. Demharter J, Bohndorf K, Michl W et al 1997 Chronic recurrent multifocal osteomyelitis: a radiological and clinical investigation of five cases. Skeletal Radiol 26: 579–588.
54. Felsberg G J, Gore R L, Scwetzer M E et al 1990 Sclerosing osteomyelitis of Garré (periostitis ossificans). Oral Surg Oral Med Oral Pathol 70: 117–120.
55. Rifai A, Nyman R 1997 Scintigraphy and ultrasonography in differentiating osteomyelitis from bone infarction in sickle cell disease. Acta Radiol 38: 139–143.
56. Wignall T A, Carrington B M, Logue J P 1998 Post-radiotherapy osteomyelitis of the symphysis pubis: computed tomographic features. Clin Radiol 53: 126–130.
57. Sugimoto H, Tamura K, Fujii T 1998 The SAPHO syndrome: defining the radiologic spectrum of diseases comprising the syndrome. Eur Radiol 8: 800–806.
58. al-Shahed M S, Sharif H S, Haddad M C et al 1994 Imaging features of musculoskeletal brucellosis. Radiographics 14: 333–348.
59. Arkun R 2004 Parasitic and fungal disease of bones and joints. Semin Musculoskelet Radiol 8: 231–242.
60. Abd El Bagi M E, Sammak B, Al Shahed M et al 1999 Rare bone infections excluding the spine. Eur Radiol 9: 1078–1087.
61. Weingardt J P, Kilcoyne R F, Russ P D, Johnston R J, Nawaz S 1996 Disseminated *Mycobacterium avium* complex presenting with osteomyelitis of the distal femur and proximal tibia. Skeletal Radiol 25: 193–196.
62. Tehranzadeh J, Ter-Oganesyan R R, Steinbach L S 2004 Musculoskeletal disorders associated with HIV infection and AIDS. Part I: infectious musculoskeletal conditions. Skeletal Radiol 33: 249–259.
63. Wyatt S H, Fishman E K 1995 CT/MRI of musculoskeletal complications of AIDS. Skeletal Radiol 24: 481–488.
64. Bureau N J, Cardinal E 2001 Imaging of musculoskeletal and spinal infections in AIDS. Radiol Clin North Am 39: 343–355.
65. Normelli H C, Aaro S I, Follin P H 1998 Vertebral hydatid cyst infection (*Echinococcus granulosus*): a case report. Eur Spine J 7: 158–161.
66. Palestro C J, Torres M A 1997 Radionuclide imaging in orthopedic infections. Semin Nucl Med 27: 334–345.
67. WHO Expert Committee on Leprosy 1998 World Health Organization Technical Report Series 874: 1–43.
68. Cossermelli-Messina W, Festa Neto C, Cossermelli W 1998 Articular inflammatory manifestations in patients with different forms of leprosy. J Rheumatol 25: 111–119.
69. Martinoli C, Bianchi S, Derchi L E 1999 Tendon and nerve sonography. Radiol Clin North Am 37: 691–711, viii.
70. Kalish R 1993 Lyme disease. Rheum Dis Clin North Am 19: 399–426.
71. Thummakul T, Wilde H, Tantawichien T 1999 Melioidosis, an environmental and occupational hazard in Thailand. Mil Med 164: 658–662.
72. Suputtamongkol Y, Hall A J, Dance D A B et al 1994 The epidemiology of melioidosis in Ubon Ratchatani, northeast Thailand. Int J Epidemiol 23: 1082–1090.
73. Rode J W, Webling D D 1981 Melioidosis in the Northern Territory of Australia. Med J Aust 1: 181–184.
74. Pui M H, Tan A P 1995 Musculoskeletal melioidosis: clinical and imaging features. Skeletal Radiol 24: 499–503.
75. McGill P E 1995 Rheumatic syndromes associated with parasites. Baillières Clin Rheumatol 9: 201–213.
76. Bocanegra T S, Vasey F B 1993 Musculoskeletal syndromes in parasitic diseases. Rheum Dis Clin N Am 19: 505–513.
77. Congenital syphilis—United States, 1998. 1999 MMWR Morb Mortal Wkly Rep 48: 757–761.
78. Reginato A J 1993 Syphilitic arthritis and osteitis. Rheum Dis Clin N Am 19: 379–398.
79. Vassilopoulos D, Chalasani P, Jurado R et al 1997 Musculoskeletal infections in patients with human immunodeficiency virus infection. Medicine 76: 284–294.
80. Sengupta S 1985 Musculoskeletal lesions in yaws. Clin Orthop 1985: 193–198.
81. De Vuyst D, Vanhoenacker F, Gielen J, Bernaerts A, De Schepper A M 2003 Imaging features of musculoskeletal tuberculosis. Eur Radiol 13: 1809–1819.
82. Yao D C, Sartoris D J 1995 Musculoskeletal tuberculosis. Radiol Clin North Am 33: 679–689.
83. Loke T K, Ma H T, Chan C S 1997 Magnetic resonance imaging of tuberculous spinal infection. Australas Radiol 41: 7–12.
84. Bhatty M A, Turner D P, Chamberlain S T 2000 *Mycobacterium marinum* hand infection: case reports and review of literature. Br J Plast Surg 53: 161–165.
85. Silverman F N 1976 Virus diseases of bone. Do they exist? The Neuhauser Lecture. AJR Am J Roentgenol 126: 677–703.

SECTION

Women's Imaging

CHAPTER 52

The Breast

Jonathan J. James, A. Robin M. Wilson and Andrew J. Evans

- Methods of examination
- Normal anatomy
- Breast pathology
- Other imaging techniques
- Breast cancer screening

Imaging is essential for accurate breast diagnosis and the early detection of breast cancer. Population screening with mammography is the only intervention proven to reduce mortality from breast cancer through early detection. Mammography and ultrasound are the first-line investigations for imaging the breast in women with breast symptoms. Magnetic resonance imaging (MRI) is established as an adjunctive diagnostic tool because of its high sensitivity for breast pathology. The combination of imaging, clinical examination and needle biopsy—known as 'triple assessment'—is the expected standard for breast diagnosis.

In recent years, there have been major advances in mammographic technology with the development of full field digital mammography (FFDM). It is expected that this will outperform conventional screen/film mammography, providing significant logistic advantages and facilitating new applications, such as computer-assisted detection (CAD).

Breast cancer is the most common malignant tumour in women in the UK, with over 40 000 diagnosed annually, over 80% in women over the age of 50. Screening aims to reduce mortality by detecting the disease at an earlier stage, before it has spread beyond the breast. Mammography can significantly reduce mortality from breast cancer, with the benefit greatest in women aged 55–70 years.

Imaging is important not only in the detection and diagnosis of breast disease but also in guiding needle biopsies. Wide use of mammography for screening has resulted in the discovery of increasingly large numbers of small lesions that are impalpable. Percutaneous image-guided biopsy is used for the diagnosis of these lesions, thus avoiding unnecessary open surgical biopsies. Even for clinically palpable abnormalities, image-guided biopsy can improve the diagnostic accuracy. Fine needle aspiration (FNA) was the first method of biopsy employed for breast diagnosis, with samples obtained for cytological assessment. In many centres FNA has been largely superseded by core needle biopsy, allowing tissue to be obtained for histological evaluation. Vacuum-assisted mammotomy (VAM) enables the sampling of larger areas of tissue, further improving diagnostic accuracy.

METHODS OF EXAMINATION

Mammography (physics, technique, equipment, digital versus screen/film)

Mammography places stringent demands on equipment and image quality. High spatial resolution is required to identify tiny structures within the breast, such as microcalcifications measuring in the order of 100 μm. Short exposure times are necessary to limit movement unsharpness. The breast is composed predominantly of fatty tissue and has a relatively narrow range of inherent densities. Consequently, special X-ray tubes are required to produce the low energy radiation necessary to achieve high tissue contrast, enabling the demonstration of small changes in breast density. However, for some examinations where the breasts are thicker or are composed of denser glandular tissue, higher energy radiation is required. In addition, radiation dose must be kept to a minimum.

X-ray tubes produce a spectrum of radiation energies, which is determined by the target and filter combination and the peak kilovoltage (kVp). A molybdenum target is used because it produces a low energy spectrum with peaks of 17.5 and 19.6 keV, providing high contrast. A tungsten target is less desirable because it produces higher energies (Fig. 52.1). The spectrum is refined further by adding a filter to reduce the proportion of radiation above and below the desired range. Commercially available target/filter combinations include molybdenum/molybdenum, molybdenum/rhodium, rhodium/rhodium, tungsten/molybdenum and tungsten/rhodium. Molybdenum/molybdenum is the most frequently used combination.

To achieve the required spatial resolution, mammography tubes must have an extremely small focal spot, 0.3 mm for routine mammography. For magnification mammography a smaller focal spot of 0.1 mm is required. Tube current should be as high as possible in order to keep exposure times short.

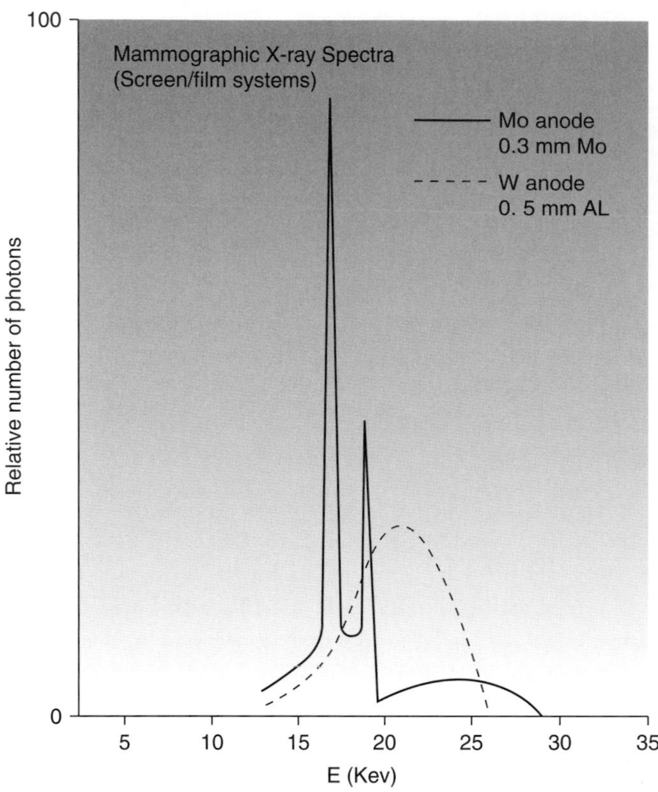

Figure 52.1 X-ray spectra obtained from a molybdenum (Mo) target tube set at 29 kVp and a tungsten (W) target tube set at 26 kVp. (From Haus A G, Metz C E, Chiles J T, Rossman K 1976 The effect of x-ray spectra from molybdenum and tungsten target tubes on image quality in mammography. Radiology 118: 705–709, with permission from the Radiological Society of North America.)

Movement unsharpness may occur when exposure times exceed 1 s. Grids are used routinely for all mammographic studies. These reduce scattered radiation and so increase contrast, especially in the dense or thick breast.

Modern mammography machines have a facility for automatic selection of target/filter combination, kVp and tube current according to breast density and the thickness of the compressed breast. In addition, automatic exposure control devices sense the amount of radiation striking the detector and terminate the exposure at a preset level.

Standard projections

There are two standard mammographic projections: a mediolateral oblique (MLO) view and a craniocaudal (CC) view (Fig. 52.2). The MLO is taken with the X-ray beam directed from superomedial to inferolateral, usually at an angle of 30–60°, with compression applied obliquely across the chest wall, perpendicular to the long axis of the pectoralis major muscle (Fig. 52.3A). The MLO projection is the only projection in which all the breast tissue can be demonstrated on a single image. A well-positioned MLO view should demonstrate the inframammary angle, the nipple in profile and the nipple positioned at the level of the lower border of the pectoralis major, with the muscle across the posterior border of the film at an angle of 25–30° to the vertical.

For the CC view, the X-ray beam travels from superior to inferior. Positioning is achieved by pulling the breast up and forward away from the chest wall, with compression applied from above (Fig. 52.3B). A well-positioned CC view

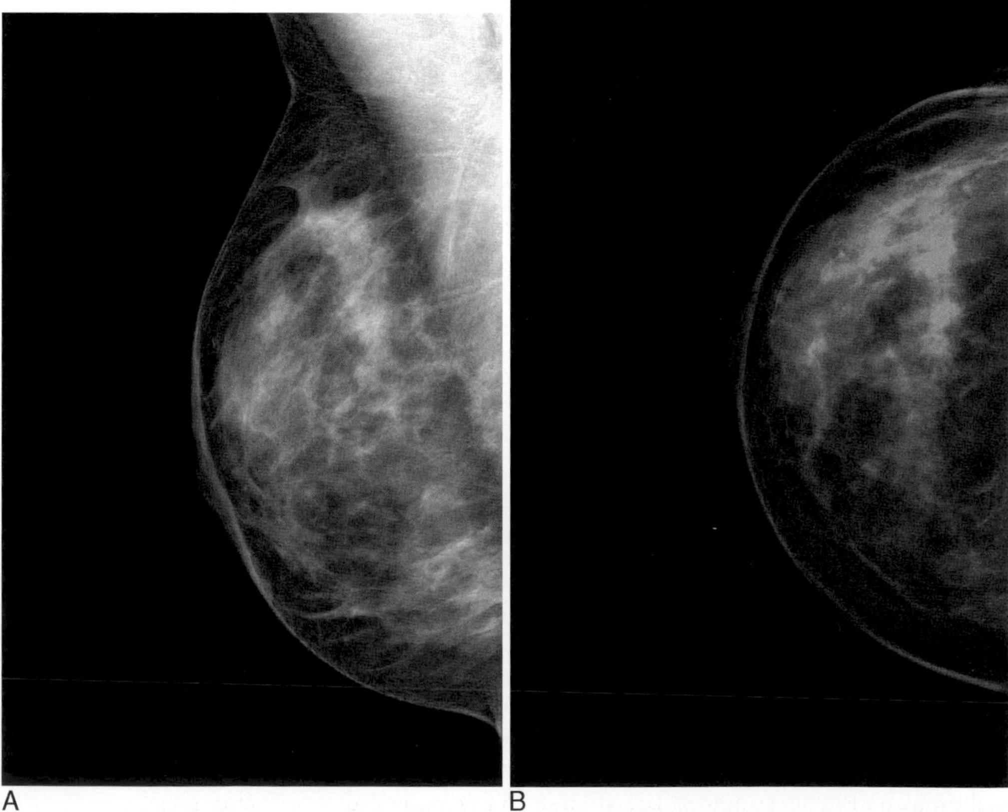

Figure 52.2 A standard set of mammograms consists of the mediolateral oblique (MLO) view (A) and the craniocaudal (CC) view (B). This normal breast contains a moderate amount of dense glandular tissue.

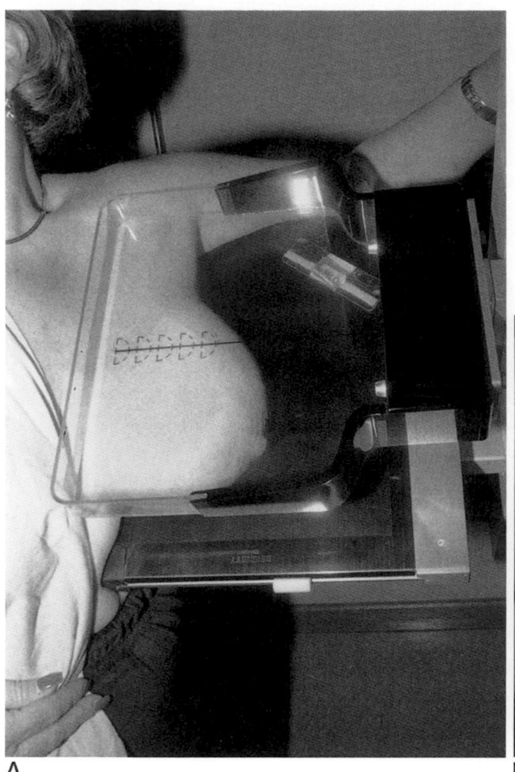

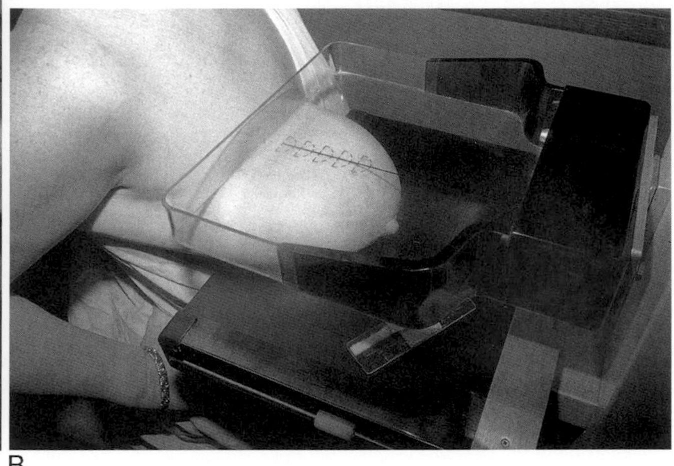

A B

Figure 52.3 Breast positioning. Positioning for the (A) mediolateral oblique and (B) craniocaudal views.

should demonstrate the nipple in profile. It should demonstrate virtually all of the medial tissue and the majority of the lateral tissue with the exclusion of the axillary tail of the breast. The pectoralis major is demonstrated at the centre of a CC film in approximately 30% of individuals and the depth of breast tissue demonstrated should be within 1 cm of the distance from the nipple to the pectoralis major on the MLO projection.

Additional projections

Supplementary views may be taken to solve specific diagnostic problems[1,2]. For example, the CC view can be rotated to visualize either more of the lateral or medial aspect of the breast compared to the standard CC projection. Localized compression or 'paddle views' can be performed. This involves the application of more vigorous compression to a localized area using a compression paddle (Fig. 52.4). These views are used to distinguish real lesions from superimposition of normal tissues and to define the margins of a mass.

A true lateral view may be used to provide a third imaging plane in order to distinguish superimposition of normal structures from real lesions or to increase the accuracy of wire localizations of non-palpable lesions. The true lateral view is performed with the mammography unit turned through 90° and a mediolateral or lateromedial X-ray beam.

Magnification views are most frequently performed to examine areas of microcalcifications within the breast, to characterize them and to establish their extent. Magnification views are typically performed in the craniocaudal and lateral projections. The magnified lateral view will demonstrate 'teacups' typical of benign microcalcifications, described later in the chapter.

Mammographic technique may need to be modified in women with breast implants. Silicon and saline implants are radio-opaque and may obscure much of the breast tissue. Consequently, mammography is of limited diagnostic value in some women. The Eklund technique can be employed to displace the implant posteriorly, behind the compression plate, maximizing the volume of breast tissue that is compressed and imaged[3]. Mammography-induced implant rupture has not been reported.

Breast compression

Compression of the breast is essential for good mammography, for the following reasons:

1 It reduces geometric unsharpness by bringing the object closer to the film.
2 It improves contrast by reducing scatter.
3 It diminishes movement unsharpness by permitting shorter exposure times and immobilizing the breast.
4 It reduces radiation dose, as a lesser thickness of breast tissue needs to be penetrated and scatter is reduced.
5 It achieves more uniform image density: a homogeneous breast thickness prevents overexposure of the thinner anterior breast tissues and underexposure of the thicker posterior breast tissues.
6 It provides more accurate assessment of the density of masses. As cysts and normal glandular tissue are more easily compressed, the more rigid carcinomas are highlighted.
7 It separates superimposed breast tissues so that lesions are better seen.

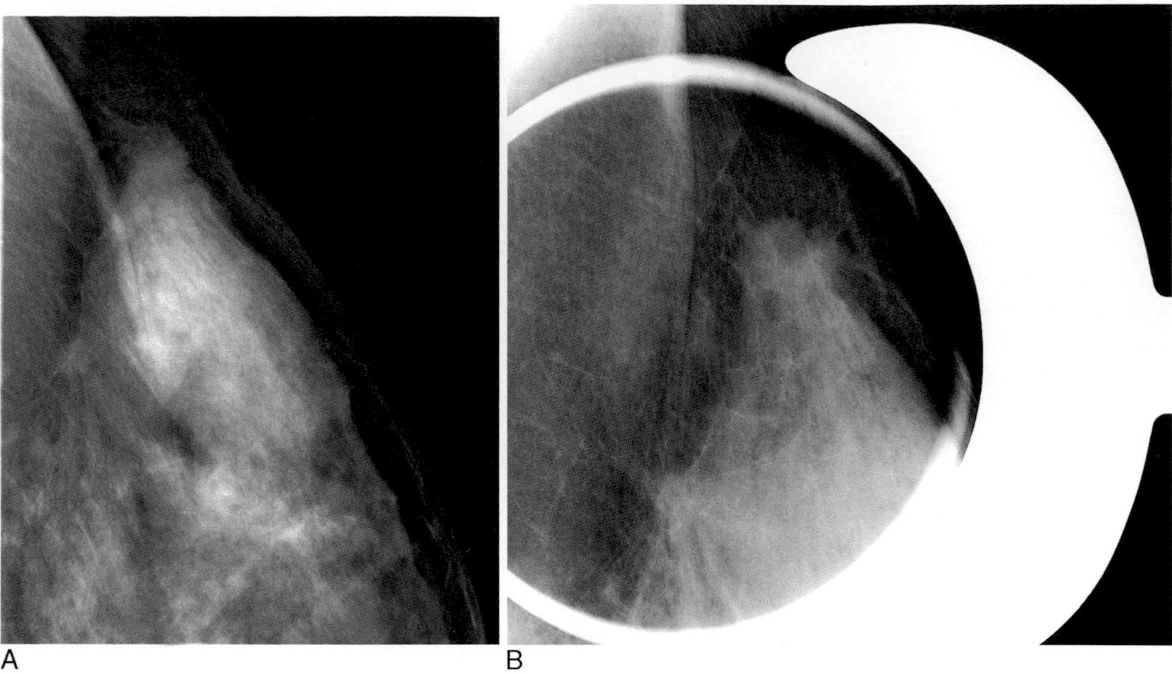

Figure 52.4 Additional Mammographic Views. (A) An area of concern was identified in the lateral aspect of the left breast on initial mammography. (B) A 'paddle view' was performed and two suspicious spiculated mass lesions were demonstrated much more clearly. Both proved to be invasive carcinomas on subsequent biopsy.

Indications for mammography

Mammography is rarely indicated before the age of 35. The main indications are:

- evaluation of breast symptoms and signs, including masses, skin thickening, deformity, nipple retraction, nipple discharge and nipple eczema
- breast cancer screening
- follow-up of patients with previously treated breast cancer
- guidance for biopsy or localization of lesions not visible on ultrasound.

Radiation dose

Mammography uses ionizing radiation to image the breast. The risks of ionizing radiation are well known and any exposure needs to be justified, with doses kept as low as possible. The radiation dose for a standard two-view examination of both breasts is approximately 4.5 mGy[4].

Dose is more of an issue in a population screening programme, where women who may never develop breast cancer are being exposed to radiation. It has been estimated that the risk of inducing a breast cancer in women screened in the United Kingdom National Health Service Breast Screening Programme (NHSBSP) is 1 in 100 000 per mGy. A risk–benefit calculation has established that the benefits of screening far outweigh the risk of inducing a cancer, with the ratio of lives saved to lives lost calculated as approximately 100:1[4].

Digital mammography systems are still undergoing evaluation, but there is evidence that they have the potential to reduce patient dose without loss of image quality.

The detector (screen/film versus digital)

Traditionally the mammographic image has been recorded on film. The film is contained within specially designed cassettes, where film with a single layer of emulsion on one side is held in intimate contact with a single intensifying screen. Screen/film radiography of other areas of the body use double emulsion film held between two intensifying screens. This allows the dose to be reduced but the resulting spatial resolution is not sufficient for mammography. The use of single screen single emulsion, together with a thinner layer of phosphor on the intensifier screen, maximizes spatial resolution.

The main advantage of digital mammography systems is the separation of image acquisition, processing and display, allowing each of these steps to be optimized. Manufacturers have developed a number of different approaches to producing a digital mammogram.

The first type of digital system developed for mammography uses photostimulable phosphor computed radiography (CR). This technology is now widely used for general radiography. An imaging plate coated with a phosphor replaces traditional screen/film cassettes. The imaging plate, stored in a conventional-looking cassette, is exposed in the usual fashion in a conventional mammography machine. A latent image is stored in the phosphor after exposure. The cassette containing the imaging plate is inserted into a reader. The imaging plate is scanned by a laser beam and light is emitted in proportion to the absorbed X-rays. The emitted light is then detected by a photomultiplier system and the resulting electrical signal is digitized to produce the image.

The second type of digital system uses a light-sensitive element called a charge couple device (CCD) as the basis for the detector. The SenoScan system (Fischer Medical Imaging) has a narrow rectangular detector consisting of a scintillator coupled to a CCD. The X-ray beam is collimated to fit the detector. When an exposure is made, the X-ray beam moves across the breast synchronously with the detector, enabling an image of the whole breast to be obtained.

A flat panel phosphor system is used as the detector for Senographe digital mammography units (GE Medical Systems). The detector consists of a phosphor layer coated onto a light-sensitive thin film transistor (TFT) array composed of amorphous silicon. Charge from the TFT array produced in response to the light emission from the phosphor is measured and digitized.

The above digital systems require multiple conversion steps in the acquisition of the image: X-ray energy is converted into light energy, which is then converted into electrical energy. Multiple conversion steps are inefficient and have the potential to degrade image quality. Systems that avoid these conversion losses are described as being more 'direct'. The Lorad Selenia digital mammography system (Hologic) uses amorphous selenium in the detector, allowing the energy of the X-ray photon to be directly converted into electrical energy. Other manufacturers are also developing detectors that allow the direct conversion of X-ray energy into an electrical signal. The Sectra Micro Dose Mammography System (Sectra, Sweden) uses a silicon dioxide detector.

Once the image is in a digital format it is possible to manipulate the appearance of the image to optimize image quality. Digital mammograms are best reported using a workstation equipped with high resolution monitors (soft-copy reporting) (Fig. 52.5). This enables the reader to quickly change the appearance of the image. Windowing can be adjusted, different processing algorithms can be applied, measurements performed, images magnified and the grey scale inverted. The latter two functions are particularly useful in the assessment of microcalcifications. It would appear that electronic magnification on the workstation is just as effective as direct magnification mammography in the detection and characterization of microcalcifications[5]. Grey scale inversion, enabling the image to be changed from white on black to black on white, is useful in identifying microcalcifications within the breast.

Digital mammography in clinical practice

It is generally believed that film readers prefer the look of digital mammograms. Different anatomical regions such as the skin, retromamillary region and dense parenchymal areas are seen better on digital than on screen/film mammograms (Fig. 52.6)[6,7]. Abnormalities such as microcalcifications and masses may be more conspicuous on digital mammograms[8]. It is important to establish whether an improvement in visualization of structures in the breast actually translates into an improvement in cancer detection rates. In view of the high financial cost of purchasing a digital mammography machine, such systems are not likely to be widely adopted if diagnostic accuracy is only equivalent to screen/film mammography.

A powerful test of the potential of digital mammography to improve cancer detection rates is in a screening setting. The first published study from North America in 2002 looked at a group of 6736 women screened with both conventional and digital mammography. Overall there was no significant difference in the cancer detection rate between the two techniques, with each technique missing cancers detected by the other[9]. Another study with a similar design performed in Scandinavia—the Oslo I study—screened 3683 women with both techniques. Again no significant difference in cancer detection rates was demonstrated between

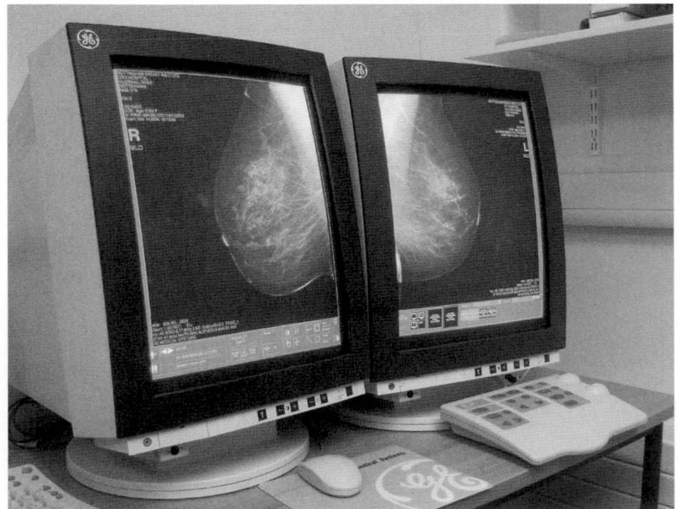

Figure 52.5 Two-monitor workstation. Images are easily manipulated by either a mouse click or the push of a button on the console.

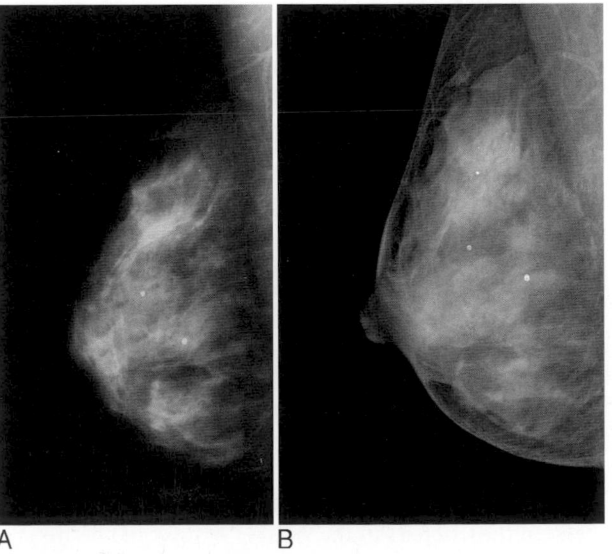

Figure 52.6 Screening mammogram of a 57-year-old, with dense breast parenchyma and scattered benign microcalcifications. This MLO view has been performed on (A) a conventional screen/film system and (B) a digital mammography system.

the two techniques[10]. More encouragingly, the larger Oslo II study, which randomized over 25 000 women to either conventional or digital mammography, has shown an increase in cancer detection in the women undergoing a digital mammogram, but this did not quite reach statistical significance ($p = 0.053$)[11].

To detect significant differences between the two techniques the population size needs to be large as the cancer detection rate in a screening population is around six per 1000 women screened. The North American Digital Mammographic Imaging Screening Trial (DMIST) enrolled 49 500 women. This study found that overall the diagnostic accuracy of digital and conventional mammography was similar. In women under the age of 50, those with dense breast parenchyma and women who were pre- or perimenopausal, digital mammography showed significantly improved diagnostic accuracy[12]. Encouragingly, it is in these groups of women that conventional screen/film mammography has been at its least sensitive for detecting breast cancer.

Digital mammography has other advantages, including the potential to improve patient throughput, as conventional mammography is labour intensive, with time taken in handling cassettes, loading/unloading film and processing. Radiographers can rapidly establish whether the examination is satisfactory before the patient leaves the department. There is a reduction in repeat examinations, as many images that initially appear inappropriately exposed can be manipulated to produce images of acceptable quality. With many hospitals becoming filmless, digital mammography equipment can interface directly with a picture archiving and communication system (PACS). Once in digital format, other advanced applications such as computer-aided detection can be used.

Computer-aided detection

Computer-aided detection (CAD) is a computer software system that is designed to aid the film reader by placing prompts over areas of concern, and to try to reduce observational oversights. CAD systems are highly sensitive for detecting cancers on screening mammograms. CAD software will correctly prompt around 90% of all cancers, with 86–88% of all masses and 98% of microcalcifications correctly marked. Specificity is much more of a problem with a high rate of false-positive prompts. The number of false prompts will vary according to the level of sensitivity at which the system is set; typically there are between two and four false prompts per study[13–15].

There is no consensus in the literature as to whether CAD improves film reader performance. Some prospective studies of the use of CAD in the screening setting have shown a significant improvement in a single film reader's performance when CAD software is applied, whereas others have shown no effect on cancer detection rates[15,16]. However, it is difficult to extrapolate the findings of these studies to the NHSBSP in the UK, where virtually all films are double read by two readers. In the context of the NHSBSP, it would be helpful to establish whether one reader using CAD could produce results equivalent to double reading and whether CAD is a more cost-effective solution to the manpower problem than training nonmedically qualified film readers.

Ultrasound (physics, technique, equipment)

Breast ultrasound requires the use of high frequency ultrasound of at least 7.5 MHz. Higher frequencies result in greater resolution. However, as the frequency increases, the ability of the ultrasound beam to penetrate to deeper breast tissue decreases. Consequently, the frequency selected has to be appropriate for the size of the breast to be examined.

The patient is examined in the supine position with the ipsilateral arm placed behind the patient's head. When imaging the outer portion of the breast it helps to turn the patient into a more oblique position. The aim is to flatten the breast tissue against the chest wall, reducing the thickness of breast tissue to be imaged.

Is best to image the breast tissue in two planes perpendicular to each other. A transverse and a sagittal plane is a common combination, but some authors advocate examining the breast in a radial and antiradial direction. The theory behind this method is that the ducts of the breast are positioned in a radial direction, running towards the nipple rather like the spokes of a bicycle wheel. Most breast cancers begin in the ducts and so tumours extending along the ductal system may be better visualized in this plane[17].

Indications for ultrasound

- Characterization of palpable mass lesions
- Assessment of abnormalities detected on a mammogram
- Primary technique for the assessment of breast problems in younger patients
- Guidance for biopsy and wire localizations

NORMAL ANATOMY

The breast consists of three types of tissue: the skin, subcutaneous adipose tissue and the functional glandular tissue. Centrally, there is the nipple–areolar complex. Collecting ducts open onto the tip of the nipple. There are sebaceous glands within the nipple–areolar complex called Montgomery's glands. Small raised nodular structures called Morgagni's tubercles are distributed over the areola, representing the openings of the ducts of Montgomery's glands onto the skin surface[18].

Deep to the nipple–areolar complex, the breast is divided into 15–25 lobes, each consisting of a branching duct system leading from the collecting ducts to the terminal duct lobular units (TDLU), the site of milk production in the lactating breast. Each duct drains a lobe made up of 20–40 lobules[18].

The breast lies on the chest wall on the deep pectoral fascia. The superficial pectoral fascia envelops the breast. Suspensory ligaments— called Cooper's ligaments—connect the two layers, providing a degree of support to the breast and giving the breast its shape (Fig. 52.7).

The number of lobules per lobe varies according to age, lactation, parity and hormonal status. At the end of reproductive life there is an increase in the amount of adipose tissue and, although the main duct system is preserved, there is considerable loss of lobular units. These changes in breast composition are manifested by changes in the breast density on mammography.

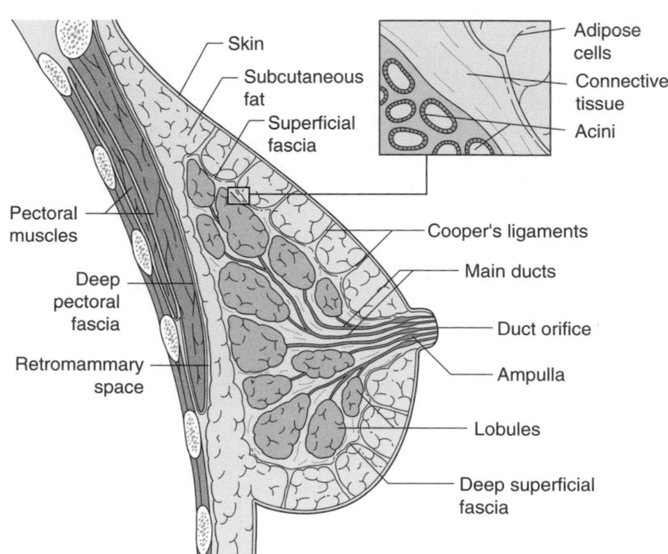

Figure 52.7 Gross anatomy of the breast.

Usually, younger women tend to have more of the dense glandular breast tissue. In older women, the mammographic density tends to decrease, with replacement of the glandular tissue by fatty tissue. However, there are young women who have very fatty-appearing breasts on mammography and older women with mammographically dense breasts. Classifications systems have been developed to describe the density of breast tissue on mammography. One of the best known is the Wolfe classification[19]:

- Wolfe N1 pattern refers to a breast containing a high proportion of fat
- Wolfe DY pattern refers to extremely dense breast tissue
- Wolfe P1 pattern refers to a predominantly fatty breast with < 25% visible glandular tissue
- Wolfe P2 pattern refers to a breast with > 25% visible glandular tissue.

There is some evidence suggesting that there is a relationship between the mammographic parenchymal pattern and the risk of developing breast cancer[20]. Women with dense breast tissue have a higher than average risk of developing breast cancer. In addition, dense breast tissue may hide abnormalities in the breast, making cancer detection more difficult. The sensitivity of mammography for detecting breast cancer is directly related to the density of the breast tissue. In general, mammography is more sensitive at detecting breast cancer in older, postmenopausal women because the breast tends to be composed of greater amounts of fatty tissue.

BREAST PATHOLOGY

Benign mass lesions

Cysts

Cysts are the most common cause of a discrete breast mass, although they are often multiple and bilateral. They are common between the ages of 20 and 50 years, with a peak incidence between 40 and 50 years. Simple cysts are not associated with an increased risk of malignancy and have no malignant potential.

On mammography they are seen as well-defined, round or oval masses. Sometimes a characteristic halo is visible on mammography (Fig. 52.8A).

Cysts can be readily diagnosed with ultrasound. They have well-defined margins, are oval or round in shape, and show an absence of internal echoes indicating the presence of fluid. The area of breast tissue behind a cyst appears bright on ultrasound (posterior enhancement) due to improved transmission on the ultrasound beam through the cyst fluid (Fig. 52.8B). When these features are present, a cyst can be diagnosed with certainty. Aspiration is easily performed under ultrasound guidance to alleviate symptoms or when there is diagnostic uncertainty. Cytology on cyst fluid is not routinely performed unless there are atypical imaging features or the aspirate is bloodstained.

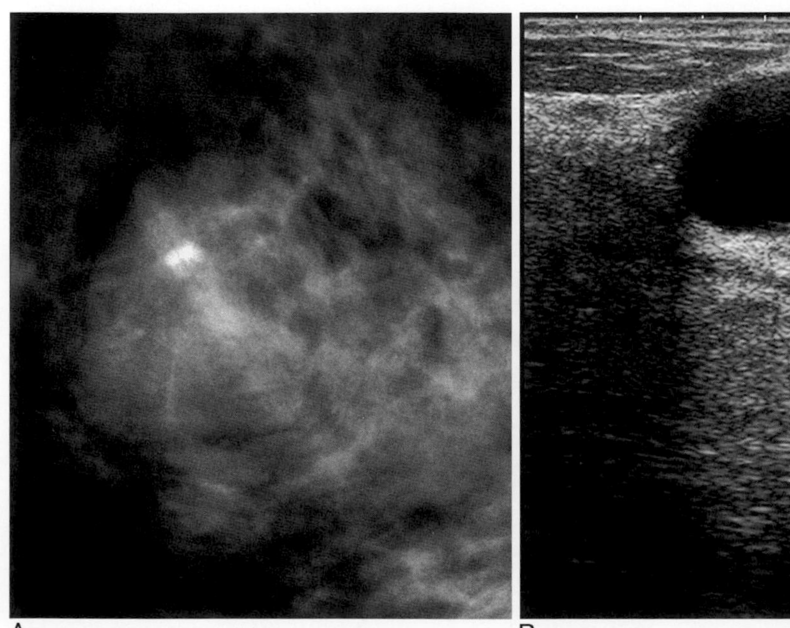

Figure 52.8 Cyst. (A) A well-defined rounded mass, with an associated lucent halo characteristic of a cyst. (B) The absence of internal echoes and the posterior enhancement of the ultrasound beam are diagnostic of a cyst.

Fibroadenomas and related conditions

Fibroadenomas are the most common cause of a benign solid mass in the breast. They present clinically as smooth, well-demarcated, mobile lumps. They are most frequently encountered in younger women with a peak incidence in the third decade. With the advent of screening, many previously asymptomatic lesions are detected.

On mammography, fibroadenomas are seen as well-defined, rounded or oval masses. In the majority of cases they are solitary, but in 10–20% they are multiple (Fig. 52.9A)[18]. Coarse calcifications may develop within fibroadenomas, particularly in older women (Fig. 52.10).

Ultrasound features have been described that are characteristic of benign masses[17]. These include hyperechogenicity compared to fat, an oval or well-circumscribed, lobulated, gently curving shape and the presence of a thin, echogenic pseudocapsule. If several of these features are present and there are no features suggestive of malignancy, then a mass can be confidently classified as benign.

Many fibroadenomas have a smooth, well-defined margin, are gently lobulated and are oval in shape (Fig. 52.9B). Most fibroadenomas are isoechoic or mildly hypoechoic relative to fat. A thin echogenic pseudocapsule may be seen. In most cases, even though the mass has benign features, percutaneous biopsy is necessary to confirm the diagnosis. However, in patients with no suspicious features in whom several benign characteristics are present, a percutaneous biopsy may be avoided[17]. One such group may be women under the age of 25, where the risks of any mass being malignant are very small.

Fibroadenomas must be distinguished from well-circumscribed carcinomas; this is done by percutaneous biopsy. Phyllodes tumour can have a similar appearance to fibroadenoma, leading to diagnostic difficulties (Fig. 52.11). The pathological characteristics can also be similar to those of large fibroadenomas. The majority of phyllodes tumours are benign, but some (less than 25%) are locally aggressive and may even metastasize[18]. When a diagnosis of phyllodes tumour is made, surgical excision must be complete with clear margins to prevent the possibility of recurrence. Many larger fibroadenomas (over 3 cm), and those that show a rapid increase in size, tend to be excised, in order to avoid missing a phyllodes tumour.

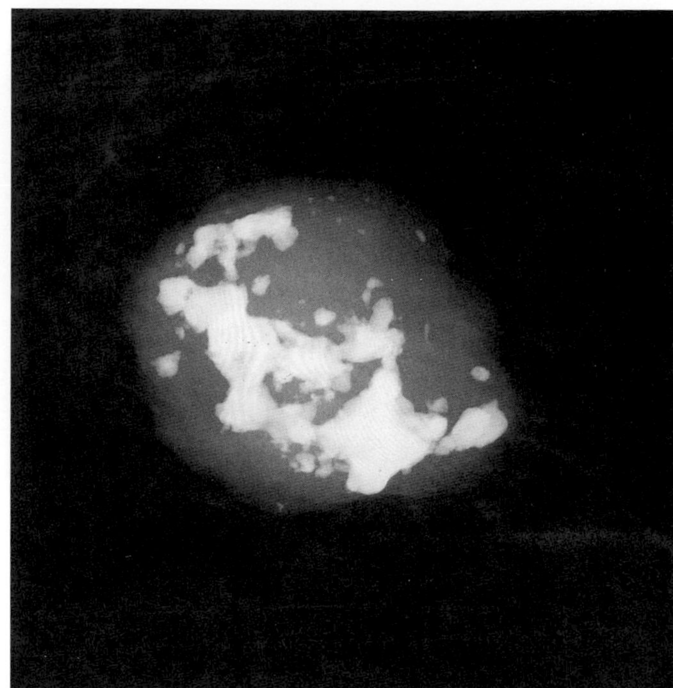

Figure 52.10 Fibroadenomas may develop coarse 'pop-corn' type calcifications.

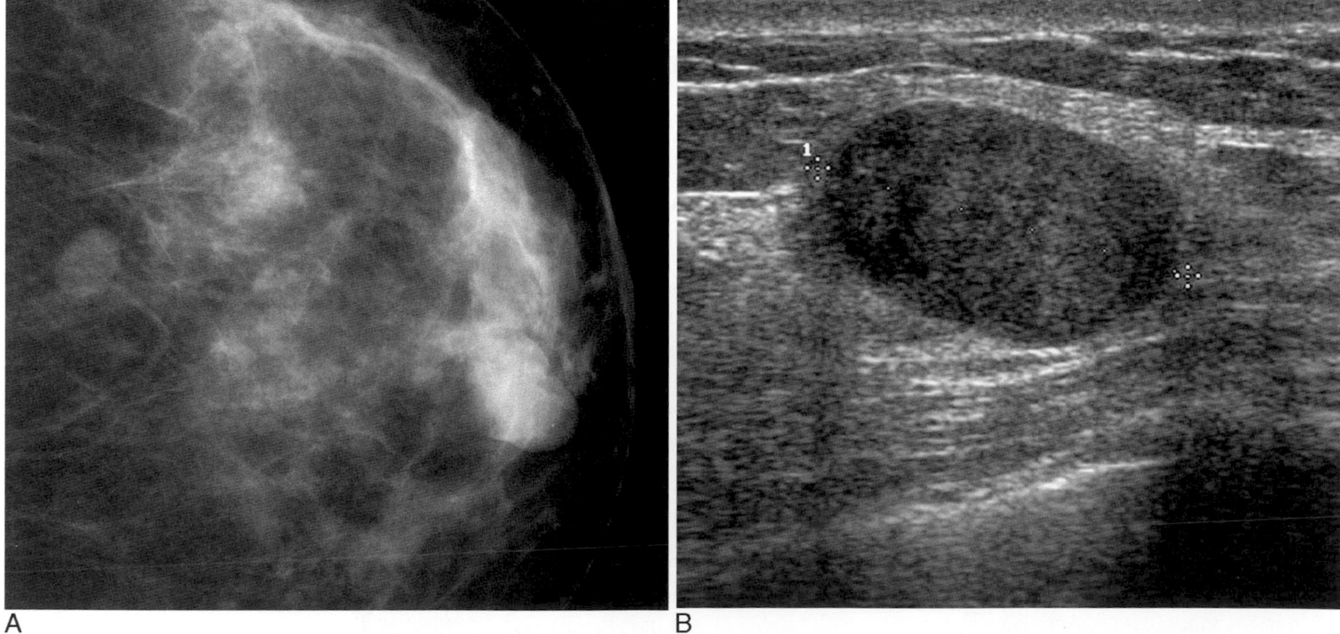

Figure 52.9 Fibroadenoma. (A) Two well-defined masses on mammography. (B) Ultrasound of the lesion nearer the nipple showed a well-defined oval mass. Both lesions were confirmed as fibroadenomas on ultrasound-guided core biopsy.

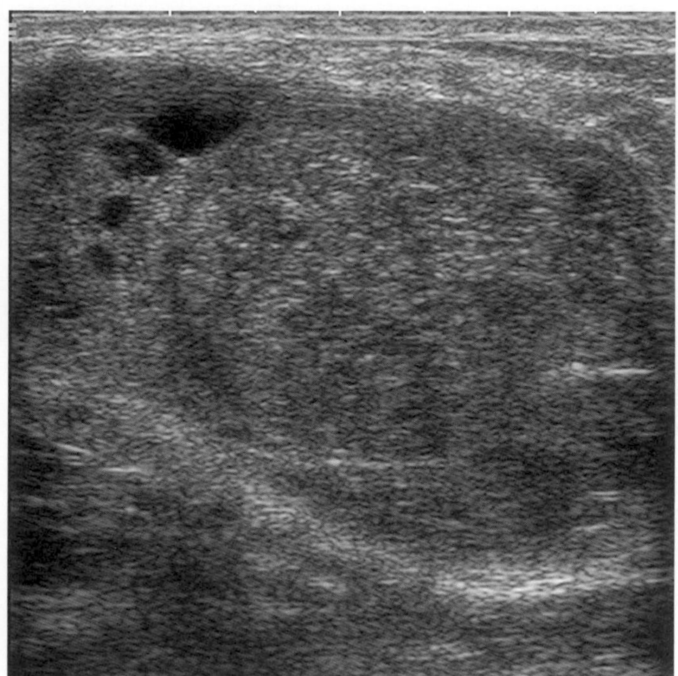

Figure 52.11 Phyllodes tumour. The presence of several cystic spaces within this large, well-defined mass suggested the possibility of a phyllodes tumour. This was confirmed on core biopsy and surgical excision.

Papilloma

Papillomas are benign neoplasms, arising in a duct, either centrally or peripherally within the breast. Many papillomas secrete watery material leading to a nipple discharge. As they are often friable and bleed easily, the discharge may be bloodstained.

On mammography, they may be seen as a well-defined mass, commonly in a retroareolar location (Fig. 52.12A). Sometimes the mass is associated with microcalcifications. On ultrasound, they typically appear as a filling defect within a dilated duct or cyst (Fig. 52.12B). On aspiration, any cyst fluid may be bloodstained. As it is impossible to differentiate papillomas from papillary carcinomas on imaging criteria, percutaneous biopsy is required.

Papillomas may be associated with an increased risk of malignancy, particularly if they are multiple or occur in a more peripheral location within the breast. Consequently, excision of papillary lesions is desirable and may be therapeutic in cases of nipple discharge. In situations where percutaneous biopsy shows no evidence of cellular atypia, then an alternative to surgical excision is piecemeal percutaneous excision using a vacuum-assisted biopsy device.

Lipoma

Lipomas are benign tumours composed of fat. They present clinically as soft, lobulated masses. Large lipomas may be visible on mammography as a radiolucent mass (Fig. 52.13A). On ultrasound their characteristic appearance is that of a well-defined lesion, hyperechoic compared to the adjacent fat (Fig. 52.13B).

Hamartoma

Hamartomas are benign breast masses composed of lobular structures, stroma and adipose tissue, the components that make up normal breast tissue. They occur at any age. On imaging they may be indistinguishable from other benign masses, such as fibroadenomas. Sometimes large hamartomas, detected on screening mammograms, are impalpable (Fig. 52.14). On mammography they classically appear as large, well-circumscribed masses containing a mixture of dense and lucent areas, reflecting the different tissue components present. Diagnostic

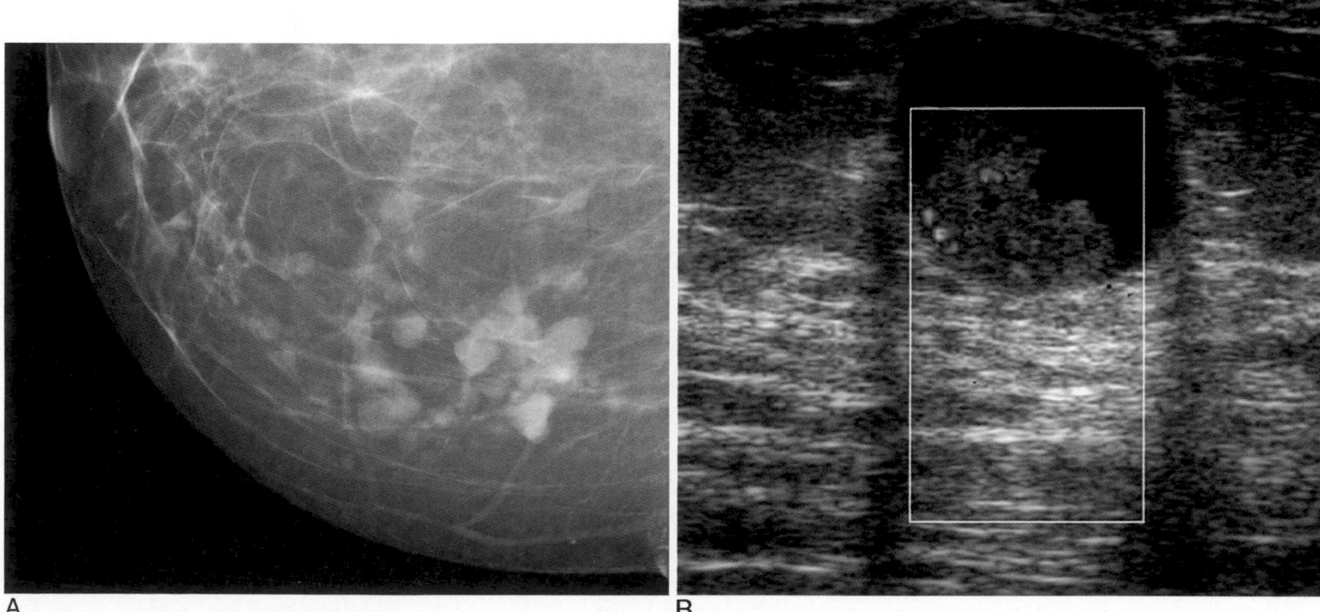

Figure 52.12 (A) **Multiple small papillomas.** Papillomas are frequently well defined on mammography, although part of the mass may have an irregular or ill-defined contour. (B) On ultrasound, the presence of a filling defect within a cystic structure suggests the diagnosis. Colour Doppler can be useful to distinguish debris within a cyst from a soft tissue mass.

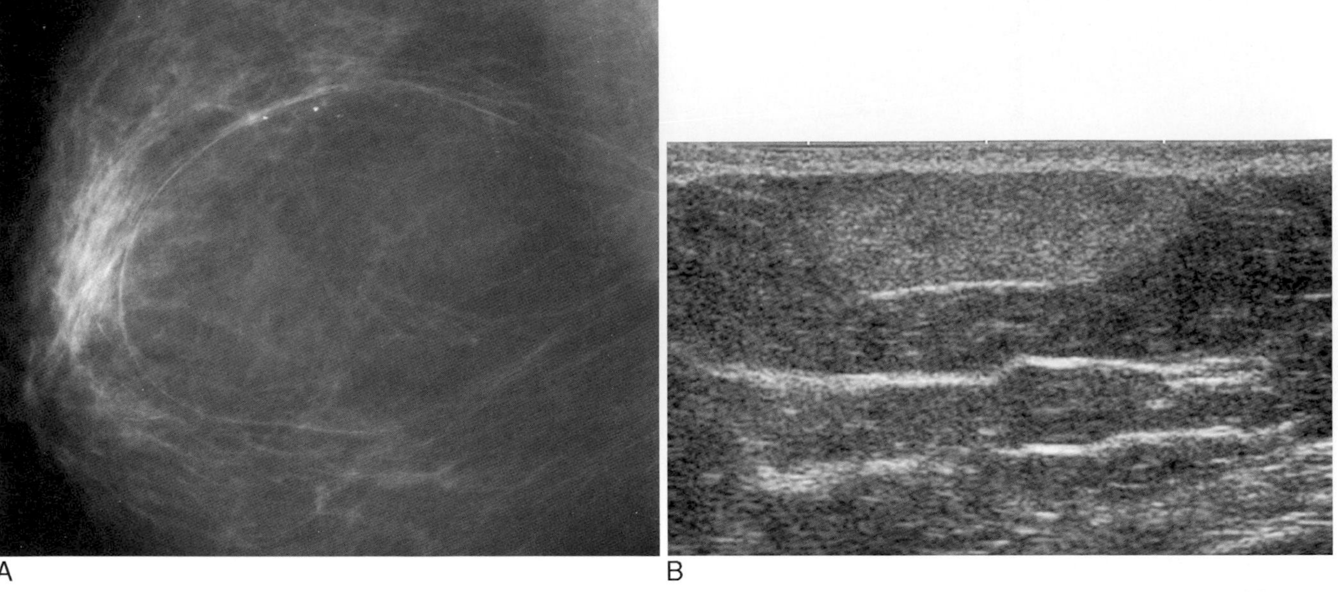

Figure 52.13 Lipoma. (A) On mammography, a lipoma may be seen as a well-defined mass of fat density, contained within a thin capsule. (B) On ultrasound, a well-defined hyperechoic lesion characteristic of a lipoma is seen.

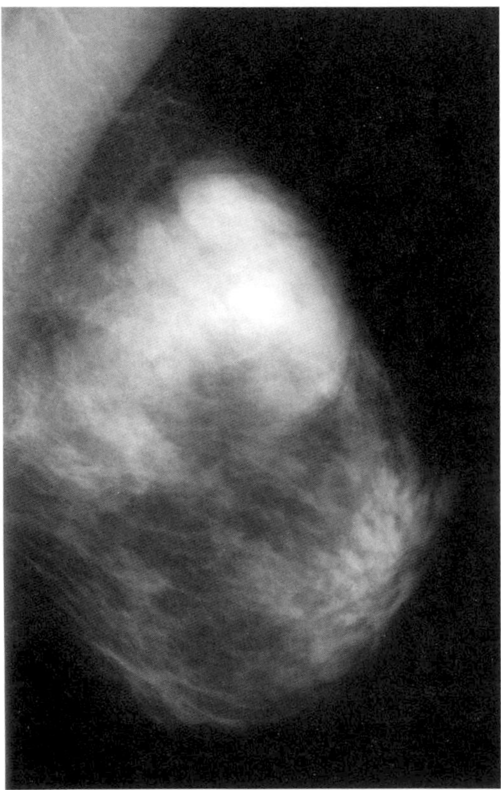

Figure 52.14 Hamartoma. Hamartomas are frequently encountered on screening mammograms as large, lobulated masses with areas of varying density reflecting the presence of elements which are of fat and soft tissue density.

difficulty may be encountered because percutaneous biopsy specimens may be reported as normal breast tissue.

Invasive carcinoma

Breast carcinomas originate in the epithelial cells that line the terminal duct lobular unit (TDLU). When malignant cells have extended across the basement membrane of the TDLU into the surrounding normal breast tissue, the carcinoma is invasive. Malignant cells contained by the basement membrane are termed noninvasive or in situ.

Classification of invasive breast cancer

There is much confusion regarding the classification of breast cancer. Some tumours show distinct patterns of growth, allowing certain subtypes of breast cancer to be identified. Those with specific features are called invasive carcinoma of special type, while the remainder are considered to be of no special type (NST or ductal NST). Special type tumours include lobular, medullary, tubular, tubular mixed, mucinous, cribriform and papillary. Different types of tumour have different clinical patterns of behaviour and prognosis. It should be understood that when a tumour is classified as of a special type this does not imply a specific cell of origin, but rather a recognizable morphological pattern[18,21].

Histological grade has implications for tumour behaviour, imaging appearances and prognosis. The morphological features on which histological grade is based are tubule formation, nuclear pleomorphism and frequency of mitoses[21]. Low-grade tumours that are well differentiated are less likely to metastasize.

Imaging appearance of invasive breast cancer

Mammography Carcinomas typically appear as ill-defined or spiculated masses on mammography (Fig. 52.15A,B). Lower-grade cancers tend to be seen as spiculated masses, due to the presence of an associated desmoplastic reaction in the adjacent stroma. Higher-grade tumours are usually seen as an ill-defined mass, but sometimes a rapidly growing tumour may appear relatively well defined, with similar appearances to a benign lesion such as a fibroadenoma (Fig. 52.15C).

Many breast cancers arise from areas of ductal carcinoma in situ (DCIS) and are associated with microcalcifications

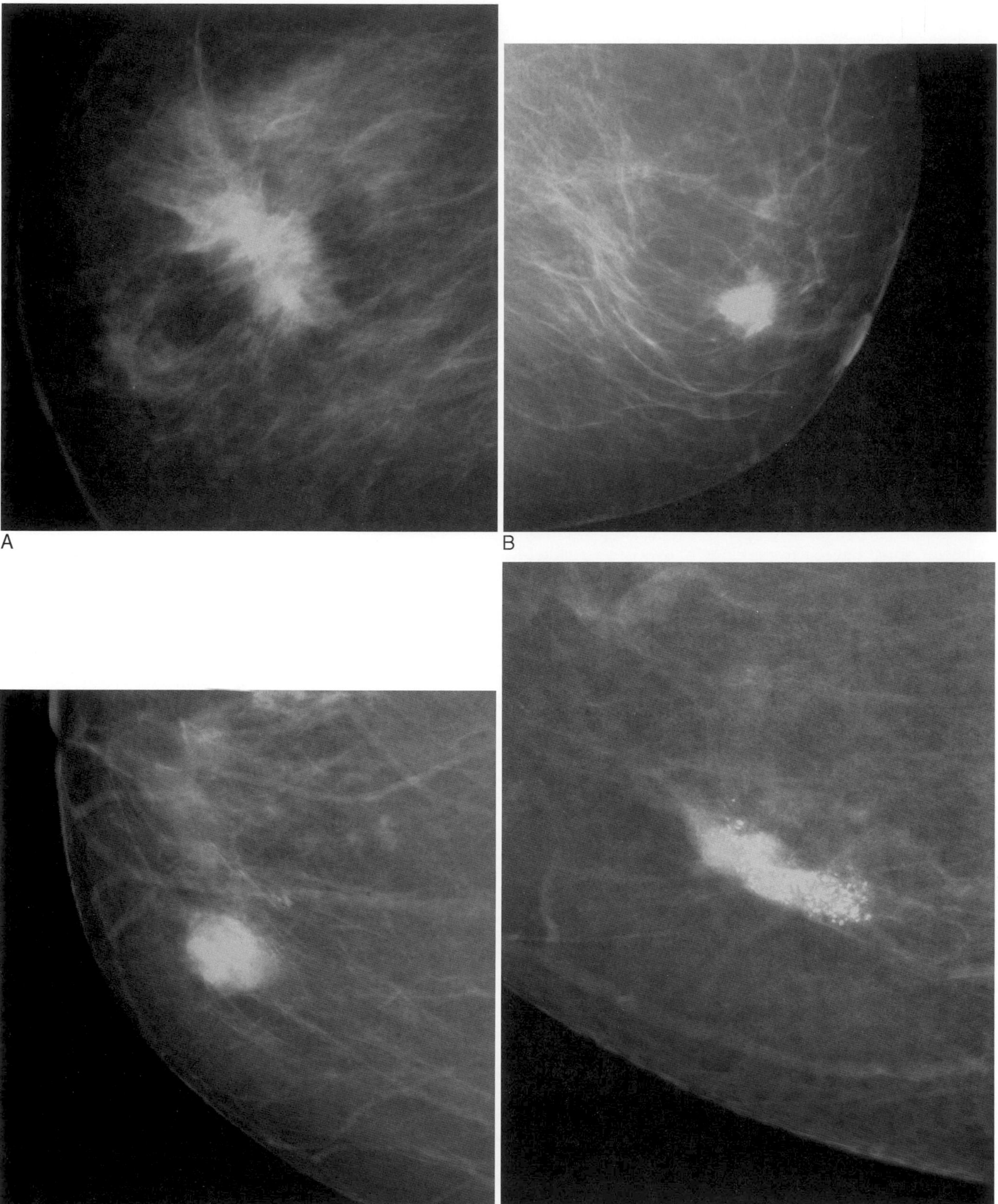

Figure 52.15 Mammographic appearances of invasive carcinoma. Spiculated and ill-defined masses are typical features of malignancy. The spiculated mass (A) and the ill-defined mass (B) were found to be ductal NST carcinomas of intermediate grade on core biopsy. (C) Sometimes high-grade tumours that exhibit rapid growth may appear more well defined. (D) Calcifications typical of high-grade DCIS may be found associated with invasive carcinomas.

on mammography (Fig. 52.15D). This is particularly true for high-grade invasive ductal carcinomas that are often associated with high-grade DCIS[22].

Special type tumours can have particular mammographic characteristics:

- Lobular carcinomas can be difficult to perceive on a mammogram due to their tendency to diffusely infiltrate fatty tissue. Compared with ductal NST tumours, lobular cancers are more likely to be seen on only one mammographic view, are less likely to be associated with microcalcifications, and are more often seen as an ill-defined mass or an area of asymmetrically dense breast tissue[23].
- Tubular and cribriform cancers often present as architectural distortions or small spiculated masses[24].
- Papillary, mucinous and medullary neoplasms may appear as new or enlarging multilobulated masses and may be well defined, simulating an apparently benign lesion[25,26].
- A small spiculated mass will be easily visible in a fatty breast, whereas even large lesions can be obscured by dense breast parenchyma.

Sometimes the only clue to the presence of an invasive tumour may be abnormal trabecular markings, known as an architectural distortion, or the presence of microcalcifications, which tend to be visible even when the breast parenchyma is dense.

The ability to perceive small or subtle cancers on a mammogram is improved by having the two standard mammographic views available and seeking out previous studies for comparison. An increase in the size of a mass or the presence of a new mass is suspicious of malignancy, whereas a lesion that remains unchanged over many years is invariably benign. Multiple masses in both breasts would favour a benign disease such as cysts or fibroadenomas.

Ultrasound There are characteristic malignant features on ultrasound[17]:

- Carcinomas are seen as ill-defined masses and are markedly hypoechoic compared to the surrounding fat (Fig. 52.16A).
- Carcinomas tend to be taller than they are wide (the anterior to posterior dimension is greater than the transverse diameter).
- There may be an ill-defined echogenic halo around the lesion, particularly around the lateral margins, and distortion of the adjacent breast tissue may be apparent, analogous to spiculation on the mammogram.
- Posterior acoustic shadowing is frequently observed, due to a reduction in the through transmission of the ultrasound beam via dense tumour tissue.

Poorly differentiated, high-grade tumours are more likely to be well defined, without acoustic shadowing (Fig. 52.16B), hence the importance of carrying out a biopsy of solid masses even when the ultrasound appearances are benign. Microcalcifications are sometimes observed, associated with high-grade tumours arising in areas of DCIS, although this is less frequently encountered than with mammography (Fig. 52.16C). Lobular carcinomas can be difficult to demonstrate on ultrasound. They may produce vague abnormalities, such as subtle alterations in echotexture, or the ultrasound findings may even be normal.

Doppler examination of malignant masses may show abnormal vessels that are irregular and centrally penetrating. In contrast, benign lesions such as fibroadenomas tend to show displacement of normal vessels around the edge of a lesion.

Ultrasound is a useful tool in the local staging of breast cancer preoperatively. It tends to be a better predictor of tumour size than mammography and may detect intraductal tumour extension. Ultrasound may also detect small satellite tumour foci not visible on mammography (Fig. 52.17).

It has long been recognized that involvement of axillary lymph nodes is one of the most important prognostic factors for women with breast cancer. Traditionally, the axilla has been staged at the time of surgery by lymph node sampling procedures, sentinel node biopsy, or clearance of the axillary lymph nodes. Surgical clearance of axillary lymph nodes is probably the 'gold standard'; however, it carries the risk of significant postoperative morbidity, with some women developing disabling lymphoedema in the arm. Ultrasound can identify abnormal nodes preoperatively that can then be biopsied percutaneously under ultrasound guidance (Fig. 52.18), allowing a preoperative diagnosis of lymph node involvement to be made in just over 40% of patients who are lymph node positive[27]. This enables the more radical axillary clearance to be targeted to those patients with a preoperative diagnosis of axillary disease, with the sampling or sentinel node procedures reserved for those patients with a much lower risk of axillary involvement.

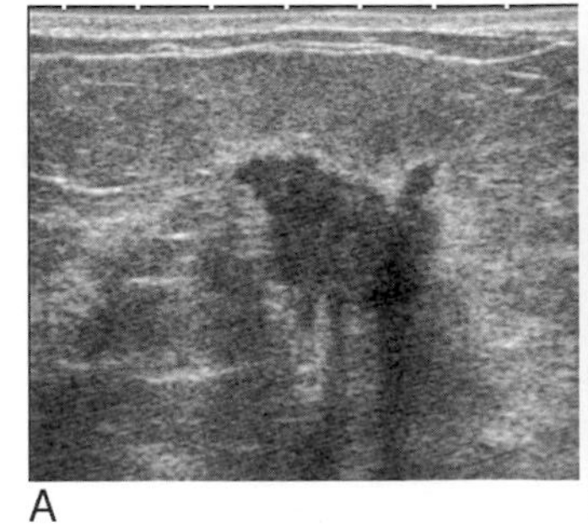

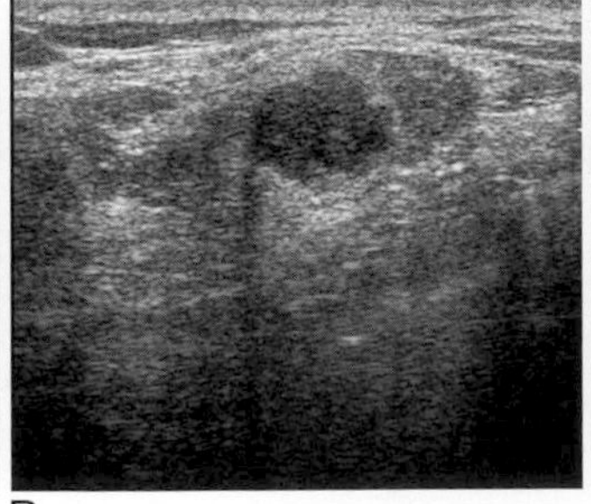

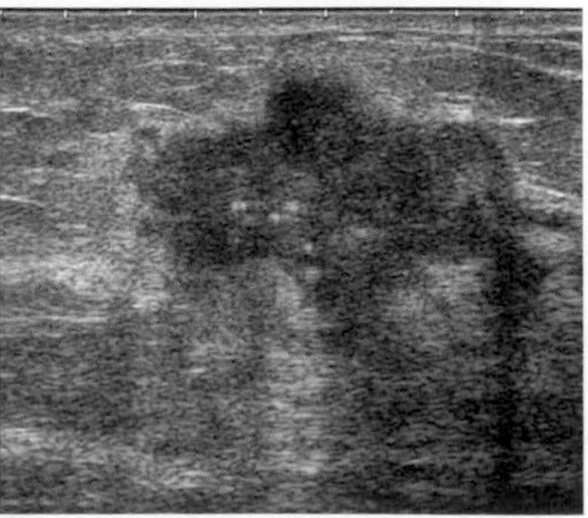

Figure 52.16 Ultrasound appearances of invasive carcinoma. (A) This irregular hypoechoic mass with acoustic shadowing and an echogenic halo is typical of a carcinoma. (B) Occasionally high-grade tumours may appear well defined, mimicking benign lesions. This shows the importance of performing a core biopsy even on apparently benign-appearing mass lesions. (C) Small echogenic foci of microcalcification associated with malignant lesions may be identified.

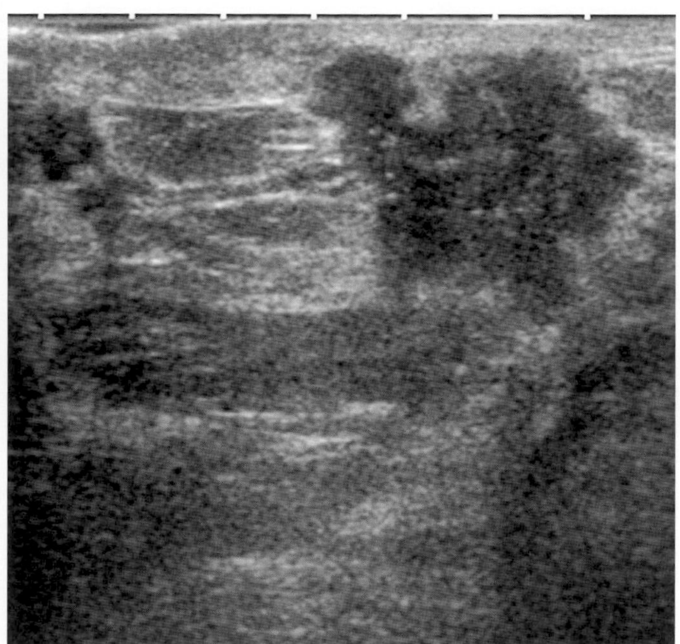

Figure 52.17 A small satellite tumour focus (on the left) is visible adjacent to the main tumour mass. A duct can be appreciated extending between the two lesions.

The differential diagnosis of malignancy

Many apparently suspicious findings seen on mammography or ultrasound can be caused by benign disease or even normal breast tissue.

The presence of a surgical scar may cause a spiculated mass or an architectural distortion (Fig. 52.19). Radiographers should be encouraged to record the presence and position of any scars when performing a mammogram to aid image interpretation by the film reader.

Infection and inflammatory processes in the breast can be mistaken for malignancy on mammography and ultrasound. Breast abscesses are typically encountered in young lactating women. Treatment is with antibiotics and aspiration of the pus, frequently under ultrasound guidance. Inflammation in a non-lactating breast is a more worrying feature, although infections and more unusual inflammatory conditions such as granulomatous mastitis can occur. Skin erythema and oedema may be caused by an underlying carcinoma, termed 'inflammatory carcinoma'. In this situation, skin thickening and oedema may be the only signs of malignancy recognized on the mammogram. In any case of unexplained inflammation, or when infection fails to resolve, percutaneous biopsy is required to make the diagnosis or exclude malignancy.

Radial scars, also called complex sclerosing lesions, can produce a spiculated lesion indistinguishable from malignancy on both mammography and ultrasound (Fig. 52.20). Many of these lesions are asymptomatic and are encountered on screening mammography. Epithelial atypia, DCIS and invasive carcinoma are found in association with radial scars.

Superimposition of normal breast tissue may produce apparent masses, distortions, or worrying asymmetric densities on mammography. These summation shadows are usually evaluated with additional mammographic views. Localized compression or paddle views are particularly helpful in deciding whether a lesion is real or just a summation shadow. Ultrasound of the area of mammographic concern can help to determine whether a lesion is truly present.

Microcalcifications

Microcalcifications are frequently encountered on routine screening mammograms. In many cases these microcalcifications turn out to be benign, but occasionally are an important feature of DCIS. Some calcifications have a characteristic

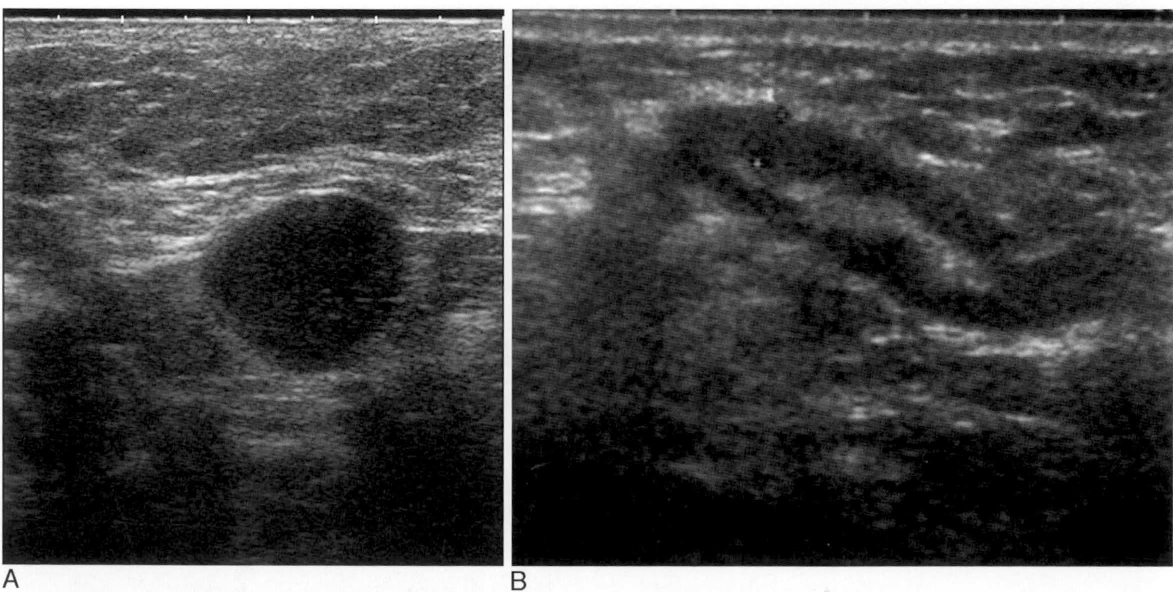

Figure 52.18 Axillary lymph nodes can be assessed on the basis of shape and the morphology of the cortex. (A) Nodes are likely to contain tumour if their longitudinal to transverse diameter is less than 2 (the node appears round rather than oval). Nodes are more likely to contain tumour if the cortex is thickened to more than 2 mm. (B) The node has a normal shape, but part of the cortex had a thickness of 3 mm. Both these axillary lymph nodes were biopsied under ultrasound guidance and found to contain tumour.

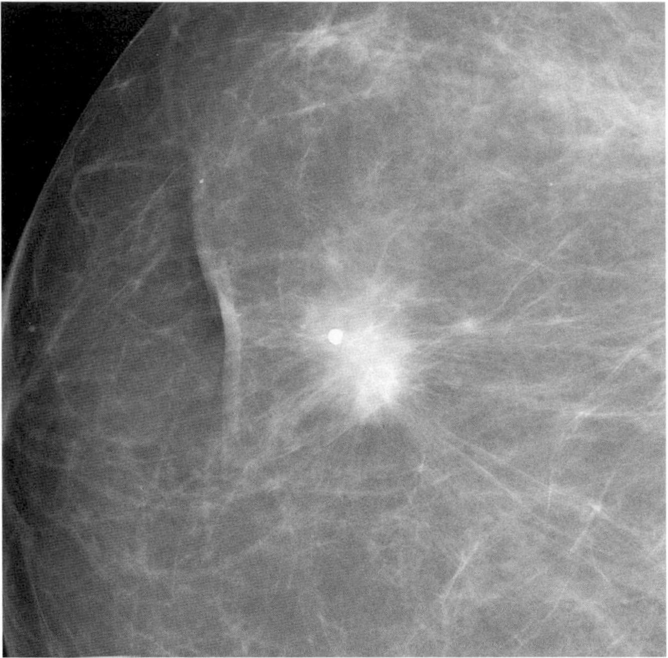

Figure 52.19 Postoperative scar. This patient had undergone a previous wide excision for a screen-detected cancer. There is associated deformity with indrawing of the skin. There is a focus of benign calcification, probably the result of fat necrosis.

benign appearance and require no further action. There is a considerable overlap between the appearance of benign and malignant microcalcifications, necessitating a percutaneous biopsy in many cases.

Benign microcalcifications

Many benign processes in the breast can cause microcalcifications, including fibrocystic change, duct ectasia, fat necrosis and fibroadenomatoid hyperplasia. Fibroadenomas and papillomas can also become calcified. Sometimes normal structures, such as the skin or small blood vessels, calcify. Calcifications can also develop in atrophic breast lobules or normal stroma.

Vascular calcifications have a characteristic 'tramline' appearance caused by calcification in both walls of the vessel (Fig. 52.21). Similarly, duct ectasia has a classical appearance that rarely causes diagnostic difficulty. In this condition, coarse rod and branching calcifications are recognized due to calcification of debris within dilated ducts. These calcifications have been described as having a 'broken needle' appearance and are usually bilateral (Fig. 52.22A). Sometimes the debris may extrude from the ducts into the adjacent parenchyma, leading to an inflammatory type reaction. Fat necrosis may then occur and the calcifications take on a characteristic 'lead-pipe' appearance (Fig. 52.22B). In many cases the diagnosis is obvious, but sometimes biopsy may be required, particularly if the calcifications are unilateral or focal.

Fibrocystic change is a common cause of microcalcifications (Fig. 52.23). On a lateral magnification view, layering of calcific fluid contained within microcysts can be appreciated, producing a characteristic 'teacup' appearance. However, in many cases, percutaneous biopsy is required to exclude DCIS.

Fat necrosis is a frequently encountered cause of benign calcifications, particularly when there is a history of trauma or previous surgery (Fig. 52.24). It may present as 'egg shell'

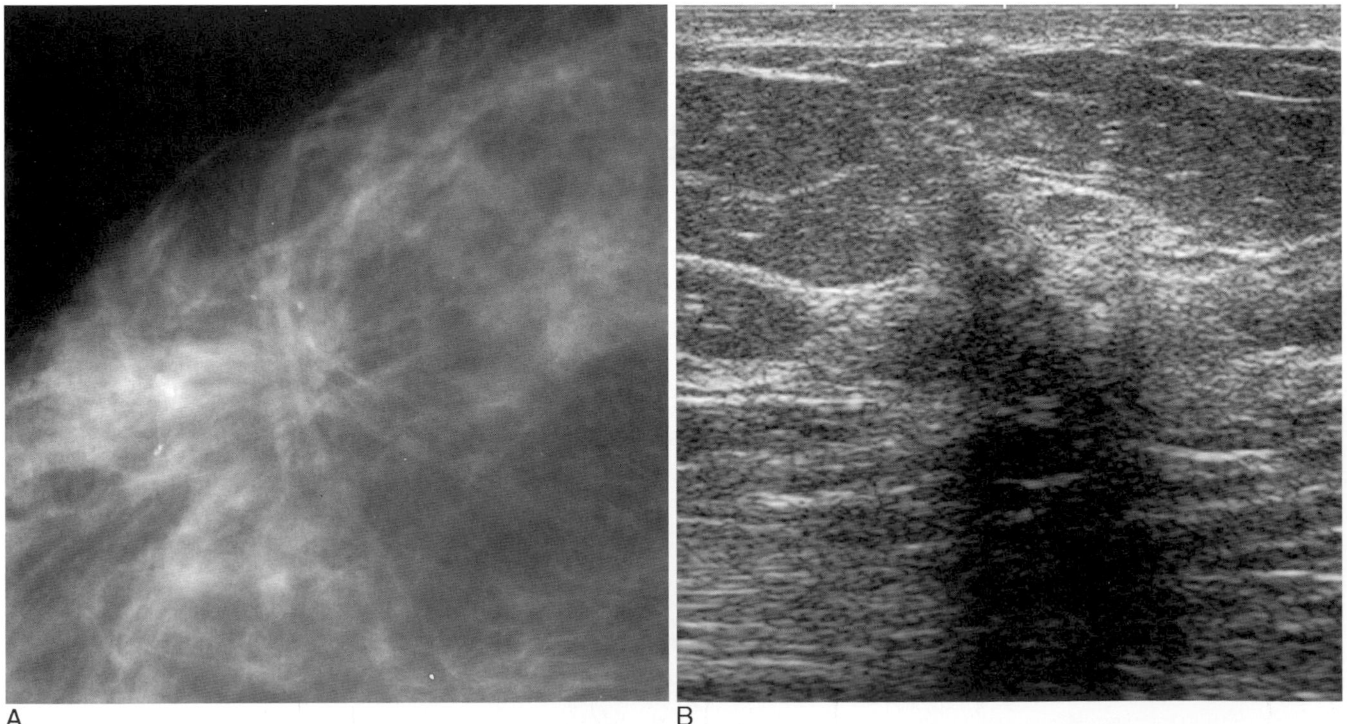

Figure 52.20 Radial scar. (A) Radial scar with a stellate appearance but no central mass. It is not possible to differentiate benign and malignant causes of parenchymal distortion on the basis of imaging alone. (B) Sometimes a radial scar can mimic a malignant lesion on ultrasound.

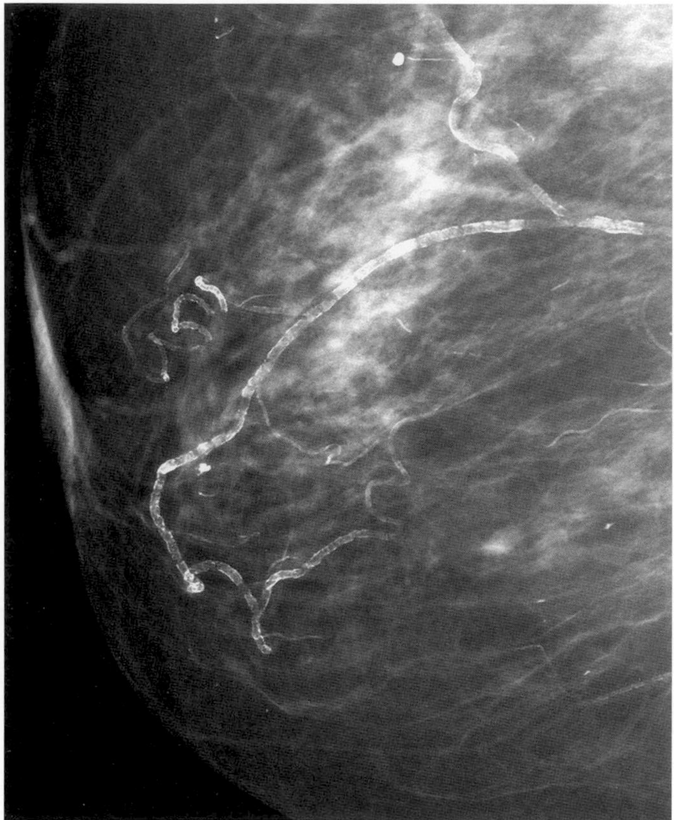

Figure 52.21 Vascular calcifications.

calcifications within the wall of an oil cyst or as coarse dystrophic calcifications associated with areas of scarring.

Fibroadenomas may become calcified, particularly after the menopause. Classically, the calcifications have a coarse, 'popcorn' appearance (Fig. 52.11). However, they can be small and punctuate, necessitating a biopsy to establish the diagnosis. Fibroadenomatoid hyperplasia is an increasingly common cause of microcalcifications detected during screening. Histologically, there are features of a fibroadenoma and fibrocystic change. There is usually no associated mass lesion and in many cases biopsy is required to exclude DCIS (Fig. 52.25).

Skin calcifications are characteristically round, well defined, have a lucent centre and are very often bilateral and symmetrical. Talcum powder or deodorants on the skin, as well as tattoo pigments, can mimic microcalcifications.

Malignant microcalcifications

Microcalcifications are found associated with invasive breast cancer and DCIS. Calcifications are more likely to be malignant if they are clustered rather than scattered throughout the breast, if they vary in size and shape (pleomorphic), and if they are found in a ductal or linear distribution. Malignant microcalcifications associated with high histological grade DCIS are classically rod shape and branch. These calcifications are known as casting or comedo microcalcifications and represent necrotic debris within the ducts, hence their linear, branching structure (Fig. 52.26). Approximately one third of malignant microcalcification clusters have an invasive focus within them at surgical excision[28]. The greater the number of flecks of

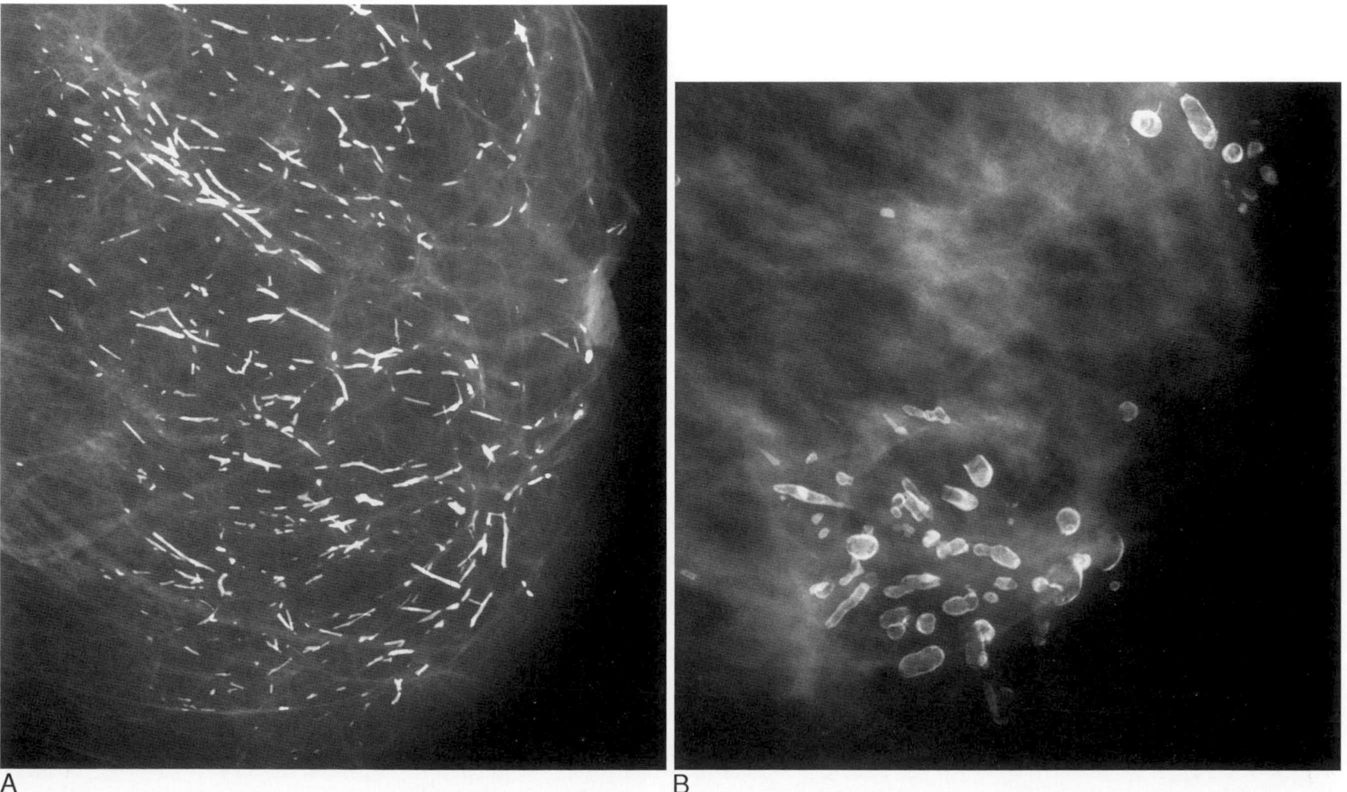

Figure 52.22 Duct ectasia. (A) Broken needle appearance, typical of duct ectasia. (B) Sometimes thicker, more localized calcifications can be seen, giving a 'lead-pipe' appearance.

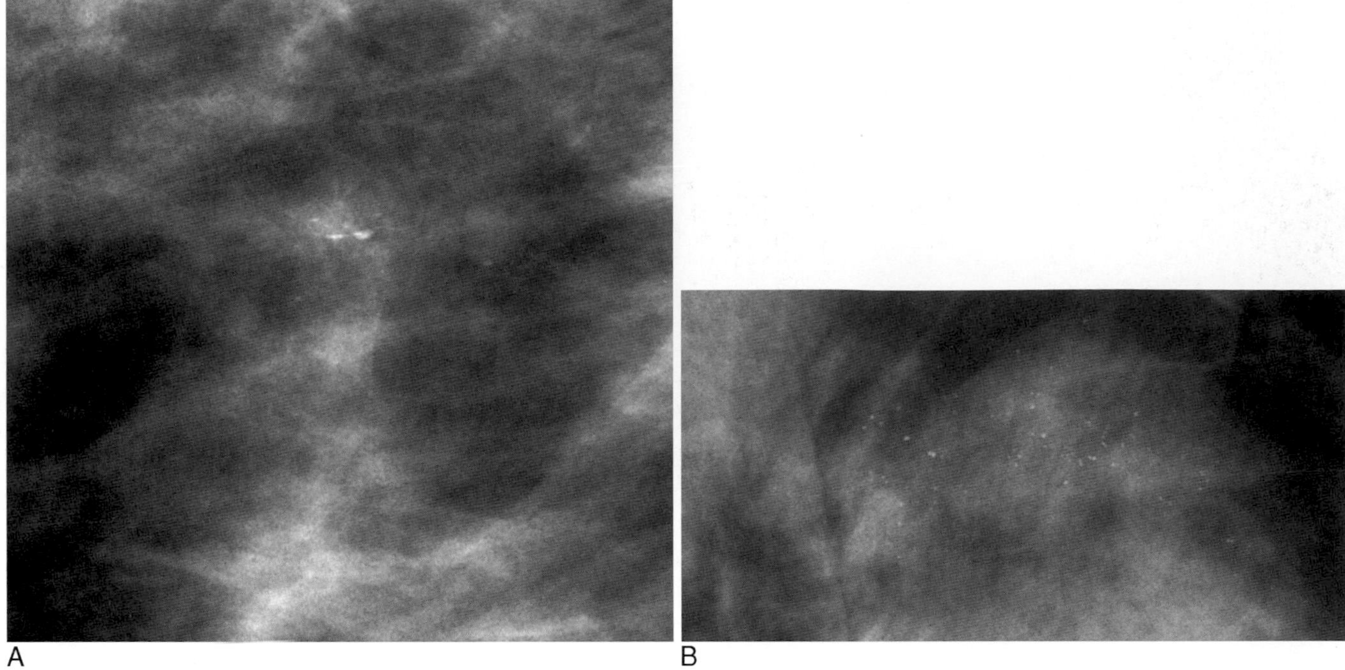

Figure 52.23 Fibrocystic change. (A) 'Teacups' representing the layering out of calcific material in the dependent portion of microcysts on a lateral magnification view. (B) As calcifications associated with areas of fibrocystic change may not exhibit this characteristic appearance, stereotactic core biopsy is required.

microcalcification associated with an area of DCIS, the greater the risk of invasive disease[28].

In the screening setting, it is often the presence of mammographically visible calcifications associated with high-grade DCIS that leads to the diagnosis of small, high-grade cancers[29]. Calcifications are much less frequently found in low-grade DCIS, as there is usually no intraductal necrosis. When they do occur, they are clustered, but otherwise have a nonspecific appearance.

The sensitivity of ultrasound for detecting DCIS is significantly lower than mammography, which is one of the reasons why ultrasound is not a useful screening test for breast cancer. However, ultrasound may be able to identify areas of microcalcifications seen on a mammogram, aiding percutaneous biopsy.

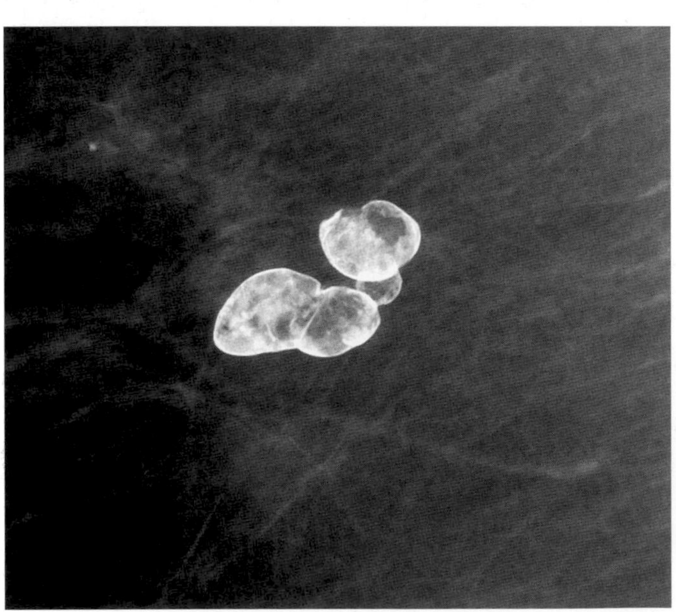

Figure 52.24 'Egg shell' calcifications of fat necrosis.

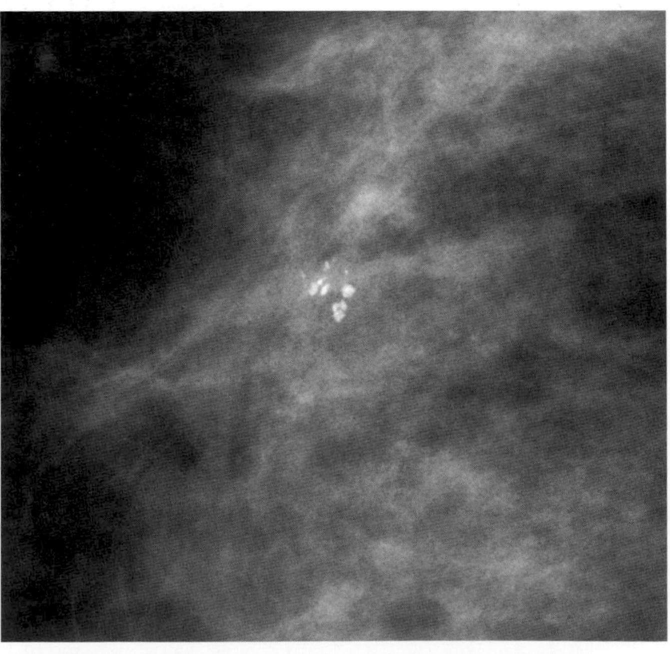

Figure 52.25 Small cluster of indeterminate microcalcifications. Stereotactic biopsy revealed fibroadenomatoid change.

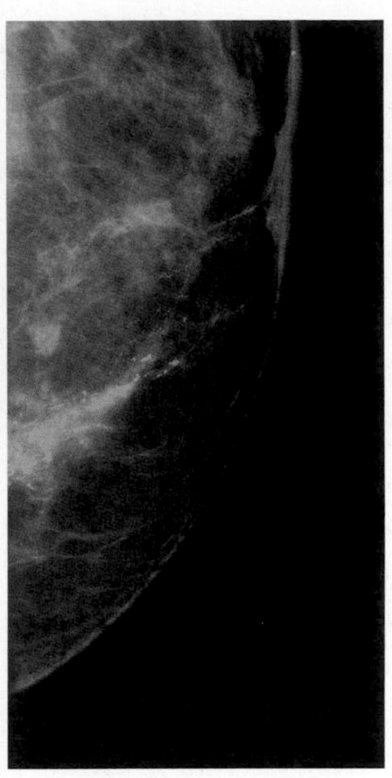

Figure 52.26 Ductal carcinoma in-situ (DCIS). Mammography shows the segmental distribution of pleomorphic microcalcifications. Granular, rod-shaped and branching calcifications can be identified. The appearances are typical of high-grade DCIS.

OTHER IMAGING TECHNIQUES

Magnetic resonance imaging

Although mammography and ultrasound remain the most frequently used techniques for imaging the breast, contrast-enhanced MRI is becoming increasingly important, largely because of its high sensitivity for detecting invasive breast cancer, which approaches 100% in many studies. There are problems with specificity, with some benign lesions and even normal breast tissue having a worrying appearance on MR imaging. The problems with specificity are compounded by limited availability of MR-guided localization and biopsy systems.

MRI is the technique of choice for assessing the integrity of breast implants. It is more accurate than mammography, ultrasound, or clinical examination in identifying implant failure. Unenhanced MRI is used to assess breast implants for complications.

Technique

Successful breast MR studies require high field strength magnets (1.5 Tesla) and the use of a dedicated breast coil. Some breast coils have inbuilt compression devices to stabilize the breast and reduce the number of slices required to cover the whole of the breast. Patients are examined in the prone position with the breast hanging down into the coil.

The intravenous injection of gadolinium-based contrast agent is required. It is the presence of abnormal vasculature within the lesion that enables detection.

Some method of eliminating the signal from fat is required as an enhancing lesion and fat display similar high signal on a T1-weighted image. Fat suppression may be active or passive: active fat suppression is typically achieved by the use of spectrally selective pulse sequences to suppress the signal from fat; passive fat suppression involves subtraction of the unenhanced images from the enhanced images. Subtraction allows faster imaging, with good spatial and temporal resolution, but it requires no patient movement between the two sets of images. New methods of active fat suppression, such as parallel imaging, including the sensitivity encoding technique (SENSE), allow fat suppression to be achieved with shorter examination times while maintaining good spatial and temporal resolution[30].

Fast, 3D gradient echo pulse sequences provide the optimum method for imaging small lesions. Temporal resolution is important because the optimum contrast between malignancy and normal breast tissue is achieved in the first 2 min following the injection of gadolinium contrast agent. Later, normal breast tissue may start to show nonspecific enhancement, masking the presence of malignancy. Other signs of malignancy, such as a rapid uptake of contrast agent followed by a 'washout' phase, may only be apparent if images are acquired dynamically every minute over a period of 6–7 min after the injection of gadolinium.

Unfortunately, increased spatial resolution (thin slices) can only be achieved at the expense of an increased examination time. Improving temporal resolution allows rapid dynamic scanning but at the expense of spatial resolution or the volume of the breast imaged. With modern equipment it should be possible to achieve a slice thickness of 3–4 mm while maintaining a temporal resolution of 60–90 s, covering the whole of both breasts.

Lesion characterization

There are two main approaches to image interpretation: the first relates to lesion morphology and the second to assessment of enhancement kinetics. The architectural features that indicate benign and malignant disease are similar to those already described for mammography and ultrasound. Benign lesions tend to be well defined with smooth margins whereas malignant lesions are poorly defined and may show spiculation or parenchymal deformity.

Malignant lesions tend to enhance rapidly following the injection of contrast agent and may show characteristic ring enhancement. Dynamic MRI enables more detailed enhancement curves to be calculated to aid characterization. Malignant lesions usually show a rapid uptake of contrast agent in the initial phase of the examination, followed by a washout or plateau in the intermediate and late periods after injection, whereas benign lesions exhibit a steady increase in signal intensity throughout the time course of the examination[31]. One of the strengths of breast MR imaging is that invasive cancer can be effectively excluded with a high degree of certainty if no enhancement is seen.

Investigators use a combination of architectural features and enhancement kinetics to differentiate benign from malignant lesions. However, there is some overlap in the enhancement characteristics of benign and malignant lesions. Sinister patterns of contrast enhancement have been observed in benign conditions, including fibroadenomas, fat necrosis and fibrocystic change. Even normal breast tissue may enhance and this enhancement is in part dependent on the phase of the menstrual cycle. Normal breast tissue is more likely to enhance during the middle of the cycle, between the sixth and seventeenth days[32].

Recent surgery or radiotherapy can interfere with image interpretation. It used to be recommended that at least 12 months should elapse between breast radiotherapy and an MRI study, but more recent work has suggested that enhancement patterns return to normal between 3 and 6 months after radiotherapy[33]. Percutaneous breast biopsy (FNA, core, or vacuum-assisted biopsy) rarely interferes with MRI interpretation.

Indications for breast MRI

Contrast-enhanced breast MRI is most frequently used for local staging of primary breast cancer. MRI is the most accurate technique for sizing invasive breast carcinomas and will sometimes show unsuspected multifocal disease in the same breast or even additional tumour foci in the contralateral breast[34]. Additional information on tumour extent can be expected in 15–30% of patients, which can lead to a change in the therapeutic approach, avoiding inappropriate breast-conserving surgery. There is an argument for breast MRI in all patients considering breast-conserving surgery. However, due to scarcity of resources and specificity issues, MRI is usually reserved for patients where estimating tumour size is proving difficult by conventional methods, including mammographically occult lesions, patients with mammographically dense breasts, and where there is significant discrepancy between size estimations at mammography, ultrasound and clinical examination.

Another group of patients who benefit from preoperative staging with MRI are those whose carcinomas have lobular features. Lobular carcinomas are more likely to be multifocal compared to ductal NST tumours. They are more difficult to detect and their size is more difficult to measure by conventional methods because of their infiltrating growth pattern. In approximately 50% of such patients MRI will show more extensive tumour (Fig. 52.27)[35].

Another important role of MRI is identifying an occult primary tumour in women presenting with malignant axillary lymphadenopathy with a normal mammogram and breast ultrasound. In this situation, MRI is highly sensitive for identifying an occult primary. MRI is also useful in the postsurgical breast, differentiating surgical scarring from tumour recurrence.

MRI can help to assess the response to treatment in women receiving neoadjuvant chemotherapy for locally advanced primary breast cancers. It can recognize nonresponders to treatment earlier than other imaging methods by demonstrating a reduction in lesion size, or a change in the enhancement pattern, with the level of enhancement reducing or taking on a more benign appearance.

MRI can be used to screen younger women with a high familial risk of breast cancer. Some of these women (e.g. known gene mutation carriers) have a lifetime risk of developing breast cancer of around 85%. In these younger women the sensitivity of mammography for detecting malignancy is low, largely due to the presence of mammographically dense breast parenchyma. Screening with MRI is superior to mammography in detecting invasive breast cancer in such women, although mammography remains more sensitive for detecting DCIS[36,37].

Pitfalls of MRI

Although the sensitivity of MRI for invasive breast cancers approaches 100%, its sensitivity for detecting DCIS is more variable. Specificity is also a problem. When MRI is used for staging breast cancer, problems arise when additional enhancing lesions are detected away from the primary tumour site, as these have to be differentiated from additional tumour foci, incidental benign lesions and areas of enhancing normal glandular breast tissue.

In such cases the architectural features of the lesion and enhancement kinetics should be assessed, and the MRI findings correlated with those of mammography. Probably most useful is a targeted, second-look ultrasound of the area. In most cases, ultrasound will identify any additional lesions and facilitate image-guided biopsy. For younger women, repeating the examination at a different phase of the menstrual cycle may exclude spontaneous hormone-induced enhancement as a cause of an additional enhancing focus. For lesions that are considered low risk, follow-up MRI after a suitable period of time is acceptable.

There is concern that the increasing use of breast MRI may result in unnecessary percutaneous biopsies or diagnostic surgery. The problems of specificity are compounded by the difficulties associated with MRI-guided biopsy and localization, as these techniques are time consuming and problematic. However, when there is no mammographic or ultrasound correlate, MRI-guided biopsy may be necessary. Dedicated biopsy coils and MRI-compatible needles are now becoming commercially available.

MRI for imaging breast implants

MRI is the technique of choice for assessing the integrity of breast implants, with a sensitivity and specificity of over 90%. When imaging breast implants, no contrast agent is required unless malignancy is suspected. Imaging should be performed in the prone position using a dedicated breast coil. The main goal is to determine whether the implant has ruptured and, if so, to establish the location of the leaked filler (usually silicon).

When implants fail, the rupture may be either intracapsular or extracapsular: intracapsular rupture occurs when silicon has escaped from the plastic shell of the implant, but is contained within the fibrous implant capsule (Fig. 52.28); signs of intracapsular rupture include the 'wavy line', 'linguini', 'key-hole' and 'salad oil' sign[38]. False-positive interpretations can be made when normal implant folds are mistaken for signs of rupture.

Extracapsular rupture is diagnosed when silicon is demonstrated outside the fibrous capsule. In this situation, free silicon, silicon granulomas, or silicon in axillary lymph nodes may be demonstrated (Fig. 52.29).

Scintimammography

Scintimammography is a nuclear medicine technique. It was developed following the observation that many breast cancers

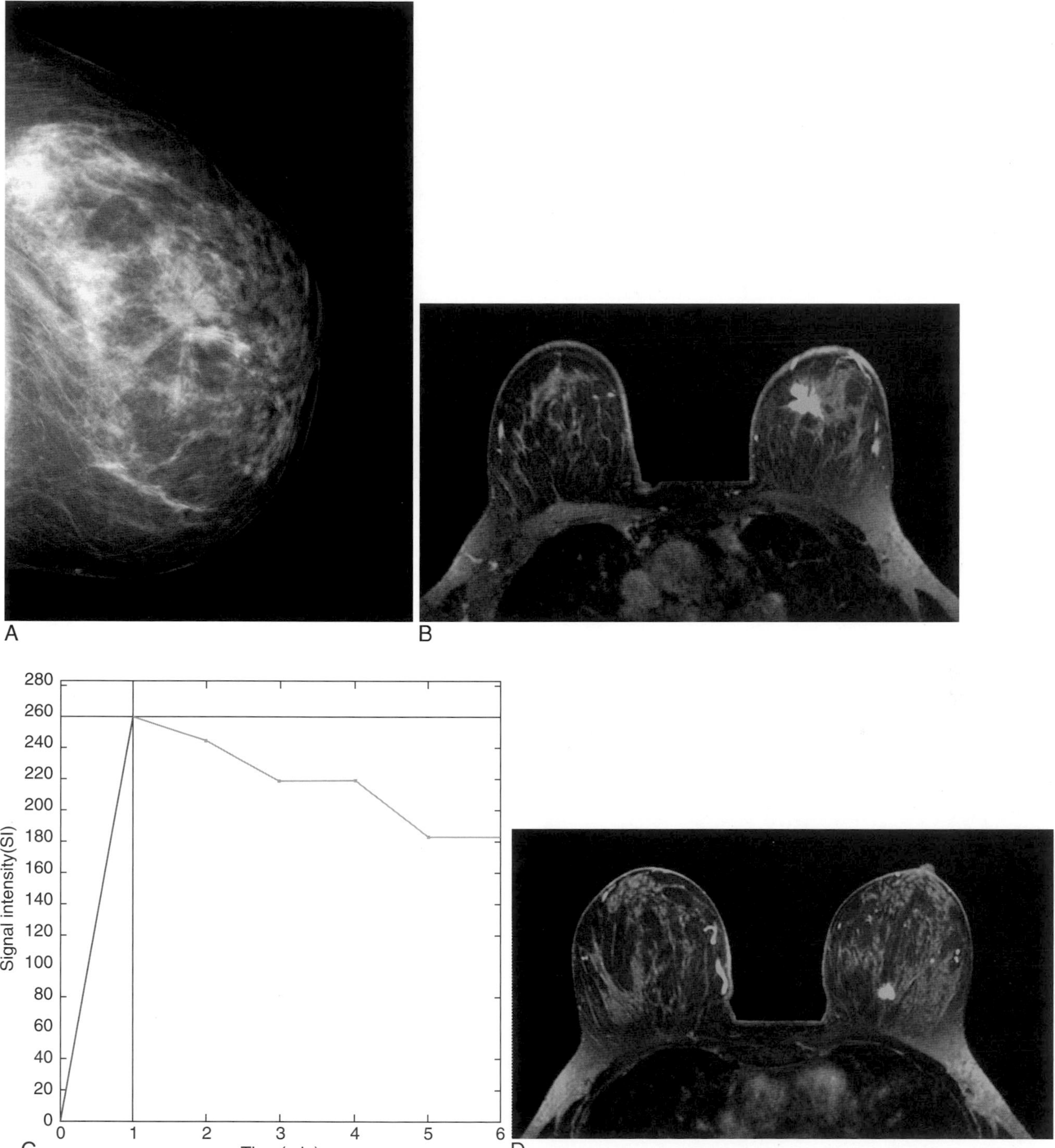

Figure 52.27 MRI for local tumour staging. This patient presented with a mass in the left breast. Mammography showed a spiculated lesion lying centrally within the breast, best appreciated on the CC view (A). Biopsy indicated a carcinoma with lobular features. MRI confirmed the presence of a malignant spiculated lesion (B) with a typically malignant enhancement curve (rapid uptake of contrast agent followed by a washout phase) (C). An additional tumour focus was identified away from the primary tumour site (D). This was confirmed at biopsy.

show uptake of isotopes used in cardiac imaging—for example, ^{99m}Tc-MIBI (Sestamibi). Indications for use overlap with those for MRI, including local staging, searching for a mammographically occult primary and detecting recurrence in the postsurgical breast. Scintimammography has failed to establish a place in routine practice due to problems with spatial resolution and its inability to detect DCIS.

BREAST CANCER SCREENING

Introduction

Breast cancer mortality in the UK is amongst the highest in the world. The causes of breast cancer are not well understood and, in the absence of any effective preventative measures, much effort and health care resources have been focused on

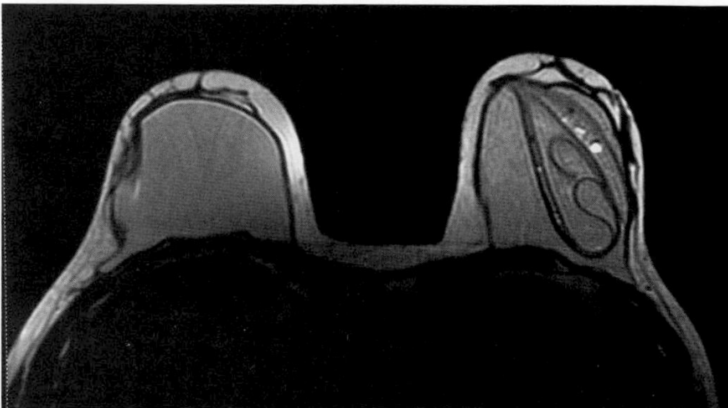

Figure 52.28 Intracapsular implant rupture. On these T2-weighted fast spin-echo images, the plastic shell of the left breast implant can be seen floating within the silicon, producing a 'wavy line' or 'linguini' sign. Note the presence of a couple of bright dots of water-like material, the 'salad oil' sign.

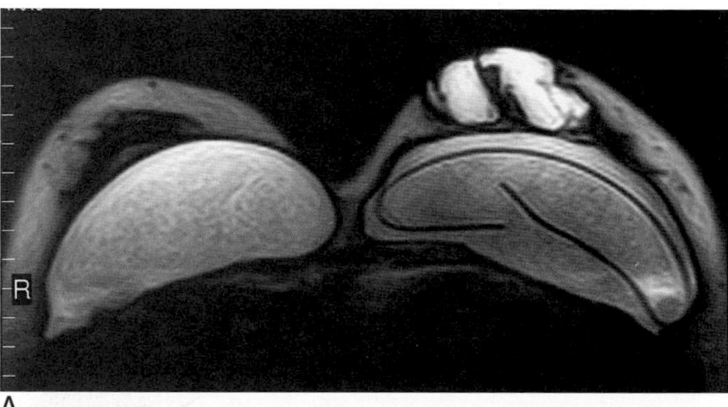

A

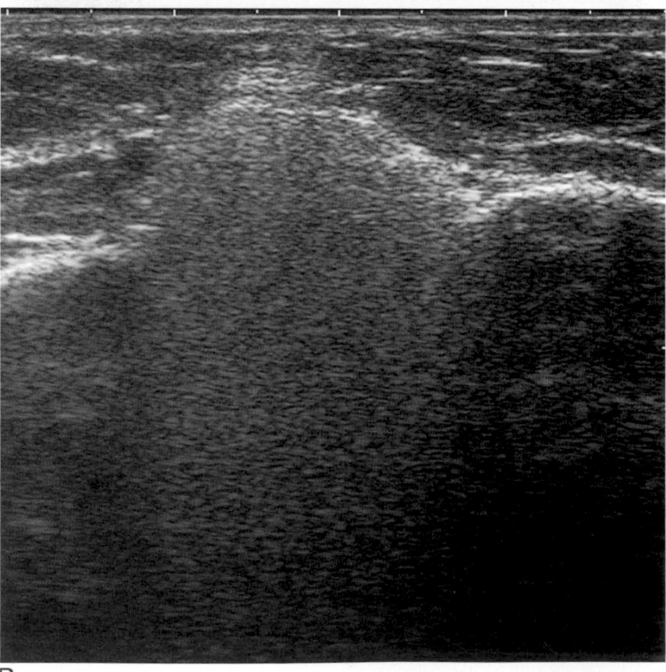

B

Figure 52.29 Extracapsular implant rupture. (A) A collection of free silicon is seen anterior to this ruptured left breast implant. (B) Ultrasound may be useful in the diagnosis of extracapsular rupture, with free silicon or silicon granulomas having a typical 'snow storm' appearance.

the quest to reduce breast cancer mortality by early detection through screening. A number of randomized controlled trials (RCTs) and case control studies carried out since the mid 1960s have shown that screening by mammography can reduce breast cancer mortality.

The UK National Health Service Breast Screening Programme was set up following the publication of the Forrest Report in 1986[39]. This document, commissioned by the UK Department of Health under the chairmanship of Professor Sir Patrick Forrest, reviewed the scientific evidence for population breast cancer screening. It recommended the immediate introduction of screening by mammography in the UK.

Within a year of publication, population breast cancer screening, free at the point of delivery, was introduced into the UK National Health Service (NHS). This was the first population-based breast screening programme in the world. Currently in the UK, breast cancer screening by mammography is provided for all women over the age of 50. Women between the ages of 50 and 70 are invited every 3 years. Women over 70 are not invited but are encouraged to attend by self referral. Two-view mammography is now used for all screens. The mammograms are read by at least one film reader, and in the majority of units the mammograms are double read.

The evidence for screening

Data from RCTs provide the strongest evidence of the efficacy of screening in reducing breast cancer mortality. The design of RCTs enables the elimination of lead-time bias. The majority of the RCTs of screening were carried out in Sweden.

The latest overview of these trials was published in 2002 and included data from Malmo, Gothenburg, Stockholm and the Ostergotland arm of the Two Counties study. Data from the Kopparberg arm of the Two Counties study was not made available. Almost a quarter of a million women were included in these studies, with approximately half being invited for screening and the other half making up the control group. The median trial time was 6.5 years and the median follow-up 15.8 years. The overall results indicated a 21% reduction in breast cancer mortality. The mortality reduction was largest in women aged 60–69 (33%).

Due to recent criticisms of RCTs of breast screening, which suggested that the overall mortality may be higher in those screened due to adverse effects of treatment, this study also looked at total cause mortality. This showed a relative risk of dying of any cause in the study arm of 0.98, which was of borderline statistical significance[40]. The precise mortality reduction attributable to screening is controversial as RCTs may underestimate the benefit of screening due to nonattendance and contamination (mammography occurring within the control group). A recent paper has suggested that regular attendance for mammographic screening may result in a 63% reduction in breast cancer deaths[41].

Which age groups should be screened?

There is definite evidence from RCTs of screening of a reduction in mortality in women aged 55–69. Previous meta-analyses have supported the introduction of screening at age 50 but these data are based on 10-year age bands. Data analysis based on 5-year age bands of screening women aged 50–55 has never shown a mortality benefit in this age group. The reasons for this are unclear but it has been postulated that this may be due to the unusual behaviour of breast cancer in perimenopausal women.

There is no evidence from RCTs to support the screening of women over the age of 70. However, the number of women over the age of 70 in these studies is low. Although the mammograms of older women are easy to read and the incidence of cancer is high, there would be a significant risk of overdiagnosis in this age group. Overdiagnosis is the detection and treatment of cancers that would not become clinically apparent or threaten life.

Meta-analysis of RCTs screening women aged 40–49 at randomization have shown a statistically significant mortality reduction of 29%[42]. Failure of the most recent meta-analysis in 2002 to show a mortality benefit in this age group may be because of the noninclusion of the Kopparberg arm of the Two Counties study. The Malmo[43] and Gothenburg[44] studies have both shown statistically significant mortality reductions in this age group. As breast cancer is only half as common in women in their forties compared with women in their fifties, some authors have suggested that presenting data in terms of percentage reduction in population mortality may be misleading. On the other hand, preventing breast cancer deaths in younger women will result in a larger number of life years gained and it has been shown that breast cancers arising in women in their forties account for 34% of life years lost to breast cancer.

The RCTs of screening were not designed to look at particular age groups and such subanalysis has been criticised. In particular, a proportion of the screening episodes occurring in women aged 40–49 at randomization actually occurred when women were over the age of 50. In addition, women in the control groups of these studies were not always screened at 50. Therefore, it is possible that part of the mortality benefit demonstrated in these women may be due to screening episodes over the age of 50.

The low cancer incidence in women under the age of 50 results in the specificity of both recall and surgical biopsy being lower than that in older women. It has been said that there is reduced mammographic sensitivity in women in their forties; however, recent data suggest that the use of two views and the high film density substantially improve sensitivity in younger women. The most important hindrance to screening younger women is the short lead-time of screening. The lead-time of screening is that time between mammographic detection and clinical presentation. The presence of this short lead-time indicates the need to screen more frequently in women under the age of 50. The ideal screening interval would be 12 months. The high frequency of screening required in younger women and the low incidence of breast cancer has led some to question the cost-effectiveness of screening in this age group. However, these disadvantages may be partly negated by the large number of life years gained per life saved.

Number of views

Mammographic screening is best performed using two views: MLO and CC. The RCT of screening with one view versus two views at prevalent round (first round) showed an increased cancer detection of 24% and a 15% lower recall rate using two views[45]. The cost per cancer detected was similar using one view or two views. Two-view screening resulted in a 54% increase in invasive cancer detection less than 10 mm in size[46]. Initial data suggest that introduction of two views at every screen has resulted in an increase in small invasive cancer detection. There is no evidence that adding physical examination at screening episodes is associated with an improvement in breast cancer mortality reduction.

Who should interpret mammographic images?

In the UK, interpretation of screening mammograms is limited to practitioners who read a high volume of images (greater than 5000 examinations per year) and it is recommended that film readers also participate in screening assessment. These recommendations are based on a number of studies that suggest the total number of mammograms read and access to regular feedback are the most important factors relating to radiologists' performance[47]. A recent study using a difficult test set (PERFORMS 2) indicated that high volume readers had a significantly increased sensitivity for detection of breast cancer compared to medium and low volume readers[48]. In the UK, there has been a national shortage of radiologists, and in particular breast screening radiologists. This had led to the introduction of radiographer film readers. Radiographers have been shown to have identical sensitivity and specificity when compared with screening radiologists once they have been trained.

How should the images be interpreted?

In independent double reading, if one of the readers requests recall, the patient is recalled without discussion. In consensus double reading, cases with disparate opinions are discussed by the two film readers and a consensus achieved. When arbitration is used, a third reader decides on whether a film recalled by one reader but not by another, necessitates patient recall. Recent data from the UK screening programme have shown that double reading with arbitration results in the best small invasive cancer detection rate and at an acceptable recall rate[49].

The screening process and assessment

Screening mammograms are carried out by female radiographers, either at static sites or using mobile vans. Attendance is best when using timed appointments, which can be changed by telephone. Approximately 5% of women are called back for assessment and such assessments are carried out by a multidisciplinary team at a static site. Breast screening assessment involves a combination of extra mammographic views, ultrasound and physical examination. Figure 52.30 is a flow diagram of the assessment process Approximately one in seven of those recalled have breast cancer. Four out of five operations provoked by screening are treatment operations for breast cancer.

Screening intervals

The interval at which a screening mammogram needs to be repeated is related to the lead-time of screening. In breast cancer the lead-time of mammographic screening is age related.

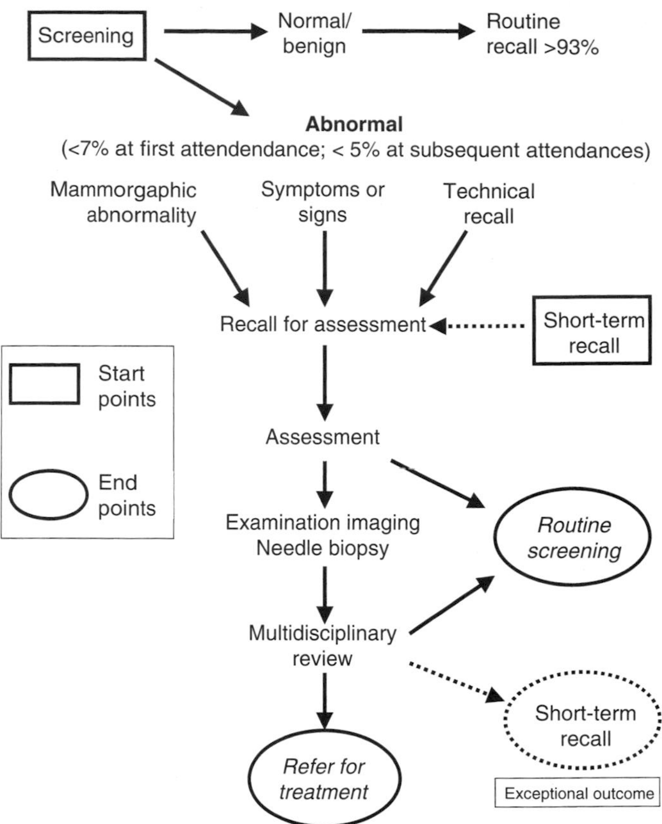

Figure 52.30 The screening assessment process. 'Start' points are enclosed in rectangles, 'end' points in ovals.

The lead-time of screening in women under the age of 50 in the Gothenburg screening trial was 2.2 years. This suggested the ideal screening interval for women under the age of 50 is either every 18 months or 12 months. The lead-time of screening for women over the age of 50 is 3–4 years. A 3-year screening interval may be appropriate. However, the UK screening programme is the only one not to use a 2-year screening interval in women over the age of 50. As there is a high rate of interval cancers in the third year after screening in the UK programme[50], shortening the screening interval in women over the age of 50 to 2 years may be beneficial.

Interval cancers

These are cancers that arise symptomatically in women who have had a normal screening mammogram before their next invitation to screening. Interval cancer analysis helps assess the effectiveness of a screening programme and enables radiologists to learn by reviewing the screening mammograms of women who later present with symptomatic cancers. Interval cancers have a prognosis similar to symptomatic cancers in the nonscreening population, which is worse than that of cancers detected at screening.

Interval cancers in the NHSBSP are now divided into three subtypes:

- Type 1 interval cancers are cancers where the previous screening mammograms show no evidence of malignancy, even in retrospect.
- Type 2 interval cancers are cancers where the previous screening mammograms show uncertain features when viewed retrospectively.
- Type 3 interval cancers are interval cancers where there are malignant features on the screening mammogram.

The mammographic features most frequently missed or misinterpreted on screening mammograms are calcification and architectural distortion[51].

How does mammographic screening reduce breast cancer mortality?

Most of the benefit of mammographic screening is due to detection of small lymph node-negative invasive cancers. Finding high-grade invasive breast cancer less than 10 mm in size is particularly useful as the prognosis of such tumours is excellent[52], whereas grade 3 invasive breast cancers presenting symptomatically have a very poor prognosis. However, some of the low-grade tubular cancers detected at screening are so indolent that a number of these lesions may never threaten life and mammographic screening in these instances may lead to overdiagnosis and overtreatment[53].

Approximately 25% of cancers detected by mammographic screening are DCIS. The merit of DCIS detection at screening is controversial. Low-grade DCIS follows an indolent course, with approximately 40% of cases eventually developing low-grade invasive breast cancer. High-grade DCIS is accepted by most authorities to be a precursor of high-grade invasive disease. The majority of DCIS detected at screening are high grade and their detection is beneficial[54].

Quality assurance (QA)

Screening mammography must utilize exemplary technique and be interpreted by highly trained film readers. This requires rigorous quality control measures and a nationally coordinated QA programme.

In the UK, local performance is monitored by regional QA teams and the data are collected centrally by the Department of Health. This is a statutory requirement and the teams are responsible for screening-unit performance monitoring and for individual performance appraisal. Some of the recent national performance figures are shown in Table 52.1. The standardized detection ratio is the actual number of cancers detected expressed as a ratio of the predicted number of cancers that need be detected to achieve a mortality reduction of 25%.

Mammography readers in the UK have a sophisticated system of personal performance assessment known as PERFORMS (performance of radiologists in mammographic screening), organized and run by an independent team. This is regarded as an educational exercise and participation is voluntary, but recommended by the Royal College of Radiologists. Each NHSBSP film reader is invited to take part annually. A test set of 120 two-view digitized copy screening mammograms, containing a mixture of normal and abnormal cases, is interpreted by the reader. The case mix is carefully selected to ensure that the cases reflect the types of subtle changes normally encountered in routine screening practice. The results

Table 52.1 UK NATIONAL HEALTH SERVICE BREAST SCREENING PROGRAMME PERFORMANCE 2001–2003

	2001/2002	2002/2003
Number of women invited	1 732 526	1 873 470
Acceptance rate (% of invited)	75.5%	74.7%
Number of women screened (invited)	1 323 968	1 400 039
Number of women screened (self referred)	137 549	123 752
Total number of women screened	1 461 517	1 541 794
Number of women recalled for assessment	77 911	79 441
Women recalled for assessment (%)	5.3%	5.2%
Number of benign biopsies	1930	1843
Number of cancers detected	10 003	10 467
Cancer detected per 1000 women screened	6.8	7.5
Number of in situ cancers detected	2132	2375
Number of invasive cancers less than 15mm	4159	4877
Standardized detection ratio	**1.22**	**1.32**

Source: NHSBSP Annual Review 2004, NHSBSP Publications, Sheffield.

are entered on to a hand-held computer and, when the task is complete, the radiologist is provided with instant feedback on performance, thus permitting immediate review of any abnormal cases the radiologist may have failed to detect or may have misclassified. Results are expressed as receiver operating characteristic (ROC) curves and include details of the types of error so that the individual can identify specific areas of weakness in detection or classification. The results are kept confidential to the individual radiologist but all participants are issued with the anonymous results of their peers to allow them to compare their performance.

Interventional breast radiology

Breast radiology requires skills in interventional techniques, particularly ultrasound and X-ray stereotactic-guided needle sampling, percutaneous excision of benign lesions and localization of abnormalities for surgical excision[54]. Eighty per cent of abnormalities detected by screening mammography are impalpable and need to be sampled using image-guided techniques. If surgery is then required, image-guided localization should be carried out. In symptomatic practice, image-guided biopsy is increasingly being used for palpable abnormalities.

Rationale for triple assessment

Needle biopsy is highly accurate in determining the nature of most breast lesions and is now used in place of open surgical biopsy. The routine use of needle biopsy in patients with benign conditions helps to avoid unnecessary surgery. In patients with breast cancer, needle biopsy provides accurate information on the nature of malignant disease, such as histological type and grade, and allows assessment of tumour biology, cell markers and genetics[54].

The methods available for breast tissue diagnosis are:

- fine needle aspiration for cytology (FNAC)
- needle core biopsy for histology (NCB)
- vacuum-assisted mammotomy (VAM)
- large core needle biopsy
- open surgical biopsy.

Fine needle aspiration for cytology and needle core biopsy

FNAC involves the manual passage of a small bore needle (usually 23 gauge) repeatedly through an abnormality to sheer off clumps of cells into the needle lumen. This is usually performed while applying suction to the aspiration needle. The aspirate is then either smeared onto a microscope slide or washed into a buffer solution ready for cytological assessment. FNAC can be performed freehand on a palpable abnormality or carried out under ultrasound or X-ray stereotactic guidance. The procedure is quick to perform and associated with minimal morbidity. However, it is associated with significant false-positive and false-negative results, is operator dependent and relies greatly on the experience and skill of the cytopathologist. For these reasons core needle biopsy is usually preferred for breast diagnosis[55,56].

Core biopsy of breast tissue is best carried out using a 14 gauge diameter needle with a 20 mm sample notch attached to an automated spring-loaded device. Smaller gauge needles give less reliable results. The needle retrieves a core of tissue, approximately 15–20 mg in weight, which is suitable for histological assessment. This technique is less operator dependent than FNAC and breast tissue histological expertise is much more widely available. Core needle biopsy is associated with fewer false-positive and false-negative results than FNAC and is the technique of choice for routine use in breast diagnosis.

The better overall performance of core biopsy compared to FNAC is illustrated in the performance of the NHS Breast Screening Programme in the UK. At the start of the programme, needle sampling by FNAC was almost universal but fewer than 10% of the 90 screening units were able to achieve the target of 70% preoperative diagnosis of breast cancer. After transferring to core biopsy, all of these units now routinely achieve greater than 90% preoperative diagnosis of breast cancer[57].

Other needle biopsy techniques

The predominant reasons for failure to achieve accurate diagnosis by needle biopsy are sampling error and failure to retrieve sufficient representative material. These problems have been largely addressed by the development of larger directional core biopsy techniques that provide much larger volumes of tissue. Some involve very large diameter core needles that remove a single tissue sample up to 20 mm in diameter. More widely used are 11 to 8 gauge vacuum-assisted needle systems that can provide multiple cores, each weighing up to 300 mg. These techniques are known as vacuum-assisted mammotomy (VAM). Some systems enable multiple cores to be retrieved without removing the needle from the breast, while others require the needle to be removed to retrieve each specimen. The former is preferred when wider sampling or removal of the entire abnormality is required.

VAM significantly improves the diagnostic accuracy for borderline breast lesions and lesions at sites in the breast difficult to biopsy using other techniques. VAM understages both in situ and invasive cancer approximately half as often as conventional core biopsy (typically 10% compared to 20%). The indications for VAM are[58]:

- very small mass lesions
- architectural distortions
- failed 'conventional' core biopsy
- microcalcifications
- papillary- and mucocele-like lesions
- diffuse nonspecific abnormality
- excision of benign lesions
- sentinel node sampling.

Core biopsy and VAM are the techniques of choice for sampling calcifications and mammographic architectural distortions. If calcification is not demonstrated on the specimens' radiograph and the histology is benign, then management cannot be based on this result as there is a high risk of sampling error; the procedure must either be repeated or an open surgical biopsy carried out.

VAM can be used for either ultrasound or X-ray stereotactic-guided biopsy. After placement in the breast, suction is applied through a double lumen needle using one lumen to aspirate the tissue into a sampling chamber while a rotating inner cannula in the second lumen is advanced to cut the specimen into the chamber. Suction is then used to retrieve the specimen from the breast while the probe stays in place, ready to obtain the next sample. Contiguous core biopsies can be obtained by rotating the probe through 360°. Unlike core biopsy, the VAM probe does not have to pass directly through the area being sampled as the suction can be used to draw the abnormality into the sampling chamber, allowing a satisfactory sample to be obtained by placing the probe close to rather than through the abnormality. The VAM technique is also preferred for biopsy of abnormalities at sites that are difficult to reach using FNA or core biopsy, such as close to the chest wall or behind the nipple. Ultrasound-guided hand-held mammotomy can be used as an alternative to surgery to completely excise benign lesions, such as fibroadenomas, and to widely sample lesions that may be associated with an increased risk of malignancy, such as radial scars and papillary lesions.

Guidance methods for breast needle biopsy

Ultrasound guidance is the method of choice for biopsy of both palpable and impalpable breast lesions, as it provides real-time visualization of the biopsy procedure and visual confirmation of adequate sampling. Between 80 and 90% of breast abnormalities that need to be biopsied are visible on ultrasound. For impalpable abnormalities not visible on ultrasound, stereotactic X-ray-guided biopsy is required. A few lesions are visible only on MRI and require MR-guided biopsy.

X-ray-guided stereotactic biopsy is used for impalpable lesions that are not visible on ultrasound. The majority of microcalcifications and mammographic architectural deformities need to be biopsied under X-ray guidance. There are two types of stereotactic equipment: add-on devices that attach to a conventional upright mammography machine and dedicated prone table devices (Fig. 52.31). Both types use a digital image receptor that permits rapid image acquisition to check needle positions while sampling. Prone table devices are expensive

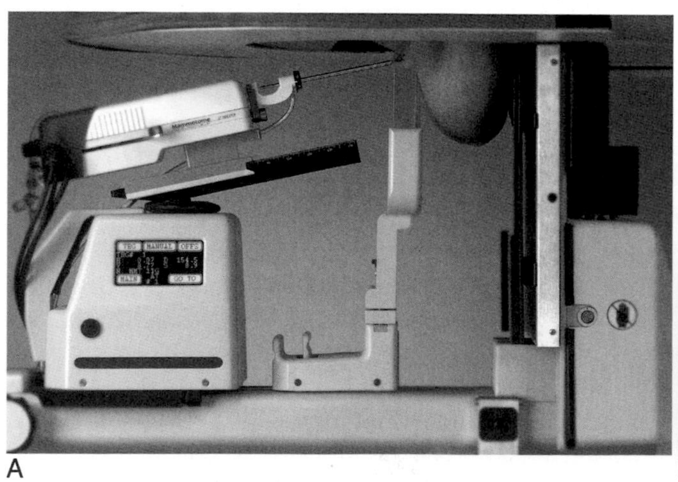
A

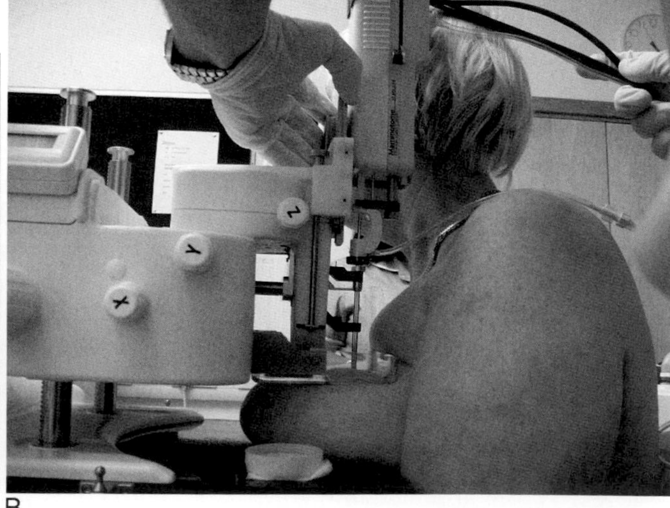

B

Figure 52.31 Breast biopsy table. (A) A prone stereotactic X-ray breast biopsy table. (B) An upright add-on breast biopsy table showing vacuum-assisted mammotomy being performed with vertical positioning of the biopsy probe.

and can only be used for breast biopsy; they require a room in the breast imaging department dedicated for this purpose. The main advantage of this type of device is that the patient cannot see the biopsy procedure while it is being done and vasovagal episodes are said to be less frequent. However, add-on devices can be attached to a mammography machine that is otherwise available for routine mammography. These are less expensive and do not require dedicated space. The two methods have equally high levels of accuracy (95% retrieval of representative material) and both are associated with low levels of morbidity and few complications. Vasovagal episodes can be minimized by giving the patient an anxiolytic agent such as sublingual lorazepam 30 min before the procedure. Upright add-on systems can also be used with the patient lying in the lateral decubitus position.

Both the add-on and prone table stereotactic devices allow precise localization of the position of the lesion by acquiring two images, 15° on either side of the central axis of the X-ray gantry. The x, y and z coordinates of the lesion are calculated from the relative positions of the target lesion on the two stereotactic images compared to a fixed reference point. These coordinates are calculated with an accuracy of less than 1 mm and the system is programmed to site the biopsy needle at the correct depth and angle to ensure that that target area is sampled. After injection of local anaesthetic, the biopsy needle is advanced into the breast via a small skin incision through a needle holder that guides it to the correct depth. Images are taken before sampling to ensure that the needle is correctly sited. Adjustments to the coordinates can be made at this stage, if necessary. Images can also be taken after the biopsy to show that the correct area has been sampled. For microcalcifications, core specimen radiography should always be performed to prove that representative material has been obtained (Fig. 52.32). If it is possible that the whole of the mammographic abnormality may have been removed by the biopsy procedure, a marker should be placed at the biopsy site to identify this site for possible further procedures or localization during surgery. A variety of metal clip and gel pellet markers are available for this purpose; combined gel and metal markers are ideal as these allow subsequent procedures to be carried out under ultrasound rather than stereotactic guidance (Fig. 52.33). Core biopsy and VAM under local anaesthesia are the preferred methods for use under stereotactic guidance. FNAC is not recommended for most stereotactic biopsies because the lesions that require this method of guidance require larger volumes of tissue to be harvested to achieve the required sensitivity and positive predictive value.

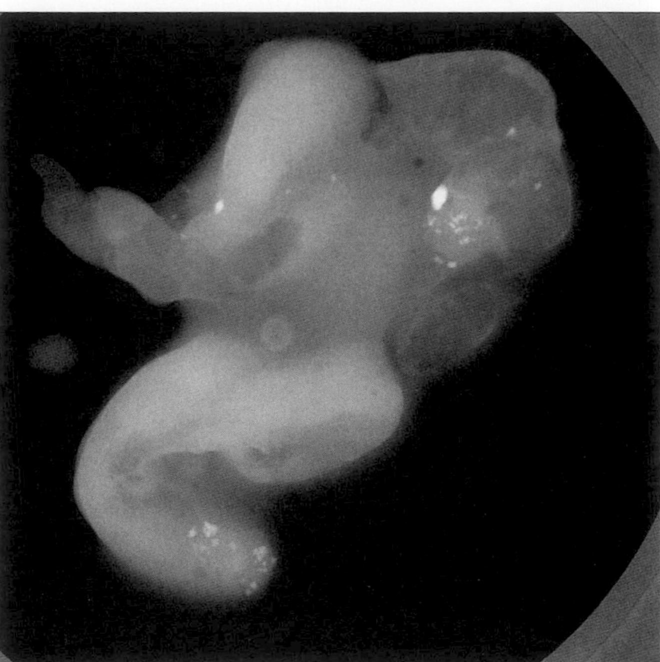

Figure 52.32 Core specimen radiography. A specimen radiograph showing a good yield of microcalcifications in several vacuum-assisted mammotomy biopsy cores.

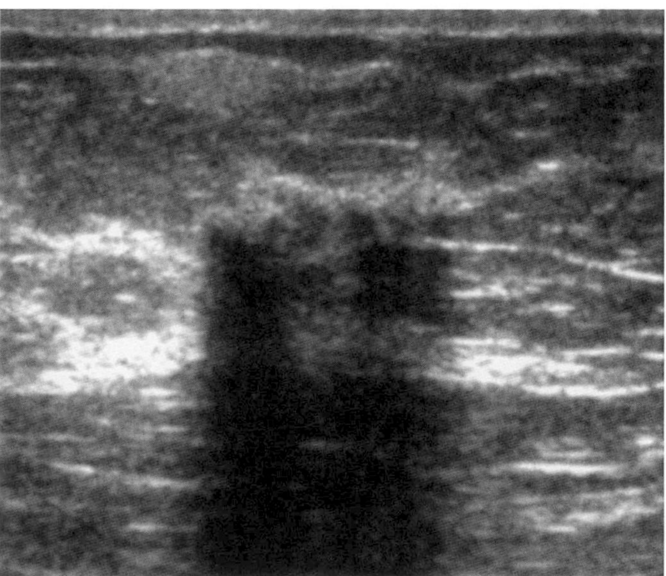

Figure 52.33 An ultrasound image of breast tissue containing gel pellets placed at the site of a stereotactic biopsy showing how the mass effect with distal shadowing allows the biopsy site to be easily identified on ultrasound.

Number of samples

Sufficient material must be obtained but it is unnecessary to cut multiple cores as a matter of routine. For ultrasound-guided biopsy where there is a suspicion of carcinoma, a minimum of two core specimens is recommended.

As stereotactic biopsy is used for abnormalities that are difficult to define on ultrasound and are therefore more difficult to sample, a minimum of five core specimens should be obtained. Ensuring that calcification is present in at least three separate cores and/or five separate flecks of calcification are retrieved from the area of suspicion will allow an accurate diagnosis to be made (Fig. 52.32)[59].

When diagnostic uncertainty remains, larger gauge (8 g) VAM can be used to obtain greater tissue volumes (approximately 300 mg per core). The larger mammotomy probe is also preferred for therapeutic removal of breast lesions such as fibroadenomas.

MR-guided biopsy

A few breast lesions are only visible on MR and therefore have to be localized and biopsied under MR guidance. A number of different approaches have been developed for this procedure using both closed and open magnets. FNA, core biopsy and VAM may all be used for MR-guided sampling.

Managing the result of needle biopsy

It is important that the result of needle breast biopsy is correlated with the imaging and clinical findings before clinical management is discussed with the patient. This is best achieved by reviewing each case at a multidisciplinary meeting at which the imaging, clinical and pathological findings are reviewed and management decisions and choices to be offered are discussed and agreed before the patient is seen to be given the results.

Preoperative localization of impalpable lesions

The purpose of preoperative needle localization is to ensure that impalpable lesions are accurately identified for the surgeon to remove completely with the required amount of surrounding tissue. Without localization, it is often necessary to remove much larger volumes of tissue than would otherwise be required, with the potential to cause unnecessary deformity of the breast. This is particularly undesirable where the lesion proves to be benign. In addition, accurate localization ensures that the surgeon can remove impalpable malignant lesions with the required amount of surrounding tissue to ensure complete excision; the usual aim is to remove a minimum of 5 mm (and preferably 10 mm) of surrounding normal breast tissue at all margins. Specimen radiography is used to confirm that the lesion has been removed and that adequate excision margins have been achieved. The specimen is orientated using radio-opaque markers to identify the margins and, where excision appears inadequate, further margin excision can be carried out at the same operation (Fig. 52.34).

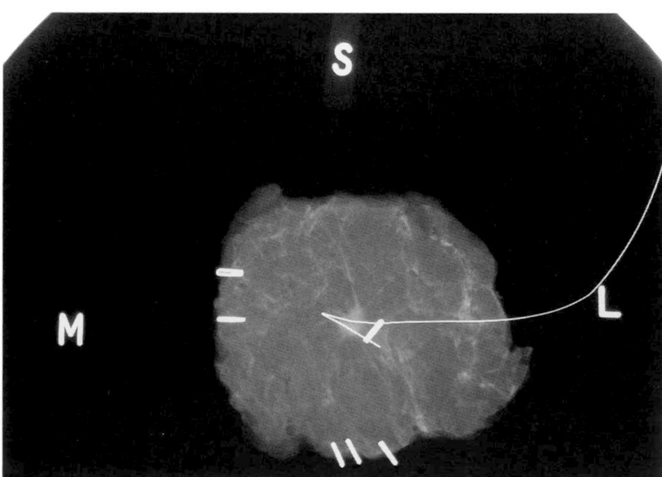

Figure 52.34 A specimen radiograph of a marker localization surgical biopsy showing the hook wire through the small mass lesion. The specimen is orientated by surgical clips showing the superior (S), lateral (L), and medial (M) margins. The radiograph shows clear margins of excision in these directions.

There are a number of methods in routine use for the localization of impalpable breast lesions for surgical removal. These include simple skin marking over the lesion, insertion of a wire, or injection of carbon dye or radioisotope-labelled colloid. The method used should be agreed in advance with the surgeon performing the operation. Localization is normally carried out on the same day as the surgery. Once the localization has been performed, the nature and accuracy of the procedure should be formally recorded and the details communicated to the surgeon. The imaging method of choice for identifying and localizing lesions is ultrasound. X-ray-guided localization is usually restricted to lesions that are not visible on ultrasound. Marking the biopsy site of lesions that initially require needle biopsy under X-ray stereotactic guidance with gel pellets allows subsequent localization for surgery to be done under ultrasound guidance (Fig. 52.33).

The techniques and skills required for image-guided localization are similar to those needed for image-guided biopsy. For superficial lesions the simplest method is to mark the skin directly over the lesion with an indelible marker pen and record the depth of the lesion from the skin surface. The majority of lesions are deeper in the breast and require the use of one or more internal markers, usually a flexible wire incorporating a retaining hook. Wires that allow the surgeon to localize the lesion without the need to follow the wire to the lesion are preferred as they allow the surgeon to choose the site of the skin incision that will provide the best cosmetic result.

The ideal wire is easy to insert, clearly visible on ultrasound and mammography, flexible enough to allow for check mammography after insertion and stable once sited to allow the lesion to be accurately identified by the surgeon. Several types of hook wire systems are available. All use an introducing needle through which the wire is advanced into the breast. For mass lesions and small clusters of microcalcification, the wire should be placed directly through the lesion or area, with the tip of the wire just beyond it. For an area of clustered calcifications, several wires may be used to 'bracket' the area to be removed by the surgeon. Check mammograms should be performed to confirm that the correct area has been localized; these should be available for the surgeon during the surgical procedure.

Impalpable lesions can be localized using radio-labelled high molecular weight colloid. This technique is known as radio-opaque lesion localization (ROLL). ^{99m}Tc-labelled colloid is injected under image guidance into the immediate vicinity of the tumour and the surgeon then localizes the lesion using a fine-tipped gamma probe. The colloid must be large enough not to diffuse away from the injection site; the type of colloid used for lung scintigraphy is ideal. A small amount of non-ionic contrast medium is mixed with the colloid so that the accuracy of the localization can be assessed, with mammography performed immediately afterwards. ROLL can be combined with radio-isotope sentinel lymph node biopsy by also injecting low molecular weight colloid that will diffuse into the lymphatic system and accumulate in the sentinel lymph nodes.

Specimen radiography

When microcalcifications are sampled by NCB or VAM, the specimens must be X-rayed to ensure that representative material has been obtained. This can be done with a conventional mammography machine or using a specially designed specimen X-ray cabinet. If there is no calcium in the specimens, further samples should be taken.

All marker localization surgical biopsies and wide local excisions should also undergo specimen radiography at the time of surgery to confirm that the lesion has been removed and that there is an adequate surrounding margin of normal breast tissue. The specimen needs to be orientated with clips or radio-opaque sutures that identify the different margins. The surgeon should be able to assess the radiograph immediately. If the lesion is not visible, or a margin is close to the lesion on this radiograph, the surgeon will usually remove additional tissue. Although calcified lesions are usually visualized radiographically with ease, noncalcified lesions may be more difficult to assess. Previously impalpable breast masses can often be appreciated by the surgeon by palpation in the excised specimen. To ensure the accuracy of histological diagnosis, it may be necessary for the radiologist to localize the lesion in the specimen for the pathologist. This localization should be performed in all cases in which the size of the specimen greatly exceeds the size of the lesion.

After the excised breast tissue is received by the pathology laboratory, it is sectioned and embedded in paraffin blocks, each about 5 mm thick. A single 4–5 mm section is obtained from each block. Even if the calcifications are confirmed on radiographs of the specimen, the pathologist may not examine the correct area in each paraffin block. In such cases, paraffin block radiography may be useful in directing the pathologist to the appropriate area for subsequent histological evaluation.

Calcium oxalate crystals may be seen on specimen radiography but not on histological section stained with haematoxylin and eosin (H&E). Such crystals are birefringent and need to be viewed using polarized light microscopy. Calcium oxalate calcifications are virtually always due to benign disease. By comparison, calcium phosphate calcifications are easily seen on H&E-stained sections. These may represent either benign or malignant disease.

REFERENCES

1. Sickles E A 1988 Practical solutions to common mammographic problems: tailoring the examination. Am J Roentgenol 151: 31–39
2. Feig S A 1988 Importance of supplementary mammographic views to diagnostic accuracy. Am J Roentgenol 151: 40
3. Eklund G W, Busby R C, Miller S H et al 1988 Improving imaging of the augmented breast. Am J Roentgenol 151: 469–473
4. Review of Radiation Risk in Breast Screening 2003 Report by a joint working party of the NHSBSP National Coordinating Group for Physics, Quality Assurance and the National Radiological Protection Board. NHSBSP Publication No 54, Sheffield
5. Hermann K, Obenauer S, Fischer U et al 2002 Significance of additional spot magnification in full-field digital mammography. Radiology 225: 268
6. Obenauer S, Luftner-Nagel S, Von Heyden D et al 2002 Screen film vs full-field digital mammography: image quality, detectability and characterisation of lesions. Eur Radiol 12: 1697–1702
7. Cowen A R, Parkin G J, Hawkridge P 1997 Direct digital mammography image acquisition. Eur Radiol 7: 918–930
8. Venta L A, Hendrick R E, Adler Y T et al 2001 Rates and causes of disagreement in interpretation of full-field digital mammography and film-screen mammography in a diagnostic setting. Am J Roentgenol 176: 1241–1248
9. Lewin J M, D'Orsi C J, Hendrick R E et al 2002 Clinical comparison of full-field digital mammography and screen-film mammography for detection of breast cancer. Am J Roentgenol 179: 671–677
10. Skaane P, Young K, Skjennald A 2003 Population-based mammographic screening: comparison of screen-film and full-field digital mammography with soft-copy reading: Oslo I study. Radiology 229: 877–884
11. Skaane P, Skjennald A 2004 Screen-film mammography versus full-field digital mammography with soft-copy reading: randomised trial in a population-based screening program: the Oslo II study. Radiology 232: 197–204
12. Pisano E D, Gatsonis C, Hendrick E et al 2005 Diagnostic performance of digital versus film mammography for breast-cancer screening. N Engl J Med 353: 1846–1847
13. Castellino R A, Roehrig J, Zhang W 2000 Improved computer-aided detection (CAD) algorithms for screening mammography. Radiology 217: 400
14. Malich A, Marx C, Facius M et al 2001 Tumour detection rate of a new commercially available computer-aided detection system. Euro Radiol 11: 2454–2459
15. Freer T W, Ulissey M J 2001 Screening mammography with computer-aided detection: prospective study of 12,860 patients in a community breast centre. Radiology 220: 781–786
16. Gur D, Sumkin J H, Rockette H E et al 2004 Changes in breast cancer detection and mammography recall rates after the introduction of a computer-aided detection system. J Natl Cancer Inst 3: 185–190
17. Stavros A T, Thickman D, Rapp C L et al 1995 Solid breast nodules: use of sonography to distinguish between benign and malignant lesions. Radiology 196: 123–134
18. Elston C W, Ellis I O 1988 The breast, 3rd edn. Churchill Livingstone, Edinburgh
19. Wolfe J N 1967 A study of breast parenchyma by mammography in the normal woman and those with benign and malignant disease. Radiology 89: 201–205
20. Brisson J, Diorio C, Masse B 2003 Wolfe's parenchymal pattern and percentage of the breast with mammographic densities. Cancer Epidemiol Biomarkers Prev 12: 728–732
21. Ellis I O, Galea M, Broughton N et al 1992 Pathological prognostic factors in breast cancer. II. Histological type. Relationship with survival in a large study with long-term follow-up. Histopathology 20: 479–489
22. Lampejo O T, Barnes D M, Smith P et al 1994 Evaluation of infiltrating ductal carcinomas with a DCIS component: correlation of the histologic type of the in-situ component with the grade of the infiltrating component. Semin Diagn Pathol 11: 215–222
23. Cornford E J, Wilson A R M, Athanassiou E 1995 Mammographic features of invasive lobular and invasive ductal carcinoma of the breast: a comparative analysis. Br J Radiol 68: 450–453
24. Stutz J A, Pinder S, Ellis I O et al 1994 The radiological appearances of invasive cribriform carcinoma of the breast. Clin Radiol 49: 693–695
25. Chopra S, Evans A J, Pinder S E et al 1996 Pure mucinous breast cancer—mammographic and ultrasound findings. Clin Radiol 51: 421–424
26. McCulloch G L, Evans A J, Yeoman L J et al 1997 Radiological features of papillary carcinoma of the breast. Clin Radiol 52: 865–868
27. Damera A, Evans A J, Cornford E J et al 2003 Diagnosis of axillary nodal metastases by ultrasound-guided core biopsy in primary operable breast cancer. Br J Cancer 89: 1310–1313
28. Bagnall M J C, Evans A J, Wilson A R M et al 2001 Predicting invasion in mammographically detected microcalcification. Clin Radiol 56: 828–832

29. Evans A J, Pinder S E, Snead D R J et al 1997 The detection of ductal carcinoma in situ at mammographic screening enables the diagnosis of small, grade 3 invasive tumours. Br J Cancer 75: 542–544
30. Friedman P D, Swaminathan S V, Smith R 2005 Technical innovation: SENSE imaging of the breast. Am J Roentgenol 184: 448–451
31. Kuhl C K, Mielcareck P, Klaschik S et al 1999 Dynamic breast MR imaging: are signal intensity time course data useful for differential diagnosis of an enhancing lesion? Radiology 211: 101–110
32. Kuhl C K, Bieling H B, Gieske J et al 1997 Healthy premenopausal breast parenchyma in dynamic contrast enhanced MR imaging of the breast: normal contrast medium enhancement and cyclical phase dependency. Radiology 203: 137–144
33. Morakkabati N, Leutner C C, Schmiedel A et al 2003 Breast MR imaging during or seen after radiation therapy. Radiology 229: 893–901
34. Fischer U, Kopka L, Grabbe E 1999 Breast carcinoma: effect of preoperative contrast-enhanced MR imaging on the therapeutic approach. Radiology 213: 881–888
35. Weinstein S P, Orel S G, Heller R et al 2001 MR imaging of the breast in patients with invasive lobular carcinoma. Am J Roentgenol 176: 399–406
36. MARIBS Study Group 2005 Screening with magnetic resonance imaging and mammography of a UK population at high familial risk of breast cancer: a prospective multicentre cohort study (MARIBS). Lancet 365: 1769–1778
37. Kriege M, Brekelmans C T M, Boetes C et al 2004 Efficacy of MRI and mammography for breast-cancer screening in women with a familial or genetic predisposition. N Engl J Med 351: 427–437
38. Middleton M S 1998 Magnetic resonance evaluation of breast implants and soft-tissue silicon. Top Magn Reson Imaging 9: 92–137
39. Forrest APM (Chairman): Working Group on Breast Cancer Screening 1986 Report to the Health Ministers of England, Wales, Scotland and Northern Ireland. HMSO, London
40. Nystrom L, Andersson I, Bjurstam N et al 2002 Long-term effects of mammographic screening: update overview of the Swedish randomised trials. Lancet 359: 909–919
41. Tabar L, Vitak B, Tony H H et al 2001 Beyond randomised controlled trials: organised mammographic screening substantially reduces breast carcinoma mortality. Cancer 91: 1724–1731
42. Hendrick R E, Smith R A, Rutledge J H et al 1997 Benefit of screening mammography in women aged 40–49: a new meta-analysis of randomized controlled trials. J Natl Cancer Inst Monogr 22: 87–92
43. Andersson I, Janzon L 1997 Reduced breast cancer mortality in women under age 50: updated results from the Malmo mammographic screening program. J Natl Cancer Inst Monogr 22: 63–68
44. Bjurstam N, Bjorneld L, Duffy S W et al 1997 The Gothenburg Breast Screening Trial. First results on mortality, incidence and mode of detection for women ages 39–49 years at randomisation. Cancer 80: 2091–2099
45. Wald N, Murphy P, Major P et al 1995 UKCCCR multicentre randomised controlled trial of one and two view mammography in breast cancer screening. Br Med J 311: 1189–1193
46. Blanks R G, Moss S M, Wallis M G 1997 Use of two-view mammography compared with one view in the detection of small invasive cancers: further results from the National Health Service breast screening programme. J Med Screen 4: 98–101
47. Elmore J G, Wells C K, Howard D H 1998 Does diagnostic accuracy in mammography depend on radiologists' experience? J Women's Health 7: 443–449
48. Esserman L, Cowley H, Eberle C et al 2002 Improving the accuracy of mammography: volume and outcome relationships. J Natl Cancer Inst 94: 369–375
49. Blanks R G Wallis M G, Moss S M 1998 A comparison of cancer detection rates achieved by breast cancer screening programmes by number of readers, for one and two view mammography: results from the National Health Service breast screening programme. J Med Screen 5: 195–201
50. Day N, McCann J, Camilleri-Ferrante C et al 1995 Monitoring interval cancers in breast screening programmes: the East Anglian experience. J Med Screen 2: 180–185
51. Burrell H, Sibbering D, Wilson A et al 1996 The mammographic features of interval cancers and prognosis compared with screen detected symptomatic breast cancers. Radiology 199: 811–817
52. Tabar L, Duffy S W, Vitak B, Chen H-H, Prevost T C 1999 The natural history of breast cancer: what have we learned from screening? Cancer 86: 449–462
53. Evans A J, Pinder S E, Burrell H C et al 2001 Detecting which invasive cancers at mammographic screening saves lives? J Med Screen 8: 86–90
54. Teh W, Evans A J, Wilson A R M 1998 Editorial. Definitive non-surgical breast diagnosis: the role of the radiologist. Clin Radiol 53: 81–84
55. Britton P D 1999 Fine needle aspiration or core biopsy. The Breast 8: 1–4
56. Britton P D, McCann J 1999 Needle biopsy in the NHS breast screening programme 1996/7: how much and how accurate? The Breast 8: 5–11
57. NHSBSP Annual Report 2004 www.cancerscreening.nhs.uk/breastscreen/publications/2004review.html
58. Guidelines for Breast Screening Assessment 2005 NHSBSP Publication No 49. www.cancerscreening.nhs.uk/breastscreen/publications/nhsbsp49.html
59. Bagnall M J C, Evans A J, Wilson A R M, Burrell H C, Pinder S E, Ellis I O 2000 When have mammographic calcifications been adequately sampled at needle core biopsy? Clin Radiol 55: 548–553

CHAPTER 53

Imaging in Obstetrics and Infertility

Laura Fender and Peter Twining

INFERTILITY

Infertility affects 14 per cent of European couples and is defined as a failure to conceive after 2 years of unprotected, regular sexual intercourse. It is estimated that 84 per cent of women conceive within 1 year of unprotected intercourse and 92 per cent after 2 years[1]. The investigation of infertility is usually commenced after 1 year but may be expedited in couples aged over 35 years or those with established predisposing conditions.

The role of imaging is two-fold. Firstly in the investigation of infertility and then in the subsequent management of patients undergoing stimulated ovulation or assisted reproduction techniques.

NORMAL CYCLE MENSTRUAL CYCLE

In order to interpret the ultrasound (US) appearances that occur with ovarian stimulation it is important to have an understanding of the physiological changes that occur to both the ovary and endometrium during a physiological menstrual cycle.

CAUSES OF INFERTILITY

There are a number of common causes of infertility and these are outlined in Table 53.1. In general there are three tests that are recommended in the primary investigation of infertility: (A) mid-luteal phase serum progesterone to assess ovulation, (B) semen analysis and (C) a test to establish tubal patency[2]. The role of routine pelvic US is not established unless there is a history suggestive of pelvic disease or recurrent first or second trimester miscarriage. This said, transvaginal pelvic US enables documentation of uterine and ovarian morphology and the physiological changes that occur through the normal and abnormal menstrual cycle (Fig. 53.1). Physiological cycles can be distinguished from insufficient or abnormal cycles by the size and development of the maturing follicles, coupled with serum oestradiol levels. Maximal follicular size is significantly smaller in insufficient cycles and the corpus luteum is more frequently absent.

Table 53.1 CAUSES OF INFERTILITY[2]

Cause	%
Sperm dysfunction	24%
Failure of ovulation	21%
Tubal damage	14%
Endometriosis	6%
Coital failure	6%
Cervical mucus dysfunction	3%
Unexplained	28%

NB: Data includes co-existing pathology

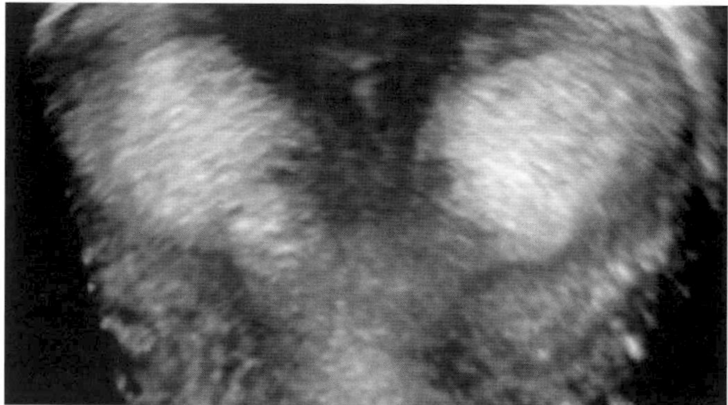

Figure 53.1 Bicornuate uterus. Three-dimensional transvaginal US demonstrating endometrium in a bicornuate uterus.

TUBAL DISEASE

Tubal disease accounts for 14 per cent of infertility and the causes include pelvic inflammatory disease, adhesions due to infection or surgery and endometriosis. Tubal patency can be proven by laparoscopy and dye, hysterosalpingography (HSG) or hysterosalpingo-contrast-sonography (HyCoSy). Laparoscopy is recommended for tubal assessment when there are known co-existing pelvic problems, such as endometriosis or pelvic inflammatory disease[3]. HSG is a reliable indicator of tubal patency, particularly of the proximal tube, and patency is confirmed at laparoscopy in 94 per cent of patients. However it should be noted that tubal occlusions demonstrated by HSG are only confirmed in 34 per cent of cases at laparoscopy[4]. Müllerian duct fusion anomalies (Fig. 53.2) and other abnormalities of the uterine cavity such as adenomyosis (Fig. 53.3) and uterine polyps (Fig. 53.4) can also be delineated. Improved pregnancy rates following HSG are well documented[5].

Tubal patency can also be confirmed by HyCoSy. Transcervical injection of US contrast media or saline and air allows real-time assessment of tubal disease and the pelvic structures. The accuracy is comparable to HSG and involves no ovarian irradiation. In addition endometrial abnormalities can also be demonstrated.

INDUCED CYCLES

Ovulation induction promotes follicle maturation and oocyte release utilizing pharmacological agents. The most commonly used agent is Clomiphene citrate, which increases follicle-stimulating hormone release at the level of the hypothalamus. It is usually given for 5 d during the mid-follicular phase and ovulation occurs 1–10 d following the final dose. Alternative ovulation induction agents include metformin and gonadotrophins.

Transvaginal US is used to track the development of follicles and the endometrial thickness so that the dose of the agent can be titrated and intercourse or insemination can be correctly timed to coincide with ovulation. Although the maturity of the oocyte can only be indirectly inferred from the size of the follicle, the US information can be coupled with oestradiol values to provide an accurate assessment of the presence or absence and number of mature follicles. It is important to look for the complications of ovulation induction such as hyperstimulation. This occurs most commonly in gonadatrophin-induced cycles. The ovary becomes enlarged, sometimes massively so, and oedematous, containing multiple immature follicles. Abdominal ascites may also be demonstrated. The hyperstimulated ovaries are prone to torsion. The signs and symptoms of ovarian hyperstimulation disorder are variable, ranging from mild abdominal discomfort, probably due to the distension of the ovarian capsule, to severe circulatory compromise and electrolyte imbalance. The more severe form, ovarian hyperstimulation syndrome (OHSS), is usually associated with massive stromal oedema of the ovary. The enlarged ovaries may be prone to torsion (Fig. 53.5). On US, patients with OHSS usually have enlarged ovaries (>10 cm) that may contain several hypoechoic areas. The hypoechoic areas may correspond to atretic follicles or to regions of haemorrhage within the ovary. The symptoms associated with OHSS usually begin 5–8 d after hCG is given, but they can be most severe in patients who actually achieve pregnancy. Recent studies have shown that hyperstimulation is unlikely in women whose ovaries contain several large (>15 mm) follicles, and tends to occur when there are several small or intermediate-sized follicles[6]. With supportive therapy, this syndrome usually regresses spontaneously.

ASSISTED REPRODUCTION TECHNOLOGY

The success of in vitro fertilization (IVF) has been due in part to the US identification of follicular maturity and subsequent transvaginal US-guided oocyte recovery techniques.

The principles of IVF involve controlled ovarian hyperstimulation using gonadotrophins. This allows several follicles to develop, as opposed to just one dominant follicle in a natural cycle, allowing for the recruitment of several oocytes.

The first stage of IVF involves the administration of a gonadotrophin-releasing hormone (GnRH) analogue to downregulate the pituitary. Follicular development is then induced through the administration of follicle-stimulating hormone (FSH). The follicles are monitored using TV US until at least three large follicles are present. Ovulation can be triggered once follicular maturity has been demonstrated by human chorionic gonadotrophin. This allows for suitable timing of ovulation so that the oocytes can be aspirated prior to the occurrence of in vivo ovulation.

Follicular aspiration is possible with a needle-guide attachment to the vaginal probe for subsequent IVF or intracytoplasmic sperm injection (ICSI). For these aspiration techniques, a long (30-cm) 18-gauge needle is used, which is scored at the tip, making it easier to visualize under US. Transvaginal sonography (TVS)-guided follicular aspiration

the placenta (Fig. 53.6). It lies within the decidua and therefore lies in an eccentric position within the uterus. It should not be confused with a pseudogestational sac in cases of ectopic pregnancy or fluid within the endometrial cavity, which lie centrally within the endometrial cavity. The gestational sac contains the embryonic disk within a small amniotic sac and the yolk sac. The yolk sac is the first structure to be visualized on TVS within the chorionic sac at 5.5 weeks' menstrual age. The yolk sac is a rounded structure with a central lucency. It should be evident once the gestational sac measures 10 mm. Visualization of the yolk sac precedes that of the embryo and amniotic sac by 3–7 d. Initially the yolk sac occupies much of the chorionic sac, though as the embryo grows it pushes the yolk sac to the side. The yolk sac degenerates at 12 weeks' LMP in normal pregnancies.

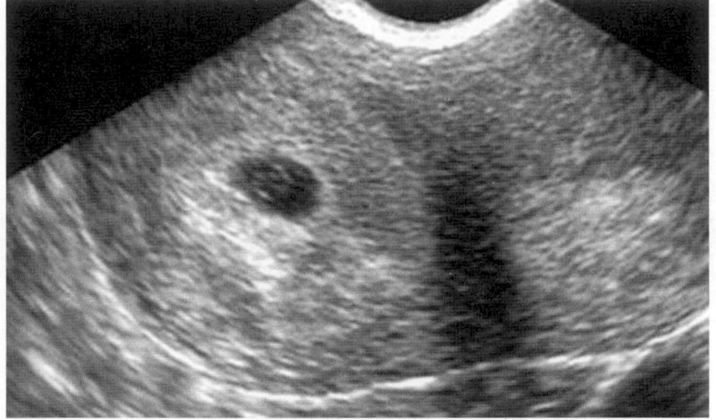

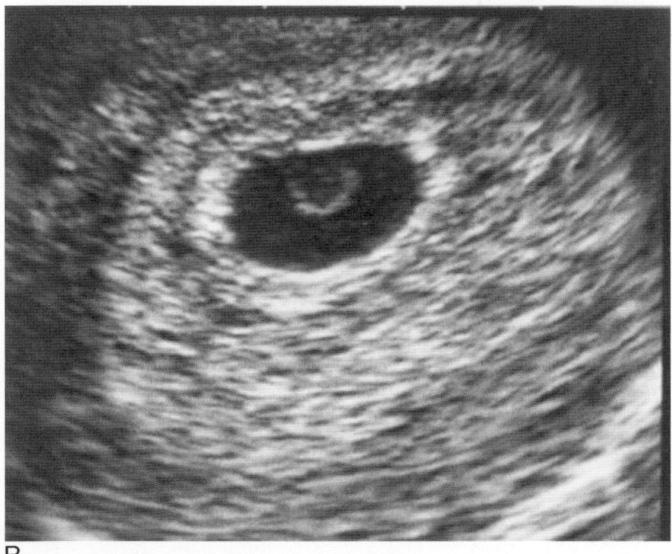

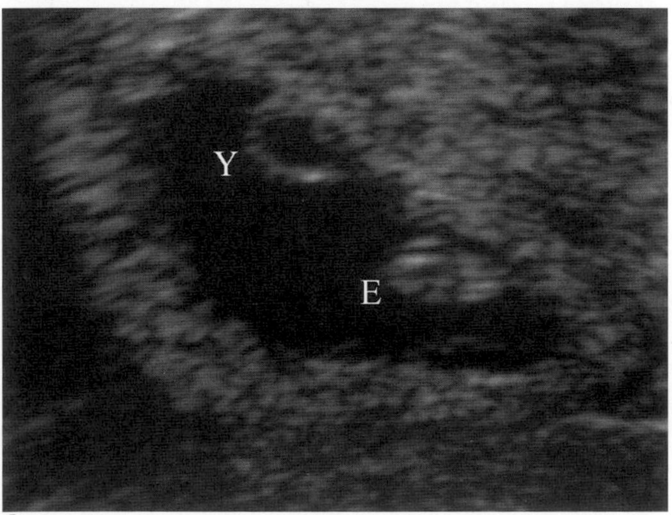

Figure 53.6 TVS of early pregnancy. (A) TVS at 6 weeks' gestation demonstrates a gestational sac and an echogenic ring within the deciduas. (B) A yolk sac is identified by 5.5 weeks' gestation as a circular echogenic ring with a central lucency. (C) Gestation sac containing a yolk sac – Y and embryo – E.

The embryo is first seen on high-resolution images as a thickening on the margin of the yolk sac. With high resolution, the heartbeat is seen as a regular flutter in the embryo, first evident at 5 mm crown to rump length (CRL) (6.2 weeks). Thus it is possible to see viable embryos without heartbeats. In such cases, a follow-up study in 5–7 d will almost always demonstrate the heartbeat in healthy embryos.

On TVS embryos should be seen at mean sac diameters (MSDs) of 18 mm. With lower resolution abdominal US, embryos should be seen with MSDs of 25 mm. The gestational sac size is useful in early pregnancy in the diagnosis of miscarriage and anembryonic pregnancies. It should be measured in three orthogonal planes and the MSD calculated by averaging these measurements.

NONVIABLE PREGNANCY

Miscarriages occur in up to 25 per cent of pregnancies. They may present with vaginal bleeding or be silent. It is important to adhere to strict guidelines when determining the viability of an early pregnancy[12] and to be familiar with the normal first trimester US landmarks.

Hypoechoic areas behind the choriodecidua may be related to retrochorionic haemorrhage. Small haematomas may resolve but larger bleeds are associated with a high rate of pregnancy loss. The gestational sac may appear irregular in outline or appear to be collapsing in a failing pregnancy. A fetal pole should be evident if the mean sac diameter is greater than 20 mm. An anembryonic pregnancy occurs when the embryo fails to form and the gestational sac remains empty with a mean sac diameter greater than 20 mm.

Embryonic demise can be diagnosed if no cardiac activity is evident in a fetal pole measuring more than 6 mm.

If uncertainty remains and the gestational sac measures less than 20 mm or the fetal pole length less than 6 mm, then a repeat examination should be performed after an interval of 7 d.

ECTOPIC PREGNANCY

The incidence of ectopic pregnancy has increased significantly in the past few decades. This is in part due to an increased incidence of pelvic inflammatory disease and assisted reproduction techniques. Based on hospital discharge data, the incidence of ectopic pregnancy has risen from 3.45 cases per 1000 pregnancies between 1966 and 1970 to 15.5 cases per 1000 pregnancies from 1994 to 1996[13].

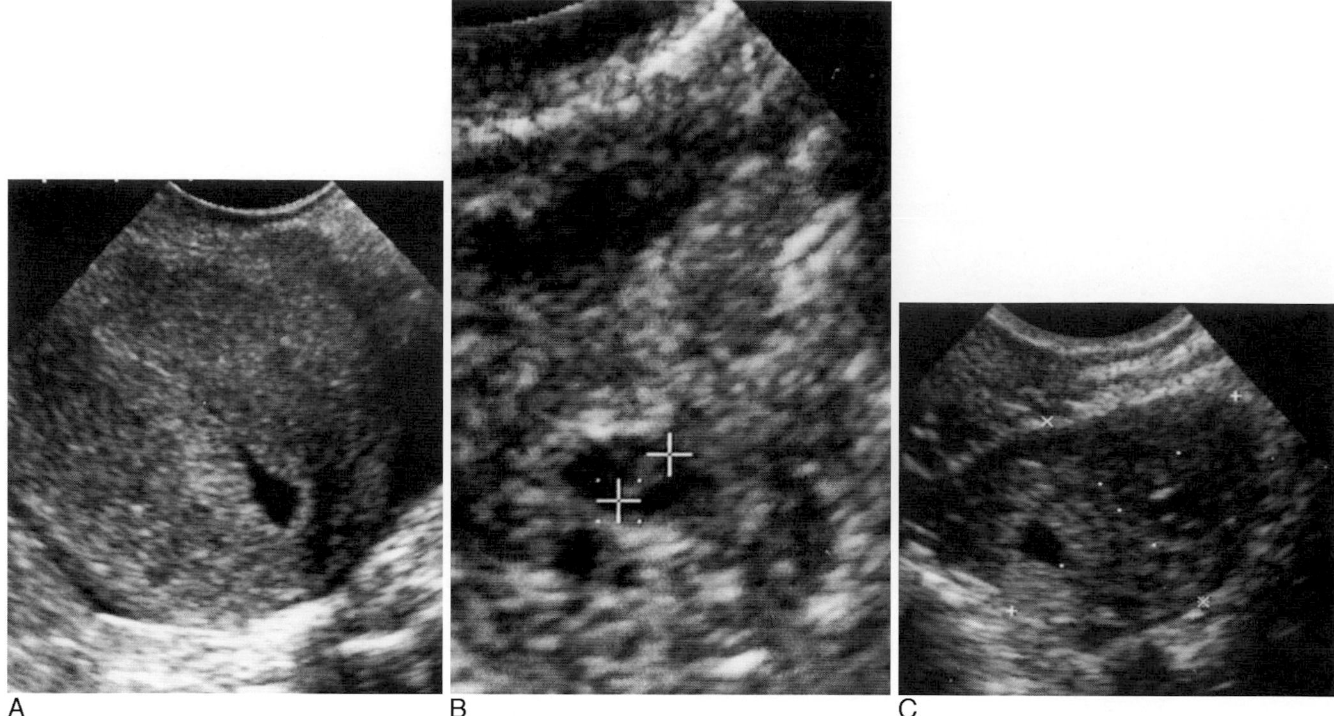

Figure 53.7 TVS of ectopic pregnancy. (A) Uterus containing an intraluminal fluid collection surrounded by a mild decidual reaction. (B) Left adnexa contains an echogenic ring containing a live embryo consistent with an unruptured ectopic pregnancy. (C) Unruptured ectopic pregnancy surrounded by blood within a distended tube.

TVS is the first-line investigation in haemodynamically stable women presenting with suspected ectopic pregnancy and is accurate in up to 90 per cent of cases[14]. Unruptured ectopic pregnancies appear as a complex adenexal mass separate from both the uterus and the ovary in 80 per cent of cases (Fig. 53.7). The mass may contain a yolk sac or evidence of an embryo, which is the only true sign of an ectopic pregnancy. A hyperechoic ring may surround a gestational sac, the doughnut or bagel sign. Following Fallopian tube rupture or tubal abortion, intraperitoneal fluid is present and is visible with the pouch of Douglas on TVS. The uterus should be examined for evidence of an intrauterine pregnancy. In a low-risk patient, with no history of pelvic inflammatory disease (PID) or infertility, the risk of a heterotopic pregnancy is one in 30 000[15], though this can increase up to 7-fold in women with predisposing risk factors[16]. The endometrial cavity may contain fluid and areas of hyperechogenicity, the so-called pseudo sac. This lies centrally within the uterine cavity and not in the usual eccentric position of a normal gestational sac.

An ectopic pregnancy can be suspected if the transvaginal US examination does not detect an intrauterine gestational sac when the β-hCG level is higher than 1000 mIU per mL. This has a positive predictive value of 86 per cent and a sensitivity of 93 per cent[17].

ESTABLISHING GESTATIONAL AGE

It is important to accurately establish the gestational age during pregnancy in order to estimate the date of delivery and to correctly time biochemical screening in the second and third trimesters. The most accurate assessment of gestational age is the crown rump length[18]. This is more accurate than the menstrual history alone or the gestational sac size.

During the second and third trimesters, fetal biometry can provide some assessment of gestational age though there is a greater scatter in distribution. The fetal head circumference, biparietal diameter and abdominal circumference can be correlated with appropriate charts[19,20].

MULTIPLE PREGNANCIES

Of twin pregnancies, 80 per cent are dizygotic. By implication two separate amniotic sacs are present in dizygotic twin pregnancies and the placentas are always dichorionic but may be fused or unfused (Fig. 53.8). The remaining 20 per cent of twin pregnancies are monozygotic twins resulting from the fertilization of one ovum followed by division of the zygote. The chorionicity and the amnionicity of a monozygotic pregnancy depends on the time of division of the zygote (Table 53.2).

The chorionicity can be assessed by US most effectively between 9 and 10 weeks' gestation. A thick membrane is seen to separate diamniotic dichorionic twins and the so-called lambda sign can be seen (Fig. 53.9). A thin membrane is evident between monochorionic diamniotic twins and no membrane at all is present in cases of rarer monoamniotic twinning (Fig. 53.10). It is important to determine the chorionicity of a twin pregnancy as monochorionic twins are associated with an increased risk of fetal malformations, prematurity and twin-to-twin transfusion syndrome.

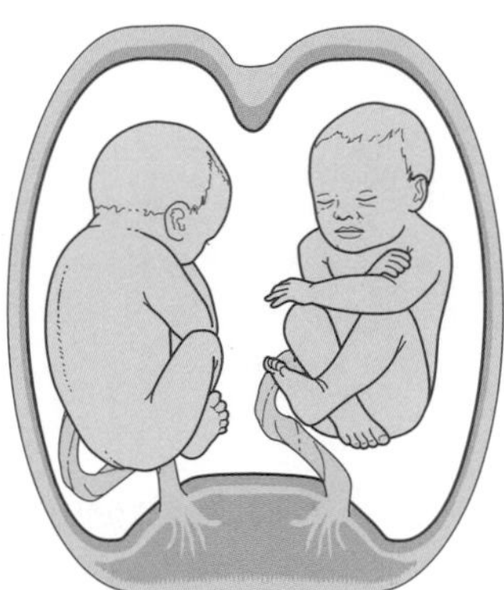

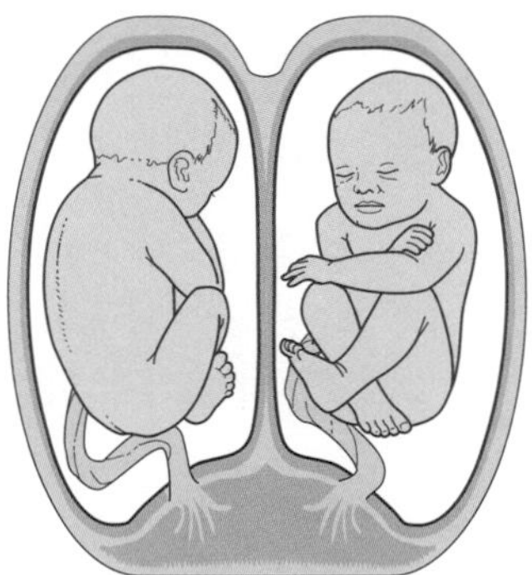

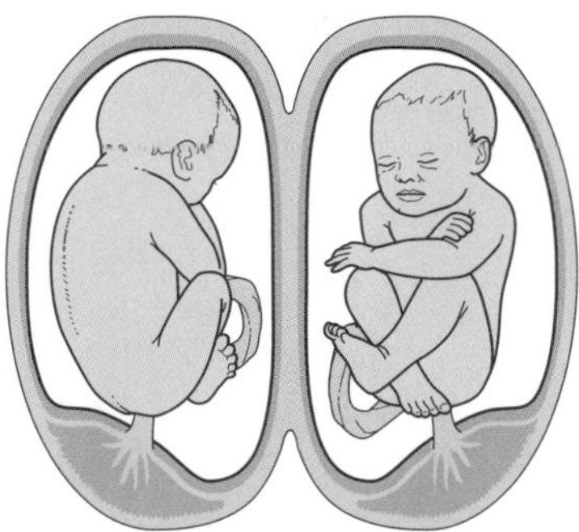

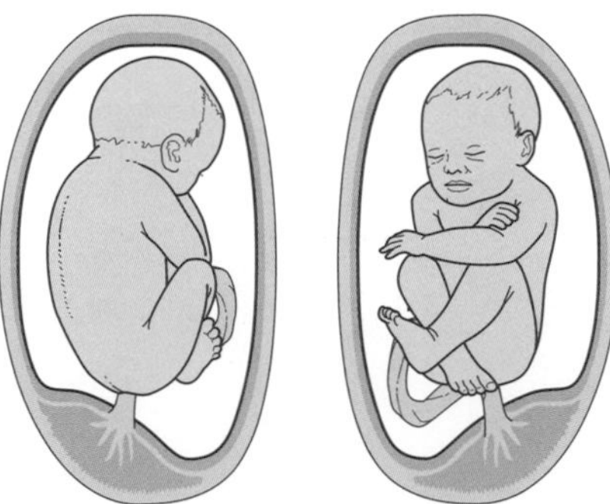

Figure 53.8 Different types of fetal membrane patterns in twinning. (From Twining P, McHugo J M, Pilling D W (eds.) 2006 Textbook of Fetal Abnormalities, 2nd edition, Churchill Livingstone.)

Table 53.2 MONOZYGOTIC TWIN TYPES

Time of division	Type of twinning
<4 d	Dichorionic diamniotic
4–8 d	Monochorionic diamniotic
8–13 d	Monochorionic monoamniotic
>13 d	Conjoined twins

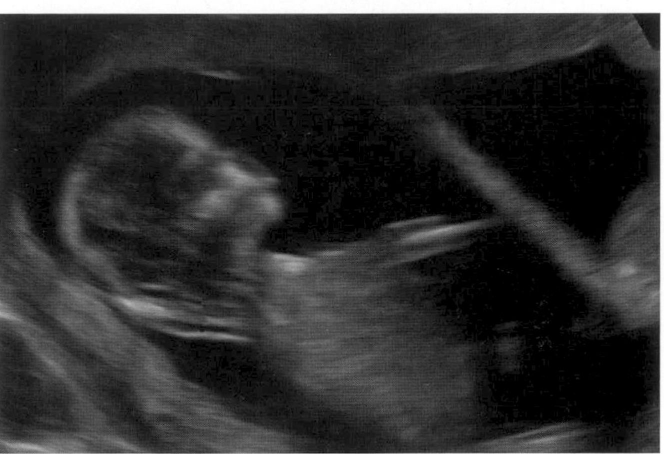
A

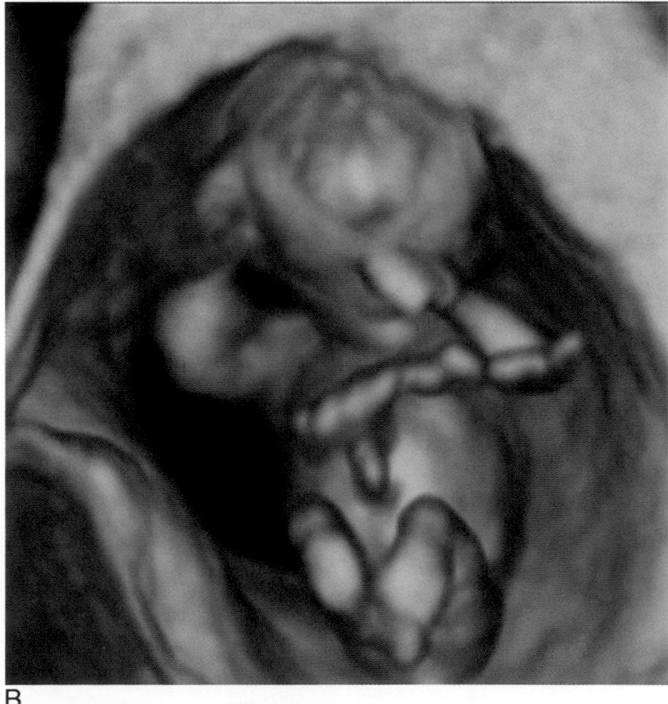
B

Figure 53.9 Dichorionic diamniotic twin pregnancy. (A) A thick membrane separates the two gestation sacs, known as the lambda sign. (B) 3D US demonstration of the lambda sign.

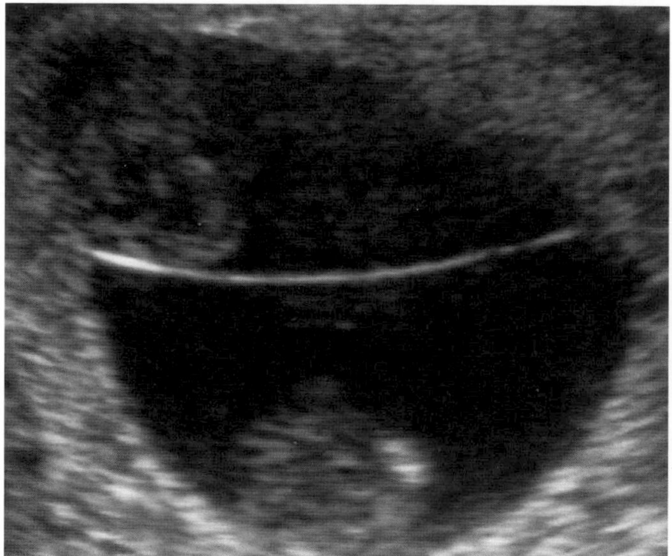

Figure 53.10 Monochorionic diamniotic twin pregnancy. A thin membrane between the two gestation sacs is shown.

NUCHAL TRANSLUCENCY SCREENING

It has been observed that there is an increase in lymphatic fluid accumulation under the skin of the fetal neck in cases of Down's syndrome[21]. The measurement of this, the nuchal translucency, can be used as a screening tool for Down's syndrome. When combined with the maternal age-related risk for trisomy 21, nuchal translucency screening detects up to 80 per cent of cases of Down's syndrome with a false-positive rate of 5 per cent[22]. The detection rate can be increased to almost 90 per cent when combined with first or second trimester biochemical screening[23].

The nuchal translucency can be measured between 11 weeks and 13 weeks 6 d (Fig. 53.11). An increase in nuchal translucency is associated not only with chromosomal abnormalities but also structural abnormalities and some rare genetic syndromes (Table 53.3). Therefore a detailed assessment of fetal anatomy should be made in the presence of a raised nuchal translucency and normal karyotype.

FIRST TRIMESTER DETECTION OF FETAL ABNORMALITIES

Fetal anomaly US is routinely performed in the UK at around 20 weeks' gestation. It has been proposed that the first trimester is the optimum time to assess the fetus along with nuchal translucency measurements. However, comparable detection rates are only obtained with TVS at this gestation period, which is not routinely available and is limited by reduced US probe manoeuverability. In addition some conditions have variable onset and may only present later in gestation.

A number of conditions are readily detected at a first trimester dating and these include anencephaly, gastroschisis and omphalocoele (Fig. 53.12).

SECOND TRIMESTER ANOMALY SCREENING

Second trimester US is widely used to detect fetal anomalies. The published sensitivity of antenatal anomaly screening varies from 34 per cent[24] to 74 per cent[25]. These studies were however conducted at a time when the standard of US equipment and expertise are not as they are today. For a full description of the range of antenatal abnormalities and their detection the reader is referred to specialist literature[26,27].

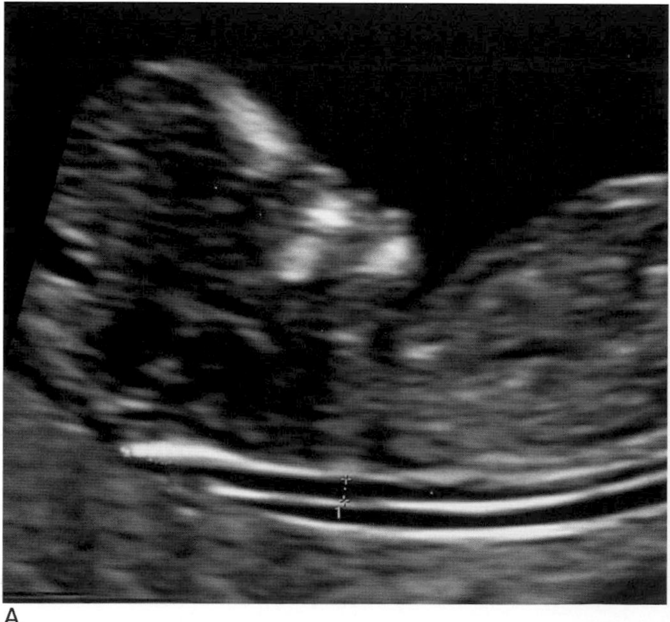

A

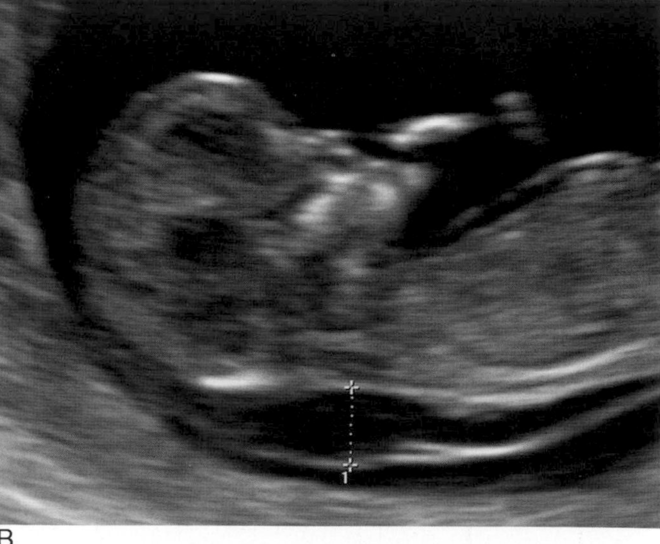

B

Figure 53.11 Nuchal translucency measurement. (A) The nuchal translucency should be measured on a magnified image of the fetal head and neck in the neutral position. The amniotic membrane is seen separate to the nuchal membrane. (B) An increased nuchal translucency associated with Down's syndrome.

Table 53.3 CAUSES OF AN INCREASED NUCHAL TRANSLUCENCY
Chromosomal abnormalities
Cardiac abnormalities
Diaphragmatic hernia
Exomphalos
Skeletal dysplasias
Noonan's syndrome
Myotonic dystrophy
Spinal muscle atrophy
Smith-Lemli-Opitz syndrome
Congenital adrenal hyperplasia
Fetal akinesia deformation sequence

Abnormalities of the central nervous system account for up to one-third of fetal malformations. The intracranial structures can be clearly visualized in the majority of patients if the correct sectional planes are obtained through the thalami, ventricles and cerebellum. The lateral ventricles should be routinely measured and should measure less than 10 mm. Associated abnormalities are present in up to 67 per cent of cases. These include neural tube defects, congenital infection and chromosomal abnormalities (Fig. 53.13).

Congenital heart defects are the most common neonatal abnormalities, with an incidence of eight per 1000 (Fig. 53.14)[28].

The sensitivity of antenatal US in detecting congenital cardiac defects is variable, with reported detection rates ranging from 4 per cent to 78 per cent[29]. The four-chamber view is the

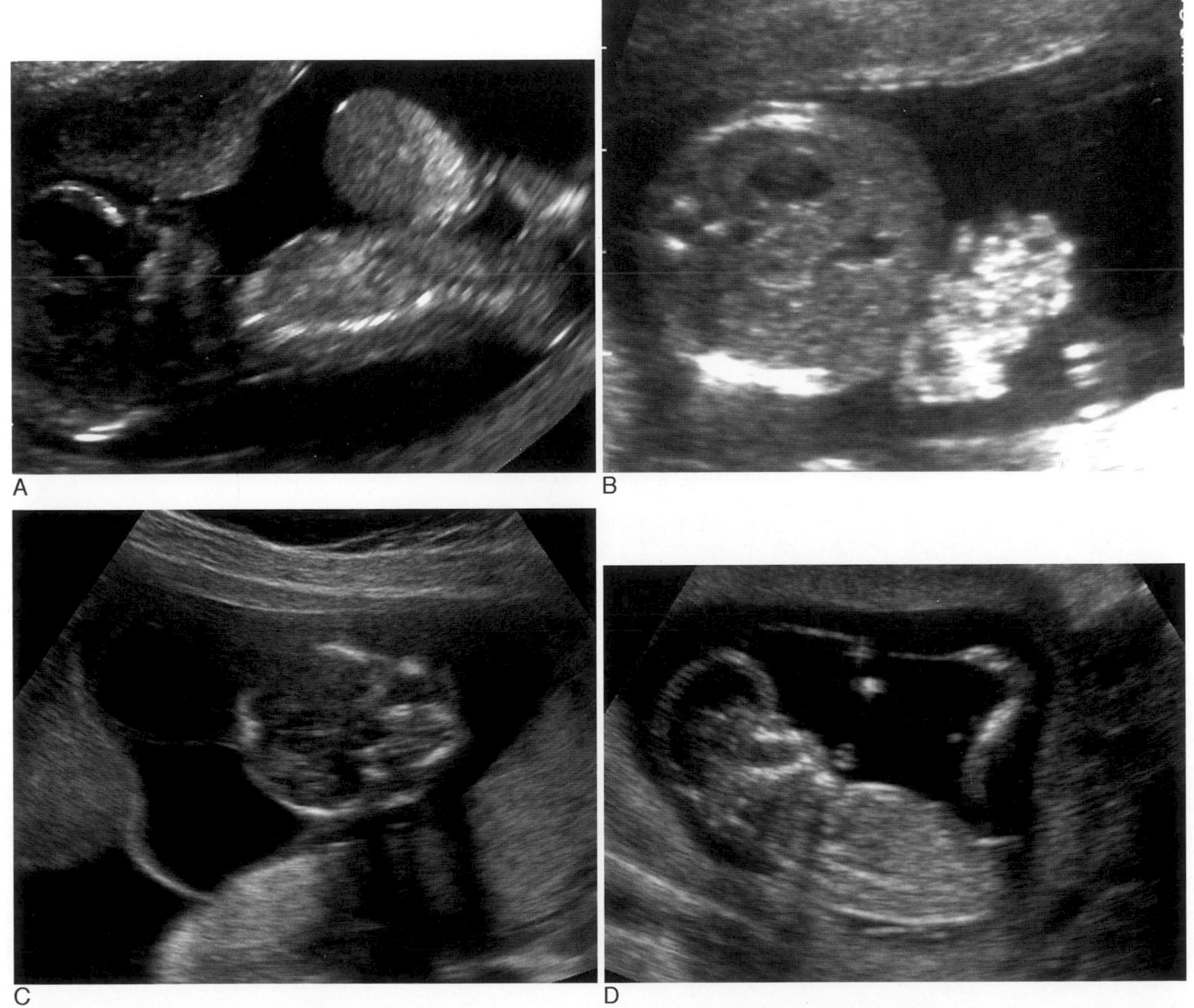

Figure 53.12 First trimester fetal anomalies. (A) Omphalocoele at 14 weeks' gestation. (B) Gastroschisis containing free loops of bowel. (C) Large septated cystic hygroma in a fetus with Turner's syndrome. (D) Anencephaly at 13 weeks' gestation. The cranium is absent and a thin membrane is present.

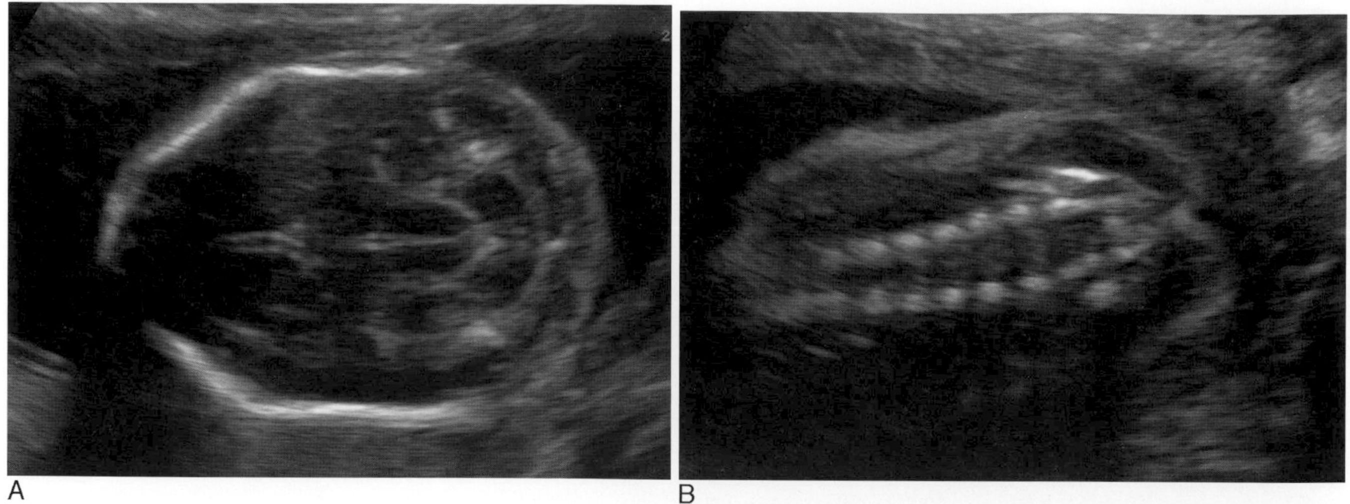

Figure 53.13 Neural tube defects. (A) Lemon-shaped skull associated with a neural tube defect. The cisterna magna is effaced due to an Arnold–Chiari malformation. (B) In the same fetus the coronal view of the lumbar shows splaying of the posterior ossification centres in a fetus with an open neural tube defect.

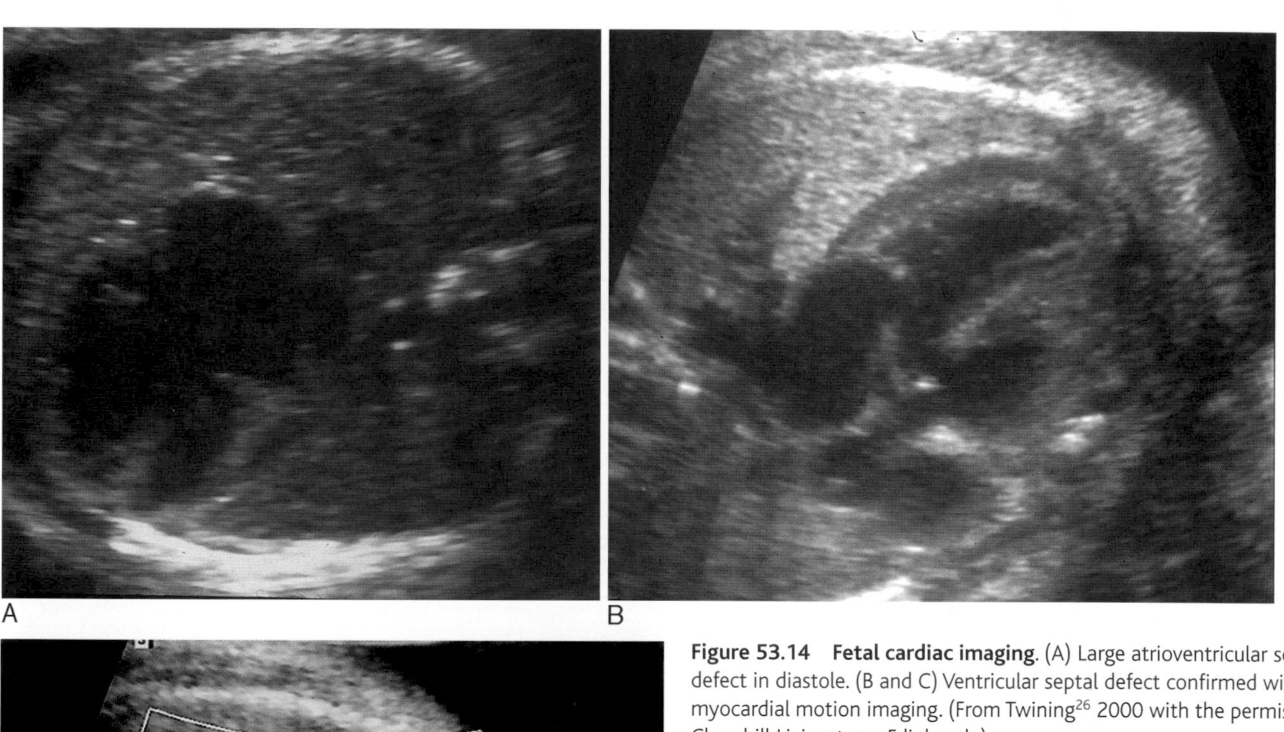

Figure 53.14 Fetal cardiac imaging. (A) Large atrioventricular septal defect in diastole. (B and C) Ventricular septal defect confirmed with myocardial motion imaging. (From Twining[26] 2000 with the permission of Churchill Livingstone, Edinburgh.)

most easily obtained view of the fetal heart and allows examination of the atrioventricular connection, ventricular septum and pulmonary veins. A number of critical cardiac anomalies such as transposition of the great arteries will have a normal four-chamber view and the detection of fetal cardiac abnormalities can be further increased by imaging the cardiac outflow tracts[30].

Space-occupying lung lesions may cause a deviation in the cardiac axis. Congenital cystic adenomatoid malformations and pulmonary sequestrations are well demonstrated by antenatal US (Fig. 53.15). They often become less apparent in the third trimester as the echogenecity of the normal, fluid-filled lung increases.

Renal tract anomalies are relatively common, accounting for 20 per cent of fetal abnormalities. The significance of antenatally detected renal abnormalities remains contentious in particular mild renal pelvis dilatation. However, severe bilateral renal abnormalities account for 10 per cent of all terminations for lethal abnormalities (Fig. 53.16).

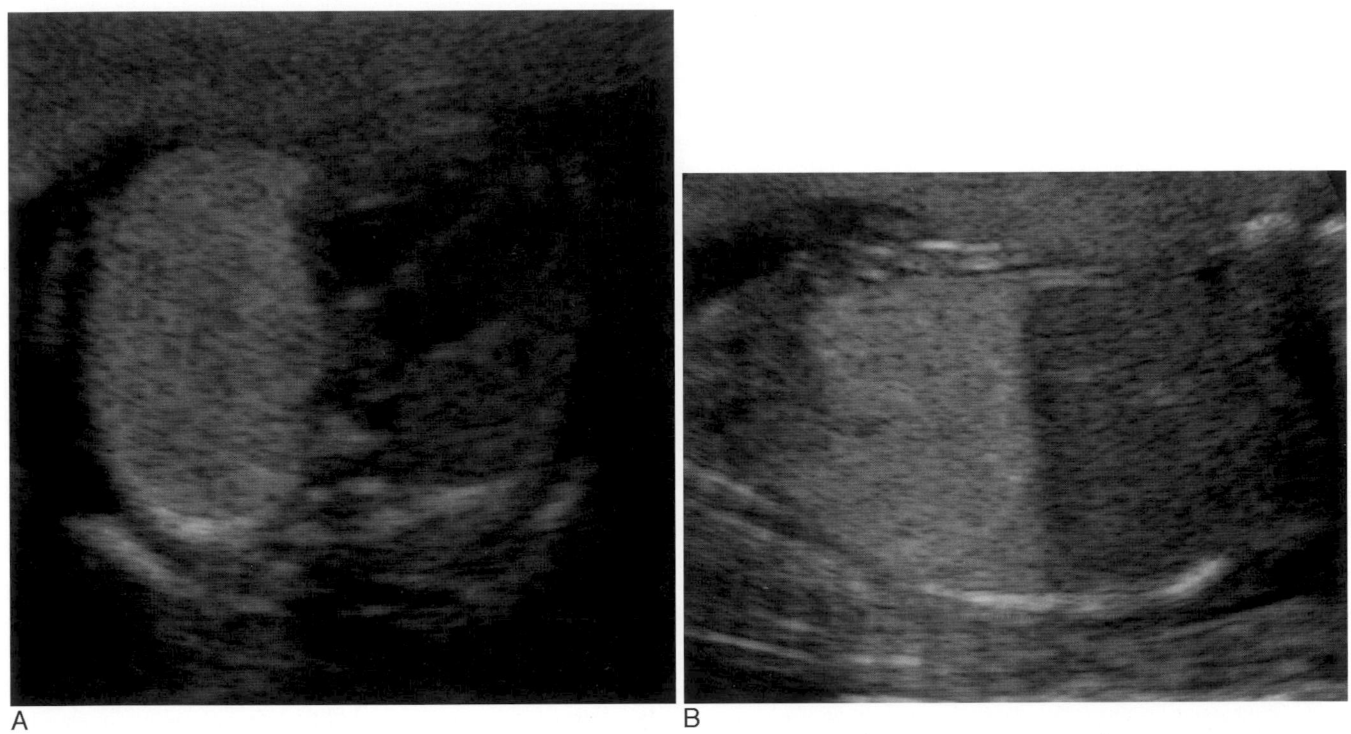

Figure 53.15 Congential cystic adenomatoid malformation. (A) Axial image through the fetal thorax shows significant deviation of the heart to the left by the hyperechoic right-sided cystic adenomatoid malformation. (B) The involvement of the whole right lower lobe is confirmed on the sagittal image.

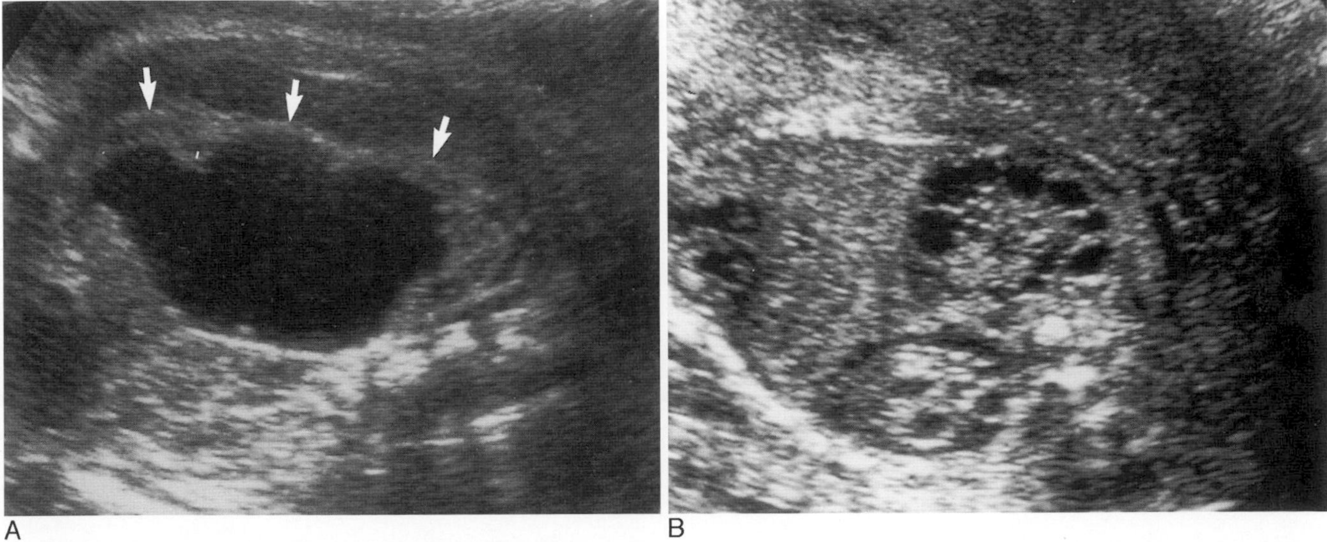

Figure 53.16 Renal abnormalities. (A) Unilateral pelvi-ureteric junction obstruction. Coronal imaging demonstrating hydronephrosis and cortical thinning. (B) Bilateral multicystic dysplastic kidney. Multiple, peripheral cortical cysts are present bilaterally. Severe oligohydramnios is present. (From Twining P, McHugo J M, Pilling D W 2000 Textbook of Fetal Abnormalities. Churchill Livingstone, Edinburgh, with the permission of Churchill Livingstone, Edinburgh.)

HYDROPS

Fetal hydrops is defined as the presence of excess fluid in more than one body cavity, such as ascites, pleural effusions and pericardial effusions (Fig. 53.17). With the introduction of prophylactic anti-D immunoglobulin, immune hydrops is no longer the most common aetiology. Chromosomal causes predominate in cases presenting before 24 weeks' gestation (Table 53.4). After this gestation period cardiac causes, including structural cardiac disease and cardiac arrthymias, account for one-quarter of cases.

US remains essential in the initial assessment of the hydropic fetus, to exclude structural abnormalities, and to assess fetal well-being using biophysical assessment and umbilical artery Doppler. Middle cerebral artery Doppler may also be useful in the assessment of the hydropic fetus. Raised peak systolic velocities in the middle cerebral artery are seen in cases of moderate to severe fetal anaemia with a sensitivity of 100 per cent[31]. Doppler of the middle cerebral artery is also a useful noninvasive tool for the assessment for fetal anaemia in monitoring patients with known red-cell alloimmunization. This removes the need for regular cordocentesis with its associated morbidity and mortality.

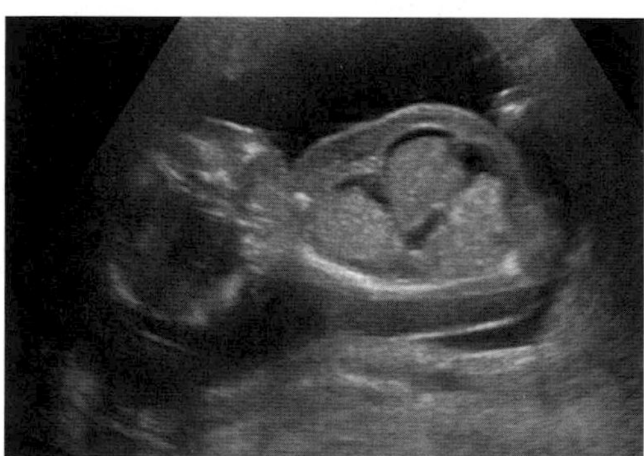

Figure 53.17 Fetal hydrops. Longitudinal view of a fetus with skin oedema, ascites and a hydrothorax.

Table 53.4 CAUSES OF NONIMMUNE HYDROPS AT LESS THAN 20-WEEKS' GESTATION

Cause	%
Chromosomal cause	65.6%
Infection	7.3%
Cardiovascular cause	2.1%
Fetal akinesia	8.3%
Multiple malformation	2.1%
Other anatomical defect	3.1%
Haematological cause	1.1%
Unknown	10.4%

(From Twining P, McHugo J M, Pilling D W (eds.) 2006 Textbook of Fetal Abnormalities, 2nd edition, Churchill Livingstone.)

THREE- AND FOUR-DIMENSIONAL ULTRASOUND

The development of three-dimensional (3D) and four-dimensional (4D) US of the fetus has received much attention for its social benefits. The clinical applications however are still evolving and the huge potential for the diagnosis of fetal abnormalities is being explored[32,33]. 3D US has already proven to be beneficial in the diagnosis of facial clefts, skeletal abnormalities and neural tube defects (Fig. 53.18). Attention is now turning to fetal cardiac applications. Recent technological advances using 4D echocardiography allow an automatic volume acquisition of the fetal heart. The 3D data can then be analyzed in different planes to examine the short- and long-axis views of the fetal heart and outflow tracts.

DISORDERS OF PLACENTATION

US has a pivotal role in the detection of placental abnormalities and determining placental site for invasive procedures such as chorionic villus sampling. In a patient with bleeding in the second or third trimester, sonography is essential to delineate placenta praevia. Placenta praevia is defined as a placenta that is partially or wholly positioned in the lower uterine segment. It should not be diagnosed before 32 weeks' gestation as the lower segment has not formed at this time. For this diagnosis, the presence of placenta covering the area of the internal cervical os should be documented by US. An overly distended urinary bladder may compress the lower uterine segment inwards, simulating the appearance of a low-lying placenta and TVS is the gold standard in the diagnosis of placenta praevia. Areas of retroplacental haemorrhage can also be evaluated sonographically. In these patients, hypoechoic areas that indent the placenta, indicating space-occupying lesions, can be identified.

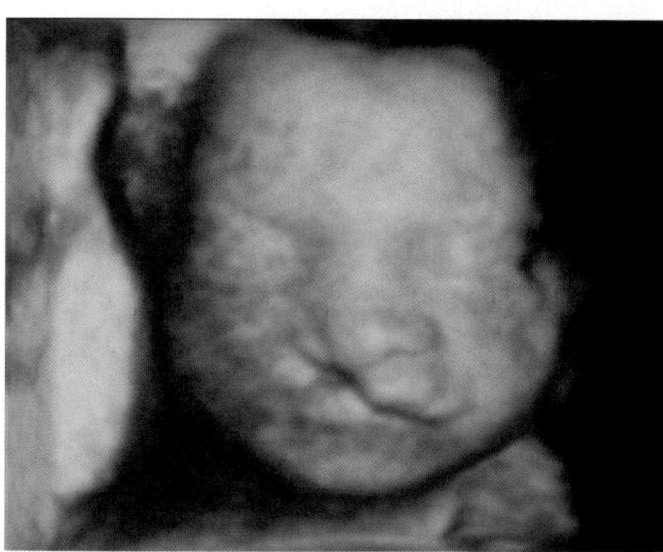

Figure 53.18 Facial cleft demonstrated on 3D US.

CERVICAL LENGTH

The incidence of preterm birth has not altered significantly in the past few decades and remains the most significant cause of neonatal morbidity and mortality with long-term sequelae for survivors. One cause of premature delivery is cervical incompetence, which is defined as the painless dilatation of the cervix and delivery without uterine contractions during the midtrimester. Cervical length is a useful tool to assess the cervix during pregnancy. Although it can be visualized by the transabdominal and transperineal route, TVS is more accurate (Fig. 53.19). TVS is more accurate in determining cervical shortening and funnelling than digital examination and may also demonstrate prolapsing membranes[34,35]. The sensitivity and positive predictive value of screening for cervical length improve in the high-risk population. Surveillance should be offered to women with the following risk factors:

- previous mid-trimester fetal loss
- previous cervical surgery or cervical manipulations
- polyhydramnios.

Cervical length measurements are also useful in predicting premature delivery in women presenting with signs of premature labour. Of women presenting with a cervical length less than 16 mm, 49 per cent deliver within 7 d[36].

Cervical cerclage is currently the treatment of choice for patients with documented cervical incompetence. The literature however is not conclusive for the benefits of cerclage when compared to bed rest alone.

FETAL MAGNETIC RESONANCE IMAGING

Fetal MRI is now a useful adjunct to US in the detection and delineation of fetal anomalies. T2-weighted single-shot turbo spin-echo sequences, such as HASTE, have rapid acquisition times, which lends itself to imaging the fetus without the need for transplacental sedation. Each slice is acquired in less than 1 s so the effects of fetal movement are reduced. Fetal MRI will not replace US as a screening tool but it is useful to clarify abnormalities detected on US and in cases such as large maternal body habitus and oligohydramnios, which limit visualization on US (Fig. 53.20). Fetal MRI has proven diagnostic benefits in cranial abnormalities[37,38] (Figs 53.21, 53.22) and also in abnormalities of the renal tract[39] (Fig. 53.23).

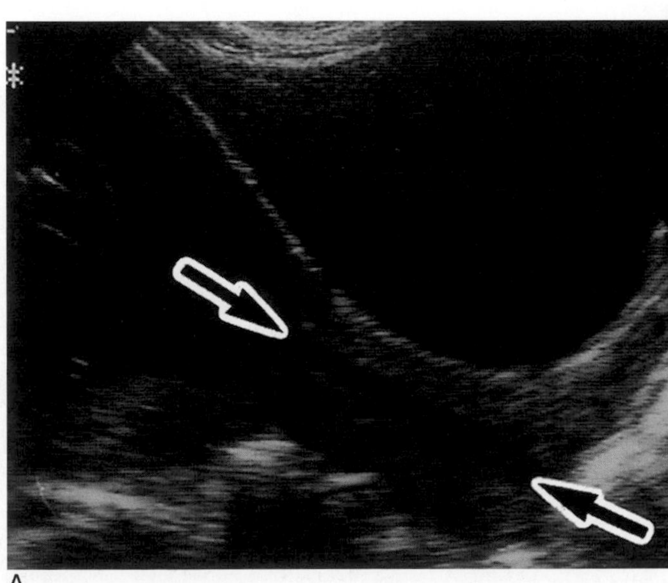
A

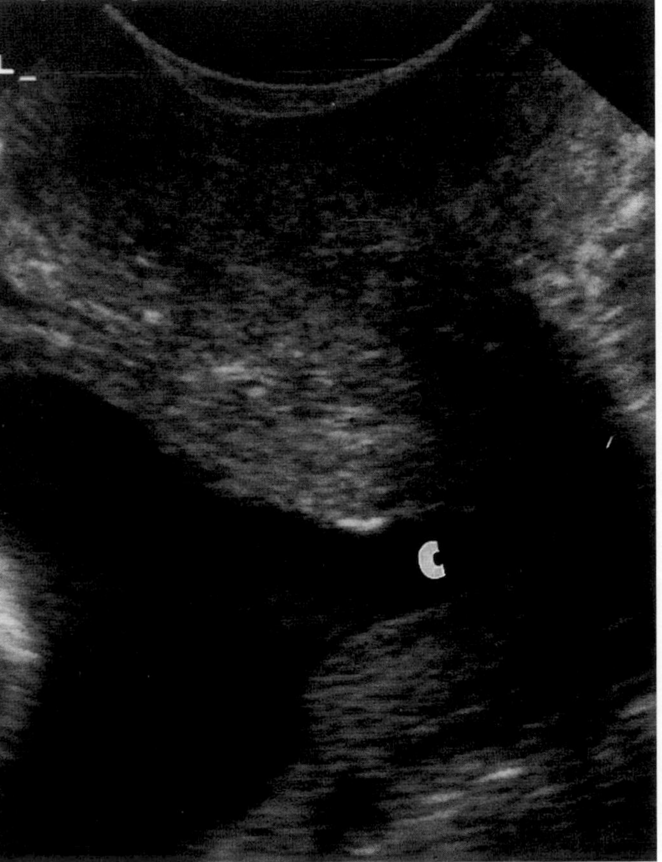

B

Figure 53.19 Cervix. (A) Normal cervix (between arrows) with hypoechoic endocervical canal. (B) Dilatation of the endocervical canal in a patient with cervical incompetence.

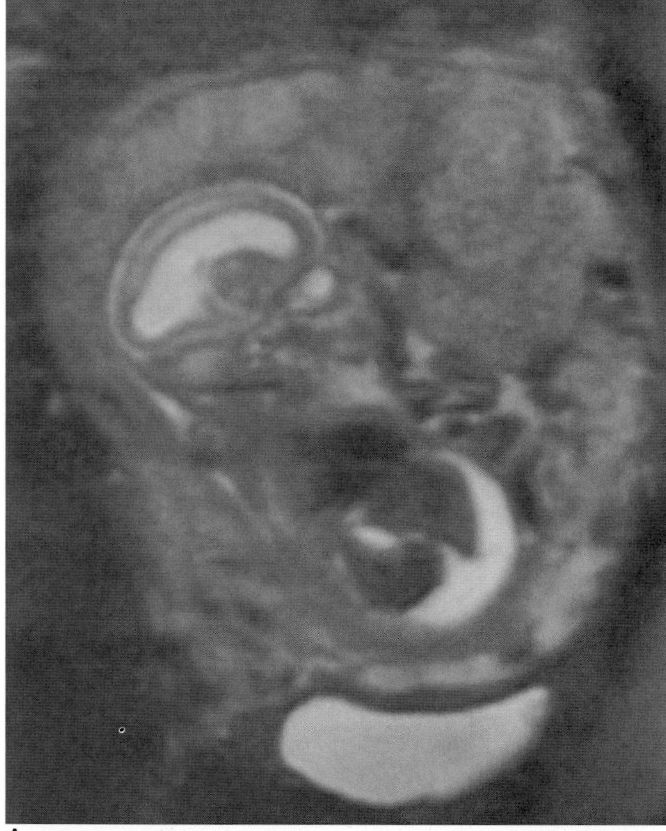
A

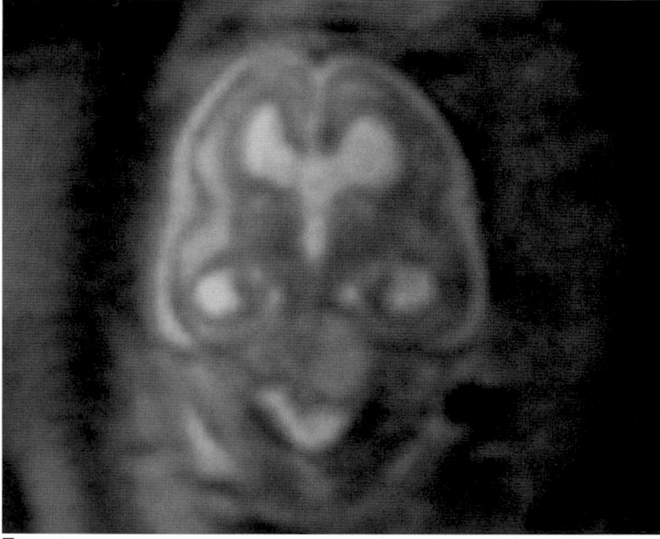
B

Figure 53.20 Congenital CMV. (A) Sagittal fetal MRI in a case with anhydramnios demonstrates fetal ascites. (B) Coronal view of the fetal brain shows high signal in the brain parenchyma consistent with cerebritis and haemorrhage in the cerebellum.

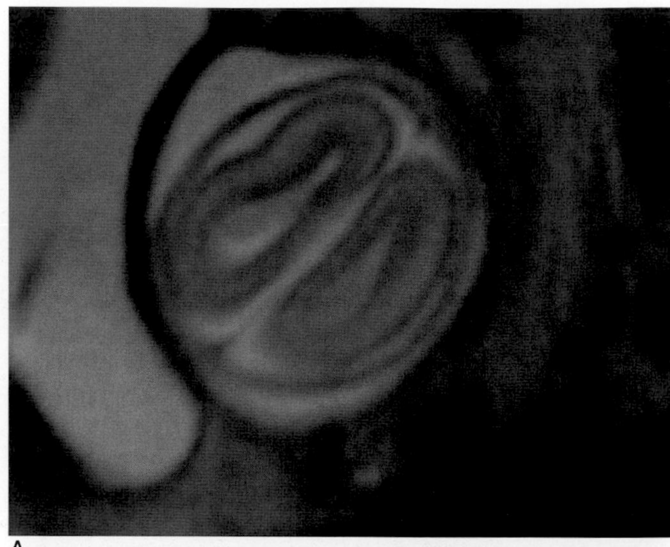
A

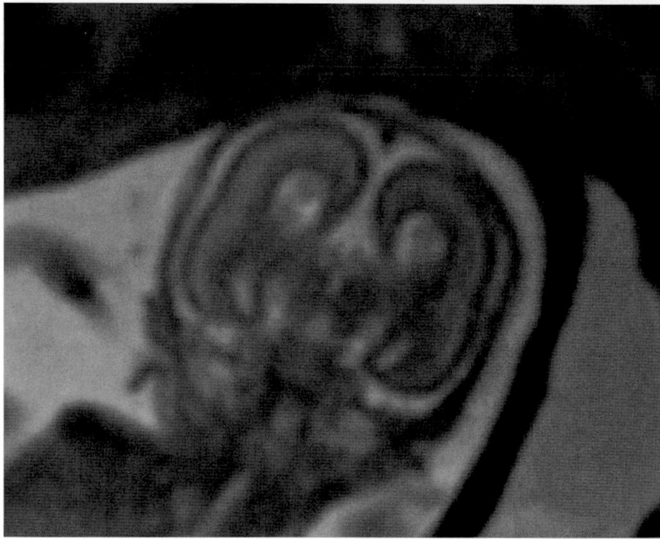
B

Figure 53.21 Agenesis of the corpus callosum. (A) Axial MRI through the fetal brain shows parallel, separated ventricles. (B) Coronal imaging confirms agenesis of the corpus callosum.

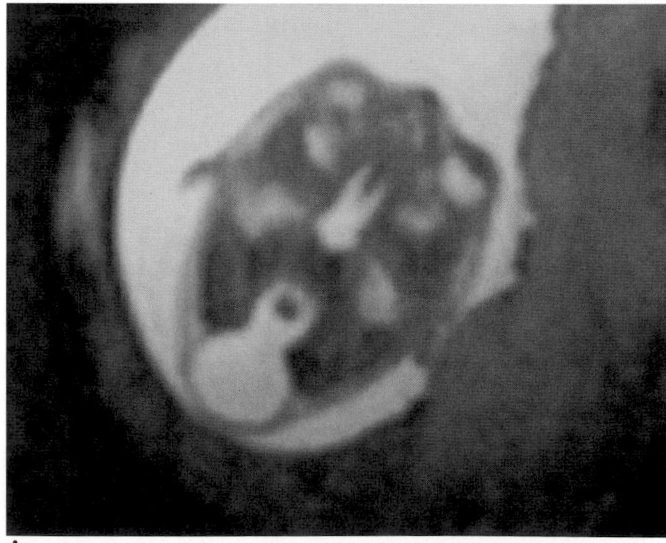
A

Figure 53.22 Occipital meningocoele. (A) Axial MRI through the cranio-cervical junction shows a large open neural tube defect.

Continued

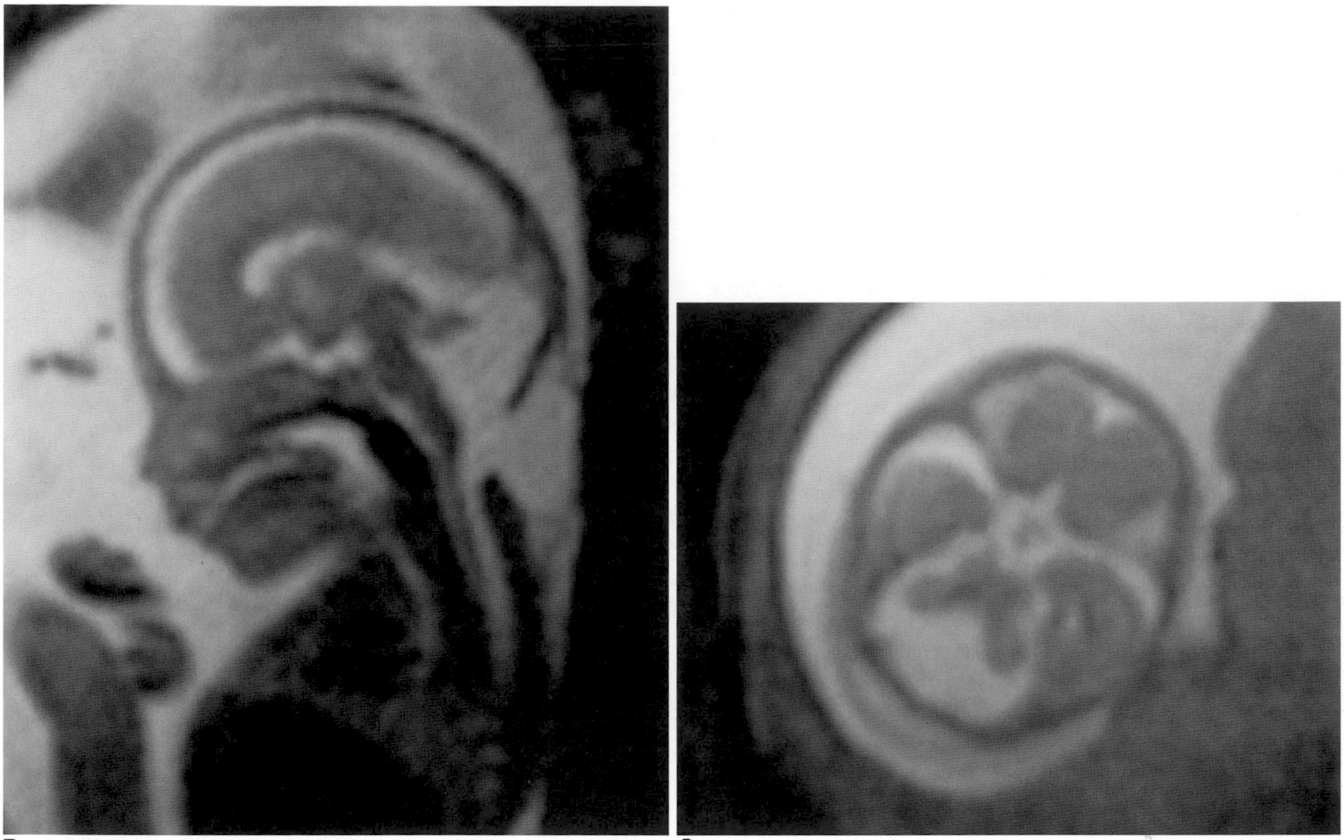

B C

Figure 53.22 Cont'd Occipital meningocoele. (B) Sagittal image showing the extent of the defect. (C) This was associated with cerebellar vermian agenesis.

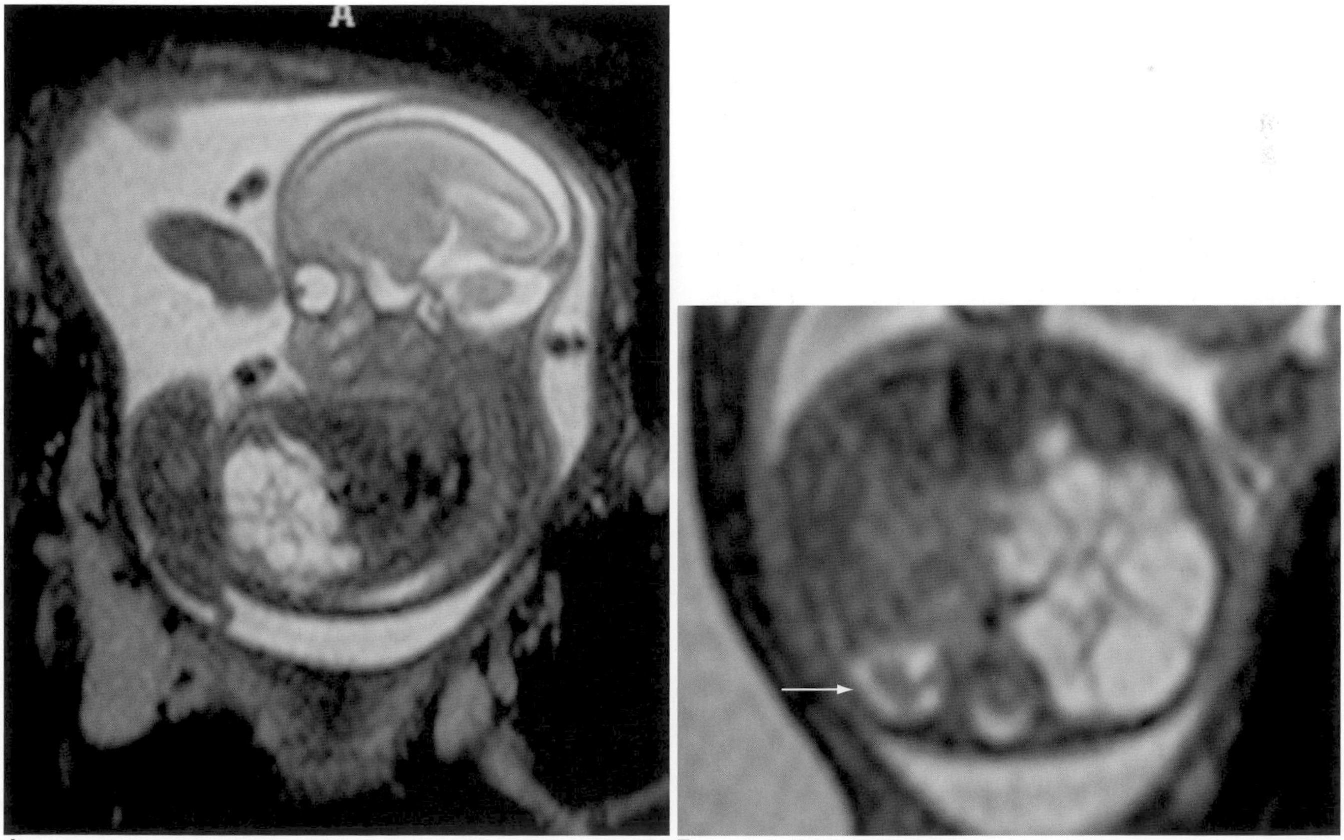

A B

Figure 53.23 Polycystic renal disease. (A) Longitudinal fetal MRI confirms the large polycystic kidney detected on US. (B) Axial MRI also shows that the contralateral kidney is dysplastic with small cortical cysts (arrow).

REFERENCES

1. te Velde E R, Eijkemans R, Habbema H D 2000 Variation in couple fecundity and time to pregnancy, an essential concept in human reproduction. Lancet 355:1928–1929
2. Hull M G, Glazener C M, Kelly N J et al 1985 Population study of causes, treatment, and outcome of infertility. Br Med J 291:1693–1697
3. National Collaborating Centre for Women's and Children's Health 2004 Fertility: assessment and treatment for people with fertility problems. Commissioned by the National Institute for Clinical Excellence. Feb
4. Swart P, Mol B W, van der Veen F, van Beurden M, Redekop W K, Bossuyt P M 1995 The accuracy of hysterosalpingography in the diagnosis of tubal pathology: a meta-analysis. Fertil Steril 64:486–491
5. Johnson N, Vandekerckhove P, Watson A, Lilford R, Harada T, Hughes E 2005 Tubal flushing for subfertility. Cochrane Database Syst Rev 18
6. Blankstein J, Shaley J, Saadon T et al 1987 Ovarian hyperstimulation syndrome: prediction by number and size of preovulatory ovarian follicles. Fertil Steril 47:597–602
7. Dellenbach P, Nisand I, Moreau L et al 1985 Transvaginal sonographically controlled follicle puncture for oocyte retrieval. Fertil Steril 44:656–662
8. Gonen Y, Casper R F, Jacobson W, Blankier J 1989 Endometrial thickness and growth during ovarian stimulation: a possible predictor of implantation in in vitro fertilization. Fertil Steril 52:446–450
9. Raga F, Bonilla-Musoles F, Casan E M, Klein O, Bonilla F 1999 Assessment of endometrial volume by three-dimensional ultrasound prior to embryo transfer: clues to endometrial receptivity. Hum Reprod 14:2851–2854
10. Steer C, Tan S, Dillon D, Mason B A, Campbell S 1995 Vaginal color Doppler assessment of uterine artery impedance correlates with immunohistochemical markers of endometrial receptivity required for the implantation of an embryo. Fertil Steril 63:101–108
11. Kupesic S, Bekavac I, Bjelos D, Kurjak A 2001 Assessment of endometrial receptivity by transvaginal color Doppler and three-dimensional power Doppler ultrasonography in patients undergoing in vitro fertilization procedures. J Ultrasound Med 20:125–134
12. Royal College of Radiologists and Royal College of Obstetricians and Gynaecologists 1995 Guidance on Ultrasound Procedures in Early Pregnancy
13. Rajkhowa M, Glass M R, Rutherford A J, Balen A H, Sharma V, Cuckle H S 2000 Trends in the incidence of ectopic pregnancy in England and Wales from 1966 to 1996. BJOG 107:369–374
14. Condous G, Okaro E, Khalid A et al 2005 The accuracy of transvaginal ultrasound for the diagnosis of ectopic pregnancy prior to surgery. Hum Reprod 20:1404–1409
15. DeVoe R W, Pratt J H 1948 Simultaneous intrauterine and extrauterine pregnancy. Am J Obst Gynecol 56:1119
16. Richards S R, Stempel L E, Carlton B D 1982 Heterotopic pregnancy: Reappraisal of incidence. Am J Obst Gynecol 142:928–930
17. Gabrielli S, Romero R, Pilu G et al 1992 Accuracy of transvaginal ultrasound and serum hCG in the diagnosis of ectopic pregnancy. Ultrasound Obstet Gynecol 2:110–115
18. Robinson H P 1973 Sonar measurement of fetal crown-rump length as means of assessing maturity in first trimester of pregnancy. Br Med J 4:28–31
19. Chitty L S, Altman D G, Henderson A, Campbell S 1994 Charts of fetal size: 2. Head measurements. Br J Obstet Gynaecol 101:35–43
20. Chitty L S, Altman D G, Henderson A, Campbell S 1994 Charts of fetal size: 3. Abdominal measurements. Br J Obstet Gynaecol 101:125–131
21. Nicolaides K H, Azar G, Byrne D, Mansur C, Marks K 1992 Fetal nuchal translucency: ultrasound screening for chromosomal defects in first trimester of pregnancy. Br Med J 304:867–869
22. Snijders R J M, Noble P, Sebire N, Souka A, Nicolaides K H 1998 UK multicentre project on assessment of risk of trisomy 21 by maternal age and fetal nuchal-translucency thickness at 10–14 weeks of gestation. Lancet 352:343–346
23. Nicolaides K H, Spencer K, Avgidou K, Faiola S, Falcon O 2005 Multicenter study of first-trimester screening for trisomy 21 in 75 821 pregnancies: results and estimation of the potential impact of individual risk-orientated two-stage first-trimester screening. Ultrasound Obstet Gynecol 25:221–226
24. Ewigman B G, Crane J P, Frigoletto F D, LeFevre M L, Bain R P, McNellis D and the RADIUS Study Group 1993 Effect of prenatal ultrasound screening on perinatal outcome. N Engl J Med 329:821–827
25. Chitty L S, Hunt G H, Moore J, Lobb M O 1991 Effectiveness of routine ultrasonography in detecting fetal structural abnormalities in a low risk population. Br Med J 303:1165–1169
26. Twining P, McHugo J M, Pilling D W 2000 Textbook of Fetal Abnormalities. Churchill Livingstone, Edinburgh
27. Nyberg D A, McGahan J P, Pretorius D H, Pilu G 2006 Diagnostic imaging of fetal anomalies. Lippincott Williams & Wilkins, New York
28. Mitchell S C, Korones S B 1971 Congenital heart disease in 56 109 births. Incidence and natural history. Circulation 43:323–332
29. Pitkin R M 1991 Screening and detection of congenital malformation. Am J Obstet Gynecol 164:1045–1048
30. Carvalho J S, Mavrides E, Shinebourne E A, Campbell S, Thilaganathan G 2002 Improving the effectiveness of routine prenatal screening for major congenital heart defects. Heart 88:487–491
31. Mari G, Deter R L, Carpenter R L et al 2000 Noninvasive diagnosis by Doppler ultrasonography of fetal anemia due to maternal red cell alloimmunization. Collaborative Group for Doppler Assessment of the Blood Velocity in Anemic Fetuses. N Engl J Med 342:9–14
32. Merz E 1998 3-D ultrasound in obstetrics and gynecology. Lippincott Williams & Wilkins, New York
33. Bega G, Lev-Toaff A, Kuhlman K, Kurtz A, Goldberg B, Wapner R 2001 Three-dimensional ultrasonographic imaging in obstetrics. J Ultrasound Med 20:391–408
34. Berghella V, Tolosa J E, Kuhlman K, Weiner S, Bolognese R J, Wapner R J 1997 Cervical ultrasonography compared with manual examination as a predictor of preterm delivery. Am J Obstet Gynecol 177:723–730
35. Iams J D, Johnson F F, Sonek J, Sachs L, Gebauer C, Samuels P 1995 Cervical competence as a continuum: a study of ultrasonographic cervical length and obstetric performance. Am J Obstet Gynecol 175 (4 Pt 1):1097–1103
36. Tsoi E, Fuchs I B, Rane S, Geerts L, Nicolaides K H 2005 Sonographic measurement of cervical length in threatened preterm labor in singleton pregnancies with intact membranes. Ultrasound Obstet Gynecol 25:353–356
37. Garel C 2003 MRI of the Fetal Brain: Normal Development and Cerebral Pathologies. Springer-Verlag, Berlin and Heidelberg GmbH & Co.
38. Griffiths P D, Paley M N, Widjaja E, Taylor C, Whitby E H 2005 In utero magnetic resonance imaging for brain and spinal abnormalities in fetuses. Br Med J 331:562–565
39. Hormann M, Brugger P C, Balassy C, Witzani L, Prayer D 2006 Fetal MRI of the urinary system. Eur J Radiol 57:303–311

CHAPTER 54

Imaging in Gynaecology

Evis Sala, Sandra Allison, Susan M. Ascher and Hedvig Hricak

- Imaging techniques
- Congenital anomalies of the female genital tract
- Infertility
- Pelvic pain
- Uterus and cervix
- The adnexa
- Vulva and vagina
- Contraception

The results of diagnostic imaging tests frequently change treatment strategies and impact our understanding of disease processes. This chapter gives a brief review of common gynaecological entities and presents indications for each imaging technique used while focusing on advances in ultrasound (US), computed tomography (CT), magnetic resonance imaging (MRI) and positron emission tomography (PET). As with any changing technological arena, imaging strategies are not static and require on-going updates and re-evaluation.

IMAGING TECHNIQUES

Ultrasound

Ultrasound (transabdominal or transvaginal) is accepted as the primary imaging technique for examining the female pelvis. Currently, the main role of ultrasound (US) in gynaecology includes evaluation of a suspected pelvic mass, evaluation of the causes of uterine enlargement, identification of endometrial abnormalities in a patient with postmenopausal bleeding and characterization of ovarian masses. It is also the primary imaging technique of choice in the evaluation of women with acute pelvic pain. In addition, ultrasound has become invaluable in guiding a wide selection of invasive procedures. For example, it is used for transabdominal and transvaginal guidance of fluid or tissue sampling, transvaginal-guided drain placement, guidance for placement of brachytherapy for cervical and endometrial malignancy and intraoperative assessment for completion of evacuation and instrument placement, especially when the anatomy is difficult to assess preoperatively.

A full bladder provides a sonic window and is mandatory for transabdominal US. It is usual to employ 3.5–5.0 MHz transducers. Transvaginal ultrasound, which is optimally performed with an empty bladder, provides greater detail of the anatomy and pathology due to the closer apposition to the pelvic organs as well as the higher frequencies of insonation (5–8 MHz). Colour, power and spectral Doppler provide additional information regarding associated vascularity.

Ultrasound has many advantages in routine pelvic imaging: it is relatively inexpensive, provides multiplanar views, is widely available and lacks ionizing radiation or contrast media. Its portability allows use in virtually any setting, including the ultrasound suite, operating room, patient bedside, or radiation therapy suite. However, US also has a number of limitations: it is operator dependent and image quality varies with patient body habitus. Although transvaginal, sonohysterography and endorectal US provide improved spatial resolution, they are not as useful as either CT or MRI in the staging of pelvic malignancies, including the evaluation of regional extent or metastatic spread.

Normal ultrasound anatomy

The normal uterus measures between 5 and 9 cm in length and is usually visualized in an anteverted position (in relation to the urinary bladder). The appearance of the endometrium changes in response to the menstrual cycle (Fig. 54.1). In the proliferative phase of the cycle, the endometrium is well defined and may measure up to 8 mm. In midcycle, the endometrium assumes a trilaminar appearance and may measure up to 12–16 mm. During the secretory phase, the layers become hyperechoic due to the increasing complexity of glandular structure and secretions. The Fallopian tubes are usually not identified unless distended with fluid.

Following menopause, the uterus may decrease in size and an endometrial thickness of 5 mm serves as a threshold for endometrial biopsy. An endometrial thickness of up to 8 mm is considered acceptable for those on hormonal therapy.

Normal ovaries are visualized in the majority of premenopausal patients. They are more readily identified on transvaginal US. The iliac vessels lie immediately posterior to the ovary

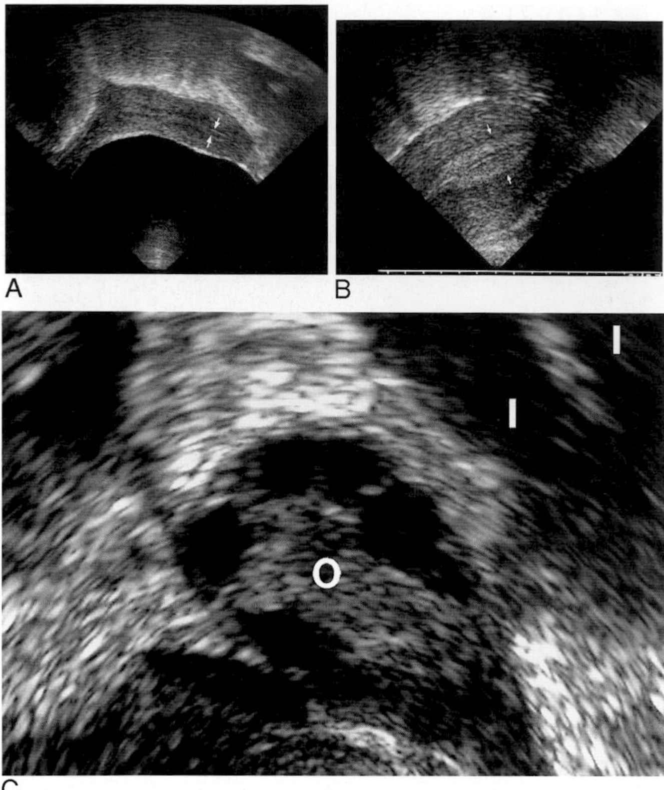

Figure 54.1 (A) Transvaginal US shows **normal endometrium** (arrows) in **proliferative phase** and (B) in **follicular phase** (arrows). (C) Sagittal transvaginal US shows a **normal ovary** (O) with follicles. Note the location of the ovary anterior and medial to the internal iliac vessels (I) within the ovarian fossa.

and assist in its identification (Fig. 54.1). A normal ovary typically measures 30 mm in any two dimensions but may measure 50 mm or more in one plane. The volume of the ovary can be estimated from the formula for an ellipsoid (0.5 × length × width × breadth) and is usually less than 10 cm^3. Follicular and luteal cysts are seen within the ovary.

Computed tomography

CT is the most commonly used primary imaging study for evaluating the extent of gynaecological malignancy and for detecting persistent and recurrent pelvic tumours. CT-guided biopsy can be used to confirm pelvic recurrence. Advantages of CT include oral and rectal contrast opacification of the gastrointestinal tract, intravenous contrast enhancement of blood vessels and viscera, fast data acquisition and high spatial resolution. Disadvantages of CT include the use of ionizing radiation (this is why it is essential to exclude the possibility of pregnancy before performing CT), degradation of image quality by body habitus or metallic hip prosthesis and the risk of morbidity and mortality associated with iodinated contrast agents. Although CT is useful in the later stages of pelvic malignancy, it often has limited utility in characterizing early-stage disease. The advent of helical (spiral) and multidetector CT (MDCT) has made it possible for images to be acquired during the arterial, capillary and venous phases of enhancement following contrast medium administration. The new generation of CT equipment provides good delineation of uterine anatomy (i.e. myometrium, endometrium, cervix and parametrium) and the major pelvic vessels. With helical and multidetector CT, reformatting of images is also possible, including the creation of 3D volume renderings.

Normal CT anatomy

CT examination displays the uterus as a triangular or ovoid soft tissue structure behind the urinary bladder (Fig. 54.2). On unenhanced images, secretions within the endometrial canal demonstrate centrally located decreased attenuation. Following intravenous (IV) contrast medium administration, the myometrium enhances, helping to delineate the endometrium. The vagina, cervix and uterine corpus can be distinguished by morphological and enhancement pattern characteristics. The uterine corpus is typically triangular, whereas the cervix is more rounded. At the level of the fornix, the vagina is seen as a flat rectangle. The broad and round ligaments can be seen coursing laterally and anteriorly, respectively. Occasionally, the uterosacral ligaments are depicted as arc-like structures extending from the cervix to the sacrum. In the premenopausal patient

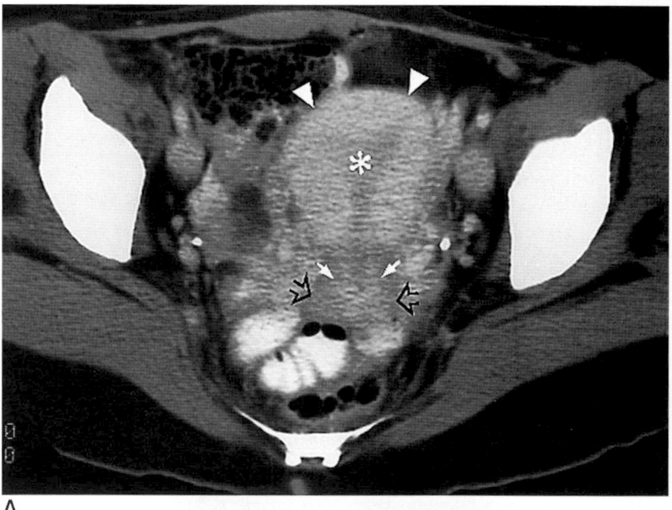

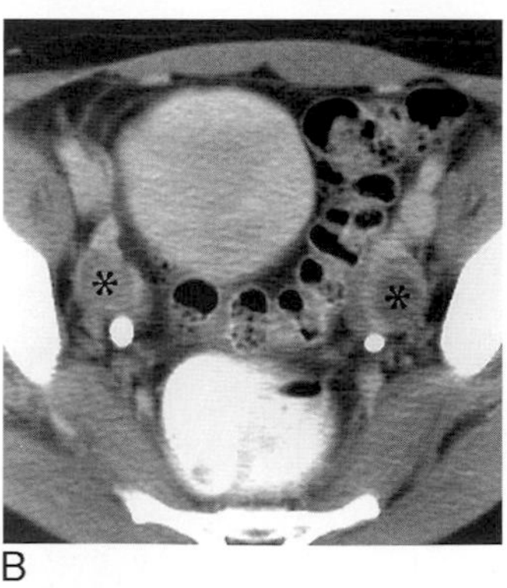

Figure 54.2 (A) **Normal uterus.** Helical CT of the normal uterus and adnexa shows the low attenuation endometrial canal (*) flanked by enhancing myometrium (arrowheads). Enhancing endocervical mucosa (short solid white arrows) surrounds the endocervical canal. The fibrous cervical stroma (open black arrows) enhances less than the uterine corpus myometrium. A physiological cyst is seen in the right ovary. (B) **Normal ovary**. Helical CT shows bilateral physiological ovarian cysts (*). The ovaries are in their expected location, anterior to the internal iliac vessels and posterior to the external iliac vessels. The zonal anatomy of the uterus is faintly defined.

the normal ovaries are routinely seen, usually posterolateral to the uterine corpus (Fig. 54.2). Their uniform soft tissue density is punctuated by small cystic regions representing follicles. In the postmenopausal patient the ovaries are small and may not be discernible.

Magnetic resonance imaging

The role of MRI in gynaecology has evolved during the last two decades. There is now a substantial body of evidence that MRI is useful in evaluating Müllerian duct anomalies and both benign and malignant conditions of the pelvis. MRI has been shown to be superior to CT in the work-up of uterine and cervical cancer and may be a useful problem-solving tool in the evaluation of ovarian cancer. In addition, there is evidence that MRI may aid the differentiation of radiation fibrosis from recurrent tumour. The accuracy of MRI assessment of lymph node invasion is similar to that of CT; both rely on size criteria to detect lymphadenopathy. In addition, MR-guided biopsies are also gaining wider clinical acceptance.

Although MRI is still relatively expensive, it has been shown to minimize costs in some clinical settings by limiting or eliminating the need for further expensive and/or more invasive diagnostic or surgical procedures. Advantages of MRI include superb spatial and tissue contrast resolution, no use of ionizing radiation, multiplanar capability and fast (i.e. breath-hold and breathing-independent) techniques. MRI is the technique of choice for patients with previous reactions to iodinated IV contrast media or impaired renal function. However, MRI is contraindicated in patients with implants such as pacemakers, neural stimulators or cochlear implants, certain vascular clips and metallic objects. Some patients may experience claustrophobia, causing difficulty in completing the examination or requiring sedative pre-medication in subsequent MR examinations.

Normal MRI anatomy

Pelvic anatomy is exquisitely demonstrated by MRI (Fig. 54.3). On T1-weighted sequences, the normal pelvic musculature and viscera demonstrate homogeneous low to intermediate signal intensity. However, it is the contrast resolution of T2-weighting that is the basis for the superb tissue characterization of MRI. On T2-weighted sequences, the uterus, cervix and vagina exhibit distinct layers of different signal intensity—the so-called zonal architecture. The endometrium yields high signal intensity on T2-weighted images. The peripheral myometrium, in comparison, is intermediate in signal intensity, higher than striated muscle. Interposed between these two layers is a narrow band of decreased signal intensity, the junctional zone (JZ), which corresponds to the innermost myometrium. Its signal properties reflect its lower water content, compared with the remainder of the myometrium, which may be a function of its decrease in extracellular matrix/unit volume. The three zones seen on MR images, however, are not identical to the different zones seen on US. The width of the endometrium (both leaflets) varies with the menstrual cycle and, on the sagittal plane of section, measures up to 3 mm in the proliferative phase and up to 7 mm in the secretory phase. In postmenopausal women not receiving exogenous hormones, uterine zonal anatomy is often indistinct and the endometrium measures less than 3 mm.

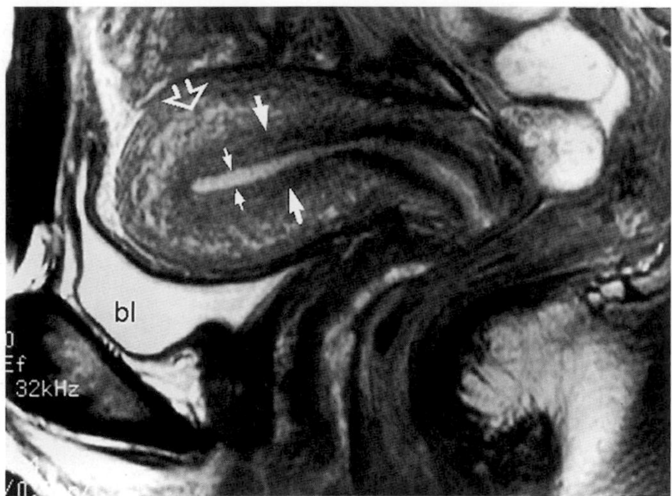

Figure 54.3 Zonal anatomy of the uterus. Sagittal T2-weighted MRI. The central, high-signal intensity stripe represents the endometrium (small arrows); the band of low signal intensity subjacent to the endometrial stripe represents the inner myometrium or junctional zone (arrows). The outer layer of the myometrium is of intermediate signal intensity (open arrow). bl = bladder.

The cervix also demonstrates zonal architecture on T2-weighted images, with the normal cervix demonstrating a central area of high signal intensity (endocervical glands and mucus) surrounded by low signal intensity stroma (elastic fibrous tissue). Around the periphery of the cervix, smooth muscle predominates, resulting in a rim of intermediate signal intensity similar to that of myometrium. Occasionally, intermediate signal intensity cervical mucosal folds (plicae palmatae) can be seen interposed between the low signal intensity cervical stroma and the high signal intensity endocervical canal. T2-weighted images of the vagina reveal two zones: the bright vaginal mucosa and the intermediate intensity vaginal wall. The ligamentous structures are identified with low signal intensity by their anatomical location. Following IV administration of paramagnetic gadolinium chelates, the zonal anatomy of the uterus is demonstrated on T1-weighted images. The endometrium and outer myometrium enhance to a greater extent than the JZ. Similarly, the inner cervical mucosa and outer smooth muscle enhance more than the fibrocervical stroma. The parametrial tissues, vaginal walls and submucosa also enhance after IV contrast medium administration.

The normal MRI appearance of the ovaries varies depending on the pulse sequence used. On T1-weighted images, the ovaries display homogeneous low to intermediate signal intensity, whereas on T2-weighted images the follicles become brighter than the surrounding stroma. The normal Fallopian tubes are not routinely seen because of their small size and tortuous course.

Positron emission tomography

PET (and PET-CT) is maturing as an imaging technique. PET takes advantage of the biochemical changes associated with malignancy that often precede and are more specific than the structural changes visualized by conventional means. Specifically, with the most commonly used glucose analogue, 2-[^{18}F]-fluoro-2-deoxy-D-glucose (FDG), PET exploits the accelerated rate of glycolysis common to neoplastic cells to image tumours. Because PET requires specialized instrumentation and a local source of positron emitters, it is not widely available and its routine use is often limited to tertiary care settings. Most work to date with PET and gynaecological malignancy has focused on cervical and ovarian cancer.

Hysterosalpingography

Hysterosalpingography (HSG) is an imaging test whereby radio-opaque contrast medium is instilled into the uterus and Fallopian tubes. It is used mainly to evaluate infertility (e.g. tubal obstruction). In the past, HSG was used for the evaluation of congenital abnormalities of the uterus but has been replaced by US and MRI. The optimal time to perform HSG is towards the end of the first week after the menstrual period, when the isthmus is most distensible and the Fallopian tubes most readily filled with contrast medium and the chance of pregnancy is small. Nonionic contrast media have little advantage compared to ionic agents but may cause less peritoneal irritation. HSG is contraindicated in pregnancy and active pelvic infection and in the pre- and postmenopausal phases. Possible complications are pain, pelvic infection, haemorrhage and vasovagal attacks.

Normal hysterosalpingography anatomy

The cervical canal is usually 30–40 mm long and tends to shorten after childbirth. It measures about one third of the entire length of the uterus and is often spindle shaped. Glandular filling often occurs in the normal cervix. The isthmus is seen as a distinct segment, narrower than the uterine body and cervical canal, in only half of all normal hysterograms. The internal os may appear as a short constriction of the lumen. The cavity of the uterine body is triangular in shape (Fig. 54.4), its walls normally regular and straight or concave. Both the average length and the intercornual diameter measure approximately 35 mm. The cornual sphincters are pear or spindle shaped and are often separated from the uterine body by a short, dark line due to a mucosal fold. The apex of each cornu opens continually to the tubal lumen. The Fallopian tubes are approximately 5 or 6 cm long, with a variable degree of tortuosity. The isthmic portion is of uniform diameter and opens laterally into the wide ampulla.

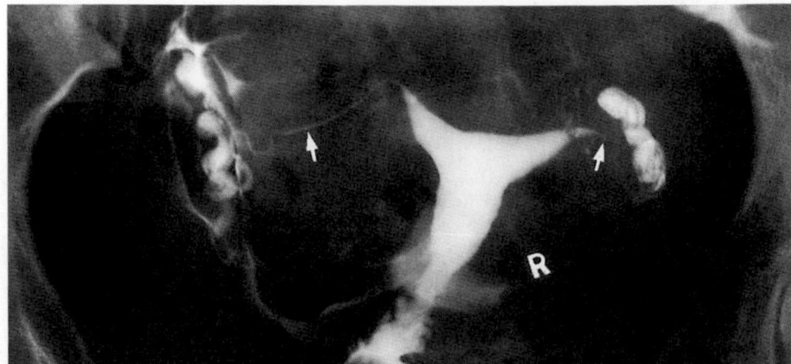

Figure 54.4 Normal hysterosalpingogram. Cervix and uterine body are delineated by contrast media. Both Fallopian tubes are shown (arrows), with early peritoneal spill.

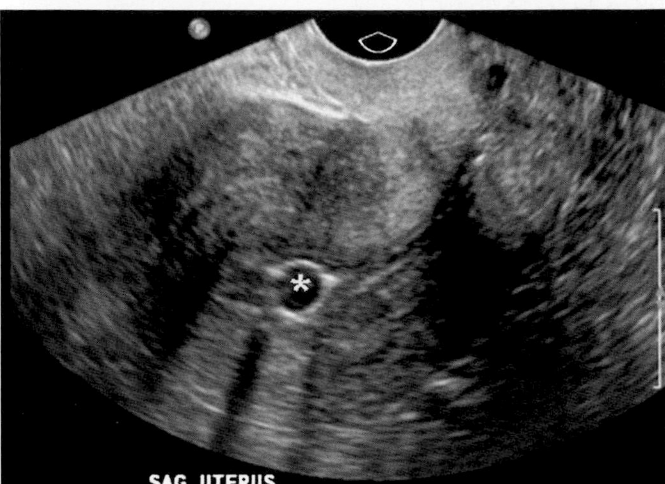

A

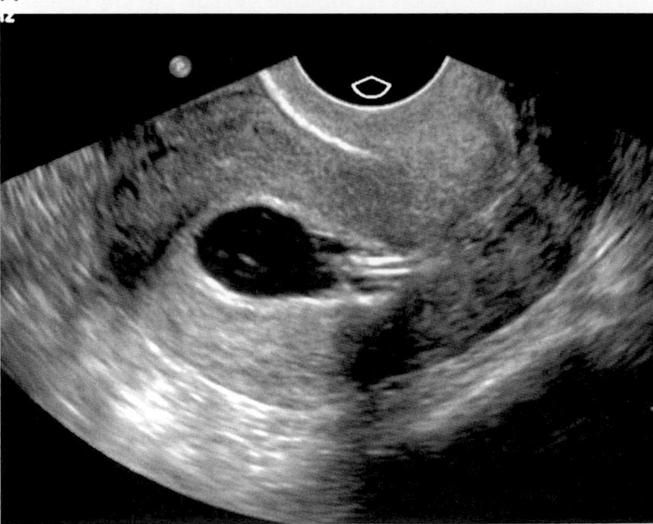

B

Figure 54.5 Sonohysterography. Sagittal transvaginal US (A) demonstrates the inflated balloon of the sonohysterographic catheter (*) within the endometrial canal. Following the instillation of 40 cc of sterile saline (B), fluid distends the endometrial canal.

Sonohysterography

This technique involves placement of a 5 F catheter through the cervix and distension of the uterine cavity with sterile saline under direct ultrasound visualization (Fig. 54.5). The procedure is well tolerated with few contraindications and virtually no complications. It can be performed rapidly on an outpatient basis without the use of ionizing radiation or contrast agent. Several studies have shown that the accuracy of US HSG exceeds that of endovaginal US alone. US HSG can make a more precise diagnosis in cases where endovaginal US only shows abnormal thickening of the endometrium and can differentiate intracavitary, endometrial and subendometrial pathology. It can therefore select and effectively triage patients to appropriate methods of endometrial sampling and direct hysteroscopic removal of pathology when appropriate. Because the single layer endometrium is visualized, focal pathology can be differentiated from diffuse endometrial conditions with increased accuracy. In the evaluation of tubal patency, the identification of free fluid in the pouch of Douglas indicates that at least one tube is patent.

CONGENITAL ANOMALIES OF THE FEMALE GENITAL TRACT

General considerations

Müllerian duct anomalies result from nondevelopment or varying degrees of nonfusion or nonresorption of the Müllerian ducts. These congenital anomalies occur in 1–15% of women. Müllerian duct anomalies are associated with menstrual disorders, infertility and obstetric complications. Renal anomalies (especially agenesis or ectopia) may be present in up to 50% of these patients. Embryologically, the uterus, the upper two thirds of the vagina and the Fallopian tubes are derived from paired Müllerian ducts. At approximately 10 weeks following conception, the ducts migrate caudally and undergo fusion and subsequent canalization. This process may be interrupted at any time. Failure of the ducts to develop leads to various types of uterine, cervical and vaginal agenesis, while absent or incomplete fusion results in didelphys or bicornuate uteri, respectively. In those instances where fusion does occur, but there is absent or incomplete resorption of the septum between the Müllerian duct components, a septate uterus will result.

Evaluation of Müllerian duct anomalies with physical examination and more traditional imaging studies (HSG and US) is often inconclusive. MRI is the most accurate imaging technique for evaluating patients with congenital anomalies, allowing both precise classification and demonstration of associated complications.

Müllerian duct anomalies

The clinical classification of Müllerian duct anomalies follows the guidelines proposed by Buttram and Gibbons/American Fertility Society. The role of imaging is to provide a detailed map of the pelvic anatomy, including the presence and extent of any anomalies. Surgical management in female patients with anatomical anomalies is aimed at preventing endometriosis and preserving fertility.

Class I: Müllerian agenesis or hypoplasia

Uterine agenesis or hypoplasia results from nondevelopment or rudimentary development of the Müllerian ducts.

A subtype of uterine agenesis is the Mayer–Rokitansky–Kuster–Hauser (MRKH) syndrome. In this syndrome, the presence of vaginal agenesis or hypoplasia with intact ovaries and Fallopian tubes is accompanied by variable anomalies of the uterus, urinary tract and skeletal system. Uterine remnants may be present. Patients with this malformation benefit from US as well as MRI. On MR images the absence or anomalies of the uterus and upper vagina, with varying degrees of development of the lower vagina, is reliably detected on a combination of sagittal and axial images (Fig. 54.6). Normal ovaries are usually present. Uterine hypoplasia is diagnosed when the uterus is small, the endometrium is atrophic and on T2-weighted MR images the myometrium is of lower than normal signal intensity.

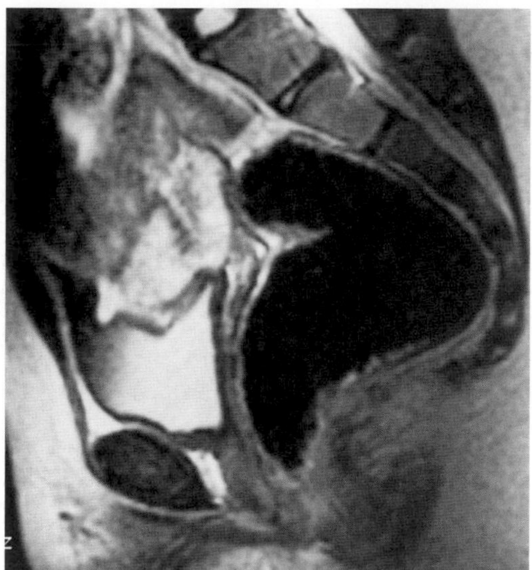

Figure 54.6 Absence of the uterus. Sagittal T2-weighted MRI shows no uterine tissue.

Class II: Unicornuate uterus

The unicornuate uterus results from nondevelopment or rudimentary development of one Müllerian duct. The other Müllerian duct is fully developed and demonstrates a 'banana-like' configuration. The role of imaging is to demonstrate:

1 the presence or absence of a rudimentary horn
2 whether or not the rudimentary horn contains endometrium
3 whether or not the rudimentary horn communicates with the main uterine cavity.

Patients with a rudimentary horn communicating with the uterine cavity might benefit from surgical removal of this rudimentary horn. On T2-weighted MR images, unicornuate uterus demonstrates a curved, elongated uterus with tapering of the fundal segment off midline (the 'banana-like' configuration). Normal uterine zonal anatomy is maintained. The rudimentary horn, when present, usually demonstrates lower signal intensity.

Class III: Uterus didelphys

Uterus didelphys results from nonfusion of the two Müllerian ducts. Two separate normal-sized uterine horns and cervices are demonstrated on T2-weighted MR images. A longitudinal vaginal septum is present in 75% of cases, occasionally complicated by transverse septa causing obstruction. The two uterine horns are usually widely separated, with preservation of the endometrial and myometrial widths. An oblique plane of imaging parallel to the long axis of the uterus is useful to delineate the uterus, whereas the axial oblique plane is useful to delineate the vaginal septum. Haemorrhage in the obstructed segment is best seen on T1-weighted images.

Class IV: Bicornuate uterus

Partial fusion of the Müllerian ducts results in the bicornuate uterus (Figs 54.7, 54.8). There is incomplete fusion of the cephalad extent of the uterovaginal horns with resorption of the uterovaginal septum. MRI shows uterine horns separated by an intervening cleft longer than 1 cm, in the external fundal myometrium. Normal zonal anatomy is seen in each horn and there is a dividing septum composed of myometrium.

Class V: Septate uterus

A septate uterus is seen when there is incomplete resorption of the final fibrous septum between the two uterine horns.

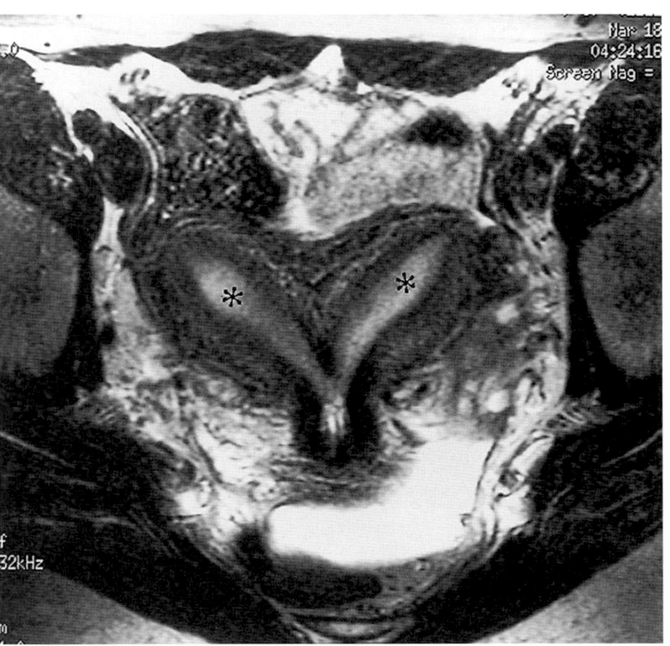

Figure 54.7 Uterus bicornuate. Coronal T2-weighted MRI demonstrating two endometrial canals (*).

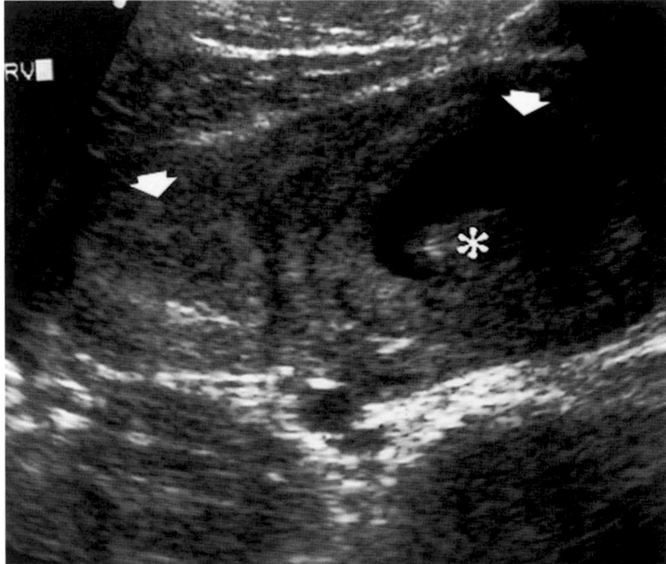

Figure 54.8 Bicornuate uterus with pregnancy in one horn. Transverse transvaginal US shows two endometrial cavities (arrows) in a patient with a bicornuate uterus. A living fetus (*) was noted in the left horn.

The septum may be partial, or it may be complete and extend to the external cervical os. The differentiation between the septate and the bicornuate uterus is clinically important. The septate uterus is associated with a higher rate of reproductive complications, with only 3% of pregnancies delivered at term. Lacking the necessary blood supply, the collagenous septum in the septate uterus cannot support a pregnancy as well as the myometrial septum in the bicornuate uterus. The abortion rate in patients with a septate uterus is twice that of patients with a bicornuate uterus. When clinically warranted, the dividing septum can be removed hysteroscopically. T2-weighted MR images taken parallel to the long axis of the uterus demonstrate a convex, flat, or concave (< 1 cm) external uterine contour and the presence of the fibrous septa[1].

Vaginal anomalies

A number of anomalies have been found in vaginas that have not developed normally. Vaginal anomalies may be categorized as follows.

Congenital absence of the Müllerian ducts (vaginal aplasia, MRKH syndrome)

The pathophysiology of vaginal absence may be either a result of failure of the vaginal plate to form, or failure of cavitation. Absence of the uterus and Fallopian tubes indicates total failure of Müllerian duct development and is known as a Mayer–Rokitansky–Kuster–Hauser (MRKH) syndrome. The presence of vaginal agenesis or hypoplasia with intact ovaries and Fallopian tubes is accompanied by variable anomalies of the uterus, urinary tract and skeletal system (Fig. 54.9). (See above section on Müllerian duct anomalies for further discussion of MRKH syndrome.)

Disorder of vertical fusion

The transverse vaginal septum prevents loss of menstrual blood and results in haematocolpos. Most patients present as teenagers with cyclical abdominal pain and a haematocolpos might be palpable within the pelvis (Fig. 54.10). In these patients a careful pelvic examination and US are helpful for diagnosis. On MRI, T2-weighted images show dilatation of the vagina with intraluminal fluid of intermediate or high signal intensity and the occasional presence of fluid/debris levels. The lower third of the vagina is replaced by low signal intensity fibrous tissue with loss of normal zonal anatomy. T1-weighted images with fat suppression confirm blood products in haematometrocolpos and associated endometriosis if present.

Disorder of lateral fusion

These patients often present with the incidental finding of a vaginal septum that is usually asymptomatic. It may first be diagnosed during pregnancy and excision will be necessary to ensure a vaginal delivery. This malformation may be missed if careful examination is not performed.

INFERTILITY

Imaging plays an important role in the evaluation of infertility. In this section we describe the use of imaging in patients

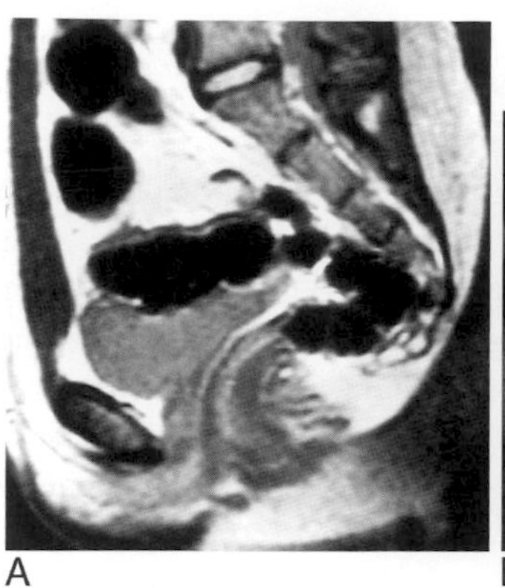

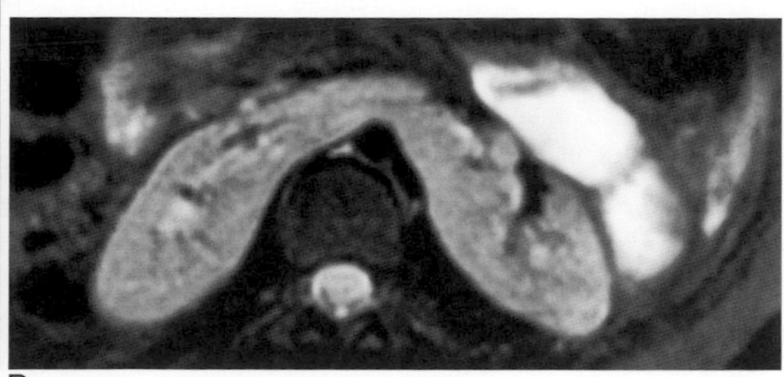

Figure 54.9 Uterine hypoplasia, horseshoe kidney. The sagittal T2-weighted MRI shows a hypoplastic uterus (A), without zonal architecture. On the axial image a horseshoe kidney is shown (B).

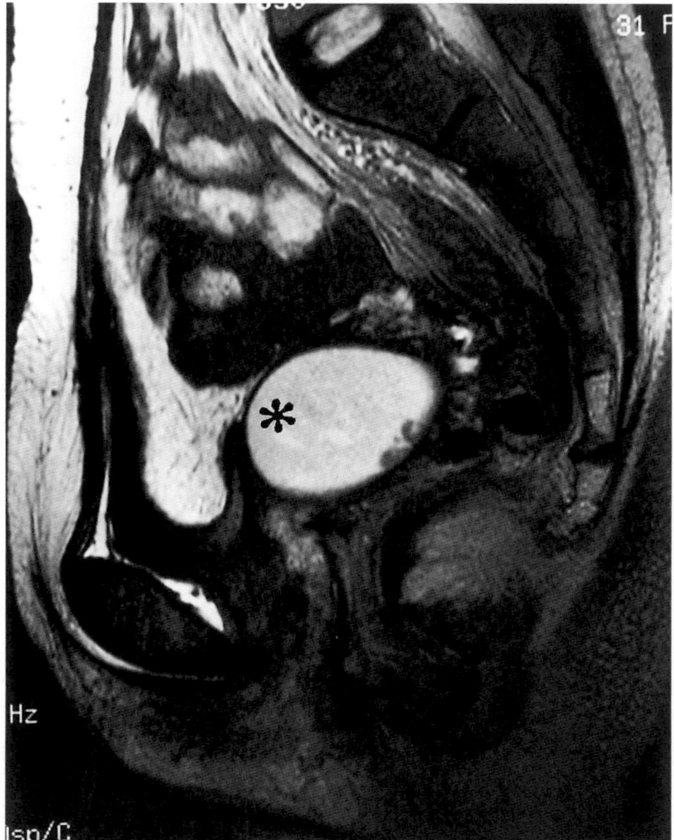

Figure 54.10 Vaginal septum. Sagittal T2-weighed MRI shows the presence of hematometra(*) caused by a transverse vaginal septum.

undergoing modern infertility treatments. The success of in vitro fertilization (IVF) has been due in part to the correct timing of ovulation and subsequent oocyte recovery that US can provide. Using transabdominal US, ovarian follicles of 3–5 mm diameter can be visualized. They appear as echo-free structures amidst the more echogenic ovarian tissue. Their rate of growth is linear and the mean diameter before ovulation is 20.2 mm (range 8–42 mm). Structures within the follicle such as the cumulus oophorus can also be visualized. Following ovulation, internal echoes appear because of bleeding. Free fluid may also be observed in the pouch of Douglas. Transvaginal US has largely replaced the transabdominal approach in infertility practice. Follicular aspiration is possible with a needle-guide attachment to the vaginal probe, as is fine needle aspiration of fluid in the pouch of Douglas. A more precise measurement of follicular size is possible and the corpus luteum is easily recognized. US is also useful for accurate timing of artificial insemination, while a postcoital test can help differentiate between inadequate sperm penetration and poor mucus production in the presence of immature follicles.

Ultrasound is also used to monitor patients on clomiphene therapy and there is good correlation between follicular diameters and plasma oestradiol concentrations. The hyperstimulation syndrome is uncommon if gonadotrophin therapy is monitored by US in conjunction with measurements of plasma oestradiol levels. The waveforms of blood flow in vessels supplying the ovaries of women undergoing IVF have also been studied using transvaginal pulsed Doppler US[2]. Certain blood flow patterns may help predict implantation failure.

MRI is valuable in the investigation of infertility where uterine or adnexal pathology is suspected. It provides a particularly high diagnostic yield in patients with dysmenorrhoea and menorrhagia[3], confidently diagnosing leiomyomas, adenomyosis and/or endometriosis. It should be part of the investigation of patients with persistent unexplained infertility awaiting costly procedures such as gamete intra-Fallopian transfer (GIFT) and IVF.

PELVIC PAIN

Chronic pelvic pain (CPP) has been described as noncyclic pelvic pain of greater than 6 months' duration that is not relieved by strong analgesics. Common causes of CPP are endometriosis, adenomyosis, leiomyomas, pelvic varices and pelvic inflammatory disease (PID). A detailed discussion of each entity is included under the anatomical area affected (e.g. uterus, adnexa).

Radiological evaluation of women with CPP often includes US and MRI. US (transvaginal and transabdominal) is considered the primary imaging technique in the evaluation of CPP, while MRI is reserved as a problem-solving tool[4].

UTERUS AND CERVIX

Benign uterine conditions

Leiomyoma

Leiomyomas are the most common uterine tumours. These benign tumours are found in up to 40% of women in their reproductive years. They are usually multiple and may be subserosal, intramural, or submucosal in location. Symptoms may be caused by the location of the leiomyoma (e.g. menorrhagia with submucosal leiomyomas) and/or their mass effect (e.g. urinary frequency caused by a large subserosal leiomyoma).

Hysterectomy has been the traditional primary treatment for debilitating leiomyomas. While hysterectomy is curative, alternative uterine-sparing procedures may be appropriate for some patients. Specifically, myomectomy has been successfully performed for many years and, more recently, transcatheter uterine arterial embolization (UAE) is being used as an alternative, less invasive therapy for symptomatic leiomyomas. Another recent, minimally invasive treatment is MR-guided high intensity focused ultrasound ablation. Diagnostic ultrasound is often the initial radiological evaluation in these patients, while MRI is usually reserved for patients with inconclusive US results or patients undergoing myomectomy, uterine embolization, or MR-guided focused ultrasound ablation. In all of these situations, MR is used to assist in appropriate selection of patients for UAE[5].

Ultrasound In most cases, US can accurately detect leiomyomas and distinguish them from extrauterine disease. Twenty per cent of small leiomyomas may be occult by ultrasound. The myomatous uterus is typically enlarged and its outline may be irregular or lobular. The most common appearance of a leiomyoma is that of a well-marginated, hypoechoic, rounded and/or oval mass within the uterine body. Depending on the proportion of smooth muscle, fibrosis and degeneration present within the myoma, the appearance may range from hypoechoic to echogenic, homogenous to heterogeneous, with or without acoustic shadowing (Fig. 54.11). Calcification when present appears as shadowing echogenic foci.

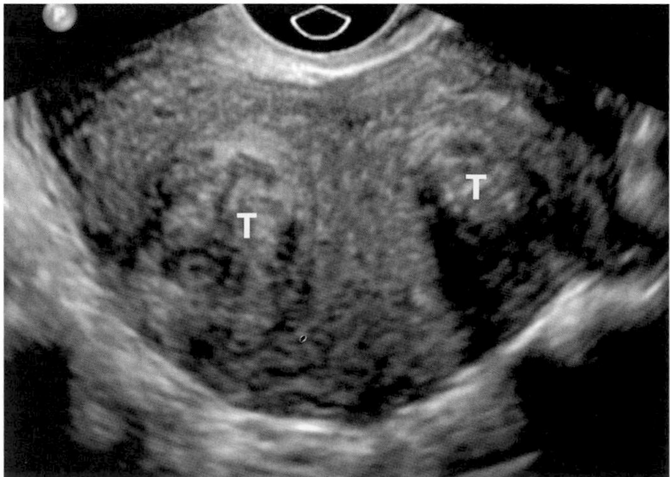

Figure 54.11 Leiomyoma, transvaginal US. Transvaginal US demonstrating hypo- to isoechoic well-defined intramural heterogeneous masses (T), the typical ultrasound appearance of leiomyomas.

Distortion of the endometrial complex is helpful in identifying a submucosal component and associated menorrhagia may cause a prominent endometrial echo. Submucosal leiomyomas may mimic endometrial lesions and US HSG may aid in making the final diagnosis, particularly in the case of a pedunculated or intracavitary leiomyoma. Special care should be taken when evaluating a pregnancy within a leiomyomatous uterus, as multiple leiomyomas increase the frequency of malposition, retained placenta and premature uterine contractions. In addition, because of hormonal influence, leiomyomas can grow during pregnancy, further compromising the fetus.

Magnetic resonance imaging is indicated when the US examination is indeterminate or limited. It allows precise determination of the size, location and number of leiomyomas. It is also very useful in differentiating a pedunculated subserosal leiomyoma from an adnexal mass[5]. MRI may help select patients for invasive treatment (myomectomy versus UAE versus hysterectomy). Additionally, MRI may be useful to monitor the success of UAE and assess its durability. The effects of hormonal therapy on leiomyomas can also be monitored.

MRI is the most accurate noninvasive diagnostic imaging investigation available so far for differentiation of a leiomyoma from adenomyosis[6]. This distinction impacts clinical management, as an accepted surgical treatment of a leiomyoma is myomectomy, whereas standard treatment of debilitating adenomyosis is hysterectomy.

On T1-weighted images, leiomyomas most commonly present as well-circumscribed, rounded lesions with intermediate signal intensity, often indistinguishable from adjacent myometrium. Optimum contrast is achieved on T2-weighted images, where the tumour is of lower signal intensity relative to the myometrium or endometrium (Fig. 54.12). The presence of calcification usually results in areas of signal void on both T1- and T2-weighted images; however, on MRI, signal void can also be produced by fast flowing blood and therefore is not as specific for calcification as it is on CT. A variety of degenerative processes can alter the characteristic appearance of a leiomyoma, making differential diagnosis more difficult. Following administration of IV contrast medium, most leiomyomas enhance less than adjacent myometrium, whereas degenerated areas may not enhance. Fat saturation T1-weighted images may be helpful in cases of haemorrhagic degeneration[5,6].

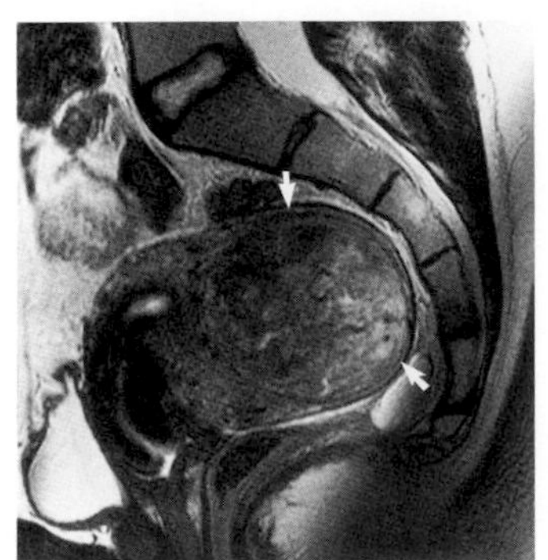

Figure 54.12 Leiomyoma, MRI. T2-weighted sagittal MRI. A subserosal leiomyoma (arrows) distends the posterior aspect of the uterus, displacing the endometrium.

Computed tomography Leiomyomas are usually an incidental finding during CT performed for other reasons. CT is not recommended for the evaluation of leiomyomas. Leiomyomas usually have a soft tissue density similar to that of normal myometrium, although necrosis or degeneration may result in low attenuation. On CT, while a contour deformity is the most common sign of a uterine leiomyoma, calcification is the most specific finding for a leiomyoma.

Hysterosalpingography Submucosal leiomyomas are particularly likely to cause distortion of the uterine cavity, whereas subserosal and small intramural leiomyomas are often associated with normal hysterographic findings. A single leiomyoma will cause a smooth and rounded filling defect on the uterine contour (Fig. 54.13). Multiple submucosal leiomyomas are associated with separate filling defects and sometimes gross distortion of the uterine cavity. HSG is no longer recommended for the evaluation of submucosal leiomyomas.

Adenomyosis

Adenomyosis is the presence of endometrial tissue within the myometrium and secondary smooth muscle hypertrophy/hyperplasia. It can be diffuse or focal. The most frequent symptoms are dysmenorrhoea and dysfunctional uterine bleeding. It is found in 15–27% of hysterectomy specimens, with an increased incidence in multiparous women. Transvaginal US is the initial imaging investigation, with MRI being reserved for indeterminate cases or those undergoing uterus-sparing surgery[6,7]. Pitfalls in the diagnosis of uterine adenomyosis include leiomyoma, endometrial carcinoma and myometrial contractions[8].

Ultrasound Transvaginal US has an accuracy of 68–86% in the diagnosis of diffuse adenomyosis. Typically, the uterus assumes an enlarged but globular configuration, often with antero-posterior asymmetry. Myometrial heterogeneity is related to the presence of endometrial implants and intervening smooth muscle hypertrophy. The implants present as diffuse echogenic nodules, subendometrial echogenic linear striations and nodules and 2–6 mm subendometrial cysts (present in 50% of cases) which represent haemorrhage within the implants. Other ultrasound features of adenomyosis include endometrial pseudowidening, poor definition of the endomyometrial junction and multiple fine areas of attenuation throughout the lesion—the 'rain shower' appearance. Colour Doppler examination demonstrates a speckled pattern of increased vascularity within the heterogeneous area[8]. While the diagnosis of diffuse adenomyosis can be suggested on transvaginal US, the findings of focal adenomyosis are hard to distinguish from leiomyoma. Because the findings may be subtle, real time or video evaluation (as opposed to static images) of women suspected of adenomyosis may be the key to making the diagnosis.

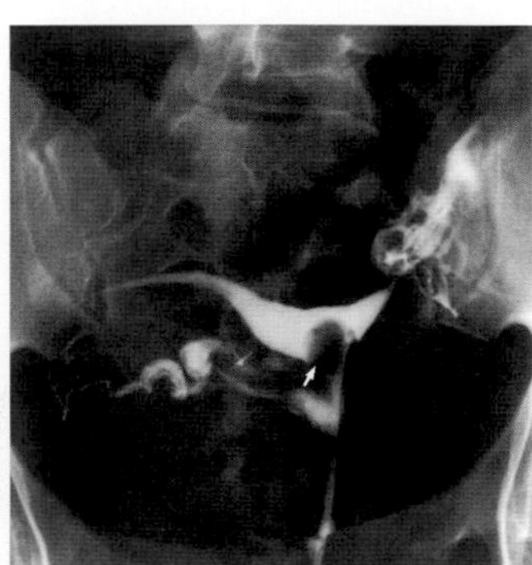

Figure 54.13 Leiomyoma, hysterosalpingogram. A submucosal leiomyoma presents as filling defect (arrow).

Magnetic resonance imaging On T2-weighted MRI, adenomyosis appears as areas of low myometrial signal intensity, which presents as focal or diffuse thickening of the JZ (Fig 54.14). When diffuse, a widened low intensity JZ >12 mm *diagnoses* disease with high accuracy, while a JZ <8 mm *excludes* disease with high accuracy. For indeterminate cases (JZ 8–12 mm), ancillary criteria are used. These include the presence of high signal intensity linear striations (finger-like projections) extending out from endometrium into myometrium on T2-weighted images and high signal intensity foci on T1-weighted images. These foci are believed to represent endometrial rests and/or small punctate haemorrhages[6,7].

Endometrial polyps

Benign endometrial polyps are common in the endometrial cavity at all ages, with their greatest prevalence after age 50. They consist of stromal cores with mucosal surfaces projecting above the level of the adjacent endometrium. Endometrial polyps must be differentiated from submucosal leiomyomas and malignant neoplasms. Pelvic US often does not reveal endometrial polyps. While MRI is diagnostic, it is rarely employed because of high cost. US HSG is highly accurate in detecting endometrial polyps, even in the setting of endometrial hyperplasia, but differentiating a broad-based polyp from a submucosal fibroid may be problematic. Polyps are typically isoechoic to and continuous with the endometrium and preserve the endomyometrial interface. They are usually homogeneous but may be centrally cystic. Colour Doppler may reveal a characteristic feeding vessel. Outpatient hysteroscopy is the technique of choice for their diagnosis.

Endometrial hyperplasia

Endometrial hyperplasia may be subdivided into cystic hyperplasia (simple), adenomatous hyperplasia (complex) and atypical hyperplasia. The main presentations are abnormal uterine bleeding, infertility and postmenopausal bleeding. The important practical considerations in the natural history of endometrial hyperplasia are coexisting endometrial carcinomas, coexisting ovarian carcinomas and the risk of progression to endometrial carcinoma. The main objective of investigating a woman found to have endometrial hyperplasia is to exclude invasive endometrial cancer or ovarian cancer. If endometrial hyperplasia has been diagnosed using an outpatient biopsy instrument, a formal examination under anaesthesia, hysteroscopy and curettage are required to palpate the adnexa and explore the endometrial and endocervical cavities.

US evaluation might reveal endometrial thickening, which may be due to endometrial hyperplasia, polyps, or carcinoma. In postmenopausal women, the threshold value for serious endometrial abnormalities on transvaginal US is 5 mm. Although there is no reliable threshold value for premenopausal

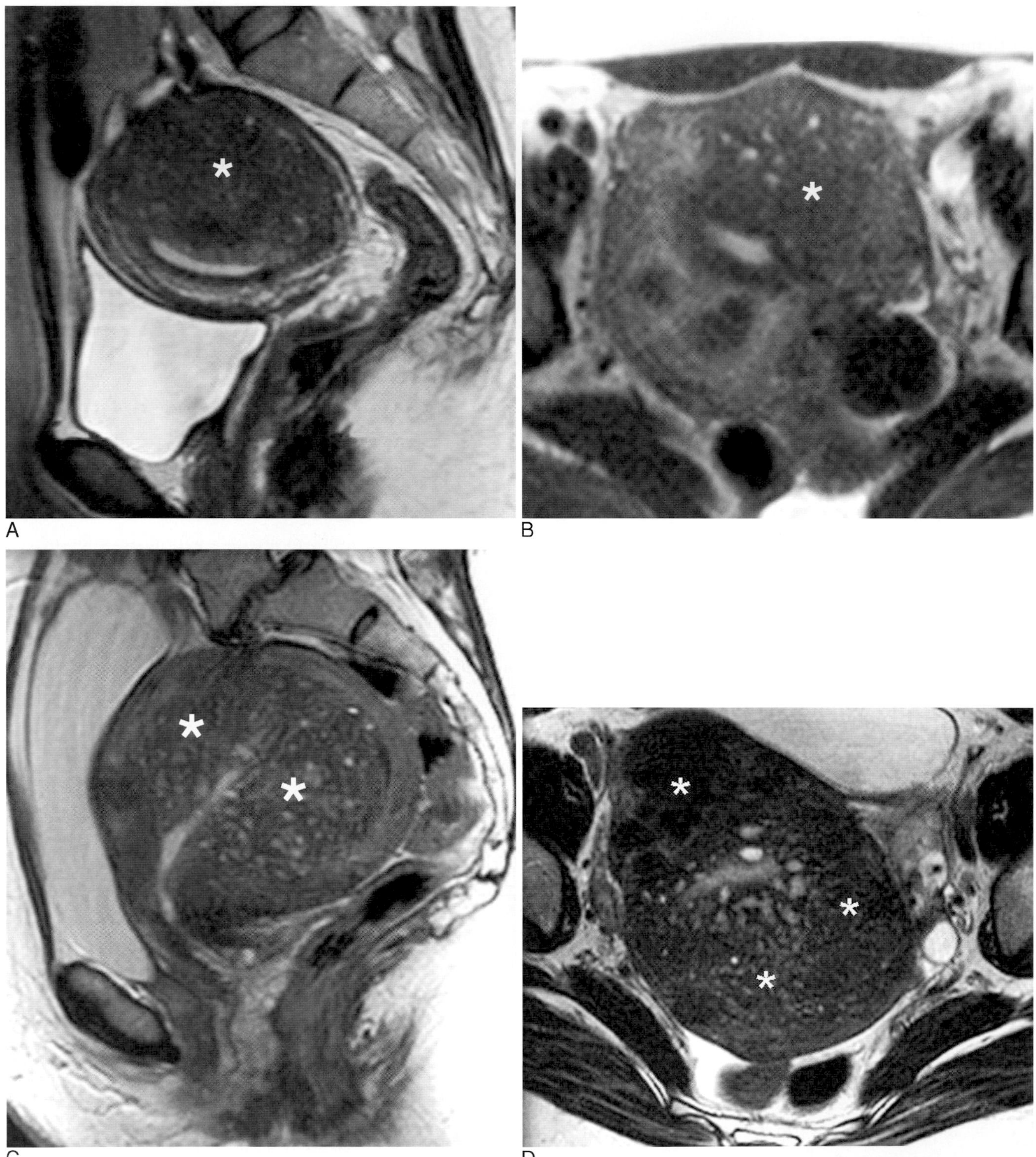

Figure 54.14 MRI, adenomyosis. Sagittal (A) and axial (B) T2-weighted MR images through the pelvis demonstrate focal junctional zone widening and multiple punctate high signal intensity foci with the areas of thickening (*, A, B) characteristic of focal adenomyosis. Sagittal (C) and axial (D) T2-weighted MR images in a different patient demonstrate widening of the entire junctional zone (*, C, D) which contains multiple foci of high signal intensity that represent endometrial rests. Appearances are typical of diffuse adenomyosis.

women, limited data in the literature suggest that endometrial thickness greater than 8 mm during the proliferative phase, or greater than 16 mm during the secretory phase, is abnormal. On US HSG endometrial hyperplasia presents as focal or, more commonly, diffuse endometrial thickening without a localized mass or abnormality. Because secretory phase endometrium may mimic hyperplasia, the timing of sonohysterography is essential to making or excluding the diagnosis. The focal form of hyperplasia may be difficult to distinguish from a broad-based polyp.

Endometrial hyperplasia usually presents as diffuse thickening of the endometrial stripe on T2-weighted images. The signal intensity of the endometrial stripe is isointense or slightly hypointense relative to normal endometrium. However, these

MRI characteristics are nonspecific and are also seen with endometrial carcinoma.

Uterine infections

Uterine infections most often occur in the puerperium. Endometritis might also be caused by septic abortion or postoperatively. Pyometra may occur in patients with cervical stenosis due to carcinoma of the cervix or following radiotherapy, or as a complication of endometritis (Fig. 54.15). The distended uterus may be identified on US or cross-sectional studies. The uniform thick-walled appearance of the distended uterus and failure to identify the uterus as a separate structure should differentiate the appearances from a pelvic abscess.

Cervical incompetence

Cervical incompetence is responsible for approximately 15% of second- and third-trimester abortions. Primary incompetence may be congenital, associated with diethylstilbestrol exposure, or caused by reduced collagen within the cervix. Secondary incompetence usually results from multiple gestations, gynaecologic/obstetric trauma, or increased prostaglandin production. US is currently the investigation of choice for diagnosing cervical incompetence during pregnancy.

A number of US parameters have been described to indicate cervical incompetence. Shortening of the cervix in the absence of any other changes may not alter the prognosis. The cervical length in normal pregnancy should measure more than 3 cm. The width of the cervical canal is by far the most reliable parameter to predict cervical incompetence and should measure less than 2 cm in the second trimester. If bulging of membranes into the cervical canal is seen, the prognosis is unfavourable[9]. US criteria for diagnosing cervical incompetence have not been established in the nongravid patient.

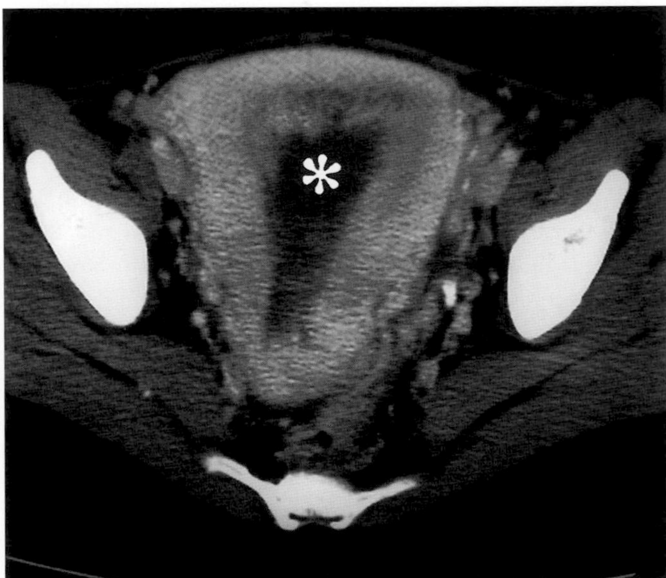

Figure 54.15 Pyometra. Helical CT shows a distended fluid-filled endometrial canal (*) in a postpartum patient with endometritis and pyometra. Without the presence of gas, it may be impossible to differentiate a pyometra from a hydrometra.

MRI offers the potential to diagnose cervical incompetence in the nonpregnant as well as the pregnant patient. Four MRI findings have been described as suggestive of cervical incompetence[10]:

- shortening of the endocervical canal (< 3 cm)
- widening of the internal cervical os (> 4 mm)
- asymmetric widening of the endocervical canal
- thinning or absence of the low signal intensity cervical stroma.

When one or more of these findings are present, cervical incompetence should be suspected.

Malignant uterine conditions

Endometrial carcinoma

Endometrial carcinoma is the fourth most common female cancer and the most common malignancy of the female reproductive tract. Due to earlier diagnosis and treatment advances, its overall mortality has decreased by 28% over the last two decades. Presenting as postmenopausal bleeding, the disease occurs most frequently in white women, with a peak incidence between the ages of 55 and 65 years. Risk factors include unopposed oestrogen intake, nulliparity, obesity, diabetes and polycystic ovarian syndrome. The prognosis of endometrial carcinoma depends on a number of factors, including stage, depth of myometrial invasion, nodal status and grade. Preoperative evaluation of prognostic factors helps in subspecialist treatment planning.

Detection, diagnosis and staging Endometrial carcinomas are typically diagnosed at endometrial biopsy or dilatation and curettage, with imaging being reserved to evaluate extent of disease. Imaging criteria for staging of endometrial cancer are based on the TNM/FIGO classification (Table 54.1).

Ultrasound Transvaginal US is superior to transabdominal US for imaging endometrial abnormalities[11]. The most common appearance of endometrial cancer is nonspecific thickening of the endometrium. While this thickening is indistinguishable from that found with hyperplasia or polyp, the diagnosis of endometrial cancer should be considered when the endometrial/myometrial junction is disrupted or the endometrial surface is irregular (Fig. 54.16). In postmenopausal women, the threshold value for serious endometrial abnormalities (i.e. endometrial carcinoma, atypical hyperplasia, or complex hyperplasia) is 5 mm. In sonohysterosalpingography, endometrial cancer may appear as an intracavitary polyp or as asymmetric thickening of the endometrial lining. Doppler and colour US have been advocated to improve endometrial carcinoma detection.

The use of US is limited to the evaluation of stage I disease with emphasis on the evaluation of the depth of myometrial invasion. For evaluation of myometrial invasion, the presence and continuity of the hypoechoic halo that surrounds the outer layer of the endometrium is assessed (i.e. intact, focally disrupted, or totally disrupted). The extent of myometrial invasion is then estimated by measuring the distance from the central lumen of the uterus to the distal junction between tumour and normal myometrium.

Table 54.1 TNM AND FIGO CLASSIFICATION FOR ENDOMETRIAL CARCINOMA

TNM	FIGO	Uterus
Tis	0	Carcinoma in situ
T1	I	Limited to the uterus
T1a	Ia	Tumour limited to endometrium
T1b	Ib	Invasion less than or equal to half of the myometrium
T1c	Ic	Invasion greater than half of the myometrium
T2	II	Invasion of cervix, but not beyond the uterus
T2a	IIA	Endocervical glandular involvement
T2b	IIB	Cervical stromal invasion
T3 and/or N1	III	Local and/or regional spread
T3a	IIIA	Tumour involves the serosa and/or adnexa and/or positive peritoneal cytology
T3b	IIIB	Vaginal involvement
T3c	IIIC	Metastatic to pelvic and/or para-aortic nodes
T4	IV	Tumour extends outside pelvis or invades bladder or rectal mucosa
T4a	IVA	Tumour invades bladder and/or bowel mucosa
M1	IVB	Distant metastasis

Computed tomography High quality pelvic CT in patients with endometrial carcinoma requires good bowel opacification. Prolonged oral and IV contrast medium are mandatory. The use of rectal contrast is optimal. The use of IV contrast serves to enhance normal myometrium and to delineate endometrial and myometrial tumours. On contrast-enhanced CT, endometrial tumour is seen as a hypodense mass relative to normal myometrium.

CT, especially MDCT, has been used for the staging of endometrial cancer. Its greatest clinical impact is in confirming parametrial and sidewall extension in stage III tumours and in detecting pelvic lymphadenopathy. Limitations of CT include a tendency to understage endometrial carcinoma because of failure to detect bowel or bladder invasion and cervical extension of the tumour.

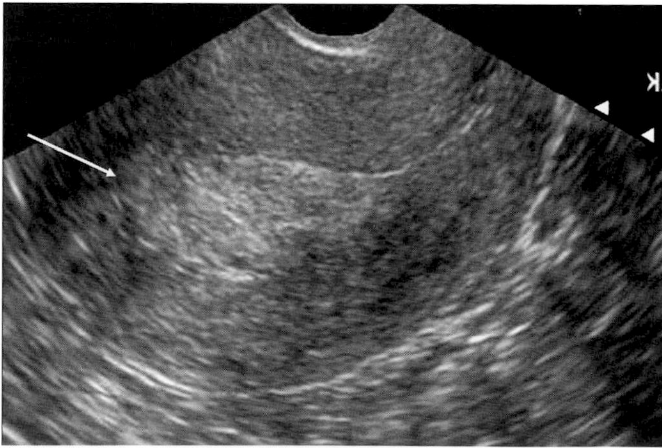

Figure 54.16 Endometrial carcinoma, transvaginal US. The endometrium is thickened and irregular in this postmenopausal patient. Near the fundus, the endometrial–myometrial junction is indistinct, indicating myometrial invasion (arrow).

Magnetic resonance imaging Dynamic contrast-enhanced MR (CEMR) imaging offers a 'one-stop' examination with the highest efficacy for pre-treatment evaluation in patients with endometrial cancer[12]. The MRI protocol includes T1-weighted axial images with a large field of view (FOV) to evaluate the entire pelvis for lymphadenopathy, T2-weighted images (small FOV) in the axial and sagittal planes and dynamic contrast-enhanced T1-weighted images (small FOV) in the sagittal and axial planes to evaluate local disease. On unenhanced T1-weighted images, endometrial carcinoma is isointense with the normal endometrium. Although endometrial cancer may demonstrate high signal intensity on T2-weighted sequences, it is more typically heterogeneous and may even be of low signal intensity. Routine use of dynamic IV contrast enhancement is necessary for state-of-the-art MR evaluation of endometrial carcinoma[12]. Following IV contrast medium administration, there is early avid enhancement of normal myometrium. Endometrial cancer enhances slower than the adjacent myometrium allowing identification of small tumours, even those contained by the endometrium. In the later phases of enhancement, tumour appears hypointense relative to the myometrium (Fig. 54.17).

MRI is significantly superior to US and CT in the evaluation of both tumour extension into the cervix and myometrial invasion. The overall staging accuracy of MRI has been reported to be between 85 and 93%. Stage I endometrial cancers include tumours confined to the corpus. Stage IA tumours (limited to endometrium) appear as a normal or widened (focal or diffuse) endometrium. An intact JZ and a band of early subendometrial enhancement (SEE) exclude deep myometrial invasion. Regardless of sequence, the tumour–myometrium interface is smooth and sharp. In stage IB disease, tumour extends less than 50% into the myometrium with associated disruption or irregularity of the JZ and SEE. If these landmarks are not present, stage IB tumour is suggested by an irregular tumour–myometrium interface. The presence of low

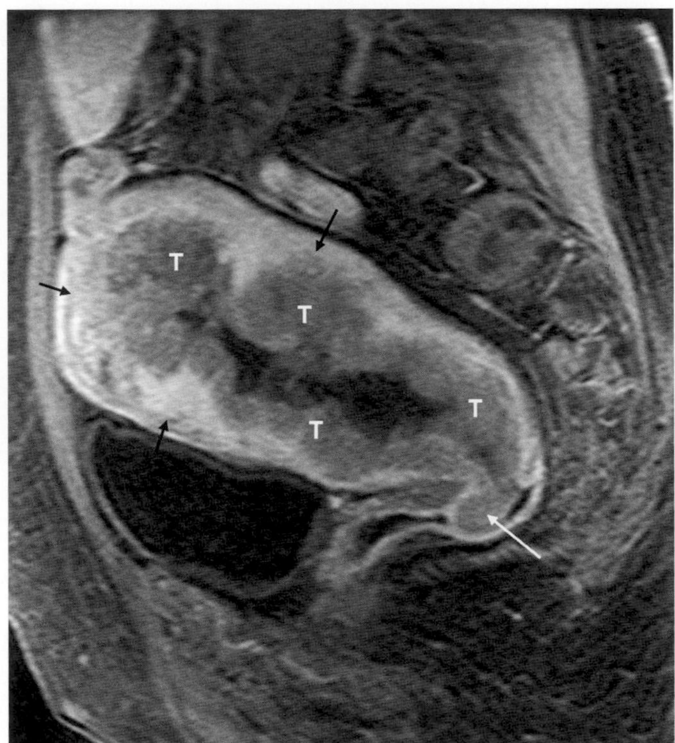

Figure 54.17 Endometrial carcinoma, MRI. Sagittal gadolinium-enhanced T1-weighted fat-suppressed MR image shows an endometrial cancer (T) with deep myometrial invasion. Note the thin rim of normal myometrium (black arrows). The disease extends to the upper third of the vagina (white arrow).

signal intensity tumour (later phases of enhancement) within the outer myometrium or beyond indicates deep myometrial invasion—stage IC disease.

Stage II includes tumour extension beyond the uterine corpus into the cervix. In stage IIA, invasion of the endocervix appears as widening of the internal os and endocervical canal with preservation of the normal low signal intensity fibrocervical stroma. Disruption of the fibrocervical stroma by high signal intensity tumour on T2-weighted images, together with disruption of normal enhancement of the cervical mucosa by low signal intensity tumour on early dynamic CEMR, indicate cervical invasion—stage IIB disease.

In stage III disease, tumour extends outside the uterus but not the true pelvis. Parametrial involvement—stage IIIA—appears as disruption of the serosa with direct extension into the surrounding parametrial fat. In stage IIIB disease, tumour extends into the upper vagina and there is segmental loss of the low signal intensity vaginal wall. In stage IIIC disease, lymphadenopathy is present. Stage IV disease is tumour that extends beyond the true pelvis or invades the bladder or rectum.

Recommended imaging approach US, especially transvaginal US, is often considered to be the primary imaging approach. The role of MRI in the work-up of a patient with endometrial malignancy includes the assessment of the depth of myometrial invasion and the accurate determination of stage in patients with an equivocal pelvic examination or a medical contraindication to surgical staging. CT is very useful in screening for lymphatic or peritoneal metastases in patients with a poorly differentiated carcinoma or sarcoma and for confirmation of stage III or stage IV disease. PET imaging is promising in the post-treatment surveillance of endometrial cancer patients[13].

Impact of imaging on treatment Endometrial cancer primarily presents at stage I (80% of cases), for which the standard treatment is total abdominal hysterectomy and bilateral salpingo-oophorectomy. The major diagnostic factors necessary for the preoperative evaluation of endometrial cancer are as follows:

1 Differentiation between stages IA and IB; this is becoming critical with increased use of medical (hormonal) treatment for stage IA disease.
2 Determination of the risk of lymph node metastasis in order to have skilled surgical consultation available (i.e. retroperitoneal lymph node sampling may be indicated). Differentiation of stage IB from stage IC has prognostic as well as morbidity implications, as stage IB patients would undergo lymph node sampling whereas stage IC patients would undergo radical lymph node surgical resection.
3 Diagnosing gross cervical invasion, which requires preoperative radiation therapy or a different treatment plan, i.e. radical hysterectomy instead of total abdominal hysterectomy.

In summary, the role of imaging is to depict noninvasively the depth of myometrial invasion and the presence of lymphadenopathy and to stage the tumour extent before treatment planning.

Uterine sarcomas (leiomyosarcomas, endometrial sarcomas, malignant mixed Müllerian tumours)

Sarcomas of the uterus are often highly malignant. They are rare, with an incidence of approximately 2 per 100 000 women over the age of 20 and account for 3–5% of all uterine cancers. Leiomyosarcomas show an extremely bizarre US configuration. The tumours are frequently very large at the time of the examination and it is difficult to determine the primary origin of the mass. MRI can provide an accurate preoperative assessment of uterine size and degree of involvement. Because uterine sarcomas commonly metastasize to the lung, chest CT should be considered for staging purposes.

Gestational trophoblastic disease

Gestational trophoblastic neoplasms include the tumour spectrum of hydatidiform mole, invasive mole (choriocarcinoma destruens) and choriocarcinoma. They arise from fetal tissue within the maternal host and are composed of both syncytiotrophoblastic and cytotrophoblastic cells. In addition to being the first and only disseminated solid tumours that have proved to be highly curable by chemotherapy, they elaborate a unique and characteristic tumour marker—human chorionic gonadotropin (hCG).

The role of imaging in gestational trophoblastic disease (GTD) has been primarily to document metastatic disease at initial diagnosis or to evaluate persistent disease. As yet, there are no specific imaging findings that allow differentiation of complete mole from invasive mole or choriocarcinoma.

Ultrasound The US appearance of GTD is most commonly a large-for-gestational-age uterus with an echogenic soft tissue mass distending the endometrial canal, punctuated by multiple small cystic spaces. In cases of complete hydatidiform mole, the small spaces correspond to the hydropic villi (Fig. 54.18)[14]. Although US has been used for the initial diagnosis of GTD and to exclude a normal intrauterine pregnancy, the findings are nonspecific and the diagnosis relies heavily on history and serology.

Computed tomography Uterine enlargement is the most common CT feature of GTD. Following administration of IV contrast medium, uterine enhancement is typically heterogeneous and focal enlargement or irregular hypodense regions may be seen within the myometrium[14]. The extrauterine manifestations of GTD are well seen on CT. Adnexal findings include bilateral ovarian enlargement by multilocular, theca lutein cysts. Locoregional spread is characterized by enhancing soft tissue density in the parametria and/or obliteration of the pelvic fat or muscle planes.

Magnetic resonance imaging On T2-weighted images, GTD is seen as a heterogeneous, predominantly high signal intensity mass that obliterates normal uterine zonal anatomy[14,15]. On T1-weighted images, it may be iso- or hyperintense to adjacent myometrium. The tumours are hypervascular and enlarged vessels in the broad ligament and the uterus are depicted as signal voids on both T1- and T2-weighted images. The tumours avidly enhance following injection of IV contrast medium.

Carcinoma of the cervix

Cervical cancer is the third most common gynaecological malignancy. Between 1960 and 1990 there was a 63% decrease in cervical cancer mortality. This improvement in mortality has been attributed to the development of the Papanicolaou smear and only minor improvement has been achieved in the survival of invasive cervical cancer. Established risk factors for cervical cancer include early sexual activity (especially with multiple partners), cigarette smoking, immunosuppression and infection with human papilloma viruses 16 and 18. Abnormal uterine bleeding (especially after intercourse) and vaginal discharge may be symptoms leading to the diagnosis. In colposcopy, a lesion may be detected and vaginal cytology is usually positive.

Staging Recommendations for diagnostic evaluation of tumour staging derive from the TNM/FIGO clinical staging system (Table 54.2). Accurate tumour staging is important not only for prognosis, but also in determining appropriate therapy. Among the various prognostic indicators, the most critical include tumour grade, tumour size, depth of stromal invasion, parametrial extension and lymph node involvement. Because of a relatively high likelihood of parametrial invasion and/or lymph node metastases, cross-sectional imaging is recommended in evaluating cervical carcinoma patients with clinical stage IB disease or greater when the primary lesion is larger than 2 cm[16,17].

Imaging techniques for detection, diagnosis and staging

Ultrasound Transabdominal US can show the presence of hydronephrosis but has a limited role in the evaluation of the local extent of cervical cancer. Transrectal and transvaginal US have been used in the assessment of local disease but are limited in the detection of parametrial disease and pelvic sidewall involvement due to poor soft tissue contrast, small FOV and operator dependence. More advanced cervical cancer can be visualized with transvaginal US. The cervix appears as an enlarged, irregular, hypoechoic mass that may mimic a cervical myoma. If tumour obstructs the endocervical canal, hydro- and/or haematometra result.

Computed tomography Typically, CT findings in cervical cancer include enlargement of the cervix. After administration of IV contrast medium, low-attenuation areas may be seen within the tumour. These regions of decreased attenuation are a function of tumour necrosis/ulceration and/or inherent differences in the attenuation between tumour and normal

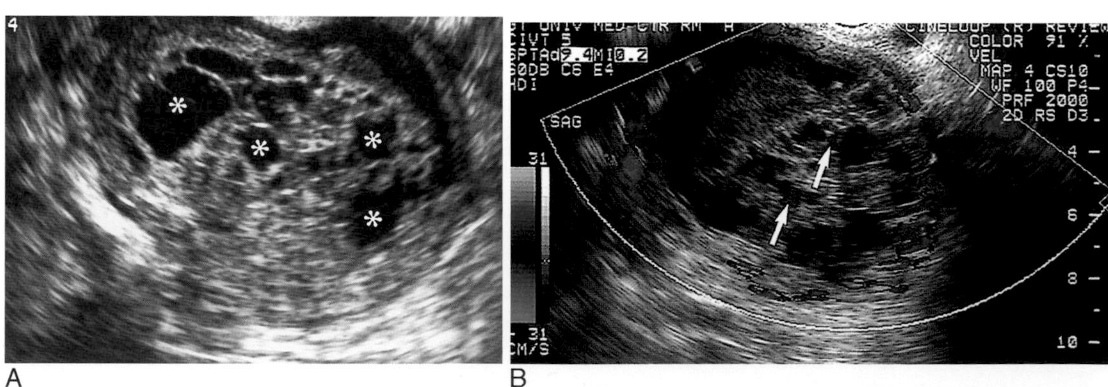

Figure 54.18 Gestational trophoblastic disease. Transverse transvaginal US (A) shows an echogenic mass with multiple cystic spaces within the endometrial cavity in a woman with a hydatidiform mole. The small cystic spaces (*, A) are felt to represent hydropic villi. Sagittal transvaginal US with colour flow (arrows, B) documents flow to the mole. Hydatidiform mole is a subtype of gestational trophoblastic disease.

Table 54.2 TNM AND FIGO CLASSIFICATION FOR CERVICAL NEOPLASM

TNM	FIGO	Cervix
Tis	0	Carcinoma in situ
T1	I	Carcinoma confined to the cervix
T1a	Ia	Invasive carcinoma identified only microscopically
		All gross lesions, even with superficial invasion, are stage Ib cancers
		Measured stromal depth should be no greater than 5 mm and no wider than 7 mm
T1a1	Ia1	Measured invasion no greater than 3 mm in depth and no wider than 7 mm
T1a2	Ia2	Measured invasion greater than 3 mm but no greater than 5 mm in depth and no wider than 7 mm
T1b1	Ib1	Clinical lesions no greater than 4 cm in size
T1b2	Ib2	Clinical lesions confined greater than 4 cm in size
T2	II	Carcinoma extending beyond cervix and involving the vagina (but not to pelvic sidewall or lower third of vagina)
T2a	IIa	Carcinoma has involved the vagina
T2b	IIb	Carcinoma has infiltrated the parametrium
T3	III	Carcinoma involving the lower third of the vagina and/or extending to the pelvic sidewall (there is no free space between the tumour and the pelvic sidewall)
T3a	IIIa	Carcinoma involving the lower third of the vagina
T3b	IIIb	Carcinoma extending to the pelvic wall and/or hydronephrosis or nonfunctioning kidney due to ureterostenosis caused by tumour
T4	IVa	Carcinoma involving the mucosa of the bladder or rectum and/or extending beyond the true pelvis
M1	IVb	Spread to distant organs

cervical tissue. Distinguishing tumour from normal cervix and parametrium may be problematic. Obstruction of the endocervical canal can result in uterine enlargement with a fluid-filled endometrial cavity. There is a consensus in the literature that the value of CT increases with higher stages of disease (Fig. 54.19) and that CT has limited value (a positive predictive value of 58%) in the evaluation of early parametrial invasion. However, CT has an accuracy of 92% in the depiction of advanced disease (Fig. 54.19).

Magnetic resonance imaging can accurately determine tumour location (exophytic or endocervical), tumour size, depth of stromal invasion and extension into the lower uterine segment[17]. MRI is the best single imaging investigation for this purpose, since it is better than either CT or physical examination in demonstrating parametrial invasion and as good as CT in detecting nodal metastases[18]. The staging accuracy of MRI ranges from 75 to 96%. The reported sensitivity of MRI in the evaluation of parametrial invasion is 69% and the specificity is 93%[17,18].

The MR imaging protocol should include T1-weighted axial images with a large FOV to evaluate the entire pelvis for lymphadenopathy and T2-weighted images in the axial and sagittal planes with a small FOV. Use of dynamic contrast-enhanced MRI is optional[16,17].

On T1-weighted images, tumours are usually isointense with the normal cervix and may not be visible. On T2-weighted images, cervical cancer appears as a relatively hyperintense mass and is easily distinguishable from low signal intensity cervical stroma.

Stage I tumours are confined to the uterus. Stage IA is defined as a microinvasive tumour that cannot be demonstrated at MRI. Stage IB carcinoma appears as a high signal intensity mass in contrast to the low signal intensity fibrocervical stroma on T2-weighted images. In stage IIA tumours, segmental disruption of the upper two thirds of the vaginal wall without parametrial invasion is demonstrated on T2-weighted images. The lack of preservation of low signal intensity cervical stroma is highly indicative of parametrial invasion—stage IIB disease (Fig. 54.20). In stage IIIA, vaginal involvement reaches the lower third of the vaginal canal without extending to the pelvic sidewall. When the tumour extends to the pelvic sidewall (pelvic musculature or iliac vessels) or causes hydronephrosis, it is defined as stage IIIB. Once tumour invades the adjacent organs such as the bladder and rectal mucosa, or distant metastasis occurs, the stage is defined as IV. Although pelvic node metastases do not change the FIGO stage, para-aortic or inguinal node metastases are classified as stage IVB.

PET Although the use of PET in the initial evaluation of cervical cancer is still under investigation, PET can be used to assess nodal disease and tumour recurrence. In the detection of metastatic lymph nodes in patients with cervical cancer, PET has been reported to have a sensitivity of 91% and a specificity of 100%, which are higher than the sensitivity (73%) and specificity (83%) of MRI[19]. PET has added value in patients with recurrent cervical cancer who undergo salvage therapy, as it can provide precise re-staging information.

Recommended imaging approach Transvaginal US has poor soft tissue contrast and thus limited value in cervical cancer detection and in the determination of stromal invasion or parametrial extension. Multidetector contrast-enhanced CT may be helpful in local staging; however, it is mainly used in advanced disease and in the assessment of lymph nodes. CT is also performed to detect distant metastases

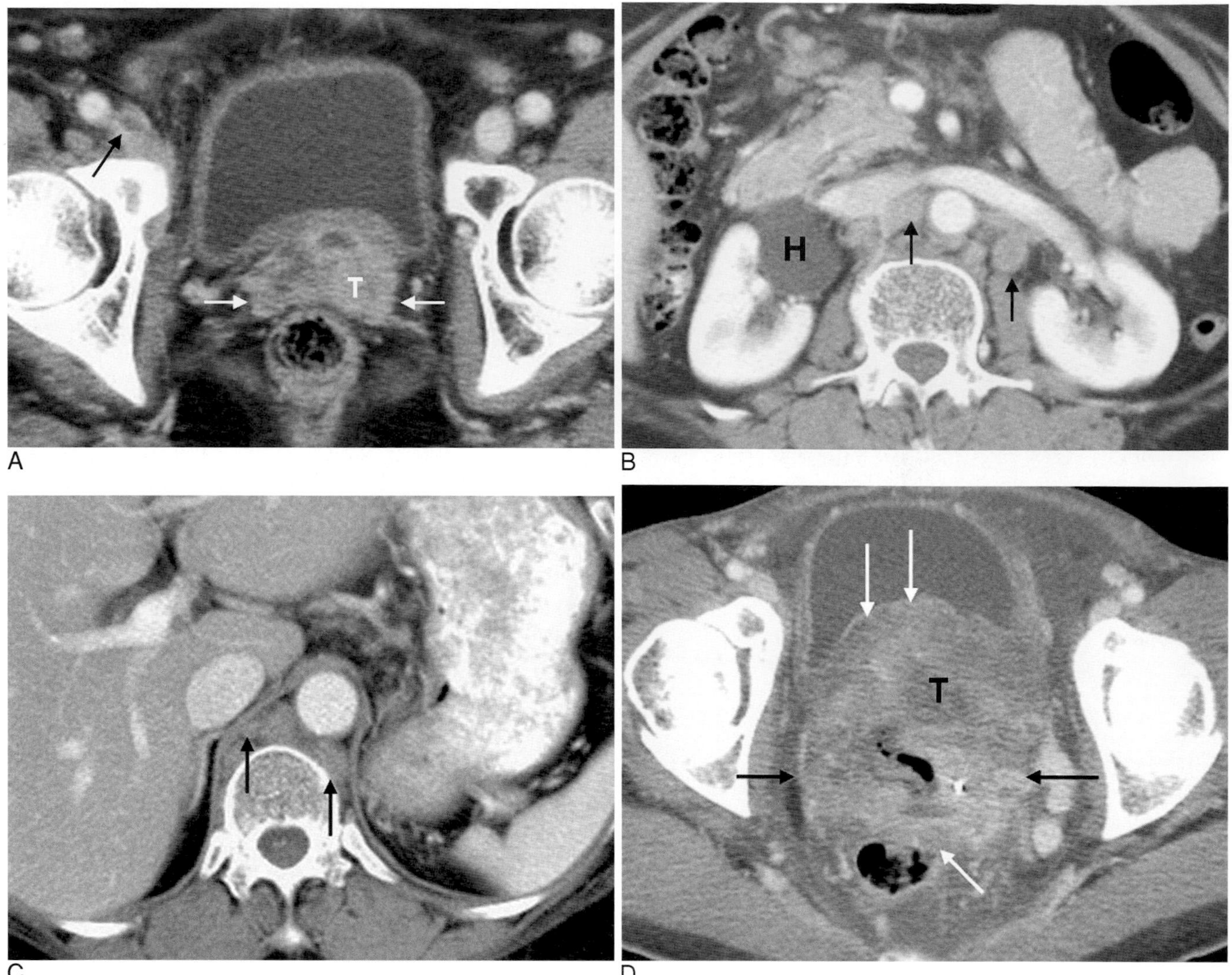

Figure 54.19 Cervical cancer, CT. Axial CT images (A–C) show a cervical cancer (T, A) which is contiguous with the adjacent parametrial fat, indicating parametrial invasion (white arrows, A). Note the presence of a filling defect within the right external femoral vein suggesting deep venous thrombosis (black arrow, A). There is bilateral para-aortic (black arrows, B) and retrocrural lymphadenopathy (black arrows, C). Also, note the presence of right hydronephrosis (H, B). Axial CT image (D) of extensive cervical cancer (T, D) in a different patient. The tumour extends to both parametria (black arrows, D) and invades the posterior aspect of the bladder (white arrows, D) and anterior rectal wall (white arrow, D).

for radiotherapy planning and for guiding interventional procedures. For locoregional staging, MRI is the method of choice because it is accurate in the determination of tumour size, location (exophytic or endocervical), depth of stromal invasion and the local extent of the tumour. As noted earlier, although the role of PET in the initial evaluation of cervical cancer is still under investigation, it can be used to assess nodal disease and tumour recurrence.

Impact of imaging on treatment The most important issue in the staging of cervical cancer is to distinguish early disease (stages I and IIA) that can be treated with surgery from advanced disease that must be treated with radiation alone or combined with chemotherapy. Imaging techniques must be directed to solve this clinically important question. Conventional radiological studies such as excretory urography, barium enema and lymphangiography have become obsolete and cross-sectional imaging, particularly CT and MRI, is now used.

THE ADNEXA

Benign ovarian conditions

Physiological cysts

Benign ovarian cysts are common, frequently asymptomatic and often resolve spontaneously. One of the most frequently seen ovarian masses is the follicular cyst. Follicular cysts are a common asymptomatic finding, usually larger than the typical preovulatory follicle and varying in size from 3 to 8 cm in diameter. These cysts represent the failure of the fluid in an incompletely developed follicle to be reabsorbed. Follow-up US is recommended in 6 weeks, preferentially immediately after menstruation. No treatment is required in the majority of cases as the cysts usually regress spontaneously in 2 months.

Two types of lutein cyst are recognized: corpus luteum and theca lutein cysts. Corpus luteum cysts are functional, non-neoplastic enlargements of the ovary, following ovulation. A persistent corpus luteum cyst may cause local pain and tenderness and either amenorrhoea or delayed menstruation, thus

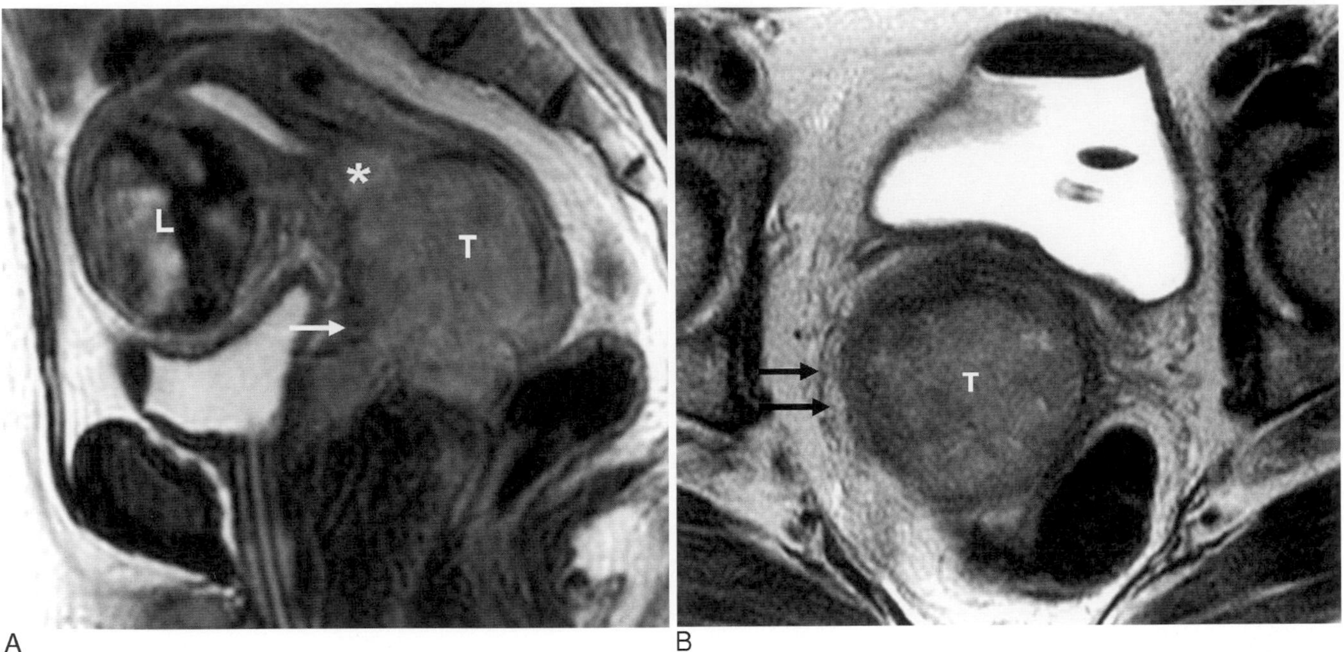

Figure 54.20 Cervical cancer, MRI. Sagittal (A) and axial (B) T2-weighted images show a large cervix cancer (T) involving the anterior fornix of the vagina (arrow, A). The tumour invades the fibrocervical stroma on the right (arrows, B). Note the tumour extends into the lower endometrial canal (*, A). Incidentally, presence of a large uterine leiomyoma (L, A) is noted.

simulating the clinical picture associated with ectopic pregnancy. Theca lutein cysts are of small to medium size, usually bilateral and filled with clear, straw-coloured fluid. These cysts are found in association with polycystic ovarian disease, hydatidiform mole, choriocarcinoma and chorionic gonadotrophin or clomiphene therapy.

Endometriosis

Endometriosis is the presence of endometrial epithelium and stroma outside of endometrium and myometrium. Common locations of endometrial tissue include ovary, uterine ligaments, Fallopian tubes, rectovaginal septum, pouch of Douglas, bladder wall and umbilicus. Endometriosis is perhaps the most prevalent cause of CPP, occurring in up to 65% of women with pelvic pain. It usually affects women of reproductive age. The clinical manifestations are variable: some patients are asymptomatic while others present clinically with dysmenorrhoea, dyspareunia, abdominal pain, dysfunctional uterine bleeding and infertility. Endometriosis is a syndrome that can present with endometriomas, adhesions, or endometrial implants. Staging of endometriosis requires a laparoscopic procedure to look for any of these elements. Although imaging is most commonly used for the diagnosis and follow-up of endometriomas, laparoscopy is the gold standard as it can provide a complete evaluation for endometrial implants in both the abdomen and pelvis. Transvaginal US is the primary imaging investigation, with MRI reserved for masses atypical on US.

Ultrasound On ultrasound, endometriomas appear as cystic masses with diffuse uniform low-level echoes (Fig. 54.21). After repeated episodes of bleeding and re-bleeding, they may develop irregular walls and echogenic mural nodules. Fluid–fluid levels or fluid–debris levels represent blood products. When the cysts have thin or thick septations, it may sometimes be difficult to differentiate them from malignant ovarian masses. US plays no role in the evaluation of endometrial implants or adhesions.

Magnetic resonance imaging Endometriomas appear hyperintense on T1-weighted images and heterogeneously hyperintense on T2-weighted images. The use of fat suppression increases the conspicuity of endometriosis (Fig. 54.21)[20]. Endometriomas larger than 1 cm are routinely seen, but imaging small implants remains problematic. Endometrial implants can be detected on MRI, but evaluation on MRI is inferior to laparoscopic staging.

Polycystic ovarian disease (Stein–Leventhal syndrome)

Polycystic ovarian disease is characterized by bilaterally enlarged polycystic ovaries, secondary amenorrhoea or oligomenorrhoea and infertility. About 50% of patients are hirsute and many are obese. Many cases of female infertility secondary to failure of ovulation are due to polycystic ovarian disease. The classic appearance on ultrasound is enlarged ovaries with echogenic central stroma and greater than 10 peripherally placed cysts less than 9 mm in diameter (Fig. 54.22).

Pelvic inflammatory disease

Pelvic inflammatory disease (PID) is defined as the acute clinical syndrome associated with ascending spread of micro-organisms from the vagina or cervix to the endometrium, Fallopian tubes and/or contiguous structures. *Chlamydia trachomatis* and *Neisseria gonorrhoeae* are probably the most prevalent sexually transmitted bacteria in the western world. Early diagnosis of PID is of paramount importance in the management of women with acute upper genital tract infection, as delay will

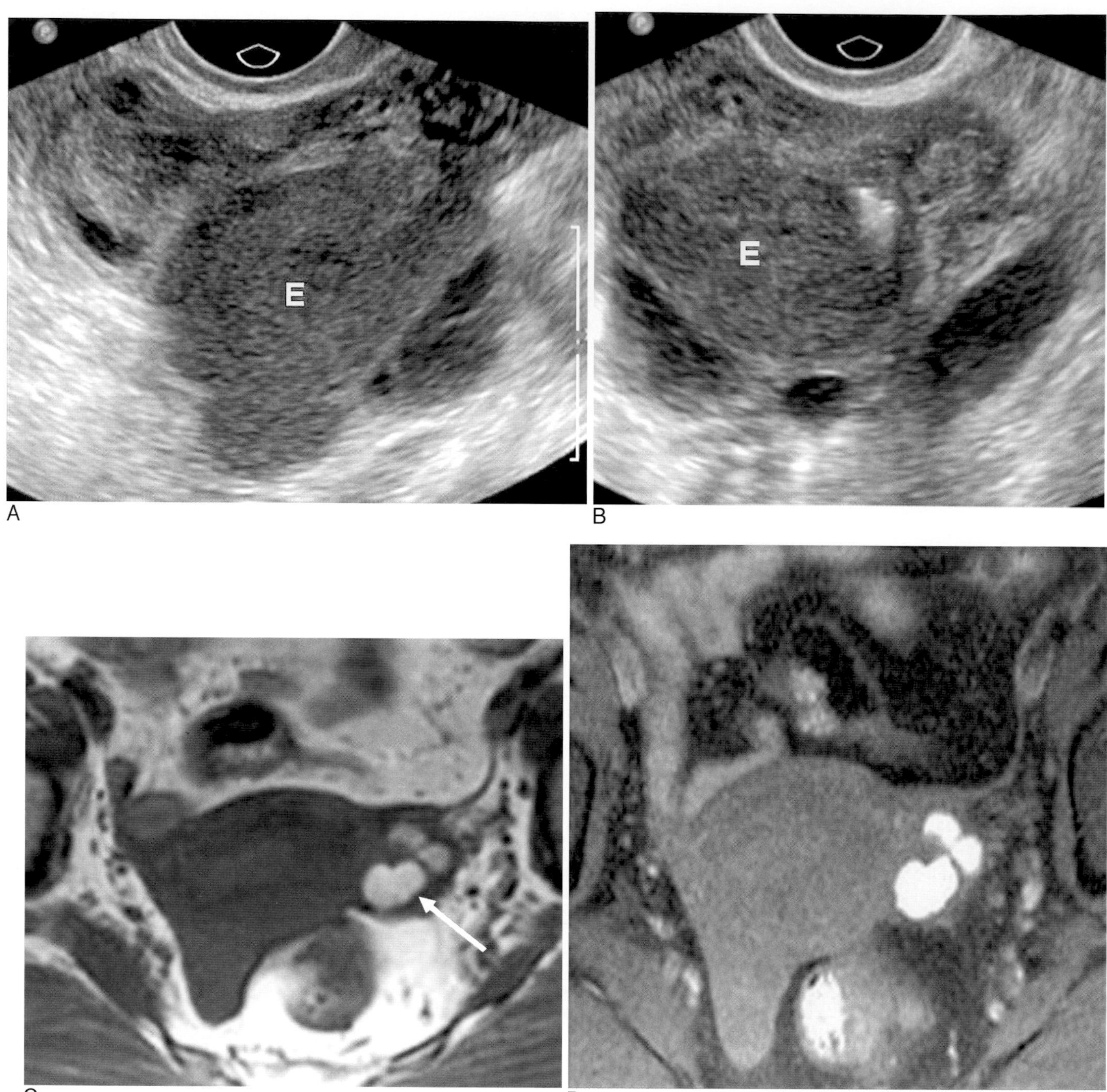

Figure 54.21 Endometrioma. Transvaginal US in sagittal (A) and coronal (B) planes demonstrates a complex cystic mass in the left ovary consistent with endometrioma (E in A, B). Although endometriomas can appear similar to haemorrhagic cysts, the irregular contour, homogeneity of the internal echoes and persistence over an extended period favours the diagnosis of endometrioma. Axial T1-weighted (C) and T1-weighted fat-suppressed MR (D) images in a different patient show multiple high signal intensity lesions within the left ovary (arrow, C), suggesting either endometriosis or haemorrhagic cysts. Note how fat suppression increases the conspicuity of haemorrhagic lesions and helps differentiate them from dermoids. Diagnosis of endometriosis was confirmed at surgery.

result in late treatment, with an attendant increased risk of complications (e.g. infertility).

Classically, women with PID present with subacute lower abdominal pain that is dull in nature and usually bilateral. They also have a fever, purulent vaginal discharge, bilateral adnexal tenderness with cervical excitation and an elevated erythrocyte sedimentation rate. A number of other gynaecological and surgical conditions where lower abdominal pain is the principal presenting complaint also mimic the clinical picture of acute PID, causing diagnostic uncertainty. Furthermore, there is evidence that in many women with acute upper genital tract infection, the condition goes unnoticed because it is atypical or asymptomatic and yet the extent of tubal damage in these women is the same as in symptomatic disease.

At US, the uterus appears slightly enlarged, more hypoechoic than normal and the uterine margins are not clearly defined.

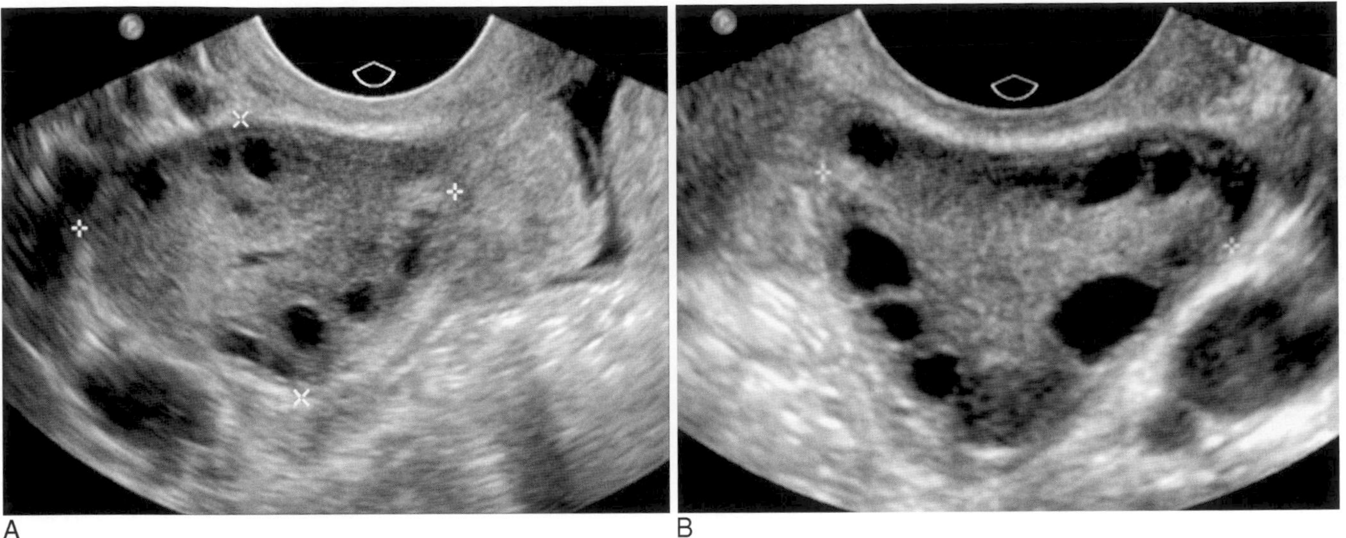

Figure 54.22 Polycystic ovaries. Sagittal (A) and transverse (B) transvaginal ultrasound of the left ovary depicting multiple subcentimetre peripherally placed follicles in enlarged ovaries with echogenic central stroma.

These early changes are often subtle and difficult to assess. The endometrial echo may be prominent due to associated endometritis, with sonolucent margins. The adnexa appear prominent and have a complex but usually symmetrical ultrasound pattern. Small amounts of fluid may be present in the peritoneal cul-de-sac. Pyosalpinx or hydrosalpinx (Fig. 54.23) as well as tubo-ovarian abscesses (Fig. 54.24) may be present due to PID-associated adhesions. Septic abortion, intrauterine manipulation and pelvic operations may also provoke a pyogenic adnexal abscess. On US, a tubo-ovarian abscess presents as an adnexal mass with a thickened echogenic wall. There may also be hypoechoic areas with associated thick and irregular septations.

On CT, an adnexal abscess is seen as a soft tissue mass with central areas of low attenuation. Thick, irregular walls are commonly present and it may be difficult to differentiate an ovarian abscess from a necrotic tumour or endometrioma based solely on the CT finding. MRI features of adnexal abscess are similarly nonspecific. Pyosalpinx and hydrosalpinx may present as a flask-shaped cystic adnexal mass that may contain faintly echogenic material due to debris. A large hydrosalpinx may be indistinguishable from an ovarian cyst. Both CT and MRI may demonstrate a serpentine cluster of cysts.

Pelvic varices

Pelvic varices are dilated veins in the broad ligament and ovarian plexus. When symptomatic, the condition is called 'pelvic congestion syndrome'. Symptoms have been described as dull, aching pain, often occurring during walking, sexual intercourse, or other activities that create increased intra-abdominal pressure. Varices are most often found in multiparous women of reproductive age. The criteria for diagnosis include venous structures greater than 4 mm in diameter, slower than 3 cm s^{-1} velocity flow and connecting arcuate veins within the myometrium.

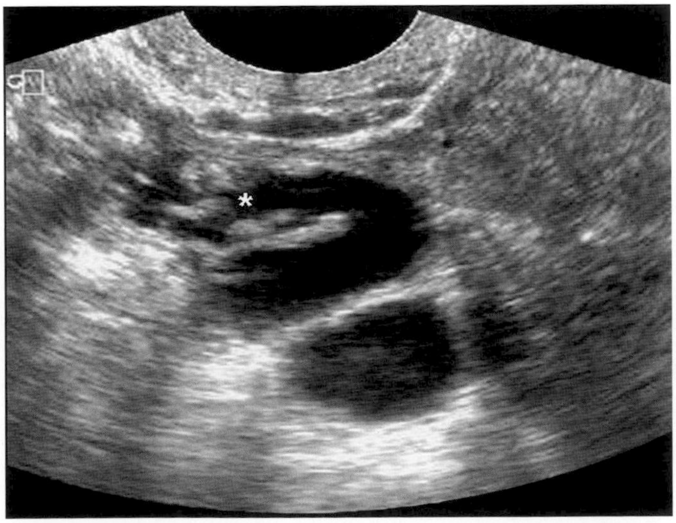

Figure 54.23 Hydrosalpinx. Sagittal transvaginal ultrasound image demonstrates a cystic lesion of tubular appearance within the pelvis. Small internally projecting nodules are compatible with the fimbriae and give the cyst (*) a 'cogwheel' appearance, typical of hydrosalpinx.

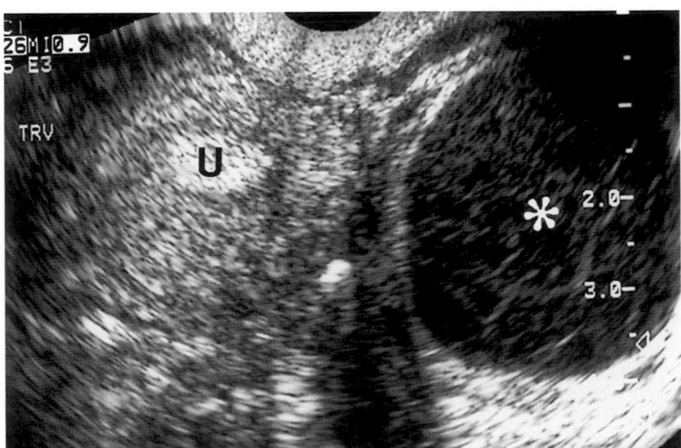

Figure 54.24 Pelvic tubo-ovarian abscess. Transverse transvaginal US shows a complex left ovarian mass (*) in a woman with pelvic pain and fever. This constellation of findings is consistent with pelvic inflammatory disease complicated by tubo-ovarian abscess. U = uterus.

Varices show on CT as serpiginous structures that enhance following administration of contrast medium. 3D T1 gradient-echo sequences performed after the IV administration of gadolinium are the most effective MR imaging sequence for demonstrating pelvic varices. Blood flow in pelvic varices appears with high signal intensity[4].

Benign tumours of the ovary

Ninety per cent of all ovarian tumours are benign, although this varies with age.

Germ cell tumours are among the most common ovarian tumours seen in women less than 30 years of age. Overall, only 2–3% of germ cell tumours are malignant.

Dermoid cysts (mature cystic teratoma) are the only benign germ cell tumours and are quite common. Dermoid cysts stem from cells that differentiate into embryonic tissues and account for around 40% of all ovarian neoplasms. They are most common in young women with a median age at presentation of 30 years.

Mature solid teratomas are rare tumours containing mature tissues just like the dermoid cysts. They must be differentiated from immature teratomas, which are malignant.

Benign epithelial tumours

The majority of ovarian neoplasms, both benign and malignant, arise from the ovarian surface epithelium.

Serous cystadenoma is the most common benign epithelial tumour and is usually a unilocular cyst with papilliferous processes on the inner surface and occasionally on the outer surface.

Mucinous cystadenoma contributes to 15–25% of all ovarian tumours and is the second most common epithelial tumour.

Endometrioid cystadenomas are often malignant and difficult to distinguish from endometriosis.

Brenner tumours account for only 1–2% of all ovarian tumours and probably arise from Wolffian metaplasia of the surface epithelium.

Sex cord stromal tumours

Theca cell tumours are almost always benign, solid and unilateral. Many produce oestrogens in sufficient quantity to provoke systemic effects, such as precocious puberty, postmenopausal bleeding, endometrial hyperplasia, or endometrial cancer.

Fibromas are uncommon tumours and present most frequently around 50 years of age. Most are derived from stromal cells and are similar to thecomas.

Sertoli–Leydig cell tumours are rare and usually of low grade malignancy. Many produce androgens and clinical signs of virilization can be seen in patients presenting with this tumour type.

Granulosa cell tumours are all malignant tumours but are mentioned here because they are generally confined to the ovary when they present and so have a good prognosis. However, they grow very slowly and recurrences are frequently diagnosed.

Ultrasound The ovaries are well imaged with transvaginal US. Changes in their appearance can be correlated with their functional status. Follicular cysts may be up to 10 cm in diameter and difficult to distinguish from other ovarian tumours unless serial ultrasound examinations are obtained, in which regression of the follicular cyst is demonstrated. The ultrasound appearance of dermoid cysts varies. The three most common appearances are: (A) a cystic mass with an echogenic nodule projecting into the lumen; (B) a predominantly echogenic mass with posterior sound attenuation owing to the presence of sebaceous material and hair; and (C) a cystic mass with fine internal echogenic lines also representing hair. A fluid–fluid level may be seen which represents sebaceous material floating on fluid. The imaging features of other benign ovarian tumours are nonspecific. Different imaging techniques are combined for ovarian lesion characterization, as discussed more extensively in the next section.

Magnetic resonance imaging The MRI appearance of simple cysts is diagnostic: low signal intensity on T1-weighted images, high signal intensity on T2-weighted images and no enhancement following the administration of IV contrast medium. The strength of MRI is its ability to characterize adnexal lesions, particularly in the case of masses that are indeterminate on US (see next section for a full discussion). Among benign lesions, MRI can also be used to diagnose dermoid cysts with confidence as the fat or sebum within the cyst parallels the signal intensity of fat on all pulse sequences. Specifically, by exploiting the processional frequency differences between fat and water protons, fat saturation techniques cause the fatty elements to lose signal and are 100% specific and 96% accurate in identifying dermoid cysts (Fig. 54.25). Additional features include fat–water chemical shift artefact, fat–fluid and/or fluid–fluid levels, layering debris, low signal intensity calcifications (e.g. teeth) and soft tissue protuberances (Rokitansky nodules or dermoid plugs) attached to the cyst wall.

Malignant ovarian conditions

Ovarian carcinoma

Ovarian neoplasms account for more cancer-related deaths than all other primary cancers of the reproductive system. In general, ovarian cancer is a disease of postmenopausal women and, occasionally, prepubescent girls. The cause of ovarian cancer is unknown, although a number of risk factors have been identified. Chronic anovulation, multiparity and a history of breast feeding seem to be protective, whereas genetic factors appear to play an important role in the development of progression of ovarian cancer. Ten per cent of ovarian

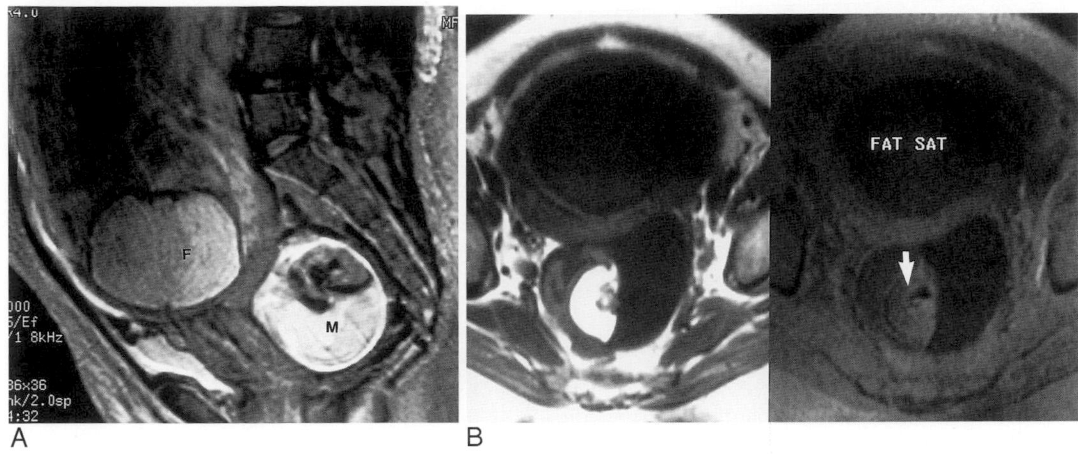

Figure 54.25 Ovarian dermoid, intrauterine pregnancy. T2-weighted sagittal (A) and T1-weighted axial (B) MRI. The sagittal image demonstrates a fetus (F) in vertex position. Situated posterior to the uterus in the cul-de-sac is a hyperintense cystic and solid, rounded mass (M). A portion of the mass is high signal on T1-weighted image and falls in signal intensity following a fat saturation pulse (arrow B). This is consistent with fat, allowing the diagnosis of dermoids to be made with confidence.

cancers are due to hereditary syndromes such as BRCA-1 and BRCA-2 mutations (risk of breast cancer) and Lynch syndrome II (risk of colon cancer). Approximately 90% of ovarian cancers are of epithelial origin. Epithelial tumours are subtyped as serous (50%), mucinous (20%), endometroid (20%), clear cell (10%), or undifferentiated (1%). Nonepithelial cancers include malignant granulosa cell tumour, dysgerminoma, immature teratoma, endodermal sinus tumour and metastases to the ovary.

Staging Cross-sectional imaging is better accepted and more commonly used in the evaluation and staging of ovarian carcinoma than for other gynaecological malignancies[21,22]. The TNM and FIGO staging systems are outlined in Table 54.3. Imaging is an adjunct to surgical staging and is becoming a valuable tool in the detection of nonresectable disease. Findings that indicate nonresectable disease include:

- in the pelvis: invasion of pelvic sidewall or urinary bladder, or urinary obstruction
- in the upper abdomen: tumour deposits greater than 1 cm in size in the gastrosplenic ligament, lesser sac, fissure for the ligamentum teres, porta hepatis, subphrenic space, small bowel mesentery, or retroperitoneal nodes above the renal hila
- distant metastases (i.e. liver, spleen, lung).

Table 54.3 TNM AND FIGO STAGING FOR PRIMARY OVARIAN CANCER

TNM	FIGO	Ovary
T1	I	Growth limited to ovaries
T1	Ia	Growth limited to one ovary, no ascites; no tumour on external surface; capsule intact
T1b	Ib	Growth limited to both ovaries, no ascites; no tumour on external surface; capsule intact
T1c	Ic	Tumour either stage Ia or Ib, but tumour on surface of one or both ovaries; or with capsule ruptured; or with ascites present containing malignant cells; or with positive peritoneal washings
T2	II	Growth involving one or both ovaries with pelvic extension
T2a	IIa	Extension and/or metastasis to the uterus or tubes
T2b	IIb	Extension to other pelvic tissue
T2c	IIc	Tumour either stage IIa or IIb but tumour on surface of one or both ovaries; or with capsule ruptured; or with ascites present containing malignant cells; or with positive peritoneal washings
T3 and/or N1	III	Growth involving one or both ovaries with peritoneal implants outside the pelvis or positive retroperitoneal or inguinal nodes
		Superficial liver metastasis equals stage III
T3a	IIIa	Tumour grossly limited to the true pelvis with negative nodes but with histologically confirmed microscopic seeding of abdominal peritoneal surfaces
T3b	IIIb	Tumour with histologically confirmed implants on abdominal peritoneal surfaces, none exceeding 2 cm in diameter
		Nodes are negative
T3c and/or N1	IIIc	Abdominal implants greater than 2 cm in diameter or positive retroperitoneal or inguinal nodes
M1	IV	Growth involving one or both ovaries with distant metastases
		If pleural effusion is present there must be positive cytology to allot a case to stage IV
		Parenchymal liver metastasis equals stage IV

Imaging techniques for detection, diagnosis and staging

Ultrasound Combined transabdominal and transvaginal US has been advocated for the detection of ovarian carcinoma. These studies provide superb morphological detail of the adnexa, allowing detection of masses before they are clinically apparent. Ultrasound features that suggest benignancy and malignancy have been well described. Although several scoring systems have been devised to predict the nature of an adnexal mass, most researchers agree that wall irregularity, thick septations (> 3 mm), papillary projections, solid components and size (> 9 cm) are suspicious for malignancy[23].

As colour and duplex US become more widely available, their potential value for differentiating benign from malignant ovarian masses is being explored (Fig. 54.26)[23]. Malignant tumours often have neovascularity that consists of blood vessels with walls that have little or no smooth muscle support. As a result, these vessels frequently have a characteristic waveform with a low resistive index (RI < 0.4) (peak systolic–end diastolic Doppler shift/peak systolic Doppler shift). A meta-analysis of the literature demonstrated that the best adnexal lesion characterization is achieved by the combined use of grey scale and colour Doppler US[24]. Assessment of adnexal masses on imaging for malignancy or benignancy is only possible if the ovaries can be visualized. This may be problematic in postmenopausal women.

Computed tomography is the most commonly performed study for the preoperative staging of a suspected ovarian carcinoma. It is particularly useful in determining the extent of cytoreductive surgery required to optimize subsequent chemotherapeutic response. Ovarian cancer is frequently bilateral (Fig. 54.27D). On CT, ovarian cancer demonstrates varied morphological patterns, including a multilocular cyst with thick internal septations and solid mural or septal components, a partially cystic and solid mass (Fig 54.27D) and a lobulated papillary heterogeneous solid mass. The outer border of the mass may be irregular and poorly defined and amorphous coarse calcifications and contrast enhancement may be seen in the cyst wall or soft tissue components[25]. It is possible to suggest the histological subtype of the epithelial cancer based on the imaging findings. Calcification suggests a serous tumour, whereas high density within the locules of a multilocular tumour is suggestive of proteinaceous fluid in a mucinous tumour. Endometroid carcinomas are associated with endometrial hyperplasia or carcinoma in 20–30% of cases.

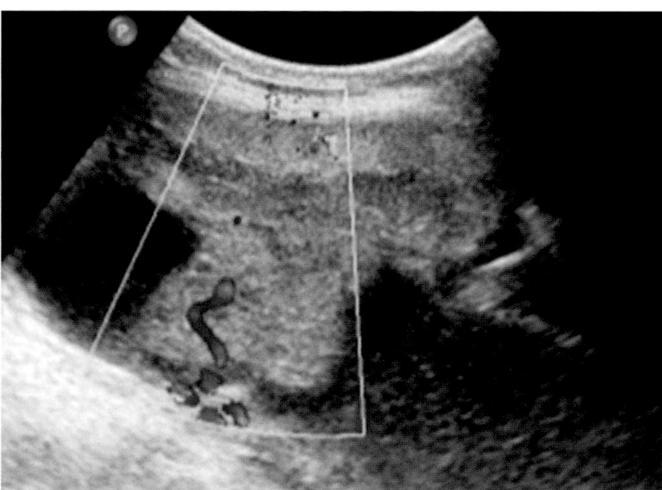

Figure 54.26 Ovarian carcinoma. Sagittal transvaginal US image demonstrates a large complex cystic mass arising from the left adnexa. The presence of flow within the solid nodule suggests malignant aetiology.

Intraperitoneal dissemination is the most common route of spread of ovarian cancer. Peritoneal implants appear as nodular or plaque-like enhancing soft tissue masses of varying size (Fig. 54.27E). Ascitic fluid may outline small implants, facilitating detection. Although peritoneal implants may occur anywhere in the peritoneal cavity, the most common sites include the pouch of Douglas, paracolic gutters, surface of the small and large bowel, greater omentum, surface of the liver (perihepatic implants) and subphrenic space. CT is useful in differentiating between subcapsular and parenchymal liver metastasis, which alters staging and therapy[26]. Ascites is a nonspecific finding but, in a patient with ovarian cancer, usually indicates peritoneal metastases[27].

In addition to peritoneal implantation, ovarian cancer also spreads by local continuity to the ovary, uterus and other pelvic organs. Surgically important features of local spread that may be detected by imaging are invasion of the pelvic sidewall, rectum, sigmoid colon, or urinary bladder. Pelvic sidewall invasion should be suspected when the primary tumour lies within 3 mm of the pelvic sidewall or when the iliac vessels are surrounded or distorted by tumour. The ovarian lymphatic vessels are another important route of metastatic spread. While enlarged nodes are likely to be involved, CT is unable to exclude disease in normal-sized nodes.

The CT appearance of ovarian metastasis is indistinguishable from that of a primary ovarian neoplasm and the stomach and colon should be carefully examined as potential primary tumour sites. Occasionally, it is not possible to determine whether the origin of a pelvic mass is ovarian or uterine on CT.

Magnetic resonance imaging The role of MRI in patients with suspected or known ovarian carcinoma is still evolving. To optimize MR detection and characterization of an adnexal mass, contrast-enhanced protocols and attention to eliminating, or at least limiting, bowel motion are needed. Both transvaginal US and contrast-enhanced MRI have high sensitivity (97% and 100%, respectively) in the identification of solid components within an adnexal mass. MRI, however, shows higher accuracy (93%)[27]. Primary and ancillary criteria for characterizing an adnexal mass as malignant have been established. Primary criteria for malignancy include: (A) size larger than 4 cm; (B) a cystic lesion with a solid component; (C) irregular wall thickness greater than 3 mm; (D) septa greater than 3 mm and/or the presence of vegetations or nodularity; and (E) a solid mass with the presence of necrosis. Ancillary criteria for malignancy include: (A) involvement of pelvic organs or sidewall; (B) peritoneal, mesenteric, or omental disease; (C) ascites; or (D) adenopathy. Utilizing unenhanced T1-, T2- and contrast-enhanced T1-weighted sequences, the presence of at least one of the primary criteria coupled with a single criterion from

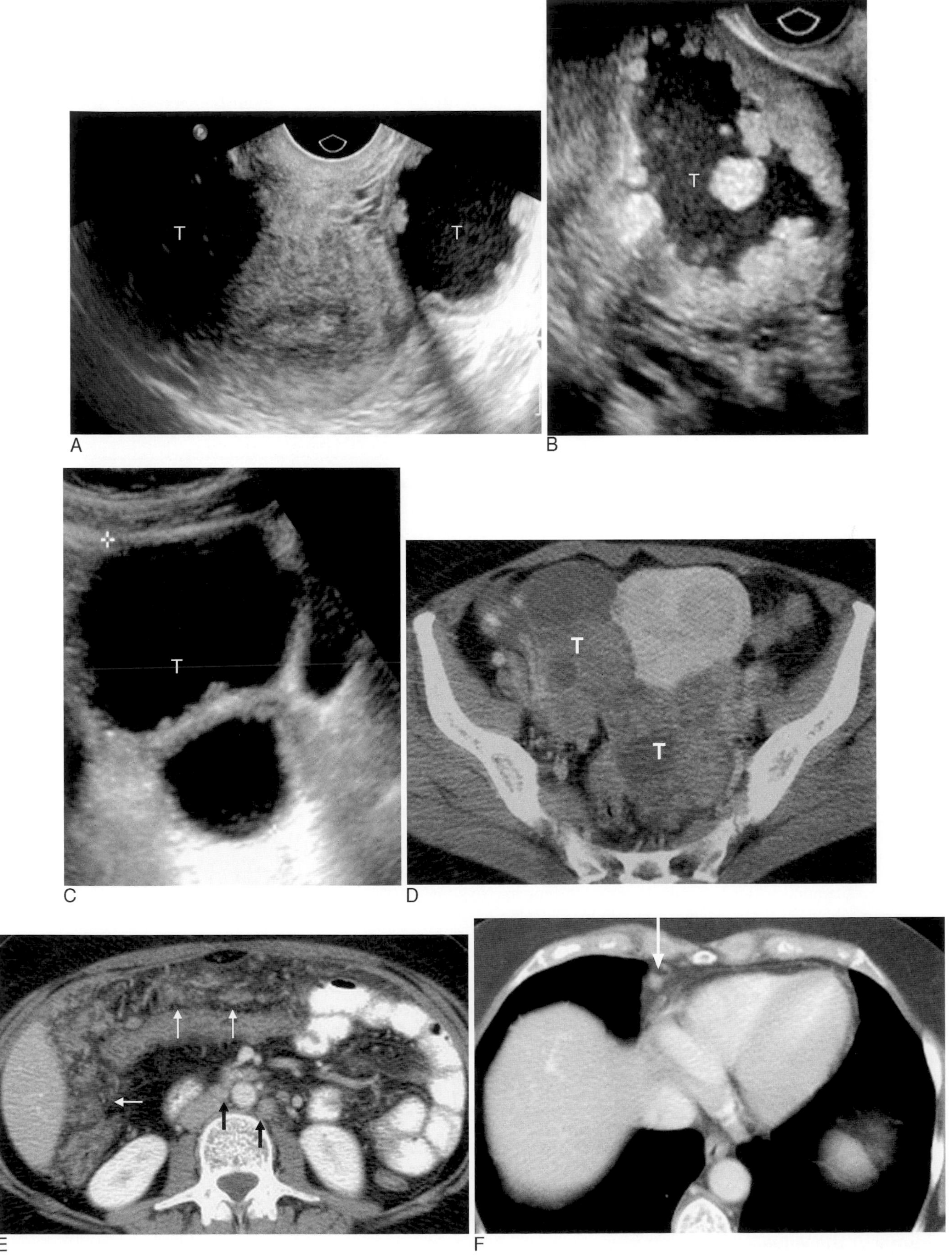

Figure 54.27 Bilateral ovarian carcinoma. Transverse (A) transvaginal ultrasound image of the pelvis shows bilateral cystic adnexal masses (T). Sagittal images of right (B) and left (C) ovaries demonstrate cystic mass (T) with mural nodularity (B) and multiple septations (C). MDCT of a different patient shows bilateral complex solid and cystic adnexal masses (T, D), highly suggestive of ovarian carcinoma, and demonstrates the presence of omental tumour implants (white arrows, E). Note also the presence of left para-aortic, interaortocaval (black arrows, E) and superior diaphragmatic (arrow, F) lymphadenopathy.

the ancillary group correctly characterizes 95% of malignant lesions[28].

MRI is very sensitive (95%) for detection of peritoneal metastases, which show delayed enhancement on contrast-enhanced MRI[29].

PET PET and PET-CT have a potential role in evaluating patients for recurrent ovarian cancer, particularly those with negative CT or MRI findings and rising tumour marker levels[30]. PET is also useful in the detection of implants difficult to assess by conventional imaging studies, such as serosal bowel implants or tumour deposits within the small bowel mesentery.

Recommended imaging approach US is the primary technique for detection and characterization of adnexal masses. MRI is a problem-solving investigation in cases of indeterminate adnexal masses and the best technique to assess pelvic sidewall invasion. Multidetector contrast-enhanced CT of the abdomen and pelvis is the imaging technique of choice for preoperative staging and for follow-up. CT is the primary technique for prediction of tumour resectability, tumour extent into the upper abdomen and related complications such as hydronephrosis and bowel obstruction. PET-CT is very valuable in the setting of recurrent disease and particularly useful for detecting tumour deposits in mesentery and bowel serosa.

Impact of imaging on treatment Early ovarian cancer is treated with comprehensive staging laparotomy, which includes transabdominal hysterectomy and bilateral salpingo-oophorectomy (TAH/BSO), omentectomy, retroperitoneal lymph node sampling, peritoneal and diaphragmatic biopsies and cytology of peritoneal washings. Advanced but operable disease is treated with primary cytoreductive surgery (debulking) followed by adjuvant chemotherapy. Patients with nonresectable disease may benefit from neoadjuvant (preoperative) chemotherapy before debulking.

Cross-sectional imaging plays a crucial role:

- in treatment planning by identifying patients with inoperable disease who may be more appropriately managed by neoadjuvant chemotherapy followed by cytoreductive surgery after tumour shrinkage
- following treatment response
- in detection of recurrent disease.

It is important to realize that second-look surgery is no longer routine and imaging diagnosis of recurrence may obviate a second-look laparotomy since secondary cytoreduction is only justified if resection is possible with no residual tumour[22,25].

VULVA AND VAGINA

Carcinoma of the vulva

Metastases from carcinoma of the vulva spread to the superficial inguinal nodes and subsequently to the deep inguinal and external iliac groups. CT and MRI are usually performed for staging of vulvar carcinoma.

Vulvar varices

These usually occur in multiparous women, often with varicose veins of the legs. Contrast medium may be injected directly into vulvar varicose veins to show their connections.

Congenital abnormalities

Abnormalities of the vagina have been described in previous sections.

Vaginal malignancies

Primary vaginal malignancies are uncommon. Metastatic tumours to the vagina are more frequent and originate most commonly from carcinoma of the endometrium and cervix, followed by melanoma and carcinoma of the colon and kidney.

CONTRACEPTION

Intrauterine contraceptive devices

The intrauterine contraceptive device (IUCD) is an effective, long-acting method of contraception, which is perhaps underrated in the developed world. It exerts a local inflammatory reaction within the cavity of the uterus, which probably interferes with the viability of both sperm and eggs in addition to inhibiting implantation. Modern copper-containing devices are effective for long periods and it is now recommended that they need to be changed only every 5 years. Using modern IUCDs, the rates for perforation and expulsion are 4–9 and 0.2 per 100 users, respectively. The incidence of both complications is increased with postpartum insertions, which should be delayed until 6–8 weeks after delivery.

Transvaginal ultrasound is the initial technique of choice in evaluating possible IUCD malposition. Most devices are echogenic on ultrasound and visualized as a linear structure within the endometrial cavity. During the examination, the presence of an intrauterine gestation is excluded and the position of the device established. The device may be identified within the myometrium. If it has been completely extruded from the uterus, a plain radiograph will establish whether it has either been expelled from the patient or lies within the pelvis. CT may accurately depict the presence of the device within the pelvic cavity. IUCDs can be safely imaged with MRI and their presence does not create artefacts that impede image interpretation[31].

REFERENCES

1. Carrington B M, Hricak H, Nuruddin R N, Secaf E, Laros R K Jr, Hill E C 1990 Mullerian duct anomalies: MR imaging evaluation. Radiology 176: 715–720
2. Baber R J, McSweeney M B, Gill R W et al 1988 Transvaginal pulsed Doppler ultrasound assessment of blood flow to the corpus luteum in IVF patients following embryo transfer. Br J Obstet Gynaecol 95: 1226–1230

3. De Souza N M, Brosens J J, Schwieso J E, Paraschos T, Winston R M 1995 The potential value of magnetic resonance imaging in infertility. Clin Radiol 50: 75–79
4. Kuligowska E, Deeds L 3rd, Lu K 3rd 2005 Pelvic pain: overlooked and underdiagnosed gynecologic conditions. Radiographics 25: 3–20
5. Murase E, Siegelman E S, Outwater E K, Perez-Jaffe L A, Tureck R W 1999 Uterine leiomyomas: histopathologic features, MR imaging findings, differential diagnosis and treatment. Radiographics 19: 1179–1197
6. Ascher S M, Jha R C, Reinhold C 2003 Benign myometrial conditions: leiomyomas and adenomyosis. Top Magn Reson Imaging 14: 281–304
7. Tamai K, Togashi K, Ito T, Morisawa N, Fujiwara T, Koyama T 2005 MR imaging findings of adenomyosis: correlation with histopathologic features and diagnostic pitfalls. Radiographics 25: 21–40
8. Reinhold C, Tafazoli F, Mehio A et al 1999 Uterine adenomyosis: endovaginal US and MR imaging features with histopathologic correlation. Radiographics 19: S147–160
9. Leitich H, Brunbauer M, Kaider A, Egarter C, Husslein P 1999 Cervical length and dilatation of the internal cervical os detected by vaginal ultrasonography as markers for preterm delivery: a systematic review. Am J Obstet Gynecol 181: 1465–1472
10. Hricak H, Chang Y C, Cann C E, Parer J T 1990 Cervical incompetence: preliminary evaluation with MR imaging. Radiology 174: 821–826
11. Arko D, Takac I 2000 High frequency transvaginal ultrasonography in preoperative assessment of myometrial invasion in endometrial cancer. J Ultrasound Med 19: 639–643
12. Manfredi R, Mirk P, Maresca G et al 2004 Local–regional staging of endometrial carcinoma: role of MR imaging in surgical planning. Radiology 231: 372–378
13. Saga T, Higashi T, Ishimori T et al 2003 Clinical value of FDG-PET in the follow up of post-operative patients with endometrial cancer. Ann Nucl Med 17: 197–203
14. Green C L, Angtuaco T L, Shah H R, Parmley T H 1996 Gestational trophoblastic disease: a spectrum of radiologic diagnosis. Radiographics 16: 1371–1384
15. Hricak H, Demas B E, Braga C A, Fisher M R, Winkler M L 1986 Gestational trophoblastic neoplasm of the uterus: MR assessment. Radiology 161: 11–16
16. Scheidler J, Heuck A F 2002 Imaging of cancer of the cervix. Radiol Clin North Am 40: 577–590, vii
17. Okamoto Y, Tanaka Y O, Nishida M, Tsunoda H, Yoshikawa H, Itai Y 2003 MR imaging of the uterine cervix: imaging–pathologic correlation. Radiographics 23: 425–445, quiz 534–535
18. Hricak H, Powell C B, Yu K K et al 1996 Invasive cervical carcinoma: role of MR imaging in pretreatment work-up: cost minimization and diagnostic efficacy analysis. Radiology 198: 403–409
19. Reinhardt M J, Ehritt-Braun C, Vogelgesang D et al 2001 Metastatic lymph nodes in patients with cervical cancer: detection with MR imaging and FDG PET. Radiology 218: 776–782
20. Woodward P J, Sohaey R, Mezzetti T P Jr 2001 Endometriosis: radiologic–pathologic correlation. Radiographics 21: 193–216; questionnaire 288–294
21. Tempany C M, Zou K H, Silverman S G, Brown D L, Kurtz A B, McNeil B J 2000 Staging of advanced ovarian cancer: comparison of imaging modalities—report from the Radiological Diagnostic Oncology Group. Radiology 215: 761–767
22. Woodward P J, Hosseinzadeh K, Saenger J S 2004 From the archives of the AFIP: radiologic staging of ovarian carcinoma with pathologic correlation. Radiographics 24: 225–246
23. Brown D L, Doubilet P M, Miller F H et al 1998 Benign and malignant ovarian masses: selection of the most discriminating gray-scale and Doppler sonographic features. Radiology 208: 103–110
24. Kinkel K, Hricak H, Lu Y, Tsuda K, Filly R A 2000 US characterization of ovarian masses: a meta-analysis. Radiology 217: 803–811
25. Coakley F V 2002 Staging ovarian cancer: role of imaging. Radiol Clin North Am 40: 609–636
26. Coakley F V, Choi P H, Gougoutas C A et al 2002 Peritoneal metastases: detection with spiral CT in patients with ovarian cancer. Radiology 223: 495–499
27. Hricak H, Chen M, Coakley F Vet al 2000 Complex adnexal masses: detection and characterization with MR imaging—multivariate analysis. Radiology 214: 39–46
28. Stevens S K, Hricak H, Stern J L 1991 Ovarian lesions: detection and characterization with gadolinium-enhanced MR imaging at 1.5 T. Radiology 181: 481–488
29. Ricke J, Sehouli J, Hach C, Hanninen E L, Lichtenegger W, Felix R 2003 Prospective evaluation of contrast-enhanced MRI in the depiction of peritoneal spread in primary or recurrent ovarian cancer. Eur Radiol 13: 943–949

SECTION 7

Neuroradiology, including the head and neck

CHAPTER 55

Skull and Brain: Methods of Examination and Anatomy

Dawn Saunders, H. Rolf Jäger, Alison D. Murray and John M. Stevens

METHODS OF EXAMINATION

Almost all neuroradiological examinations consist of cross-sectional imaging with computed tomography (CT) and magnetic resonance imaging (MRI). Plain radiography is assuming a historical role, but general radiologists and neuroradiologists still need to be familiar with the appearances of plain radiographs of the skull. Vascular grooves and other bony landmarks are shown well by skull radiographs and remain part of the core knowledge required in professional examinations. Knowledge of these structures is also useful for the interpretation of more advanced imaging techniques, such as CT and MRI of the skull base and pituitary region. For these reasons much of the original section on plain radiography is retained in this edition.

The technical principles of CT and MRI and radionuclide studies are covered elsewhere. This chapter discusses only specific issues concerning their application to the imaging of the brain, covering advanced imaging methods such as MR diffusion and MR perfusion imaging and functional imaging with MRI, positron emission tomography (PET), and single-photon emission computed tomography (SPECT).

Noninvasive vascular imaging techniques, such as MR angiography (MRA) and CT angiography (CTA) compete now with intra-arterial cerebral angiography, replacing it for many indications. The technical principles of invasive and noninvasive imaging of the extra- and intracranial vessels are discussed and followed by an overview of the vascular anatomy.

PLAIN RADIOGRAPHY

General considerations

Skull radiography has been replaced by axial imaging methods such as CT and MRI but may still be used on occasions. Scrupulous patient positioning is essential and high-definition films in grid cassettes (24–40 lines cm^{-1}) are preferred. Tube voltages of 50–90 kVp are employed, with a focal spot no larger than 0.6 mm and a film-focus distance of 90 cm. An isocentric skull unit is desirable. Recommendations in this chapter are based on those of the 1961 Commission on Neuroradiology of the World Federation of Neurology, with certain modifications suggested by du Boulay[1].

Lines[2]

1 The *anthropological base line* is drawn from the lower margin of the orbit to the superior border of the external auditory meatus (EAM) known as Reid's or Frankfurt line; or from the outer canthus to the centre of the meatus: orbitomeatal (OM) line.

2 The *auricular line*: perpendicular to the above, drawn vertically through the EAM.
3 The *interpupillary line*: through both pupils, perpendicular to the median sagittal plane (see below).

Planes

1 The *medial sagittal plane* is the anatomical midline.
2 The *horizontal (Frankfurt) plane* contains both anthropological base lines; it is perpendicular to the above. A corresponding orbitomeatal plane includes both orbitomeatal lines.
3 The *frontal biauricular (coronal) plane*: perpendicular to both the preceding planes, passing through the EAM.

The full 'skull series' includes the four views described below.

Lateral projection (Fig. 55.1)

With the midsagittal plane parallel to the detector plate, a horizontal beam is centred 25 mm anterior to the EAM and 10 mm above the orbitomeatal line with the patient supine or sitting, thus placing the sella turcica in the centre of the beam. The anterior clinoid processes and the orbital roofs on the two sides should be superimposed.

Posteroanterior (occipitofrontal, OF) projection (Fig. 55.2)

The midsagittal and orbitomeatal planes are perpendicular to the plate: this is achieved by resting the nose and forehead on the cassette. The tube is angled 20 degrees caudally, with the beam centred on the nasion. A fronto-occipital (anteroposterior [AP]) projection should not be used as it causes magnification and blurring of the more important anterior structures. The petrous ridges should be projected at or near the inferior orbital margins.

Half-axial anteroposterior (Towne's) projection (Fig. 55.3)

The median sagittal plane is again perpendicular to the plate. Placing the occiput on the cassette, with the orbitomeatal or anthropological line perpendicular to it, and angling the tube 30 degrees caudally gives an effective caudal angulation of 25–40 degrees. The beam is centred on the foramen magnum. Lateral rotation is assessed as described earlier.

Submentovertical (base) projection (Fig. 55.4)

With the patient supine, the neck is fully hyperextended by placing a thick pillow or bolster under the shoulders so that the anthropological line is parallel with the plate; the median sagittal plane is again perpendicular to it. The beam is centred on the bi-auricular line, halfway between the angles of the mandible. A satisfactory radiograph shows no rotation and the angles of the mandibles lie just anterior to the middle ear cavities.

Anatomy

The standard projections are shown in Figures 55.1–55.4 and the detailed radioanatomy of the pituitary fossa in Figure 55.5. For anatomical purposes, the basal portion of the skull is divided into three fossae.

The anterior cranial fossa lies above the orbital roofs, anterior to the ridge formed by the greater and lesser wings of the sphenoid. It contains the frontal lobes and the olfactory bulbs and tracts.

The middle cranial fossa lies posteroinferior to the sphenoid ridge, on either side of the basisphenoid, and is bounded laterally by the squamous temporal bone and posteroinferiorly by the petrous ridge. It contains the temporal lobe and should not be confused with the temporal fossa, which is the extracranial space deep to the zygomatic arch.

The posterior cranial fossa comprises all the space below the tentorium or the centrally placed tentorial hiatus and above the foramen magnum. It is bounded anteriorly by the clivus (basisphenoid and basiocciput) in the midline, anterolaterally by the posterior surface of the petrous bone, and elsewhere by the occipital bone. Superolaterally its extent is indicated on skull radiographs by the groove for the transverse venous sinus, but in the midline the apex of the tentorium lies almost at the level of the pineal. Marked variations in the shape of the tentorium (e.g. the straight sinus can be

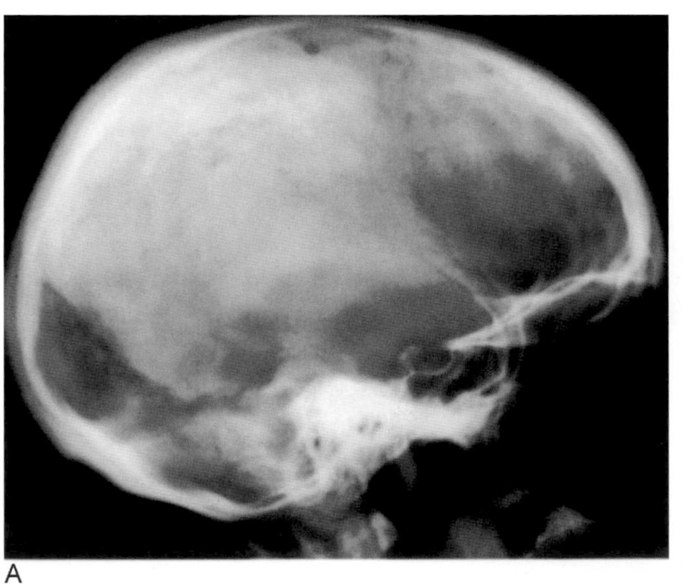

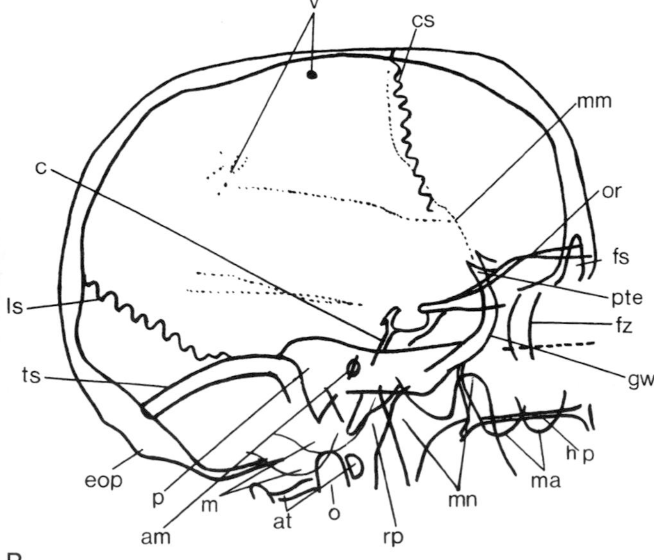

Figure 55.1 Lateral radiograph and diagram of the skull. (For key, see Figure 55.4)

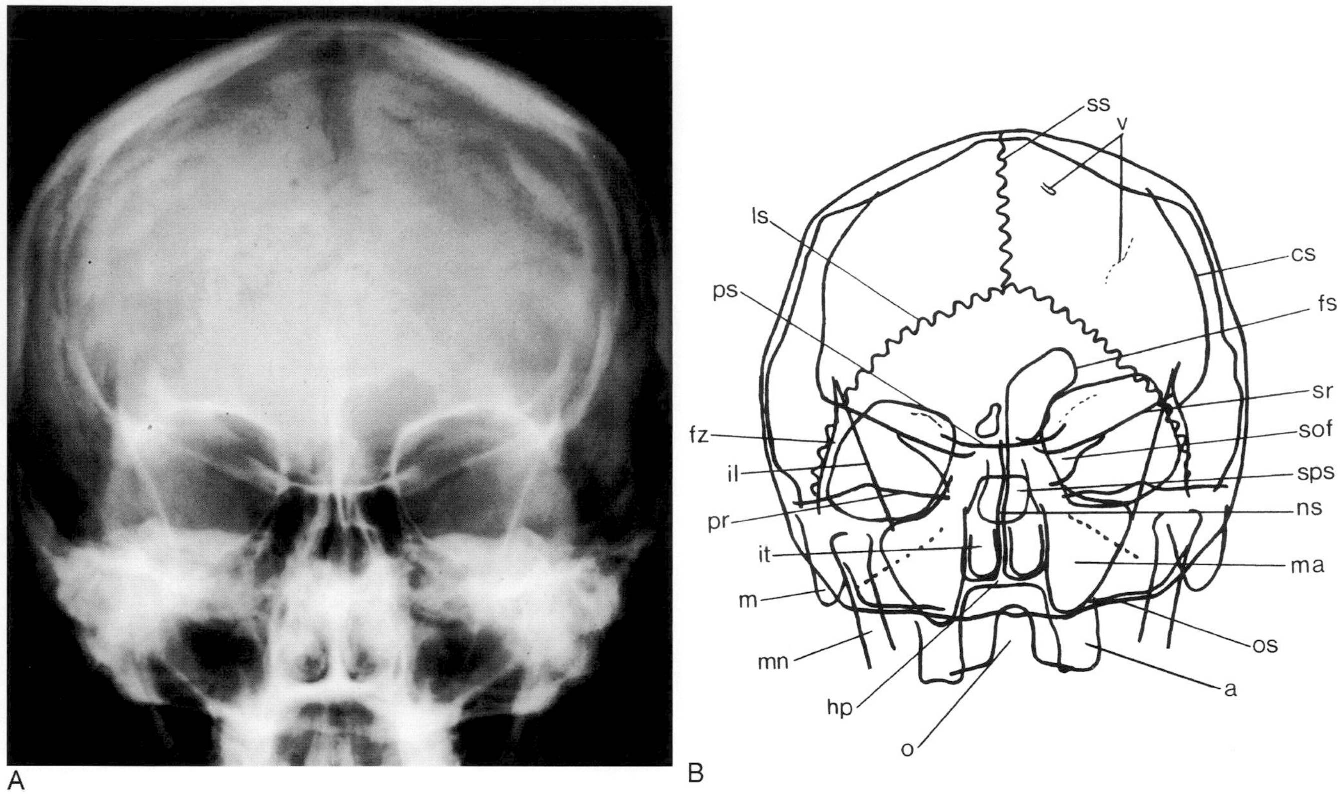

Figure 55.2 Occipitofrontal radiograph and diagram of the skull. (For key, see Figure 55.4)

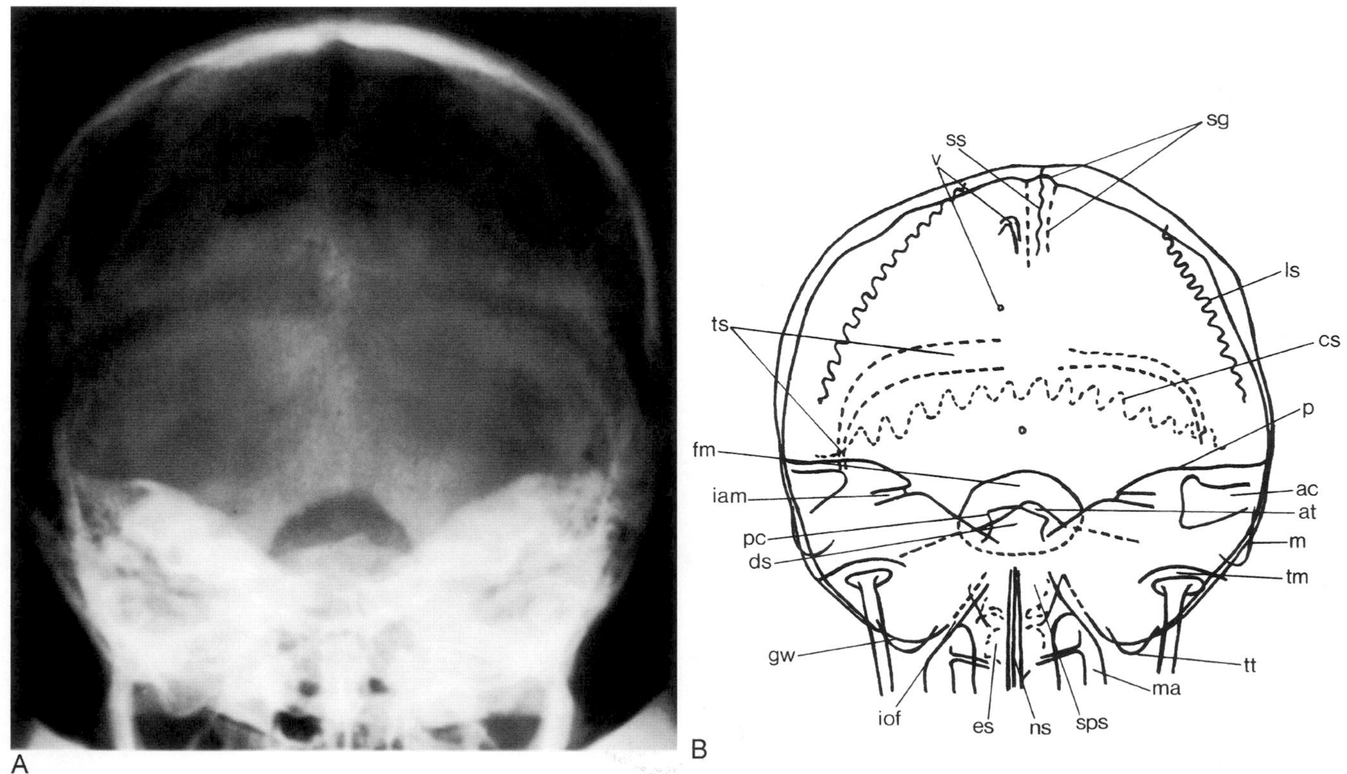

Figure 55.3 Half-axial (Towne's) radiograph and diagram of the skull. (For key, see Figure 55.4)

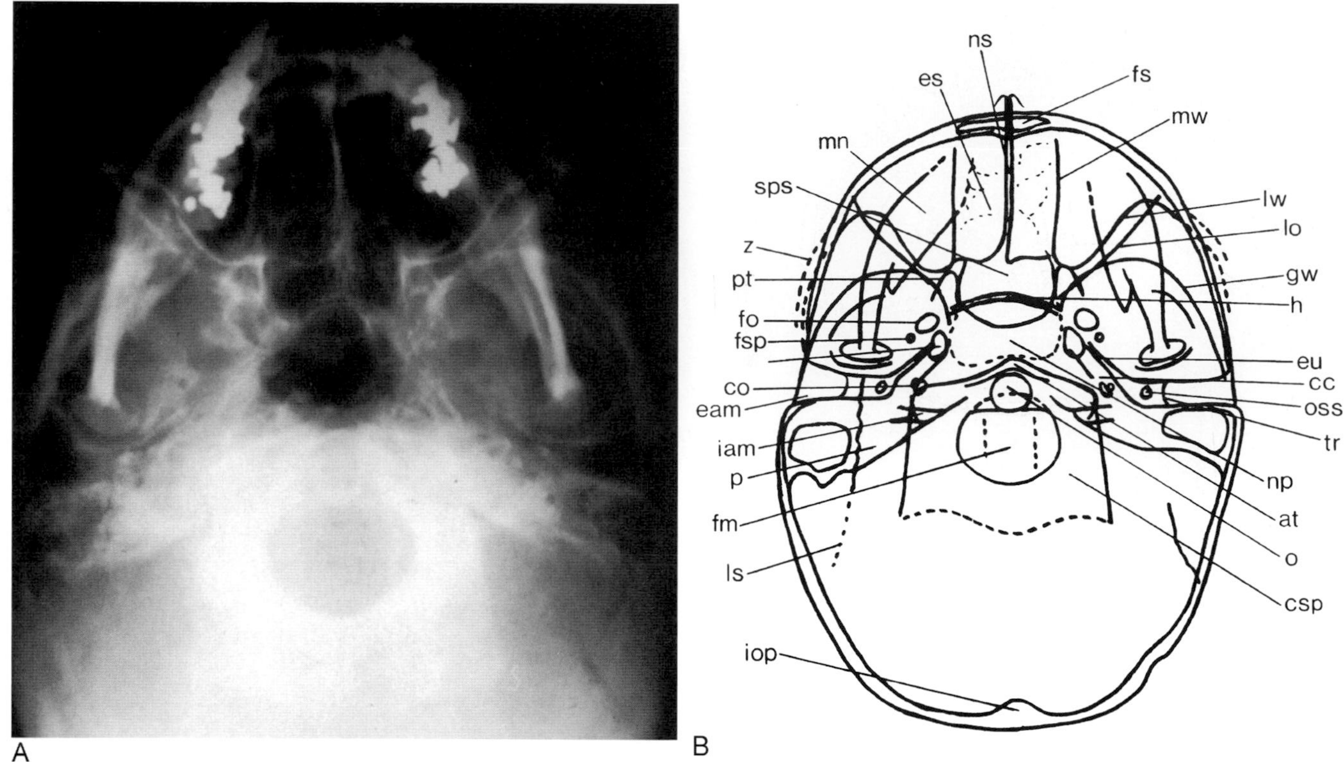

Figure 55.4 Submentovertical radiograph and diagram of the skull. *Key for Figures 55.1–55.4:* a = alveolus, ac = air cells in petrous bone, at = atlas, c = clivus, cc = carotid canal, co = cochlea, cs = coronal suture, csp = cervical spine, ds = dorsum sellae, eam = external auditory meatus (superimposed on lateral projection), eop = external occipital protuberance, es = ethmoid sinus, eu = Eustachian tube, fm = foramen magnum, fo = foramen ovale, fs = frontal sinus, fsp = frontal spinosum, fz = frontozygomatic synostosis, gw = greater wing of sphenoid bone, h = hyoid bone, hp = hard palate, iam = internal auditory meatus (superimposed on lateral projection), il = innominate line, iof = inferior orbital fissure, iop = internal occipital protuberance, it = inferior turbinate, lo = lateral wall of orbit, ls = lambdoid suture, lw = lateral wall of maxillary antrum, m = mastoid process, ma = maxillary antrum, mm = groove for middle meningeal artery, mn = mandible, mw = medial walls of orbit and maxillary antrum (superimposed), np = nasopharynx, ns = nasal septum, o = odontoid, or = roof of orbit, os = occipital squame, oss = ossicles (auditory), p = petrous bone, pc = posterior clinoid process, pr = petrous ridge, ps = planum sphenoidale, pt = pterygoid plates, pte = pterion, rp = retropharyngeal soft tissue, sg = groove for superior sagittal sinus, sof = superior orbital fissure, sps = sphenoid sinus, sr = sphenoid ridge, ss = sagittal suture, tm = temporomandibular joint, tr = tympanic ring, ts = groove for transverse sinus, tt = temporal tubercle, v = venous markings, z = zygomatic arch.

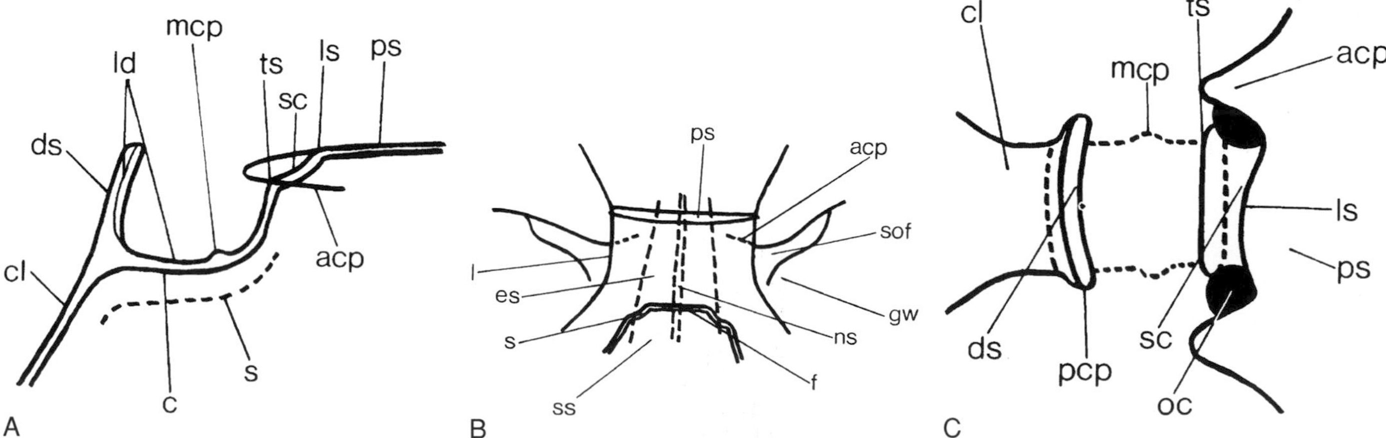

Figure 55.5 Diagram of the sellar region. (A) Lateral projection; (B) frontal projection; (**C**) from above. acp = anterior clinoid process, c = cortical bone lining sphenoid sinus, cl = clivus, ds = dorsum sellae, es = ethmoid sinus, f = floor of sella turcica, gw = greater wing of sphenoid, l = lamina papyracea, ld = lamina dura (cortical bone lining sella turcica), ls = limbus sphenoidale, mcp = middle clinoid process (inconstant), ns = nasal septum, oc = optic canal, pcp = posterior clinoid process, ps = planum sphenoidale, s = carotid sulcus, sc = sulcus chiasmaticus, sof = superior orbital fissure, ss = sphenoid suture, ts = tuberculum sellae.

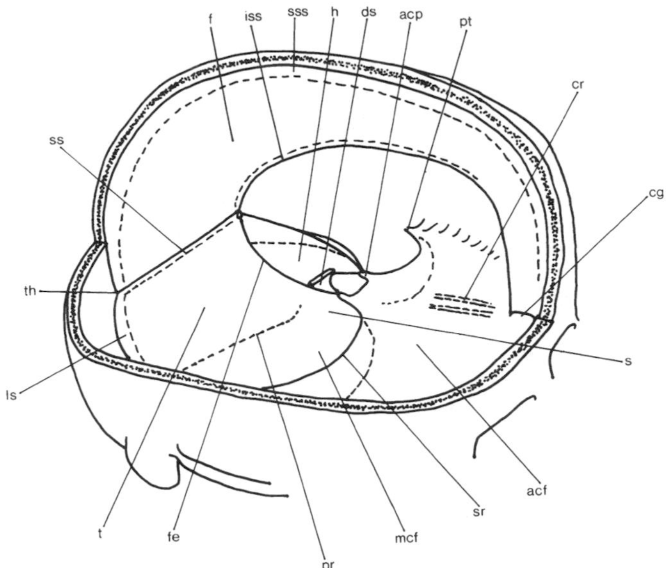

Figure 55.6 The cranial fossae and dural reflections. The right side of the cranial vault has been removed, as have all the cranial contents apart from the dura mater. acf = floor of the anterior cranial fossa (= orbital roof), acp = anterior clinoid process, cg = crista galli, cr = cribriform plate region, ds = dorsum sellae, f = falx cerebri, fe = free edge of the tentorium, h = tentorial hiatus, iss = inferior sagittal sinus, ls = lateral (transverse) sinus, mcf = middle cranial fossa, pr = petrous ridge, pt = pterion, s = cavernous sinus, sr = sphenoid ridge, ss = straight sinus, sss = superior sagittal sinus, t = tentorium, th = torcular Herophili (confluence of the dural venous sinuses).

almost vertical or nearly horizontal) make plain radiographic assessment of the size of the posterior fossa unreliable. It contains the brainstem, cerebellum, fourth ventricle, lower cranial nerves and vertebro-basilar arterial tree.

The major components of the cranial cavity defined by the dural structures are shown schematically in Figure 55.6. The base of the skull is perforated by a number of foramina and canals (the latter being longer than the former) (Table 55.1). Causes of physiological intracranial calcification are listed in Table 55.2.

CROSS-SECTIONAL IMAGING TECHNIQUES

Computed tomography

Routine CT examinations of the brain and specific areas

Brain computed tomography The routine study of the head is made in the axial plane. Some centres prefer to angle the plane so that it is parallel to the orbital roof, and therefore the routine examination does not include the eye. Others image parallel to the cantho-meatal line, which then includes the orbital contents. Slice thickness was originally 5–10 mm for the supratentorial compartment and 5 mm or less for the posterior fossa, mainly in an attempt to reduce beam-hardening artefact. But multidetector CT can provide thinner cuts and many more options, including multiplanar reconstructions. Window widths and levels are set to maximize contrast between grey and white matter, and are kept constant from patient to patient. Head injury examinations should be reviewed using a bone reconstruction algorithm.

Pituitary region Here thinner sections are used, usually 2–3 mm, and smaller fields of view. Imaging can be in the axial plane, with multi-planar reformatting to generate views in the coronal plane if deemed appropriate. Many centres prefer imaging in the direct coronal plane, with the patient prone and head maximally extended, which is not always possible. The preliminary digital CT radiograph is used to select the most favourable plane to avoid metallic dental work projecting artefact into the field of interest. IV contrast medium is given (see later).

Craniocervical junction This region is best examined by MRI. Therefore this investigation is not routine, but can be invaluable in unravelling complex skeletal anomalies in the region, and checking the integrity of bone in erosive or destructive processes prior to excisions or stabilization procedures. Thin sections are necessary and high-resolution bone review algorithms. The axial plane is appropriate, using 2 mm or less slice thickness in either spiral or multislice modes. Multi-planar reformatting and occasionally shaded surface rendering can be extremely helpful in interpretation.

Orbits and petrous bones These special areas are covered in dedicated chapters.

Intravenous contrast medium

A plain unenhanced study always should be performed first. IV contrast enhancement shows areas of blood–brain barrier breakdown within the brain, which is a very nonspecific phenomenon; it can make small lesions much more conspicuous. Some centres still insist on IV contrast medium for all CT examinations of the head but most centres are more selective. Guidelines for contrast medium use include: (A) when plain CT is abnormal and there is a reasonable expectation that enhancement may improve diagnostic accuracy; (B) when lesions are suspected close to the skull base or in the posterior fossa (this includes pituitary and imaging for visual failure); (C) when staging for carcinomas known frequently to metastasize to the brain; (D) when suspecting focal intracranial infections; and (E) when meningeal disease is suspected such as may be caused by sarcoidosis or metastases (e.g. cranial nerve palsies, especially if multiple).

An IV injection of iodinated contrast medium licensed for intravascular use, at dose equivalents of 15–30 g of iodine generally are given; some clinics use two or even three times that dosage. Most units now prefer to inject through indwelling cannulae rather than ordinary needles, so that IV access is assured should an adverse reaction occur. Life-support equipment and medical staff trained in its use should be nearby.

Anatomy on CT

The electron density of grey matter is slightly greater than white, and adequate images should allow clear differentiation of the larger grey and white matter areas of cerebral hemispheres and cerebellum. Usually only the decussation of the superior cerebellar peduncles can be differentiated in the brainstem, which is located in the lower midbrain. The boundaries of brain to cerebrospinal fluid (CSF) are clearly defined, and those of bone to soft tissue are even better. General anatomy is

Table 55.1 THE CRANIAL FORAMINA AND CANALS

Foramen/canal	Site	From	To	Contents	Size	Best projection	Notes
Optic canal	Basisphenoid	Orbital apex	Middle cranial fossa	Optic nerve and sheath; ophthalmic artery	6 mm diameter 8 mm long	Optic canal view	1 mm difference in size suspicious; keyhold and figure of eight variants
Superior orbital fissure	Between greater & lesser wing of sphenoid	Orbital apex	Middle cranial fossa	III, IV, V^1, VI; superior ophthalmic vein; middle meningeal artery branch	Very variable	Occipitofrontal	Thin greater wing may stimulate erosion of lower border
Foramen rotundum	Greater wing of sphenoid	Middle cranial fossa	Pterygopalatine fossa	V^2, artery of the foramen rotundum	3–4 mm diameter	Occipitofrontal	May be surrounded by extensive sphenoid sinus
Pterygoid (vidian) canal	Body of sphenoid, lateral to f. rotundum	Foramen lacerum	Pterygopalatine fossa	Vidian nerve and artery	Smaller than f. rotundum	Occipitofrontal	
Foramen ovale	Greater wing of sphenoid, posteriorly	Middle cranial fossa	Infratemporal fossa	V^3, accessory meningeal artery; veins	5 × 9.5 mm	Submento-vertical	Frequently poorly seen on one or both sides. May be confluent with f. spinosum
Foramen spinosum	Greater wing of sphenoid, posterolateral to f. ovale	Middle cranial fossa	Infratemporal fossa	Middle meningeal artery	2.5–3 mm, rarely 5 mm	Submento-vertical	May be double
Carotid canal	Petrous temporal	Skull base	Middle cranial fossa, above f. lacerum	Internal carotid artery and sympathetic plexus	6–9 mm diameter; 1.5 cm+ in length	Submento-vertical	Runs postero-medial to Eustachian tube; rarely passes through middle ear; absent in aplasia of internal carotid artery
Internal auditory meatus	Petrous temporal	Posterior cranial fossa	Inner ear	VII, VIII and dural sheath; internal auditory artery	5–6 mm in height	Perorbital	Height difference of 2 mm + is suspicious
Jugular foramen	Between petrous temporal and basiocciput	Posterior cranial fossa	Extracranial jugular fossa	Pars nervosa; IX, inferior petrosal sinus; pars vascularis; X, XI, internal jugular vein and ascending pharyngeal and occipital artery branches	11 × 17 mm; right often larger	Under-tilted submentovertical	Pars nervosa and vascularis may be separate
Foramen magnum	Basiocciput	Posterior cranial fossa	Cervical spinal canal	Medulla oblongata, meninges and ligaments; XI (spinal root); vertebral and spinal arteries and veins	30 × 35 mm	Lateral; submentovertical	Shape very variable
Hypoglossal (anterior condylar) canal	Occipital condyle	Foramen magnum	Medial to jugular fossa	XII; branch of ascending pharyngeal artery	5 mm diameter	Reversed Stenvers: Stockholm 'C'	

demonstrated in Figure 55.7. Anatomy of the skull base on CT with bone window settings is shown in Figure 55.8.

SPECIAL TECHNIQUES

Computed tomography cisternography

This test is rarely performed these days, as its only indication is to identify the site of CSF leaks before operative closure. An important requirement is that the patient is actually leaking at the time of the examination, and many workers apply pressure to the neck by hand to temporarily occlude both jugular veins for 4 or 5 min before the study, to encourage active leakage. Water-soluble contrast medium (licensed for intrathecal use, e.g. iohexol) is instilled by lumbar puncture; a concentration of 240 mg ml^{-1} and of about 10 ml are usually more than adequate. Head-down tilting with the patient on their side ensures cranial penetration. Generally it is best to start

Table 55.2 PHYSIOLOGICAL INTRACRANIAL CALCIFICATION
Pineal gland (60 per cent of adults)
Habenular commissure (30 per cent)
Choroid plexus (10 per cent)
Dura mater falx cerebri (7 per cent) and superior sagittal sinus
Tentorium dural plaques (frequently parasagittal)
Petroclinoid (12 per cent) and interclinoid ligaments
Diaphragm sellae
Pituitary gland (rare)[2]
Carotid arteries (in elderly patients)

imaging in the direct coronal plane with the patient prone, as leaking is likely to be maximal in this position. Jugular vein compression is applied at this stage just before imaging if there is doubt about leaking. Thin sections (1–2 mm) on high-resolution modes and smaller fields of view are made through the general area of suspected leakage (which often is already known). A normal CT cisternogram with its anatomical landmarks is shown in Figure 55.9. An axial series with the patient supine often is performed as well, especially if CSF leakage is profuse; if leakage is very profuse, rapid axial imaging in the supine plane may be required initially.

Xenon computed tomography

There are two fundamentally different methods on how CT can be used to assess cerebral blood perfusion. One uses the inhalation of xenon, the other a bolus injection of an iodinated contrast medium[3,4].

Xenon is a stable gas that has an atomic number close to iodine and therefore attenuates the X-ray beam in a similar fashion. Unlike iodine, xenon is freely diffusable and penetrates the blood–brain barrier. Current set-ups for xenon CT consist of the inhalation of a gas containing 28 per cent xenon during sequential acquisition of CT images over a period of approximately 6 min[3]. The distribution of xenon in the brain depends on the regional blood flow and is slightly quicker in grey matter than in white matter. The change of the Hounsfield numbers (CT numbers) over time

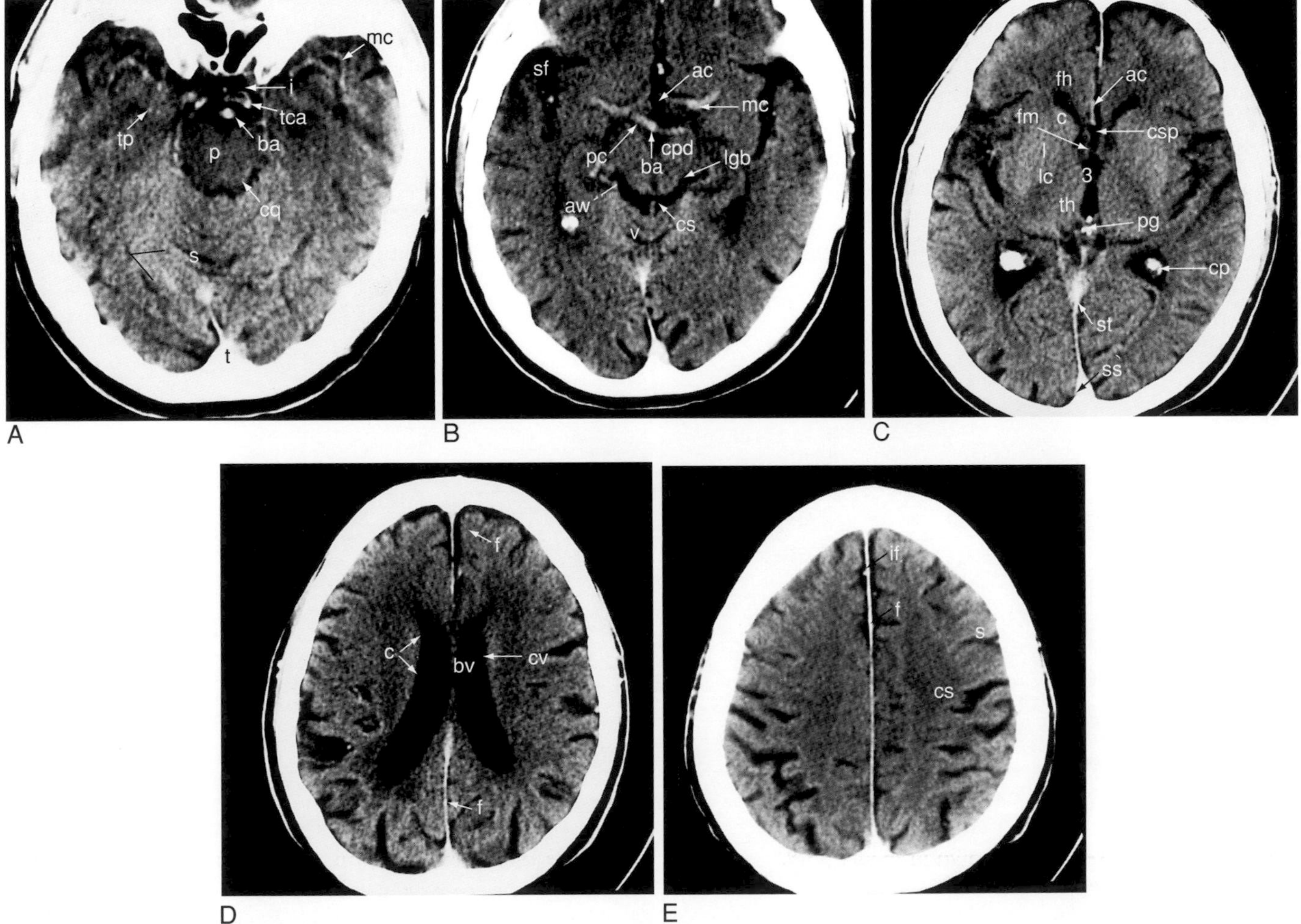

Figure 55.7 (A–E) **Normal contrast-enhanced CT anatomy.** 3 = third ventricle, ac = anterior cerebral artery, ba = basilar artery, bv = body of lateral ventricle, c = caudate nucleus, cc = corpus callosum (genu), cp = choroids plexus, cpd = cerebral peduncle, cq = colliqulus, cs = centrum semiorale, csp = cave of septum pellucidum, cv = internal cerebral vein, f = falx, fh = frontal horn of lateral ventricle, fm = foramen of Monro, i = infundibulum of pituitary, ic = internal capsule, if = intracerebral fissure, l = lateral sulcus, lgb = lateral geniculate body, mc = middle cerebral artery, o = white matter tracts, p = pons, pc = posterior cerebral artery, pg = pineal gland, s = sulcus, sf = sylvian fissure, sp = septum between lateral ventricles, st = straight sinus, ss = sagital sinus, tca = terminal carotid artery, th = thalamus, tp = temporal horn, tr = trigone of lateral ventricle.

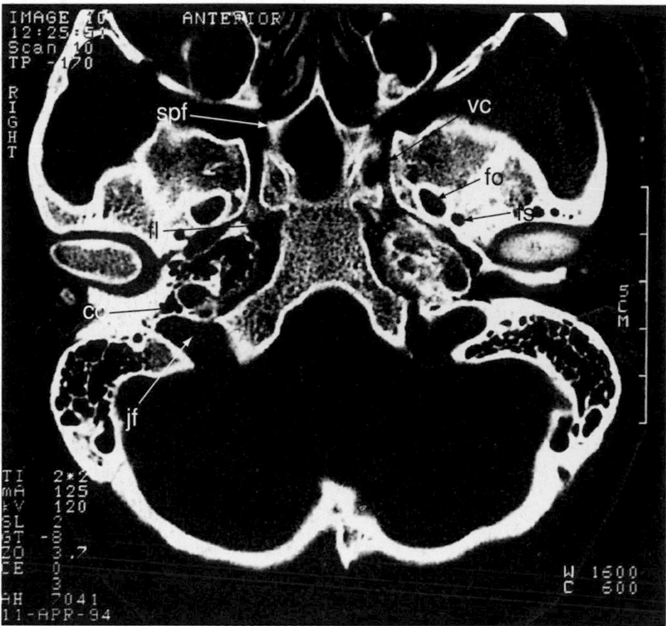

Figure 55.8 CT. Base of skull. Thin-section (1.5 mm) slice showing the important foramina at the skull base. cc = carotid canal, fo = foramen ovale, fl = foramen lacerum, fr = foramen rotundum, fs = foramen spinosum, fv = vidian canal, jf = jugular foramen, spf = sphenopalatine foramen.

during inhalation of xenon forms the basis of blood flow calculations, which are usually displayed as colour maps. The washout of xenon occurs relatively rapidly, allowing a repeat examination after 15–20 min. A disadvantage of this method is that any patient movement during the 6-minute period of imaging causes misregistration of data. Xenon uptake may also be impaired in patients with severe pulmonary disease.

Perfusion computed tomography

The second technique of CT perfusion imaging tracks transient attenuation changes in the blood vessels and brain parenchyma during the first-pass passage of an intravenously injected contrast medium, similar to MR perfusion imaging (see later). A series of images is acquired at a predetermined level with a temporal resolution of one image every 1 or 2 s. The passage of the contrast-medium bolus causes a transient increase in Hounsfield units, which is proportional to the iodine concentration in the perfused tissue. Maps of cerebral blood volume (CBV), mean transit time (MTT) and cerebral blood flow (CBF) can be obtained from a pixel-by-pixel analysis of the density changes over time. Although absolute quantification of CBF is theoretically possible with this method, because of the linear relationship between iodine concentration and Hounsfield numbers, there remains some doubt about its accuracy in practice. Blood flow measurements of cortical grey matter using the bolus perfusion technique were systematically lower compared to data of xenon CT studies[4].

MAGNETIC RESONANCE IMAGING

Routine sequences and imaging protocols

Routine brain magnetic resonance imaging

A dedicated head coil is essential for most indications. This is performed in the axial plane, baseline as for CT. Section thicknesses of 4–5 mm are adequate throughout the head. A standard study usually consists of a sagittal scout multislice acquisition using a fast gradient echo sequence, with T1-weighted contrast, followed by an axial dual-echo multislice series providing balanced (proton density) contrast on the first echo and T2-weighted contrast on the second (Fig. 55.10). Optimal timings,

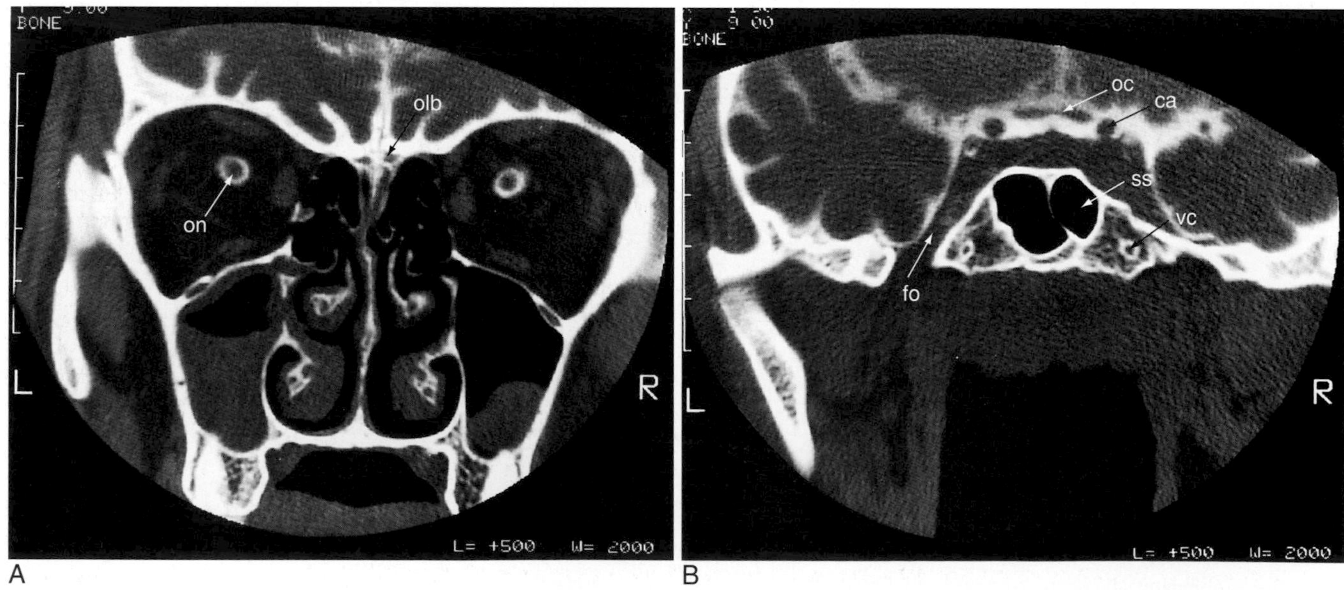

Figure 55.9 CT cisternography. Thin-section (1.5 mm) slices at the (A) level of the olfactory grooves and (B) foramen ovale. The intrathecal contrast outlines the subarachnoid space and extends into the optic nerve sheaths, outlining the optic nerves. ca = carotid artery, fo = foramen ovale, oc = optic chiasm, ob = olfactory bulb, on = optic nerve, ss = sphenoid sinus, vc = vidian canal.

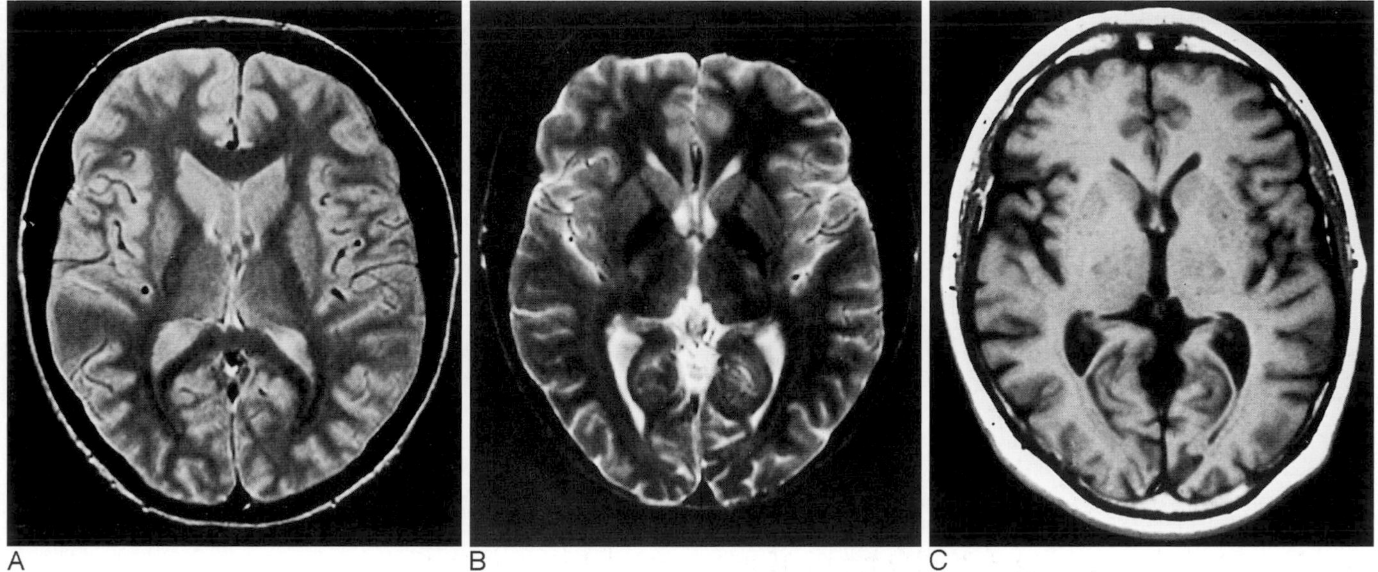

Figure 55.10 Conventional MRI. (A) Fast spin-echo proton density (TR/TE = 3000/20). (B) Fast spin-echo T2-weighted (3000/90). (C) Spin-echo T1-weighted images (400/14).

matrix sizes and fields of view vary between machines. The coronal plane is preferred for the dual-echo acquisition in patients with epilepsy and may be added if judged useful in other situations. A sagittal T2-weighted acquisition may aid detection of corpus callosum involvement in multiple sclerosis, which frequently is in the clinical differential diagnosis. Most units substitute a FLAIR (fluid-attenuated inversion recovery) sequence for the proton density-weighted acquisition in their routine examination[5]. Gradient-recalled susceptibility-weighted acquisitions can be useful on occasions to emphasize the presence of blood products in potentially haemorrhagic lesions.

Strategies to reduce acquisition time at the expense of image quality may be necessary in restless and claustrophobic patients. Most modern equipment has the capability of fast and very fast acquisitions over a few seconds. Multislice modes utilize gradient echos, but single-slice fast spin-echo techniques can be a satisfactory alternative in some cases.

Contraindications to MRI are discussed in Chapter 5.

Special areas

The **pituitary gland** is studied at higher resolution using smaller fields of view, usually with T1-weighted contrast, with contiguous acquisitions in both sagittal and coronal planes. High-resolution modes and thin sections (2–3 mm) are desirable for examining the posterior fossa cisterns, middle and inner ears and the craniocervical junction using acquisitions emphasizing T2-dependent contrast.

Intravenous magnetic resonance contrast medium

As with CT, many units use this routinely, but most are more selective. An unenhanced T1-weighted acquisition is essential first, as with CT. An IV injection of around 10 ml of one of the few MR contrast agents (e.g. gadolinium DTPA) currently licensed for intravascular use is made, imposing a far lower solute load than needed for CT. Similar precautions in case of adverse reactions should be taken, however. Indications for selective use are entirely similar to CT.

ANATOMY (Fig. 55.11)

Grey white matter contrast, and contrast within and between different white matter regions, is far greater on MRI than on CT. A major contribution to this contrast is myelin density, increases in which generally lower signal intensity, though the effect is more complex with T1-weighted contrast where signal is increased in all but the most densely myelinated and compacted tracts. Contrast discrimination within the brain and brainstem generally is greatest on mainly proton density-weighted images: T2-dependent contrast is present as well and signal-to-noise is significantly higher in the first than second echo of a dual-echo acquisition.

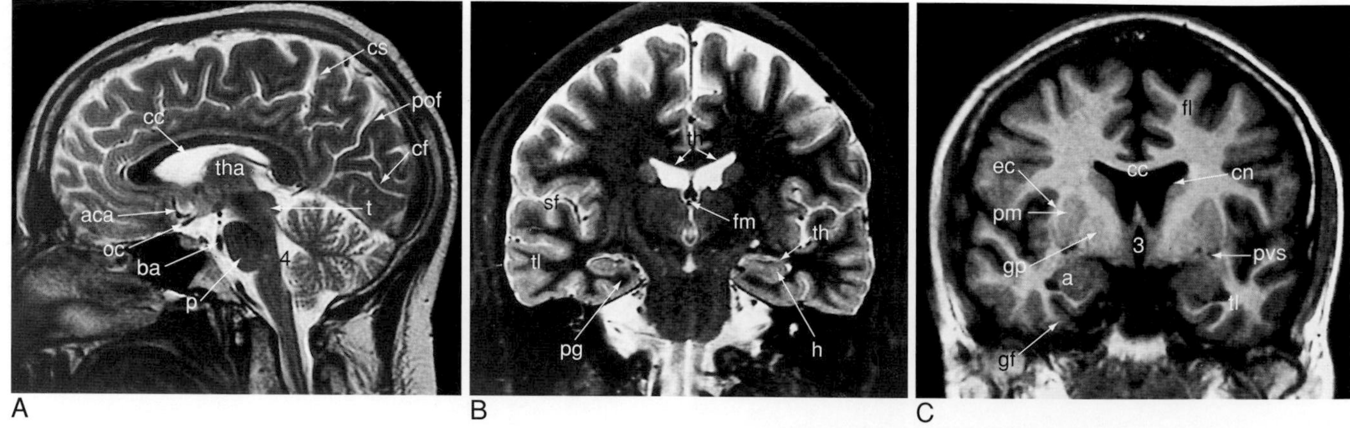

Figure 55.11 Normal MRI. T2-weighted sagittal images through the midline (A). Coronal T2-weighted images through the hippocampi (B). Coronal T1-weighted images through the level of the third ventricle (C). 3,4 = third and fourth ventricle, a = amygdala, aca = anterior cerebral artery, ba = basilar artery, cc = corpus callosum, cf = calcarine fissure, ch = cerebellar hemisphere, cn = caudate nucleus, cs = central sulcus, ec = external capsule, fh = frontal horn, fl = frontal lobe, fm = foramen of Munro, gf = gyrus fusiformis, gp = globus pallidus, h = hippocampus, mca = middle cerebral artery, oc = optic chiasm, oh = occipital horn, p = pons, pg = parahippocampal gyrus, pm = putamen, pof = parieto-occipital fissure, pvs = perivascular spaces, sf = sylvian fissure, t = tectal plate, th = temporal horn, tha = thalamus, tl = temporal lobe.

ADVANCED MAGNETIC RESONANCE IMAGING

MAGNETIC RESONANCE DIFFUSION IMAGING

Diffusion-weighted MRI exploits the presence of random motion (Brownian motion) of water molecules to produce image contrast, thereby providing information not available on standard T1- or T2-weighted images. This is achieved by applying a pair of diffusion sensitizing gradients symmetrically around a 180 refocusing RF pulse of a T2-weighted MR sequence. Mobile molecules acquire phase shifts, which prevent their complete rephasing and result in signal loss. The loss of signal is proportional to the degree of microscopic motion that occurs during the pulse sequence[6]. On diffusion-weighted images, regions of relatively stationary water molecules appear much brighter than areas with a higher molecular diffusion. The degree of phase shift and signal loss depends also on the strength and duration of the diffusion sensitizing gradient, which is expressed by the 'b-value'. B-values used for imaging of acute stroke lie typically around 1000 s mm^{-2}. Quantitative analysis of the apparent diffusion coefficient (ADC) requires sequences with at least two different b-values and additional postprocessing. ADC maps are solely based on differences of tissue diffusion, independent of any T2 effects[7]. The ADC in the normal brain ranges from $2.94 \times 10^{-3} mm^2 s^{-1}$ for CSF to $0.22 \times 10^{-3} mm^2 s^{-1}$ for white matter; grey matter lies in between with a ADC of $0.76 \times 10^{-3} mm^2 s^{-1}$[8]. Areas with a decreased ADC appear dark on ADC maps, which is the converse to diffusion-weighted images where areas of decreased diffusion appear bright[7].

A further feature of diffusion in the brain is its directional dependence, or anisotropy. This is particularly prominent in compacted white matter tracts, and least evident in grey matter. Diffusion tension imaging (DTI) explores anisotropy from six to nine directions and is capable of generating notionally invariant values, which characterize anisotropy on a pixel-by-pixel basis.

Magnetic resonance perfusion imaging

MR perfusion imaging exploits magnetic susceptibility effects within the brain tissue during the first pass of an intravenously injected gadolinium-based contrast agent. During its first pass through the brain, the contrast medium causes a transient signal drop on T2*-weighted (susceptibility-weighted) MRI[8] (see Chapter 8 for images). Images are typically acquired with a temporal resolution of one image every 1–2 s, similar to CT perfusion. The use of singleshot echoplanar imaging (EPI) however, allows multislice imaging with full-brain coverage. MR perfusion imaging is, however, at present only semiquantitative and cannot provide absolute values[9]. A newer MR perfusion technique, arterial spin labelling, that does not require exogenous contrast medium, is currently being developed particularly at higher field strengths, but is not yet robust enough for clinical use[10].

The sequential changes in signal intensity can be plotted as a time–signal intensity curve of a chosen region of interest or reproduced as pixel-based colour maps. Summary parameters are then generated by the manufacturer's software. The relative cerebral blood volume (rCBV) is proportional to the area under the curve on the time–signal intensity graph. Other measurements that can be derived are arrival time (T_0), time to peak (Tp) and mean transit time (MTT) of the gadolinium bolus. Using tracer kinetics, the rCBF can be estimated by dividing the relative blood volume by the mean transit time (rCBF = rCBV divided by MTT). In the absence of absolute quantification of the CBF, comparison with the contralateral hemisphere provides the easiest way to analyse MR perfusion images. This becomes, however, problematic if the perfusion of the contralateral hemisphere is not normal, as in the presence of bilateral carotid artery disease[11].

Magnetic resonance spectroscopy

Magnetic resonance spectroscopy (MRS) is a noninvasive in vivo method that allows the investigation of biochemical changes in both animals and man. Histochemical and cell culture studies have shown that specific cell types or structures have metabolites that give rise to ^{1}H-MRS peaks. A change in the resonance intensity of these marker compounds may reflect loss or damage to a specific cell type. The acquisition of long echo time data (TE = 270 ms, TR = 3 ms) allows the detection of *N*-acetylaspartate (NAA), creatine (Cr/PCr) and choline (Cho) in normal brain, and lactate in areas of abnormality. The methyl resonance of NAA produces a large sharp peak at 2.01 p.p.m. and acts as a neuronal marker as it is almost exclusively found in neurons in the human brain, where it is found predominantly in the axons and nerve processes[12]. The creatine peak (3.03 p.p.m.) arises from both phosphocreatine- and creatine-containing substances in the cell and choline (3.22 p.p.m) is thought to arise from choline-containing substances in the cell membrane.

The acquisition of short echo time data (TE = 30 ms, TR = 2 s) has become the standard spectroscopy sequence and has the advantage of reduced effects from T2 losses and therefore provides spectra with better signal to noise. In addition, it detects additional resonances from metabolites with complex MR spectra such as myo-inositol, glutamate and glutamine (Chapter 8). Whilst providing more information, the broad background signal consisting of low concentration metabolites, and macromolecules and lipids, increases the difficulty of peak area estimation[13].

FUNCTIONAL IMAGING TECHNIQUES

A variety of different techniques are available for functional brain imaging. Those most widely used are SPECT, PET and functional magnetic resonance imaging (fMRI).

Single-photon emission computed tomography

SPECT images are formed from detection of gamma rays emitted during radionuclide decay as part of a nuclear medicine examination. Gamma rays or photons are detected by a gamma camera which, if rotated about the patient's head, allows reconstruction of tomographic slices of distribution of activity in that part of the patient. Radionuclide imaging of the brain requires radiopharmaceuticals that cross the blood–brain barrier. SPECT may be used to produce images of a rCBF using the radiopharmaceuticals ^{133}Xe, ^{123}I isopropyl iodoamphetamine (IMP), ^{99m}Tc ethyl cysteinate dimer (ECD) or ^{99m}Tc hexamethylpropylene amine oxide (HMPAO) (Fig. 55.12). Clinical applications include dementia, cerebrovascular disease, epilepsy, encephalitis and head injury. SPECT can also be used to image uptake at neurotransmitter receptors using various radiopharmaceuticals usually labelled with ^{123}I. Many different SPECT radiopharmaceuticals are taken up into intracranial tumours,

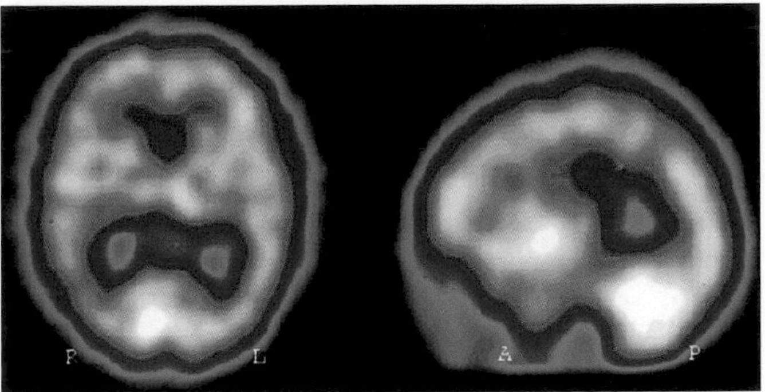

Figure 55.12 SPECT. Normal ^{99m}Tc HMPAO SPECT of the brain, axial (L) and sagittal (R) images.

including ^{201}Tl chloride, ^{99m}Tc MIBI, ^{123}I α-methyl tyrosine and ^{111}In octreotide. Because of the requirement for lead collimation, SPECT has inherently poorer resolution than PET and absolute quantitation is not possible. However, in its favour, SPECT is available in most nuclear medicine departments, is relatively inexpensive and has good patient acceptability.

Positron emission tomography

Positron emission tomography (PET), like SPECT, produces tomographic images. Positron-emitting radioisotopes decay by emission of positrons, or positively charged electrons. These quickly combine with an adjacent electron in an annihilation reaction with the emission of two high-energy gamma rays in opposing directions. Detection of these simultaneously emitted photons allows calculation of their site of origin and, therefore, a map of radiopharmaceutical distribution in the patient. PET can be used to study different physiological processes in the brain.

A cyclotron is required to generate positron-emitting isotopes that can be made from a variety of biologically interesting compounds, such as ^{18}F, ^{11}C, ^{13}N and ^{15}O. Physiological parameters can be derived, for example, cerebral glucose uptake, using ^{1,8}fluorodeoxyglucose (FDG), oxygen metabolism, using $^{15}O_2$ or ^{11}CO and rCBF using $H_2{}^{15}O$. PET rCBF studies can be used to study cortical activation during 'brain tasks' such as finger tapping or visual stimulation. The area of cerebral cortex responsible for a particular function demonstrates slightly increased rCBF during activation. A number of radiopharmaceuticals are available for PET receptor imaging. FDG, ^{11}C methionine and ^{1,8}Fα-methyl tyrosine are used for tumour imaging.

Disadvantages of PET compared with SPECT are its limited availability and high cost due to the necessity of a cyclotron close to the PET unit. PET has the advantage over SPECT and fMRI of enabling absolute quantitation of, for example, CBF, provided arterial blood sampling is performed. Compared with fMRI the main disadvantages of PET are limited availability and ionizing radiation, limiting the number of repeat studies in any one patient.

FUNCTIONAL MAGNETIC RESONANCE IMAGING

Functional MRI techniques can also be used to study cortical activation. The most commonly applied technique is measurement of a tiny increase in signal intensity on T2*-weighted acquisitions in the relevant cortex during neuronal activation. This occurs as a result of the magnetic susceptibility effects of oxyhaemoglobin. Oxyhaemoglobin is diamagnetic while deoxyhaemoglobin is paramagnetic. During cortical activation there is an increase in rCBF and thus an increase in oxygen delivery to the activated brain, which exceeds the local oxygen metabolic requirement. There is, therefore, a net increase in oxyhaemoglobin concentration in the venules and veins in the vicinity of the activated brain, which results in a tiny increase in MR signal, the so called *b*lood *o*xygenation *l*evel *d*ependent or, BOLD effect. The magnitude of this MR signal change is field dependent, being greater at higher field strengths. Nevertheless, it is a tiny signal and quantitative comparison must be made between the MR signal during the resting state and the activation state during multiple repetition in order to detect activation.

Major advantages of fMRI over PET are the lack of ionizing radiation and higher temporal resolution. However, due to the haemodynamic response time, fMRI will never approach the time resolution of electrophysiological methods such as EEG. Another significant limitation of fMRI is that the magnitude of the MR signal change is not directly proportional to rCBF change and therefore absolute quantification is not possible. For activation purposes this is not an important limitation as it is relative changes during activation tasks that are important. Although fMRI is being increasingly used for brain mapping, the technique has limited clinical applications and is used primarily for the identification of eloquent cortex, particularly the motor strip, prior to surgery in patients with structural lesions and arteriovenous malformations[14].

VASCULAR IMAGING

TECHNIQUES

Intra-arterial catheter angiography has been the mainstay for the investigation of neurovascular diseases in the past. Its role is changing with continuous advances in noninvasive vascular imaging, which include Doppler sonography, magnetic resonance angiography and CT angiography. These noninvasive techniques have replaced intra-arterial angiography for a number of diagnostic indications.

This section discusses the techniques of vascular imaging (invasive and noninvasive) before giving a brief overview of vascular neuroanatomy, mostly illustrated with intra-arterial angiograms but equally applicable to the noninvasive techniques.

Conventional intra-arterial angiography techniques of catheterization[15,16]

General principles and basic arteriographic techniques are described elsewhere.

Most diagnostic cerebral angiography can be performed under local anaesthesia. General anaesthesia is indicated in very anxious or restless patients and if interventional endovascular procedures are planned to follow the diagnostic study.

The **transfemoral route** is now almost exclusively used for catheterization of the cerebral vessels and puncture of the axillary artery or direct puncture of the carotid artery are only rarely performed. Insertion of a femoral sheath is not necessary for straightforward cases, but may be useful in more complex cases where a change of catheter during the procedure is anticipated, and is mandatory for interventional procedures.

A variety of catheters are available for catheterization of the carotid and vertebral arteries and the choice of catheter is largely a personal one. The most frequently used catheters are 4F or 5F with a tapered J-shaped tip; some neuroradiologists prefer more complex shapes such as a Mani catheter. In elderly or hypertensive patients, the aortic arch and great vessels are often ectatic and tortuous. In such cases it is best to use a reverse curve catheter, such as a Sidewinder catheter. The use of hydrophilic guidewires greatly facilitates catheterization of the cerebral vessels. It is important to choose a guidewire of the appropriate size, occupying the lumen of the catheter. The choice of a guide that is too small facilitates reflux of blood into the catheter, which can clot and be the source of embolic complications. For catheterization of the carotid and vertebral arteries the surgeon should always lead with a soft-tipped guidewire and advance the catheter over the wire, in order to avoid trauma to the intima.

Most intracranial abnormalities require selective internal carotid and/or vertebral artery injections, depending on the clinical problem. Common carotid artery injection can, however, be performed in elderly patients and those with significant atheromatous disease at the carotid bifurcation. If the latter is suspected, the carotid bifurcation should be visualized under fluoroscopy or with an angiographic run, before advancing the guidewire into the internal carotid artery. The left vertebral artery is larger or of equal size than the right vertebral artery in approximately 75 per cent and therefore represents the first-line approach to angiography of the posterior circulation. Should the left vertebral artery appear to be absent, it probably arises from the arch of the aorta between the left common carotid and subclavian arteries. Very rarely neither vertebral artery can be catheterized, and under these circumstances the subclavian artery can be injected during inflation of a blood pressure cuff, which reduces flow of contrast medium and blood down the arm.

External carotid artery catheterization is necessary for head and neck lesions in intracranial lesions with a potential meningeal supply (such as meningiomas or cerebral arteriovenous malformations [AVMs] and dural fistulae). The origin of the external carotid artery lies anterior and medial to that of the internal carotid artery in the majority of cases.

Once the catheter has been positioned in the appropriate vessel, a double-flush technique, withdrawing blood into one syringe and saline flushing from another, is used to minimize the risks of embolism.

Non-ionic low-osmolality contrast media is recommended for cerebral angiography. For a modern digital angiography system, using a concentration of 150 mg I ml^{-1} is sufficient in the case of internal carotid or vertebral artery injections. A higher concentration of contrast medium (up to 300 mg I ml^{-1}) may be necessary for common carotid artery injections and high-flow lesions, such as large AVMs.

Injection of contrast medium into the external carotid artery is uncomfortable in a number of patients. If the procedure is performed under a local anaesthetic, it is best to warn the patient of a hot feeling in the face and 'funny taste' in the mouth. Similarly, patients should be warned prior to a vertebral artery injection that they might experience flashing lights in the eyes.

Contrast medium can be injected manually or with an automatic pump (6–8 ml of contrast medium at a rate of 3–4 ml s^{-1} for internal carotid and vertebral artery injections when using digital subtraction angiography [DSA]); less forceful and lower-volume injections are needed in the external carotid artery and its branches.

Technique of image acquisition

Nowadays, cerebral angiography is carried out on a DSA system. Modern digital systems provide an image resolution of 1024 × 1024 pixels and good-quality digital fluoroscopy with additional features such as 'road mapping', which is useful for superselective catheterization with microcatheters during interventional procedures.

Standard radiographic projections for carotid angiography include a lateral projection, centred on the pituitary fossa, and an AP view with the petrous ridge projected approximately over the roof of the orbit. Ipsilateral anterior oblique views are routinely performed for the investigation of aneurysms in subarachnoid haemorrhage and a number of additional views such as an occipitomental or periorbital view may be necessary. Three standard projections are employed for the vertebral angiogram: lateral, half-axial (Towne's), and AP, with the petrous ridge superimposed on the lower border of the orbit.

A biplane angiography unit is of major advantage in neuroangiography. It allows simultaneous acquisition of two projections (such as AP and lateral or two oblique views) during a single injection. This reduces the number of contrast medium injections and thereby the risk of catheter-related complications.

Two major technical advances in digital angiography are rapid-frame-rate acquisition (up to 30 images s^{-1}) and three-dimensional (3D) rotational angiography. Routine cerebral angiography is carried out with a frame rate of 2 or 3 images s^{-1} for the arterial phase and 1–2 images s^{-1} for the venous phase. The investigation of AVMs benefits from a higher frame rate in the arterial phase, in the order of 6 images s^{-1}. Occasionally a higher frame rate (15 frames s^{-1}) can be used to analyze the haemodynamics in high flow lesions or certain types of aneurysms[17].

3D rotational angiography involves image acquisition with a precisely calibrated rotating X-ray tube (describing an 180-degree arc) before and during pump injection of contrast medium. This allows the acquisition of volumetric datasets, which are post-processed on a computer workstation. Following removal of the bony structures, high-resolution images of the cerebral vessels can be manipulated in different ways and viewed from any angle. This obviates the need for multiple angiographic runs and has proved very useful in the planning of endovascular treatment of aneurysms, providing a 3D view of the aneurysm morphology and its neighbouring vessels[18].

Indications

Owing to the advent of new noninvasive imaging techniques, particularly computed tomographic angiography (CTA), the indications for intra-arterial cerebral angiography are changing. In departments where CTA is routinely used, cerebral angiography is used to resolve discrepancies between two noninvasive methods and as an integral part of endovascular interventional procedures. It may be used for the investigation of aneurysms in subarachnoid haemorrhage, cerebral AVMs and carotid artery disease to confirm a significant stenosis suspected on noninvasive imaging. Preoperative angiography is sometimes performed in glomus jugulare tumours and meningiomas to assess tumour vascularity, and is frequently combined with preoperative embolization in very vascular tumours[19].

Contraindications

There are very few absolute contraindications to cerebral angiography, but since it is not without risk, it should *never* be carried out if it is clear that the results will not influence management. A well-documented history of untoward reactions to contrast media is a relative contraindication. Intra-arterial angiography is now increasingly used in the context of thrombolytic treatment of acute stroke[20]. Treatment with anticoagulant drugs does not contraindicate arteriography, provided the prothrombin level is within the normal therapeutic range.

Complications

Local and general complications of arteriography are discussed in Chapter 6.

Specific risks of catheterization of the aortic arch or cervical arteries include cerebral embolism and damage to the arteries by the catheter or guidewire, which include spasm, thrombosis and dissection. A previous study showed that the stroke risk of arch aortography and DSA is similar to that of selective injections, which suggests that the risk is mainly due to embolism from catheter or guidewires[21]. Reported risks of cerebral angiography in studies published over the last 15 years vary from 0.5–2.3 per cent[22–24]. The North American Asymptomatic Carotid Stenosis trial (ACAS) identified the risk of significant disabling stroke as being 1.2 per cent, which was similar to the stroke risk of carotid endarterectomy in asymptomatic patients[25].

A recent, retrospective study of 454 patients mainly investigated for suspected aneurysms or AVMs (with one-third of the studies performed in the acute stage of intracranial haemorrhage), showed an overall neurological complication rate of 2.3 per cent with persistent neurological deficits in 0.4 per cent[24].

COMPUTED TOMOGRAPHY ANGIOGRAPHY (Fig. 55.13)

Selective imaging of blood vessels with CT has become possible with the introduction of spiral CT systems[26]. The technical principles of spiral CT data acquisition are explained in Chapter 4. For CTA, a volumetric dataset is acquired during the vascular phase of an iodinated contrast, which is injected intravenously. The data acquisition time and amount of contrast medium used depend on the area to be covered and choice of slice collimation and table speed. Earlier spiral CT systems offered only a limited area coverage (such as the carotid bifurcation or circle of Willis), due to X-ray tube heating limits. The quality of CTA has dramatically improved with the introduction of multidetector CT[27] with improved area coverage and spatial resolution. Modern multidetector-CT machines are able to cover an area from the carotid bifurcation up to the circle of Willis or the entire intracranial circulation from the skull base to the vertex with a single data acquisition.

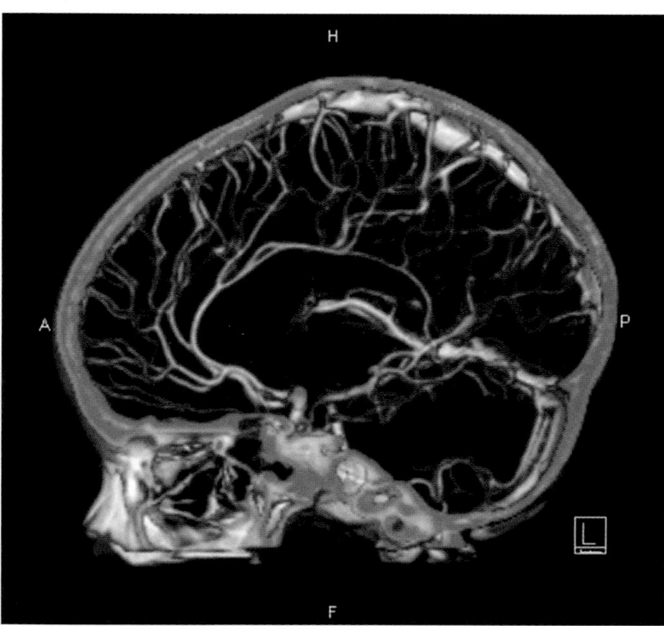

Figure 55.13 CTA 3D volume-rendered CTA. The arterial anatomy is well visualized. Filling of the internal cerebral venous and venous sinuses is also seen.

Timing of data acquisition in relation to the administration of contrast medium is critical for maximum arterial opacification. The operator can either set a standard delay or use an automating bolus detection system, which is available on most machines. Recommended standard delays between the start of the injection and image acquisition are 12 s for examination of the extracranial and 15 s for examination of the intracranial vessels[28]. Automated bolus detection is, however, more satisfactory because it adjusts for individual variations in circulation time. Injection rates and volumes vary with the cannula size, number of slices and cardiac output. Typical volumes of 100–120 ml contrast medium are given at a rate of 3–5 ml s^{-1}.

The quality of CT angiograms depends heavily on post-processing of the image data. Enhanced blood vessels are extracted from a 3D dataset by applying specific density thresholds. The vessels can then be displayed as 2D projectional images, which resemble conventional angiograms, or as 3D surface-rendered structures. Separation of vessels running close to bone (near the skull base and cranial vault may be difficult. These difficulties can be at least partially resolved by using thick-section multiplanar reformats (which can be angled in such a way to exclude bone) and by interactive viewing of the source data[29].

CTA has been used successfully for the evaluation of carotid artery stenosis[30,31], carotid artery dissection[32], intracranial vascular occlusion[33] and intracranial aneurysms[34,35]. CTA for the assessment of cerebral AVM is subject to ongoing research; their complex structure needs more sophisticated post-processing and interactive viewing[36].

CTA can also be used to examine the cerebral venous system (CT venography), its main application being suspected dural sinus thrombosis[37].

The **advantages of CTA** over MRA are that it can be used in claustrophobic patients and patients with cardiac pacemakers, or other implants that preclude MR data acquisition. Its disadvantages are the use of ionizing radiation and iodinated contrast media.

MAGNETIC RESONANCE ANGIOGRAPHY

MRA has progressed rapidly in the last decade. Its basic principles are outlined in Chapter 6. Traditionally, MRA has been performed without administration of an exogenous contrast medium, relying on inflow of unsaturated spin (time-of-flight [TOF] MRA) or accumulation of phase shifts proportional to the flow velocity (phase contrast MRA)[38]. More recently, MRA has been used in conjunction with the injection of gadolinium-based contrast media (contrast-enhanced MRA)[39]. Both non-enhanced and enhanced MRA techniques benefited from the development of high-performance gradients allowing shorter repetition (TR) and echo (TE) times as well as software developments such as zero-filled interpolation processing. Both TOF and phase contrast techniques can be performed with a 2D or 3D data acquisition[40]. 2D-TOF or 3D-TOF MRA of the neck vessels have limitations in areas of turbulent or slow flow, which may remain undetected due to intravoxel dephasing[41,42]. This can simulate the presence or exaggerate the degree of carotid artery stenoses.

For imaging of the intracerebral vessels, 3D-TOF MRA is the technique of choice[43]. A single slab 3D-TOF aquisition is adequate for imaging the circle of Willis, but coverage of a larger part of the intracranial circulation requires three or four multiple overlapping slabs (MOTSA technique) (Fig. 55.14). Data are usually displayed as maximum intensity projections, but inspection of the source data should always be performed to resolve difficult cases or to confirm the suspicion of an artefact[43]. Intracranial 3D-TOF MRA has been successfully used for the detection of aneurysms (with a high sensitivity for aneurysms larger than 5 mm)[44–46], assessment of intracranial stenosis and, to a limited extent, AVMs[47].

Phase contrast MRA is based on the detection of phase shifts generated by a flow-encoding gradient. The phase shift is proportional to the velocity of blood, and care must be taken to choose an appropriate 'velocity window' depending on the area studied. Typical velocity parameters are 10–20 cm s^{-1} for dural sinuses and 50–60 cm s^{-1} for major cerebral arteries. Although generally inferior to 3D MRA, it is more sensitive for detection of slow flow (with the appropriate velocity encoding) and can therefore be used for imaging cerebral veins[48]. It does not suffer from T1-contamination artefact and it can provide information about the direction of blood flow. 3D phase contrast MRA can also be used to show the direction of collateral blood flow across the circle of Willis (Fig. 55.15) with significant differences between normal volunteers and patients with carotid artery occlusion[49].

The administration of a gadolinium-based contrast medium has been shown to have some benefit in conjunction with intracranial 3D-TOF MRA for conditions such as AVMs and intracranial stenoses[50,51]. The acquisition of 3D gradient-echo

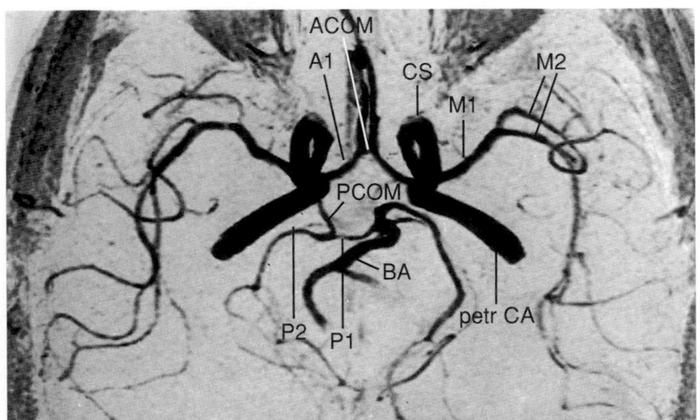

Figure 55.14 3D TOF MRA of the intracranial circulation: axially collapsed maximum intensity projection. A1 = precommunicating segment of anterior cerebral artery, ACOM = anterior communicating artery, BA = basilar artery, CS = carotid siphon, M1 = first (horizontal) segment of middle cerebral artery, M2 = M2 segments of middle cerebral artery, P1 = precommunicating segment of posterior cerebral artery, P2 = P2 segment of posterior cerebral artery, PCOM = posterior communicating artery, petr CA = petrous segment of ICA.

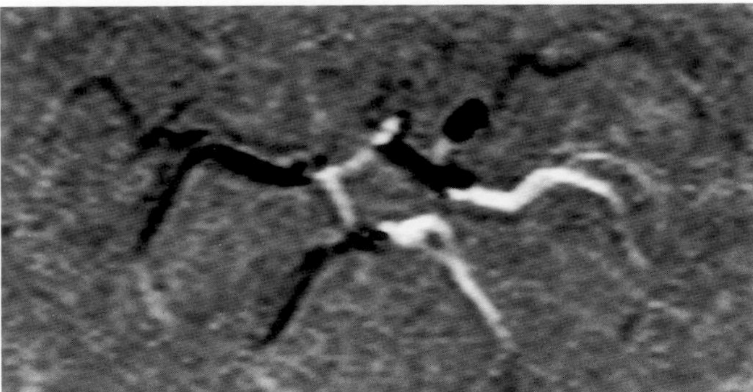

Figure 55.15 Phase contrast MRA of circle of Willis. Phase contrast MRA allows encoding of the flow direction. Here the flow-encoding direction is right (R) to left (L): flow in this direction appears white, whereas flow in the opposite direction (towards the right) appears black.

images, during the first pass of a contrast medium bolus, represents a relatively recent development. Demonstration of vascular structures with this technique depends on the T1 shortening of blood and not on inflow or phase-shift effects[39] (Fig. 55.16). Contrast-enhanced MRA of the carotid arteries does not suffer from artificial signal loss due to turbulent and slow flow (like the TOF techniques) and initial results show that it compares favourably with intra-arterial angiography[52]. Applications of this method for imaging intracranial vessels are emerging[53].

Doppler ultrasound

Technical principles and Doppler US and its use in the assessment of the carotid artery stenosis are discussed in Chapter 3.

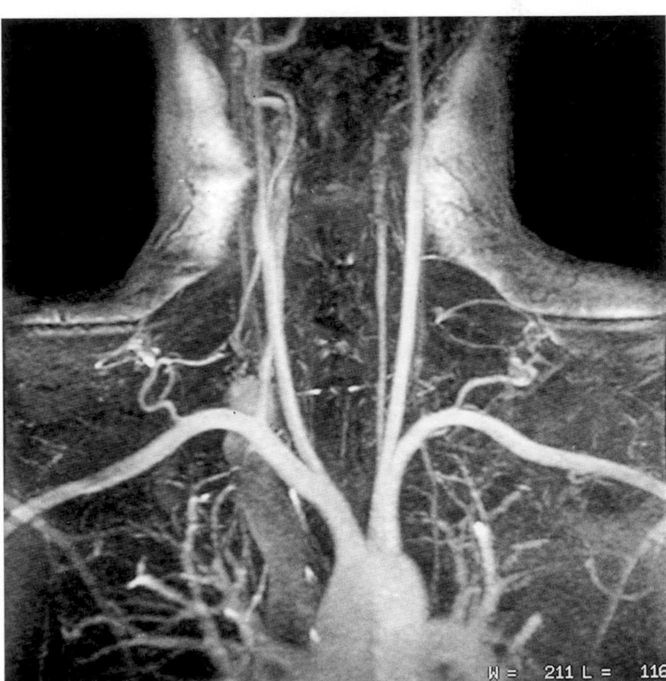

Figure 55.16 Contrast-enhanced MRA of aortic arch. A 3D gradient-echo sequence has been acquired during the first pass of an intravenously injected gadolinium bolus. It shows the origins of the great vessels. Note also that there is background opacification of the pulmonary vessels.

ANATOMY OF CEREBRAL ARTERIES AND VEINS[16]

INTRACRANIAL ARTERIES

The internal carotid arteries supply the anterior cerebral circulation and the vertebral and basilar arteries supply the posterior circulation. The external carotid arteries supply most extracranial head and neck structures (except the orbits) and make an important contribution to the supply of the meninges. There are numerous anastomoses between the external carotid arteries and the anterior and posterior circulation.

Anterior circulation

The right common carotid artery is the first main branch of the innominate or brachiocephalic artery and the left common carotid artery is the second main branch of the aortic arch (Fig. 55.17). Each common carotid artery runs within a fascial plane, the carotid sheath, lateral to the vertebral column, and bifurcates between the level of the third and fifth cervical vertebrae into external and internal carotid arteries. At the bifurcation, the internal carotid lies usually posterior and lateral to the external carotid artery.

Internal carotid artery[16,54,55]

The internal carotid artery can be divided into a number of segments between the carotid bulb and its bifurcation into middle and anterior cerebral arteries. Unfortunately there are several classification systems, some numbering the segments with the direction of blood flow and others against it[54]. Until a consensus is reached, it is best to use anatomical names for the internal carotid artery segments. A simplified anatomical division distinguishes between cervical, petrous, cavernous and supraclinoid segments of the internal carotid artery[56].

No named branches arise from the cervical segment of the internal carotid artery. The petrous segment is intraosseous. It begins at the carotid canal where the artery enters the skull base. The internal carotid artery then runs forward and medially in the foramen lacerum and lies extradurally until it reaches the petrolingual ligament; after this it becomes the cavernous segment, which gives off several important branches. After leaving the cavernous sinus, it pierces the dura and enters the subarachnoid space at the level of the anterior clinoid process, after which it becomes the supraclinoid segment. The carotid siphon is formed by the cavernous and supraclinoid segments. The supraclinoid segment terminates, dividing into the anterior and middle cerebral arteries (Fig. 55.18).

The principal branches of the cavernous segment are:

1 The *posterior trunk (meningohypophyseal artery)* arises posteriorly from the superior aspect of the first bend of the cavernous segment and gives off branches to the pituitary gland and tentorium cerebelli (marginal tentorial artery).
2 The *inferolateral trunk* arises more anteriorly and laterally from the horizontal portion of the cavernous segment. It supplies the third, fourth and fifth cranial nerves and has important anastomoses with the external carotid system: with the maxillary artery through the foramen rotundum and ovale and with the middle meningeal artery through the foramen spinosum.

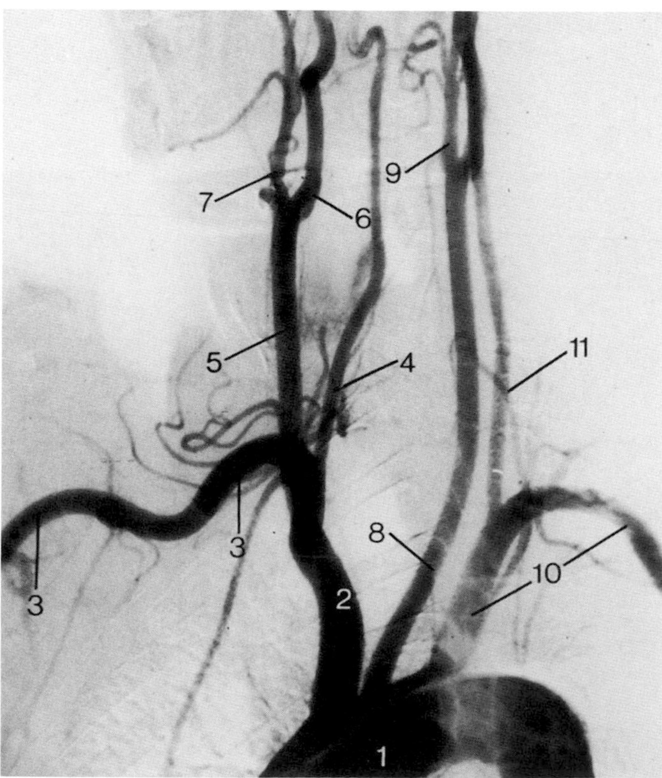

Figure 55.17 Arch aortogram, left anterior oblique projection, arterial phase, 1 = arch of aorta, 2 = innominate (brachiocephalic) artery, 3 = right subclavian artery, 4 = right vertebral artery, 5 = right common carotid artery, 6 = right internal carotid artery, 7 = right external carotid artery, 8 = left common carotid artery, 9 = left external carotid artery, 10 = left subclavian artery, 11 = left vertebral artery.

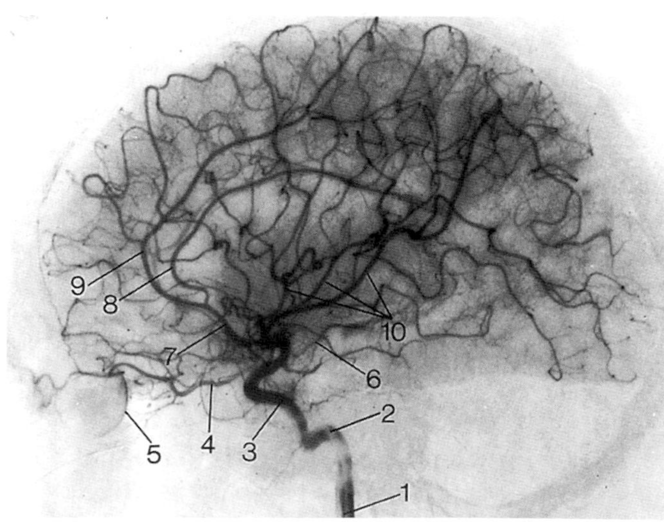

Figure 55.18 Internal carotid arteriogram; lateral projection, arterial phase. 1 = cervical portion of internal carotid artery, 2 = petrous portion, 3 = cavernous portion (siphon), 4 = ophthalmic artery, 5 = choroidal (ophthalmic) crescent, 6 = anterior choroidal artery, 7 = anterior cerebral artery, 8 = pericallosal artery, 9 = callosomarginal artery, 10 = middle cerebral artery branches.

The principal branches of the supraclinoid segment are:

1 The *ophthalmic artery* is usually given off just after the carotid artery leaves the cavernous sinus, but its origin is variable and it can sometimes arise from the middle meningeal artery.

2 The *posterior communicating artery* arises posteriorly from the distal loop of the siphon, to link the internal carotid artery with the posterior cerebral artery, which arises normally from the posterior (vertebral) circulation. It is extremely variable in size and, when small, inconstantly opacified by carotid injection. The posterior cerebral artery can arise directly from the internal carotid artery, which is called a 'fetal arrangement'.

3 The *anterior choroidal artery* arises just distal to the posterior communicating artery and runs posterosuperiorly and laterally. It is an important artery that supplies the posterior limb of internal capsule, cerebral peduncle and optic tract, medial temporal lobe and choroid plexus.

Anterior cerebral artery[16,57–60]

The anterior cerebral artery is divided into three anatomical segments: the horizontal or precommunicating segment (A1), vertical or postcommunicating segment (A2), and distal ACA including cortical branches (A3).

The **A1 segment** runs beneath the frontal lobe of the brain and courses over the optic nerves and chiasm to the midline, where it is joined to the contralateral A1 segment by the anterior communicating artery. The A1 segment gives rise to a variable number of perforating branches, the medial lenticulostriate arteries. The recurrent artery of Huebner is the largest of the perforating branches and may arise from the A1 or A2 segment. It derives its name from the fact that it doubles back on its parent artery at an acute angle to join the lenticulostriate vessels. A common anatomical variation is hypoplasia or aplasia of the A1 segment, in which case the distal segments fill preferentially from the other side via the anterior communicating artery. Other variations include a fusion of the A2 segment in the midline to give a single 'azygos' anterior cerebral artery, which then supplies both hemispheres.

The **A2 segment** turns upwards, gives off a frontopolar branch and divides, at the level of the genu of the corpus callosum, into the callosomarginal and pericallosal arteries, which are the A3 segments. The former lies in the cingulate sulcus and the latter course along the posterior aspect of the corpus callosum, which it supplies. Cortical branches of the callosomarginal artery supply the medial frontal lobe (frequently as far back as the Rolandic fissure), whereas cortical branches of the pericallosal artery supply the medial parietal lobe.

Middle cerebral artery[16,59,60]

The middle cerebral artery is divided into four anatomical segments: the horizontal segment (M1), insular segment (M2), opercular segment (M3) and cortical branches (M4 segments). Medial and lateral lenticulostriate arteries are perforating branches that arise from the M1 segment (Fig. 55.19); they supply the basal ganglia and capsular region.

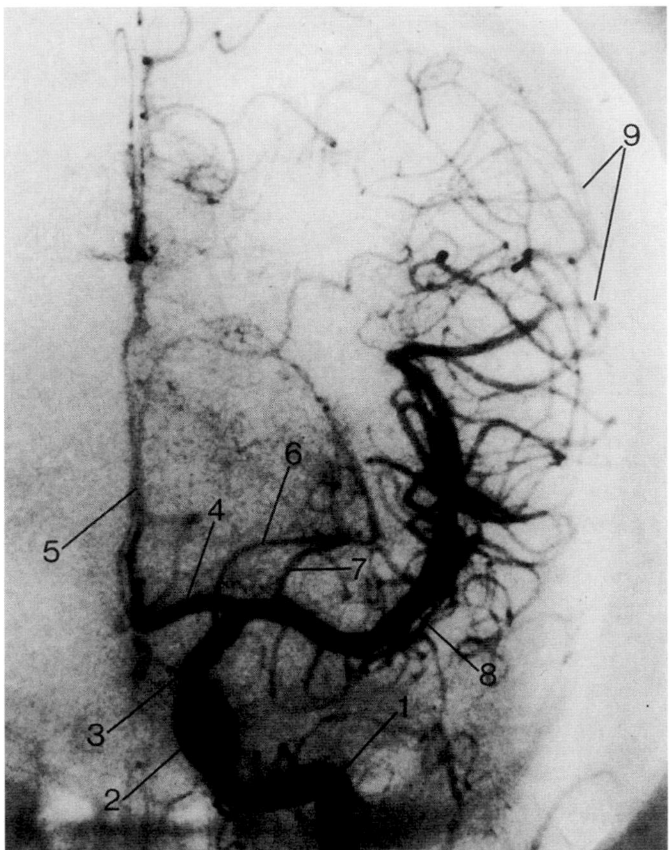

Figure 55.19 Internal carotid arteriogram: AP projection, arterial phase. 1 = petrous segment of internal carotid artery, 2 = cavernous portion, 3 = supraclinoid (subarachnoid) portion, 4 = anterior cerebral artery precommunicating segment, lying above the pituitary fossa, 5 = pericallosal and callosomarginal arteries, superimposed, lying in the midline, 6 = anterior choroidal artery, 7 = lenticulostriate artery, 8 = major divisions of the middle cerebral artery, 9 = cortical branches, which extend to the cranial vault.

The M1 segment runs in the Sylvian fissure and gives off an anterior temporal artery of variable size before dividing into two or three main trunks (M2 segments). Its branches run over the frontoparietal and temporal opercula (M3 segments). The characteristic loops formed by the upward and downward course of the insular and opercular segments form a straight line on the lateral projection, which represents the upper border of the 'Sylvian triangle', its inferior border being formed by main middle cerebral artery trunk. The 'Sylvian point' is the highest and most medial point where the angular artery turns inferolaterally to exit the Sylvian fissure. Displacement of these landmarks has been used in the past to locate cerebral mass lesions; they are now largely of historical interest.

The cortical branches (M4 segments) of the middle cerebral artery are variable and complex, but temporal, ascending frontoparietal, parietal, angular and posterior temporal branches can usually be identified (Figs 55.18, 55.19) and supply most of the lateral surface of the cerebral hemisphere, excluding a narrow superomedial strip supplied by the anterior and posterior cerebral arteries.

Posterior circulation[15,16,59] (Figs 55.20, 55.21)

Vertebro-basilar system

The **right and left vertebral arteries** usually arise as the first branches of the corresponding subclavian arteries. Each then enters the foramen transversarium of the sixth cervical vertebra, and runs directly upwards in the bony vertebral canal formed by these foramina before arching laterally then medially around the anterior arch of the atlas behind the lateral mass of the atlas to pierce the dura mater and enter the subarachnoid space at the level of the foramen magnum, subsequently fusing with its fellow behind the clivus and in front of the lower pons, to give rise to the midline basilar artery.

The vertebral arteries give muscular branches, which frequently anastomose with those of the ascending pharyngeal and occipital arteries, and they commonly furnish important feeding vessels to the cervical spinal cord. One of the vertebral arteries often gives off the posterior meningeal artery, which passes upwards through the foramen magnum to run posteriorly in the midline on the dura mater of the occipital bone. Soon after entering the cranial cavity, each vertebral artery gives off a posterior inferior cerebellar artery, which runs around the medulla oblongata, looping under the olive, to lie near its fellow in the midline behind the medulla, before running posteriorly above the cerebellar tonsil, where it lies close to the roof of the fourth ventricle, and continuing on the undersurface of the cerebellum as the inferior vermian artery. The posterior inferior cerebellar artery also gives off tonsillar and hemispheric branches.

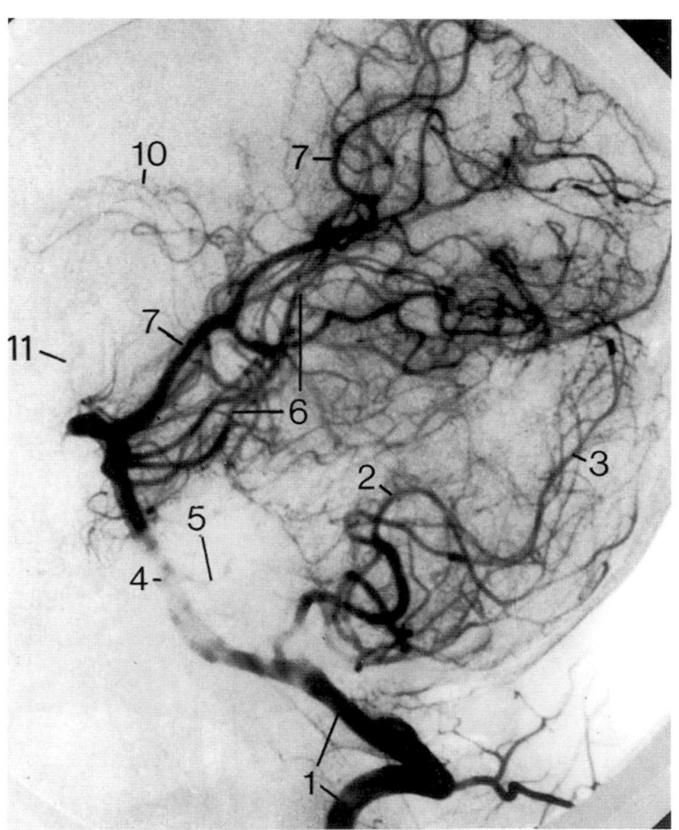

Figure 55.20 Vertebral angiogram. Lateral projection, arterial phase. *Key for Figures 55.20 and 55.21:* 1 = vertebral artery, 2 = posterior inferior cerebellar artery, 3 = inferior vermian branch, 4 = basilar artery, 5 = anterior inferior cerebellar artery, 6 = superior cerebellar artery (duplicated on left), 7 = posterior cerebral arteries, 8 = posterior temporal branches, 9 = internal occipital and calcarine branches, 10 = posterior choroidal arteries, 11 = thalamoperforating arteries, 12 = filling of middle cerebral arterial branches via posterior communicating artery.

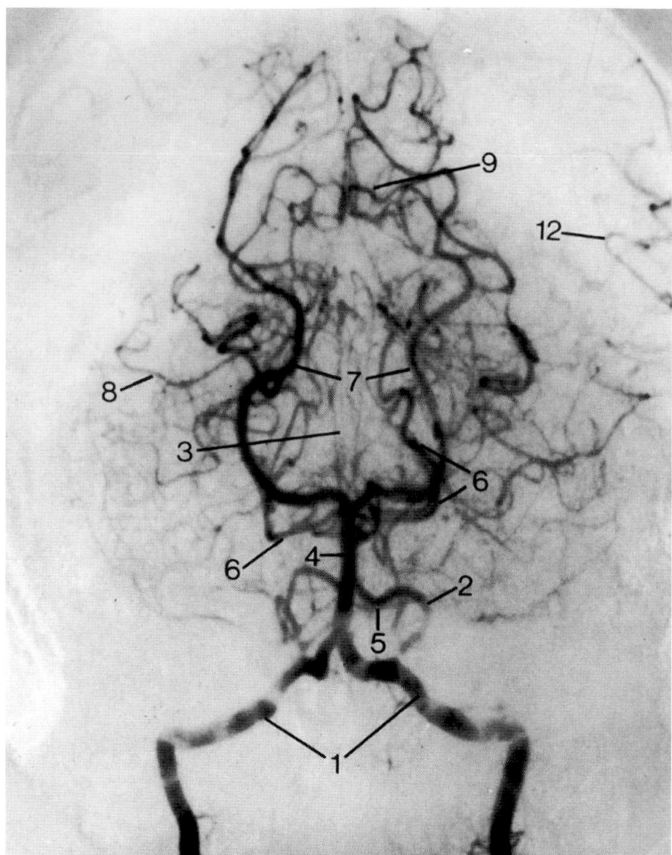

Figure 55.21 Vertebral angiogram. Half-axial projection, arterial phase. (For Key, see Fig. 55.20 caption.)

The vertebral arteries are commonly unequal in size; when this is the case, the left is usually the larger, but the right is of greater calibre in about one-fifth of cases. When one of the arteries is very small, it frequently supplies only the ipsilateral posterior inferior cerebellar artery territory, which is called a PICA termination of the vertebral artery.

The **basilar artery** runs superiorly on the anterior surface of the pons and gives off anterior inferior cerebellar, superior cerebellar and posterior cerebral arteries on both sides. Terminating just above the tip of the dorsum sellae, it generally shows a slight anterior convexity and deviates from the midline following the curve of the dominant vertebral artery; its form is sufficiently variable, especially in the elderly, to render assessment of lateral or posterior displacement difficult.

The **anterior inferior cerebellar arteries** arise close to the origin of the basilar artery and run laterally on the pons and anteroinferior surface of the cerebellum. They loop in the cerebellopontine angle, and supply the surrounding structures, their branches including the internal auditory arteries, to the nerves in the internal auditory meatus. The cerebellar branches anastomose with those of the posterior inferior cerebellar artery and there is frequently a reciprocal relationship:

if the posterior artery is small on one side, the corresponding anterior artery is larger, branching more extensively, and vice versa.

The **superior cerebellar arteries** arise several millimetres below the posterior cerebral arteries that are the terminal branches of the basilar artery, from which they are separated by the tentorium cerebelli. The superior cerebellar arteries are frequently duplicated, in which case the individual vessels are smaller. They pass around the brainstem to fan out over the superior surface of the cerebellar hemispheres, while their main trunks run back over the superior vermis, giving a precentral branch that passes down between the roof of the fourth ventricle and the central lobule of the cerebellum.

POSTERIOR CEREBRAL ARTERIES

The bifurcation of the basilar arteries can appear either V-shaped (caudal fusion of the posterior cerebral arteries) or T-shaped (cranial fusion of the cerebral arteries). It can also be asymmetrical with a caudal fusion on one side and a cranial fusion on the other. Basilar tip aneurysms are much more frequently associated with a caudal fusion than with a cranial fusion of the posterior cerebral arteries[61].

After bifurcating, the basilar artery gives rise to the two posterior cerebral arteries, each of which has four segments. P1 is the precommunicating segment before which it joins with the posterior communicating arteries to become the P2 or 'ambient' segment and P3 or 'quadrigeminal' segment, named after the basal cistern in which it runs. The P4 segment is the terminal segment of the posterior cerebral artery, which includes the occipital and inferior temporal branches. There is reciprocity in calibre of the precommunicating (P1) segments of the posterior cerebral arteries and the posterior communicating arteries: if the latter are large and the main source and give rise to a so-called fetal origin of the posterior cerebral artery, the P1 segments may be so small that little or no distal filling is seen on vertebral arteriography. The appearances are commonly asymmetrical.

The posterior communicating arteries give off the anterior thalamoperforating arteries, and the P1 segment the posterior thalamoperforating and thalamogeniculate arteries, which pass posterosuperiorly into the interpeduncular fossa to enter the posterior perforated substance. The medial posterior choroidal artery arises from the P2 segment and passes around the midbrain, then superiorly, over the pulvinar of the thalamus to reach the third ventricle. Two or more lateral posterior choroidal arteries arise also from the P2 segment and follow a similar course, but lie more posteriorly on the lateral view.

Cortical branches arise from the P2 segment (anterior and posterior temporal arteries) and form the P4 segment, which divides into a group of the inferior temporal arteries supplying a considerable portion of the inferior surface of the temporal lobe and the parieto-occipital and calcarine branches, supplying the medial surface of the occipital lobe, including the visual cortex.

External carotid artery[15,16,62,63]

The major branches of the external carotid artery are shown in Figure 55.22; in general they are named simply for their territory of supply. They are best examined using the lateral projection. The first, anterior branch, the superior thyroid artery, may arise from the terminal common carotid artery. The lingual and facial arteries also arise anteriorly, sometimes from a common trunk, and run forwards, the former deep to and the latter lateral to the mandible. In addition to the structures from which they take their names, they also supply the salivary glands. The ascending pharyngeal artery (Fig. 55.23) runs vertically upwards (often obscured on common carotid

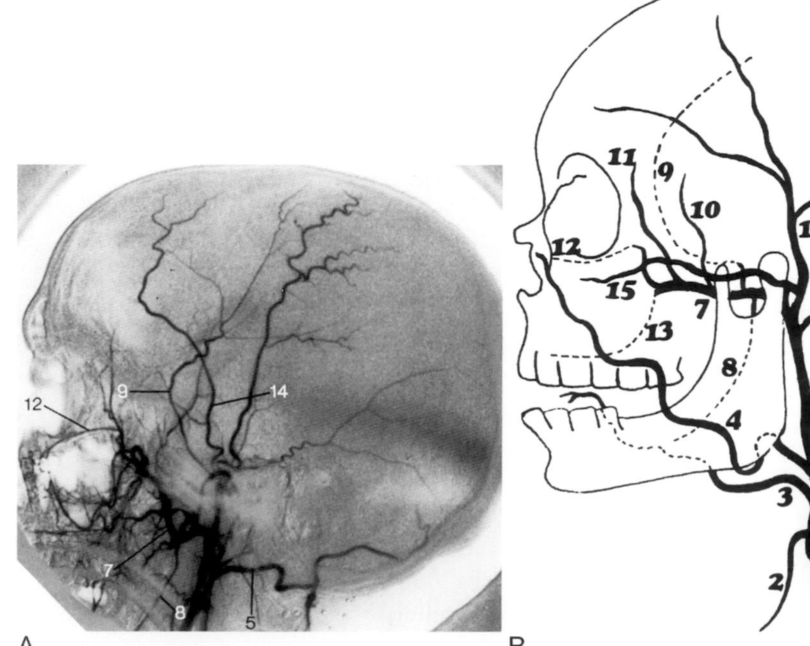

Figure 55.22 External carotid artery. Proximal injection. Radiograph (A) and diagram (B) of principal branches. (For key, see Fig. 55.24 caption.)

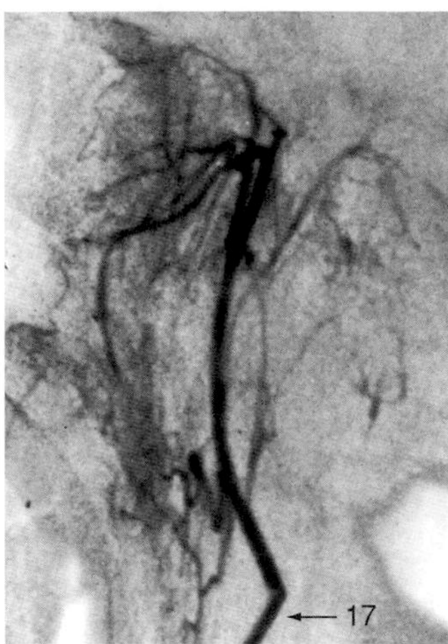

Figure 55.23 (Left) **Injection of the ascending pharyngeal artery.** (For key, see Fig. 55.24 caption.)

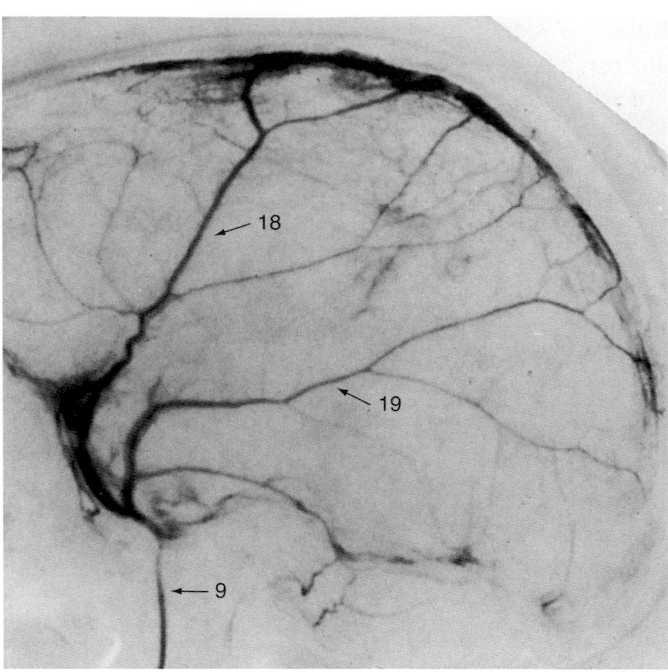

Figure 55.24 (Right) **Injection of the middle meningeal artery.** *Key for Figures 55.22–55.24*: 1 = internal carotid artery, 2 = superior thyroid artery, 3 = lingual artery, 4 = facial artery, 5 = occipital artery, 6 = posterior auricular artery, 7 = internal maxillary artery, 8 = inferior dental artery, 9 = middle meningeal artery MMA, 10 = middle deep temporal artery, 11 = anterior deep temporal artery, 12 = infraorbital artery, 13 = descending (greater) palatine artery, 14 = superficial temporal artery, 15 = transverse facial artery, 16 = common carotid artery, 17 = ascending pharyngeal artery, 18 = anterior branch of the MMA, 19 = posterior branch of the MMA.

injections by the much larger internal carotid artery), giving fine branches to the pharynx, the dura mater of the posterior cranial fossa and, in many individuals, to the posterior lobe of the pituitary gland.

Posterior branches include the occipital artery, through which the carotid system frequently communicates with the vertebral arteries. The artery supplies muscles, scalp and, via a petromastoid branch, the dura mater. The posterior auricular artery is often very small. The terminal branches of the external carotid artery are the internal maxillary and superficial temporal arteries. The former turns forwards, deep to the mandible, giving inferior dental, middle meningeal, deep temporal, accessory meningeal, sphenopalatine, infraorbital and descending palatine branches. Of these, the middle meningeal artery (Fig. 55.24) is of particular radiological interest; it runs superiorly, often appearing to cross the superficial temporal artery on the lateral projection, through the foramen spinosum, where it makes an angular forward bend to run in a smooth curve around the greater wing of the sphenoid and up over the convexity to the midline at the vertex. It gives a posterior branch that runs backwards across the squamous temporal bone towards the lambda. Supplying the dura mater and the inner table of the skull, the middle meningeal artery may also give off the ophthalmic artery; conversely, it may arise as a recurrent branch of the latter.

The superficial temporal artery is the main feeder to the scalp. It gives off a very proximal major branch, the transverse facial artery, which runs forwards parallel with the zygomatic arch, the branches over the cranium, with a more tortuous course than that of the middle meningeal artery.

Anastomotic pathways[16,43,64,65]

There are three main categories of collateral supply to the brain: extracranial–intracranial anastomoses, the circle of Willis and leptomeningeal collaterals. The extracranial–intracranial collaterals are actual or potential anastomotic connections between branches of the external carotid artery and the internal carotid or vertebral arteries. These play a role in chronic cerebrovascular occlusive disease and their knowledge is of importance for interventional endovascular procedures.

Principal anastomoses between the external and internal carotid artery are:

- facial artery
- middle meningeal artery
- ophthalmic artery
- superficial temporal artery
- artery of foramen rotundum
- vidian artery
- carotid siphon

Principal anastomoses between the external and posterior circulation are:

- occipital artery
- ascending pharyngeal artery
- vertebral artery

The circle of Willis[65] plays a critical role as a collateral supply in acute and chronic cerebrovascular occlusive disease and during balloon occlusion of one of the internal carotid arteries. Its anterior part is formed by the distal internal carotid arteries, precommunicating segments of the anterior cerebral arteries (A1 segments), and anterior communicating artery; its posterior part is formed by the distal basilar artery, precommunicating segments of the posterior cerebral arteries (P1 segments), and posterior communicating arteries. The A1 segments course above the optic nerves and the posterior communicating arteries course below the optic tracts.

The circle of Willis is well demonstrated with axial projections of MR angiograms and phase contrast MRA can provide information about the flow direction in its various components (see Figs 55.14, 55.25). A complete circle of Willis is only found in about 40 per cent of people and various segments of the circle may be sufficiently small or absent to be ineffective as a collateral channel. Common variations include absence or hypoplasia of one of the A1 segments and of one or both posterior communicating arteries. Another common variation is a fetal origin of the posterior cerebral artery from the internal carotid artery, which occurs in 20–30 per cent and is often associated with hypoplasia of the P1 segment on that side.

There are other developmental connections between the anterior (carotid) and posterior (vertebrobasilar) circulation that may persist into adult life (Fig. 55.26, Table 55.3); of these only the trigeminal artery is encountered with any frequency, but is found in less than 1 per cent of normal people.

Leptomeningeal (pial) collaterals are end-to-end anastomoses between distal branches of the intracerebral arteries that can provide collateral flow across vascular watershed zones. These are highly variable and are of great importance in acute occlusion of intracerebral vessels.

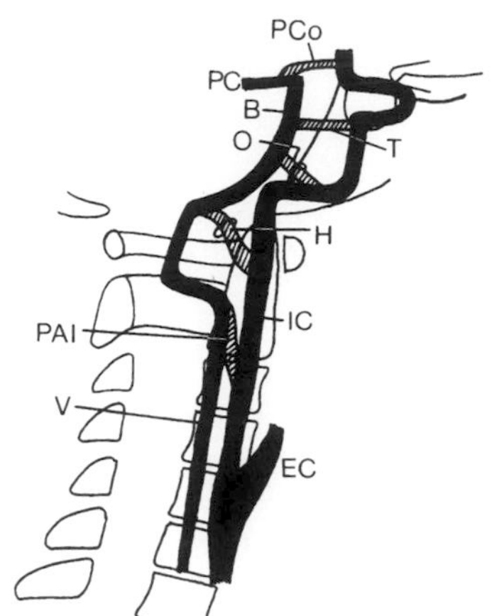

Figure 55.26 Persistent caroticovertebral connections. B = basilar artery, EC = external carotid artery, H = hypoglossal artery, IC = internal carotid artery, O = otic artery, PAI = pro-atlantal intersegmental artery, PC = posterior cerebral artery, PCo = posterior communicating artery, T = trigeminal artery, V = vertebral artery.

Table 55.3 PERSISTENT CAROTICOVERTEBRAL ANASTOMOSES

Artery	Origin	Termination	Route
Pro-atlantal	Cervical internal	Vertebral artery	Via foramen intersegmental carotid artery magnum
Hypoglossal	Internal carotid	Vertebral artery	Via hypoglossal artery canal
Otic	Petrous internal	Basilar artery	Via internal (exceptionally rare) carotid artery auditory meatus
Trigeminal	Precavernous	Basilar artery	Transdural internal carotid artery

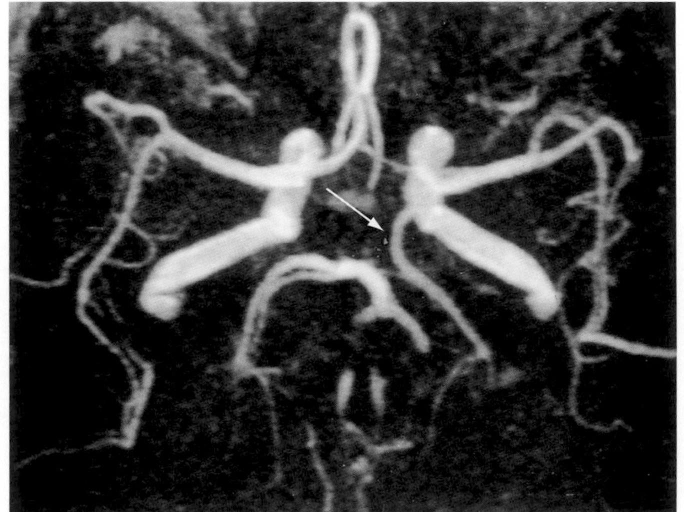

Figure 55.25 Fetal origin of the posterior cerebral artery. A 3D TOF MRA of the circle of Willis shows a fetal origin of the left posterior cerebral artery (arrow), which arises from the left internal carotid artery and is associated with hypoplasia of the left P1 segment.

INTRACRANIAL VEINS[16,66,67]

Dural sinuses

The dural sinuses run within the major dural septa: the superior sagittal sinus between the layers of the upper part of the falx cerebri and the inferior sagittal sinus in the lower border of the falx, running backwards to join the great vein of Galen. The straight sinus is formed by the confluence of the vein of Galen and inferior sagittal sinus and runs downwards in the junction of the falx cerebri and tentorium cerebelli towards the torcular Herophili. The transverse (or lateral) sinuses run in the outer border of the tentorium itself, where it attaches to the vault. They appear frequently asymmetrical in size and the right is usually the dominant one. They become the sigmoid sinuses as they turn downward behind the lateral portions of the petrous bones to discharge into the internal jugular veins, which run in the lateral portion (the pars vascularis) of the jugular foramina.

The superior petrosal sinuses extend from the cavernous sinus to the sigmoid sinuses and run along the attachment of the tentorium cerebelli to the petrous ridge. The inferior petrosal sinuses connect the cavernous sinus to the jugular bulb and run in a groove between the petrous apices and clivus. The disposition of the inferior petrosal sinuses is highly variable, which has practical implications for inferior petrosal sampling, a procedure sometimes performed to lateralize pituitary microadenomas.

Cerebral veins (Figs 55.27, 55.28)

Angiographically, these consist of two groups: the deep, sub-ependymal veins and the cortical veins. The former are rather constant, while the latter are extremely variable. In the angiographic series, the cortical veins fill before the deep ones, and usually from frontal to occipital, but deviations from this pattern are not necessarily abnormal. The deep and superficial groups are in fact joined by fine medullary veins, which run a straight course, perpendicular to the surface of the brain.

Deep veins

The septal veins course directly posteriorly on either side of the midline, on the septum pellucidum, to join the thalamostriate veins as the latter run anteromedially across the floor of the lateral ventricle. They meet at the posterior lips of the foramina of Monro forming the venous angle, from which the internal cerebral veins run posteriorly on the roof of the third ventricle, near the midline. All the aforementioned veins are paired bilateral structures, as are the basal veins (of Rosenthal), which arise in the region of the choroidal fissures and course posterosuperiorly around the midbrain.

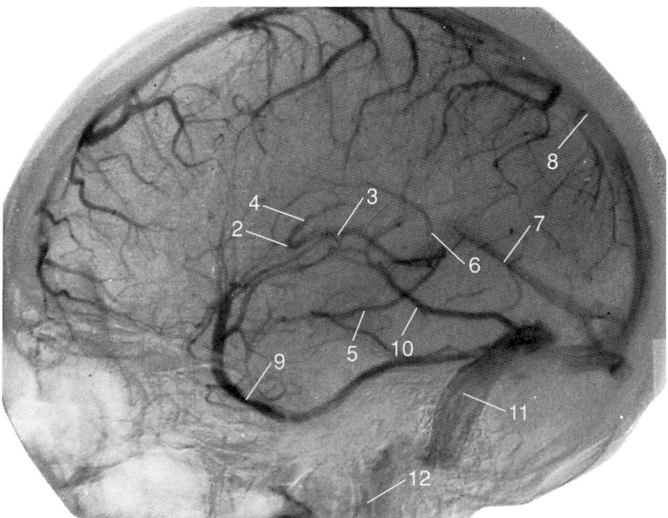

Figure 55.27 Venous phase of internal carotid arteriogram. Lateral projection. 1 = septal vein, 2 = venous angle indicating the foramen of Monro, formed by junction of 3 = internal cerebral vein and 4 = thalamostriate vein, 5 = basal vein (of Rosenthal), 6 = great vein of Galen, 7 = straight sinus, 8 = superior sagittal sinus, 9 = superficial middle cerebral vein, 10 = temporoparietal cortical vein (inferior anastomotic vein of Labbé), 11 = lateral sinus, 12 = internal jugular vein.

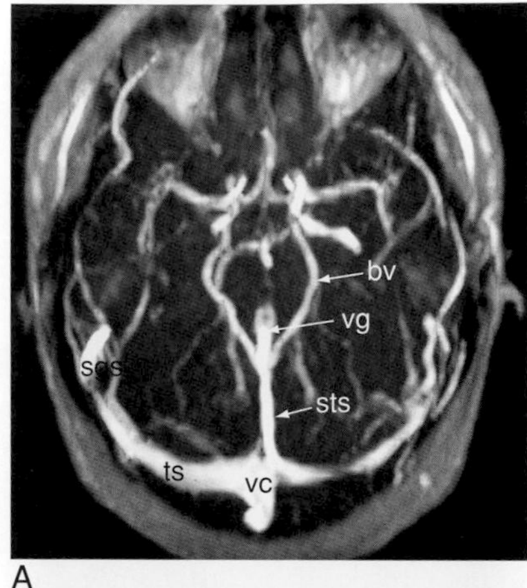

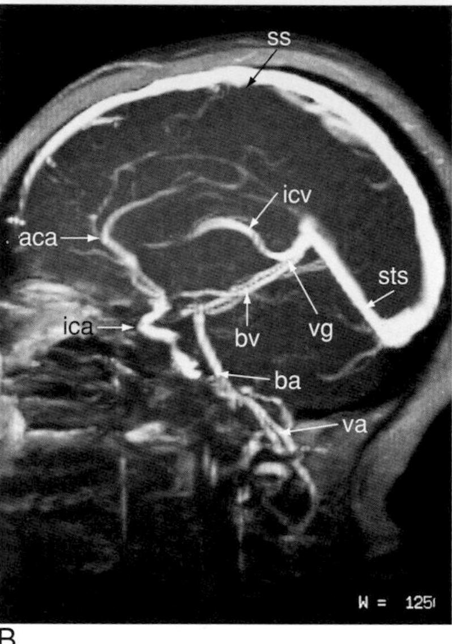

Figure 55.28 B3D TOF MR venogram in axial (A) and sagittal (B) plane. Note that arteries can sometimes also be seen on MR venograms. aca = anterior cerebral artery, ba = basilar artery, bv = basal vein of Rosenthal, ica = internal cerebral artery, icv = internal cerebral vein, sgs = sigmoid sinus, smcv = superficial middle cerebral vein, sts = straight sinus, ss = sagittal sinus, ts = transverse sinus, va = vertebral artery, vc = venous confluence, vg = vein of Galen.

The confluence of both internal cerebral and both basal veins gives rise to the unpaired great vein of Galen, which lies in the quadrigeminal cistern and shows a characteristic upward concavity as it delineates the posterior end of the corpus callosum before discharging into the straight sinus.

Because of their constant relationships to the ventricular system, and the fact that they generally become visible at the point at which they reach the ependyma, the deep cerebral veins are an indicator of the size and shape of the lateral ventricles. The spread of the thalamostriate veins on the AP projection indicates the size of the central part of the lateral ventricles. Displacement of the deep cerebral veins from the midline is seen with posteriorly placed masses, whereas anterior masses cause displacement of the anterior cerebral arteries.

Superficial veins

Cortical veins can be divided into three main groups. The largest numbers drain upwards and medially to the superior sagittal sinus.

Veins in the inferior frontoparietal and temporal regions drain to the superficial middle cerebral vein, thence to the sphenoparietal sinus. Inferior parietal, posterior temporal and occipital veins drain directly to the transverse sinuses. Two large cortical veins running posterosuperiorly across the parietal lobe to the superior sagittal sinus and posteroinferiorly over the temporal lobe to the transverse sinus are the superior and inferior anastomotic veins (of Trolard and Labbé, respectively); it is uncommon for both to be well developed.

Posterior fossa veins (Figs 55.29, 55.30)

The anatomy of the posterior fossa veins is very variable. There are three principal drainage pathways: the vein of Galen, the superior petrosal sinus and direct tributaries into the transverse and straight sinuses.

The pontomesencephalic veins outline the midbrain and brainstem. The anterior and lateral pontomesencephalic veins are connecting channels of a plexus of small veins, closely applied to the anterior surface of the pons.

The precentral cerebellar vein and superior cerebellar vein outline the anterior and posterior aspects of the superior cerebellar vermis, respectively. They enter the vein of Galen either jointly or separately. The inferior vermian veins are paired paramedian vessels that enter the straight sinus or anastomose with the superior vermian vein. The cerebellar hemispheres are drained by hemispheric veins that usually enter the transverse sinuses.

The petrosal veins course anterolaterally below the trigeminal nerves to enter the superior petrosal sinuses just above the internal auditory meatus. They receive numerous tributaries from the cerebellum, pons and medulla and inner ear.

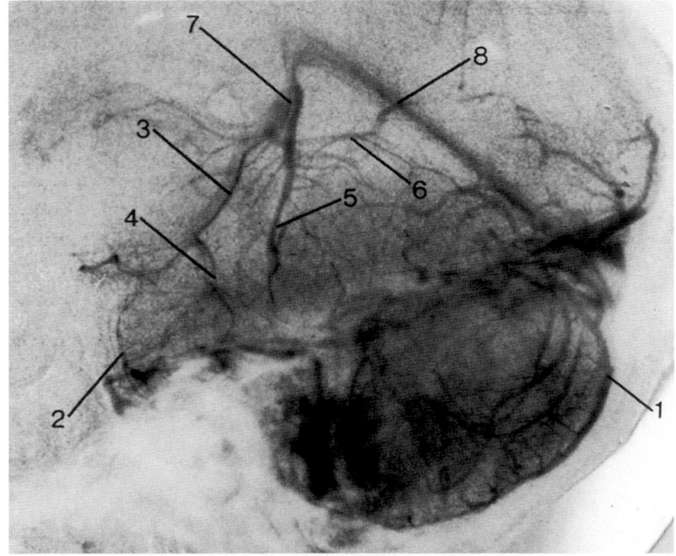

Figure 55.29 Vertebral angiogram. Lateral projection, venous phase. (For key, see Fig. 55.30 caption.)

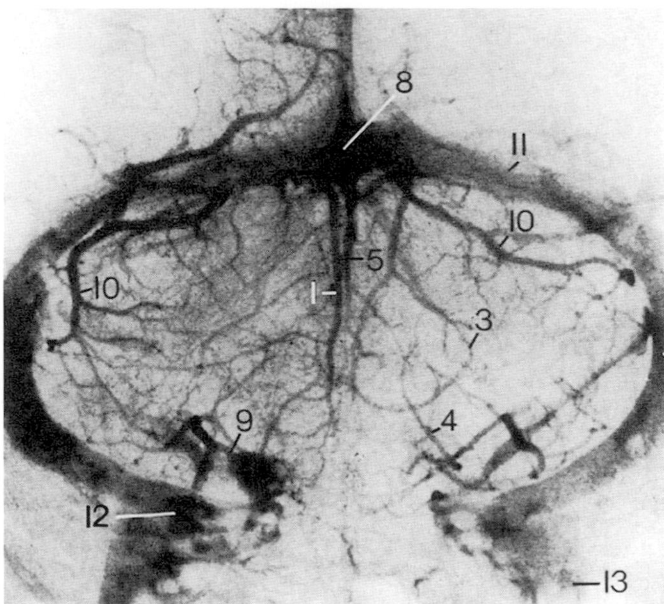

Figure 55.30 Vertebral angiogram. Half-axial projection, venous phase. *Key for Figures 55.29–55.30*: 1 = inferior vermian vein, 2 = anterior pontomesencephalic vein, 3 = posterior mesencephalic vein, 4 = lateral mesencephalic vein, 5 = precentral cerebellar vein, 6 = superior vermian vein, 7 = great vein of Galen, 8 = straight sinus, 9 = petrosal vein, 10 = cerebellar hemispheric veins, 11 = transverse sinus, 12 = sigmoid sinus, 13 = internal jugular vein. Note the normal asymmetry of the posterior fossa.

REFERENCES

1. Du Boulay E 1980 Principles of X-ray diagnosis of the skull. Butterworth, London, pp 1–28
2. Newton T, Potts G 1971 Radiology of the skull and brain: The Skull, vol. 1, Mosby, St Louis
3. Jungreis C A, Yonas H, Firlik A D, Wechsler L R 1999 Advanced CT imaging (functional CT). Neuroimaging Clin North Am 9: 455–464
4. Koening M, Klotz E, Luka B, Vanderink D, Spittler J, Heuser L 1998 Perfusion CT of the brain: diagnostic approach for early detection of ischaemic stroke. Radiology 209: 85–93
5. Okuda T, Korogi Y, Shigematsu Y et al 1999 Brain lesions: when should fluid-attenuated inversion-recovery sequences be used in MR evaluation. Radiology 212: 793–798
6. Beauchamp N, Ulug A, Passe T, Zijl P V 1998 MR diffusion imaging in stroke: review and controversies. Radiographics 18: 1269–1283
7. Provenzale J, Sorensen G 1999 Diffusion-weighted MR imaging in acute stroke: theoretic considerations and clinical applications. Am J Roentgenol 173: 1459–1467
8. Yoshiura T, Wu O, Sorensen A 1999 Advanced MR techniques. Diffusion MR imaging, perfusion MR imaging, and spectroscopy. Neuroimaging Clin North Am 9: 439–453
9. LeBihan D 1995 Diffusion and Perfusion Magnetic Resonance Imaging: Applications to Functional MRI. Raven Press, New York, pp 365
10. Duyn J H, van Gelderen P, Talagala L, Koretsky A, de Zwart J A 2005 Technological advances in MRI measurement of brain perfusion. J Magn Reson Imaging 22: 51–53
11. Keston P, Murray A D, Jackson A 2003 Cerebral perfusion imaging using contrast-enhanced MRI. Clin Radiol 58: 505–513
12. Tallan H, Moore S, Stein W 1956 N-acetyl-L-aspartic acid in brain. J Biochem 219:257–264

13. Saunders D, Howe F, van den Boogart A, Griffiths J, Brown M 1997 Discrimination of metabolites from lipid and macromolecule resonances in cerebral infarction in humans using short echo proton spectroscopy. J Magn Resonance Imag 7: 1116–1121
14. Dillon W, Robert T 1999 The limitations of functional MR imaging: a caveat. Am J Neuroradiol 20: 536
15. Morris P (ed) 1997 Practical Neuroangiography, vol. 1. Williams & Wilkins, Baltimore, pp 1–408
16. Osborn A G 1999 Diagnostic cerebral angiography, 2nd edn. Lippincott Williams & Wilkins, Washington, pp 462
17. Tenjin H, Asakura F, Nakahara Y et al 1998 Evaluation of intraneurysmal blood velocity by time-density curve analysis and digital subtraction angiography. Am J Neuroradiol 19: 1303–1307
18. Anxionnat R, Bracard S, Macho J et al 1998 3D angiography. Clinical interest. First applications in interventional neuroradiology. J Neuroradiol 25: 251–262
19. Probst E N, Grzyska U, Westphal M, Zeumer H 1999 Preoperative embolization of intracranial meningiomas with a fibrin glue preparation. Am J Neuroradiol 20: 1695–1702
20. Ng P P, Higashida R T, Cullen S P, Malek R, Dowd C F, Halbach V V 2004 Intraarterial thrombolysis trials in acute ischemic stroke. J Vasc Interv Radiol 15 (1 Pt 2): S77–S85
21. Stevens J M, Barter S, Kerslake R, Schneidau A, Barber C, Thomas D J 1989 Relative safety of intravenous digital subtraction angiography over other methods of carotid angiography and impact on clinical management of cerebrovascular disease. Br J Radiol 62: 813–816
22. Willinsky R A, Taylor S M, TerBrugge K, Farb R I, Tomlinson G, Montanera W 2003 Neurologic complications of cerebral angiography: prospective analysis of 2,899 procedures and review of the literature. Radiology 227:522–528. Epub 2003 Mar 13
23. Heiserman J E, Dean B L, Hodak J A, Flom R A, Bird C R, Drayer B P 1994 Neurologic complications of cerebral angiography. Am J Neuroradiol 15: 1401–1407
24. Leffers A, Wagner A 2000 Neurologic complications of cerebral angiography. Acta Radiol 41: 204–210
25. National Institute of Neurological Disorders and Stroke 1995 Carotid endarterectomy for patients with asymptomatic internal carotid artery stenosis. J Neurol Sci 129: 76–77
26. Napel S 1995 Principles and techniques of 3D spiral CT angiography. In: Fishman E, Jeffrey B (eds) Spiral CT: Principles, Techniques and Clinical Applications. Raven Press, New York, pp 167–182
27. Rubin G D, Shiau M C, Schmidt A J et al 1999 Computed tomographic angiography: historical perspective and new state-of-the-art using multi detector-row helical computed tomography. J Comput Assist Tomogr 23 (suppl 1): S83–S90
28. Provenzale J, Beauchamp N 1999 Recent advances in imaging of cerebrovascular disease. Radiol Clin North Am 37: 467–488
29. Velthuis B K, Leeuwen M S, Witkamp T D, Boomstra S, Ramos L, Rinkel G J E 1997 CT angiography: source images and post-processing techniques in the detection of cerebral aneurysms. Am J Roentgenol 169: 1411–1417
30. Link J, Brossmann J, Grabener M et al 1996 Spiral CT angiography and selective digital subtraction angiography of internal carotid artery stenosis. Am J Neuroradiol 17: 89–94
31. Leclerc X, Godefroy O, Lucas C et al 1999 Internal carotid arterial stenosis: CT angiography with volume rendering. Radiology 210: 673–682
32. Leclerc X, Godefroy O, Salhi A, Lucas C, Leys D, Pruvo J P 1996 Helical CT for the diagnosis of extracranial internal carotid artery dissection. Stroke 27: 461–466
33. Wong K S, Liang E Y, Lam W W, Huang Y N, Kay R 1995 Spiral computed tomography angiography in the assessment of middle cerebral artery occlusive disease. J Neurol Neurosurg Psychiatry 59: 537–539
34. Tipper G, U-King-Im JM, Price S J et al 2005 Detection and evaluation of intracranial aneurysms with 16-row multislice CT angiography. Clin Rad 60: 565–572
35. Karamessini M T, Kagadis G C, Petsas T et al 2004 CT angiography with three-dimensional techniques for the early diagnosis of intracranial aneurysms. Comparison with intra-arterial DSA and the surgical findings. Eur J Radiol 49: 212–223
36. Jäger H R, Grieve J, Moore E, Kitchen N, Taylor W 1999 Comparison of CTA and intra-arterial DSA in patients with cerebral AVMs. Neuroradiology 41: 227–228
37. Casey S O, Alberico R A, Patel M et al 1996 Cerebral CT venography. Radiology 198: 163–170
38. Graves M J 1997 Magnetic resonance angiography. Br J Radiol 70: 6–28
39. Leclerc X, Gauvrit J Y, Nicol L, Pruvo J P 1999 Contrast-enhanced MR angiography of the craniocervical vessels: a review. Neuroradiology 41: 867–874
40. Isoda H, Takehara Y, Isogai S et al 1998 Technique for arterial-phase contrast-enhanced three-dimensional MR angiography of the carotid and vertebral arteries. Am J Neuroradiol 19: 1241–1244
41. Anderson C, Saloner D, Tsuruda J 1990 Artifacts in maximum-intensity-projection display of MR angiograms. Am J Roentgenol 154: 623–629
42. Ozsarlak O, Van Goethem J W, Maes M, Parizel P M 2004 Angiography of the intracranial vessels: technical aspects and clinical applications. Neuroradiology 46: 955–972. Epub 2004 Dec 4
43. Barboriak D, Provenzale J 1998 MR arteriography of intracranial circulation. Am J Roentgenol 171: 1469–1478
44. Ida M, Kurisu Y, Yamashita M 1997 MR angiography of ruptured aneurysms in acute subarachnoid hemorrhage. Am J Neuroradiol 18: 1025–1032
45. Jäger H R, Mansmann U, Hausmann O, Partzsch U, Moseley I F, Taylor W J 2000 MRA versus DSA in acute subarachnoid haemorrhage: a blinded multireader study of prospectively recruited patients. Neuroradiology 42: 313–326
46. Oelerich M, Lentschig M G, Zunker P, Reimer P, Rummeny E J, Schuierer G 1998 Intracranial vascular stenosis and occlusion: comparison of 3D time-of-flight and 3D phase-contrast MR angiography. Neuroradiology 40: 567–573
47. Jäger H, Grieve J 2000 Advances in non-invasive imaging of intracranial vascular disease. Ann R Coll Surg Engl 82: 1–5
48. Liauw L, Buchem M, Spilt A et al 2000 MR angiography of the intracranial venous system. Radiology 214: 678–682
49. Ross M R, Pelc N J, Enzmann D R 1993 Qualitative phase contrast MRA in the normal and abnormal circle of Willis. Am J Neuroradiol 14: 19–25
50. Yano T, Kodama T, Suzuki Y, Watanabe K 1997 Gadolinium-enhanced 3D time-of-flight MR angiography. Acta Radiol 38: 47–54
51. Jung H W, Chang K H, Choi D S, Han M H, Han M C 1995 Contrast-enhanced MR angiography for the diagnosis of intracranial vascular disease: Optimum dose of gadopentate dimeglumine. Am J Roentgenol 165: 1251–1255
52. Remonda L, Heid O, Schroth G 1998 Carotid artery stenosis, occlusion and pseudo-occlusion: first-pass gadolinium-enhanced, three-dimensional MR angiography-preliminary study. Radiology 209: 95–102
53. Isoda H, Takehara Y, Osogai S et al 2000 Software-triggered contrast-enhanced three-dimensional MR angiography of the intracranial arteries. Am J Roentgenol 174: 371–375
54. Morris P 1997 The internal carotid artery. In: Morris P (ed.) Practical neuroangiography. Williams and Wilkins, Baltimore, pp 117–163
55. Willinsky R, Lasjaunias P, Berenstein A 1987 Intracavernous branches of the internal carotid artery [ICA]: comprehensive review of their variations. Surg Radiol Anat 9: 201–215
56. Osborn A 1994 Diagnostic neuroradiology. In: Patterson A (ed.) Diagnostic Neuroradiology, vol. 1. Mosby-Year Book, St Louis, pp 1–936
57. Perlmutter D, Rhoton A L 1976 Microsurgical anatomy of the anterior cerebral-anterior communicating-recurrent artery complex. J Neurosurg 45: 259–271
58. Perlmutter D, Rhoton A L 1978 Microsurgical anatomy of the distal anterior cerebral artery. J Neurosurg 49: 204
59. Lasjaunias P, Berenstein A 1990 Surgical Neuroangiography, Functional Vascular Anatomy of Brain, Spinal Cord and Spine, 1st edn, vol 3. Springer-Verlag, Berlin, pp 1–337

60. Gibo H, Carver C C, Rhoton A L, Lenkey C, Mitchell R J 1981 Microsurgical anatomy of the middle cerebral artery. J Neurosurg 54: 151–169
61. Campos C, Churojana A, Rodesch G, Alvarez H, Lasjaunias P 1998 Basilar tip aneurysms and basilar tip anatomy. Intervent Neuroradiol 4: 121–125
62. Lasjaunias P L, Choi I S 1991 The external carotid artery: functional anatomy. Rev Neuroradiol 4 (suppl 1): 39–45
63. Williams P L 1995 Carotid system of arteries. In: Gray's Anatomy, 38th edn. Churchill Livingstone, New York, pp 1513–1523
64. Helgertner L, Szostek M, Malek A K, Staszkiewicz W 1994 Collateral role of the external carotid artery and its branches in occlusion of the internal carotid artery. Int Angio 13: 5–9
65. Wolpert S M 1997 The circle of Willis. Am J Neuroradiol 18: 1033–1034
66. Curé J K, Van Tussel P, Smith M T 1994 Normal variant anatomy of the dural venous sinuses. Semin Ultrasound CT MR 15: 499–519
67. Carpenter A 1996 Cerebral veins and venous sinuses. In: Carpenter's Human Neuroanatomy, 9th edn. Williams and Wilkins, Media, PA, pp120–128

FURTHER READING

Atlas S 1996 Magnetic resonance imaging of the brain and spine. In: Atlas S (ed.) 2nd edn, Lippincott-Raven, New York, pp 1–1675

Beauchamp N, Ulug A, Passe T, Van Zijl P 1998 MR diffusion imaging in stroke: review and controversies. Radiographics 18: 1269–1283

De Deyn P P, Dierckx R A, Alave A, Pickut B A (eds) 1997 A Textbook of SPECT in Neurology and Psychiatry. John Libbey, London

Frackowiak R S J, Friston K J, Frith C D, Dolan R J, Mazziotta J C 1997 Human Brain Function. Academic Press, London

Keats T 1996 Atlas of Normal Roentgen Variants That May Stimulate Disease. Mosby 6th edn.

Lasjaunias P, Berenstein A 1990 Surgical Neuroangiography, Functional Vascular Anatomy of Brain, Spinal Cord and Spine, 1st edn, vol 3. Springer-Verlag, Berlin, pp 1–337

Ockner J, Nesbit G 1999 Angiographic evaluation and correlative anatomy. Neuroimaging Clin North Am 9: 475–490

Osborn A G 1999 Diagnostic cerebral angiography, 2nd edn. Lippincott Williams & Wilkins, Washington

CHAPTER 56

Benign and Malignant Intracranial Tumours in Adults

H. Rolf Jäger, Gisele Brasil Caseiras and Philip M. Rich

RADIOLOGICAL INVESTIGATIONS IN INTRACRANIAL TUMOURS

Plain radiographic findings in brain tumours are of historical interest, but radiologists should still be familiar with signs of raised intracranial pressure (ICP) such as erosion of the lamina dura of the dorsum sellae, or a 'J-shaped' sella. Skull radiography may also demonstrate tumour calcification and enlargement of middle meningeal artery grooves in meningiomas.

The use of diagnostic catheter angiography for brain tumours has dramatically decreased with the advances in cross-sectional imaging. It is occasionally performed to assess the vascular supply of meningiomas pre-operatively. Otherwise it is now mostly performed in conjunction with pre-operative or palliative tumour embolizations or intra-arterial chemotherapy for treatment of high-grade gliomas.

Magnetic resonance imaging (MRI) is the preferred investigation of patients with suspected intracranial tumours. It provides a better soft-tissue differentiation and tumour delineation than CT and advanced MR imaging techniques, such as diffusion-weighted (DWI) and perfusion-weighted (PWI) imaging and MR spectroscopy (MRS), allow the assessment of physiological and metabolic processes.

COMPUTED TOMOGRAPHY

Most clinically symptomatic brain tumours are detectable on CT, by virtue of mass effect and/or altered attenuation. Intra-axial tumours are usually of low attenuation on non-enhanced CT images. High attenuation areas within a tumour indicate tumour calcification or recent intratumoural haemorrhage. Tumours frequently exhibiting these two features are listed in Table 56.1.

Bone-window settings can reveal bone erosion or hyperostosis, associated with extra-axial tumours.

Contrast-enhancement improves the visualization of strongly enhancing mass lesions such as menigiomas, neuromas, metastases and certain types of glial tumours.

More recently CT perfusion has emerged as a technique to assess the relative blood volume (rCBV) and permeability

Table 56.1 COMMONLY CALCIFIED AND HAEMORRHAGIC LESIONS

Commonly calcified lesions	Commonly haemorrhagic lesions
Oligodendrogliomas (90%)	GBM (grade 4 glioma)
Choroid plexus tumours	Oligodendroglioma
Ependymoma	
Central neurocytoma	Metastases
Meningioma	– Melanoma
Craniopharyngioma	– Lung
Teratoma	– Breast
Chordoma	

changes in brain tumours[1]. Compared with MR perfusion techniques it has still limited area coverage despite progress in multi-detector technology. It has, however, the advantage of a direct relationship between the CT attenuation coefficient and contrast material concentration in tissue.

MAGNETIC RESONANCE IMAGING

STRUCTURAL MRI

The MRI protocol for structural tumour imaging should include T2-weighted (T2W), fluid-attenuated recovery (FLAIR) sequence and T1-weighted (T1W) images before and after injection of a gadolinium-based contrast medium.

Most tumours appear hypointense on T1W and hyperintense on T2W and FLAIR images. The latter provide a particularly good contrast between normal brain tissue and glial tumours and show signal loss in cystic tumour components[2]. Highly cellular tumours such as lymphomas and primitive neuroectodermal tumours have decreased water content and therefore appear relatively hypointense on T2W images. Intratumoural haemorrhage or calcification are also hypointense on T2W images and become more conspicuous on T2*W images, where magnetic susceptibility effects are stronger. Hyperintensities on T1W images can be due to haemorrhage, calcification, melanin (in metastatic melanomas) or fat.

Enhancement with gadolinium is seen in vascular extra-axial tumours such as meningiomas and in intra-axial tumours, which disrupt the blood–brain barrier. This is generally a feature of high-grade intra-axial tumours, but can also be present in certain low-grade tumours, such as pilocytic astrocytomas and WHO grade II oligodendrogliomas. The visibility of contrast enhancement on MR can be improved by magnetization transfer imaging, by doubling or tripling the gadolinium dose[3], or by using high relaxivity gadolinium compounds[4].

PHYSIOLOGY-BASED MR IMAGING

DWI, PWI, MRS and functional MRI (fMRI) with blood oxygen level dependent (BOLD) imaging provide information about physiological and metabolic processes not available on standard MRI. Much of the recent progress in tumour imaging is based on the use of these methods, which are now increasingly implemented in clinical practice[5–8].

MR PERFUSION IMAGING

Dynamic susceptibility-weighted contrast-enhanced (DSC) MR imaging is the most widely used technique of PWI in brain tumours. It offers the possibility to assess the density of blood vessels within a tumour and provides an indirect measure of tumour neovascularity, an important feature of malignant tumours[5,8,9]. It differs from contrast enhancement, which is an indicator of vascular endothelial (blood–brain barrier) integrity. rCBV measurements derived from PWI correlate closely with angiographic and histological markers of tumour vascularity[10], and also with the expression of vascular endothelial growth factor (VGEF) in tumours[11], an important determinant of angiogenesis. High-grade glial tumours tend to have higher rCBV values than low-grade tumours and PWI significantly increases the specificity and sensitivity of conventional MRI in the classification of gliomas. MRP can be preformed using a spin-echo or gradient-echo technique. The latter is influenced by vessels of a larger size and has been shown to be superior in discriminating low-grade from high-grade gliomas[12]. Maps of rCBV may also be a useful adjunct for stereotactic tumour biopsies, and can help to direct tissue sampling towards areas with maximal angiogenesis.

PERMEABILITY IMAGING (K^{TRANS})

Microvascular permeability of brain tumours can be quantified by measuring the transfer coefficient K^{TRANS}, which is influenced by endothelial permeability, vascular surface area and flow. In can be measured using a T1W steady-state or a first-pass T2*W gradient-echo technique. The former has a higher spatial resolution and is more accurate but requires longer acquisition times and more complicated post-processing; the latter can be combined with DSC perfusion imaging. K^{TRANS} correlates with tumour grade and might be even more sensitive than rCBV measurements for glioma grading[13].

MR DIFFUSION IMAGING

Diffusion-weighted imaging (DWI) measures Brownian motion of water molecules within the tissue. Isotropic- trace-weighted DW images are obtained by measuring the signal loss on typically T2W images following the application of diffusion gradients. The signal loss depends on several factors including the gradient strength and apparent diffusion coefficient (ADC), which describes water diffusibility in tissue. The more mobile the water molecules are, the higher the ADC and the greater the signal loss on DW images[8]. Trace-weighted DW images are to some degree still dependent on T2 effects, which can lead to T2 shine-through artefacts, whereas ADC maps provide a quantitative voxel-by-voxel representation of water movement.

Visual inspection of trace-weighted DW images plays a limited role in the diagnosis of brain tumours. It may be useful to identify lesions with severely restricted diffusion, such as acute infarcts or abscesses, which can occasionally mimic brain tumours on standard MRI. More detailed analysis of brain tumours requires measurement of the ADC, which is an indicator of disruption of tissue microstructure, cellular density and matrix composition in tumours. ADC measurements correlate inversely the histological cell count of gliomas[14] and positively with the presence of hydrophilic substances in the tumour matrix[15]. DWI and ADC measurements assess the overall freedom of water-movement whereas diffusion tensor imaging (DTI) provides additional information about the direction of water diffusion[16]. The tendency of water to move in some directions more than others is called anisotropy and can be quantified using parameters such as fractional anisotropy (FA). Compact white matter tracts show normally a high degree of anisotropy, which can be lost if they are infiltrated by tumour cells, which destroy the ultrastructural boundaries formed by myelin sheaths.

Post-processing of DTI allows the depiction of important white matter tracts and their connections (tractography), which can be displayed in direction-encoded colour images. Tractography is useful in the pre-operative assessment of brain tumours and can differentiate between displacement and infiltration of white matter tracts[17].

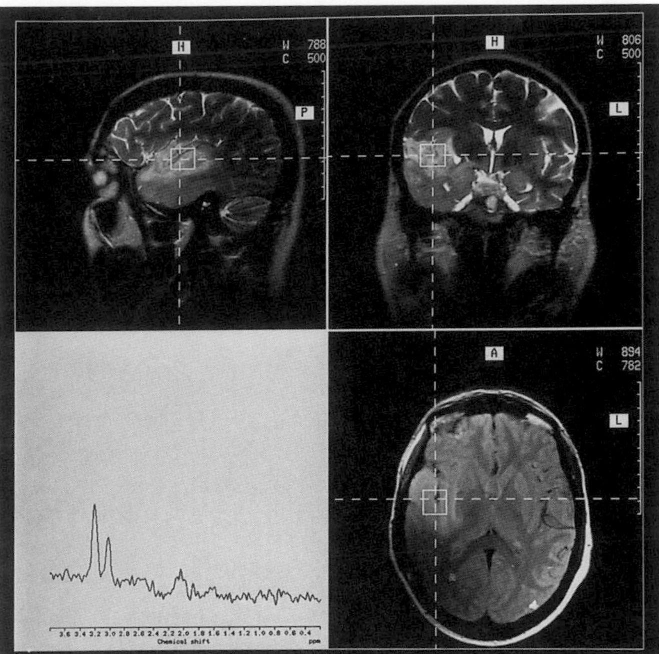

Figure 56.1 Proton magnetic resonance spectroscopy. The choline peak (3.22 p.p.m.) is elevated, the creatine peak (3.03 p.p.m.) is low and the *N*-acetyl aspartate peak (2.01 p.p.m.) is nearly undetectable; characteristic spectroscopic appearance of gliomas (CHO = choline, PCr/Cr = creatine, NAA = *N*-acetylaspartate).

MR SPECTROSCOPY

Proton MR spectroscopy (MRS) analyses the biochemistry of a brain tumour and provides semiquantitative information about major metabolites[7,18]. A common pattern in brain tumours is a decrease in *N*-acetylaspartate (NAA), a neuron-specific marker, and creatine (Cr) and an increase in choline (Cho), lactate (Lac), lipids (L) (Fig. 56.1). The concentration of Cho is a reflection of the turnover of cell membranes (due to accelerated synthesis and destruction) and is more elevated in regions with a high neoplastic activity. Lactate (Lac) is the end product of nonoxidative glycolysis and a marker of hypoxia in tumour tissue. This is of increasing interest as tumour hypoxia is now recognized as a major promoter of tumour angiogenesis and invasion. Lac is probably associated with viable but hypoxic tissue, whereas mobile lipids are thought to reflect tissue necrosis with breakdown of cell membranes.

The choice of echo time (TE) is an important technical consideration for performing MRS. It can be short (20–40 ms), intermediate (135–144 ms) or long (270–288 ms). MRS with a short TE has the advantage of demonstrating additional metabolites, which may improve tumour characterization, such as myo-inositol, glutamate/glutamine (Glx) and lipids but is hampered by baseline distortion and artefactual NAA peaks. Intermediate echo times have a better defined baseline and quantification of NAA and Cho is more accurate and reproducible. Long echo times lead to a decrease of signal to noise.

MRS is presently a sensitive but not very specific technique. Single voxel acquisition provides good-quality spectra but is prone to sampling errors. Chemical shift imaging is technically more demanding but covers a larger volume of tissue.

FMRI

Blood oxygen level-dependent (BOLD) imaging detects changes in regional cerebral blood flow during various forms of brain activity. Paradigms using motor tasks, language and speech productions and memory are able to show activation of relevant cortical areas (Fig. 56.2). The main use of fMRI in tumour imaging is the pre-operative localization of eloquent cortical regions that may have been displaced, distorted or compressed by the tumour[18]. This can improve the safety of surgery and allow for a more radical resection. If possible fMRI should be combined with MR tractography in order to minimize intra-operative injury to white matter tracts connected to eloquent cortical areas.

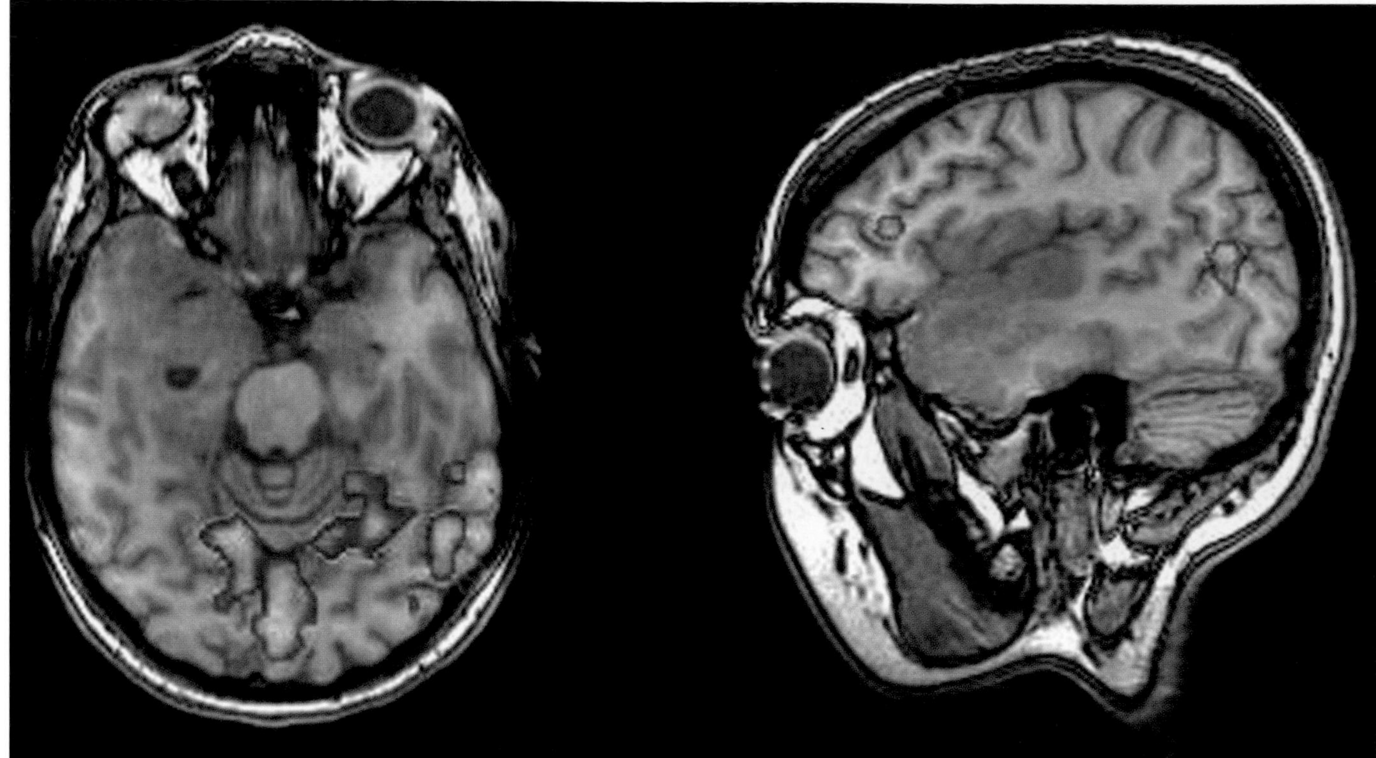

Figure 56.2 fMRI in a patient with a right peri-insular and temporal lobe tumour. Images acquired during a picture-naming task show activation in the visual cortex and in the right Broca's area, which lies outside the tumour.

CLASSIFICATION OF INTRACRANIAL TUMOURS

There are several ways of classifying brain tumours: primary versus secondary, intra-axial (arising from the brain parenchyma) versus extra-axial (arising from tissues covering the brain, such as the dura) and various regional classifications (supratentorial, infratentorial, intraventricular, pineal region and sellar region tumours).

The World Health Organization (WHO) classification of intracranial tumours is a universally accepted histological classification of brain tumours. It was extensively revised in 1993 and updated in 2000, stratifying neoplasms by their overall biological potential[19,20]. The WHO classification no longer relies on standard pathological features alone but includes information from immunochemistry and molecular tumour profiling. An outline of this classification is given in Table 56.2.

Intra-axial tumours, which conform largely to the tissue types 1, 4 and 5 and 9, will be discussed first, followed by extra-axial tumours corresponding to the tissue types 2, 3, 6, 7 and 8.

Table 56.2 ABBREVIATED WHO CLASSIFICATION OF BRAIN TUMOURS

1.	Tumours of neuroepithelial tissue	4	Lymphoma and haemopoetic tumours
1.1	Astrocytic tumours	5	Germ cell tumours
1.2	Oligodendroglial tumours	5.1	Germinoma
1.3	Ependymal tumours	5.2	Teratoma
1.4	Mixed gliomas	5.3	Choriocarcinoma
1.5	Choroid plexus tumours	6	Cysts and tumour-like conditions
1.6	Uncertain origin	6.1	Rathke's cleft cyst
1.7	Neuronal and mixed neuronal-glial tumours	6.2	Epidermoid cyst
1.8	Pineal tumours	6.3	Dermoid cyst
1.9	Embryonal tumours	6.4	Colloid cyst
2	Tumours of cranial and spinal nerves	7	Tumours of the sellar region
2.1	Schwannoma	7.1	Pituitary adenoma
2.2	Neurofibroma	7.2	Craniopharyngioma
3.	Tumours of the meninges	8	Local extension from regional tumours
3.1	Meningioma	9	Metastases
3.2	Mesenchymal tumours (incl. haemangiopericytoma)		

INTRA-AXIAL TUMOURS

NEUROEPITHELIAL TUMOURS

Neuroepithelial tumours account for 50–60 per cent of all primary brain tumours and represent a broad spectrum of neoplasms arising from or sharing morphological properties of neuroepithelial cells. They include glial neoplasms; choroid plexus tumours; tumours with predominant neuronal phenotype (ganglioglioma, dysembryoplastic neuroepithelial tumour and neurocytoma); pineal tumours and embryonal tumours (neuroectodermal tumours, medulloblastoma).

Gliomas

Gliomas are the commonest neuroepithelial tumours. There are three types, distinguished depending on the cell type they originate from: atrocytomas, oligodendrogliomas and oligoastrocytomas[21].

Astrocytic tumours

Astrocytomas account for approximately 75 per cent of glial tumours. The WHO classification distinguishes four histological grades, ranging from the benign pilocytic astrocytomas (grade I) to glioblastoma multiforme (GBM) (grade IV), which is the most malignant astrocytic tumour. The incidence of the various types of astrocytic tumours varies with age. In children, most of these are relatively benign tumours (pilocytic or low-grade astrocytomas); in young adults low-grade astrocytomas predominate, whereas anaplastic astrocytomas have a peak incidence around 40 years and GBM usually occurs after 40 years[21].

WHO grade I is now reserved for pilocytic astrocytomas. These are well-circumscribed, potentially resectable lesions with a low proliferative potential and a predilection for the posterior fossa (Fig. 56.3). They are primarily seen in children and are rare in adults. Pilocytic atrocytomas have usually a significant cystic component and show enhancement that can be nodular or ring-like. Infratentorial pilocytic astrocytomas in adults are frequently mistaken for haemangioblastomas, which have a similar appearance and represent the commonest primary intra-axial tumour below the tentorium cerebelli in adults. About 20 per cent of haemangioblastomas occur in association with von Hippel–Lindau disease. Typical CT and MR appearance is of a cystic mass with an enhancing mural nodule. Some haemangioblastomas may, however consist of only solid components, which enhance strongly, whereas others may appear mainly cystic without significant enhancement.

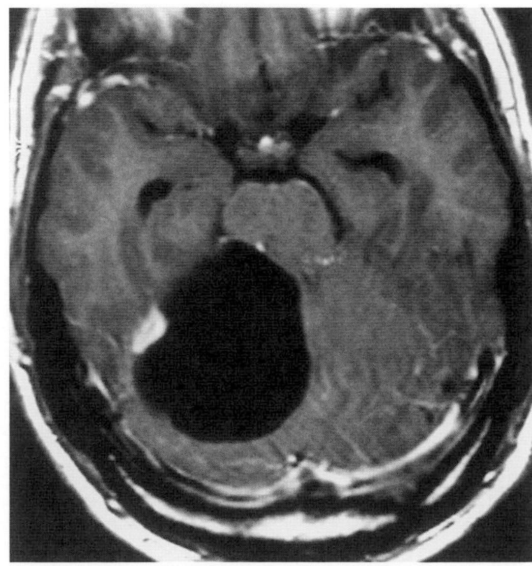

Figure 56.3 Cerebellar pilocytic astrocytoma. Axial T1W post-gadolinium MRI. There is a cystic lesion in the cerebellum with a small, enhancing mural nodule but otherwise nonenhancing cyst wall. The fourth ventricle is compressed causing hydrocephalus (note enlargement of the temporal horns). The differential diagnosis of this lesion is a cerebellar haemangioblastoma.

Diffuse astrocytomas WHO grade II are infiltrating low-grade tumours that occur typically in the hemispheres of young adults, involving cortex and white matter. They have less well-defined borders than pilocytic astrocytomas and contrast enhancement is usually absent. WHO grade II astrocytomas show a low mitotic activity but have a propensity to progress to a higher histological grade. They have variable mass effect, appear iso- or hypodense on CT and show areas of calcification in up to 20 per cent. MRI (and specifically a FLAIR sequence) is better in defining the extent of the low-grade gliomas (Fig. 56.4), which are hyperintense on T2W images and FLAIR images and hypo/isointense on T1W images.

Anaplastic astrocytomas (WHO grade III) are high-grade gliomas with an increased mitotic activity and raised immunohistochemical proliferation indices. According to the revised WHO classification of 2000, presence of a single mitosis is, however, no longer a distinguishing criterion between grade II and grade III astrocytomas[20]. Anaplastic astrocytomas show usually contrast enhancement, and infiltration of the peritumoural tissues is more extensive than in grade II lesions[22,23]. They may also be accompanied by vasogenic oedema (Fig. 56.5).

Pleomorphic xanthoastrocytoma (PXA) arises near the surface of the cerebral hemispheres and is frequently cystic. The tumour may enhance strongly and is usually associated with little or no oedema. Despite its fat content, it is T1 hypointense and T2 hyperintense on MRI[31]. PXA may be WHO grade II or III, depending on its proliferation rate[24].

GBM (WHO grade IV) shows poorly differentiated, often highly pleomorphic glial tumour cells with vascular proliferation and necrosis. It has the worst prognosis but is unfortunately also the commonest primary intracranial neoplasm in adults[25]. These rapidly growing, highly mitotic tumours may arise from pre-existing lower grade astrocytomas or occur de novo (particularly in older patients)[21]. Vasogenic oedema and contrast enhancement are usually much more extensive than in anaplastic astrocytomas. Tumour necrosis is a hallmark of GBM and appears on MRI as areas of non-enhancing T1 hypointensity, frequently surrounded by irregularly enhancing regions of active mitosis. Intratumoural haemorrhage contributes to the heterogeneous MR appearance of GBM with areas of high signal on T1W images and low signal on T2W images. A small number of GBMs may show evidence of subarachnoid seeding.

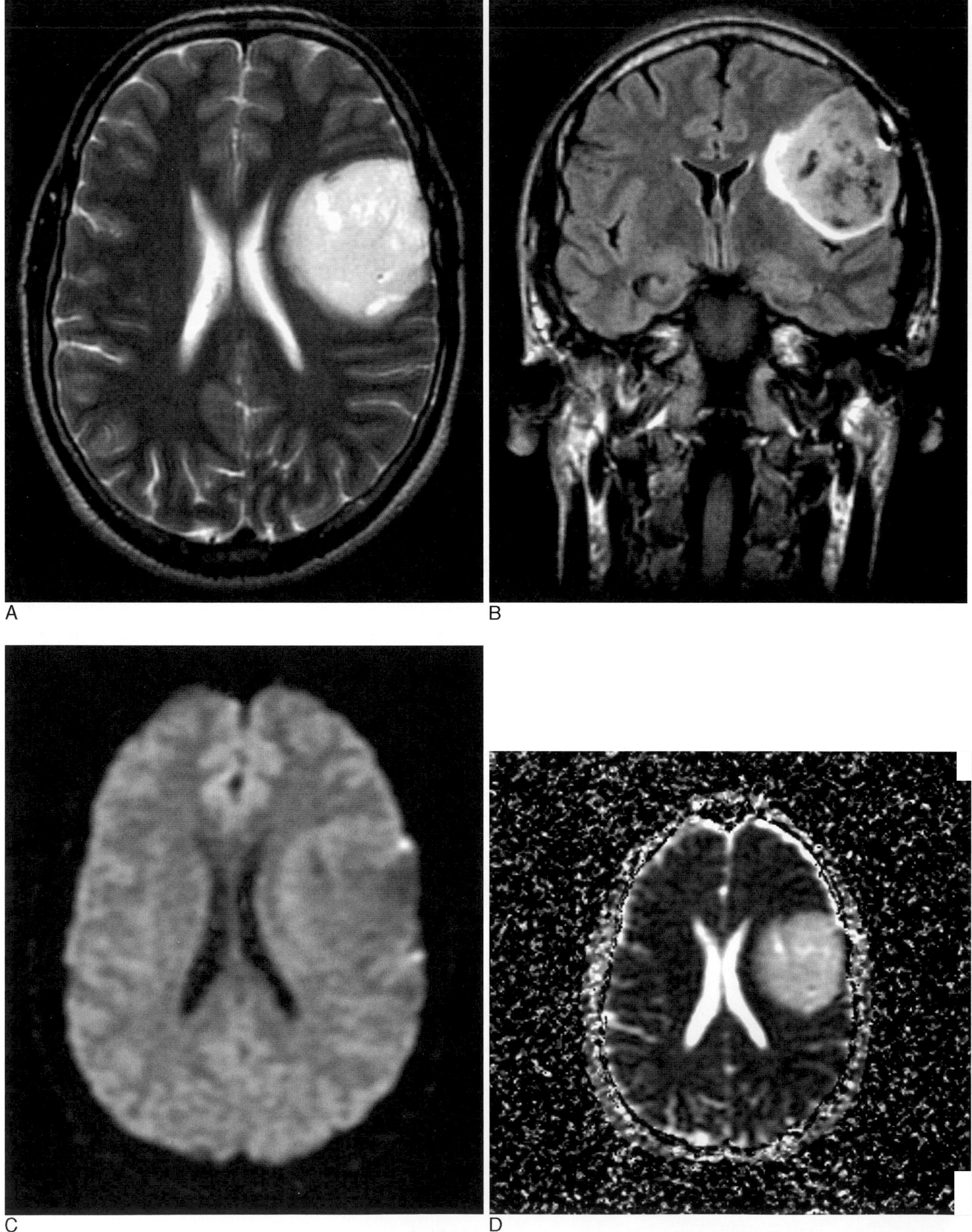

Figure 56.4 WHO grade II astrocytoma. Axial T2W (A), FLAIR (B) images showing a left frontal hyperintense mass lesion with well-defined borders and small cystic areas. On the trace-weighted DW image (C) the tumour is not very conspicuous as T2 effects and diffusion effects cancel each other out. On the ADC map (D) the glioma is easily identified as an area of increased diffusivity compared to normal brain parenchyma.

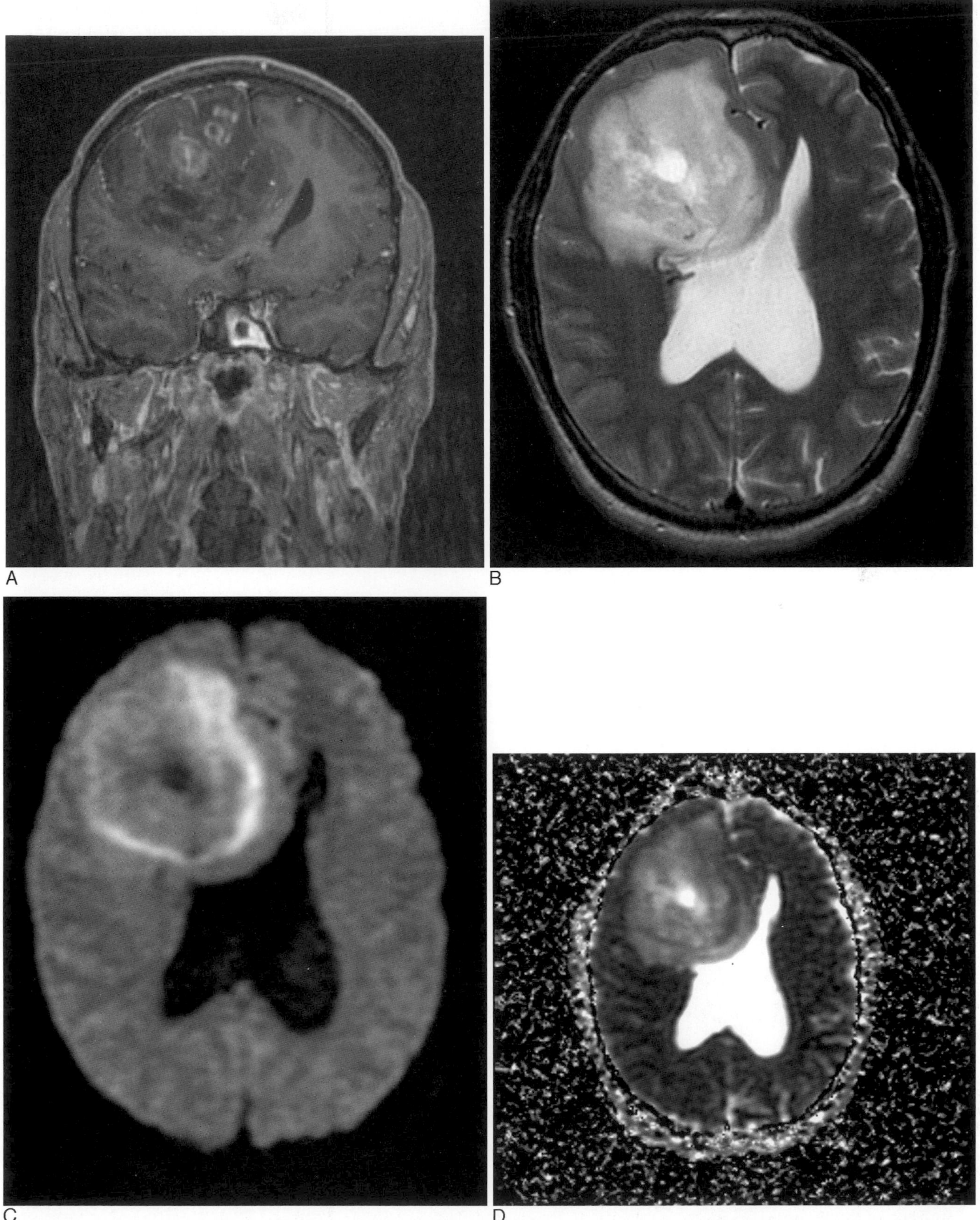

Figure 56.5 WHO grade III astrocytoma. Coronal T1W post-contrast image (A) of a frontal irregularly enhancing mass with some cystic areas, which appears heterogeneous on T2W images (B). The latter also shows associated vasogenic oedema at the posterior margin of the tumour. There is marked mass effect with midline shift. The trace-weighted DW images (C) and ADC map (D) appear heterogeneous with cystic areas and more restricted diffusion peripherally.

Oligodendrogliomas

Oligodendrogliomas account for 10–15 per cent of all gliomas, and occur predominantly in adults. They are diffusely infiltrating neoplasms that are found almost exclusively in the cerebral hemispheres, most commonly in the frontal lobes, and typically involve subcortical white matter and cortex (Fig. 56.6). The WHO classification distinguishes between WHO grade II (well-differentiated low-grade) and WHO grade III (anaplastic high-grade) oligodendrogliomas. The former are slowly growing tumours with rounded homogenous nuclei; the latter have increased tumour cell density, mitotic activity, microvascular proliferation and necrosis. Both low- and high-grade oligodendral tumours express proangiogenic mitogens and may contain regions of increased vascular density with finely branching capillaries that have a 'chicken wire' appearance. This contributes to their appearance on contrast-enhanced MRI and MRP. Up to 90 per cent of oligodendrogliomas contain visible calcification on CT, which can be central, peripheral or ribbon-like[26].

On MRI, areas of calcification may be more difficult to appreciate due to the variable appearance of calcification. Intratumoural calcification appears typically T2 hypo- and T1 hyperintense but intratumoural haemorrhage, which occurs uncommonly in oligodendrogliomas, may have a similar appearance. Contrast enhancement is variable and often heterogeneous. Unlike in astrocytomas, contrast enhancement is not a reliable indicator of tumour grade in oligodendrogliomas. WHO grade II tumours do not infrequently exhibit some contrast enhancement whereas WHO grade III oligodendrogliomas may not enhance[27]. Low-grade oligodendrogliomas may also have an elevated rCBV on PWI[28] (Fig. 56.7). The identification of oligodendroglial tumour with loss of chromosomes 1p and 19q has become important as these subtypes show a better response to chemotherapy. Oligodendrogliomas with 1p/19q loss appear to have a significantly higher rCBV than those with intact 1p and 19q[29]. Conventional MR images may provide a further clue to the oligodendroglioma genotype. Tumours with intact1p/19q show more homogeneous signal on T1W and T2W images and have sharper borders than the tumours with chromosome deletions[30].

MRS of low-grade tumours with oligodendral elements shows increased levels of myo-inositol/glycine as well as glutamine and glutamate[7].

Physiological MR imaging in the differential and grading diagnosis of glial tumours

Recent studies demonstrated that PWI and DWI can help to differentiate low-grade astrocytic from low-grade oligodendroglial tumours. WHO grade II oligodendrogliomas have significantly higher rCBV than WHO grade II astrocytomas with median values of 3.68 versus 0.92, respectively[28]. This concurs with the histological findings of regions with increased vascular density seen in oligodendrogliomas. Using a method of histogram analysis of all intra-tumoural ADC measurements, oligodendrogliomas were shown to have significantly lower ADC values than atrocytomas, which is probably a reflection of their higher cellular density and different tumour matrix composition[31]. Several studies have investigated the potential of advanced MR imaging to distinguish between low- and high-grade gliomas.

Formation of new blood vessels (angiogenesis) represents an important aspect of tumour progression and growth and the microvascular density in glial tumours correlates with histological tumour grade. MR perfusion imaging is a noninvasive method of assessing the tumour microvasculature. Sugahara et al[10] found mean maximum rCBV values of 7.32, 5.84 and 1.26 for glioblastomas, anaplastic astrocytomas and low-grade gliomas, respectively, which correlate closely with the findings of other investigators[32]. A recent study of 160 primary cerebral gliomas showed that rCBV measurements significantly increased the sensitivity and positive predictive value of conventional MR imaging in glioma grading[33]. PWI had a sensitivity of 95 per cent and positive predictive value of 87 per cent for distinguishing low-grade from high-grade gliomas when an rCBV threshold of 1.75 was used[33]. A separate study of low-grade gliomas demonstrated rCBV values above 1.75 to be associated with a more rapid tumour progression[34].

The role of DWI in differentiating high-grade from low-grade gliomas is more controversial. Initial reports were

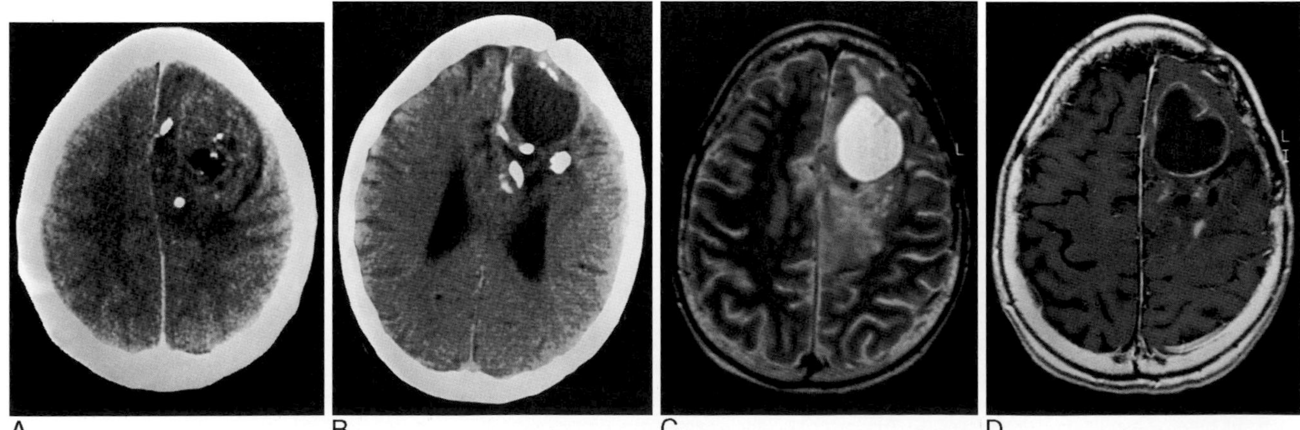

Figure 56.6 Oligodendroglioma. CT after IV contrast medium (A) shows a large left frontal tumour that involves the cortex. It is predominantly solid with irregular enhancement, but there are also cysts and coarse calcification. Follow-up after 2 years with CT (B), T2W MRI (C) and T1W post-contrast MRI (D) shows more extensive cyst formation and calcification than on the first scan. The calcification is much less apparent on MRI and appears as nonspecific low signal areas. Posterior infiltration of the tumour is, however, best seen on MRI (C). Note that the patient had undergone a left frontal craniotomy after the first CT.

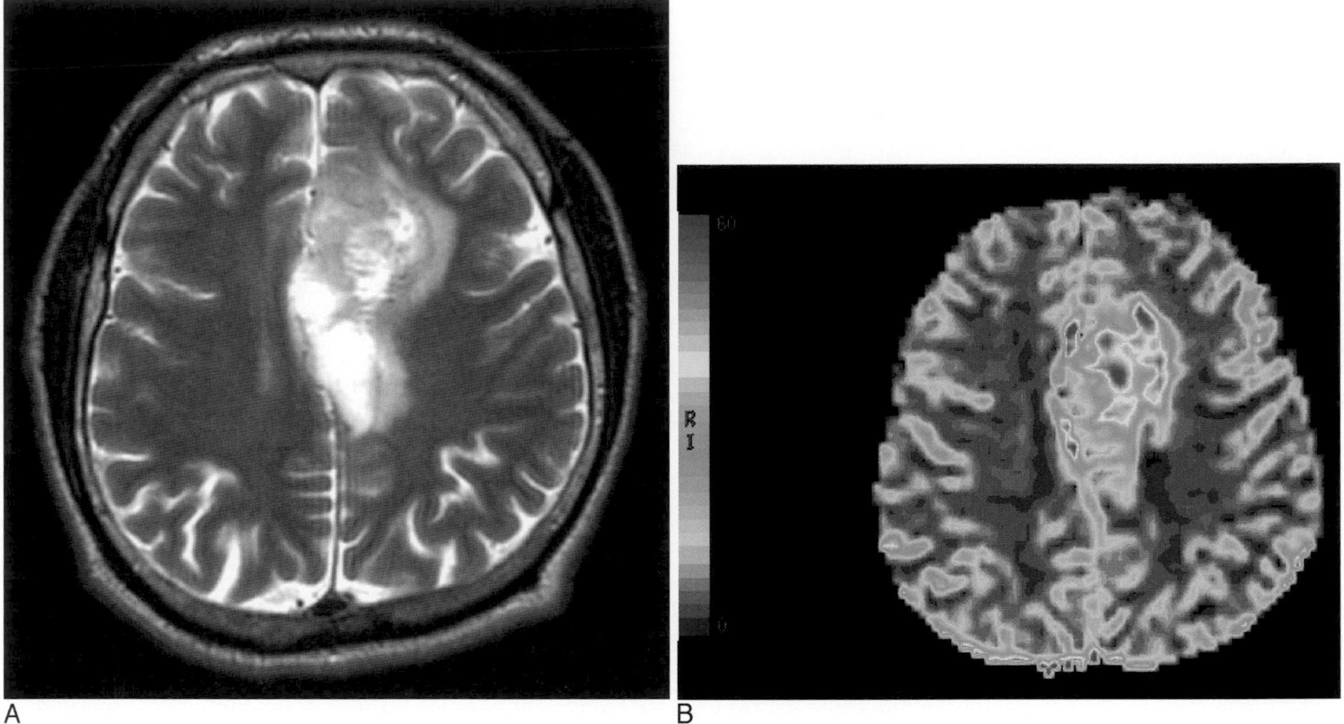

Figure 56.7 WHO grade II oligodendroglioma. Axial T2W image (A) and colour rCBV map (B) showing areas of increased rCBV (yellow and red areas) within the inhomogenous left frontal tumour.

encouraging by showing lower ADC measurements in high-grade lesions[14,32]. This could be accounted for by the increased cellularity and lesser content of hydrophylic components in the extracellular matrix of high-grade tumours. Subsequent studies failed, however, to demonstrate significant ADC differences between glioma grades[35]. The role of ADC measurements in predicting the glioma grade remains at present unclear and appears less promising than the rCBV measurements.

The role of MRS in glioma grading is also subject to debate and remains currently investigational. Low-grade tumours have generally lower Cho levels than high-grade tumours, and lipid and lactate levels correlate with necrosis present in high-grade neoplasms. A threshold value of 1.56 for the Cho/Cr ratio produced a 75.8 per cent sensitivity and 47.5 per cent specificity for differentiating high- from low-grade gliomas[7].

Radiation necrosis is a late complication of radiotherapy or gammaknife surgery, and can present as an enhancing mass lesion, difficult to distinguish from recurrent tumour on conventional imaging. PWI and DWI may help to distinguish between radiation necrosis and tumour recurrence. In radiation necrosis the enhancing lesion has a low rCBV, which tends to be high in tumour recurrence as a consequence of increased new vessel formation[8]. ADC measurements of the enhancing components in recurrent tumour are significantly lower than in radiation necrosis[36], mirroring the higher cellular density in recurrent neoplasm.

Investigation of peritumoural regions with physiology-based MR techniques may be just as important as the assessment of the tumour itself. Differences in the peritumoural tissues of low-grade and high-grade gliomas have been demonstrated with DWI, PWI or MRS[8,23,37–39]. The peritumoural regions of high-grade gliomas show a more marked decrease in ADC, fractional anisotropy and NAA and increase in rCBV compared to low-grade tumours. This is a reflection of the more invasive nature of these tumours, which infiltrate the adjacent brain tissue along vascular channels, leading to an rCBV increase; destroy ultrastructural boundaries with a consequent decrease in ADC and FA; and replace normal brain tissue, resulting in a drop of NAA. Metastases on the other hand are surrounded by 'pure' vasogenic oedema, which contains no infiltrating tumour cells. These peritumoural regions in metastases therefore show no increase in rCBV or decrease in FA.

Tumours of predominantly neuronal cell origin

These include gangliocytomas, gangliogliomas, dysembryoplastic neuro-epithelial tumours (DNETs) and central neurocytomas. The latter is discussed under the section 'Intraventricular tumours' below.

Gangliogliomas and gangliocytomas are slow-growing tumours with a low malignant potential, which occur preferentially in young adults and in the temporal lobe presenting with epilepsy. Gangliogliomas contain a mixture of neural and glial elements with neoplastic large ganglion cells; gangliocytomas have only neuronal elements. CT and MRI show peripherally located mixed solid/cystic lesions that commonly calcify. Enhancement can be variable and is often peripheral.

Dysembryoplastic neuroepithelial tumours (DNETs) are highly polymorphic tumours that arise during embryogenesis. They are preferentially located in the supratentorial cortex and frequently manifest through intractable complex partial seizures. DNETs are usually hypodense on CT and T1-hypointense and T2-hyperintense on MRI. Small intratumoural cysts may be present and cause a 'bubbly' appearance (Fig. 56.8) Calcification is seen in about 25 per cent but enhancement is uncommon. Thinning of the overlying bone is present in approximately half of the cases, reflecting the extremely slow growth of these tumours, which allows bone remodelling to occur[40].

Pineal region tumours

Pineal region tumours account for approximately 1 per cent of intracranial tumours in adults, whereas they represent 10 per cent of all paediatric brain tumours. They present either with obstructive hydrocephalus secondary to aqueduct compression or with problems with eye movements and accommodation, due to compression of the underlying tectal plate. More than half of all pineal region tumours are of germ cell origin (germinoma, teratoma, yolk sac tumours and choriocarcinoma)[41]. The diagnosis of a germ cell tumour is often made by the presence of marker proteins (such as α-fetoprotein or chorionic gonadotropin) in the cerebrospinal fluid.

Germinomas are usually rounded, and often grey matter isointense on standard MRI. They show marked, homogeneous contrast enhancement and virtually never calcify. Germinomas may be multifocal (the second commonest site being the hypothalamic region) or show diffuse subependymal and subarachnoid spread, best appreciated on contrast-enhanced T1W images[42].

Teratomas appear more lobulated and inhomogeneous on CT and MRI, reflecting fat content and calcification. The margins of these tumours are often irregular.

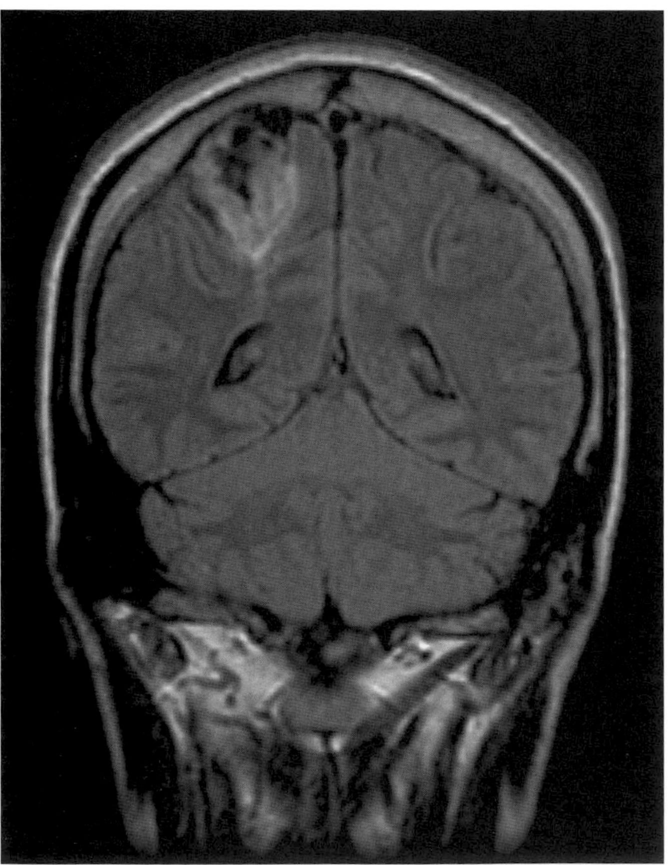

Figure 56.8 Coronal FLAIR of a dysembryoplastic neuro-epithelial tumour (DNET) showing a right parietal, pyramidal-shaped, predominantly cortically based, tumour. It has peripheral cystic areas and a linear area of hyperintensity extends towards the right lateral ventricle.

The remaining pineal region tumours are of pineal cell (pineoblastomas, pineocytomas) or glial origin (astrocytomas). Pineocytomas are histologically benign tumours that lack specific imaging features and are therefore difficult to differentiate from other pineal region neoplasms. Pineoblastomas belong to the group of primitive neuroectodermal tumours (PNETs), and behave like cerebellar medulloblastomas, with frequent seeding via the CSF. They tend to be of low signal intensity on T2W images and can appear bright on DWI. Benign pineal cysts are common and must be differentiated from pineal tumours. They are smooth and well defined and can exhibit rim enhancement. Their signal on T1W, proton density-weighted and FLAIR images may be higher than CSF due to their protein content. They do not, however, cause hydrocephalus or a midbrain syndrome.

Embryonal tumours

These are also called PNETs (primary neuro-ectodermal tumours) and represent high-grade (WHO grade IV) tumours of neuro-ectodermal origin, which include medulloblastomas and the aforementioned pineoblastomas. Medulloblastomas are the commonest posterior fossa tumour in children and arise classically from the super medullary velum at the roof of the 4th ventricle (Fig. 56.9). PNETs have a high cellular density and appear therefore hyperdense on CT, hyperintense on DWI and of intermediate to low density on T2W images. A strong (3–4-fold) elevation of Cho and Lip on MRS is also an expression of the high cellularity and cell turnover of these tumours[7]. PNETs enhance with IV contrast medium and have a propensity for dissemination in the subarachnoid space with leptomeningeal deposits. Staging of these tumours therefore requires a contrast-enhanced MRI of the entire neuroaxis[23].

LYMPHOMAS

Primary cerebral lymphoma (PCL) has tripled in incidence over the past 2 decades[23]. This is partly due to a rise in patients with AIDS but PCL has also increased in immunocompetent patients. PCL appears as a single (less frequently multiple) lobulated enhancing mass, often abutting an ependymal or meningeal surface and involving basal nuclei. Enhancement is uniform in immunocompetent patients and ring-like in immunocompromised patients, in whom PCL frequently contains areas of central necrosis. The high cellular density and nucleus-to-cytoplasm ratio make PCL appear hyperdense on CT and hypointense on T2W images (Fig. 56.10). The ADC of PCL is lower than in gliomas[43] or toxoplasmosis[44], which is an important differential diagnosis in immunocompromised patients. PCL grows in an angiocentric fashion around existing blood vessels without extensive new vessel formation. Perfusion-weighted MRI therefore shows only a modest increase in rCBV, much less marked than in high-grade gliomas, where angiogenesis is a prominent feature[23].

A characteristic finding is rapid resolution of the tumour following administration of steroids and/or radiotherapy. Diffuse meningeal involvement is more common in secondary lymphoma and relatively rare in PCL.

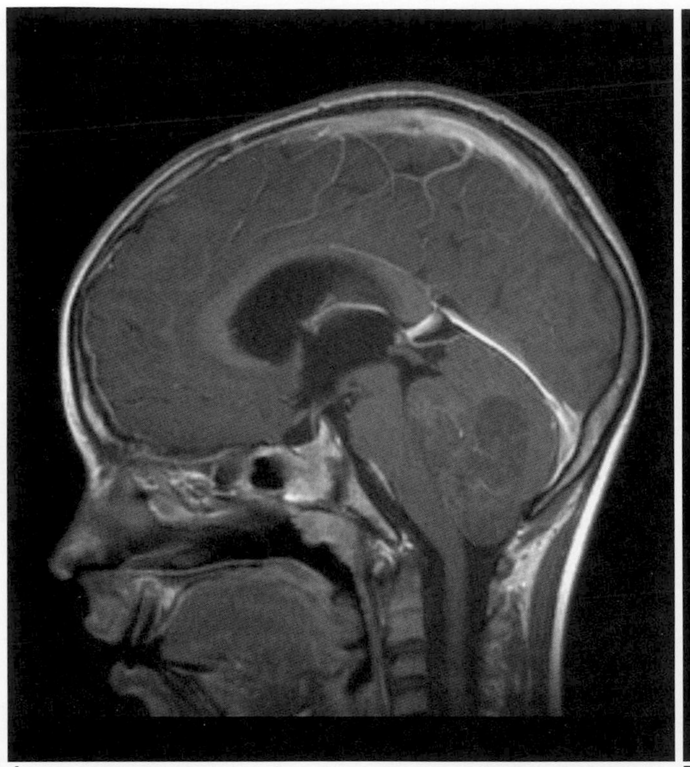

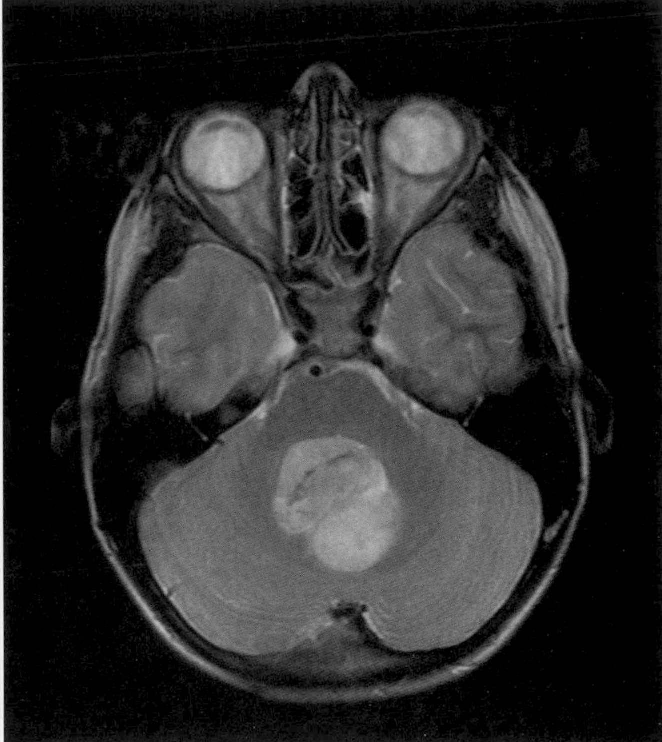

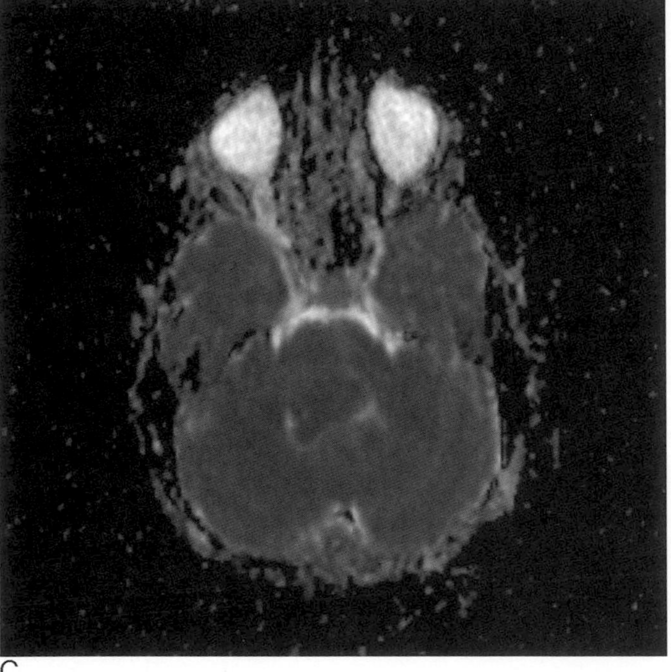

Figure 56.9 Medulloblastoma. Sagittal gadolinium-enhanced T1W (A), axial T2W images (B) and ADC map (C) demonstrate a heterogeneously enhancing mass posterior to the 4th ventricle, which is obliterated. The increased cellularity of this tumour is reflected by its relative hypointensity on the ADC map. (Courtesy of Dr R. Gunny.)

METASTASES

The primary neoplasms that most commonly metastasize to the brain are carcinoma of the lung, breast and malignant melanoma (Fig. 56.11). Generally, metastases appear as multiple rounded lesions with a tendency to seed peripherally in the cerebral substance, at the grey/white matter junction. They can, however, occur anywhere in the cerebrum, brainstem or cerebellum and can also spread to the meninges. Metastases are characterized by oedema in the surrounding white matter, which appears dark on trace-weighted DWI and is often

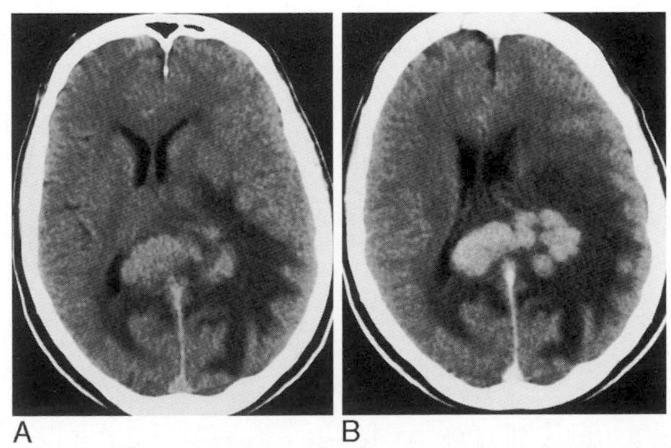

Figure 56.10 Primary cerebral lymphoma. CT before (A) and after IV contrast medium (B). An irregular mass that is hyperdense to grey matter expands the splenium of the corpus callosum and extends into the left hemisphere. It is surrounded by extensive white matter oedema and enhances avidly with contrast.

disproportionate to the size of the tumour itself. On T2W images, the neoplastic nodule may blend with the surrounding oedema, giving a picture of widespread vasogenic oedema and obscuring the diagnosis. Most metastases enhance strongly with IV contrast medium, either uniformly, or ring-like if the metastasis has outgrown its blood supply. Most metastases from lung and breast are similar in density to normal brain parenchyma on CT, but some types are spontaneously dense, particularly deposits from malignant melanoma[45].

Haemorrhage occurs in about 10 per cent of metastases, resulting in high signal on T1W images and high or low signal on T2W images. Similar signal characteristics can also occur in nonhaemorrhagic metastases from melanoma, due to the paramagnetic properties of melanin. Small metastases and those that are not made conspicuous by surrounding oedema are often only detected on contrast-enhanced studies. Increasing the contrast dose or relaxivity of gadolinium compounds can improve the sensitivity for detection of metastases on MRI[3].

Advanced MRI methods can also contribute towards diagnosis and differential diagnosis of metastases. DWI may help to predict the histology of metastases. Well-differentiated adenocarcinoma metastases are hypointense on trace-weighted DWI, whereas small cell and neuroendocrine metastases are hyperintense, due to their higher cellularity[46,47]. On standard MRI it may occasionally be difficult to distinguish a single metastasis from a glioma. PWI and MRS of the peritumoural rather than intratumoural region were shown to be useful in differentiating the two, as mentioned earlier.

DWI is helpful to differentiate cystic metastasis (Fig. 56.12) from cerebral abscesses (Fig. 56.13)[47]. The latter contain more

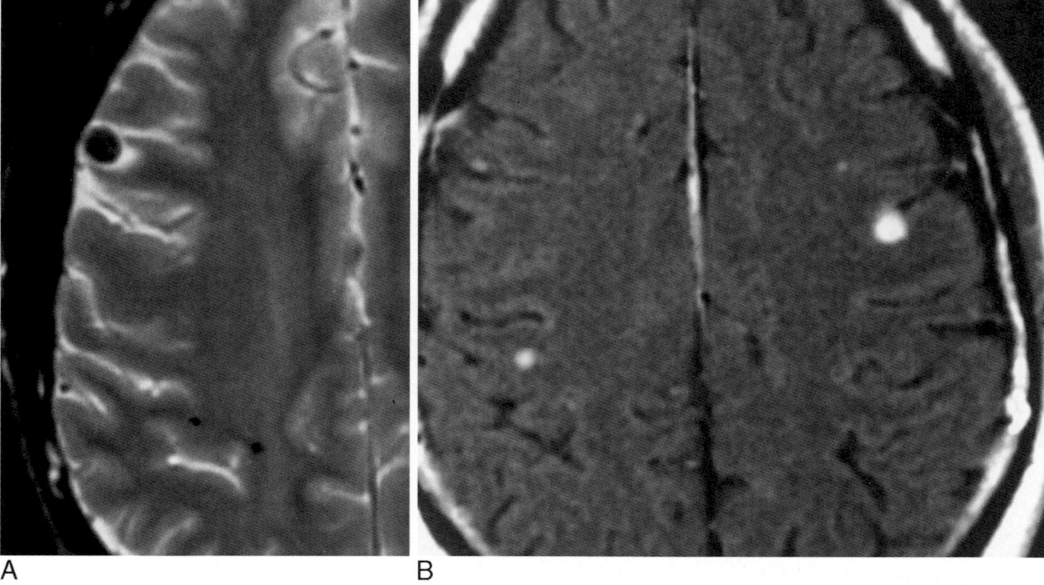

Figure 56.11 Metastases: (A) melanoma (MRI): axial T2W (2000/80). There are at least three foci of signal hypointensity in the right hemisphere, the largest in the right posterior frontal cortex and the others deeper in the subcortical parietal region. This T2 shortening is attributable to melanin. (B) Axial post-contrast T1W with magnetization transfer (650/16). At a slightly different level, this post-contrast study discloses at least four rounded hyperintense metastatic deposits, all in the cortex or subcortical regions.

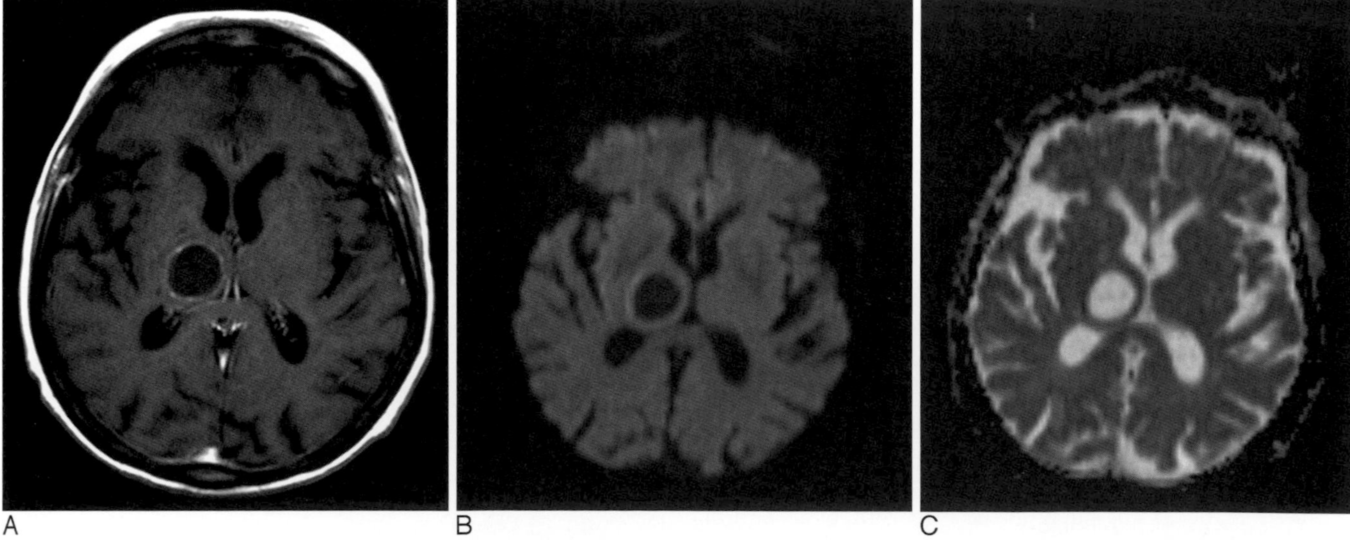

Figure 56.12 Cystic metastasis from CA breast. Axial T1W post-contrast image (A) demonstrates a peripherally enhancing, centrally necrotic lesion in the right thalamus. The lesion appears dark on the trace-weighted DW image (B) and bright on the ADC map (C), which is consistent with a relatively unrestricted diffusion in the center of the mass.

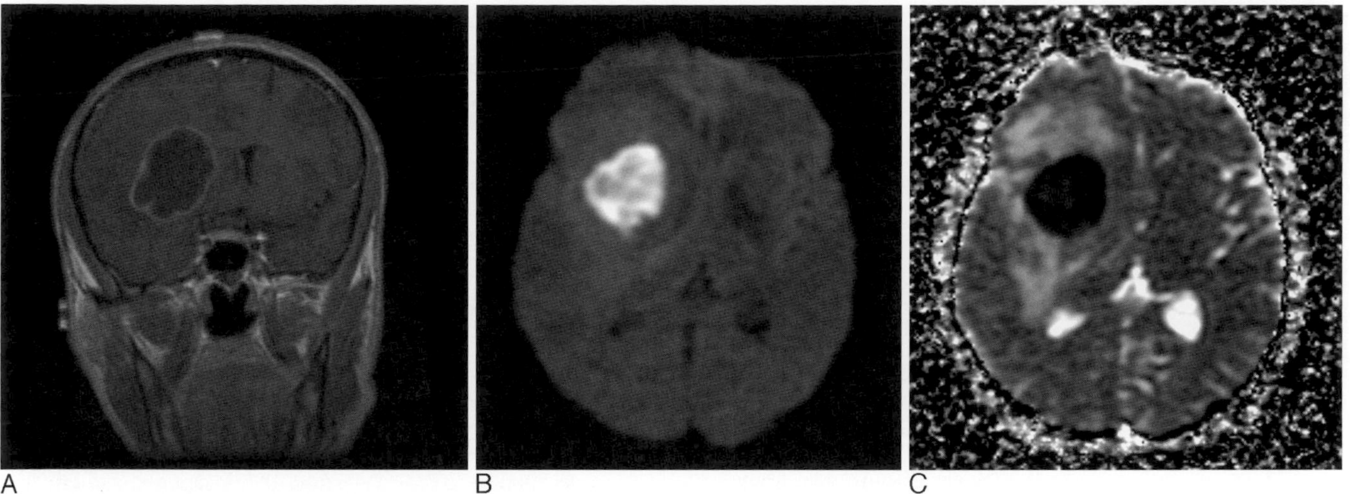

Figure 56.13 Brain abscess. T1W post-contrast image (A) shows a cystic lesion with an enhancing rim centred on the region of the right basal ganglia. The trace-weighted DW image (B) shows a hyperintense lesion that appears markedly hypointense on the ADC map (C), and is distinct from the surrounding hyperintense vasogenic oedema. These features indicate severely restricted diffusion in the abscess cavity.

viscous fluid and pus and show a more marked restriction of water diffusion than necrotic tumours. Abscesses appear therefore bright on trace-weighted DWI and dark on ADC maps.

INTRAVENTRICULAR TUMOURS

Approximately one-tenth of all primary intra-axial brain tumours involve the ventricular system. The precise anatomical location of the tumour within the ventricles often provides an important clue to the nature of the lesion. Common intraventricular tumours and cysts and their sites of predilection are summarized in Table 56.3. Intraventricular tumours arising from neuro-epithelial tissue (ependymomas, central neurocytoma and choroid plexus tumours) are discussed first.

Ependymomas

Ependymomas arise from neoplastic transformation of the ependyma and account for about 5 per cent of adult primary brain tumours, being twice as frequent in children. Ependymomas are usually intraventricular, although extraventricular rests of ependymal cells may give rise to hemisphere tumours. Supratentorial tumours occur in young adults and fourth ventricular ependymomas (Fig. 56.14), which frequently extend through the foramina of Magendie and Luschka and have two age peaks: at 5 and 35 years of age. They are well-demarcated, lobulated mass lesions that show calcification on CT in over 50 per cent and are of mixed signal intensity on MRI (predominantly hyperintense on T2W and iso- to hypointense on T1W images). MRI may demonstrate small cysts but calcification is less conspicuous than on CT. Enhancement is mild to moderate and often heterogeneous.

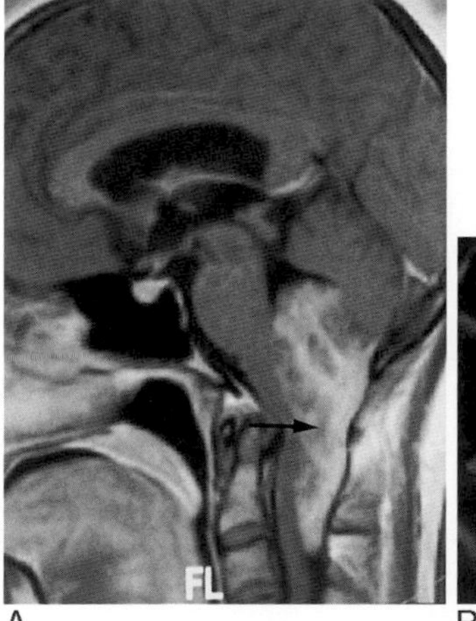

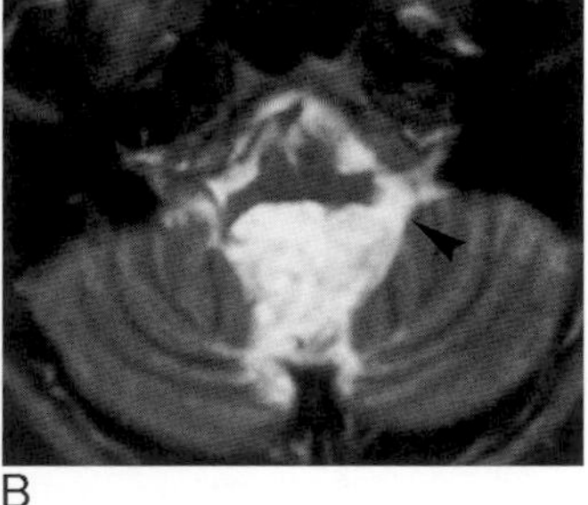

Figure 56.14 Ependymoma of the fourth ventricle. Sagittal gadolinium-enhanced T1W (A) and axial T2W (B) MRI. A heterogeneously enhancing mass (arrow) fills the lower half of the fourth ventricle and extends through the foramina of Lushka (arrowhead) and Magendie to lie posterior to the medulla oblongata and upper cervical spinal cord, which are compressed from behind. There is obstructive hydrocephalus.

Table 56.3 INTRAVENTRICULAR LESIONS

Tumour	Typical site
Colloid cyst	Foramen of Monro/third ventricle
Meningioma	Trigone of lateral ventricle
Choroid	Fourth ventricle
Ependymoma	Lateral ventricle (more common in children) and fourth ventricle
Neurocytoma	Lateral ventricles (involving septum pellucidum)
Metastases	Lateral ventricles, ependyma and choroid plexus

Central neurocytomas

Central neurocytomas are slow-growing intraventricular tumours of purely neuronal origin[48]. Before the advent of immunohistological methods they were frequently misdiagnosed as subependymal oligodendrogliomas. These relatively benign tumours occur predominantly in the second and third decades of life, and represent probably the commonest lateral ventricular masses in this age group. They typically arise from the septum pellucidum and occupy the frontal horns and bodies of the lateral ventricles, and sometimes extend through the foramen of Monro. CT frequently shows calcification and small cysts. MRI shows a heterogeneously enhancing mixed-signal intensity mass containing septated cysts, susceptibility artefact from calcification and grey-matter-isointense nodules (Fig. 56.15). Obstructive hydrocephalus is common.

Choroid plexus tumours

Choroid plexus papillomas are much more common than choroid plexus carcinomas (Fig. 56.16). The location and incidence of choroid plexus papillomas varies with age. They are relatively more common in childhood (3 per cent of primary brain tumours), presenting as a 'cauliflower-like' mass in the trigone of the lateral ventricle. In adults, papillomas are less common, and occur predominantly in the fourth ventricle. CT shows an iso- to hyperdense mass with punctate calcification and homogeneous enhancement. On MRI the papillomas appear as lobulated, intraventricular masses of heterogeneous, predominantly intermediate signal intensity on both T1W and T2W images, with intense contrast enhancement. Angiography, which is now rarely indicated, shows a highly vascular mass supplied predominantly by the anterior and posterior choroidal arteries. Choroid plexus carcinomas are rare, highly malignant tumours that invade the adjacent brain parenchyma to a greater degree than papillomas.

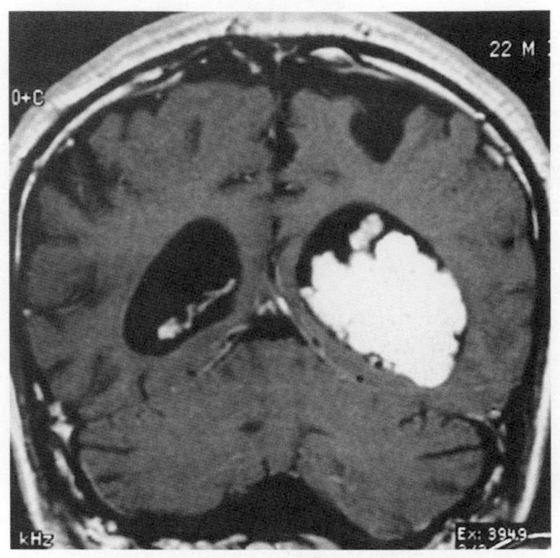

Figure 56.16 Choroid plexus papilloma. Coronal T1W post-gadolinium MRI. There is a lobulated, strongly enhancing tumour in the trigone of the left lateral ventricle. Both lateral ventricles are dilated due to hydrocephalus associated with this tumour.

Colloid cysts

These benign lesions occur exclusively at the paraphysis, which lies in the posterior lip of the foramen of Monro, between the third and lateral ventricles. They tend to cause hydrocephalus, by intermittently or continuously obstructing the outflow of cerebrospinal fluid from the lateral ventricles and are smooth, spherical lesions that are characteristically hyperdense on unenhanced CTs (Fig. 56.17). Their MR appearance varies depending on the cyst content (calcium, cholesterol, haemosiderin); some can have similar signal to CSF, but most are of high signal on T1W and on T2W images.

Meningiomas

This is the commonest cause of a mass in the trigone of the lateral ventricle after the first decade of life. The CT and MRI appearances are similar to those of extraventricular meningiomas (see later): a well-defined, globular lesion that is usually hyperdense on CT and may give similar signal to cerebral

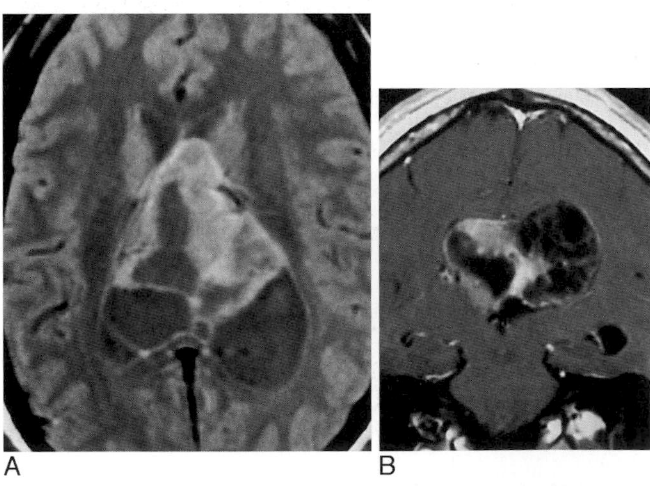

Figure 56.15 Central neurocytoma. Axial proton density (A) and coronal T1W post-gadolinium (B) MRI. A partly cystic, multi-septated, enhancing mass, which is related to the septum pellucidum, fills the bodies of both lateral ventricles and causes hydrocephalus with dilatation of the left temporal horn.

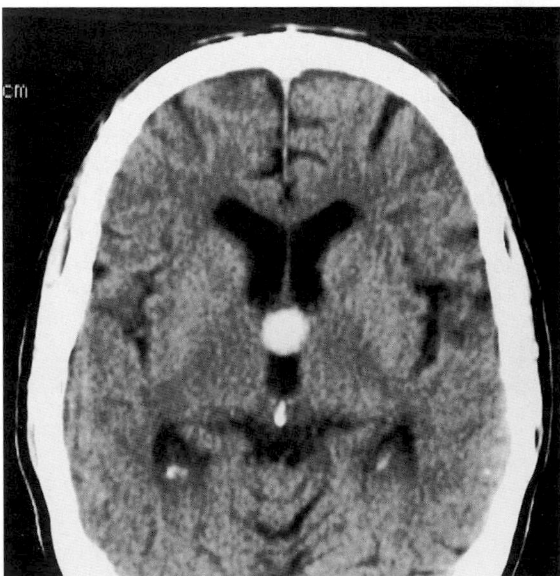

Figure 56.17 Colloid cyst. Unenhanced CT. There is a dense, rounded mass in the region of the foramen of Monro causing enlargement of the lateral ventricles, and indenting the anterior aspect of the third ventricle.

cortex on T1W and T2W images. They usually show marked contrast enhancement on CT and MRI.

EXTRA-AXIAL TUMOURS

Primary extra-axial neoplasms arise from the meningothelial arachnoidal cells (meningiomas), mesenchymal pericytes (haemangiopericytoma) or cranial nerves (schwannomas, neurofibromas) and include developmental cysts or tumour-like lesions (epidermoid and dermoid cysts). Metastatic involvement of the meninges and tumours in specific regions (around the sella turcica and skull base) are discussed separately. Overall, meningiomas represent the commonest non-glial intracranial neoplasm, accounting for approximately 20 per cent of all primary intracranial tumours. Multiple meningiomas and cranial nerve tumours are found in neurofibromatosis type 2. Extra-axial lesions occur much more frequently in adults than in children and account for the majority of primary infratentorial tumours in adults, with three lesions sharing a predilection for the cerebellopontine region: vestibular schwannoma, meningioma and epidermoid cysts.

When analysing an extra-axial lesion, it is important to pay attention to associated bone changes: meningiomas tend to induce a hyperostotic bone reaction, whereas dermoid cysts and schwannomas tend to cause bone thinning resulting in enlargement of, for example, the middle cranial fossa or internal auditory meatus. Other features distinguishing extra- from intra-axial mass lesions are 'buckling' and medial displacement of the grey–white matter interface, a CSF cleft separating the base of the mass from adjacent brain and a broad base along a dural or calvarial surface[37].

Meningiomas

Meningiomas originate from arachnoid cell rests, related to arachnoid granulations of the dura mater and may assume a spherical, well-circumscribed shape or be flat, infiltrating ('en plaque') lesions[49]. There are several histological types of meningioma including meningothelial, fibrous/fibroblastic, transitional and psammomatous tumours. Most of them correspond to WHO grade I. Meningiomas with atypical features such as increased mitotic activity, patternless growth and necrosis correspond to grade II (atypical) or grade III (anaplastic meningioma), depending on the extent of these features[20].

Of meningiomas, 90 per cent are supratentorial arising, in decreasing order of frequency, from the parasagittal region, cerebral convexities, sphenoid ridge and olfactory grove. Infratentorial meningiomas are most frequently located on the posterior surface of the petrous bones and clivus and can mimic acoustic neuromas. Bone sclerosis is in favour of meningioma and enlargement of the internal auditory meatus is much more common in neuroma.

On CT, 60 per cent of meningiomas are spontaneously hyperdense and up to 20 per cent contain calcification. Enhancement on CT is usually intense and uniform (Fig. 56.18). Hyperostosis, best seen on bone window settings, indicates the site of the tumour attachment to the meninges.

On MRI, meningiomas appear frequently isointense to cerebral cortex on both T1W and T2W images and may be difficult to detect without IV contrast medium. Meningiomas can have 'capping cysts' of similar MRI signal intensity to CSF. As on CT, meningiomas enhance vividly and homogeneously, except for the uncommon cystic and very densely calcified tumours. There may also be a linear, contrast-enhancing 'dural tail' extending from the tumour along the dura mater.

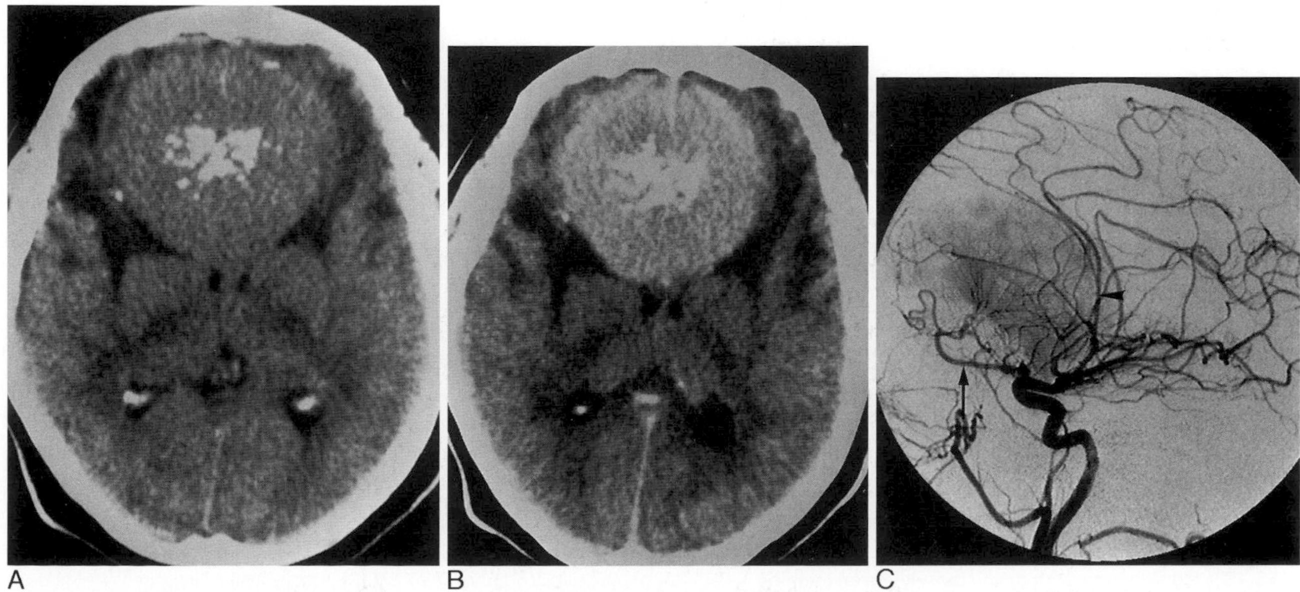

Figure 56.18 Subfrontal meningioma. CT before (A) and after (B) IV contrast medium, and lateral projection of common carotid arteriogram (C). There is a large circumscribed mass in the anterior cranial fossa that is isodense to normal grey matter, contains foci of calcification centrally and enhances homogeneously. There is oedema in the white matter of both frontal lobes and posterior displacement and splaying of the frontal horns of the lateral ventricles. On the arteriogram (C) the mass is delineated by a tumour blush and there is posterior displacement of the anterior cerebral arteries (arrowhead), mirroring the mass effect seen on CT. The ophthalmic artery is enlarged as its ethmoidal branches supply the tumour (arrow).

The 'dural tail sign', once thought to be pathognomonic for meningioma (Fig. 56.19) can also be seen with other tumours such as schwannoma or metastasis.

Vasogenic oedema is not infrequently associated with meningiomas. The extent of the vasogenic oedema does not correlate with the size of the meningioma and, as with metastases, even small lesions can cause quite extensive oedema[50,51]. Meningiomas abutting the superior sagittal or transverse sinuses can compress or invade these venous structures. The distinction between compression and occlusion is important for preoperative planning, and can be made by magnetic resonance or computed tomography angiography (MRA and CTA, respectively).

Physiological MR imaging methods are also of help in the diagnosis of meningiomas. DWI shows differences between typical and atypical meningiomas: the latter have lower ADC values than the former[52]. MRS may show an alanin peak, which is characteristic for a meningioma but this is seen in less than 50 per cent of cases[7]. Meningiomas have usually a markedly elevated rCBV on PWI (Fig. 56.19C), which can be used to differentiate from dural metastases, which tend to have a lower rCBV[53]. Angiography is occasionally performed for pre-operative assessment of the blood supply, and can be combined with pre-operative embolization, to reduce the blood loss during operation.

The cardinal angiographic findings are supplied from meningeal vessels and a dense, homogeneous, persistent blush. Parasitization of cortical vessels by tumours over the cerebral convexity or of branches of the ophthalmic artery by subfrontal masses is not rare (Fig. 56.18.C).

Haemangiopericytomas enter into the differential diagnosis for meningiomas. Features suggestive of a haemangiopericytoma rather than meningioma, are a lobulated (rather than spherical) dural-based mass, absence of calcification and hyperostosis and multiple areas of flow void on MRI, reflecting the high vascularity of these tumours[54].

Cranial nerve sheath tumours

Cranial nerve sheath tumours, originating from cranial nerves, account for 6–8 per cent of primary intracranial tumours. Most are benign neoplasms arising from Schwann cells ('schwannomas') of the nerve sheaths. Schwannomas arise eccentrically from the sheath and compress the parent nerve rather than invading it. All cranial nerves except I (olfactory) and II (optic), which are white matter tracts of the cerebrum, have nerve sheaths; however schwannomas usually grow on the sensory nerves, most frequently from the superior vestibular division of the vestibulocochlear nerve ('acoustic neuroma') and, with decreasing frequency, from the trigeminal, glossopharyngeal and lower cranial nerves. Pure motor cranial nerves rarely form schwannomas. Multiple cranial nerve schwannomas are found in neurofibromatosis type 2 and bilateral vestibular schwannomas are pathognomonic of this condition. Neurofibromas are benign tumours, composed of fibroblasts, reticulin and a mucoid matrix in addition to Schwann cells. Cranial nerve tumours are T1 iso/hypointense and T2 hyperintense, and larger lesions often contain areas of cystic degeneration (Fig. 56.20). Cranial nerve tumours almost invariably show marked enhancement with IV contrast medium, which is solid in two-thirds and ring-like or heterogeneous in one-third of cases.

Acoustic or, more accurately, vestibular schwannomas account for over 80 per cent of cerebellopontine lesions and widen the internal auditory meatus (IAM) if large enough. MRI is much more sensitive than CT for the detection of small vestibular schwannomas. High-resolution, thin-section, T2W fast spin-echo images of the posterior fossa shows the 7th and 8th nerves in detail (Fig. 56.21) and can detect small tumours causing focal nerve thickening. If the findings are equivocal, gadolinium-enhanced images refute or confirm the suspicion of a tumour.

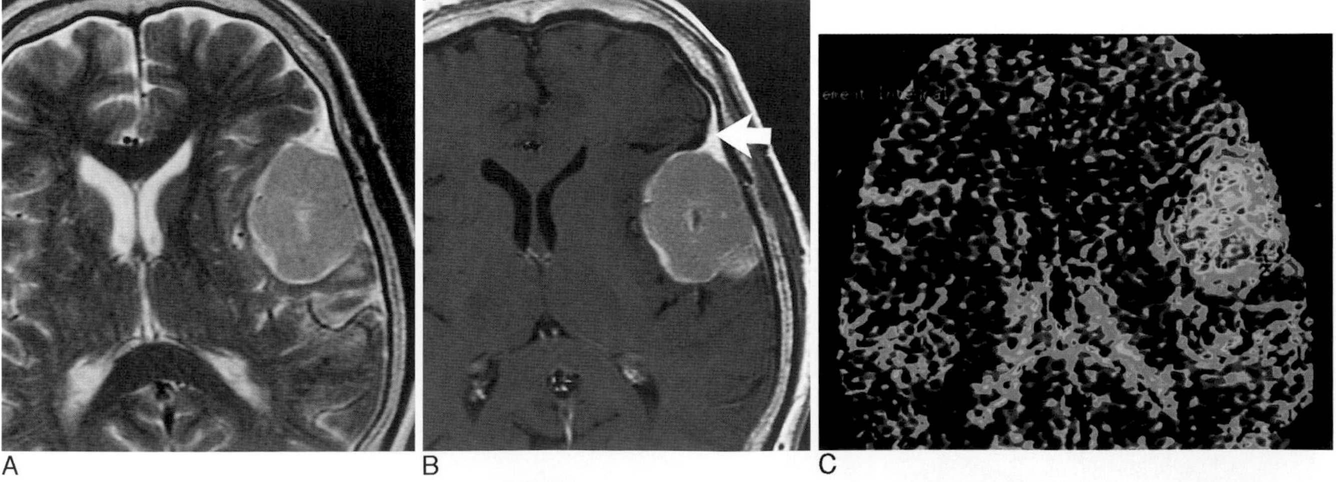

Figure 56.19 Meningioma with perfusion-weighted imaging. Axial T2W (A), gadolinium-enhanced T1W (B) and perfusion-weighted (C) MRI. A grey-matter isointense mass deeply indents the left cerebral convexity (A). Its broad dural base, the surrounding displaced cerebral sulci and the small pial vessel between the tumour and the brain surface (arrowhead) are all features of an extra-axial lesion. The tumour enhances and there is a 'dural tail' (arrow) (B), which is a frequent radiological finding in meningioma, but is not pathognomonic (see Fig 56.24). Perfusion-weighted MRI (C): a colour map of the relative cerebral blood volume (rCBV) shows increased blood volume of the tumour compared to normal cortex and white matter, confirming its highly vascular nature.

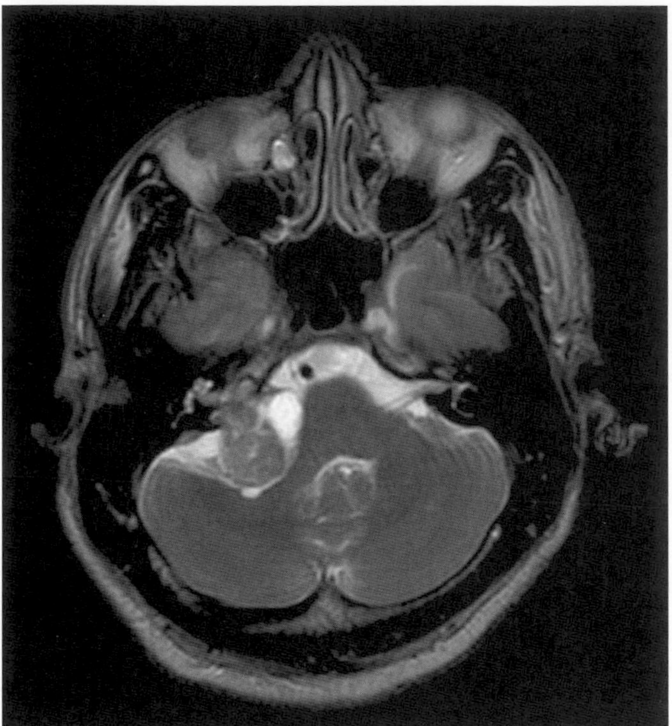

Figure 56.20 Cystic vestibular schawannoma. T2W image reveals a large right cerebellopontine angle tumour with a medial cystic component. The mass extends into and expands the internal auditory meatus and distorts the right middle cerebellar peduncle.

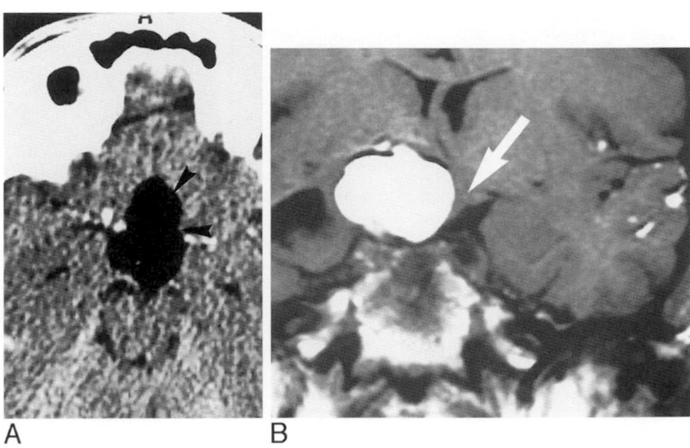

Figure 56.22 Suprasellar dermoid tumours. CT (A). There is a midline, fat density tumour (arrowheads) occupying the suprsasellar region. (B) Coronal T1W MRI of a different patient with a ruptured dermoid tumour. There is a lobulated high signal mass in the chiasmatic cistern compressing and displacing the optic chiasm to the left (arrow). Fat globules, which have spilled into the subarachnoid space, are seen as high signal foci in the left Sylvian fissure. The patient has had previous surgery via a right temporal approach, causing right temporal atrophy and enlargement of the right temporal horn.

Epidermoid and dermoid tumours

Epidermoid and dermoid cysts, or 'pearly tumours', result from inclusion of ectodermal elements during the closure of the neural tube. Intracranial dermoid cysts lie usually near the midline and contain all skin elements, including fat, which is why they appear to be of very low density on CT and high signal intensity on T1W images (Fig. 56.22). They may rupture and release fat globules, which float in the CSF space.

Epidermoid cysts can be central (chiasmatic and quadrigeminal plate cisterns) or eccentric (cerebellopontine angle, middle cranial fossa, Sylvian fissure). Although present at birth, these lesions grow slowly by accumulating desquamated epithelium and conform to the shape of the portion of the subarachnoid space they occupy, sometimes invaginating into the brain parenchyma. On CT and standard T1W and T2W images, epidermoid cysts are non-enhancing lesions of similar density or signal intensity to CSF. They have to be differentiated from arachnoid cysts, which have better defined margins and cause bone thinning. DWI is very helpful to distinguish epidermoid tumours from arachnoid cysts (Fig. 56.23): water diffusion is markedly restricted in epidermoid tumours (which appear bright on DWI) but not in arachnoid cysts, which have similar signal characteristics to CSF.

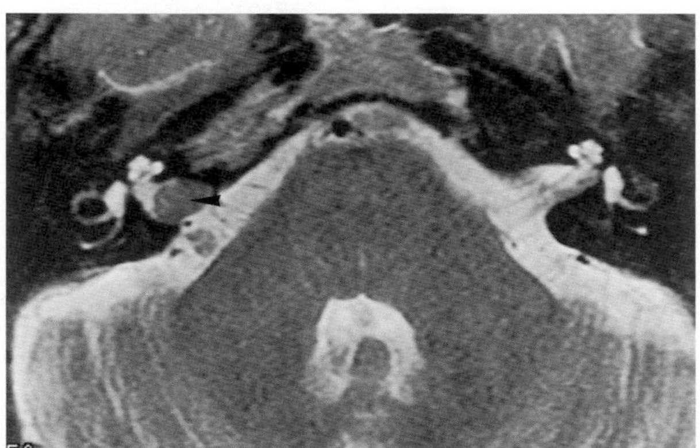

Figure 56.21 Vestibular schwannoma (Acoustic neuroma). Axial, high-resolution T2W MRI. There is a small soft-tissue mass (arrowhead) in the right internal auditory meatus, which is only minimally expanded. The normal 7th and 8th nerves on the left are clearly demonstrated.

Meningeal metastases

Meningeal metastases may involve the pachymeninges (dura mater), leptomeninges (arachnoid and pia mater) or both. Contrast-enhanced MRI is much more sensitive than contrast-enhanced CT for detection of metastatic meningeal involvement. Carcinomatosis of the dura mater, common in carcinoma of the breast, manifests itself as focal curvilinear or diffuse contrast enhancement closely applied to the inner table of the skull, which does not follow the convolutions of the gyri. Focal segmental lesions may be difficult to distinguish from en plaque meningioma (Fig. 56.24). Leptomeningeal carcinomatosis produces linear or finely nodular contrast enhancement of the surface of the brain, extending into the sulci and following the convolutions of the brain. It may be indistinguishable from infective meningitis or sarcoidosis. Leptomeningeal disease is commonly seen in leukaemia, lymphoma and breast or lung cancer.

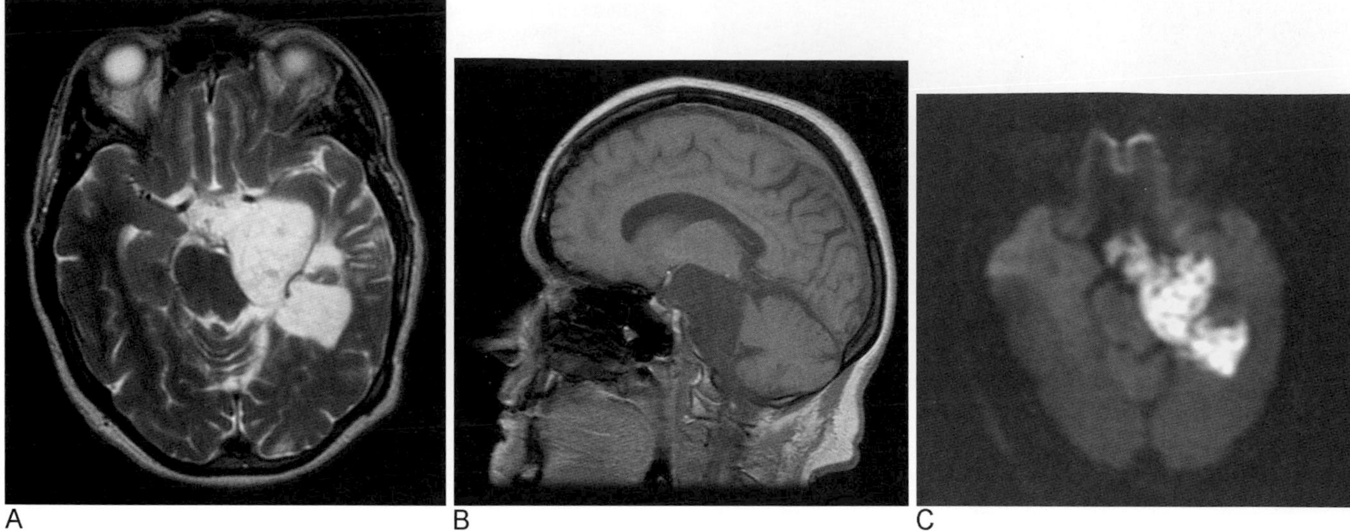

Figure 56.23 Epidermoid tumour. Axial T2W image (A) and sagittal gadolinium-enhanced T1W image (B) shows a large nonenhancing lesion of similar signal intensity to CSF, which occupies the chiasmatic and ambient cisterns, and distorts the medial aspect of the left temporal lobe. On the trace-weighted DW image (C) the lesion appears markedly hyperintense, indicating restricted diffusion.

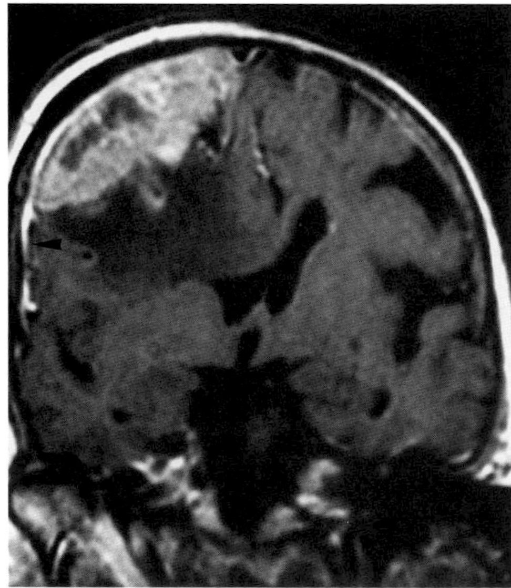

Figure 56.24 Dural metastasis from breast carcinoma. Coronal T1W post-contrast MRI. There is a heterogeneously enhancing mass with an irregular surface that arises from the dura over the right cerebral convexity. It displaces the underlying brain and causes considerable low signal oedema within it. There is a dural 'tail' extending away from the tumour (arrowhead).

SKULL BASE TUMOURS

Tumours of the skull base include a large pathological spectrum, such as metastases, myeloma/plasmacytoma, meningioma, caudally extending pituitary adenomas, direct extension of nasopharyngeal malignancies as well as tumours and inflammatory lesions arising in the paranasal sinuses. Two specific lesions of the central and posterior skull base are discussed later: chordoma and glomus jugulare tumours.

Chordomas

Chordomas originate from malignant transformation of notochordal cells and their most frequent location in the skull base is the spheno-occipital synchrondrosis of the clivus, followed by the basiocciput and petrous apex: tumours away from the midline are considerably less common. These tumours present usually with pain and lower cranial nerve palsies. They cause bone destruction and contain calcification, both of which are well demonstrated on CT with bone windows. On MRI the tumours exhibit mixed, heterogeneous signal[55], and may have a 'soap-bubble' appearance (Fig. 56.25). The solid components show variable, but often marked contrast enhancement. Fat-suppressed T1W spin-echo sequences are particularly helpful for demonstrating the extent of the tumour and distinguishing pathological enhancement from the high signal of adjacent clival fat. The differential diagnosis includes chondrosarcoma, metastasis and nasopharyngeal carcinoma.

Glomus jugulare tumours

Glomus jugulare tumours (chemodectomas) arise from paraganglion cells, the precursors of the chemo- and baroreceptors of the great vessels. The most common site is the jugular bulb and their presentation is with pulsatile tinnitus, deafness, vertigo and lower cranial nerve palsies. The tumour causes bone destruction with enlargement of the pars vasorum of the jugular foramen, well demonstrated on CT. The tumour, which fills the expanded foramen, gives high signal on T2W images. Glomus jugulare tumours enhance intensely with IV contrast medium and, because of their extreme vascularity, they tend to show areas of flow void that correspond to dilated vessels (Fig. 56.26). These tumours frequently obstruct the internal jugular vein, which may show signal changes indicative of thrombosis.

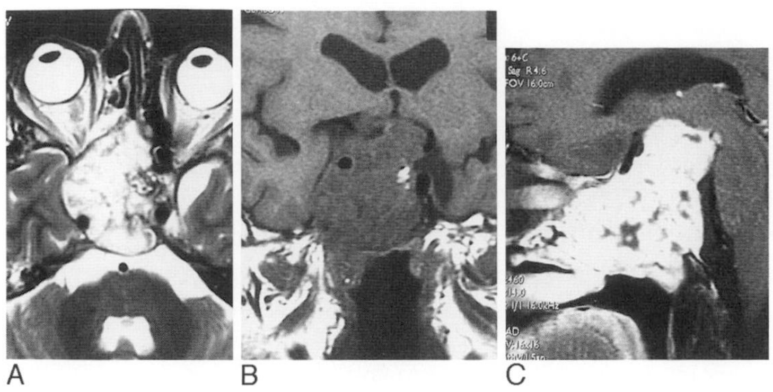

Figure 56.25 Clivus chordoma. Axial T2W (A), coronal T1W (B) and sagittal T1W post-gadolinium (C) MRI. A large mass has destroyed the clivus and extends superiorly compressing the midbrain and hypothalamus. It invades the right cavernous sinus, encasing the internal carotid artery, and extends into the nasopharyngeal soft tissues, posterior ethmoid air cells and optic canals. Tumour also projects into the pontine cistern but appears restrained by dura. The mass returns mixed signal and there is irregular enhancement following contrast injection.

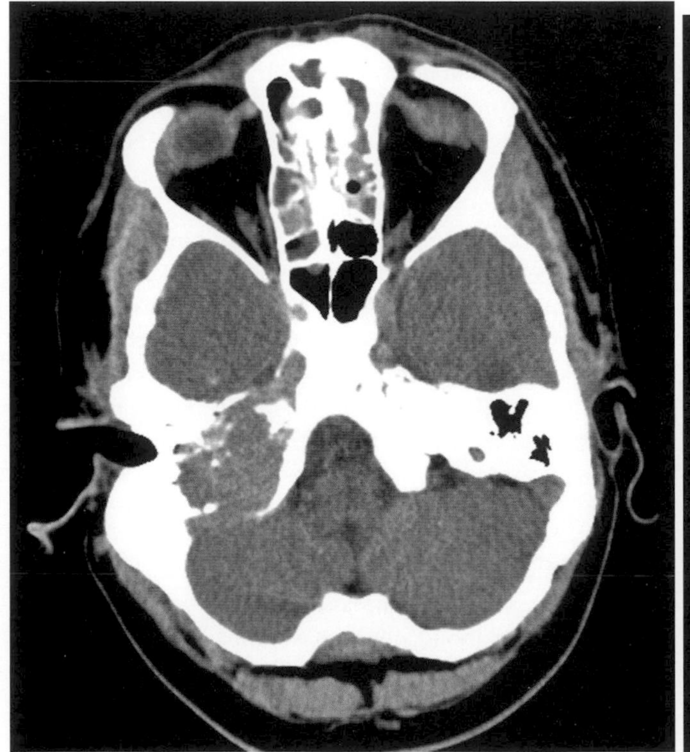

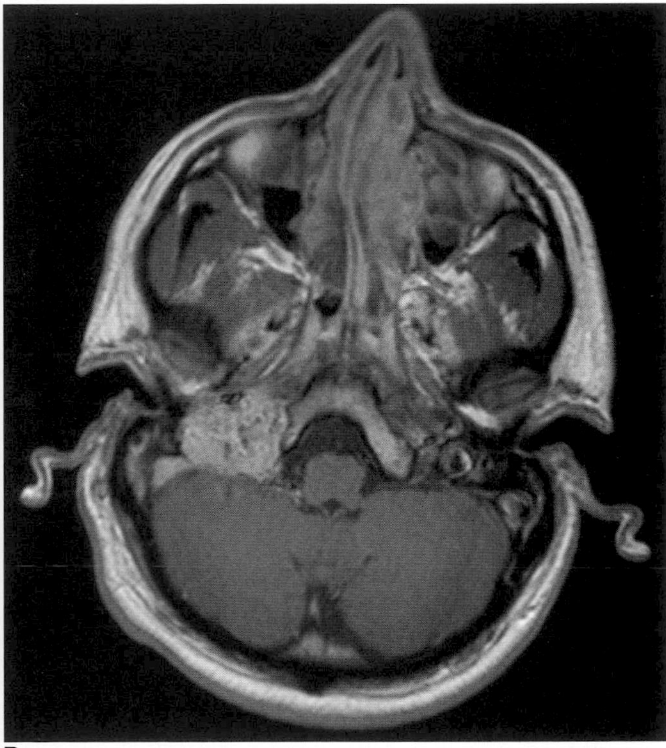

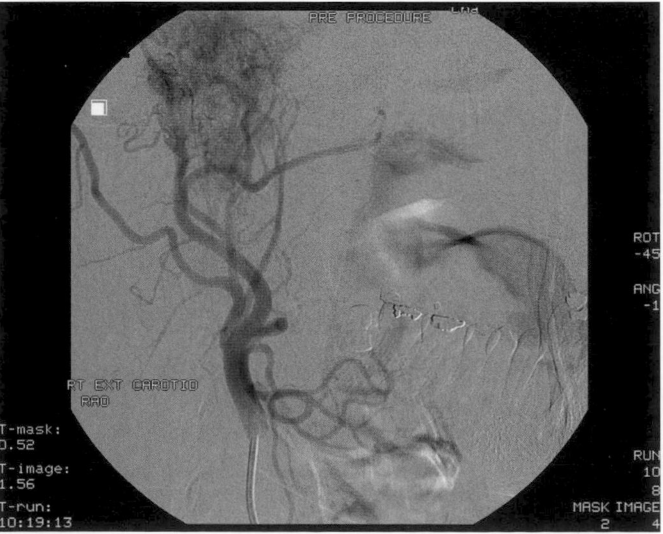

Figure 56.26 Glomus jugulare tumour. An axial CT (A) demonstrates expansion of the right jugular foramen and bone destruction in the adjacent petrous bone by a mass that is markedly enhancing on axial T1W post-contrast images (B). The mass contains areas of flow voids, corresponding to the dilated tumour vessels seen on the right external carotid artery angiogram (C). (Courtesy of Dr M. Adams.)

PITUITARY REGION TUMOURS

The region of the sella turcica contains many different tissues that have a propensity to undergo neoplasia[55] and the differential diagnosis for sellar and parasellar masses is indeed large (Table 56.4). In addition to tumours, non-neoplastic lesions such as arachnoid cysts or giant aneurysms have to be considered.

Pituitary adenomas

Pituitary adenomas are the most common neoplasms in the sellar region. They are classified as microadenomas (diameter < 1 cm) and macroadenomas (> 1 cm). They become symptomatic either because of their endocrine activity (microadenomas and functioning macroadenomas) or by the mass effect they exert (nonfunctioning macroadenomas), usually manifest by visual symptoms secondary to compression of the optic nerves and chiasm. Nonfunctioning microadenomas are not uncommon and can be found incidentally on MRI studies performed for other reasons.

MRI is the investigation of choice for the detection of microadenomas. The standard protocol should include 3-mm thick coronal and sagittal T1W images through the pituitary gland before and after IV gadolinium. It is desirable to perform a fat-saturated T1W sequence after administration of IV contrast medium to eliminate high signal from fat in the clivus and clinoid processes, which could be mistaken for enhancement. The conspicuity of microadenomas can be increased by performing dynamic pituitary MRI (Fig. 56.27), which involves the acquisition of a series of rapid images with a time interval of approximately 10–15 s and exploits the time differences in enhancement between the adenoma and normal gland[56].

Functioning microadenomas can produce prolactin (prolactinomas), ACTH (in Cushing's disease) or growth hormone (eosinophilic microadenomas). Prolactinomas are the most common functioning microadenomas and tend to arise laterally within the anterior lobe of the pituitary gland. They may depress the floor of the sella turcica or expand one side of the gland, causing a subtle upwardly convex bulge and contralateral displacement of the infundibulum. Microadenomas are best shown on contrast-enhanced images and usually enhance later and/or to a lesser degree than normal pituitary tissue.

The primary treatment of prolactin-secreting microadenomas is medical and the role of imaging in cases of hyperprolactinaemia is therefore mainly to exclude a macroadenoma. Precise localization of the microadenoma is, however, important in ACTH and thyroid-stimulating hormone (TSH)-producing adenomas, which are treated surgically. If MRI is not conclusive, petrosal venous sampling may be necessary to lateralize an adenoma in pituitary-driven Cushing's disease. Eosinophilic microadenomas can cause enlargement of the sella along with other features of acromegaly.

Macroadenomas balloon the pituitary fossa and can have a suprasellar component or extend inferiorly into the sphenoid sinus and clivus. Suprasellar extension leads first to elevation, then to compression of the optic chiasm and intracranial optic nerves and a large tumour may compress brain parenchyma, often in the region of the hypothalamus. Most macroadenomas are isointense with brain parenchyma on unenhanced T1W images and hyperdense on CT. Administration of IV contrast may show uniform or heterogenous enhancement and facilitates the detection of cavernous sinus invasion[57]. Macroademomas may contain cystic or haemorrhagic components. Acute haemorrhage into a pituitary macroademona can lead to rapid expansion of the gland resulting in acute compression of the optic chiasm (pituitary apoplexy). Haemorrhage appears hyperintense on non-enhanced T1W images (Fig. 56.28) and, in the acute stage, hyperdense on CT.

Craniopharyngiomas

Craniopharyngiomas are suprasellar tumours that occur most frequently in childhood, but may arise in adult life, and have a second peak of incidence at about the 6th decade. Symptoms

Table 56.4 PRIMARY TUMOURS IN THE SELLAR AND PARASELLAR REGION

Tumour	Typical features
Pituitary macroadenoma	Enlarged sella turcica, strong enhancement, sometimes haemorrhage
Meningioma	Broad dural base, enhancement along planum sphenoidale
	Hyperostosis, 'blistering' of sphenoid sinus
Schwannoma	T1-hypo- and T2-hyperintense, strong (e.g. of fifth nerve) enhancement
Chordoma	Bone destruction on CT, heterogeneous signal and enhancement on MRI
Chondrosarcoma	Bone destruction and calcification on CT, T2 hyperintense on MRI
Crangiopharyngioma	Calcification, cysts, nodular enhancement
Rathke's cleft cyst	T1-hyperintense on MRI, smooth peripheral enhancement
Dermoid	Hypodense on CT and T1 hyperintense on MRI
Epidermoid	Isodense to CSF on CT and isointense to CSF on T1 and T2 weighting, brighter than CSF on FLAIR and DWI
Tuber cinerum	Grey matter isointense on T1 weighting and T2 hamartoma hyperintense
Optic glioma	Thickening of chiasm, spread along optic pathways
Germ cell tumours	Located in midline, intense enhancement; can be synchronous with pineal germinomas

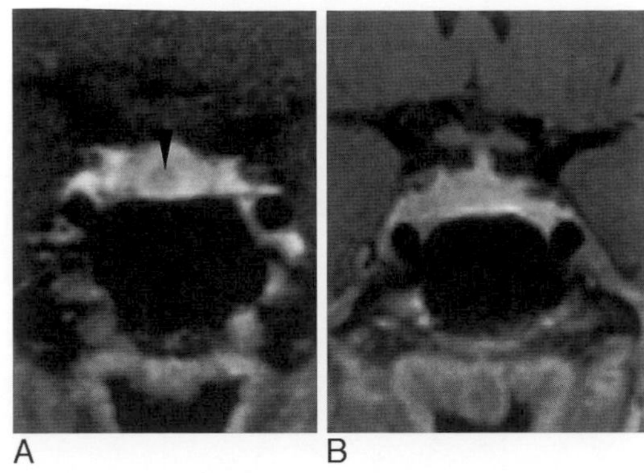

Figure 56.27 Dynamic contrast-enhanced MRI of pituitary adenoma. Dynamically enhanced thin-section coronal T1W images of the pituitary gland. Images were acquired at 15-s intervals following injection of gadolinium. The scan at 90 s (A) reveals a microadenoma (arrowhead) to the right of the midline, which has enhanced to a lesser degree than the surrounding normal pituitary tissue at this stage. On the conventional enhanced MRI, acquired over 4 min (B), the enhancement of the lesion is similar to the rest of the gland.

are due to compression of the optic chiasm or to raised intra-cerebral pressure (ICP) secondary to obstruction of the foramen of Monro.

They arise from epithelial remnants of Rathke's pouch, from which the anterior pituitary develops, and can be cystic, solid or mixed cystic/solid (Fig. 56.29). Craniopharyngiomas tend not to expand the pituitary fossa unless they become very large (a differentiating feature from pituitary macroadenomas).

The MRI appearances differ according to the histological type[58]. The adamantinous type, more commonly occurring in children, is more likely to have large T1 hyperintense cystic components, whereas the squamous-papillary type, which is more frequent in adults, is more likely to be predominantly solid and associated cysts return low signal on T1W images, similar to CSF.

The solid components of craniopharyngiomas show intense contrast enhancement and may be partially calcified.

Rathke's cleft cysts

Symptomatic Rathke's cleft cysts are much less common than craniopharyngiomas but asymptomatic lesions are relatively commonly found at postmortem. The cysts usually lie within the pituitary gland, although others are found adjacent to the infundibulum, above the sella. On MRI they appear frequently as T1 hyperintense cysts but may also exhibit similar signal characteristics to CSF. Rathke's cysts do not usually enhance following IV contrast medium, although enhancement of the cyst wall is possible.

Other sellar region tumours

Parasellar meningiomas can arise from the dura mater of the cavernous sinus or the tuberculum, dorsum or diaphragma sellae (Fig. 56.30). Clinical presentation is with cranial nerve palsies or visual symptoms. Parasellar meningiomas are strongly enhancing masses that expand the cavernous sinus and frequently encase and narrow of the cavernous portion of the internal carotid arteries. Suprasellar meningiomas often show a forward extension along the dura mater of the anterior cranial fossa and are associated with dilatation ('blistering') of the sphenoid sinus. Intracranial extension of optic nerve sheath meningiomas characteristically involves the planum shenoidale.

Optic nerve gliomas are astrocytic tumours, which occur in childhood and may involve the optic nerves, optic chiasm and optic tracts (Fig. 56.31). These tumours can be associated with NF 1 but chiasmic tumours are more frequently seen in patients who do not have NF 1[59].

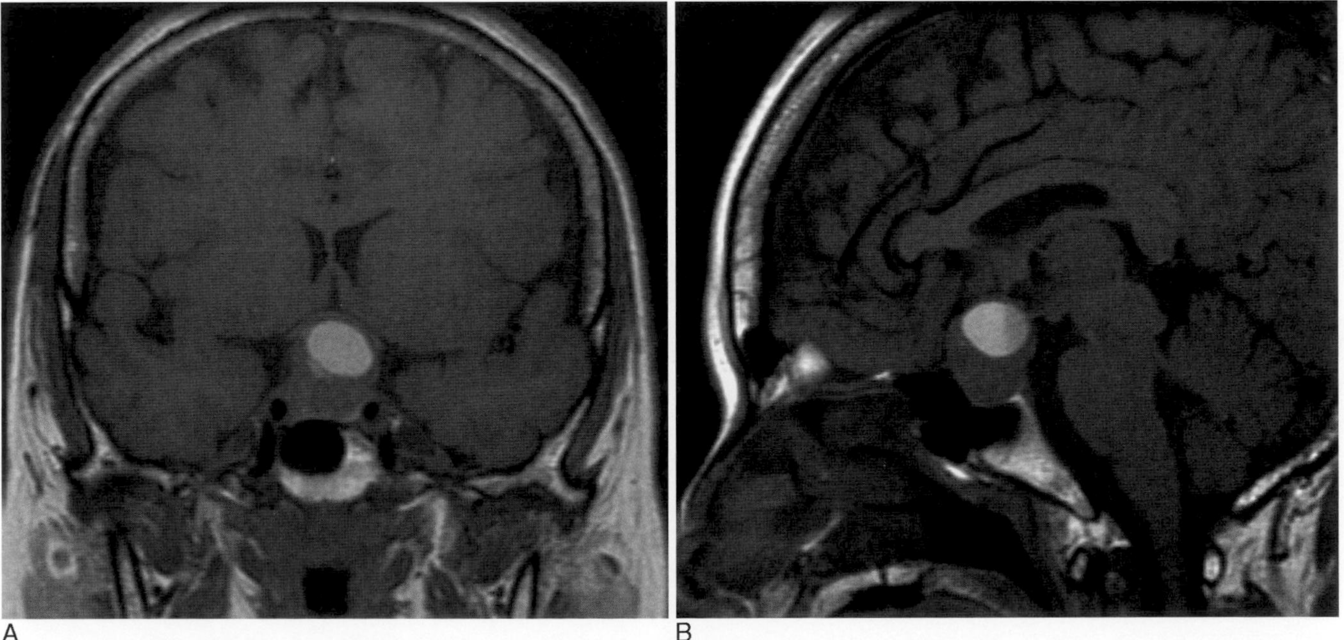

Figure 56.28 Pituitary apoplexy due to haemorrhage into a pituitary macroadenoma. Coronal (A) and sagittal (B) T1W images demonstrate a hyperintense area at the superior aspect of the tumour that contains a fluid level and it is consistent with a recent intratumoural haemorrhage. The optic chiasm is stretched across the apex of the mass.

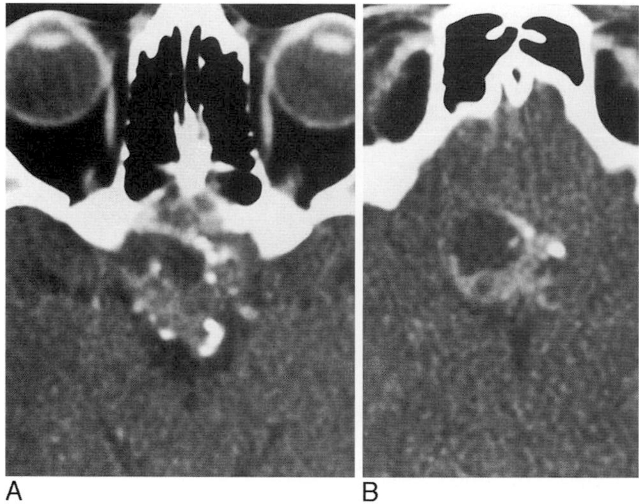

Figure 56.29 Craniopharyngioma. CT following IV contrast medium. There is a partly calcified, partly cystic lesion in the suprasellar region. There is inhomogenous enhancement of the solid tumour components.

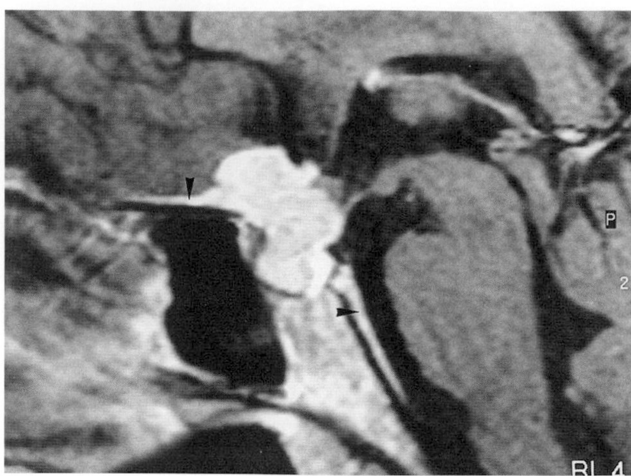

Figure 56.30 Suprasellar meningioma. Sagittal T1W post-gadolinium MRI. A lobulated, enhancing suprasellar mass arises from the region of the tuberculum sellae and extends down into the pituitary fossa displacing the pituitary stalk posteriorly. Enhancing dural 'tails' (arrowheads) can be seen extending over the planum sphenoidale and clivus.

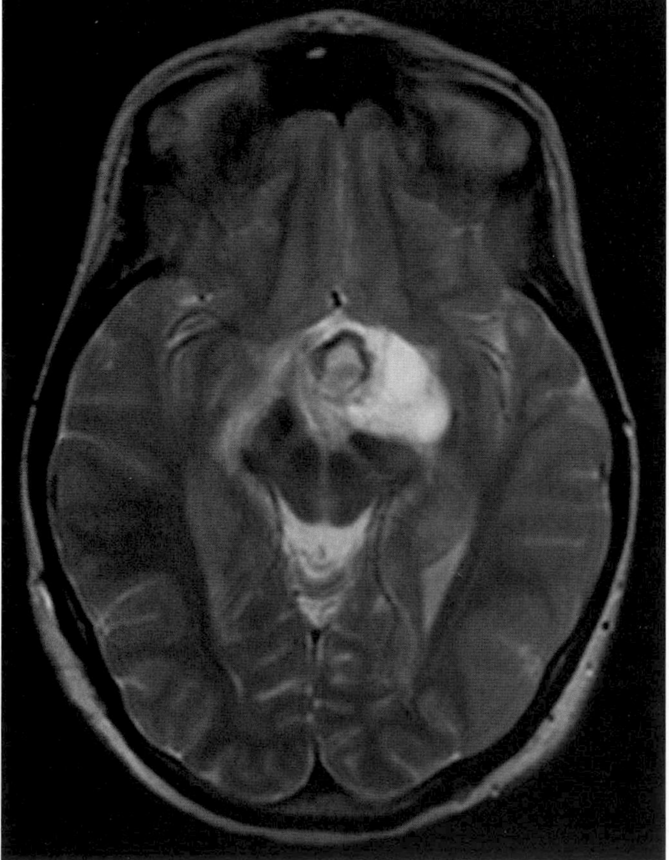

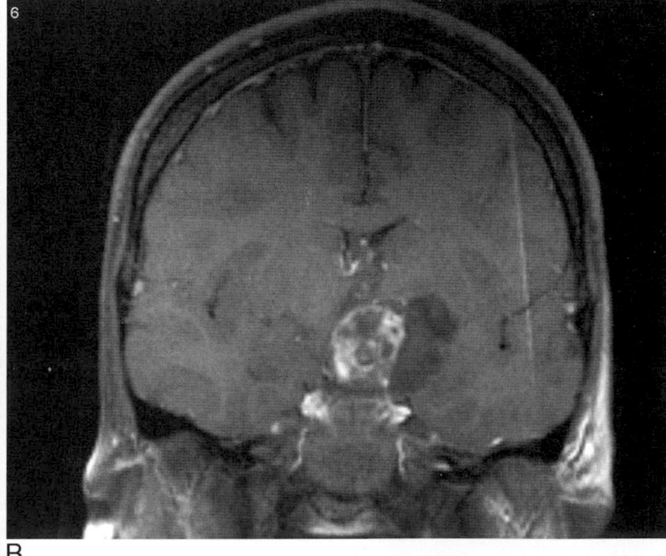

Figure 56.31 Intra-cranial optic nerve glioma in a patient without NF1. T2W (A) and T1W post-contrast images (B) show an inhomogeneous enhancing mass occupying the chiasmatic cistern, which is inseparable from the optic chiasm. The mass invaginates the left temporal lobe medially and the T2W image (A) shows extension of abnormal signal into the right optic tract.

Metastases, particularly from breast carcinoma, can cause thickening of the pituitary stalk and can present with diabetes insipidus. Similar appearances may be seen in histiocytosis and sarcoidosis.

REFERENCES

1. Hoeffner E G, Case I, Jain R et al 2004 Cerebral perfusion CT: technique and clinical applications. Radiology 231:632–644
2. Bynevelt M, Britton J, Seymour H, MacSweeney E, Thomas N, Sandhu K 2001 FLAIR imaging in the follow-up of low-grade gliomas: time to dispense with the dual-echo? Neuroradiology 43:129–133
3. Yuh W, Maley J 1999 Contrast dosage in the neuroimaging of brain tumors. Principles and indications. MRI Clin N Am 6:113–124
4. Essig M 2006 MR imaging of CNS tumors: are all contrast agents created the same? Neuroradiology 48(Suppl 1):3–8
5. Cha S 2004 Perfusion MR imaging of brain tumors. Top Magn Reson Imaging 15:279–289
6. Cha S 2006 Update on brain tumor imaging: from anatomy to physiology. AJNR Am J Neuroradiol 27:475–487
7. Law M 2004 MR spectroscopy of brain tumors. Top Magn Reson Imaging 15:291–313
8. Provenzale J M, Mukundan S, Barboriak D P 2006 Diffusion-weighted and perfusion MR imaging for brain tumor characterization and assessment of treatment response. Radiology 239:632–649
9. Folkman J 1997 Angiogenesis and angiogenesis inhibition: an overview. Department of Surgery, Children's Hospital, Boston. E X S 79:1–8
10. Sugahara T, Koroghi Y, Kochi M et al 1998 Correlation of MR imaging-determined cerebral blood maps with histologic and angiographic determination of vascularity of gliomas. AJR Am J Roentgenol 171:1479–1486
11. Maia A C Jr, Malheiros S M, da Rocha A J et al 2005 MR cerebral blood volume maps correlated with vascular endothelial growth factor expression and tumor grade in nonenhancing gliomas. AJNR Am J Neuroradiol 26:777–783
12. Sugahara T, Korogi Y, Kochi M, Ushio Y, Takahashi M 2001 Perfusion-sensitive MR imaging of gliomas: comparison between gradient-echo and spin-echo echo-planar imaging techniques. AJNR Am J Neuroradiol 22:1306–1315
13. Cha S, Yang L, Johnson G et al 2006 Comparison of microvascular permeability measurements, K(trans), determined with conventional steady-state T1-weighted and first-pass T2*-weighted MR imaging methods in gliomas and meningiomas. AJNR Am J Neuroradiol 27:409–417
14. Sugahara T, Korogi Y, Kochi M et al 1999 Usefulness of diffusion-weighted MRI with echo-planar technique in the evaluation of cellularity in gliomas. J Magn Reson Imaging 9:53–60
15. Sadeghi N, Camby I, Goldman S et al 2003 Effect of hydrophilic components of the extracellular matrix on quantifiable diffusion-weighted imaging of human gliomas: preliminary results of correlating apparent diffusion coefficient values and hyaluronan expression level. AJR Am J Roentgenol 181:235–241
16. Le Bihan D, Mangin J F, Poupon C et al 2001 Diffusion tensor imaging: concepts and applications. J Magn Reson Imaging 13:534–546
17. Field A S, Alexander A L 2004 Diffusion tensor imaging in cerebral tumor diagnosis and therapy. Top Magn Reson Imaging 15:315–324
18. Vlieger E J, Majoie C B, Leenstra S, Den Heeten G J 2004 Functional magnetic resonance imaging for neurosurgical planning in neurooncology. Eur Radiol 14:1143–1153
19. Kleihues P, Burger P, Scheithaur B 1993 The new WHO classification of brain tumours. Brain Pathol 3:255–268
20. Kleihues P, Louis D N, Scheithauer B W et al 2002 The WHO classification of tumors of the nervous system. J Neuropathol Exp Neurol 61:215–225; discussion 226–229
21. Behin A, Hoang-Xuan K, Carpetier A F, Delattre J Y 2003 Primary brain tumours in adults. Lancet 361:323–331
22. Wilms G, Demaerel P, Sunaert S 2005 Intra-axial brain tumours. Eur Radiol 15:468–484
23. Young R J, Knopp E A 2006 Brain MRI: tumor evaluation. J Magn Reson Imaging 24:709–724
24. Patel M R, Tse V 2004 Diagnosis and staging of brain tumors. Semin Roentgenol 39:347–360
25. Nelson S J, Cha S 2003 Imaging glioblastoma multiforme. Cancer J 9:134–145
26. Ricci P 1999 Imaging of adult brain tumors. Neuroimaging Clin North Am 9:651–669
27. White M L, Zhang Y, Kirby P, Ryken T C 2005 Can tumor contrast enhancement be used as a criterion for differentiating tumor grades of oligodendrogliomas? AJNR Am J Neuroradiol 26:784–790
28. Cha S, Tihan T, Crawford F et al 2005 Differentiation of low-grade oligodendrogliomas from low-grade astrocytomas by using quantitative blood-volume measurements derived from dynamic susceptibility contrast-enhanced MR imaging. AJNR Am J Neuroradiol 26:266–273
29. Jenkinson M D, Smith T S, Joyce K A et al 2006 Cerebral blood volume, genotype and chemosensitivity in oligodendroglial tumours. Neuroradiology 48:703–713
30. Jenkinson M D, du Plessis D G, Smith T S, Joyce K A, Warnke P C, Walker C 2006 Histological growth patterns and genotype in oligodendroglial tumours: correlation with MRI features. Brain 129:1884–1891
31. Tozer D J, Jager H R, Danchaivijitr N et al 2006 Apparent diffusion coefficient histograms may predict low-grade glioma subtype. NMR Biomed 20: 49–57
32. Yang D, Korogi T, Sugahara T et al 2002 Cerebral gliomas: prospective comparison of multivoxel 2D chemical-shift imaging proton MR spectroscopy, echoplanar perfusion and diffusion-weighted MRI. Neuroradiol 44:656–666
33. Law M, Yang S, Wang H et al 2003 Glioma grading: sensitivity, specificity, and predictive values of perfusion MR imaging and proton MR spectroscopic imaging compared with conventional MR imaging. AJNR Am J Neuroradiol 24:1989–1998
34. Law M, Oh S, Babb J S et al 2006 Low-grade gliomas: dynamic susceptibility-weighted contrast-enhanced perfusion MR imaging – prediction of patient clinical response. Radiology 238:658–667
35. Catalaa I, Henry R, Dillon W P et al 2006 Perfusion, diffusion and spectroscopy values in newly diagnosed cerebral gliomas. NMR Biomed 19:463–475
36. Hein P A, Eskey C J, Dunn J F, Hug E B 2004 Diffusion-weighted imaging in the follow-up of treated high-grade gliomas: tumor recurrence versus radiation injury. AJNR Am J Neuroradiol 25:201–209
37. Chiang I C, Kuo Y T, Lu C Y et al 2004 Distinction between high-grade gliomas and solitary metastases using peritumoral 3-T magnetic resonance spectroscopy, diffusion, and perfusion imagings. Neuroradiology 46:619–627
38. Provenzale J M, McGraw P, Mhatre P, Guo A C, Delong D 2004 Peritumoral brain regions in gliomas and meningiomas: investigation with isotropic diffusion-weighted MR imaging and diffusion-tensor MR imaging. Radiology 232:451–460
39. Stadlbauer A, Ganslandt O, Buslei R et al 2006 Gliomas: histopathologic evaluation of changes in directionality and magnitude of water diffusion at diffusion-tensor MR imaging. Radiology 240:803–810
40. Stanescu Cosson R, Varlet P, Beuvon F et al 2001 Dysembryoplastic neuroepithelial tumors: CT, MR findings and imaging follow-up: a study of 53 cases. J Neuroradiol 28:230–240
41. Tien R D, Barkovich A J, Edwards M S 1990 MR imaging of pineal tumors. AJR Am J Roentgenol 155:143–151
42. Sumida M, Uozumi T, Kiya K et al 1995 MRI of intracranial germ cell tumours. Neuroradiology 37:32–37
43. Guo A C, Cummings T J, Dash R C, Provenzale J M 2002 Lymphomas and high-grade astrocytomas: comparison of water diffusibility and histologic characteristics. Radiology 224:177–183
44. Camacho D L, Smith J K, Castillo M 2003 Differentiation of toxoplasmosis and lymphoma in AIDS patients by using apparent diffusion coefficients. AJNR Am J Neuroradiol 24:633–637

45. Young R J, Sills A K, Brem S, Knopp E A 2005 Neuroimaging of metastatic brain disease. Neurosurgery 57:S10–S23; discusssion S11–S14
46. Hayashida Y, Hirai T, Morishita S et al 2006 Diffusion-weighted imaging of metastatic brain tumors: comparison with histologic type and tumor cellularity. AJNR Am J Neuroradiol 27:1419–1425
47. Guzman R, Barth A, Lovblad K O et al 2002 Use of diffusion-weighted magnetic resonance imaging in differentiating purulent brain processes from cystic brain tumors. J Neurosurg 97:1101–1107
48. Zhang D, Wen L, Henning T D et al 2006 Central neurocytoma: clinical, pathological and neuroradiological findings. Clin Radiol 61:348–357
49. Drevelegas A 2005 Extra-axial brain tumors. Eur Radiol 15:453–467
50. Vaz R, Borges N, Cruz C, Azevedo I 1998 Cerebral edema associated with meningiomas: the role of peritumoral brain tissue. J Neuro-oncol 36:285–291
51. Zee C S, Chin T, Segall H D, Destian S, Ahmadi J 1992 Magnetic resonance imaging of meningiomas. Semin Ultrasound CT MR 13:154–169
52. Filippi C G, Edgar M A, Ulug A M, Prowda J C, Heier L A, Zimmerman R D 2001 Appearance of meningiomas on diffusion-weighted images: correlating diffusion constants with histopathologic findings. AJNR Am J Neuroradiol 22:65–72
53. Kremer S, Grand S, Remy C et al 2004 Contribution of dynamic contrast MR imaging to the differentiation between dural metastasis and meningioma. Neuroradiology 46:642–648
54. Chiechi M V, Smirniotopoulos J G, Mena H 1996 Intracranial hemangiopericytomas: MR and CT features. AJNR Am J Neuroradiol 17:1365–1371
55. Simonetta A 1999 Imaging of suprasellar and parasellar tumors. In: Ricci P (ed.) Neuroimaging Clinics of North America. Philadelphia: W B Saunders Company, pp 717–732
56. Bartynski W S, Lin L 1997 Dynamic and conventional spin-echo MR of pituitary microlesions. AJNR Am J Neuroradiol 18:965–972
57. Cottier J, Destrieux C, Brunereau L et al 2000 Cavernous sinus invasion by pituitary adenoma: MR imaging. Radiology 215:463–469
58. Sartoretti-Schefer S, Wichmann W, Aguzzi A, Valavanis A 1997 MR differentiation of adamantinous and squamous-papillary craniopharyngiomas. AJNR Am J Neuroradiol 18:77–87
59. Kornreich L, Blaser S, Schwarz M et al 2001 Optic pathway glioma: correlation of imaging findings with the presence of neurofibromatosis. AJNR Am J Neuroradiol 22:1963–1969

CHAPTER 57

Cerebrovascular Disease and Nontraumatic Intracranial Haemorrhage

Philip M. Rich, H. Rolf Jäger

There have been exciting recent advances in cerebrovascular imaging, particularly for acute ischaemic stroke and noninvasive angiography. This has been driven by the desire to rapidly identify candidates for thrombolysis for whom 'time is brain', and a generally more interventional approach to stroke management, which seems to be associated with better outcomes.

This chapter begins with a discussion of ischaemic stroke, including imaging strategies in the hyperacute stage, when thrombolysis may be appropriate. Subsequent sections cover spontaneous intracranial haemorrhage, aneurysms and vascular malformations. Traumatic intracranial haemorrhage is discussed elsewhere.

CEREBRAL ISCHAEMIA

Stroke is the clinical syndrome of a sudden neurological deficit of vascular origin. Ischaemic and haemorrhagic stroke cannot be distinguished clinically and around 30 per cent of patients presenting with a stroke-like episode have a nonvascular cause[1], hence the importance of diagnostic imaging. After exclusion of subarachnoid haemorrhage (SAH), ischaemia accounts for 85 per cent of strokes and spontaneous intracranial haemorrhage for 15 per cent[2].

Ischaemic stroke may be caused by atherothrombotic arterial occlusion, or embolism from carotid or vertebral artery atheroma or the heart. Cervical arterial dissection, vasculitis, venous thrombosis and substance abuse also cause stroke and rarely in adults stroke-like episodes are due to metabolic disorders such as mitochondrial cytopathies.

A **transient ischaemic attack** (TIA) by definition resolves within 24 h. This includes amaurosis fugax, a transient loss of vision in one eye. The risk of stroke following a TIA is higher than previously thought, maybe up to 8 per cent in the first week and 12 per cent within a month[3], and even more in those awaiting endarterectomy for a symptomatic carotid stenosis[4]. These figures do not allow for mild TIAs that go unrecognized but even so a recent TIA should now prompt urgent investigation for treatable risk factors including cervical arterial stenoses. Implementation of such a policy has major resource implications but this may be offset if strokes are prevented.

The role of stroke imaging has shifted away from merely excluding haemorrhage and nonvascular causes and towards the identification of early ischaemia and the differentiation of viable from irreversibly damaged tissue: the concept of the ischaemic penumbra, which will be discussed later. Advanced magnetic resonance imaging (MRI) techniques have been the cornerstone of this approach, particularly perfusion and diffusion-weighted imaging (DWI) but the advent of multi detector computed tomography (MDCT) provides a reasonable alternative[5].

The rapidly enlarging literature on advanced techniques should not distract us from the importance of properly performed and interpreted basic imaging. Unenhanced brain CT remains the workhorse of stroke imaging in most institutions and its enduring value should not be diminished, particularly because it is readily available and easy to use in critically ill patients. The additional value of some newer techniques has yet to be proven in randomized trials. This may change as more is learnt about how imaging can be used to predict outcome from strokes and treatment. It seems likely this will come via MRI, which has a greater inherent capacity than CT to measure different tissue parameters.

IMAGING OF CEREBRAL ISCHAEMIA

Pathophysiological considerations[6–8]

Angiography and perfusion studies show flow abnormalities immediately after onset. Cerebral autoregulation responds to a fall in cerebral perfusion pressure (CPP) with vasodilatation and recruitment of collateral vessels, thus increasing cerebral blood volume (CBV) and reducing resistance, in order to maintain cerebral blood flow (CBF). After the vessels are fully dilated the autoregulatory system cannot properly respond to any further reduction in CPP and therefore both CBF and CBV start to fall.

Oxygen extraction goes up to compensate, but once this is maximal any further fall in CBF causes cellular dysfunction. A CBF of around 23 ml $100\,g^{-1}$ min^{-1} causes a reversible neurological deficit. Electrical activity ceases below about 18–20 ml $100\,g^{-1}$ min^{-1}. Such tissue remains viable but infarction is likely if perfusion is not restored. At 10–15 ml $100\,g^{-1}$ min^{-1}, failure of energy-dependent membrane pumps leads to a shift of sodium and water into cells causing swelling of neurons and cytotoxic oedema, shown earliest on MR diffusion-weighted imaging (DWI) as restriction of water diffusion, but it can also produce subtle signs on CT. This degree of perfusion compromise results in an infarct much more rapidly.

In time, structural breakdown of the blood–brain barrier occurs due to ischaemic damage to capillary endothelium. Leakage of intravascular fluid and protein into the extracellular space and later net influx of water to the infarcted area cause vasogenic oedema.

Clinical outcome depends on the arterial territory involved and the adequacy of collateral blood supply[9]. Proximal occlusions cause infarcts of an entire arterial territory unless sufficient collateral circulation exists, in which case there may be deep infarcts with sparing of overlying cortex. Emboli or occlusion of terminal branches cause cortical infarcts. Perforator vessel occlusions cause lacunar infarcts (see small vessel disease later).

Most carotid territory infarcts involve the middle cerebral artery. Anterior cerebral artery (ACA) collateral flow is generally excellent and emboli relatively rare. The commonest cause of ACA infarcts is vasospasm following subarachnoid haemorrhage. The basilar artery supplies the posterior cerebral arteries unless the posterior communicating artery is large, in which case emboli from the carotid circulation may enter their territory. Brainstem infarcts are commonly due to occlusion of short perforating vessels. A combination of infratentorial, thalamic and occipital infarcts suggests an occlusion of distal basilar artery, or 'top of the basilar' syndrome[10]. Multiple infarcts in different arterial territories suggest a cardiac rather than a carotid source of emboli, or haemodynamic strokes due to hypotension if the distribution conforms to the arterial border zones.

Imaging

This account is intentionally directed towards very early stroke imaging and thrombolysis, reflecting the many recent publications on this subject. It is acknowledged that the great majority of stroke patients are not managed in this way, and many never have any imaging other than unenhanced brain CT. However the fundamental concepts are applicable to all stroke patients.

Structural imaging

A dense artery is the earliest detectable change on CT. As it is caused by fresh thrombus occluding the vessel it can be seen at the onset of the ictus (Fig. 57.1). Thrombus may rapidly disperse so this sign is not always present. When found in the proximal MCA it correlates with large infarcts, although it has a better prognosis if limited to an MCA branch within the Sylvian fissure[11] (Fig. 57.2). MCA calcification can mimic this sign but is often bilateral. The basilar artery may also appear dense in the case of posterior circulation infarcts particularly the 'top of basilar' syndrome (Fig. 57.3).

Thrombus may cause loss of a normal arterial flow void on MRI. However arterial high signal may be seen in a patent vessel on FLAIR MRI due to altered flow, a useful qualitative sign of reduced perfusion when the parenchyma usually still

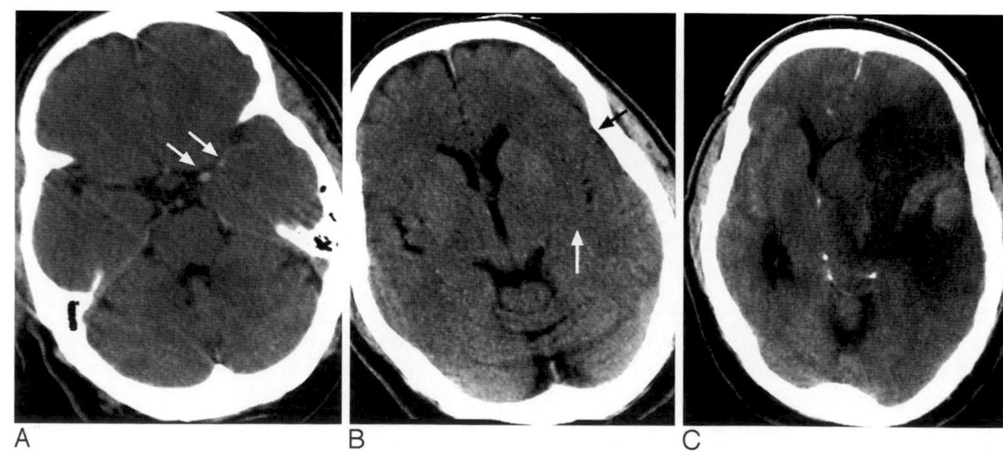

Figure 57.1 Large MCA territory infarct on CT. (A) Acute left middle cerebral artery thrombus appears dense (arrows). (B). Grey-white differentiation is lost around the left putamen and insular cortex (white arrow) and there is mild effacement of the Sylvian fissure (black arrow), early signs of an MCA territory infarct. The 'insula ribbon' and lentiform nucleus appear normal on the right. (c) Three days later there is malignant oedema and haemorrhagic transformation (higher density areas).

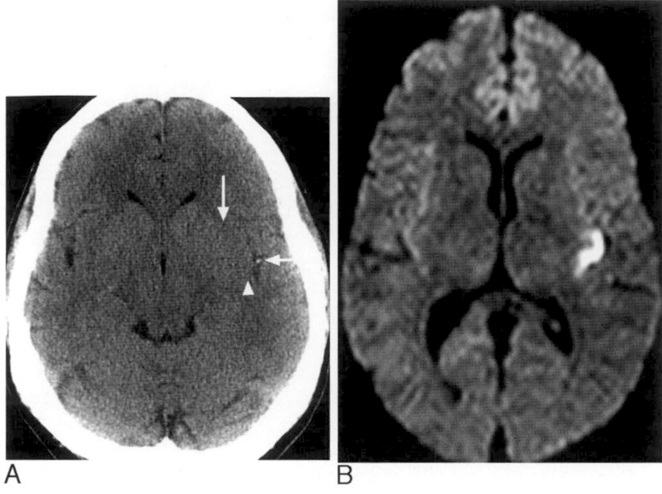

Figure 57.2 Sylvian 'dot' sign. (A) CT shows dense MCA branch due to occlusive acute thrombus (short arrow). There is very subtle loss of grey-white differentiation between the insular cortex and lateral border of putamen posteriorly (arrowhead), whereas more anteriorly it is preserved (long arrow). (B) DWI confirms a small acute cortical infarct adjacent to the thrombosed vessel.

appears normal[12](Fig. 57.4A). Intravascular enhancement due to sluggish flow in affected vessels may be seen on contrast-enhanced CT and MRI in the first few days after an infarct, becoming less obvious towards the end of the first week[13] (Fig. 57.4B).

The early parenchymal signs on CT are reduced grey matter density and brain swelling, manifest as effacement of sulci. These changes are traditionally thought to reflect cytotoxic oedema, which reduces the Hounsfield number of grey matter so it is indistinguishable from adjacent white matter. In early MCA infarcts this causes a reduction in clarity of the margins of the lentiform nucleus and cortex, particularly in the insula (Figs 57.1, 57.2).

The equivalent MRI signs are cortical swelling and T1/T2 prolongation, more obvious on T2-weighted sequences, particularly FLAIR. T2 hyperintensity is often absent or very subtle in infarcts only a few hours old[14], suggesting that early parenchymal low density on CT may be due to abnormal perfusion (reduced CBV) rather than oedema[5]. Furthermore brain swelling on CT without accompanying low density does not always progress to infarction. Such cases may also be due to abnormal perfusion, but a compensatory increase in CBV rather than a reduction[15]. Thus whilst it is generally accepted that swelling with obvious low density on CT is an indication of infarction, perhaps subtle low density or swelling without low density are sometimes signs of compromised perfusion that may be reversible, particularly the latter (see earlier).

Hypodensity on early CT examinations affecting more than 50 per cent of the MCA territory is associated with a high mortality rate[16]. Greater than one-third involvement is commonly a contraindication to thrombolysis (although the increased mortality in this group does not reach statistical significance[17]). The subtle early CT signs of ischaemia are easily overlooked and it can be difficult to accurately estimate percentage involvement of a vascular territory, particularly for less experienced observers. The sensitivity of CT for infarcts has been reported to be only 30 per cent at 3 h[18] and 60 per cent at 24 h. A post hoc expert review of CT studies in the European Cooperative Acute Stroke Study (ECASS) showed that the initial 'on site' interpretation had overlooked an early infarct in 11 per cent of the patients[19].

These difficulties led to the development of the Alberta Stroke Program Early CT Score (ASPECTS)[20]. In this simple rating scale the affected middle cerebral artery territory is divided into ten segments, namely: internal capsule, caudate nucleus, lentiform nucleus, insula and six segments for cortical areas (Fig. 57.5). One point is lost for each area that shows early ischaemic changes of swelling or reduced attenuation, a lower total score carrying a worse prognosis. ASPECTS

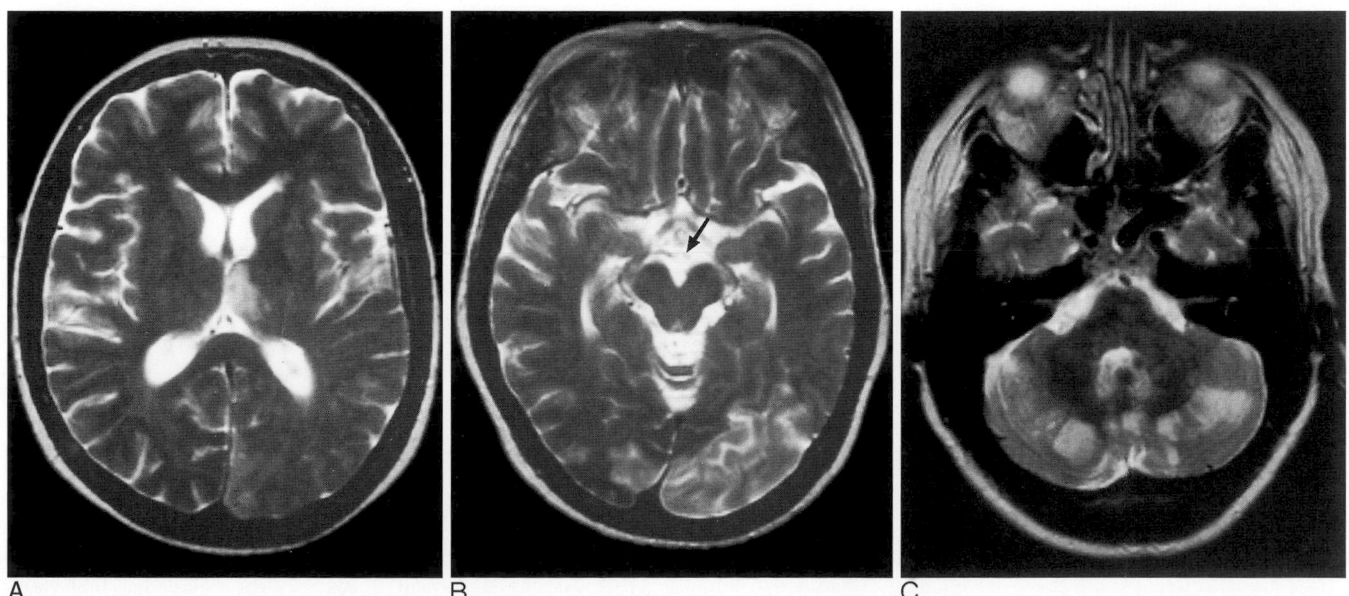

Figure 57.3 'Top of the basilar' syndrome. T2-weighted MRI shows multiple infarcts in the basilar and posterior cerebral artery territories including the left thalamus (A), both occipital lobes (B), and cerebellar hemispheres (C). Note the absence of flow void in the distal basilar artery in B (arrow).

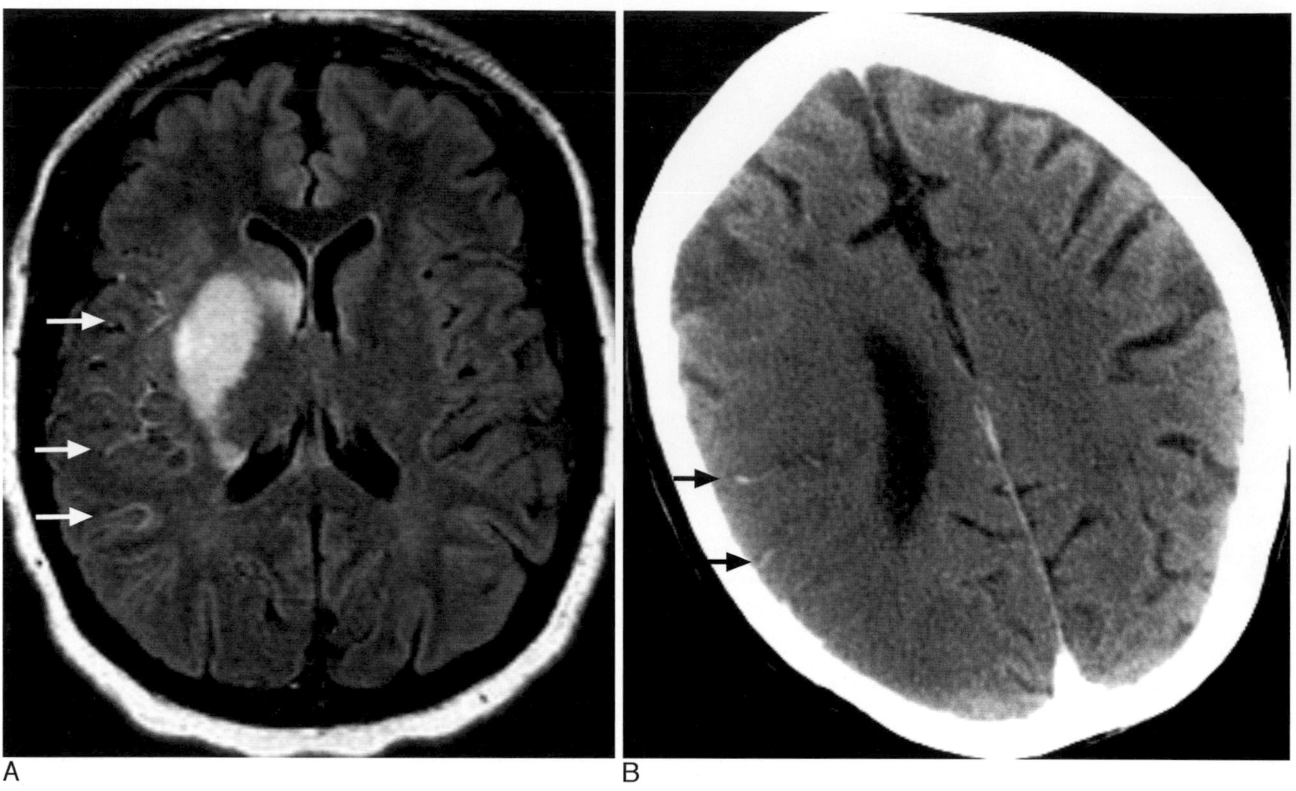

Figure 57.4 Vascular signs in acute infarcts. (A) FLAIR axial image of an acute right striatocapsular infarct. Note asymmetrical high signal returned from patent right MCA cortical branches due to compromised flow (arrows). (B) Contrast-enhanced CT shows early infarct changes of mild low density and local swelling in posterior part of right MCA territory. There is asymmetrical enhancement of MCA cortical branches because of sluggish flow (arrows).

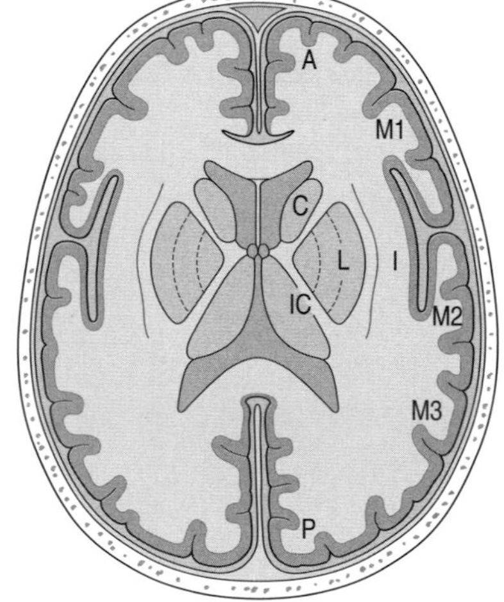

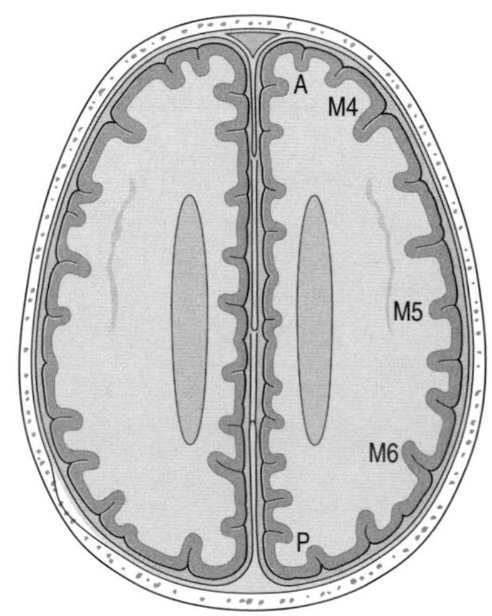

Figure 57.5 ASPECTS for early ischaemic change on CT (from Barber P A, Demchuk A M, Zhang J et al 2000 Validity and reliability of a quantitative computed tomography score in predicting outcome of hyperacute stroke before thrombolytic therapy. Lancet 355:1670–1674 with permission from Elsevier). A = anterior circulation; P = posterior circulation; C = caudate; L = lentiform; IC = internal capsule; I = insular ribbon; M1 = anterior middle cerebral artery (MCA) cortex; M2 = MCA cortex lateral to insular ribbon; M3 = posterior MCA cortex; M4, M5 and M6 are anterior, lateral and posterior MCA territories immediately superior to M1, M2 and M3, rostral to basal ganglia. Subcortical structures are alotted 3 points (C, L and IC), MCA cortex is alotted 7 points (insular cortex, M1, M2, M3, M4, M5 and M6). A point is lost for each area that shows early ischaemic change (low density or swelling). The range of scores is 0–10, representing an infarct of the entire territory and normal findings, respectively.

can be used to predict outcome and risk of post-thrombolysis haemorrhage[20]. It correlates well with DWI findings at presentation[21] and facilitates more accurate interpretation of emergency CT by nonexperts[22]. Even in patients not suitable for thrombolysis it seems intuitive that a methodical approach such as ASPECTS is likely to increase accuracy of CT interpretation, at least for supratentorial events. Brainstem infarcts are notoriously difficult to detect by CT at any stage after onset, even using the most modern CT equipment.

In the **subacute phase** there is structural breakdown and blood–brain barrier disruption. Fluid leaks into the extracellular space causing low attenuation on CT and T2 hyperintensity on MRI that involves both grey and white matter in large infarcts. The severity and duration of brain swelling depends on infarct size. It usually increases during the first week, persists during the second week and then regresses. Other diagnoses such as tumour or infection should be considered if there is extensive white matter oedema without cortical involvement or prolonged brain swelling.

Contrast enhancement on CT and MR due to blood–brain barrier disruption is common in the subacute stage; indeed on MRI it occurs in almost all cases by the end of the first week[13] and persists for several months. The pattern is variable and therefore not always specific, however gyriform enhancement, if present, is most characteristic of a cortical infarct. Lack of enhancement of large cortical lesions on MRI suggests alternative diagnoses such as low-grade glioma.

CT has a much higher sensitivity than spin-echo MRI for the detection of acute haemorrhage, the main differential diagnosis of ischaemic stroke. However the T2*-weighted gradient echo sequence has equivalent sensitivity or better than CT. Gradient echo imaging also detects the haemosiderin that can persist for years following a haemorrhage[23–25]. Establishing the diagnosis of an old haemorrhage is not possible with CT, since blood clots become hypodense within a few weeks and old haemorrhagic cavities can resemble infarcts.

Haemorrhagic transformation due to secondary bleeding into reperfused ischaemic tissue occurs during the first 2 weeks. It is shown in up to 80 per cent of infarcts on MRI[26], appearing hyperintense on T1-weighted and hypointense on T2-weighted images. It is often seen in the basal ganglia and cortex, where it can assume a gyriform pattern (Fig. 57.6 and see Fig. 57.1C). The occurrence and severity of haemorrhagic transformation correlates with the size of the infarct and degree of contrast enhancement in the early stage[26].

The final stage of an infarct is encephalomalacia and atrophy, causing enlargement of adjacent sulci and ventricles. The density on CT and signal intensity on MRI approaches that of CSF. Wallerian degeneration is sometimes visible as faint T2 hyperintensity in the ipsilateral corticospinal tract and asymmetrical brainstem atrophy.

Proton magnetic resonance spectroscopy (MRS) of cerebral infarcts shows the appearance of lactate, while N-acetylaspartate (NAA), a neuronal marker, and total creatine are reduced compared to the contralateral hemisphere (Fig. 57.7). Longitudinal studies have shown progressive reduction of NAA suggesting that ischaemic injury continues for more than a week following infarction[27]. However since the advent of DWI, MRS is not required to diagnose an acute infarct. Furthermore it requires the subject to keep still for several minutes, which is not always possible in acute stroke patients who may be confused and restless.

Vascular imaging

Catheter angiography has been the traditional way of investigating intracranial vessel occlusions and collateral pathways and is still used for intra-arterial thrombolysis. Noninvasive angiography by US, CTA or MRA is preferable for other patients. CTA can be performed as part of the same examination as perfusion imaging with separate IV infusions of contrast medium. No delay is necessary between the two acquisitions. A three-dimensional (3D) time-of-flight technique is preferred for MR angiography.

Advanced techniques—perfusion and diffusion imaging

Currently perfusion imaging for acute stroke patients is most conveniently achieved using dynamic bolus tracking techniques, either perfusion CT (CTP) or perfusion-weighted MRI (PW-MRI)[28,29]. Unlike other techniques the perfusion data is acquired in under a minute on the same machine (CT or MR) used to acquire diagnostic brain images. Other modalities used for perfusion imaging clinically or in research include xenon CT, arterial spin labelling MRI, transcranial Doppler US, single-photon emission CT (SPECT) and positron emission tomography (PET). Their various strengths and weaknesses are explored in a recent review[28].

PW-MRI produces maps of time-to-peak contrast (TTP), mean transit time (MTT), CBV and CBF (CBF=CBV/MTT). TTP provides a qualitative overview of brain perfusion. A threshold of 4 s delay seems to indicate tissue at risk and correlates with a CBF of under 20 ml $100\,g^{-1}$ min^{-1}[30]. However proximal vessel stenosis can delay TTP even if CBF via collaterals is normal and tissue viability not threatened. As outlined earlier, within an area of prolonged MTT (or TTP), moderate ischaemia may cause increased CBV, however reduced CBV indicates inadequate collateral supply and high risk of infarction. On perfusion imaging a CBV deficit seems to be the best predictor of initial infarct size (and final size if successfully reperfused). The MTT and CBF indicate tissue at risk[5], in other words the final infarct volume unless reperfusion occurs,

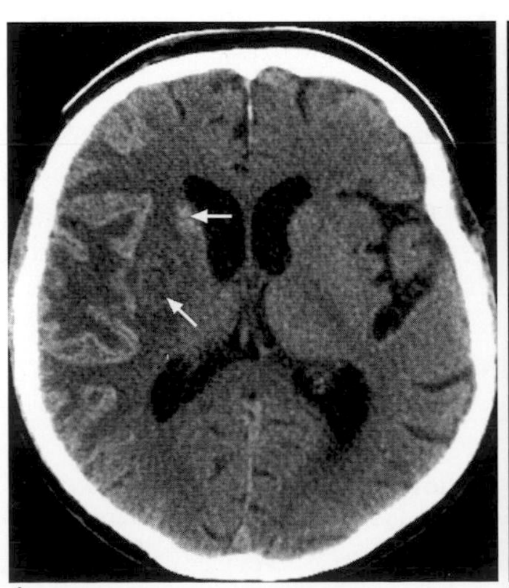
A

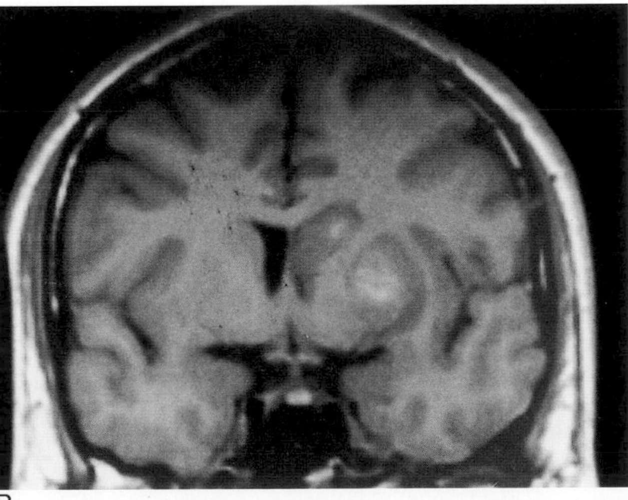
B

Figure 57.6 Haemorrhagic transformation. (A) Unenhanced brain CT 2 weeks after a large right MCA territory infarct shows a gyriform pattern of haemorrhagic transformation in right cerebral cortex. There is also haemorrhage in the basal ganglia (arrows). (B) Coronal T1-weighted image shows swelling and signal alteration of the caudate and lentiform nuclei. Sparing of the cortex is due to adequate leptomeningeal collateral circulation. The central T1-hyperintense area within the infarct indicates haemorrhagic transformation.

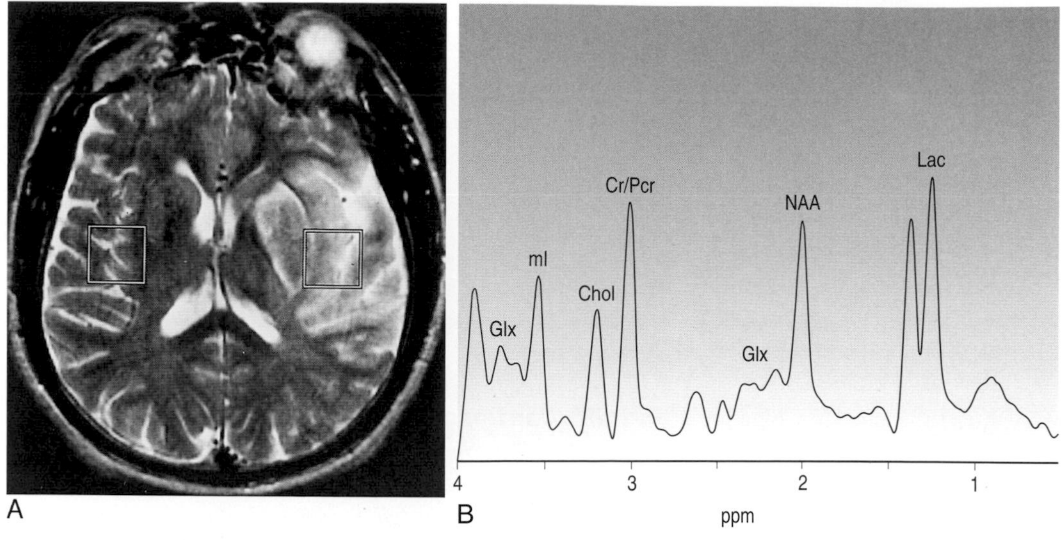

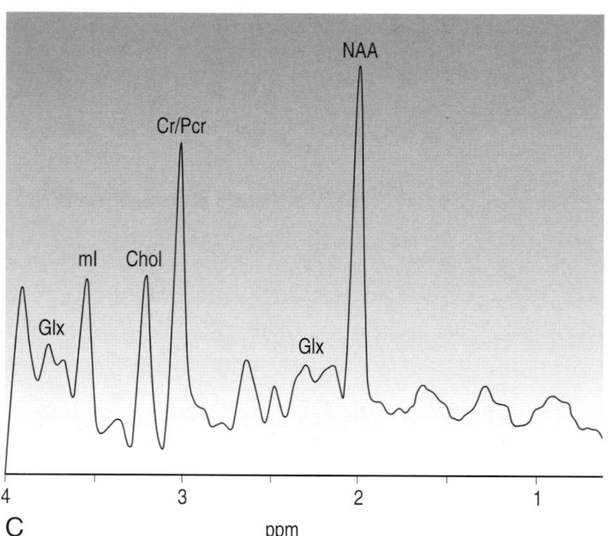

Figure 57.7 MR spectroscopy in acute stroke. (A) Axial T2-fast spin-echo image (TR/TE = 3500/95) of a 55-year-old male stroke patient at 14 h from stroke onset, to show the positions of voxels within the infarct and contralateral hemisphere. (B) Proton spectrum (TR 2000/TE 30 ms) acquired at time of presentation on a 1.5 T MR system. The total creatine (3.03 p.p.m.) and choline (3.22 p.p.m.) are reduced, the NAA peak (2.01 p.p.m.) is almost absent and there is a large lactate doublet at 1.33 p.p.m. compared to the contralateral hemisphere. (C) Normal spectrum acquired from the contralateral hemisphere. Resonance peaks are lactate (Lac), N-acetyl aspartate (NAA), creatine (Cr/Pcr), myoinositol (ml), and glutamate and glutamine (Glx).

either naturally or following medical intervention. CBV in the infarcted region increases in the subacute stage[31], often associated with vessel recanalization, followed by a decrease later (Fig. 57.8).

Absolute CBF levels may allow more accurate prognostication and treatment targeting, however quantitative data is not readily obtained from PW-MRI. This does not seem to be a major problem in acute stroke, MRI usually adequately defining hypoperfused brain relative to a normal contralateral hemisphere. However it may have implications if there are bilateral or multifocal deficits, for example in bilateral severe carotid stenoses or vasospasm following subarachnoid haemorrhage. Calculated arterial input functions may make MR data more quantitative in due course. Quantitative perfusion data can be obtained from CTP or arterial spin-labelled MRI techniques, although at the moment the latter takes longer to acquire than contrast-enhanced perfusion MRI.

The whole brain is covered on PW-MRI whereas CTP only allows partial coverage, although this will increase with more modern MDCT systems. However this technical limitation does not seem to significantly affect the practical application of CTP in most cases.

Perfusion imaging, including PET, is also used for elective assessment of haemodynamic reserve and stroke risk (Fig. 57.9). For example perfusion may be normal at rest despite a significant carotid stenosis but show reduced blood flow following acetazolamide challenge, which is the reverse of normal[32,33]. SPECT with ^{99m}Tc HMPAO or ECD will show a perfusion defect as soon as vascular occlusion occurs, although care must be taken in interpretation of HMPAO SPECT studies 10 days or more after the onset of stroke due to hyperfixation of the radiopharmaceutical in infarcted tissue[34]. Quantitation of the degree of ischaemia using HMPAO SPECT will predict risk of intracranial haemorrhage following intra-arterial thrombolysis[35].

DWI has a pre-eminent role in acute stroke imaging due to its high sensitivity in the first few hours after infarction, when T2-weighted images are usually normal. DWI should be interpreted in conjunction with an apparent diffusion coefficient (ADC) map, which is derived from the DWI data and in the clinical environment is displayed as a grey scale 'image' for ease of use (Fig. 57.10). Restricted diffusion in acute infarcts (low ADC) returns high signal on DWI and appears dark on the ADC map. After 5–14 d, loss of structural integrity results in

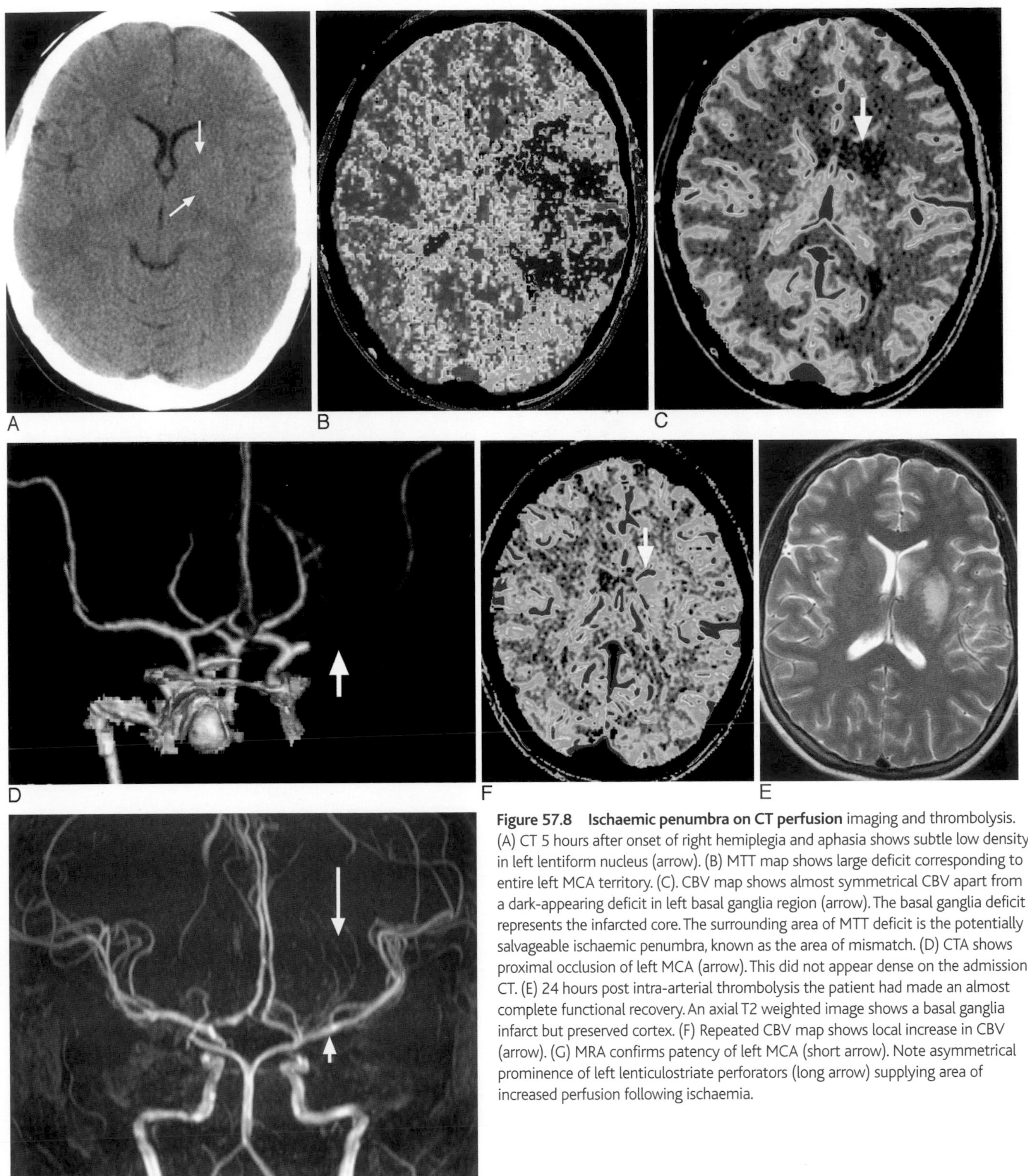

Figure 57.8 Ischaemic penumbra on CT perfusion imaging and thrombolysis. (A) CT 5 hours after onset of right hemiplegia and aphasia shows subtle low density in left lentiform nucleus (arrow). (B) MTT map shows large deficit corresponding to entire left MCA territory. (C). CBV map shows almost symmetrical CBV apart from a dark-appearing deficit in left basal ganglia region (arrow). The basal ganglia deficit represents the infarcted core. The surrounding area of MTT deficit is the potentially salvageable ischaemic penumbra, known as the area of mismatch. (D) CTA shows proximal occlusion of left MCA (arrow). This did not appear dense on the admission CT. (E) 24 hours post intra-arterial thrombolysis the patient had made an almost complete functional recovery. An axial T2 weighted image shows a basal ganglia infarct but preserved cortex. (F) Repeated CBV map shows local increase in CBV (arrow). (G) MRA confirms patency of left MCA (short arrow). Note asymmetrical prominence of left lenticulostriate perforators (long arrow) supplying area of increased perfusion following ischaemia.

increased water mobility and the imaging appearance reverses to low signal on DWI and bright on the ADC map[36,37]. Between the two states is a transition period of DWI 'pseudo-normalization', during which small infarcts can be masked. Larger lesions will still be obvious on structural images. Prolonged restriction of diffusion in small white matter infarcts lasting several weeks has been reported, the explanation for which is not entirely clear[38].

Chronic lesions with very long T2 relaxation times may appear high signal on DWI due to 'T2 shine through', but in comparison to acute infarcts they will also appear bright on the ADC map. Another potential pitfall of DWI is acute haemorrhage,

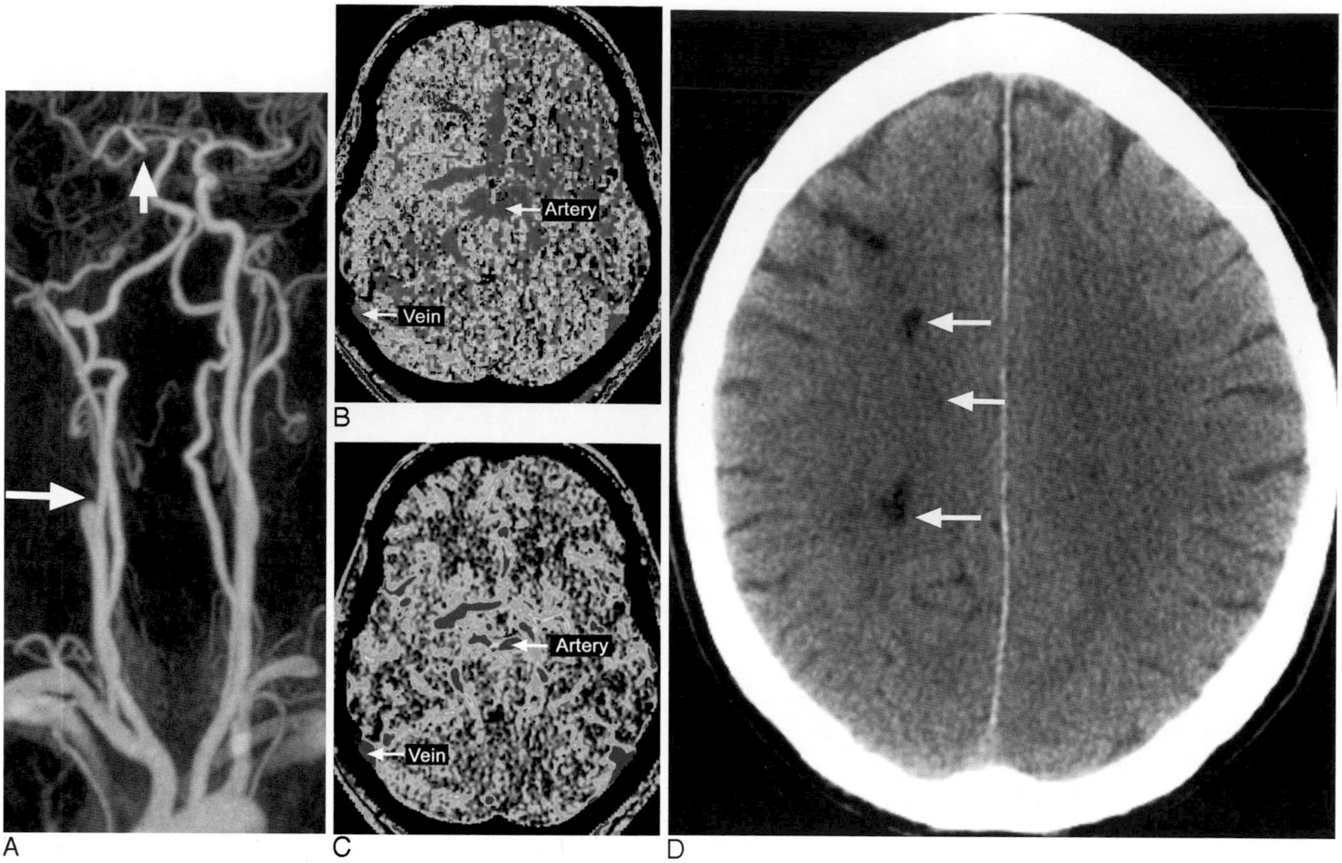

Figure 57.9 Autoregulatory response to chronic ischaemia on CT perfusion imaging. (A) CEMRA shows right internal carotid artery (ICA) occluded from its origin (long arrow). There is intracranial reconstitution via the circle of Willis (short arrow). Note the entire arterial tree from the aortic arch to the circle of Willis is shown on a single examination. (B) MTT is prolonged throughout right ICA territory. (C) CBV appears symmetrical. Measured regions of interest showed slight relative increase in the right frontal lobe due to opening of collateral pathways and vasodilatation responding to a reduction in perfusion pressure. (D) CT shows small mature watershed infarcts (arrows) but the majority of the right ICA territory is preserved.

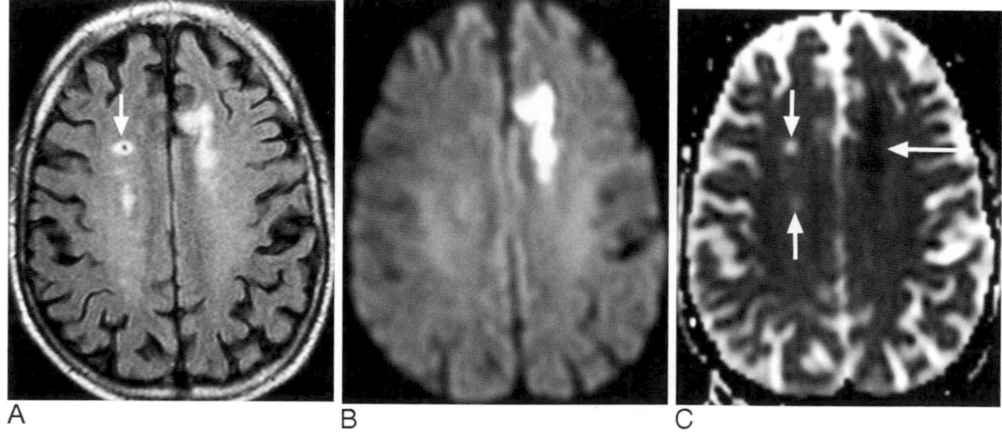

Figure 57.10 New and old infarcts on DWI. (A) FLAIR shows high signal ischaemic change of indeterminate age in both frontal lobes. There is a small mature lacunar infarct on the right with a low signal central cavity (arrow). (B) DWI shows an acute high signal lesion on the left. (C) The ADC map confirms the left-sided lesion is acute (dark indicates low ADC; long arrow). The infarcts on the right are bright, indicating increased ADC and therefore older lesions (short arrows).

which can return high signal resembling an infarct. However there is often also a low signal margin produced by susceptibility effects[39]. Analysis of other sequences should indicate the correct diagnosis.

The CBV deficit on perfusion CT and extent of low density on CT angiogram source images (CTA-SI) both correlate sufficiently well with DWI lesion size to make them practical CT surrogates for DWI[40] (Fig. 57.8). The explanation for low density on CTA-SI may lie in a reduced CBV rather than cytotoxic oedema (see earlier)[17].

Imaging strategies in acute stroke

Only neuroimaging can accurately identify patients with haemorrhage or a nonvascular diagnosis. Exclusion of haemorrhage allows aspirin to be prescribed, which is beneficial if commenced within 48 h[41]. In principle it seems preferable that either CT or MR (usually CT) is performed at the time of admission or as soon as possible afterwards so the correct diagnosis is established. Economic as well as medical arguments have been advanced to justify this approach[42,43] and it is accepted practice in many countries, although implementing such a policy where it is not already in place has significant implications for local resources and work patterns. Patients on anticoagulation should have urgent imaging so it can be reversed if they have had a haemorrhagic stroke. Other reasons for urgent neuroimaging include: a history of immunosuppression or malignancy as such patients may have a cerebral infection or tumour; depressed conscious level; and a suspected posterior cranial fossa haematoma that may require surgical evacuation.

CT is usually the first-line investigation, being more widely available outside routine working hours and generally regarded as a 'simpler' technique, although in fact early infarcts are much easier to detect on DWI, particularly for the inexperienced observer. Other advantages of DWI over CT include the demonstration of a new infarct on a background of chronic ischaemic damage (Figs 57.10, 57.11) and importantly the correct diagnosis of a transient ischaemic attack, which indicates a high short-term risk of stroke. Abnormalities may be shown on DWI following a TIA, particularly if there is a motor deficit, aphasia or an event lasting more than 1 h, although lesions may be transient[44]. The presence of a lesion confirms a cerebrovascular substrate and the location indicates the vascular territory involved.

In general MRI more clearly shows the extent of ischaemic change, the anatomical distribution and to some degree allows a better estimation of type of stroke and age of different lesions (large or small vessel, embolic, hypoperfusion).

Cervical and sometimes intracranial angiography is often important after stroke and in most circumstances conventional catheter angiography has been replaced by noninvasive

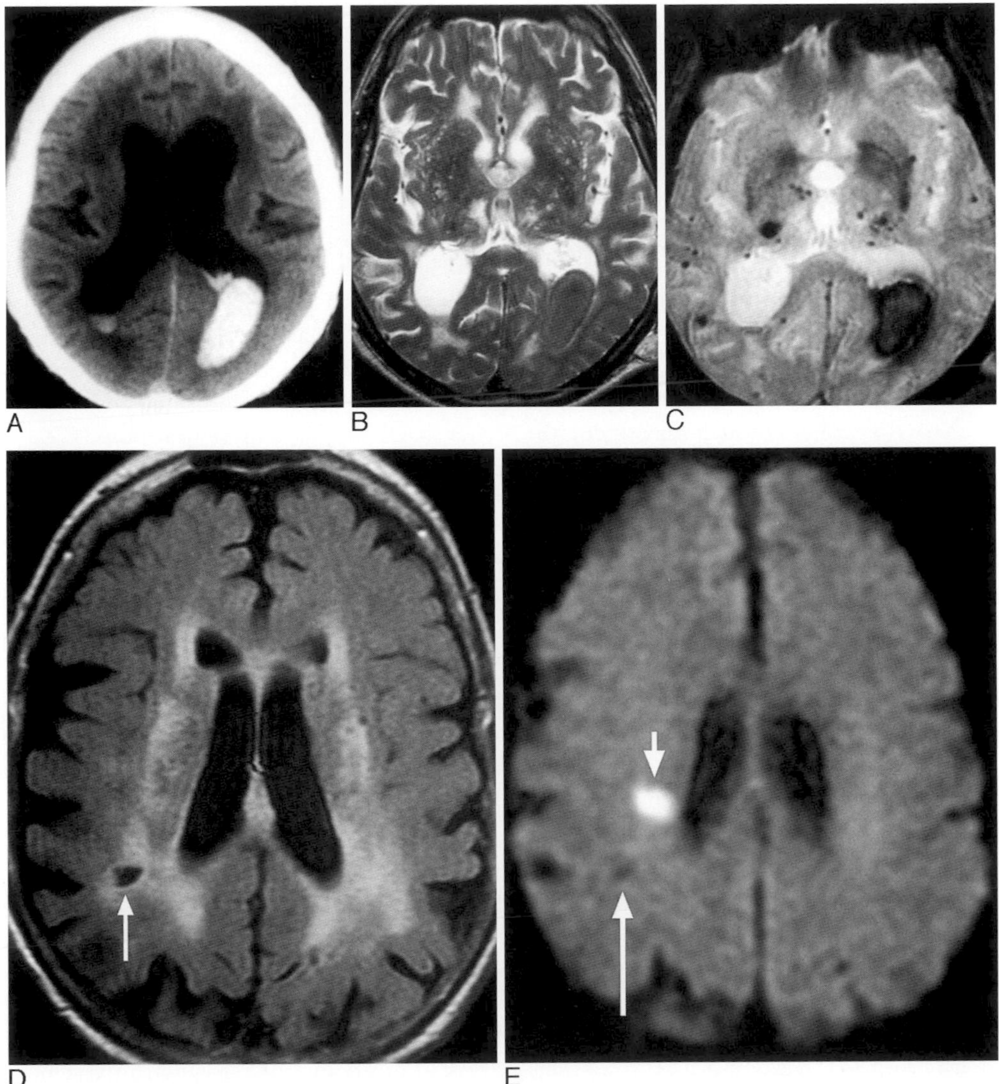

Figure 57.11 Small-vessel disease. (A) On CT there is diffuse cerebral white matter low density (leukoaraiosis) indicating small vessel disease. There is an acute haematoma in the left lateral ventricle with a small blood level in the dependent part of the right occipital horn. (B) The acute intraventricular blood returns low signal on an axial T2-weighted image. There are high signal foci due to small infarcts and widened perivascular spaces in the thalami and basal ganglia. (C) Axial gradient echo image shows the acute intraventricular blood as low signal. There are also numerous low signal foci in the deep nuclei and cerebral hemispheres. These are old areas of haemosiderin staining known as microbleeds. Note they are not visible on CT. (D). Axial FLAIR of a different patient shows diffuse high signal indicating small vessel ischaemic change in deep and periventricular cerebral white matter. There is a mature lacunar infarct in the right parietal lobe (arrow). (E). Axial DWI shows an acute infarct as high signal (short arrow) and the mature lacune as low signal (long arrow). Only DWI can differentiate the acute infarct from the surrounding signal abnormality.

methods. Doppler ultrasonography is simple to perform at the bedside, although it is operator dependent and does not clearly show arterial segments that are anatomically inaccessible or heavily calcified. CTA or MRA allows a full survey including the aortic arch and cervical vessels, circle of Willis and major intracranial arteries. CTA is quicker to perform than MRA but requires more time at the workstation to properly interpret. These techniques will be discussed further later.

The concept of the ischaemic penumbra is central to under-standing current thinking on the interrelationship between early stroke pathophysiology, treatment and imaging (Fig. 57.8). In the hyperacute stage there may be a discrepancy in the size of lesions shown separately on DWI and perfusion imaging. In this model the ischaemic zone consists of two areas: the core of restricted diffusion (or CT CBV deficit) already infarcted surrounded by an underperfused penumbra representing salvageable ischaemic tissue liable to infarct without early spontaneous or therapeutic recanalization. If the penumbra is larger than the core the difference between the two is the area of mismatch. A matched defect (i.e. the two areas coincide) is assumed to indicate a completed infarct without areas of reversibility.

This view has been complicated by a realization that restricted diffusion may be reversible in the earliest period after onset[36,45,46] and the penumbral perfusion defect may include areas of benign oligaemia as well as tissue at risk[47]. It appears likely that diffusion can already be impaired if the blood flow lies between 10–20 ml $100\,g^{-1}\,min^{-1}$, above the threshold for irreversible ischaemia. Interestingly this implies low density on CT may sometimes be more specific for infarction than DWI signal change assessed visually, although quantifying the ADC increases specificity for infarcts in patients with strokes or TIAs[48].

Relatively few stroke patients are currently offered thrombolysis. Acute stroke imaging protocols are designed to rapidly obtain the necessary anatomical, vascular and functional information, using CT (unenhanced CT brain, perfusion imaging and CTA) or MRI (usually with scout, FLAIR, gradient-echo, DWI, intracranial MRA and perfusion imaging). Treatment options include IV or intra-arterial thrombolysis and mechanical clot disruption.

Management strategies vary but frequently IV thrombolysis is given within 3 h of symptom onset as soon as haemorrhage or an obvious large infarct has been excluded. Because early DWI lesions may reverse, some thrombolysis centres treat patients presenting within 3 h, even if perfusion imaging shows a matched defect. Intra-arterial thrombolysis or mechanical disruption may be attempted if the patient does not rapidly improve and a proximal vessel occlusion is shown angiographically or as a dense artery on CT. Beyond 3 h restricted diffusion is less likely to be reversible so thrombolysis is usually only appropriate if there is mismatch and many centres opt for primary intra-arterial treatment if there is also a proximal vessel occlusion.

There is little randomized evidence to support some of these therapeutic manoeuvres and they are performed at the risk of provoking catastrophic intracranial haemorrhage. The published literature includes arguments for and against the use of CT or MRI and various treatment strategies, although in practice much still depends on local scanner access and available expertise[5,8,17,29,49]. It is noteworthy that the US Food and Drug Administration's approval for the use of recombinant tissue plasminogen activator in acute ischaemic stroke was based on a trial that selected patients with unenhanced CT alone[50]. A recent UK Cochrane Collaboration review acknowledged the net benefit of thrombolysis in acute stroke but in somewhat guarded terms with emphasis on the risk of haemorrhage and suggested that further randomized trials were required[51]. Hopefully further research and experience with advanced imaging will refine patient selection for this important but hazardous treatment.

Other patterns of cerebrovascular disease

Small vessel ischaemic disease (Fig. 57.11)

Cerebral white matter small vessel disease is the norm in older people. More than 95 per cent of those over 65 years of age have white matter lesions on MRI, usually limited in extent[52]. More severe ischaemic damage is associated with cognitive impairment and gait disturbance. Risk factors include age, hypertension and elevated glycated haemoglobin levels[52,53]. The basal ganglia are often also involved.

Arterioles of the long penetrating arteries become occluded, the outcome probably depending on vessel size. Occlusion of a large vessel causes a lacunar infarct; blockage of smaller arterioles results in ischaemic demyelination and gliosis. Although highly variable in extent, it affects predominantly the periventricular and deep cerebral white matter, basal ganglia and ventral pons. CT shows white matter hypodensities ('leukoaraiosis') but MRI, particularly FLAIR, is much more sensitive. There may be cavities indicating lacunar infarcts.

DWI will confirm the site of an acute subcortical infarct even if there is widespread pre-existing ischaemic change. New infarcts develop every few months in small vessel disease and are clinically silent unless they arise in eloquent areas, although they will be shown on fortuitously timed DWI[54]. It is important to realize that these white matter changes are nonspecific and similar appearances may be encountered in vasculitis[55].

Foci of old haemorrhage known as microbleeds occur with small vessel disease. They are common in ischaemic stroke patients, occurring in up to 26 per cent[56], but they are also present in around 6 per cent of asymptomatic older people, associated with age, hypertension and radiological extent of small vessel disease[57]. They are a marker of vascular fragility in hypertensive small vessel disease, their distribution mirroring symptomatic haemorrhages[58,59]. At present it is not clear if they should be a contraindication for anticoagulant or antiplatelet therapy, or whether they increase the risk of post thrombolysis haemorrhage[60,61]. The susceptibility effect of haemosiderin reveals their presence on T2-weighted gradient-echo MRI, spin-echo sequences being much less sensitive. Microbleeds are not visible on CT.

Global cerebral hypoperfusion and anoxia (Fig. 57.12)

Inadequate oxygen supply to the entire brain can be the consequence of severe hypotension or impaired blood oxygenation. Global hypoperfusion can result in watershed infarcts, shown as wedge-shaped lesions in the frontal and/or parietal lobes at the margins of anterior and middle and middle and posterior cerebral artery territories, respectively. DWI can be especially useful, as the early signs on CT or MRI are rendered even subtler by their frequently symmetrical distribution. Anoxia due to defective blood oxygenation such as in carbon monoxide poisoning tends to cause infarcts in sensitive regions, for example the basal ganglia.

Venous infarcts

Causes of cerebral venous thrombosis include trauma, infection (particularly subdural empyema) and hypercoagulability disorders including those due to oral contraceptives. Venous infarcts do not conform to arterial territories and are often haemorrhagic and multifocal. The superior sagittal sinus is most commonly involved, which can lead to bilateral parasagittal infarcts. Isolated occlusion of the transverse sinus or the deep cerebral veins can occur (Fig. 57.13). On unenhanced CT acute thrombosis will cause a venous sinus to appear expanded and hyperdense. IV contrast medium causes more intense enhancement of the walls of the sinuses than of their contents, the so-called 'delta sign' (Fig. 57.14). MRI shows lack of flow void in the affected sinuses but normal slow flowing blood may appear bright, simulating a thrombus and acute thrombus can appear hypointense on spin-echo images mimicking a flow void (Fig. 57.13). Therefore structural MRI is not always reliable for the exclusion of venous occlusion, particularly if chronic, and a phase-contrast MR venogram (MRV) is usually acquired, which depicts only flow and not thrombus. A low-velocity encoding (VENC) is chosen to demonstrate venous flow. CT venography is a satisfactory alternative if MRV is unavailable or equivocal[62]. Using a combination of structural images, MR and CT venography, there is very little need to resort to DSA to confirm the diagnosis of venous thrombosis.

Other pathology

A variety of conditions can mimic infarcts, including tumours, inflammatory conditions, in particular cerebritis or encephalitis and sometimes an early presentation of multifocal leukoencephalopathy. Knowledge of the distribution of vascular territories and attention to clinical details and radiological signs are helpful in distinguishing these conditions from an infarct. In many cases modern imaging and expert neuroradiological review will provide the answer. Follow-up imaging is sometimes useful and variance from the usual pattern of infarct evolution should prompt a review of the diagnosis.

Angiography in ischaemic stroke

Most vascular studies in patients with ischaemic stroke or TIAs are carried out for secondary prevention of strokes and primarily concern the extracranial vessels. Intracranial arterial imaging may be obtained in the acute phase if thrombolysis is an option (see earlier). Intracranial studies may also be appropriate in black and oriental stroke patients, who have a higher incidence of intracranial arterial stenosis than white patients, the reverse being the case for extracranial disease[63].

Imaging of extracranial vessels (Fig. 57.16)

Atheroma can occur at vessel origins (including vertebral arteries), at the carotid bifurcation, and in the distal course of internal carotid or vertebral arteries. The carotid bifurcation is the commonest site.

The North America Symptomatic Carotid Endarterectomy Trial[64] and European Carotid Surgery Trial[65] found patients with symptomatic 70–99 per cent stenosis of the internal carotid artery benefited from surgery. Stenosis measurements in these trials were performed on conventional catheter angiograms, using slightly different methods,

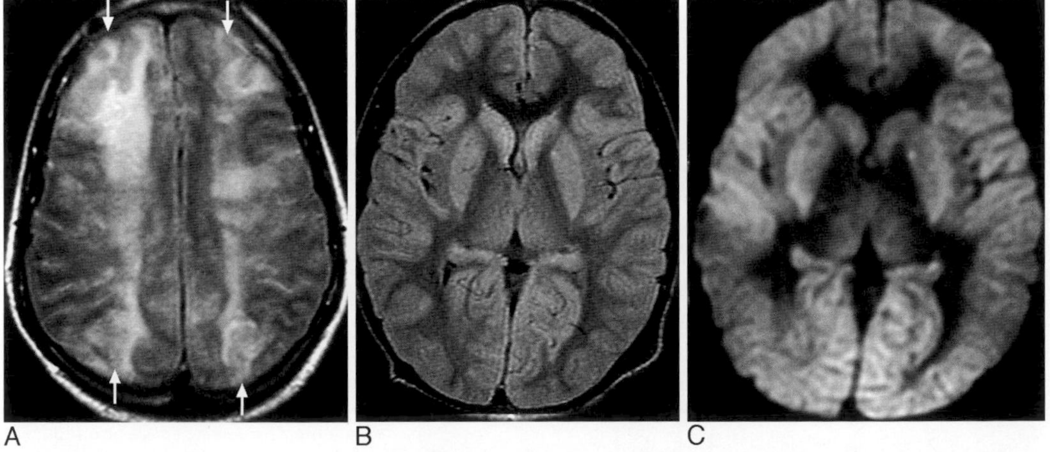

Figure 57.12 Global hypoperfusion. (A) Acute watershed infarcts and diffuse brain swelling on FLAIR axial image after a cardiac arrest (arrows). (B) FLAIR axial image in a different patient with a generalized hypoxic ischaemic brain insult after self-hanging shows diffuse high signal that could be mistaken for normal because of the perfectly symmetrical appearance. (C) DWI shows diffuse grey matter restricted diffusion markedly different from white matter signal intensity, alerting the observer that the scan is abnormal despite its symmetry. Obvious grey-white differentiation is not a normal feature of DWI (see Figs 57.2B, 57.11E).

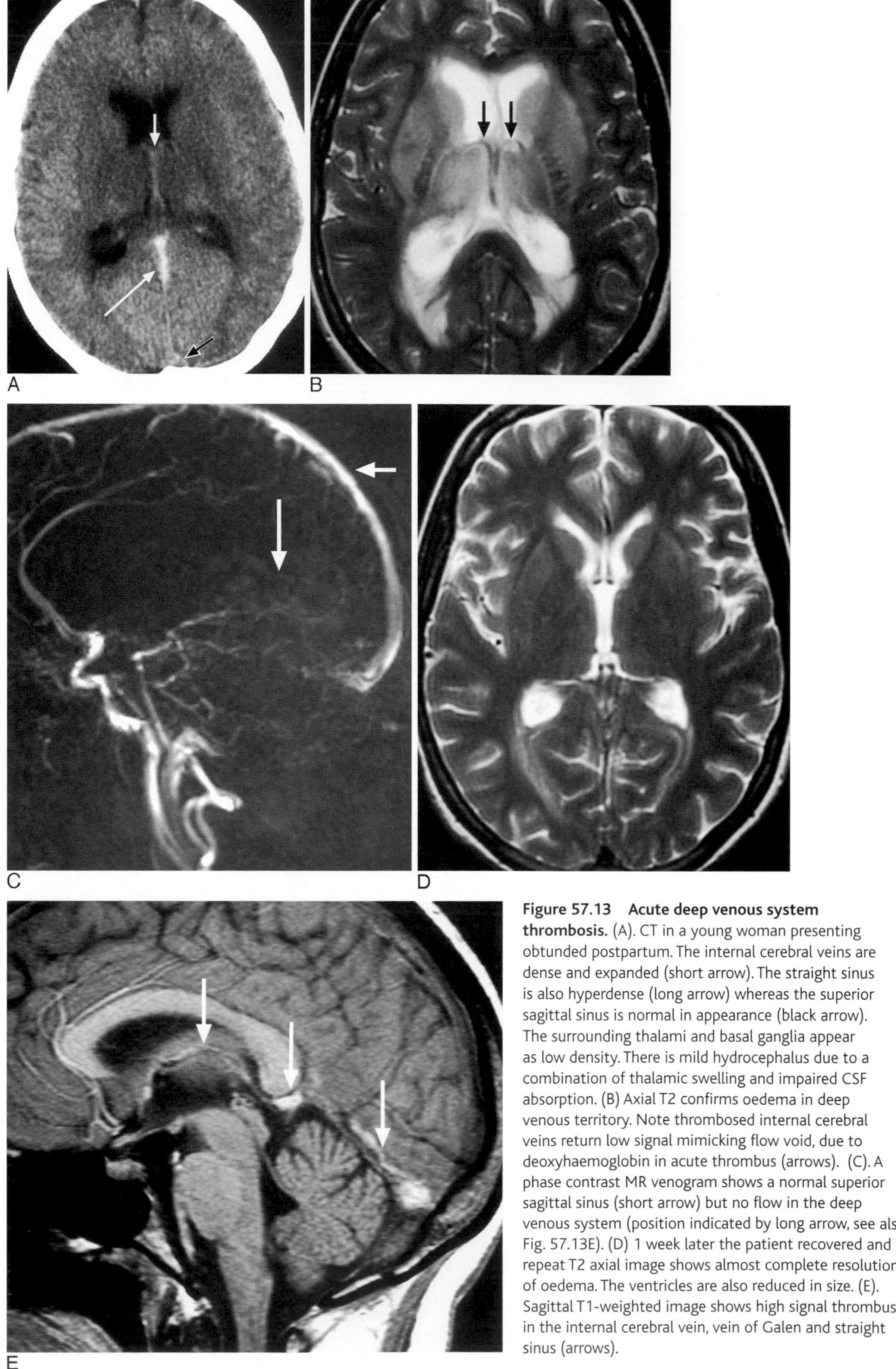

Figure 57.13 Acute deep venous system thrombosis. (A). CT in a young woman presenting obtunded postpartum. The internal cerebral veins are dense and expanded (short arrow). The straight sinus is also hyperdense (long arrow) whereas the superior sagittal sinus is normal in appearance (black arrow). The surrounding thalami and basal ganglia appear as low density. There is mild hydrocephalus due to a combination of thalamic swelling and impaired CSF absorption. (B) Axial T2 confirms oedema in deep venous territory. Note thrombosed internal cerebral veins return low signal mimicking flow void, due to deoxyhaemoglobin in acute thrombus (arrows). (C). A phase contrast MR venogram shows a normal superior sagittal sinus (short arrow) but no flow in the deep venous system (position indicated by long arrow, see also Fig. 57.13E). (D) 1 week later the patient recovered and a repeat T2 axial image shows almost complete resolution of oedema. The ventricles are also reduced in size. (E). Sagittal T1-weighted image shows high signal thrombus in the internal cerebral vein, vein of Galen and straight sinus (arrows).

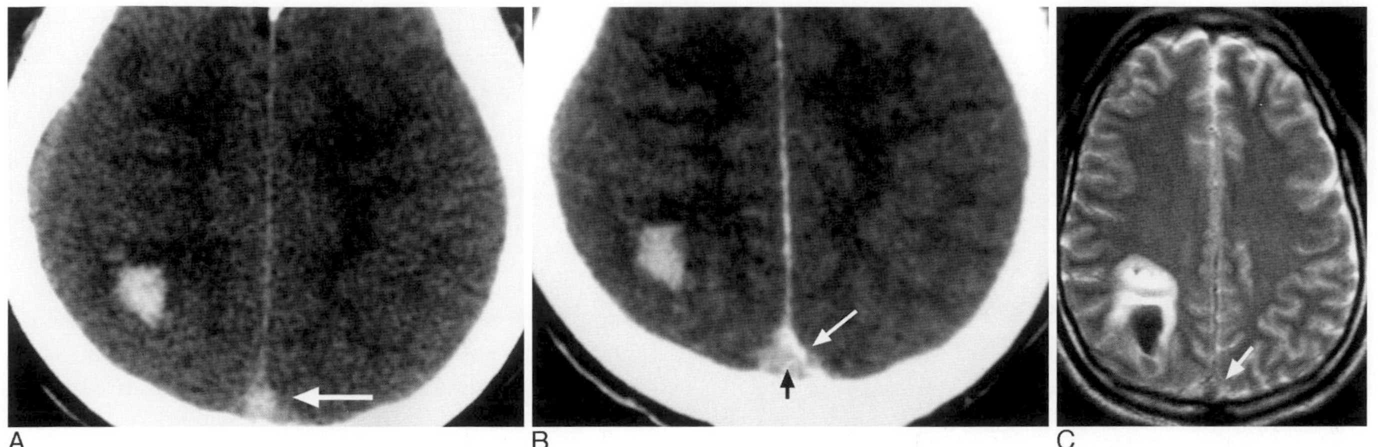

Figure 57.14 Delta sign in superior sagittal sinus thrombosis. (A) Young man with a seizure after several days of headaches. An unenhanced CT shows a small right parietal acute haematoma. The superior sagittal sinus is occluded by acute thrombus. It appears expanded and the same density as the intraparenchymal clot (arrow). (B) Contrast-enhanced CT shows the dura around the sinus (long arrow) is higher density than the lumen (short arrow). This is the 'delta sign', although in acute sinus thrombosis the unenhanced CT alone may indicate the correct diagnosis, as in this case. (C) T2-weighted MRI shows the recent haematoma. Note the superior sagittal sinus returns intermediate signal rather than flow void (arrow).

which are illustrated in Fig. 57.15. Surgery also reduces the risk of stroke in asymptomatic carotid stenosis of 70 per cent or more as measured by US[66]. Symptomatic 50–69 per cent stenoses may be a suitable target for intervention but in both cases the benefits are smaller and the advantages of surgery could more easily be outweighed by poor patient selection or excess morbidity from surgery (or angiography) in comparison with trial centres[67]. Carotid intervention should not be considered for a stenosis of less than 50 per cent regardless of symptoms.

Since these trial results were published there has been tremendous progress in noninvasive vascular imaging, a great attraction of which, apart from ease of use, is avoidance of the small but definite risk of stroke associated with catheter angiography, which for steno-occlusive cerebrovascular disease approaches 1 per cent in most published series[68].

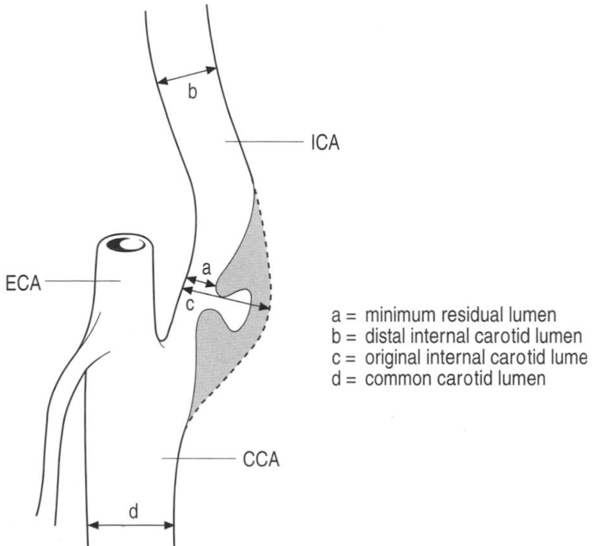

Figure 57.15 Different ways of measuring percentage of carotid artery stenosis (adapted from[86]): a) NASCET method = [1–(a/b)] × 100; b) ESCT method = [1–(a/c)] × 100; common carotid method = [1–(a/d)] × 100.

A review of Doppler US, spiral CTA and time-of-flight (TOF) MRA showed similar accuracy of all three techniques, with US showing the best correlation with DSA. Combining two or three noninvasive techniques improved accuracy[69]. However TOF MRA is a flow-sensitive technique prone to artifactual signal loss due to changes in vessel orientation and high-grade stenoses. It has been superseded by contrast-enhanced MR angiography (CEMRA). Multidetector CT also represents a technical advance, with each new generation scanner offering higher resolution than the last at shorter examination times. CEMRA and CTA both allow a full assessment of the arterial tree from the aortic arch to the circle of Willis and beyond, which is not possible on US or usually on TOF MRA.

There is good correlation between CEMRA, four-detector row CTA and Doppler US for the assessment of symptomatic carotid bifurcation stenosis[70]. CEMRA also compares well with DSA for assessment of carotid and vertebral artery disease[71,72]. A tendency for carotid stenosis to be exaggerated on CEMRA has been reported. Vessel narrowing can be underestimated on DSA if plaque is partially obscured on frames acquired when contrast density is maximal[71]. Using a fast frame rate in different projections or inspecting the source images from rotational angiography may avoid this. The length of an occlusion can be exaggerated on CEMRA if the vessel partially fills by retrograde flow on late frames of a DSA. This may be avoided in the future with time-resolved MRA techniques[72].

The nonvertical segments of tortuous vertebral artery origins can appear narrowed on CEMRA, although the true lumen diameter can often be appreciated on source images. In practice even CEMRA and CTA combined sometimes fail to adequately resolve vertebral artery origins; in such cases catheter angiography is definitive. Review of CTA should include assessment of any stenosis in the axial plane in addition to reconstructed images and this is particularly helpful in differentiating between string flow and occlusion, often a difficult judgement on other

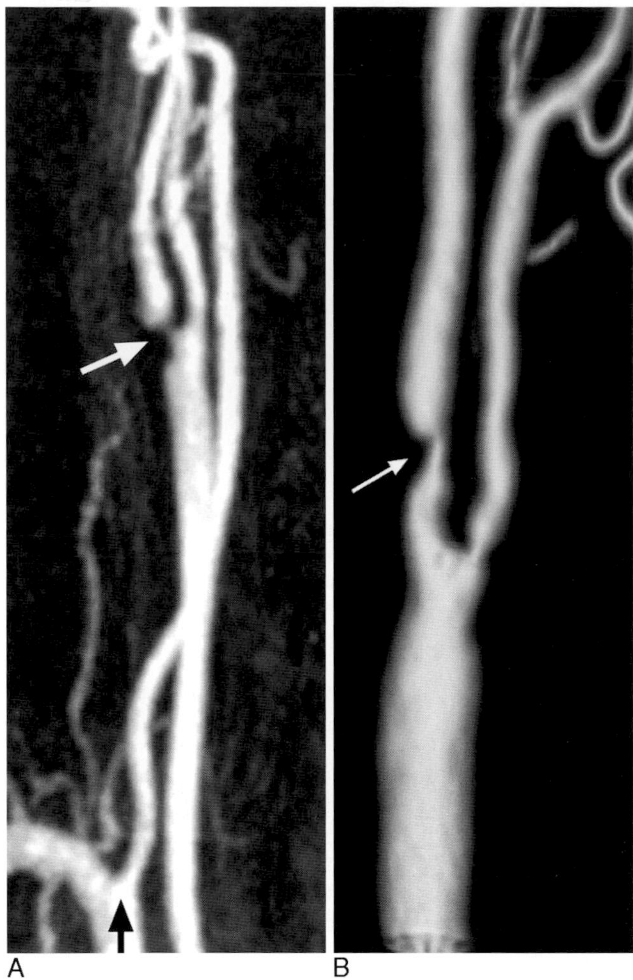

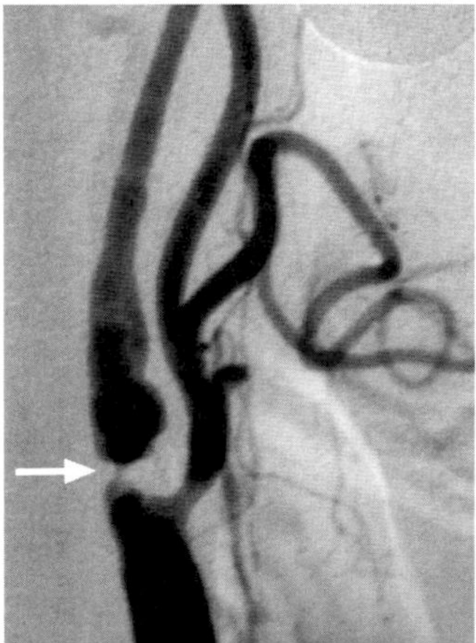

Figure 57.16 Carotid bifurcation atheroma. Examples of internal carotid artery stenoses (arrows) from different patients on (A) CEMRA MIP, (B) CTA volume rendering and (C) DSA. Note the right vertebral artery origin is clearly demonstrated in A (black arrow).

modalities. Calcified plaque exaggerates stenoses on MIPs; carefully windowed minimum thickness multiplanar reformat (MPR) images are likely to be a better guide in such circumstances.

Inevitably there are local variations but many centres opt to combine more than one technique to improve accuracy, for example US plus CEMRA, with CTA used as a problem-solving tool if there is discrepancy. DSA is still occasionally necessary if other techniques are inconclusive and it currently remains the investigation against which others are judged. It shows sequential opacification of the arterial tree, including collateral pathways and steal phenomena. However excessive use of DSA reduces the benefit of carotid revascularization by exposing the patient population to the additional stroke risk of the investigation. Decision making is even more finely balanced for patients with an asymptomatic stenosis[70].

Irregularity due to atheroma must be differentiated from catheter-induced spasm (Fig. 57.17), fibromuscular dysplasia and spontaneous or iatrogenic dissection. Fibromuscular dysplasia causes extensive, concentric corrugation of the artery, frequently bilateral and rarely extending above the skull base (Fig. 57.18). There may be associated renal artery stenosis. Dissection of the cervical arteries is an important cause of stroke, particularly in younger patients. It can be diagnosed acutely with MRI, which shows an expanded artery with high signal intramural haematoma around a narrow, often eccentric signal void indicating the true lumen. Internal carotid artery dissection often involves the vessel just below the skull base and may be identified on the lowermost routine axial T2-weighted images through the brain, without the need for additional special sequences. If not it is

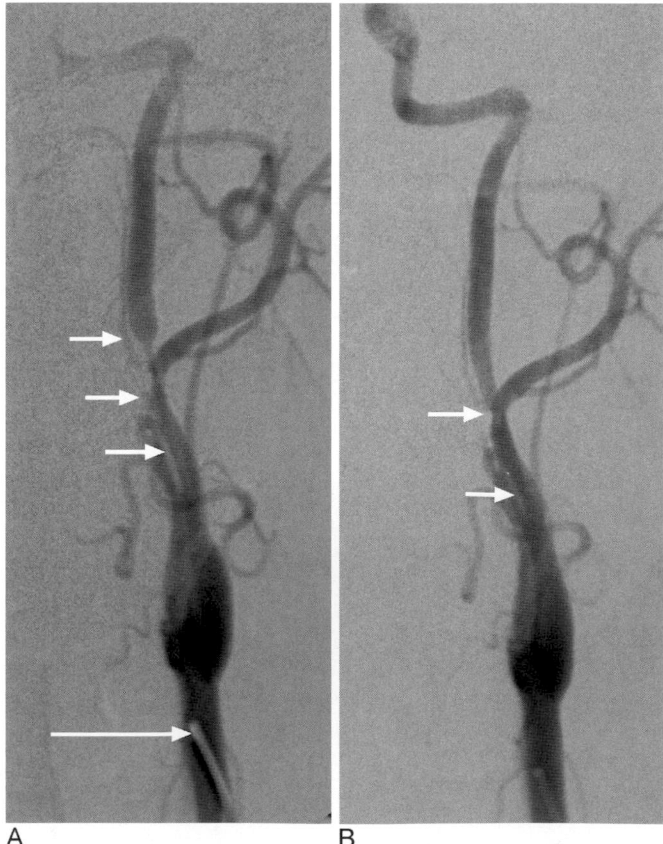

Figure 57.17 Catheter-induced arterial spasm. (A) Elective arteriogram following aneurysm coiling 6 months earlier. AP view of left internal carotid artery shows marked spasm in response to selective catheterization (short arrows). The catheter was withdrawn into the common carotid artery before this run (long arrow). (B) Four minutes later the spasm has almost resolved (arrows).

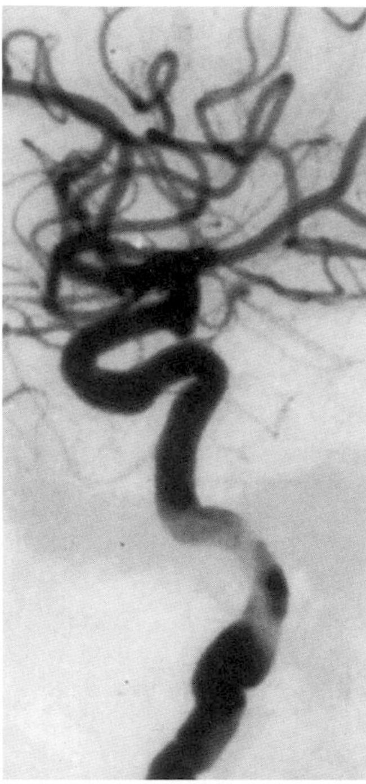

Figure 57.18 Fibromuscular dysplasia; internal carotid arteriogram, lateral projection. The cervical portion of the artery shows regular concentric corrugations: appearances were similar on the other side.

usual to employ fat-suppressed T1- or T2-weighted axial sequences through the neck. In practice vertebral artery dissection is more difficult to diagnose in this way, perhaps because these signs are harder to detect in a smaller vessel (Fig. 57.19).

Signs of dissection on angiography include a tapered stenosis or occlusion of the true lumen ('rat's tail'), which in the internal carotid arteries often starts at or just above the carotid bifurcation and sometimes extends intracranially. An intraluminal flap may be visible. Imaging at fast frame rates may show differential opacification and contrast washout in the true and false lumens if they are both patent. Many of these features can be shown on MRA or CTA and the diagnosis can often be made without recourse to DSA. CTA has shown promise in the noninvasive diagnosis of vertebral artery dissection[73]. The source images and MPRs may show an eccentric lumen within an enlarged vessel analogous to the appearance on axial MRI (Fig. 57.19).

Internal carotid artery dissection may also be diagnosed using Doppler US (see Ch. 3).

Finally within this section, cross-sectional imaging (MRI, CTA and US) is being used to image atheromatous plaque in the hope that characteristics such as lipid content might help to predict stroke risk and guide therapy[74]. These are largely still

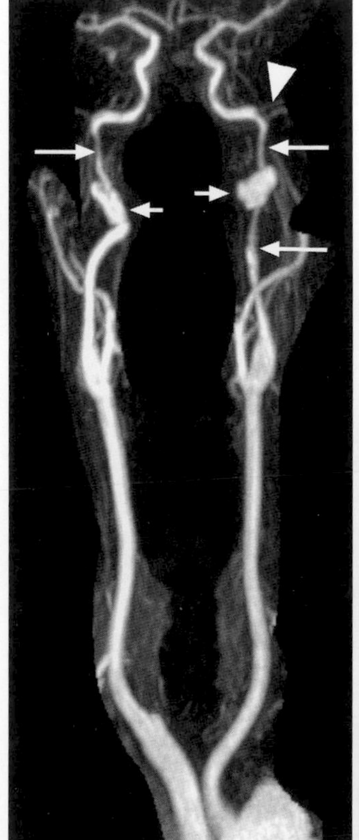

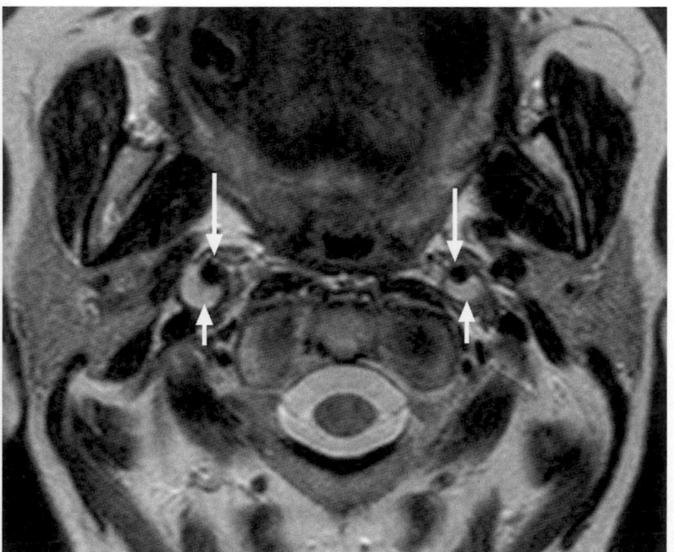

Figure 57.19 Diagnosis of cervical arterial dissection on MRA and CTA. (A) CEMRA in a 50-year-old man with left-sided neck pain and a right Horner's syndrome after cervical manipulation (vertebral arteries removed for clarity). There are bilateral ICA dissections with irregular narrowing (long arrows), extending into the proximal petrous canal on the left (arrowhead). There are also pseudoaneurysms on both sides (short arrows). (B) Axial T2-weighted image through the neck at C2 level in a different patient. On both sides there is high signal mural thrombus (short arrows) with eccentric flow void indicating the position of the true lumen (long arrows). The appearance is diagnostic of ICA dissections.

Continued

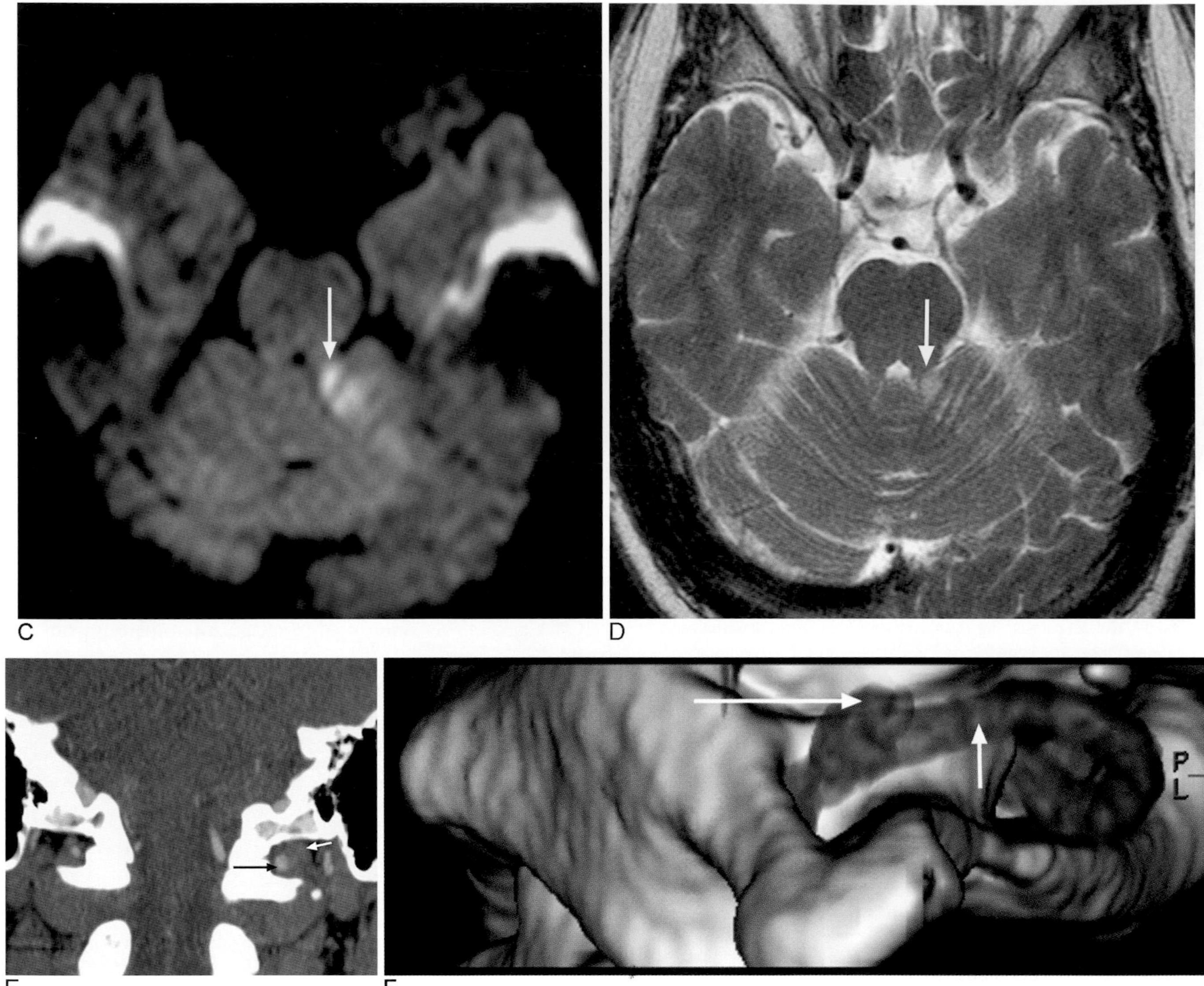

Figure 57.19, Cont'd (C) DWI in a different patient shows a small left superior cerebellar infarct (arrow), which would be easily overlooked on D, the corresponding T2-weighted image (arrow). (E) Coronal reformat from CTA shows expanded left vertebral artery at C1 with mural thrombus (short arrow) and eccentric enhancing lumen (long arrow), analogous to the MRI appearance in B. (F) Volume rendering from the same examination shows the left vertebral artery (short arrow) as it passes around the left lateral mass of C1, viewed from the left and slightly in front. A small pseudoaneurysm is shown (long arrow).

research techniques at present. DSA can show plaque ulceration but no information can be derived regarding composition of plaque or arterial wall.

Imaging of intracranial vessels

In addition to stroke (see earlier) and haemorrhage (see later), intracranial vessels are sometimes imaged for suspected cerebral vasculitis. This heterogeneous group of inflammatory diseases mainly affects smaller parenchymal and leptomeningeal vessels. Conditions that cause cerebral vasculitis, other than primary (isolated) angiitis of the central nervous system, include infection, malignancy, radiotherapy, cocaine ingestion and autoimmune diseases such as systemic lupus erythematosus, polyarteritis nodosa, giant cell arteritis and Sjögren's syndrome.

High-resolution intra-arterial angiography is superior to MRA and CTA, particularly for smaller, more peripheral vessels. Angiographic signs suggesting a vasculitis include stenoses, occlusion, thromboses or arterial beading, although they are not specific (Fig. 57.20). Angiography is frequently negative and it should not be regarded as the gold standard investigation; a brain or meningeal biopsy is often necessary to make a firm diagnosis.

Moya moya

Moya moya is Japanese for 'puff of smoke', describing the angiographic appearance of dilated collateral vessels that develop secondary to progressive occlusion of the supraclinoid internal carotid arteries. Moya moya represents an idiopathic arteriopathy

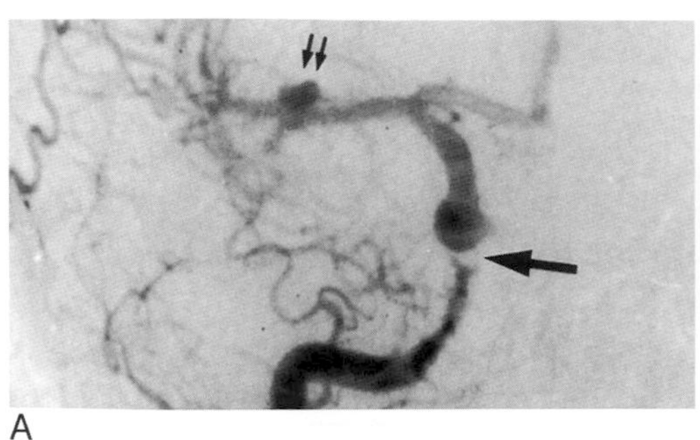

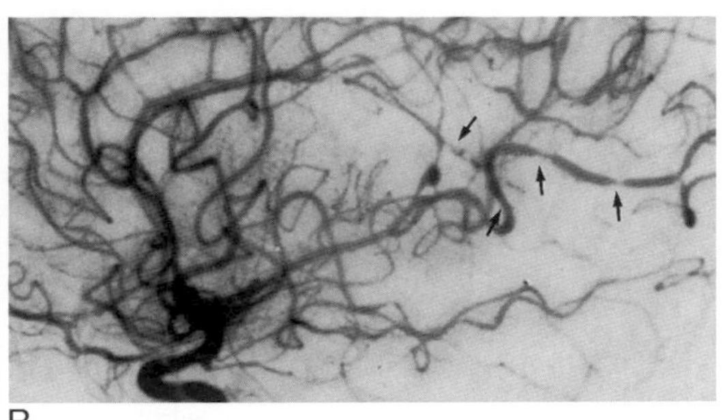

Figure 57.20 Arteritis caused by septic emboli of cardiac origin. (A) Common carotid arteriogram, anteroposterior projection. Filling defects are seen (arrows), many vessels are irregular and under filled, and the middle cerebral artery bears a mycotic aneurysm (double arrows). (B) Beaded appearance of cortical arteries (arrows), lateral projection.

mainly seen in Japan and the Pacific Rim. In advanced cases there may be extensive dural, leptomeningeal and pial collateral circulation. The characteristic vascular changes can also be shown on MRA or CTA and MRI may show associated infarcts. A moya moya-like pattern may be found in other conditions such as sickle cell disease, Down's syndrome, previous radiotherapy or tuberculous meningitis and Type 1 neurofibromatosis[75].

NONTRAUMATIC INTRACRANIAL HAEMORRHAGE

Intracranial haemorrhage may be traumatic or spontaneous (nontraumatic) and is described anatomically as intraparenchymal, intraventricular, subarachnoid, subdural, or extradural. Common causes of spontaneous haemorrhage include hypertension, amyloid angiopathy, aneurysms and various vascular malformations.

SUBARACHNOID HAEMORRHAGE

Spontaneous SAH is due to a ruptured arterial aneurysm in 70–80 per cent of patients and an arteriovenous malformation in about 10 per cent. In the remaining approximately 15 per cent, no underlying cause is found on angiography, which is more likely when the subarachnoid blood is confined to the perimesencephalic area. Patients with a nonaneurysmal perimesencephalic SAH (who by definition have a negative angiogram) have a very good long-term prognosis[76]. The risk of further bleeding is thought to be no higher than that in the general population. Variations in venous anatomy found with this pattern of SAH suggest a venous origin[77].

Appearance on CT and MRI

CT is positive for SAH in 98 per cent within 12 h of onset[78] but this falls to less than 75 per cent by the third day[79]. Recent SAH causes increased density of the cerebrospinal fluid (CSF) spaces on CT, assuming sufficient elevation of the CSF haematocrit (Fig. 57.21). Most aneurysms are located on or close to the circle of Willis and blood is therefore seen in the basal cisterns, although the entire intracranial subarachnoid space

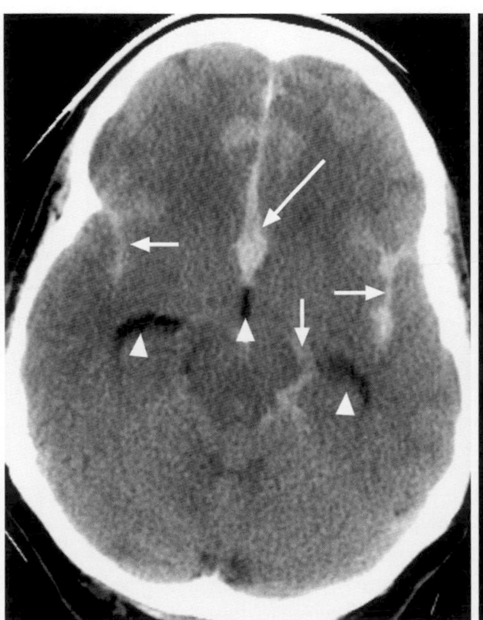

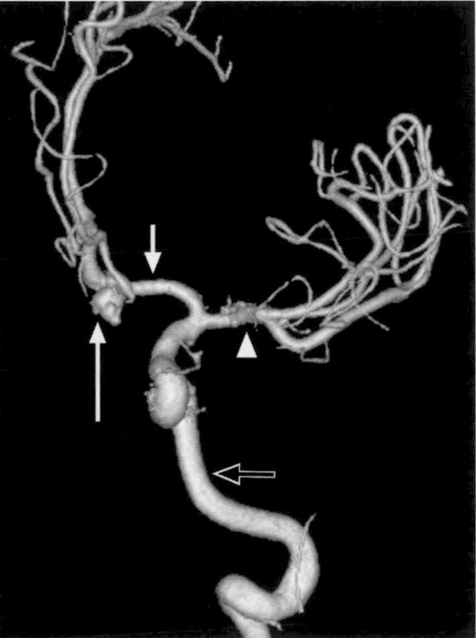

Figure 57.21 Anterior communicating artery aneurysm rupture. (A) CT shows diffuse subarachnoid haemorrhage (short arrows) and a small haematoma in the septum pellucidum indicating the likely source is an aneurysm of the anterior communicating artery (long arrow). The temporal horns of the lateral ventricles and anterior recesses of the third ventricle are enlarged (arrowheads) due to secondary communicating hydrocephalus, an extremely common finding in acute SAH. (B) A 3D angiogram shows a lobulated aneurysm in the predicted location (long arrow). The left proximal anterior cerebral artery (short arrow), middle cerebral artery (arrowhead) and internal carotid artery (open arrow) are clearly shown.

may be opacified and intraventricular blood is common. In some cases surrounding clot indicates the aneurysm location. A lumbar puncture should be performed when there is a strong clinical suspicion of SAH but negative CT.

Spin-echo MRI sequences are unreliable in SAH but using a T2* gradient-echo or FLAIR sequence (Fig. 57.22), sensitivities of 94–100 per cent and 81–87 per cent can be achieved in the acute (less than 4 d) and subacute (more than 4 d) periods, respectively[80]. However FLAIR is less sensitive at low CSF red blood cell concentrations following normal CT[81]. The susceptibility effects of para-magnetic iron cause low signal on gradient echo sequences; on FLAIR the CSF appears high signal due to the presence of increased protein. FLAIR may remain positive for at least 45 d after a haemorrhage[82], at a time when the blood has long since become invisible on CT.

Therefore MRI may be used to diagnose SAH following normal CT, but a lumbar puncture should still be performed following a negative CT and MRI in someone with a high clinical suspicion of SAH. Supplemental inspired oxygen[83] and contrast medium leakage into the subarachnoid space after an acute infarct[84] can both cause the CSF to return high signal on FLAIR and CSF flow is a common cause of artifactual high signal in daily practice.

CT and MRI may also show a number of complications in patients with SAH, of which communicating hydrocephalus and ischaemia secondary to vasospasm are the most important. It is very common to see mild dilatation of the ventricles, particularly the temporal horns, at diagnosis. Indeed it may be a useful clue to the diagnosis if the presence of blood is not obvious. It usually resolves over several days, but may progress and necessitate a ventricular drain or shunt. Vasospasm usually occurs between 4 and 11 d after the haemorrhage and is a significant cause of morbidity during this period[85]. It is more likely if the initial CT shows a large amount of subarachnoid blood.

MRI in chronic repeated SAH may show evidence of superficial siderosis with haemosiderin staining of the leptomeninges, particularly around the midbrain and in the posterior fossa. Such patients often present with symptoms related to the lower cranial nerves, ataxia or gradual cognitive decline (Fig. 57.23).

CEREBRAL ANEURYSMS

Cerebral aneurysms may be saccular, fusiform, or dissecting[86]. Fusiform aneurysms can be regarded as an extreme form of focal ectasia in arteriosclerotic disease. Intracranial aneurysms can also develop following an arterial dissection. However the majority are saccular aneurysms, which are usually round or lobulated and arise from arterial bifurcations. Giant aneurysms by definition measure over 25 mm in diameter and account for approximately 5 per cent of all cerebral aneurysms. They often contain layers of organized thrombus. Aneurysms tend to present with SAH or mass effect on adjacent structures, most commonly a posterior communicating artery aneurysm causing a third nerve palsy.

Increasingly saccular aneurysms are discovered incidentally on scans for other indications and this represents a management problem. A recent large-scale study suggests that the annual risk of haemorrhage from small incidental aneurysms is substantially lower than previously thought and the risks of elective intervention higher[87,88]. Current data indicates that there is no benefit from treating aneurysms of

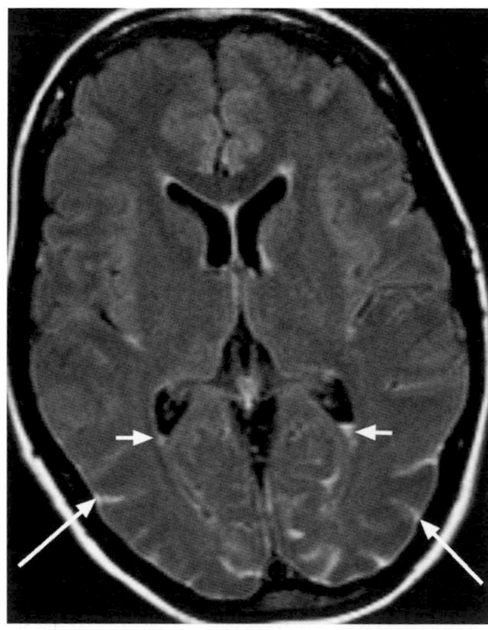

Figure 57.22 Subarachnoid haemorrhage on FLAIR. Blood is shown as high signal in occipital sulci (long arrows) and layered in the occipital horns of both lateral ventricles (short arrows).

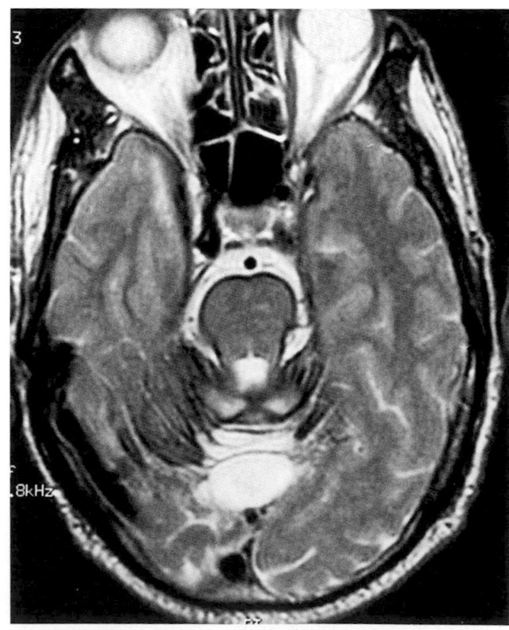

Figure 57.23 Superficial siderosis. Axial T2-weighted image shows the pons, mesial temporal lobes and cerebellar folia are outlined by a low signal intensity haemosiderin rim indicating repeated SAH.

the anterior circulation 7 mm or less in diameter regardless of the patient's age, if there is no prior history of SAH. The difference between the risks of haemorrhage and treatment may favour intervention for larger or posterior circulation aneurysms, depending on aneurysm size and remaining life expectancy[88].

Around 90 per cent of intracranial aneurysms arise from the carotid circulation, the remaining 10 per cent from vertebral or basilar arteries[86]. The anterior and posterior communicating arteries give rise to approximately one-third each of all intracranial aneurysms, with another 20 per cent from middle cerebral arteries and 5 per cent from the basilar termination. The remainder arises from other vessel origins and bifurcations.

A clot in the septum pellucidum, possibly extending into one or other frontal lobe, is virtually diagnostic of an aneurysm of the anterior communicating artery (Fig. 57.21). Aneurysms of the distal anterior cerebral artery related to pericallosal branches are less common. Aneurysms of the MCA bleed into the Sylvian fissure, sometimes with a clot in the temporal lobe. Aneurysms of the posterior communicating artery (which arise from the internal carotid artery at the origin of this vessel) are a frequent cause of SAH but can also present with isolated third nerve palsy due to pulsatile pressure on the nerve. Other relatively common sites of aneurysms of the internal carotid artery are the origin of the ophthalmic and anterior choroidal arteries and its terminal bifurcation.

Aneurysms of the posterior circulation are commonly located at the basilar artery bifurcation and if they rupture blood may be seen in the interpeduncular fossa, brainstem or thalamus; prognosis is frequently poor. The second commonest site in the posterior circulation is at the origin of one of the posterior inferior cerebellar arteries. They often haemorrhage into the ventricular system via the fourth ventricle and downwards into the spinal subarachnoid space.

Larger aneurysms are shown on CT and MRI. On CT they appear as rounded enhancing lesions. Giant aneurysms have an enhancing lumen and a wall of variable thickness that often contains laminated thrombus and may be calcified. On spin-echo MRI sequences a patent aneurysm appears as an area of flow void. Areas of increased signal intensity within the aneurysm may represent mural thrombus or turbulent, slow flow.

Surrounding white matter oedema suggests a mycotic aneurysm, particularly if very extensive. Mycotic aneurysms are caused by septic emboli and tend to occur peripherally, typically on the branches of the MCA. They commonly present with haemorrhage, usually with a peripheral intraparenchymal clot, which, while not specific, is highly suggestive of such a lesion in a patient with known septicaemia or bacterial endocarditis (Figs 57.20, 57.24).

Angiography in subarachnoid haemorrhage and intracranial aneurysms

Until recently SAH was an incontestable indication for intra-arterial angiography but this has changed with improved CT technology. Early CTA studies produced inconsistent results but in expert hands a very high sensitivity for aneurysm detection can now be achieved. A comparative study of spiral CTA, DSA and surgical findings for small aneurysms less than 5 mm in diameter found that CTA outperformed DSA, with sensitivities of 98–100 per cent and 95 per cent, respectively[89]. In neurovascular centres CTA is now at least the equal of two-dimensional (2D) DSA for the diagnosis and anatomical assessment of aneurysms[90] (Fig. 57.25).

It is essential to methodically review source images on a workstation, in addition to MPRs and MIPs in multiple planes and 3D renderings. Particular care should be taken close to the skull base, where adjacent bone may reduce the conspicuity of small aneurysms. CTA images can be degraded by vasospasm or inadequate opacification if the images are not acquired during the arterial phase of contrast enhancement. It is apparent on visual inspection when this is the case. The images can be rotated in multiple planes (like in 3D rotational DSA, see Fig. 57.21) allowing better demonstration of an aneurysm and its neck than sometimes achieved on DSA, especially since overlying vessels can be 'removed'. In patients subsequently undergoing catheter angiography CTA image rotation allows prior selection of optimal projections. There are occasions when aneurysms are masked by superimposition on DSA but visible on a CTA.

However the greatest benefit of CTA is its ease of use. It takes only a few minutes to prepare the patient and plan the examination and on a 16-detector CT system the whole head is imaged in less than 10 s. This is ideal in patients with SAH, who are often restless and unwell. Unenhanced cranial CT and perfusion data can be acquired during the same examination if necessary. It avoids the need for an arterial puncture and the risk of ischaemic stroke from catheter angiography, admittedly extremely small if SAH is the indication for the procedure. Patient preference has been shown for CTA over MRA or DSA in the investigation of carotid stenosis[69] and it is reasonable to assume that the same applies to aneurysm patients.

CTA can now be viewed as a complementary investigation to DSA, the latter being reserved for problem solving or in some centres dispensed with altogether as a diagnostic investigation[90]. It seems superficially attractive to consider devolving CTA to the general hospital environment. However accurate interpretation requires experience in neurovascular radiology and CTA is part of the overall care of SAH patients, which is currently delivered in a neuroscience environment.

The sensitivity of MRA for prospective detection of aneurysms larger than 5 mm is 77–94 per cent, varying with observer experience, but it is much less sensitive for aneurysms smaller than 3 mm[91–93]. Like CTA, MRA images can be rotated and may show aneurysms missed on DSA[94]. Recent SAH may cause image degradation on TOF MRA due to T1 shortening from haemorrhage. Giant aneurysms are rarely visualized in their full extent on 3D TOF MRA because of slow and turbulent flow in their fundus. The lumen is properly opacified on CTA, which also shows mural thrombus and the aneurysm wall. MRA is a reasonable first-line option for elective imaging of aneurysms, although its modest sensitivity for smaller aneurysms should be borne in mind. It is also used for following coiled aneurysms. CTA is now preferable in acute SAH.

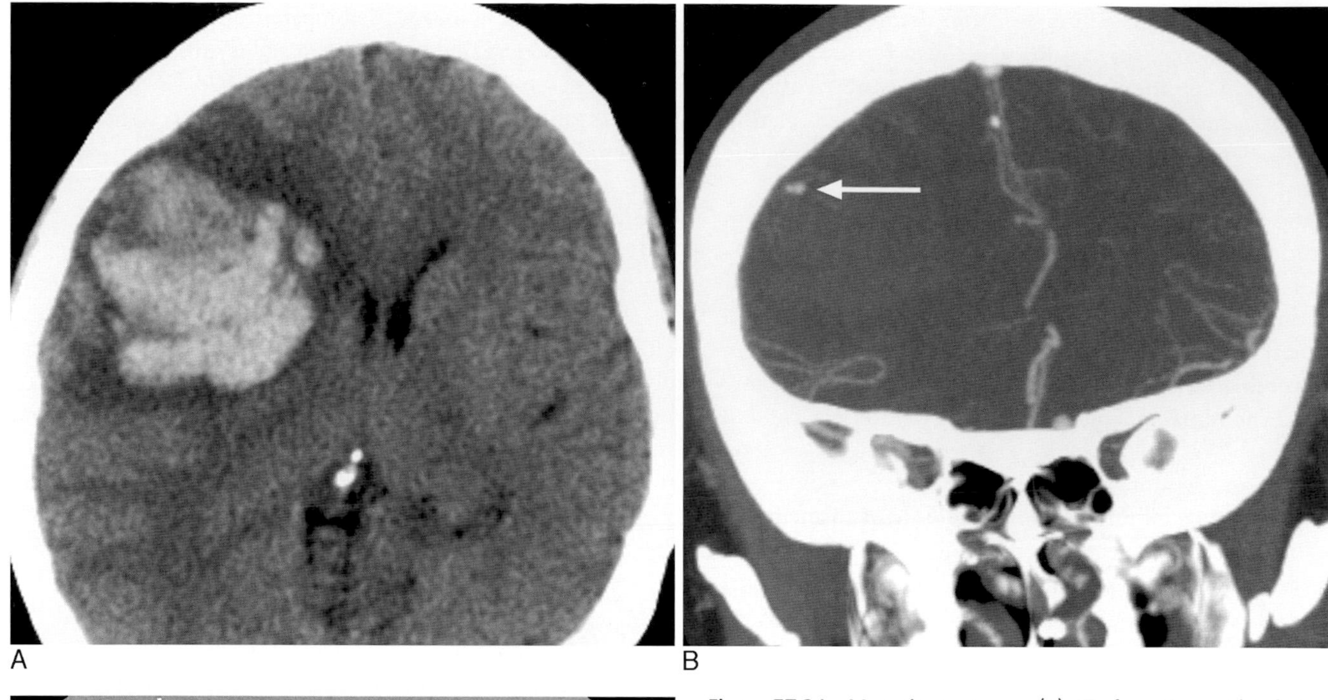

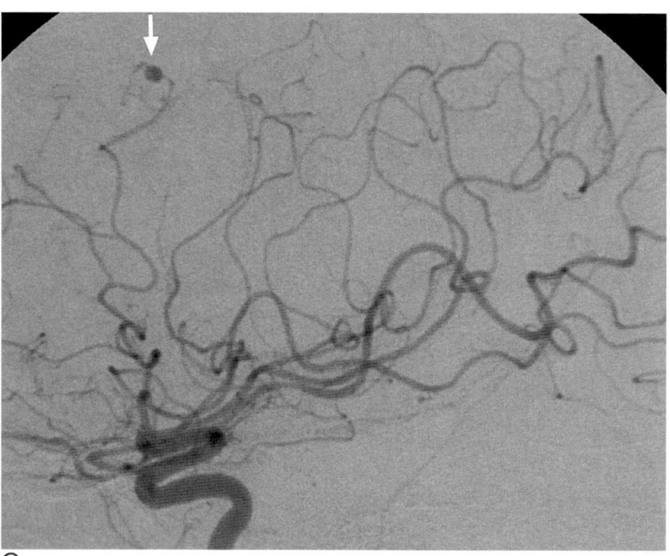

Figure 57.24 Mycotic aneurysm. (A) CT of a patient with infective endocarditis shows an acute right frontal intraparenchymal haemorrhage. (B) Coronal MIP from a CTA shows pooling of contrast at the periphery of the haematoma, suggesting an aneurysm (arrow). (C) Lateral right ICA arteriogram confirms a peripheral mycotic aneurysm (arrow).

Practice varies in patients with a negative CTA following SAH. There is a body of opinion that a single technically adequate CTA is sufficient following a classical perimesencephalic SAH[95]. Some institutions now rely solely on CTA for all diagnostic imaging in SAH. However in many centres it remains routine practice to confirm a negative CTA result with DSA, which is also used if for any reason aneurysm anatomy is not adequately displayed on CTA.

Traditionally a 'four vessel' catheter angiogram was performed because up to 20 per cent of aneurysms are multiple. This involves bilateral common or internal carotid injections and one or both vertebral arteries depending on whether reflux of contrast medium displays the contralateral posterior inferior cerebellar artery origin. If a dural fistula is a possibility the external carotid arteries should also be injected. A standard examination comprises sufficient projections to resolve all vessels without superimposition and demonstrates the anatomy of any aneurysms and adjacent arteries. It can be difficult to decide which aneurysm has ruptured if more than one is found and cross-sectional imaging shows a symmetrical distribution of blood (or if SAH was diagnosed by lumbar puncture after a negative scan). Ruptured aneurysms often have an irregular shape and may show a 'nipple' indicating the site of rupture. Alternatively the larger of multiple aneurysms is frequently incriminated, but this is not a very reliable rule.

It is justifiable to perform a limited angiogram when the territory of the bleed is indicated from cross-sectional imaging, particularly if remote vessels are normal on CTA or the patient is elderly or very sick. Angiography should be performed as soon as possible following SAH since the aneurysm re-bleed rate is greatest during the first 48 h and vasospasm can adversely affect the quality of angiograms performed several days after the haemorrhage. If a negative angiogram is marred by vasospasm, a repeat study is indicated.

Three-dimensional angiography reduces the need for multiple angiographic runs and provides high-resolution 3D

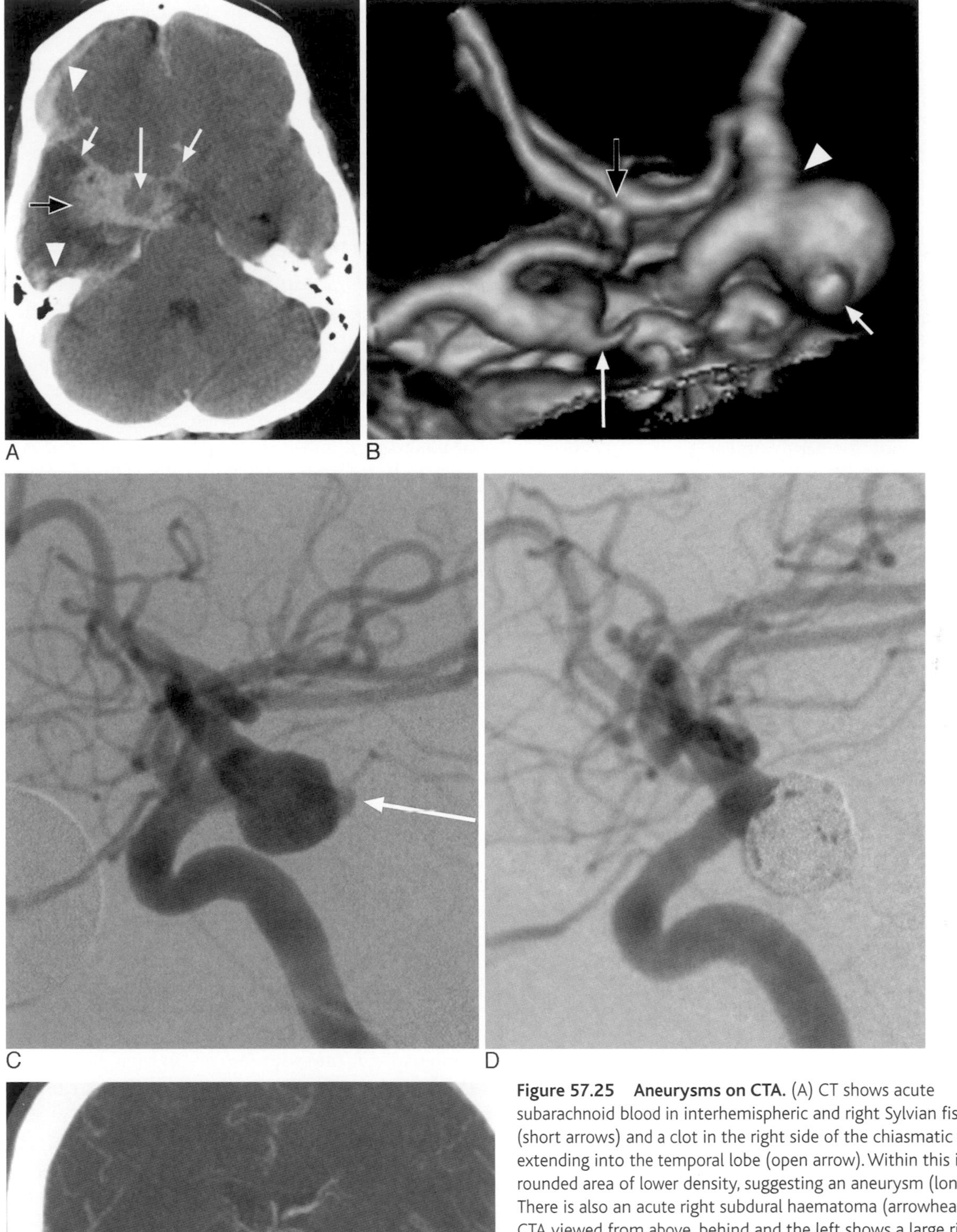

Figure 57.25 Aneurysms on CTA. (A) CT shows acute subarachnoid blood in interhemispheric and right Sylvian fissures (short arrows) and a clot in the right side of the chiasmatic cistern extending into the temporal lobe (open arrow). Within this is a rounded area of lower density, suggesting an aneurysm (long arrow). There is also an acute right subdural haematoma (arrowheads). (B) CTA viewed from above, behind and the left shows a large right distal ICA aneurysm arising at the level of the posterior communicating artery (not visible as anatomically hypoplastic). The neck is clearly shown (arrowhead) and there is a small lobule (short arrow) on the fundus possibly indicating the site of rupture. Note the left posterior communicating (long arrow) and anterior communicating arteries (open arrow). The decision to treat by endovascular coiling was based on this examination. (C, D) Lateral right ICA arteriograms from coiling procedure, immediately before and after occlusion of the aneurysm. Note confirmation of aneurysm anatomy as shown on CTA, including terminal lobule (arrow). (E) Coronal MIP from CTA in a different patient with a complex right middle cerebral artery aneurysm. Note the anatomical detail of separate lobules and artery arising from the neck of the superior aneurysm (arrow).

images of the proximal cerebral vessels that show the relationship of an aneurysm to adjacent vessels, although CTA often provides similar information (Figs 57.21, 57.25). Manipulation at the workstation permits the image to be rotated and viewed from any angle.

Aneurysms can be treated by surgical clipping or endovascular coiling (Fig. 57.25). The latter is performed via a microcatheter placed in the aneurysm sac through which a number of electrically detachable platinum coils are deployed. A multicentre randomized comparison of surgical clipping and endovascular coiling showed superior outcomes at 1 year for coiling over clipping (death or dependency 23.5 per cent vs. 30.9 per cent; absolute risk reduction 7.4 per cent). This difference was maintained at 7 years with a lower risk of epilepsy but more episodes of re-bleeding in the coiled group[96]. There is still a role for surgical clipping if the anatomy of the aneurysm is unfavourable for endovascular treatment.

INTRACEREBRAL HAEMORRHAGE

Nontraumatic intracerebral haemorrhage in older people is frequently from rupture of a small perforating vessel due to hypertension. The preferential sites of hypertensive haemorrhage are the basal ganglia, thalamus and pons. Larger hypertensive bleeds in the basal ganglia often extend into the ventricles or Sylvian fissure. Peripheral or lobar haemorrhages in the elderly are suggestive of amyloid angiopathy, particularly if they are multifocal[97] and accompanied by microbleeds elsewhere, best shown on T2 gradient-echo imaging. Primary or secondary brain neoplasms may also cause intracerebral haemorrhage.

Haemorrhage may also be due to vascular malformations and 'recreational' drugs such as cocaine and ecstasy[98]. Intracranial haemorrhage due to aneurysms is usually associated with SAH, but very occasionally a ruptured aneurysm can cause an apparently isolated intracerebral clot (particularly if the surrounding subarachnoid space has been 'sealed off' by preceding SAH). Other causes include coagulopathies, anticoagulation, vasculitis, venous infarcts and haemorrhagic transformation of arterial infarcts.

Appearance on CT and MRI

Intracerebral haemorrhage is reliably detected on CT, appearing as increased density. Calcified or highly proteinaceous material and contrast enhancement of tumours can reach a similar density to fresh blood clot, but the clinical context or correlation with unenhanced images should prevent confusion. An acute intracerebral clot is usually of fairly homogeneous density. Hyperacute unclotted blood will appear less dense, which may cause a blood–fluid level to be visible. This appearance is most commonly due to haemorrhage from coagulopathies (usually anticoagulant medication). Very rarely in severely anaemic patients with a haematocrit level below 20 per cent haematomas can be isodense to the surrounding brain[99]. Deep or extensive haemorrhage may leak into the ventricles, forming a haematoma, or a blood–fluid level in the occipital horns, which are dependent with the patient supine.

There is typically only a fine rim of low density around a fresh clot and extensive oedema at presentation suggests an underlying neoplasm. Other features favouring a neoplastic haemorrhage are a more complex structure, extensive surrounding vasogenic oedema in the acute phase and enhancing areas not immediately adjacent to the blood clot. In some cases the diagnosis can only be made after follow-up studies.

Over the course of several days, an untreated haematoma becomes less dense, from the periphery towards the centre and therefore appears smaller. The timing depends on the size of the clot. Small haemorrhages can look identical to infarcts on CT by 8–9 d, which clearly has important treatment ramifications[42]. MRI will distinguish between the two. Vasogenic oedema may develop in the surrounding white matter and should contrast medium be given at this stage, it usually produces a halo of enhancement. After several weeks, the blood products become hypodense and are eventually absorbed to leave a focal cavity or area of atrophy.

The MRI appearance of intracerebral haemorrhage changes over time as red cells lyse and haemoglobin degrades, ultimately taken up by macrophages as haemosiderin[100] (Fig. 57.26 and Table 57.1). Factors such as protein and water content, fibrin formation and clot retraction can alter the sequence and timing of changes in appearance on MRI.

Gradient-echo imaging is much more sensitive to the magnetic field inhomogeneities induced by paramagnetic blood products than spin-echo sequences and this applies to both acute and old haemorrhage (deoxyhaemoglobin and haemosiderin, respectively) (Fig. 57.11).

Angiography in intracerebral haemorrhage

The indications for angiography in intracerebral haemorrhage are determined by clinical factors as much as imaging appearance. It is unlikely a treatable vascular abnormality will be found in a basal ganglia bleed in an elderly hypertensive patient whereas a haemorrhage in the same location in a young, normotensive patient warrants further investigation with angiography to exclude an AVM. It is also noteworthy that some 'recreational' drugs are associated with aneurysm formation and rupture so angiography is often appropriate in such patients. The timing of angiography depends on the size and mass effect of the haematoma. Occasionally urgent angiography is required before surgical evacuation of a haematoma. Otherwise it is usually preferable to defer angiography until the haematoma has resolved because smaller vascular lesions can be compressed by an acute haematoma and not be apparent angiographically.

CTA seems to be a reasonable alternative to DSA in the emergency setting for the detection of ruptured AVMs and aneurysms, and it is certainly much easier and quicker to perform in very sick patients. However it is not yet established that a small arteriovenous fistula or malformation can be reliably excluded using CTA so DSA is still preferred for elective investigation of such patients. The same reservation applies to MRA although the dynamic gadolinium bolus technique of MR DSA, which is time resolved, has produced some interesting early results in patients with large dural AVFs[101]. It remains to be seen if spatial resolution improves sufficiently to increase the sensitivity of MRA to clinically useful levels.

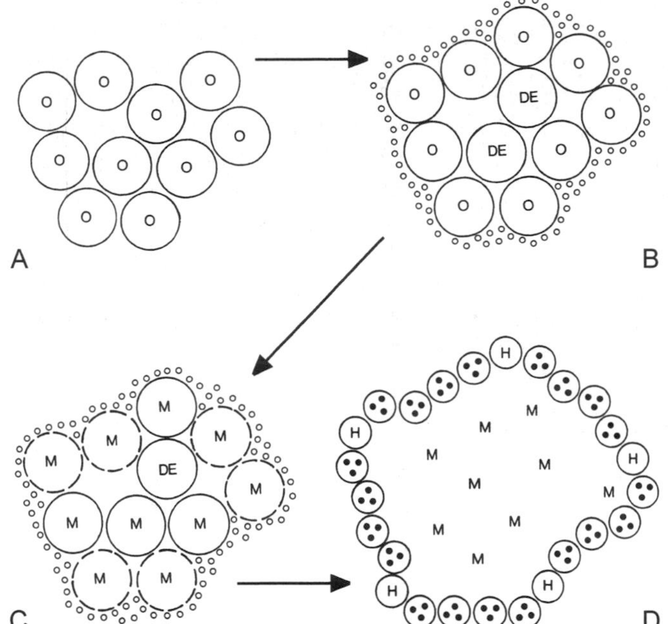

Figure 57.26 Cerebral haemorrhage: a simplified explanation of serial MRI signal changes. (A) Red cells containing oxyhaemoglobin (O), which gives signal similar to brain on both T1 and T2 weighting, are extravasated. (B) The oxyhaemoglobin in some of the cells at the centre of the clot is converted to deoxyhaemoglobin (DE), giving lower signal on T1-weighted images. The clot is now surrounded by a variable amount of cerebral oedema (small circles), which gives non-specific increased signal on T2-weighted images. (C) Most of the haemoglobin is now converted to methaemoglobin (M), which gives high signal on both T1- and T2-weighted images: however, lower signal due to the continued presence of deoxyhaemoglobin (DE) may still be evident centrally. Progressive lysis (interrupted outline) of the red cells is occurring. Surrounding oedema may become more extensive. (D) The red cells have now broken down, leaving a post-haemorrhagic cyst. This still contains methaemoglobin (M), and returns high signal on all the commonly used sequences. The oedema around the clot has resolved, but the macrophages (circles with three engulfed particles) which surround the cavity contain haemosiderin granules (H) which, because of susceptibility effects, give markedly reduced signal with T2 weighting and, to a lesser extent, on T1-weighted images. Persistence of high signal from methaemoglobin and low signal from haemosiderin is variable, but in some patients these effects can be seen for many months after documented bleeding.

ARTERIOVENOUS MALFORMATIONS

Intracranial vascular malformations can be classified according to the presence or otherwise of arteriovenous shunting[102]. The former comprises cerebral (or subpial) arteriovenous malformations (AVMs) and dural fistulae; the latter includes developmental venous anomalies (DVAs), cavernous angiomas ('cavernomas') and capillary telangiectasias. Intra-arterial angiography is still the method of choice for the investigation of cerebral AVMs and dural fistulae. Only occasionally is it necessary to confirm a DVA angiographically as the MRI appearance is usually characteristic. Cavernous angiomas and telangiectasias are angiographically occult or 'cryptic' vascular malformations.

Cerebral (subpial) AVMs are probably congenital anomalies consisting of direct arteriovenous shunts without a normal intervening capillary bed. Some are essentially fistulous; others have a plexiform nidus or a combination of the two. They lie within the brain substance or cerebral sulci and are supplied by branches of the internal carotid artery or vertebrobasilar system, sometimes recruiting additional supply from meningeal arteries. Cerebral haemorrhage is the commonest clinical presentation, others being epilepsy, headache or focal neurological deficit.

They are usually detectable on CT or MRI as serpiginous areas of high density (with marked contrast enhancement) or mixed signal, respectively. CT may show calcification and the MR signal comprises areas of flow void and high signal, which may represent thrombosis or flow-related enhancement. There may be haemorrhage at different stages of evolution. AVMs may be surrounded by areas of ischaemic damage that are low attenuation on CT and hyperintense on T2-weighted MRI. Dilated feeding arteries and early opacification of draining veins are the angiographic hallmarks of these lesions.

Dural arteriovenous fistulae are direct shunts between branches of the external carotid artery or meningeal branches of the cerebral vessels and dural sinuses. They are thought to be acquired and may be due to prior venous thrombosis. The clinical presentation depends on their location and venous drainage pattern[103]. Lesions shunting into the cavernous sinus commonly present with proptosis. Shunting into the transverse or sigmoid sinus may cause pulsatile tinnitus. Intracranial haemorrhage, which may be intracerebral, subarachnoid or subdural, usually occurs in lesions that reflux into cortical veins. They may go undetected on MRI or CT unless there are enlarged dural sinuses or cortical veins. MRA or CTA may show abnormal vessels more clearly but intra-arterial angiography is still required to make a definitive diagnosis.

Angiography for an AVM or dural fistula should include injections of all possible feeding vessels using a high frame rate to improve delineation of the nidus, which otherwise can be obscured by overlying veins in rapidly shunting lesions. There may be associated aneurysms, either on the feeding arteries or within the nidus and venous drainage may be via deep and/or superficial systems. There may be venous varices or stenoses (Figs 57.27, 57.28). There is an increased risk

Table 57.1 MR SIGNAL CHARACTERISTICS OF INTRACEREBRAL HAEMORRHAGE (ACCORDING TO BRADLEY[100])

Stage	Form of haem iron	T1-weighted MRI	T2-weighted MRI
Hyperacute (first few hours)	Oxyhaemoglobin	Iso- or hypointense	Slightly hyperintense
Acute (1–3 d)	Deoxyhaemoglobin	Slightly hypointense	Hypointense
Early subacute (3–7 d)	Intracellular methaemoglobin	Hyperintense	Hypointense
Late subacute (1–4 weeks)	Extracellular methaemoglobin	Hyperintense	Hyperintense
Chronic	Haemosiderin	Iso- or hypointense	Markedly hyperintense

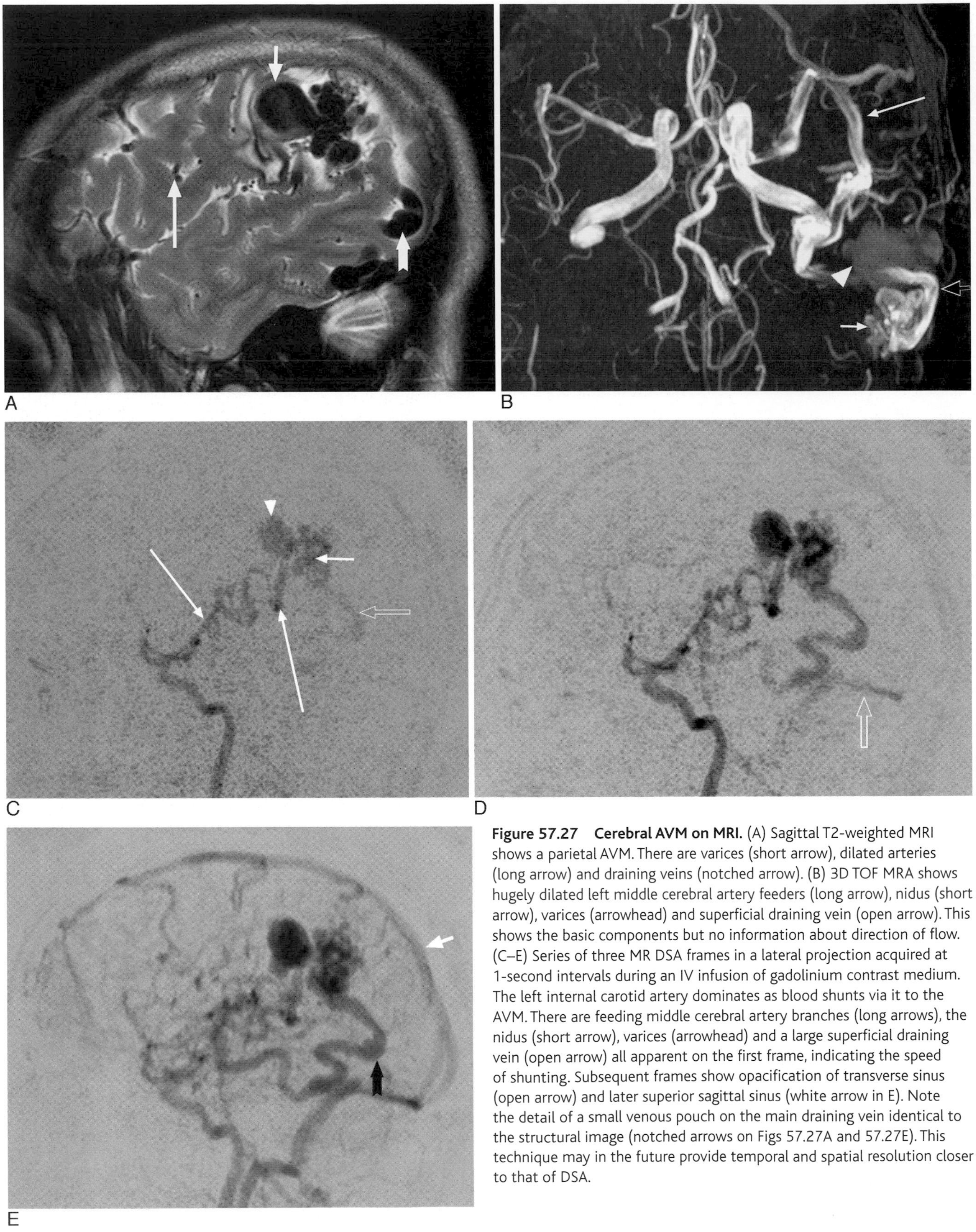

A

B

C

D

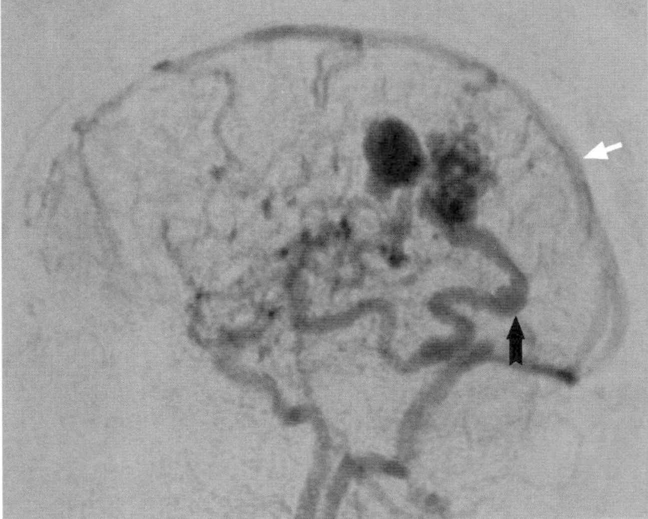

E

Figure 57.27 Cerebral AVM on MRI. (A) Sagittal T2-weighted MRI shows a parietal AVM. There are varices (short arrow), dilated arteries (long arrow) and draining veins (notched arrow). (B) 3D TOF MRA shows hugely dilated left middle cerebral artery feeders (long arrow), nidus (short arrow), varices (arrowhead) and superficial draining vein (open arrow). This shows the basic components but no information about direction of flow. (C–E) Series of three MR DSA frames in a lateral projection acquired at 1-second intervals during an IV infusion of gadolinium contrast medium. The left internal carotid artery dominates as blood shunts via it to the AVM. There are feeding middle cerebral artery branches (long arrows), the nidus (short arrow), varices (arrowhead) and a large superficial draining vein (open arrow) all apparent on the first frame, indicating the speed of shunting. Subsequent frames show opacification of transverse sinus (open arrow) and later superior sagittal sinus (white arrow in E). Note the detail of a small venous pouch on the main draining vein identical to the structural image (notched arrows on Figs 57.27A and 57.27E). This technique may in the future provide temporal and spatial resolution closer to that of DSA.

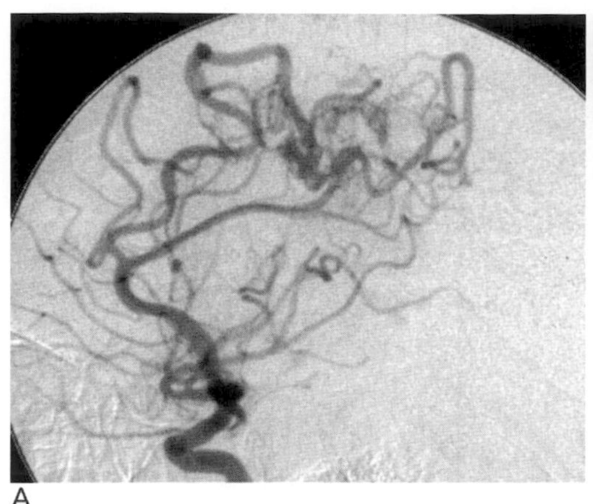
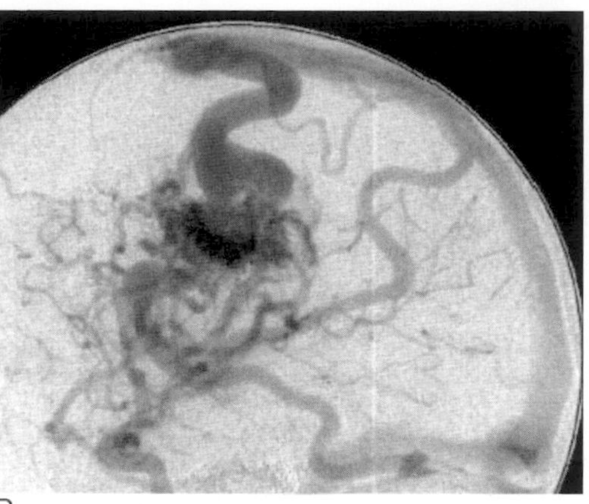

Figure 57.28 Cerebral AVM on DSA. (A) Arterial and (B) venous phase of DSA in a patient with a cerebral AVM. The AVM is fed by branches of the anterior and middle cerebral arteries and the venous drainage is predominantly superficial into the superior sagittal and transverse sinuses.

of haemorrhage in the presence of intranidal aneurysms, a single draining vein, deep venous drainage and venous stenoses[104,105]. CTA and MRA show the components of an AVM[94] but they currently lack the spatial resolution of intra-arterial angiography and do not produce sequential images necessary to judge transit time and direction of flow through the constituent vessels. In due course MR DSA may go some way to providing this information[101] (Fig. 57.27).

The treatment options for cerebral AVMs include surgery, radiosurgery and endovascular embolization. More than one technique may be used in combination.

Cavernous angiomas are mulberry-like lesions consisting of vascular spaces with little intervening tissue and haemorrhage of different ages. The incidence of clinically symptomatic haemorrhage remains uncertain, but is less frequent than with cerebral AVMs or dural fistulae. A previous bleed and infratentorial location are the main prognostic factors for recurrent haemorrhage. Lesions in or close to the cerebral cortex may cause epilepsy. They are occasionally intraventricular or arise on a cranial nerve. They appear as relatively well-defined, dense or calcified lesions on CT, which may show patchy contrast enhancement. On MRI they appear multilobular with mixed signal intensity centrally surrounded by a dark haemosiderin rim[106] (Fig. 57.29). Not surprisingly gradient-echo sequences are the most sensitive. They may be multiple, particularly in familial cases[107]. In many clinical situations the discovery of a cavernoma represents an incidental finding.

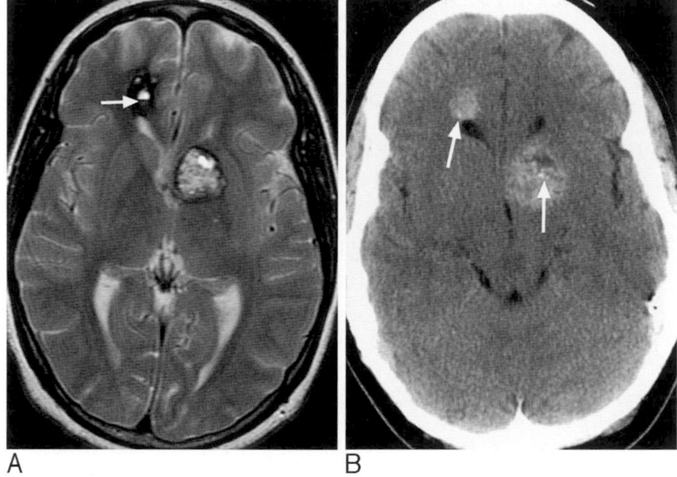

Figure 57.29 Cavernous haemangioma. (A) T2-weighted axial image showing typical mixed signal intensity lesions. High signal is due to methaemoglobin and the low signal intensity rim of haemosiderin indicates an old haemorrhage. The 'popcorn' appearance of the larger lesion is typical of a 'cavernoma'. Note the blood–fluid level in the smaller lesion (arrow). (B) Unenhanced CT of the same patients shows the lesions to be predominantly high density with tiny foci of calcification (arrows).

Developmental venous anomalies are not malformations but represent a benign variation in venous drainage. They may be found with cavernomas. They consist of radially arranged, dilated transmedullary veins that have a typical 'caput medusa' appearance on the venous phase of conventional angiograms (Fig. 57.30). They may drain into the superficial or deep venous system. They are readily diagnosed by contrast-enhanced CT or MRI[106].

Capillary telangiectasias are benign nests of dilated capillaries with normal brain tissue in between. They are usually found on postmortem examinations and are occasionally visible on MRI as areas of very subtle T2 hyperintensity or ill-defined enhancement. They do not cause haemorrhage.

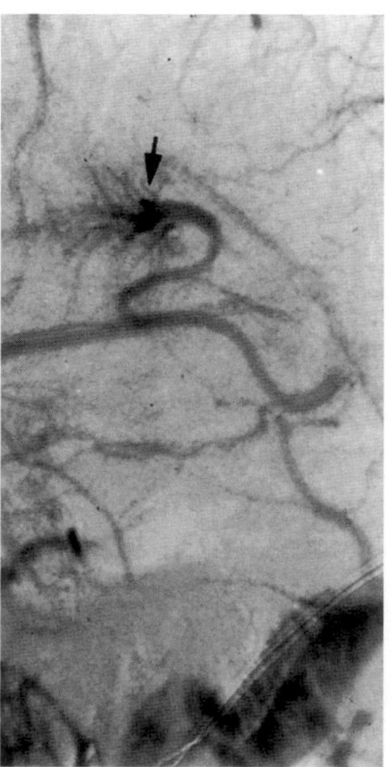

Figure 57.30 Developmental venous anomaly (DVA) (arrow) draining into a large thalamostriate vein. Internal carotid arteriogram, lateral projection, venous phase.

SUBDURAL AND EXTRADURAL HAEMORRHAGE

Acute subdural and extradural haematomas are almost always post-traumatic and are considered in Chapter 59.

Occasionally rupture of a cerebral aneurysm may cause an **acute subdural haematoma**, most frequently a posterior communicating artery aneurysm lying next to the free edge of the tentorium cerebelli. A dural arteriovenous fistula may also bleed into the subdural space. Angiography is therefore indicated following a spontaneous acute subdural haematoma.

Chronic subdural haematomas represent a different entity. These are frequently bilateral and occur in elderly patients or alcoholics with underlying brain atrophy, patients on anticoagulants or following shunting for hydrocephalus. The underlying mechanism is thought to be leakage from bridging cortical veins following minor trauma. They may present with increasing confusion and a reduction in conscious level. Burr holes for drainage of a chronic subdural collection, sometimes under a local anaesthetic, is one of the few neurosurgical operations performed on the very elderly.

On CT they appear to be of lower density than the brain but may contain areas of high density, or even fluid levels, due to more recent haemorrhage. The MRI appearance evolves in a similar pattern to intraparenchymal haemorrhage. Chronic subdural haematomas continue to give high signal on T2-weighted images, while returning low signal on T1-weighted images, without becoming isointense to CSF, because of their higher protein content. Repeated episodes of bleeding can produce variable changes of signal intensity (Fig. 57.31) analogous to the variable density changes on CT. A pseudomembrane, which forms around chronic subdural haematomas, may show marked contrast enhancement or haemosiderin staining.

Shallow subdural fluid collections and occasionally overt haemorrhage may also develop around the cerebral hemispheres and cerebellum secondary to mild brain descent in the low CSF volume syndrome[108]. In this condition patients usually present with postural headache that is worse on standing and relieved by lying down. There is sometimes a history of vigorous Valsalva, lumbar puncture or other spinal intervention. The MRI features, other than subdural collections, are diffuse dural thickening shown best on FLAIR or contrast-enhanced T1-weighted images and mild cerebellar ectopia. These changes resolve after successful treatment.

ACKNOWLEDGEMENT

Dr Andrew Carne (Department of Radiology, St George's Hospital, London UK) for his technical expertise during the preparation of images for this chapter.

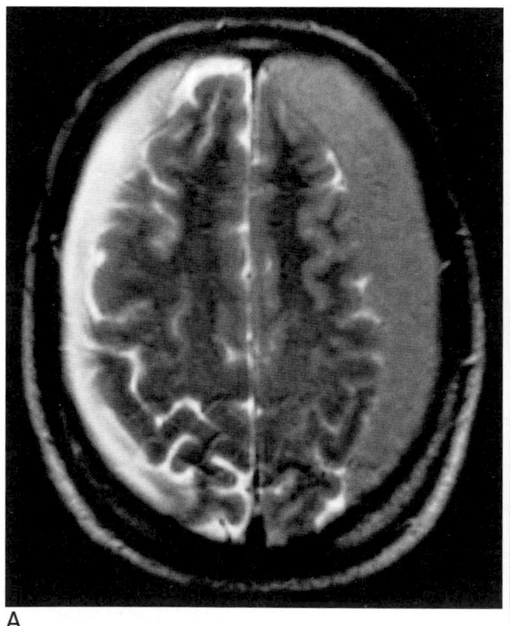
A

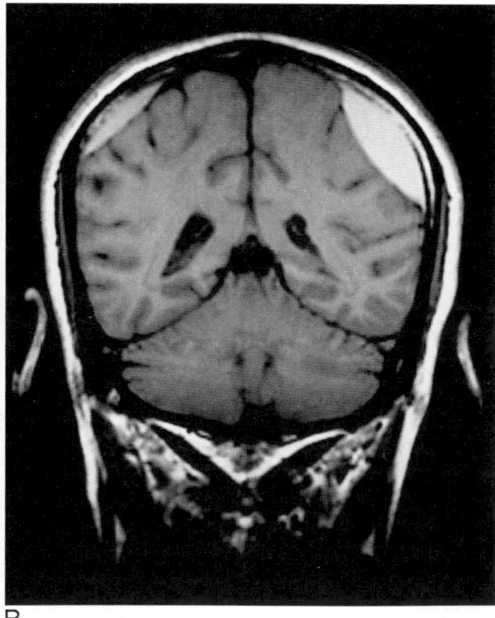
B

Figure 57.31 Subdural haematomas. (A) Axial T2-weighted and (B) coronal T1-weighted MRI of bilateral spontaneous subdural haematomas of different ages. The left-sided collection is a few days old (early subacute stage) and is of low signal on T2 weighting and high signal on T1 weighting. The right-sided collection is a few weeks old (late subacute stage) and appears of high signal on both sequences, but it appears less bright on the T1-weighted sequence than the more recent contralateral collection (see Table 57.1).

REFERENCES

1. Blight A, Pereira A C, Brown M M 2000 A single consultation cerebrovascular disease clinic is cost effective in the management of transient ischaemic attack and minor stroke. J R Coll Physicians Lond 34: 452–455
2. Bath P, Lees K 2000 Acute stroke. Br Med J 320: 920–992
3. Lovett J K, Dennis M S, Sandercock P A G et al 2003 Very early risk of stroke after a first transient ischemic attack. Stroke 34: e138–e140
4. Fairhead J F, Mehta Z, Rothwell P M 2005 Population-based study of delays in carotid imaging and surgery and the risk of recurrent stroke. Neurology 65: 371–375
5. Zimmerman R D 2004 Stroke wars: Episode IV. CT strikes back. AJNR Am J Neuroradiol 25: 1304–1309
6. Ueda T, Yuh W, Taoka T 1999 Clinical application of perfusion and diffusion MR imaging in acute ischemic stroke. J Magn Reson Imaging 10: 305–309
7. Markus H S 2004 Cerebral perfusion and stroke. J Neurol Neurosurg Psychiatry 75: 353–361

8. Halpin S F S 2004 Brain imaging using multislice CT: a personal perspective. Br J Radiol 77: 20–26
9. Liebeskind D S 2003 Collateral circulation. Stroke 34: 2279–2284
10. Caplan L R 1980 'Top of the basilar' syndrome. Neurology 30: 72–79
11. Barber P A, Demchuk A M, Hudon M E et al 2001 Hyperdense Sylvian fissure MCA 'dot' sign: a CT marker of acute ischemia. Stroke 32: 84–88
12. Toyoda K, Masahiro I, Fukuda K 2001 Fluid-attenuated inversion recovery intra-arterial signal: an early sign of hyperacute cerebral ischemia. AJNR Am J Neuroradiol 22:1021–1029
13. Karonen J O, Partanen P L K, Vanninen R L et al 2001 Evolution of MR contrast enhancement patterns during the first week after acute ischemic stroke. AJNR Am J Neuroradiol 22: 103–111
14. Mullins M E, Schaefer P W, Sorensen A G et al 2002 CT and conventional and diffusion-weighted MR imaging in acute stroke: study in 691 patients at presentation to the emergency department. Radiology 224: 353–360
15. Na D G, Kim E Y, Ryoo J W et al 2005 CT sign of brain swelling without concomitant parenchymal hypoattenuation: comparison with diffusion- and perfusion-weighted MR imaging. Radiology 235: 992–998
16. Kummer R, Meyding-Lamade U, Forsting M et al 1994 Sensitivity and prognostic value of early CT in occlusion of the middle cerebral artery trunk. AJNR Am J Neuroradiol 15: 9–15
17. Demchuk A M, Coutts S B 2005 Alberta stroke program early CT score in acute stroke triage. Neuroimag Clin N Am 15: 409–419
18. Bryan R N, Levy L M, Whitlow W D et al 1991 Diagnosis of acute cerebral infarction: comparison of CT and MR imaging. AJNR Am J Neuroradiol 12: 611–620
19. Hacke W, Kaste M, Fieschi C et al 1995 Intravenous thrombolysis with recombinant tissue plasminogen activator for acute hemispheric stroke. The European Cooperative Acute Stroke Study (ECASS). JAMA 274:1017–1025
20. Barber P A, Demchuk A M, Zhang J et al for the ASPECTS study group 2000 Hyperacute stroke: the validity and reliability of a novel quantitative CT score in predicting outcome prior to thrombolytic therapy. Lancet 355: 1670–1674
21. Barber P A, Hill M D, Eliasziw M et al 2005 Imaging of the brain in acute ischaemic stroke: comparison of computed tomography and magnetic resonance diffusion-weighted imaging. J Neurol Neurosurg Psychiatry 76:1528–1533
22. Coutts S B, Demchuk A M, Barber P A, et al 2004 Interobserver variation of ASPECTS in real time. Stroke 35: e103–e105
23. Liang L, Korogi Y, Sugahara T et al 1999 Detection of intracranial hemorrhage with susceptibility-weighted MR sequences. AJNR Am J Neuroradiol 20: 1527–1534
24. Fiebach J B, Schellinger P D, Gass A et al 2004 Stroke magnetic resonance imaging is accurate in hyperacute intracerebral haemorrhage: a multicenter study on the validity of stroke imaging. Stroke 35: 502–506
25. Kidwell C S, Chalela J A, Sayer J L et al 2004 Comparison of MRI and CT for detection of acute intracerebral haemorrhage. JAMA 292: 1823–1830
26. Mayer T E, Schuffe-Altedorneburg G, Droste D W et al 2000 Serial CT and MRI of ischaemic cerebral infarcts: frequency and clinical impact of haemorrhagic transformation. Neuroradiology 42: 233–239
27. Saunders D E, Howe F A, van den Boogart A et al 1995 Continuing ischaemic damage following acute middle cerebral artery infarction in man demonstrated by short echo proton spectroscopy. Stroke 26: 2272–2276
28. Wintermark M, Sesay M, Barbier E et al 2005 Comparative overview of brain perfusion imaging techniques. Stroke 36: e83–e99
29. Schellinger P D 2005 The evolving role of advanced MR imaging as a management tool for adult ischemic stroke: A Western-European perspective. Neuroimag Clin N Am 15: 245–258
30. Sobesky J, Weber O Z, Lehnhardt F-G et al 2004 Which time-to-peak threshold best identifies penumbral flow? A comparison of perfusion-weighted magnetic resonance imaging and positron emission tomography in acute ischemic stroke. Stroke 35: 2843–2847
31. Kim J H, Shin T, Chung J D et al 1998 Temporal pattern of blood volume change in cerebral infarction: evaluation with dynamic contrast-enhanced T2-weighted MR imaging. AJR Am J Roentgenol 170: 765–770
32. Guckel F J, Brix G, Schmiedek P et al 1996 Cerebrovascular reserve capacity in patients with occlusive cerebrovascular disease: assessment with dynamic susceptibility contrast-enhanced MR imaging and the acetazolamide stimulation test. Radiology 201: 405–412
33. Kuwabara Y, Ichiya Y, Sasaki M 1998 PET evaluation of cerebral hemodynamics in occlusive cerebrovascular disease pre- and postsurgery. J Nucl Med 39: 760–765
34. Sperling B, Lassen N 1999 Cerebral blood flow by SPECT in ischaemic stroke. In: Deyn P D, Diercks R, Alave A, Pickut B (eds) A Textbook of SPECT in Neurology and Psychiatry. John Libbey, London
35. Alexandrov A, Masdeu J, Devous S 1997 Brain single-photon emission CT with HMPAO and safety of thrombolytic therapy in acute ischemic stroke. Stroke 28: 1830–1834
36. Provenzale J, Sorensen G 1999 Diffusion-weighted MR imaging in acute stroke: theoretic considerations and clinical applications. AJR Am J Roentgenol 173: 1459–1467
37. Burdette J 1998 Cerebral infarction: time course of signal intensity changes on diffusion-weighted images. AJR Am J Roentgenol 171: 791–795
38. Geijer B, Lindgren A, Brockstedt S et al 2001 Persistent high signal on diffusion weighted MRI in the late stages of small cortical and lacunar ischaemic lesions. Neuroradiology 43: 115–122
39. Morita N, Harada M, Yoneda K et al 2002 A characteristic feature of acute haematomas in the brain on echo-planar diffusion-weighted imaging. Neuroradiology 44: 907–911
40. Schramm P, Schellinger P D, Klotz E et al 2004 Comparison of perfusion computed tomography and computed tomography angiography source images with perfusion-weighted imaging and diffusion-weighted imaging in patients with acute stroke of less than 6 hours' duration. Stroke 35: 1652–1657
41. Chen Z M, Sandercock P A G, Pan H C, et al, on behalf of the CAST and IST collaborative groups 2000 Indications for early aspirin use in acute ischaemic stroke. A combined analysis of 40,000 randomised patients from the Chinese Acute Stroke Trial and the International Stroke Trial. Stroke 31:1240–1249
42. Wardlaw J M 2002 Recent developments in imaging of stroke. Imaging 14: 409–419
43. Wardlaw J M, Farrell A J 2004 Editorial: Diagnosis of Stroke on Neuroimaging. Br Med J 328: 655–656
44. Cristomo R A, Garcia M M, Tong D C 2003 Detection of diffusion-weighted MRI abnormalities in patients with transient ischaemic attack. Stroke 34: 932–937
45. Yuh W, Ueda T, White M et al 1999 The need for objective assessment of the new imaging techniques and understanding the expanding roles of stroke imaging. AJNR Am J Neuroradiol 20: 1779–1784
46. Latchaw R 1999 The roles of diffusion and perfusion imaging in acute stroke management. AJNR Am J Neuroradiol 20: 957–959
47. Kidwell C S, Alger J R, Saver J L 2003 Beyond mismatch. Evolving paradigms in imaging the ischemic penumbra with multimodal magnetic resonance imaging. Stroke 34: 2729–2735
48. Winbeck K, Bruckmaier K, Etge T et al 2004 Transient ischemic attack and stroke can be differentiated by analyzing early diffusion-weighted imaging signal intensity changes. Stroke 35: 1095–1099
49. Liebeskind D S, Kidwell C S on behalf of UCLA thrombolysis investigators 2005 Advanced MR imaging of acute stroke: the University of California at Los Angeles endovascular therapy experience. Neuroimag Clin N Am 15: 455–466
50. National Institute of Neurological Disease and Stroke rt-PA Study Group 1995 Tissue plasminogen activator for acute ischaemic stroke. N Engl J Med 355; 1581–1587
51. Wardlaw J M, del Zoppo G, Yamaguchi T et al 2005 Thrombolysis for acute ischaemic stroke. The Cochrane Database of Systematic Reviews Issue 4
52. Longstreth W T, Manolio T A, Arnold A et al for the Cardiovascular Health Study Collaborative research group 1996 Clinical correlates of

white matter findings on cranial magnetic resonance imaging of 3301 elderly people. Stroke 27: 1274–1282

53. Murray A D, Staff R T, Shenkin S D et al 2005 Brain white matter hyperintensities: Relative importance of vascular risk factors in nondemented elderly people. Radiology 237: 251–257
54. O'Sullivan M, Rich P M, Barrick T R et al 2003 Frequency of subclinical lacunar infarcts in ischemic leukoaraiosis and CADASIL. AJNR Am J Neuroradiol 24: 1348–1354
55. Pomper M, Miller T, Stone H et al 1999 CNS vasculitis in autoimmune disease: MR imaging findings and correlation with angiography. AJNR Am J Neuroradiol 20: 75–85
56. Kwa V I, Franke C L, Verbeeten B Jr 1998 Silent intracerebral microhemorrhages in patients with ischemic stroke. Amsterdam Vascular Medicine Group. Ann Neurol 44: 372–377
57. Roob G, Schmidt R, Kapeller P et al 1999 MRI evidence of past cerebral microbleeds in a healthy elderly population. Neurology 52: 991–994
58. Lee S H, Kwon S J, Kim K S et al 2004 Cerebral microbleeds in patients with hypertensive stroke. Topographical distribution in the supratentorial area. J Neurol 251: 1183–1189
59. Lee S H, Kwon S J, Kim K S et al 2004 Topographical distribution of pontocerebellar microbleeds. AJNR Am J Neuroradiol 25: 1337–1341
60. Kakuda W, Thijs V N, Lansberg M G et al 2005 Clinical importance of microbleeds in patients receiving IV thrombolysis. Neurology 65: 1175–1178
61. Kidwell C S, Saver J L, Villablana J P et al 2002 Magnetic resonance imaging detection of microbleeds before thrombolysis. Stroke 33: 95–98
62. Ozsvath R R, Casey S O, Lustrin E S et al 1997 Cerebral venography: comparison of CT and MR projection venography. AJR Am J Roentgenol 169: 1699–1707
63. Caplan L R, Gorelick P B, Hier D B 1986 Race, sex and occlusive cerebrovascular disease: a review. Stroke 17: 648–655
64. North American Symptomatic Carotid Endarectomy trial collaborators 1991 Beneficial effect of carotid endarterectomy in symptomatic patients with high grade carotid stenosis. N Engl J Med 325: 445–453
65. European Carotid Surgery Trialists' collaborative group 1991 MRC European carotid surgery trial: interim results for symptomatic patients with severe (70–99%) or with mild (0–29%) carotid stenosis. Lancet 337: 1235–1243
66. Halliday A, Mansfield A, Marro J et al 2004 Prevention of disabling and fatal strokes by successful carotid endarterectomy in patients without recent neurological symptoms: randomised controlled trial. Lancet 363: 1491–1502
67. Chaturvedi S, Bruno A, Feasby T et al Carotid endarterectomy – An evidence based review. Neurology 65: 794–801
68. Executive Committee for the Asymptomatic Carotid Atherosclerosis (ACAS) Study 1995 Endarterectomy for asymptomatic carotid artery stenosis. JAMA 273: 1421–1428
69. Patel S G, Collie D A, Wardlaw J M et al 2002 Outcome, observer reliability, and patient preferences if CTA, MRA, or Doppler ultrasound were used, individually or together, instead of digital subtraction angiography before carotid endarterectomy. J Neurol Neurosurg Psychiatry 73: 21–28
70. Nonent M, Serfaty J-M, Nighoghossian N et al 2004 Concordance rate differences of 3 noninvasive imaging techniques to measure carotid stenosis in clinical routine practice: results of the CARMEDAS multicenter study. Stroke 35: 682–686
71. Cosottini M, Pingitore A, Puglioli M et al 2003 Contrast-enhanced three-dimensional magnetic resonance angiography of atherosclerotic internal carotid stenosis as the noninvasive imaging modality in revascularization decision making. Stroke 34: 660–664
72. Yang C W, Carr J C, Futterer S F et al 2005 Contrast-enhanced MR angiography of the carotid and vertebrobasilar circulations. AJNR Am J Neuroradiol 26: 2095–2101
73. Chen C-J, Tseng Y-C, Lee T-H et al 2004 Multisection CT angiography compared with catheter angiography in diagnosing vertebral artery dissection. AJNR Am J Neuroradiol 25: 769–774
74. Fayad Z A, Guest editor 2002 Imaging of atherosclerosis. Neuroimaging Clinics of North America 12(3)
75. Barkovich A J 2005 Pediatric Neuroimaging, 4th edn. Lippincott Williams & Wilkins, USA p. 906
76. Rinkel G J, Wijdicks E F, Hasan D et al 1991 Outcome in patients with subarachnoid haemorrhage and negative angiography according to pattern of haemorrhage on computed tomography. Lancet 338: 964–968
77. van der Schaaf I C, Velthius B K, Gouw A et al 2004 Venous drainage in perimesencephalic haemorrhage. Stroke 35:1614–1618
78. van der Wee N, Rinkel G J, Hasan D et al 1995 Detection of subarachnoid haemorrhage on early CT: is lumbar puncture still needed after a negative scan? J Neurol Neurosurg Psychiatry 58: 357–359
79. Adams Jr H P, Kassell N F, Torner J C et al 1983 CT and clinical correlations in recent aneurysmal subarachnoid hemorrhage: a preliminary report of the Cooperative Aneurysm Study. Neurology 33: 981–988
80. Mitchell P, Wilkinson I D, Hoggard N et al 2001 Detection of subarachnoid haemorrhage with magnetic resonance imaging. J Neurol Neurosurg Psychiatry 70: 205–211
81. Mohamed M, Heasely D C, Yagmurlu B et al 2004 Fluid-attenuated inversion recovery MR imaging and subarachnoid hemorrhage: Not a panacea. AJNR Am J Neuroradiol 25: 545–550
82. Noguchi K, Ogawa T, Seto H, et al 1997 Subacute and chronic subarachnoid hemorrhage: diagnosis with fluid-attenuated inversion-recovery MR imaging. Radiology 203: 257–262
83. Deliganis A V, Fisher D J, Lam A M et al 2001 Cerebrospinal fluid signal intensity increase on FLAIR MR images in patients under general anesthesia: the role of supplemental O_2. Radiology 218: 152–156
84. Dechambre S D, Duprez T, Grandin C B et al 2000 High signal in cerebrospinal fluid mimicking subarachnoid haemorrhage on FLAIR following acute stroke and intravenous contrast medium. Neuroradiology 42: 608–611
85. Kassell N F, Sasaki T, Colohan A R T et al 1985 Cerebral vasospasm following aneurysmal subarachnoid hemorrhage. Stroke 16: 562–572
86. Osborn A G 1999 Diagnostic cerebral angiography, 2nd edn. Lippincott Williams & Wilkins, Washington, p. 462
87. Wiebers D O, Whisnant J P, Huston J 3rd et al 2003 International Study of Unruptured Intracranial Aneurysms Investigators. Unruptured intracranial aneurysms: natural history, clinical outcome and risks of surgical and endovascular treatment. Lancet 362:103–110
88. Vindlacheruvu R R, Mendelow A D, Mitchell P 2005 Risk-benefit analysis of the treatment of unruptured intracranial aneurysms. J Neurol Neurosurg Psychiatry 76: 234–239
89. Villablanca J P, Jahan R, Hooshi P et al 2002 Detection and characterisation of very small cerebral aneurysms by using 2D and 3D helical CT angiography. AJNR Am J Neuroradiol 23: 1187–1198
90. Hoh B L, Cheung A C, Rabinov J D et al 2004 Results of a prospective protocol of computed tomographic angiography in place of catheter angiography as the only diagnostic and pretreatment planning study for cerebral aneurysms by a combined neurovascular team. Neurosurgery 54: 1329–1340
91. Huston J, Nichols D A, Luetmer P H et al 1994 Blinded prospective evaluation of sensitivity of MR angiography to known intracranial aneurysms: importance of aneurysm size. AJNR Am J Neuroradiol 15: 1607–1614
92. Atlas S, Sheppard L, Goldberg H I et al 1997 Intracranial aneurysms: detection and characterization with MR angiography with use of an advanced postprocessing technique in a blinded-reader study. Radiology 203: 807–814
93. Ida M, Kurisu Y, Yamashita M 1997 MR angiography of ruptured aneurysms in acute subarachnoid hemorrhage. AJNR Am J Neuroradiol 18: 1025–1032
94. Jager H R, Grieve J P 2000 Advances in non-invasive imaging of intracranial vascular disease. Ann R Coll Surg Engl 82:1–5
95. Ruigrok Y M, Rinkel G J, Buskens E et al 2000 Perimesencephalic hemorrhage and CT angiography: A decision analysis. Stroke 31: 2976–2983

96. Molyneux A J, Kerr R S C, Yu L-M et al 2005 International subarachnoid aneurysm trial (ISAT) of neurosurgical clipping versus endovascular coiling in 2143 patients with ruptured intracranial aneurysms: a randomised comparison of effects on survival, dependency, seizures, rebleeding, subgroups, and aneurysm occlusion. Lancet 366: 809–817
97. Greenberg S M 1998 Cerebral amyloid angiopathy: prospects for clinical diagnosis and treatment. Neurology 51: 690–694
98. McEvoy A, Kitchen N, Thomas D 2000 Intracerebral haemorrhage in young adults: the emerging importance of drug abuse. Br Med J 320: 1322–1324
99. Gaskill-Shipley M 1999 Routine CT evaluation of acute stroke. Neuroimaging Clin North Am 9: 411–422
100. Bradley W G Jr 1994 Hemorrhage and hemorrhagic infections in the brain. Neuroimaging Clin North Am 4: 707–732
101. Coley S C, Romanowski C A J, Hodgson T J et al 2002 Dural arteriovenous fistulae: non-invasive diagnosis with dynamic MR digital subtraction angiography. AJNR Am J Neuroradiol 23: 404–407
102. Valavanis A 1996 The role of angiography in the evaluation of cerebral vascular malformations. Neuroimaging Clin North Am 6: 679–704
103. Rodesch G, Lasjaunias P 1992 Physiopathology and semeiology of dural arteriovenous shunts. Rivista di Neuroradiologia 5: 11–21
104. Meisel H J, Mansmann U, Alvarez H et al 2000 Cerebral arteriovenous malformations and associated aneurysms: analysis of 305 cases from a series of 662 patients. Neurosurgery 46: 793–800
105. Mast H, Young W L, Koennecke H C et al 1997 Risk of spontaneous hemorrhage after diagnosis of cerebral arteriovenous malformation. Lancet 350: 1065–1068
106. Wilms G, Demaerel P, Bosmans H et al 1999 MRI of non-ischemic vascular disease: aneurysms and vascular malformations. Eur Radiol 9: 1055–1060
107. Brunereau L, Labauge P, Tournier-Lasserve E et al 2000 Familial form of intracranial cavernous angioma: MR imaging findings in 51 families. Radiology 214: 209–216
108. Goadsby P J, Boes C 2002 New daily persistent headache. J Neurol Neurosurg Psychiatry 72 (suppl 2): ii6–ii9

CHAPTER 58

Cranial and Intracranial Disease: Infections, AIDS, Inflammatory, Demyelinating and Metabolic Diseases

Daniel J. Scoffings and John M. Stevens

INTRACRANIAL INFECTIONS

Intracranial infections take the following forms:

- **Cerebritis**: focal, usually pyogenic infection, without a capsule or pus formation
- **Abscess**: a focal, encapsulated, pus-containing cavity
- **Empyema**: an abscess that forms in an enclosed space (or potential space), e.g. sub- or extradural
- **Granuloma**: a focal, more or less encapsulated, inflammatory lesion, usually chronic, without pus formation
- **Encephalitis**: direct infection of the brain, usually viral and often diffuse
- **Meningitis**: infection of the meninges, which may be suppurative or granulomatous
- **Osteomyelitis** of the skull may also occur; infections of the paranasal sinuses are discussed elsewhere.

BRAIN ABSCESS

In immunocompetent patients most brain abscesses are bacterial, streptococci accounting for the majority. In 20–40 per cent no causative organism is identified. Brain abscesses arise by haematogenous dissemination, penetrating trauma or direct spread from contiguous infection. The site of an abscess depends on its cause; frontal sinusitis will result in an abscess in or beneath the adjacent frontal lobe, whilst mastoiditis will give rise to a temporal lobe or cerebellar lesion. Blood-borne infection can occur anywhere in the brain, but has a predilection for the territory of the middle cerebral arteries, particularly the frontoparietal region. A thorough search for a predisposing factor should be made; a cardiac cause is frequently overlooked (occult endocarditis and septal defects). Abscesses are frequently subcortical or periventricular. Four stages of development are described: early and late cerebritis and early and late capsule formation. Patients present with fever (in 50 per cent), headache and focal neurological deficits. Brain abscesses are multiple in 10–50 per cent[1].

On computed tomography (CT), cerebritis appears as ill-defined low attenuation and shows thick ring enhancement that may progress centrally on delayed images. With capsule formation the abscess shows central low attenuation, because of pus or necrotic debris and a rim of slightly higher attenuation surrounded by low attenuation vasogenic oedema. After contrast medium, a ring of enhancement corresponds to the capsule. The enhancing rim typically has a smooth inner margin and shows thinning of its medial aspect[2] (Fig. 58.1). In comparison to cerebritis, the centre of the abscess never enhances on delayed images. The degree of enhancement is diminished in patients who are immunocompromised or are on corticosteroid therapy[3]. Abscesses rarely contain gas, most often caused by surgical intervention or communication with a cranial air-space, rarely because of a gas-forming organism.

On magnetic resonance imaging (MRI), the signal of the abscess centre is between that of cerebrospinal fluid (CSF) and white matter on T1-weighted (T1W) images, and iso- or slightly hyperintense to CSF on T2-weighted (T2W) images. On T2W images the abscess rim is relatively hypointense; it may be slightly hyperintense to white matter on T1W images[4]. The pattern of rim enhancement is similar to that shown by CT. Surrounding vasogenic oedema is of low signal on T1W and high signal on T2W images. The abscess centre is high signal on diffusion-weighted imaging (DWI) and low signal on maps of apparent diffusion coefficient (ADC), because of restricted diffusion in the viscous pus[5] (Fig. 58.2).

Though typical, the appearance of a brain abscess as a rim-enhancing mass is nonspecific and may be mimicked by

Figure 58.1 Cerebral abscess. CT: Low attenuation central abscess cavity surrounded by an enhancing rim and white matter vasogenic oedema. The medial aspect of the enhancing rim is subtly thinned.

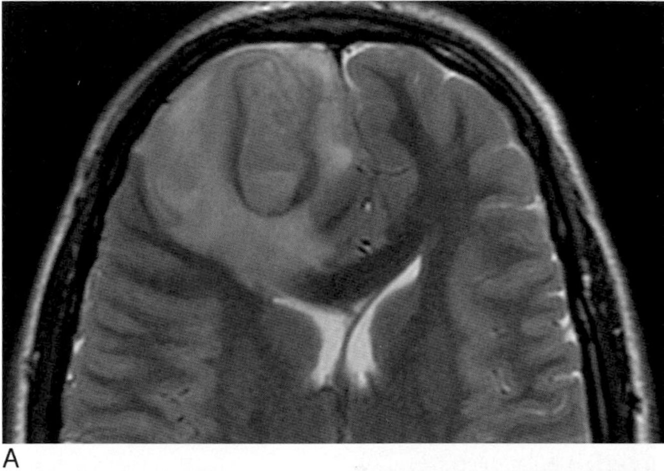

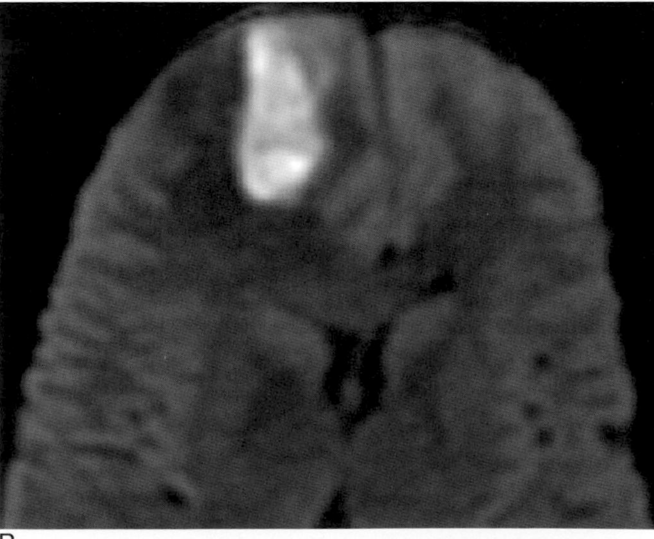

Figure 58.2 Streptococcal abscess due to penetrating trauma. MRI. (A) Axial T2W fast spin-echo image. Note low signal of the abscess capsule and extensive high signal perilesional oedema. (B) Diffusion-weighted image shows high signal in the abscess centre, indicating restricted diffusion.

metastasis, glioblastoma, resolving haematoma or subacute infarct. A thick, irregular rind of enhancement is more suggestive of tumour. Abscesses are more likely to show small satellite lesions. Despite initial hopes that restricted diffusion would reliably distinguish abscess from tumour, reduced ADC has been subsequently reported in metastases and glioblastomas. Dynamic contrast-enhanced perfusion MRI may help distinguish between brain abscess and tumour; abscesses have a lower relative cerebral blood volume in their enhancing rim than gliomas[6].

The management of brain abscesses can require both medical and neurosurgical therapy. CT diagnosis has been responsible for a marked reduction in the mortality of brain abscesses. Follow-up imaging is recommended at biweekly intervals or when new symptoms arise. Sufficient treatment is indicated by resolution of rim enhancement or disappearance of the low signal rim on T2W images. Treatment response may be better assessed with DWI than conventional MRI; low signal on DWI correlates with a good clinical response whilst increasing signal implies reaccumulation of pus[5].

Fungal cerebral abscesses are seen most typically in immunocompromised patients. They are radiologically similar to pyogenic abscesses (Fig. 58.3) but more likely to show areas of haemorrhage.

INTRACRANIAL EMPYEMA

Intracranial empyema is usuaully caused by spread of infection from the paranasal sinuses or ears. Trauma, meningitis and complications of intracranial shunts are additional causes. Empyemas are more often subdural than extradural, but both may coexist[7]. An empyema may accompany a cerebral abscess and, if unrecognized, delay response to treatment.

CT typically shows a thin fluid collection, slightly denser than CSF, overlying a convexity or in the interhemispheric fissure. Enhancement of the margin of the empyema is characteristic; IV contrast medium is therefore recommended when this diagnosis is suspected. MRI is more sensitive, showing an extracerebral lesion with prolonged T1 and T2. Contrast enhancement may be considerable. Empyemas tend to be loculated, multiple or complex (Fig. 58.4).

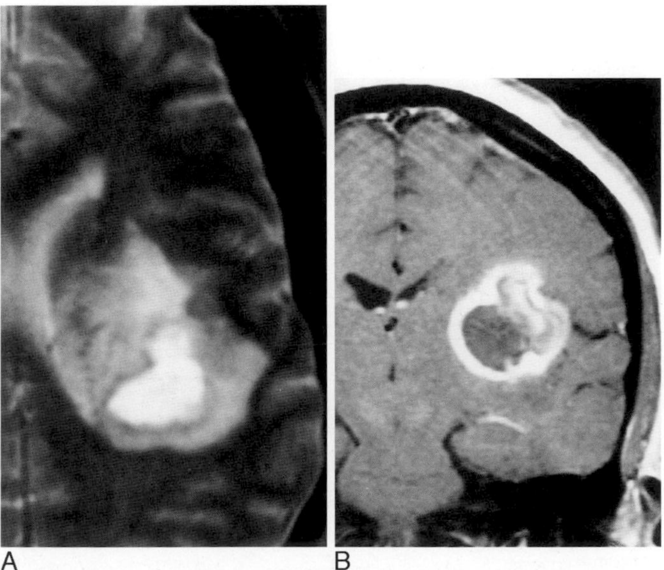

Figure 58.3 Fungal abscess in a 48-year-old diabetic patient. MRI. (A) Axial T2W image. Central high-signal abscess cavity with surrounding vasogenic oedema. (B) Coronal post-gadolinium T1W image. Large multiloculated abscess cavity with enhancement of the capsule and abscess wall. Note relative thinness of the medial wall compared with the thicker, more irregular, lateral component. Mild mass effect is evident.

VENTRICULITIS

Ventriculitis is uncommon. Causes include trauma, intraventricular rupture of an abscess, shunt infection and haematogenous spread of infection to the ependyma or choroid plexus. On MRI (Fig. 58.5) the most frequent finding is intraventricular debris, seen as increased signal on fluid-attenuated inversion recovery (FLAIR) and DWI sequences. Periventricular and subependymal high signal and enhancement of the ventricular margins are less common[8].

TUBERCULOSIS

Involvement of the central nervous system occurs in 5 per cent of cases of tuberculosis, and is especially common in patients younger than 20 years. The chest radiograph is abnormal in 45–60 per cent[1]. Tuberculous meningitis is the most frequent manifestation and tends to involve the basal leptomeninges. CT shows obliteration of the basal cisterns by isodense or slightly hyperdense exudate, which shows diffuse enhancement with IV contrast medium. The most useful CT criteria of abnormal basal meningeal enhancement are: (A) linear enhancement of the middle cerebral artery cisterns; (B) obliteration by contrast of the CSF spaces around normal vascular enhancement; (C) Y-shaped enhancement at the junction of the suprasellar and middle cerebral artery cisterns and (D) asymmetry of enhancement[9]. The meningeal exudate obstructs CSF resorption and causes communicating hydrocephalus; this is seen in 50 per cent of adults and 85 per cent of children[1]. Infarctions of the basal ganglia and internal capsules can occur, caused by an arteritis of the penetrating arteries at the base of the brain. With healing, meningeal calcification may rarely be seen.

MRI (Fig. 58.6) depicts the basal meningeal enhancement, hydrocephalus and basal ganglia infarcts with greater sensitivity than CT. The differential diagnosis includes fungal meningitis, sarcoid and carcinomatous meningitis.

Tuberculomas (parenchymal granulomas) occur most often at the corticomedullary junction. On CT they appear as small, rounded lesions isodense or hypodense to brain, with variable amounts of surrounding oedema. Enhancement is homogeneous when lesions are solid and shows rim enhancement when central caseation or liquefaction occurs. The 'target sign' of central high attenuation with rim enhancement is not pathognomonic for tuberculoma. On MRI small tuberculomas show prolonged T1 and T2; caseation results in low signal on

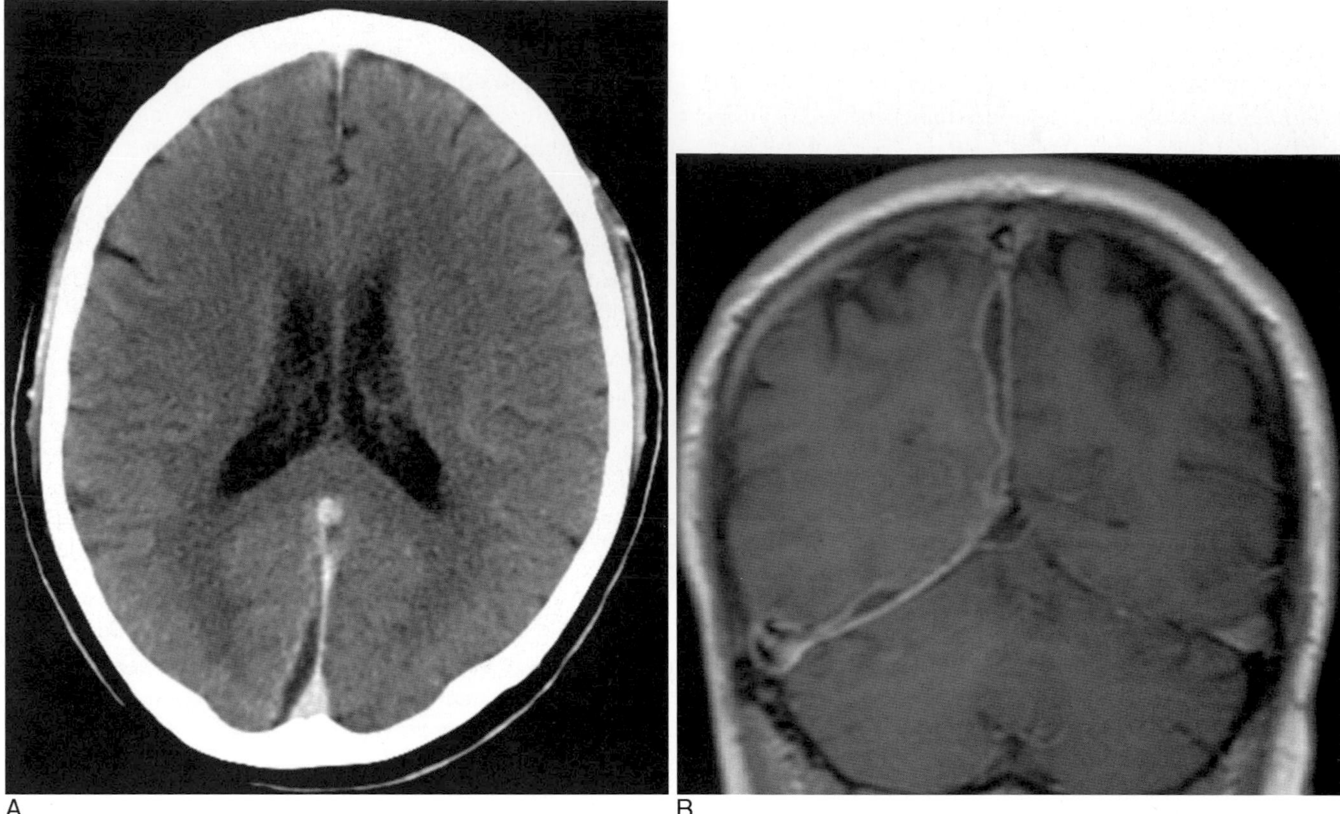

Figure 58.4 Subdural empyema. (A) Axial contrast-enhanced CT shows a low attenuation subdural fluid collection abutting the posterior falx with peripheral enhancement. (B) Coronal T1W post-gadolinium MRI shows the empyema is loculated and also extends along the right tentorial leaflet.

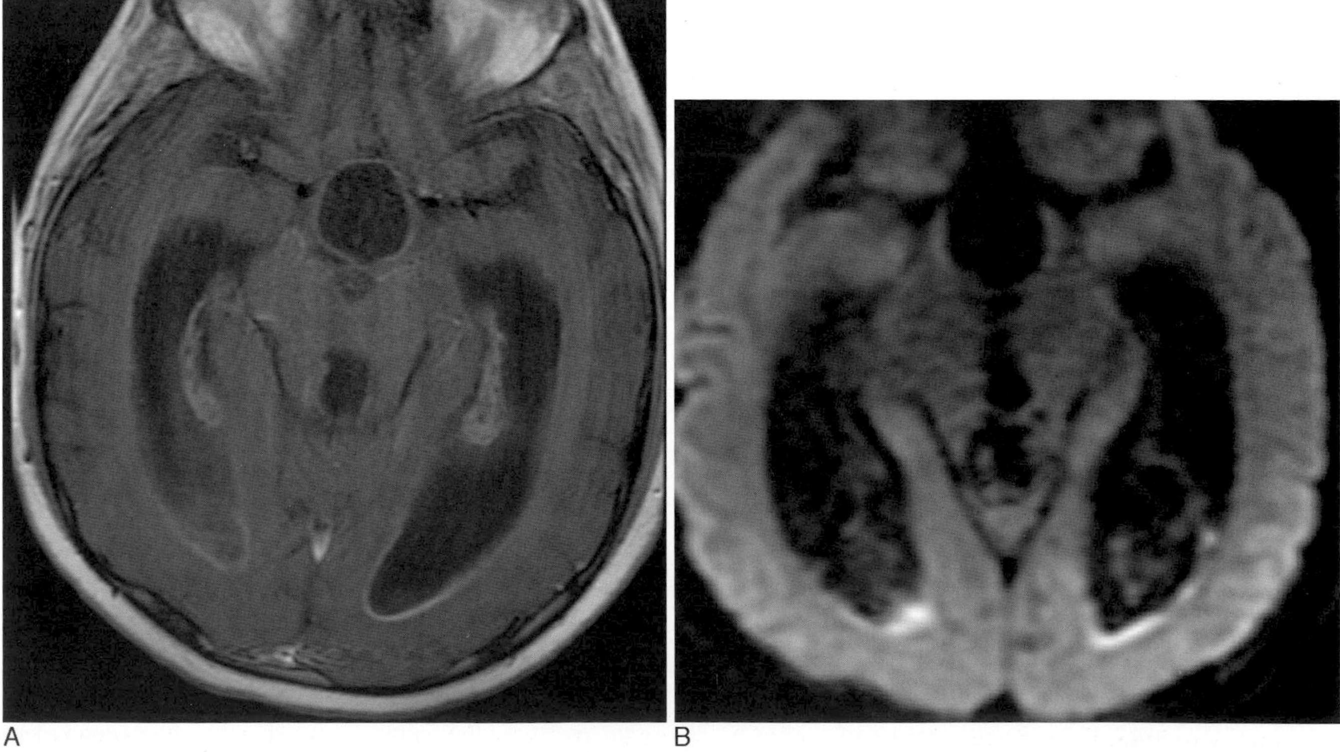

Figure 58.5 Ventriculitis: MRI. (A) Subependymal enhancement, most marked posteriorly, extends along the margins of the dilated ventricles. (B) Diffusion-weighted image shows restricted diffusion as high signal.

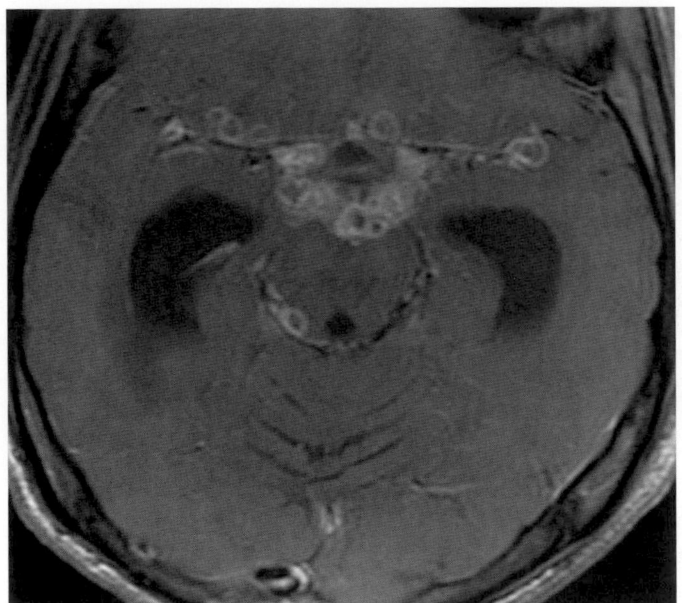

Figure 58.6 Tuberculous meningitis. Contrast-enhanced T1W MRI shows basilar meningeal enhancement, and multiple ring-enhancing tuberculomas in the suprasellar and ambient cisterns and the medial Sylvian fissures. Marked dilatation of the temporal horns indicates hydrocephalus.

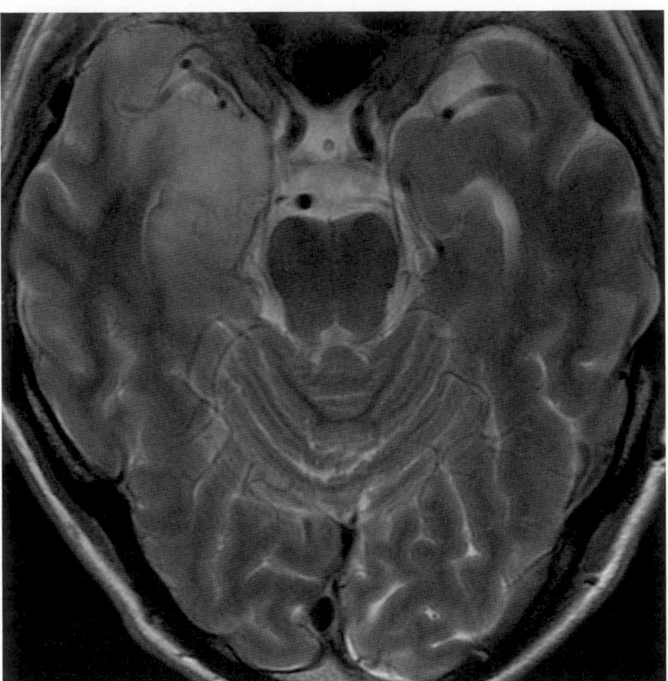

Figure 58.7 Herpes simplex encephalitis. Axial T2W MRI shows swelling and high signal in the anteromedial right temporal lobe with normal appearance on the left.

T2W images. Tuberculomas may calcify when healed, but, as with meningeal disease, this is uncommon.

Tuberculous abscesses are uncommon; they may resemble tuberculomas but are usually larger with a thinner enhancing rim[10].

ENCEPHALITIS

Most encephalitides are caused by diffuse inflammation of the brain parenchyma by viral infection. Other causes include tick-borne bacterial infection, post-infectious autoimmune disorders and paraneoplastic limbic encephalitis.

Herpes encephalitis

Herpes simplex type 1 is the most frequent cause of viral encephalitis (Fig. 58.7) in adults and is often fatal without treatment. It results from reactivation of latent infection in the trigeminal ganglion, or re-infection by the olfactory route. CT appears normal in the first 3–5 days after onset before showing low attenuation in the antero-medial temporal lobe, with or without involvement of the insula and orbital surface of the frontal lobe. Haemorrhage is seen as a late feature and not usually a prominent finding. Enhancement may be patchy or gyriform. MRI is more sensitive; T2W and FLAIR sequences show high signal within 2 d of onset[11]. The abnormal signal is mainly cortical, with secondary involvement of the subjacent white matter. MRI is also more sensitive than CT to haemorrhagic foci. DWI shows cortical hyperintensity with greater sensitivity than conventional MRI[12]. Cerebral blood flow, measured by perfusion CT or SPECT, is increased in the acute phase[13].

Neonatal herpes simplex encephalitis is caused by intrapartum infection with herpes simplex virus type 2. Imaging shows patchy white matter oedema and cortical areas of increased density on CT and low signal on T2W MRI. Lesions progress to areas of multicystic encephalomalacia.

Acute disseminated encephalomyelitis

Acute disseminated encephalomyelitis (ADEM) is a monophasic demyelinating disorder that occurs after vaccination or a viral illness. It has a fulminant course, results in encephalopathy and focal neurological deficits, and usually resolves without long-term sequelae. MRI typically shows multiple, large, irregular T2-hyperintense lesions in the subcortical white matter, cerebellum or brainstem[14]. Lesion enhancement is variable. Lesions of the thalamus, basal ganglia and spinal cord occur infrequently.

Acute haemorrhagic leukoencephalopathy

This aggressive variant of ADEM is frequently fatal within 1 week of onset. Appearances are similar to ADEM but with more oedema and mass effect, and small haemorrhages[15].

Subacute sclerosing panencephalitis

Usually caused by the measles virus, this process characteristically produces cerebral atrophy in addition to low CT attenuation and increased MRI relaxation times in the white matter[16]. However, the diagnosis is made from clinical and electroencephalogram (EEG) features rather than radiologically.

MENINGITIS

CT is usually normal in uncomplicated pyogenic meningitis, but it is useful for detecting complications such as hydrocephalus, subdural effusion, abscess or cerebral infarction. MRI may show sulcal high signal on FLAIR images but this is nonspecific and is also seen with subarachnoid haemorrhage and leptomeningeal metastases[17]. Meningeal enhancement is more sensitive; contrast-enhanced FLAIR may be better than contrast-enhanced T1W imaging in its depiction[18].

PARASITIC INFESTATIONS

Neurocysticercosis has varied imaging appearances depending on the developmental stage of the larva. Four stages are recognized and lesions in different stages may be seen concurrently. Cysticerci are ovoid cysts that contain an invaginated larval head, or scolex. Intracranial cysticerci are most frequent at the corticomedullary junction; intraventricular and racemose subarachnoid lesions also occur. In the vesicular stage the parasite is alive and incites little or no perilesional oedema. The cyst is isointense to CSF, the scolex isointense to white matter (Fig. 58.8). Enhancement is minimal or absent. In the colloidal vesicular stage the larva dies and lesions show ring enhancement with surrounding oedema. Cyst retraction in the granular nodular stage results in small enhancing nodules with mild oedema. Finally, in the nodular calcified stage, the lesions calcify. Subarachnoid cysticerci, which usually lack a scolex, may cause obstructive hydrocephalus[19].

Hydatid cysts are most often solitary and found in the middle cerebral artery territory. CT and MRI show a well-defined spherical lesion with the attenuation and signal characteristics of CSF. The cyst wall is hypointense on T2W images. Enhancement and perilesional oedema are seen only if the cyst is superinfected. Fewer than 1 per cent of cysts calcify[20].

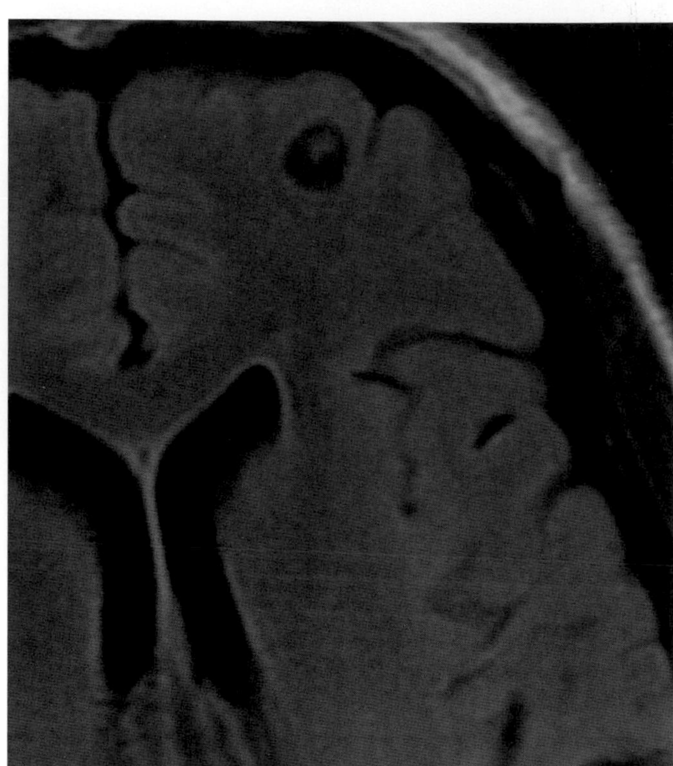

Figure 58.8 Cysticercosis: Axial FLAIR image shows a left frontal lobe cysticercus in the vesicular stage. Note the scolex surrounded by cyst fluid isointense to CSF. There is no perilesional oedema.

HIV INFECTION AND AIDS

After the lung, the central nervous system (CNS) is the organ most frequently affected by the human immunodeficiency virus (HIV). Postmortem studies show CNS abnormalities in up to 70 per cent of acquired immune deficiency syndrome (AIDS) patients. Neurological symptoms in HIV infection and AIDS occur because of opportunistic infections, the effects of HIV itself, and adverse effects of therapy. Highly active antiretroviral therapy (HAART) has decreased both mortality rates and the incidence of opportunistic infections in HIV-infected patients. Initial symptoms may be nonspecific and neurological signs difficult to elicit. Serology is often unhelpful because many opportunistic infections are reactivations of previous infections and the patient may not mount an immune response. Neuroimaging is thus a fundamental part of the assessment of HIV-infected patients with suspected CNS disease.

Asymptomatic HIV-infected patients have MRI abnormalities in only 20 per cent[21]. Abnormalities are increasingly common with significant immune suppression, in the later stages of disease and as patients live longer.

Diseases affecting the CNS that have been described in HIV infection and AIDS are listed in Table 58.1, roughly grouped according to the likelihood of encountering such cases in radiological practice. This may be modified according to the HIV risk group of the patient: for example, CNS tuberculosis is most often seen in those with a history of IV drug misuse.

MRI is more sensitive than CT in evaluating HIV-infected patients with suspected CNS disease, and as such is the imaging investigation of choice. Small lesions, and cortical or subcortical lesions, are shown with greater sensitivity by FLAIR than T2W images[22]. Whilst IV contrast medium improves the characterization of lesions, it infrequently reveals lesions that are not visible on unenhanced images and the clinical value of its routine use is unproven[23].

The commonest AIDS-related diseases seen on MRI may be classified according to simple radiological patterns (Table 58.2). The following text will discuss in more detail the typical and atypical manifestations of the more common CNS diseases.

HIV ENCEPHALOPATHY

HIV-associated cognitive-motor complex (also termed HIV encephalopathy, HIV-associated dementia or AIDS dementia complex) presents with cognitive impairment, behavioural change and motor symptoms. The clinical picture is of a subcortical dementia with slowness, forgetfulness and apathy. The prevalence of HIV encephalopathy is 10–20 per cent of AIDS

Table 58.1 CNS DISEASE IN HIV INFECTION/AIDS

Commonest	Less common	Rarest reported
HIV encephalopathy	Mycobacterial (TB/MAC)	Syphilis
Toxoplasmosis	*Candida*	*Nocardia**
Primary lymphoma	Cytomegalovirus	Histoplasmosis*
PML	Herpes simplex	Aspergillosis
Cryptococcosis	Varicella zoster	Mucormycosis
	Infarcts	Coccidioidomycosis
	Metastatic lymphoma	Amoebiasis
		Trypanosomiasis
		Protothecosis
		Measles
		Adenovirus
		Kaposi's sarcoma
		Metastatic carcinoma
		Metabolic encephalopathy

*Higher incidences in North America

cases and is rising as patients live longer. The incidence has halved since the introduction of HAART.

Multinucleate giant cells and microglial nodules characterize HIV encephalitis, the pathological correlate of HIV encephalopathy. Myelin loss, macrophage infiltration and gliosis are also seen. HIV encephalitis occurs because of cerebral infection with HIV.

The commonest imaging finding in HIV encephalopathy is cerebral atrophy, the extent of volume loss correlates with cognitive impairment[24]. White matter lesions in the centrum semiovale and periventricular regions are the next most frequent abnormality. These appear as areas of low attenuation on CT, and T2-prolongation on MRI, which lack mass effect and do not enhance[25]. The white matter changes tend to progress with time, becoming diffuse and confluent. Atrophy and white matter lesions can coexist or occur independently of one another (Fig. 58.9).

MR spectroscopy (MRS) shows decreased N-acetyl aspartate (NAA), reflecting neuronal loss, increased choline, a marker of membrane turnover, and increased myoinositol, a glial cell marker. These abnormalities can be detected in patients with normal MRI. Cognitively normal HIV-infected patients may also show increased choline and myoinositol, but little or no change in NAA. The spectroscopic abnormalities can reverse with HAART[26].

PET and SPECT may show hypermetabolism in the basal ganglia and thalami in patients with a normal MRI; these abnormalities correlate with neuropsychiatric measures of dementia. In advanced disease cortical hypometabolism is seen. Although the sensitivity of these techniques is high, the specificity is undetermined and the role in clinical practice is not established.

Diffusion tensor MR imaging (DTI) shows reduced whole-brain fractional anisotropy (FA) in cognitively impaired HIV-infected patients. The reduction in FA correlates with the severity of cognitive impairment[27].

Patients receiving HAART may show stabilization or even regression of MRI abnormalities. Early follow-up imaging may show lesion progression but this is not indicative of treatment failure[28].

Table 58.2 COMMON TYPICAL MRI PATTERNS IN HIV-RELATED CNS DISEASE

Focal parenchymal
+mass +enhancement
Toxoplasmosis
Lymphoma
Tuberculosis
Candida
Others—histoplasmosis, aspergillosis, coccidioidomycosis
+mass −enhancement
Cryptococcomas
−mass +enhancement
Diffuse toxoplasmosis
Viral encephalitides—HSV, CMV
Infarcts—± VZV arteritis
−mass −enhancement
PML
Diffuse parenchymal
HIV encephalopathy
Meningitis/meningeal disease
HIV meningo-encephalitis
Cryptococcosis
Metastatic lymphoma
Viral meningitis
Ventriculitis
CMV necrotizing ventriculitis
Basal ganglia
+mass
Toxoplasmosis
Cryptococcosis
−mass
Metabolic encephalopathy
White-matter disease
Small nonspecific focal white-matter hyperintensities on T2W
HIV encephalopathy
PML
Viral encephalitis—CMV
Myelopathy
CMV
VZV
Vacuolar myelopathy

CMV = cytomegalovirus; VZV = Varicella zoster virus; HSV = Herpes simplex virus.

CEREBRAL TOXOPLASMOSIS

Toxoplasmosis is the commonest cause of a cerebral mass lesion in AIDS and also the most treatable. It results from reactivation of latent infection by *Toxoplasma gondii*, for which the definitive host is the cat. Patients present subacutely with headache, fever, confusion, personality change and focal

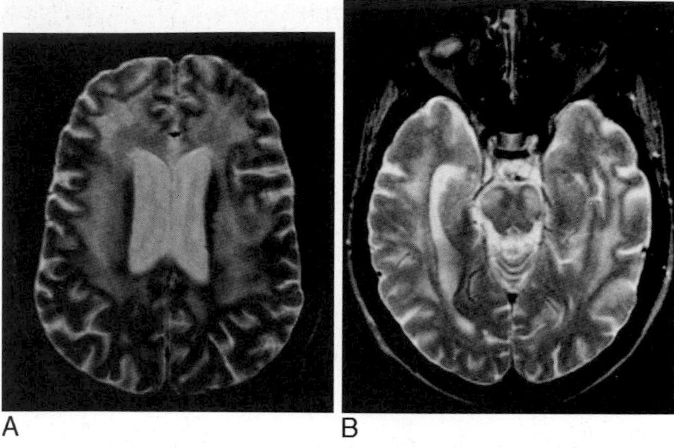

Figure 58.9 Advanced HIV encephalopathy. Axial T2W image. There is diffuse confluent and symmetrical abnormal high signal returned from the white matter of the cerebral hemispheres (A), which is also extending into the brainstem to involve the cerebral peduncles (B). In this patient there is also generalized atrophy. Features that help to differentiate HIV from PML are the symmetry of the changes and the lack of signal abnormalities on T1W images (cf. Fig. 58.17).

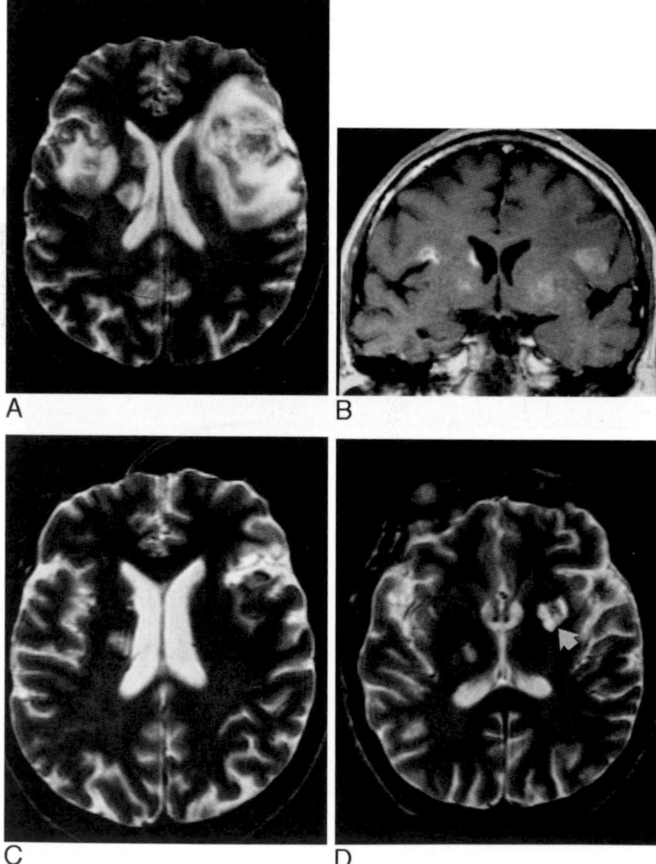

Figure 58.10 Typical toxoplasma abscesses and response to treatment. Transverse T2W images (A, C, D) and coronal T1W image (B). Multiple masses of varying sizes with a propensity to involve the basal ganglia and corticomedullary junction and associated with perilesional oedema may occur (A). High signal seen on the T1W images is due to haemorrhage (B). In response to therapy for toxoplasma (C, D), the size of the lesions and the surrounding oedema are reduced. Responding lesions may show increased intensity on T2W images and some show a surrounding low signal rim due to haemosiderin (arrow).

neurological deficits. Histopathology shows a multifocal haemorrhagic necrotizing encephalitis with the development of organizing abscesses.

Imaging typically shows multiple lesions, 1–4 cm across, at the corticomedullary junction and in the basal ganglia (Fig. 58.10). Single lesions and lesions in the brainstem or cerebellum are uncommon. The lesions show ring or nodular enhancement with associated oedema and mass effect[29] (Fig. 58.11). Enhancement may be diminished or absent in severely immunocompromised patients. MRI is more sensitive than CT to foci of haemorrhage within the lesions. The principal differential diagnosis is from primary CNS lymphoma, which can appear identical and can coexist in the same patient (Fig. 58.12).

In comparison to pyogenic abscesses cerebral toxoplasmosis is hypointense to white matter on DWI, indicating no restriction of diffusion[30].

A diffuse form of toxoplasmosis is not infrequent at postmortem examination. It appears as ill-defined foci of T2 prolongation at the corticomedullary junction, with mild and patchy enhancement.

Lifelong treatment is necessary, usually with pyrimethamine and sulfadiazine. Most lesions show reduced enhancement, oedema and mass effect within 2–4 weeks. Small lesions may heal completely whilst larger lesions can show persistent enhancement for more than 2 years on maintenance therapy.

PRIMARY CEREBRAL LYMPHOMA

Primary cerebral lymphoma is the AIDS-defining diagnosis in 5 per cent of patients. The incidence has reduced in the era of HAART. Most patients present with rapid progression of confusion, lethargy, memory loss and focal neurology.

Cerebral lymphoma is often multifocal in AIDS; lesions are commonest in the cerebral white matter but also occur in the basal ganglia, corpus callosum and ventricular margins (Figs 58.13, 58.14). Lesions abut the ependyma, leptomeninges or both in 75 per cent.

Imaging shows well-defined round or oval lesions of high attenuation on unenhanced CT, and lower signal intensity than grey matter on T2W MRI. This reflects the dense cellularity of lymphoma. Lesions have relatively little mass effect and oedema for their size[31]. Haemorrhage is unusual and calcification seen only after treatment. Enhancement is typical, often in a smooth or nodular ring surrounding a zone of central necrosis, in contrast to the solid enhancement seen in immune-competent patients.

Whilst they can be indistinguishable, there are some features that favour a diagnosis of lymphoma over toxoplasmosis. A single enhancing mass lesion in AIDS is more likely to be lymphoma, as are larger lesions and those with central low intensity on T2W images. Subependymal spread is a feature of lymphoma but is not seen in toxoplasmosis[32].

Thallium-201 SPECT and **FDG-PET** show greater uptake in lymphoma than toxoplasmosis though this is unreliable in lesions smaller than 2 cm[33]. Although lymphoma sometimes shows restricted diffusion, ADC values often overlap with those of toxoplasmosis, limiting the value of DWI in distinguishing between the two[34].

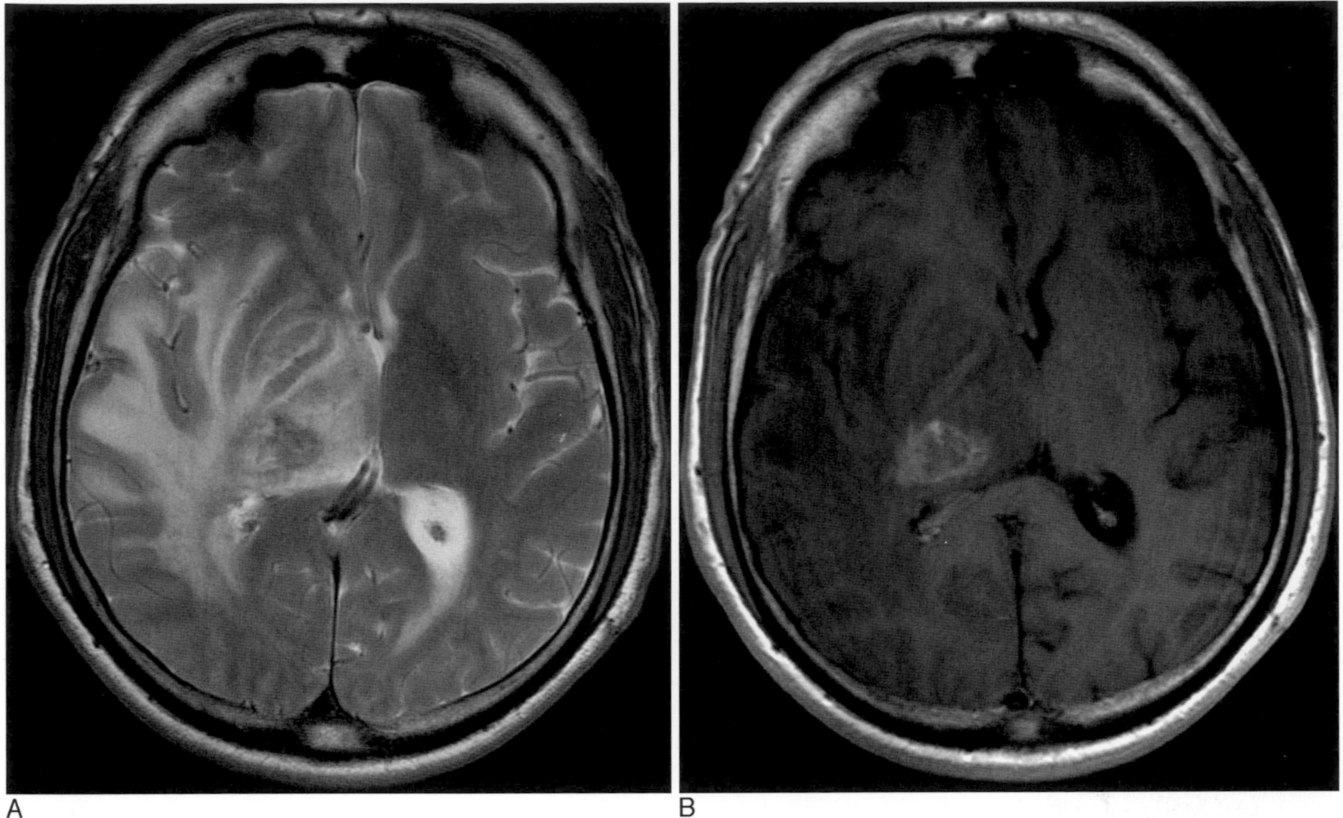

Figure 58.11 Enhancement in toxoplasmosis. (A) Axial T2W and (B) gadolinium-enhanced T1W images. Toxoplasma abscess in the right thalamus shows extensive surrounding vasogenic oedema and irregular peripheral enhancement.

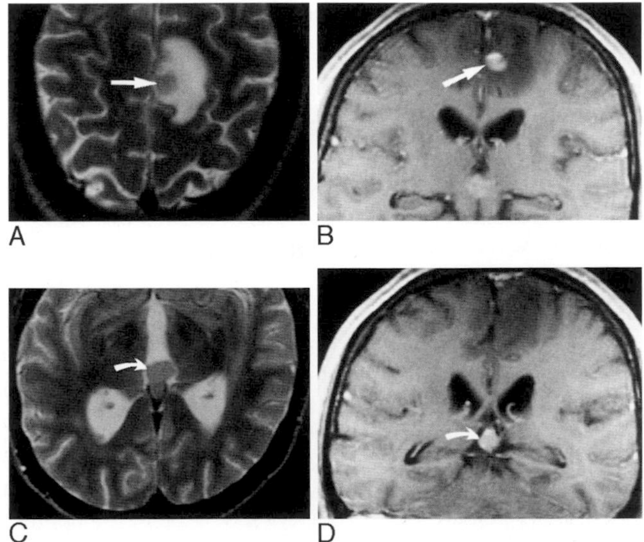

Figure 58.12 Coexistent lymphoma and toxoplasmosis. Transverse T2W spin-echo images (A, C) and enhanced coronal T1W spin-echo image. Dual or triple disease processes frequently occur in AIDS-related neurological disease. In this patient cerebral toxoplasmosis (A, B – arrow) and lymphoma involving the pineal (C, D – curved arrows) were confirmed at postmortem.

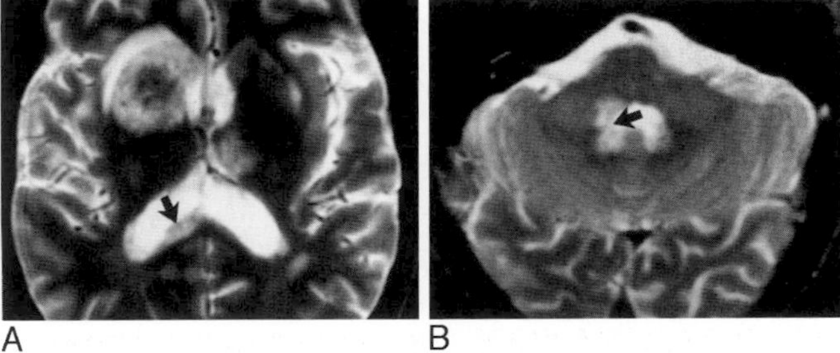

Figure 58.13 Multifocal primary cerebral lymphoma. Transverse T2W spin-echo image. Multiple masses, most of which show mixed signal intensity on T2W images, are present; like multiple toxoplasmosis, they involve the basal ganglia. However, subependymal tumour spread is clearly seen around the lateral and the 4th ventricles (arrows), which favours the diagnosis of lymphoma.

Metastases from systemic lymphoma typically involve the meninges (Fig. 58.15); parenchymal disease without leptomeningeal involvement is rare.

Lymphoma may respond dramatically to radiotherapy and/or corticosteroids but usually the prognosis is poor, HAART has prolonged median survival from 2–8 months.

CRYPTOCOCCOSIS

This is the second commonest opportunistic CNS infection in AIDS. Patients most often present with headache, fever and altered mental state. The earliest imaging manifestation is dilatation of perivascular spaces, most often in the basal ganglia but also in the brainstem and cerebral white matter (Fig. 58.16). These spaces are distended by mucoid material, organisms and inflammatory cells, and appear as multiple small foci of high signal on T2W images[35]. With disease progression cryptococcomas develop at these sites, forming lesions 3 mm to several cm in size. Cryptococcomas are of low to intermediate signal

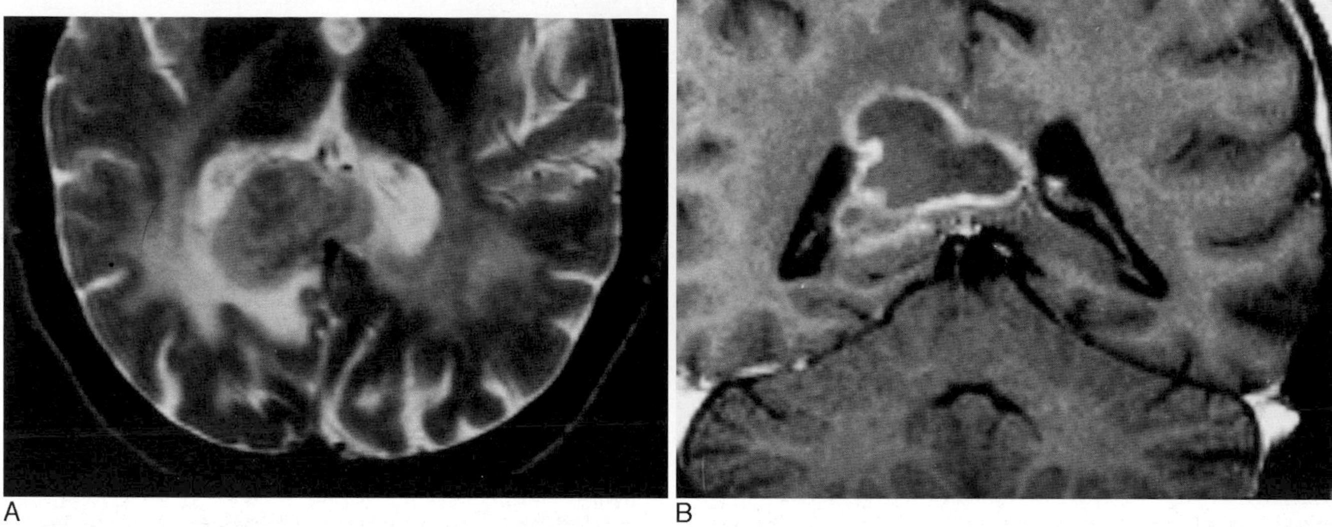

Figure 58.14 Primary cerebral lymphoma involvement of the corpus callosum. Transverse T2W spin-echo image (A) and coronal enhanced T1W spin-echo image (B). Lymphomatous masses may involve the corpus callosum, as in this patient who had multifocal primary cerebral lymphoma. Rim enhancement of the mass is seen.

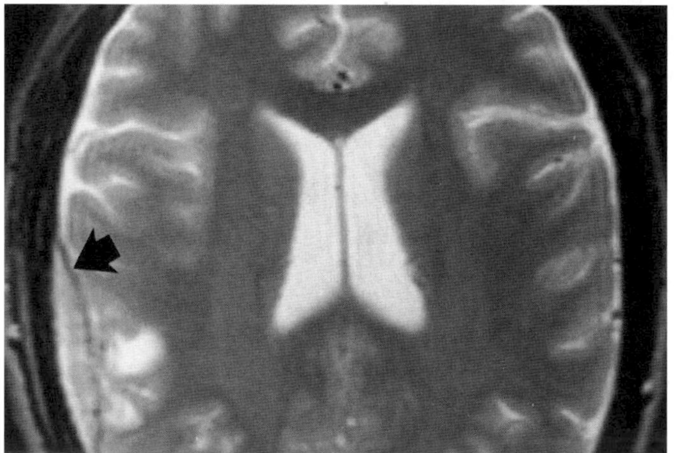

Figure 58.15 Metastatic lymphoma. Transverse T2W spin-echo image. The lymphomatous deposit is based on, and is lifting, the dura (arrow). There is oedema in the underlying brain substance, which is displaced.

on T1W and high signal on T2W images, lack surrounding oedema and do not show restricted diffusion[36]. Enhancement of cryptococcomas or the leptomeninges is rare because these patients are profoundly immunocompromised.

PROGRESSIVE MULTIFOCAL LEUKOENCEPHALOPATHY

Progressive multifocal leukoencephalopathy (PML) is a central demyelinating disease resulting from the reactivation of a latent infection of oligodendrocytes by JC polyomavirus. Eighty per cent of adults show serological evidence of prior exposure to the JC virus. The incidence of PML is about 4–5 per cent of AIDS cases; it is the AIDS-defining illness in about 1 per cent. Clinically, limb weakness is the commonest presentation, with an insidious onset and a progressive course involving visual field defects, speech abnormalities, ataxia and dementia. Pathologically, there is demyelination, astrocytosis and oligodendrocytes with intranuclear inclusions. Lesions can occur in any part of the brain but are commonest in the parieto-occipital regions. MRI shows multifocal, asymmetric bilateral white matter lesions that are of high signal on T2W and low signal on T1W images (Fig. 58.17). Extension to the subcortical U-fibres gives the lesions a characteristic 'scalloped' appearance. Apparent involvement of the basal ganglia can occur when lesions affect the white matter tracts that course through this site. Rarely, lesions may show mild mass effect and peripheral enhancement; restricted diffusion can be observed in areas of active disease progression[37].

TUBERCULOSIS (See earlier in this Chapter)

Intracranial tuberculosis is mostly seen amongst IV drug misusers. The radiological manifestations are similar to those in immunocompetent patients, hydrocephalus and meningeal enhancement being the commonest. Parenchymal lesions, in the form of tuberculomas and abscesses, are more frequent in HIV infection[10].

CANDIDIASIS

Although mucocutaneous candidiasis is common in HIV-infected patients, CNS involvement is rare. Haematogenous dissemination results in meningitis and/or cerebral abscesses. Imaging appearances are nonspecific; clinical confirmation is dependent on CSF analysis or brain biopsy.

INCIDENTAL WHITE-MATTER HYPERINTENSITIES

Focal white-matter hyperintensities, often multiple, are seen in up to 26 per cent of HIV-positive patients and up to 24

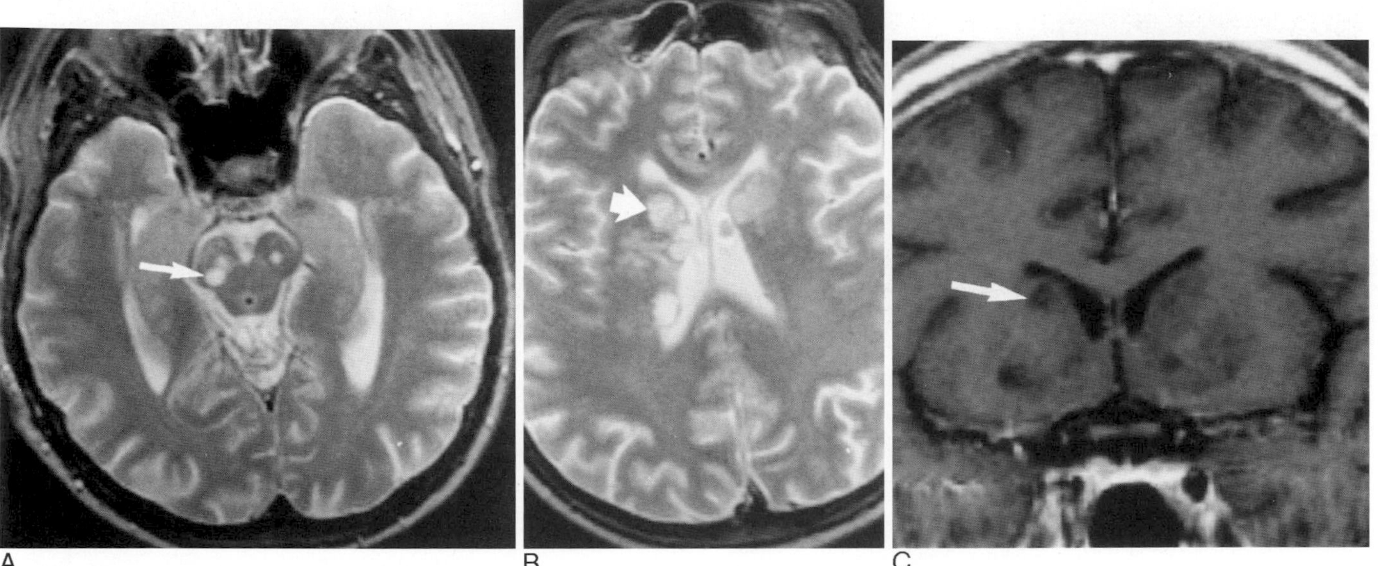

Figure 58.16 Cryptococcomas. Transverse T2W spin-echo images (A, B) and coronal T1W spin-echo image (C). Expanded Virchow-Robin spaces (arrow) of high signal on T2 and low on T1 are seen in the brainstem and the basal ganglia, so that the ganglia look like 'Swiss cheese'.

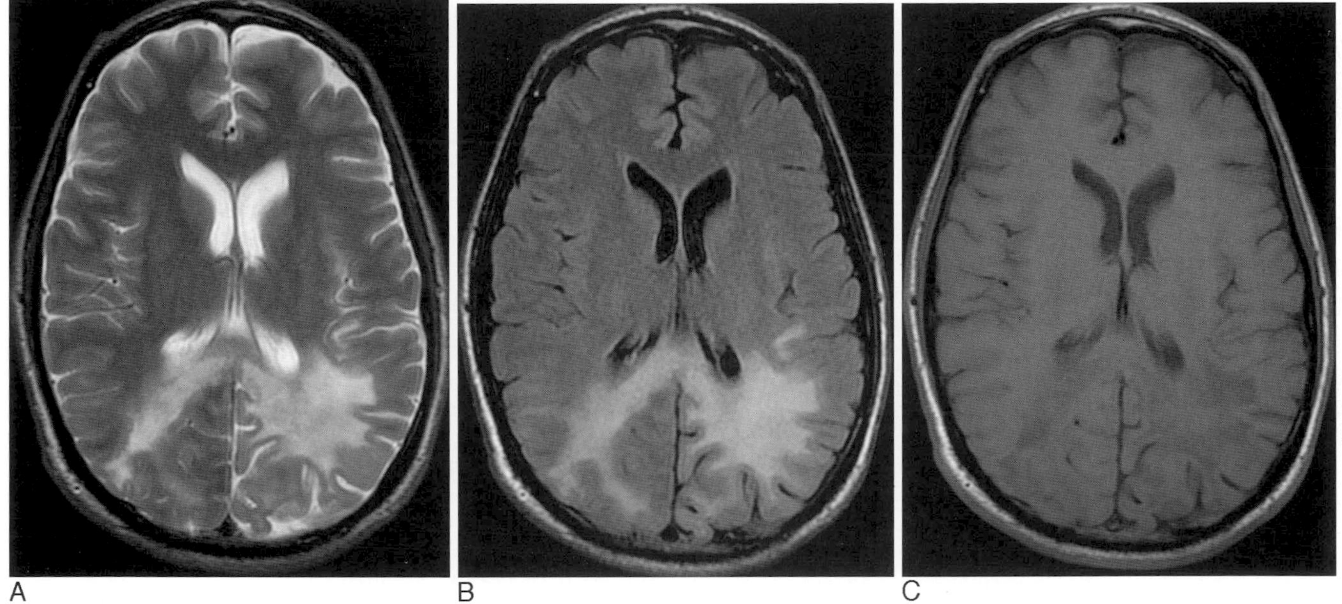

Figure 58.17 Progressive multifocal leukoencephalopathy. Axial T2W fast spin-echo image (A), FLAIR (B) and T1W spin-echo image (C). Asymmetrical signal abnormalities in the parieto-occipital white matter of both hemispheres extend to the subcortical U-fibres. There is no mass effect associated with the lesions.

per cent of seronegative men of matched ages. No associations with neurological abnormalities, CD4 count, or vascular risk factors have been identified. These lesions are probably incidental and of no clinical significance[38].

HERPES VIRUSES

Cytomegalovirus, herpes simplex and varicella zoster viruses can cause encephalitis, necrotizing ventriculitis (Fig. 58.18), and myelitis in AIDS. In encephalitis imaging may be normal, show nonspecific white matter lesions or focal enhancing lesions. Ependymal enhancement occurs with ventriculitis; myelitis manifests as nonspecific swelling and signal change in the spinal cord[39].

CEREBROVASCULAR DISEASE

Cerebral infarcts occur in fewer than 5 per cent of AIDS patients. Causes include infective vasculitis (CMV, varicella zoster or tuberculosis) and embolism from HIV cardiomyopathy. HIV also causes a dilating vasculopathy that results in fusiform aneurysms of the intracranial vessels[40].

HISTOPLASMOSIS

Histoplasmosis occurs in up to 5 per cent of AIDS patients in areas where *Histoplasma capsulatum* is endemic. CNS manifestations include meningitis with involvement of adjacent vessels,

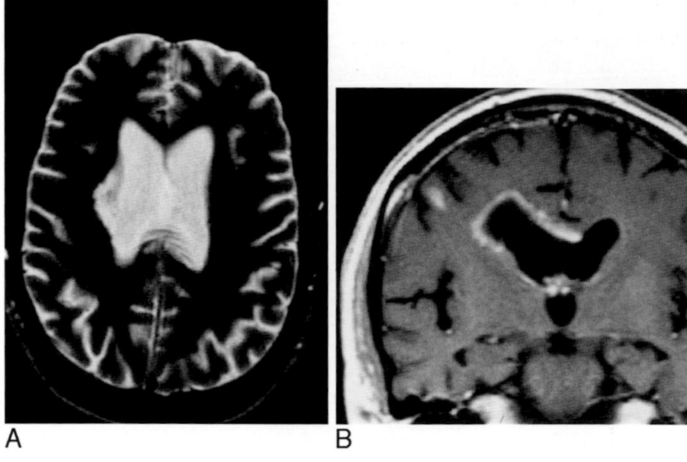

Figure 58.18 Herpes simplex ventriculitis. Transverse T2W spin-echo image (A) and coronal T1W spin-echo image (B) after IV contrast medium. The necrotic right-sided periventricular lesion shows central low signal on T1 and high on T2 with peripheral enhancement. Enhancement of the periventricular tissues (note the involvement of the corpus callosum) is also present in this case.

and single or multiple abscesses. Imaging may show meningeal enhancement, cerebral infarcts, or focal enhancing lesions with mass effect and oedema[39].

NEUROSYPHILIS

CNS involvement can occur at any stage of syphilis, in HIV-infection its course may be more aggressive. Meningovascular syphilis causes a small-vessel endarteritis that appears as arterial segmental 'beading' on angiography, with associated infarcts in the basal ganglia. Cerebral gummas are rare, typically arise from the meninges, and appear as mass lesions with variable MR signal characteristics and enhancement[41].

SPINAL CORD DISORDERS[42]

AIDS-associated vacuolar myelopathy presents insidiously and progresses to severe paraparesis; the thoracic cord is most often affected. MRI is usually normal or shows nonspecific changes such as diffuse symmetrical signal abnormalities in the cord. Primary HIV myelitis is rare and presents acutely with paraparesis and a sensory level; MRI shows multifocal asymmetrical signal change in the cord. Other diseases affecting the spinal cord in AIDS include herpes virus infections (Fig. 58.19), toxoplasmosis and tuberculosis.

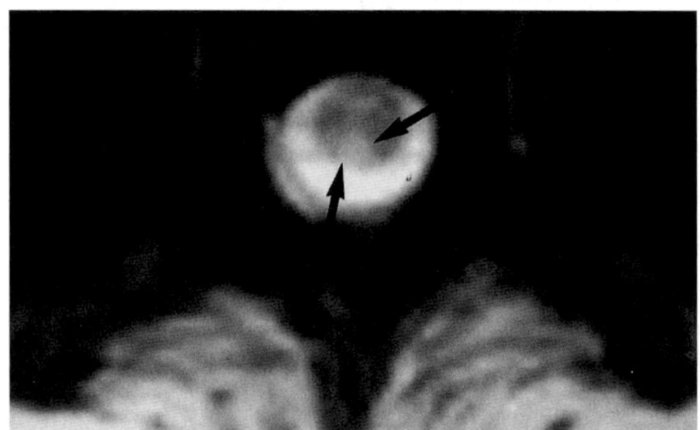

Figure 58.19 Herpes zoster cord myelitis. Axial T2W gradient echo at level of T8. Following an attack of shingles in a T8 distribution, this patient developed cord symptoms. Focal high signal is seen involving the dorsal columns (arrows).

DEMYELINATING, METABOLIC AND NONSPECIFIC INFLAMMATORY DISORDERS

There are innumerable diseases in which myelin is formed abnormally or is destroyed. Most such familial and metabolic disorders occur in infancy and childhood with nonspecific imaging findings. The reader is referred elsewhere for an account beyond the scope of this chapter[43].

Congenital leukodystrophies usually manifest in childhood, though adrenoleukodystrophy (ALD) and Krabbe's disease may not present until adulthood. White matter lesions in the leukodystrophies are typically symmetrical, manifest on CT as low attenuation, and on MRI as increased signal on T2W images and often less extensive decreased signal on T1W images. ALD usually begins posteriorly, and Krabbe's disease often involves the pyramidal tracts.

The **aminoacidurias** and **mitochondrial cytopathies** affect grey as well as white matter or instead of white matter. Some mitochondrial disorders may not present until late adulthood. A striking feature is infarct-like lesions in the basal ganglia and cortex that are not confined to vascular territories and may be transient.

WILSON'S DISEASE

Mutations in the *ATP7B* gene, which encodes a copper transporter, cause Wilson's disease. Copper first accumulates in the liver and then the brain, producing multifocal necrosis. The commonest MRI finding is high signal in the putamen on T2W images; lesions also occur in the pons, midbrain, cerebellum and subcortical white matter. Lesions initially show restricted diffusion[44] and diminish in size with copper chelation.

Some patients with hepatic failure develop symmetrical lesions in basal ganglia and cerebral white matter, a notable feature being increased signal in basal ganglia on T1W images.

INTESTINAL ENCEPHALOPATHIES

Ataxia is the commonest neurological complication of coeliac disease; MRI shows cerebellar atrophy in 79 per cent and non-specific white matter lesions in 19 per cent[45]. Bilateral calcification in the parieto-occipital cortex, associated with seizures, has also been reported in coeliac disease[46]. Intracranial venous and dural sinus thrombosis may occur, especially in ulcerative colitis.

MULTIPLE SCLEROSIS

Multiple sclerosis (MS) is an inflammatory disease of the CNS characterized pathologically by demyelination and axonal injury. Relapsing-remitting MS is the commonest form: patients experience episodic neurological deficits with intervening partial or complete recovery. The diagnosis requires evidence of dissemination of lesions in space and time, and is primarily clinical. Paraclinical studies including CSF analysis, visual evoked responses and MRI can be used to support the diagnosis[47] (Table 58.3).

Lesions can occur anywhere in the CNS but are commonest in the periventricular white matter. Typical lesions are ovoid, with the long axis orientated perpendicular to the ventricle wall (Fig. 58.20). Such lesions are better shown by proton density and FLAIR than T2W images because of increased lesion-to-CSF contrast. Lesions of the corpus callosum, both at the callososeptal interface and subcallosal striations, are characteristic, and best shown on sagittal FLAIR images. FLAIR is less sensitive than T2W imaging for infratentorial lesions, which tend to occur in the brainstem and middle cerebellar peduncles (Fig. 58.21). Spinal cord involvement is common; lesions are generally less than two vertebral segments long and aligned with the long axis of the cord.

Acute lesions can show solid or ring enhancement with IV gadolinium, which can persist for up to 3 months but generally resolves within weeks. Occasionally, large acute lesions with associated oedema and mass effect can mimic glioma (Fig. 58.22). The enhancement in such cases of tumefactive MS often forms an incomplete ring[48].

Lesions show reduced magnetization transfer ratio (MTR), reflecting decreased amounts of myelin. MTR is also reduced in normal-appearing white matter of MS patients compared with controls. This ‘occult’ tissue damage can also be detected by diffusion tensor imaging, which shows reduced fractional anisotropy[49].

Most MS lesions seem asymptomatic; disability correlates poorly with T2 lesion load but rather better with the number of low signal lesions on T1W MRI (‘black holes’). Better correlation with disability has also been found with brain and spinal cord atrophy, which develops later in the disease.

The differential diagnosis for the imaging appearance of MS includes ADEM, vasculitis (e.g. lupus, anti-phospholipid syndrome, Behçet’s disease), sarcoidosis and white matter lesions associated with small vessel ischaemia. These latter processes tend to spare the subcortical U-fibres, which are affected by MS lesions.

OSMOTIC MYELINOLYSIS[50]

Precipitous correction of severe hyponatraemia can cause acute demyelination in the central pons, and also in extrapontine sites such as the cerebellum, subinsular regions, basal ganglia and thalami. MRI is often normal initially, before showing swelling and high signal in the basal pons on T2W images. DWI is more sensitive in the acute stage, showing restricted diffusion as early as 24 h.

Table 58.3 MRI CRITERIA TO DEMONSTRATE LESION DISSEMINATION IN SPACE AND TIME

1.1.1 Dissemination in space

Three of the following:

1. At least one gadolinium-enhancing lesion or nine T2 hyperintense lesions if there is no gadolinium-enhancing lesion
2. At least one infratentorial lesion
3. At least one juxtacortical lesion
4. At least one periventricular lesion

Note: A spinal cord lesion can be considered equivalent to a brain infratentorial lesion: an enhancing spinal cord lesion is considered to be equivalent to an enhancing brain lesion, and individual spinal cord lesions can contribute together with individual brain lesions to reach the required number of T2 lesions.

1.1.2 Dissemination in time

There are two ways to show dissemination in time using imaging:

1. Detection of gadolinium enhancement at least 3 months after the onset of the initial clinical event, if not at the site corresponding to the initial event.
2. Detection of a *new* T2 lesion if it appears at any time compared with a reference scan done at least 30 days after the onset of the initial clinical event.

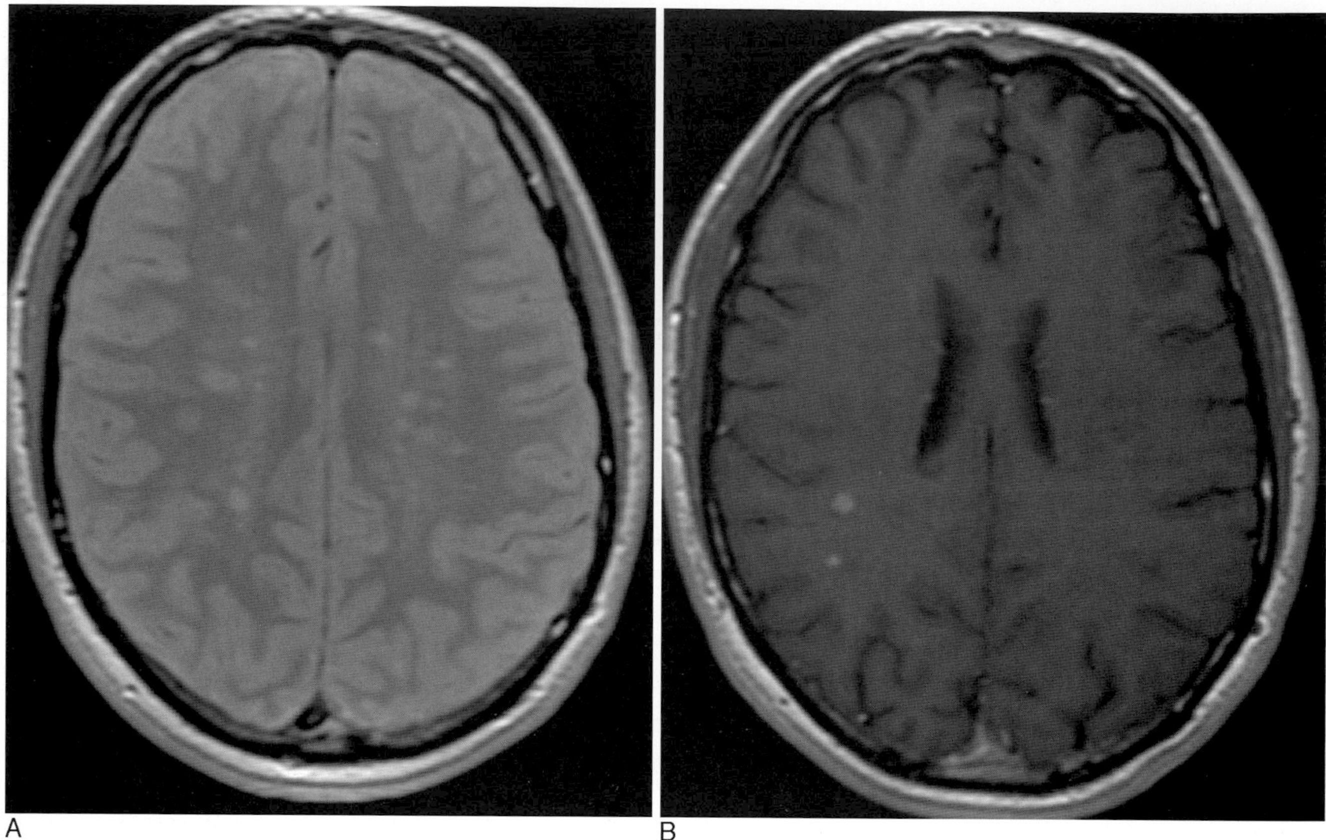

Figure 58.20 Multiple sclerosis. (A) Axial proton density and (B) gadolinium-enhanced T1W images show multiple lesions in the periventricular white matter, two of which are in the acute phase and enhance.

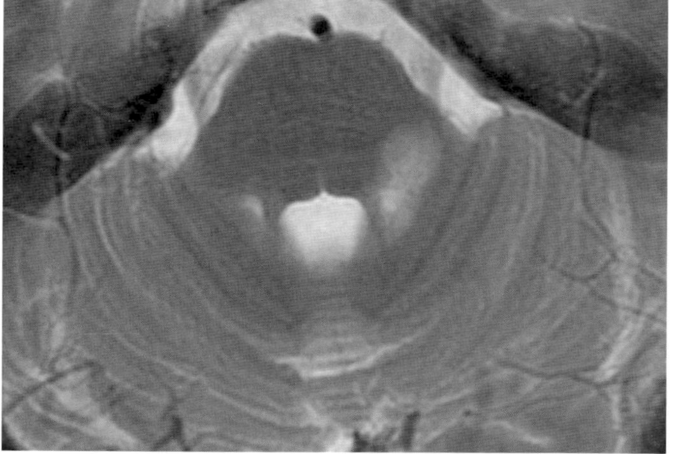

Figure 58.21 Infratentorial MS lesion. Axial T2W fast spin-echo image shows a typical MS lesion in the left middle cerebellar peduncle.

SARCOIDOSIS[51]

Symptomatic CNS involvement occurs in 5 per cent of patients with this multi-system granulomatous disorder; MRI is the investigation of choice for assessment. Meningeal disease is the most frequent finding; dural thickening and masses that can mimic meningioma, and enhancement of the basal and suprasellar meninges are well-recognized. Small enhancing granulomas are usually located superficially in brain parenchyma bordering the basal cisterns. Nonenhancing lesions in the periventricular white matter and brainstem are common and can mimic MS. Less often, subependymal granulomatous infiltration causes hydrocephalus.

In over 80 per cent of established cases the chest radiograph is abnormal. About 70 per cent of cases have skin, or visceral involvement, especially the liver.

BEHÇET'S DISEASE[52]

CNS involvement most often occurs as a chronic meningoencephalitis. Lesions tend to occur in the brainstem, diencephalon, basal ganglia and deep hemispheric white matter, and may resemble those of MS. Brainstem atrophy is seen in chronic cases.

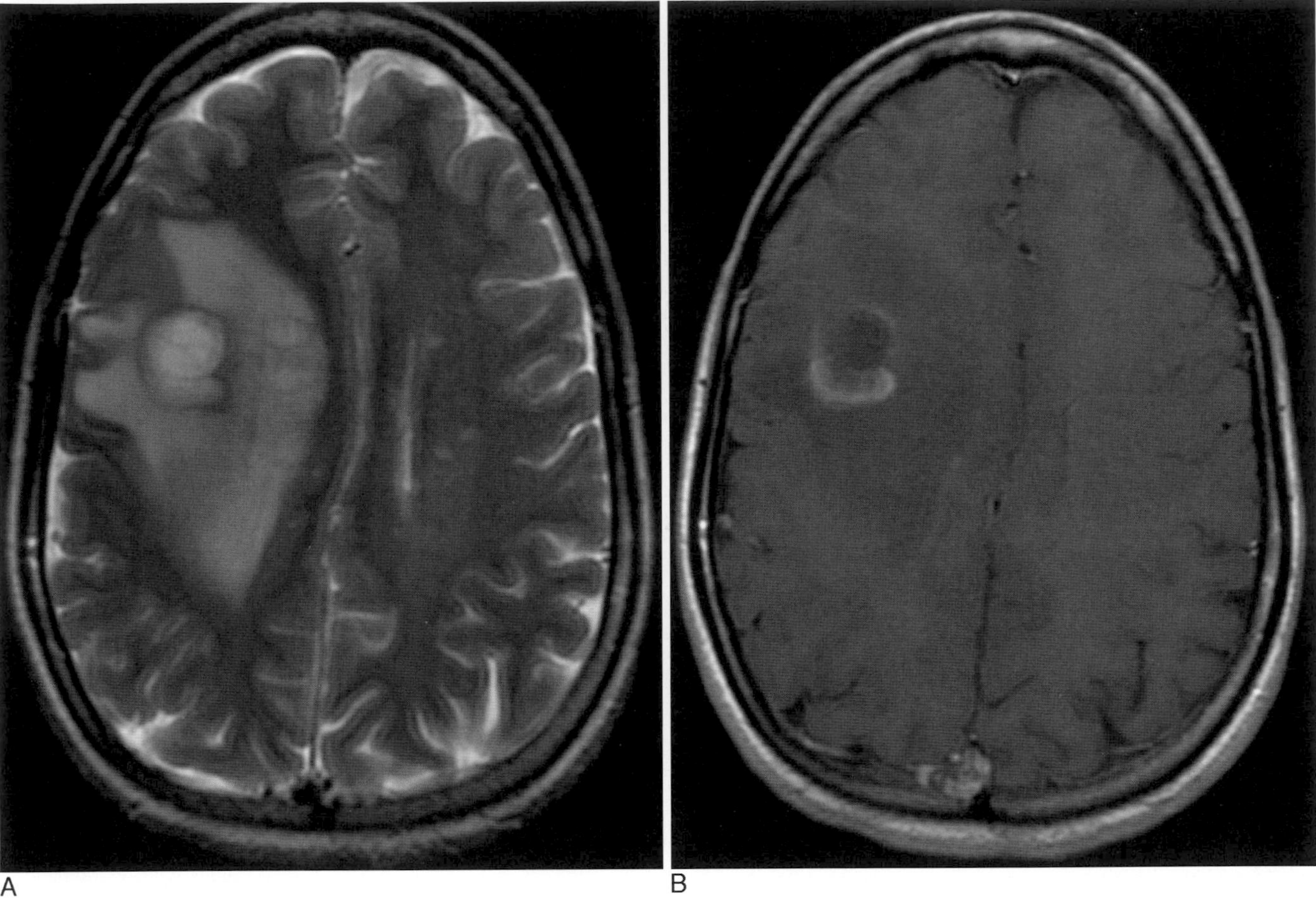

Figure 58.22 Tumefactive MS. (A) Axial T2W fast spin-echo and (B) gadolinium-enhanced T1W spin-echo images show a large MS plaque with considerable associated oedema in the right frontal lobe. Note the smaller periventricular lesions on the T2W image, and the 'open ring' of contrast enhancement.

REFERENCES

1. Roos K L 2005 Principles of neurologic infectious disease. McGraw Hill, New York
2. Stevens E A, Norman D, Kramer R A et al 1978 Computed tomographic brain scanning in intraparenchymal pyogenic abscesses. Am J Roentgenol 130:111–114
3. Enzmann D R, Britt R H, Placone R 1983 Staging of human brain abscesses by computed tomography. Radiology 146:703–708
4. Haimes A, Zimmerman R D, Morgello S et al 1989 MR imaging of brain abscesses. Am J Roentgenol 152:1073–1085
5. Cartes-Zumelzu F W, Stavrou I, Castillo M et al 2004 Diffusion-weighted imaging in the assessment of brain abscess therapy. Am J Neuroradiol 25:1310–1317
6. Holmes T M, Petrella J R, Provenzale J M 2004 Distinction between cerebral abscesses and high-grade neoplasms by dynamic susceptibility contrast perfusion MRI. Am J Roentgenol 183:1247–1252
7. Rich P M, Deasy N P, Jarosz J M 2000 Intracranial dural empyema. Br J Radiol 73:1329–1336
8. Fujikawa A, Tsuchiya K, Honya K et al 2006 Comparison of MRI sequences to detect ventriculitis. Am J Roentgenol 187:1048–1053
9. Pryzbojewksi S, Andronikou S, Wilmhurst J 2006 Objective CT criteria to determine the presence of abnormal basal enhancement in children with suspected tuberculous meningitis. Paediar Radiol 36:687–696
10. Bernaerts A, Vanhoenacker F M, Parizel P M et al 2003 Tuberculosis of the central nervous system: overview of neuroradiological findings. Eur Radiol 12:1876–1890
11. Tien R D, Feisberg G J, Osumi A K 1993 Herpesvirus infections of the CNS: MR findings. Am J Roentgenol 161:167–176
12. Küker W, Nägele T, Schmidt et al 2004 Diffusion-weighted MRI in herpes simplex encephalitis: a report of three cases. Neuroradiology 46:122–125
13. Marco de Lucas E, Gonzalez Mandly A, Gutierrez A et al 2006 Computed tomography perfusion usefulness in early imaging diagnosis of herpes simplex encephalitis. Acta Radiol 47:878–871
14. Singh S, Alexander M, Korah I P 1999 Acute disseminated encephalo-pmyelitis: MR imaging features. Am J Roentgenol 173:1101–1107
15. Gibbs W N, Kreidie M A, Kim R C et al 2005 Acute haemorrhagic leukoencephalitis: neuroimaging features and neuropathologic diagnosis. J Comp Assist Tomogr 29:689–693
16. Ozturk A, Gurses C, Baykan B et al 2002 Subacute sclerosing panencephalitis: clinical and magnetic resonance imaging evaluation of 36 patients. J Child Neurol 17:25–29
17. Kamran S, Bari Bener A, Alper D et al 2004 Role of fluid-attenuated inversion recovery in the diagnosis of meningitis: comparison with contrast-enhanced magnetic resonance imaging. J Comp Assist Tomogr 28:68–72
18. Splendani A, Puglielli E, De Amicis R et al 2005 Contrast-enhanced FLAIR in the early diagnosis of infectious meningitis. Neuroradiology 47:591–598
19. Noujaim S E, Rossi M D, Rao S K et al 1999 CT and MR imaging of neurocysticercosis. Am J Roentgenol 173:1485–1490
20. Tüzün M, Hekimoglu B 1998 Hydatid disease of the CNS: imaging features. Am J Roentgenol 171:1497–1500
21. Post M J D, Berger J R, Duncan R, Quencer R M, Pall L, Winfield D 1993 Asymptomatic and neurologically symptomatic HIV-seropositive subjects: results of long term MR imaging and clinical follow-up. Radiology 188:727–733

22. Thurnher M M, Thurnher S A, Fleischmann D et al 1997. Comparison of T2-weighted and fluid-attenuated inversion recovery fast spin-echo MR sequences in intracerebral AIDS-associated disease. Am J Roentgenol 18:1601–1609
23. Malcolm P N, Howlett D C, Saks A et al 1999 MRI of the brain in HIV-positive patients: what is the value of routine intravenous contrast medium? Neuroradiology 41:687–695
24. Patel S H, Kolson D L, Glosser G et al 2002 Correlation between percentage of brain parenchymal volume and neurocognitive performance in HIV-infected patients. Am J Neuroradiol 23:543–549
25. Post M J D, Tate L G, Quencer R M et al 1988 CT, MR and pathology in HIV encephalitis and meningitis. Am J Roentgenol 151:373–380
26. Chang L, Ernst T 2005 Physiological MR to evaluate HIV-associated brain disorders. In: Gillard J, Waldman A, Barker P Clinical MR Neuroimaging: Diffusion, Perfusion and Spectroscopy. Cambridge University Press, Cambridge pp 460–478
27. Ragin A B, Storey P, Cohen B A et al 2004 Whole brain diffusion tensor imaging in HIV-associated cognitive impairment. Am J Neuroradiol 25:195–200
28. Thurnher M M, Schindler E G, Thurnher S A et al 2000 Highly active antiretroviral therapy for patients with AIDS dementia complex: effect on MR imaging findings and clinical course. Am J Neuroradiol 21:670–678
29. Post M J D, Kursunoglu S J, Hensely G T et al 1985 Cranial CT in acquired immunodeficiency syndrome: spectrum of diseases and optimal contrast enhancement technique. Am J Roentgenol 145:929–940
30. Camacho D L A, Smith J K, Castillo M 2003 Differentiation of toxoplasmosis and lymphoma in AIDS patients by using apparent diffusion coefficients. Am J Neuroradiol 24:633–637
31. Koeller K K, Smirniotopoulos J G, Jones R V 1997 Primary central nervous system lymphoma: radiologic–pathologic correlation. Radiographics 1497–1526
32. Dina T S 1991 Primary central nervous system lymphoma versus toxoplasmosis in AIDS. Radiology 179:823–828
33. Young R J, Ghesani M V, Kagetsu N J et al 2005 Lesion size determines accuracy of thallium-201 brain single-photon emission tomography in differentiating between intracranial malignancy and infection in AIDS patients. Am J Neuroradiol 26:1973–1979
34. Schroeder P C, Post M J, Oschatz E et al 2006 Analysis of the utility of diffusion-weighted MRI and apparent diffusion coefficient values in distinguishing central nervous system toxoplasmosis from lymphoma. Neuroradiology 48:715–720
35. Miszkiel K A, Hall-Craggs M A, Miller R F et al 1996 The spectrum of MRI findings in CNS cryptococcosis in AIDS. Clin Radiol 51:842–850
36. Ho T L, Lee H J, Lee K W et al 2005 Diffusion-weighted and conventional magnetic resonance imaging in cerebral cryptococcoma. Acta Radiol 46:411–414
37. Küker W, Mader I, Nägele T et al 2006 Progressive multifocal leukoencephalopathy: value of diffusion-weighted and contrast-enhanced magnetic resonance imaging for diagnosis and treatment control. Eur J Neurol 13:819–826
38. McArthur J C, Kumar A J, Johnson D W et al 1990 Incidental white matter hyperintensities on magnetic resonance imaging in HIV infection. Multicenter AIDS cohort study. J Acq Immun Def Synd 3:252–259
39. Berger J R, Cohen B A 2005 Opportunistic infections of the central nervous system in AIDS In: Gendelman H E, Grant I, Everall I P et al The Neurology of AIDS, 2nd edn. Oxford University Press, Oxford, pp 485–491
40. Corr P D 2006 Imaging of cerebrovascular and cardiovascular disease in AIDS patients. Am J Roentgenol 187:236–241
41. Brightbill T C, Ihmedian I H, Post M J D et al 1995 Neurosyphilis in HIV-positive and HIV-negative patients: neuroimaging findings. Am J Neuroradiol 16:703–711
42. Thurnher M M, Post M J, Jinkins J R 2000 MRI of infections and neoplasms of the spine and spinal cord in 55 patients with AIDS. Neuroradiology 42:551–563
43. Barkovich A J 2005 Pediatric neuroimaging, 4th edn. Lippincott Williams & Wilkins, Baltimore
44. Sener R N 2003 Diffusion MR changes associated with Wilson disease. Am J Neuroradiol 24:965–967
45. Hadjivassiliou M, Grunewald R, Sharrack B et al 2003 Gluten ataxia in perspective: epidemiology, genetic susceptibility and clinical characteristics. Brain 126:685–691
46. Pfaender M, D'Souza W J, Trost N et al 2004 Visual disturbances representing occipital epilepsy in patients with cerebral calcifications and coeliac disease: a case series. J Neurol Neurosurg Psychiatry 75:1623–1625
47. Polman C H, Reingold S C, Edan G et al 2005 Diagnostic criteria for multiple sclerosis: 2005 revisions to the 'McDonald criteria.' Ann Neurol 58:840–846
48. Pretorius P M, Quaghebeur G 2003 The role of MRI in the diagnosis of MS. Clin Radiol 58:434–448
49. Ye G 2006 Multiple sclerosis: the role of MR imaging. Am J Neuroradiol 27:1165–1176
50. Martin R J 2004 Central pontine and extrapontine myelinolysis: the osmotic demyelination syndrome. J Neurol Neurosurg Psychiatry 75: iii22–iii28
51. Christoforidis G A, Spickler E M, Recio M V et al 1999 MR of CNS sarcoidosis: correlation of imaging features to clinical symptoms and response to treatment. Am J Neuroradiol 20:655–669
52. Akman-Demir G, Bahar S, Coban O et al 2003 Cranial MRI in Behçet's disease: 134 examinations of 98 patients. Neuroradiology 45:851–859

CHAPTER 59

Cranial and Intracranial Disease: Trauma, Cerebrospinal Fluid Disturbances, Degenerative Disorders and Epilepsy

John M. Stevens

TRAUMA TO THE SKULL AND BRAIN

HEAD INJURY

Head injuries are either open (penetrating) or closed (non-penetrating), the latter being far the more common in civilian practice. The main indication for imaging is suspected intracranial haemorrhage where prompt neurosurgical evacuation may modify outcome. Because it shows haemorrhage particularly well, computed tomography (CT) generally is recommended in preference to magnetic resonance imaging (MRI) for this purpose. Furthermore CT is more widely available on a 24-h basis and is easier to perform following major trauma. Thus there are clear recommendations from the Royal College of Radiologists[1] and the National Institute of Clinical Excellence (NICE)[2,3] about the indications for and appropriate timing of CT following trauma. During the subsequent clinical course, imaging may be required to assess neurological deterioration or other complications, or perhaps failure to improve, and later to make a final assessment of overall damage for long term prognosis. For many of these less acute indications, MRI may be preferred. Despite the numerous published guidelines for imaging of the head and cervical spine in trauma, they are only guidelines and many individual brain injury units have their own variations. The principles behind these, however, are simply the application of common sense on a case by case basis.

Skull fractures

Detection of fractures of the cranial vault by plain radiography of the skull is now appreciated to be less useful in assessing the probability of intracranial haemorrhage than had been previously suggested. Clinical assessment appears to be a better guide and this, in turn, guides the need for CT. Thus the role of skull radiography has greatly diminished. In any event simple linear fractures are often of little consequence in themselves. Like fractures elsewhere, these may be simple or comminuted. They sometimes branch, and must be distinguished from vascular markings (Fig. 59.1), including the groove in the squamous temporal bone caused by a deep temporal artery[4]. Acute fractures are usually straighter, more angulated, more radiolucent and do

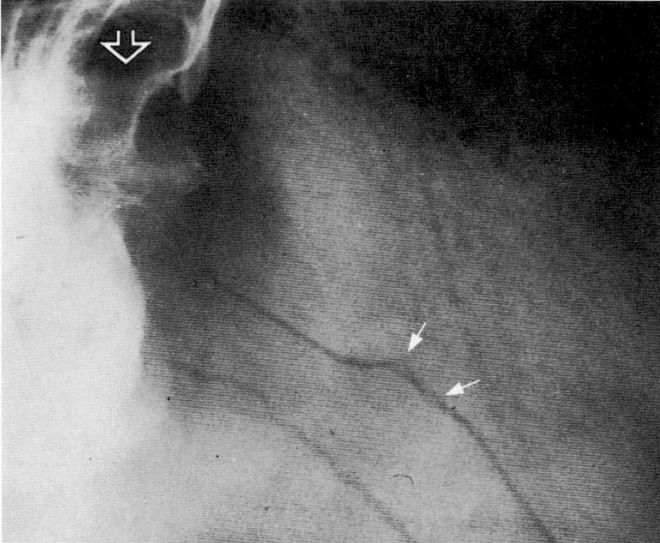

Figure 59.1 Bilateral vault fracture, with fluid level in sphenoid sinus (open arrow). Two fracture lines are seen; the more anterior (upper on this radiograph) is better defined and is therefore on the side nearer the radiographic plate. Apparent islands of bone within (small arrows) are typical of an acute fracture. This radiograph has been obtained with the patient in the supine brow up position.

not have corticated margins. A fracture passing through a sinus or air cell is effectively compound, and of much greater potential significance than a simple fracture. A compound fracture is one in which the cranial cavity is in real or potential communication with the exterior. Depressed fractures (Fig. 59.2) are usually comminuted and often compound; bone fragments embedded in brain substance often are removed or relocated to reduce the risk of post-traumatic epilepsy. Acuteness of the fracture may be determined by demonstrating overlying scalp swelling on CT. Fractures of the skull base are important because of bleeding or leakage of cerebrospinal fluid (CSF); air and fluid within the sphenoid sinus may indicate that the leptomeninges have been torn. CT is extremely helpful in assessment of fractures of the skull base, including the petrous bone, where it may also reveal ossicular dislocation, a treatable cause of traumatic hearing loss.

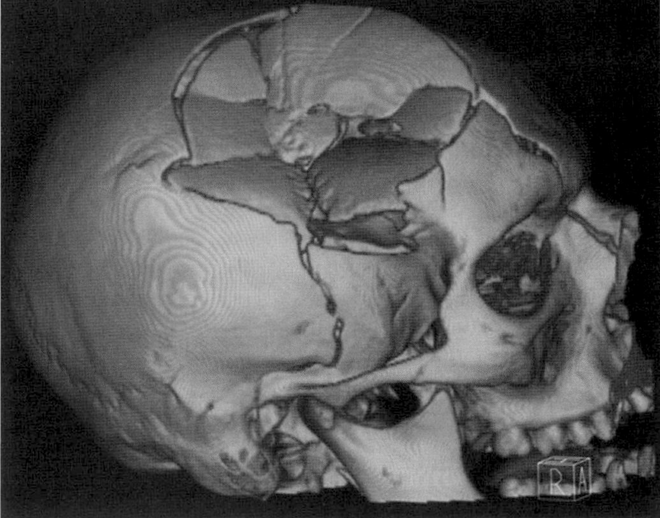

Figure 59.2 Stellate comminuted depressed fracture produced by a direct blow. CT volume rendered Image.

Growing fractures (leptomeningeal cysts) usually occur after severe head injuries early in life[4]. The dura mater underlying a linear fracture is torn, often with laceration of the underlying brain. Exposure of the remodelling bone to pulsation of the CSF results in progressive widening of the fracture line over weeks or months.

Traumatic haemorrhage

Trauma may cause bleeding into the scalp, between the cranial vault and the dura mater (extradural—but also termed epidural), between the dura and arachnoid mater (subdural), or into the subarachnoid space, brain or ventricular system. The aim of imaging in the acute stage is to identify patients with intracranial bleeding requiring surgery; they represent less than 1% of patients with well-documented head injury. CT is the imaging procedure of choice, rather than MRI, as haematomas are about the most readily recognizable abnormality on plain CT.

Extradural haemorrhage

The **acute extradural (or epidural) haematoma** is a relatively stereotyped lesion (Figs 59.3 and 59.4). Because the dura mater tends to adhere to the skull, the haematoma is seen on CT sections as a biconvex dense area immediately beneath the skull vault, convex towards both the brain and the vault. The temporoparietal convexity is the most common site, in which lesions are easily detected on axial sections. The haematoma often lies beneath a fracture of the squamous part of the temporal bone. They tend not to cross cranial sutures. Areas of low density within them may indicate continuing bleeding (Fig. 59.4), and add further urgency to the assessment. Frontal, vertical and posterior cranial fossa collections (Fig. 59.5) can be difficult to diagnose; coronal images may be required. Even then, shallow extradural haematomas may be overlooked,

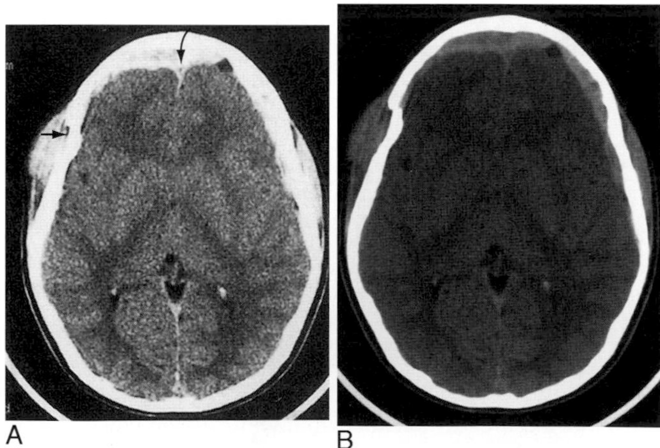

Figure 59.3 (A, B) **Depressed skull fracture with extradural haematomas;** CT. Axial 'brain and bone windows' demonstrate the right temporal bone depressed several millimetres with an evident fracture line (arrow) anteriorly. Soft tissue contusion overlying the fracture is also noted. A large extradural collection (curved upper arrow) anteriorly crosses the midline and displaces the falx posteriorly, and there is a second contiguous left frontal extradural collection as well. Other images (not shown) demonstrated bilateral skull fractures. Note the generalized cerebral swelling with complete effacement of the frontal horns.

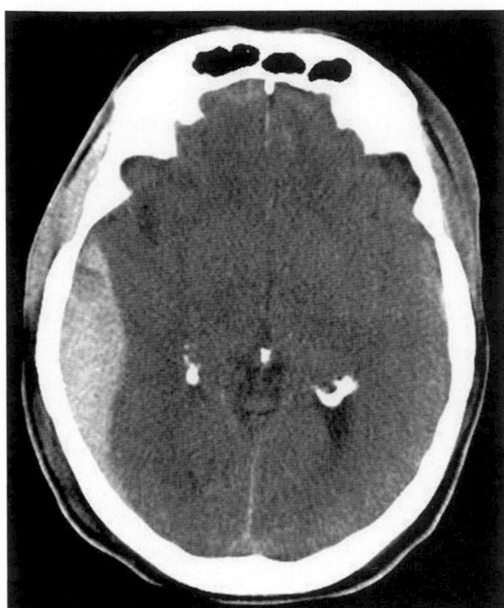

Figure 59.4 Acute extradural haematoma. CT. Large biconvex right temporal extradural collection. Note the effacement of the right occipital horn and subtle displacement of the calcified choroid plexus within. There is also a small focus of active/fresh bleeding causing a small round lucency within the high attenuation of the haematoma, close to the expected site of the middle meningeal artery. (Courtesy of Dr Dan Scoffings).

especially when adjacent to contused or haemorrhagic brain. Wide window CT images may help distinguish the intermediate density of the clot from bone and underlying brain. The underlying brain is displaced, but often appears intrinsically normal. MRI can be helpful on occasions (Fig. 59.6).

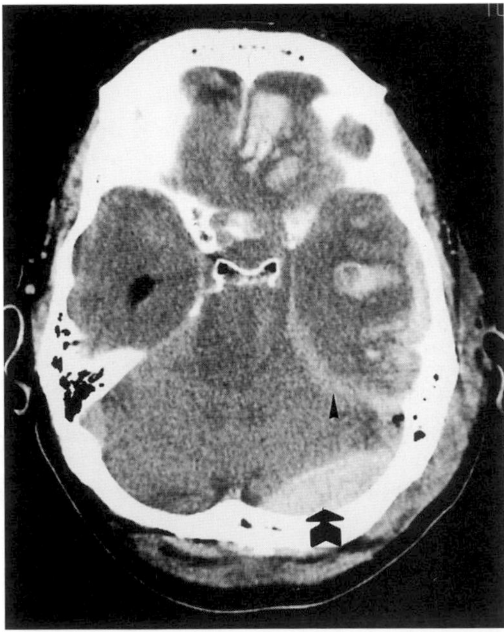

Figure 59.5 Trauma. CT. A biconvex density of blood over the left cerebellar hemisphere indicates an extradural haematoma (thick arrow). A crescent of fresh subdural blood spreads over the left temporal lobe and tracks along the tentorium in a comma shaped fashion (arrowhead); this feature differentiates it from an extradural. Typical sites of haemorrhagic contusions are also seen; gyrus recti and temporal lobe.

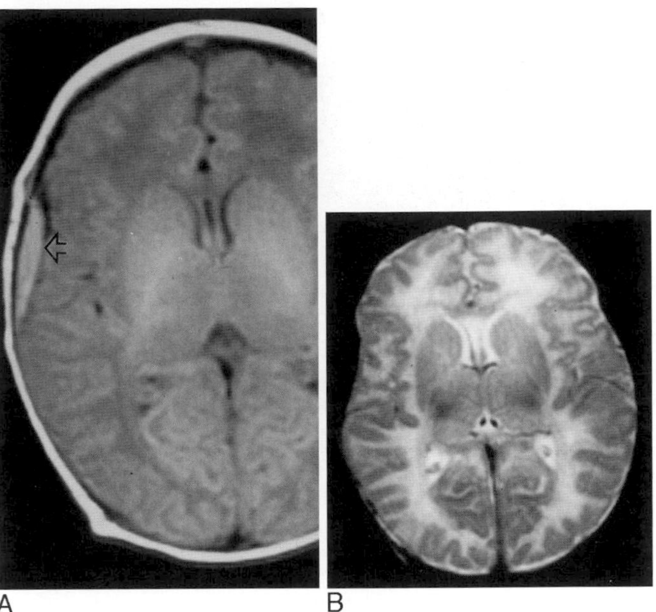

Figure 59.6 Acute extradural haematoma. MRI in a neonate with traumatic delivery. (A) Axial T1-weighted image (750/16). Slightly hyperintense epidural collection (arrow) in the right temporal region. (B) Axial T2-weighted image (3000/120), epidural collection is hypointense and is invisible except for deformation of the underlying cortex. This is the MR signature of deoxyhaemoglobin.

Subdural haemorrhage

Subdural bleeding is often, but not always, associated with damage to the brain, and arises from rupture of veins which cross the subdural space; vault fractures are much less commonly present in patients with subdural haematomas than extradural bleeds.

Subdural haematomas are seen most commonly over the cerebral convexities, under the temporal and occipital lobes, or along the falx cerebri. They lie in the virtual space between the dura and arachnoid maters and may be extensive. This is because the blood within them, while under less pressure, is less restricted and tends to spread out over the surface of the brain; bleeding may even extend over an entire cerebral hemisphere. They may follow minor head injuries, and sometimes seem to develop spontaneously, especially in the elderly and in patients with haematological abnormalities. In such situations they are often diagnosed during the investigation of persistent headache, or perhaps transient but repetitive focal neurological deficits. Large ones requiring operative evacuation are usually associated with a reduced conscious state of the patient.

On axial CT and MRI, the cerebral surface typically is concave (Fig. 59.7), but on coronal images may appear more convex. Acute lesions are usually hyperdense on CT, but mixed density is also common. They become progressively less dense over time, and typically end up of similar density to CSF within a few weeks or months. During this evolution there is often a period when the attenuation of the haematoma is similar to that of cerebral tissue; the resulting 'isodense subdural' haemotoma[6] can be difficult to identify (Fig. 59.8) and is a well recognized pitfall on CT which continues to cause problems[7]. MRI is better at making this diagnosis when these lesions are of some longstanding. Most resolve spontaneously with time, but some

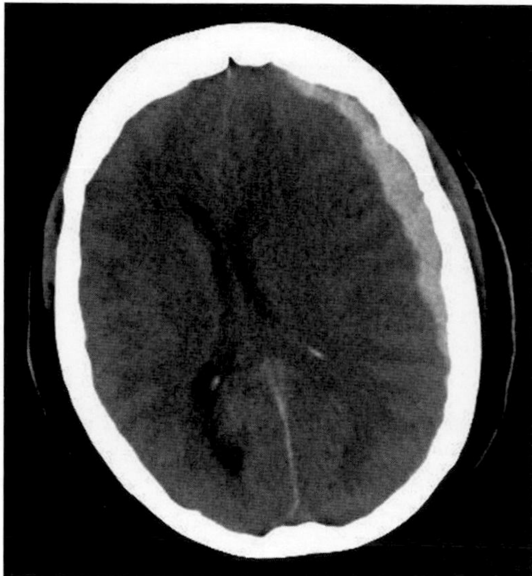

Figure 59.7 Acute subdural haematoma. CT. Heterogeneous density of irregular shape occupies extra-axial space overlying the left cerebral convexity. There is quite severe mass effect exhibited by effacement of convexity sulci, narrowing of the left sided ventricular system and midline shift. (Courtesy of Dr Dan Scoffings.)

persist, sometimes for years. Occasionally these lesions enlarge progressively at a variable, but usually slow, rate and eventually may require evacuation. The high morbidity of these lesions, particularly in the aged, is due in large part to the associated swelling, contusion or laceration of the underlying brain. It is often evident that midline displacement is greater than would be accounted for by the mass of the haematoma alone. Dilatation of the contralateral ventricle is a bad prognostic sign.

The interhemispheric subdural haematoma extends along the falx cerebri and may spread onto the tentorium, giving a characteristic comma shape on axial CT sections (see Fig. 59.5).

Coronal CT sections may be useful in distinguishing supra- and infra-tentorial bleeding. Sub- or extra-dural collections low in the posterior cranial fossa, which may be life-threatening, may be overlooked, and the presence of unexplained hydrocephalus after acute head injury should prompt thorough examination of that region.

The CT attenuation of the blood in a subacute subdural haematoma slowly decreases: as a rule of thumb, it remains denser than the brain for 1 week, and is less dense after 3 weeks (Fig. 59.9). There is thus an interim period of up to 2 weeks when it may be 'isodense' with brain (see Fig. 59.8). Not all isodense haematomas are subacute: an acute bleed can be isodense in a very anaemic patient, and if there is continued leakage of venous blood, a chronic haematoma may not be of low density. Indirect signs may then be crucial: midline shift, with compression of the ipsilateral ventricle; contralateral ventricular enlargement; effacement of cerebral sulci, and medial displacement of the junction between the white and grey matter ('buckling'). Some of these signs may be absent if there are bilateral collections; the frontal horns may then lie closer together than normal, giving a 'rabbit's ear' configuration (see Fig. 59.8). Intravenous contrast medium, by highlighting the vessels on the surface of the brain, may remove any doubts about the extracerebral location of the lesion. The increasing use of MRI for nonacute problems should help overcome this diagnostic problem in the future.

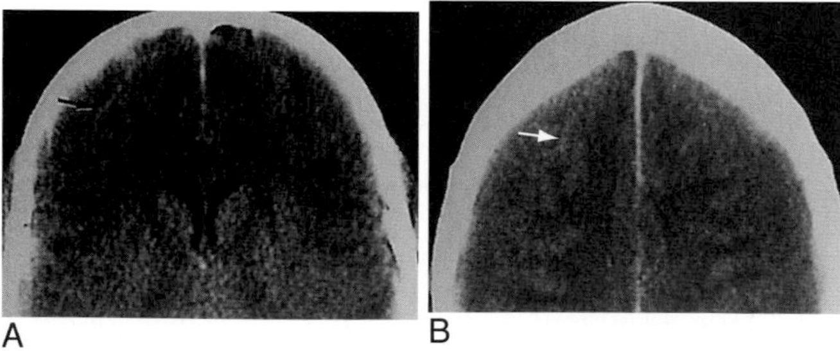

Figure 59.8 Bilateral isodense subdural haematomas on contrast-enhanced CT. The ventricles (A) are slit-like and displaced medially, giving a 'rabbit's ears' appearance. A higher section (B) indicates that the normal grey–white interface lies too near the midline; the cortex appears abnormally thick. On close inspection, both sections show cortical vessels (arrows) displaced away from the cranial vault.

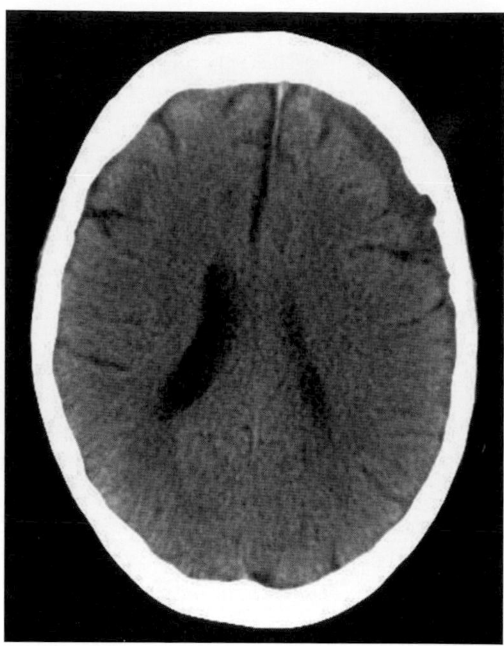

Figure 59.9 Subacute left subdural haematoma: CT. The lesion is of lower attenuation than brain tissue but denser than CSF. The underlying sulci are somewhat effaced and the left ventricle is compressed. (Courtesy of Dr Dan Scoffings.)

Chronic subdural collections are usually biconvex. Their density is less than that of brain, approaching that of CSF. Fluid–fluid levels may be seen between denser blood elements in the more dependent portions and serous fluid above, particularly if haemorrhage has been repeated. The membrane on their deep surface frequently shows contrast enhancement.

PRIMARY CEREBRAL DAMAGE IN CLOSED HEAD INJURY

This is commonly associated with intracerebral haemorrhage, usually small and multifocal. An important feature is that the haemorrhages tend to enlarge and become more conspicuous over the initial few days after injury.

Primary cerebral damage may be described as either superficial or deep. Interestingly these patterns of injury usually are mutually exclusive. Deep damage generally is considered to occur more commonly in high speed accidents and to have a worse prognosis, but exceptions are encountered quite frequently, and as in all forms of head injury, prognosis must be guarded in the initial few months following the injury.

Superficial primary cerebral damage

This consists of cerebral contusions (see Fig. 59.5) and cortical lacerations. The underlying white matter also usually is damaged to a variable extent. The lesions usually are quite extensive, and typically involve the inferior parts of the frontal lobes and the anterior parts of the temporal lobes, but they can be found elsewhere. The mechanism is rotation of the brain with respect to the skull, especially the sphenoid ridges and the anterior cranial fossa. The term contra coup contusion often is used because commonly this type of cerebral damage lies diametrically opposite the site of impact, as defined by skull fracture or scalp haematoma. However, the cause is rotation, not linear acceleration of the brain. On CT, contusion appears as superficial low density areas with mild to moderate mass effect, which tends to increase a little in the initial days and subsequently contracts into a region of focal atrophy and sometimes cavitation. Multiple, usually small hyperdense haemorrhages are often present within the low density areas in the early stages. On MRI, they appear as mixed signal lesions, later contracting to regions of persistent mainly cortical cerebral damage. MRI is not much more sensitive in assessing the extent of contusions than CT.

Deep primary cerebral damage

This pattern of injury is considerably less common. The mechanism here is differential rates of rotational acceleration within brain substance itself, producing shearing forces which damage axons and microvasculature. The injury is microscopic and may not be detected at all by CT or MRI, unless diffuse atrophy subsequently develops in the brain. Its presence is most often recognized on imaging by the presence of so-called marker lesions. These probably represent small areas of microvascular damage with haemorrhage or infarction, but they are a reliable guide to the presence of diffuse axonal injury, though not to its extent. They are small multifocal lesions, and tend to occur in more or less characteristic sites: high parasagittal cerebral white matter, corona radiata, posterior corpus collosum and subcortical white matter almost anywhere. They usually are not visible on CT unless haemorrhagic; many more may be on MRI, whether haemorrhagic or not. Susceptibility-weighted MRI (T2 'star' acquisitions) often shows still more lesions, even long after the event, as small dark patches of haemosiderin. Characteristically the surrounding brain appears normal. Quantitative diffusion tensor imaging has been considered to demonstrate the axonal damage in a few reported cases, but only when it has been exceptionally severe.

When the vascular component of the shearing injury is severe there may be larger haemorrhages in the basal ganglia and elsewhere, a pattern sometimes termed diffuse axonal injury of the brain.

Primary brainstem injuries

These usually only occur with deep cerebral damage. The most common is a haemorrhagic lesion in the dorsolateral midbrain. Another is the pontomedullary rent, usually not compatible with life and therefore rarely seen on imaging.

OTHER TYPES OF INTRACRANIAL HAEMORRHAGE AFTER CLOSED HEAD INJURY

Subarachnoid haemorrhage

Head injury is probably the most common cause overall of subarachnoid haemorrhage. It commonly accompanies superficial cerebral damage, but may be minor and inconspicuous and is usually not recognized radiologically or clinically.

Intraventricular haemorrhage

When isolated, intraventricular haemorrhage usually seems to be the result of tears in the attachments of the septum pellucidum to the corpus callosum.

Isolated large intracerebral haemorrhage

Although rare, intracerebral haemorrhage is encountered from time to time and is often a source of diagnostic confusion. Cerebral angiography may show a false aneurysm.

SECONDARY CEREBRAL DAMAGE WITH CLOSED HEAD INJURY

This results mainly from the effects of raised intracranial pressure, local pressure cones and fluctuations in systemic blood pressure and blood oxygen saturation.

A common serious problem in the initial 2 or 3 d after a major head injury is diffuse cerebral swelling due to a increase in the cerebral blood volume, appropriately referred to as hyperaemic brain swelling, and less appropriately as brain oedema. It is a potent cause of raised intracranial pressure in this period and may trigger drastic neurosurgical decompression by wide craniectomies. The appearance of brain substance on CT and MRI is not affected, so it is not directly recognizable by imaging alone.

Secondary cerebral damage consists of infarctions and brainstem haemorrhage. Infarcts most commonly occur in the cortical distributions of one or both posterior cerebral arteries, and haemorrhages are most often found in the ventral mid brain and upper ponds. Both probably, but certainly the latter, are due to pressure cones across the tentorial incisura.

OTHER COMPLICATIONS WITH CLOSED HEAD INJURIES

Hydrocephalus requiring shunting is an uncommon complication and generally is of a communicating type.

Cerebrospinal fluid fistulae are associated with skull base fractures and may present with otorrhoea or rhinorhhoea. Most heal within 10 d or so, but a small number may persist or become intermittent, and eventually require surgical repair. Detailed imaging may be necessary to identify the site of the leak[8]. CSF leaks are associated with intracranial air, which may be extradural if the meninges are intact, or if they are torn, subarachnoid or intraventricular. These are often referred to as aerocoeles or pneumocephalus.

Cranial nerve palsies are usually associated with skull base fractures and are immediate and permanent. Delayed cranial nerve palsies also may occur in the absence of fracture and may be reversible. Virtually any nerve or branch that traverses the skull base can be involved.

An arteriovenous fistula may be an immediate or a delayed complication (Fig. 59.10). The most common occurs between the internal carotid artery and the cavernous sinus[9], and is termed a direct carotid cavernous fistula. These usually are torrential, and may require urgent endovascular treatment to preserve vision, sometimes at a time when the overall outcome is in the balance. Alternatively they may be chronic and the patient may present with an alarming engorged exophthalmos.

Penetrating head injuries

Although uncommon, such injuries are increasing in frequency in civilian practice. Appearances on imaging vary with the penetrating agent and the trajectory of the cerebral penetration. Intracerebral haemorrhage usually dominates the appearances on imaging. Direct vascular injury is more common than in closed head injury, resulting in larger haemorrhages and more frequent false aneurysms.

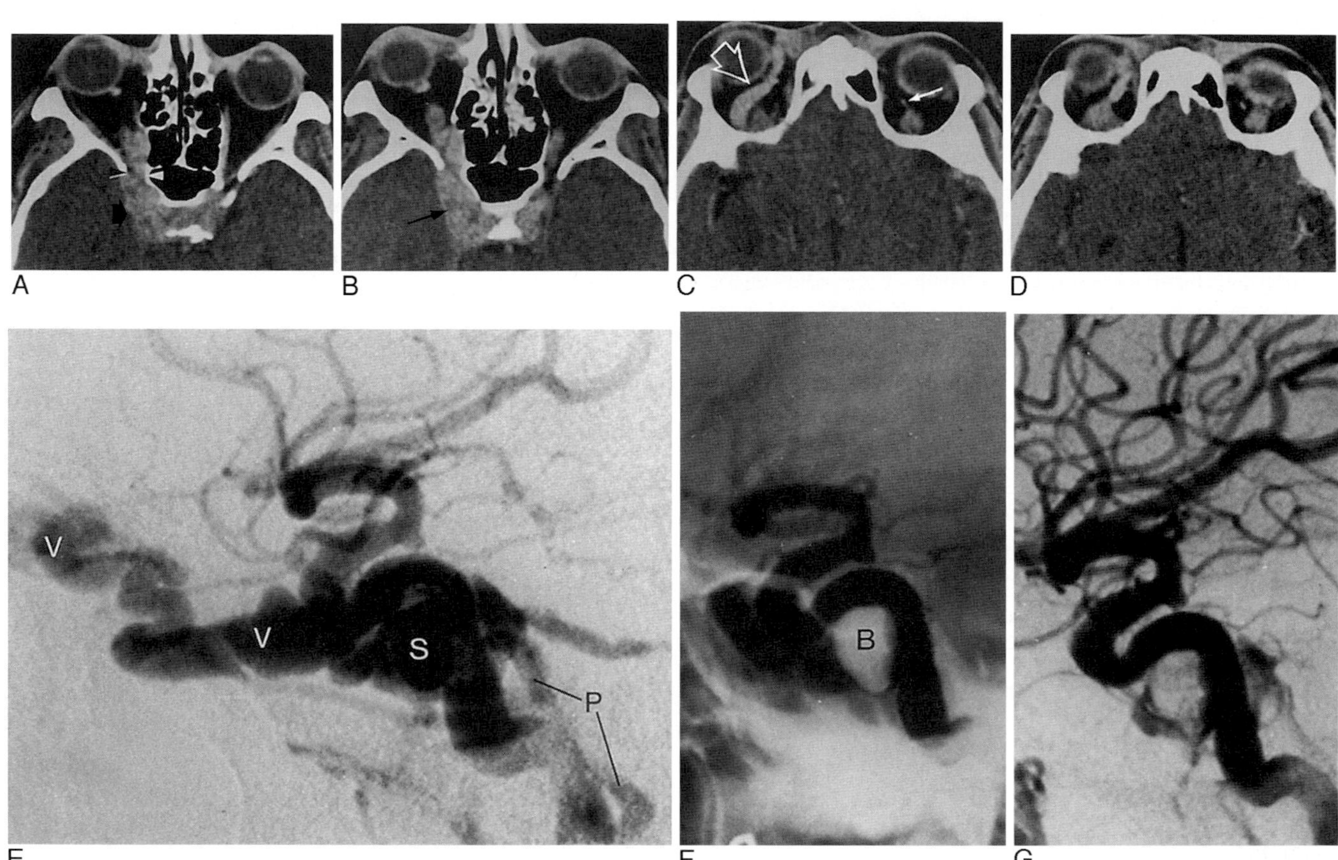

Figure 59.10 Post-traumatic caroticocavernous fistula. (A–D) Axial contrast-enhanced CT: the right cavernous sinus (A, arrow) is enlarged, and a large enhancing mass runs forwards into the orbit through a widened superior orbital fissure (A, arrowheads). A sigmoid structure (C, open arrow) in the upper part of the right orbit represents the greatly dilated superior ophthalmic vein (cf. normal left side in C, small white arrow). Some of the extraocular muscles are thicker than on the left, and there is marked right proptosis. (E) Intra-arterial DSA, lateral projection, arterial phase, following injection into the right internal carotid artery. Contrast medium floods into the cavernous sinus (S), and drains anteriorly into a grossly dilated superior ophthalmic vein (V); there is also shunting posteriorly and via the inferior petrosal sinus (P). Intracranial arterial filling is poor. (F, G) After therapeutic detachment of a balloon (B) in the cavernous sinus (F, lateral projection), shunting particularly anteriorly, is greatly reduced, and intracranial filling much improved (G).

DISEASES OF THE SKULL—BONE DISEASE

Fibrous dysplasia

In the skull, fibrous dysplasia takes two main forms. The sclerotic form is the commoner of the two, especially in the polyostotic version of the disease[10]: it involves the base and/or facial skeleton, which are expanded and dense, sometimes showing the classical featureless 'ground-glass' pattern (Fig. 59.11). This is the most common cause of 'leontiasis ossea'. In meningiomas, which represent the important differential diagnostic consideration, sclerosis is often more marked than expansion, and extension from the sphenoid bones into the facial skeleton is much less common. Lower density areas, representing cysts or fibrotic masses, within the sclerotic bone are strong evidence

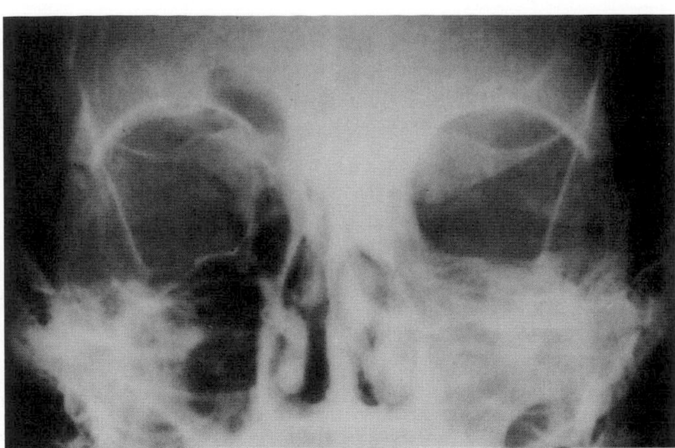

Figure 59.11 Fibrous dysplasia of the skull base. Dense 'ground glass' appearance, with loss of the normal bone texture, extending from the nasion to the clivus into the sphenoid wings on both sides, and into the left maxilla.

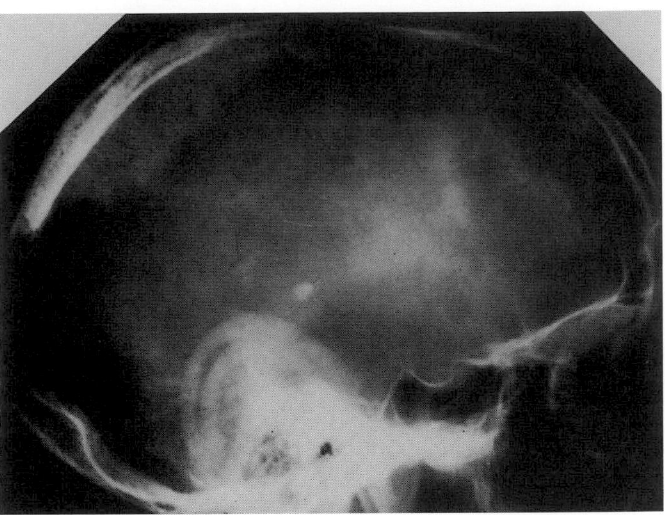

Figure 59.12 Osteoporosis circumscripta (Paget's disease). Extensive loss of bone density affects the lower part of the cranial vault; the margin between abnormal and normal bone is characteristically sharp, as seen in the upper posterior parietal region.

in favour of fibrous dysplasia. Malignant transformation may cause ragged osteolysis.

The cystic form of fibrous dysplasia, often an incidental finding, usually produces a small lesion of the skull vault, expanding the outer table and giving a 'blistered' appearance. Here the differential diagnosis is from epidermoid, which has finer, better defined borders and a more homogeneously radiolucent centre.

Paget's disease

This condition, of unknown aetiology, is rare before middle age. It affects men more than women, and familial and strong geographical variations in prevalence are also noted. The skull is involved in about two-thirds of cases presenting clinically.

A mixture of sclerosis and lysis is most commonly seen, and unless the condition is revealed incidentally, radiological changes are often advanced by the time of diagnosis. An early change is a spotty 'cotton-wool pledget' increase in density of the bone, which also becomes thicker. The middle and outer tables are most affected and thickened with course trabeculation. Generalized thickening of the vault may, however, be the first manifestation.

Osteoporosis circumscripta may progress to the type described above and is frequently found in association with skeletal Paget changes. A portion of the vault is demineralized, sometimes profoundly so, from the base upwards, with a very sharp border between normal and abnormal bone (Fig. 59.12). Striking resolution can occur with therapy[11] or the lesion may progress to classical changes of Paget's disease.

Complications include:

- **Basilar invagination**, due to softening of bone; this occurs in about a third of cases, and can lead to a 'Tam O'Shanter' deformity (Fig. 59.13).
- **Narrowing of basal foramina**, producing cranial nerve lesions, especially deafness, and occasionally compression of the medulla oblongata or upper spinal cord.

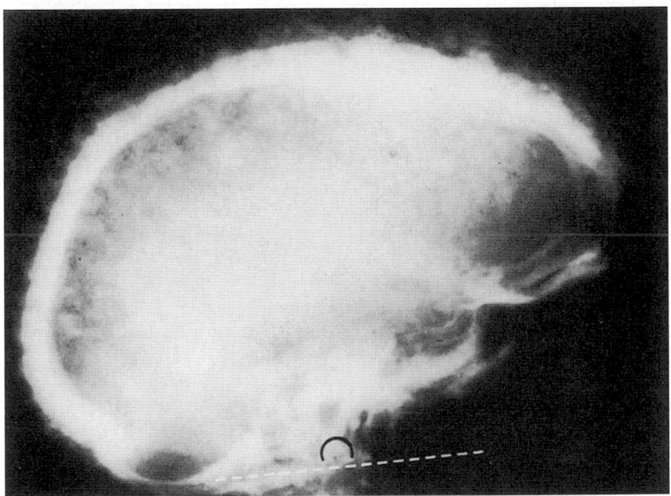

Figure 59.13 Advanced Paget's disease, with basilar invagination. Skull lateral projection: gross thickening and alteration of bone texture affects the entire skull. Basilar invagination is manifest as extension of the odontoid peg (outlined in black) above Chamberlain's line (dotted line).

- **Malignancy**: osteo- or fibro-sarcomas, which are otherwise extremely rare, arise in about 1% of patients with cranial Paget's disease, and generally manifest as irregular bone destruction.

Imaging reveals a thickened vault, which may appear irregular due to patchy sclerosis. Basilar invagination is readily recognized on sagittal MRI, and can be appreciated on axial images if the entire clivus is seen on one normally angled section, or if the ring of bone surrounding the foramen magnum appears to lie at the centre of the posterior fossa.

Tumours of the skull vault

Primary tumours of many kinds can arise in the cranial vault, but most are exceedingly rare.

Haemangioma

Haemangioma of the vault sometimes presents as a lump on the head or local tenderness. It is typified by a well-circumscribed area of punctate or stellate rarefaction without expansion (Fig. 59.14). Prominent vascular grooves may be present in the vicinity and external carotid arteriography sometimes shows a blush. The tumour is not progressive and treatment is not generally required.

Epidermoids

Characteristically, intraosseous epidermoids are well-corticated lesions of the vault, which may expand the inner and outer tables away from each other. Rarely, this appearance may be mimicked by neurofibromas or dermoids.

Osteomas

Osteomas are benign condensations of cortical bone which may project external to the skull (exostosis) or towards the cranial cavity (enostosis). Differential diagnosis includes meningioma and fibrous dysplasia; osteomas are typically denser and more circumscribed and do not show abnormal bone texture. Treatment is not usually required.

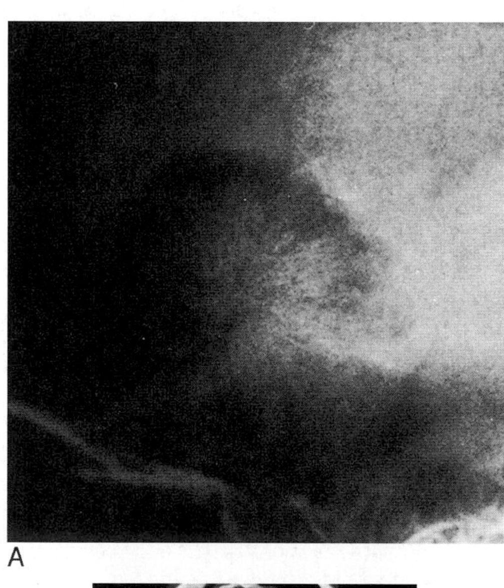
A

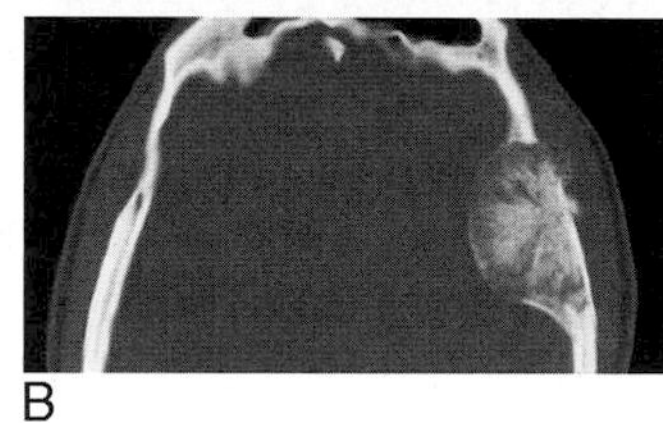
B

Figure 59.14 Haemangioma of skull vault. (A) Lateral skull and (B) CT, bone windows. The well defined lucency in the parietal bone has a typical 'spoke wheel' appearance due to prominent vascular impressions.

Tumours

Tumours of the skull are usually secondary. Local invasion from a superficial tumour, such as a nasopharyngeal or basal cell carcinoma, may occur. Metastases are common in disseminated malignancy; their characteristics are similar to those found in other bone sites: irregular lysis and/or sclerosis, and multiplicity (Fig. 59.15). In children, focal osteolytic skull defects are a common manifestation of Langerhans' cell type histiocytosis.

Thinning of the parietal bones

An uncommon condition of completely unknown aetiology is bilateral symmetrical thinning of the parietal bones, occurring in elderly patients and more common in men. It does not appear to be related either to generalized bone disease or to cerebral disease, although there may be an increase in deafness.

The plain radiological appearance is diagnostic, but may be misinterpreted if the observer is unaware of this condition. There is very marked thinning of the outer table and diploe of the superior portions of both parietal bones. On lateral radiography the markedly thinned bone is well seen, often with a sharp curved inferior border. Although commonly seen in the days of skull radiography, this condition is less widely appreciated on CT.

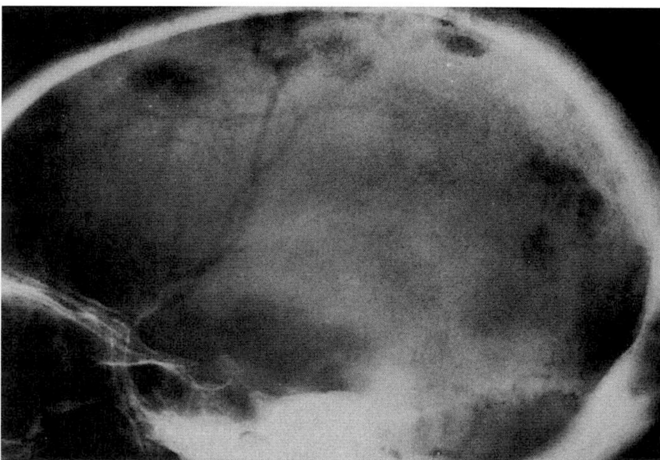

Figure 59.15 Metastases from carcinoma of the breast; plain skull radiograph, lateral projection. Numerous irregular lytic defects in the cranial vault are associated with large vascular grooves.

DISTURBANCES OF THE CEREBROSPINAL FLUID CIRCULATION

In simple terms, CSF is produced within the ventricles by the choroid plexuses, and absorbed at the cranial vertex and in the spinal canal via arachnoid villi. Reduced absorption results in hydrocephalus, 'water on the brain'. The American neurosurgeon Walter Dandy noted that dye introduced into the ventricles reached the spinal subarachnoid space in some hydrocephalic patients with what he therefore termed 'communicating hydrocephalus', but failed to do so in those with 'noncommunicating' or 'obstructive' hydrocephalus. The most common identified abnormality in children presenting with large heads and hydrocephalus is aqueduct stenosis (Fig. 59.16); most causes of obstructive hydrocephalus are referred to in

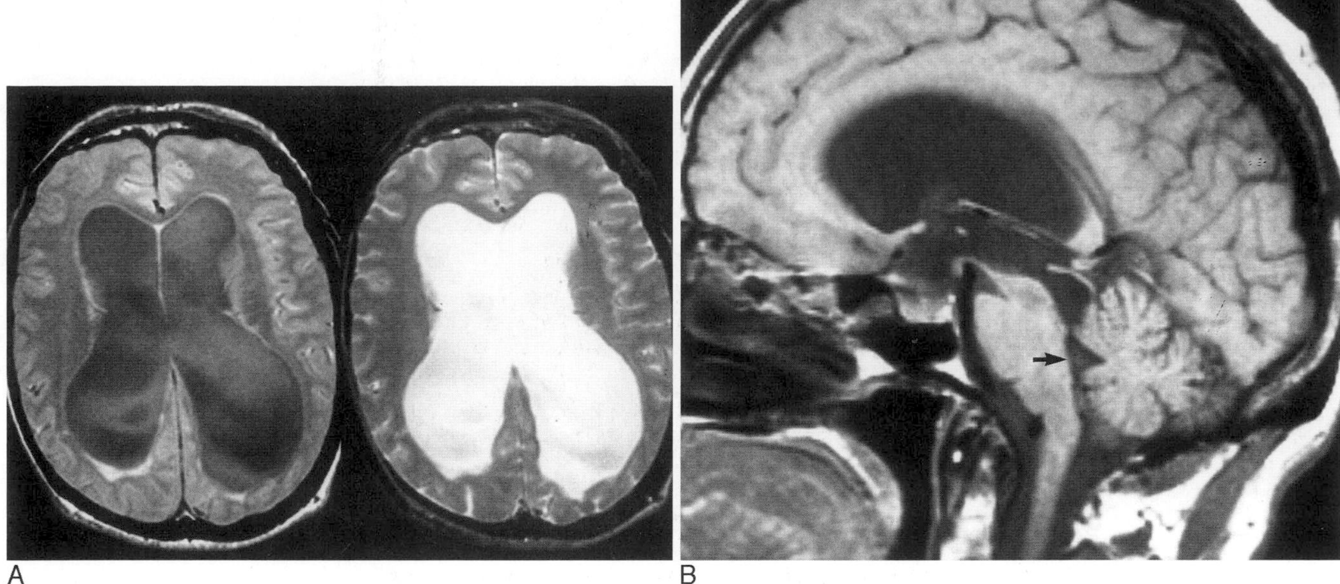

Figure 59.16 Hydrocephalus secondary to aqueduct stenosis: MRI. (A) Axial proton density and T2-weighted images. Marked enlargement of the lateral ventricles, with a thin 'halo' of interstitial oedema. Heterogeneity of the fluid signal within the ventricles is due to pulsatile artefact. (B) Sagittal T1-weighted image demonstrating massive enlargement of lateral ventricles, outpouching of the suprasellar recesses of the third ventricle impinging upon the sella, and 'ventricularization' of the proximal aqueduct just above the level of obstruction and above the fourth ventricle. Note the normal size and configuration of the fourth ventricle (arrow).

other sections of this book. Very rarely, as in papilloma of the choroid plexus, hydrocephalus is due to excessive production of fluid. There is recent interest in the concept of often unrecognized venous sinus thrombosis being a contributory factor[12].

COMMUNICATING HYDROCEPHALUS

In this variety of hydrocephalus, the barrier to absorption of CSF is distal to the foramina of Magendie and Luschka: usually at the tentorial hiatus within the basal cisterns or over the cerebral convexity.

In adults, intracranial pressure may be raised, but lumbar CSF pressure can be normal in 'normal pressure hydrocephalus'. Major causes of communicating hydrocephalus are trauma, subarachnoid haemorrhage and infection, but in a small number of cases the causative factor is not identified; spinal tumours are occasionally incriminated.

At CT or MRI, the hallmark of communicating hydrocephalus is ventricular dilatation, often marked and generalized, although the fourth ventricle may be spared. In young children the occipital horns are often most affected, but in adults enlargement of the frontal and temporal horns is more striking. Interstitial cerebral oedema is variable. The basal cisterns and fissures are sometimes prominent, but the cerebral sulci are characteristically not enlarged; they may be small.

In adults presenting with dementia, the major alternative cause of ventricular enlargement is cerebral atrophy. The differentiation may seem important, because patients with communicating hydrocephalus have been reported to show a dramatic response to shunting procedures, whereas primary neuronal degeneration and vascular dementia are essentially untreatable. However, differentiation both clinically and by imaging is difficult and the subject remains controversial. Cisternography, with radionuclides or water-soluble contrast medium and CT, has been employed in such cases; and more recently MRI using flow-sensitive sequences has shown differences in the pattern of movement of the ventricular fluid. Correlation with the results of surgery for any of these is disappointing, most workers now conceding that the best that can be hoped for is a modest improvement in gait, which nonetheless may be significant for care needs.

Ventricular shunting procedures

Imaging procedures, such as ultrasound (US) in infants and CT or MRI in adults, are often employed to assess the size of the cerebral ventricles following shunting procedures for communicating or obstructive hydrocephalus. A satisfactory result is indicated by reversion of ventricular size towards normal and, on CT or MRI, a disappearance of interstitial cerebral oedema. Patency of third ventricle ventriculostomy can be adequately assessed by cardiac gated cine-phase contrast MRI.

Complications

Those that may be detected include:

- **Malfunction** of the shunt, with failure of the hydrocephalus to resolve. This can simply be because of discontinuity in the extracranial shunt tubing, best assessed by plain radiographs; ventriculo-peritoneal shunts can also lead to a loculated intra-abdominal fluid collection, best assessed by US.
- **Incorrect placement** of the intraventricular catheter.
- **Haemorrhage,** intraventricular, intracerebral or extracerebral.
- **Subdural effusions**, of low density on CT from the outset, which are not uncommon.
- **Infection:** ventriculitis, abscess or subdural empyema.

DEGENERATIVE DISORDERS

GENERAL ASPECTS

These comprise a heterogeneous group of conditions, some common, others rare; their pathological hallmarks are neuronal or axonal degeneration and gliosis. Clinically they are characterized mainly by progressive cognitive decline and movement disorders. The pathological changes are distributed uniformly in some diseases and, in others, nonuniformly—often with characteristic predilection to involve certain regions or structures. Traditionally these diseases are defined in terms of clinical syndromes, believed to reflect the distribution of neuronal damage. In recent years great strides have been made towards unraveling the genetic and molecular basis of some of these conditions which will, in time, become much more precisely defined.

Most of these conditions are currently untreatable, but soon this is expected to change, fuelling a research drive to achieve precise clinical diagnosis early, before too much irreversible damage has occurred. Since it is in the early stages that clinical diagnosis often is most difficult, the search is on for surrogate markers and functional neuroimaging offers considerable promise. In the advanced case, CT and MRI will show atrophy in involved regions and perhaps signal change. In some diseases, but usually only in a minority of cases, the pattern of atrophy can have positive predictive value in the face of clinical ambiguity. Nevertheless, it is still the case that the main role of structural imaging is to exclude other causes, which clinically may resemble degeneration, such as neoplasms or hydrocephalus. The positive yield is vanishingly small, but CT or MRI are recommended at least once in the clinical course, repeated only if intercurrent disease is suspected.

An important feature of the degenerative diseases is that they are progressive, and rate of change exceeds that of normal ageing[13]. It is because structural imaging at one point in time is so often unhelpful that many believe functional imaging has a major role.

THE DEMENTIAS

These generally are diseases of the ageing population. After the age of about 50 years the normal brain loses mass and volume at a variable rate, perhaps averaging about 0.1–0.3% per year. Recent advances in quantitative assessment of brain volume have allowed considerable progress in the early diagnosis and assessment of dementias.

Alzheimer's disease

This is the most common cause of primary degenerative dementia, and its incidence increases with age, rising sharply over 70 years. It is a generalized disorder, although in its early stages it may affect the medial part of the temporal lobe, especially the hippocampus, more than elsewhere. The clinical problem often is to distinguish Alzheimer's disease (AD), a disorder which usually progresses to complete disability within 2–5 years, from the far more benign age related memory loss.

Structural imaging

This is usually normal, although occasionally accentuated atrophy medially in the temporal lobe is indicated by widening of the perihippocampal CSF spaces, which should be both bilateral and symmetrical[14]. There is now much greater understanding of the rate of volume change in many of the dementias[15], especially in the hippocampus[16] following the seminal work in this area using MRI[13]. Such studies require meticulous positioning and registration so that subtle volume losses over time can be appreciated.

Functional imaging

In established disease, characteristic symmetrical posterior temporal and parietal perfusion defects on regional cerebral blood flow (rCBF) SPECT have a predictive value for the diagnosis of AD of over 80%[17] (Fig. 59.17), and the severity of rCBF reduction correlates with the degree of cognitive decline[18]. Perfusion defects are not simply the result of cerebral atrophy, but are greater than can be explained by any atrophy demonstrated on anatomical imaging with CT or MRI. Similarly, [^{18}F]deoxy-D-glucose (FDG)-positron emission tomography (PET) studies show reduced glucose uptake that is not explained by atrophy[19]. Receptor imaging using radioligands for central benzodiazepine receptors has shown a similar distribution of deficits in AD[20].

Frontotemporal dementia

These comprise less than 10% of the primary degenerative dementias. They include Pick's disease. Behavioural, motor or speech disorders tend to dominate the early clinical stages rather than memory loss[21]. Discrimination from a psychiatric disorder often is the clinical issue. Structural imaging is abnormal in up to over 50% of clinically definite cases, and may confirm the diagnosis in situations of clinical ambiguity; imaging is less often helpful in the purely frontal lobe syndromes, such as primary progressive aphasia. Thin section volumetric coronal MRI seems the optimal acquisition to achieve the best positive predictive value, and interpretation may require attention to detail if more subtle changes are to be detected.

MRI and even CT show atrophy in the anterior and medial parts of the temporal lobe, which usually is *markedly asymmetric* (right or left) (Fig. 59.18), and diminishes posteriorly. Asymmetric frontal lobe atrophy may also be present.

Functional imaging

Perfusion deficits on rCBF SPECT are predominantly frontal and anterior temporal with preserved perfusion posteriorly. Reduced frontal perfusion is not specific to frontotemporal dementia and can occur in a variety of other conditions, such as schizophrenia, depression, human immunodeficiency virus

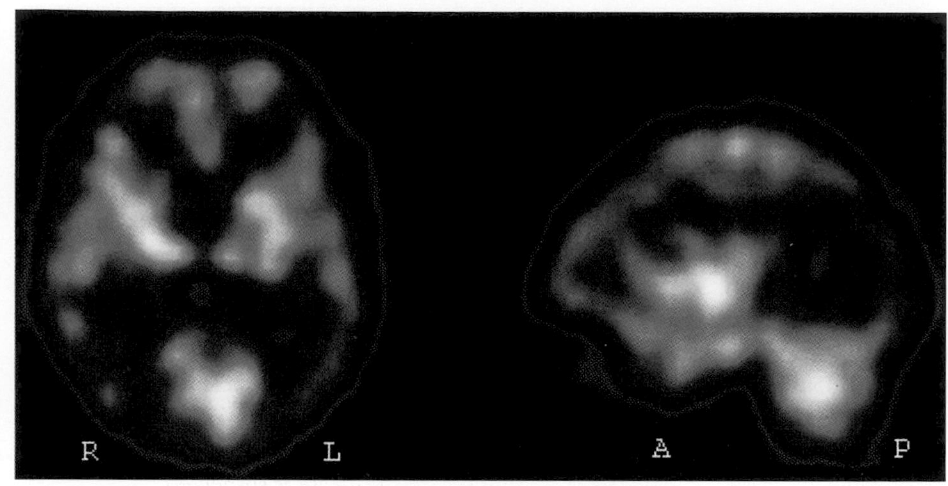

Figure 59.17 Axial (L) and sagittal (R) ^{99m}Tc HMPAO SPECT in Alzheimer's disease showing typical perfusion defects in the posterior temporal and parietal regions.

(HIV) encephalopathy, Creutzfeldt–Jacob disease (CJD) and in some cases of AD[22].

Lewy body dementia

Lewy body dementia is now recognized as the second most common degenerative dementia after AD and it accounts for approximately 20% of all dementia. Neither structural imaging nor rCBF SPECT can reliably distinguish between Lewy body dementia and AD on subjective assessment, as posterior temporoparietal defects occur in both. However, reduced frontal perfusion with HMPOA SPECT and reduced uptake in the cerebellum and visual cortex with FDG-PET is seen in Lewy body dementia compared with AD[23].

Vascular dementia

This is the clinical diagnosis in about 20% of all dementias. Evidence of ischaemic damage on CT or MRI is mandatory for diagnosis, but such changes, especially in the white matter,

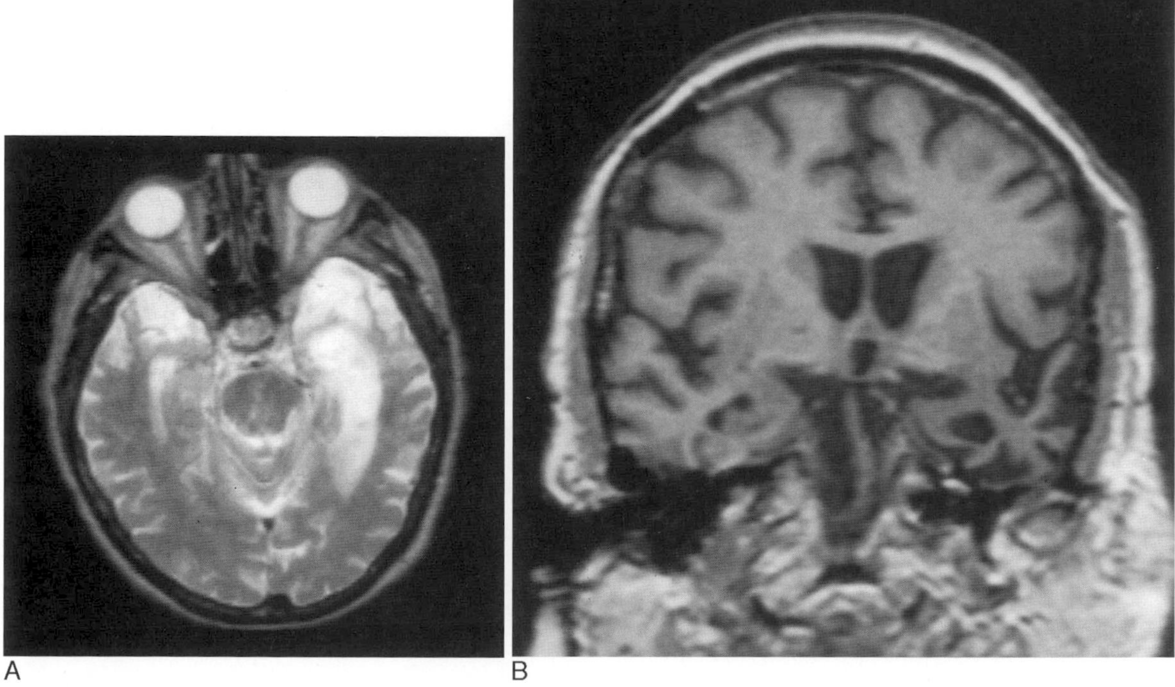

Figure 59.18 Pick's disease. (A) Axial T2-weighted images and (B) coronal T1-weighted images (from a volumetric acquisition) showing severe rather generalized mainly anterior temporal lobe atrophy, most marked on the left side. Such severe change needs to be distinguished from other causes of brain damage such as head injury and encephalitis. Lack of past history should be decisive, but the pattern of atrophy is usually sufficiently characteristic to distinguish between these conditions.

are very common in elderly nondemented subjects and there are no reliable imaging criteria to distinguish between the two. Functional imaging typically shows patchy, cortical and basal ganglia perfusion defects, but it may not always reliably distinguish between vascular dementia and frontotemporal dementia[17].

Prion diseases

These mainly comprise CJD (sporadic, iatrogenic, familial) and very recently in Europe (especially in the UK) new variant CJD (nvCJD). Rapidly progressive dementia, often with myoclonus, is the usual clinical picture, often preceded by behavioural disturbances, especially in nvCJD. Structural imaging usually appears normal in early stages, but rapidly progressive atrophy soon develops. Symmetrical increases in signal in the putamen and caudate nuclei may be shown by MRI in about 10% of sporadic CJD, and in the posterior part of the thalami in over 50% of nvCJD; when present, these signs can have considerable positive predictive value[24].

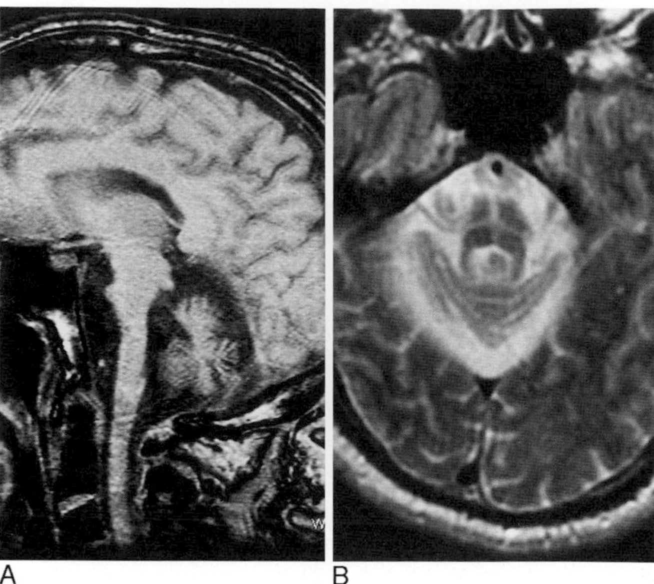

Figure 59.19 Multiple system atrophy, cerebellar type (ponto-olivocerebellar atrophy). (A) Sagittal T1- and (B) axial T2-weighted MR images showing marked atrophy of the ventral part of the pons and of the 'pontine nuclei' and their axons; on axial images signal change as well as atrophy give rise to a 'hot-cross bun' appearance, the darker areas representing the preserved corticospinal and lemniscal pathways.

MOVEMENT DISORDERS

Idiopathic Parkinson's disease and Parkinsonian syndromes

Structural imaging has little role here except to exclude other diseases and to demonstrate the extent of the atrophy (Fig. 59.19). Functional imaging provides insights into disease mechanisms in research settings, but the diagnosis still remains mainly clinical. Receptor imaging of the dopaminergic system continues to be widely studied in idiopathic Parkinson's disease and other movement disorders. New functional imaging techniques continue to evolve in this area; some now offer insights into controlling symptoms and future therapeutic innovations.

EPILEPSY

Recent onset seizures

It is recommended by various bodies[1] and by NICE[25] that anyone who has an unprovoked seizure should have brain MRI. Intravenous contrast medium is not required routinely even with focal seizures. A progressive cause such as neoplasia will be found in only about 6%, but in countries where tuberculosis and cysticercosis are common, it can be as high as over 50%. Standard MRI examinations are all that are required in this context.

Chronic epilepsy

These patients have repeated seizures, usually over years, which usually are well controlled by drug treatment. There may be no detectable underlying structural lesion (cryptogenic epilepsy), or a variety of usually nonprogressive lesions, some of which are rare or do not occur in other contexts. These may be grouped as:

- **scars**—infarcts, trauma
- **vascular lesions**—cavernomas, arteriovenous malformations
- **malformation of cortical development**—various, but especially focal cortical dysplasia, cortical hamartomas (tuberous sclerosis) and neuronal heterotopias (Fig. 59.20)
- **neoplasms**—grade I tumours usually containing mixed glial and neuronal elements: gangliogliomas, dysplastic neuroepithelial tumour
- **hippocampal sclerosis**—by far the most common and associated with temporal lobe epilepsy (TLE), the most common of the partial epilepsies (Fig. 59.21).

Structural imaging[26]

In patients with drug-resistant epilepsy, excision of a structural lesion may cure the epilepsy or at least improve seizure control. Focal excision of normal cortical tissue on the other hand, generally does not. The structural lesions associated with chronic epilepsy are shown with great sensitivity by modern MRI, and it is highly likely that any focal cortical excision in MRI-negative patients will yield histologically normal tissue. In most centres this has led to an appropriate emphasis on structural imaging with MRI in preoperative assessment, with resort to functional imaging only when further clarification is required.

Routine MRI is usually adequate to detect most lesions, and it is here that T2-weighted lesions with fat suppression (e.g. FLAIR) and high resolution volume acquisitions can be particularly helpful in drawing attention to small cortical abnormalities which may otherwise have gone unnoticed (Fig. 59.22). Acquisition in the coronal plane is mandatory to detect hippocampal sclerosis.

The signs of hippocampal sclerosis on MRI are (1) volume loss and (2) increased signal on T2-weighted images

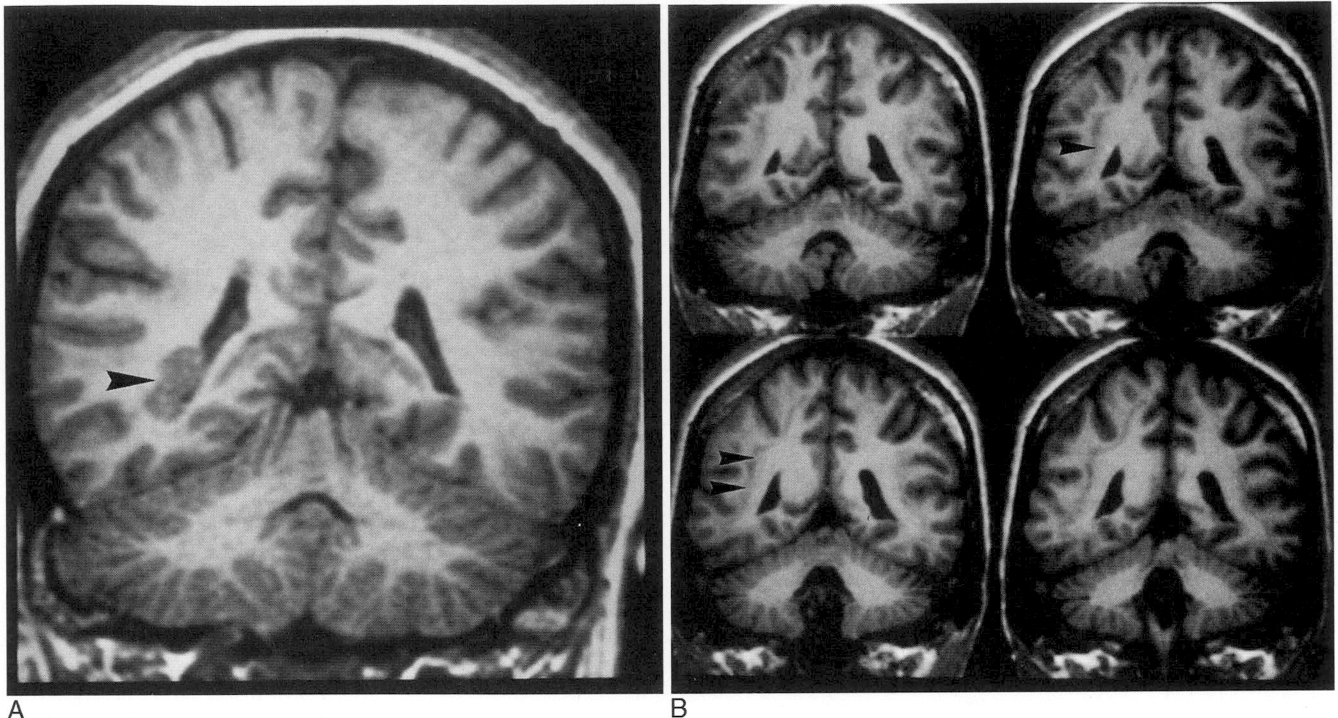

Figure 59.20 Neuronal heterotopia. Coronal T1-weighted images from a volumetric acquisition; slice thickness is 1.5 mm. (A) Subependymal (nodular) heterotopia (arrowhead), (B) laminar heterotopia (arrowheads).

(see Fig. 59.21). Outside specialized units, it is signal change that is easiest to detect and most reliable, but it may be important to ensure that the brighter hippocampus is not the larger because then the pathology would not be hippocampal sclerosis. Volume loss therefore is more specific, but it is detected reliably only by thin section volumetric acquisitions in the coronal plane and requires considerable attention to detail[26].

Functional imaging

MRI and ictal scalp electroencephalography (EEG) can be discordant or negative in up to 40% of potentially pre-operative

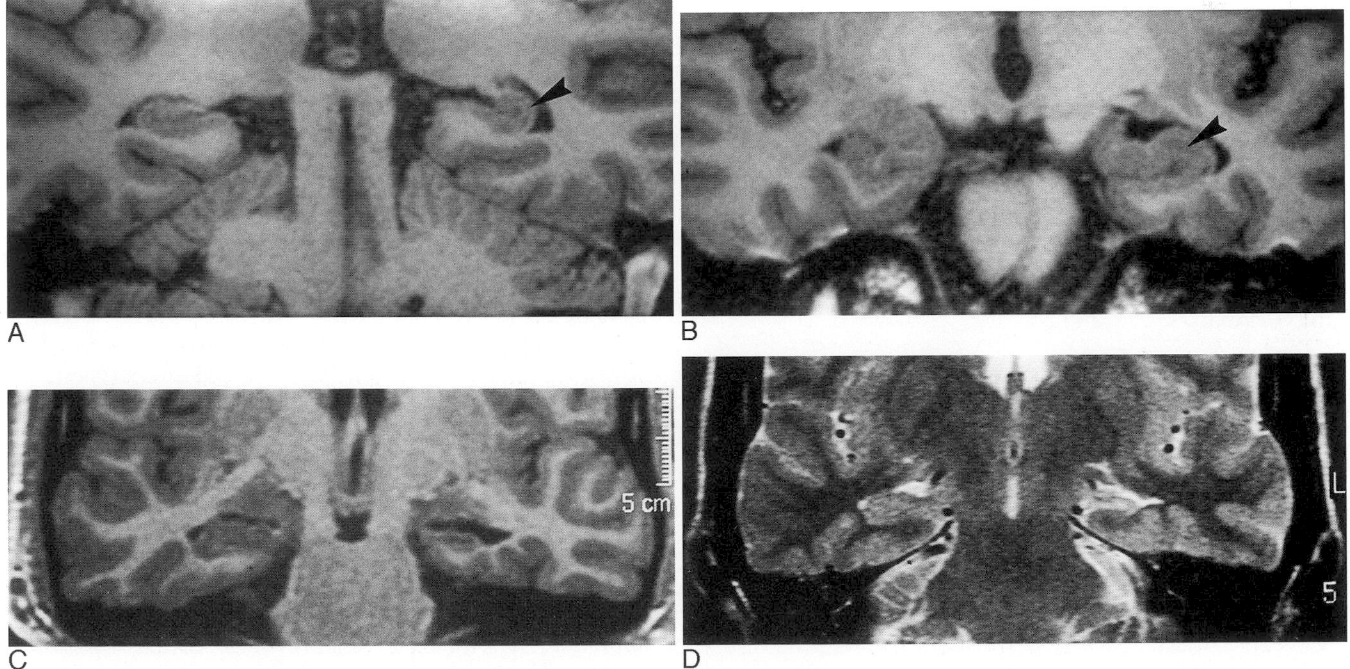

Figure 59.21 Diagnosis of hippocampal sclerosis. (A, B) Normal hippocampus (arrow heads). (A) Body, (B) head. Coronal T1-weighted MRIs from a volumetric acquisition; slice thickness is 1.5 mm. Asymmetry is due to asymmetrical position of each slice with respect to the hippocampus which is essentially unavoidable and usually appears more marked in the head region. (C) T1- and (D) T2-weighted images through the temporal lobes. In (C) the left hippocampus is smaller than the right and (D) is of higher signal. Images (C and D, Courtesy of Dr P. Rich.)

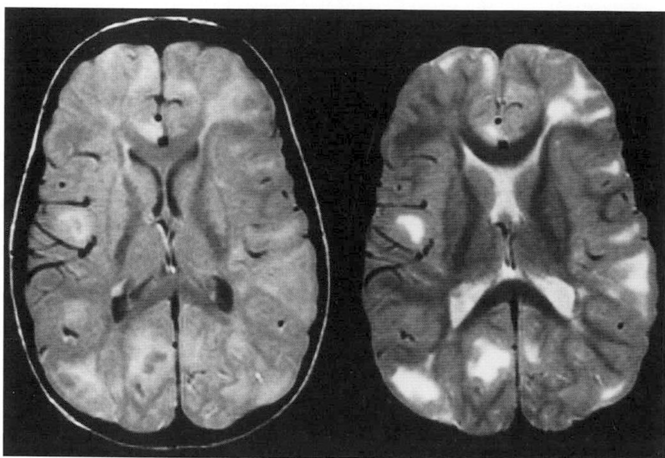

Figure 59.22 Tuberous sclerosis in a 5-year-old girl with seizures; MRI. Proton density and T2-weighted images (2000/40, 2000/80). Multiple cortical and subcortical hyperintensities represent tubers, with associated demyelination. A single hyperintense subependymal nodule is visible in the right trigone.

cases. Options for further noninvasive investigation include magnetic resonance spectroscopy (MRS), PET/CT, rCBF SPECT, FDG-PET and ^{11}C-flumazenil PET. There is still no clear evidence as to which of these tests is best and most are the subject of ongoing research. Localization of extratemporal epileptogenic foci is less successful with all investigations, including structural MRI.

Calcification of the basal ganglia

Calcification is frequently revealed by CT in normal, older people. Causes include hypoparathyroidism, pseudohypoparathyroidism and mitochondrial cytopathy, but most cases are idiopathic and disturbances of calcium metabolism are so rare that biochemical testing is performed only if indicated by other features; some cases are familial (Fahr's syndrome). In many of these conditions, MRI may show much more extensive increased signal on T1-weighted images than revealed by CT. This is believed to be due to T1 shortening in the hydration shells enclosing microscopic crystal deposits.

ACKNOWLEDGEMENTS

In the previous editions, Alison D. Murray, Dawn Saunders and Barton Lane all contributed handsomely.

REFERENCES

1. Royal College of Radiologists 2007 Making the best use of a department of clinical radiology: guidelines for doctors. London, RCR
2. National Institute for Clinical Excellence 2003 Head injury: guidelines. London, NICE http://www.nice.org.uk/guidance/CG4/guidance/pdf/English/download.dspx
3. Mayor S 2003 NICE recommends greater use of CT imaging for head injuries. BMJ 326: 1414
4. Du Boulay G H 1980 Principles of X-ray diagnosis of the skull. Butterworth, London.
5. Kingsley D P E, Till K, Hoare R D 1978 Growing fractures of the skull. J Neurol Neurosurg Psychiatry 41: 312–318
6. Naidich T P, Moran C J, Pudlowski R M, Naidich J B 1979 CT diagnosis of isodense subdural hematoma. In: Thompson R A, Green J R (eds) Adv Neurol 22: 73–105
7. Boviatsis EJ, Kouyialis AT, Sakas DE. 2003 Misdiagnosis of bilateral isodense chronic subdural haematomas. Hosp Med 64: 374–375.
8. Avdin K, Guven K, Sencer S, Jinkins JR, Minareci O 2004 MRI cisternography with gadolinium-containing contrast medium: its role, advantages and limitations in the investigation of rhinorrhoea. Neuroradiology 46: 75–80
9. Peeters F L M, Kroger R 1979 Dural and direct cavernous sinus fistulas. Am J Roentgenol 132: 599–606
10. Liakos G M, Walker C B, Carruth J A S 1979 Ocular complications of craniofacial fibrous dysplasia. Br J Ophthalmol 63: 611–616
11. Dodd G W, Ibbertson H K, Fraser T R C, Holdaway I M, Wattie D 1987 Radiological assessment of Paget's disease of bone after treatment with the biphosphonates EHDP and APD. Br J Radiol 60: 849–860
12. Higgins J N, Gillard J H, Owler B K, Harkness K, Pickard J D 2004 MR venography in idiopathic intracranial hypertension: unappreciated and misunderstood. J Neurol Neurosurg Psychiatry 75: 621–625
13. Fox N, Freeborough P, Rossor M N 1996 Visualisation and quantification of rates of atrophy in Alzheimer's disease. Lancet 348: 94–97
14. De Leon M, Golomb J, George A et al 1993 The radiological prediction of Alzheimer's disease: the atrophic hippocampal formation. Am J Neuroradiol 14: 897–906
15. Schott J M, Price S L, Frost C, Whitwell J L, Rossor M N, Fox N C 2005 Measuring atrophy in Alzheimer disease: a serial MRI study over 6 and 12 months. Neurology 65: 119–124
16. Fox N L, Warrington E, Freeborough H P et al 1996 Presymptomatic hippocampal atrophy in Alzheimer's disease. A longitudinal MRI study. Brain 119: 2001–2007
17. Duara R, Barker W, Luis C A 1999 Frontotemporal dementia and Alzheimer's disease. Differential diagnosis. Dement Geriatric Cogn Disord 10 (Suppl 1): 37–42
18. Bartenstein P, Minoshima S, Hirsch C et al 1997 Quantitative assessment of cerebral blood flow in patients with Alzheimer's disease by SPECT. J Nucl Med 38: 1095–1101
19. Ibáñez V, Pietrini P, Alexander GE et al 1998 Regional glucose metabolic abnormalities are not the result of atrophy in Alzheimer's disease. Neurology 50: 1585–1593
20. Varrone A, Soricelli A, Postiglione A et al 1997 Benzodiazepine receptor distribution in Alzheimer's disease with ^{123}I-iomazenil SPECT. In: De Deyn P P, Dierckx R A, Alave A, Pickut B A (eds) A textbook of SPECT in neurology and psychiatry. John Libbey, London, pp 45–48
21. Neary D, Snowden J S, Gustafson L et al 1998 Frontotemporal lobar degeneration: a consensus on clinical diagnostic criteria. Neurology 51: 1546–1554
22. Pickut B A, Saerens J, Mariën P et al 1997 SPECT in the differential diagnosis of frontal lobe type dementia and dementia of the Alzheimer type. In: De Deyn P P, Dierckx R A, Alave A, Pickut B A (eds) A textbook of SPECT in neurology and psychiatry. John Libbey, London, pp 3–10
23. Defebvre L J P, Leduc V, Duhamel A et al 1999 Technetium HMPAO SPECT study in dementia with Lewy bodies, Alzheimer's disease and idiopathic Parkinson's disease. J Nucl Med 40: 956–962
24. Coulthard A, Hall K, English P T et al 1999 Quantitive analysis of MRI signal intensity in new variant Creutzfeldt–Jacob disease. Br J Radiol 72: 742–748
25. National Institute for Clinical Excellence 2004 Epilepsy. London, NICE http://www.nice.org.uk/CG020
26. Stevens J M 1999 Imaging in epilepsy. Revista di Neuroradiologia 12 (Suppl): 57–62

CHAPTER 60

The Spine

John M. Stevens, Philip M. Rich and Adrian K. Dixon

METHODS OF EXAMINATION

Many techniques are available for the investigation of diseases of the spine and its contents. However, all have been superseded by magnetic resonance imaging (MRI): this is now so widely available in most countries that other neuroradiological investigations of the spine are considered only when MRI is either contraindicated or difficult to perform. The one major exception is trauma and multidetector computed tomography (CT) provides exquisite anatomical information and multiplanar viewing on a workstation of the isometric data set. Indeed many spinal lesions now come to light through CT for unrelated symptoms.

PLAIN RADIOGRAPHY OF THE SPINE

Plain radiography is still widely used but cannot really be justified any longer as a definitive investigation. However, there are a few situations where plain radiographs remain helpful, the most significant being the localization of trauma and evaluation of instability.

Cervical spine

Anteroposterior and lateral views

These are the standard views although a lateral view with the neck held in the maximal flexion that the patient can manage comfortably is often required (e.g. rheumatoid arthritis). These views may be difficult to acquire following trauma with the patient supine; here it is essential to see the alignment at C7/T1. Figure 60.1 illustrates the importance of high-quality radiography.

Oblique view

These views display the foramina; those displayed en face are those *away* from which the head is rotated (cf. lumbar spine). To avoid confusion, each oblique projection must show both right and left side markers. Again the need for such views is questionable in the era of MRI.

Thoracocervical spine

Anteroposterior views

These are good for demonstrating overall alignment (in scoliosis), vertebral collapse and the integrity of the pedicles (possible metastasis).

Lateral view

This is best obtained as a 'swimmer's view' with one arm elevated above the head and the other down by the side. Following trauma in thick-set individuals, attention to this view may prevent a referral for CT or MRI.

Thoracic spine

Anteroposterior and lateral views

If there is a scoliosis, the convexity is placed nearer the radiograph so that the divergent rays are more nearly parallel to the disc spaces. The patient may breathe gently during the exposure, blurring out the rib cage.

Lumbar spine

Anteroposterior view

Flexion of the hips and knees will reduce the lumbar lordosis.

Lateral view

Again convexity of any scoliosis is nearer the radiograph.

Anteroposterior oblique view

The pedicles can be shown en face at 30–40 degrees of obliquity and neural foramina *towards* which the trunk is rotated. This can help in possible spondylolisthesis

Lumbosacral spine

Anteroposterior and lateral views

The lowest disc space is often best assessed separately (by a coned rather overexposed image) from the remainder of the lumbar spine. The sacroiliac joints are best seen on a PA view, where the diverging beam is more aligned to the joints.

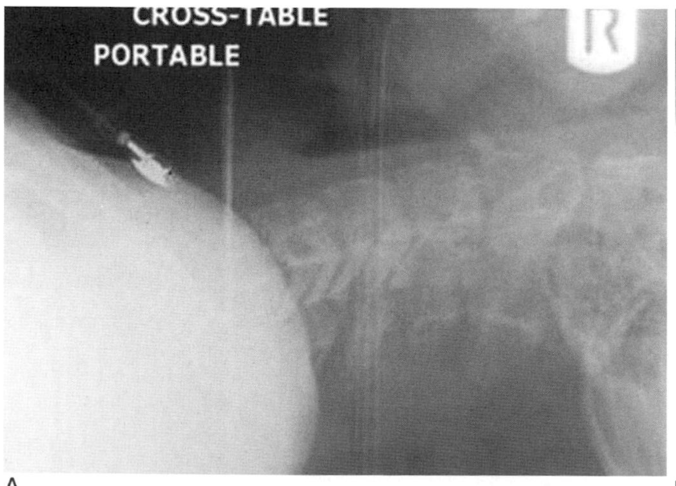

A

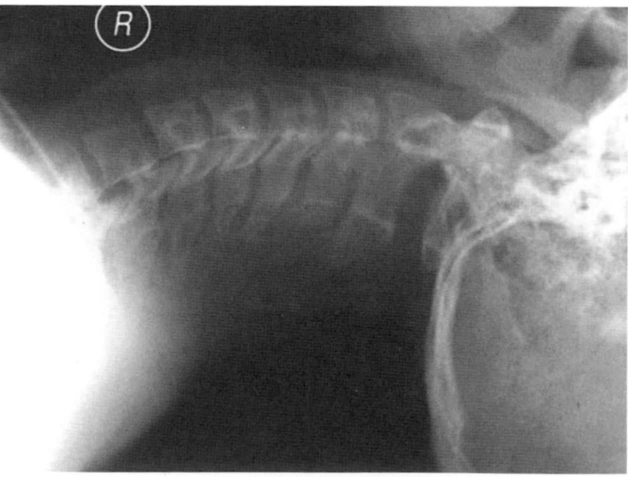

B

Figure 60.1 Lateral plain radiograph of the cervical spine. Patient being examined in the resuscitation unit following trauma. Shoot-through lateral radiographs with the patient supine. (A) Initial attempt. (B) Second radiograph with much improved radiographic positioning allowing demonstration of normal alignment including the all important C7/T1 junction.

ANATOMY

Some developmental anomalies are very common but most are without clinical significance.

SPINA BIFIDA

A wide or narrow midline defect of the posterior arch of the atlas occurs in 6 per cent of the normal population, and of the anterior arch in about 2 per cent. Sometimes both defects coexist, resulting in a bifid atlas[1]. Failure of fusion of the neural arch of L5 or S1 is even more common, occurring in 20 per cent or more of some populations[2]. The defect, known as spina bifida occulta when there are no other features, is nearly always narrow and asymmetric.

INTERVERTEBRAL FUSIONS

These usually occur only in the cervical region. Generally only one level is involved, C2/3 being the commonest, and this is frequently associated with occipital assimilation of the atlas[3] (Fig. 60.2). The AP diameter of congenitally fused vertebrae is often smaller than that of other vertebrae in the region.

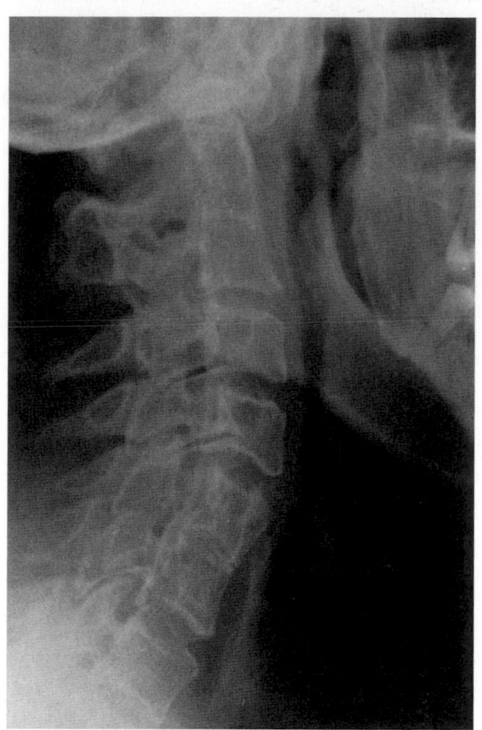

Figure 60.2 Lateral plain radiograph of the cervical spine showing the commoner intervertebral fusions: occiput – C1, C2–3 and C6–7.

TRANSITIONAL VERTEBRAE

Complete or partial fusion of L5 with the sacrum is seen in more than 6 per cent of the normal population. One or both transverse processes of L5 are enlarged, and the L5–S1 disc space is narrow[4]. Rudimentary twelfth ribs are usually identifiable. A true extra lumbar vertebra due to lumbarization of S1 is less frequent. The main significance of transitional lumbosacral or thoracolumbar vertebrae is that they may result in a level being wrongly identified pre-operatively. The level of the iliac crests provides a useful landmark; they usually correlate with the L4/5 disc.

Cervical ribs involving the seventh cervical vertebra also occur in about 6 per cent of the normal population. Oblique or lordotic projections and apical chest views may aid good demonstration. A useful feature for differentiating short first ribs from cervical ribs is that the transverse processes of T1 tend to be directed superiorly.

MAGNETIC RESONANCE IMAGING

Spatial resolution is a crucial consideration in the spine. Since the signal intensities of disc, bone, cerebrospinal fluid (CSF), spinal cord and epidural fat are very different on most sequences, it is possible to compromise on contrast resolution in the interest of spatial resolution in many applications of spinal MRI. Faster sequences are also possible and speed and throughput are not only economic considerations but also appreciated by patients. All such innovations are easier at high field strength – 1.5 T seems optimal for most applications.

VOLUMETRIC (3D) ACQUISITIONS

The deployment of fast imaging techniques has permitted three-dimensional (3D) spatial encoding within a few minutes. The result is multiple contiguous images, no interslice gaps and section thicknesses down to 1 or 2 mm. This is helpful in the evaluation of the intervertebral foramina in the cervical region. However, the best images of the spinal cord are usually obtained from slightly thicker slices (Fig. 60.3).

FAST SPIN-ECHO

In fast spin-echo (FSE) several phase-encoding steps are made at each excitation instead of just one, which greatly reduces acquisition times and permits use of much larger matrices, resulting in twice the resolution in even shorter data acquisition periods. The penalties are slight loss of contrast and increased sensitivity to physiological motion (Fig. 60.4).

FLUID ATTENUATION INVERSION RECOVERY

Fluid attenuation inversion recovery (FLAIR) sequences offer improved lesion detection by permitting heavily T2-weighted

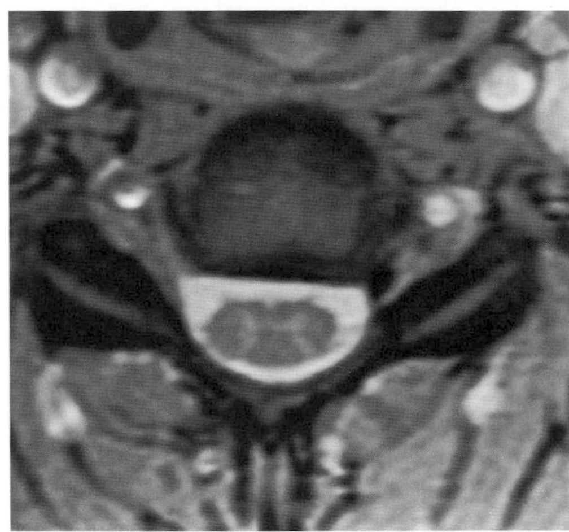

Figure 60.3 Axial MR image. Axial MRI cervical spine at C5–6, from a gradient-recalled multislice acquisition, slice thickness 4 mm. The internal structure of the spinal cord (surrounded by the white CSF) is quite well shown.

(T2W) acquisitions to be accomplished with suppression of all signal from cerebrospinal fluid. This removes motion artefact from CSF, the CSF appearing paradoxically as signal void on heavily T2W images. However, cysts and cystic lesions within the spinal cord also appear as signal voids. Most other lesions appear as high intensity. Imaging with FLAIR used to be slow and its resolution was low (see ref 14); however, new or fast FLAIR programmes now enjoy widespread clinical use, but sensitivity for detecting lesions in cord substance has been disappointing (see ref 15), and standard spin-echo techniques so far are preferable.

PHASED-ARRAY COILS

Spinal imaging requires surface coils, and the phased-array configuration enables data to be acquired simultaneously from up to four surface coils in series. This permits imaging of the entire spinal cord over one acquisition period and greatly reduces imaging time. Vertebral level counting, often difficult using single coils in the thoracic region, also becomes simpler (Fig. 60.5).

A wide variety of post-processing options has also become available on most workstations. These permit multiplanar reformatting in real time, 3D surface rendering, colour coding and many others. The ability to reconstruct in a curved plane is potentially useful in scoliosis, but its value is limited because most major curvatures occur in more than one plane. In many ways such functions are more relevant to CT than MRI.

MOTION ARTEFACTS

These are generated by pulsatile motion of the CSF. This motion has been documented and recently quantified by MRI. At C2/3, inferior movement is estimated at about 0.65 mm during systole[5]. MRI has shown that the primary driving force behind intracranial and spinal CSF flow is expansion of the brain during systole. The spinal cord and brainstem also descend slightly on systole and oscillate anteroposteriorly[6].

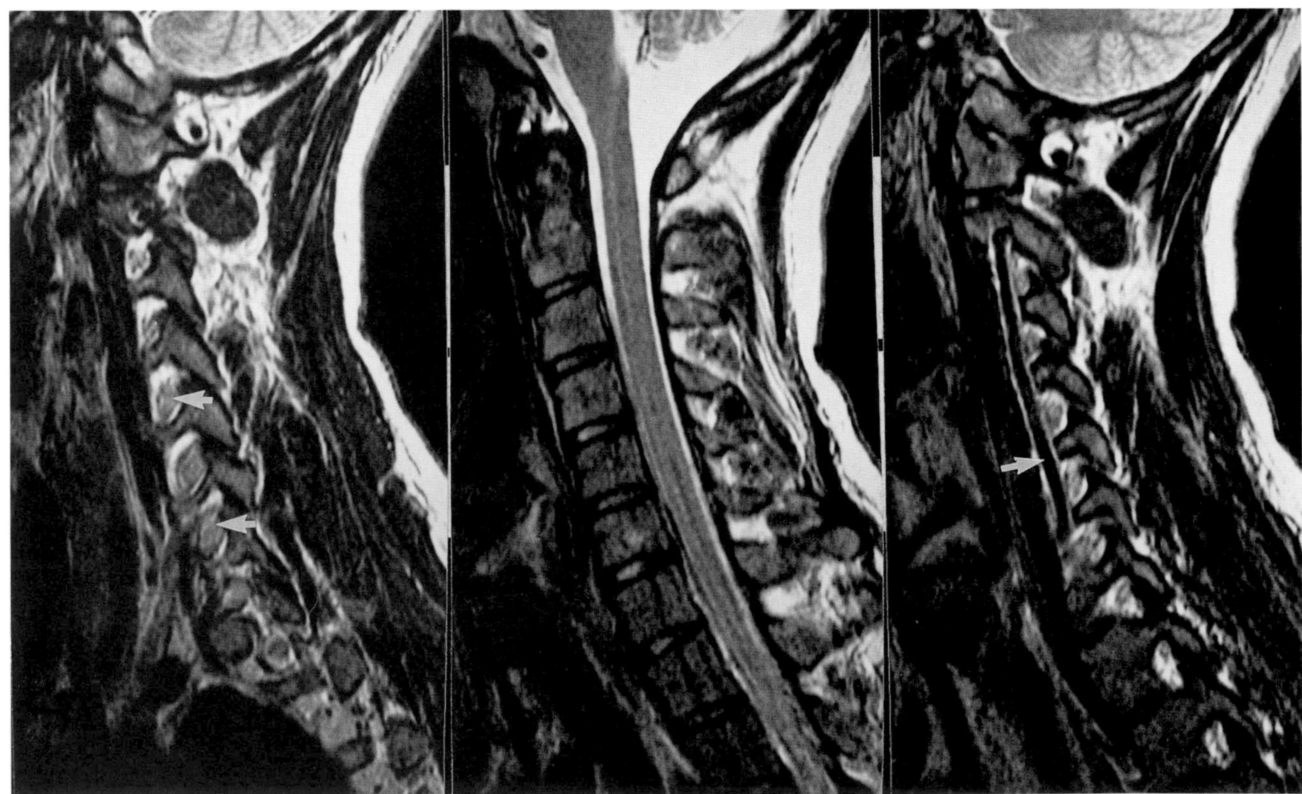

Figure 60.4 Fast spin-echo MRIs of the cervical spine from a multislice (2D) sagittal series (TR 4000 ms, TE 80, matrix 512 × 256). The vertebral artery (arrow, right image), the intervertebral canals and dorsal root ganglia (arrows in left image) are shown well, but the spinal cord image (centre) is degraded by motion artefact.

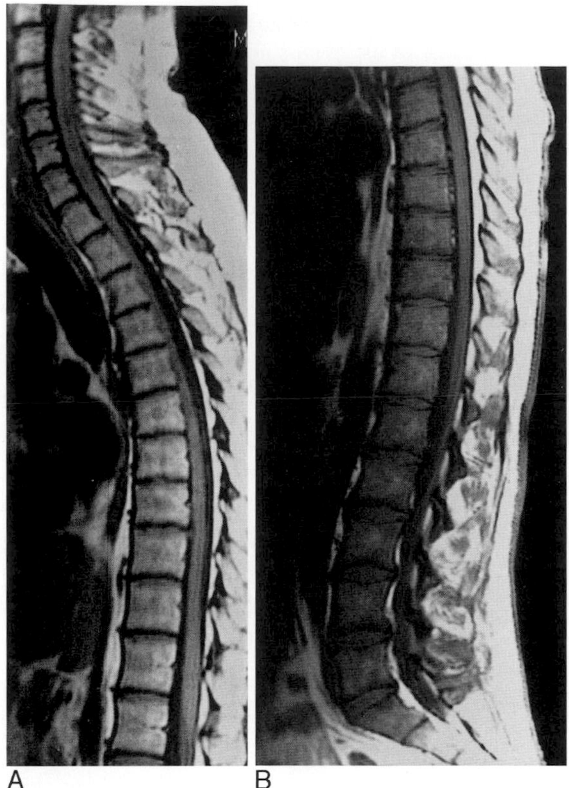

Figure 60.5 Spinal MRI using phased-array coils (spin-echo, TR 600 ms, TE 20). Two coil configurations: (A) cervical and thoracic. (B) Thoracic and lumbar.

In classic studies, Rubin and Enzmann[7] showed how such motion generates linear artefacts parallel to the spinal cord/CSF interface in the phase-encoding direction, producing signal variation in the spinal cord image that could be misinterpreted as an intramedullary lesion. Areas of turbulent CSF flow related to subarachnoid septa can result in signal variation simulating intradural masses or enlarged vessels, particularly in the thoracic spine.

Many strategies have been developed to minimize these problems, including altering the direction of the phase-encoding gradient, application of additional motion-nulling gradients and cardiac gating. Spatial presaturation is used to suppress signal arising from moving structures such as the heart.

Truncation artefacts are generated at boundaries by image processing. They are particularly significant at the CSF/spinal cord interface. Such an artefact is one possible cause of the band of high or low signal seen near the centre of the spinal cord in some midsagittal images. It is also one of several sources of error in defining the position of the cord/CSF boundary. The physical dynamics of this boundary are more complex than in CT.

Susceptibility effects are another important source of error, generated in particular by gradient-recalled echo techniques. Phantom studies have demonstrated that both electronic and caliper measurements of the midsagittal diameter of the spinal cord can be artificially reduced by over 2 mm in the phase-encoding direction, creating a spurious impression of a spinal cord flattening or exaggerating the degree of compression shown[8].

Metallic artefacts can be particularly destructive. Many spinal operations utilize metal stabilization devices and patients often require postoperative imaging at some stage. Ferromagnetic materials generate major local artefacts and usually render imaging of the spinal canal impossible. Tiny fragments from drills, invisible on plain radiographs, may also result in devastating artefacts[9]. Design of implants is also important; numerous titanium devices are now available and it is hoped that these will prove acceptable in the long term[10].

CONDUCT OF MRI EXAMINATION

Details of optimal pulse sequence, coil type and strategies for motion suppression are specified by individual manufacturers; the general principles, however, are the same for all equipment. The following is a guide only.

Some centres make an effort to reduce the number of sequences used routinely in the interests of saving time. The saving of even a few minutes per patient by omitting one sequence may become significant. Even with well-designed protocols, some patients will have to be recalled for additional sequences.

Cervical spine

MRI usually begins with a fast coronal multislice sequence as a localizer. The optimal sagittal plane for the cervical spine is selected from this series, and a multislice high-resolution sagittal series planned. Optimal sequences use matrix sizes of 512 × 256, with spatial presaturation applied over the larynx and carotid arteries. Two sagittal data acquisitions are planned, one strongly T1 weighted and the other T2 weighted. At these matrices, fast spin-echo techniques are required; artefact from CSF motion can be a problem.

Axial images are planned from the sagittal data sets, to demonstrate levels of clinical concern or structural abnormality. On modern systems thin T2W images usually suffice, although they may overestimate the degree of compression. The protocol used depends on the clinical problem. In neuroradiology this is usually myelopathy, radiculopathy (often simply arm pain), or both.

For myelopathy, a 2D multislice protocol is usually preferable, especially if intrinsic disease such as demyelination is being sought. In the latter, T2 weighting is essential and the best signal-to-noise ratio and shortest acquisition times are often achieved using a gradient-recalled echo technique. Axial fast spin-echo techniques are not usually satisfactory because of unsuppressed CSF motion.

When evaluating the degree of cord compression, demonstration of internal structure is less important, and thinner sections can be used to improve precision; a T1-weighted (T1W) spin-echo sequence may be the best option to reduce the possibility of overestimating the degree of compression.

When evaluating radiculopathy, the spinal root canals need to be targeted. The best option is a volumetric (3D) acquisition obtained in the axial plane with a T2W gradient-recalled echo sequence data set covering the spine from about C2 to T1–2. Multiplanar reformatting along and orthogonal to the root canals can be performed if so desired.

Thoracic spine

The MRI examination proceeds much as for the cervical spine, the commonest indication being a myelopathy. Spatial presaturation is necessary to exclude the heart, and as far as possible the aorta. Cardiac gating via a digital pulse monitor may be desirable. As in the cervical spine, CSF movement is a significant problem (Fig. 60.6) and fast spin-echo techniques are not usually satisfactory in the axial plane.

Lumbar spine

Again, the MRI procedure is similar to that followed for the cervical spine. CSF motion is minimal in this region, so fast spin-echo techniques can be used to good advantage even in the axial plane, allowing excellent visualization of the cauda equina (Fig. 60.7).

The emphasis of the examination is influenced by the clinical problem. For disc disease and entrapment neuropathies, after the standard T1W and T2W high-resolution sagittal multislice acquisitions, an axial 2D multislice protocol is usually optimal, orientating the slice plane to that of the abnormal or clinically relevant discs, aiming to cover from pedicle to pedicle. The increasing spatial resolution on T2 weighting provided by modern MR systems makes the T1 axial sequence less necessary.

For the postoperative lumbar spine, a more elaborate protocol is recommended. Sagittal T1W and T2W multislice sequences are made, followed by axial T1W images through the levels of interest. This is followed by a high-resolution fast spin-echo axial series through the same or more extended levels, to optimize detection of arachnoiditis as a cause for failed lumbar disc surgery. Then Gd-DTPA is given intravenously, and another T1W axial multislice series acquired, in the same positions as the first using fat signal suppression. This sequence optimizes the evaluation of postoperative scarring so that it can be distinguished more easily from fragments of degenerate fibrocartilage (Fig. 60.8).

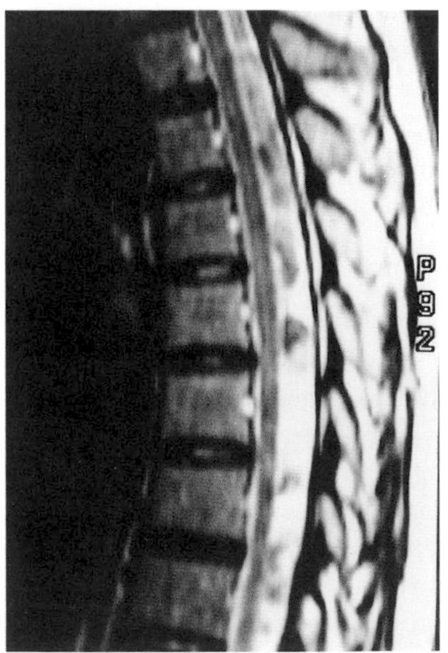

Figure 60.6 Sagittal MRI of thoracic spine using phased-array coils and a fast spin-echo technique (TR 4000 ms, TE 80), slice thickness 3 mm. Turbulent CSF flow posterior to the spinal cord is generating irregular areas of signal loss, simulating intradural masses.

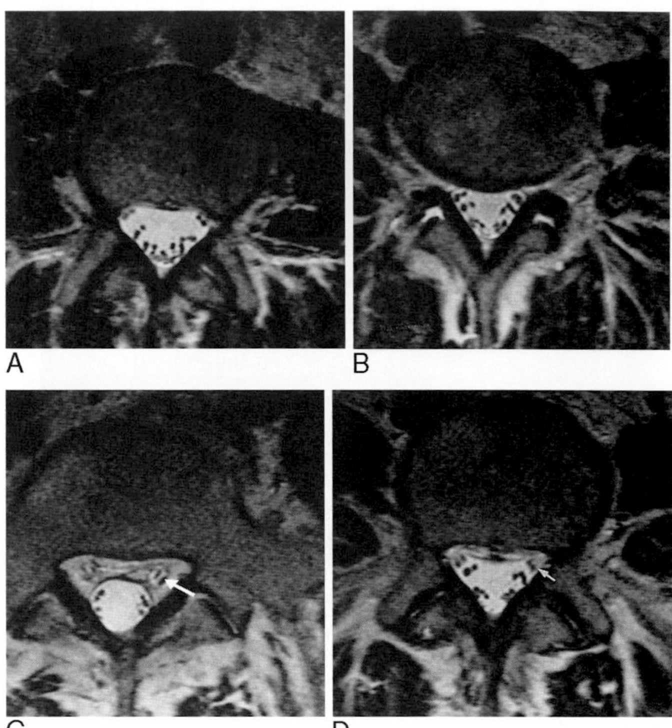

Figure 60.7 High-resolution axial MRI of the lumbar spine using a fast spin-echo multislice technique (TR 4000 ms, TE 80, matrix 512 × 256, slice thickness 4 mm). The normal distribution of the intradural roots is well shown in this series. (A) L3. (B) L3–4 disc. (C) 6 mm below B. (D) L5. The rootlets at each nerve line up in the posterolateral part of the thecal sac and leave via their root sheaths in an anteroposterior orderly sequence. Arrow in (C) = roots entering the L4 root sheaths; arrow in (D) = roots visible within the L5 root sheaths. CSF yields high signal (white).

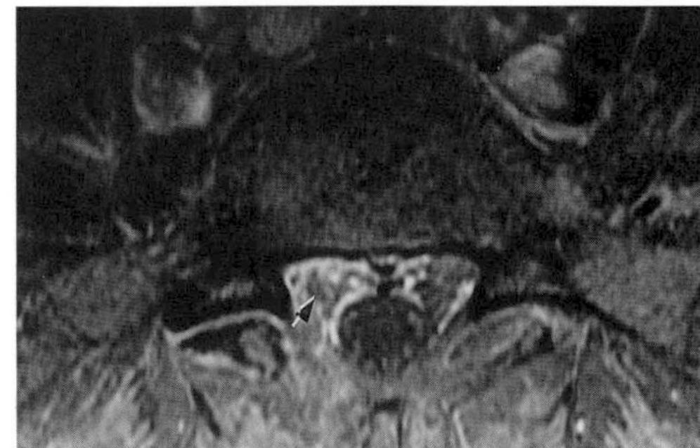

Figure 60.8 Axial MRI just below the L5–S1 disc, using a spin-echo acquisition (TR 600 ms, TE 20) with fat suppression. IV gadolinium has been given. The patient had had a right partial hemilaminectomy 18 months earlier. The right L5 root is shown embedded in enhancing scar tissue (arrowhead).

COMPUTED TOMOGRAPHY OF SPINE

CT is still sometimes used for lumbar disc disease and is essential in the evaluation of fractures. Adequate assessment of intradural structures still may require intrathecal contrast medium, though adequate visualization of the spinal cord to exclude compression usually can be achieved without intrathecal contrast medium on modern equipment.

POSITIONING

Spinal CT is usually carried out in the supine position, with the spinal column as perpendicular to the plane of section as possible. The neck is moderately flexed to reduce the normal cervical lordosis but artefacts from dental fillings may limit this. Gantry tilt and flexion of the hips was useful in the past but has been superseded by multiplanar reconstructions.

A digital radiograph ('scanogram', 'scout film') of the region to be studied is *mandatory* for selection of the levels to be examined and for retrospective localization of abnormalities. CT machines are now so fast that the patient can be instructed not to breathe or swallow during the data acquisition.

The slice thickness depends on the clinical problem. Soft-tissue contrast is better on thicker slices. Sections 2–3 mm thick are appropriate for investigating lumbar disc disease. With modern multidetector systems, a volume of data is acquired; the workstation then allows virtually infinite viewing options. When soft-tissue contrast is less important, the thinnest possible sections may be selected and images reconstructed using a bone review algorithm. This provides maximum resolution of skeletal structures. This is also appropriate for most post-myelography CT. Various post-processing techniques allow graphic 3D images (Fig. 60.9).

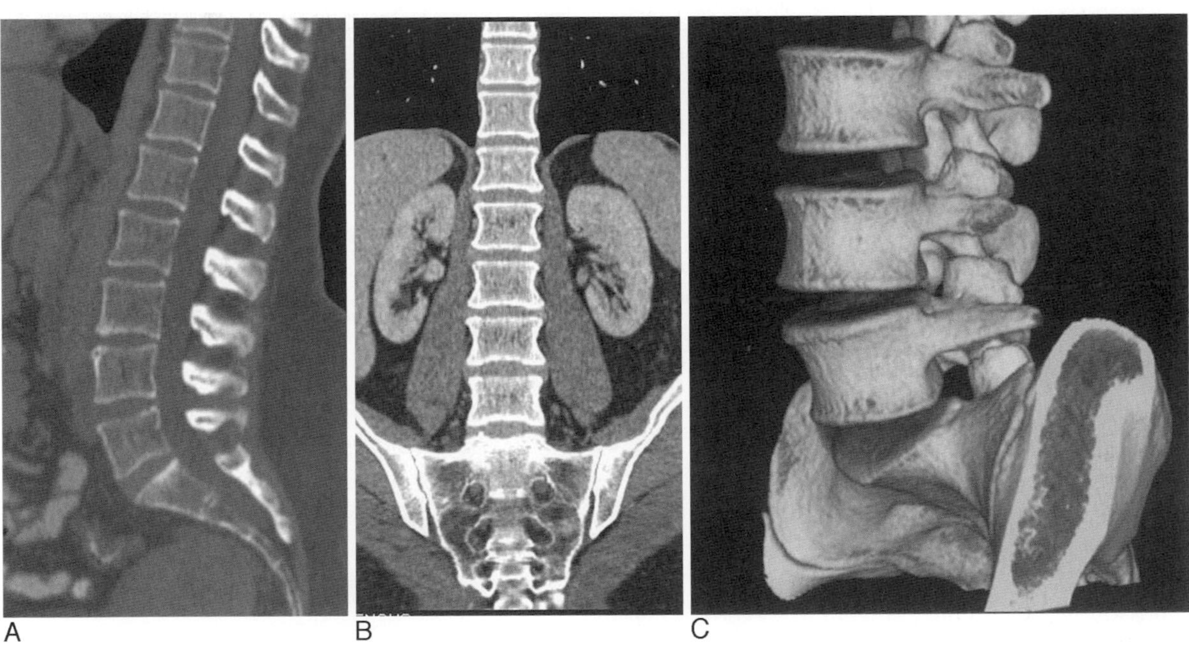

Figure 60.9 Series of lumbar spine mutiplanar reformatted CT images showing (A) Sagittal reformat showing minor degenerative changes anteriorly on either side of the slightly narrow L3/4 disc. (B) Curved coronal reformat of the image in A demonstrating the entire 'straightened' lumbosacral spine; note how this has overcome the lumbar lordosis and the sacral curvature. (C) Surface shaded 3D reconstruction of another patient.

NORMAL ANATOMY

VERTEBRAE

The thin rim of compact cortical bone is shown well by both CT and MRI. The trabecular pattern of cancellous bone is best shown by high-resolution CT but may also be shown to some extent by good-quality MRI. Vascular channels are often visible, and may simulate undisplaced fractures on CT, but do not usually cause difficulty on MRI.

Bone marrow is shown by MRI. Vertebral marrow is haemopoietic, but fatty marrow is usually present as well, constituting up to 50 per cent of spinal marrow volume in adults and increasing with age. Fatty marrow usually predominates in specific areas of the vertebral body, namely adjacent to the vertebral end-plates and around the basivertebral veins in the central parts of the vertebral body. However, there is great variability, and unusually patchy replacement of red by fatty marrow may be normal. Marrow signal is more uniform, and much less influenced by fat, in children[11].

Sclerotic bands are often visible at sites of fusion between vertebral components. These are seen most often at the neurocentral junctions, and in the axis. In the latter, these may be three in number: (A) a V-shaped band just below the apex of the dens; (B) a midsagittal band in the rest of the dens; (C) a horizontal plate within the body of the axis demarcating the body of C1 from the body of C2. Remnants of the subdental synchondrosis itself may persist throughout life, and it is common for the normal dens to appear to consist of diffusely denser bone than other vertebral bodies.

Cortical bone is thicker in the neural arches and their appendages than in the bodies. The spinal canal is widest and almost circular at C1, and usually narrows in the mid-cervical levels and slightly widens in the lower, becoming more triangular in shape[12]. In the thoracic region the canal is almost circular and becomes wider and more triangular, especially in the lower lumbar spine. Although there is considerable individual and regional variation, it is intuitive that an intrinsically narrow canal provides little margin to cope with the inevitable degenerative changes of later life. In the lumbar spine an AP diameter of 11.5 mm or less is worrying[13] and an AP diameter of 15 mm plus seems ideal. Of course precise measurements should not constitute the basis of decision making and in some ways cross-sectional areas are more relevant[14]; in the lumbar spine the cauda equina occupies about 50 mm^2 and 100 mm^2 is probably needed for reasonable CSF flow.

The posterior intervertebral joints are essentially planar in the cervical and thoracic region, and slightly concavo-convex in the lumbar. Maximal rotation of the spine occurs in the thoracic facets. Articular surfaces constitute most of the lateral masses of the cervical vertebrae, but are carried by well-defined articular processes in the thoracic and especially in the lumbar region. Interarticular parts of the laminae can be defined in the lumbar region, and also in the axis. The synovial joint spaces often contain fat, especially near their margins, the fat lying within synovial fringes projecting into the joint cavities. The bone underlying the articular surface of the lateral mass of the axis is thinned focally by the underlying tortuous vertebral artery.

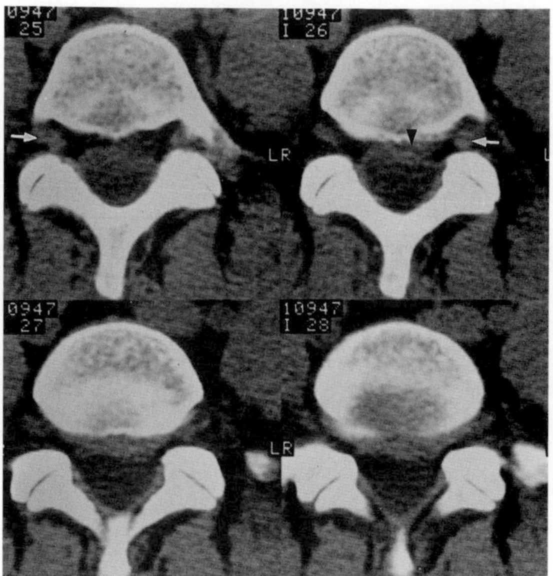

Figure 60.10 Series of four axial CT sections through the lumbar spine extending down to the L4–5 intervertebral disc, showing the intervertebral foramina and contained L4 spinal nerves (arrows). The L4–5 disc is protruding slightly on the left side (black arrowhead).

INTERVERTEBRAL DISCS

Disc structure is well shown only in the lumbar region, where the discs are largest. On CT they show an amorphous texture and a relatively high soft-tissue density, usually clearly distinguishable from the fluid-filled thecal sac, extradural roots and vessels and epidural fat (Fig. 60.10). Internal structure and maturation with age are much better shown by MRI (Fig. 60.11).

Maturation involves both the nucleus pulposus and annulus fibrosus independently, but usually concomitantly. The annulus thickens due to progressive acquisition of concentric layers of dense, organized collagen, and the nucleus pulposus acquires a transverse plate of dense collagenous tissue that bisects it into upper and lower halves. The sharp distinction in children between the more fibrous outer and the less fibrous inner component diminishes with age[15].

The disc margins may normally bulge up to 2–3 mm beyond the vertebral margins, especially in children. The posterior surface is normally flat or concave, not convex (except at L5/S1).

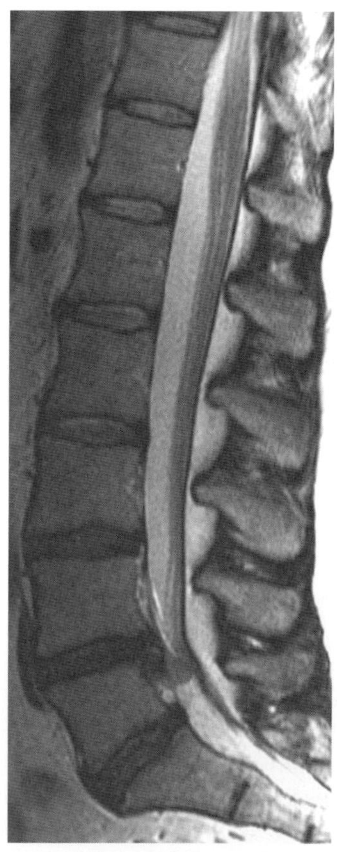

Figure 60.11 Midline sagittal T2W MRI of the lumbar spine with good demonstration of conus (normal) and cauda equina. The intervertebral discs down to L2/3 are relatively normal with degenerate discs between L3 and S1. At L4/5 there is extensive herniation of disc material, which is migrating caudally and extending posteriorly through the posterior longitudinal ligament.

INTERVERTEBRAL FORAMINA

These are best considered as spinal nerve root canals, of which the interpedicular foramen is only a part.

In the C3–7 region, the inferior boundary of each canal is the superior concavity of the transverse process, which cradles the dorsal root ganglion posterior to the foramen transversarium (Figs 60.3, 60.4). The canals are oriented anterolaterally, but nearer the coronal than sagittal plane[16]. They are only about 5 mm wide in normal people, and can be difficult to image well. Axial images on CT or MRI should be as thin as possible. Volumetric MR acquisitions allow the data to be reformatted in planes parallel and transverse to the canals for full evaluation. However, images acquired in the sagittal plane usually also show the canals quite well, with the ganglia within.

In the thoracic region the spinal root canals are short and well seen on images acquired in the sagittal plane. In the lumbar region the root canals are best considered as consisting of two parts: the lateral recess, which lies medial to the superior articular facet and pedicle in the lateral extremity of the spinal canal, and the infrapedicular part. The contents of the intervertebral foramen, which are visible on MRI (and some on CT), are epidural fat and fasciae, radicular arteries and veins, the emerging nerve roots and the dorsal root ganglia[14,17,18].

LIGAMENTS AND EPIDURAL SOFT TISSUES

The dura mater is in direct contact with the posterior longitudinal ligament throughout most of the spinal canal. The posterior longitudinal ligament blends with the intervertebral discs, but between the discs it is separated from the concave posterior surface of the vertebral bodies by the anterior epidural space. This contains fat, the basivertebral veins and the anterior internal vertebral veins, and is divided into left and right compartments by a tough midline septum that influences the course of disc herniations[19]. This epidural space is well developed only in the lumbar region.

Laterally, the dura mater is usually in contact with the medial extremity of each pedicle, although epidural fat may intervene. Below and between the pedicles, the dura is in contact with the epidural fat in continuity with the intervertebral foramina. Posteriorly, the dura mater is usually loosely attached to the anterior cortex of the spinous processes. Between the upper margins of this cortex there are wedges of epidural fat separating the dura from the laminae, posterior joints and ligamenta flava, sometimes called the interlaminar fat pad[14,18] (see Fig. 60.11).

In kyphotic regions (usually the thoracic region) the dura is frequently separated from all the posterior elements of the spinal canal by a layer of epidural fat that may be more than 5 mm thick over the most kyphotic region; this normal appearance has been misinterpreted as idiopathic epidural lipomatosis in some clinical contexts. The volume of the spinal canal occupied by epidural fat can vary greatly, and the dura may be separated from all walls of the canal by fat.

SPINAL CORD

The upper spinal cord may be shown by plain CT, especially in children, but detailed display of the anatomy of the surface of the cord by CT requires intrathecal contrast medium.

Assessment of the size and shape of the cord is, at least in theory, easier to achieve on CT myelography than on MRI. With CT, the boundary can be defined by using the most appropriate window settings, determined from a histogram[20]. Conditions are more difficult to optimize on MRI, where boundaries can be displaced artefactually and there is more variability in the histogram.

The normal internal structure of the cord is shown only by MRI; thicker sections (3–4 mm) usually optimize this, and the butterfly-shaped grey matter is shown on both T1W and T2W images (see Fig. 60.3). Midsagittal MRI of the cord often shows a thin longitudinal band in the centre of the cord, or slightly anterior to centre, which is usually mainly or exclusively a truncation artefact, but in some images it may represent the grey commissure.

The size of the spinal cord can be quantified by several measurements, probably the most robust being cross-sectional area, but wide variation between the mean values in published normative data emphasizes the practical difficulties involved.

SPINAL NERVES

High-resolution techniques are necessary to demonstrate the intradural rootlets emerging from the spinal cord and the larger roots of the cauda equina. Thin T2W images on modern machines show the rootlets, which coalesce to form anterior and posterior roots that penetrate the dura through separate ostia; these form CSF-filled pouches, the lateral extremities of which are often called the subarachnoid angles of the root sheaths. The sheaths end proximal to the dorsal root ganglia. Eccentric cystic expansions of the root sheaths are common at all levels, and are often called perineural cysts and sometimes Tarlov cysts[21]. They may enlarge an intervertebral or sacral foramen; they are particularly frequent, and are largest, on the S2 roots. It remains debatable as to whether these can contribute to symptoms[22].

The roots of the cauda equina appear as bilateral, often circular bunches near the conus medullaris, as a crescentic aggregate in the posterior part of the thecal sac in the midlumbar spine, and lateral and very peripheral at L5. The roots inferior to S1 are smaller, and often very peripheral, making them difficult to see. Some variation and asymmetry in distribution of roots is acceptable. In the lumbar region, the anterior and posterior roots align in the lateral extremity of the thecal sac. For spinal nerves L1–L5, they run in the subarticular part of the spinal root canal (the lateral recess) and cross the disc space within the thecal sac, emerging with their sheaths near the lower margins of the pedicles of the same number. The first sacral nerve usually leaves the thecal sac above the L5–S1 disc, which it crosses usually enclosed in the longest of the lumbar root sheaths to reach the S1–S2 foramen; variations in anatomy may contribute to the variations in symptoms found between patients with similar disc lesions. See also conjoined roots below. The dorsal root ganglia are readily identified at all levels on MRI, but usually only in the lumbar region by plain CT. The anterior roots and rootlets can be identified using high-resolution MRI. The dorsal root ganglia enhance strongly after IV contrast medium, while normal intradural roots do not, or perhaps only minimally.

MYELOGRAPHY

This is rarely indicated nowadays in well-equipped imaging departments, because it is invasive and less informative than MRI. It is only contemplated when MRI is unavailable or contraindicated, or is unsatisfactory due to patient tolerance or unusual shape, such as limb contractures or severe scoliosis.

Until the late 1970s, the only contrast agents available were iophendylate oil (Myodil, Pantopaque), which led to considerable long-term arachnoiditis, and air or carbon dioxide. Now there are numerous non-ionic water-soluble contrast media available for intravascular use, but many have not been licensed for intrathecal use. The rate of absorption from the subarachnoid space is extremely variable, but the mean half-life in the body is about 12 h, so that 80–90 per cent is excreted via the kidneys within 24 h. Neurotoxicity is low but not negligible. The maximum concentration recommended for intrathecal use is 300 mg I ml^{-1}, up to a maximum dose of 3 g of iodine. Contrast medium is usually introduced by lumbar puncture using a small 22-gauge needle, L2–3 or L3–4 being the levels to use routinely. The easiest position in which to perform a lumbar puncture is with the patient sitting. However, many experienced myelographers prefer the prone position, with a folded pillow or bolster placed under the abdomen. From this position the patient does not need to be moved before commencing the actual myelogram and it is easy to check the position of the needle with fluoroscopy if the puncture proves difficult. The lateral decubitus position is less often preferred but sometimes it is the only position possible. With the advent of MRI and reduced need for myelography, lateral cervical puncture is rarely performed. Few radiologists outside the major neuroradiological centres will have any experience of it and there is always the potential risk of damage to the spinal cord. Contrast medium dilutes at a variable rate, and in a total study, the first region to be examined is usually demonstrated best.

In lumbar myelography the patient is placed prone and the table tilted 45 degrees or more in the head-up position to ensure that the thecal sac is completely filled by contrast medium. Anteroposterior paired 10–15 degrees and 30–40 degrees oblique projections are made, followed by lateral views, which should include most of the sacral canal. Cervical and thoracic myelography are rarely performed nowadays and should only be carried out at specialist centres where radiologists are skilled in these procedures.

A myelogram demonstrates the spinal subarachnoid space, which in normal subjects delineates the position of the spinal dura mater. Sometimes spinal nerves at adjacent levels penetrate the dura at a single intervertebral level (conjoined roots). One root sheath is missing at the adjacent intervertebral level, and the thecal sac sometimes shows a long, smooth lateral concavity so that simulation of an elongated epidural mass can be close. However, the resulting conjoined root sleeves are large, and the composite roots are usually clearly visible. The commonest roots to be conjoined are L5 and S1, but sometimes the L4–5 roots are involved and rarely other levels (Fig. 60.12).

SPECIAL SITUATIONS

Myelography can be difficult in certain situations and it is, unfortunately, in just these situations that MR may be problematic and myelography most likely to be considered! In severe multilevel degeneration in the lumbar spine, the spinous processes may remain closely applied to one another no matter how hard the operator tries to separate them by spinal flexion. In these circumstances it is easiest to use an oblique approach to the spinal canal for which fluoroscopic guidance is essential. Spinal stenosis most commonly involves the lower lumbar region, especially L4–5 and L3–4. Therefore it is preferable to perform the lumbar puncture at L2–3, or at L5–S1.

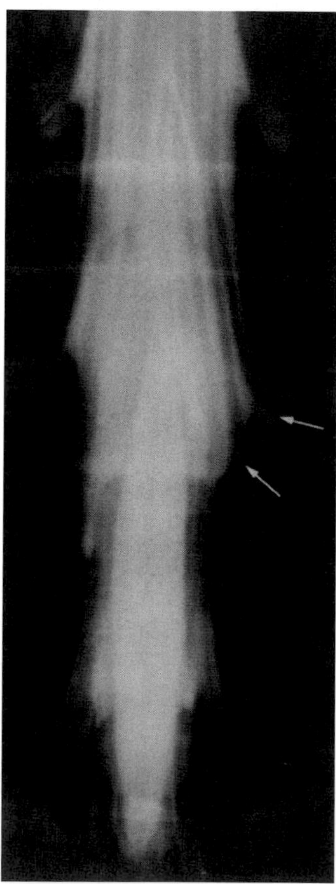

Figure 60.12 Lumbar myelogram, anteroposterior projection showing a relatively common anatomical variant: conjoined nerve roots. The left L4 and L5 roots penetrate the dura mater (arrows) close to the pedicle of L4, resulting in marked asymmetry. Apparent absence of the right L5 root sheath could be confused with compression.

Following laminectomy, the myelographer is advised to avoid attempting to enter the spinal canal through a laminectomy scar wherever possible, even though the available space may seem inviting. Postoperative infection can be chronic and occult, and adhesion of neural structures and arachnoiditis at such sites may be sufficiently common for attempts at puncture to be an excruciatingly painful experience for the patient. It is best to puncture one or two interspaces away from a lumbar laminectomy, even if this means at L1–2. The operator should avoid making a puncture through defects in the neural arches, because the spinal cord may be low and tethered posteriorly in the vicinity of such defects.

COMPLICATIONS OF MYELOGRAPHY

Lumbar puncture

Between 10 per cent and 35 per cent of patients suffer from headache following simple lumbar puncture. It is generally attributed to loss of spinal fluid through the needle puncture hole. There is evidence that the incidence and severity are reduced if small-gauge needles are used. Infection associated with the puncture is very rare. There have also been reports of intraspinal haemorrhage from lumbar puncture, especially epidural haematomas[23], and myelography should not be performed in patients with abnormal haemostasis.

Contrast medium ultimately penetrates the Virchow–Robin spaces and freely enters the interstitium of the cerebral cortex, even after lumbar myelography. Side effects do not appear to be reduced by keeping the patient recumbent for a few hours after the myelogram. Back pain and radicular pain occur in up to 30 per cent of cases, sometimes exacerbating presenting symptoms. This is usually only transient, lasting not more than an hour or two.

Even with the contrast agents now available, a slight increase in CSF protein with an appearance of few white cells occurs in some cases. Intradural inflammation virtually always used to occur after iophendylate (Myodil) oil myelography, resulting in intradural adhesions recognizable on subsequent water-soluble myelography in 70 per cent of cases[24]. It is now known that Myodil was the major cause of arachnoiditis after all forms of lumbar disc surgery, not the surgery itself. Adhesive arachnoiditis has *not* been observed after the clinical use of the non-ionic water-soluble contrast media now available.

SPINAL ANGIOGRAPHY

CT angiography can be used as a preliminary screen but formal spinal angiography[25] may be needed for a few specific situations and such procedures should generally be carried out in specialist centres where the radiologists are experienced in the procedure. Indications for spinal arteriography include suspected angiomatous malformations or vascular tumours of the spinal cord, meninges or vertebral column. It may follow negative cerebral angiography in the investigation of subarachnoid haemorrhage. Therapeutic embolization may be carried out. Some neurosurgeons require demonstration of major arterial supply to the spinal cord before any surgery that might compromise them (scoliosis correction or costotransversectomy for thoracic disc protrusion, etc.)

Since angiography is a costly time-consuming procedure with definite morbidity, no patient should be submitted to it if no action will be taken as a result of the findings. Patients considered unfit for surgery should not have spinal angiography. Nearly always, a positive MRI or myelogram should precede the angiographic search for a spinal cord tumour or arteriovenous malformation. Complications include deterioration in clinical myelopathy, relatively common but usually transient; permanent cord damage is rare.

ANATOMY

The spinal cord is supplied via three main longitudinal arterial axes: the midline anterior spinal artery and two posterolateral spinal arteries[26] (Figs 60.13 and 14). In the cervical region, these arteries arise from the vertebral and deep cervical arteries, themselves branches of the subclavian arteries, while more inferiorly they arise from the posterior intercostal or lumbar arteries. At each vertebral level, a radicular artery runs alongside the nerve root, and some of these, the radiculomedullary arteries, continue to the spinal cord and constitute the major sources of blood for the anterior or posterior spinal arteries.

One major radiculomedullary artery (Adamkiewicz) is found in the thoracolumbar region; its level of origin is variable, but it is usually on the left side, between T8 and L1–2 (Fig. 60.15). The number and origins of the posterior radiculomedullary arteries vary, and occasionally a single posterior intercostal artery will give rise to both anterior and posterior radiculomedullary branches. In the cervical region, anterior radiculomedullary arteries arise at every vertebral level, but they vary considerably in size and importance.

The anterior spinal artery is by far the most important of the axes, because it supplies the major portion of the cord substance, including the motor cells of the anterior horns. It gives off tiny sulcocommissural arteries that run into the cord; they are not visible at angiography unless pathologically enlarged.

Arteries supplying the vertebral column also arise at each vertebral level; their study involves catheterization of the same vessels as arteriography of the spinal cord.

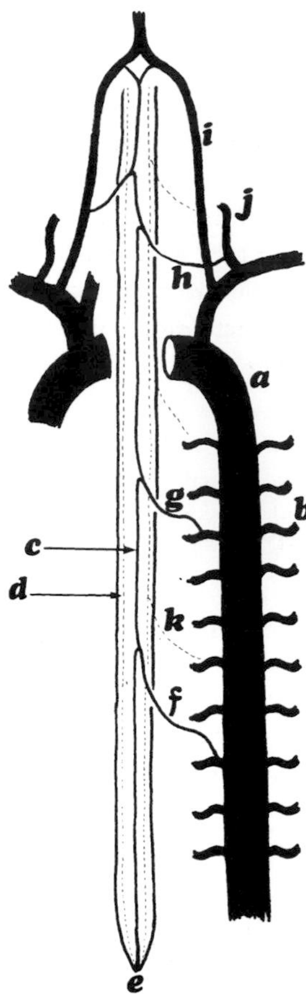

Figure 60.13 The spinal arteries and their feeding vessels. a = aorta, b = intercostal artery, c = anterior spinal artery, d = posterolateral spinal artery, e = anastomosis at conus medullaris, f = arteria radicularis magna (of Adamkiewicz), g = thoracic and h = cervical radiculomedullary arteries, i = vertebral artery, j = deep cervical artery.

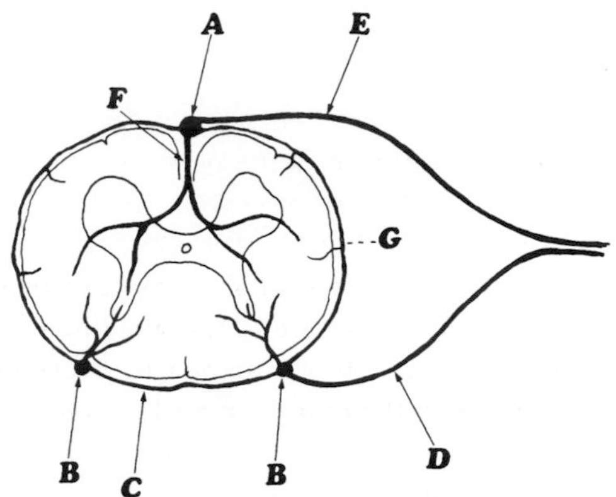

Figure 60.14 Blood supply of the spinal cord. A = anterior spinal artery, B = posterolateral spinal arteries, C = posterior anastomotic artery, D = posterior and E = anterior radiculomedullary arteries, F = sulcocommissural arteries, G = lateral anastomotic artery.

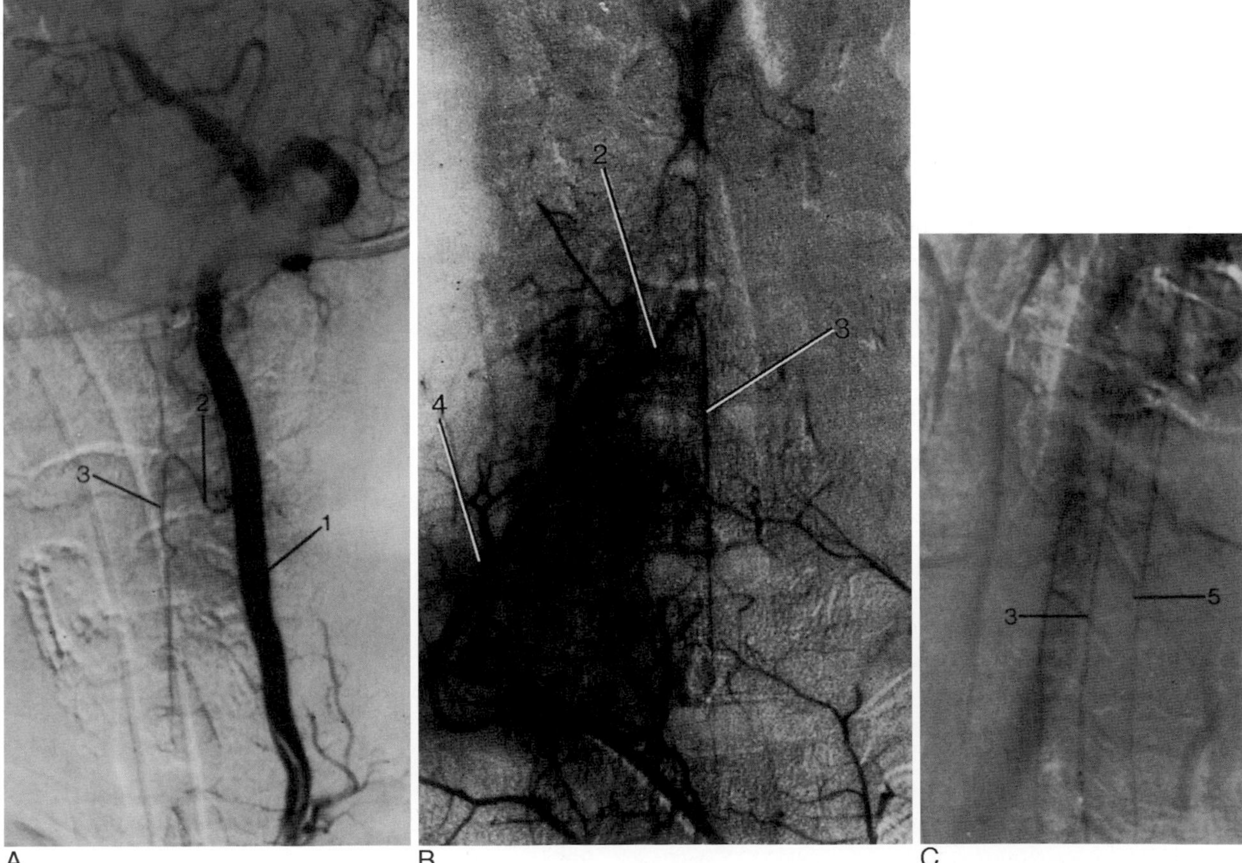

Figure 60.15 Anterior spinal artery (3) in cervical region, fed (A) from vertebral artery (1), and (B) from a deep cervical artery (4), via radiculomedullary arteries (2). The posterior spinal artery (5) is also opacified in the lateral projection (C).

DISCOGRAPHY

Discography is still employed in some orthopaedic centres, though mainly as a diagnostic preliminary before spinal fusion for the treatment of back pain or neck pain, rather than neural compression syndromes. Although special apparatus has been devised to perform the test, it is simply performed by inserting a 22-gauge spinal needle into the centre of a disc under fluoroscopic control from an oblique approach, anteriorly in the neck and posteriorly in the lumbar spine. The spinal canal and intervertebral canals are avoided. A small amount of non-ionic contrast medium is injected into the central part of the disc (the nuclear 'cavity') and anteroposterior and lateral radiographs obtained. The test is sometimes followed by CT.

Discography can be an unpleasant, painful experience for the patient. Artefacts due to inaccurate placement of the needle in the nuclear cavity, or leakage of contrast medium along the needle track, are frequent. Advocates claim that it usually provokes specific pain when the appropriate disc is injected, and may indicate tears in the annulus fibrosus that would not have been shown by any other technique. There is significant uncertainty associated with both these claims.

RADIOLOGICAL DIAGNOSTIC APPROACH TO COMMON CLINICAL SPINAL PROBLEMS

Clinical problems may be divided into acute and chronic presentations.

ACUTE PRESENTATIONS

1 Back pain
2 Root syndromes
3 Spinal cord lesions.

Acute back pain

Acute back pain and many cases of acute extremity pain of presumed spinal origin are not generally investigated radiologically; rest and conservative treatment are tried first. Plain radiographs may, however, be indicated in cases of pain following significant trauma, and in patients known to develop spinal lesions, such as those with metastatic disease or on steroid therapy. Increasingly MR is being used as the initial investigation for all forms of spinal disease and at an earlier stage in the diagnostic sequence, especially for those clinical situations 'red flagged' by guidelines[27].

Acute root syndromes

Acute lower motor neurone weakness of one arm is uncommonly due to spinal disease in the absence of trauma. Nerve root avulsion is generally not investigated radiologically in the acute stage, but may subsequently require high-resolution MRI. Lumbosacral disc protrusion may present with acute sciatic nerve root compression that is predominantly motor, giving an acute foot drop; acute unilateral leg pain or loss of sphincter function may be present. Although plain CT is nearly as good as MRI at identifying extradural disc protrusion, MRI has become the preferred investigation.

Acute lesions of spinal cord

Acute traumatic lesions of the spinal cord are often definitive and permanent. Careful clinical assessment in the early stages may, however, indicate a partial lesion with potential for some recovery. Most patients with major trauma now undergo CT, which may be definitive; MRI may be indicated, especially if plain radiographs and CT are normal.

An acute nontraumatic lesion of the spinal cord is assumed to be compressive until proven otherwise and is a medical emergency, since the degree of recovery may be related to the speed of diagnosis and treatment. A chest radiograph is mandatory, since many cases are neoplastic or infective. Plain radiographs are often still obtained, but MRI of the clinically involved region – and preferably of the whole spine if metastatic disease is suspected – is much the preferred investigation and usually will be all that is required. Water-soluble myelography by the lumbar route supplemented by CT may be necessary if MRI cannot be obtained.

Spinal angiography is not indicated unless other imaging findings indicate the presence of a highly vascular lesion. There is probably nothing to be lost in delaying angiography until the acute stage has passed.

CHRONIC PRESENTATIONS

1 Pain
2 Root compression syndromes
3 Cord lesions.

Chronic pain

Chronic pain is still widely investigated by plain radiographs, which provide a rapid, cheap overall picture. However plain radiographs are usually noncontributory[28]. Increasingly MRI is being used at the outset.

Root compression syndromes

In chronic sciatica, MRI is the preferred investigation. Myelography may occasionally help to identify the worst affected level in cases with multilevel disease, although most surgical decisions are now made on the basis of noninvasive tests alone. When pain in the arm or shoulder is thought to be of spinal origin, plain radiographs of the cervical spine are appropriate. They may show evidence of degenerative disease, cervical ribs or, more rarely, evidence of neoplasm or infection. Most patients with cervical spondylosis are treated conservatively, although MRI may be required to make therapeutic decisions.

Chronic cord lesions

Three main groups may be identified: extramedullary compressive lesions, intramedullary space-occupying lesions (mostly tumours and syringomyelia) and inflammatory or vascular disease.

Chronic compressive lesions are often cervical: spondylosis and cervical disc disease are the most frequent. They are increasingly being investigated by MRI rather than plain radiography. Intrinsic space-occupying lesions of the spinal cord are rarely evidenced by plain radiographs, but the detection of craniocervical anomalies may orientate the diagnosis towards syringomyelia. MRI is the definitive procedure, including views of the craniocervical junction. If inflammatory or demyelinating cord disease is suspected, MRI of the brain may provide valuable evidence of associated lesions, in addition to MRI of the spine. If MRI is negative, it is extremely unlikely that angiography will be revealing; even demonstration of anterior spinal artery occlusion is unreliable.

DISEASE PROCESSES AFFECTING THE SPINE

CONGENITAL LESIONS

The commonest congenital malformation found in adults involves the caudal part of the neural tube. A useful descriptive term is lipomyelomeningodysplasia, which emphasizes the varying elements. Other conditions result in a dorsal dermal sinus that runs from a skin dimple to the spinal canal, some terminating in intraspinal dermoids or epidermoids. The neurenteric canal or adhesion may persist, or form at other levels such as the upper cervical region, resulting in neurenteric cysts along the connection between the foregut and spinal canal; a persistent cutaneous communication results in a dorsal enteric fistula. Aberrant neuro-entodermal adhesions are probably also the origin of diastematomyelia. Finally, excessive retrogressive differentiation can lead to varying degrees of sacral and sacrolumbar dysgenesis, often referred to as the caudal regression syndromes.

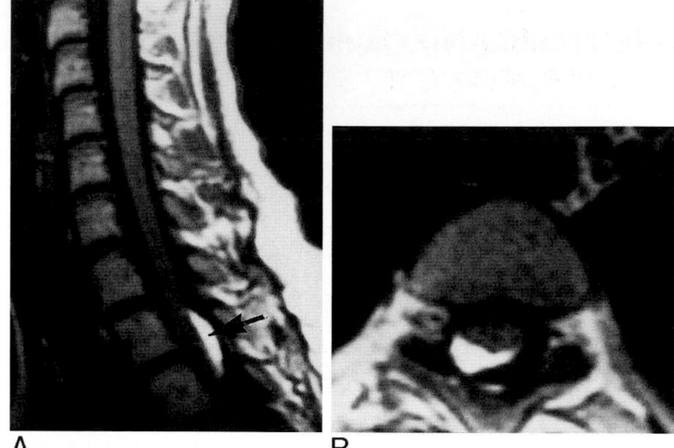

Figure 60.16 Intramedullary lipoma (arrow) with intact dura in upper thoracic. Sagittal (A) and axial (B) T1W MRIs.

SPINAL MALFORMATIONS

Intramedullary lipoma

This consists of a mass of adipose tissue located mainly between the posterior columns of the spinal cord. A tongue-like extension along the central canal is often found, in keeping with its embryogenesis. The overlying dura mater usually is intact and the lipoma entirely intradural; however, there may be a dural defect to which cord and lipoma become adherent. Such lesions occur most often near the thoracocervical or craniovertebral junctions (Fig. 60.16). CT and MR demonstrate the fatty nature of the tumour. Nonfatty elements also may be present, resulting in a heterogeneous appearance.

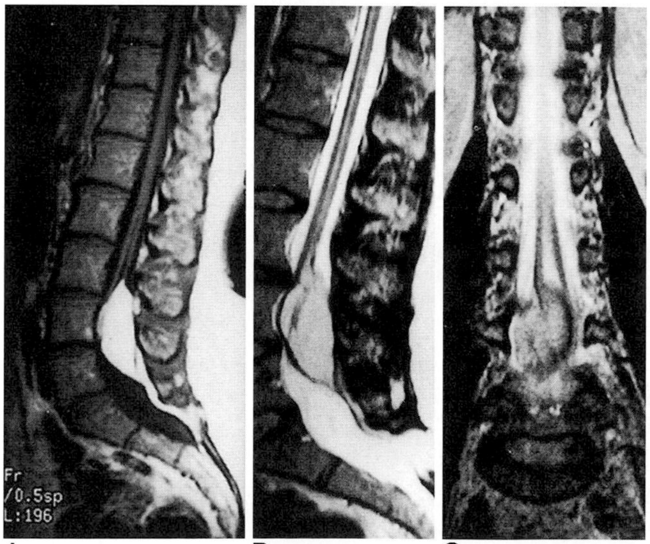

LIPOMYELOMENINGODYSPLASIAS

These represent a spectrum of abnormalities ranging from an abnormally low location of the conus medullaris with minimal or even absent lipoma, to massive lipomatous formations involving all elements of the spinal and adjacent subcutaneous tissues (Fig. 60.17). The abnormality may not be apparent clinically, hence the term occult spinal dysraphism. Unlike myelocele, Chiari malformation is present in only about 6 per cent. Patients frequently present in adult life, sometimes only with back pain and minimal neurological signs.

Figure 60.17 Lipomyelomeningodysplasia. Sagittal (A) T1- and fast spin-echo (B) T2W and coronal (C) T2W images showing the lipoma, low position of the spinal cord and a cavity in the distal spinal cord.

Plain radiographs often reveal varying degrees of nonfusion of one or more neural arches and variable expansion of the spinal canal; such incidental findings do not necessitate further investigation unless there are relevant clinical features. Even malformations involving the spinal cord may remain asymptomatic, and the efficacy of prophylactic operations to release tethering remains unclear.

MR is the optimal investigation although ultrasound (US) has been advocated in children; MR demonstrates all aspects of the abnormalities including the origin of nerve roots and associated lesions such as cysts in the spinal cord. In over 80 per cent, the spinal cord terminates at or below the level of the third lumbar vertebra, and usually is tethered to the dorsal aspect of the dura, where it fuses with the fatty tumour. Nerve roots issuing from an apparently thickened filum terminale indicate that it contains significant nervous tissue and therefore should not be divided surgically.

NEURENTERIC AND OTHER DEVELOPMENTAL CYSTS

Intraspinal neurenteric cysts are intradural, usually unilocular cysts lined by gastrointestinal or bronchial epithelium that occur in either the cervical (often near the craniovertebral junction) or lower thoracic regions[29]. They compress the spinal cord (usually the anterior aspect) and may invaginate into its substance; occasionally the cord is split into two halves as in diastematomyelia. Plain radiography may show focal expansion of the spinal canal, and thoracic lesions in particular may be associated with butterfly or hemivertebra. On MRI the cyst contents usually yield a slightly higher signal than cerebrospinal fluid, on T1- as well as T2W images, but are clearly demarcated from cord substance.

Dermoid and epidermoid cysts are rounded intradural and sometimes intramedullary lesions. Imaging may demonstrate fat within them and calcification. They may be associated with other forms of dysraphism, and in about 20 per cent a dorsal dermal sinus can be traced running obliquely downwards from the lesion to a skin dimple on the lower back, which also may be a source of intradural sepsis[30].

Ependymal cysts usually occur with other types of dysraphism. They represent little more than focal dilatations of the central canal of the spinal cord, and usually appear as swelling near the lumbar enlargement.

DIASTEMATOMYELIA

The spinal cord is split into two usually unequal hemicords, each with a central canal and anterior spinal artery, but giving rise to only ipsilateral spinal roots. Any level can be involved, including the filum terminale and medulla oblongata, but most are thoracic[31]. The cleavage usually extends over several segments and only rarely the hemicords do not re-unite caudally. The hemicords are enclosed in a common dural tube in 50 per cent of cases, usually in the cervical region, but in the remainder each is enclosed within its own dural tube, a bony or cartilaginous spur arising from malformed lamina often lying between them. Abnormal traction may be exerted by such a spur at the point of reunion of the hemicords. Clinical abnormalities are often absent, but in some symptomatic cases progression apparently was halted by excision of tethering spurs.

Plain radiographs in the region of the abnormality usually show focal expansion of the spinal canal, narrow intervertebral disc spaces and varying degrees of laminar dysplasia and fusion. This combination is very suggestive of the diagnosis, whether or not a bony spur is shown. MRI (and post-myelography) CT show the anatomy well; even plain CT may be diagnostic in some circumstances (Fig. 60.18).

CHIARI MALFORMATIONS

These represent a group of abnormalities characterized by dislocation of the hindbrain into the spinal canal. Chiari described four types, but his types III and IV are rare and the Chiari II is seen mainly in paediatric practice. The Chiari I lesion is not really a malformation at all: it may be acquired in conditions associated with raised intracranial pressure (tumours, venous hypertension), lowered intraspinal pressure (lumboperitoneal shunts) and conditions that diminish the volume of the posterior fossa (craniosynostosis, basilar investigation). It may develop during the first 3 years of life[32] in the absence of any cause other than probable slower growth of the posterior fossa relative to the hindbrain during this period when both are growing most rapidly. The Chiari I lesion used to be distinguished from coning, by the shape of the herniated tonsils, which were said to be rounded in coning and pointed in Chiari, but it is now clear that both pointed tonsils and medullary elongation may be found in situations associated with coning, and that there are no grounds for distinguishing between the two conditions.

Chiari type I lesion (cerebellar ectopia)

This is defined as descent of the otherwise normal cerebellar hemispheres below the foramen magnum, usually involving the tonsils. However, in about 50 per cent, the other component of the hindbrain, the medulla oblongata, shows elongation of the segment between the ponto-medullary junction and dorsal column nuclei, the obex of the fourth ventricle coming to lie in the cervical canal, where it may or may not be overlain by the cerebellar tonsils, the prevalence of medullary elongation increasing with increasing tonsil descent.

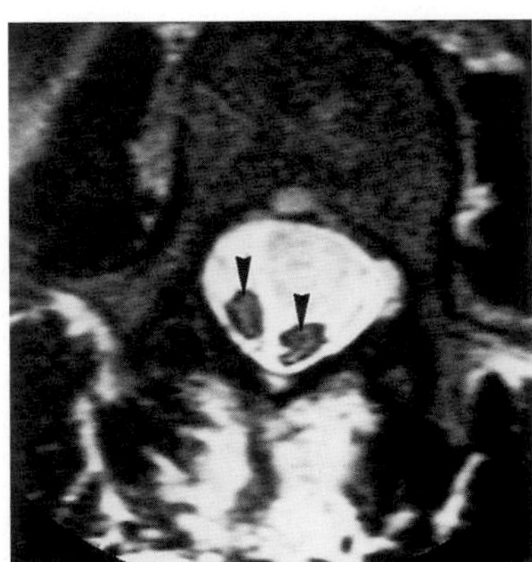

Figure 60.18 Diastematomyelia. An axial T2W fast spin-echo sequence showing two almost equal-sized hemicords (arrowheads) in a common thecal sac at L3.

Elongation is sufficient to produce a kink on the posterior surface of the medulla oblongata in about 15 per cent, where the tail of the fourth ventricle rolls down over the upper one or more segments of the spinal cord (Fig. 60.19). The prevalence of the Chiari type I lesion in the normal population has been considerably overestimated on MRI, and is probably under 1 per cent[33].

Chiari type II malformations

In these malformations the cerebellum is dysplastic. The inferior vermis is everted rather than inverted, so the nodulus becomes the most inferior part of the cerebellum and the fourth ventricle is reduced to a coronal cleft. The cerebellar herniation then consists mainly of the inferior vermis. The medulla oblongata is invariably elongated, usually enough to become kinked. Hydrocephalus and dysplasia of the cerebral hemispheres, cranial vault and meninges are frequent. A meningomyelocele is present in 98 per cent or more of cases, and may play an important role in embryogenesis[34].

These hindbrain abnormalities may be associated with compression and progressive degeneration in parts of the brainstem, cerebellum and upper spinal cord. In Chiari type I malformations, symptoms commonly do not appear until adult life, and about 50 per cent of symptomatic cases are associated with syringomyelia. Syringomyelia occurs most commonly when the cerebellar tonsils lie between the neural arches of C1 and C2, whereas cerebellar syndromes predominate when the tonsils lie lower than the neural arch of C2[35]. The outcome of foramen magnum decompression is significantly adversely affected by increasing descent of the tonsils[35].

In the type I lesion, plain radiographs are usually normal. In up to 15 per cent, occipitalization of the atlas and basilar invagination are present, and hindbrain herniation is present in over 50 per cent of cases of symptomatic basilar invagination[36]. By far the most convenient way to demonstrate these hindbrain abnormalities is by MRI. However, descent of the cerebellum through the foramen magnum of up to 3 mm seems to be present in up to 20 per cent of normal subjects on midsagittal MRI sections of 4 mm or more in thickness, due to the shape of the foramen magnum and partial volume effects in which the more laterally placed biventral lobules are included in the image when the vallecula is small[33]. MRI in the coronal plane is more reliable, and the identification of associated features, such as elongation of the upper medulla, can also be helpful.

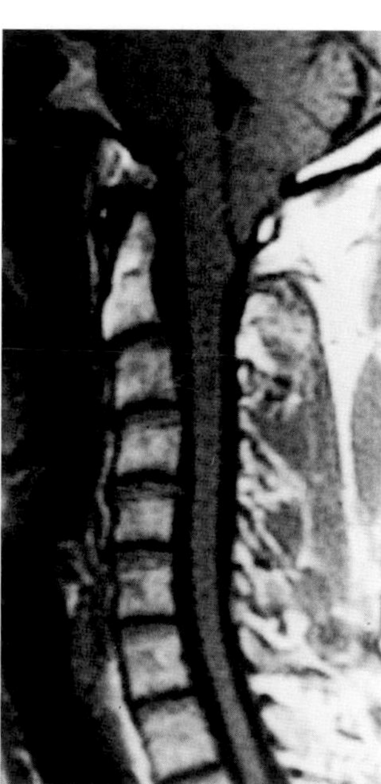

Figure 60.19 Chiari type 1 malformation. T1W sagittal image showing the cerebellar tonsils extending just caudal to the neural arch of C1, and elongation and kinking of the medulla oblongata.

MENINGOCELES

Varying degrees of dural ectasia usually accompany the spinal dysraphisms. Both generalized and focal dural ectasia may occur in systemic disorders such as neurofibromatosis, Ehlers–Danlos and Marfan's syndromes. It may occur in erosive arthropathies, especially ankylosing spondylitis[37], where focal ectasia sometimes forms pockets or saccules invaginating into the walls of the spinal canal, including the vertebral bodies and neural arches. Such lesions also occur idiopathically.

Anterior sacral meningocele

This lesion consists of a unilocular, complex lobular or even multilocular presacral cystic mass, containing CSF, which communicates with the intraspinal subarachnoid space.

There is a large usually eccentric anterior defect in the lower part of the sacrum, and the sacral canal is expanded. Varying degrees of sacral and coccygeal agenesis may be associated. On plain radiographs, the eccentric anterior sacral defect gives the remaining part of the sacrum a pathognomonic scimitar appearance. The pelvic mass may be shown by US, CT or MRI, the latter invariably demonstrating communications with the sacral canal.

Occult intrasacral meningocele is a variant of this condition. The sacral canal is expanded by a meningocele that lies below the normal level of termination of the thecal sac. There is no anterior sacral defect and no intrapelvic extension.

Lateral thoracic meningocele

This lesion commonly presents as a paravertebral mass on CXR. It is commonly solitary and usually is found on the right; 70–85 per cent is associated with neurofibromatosis. There is typically an angular kyphoscoliosis towards the side of the meningocele, and pressure erosion of the margins of the relevant intervertebral foramen is evident.

Anterior thoracic meningocele with ventral herniation of spinal cord

This is an increasingly recognized condition very occasionally providing explanation for an otherwise unexplained chronic thoracic myelopathy in adults[38]. It is most readily recognized on midsagittal MRI of the thoracic spine, where the spinal cord is displaced anteriorly in contact with a vertebral body at or very near an intervertebral disc, commonly at about T6. The meningocele may not be easy to show on axial images. Appearances are often misinterpreted as an intradural arachnoid cyst displacing the spinal cord anteriorly, from which the condition needs to be distinguished.

VERTEBRAL FUSION ANOMALIES

These usually are determined very early in development. The intervertebral discs are narrow and partly bridged by regions where disc material never developed. Fused segments usually also show varying degrees of hypoplasia, and when multiple segments are involved, marked dysplasias such as hemivertebrae are also often present. The term Klippel–Feil syndrome is appropriate when the cervical region is predominantly involved. When only the thoracic spine (which is much more rare), spondylothoracic and spondylocostal dysplasia are more appropriate terms[39,40]. Other organ systems may be involved, including neural tube and visceral abnormalities.

SKELETAL DYSPLASIAS

Achondroplasia

Neurological complications are present in 40–50 per cent of cases, the average age of onset being 38 years, rarely under 15 years[40]. The spinal canal is congenitally narrow and the narrowing is progressive due to degenerative changes and an exaggerated lumbar lordosis. In over 60 per cent of cases, neural compression occurs in the thoracolumbar region, most often of the cauda equina; it is generalized in only 10 per cent. In the remainder, compression occurs mainly in the cervical spine or at the foramen magnum, the latter accounting for virtually all the childhood and especially neonatal presentations.

The mucopolysaccharidoses

In the Morquio-Brailsford type (MPS-IV), ligament laxity results in instability and subluxations at the atlanto-axial joint and thoracolumbar junction; the former may require arthrodesis[41]. Ligamentous thickening is severe in about 50 per cent and is the main cause of upper spinal cord compression. Especially marked and extensive thickening of the dura and extradural tissues has been described in Hurler–Schiei and Maroteaux-Lamy diseases.

Spondyloepiphyseal dysplasia

Vertebrae are flattened and enlarged in an AP dimension, especially in a thoracic kyphosis. Severe scoliosis may be present. Neurological complications are uncommon, and usually arise from atlanto-axial instability associated with abnormal ossification of the dens similar to MPS-IV, but usually lacking the soft-tissue thickening. Multiple epiphyseal dysplasia, pseudo-achondroplasia and chondrodysplasia calcificans are also conditions that may have this feature[41].

NEUROFIBROMATOSIS

This disease is transmitted as an autosomal dominant disorder, but 50 per cent of cases lack a family history. The type I form is usually associated with skeletal dysplasia. About 50 per cent have a scoliosis that can be very severe, about 10 per cent have dysplastic vertebrae (often consisting of one or more absent or hypoplastic pedicles) and about 10 per cent have dural ectasia. A small number of cases show subluxations, usually involving C1/2 or C2/3.

Spinal compression develops in about 16 per cent of cases. A myelopathy developing in childhood may be more likely to be due to spinal deformity than to a neurofibroma or other tumour[39].

SPINAL INSTABILITY

Craniovertebral junction

Isolated atlanto-axial instability is occasionally encountered and may be associated with spinal cord compression. It occurs in about 30 per cent of patients with Down's syndrome. About 70 per cent of cases are associated with an os odontoideum (Fig. 60.20), and most of the remainder with cranial assimilation of the atlas, which is combined with a C2/3 intersegmental fusion in about 70 per cent of cases. Os odontoideum should probably no longer be regarded as a segmentation anomaly, but rather as abnormal ossification of the dens, secondary to instability and abnormal local stress. Congenital hypoplasia of the dens usually is a misdiagnosis, an os odontoideum in fact being present but overlooked because it is not ossified, small or malplaced. True hypoplasia of the dens only occurs in association with more complex fusion anomalies, especially those that restrict rotation at C1/2[36].

Spondylolysis

Truly congenital spondylolysis is uncommon. It is often associated with other defects, such as absent pedicles, absent superior articular facet, hypoplastic laminae with deviation of the spinous process and hypertrophy of the contralateral pedicle. Such abnormalities may be found in the cervical and lumbar regions, and usually are not associated with neurological symptoms, unless severe subluxation is present, such as sometimes occurs at C2 or C3. The spondylolytis defects, which are relatively common at the lumbosacral junction, especially in young adults, probably originate as stress fractures through the interarticular part of the laminae, resulting in a usually hypertrophic pseudarthrosis. The anatomy is well shown on high-resolution axial and sagittal MRI, or multiple thin-slice CT with reformatting. Special imaging planes may be helpful[42].

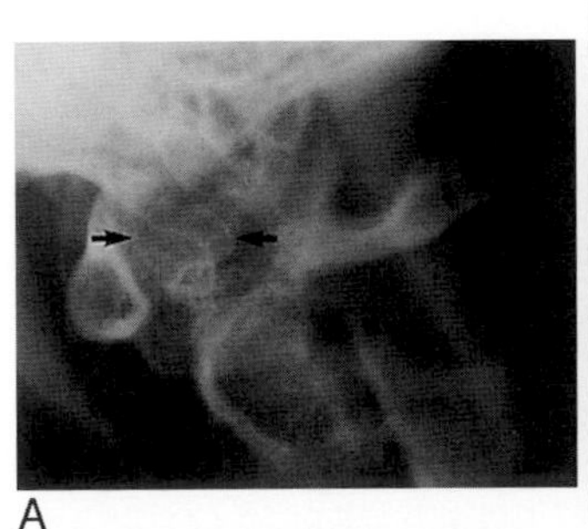
A

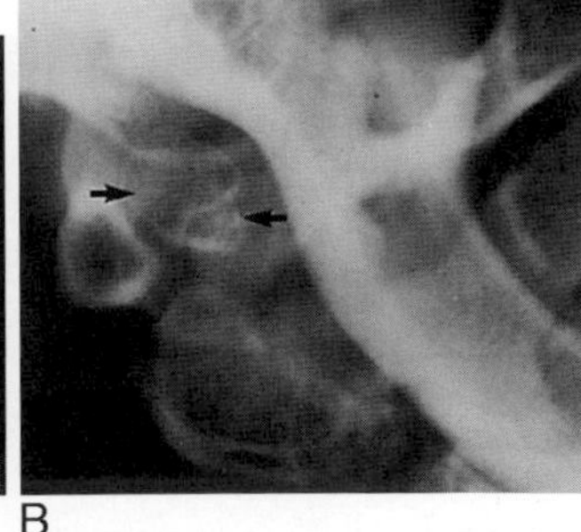
B

Figure 60.20 **Os odontoideum** (os mobile) (arrows) and atlanto-axial instability: cervical myelogram, lateral projections. There was no history of trauma. The pattern of instability, with posterior atlanto-axial subluxation in extension (B), reduced in flexion (A), is common.

INTRASPINAL ARACHNOID CYST

Extradural arachnoid cysts arise from defects in the dura mater, either congenital or inflammatory (e.g. ankylosing spondylitis); intradural arachnoid cysts arise from arachnoidal duplications or spinal arachnoiditis. Symptoms of pain or neurological disability may arise when the spinal cord or cauda equina are compressed, bearing in mind that size and intracystic pressure may vary considerably; occasionally the spinal cord or roots have herniated through a dural defect and become entrapped. Plain radiographs may show expansion of the spinal canal when the cyst is extradural. MRI shows these lesions well. Signal from fluid in the cyst, and often from the subarachnoid space below it, is usually higher than from CSF elsewhere due to reduced mobility. Effects on the spinal cord are shown, namely compression and rarely myelomalacia or syringomyelia. Small herniations of neural tissue through the dural defects may require thin imaging sections and high-resolution imaging techniques to show them. Aspiration and drainage of arachnoid cysts compressing the spinal cord may be accompanied by immediate and dramatic improvement in clinical condition[43].

Care must be exercised not to overdiagnose intradural arachnoid cysts in the thoracic region. The retromedullary subarachnoid space in the thoracic spine is commonly wide, and partly loculated by usually incomplete septae; the spinal cord usually is closely applied to the anterior margin of the bony canal and may have a flattened appearance over an exaggerated kyphosis.

Perineural arachnoid cysts (Tarlov cysts) occur commonly in the sacrum, especially on the second sacral root. They can be large, multiple and are often associated with eccentric pressure erosion of the sacral canal and are well shown by MRI. Clinical significance, even of large cysts, is doubtful[22].

SYRINGOMYELIA

The term 'syringomyelia' describes conditions in which there is a cavity within the spinal cord, lined mainly by glial tissue and containing fluid that is similar or identical with CSF. It is associated with a number of distinct pathological processes, including cerebellar ectopia and trauma[44]. Whatever the cause, the cavity seems capable of propagating, probably due to hydrodynamic forces, into normal cord tissue. Usually it involves many segments or the whole spinal cord, but sometimes smaller isolated cavities are found confined to only a few spinal segments, often referred to as fusiform syrinx. The cervical cord is involved most often, although occasionally only the thoracic cord. Only about 10 per cent of cysts extend cranial to C2, where they split into two or deviate to right or left in a plane ventral to the floor of the fourth ventricle. Small cavities usually involve the bases of the posterior columns, and commonly the central cord canal for part of their extent; larger cavities are associated with more extensive loss of cord substance. Double cavities are sometimes present and individual cavities may be multilocular. The spinal cord is enlarged in about 80 per cent, normal in size in 10 per cent and diffusely atrophic in 10 per cent. The size of the spinal cord may vary in response to posture and respiration. Size variation usually is not associated with changes in clinical state, nor does the severity of clinical disability relate to the size of the cyst and remaining cord substance[45].

Between 70 per cent and 90 per cent of cases of syringomyelia are associated with cerebellar ectopia, the cerebellar tonsils usually lying at the level of C1 or between C1 and C2[35]. It is postulated that intermittent obstruction of the outlets of the fourth ventricle and of CSF flow across the foramen magnum, combined with a patent communication between the fourth ventricle and the central canal of the spinal cord, together produce secondary degeneration of cord substance by causing intermittent distension of the central canal[46]. The term syringohydromyelia is often used for this type of cord cavitation. However, this hypothesis has some problems and does not explain all aspects; alternative hypotheses exist[47].

Other causes of cavitation of the spinal cord can result in appearances indistinguishable from syringohydromyelia. These include intramedullary tumours, chronic spinal cord compression, spinal cord trauma and arachnoiditis. Acute transverse myelitis, infection agents and other inflammatory processes such as sarcoidosis, can result in colliquative necrosis (myelomalacia), which may organize into cavities that propagate into normal cord substance. Finally in about 10–20 per cent of patients with spinal cord cavities, no cause or association can be found.

On plain radiography, the spinal canal appears expanded in 30–40 per cent of cases, especially in the cervical region, the highest frequency being in children with Chiari-associated syringomyelia[48]. Scoliosis often occurs and may be the presenting feature[49].

Syringomyelia and its cause usually are shown well by MRI. The cavity is well circumscribed and of uniformly abnormal signal, often showing prominent transverse ridges in its wall. In general, the cyst fluid yields a similar signal to CSF on T1W and T2W images (Fig. 60.21). On T2W and other types of images, the signal is more variable; pulsatile cysts show flow-related signal changes, nonpulsatile cysts do not[50]. Dynamic MRI, using phase contrast or bolus-tracking techniques, has been used to study CSF movement especially at foramen magnum level[51]. Mainly in post-traumatic syringomyelia, T2W images have shown a striking increase in signal from the full thickness of an otherwise normal cord or medulla oblongata well beyond the visible extent of the cavity, probably reflecting the extent of actual cord damage. Care must be taken not to exclude an underlying tumour, although these are usually obvious (e.g. Fig. 60.22).

On MRI, moderate correlation is found between the presence and location of the cavity and clinical features, but *not* between clinical severity and size of the syrinx relative to remaining cord substance, *or* with its degree of distension[45,52,53]. MRI is good for monitoring the mechanical success of operative strategies[54], of which three are in current use, the third being new and controversial, deriving from an alternative theory of causation: (A) foramen magnum decompression; (B) syringo-subarachnoid, peritoneal or pleural shunting; (C) lumbo-peritoneal shunting[55,56]. All seem equally effective, obtaining and

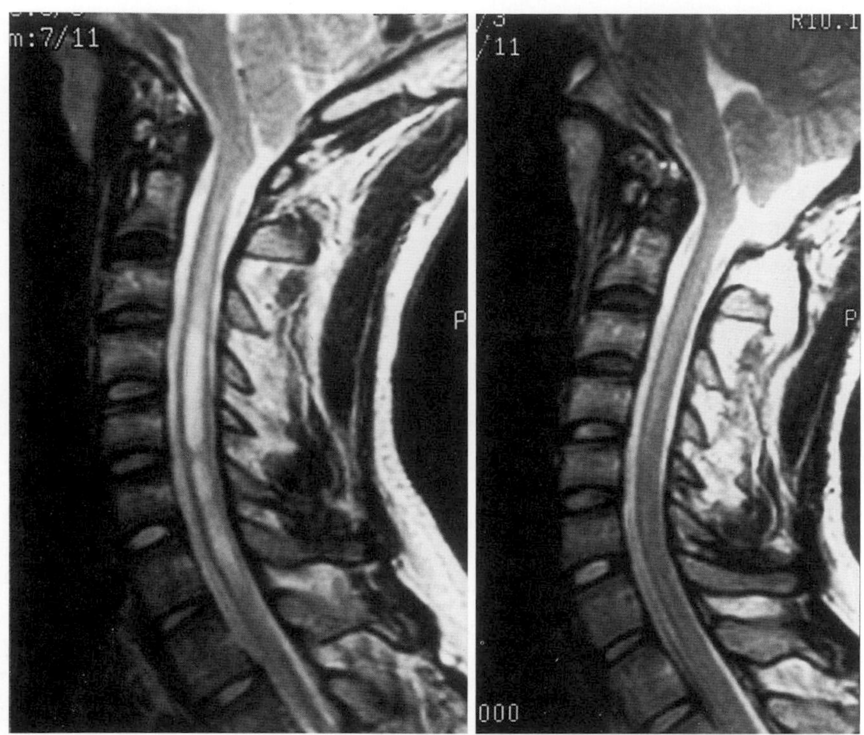

Figure 60.21 Syringomyelia. (A) Mid-sagittal T2W MR showing mild cerebellar ectopia and a syrinx within the spinal cord. (B) 1 year later, after decompression at the foramen magnum.

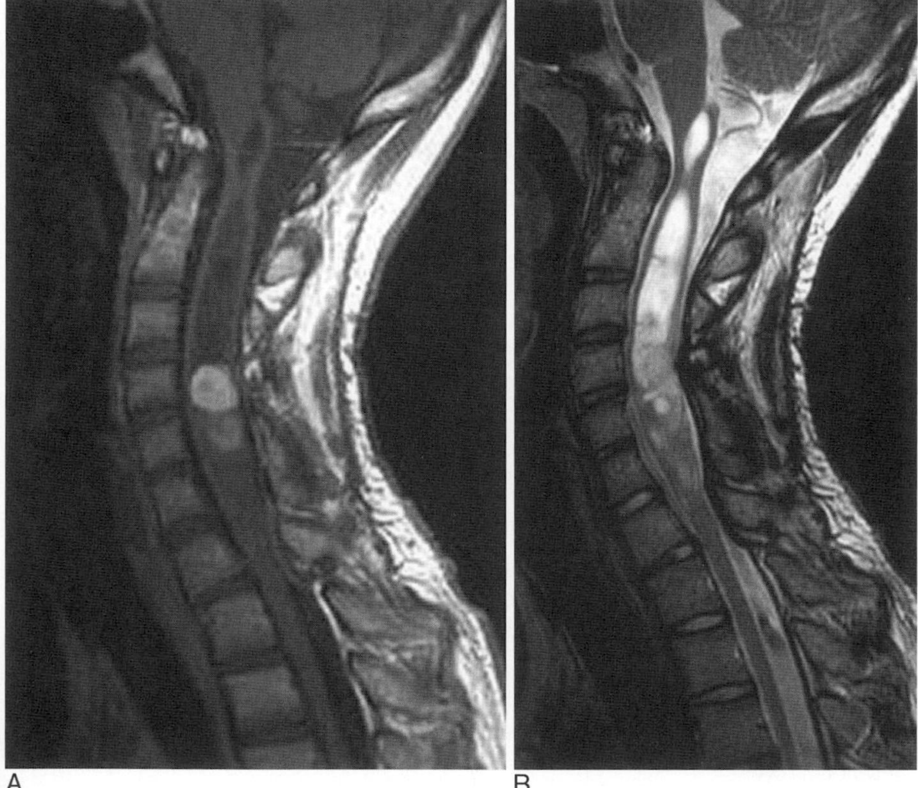

Figure 60.22 Syringomyelia associated with astrocytoma. (A) Sagittal T1W and (B) T2W MR images showing expanded fluid-filled syrinx associated with a lesion of mixed signal intensity at the C4/5 level. Note also the deformities in the vertebral bodies and posterior elements between C3 and C7. (Courtesy of Dr Justin Cross.)

generally maintaining collapse of the syrinx in 70–80 per cent of cases. Unfortunately, however, clinical outcome and extension of cord cavitation on interval images seem to bear no relation to whether the cavity remains collapsed or not[54].

Although rarely performed nowadays, standard myelography did provide interesting information about this condition. Symmetrical, smooth fusiform expansion of the spinal cord usually in the cervical region is shown, usually terminating at C2. However, in about 20 per cent of cases, the spinal cord appears normal or small. When small, the cord is usually flattened in the sagittal plane. Rotating the patient from the prone to supine position may cause considerable changes in cord size and shape. On postmyelography CT, contrast medium should enter all intramedullary cavities, though at a variable rate.

DEGENERATIVE SPINAL DISEASE

Degeneration of some intervertebral discs is identifiable in virtually everyone over the age of 60 years. It is seen most frequently at multiple levels in the cervical region, at L4/5 and L5/S1 and in the upper lumbar and lower thoracic spine. Mobility of involved segments is related to the propensity to develop degenerative change; discs adjacent to fused spinal segments, from whatever cause, are especially vulnerable.

Degeneration is closely associated with fissuring of the annulus fibrosus, usually radial[57]. The central part of the disc becomes less hydrated, loses volume and its structure disintegrates into disorganized collagen. Transverse fissures may develop, which may intermittently fill with gaseous nitrogen during movement and at other times are filled with fluid (Fig. 60.23).

The annulus fibrosus normally may bulge diffusely a little beyond the vertebral margins, especially in children. However, bulging of more than 2–3 mm is usually associated with loosening of the concentric layers of the annulus fibrosus, or radial fissures and accelerated dehydration of the nucleus.

Protrusions are focal bulges of the annulus fibrosus associated with radial tears. These can occur from any part of the disc circumference. The commonest are posterior and consist of the following types: (A) posterolateral, the commonest (Figs 60.24 and 60.25); (B) duffuse; (C) midline posterior (this term is used instead of 'central', which can be confused with nuclear herniations into the vertebral bodies); (D) lateral, which is lateral to the spinal canal (Fig. 60.26), and can involve the dorsal root ganglion in the intervertebral foramen and (E) far lateral, beyond the foramen and often affecting ventral rami.

Herniations are fibrocartilaginous masses attached to, but lying outside the annulus fibrosus. These usually extend cranial or caudal to the disc in the anterior epidural space as migratory fragments usually pass one or other side of the midline septum (see Fig. 60.24). In about 10 per cent, the herniation extends through the posterior longitudinal ligament or its lateral membrane[58] and, rarely, sequestrated fragments detach and become freely mobile. The dura itself may be penetrated, usually near a root sheath, and the intradural fragment can closely simulate a neurinoma.

Reactive changes occur in the vertebral bodies, both in the peripheral disc margin (osteophytes) and in the cancellous bone adjacent to the vertebral end-plates. In the cervical spine, osteophytes on the disc margins commonly involve the spinal canal; associated enlargement of the uncinate processes of the cervical vertebrae encroaches mainly on the intervertebral canals. Osteophytes generally reduce the range of movement and may result in spontaneous fusion. Elsewhere in the spine,

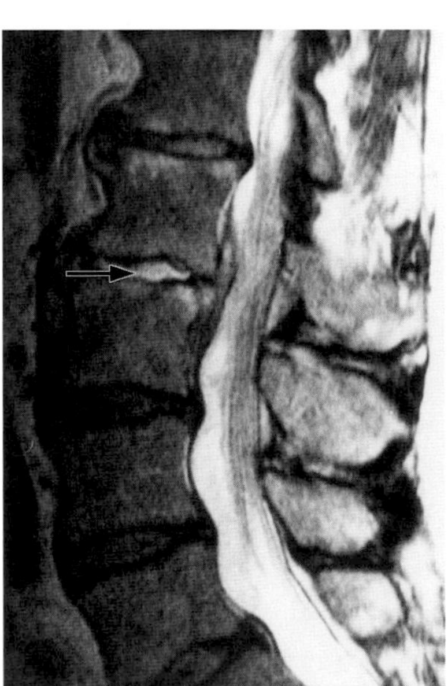

Figure 60.23 High signal intensity degenerate disc. Sagittal T2W fast spin-echo MRI of the lumbar spine showing high signal (black arrow) throughout most of a degenerate disc (between L2 and L3) associated with an irregular posterior protrusion of disc material. There is no bone destruction or reactive change in the adjacent vertebrae. This disc was not infected.

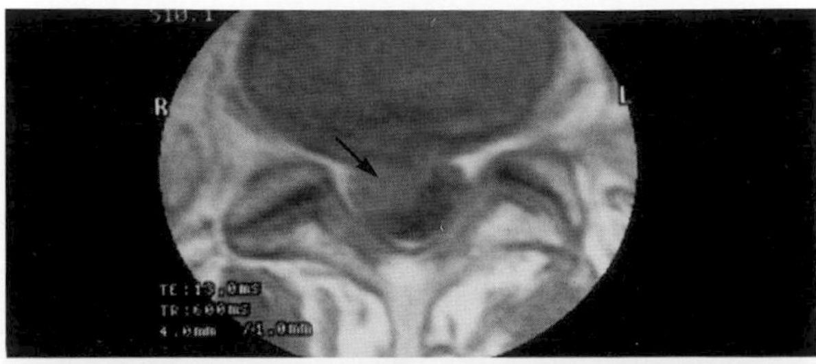

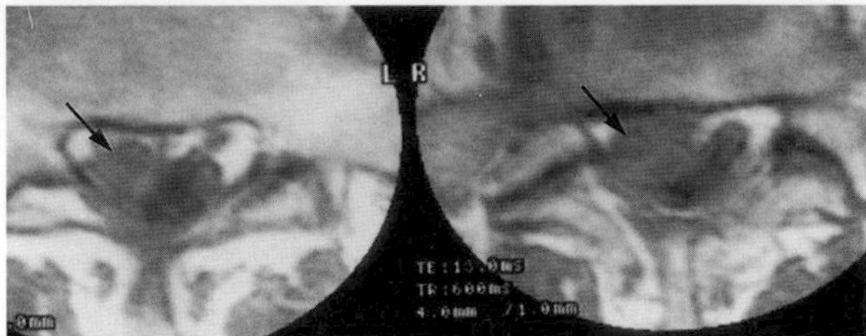

Figure 60.24 Posterolateral disc protrusion with migratory fragment (arrow). Three axial T1W MRI images at and just below the L5/S1 disc showing the large extruded and migratory disc fragment (arrow) compressing the thecal sac and right S1 root.

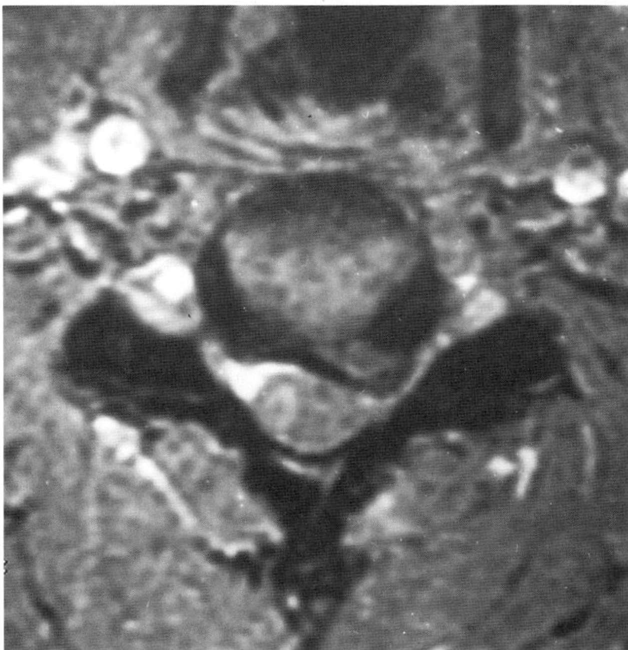

Figure 60.25 Axial MR image of the cervical spine in a patient with brachalgia at the C4/5 level. There is a left-of-centre posterior disc lesion impinging on the spinal cord and the left C5 roots.

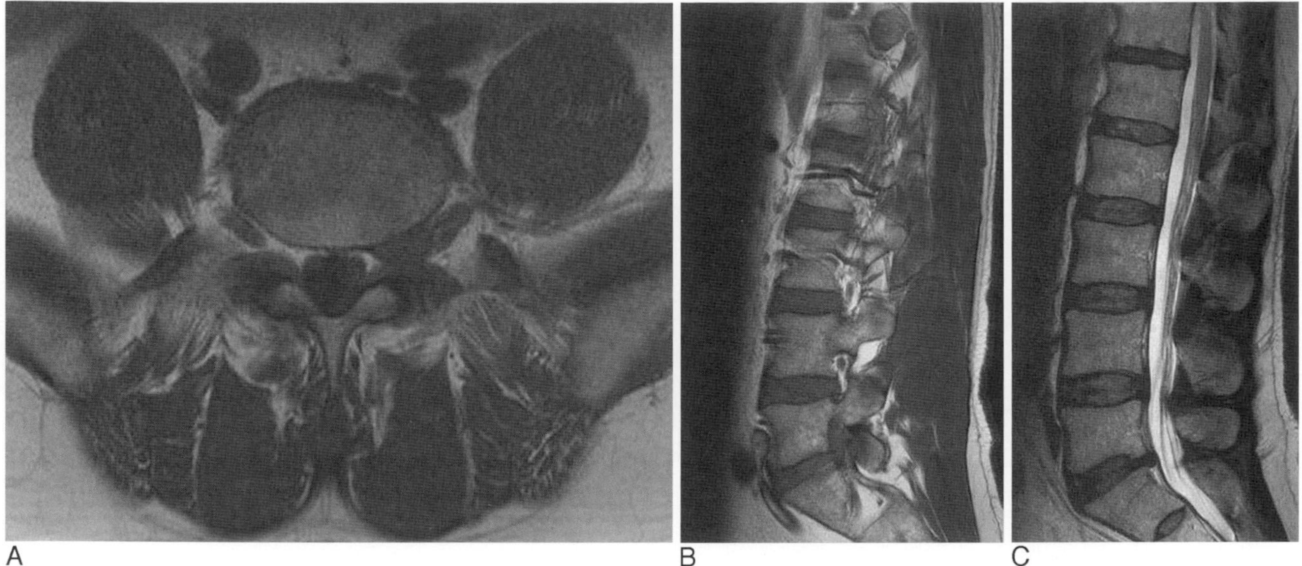

Figure 60.26 Lateral posterior disc protrusion. (A) On the axial T1W MR image there is a large lateral L5/S1 protrusion distorting the left dorsal root ganglion and ventral ramus. (B) On the para-sagittal T1W MR image the left L5 foramen is filled with disc material. (C) Note how deceptively and relatively normal the midline sagittal T2W image appears in this patient. Note also how a lateral disc affects the ventral ramus cranial to the affected disc – unlike the usual disc lesion that affects the root that will emerge at the more caudal level.

disc-related osteophytes usually do not involve the spinal canal, even when large.

Modic described three types of reactive changes in the cancellous bone adjacent to the vertebral end-plates: (type 1) in the acute stage of disc disease there is invasion of the cancellous spaces by fibrovascular reactive tissue; in time this leads to (type 2) fatty replacement of red marrow; eventually this leads to (type 3) bony sclerosis[59]. These changes are exquisitely shown by MRI: (A) type 1 changes yield low signal on T1W and high on T2W; (B) type 2 changes yield high signal on T1W and T2W (unless fat suppressed, when they will yield low signal); (C) type 3 changes yield low signal on all sequences. The vertebral end-plates may fracture and displace into the vertebral body, but the dense compact bone is not destroyed. Occasionally the end-plates become very irregular and the degenerative process progresses to a destructive disco-vertebral lesion, which may simulate many features of infective spondylitis. The key differentiation is the signal intensity of the disc on T2W – in degenerative change it will be low, whereas in infection it should be high.

POSTERIOR JOINTS AND LIGAMENTS

Osteoarthritic changes

Osteoarthritic changes develop in the facet joints at all levels, usually in close association with concomitant degeneration in the intervertebral disc. These result in hypertrophy of the articular processes and remodeling, and fragmentation of articular surfaces. The capsule thickens along with accessory ligaments. Because the disc space is narrowed, the flaval ligament thickens and buckles. All these changes encroach on the posterolateral aspect of the spinal canal and on the intervertebral foramina; remodelling and fragmentation can result in facet instability, usually causing anterior slip of the superior on the inferior vertebra[60].

Disruption of the collagen and elastin fibres of the accessory and capsular ligaments may result in infiltration by fibrovascular tissue. Sometimes focal or even diffuse cartilaginous or osseous metaplasia occurs. Myxomatous degeneration develops in the capsular ligaments of the posterior joints, which sometimes becomes invaded by hypertrophic and often haemorrhagic synovial tissue continuous with that of the joint. All of the above changes combine to create degenerative spinal stenosis (Fig. 60.27).

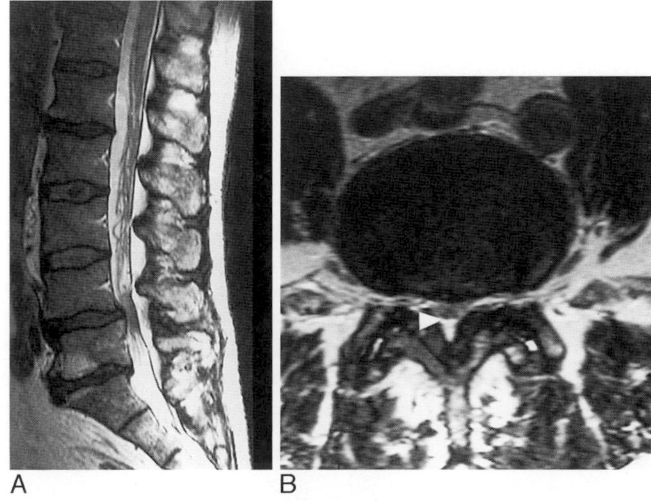

Figure 60.27 Degenerative spinal canal stenosis. Sagittal (A), and axial (B) T2W MRI of the lumbar spine showing a severe spinal canal stenosis at L4–5 with evidence of compression of the cauda equina, namely obliteration of CSF signal from the thecal sac at the site of compression (white arrowhead) and some redundant coiling of intrathecal spinal roots above.

Ossification of the posterior longitudinal ligament (OPLL) involves the mid- and lower cervical region in over 90 per cent of cases. Other ligaments are involved in only 7 per cent and a genetic propensity is present, especially in Japanese men[61]. Diffuse, segmental and mixed forms are recognized, the segmental type needing to be distinguished from posterior osteophytes. The dense bony mass can be adherent to the dura mater, unlike ordinary osteophytes, and surgical removal is often difficult. Other spinal regions can be involved, and extensive degeneration with exuberant anterolateral ossification, sometimes referred to as diffuse idiopathic skeletal hyperostosis (DISH), may also be associated with OPLL[61] (Fig. 60.28).

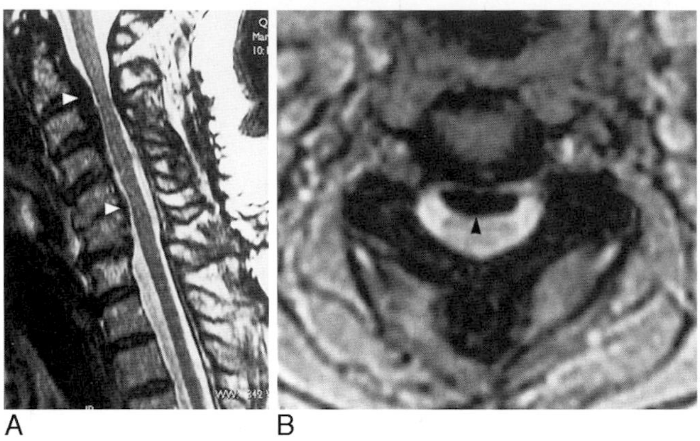

Figure 60.28 Ossification of the posterior longitudinal ligament. Sagittal (A) and axial (B), T2W MRIs of the cervical spine showing mild spinal cord compression by the thickened anteriorly located posterior longitudinal ligament (white arrowheads) within the spinal canal (black arrowhead).

Ossification of ligamentum flavum

Small tongues of ossification commonly extend into these ligaments from the superior borders of the laminae. Much more rarely, a hypertrophic bony mass or masses occur that encroach on the spinal canal; this has been reported most often in or near the thoracolumbar junction, but can occur anywhere[62].

Synovial cysts

These are uncommon lesions attached to the capsule of the posterior joints. Although they may consist mainly of degenerating synovium, and contain fluid that communicates with joint cavity, frequently they are cartilaginous or myxomatous, and solid rather than cystic. They have been confused with migratory disc fragments from which they should be distinguished by their attachment to the joints, and organized haematomas, because they may contain blood products. They usually occur only in the lower lumbar, or mid- and lower cervical regions[63] (Fig. 60.29).

Retro-odontal pseudotumour

The transverse ligament of the atlas and associated ligaments are commonly thickened in the ageing population, and often contain calcification. Rarely, the thickening has been so marked as to simulate a lesion such as meningioma. The masses usually consist of fragmented ligament and degenerate fibrocartilage, and they have also been confused with migratory disc material[64].

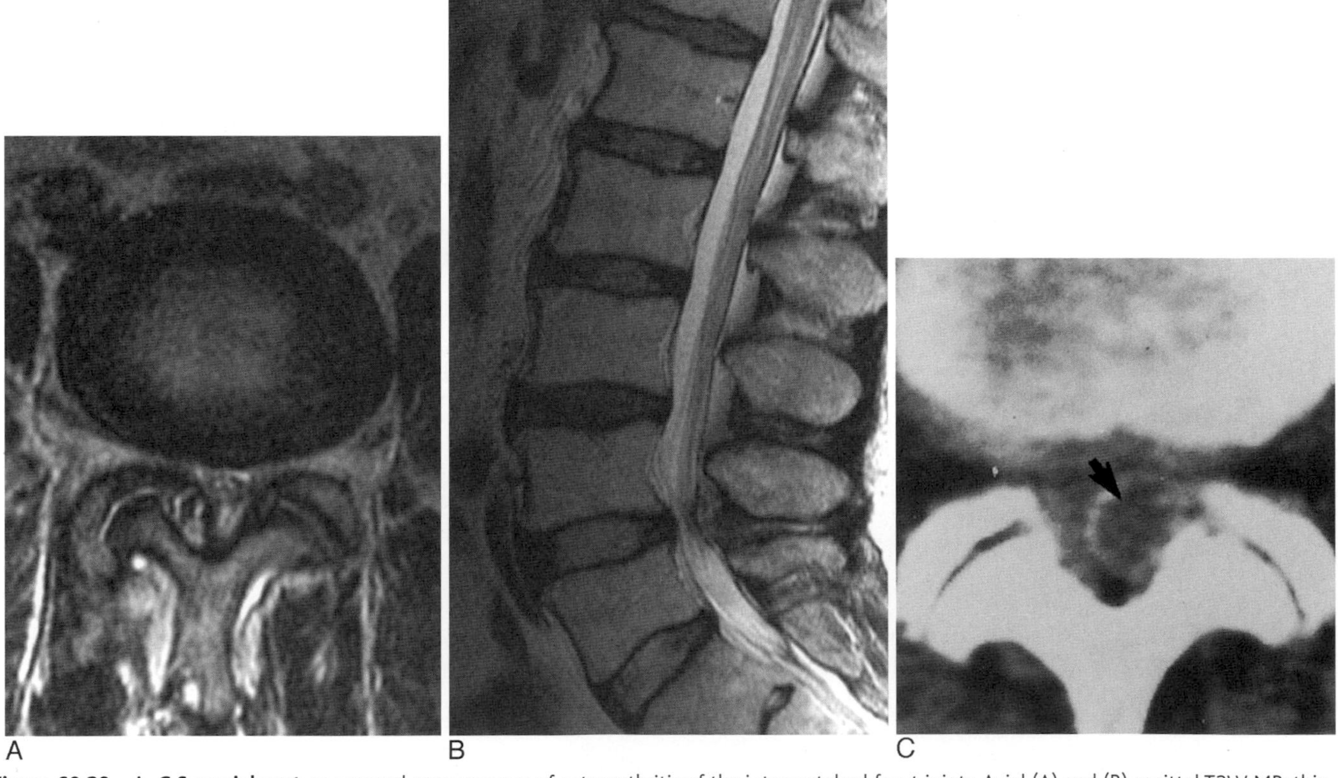

Figure 60.29 A–C Synovial cyst: an unusual consequence of osteoarthritis of the intervertebral facet joints. Axial (A) and (B) sagittal T2W MR: this lesion of the right L4/5 facet is displacing the flaval ligament and compressing the thecal sac. There is often secondary spinal stenosis at the affected level, as in this case. (C) CT of another patient. Here the lesion arises from a degenerate left-sided facet joint. They are sometimes misinterpreted as an intraspinal tumour, but involvement of the joint is characteristic.

INVOLVEMENT OF NEURAL STRUCTURES

All these degenerative processes can result in damage to the spinal cord and spinal roots, due mainly or entirely to mechanical compression. However, the severity of compression is not related linearly to the degree of damage, nor to its clinical effects. Indeed osteophytes in the cervical region are sufficient to cause up to moderate spinal cord compression in about 30 per cent of asymptomatic persons over 50 years of age[65,66] and disc protrusions in the lumbar spine sufficient to interfere with spinal nerve roots in nearly 40 per cent of asymptomatic persons[67].

Spinal cord

In the cervical region, compression is usually intermittent, or intermittently accentuated by neck movement. Cord substance is relatively inelastic, and retains the impression of deforming agents when not in direct contact[68]. Most often, damage is sustained only when the sagittal diameter of the cord is reduced by more than 50 per cent (Fig. 60.30); pathologically this damage consists of central necrosis involving mainly grey matter, and demyelination associated with axonal damage located mainly deep within the posterior and lateral columns. The mechanism is likely to be either shearing injury to axons in white matter, and to cord microvasculature in the deeper grey matter, analogous to closed head injury[69,70], or to compression-induced intermittent ischaemic damage[71]. It has a distinct propensity to be progressive, and shearing stresses in particular are generated from anterior deforming agents alone, such as a focal angular kyphosis without the necessity for an anteroposterior squeeze[72].

In the thoracic region, far greater compression is tolerated without the cord being damaged, presumably because of reduced mobility of this part of the spine. The cord frequently becomes focally moulded around the usually calcified fibrocartilaginous masses, which can occupy up to 60 per cent of the spinal canal and be associated with no clinical abnormality[73].

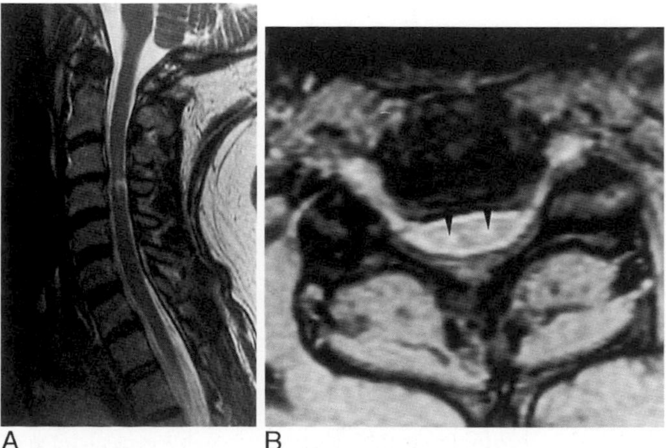

Figure 60.30 Cervical spondylotic myelopathy with myelomalacia. Sagittal (A) and axial (B), T2W MR images showing only moderate compression of the spinal cord at C3–4 level, and focal increased signal in the cord substance indicating that damage has occurred. On axial images this often has the appearance of 'snake eyes' (black arrowheads) within the spinal cord.

Spinal roots

In the cervical region, the spinal roots are compressed usually by osteophytes or fibrocartilaginous masses within or close to the entrance of the intervertebral canals. Clinical correlation is close only when these are also large enough to compress the spinal cord (see Fig. 60.30). In the lumbar region, roots usually are compressed by posterolateral disc protrusions or migrating migratory fragments in the anterior epidural space; the root that crosses the abnormal disc to reach the next inferior intervertebral foramen is usually involved, lying in the lateral extremity of the spinal canal under cover of the articular facet and within the thecal sac (except for S1 roots, which usually leave the dura cranial to the L5/S1 disc). The rarer far lateral posterior protrusions compress the dorsal root ganglion ventral ramus exiting *cranial* to the disc within the intervertebral foramen (see Fig. 60.26).

Osteo-arthritic changes in the posterior joints encroach on the lateral part of the spinal canal, and usually displace the dura and its contained root towards the centre of the canal, but occasionally the most laterally lying roots are sufficiently tethered by their sheaths to become entrapped (lateral canal entrapment). The intervertebral foramen becomes distorted and narrowed, and when severe and especially when subluxation is also present, the dorsal root ganglion may be compressed. The cauda equina as a whole may be compressed by large midline disc protrusions, or by posterior and bilateral posterolateral hypertrophic changes in bone and ligaments, usually in combination. Spinal stenosis is usually significant when there is room for only roots and not CSF, and frequently this is accompanied by redundant tortuosity of roots as a consequence of focal entrapment and stretching of these roots, which have a long intradural course (Figs 60.16, 60.19). It is only when these features are present that association with clinical cauda equina syndrome is consistently seen.

Natural history

The clinical conditions associated with degenerative lesions of the spine are: cervical spondylotic myelopathy and radiculopathy, sciatica and regional pain syndromes. Whilst relentless progression to severe disability occasionally occurs, much more often clinical features improve or resolve spontaneously in all three conditions. It is now accepted that possibly 60–70 per cent of intraspinal fibrocartilaginous masses of discogenic origin diminish in size or disappear spontaneously over a few weeks or months[74], although other much rarer conditions that can simulate migratory disc fragments, such as epidural varices and haematomas, may contribute to these figures. It has been claimed that cervical osteophytes regress after successful interbody fusion, but this has been refuted[75]. Reduction in cord cross-sectional area by more than 50–60 per cent (down to around 40 mm^2) is associated with poor operative outcome in cervical spondylotic myelopathy, with or without operative intervention[76].

IMAGING

Many of the processes discussed in the preceding section are shown on plain radiographs, namely sclerosis, osteophytes, disc space narrowing, calcified or ossified disc material and ligaments and gaseous nitrogen. A minimum midsagittal diameter of the cervical canal of less than 10 mm (tube-film distance around 2 m) indicates that cord compression is probably present. Alignment abnormalities are well shown on plain radiographs, which also show reducibility of subluxations determined by flexion and extension views.

On unenhanced CT in the lumbar region, annular bulges and protrusions, nuclear herniations and migratory fragments, enlarged degenerate ligaments and synovial cysts are usually well shown. These materials usually attenuate X-rays similar to disc substance. Calcification is uncommon; bubbles of nitrogen escaping from the disc via a tear in the annulus and entering the anterior epidural space are well shown only by CT.

Spinal canal narrowing by osteoarthritis and soft-tissue thickening is well documented by CT, and usually it is possible to tell which roots are entrapped laterally[77]. The cross-sectional area of the canal can be measured electronically; wide window settings are needed and only measurements of about 100 mm^2 or less show a consistent association with clinical cauda equina entrapment[13].

In the cervical and thoracic regions, plain CT is of less value and generally is not recommended. However, the anatomy of osteophytes is well shown, and many thoracic disc protrusions are calcified.

MRI is the optimal investigation, because effects on neural structures are shown best. The MR signal returned from degenerate discs is usually lower than from healthy discs and best appreciated on T2W images. Occasionally, signal is paradoxically higher than from healthy discs on T1W images, perhaps due to calcium precipitation, and signal may also be higher on T2W images due to the presence of fluid-filled clefts (see Fig. 60.23). The latter appearance needs to be distinguished from infective discitis (see later), especially when it is associated with reactive changes in the adjacent vertebrae; in degeneration, high signal is not uniform throughout the whole disc, and the dark band of cortical bone of the vertebral end-plates is intact though not necessarily undistorted. Tears in the external layers of the annulus fibrosus may be visible as high signal foci on T2W images. Signal from degenerate fibrocartilage within the spinal canal is quite variable on T2W images, and it is common for migratory fragments to be conspicuously brighter than the nucleus of the disc of origin. Migratory fragments can be simulated by the much rarer epidural varices or haematoma[78].

Reactive changes in the cancellous bone of the adjacent vertebral bodies also return variable signal reflecting their composition: fibrovascular infiltrates (dark on T1W, bright on T2W images), fatty replacement of red marrow (bright on T1, dark or bright on T2), sclerosis (dark on all images)[59]. Osteophytes show a similar variability in internal structure, although mostly they are sclerotic.

Compression of the spinal cord is well shown. This generally is assessed best on axial imaging, but cord flattening may be artefactually exaggerated on T2W and gradient-recalled echo images. Distortion of cord shape may be due to compression alone, or reflect underlying structural damage; when congruous with the shape of the deforming agent, it is probably due to compression and will retain the impression of an impinging agent, even when contact is removed[68]. Structural damage is usually reflected by signal change within the substance of the spinal cord, and when present, clinical myelopathy usually is also present (Fig. 60.30). Signal change usually is focal and occurs at or slightly caudal to the site of compression. When the distribution can be determined on axial images, it usually seems to involve mainly central areas[70], and often has the appearance of bilateral lesions, sometimes likened to snakes' or cats' eyes; occasionally these appearances extend over many cord segments. These changes are detected most sensitively by T2W images, and that they do not always indicate permanent damage is demonstrated by their frequent disappearance after decompressive surgery with good outcome; however they usually persist when clinical recovery is minimal or absent[79].

The spinal nerves are directly shown, and the dorsal root ganglion can often be distinguished from the compressing agent even when entrapped. The ganglia are affected by far lateral disc protrusions, and a ganglion flattened by compression from below may seem enlarged on axial images. Abnormal enhancement has been observed in compressed roots after IV contrast medium, usually focal and mainly extradural, but occasionally extending intradurally for several centimetres[80].

Myelography is still occasionally requested when multi-level disease is present or MR impossible. Disc protrusions present as indentations of the anterior surface of the thecal sac opposite the disc space; root sheaths of the spinal nerves usually fill normally but are deviated and may appear flattened. Disc herniations are generally larger, and the root sheath exiting from the intervertebral foramen below usually is obliterated. The indentation of the thecal sac is nearly always maximal opposite the level of the disc. Most far lateral posterior disc protrusions will *not* be shown; these constitute around 10 per cent of disc lesions causing entrapment neuropathies. In lateral recess stenosis the theca usually is displaced medially away from the lateral extremity of the spinal canal, resulting in a constricted or wasted appearance of the thecal sac. Postmyelography CT in the cervical region depicts most accurately the degree of compression of the spinal cord, which can be both under- and overestimated by myelography alone.

THE POSTOPERATIVE SPINE

Lumbar disc surgery involves part or complete laminectomy for access, partial facetectomy to free the lateral recess and removal of accessible disc material from spinal canal and disc space, in varying combinations. With improved preoperative imaging, microdiscectomy procedures are increasingly used; these require smaller and smaller laminectomies. However all surgery results in some epidural granulations that eventually mature into fibrous tissue. The importance of this as a cause of recurrent symptoms after operation has been greatly diminished by imaging studies in which both the prevalence and severity of these processes have been shown to be entirely similar in patients who are pain-free after operation[81]. However, it is still useful to distinguish these reactive processes from recurrent or residual disc material, the presence of which continues to be an indication for re-operation[82].

Pseudo-meningoceles sometimes occur, implying that dura was breached during surgery; they usually are not of clinical relevance, but may need to be distinguished from abscess in which communication with the thecal space is not shown. Lumbar disc surgery had long been considered a common cause of lumbosacral adhesive arachnoiditis, but this was largely due to the pre-operative myelography with oil-based contrast medium iophendylate (Myodil, Pantopaque)[83].

In the cervical region the operation most often performed is anterior spinal fusion, usually combined with a discectomy and removal of osteophytes. Usually either a dowel-shaped (Cloward) or disc-shaped (Smith-Robinson) bone graft from the iliac crest, or an osteoconductive polymer is hammered into the disc space. Sometimes anterior plates or cases are used. The graft should be flush with the anterior surface of the spinal column, the disc space should not be too distracted and the normal spinal curvature should be maintained. In multilevel disease, an extensive laminectomy may be performed, but because this often results in a progressive cervical kyphosis, the operation of laminoplasty has been devised, which widens the sagittal diameter of the spinal canal but removes little or no bone. The latter is often preferred in OPLL, because adequate decompression from the anterior approach can be difficult to achieve in this condition.

Plain radiographs may contribute little to the evaluation of the postoperative lumbar spine and, following microdiscectomy, even the operative level can be difficult to identify. However they remain useful in the cervical region to evaluate the stability of a spinal fusion (Fig. 60.31), effectiveness of laminoplasty, or severity of postlaminectomy kyphosis.

MRI is the optimal investigation for evaluating the postoperative lumbar spine (Figs 60.32 and 60.33). Recurrent or residual disc material is distinguished reliably from epidural scar and granuloma on post-gadolinium-enhanced images by lack of enhancement[82], though disc material is often surrounded by enhancing matter.

Enhancement of scar diminishes over 2 years, but generally persists for many years[82]. Arachnoiditis may be confined to the operation site or be more generalized, and all roots across the involved regions are usually involved[83]. Rarely one or more roots enhance even intradurally, and often this is the symptomatic and formerly compressed root[80].

In the cervical region, the discectomy may simulate discovertebral spondylitis, an appearance that may persist for many months. Persistent compression and degenerative changes in the spinal cord may be shown, and sometimes an alternative diagnosis is established by this study, such as multiple sclerosis. Signal change in damaged spinal cord usually regresses when functional outcome is good, but it generally persists when it is poor[84].

SPINAL TUMOURS

Spinal tumours occur in extradural, intradural extramedullary and intramedullary compartments. For each compartment, the pattern of radiological abnormality is usually distinctive. A list of the more common lesions occurring in each compartment is shown in Table 60.1.

EXTRADURAL TUMOURS

The most common extradural tumours are metastases. These usually involve the vertebral bodies and neural arches, but malignant infiltration may spread widely in the epidural space without local bony involvement. Other disseminated malignancies such as myeloma and lymphoma are indistinguishable. Primary bone tumours are less common. Those most often responsible for spinal cord compression are aneurysmal bone cyst, benign osteoblastoma, chordoma and giant cell tumour, the latter occurring mainly in the sacrum, but also in the upper thoracic or upper cervical regions (see Figs 60.34–60.37).

Plain radiographs often show evidence of focal bone destruction, and sometimes vertebral collapse; paraspinal masses may be visible, especially with myeloma and extradural neurogenic tumours. Plain CT is far more sensitive at identifying bone destruction, which is not surprising because between 50 per cent and 60 per cent of vertebral body bone

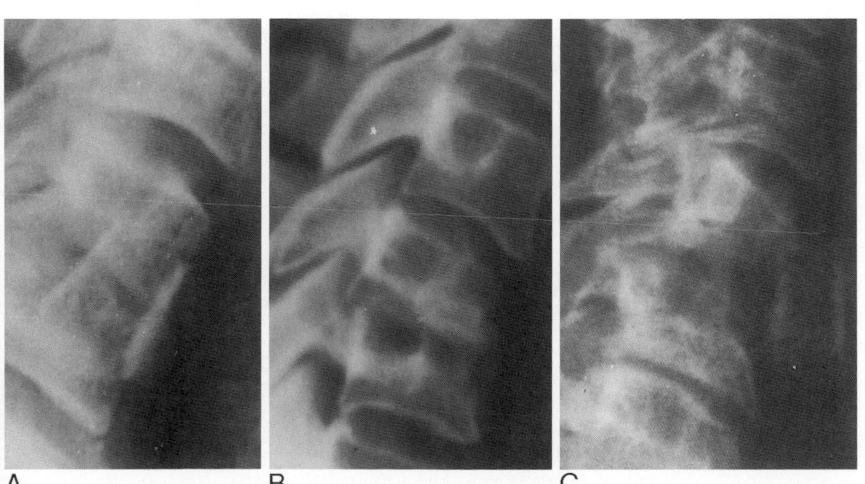

Figure 60.31 Cloward's anterior spinal fusion: postoperative radiographs in three cases. (A) Satisfactory appearances. (B) The vertebral bodies adjacent to the fusion have partially collapsed, resulting in an angular kyphosis. (C) The bone graft has been extruded anteriorly and the upper vertebra has slipped forwards; the spinal canal remains compromised.

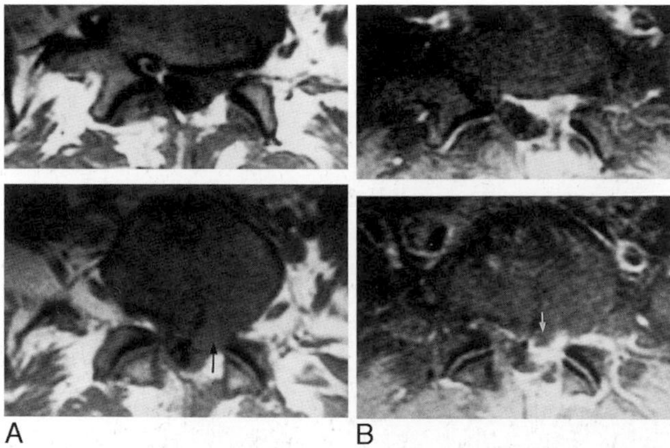

Figure 60.32 Epidural scar and residual/recurrent disc protrusion. (A) Axial T1W MRI just below (above) and through (below) the L4/5 disc, showing a large epidural mass (black arrow) on the left side. (B) Images at similar levels made after IV gadolinium and using fat presaturation, showing marked enhancement of most of the epidural mass, but also a central non-enhancing region in contact with the discal margin (arrow). At operation, recurrent disc material was found at this site, embedded in dense fibrous tissue.

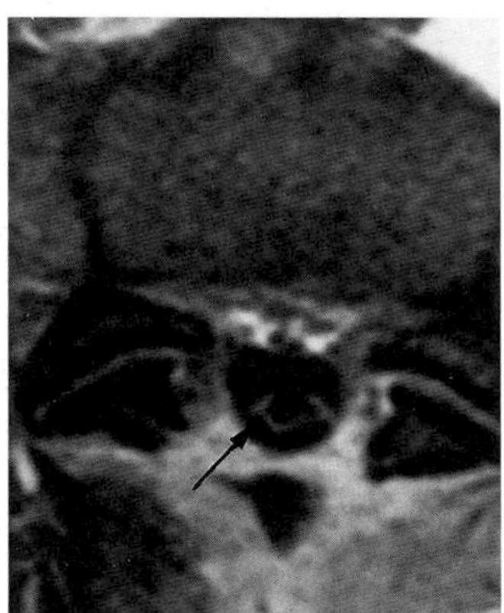

Figure 60.33 Extraspinal wound abscess and infected pseudo-meningocele. Axial T1W image at L4/5 made with fat presaturation and IV gadolinium showing a low signal cavity surrounded by a very thick white wall of granulation tissue. Operation revealed a cavity containing fluid infected by *Staphylococcus aureus*. These appearances can be mimicked by sterile postoperative pseudo-meningoceles.

mass needs to be destroyed before it becomes evident on plain X-rays. This is particularly true of lesions involving the sacrum. However, the extent of the involvement of the spinal canal is often not shown adequately by plain CT. MRI clearly demonstrates bone destruction and malignant infiltration, intra- and extraspinal masses and spinal cord compression. The entire spinal canal should be examined to reveal the full extent of the disease, and phased array coils are optimal. Although myelography is rarely performed nowadays, the most characteristic feature of an extradural lesion is displacement of the thecal sac *away from* the bony walls of the spinal canal. When major resections are planned, angiography may be requested to identify the position of the major radiculomedullary arteries. Percutaneous biopsy is often necessary when the diagnosis is not known or there is doubt about tumour transformation (e.g. in lymphoma). As in other situations, it may be performed under fluoroscopic guidance, but CT provides optimal guidance, despite the advances in MRI intervention.

Table 60.1 ANATOMICAL LOCATION OF SPINAL LESIONS
Extradural
Benign
Disc prolapse
Haematoma
Abscess
Neurofibroma
Osteochondroma
Dermoid/epidermoid
Vertebral body tumours:
Haemangioma
Osteoclastoma
Aneurysmal bone cyst
Paget's disease
Malignant
Metastases
Lymphoma
Myeloma
Sarcoma
Chordoma
Intradural/extramedullary
Neurofibroma
Meningioma
Dermoid/epidermoid
Lipoma also medullary
Ependymoma
Metastases in CSF:
Medulloblastoma
Ependymoma
Melanoma
Carcinoma
Intramedullary
Tumours:
Ependymoma
Astrocytoma
Glioblastoma
Developmental tumours
Haemangioblastoma
Syringomyelia
Myelitis
Abscess/granuloma
Haematomyelia

INTRADURAL EXTRAMEDULLARY TUMOURS

Neurinomas and meningiomas are by far the commonest lesions in this intradural extramedullary location. Significant extradural components are present in about 7 per cent of meningiomas and 30 per cent of neurinomas. Over 80 per cent of meningiomas occur in the thoracic region in middle-

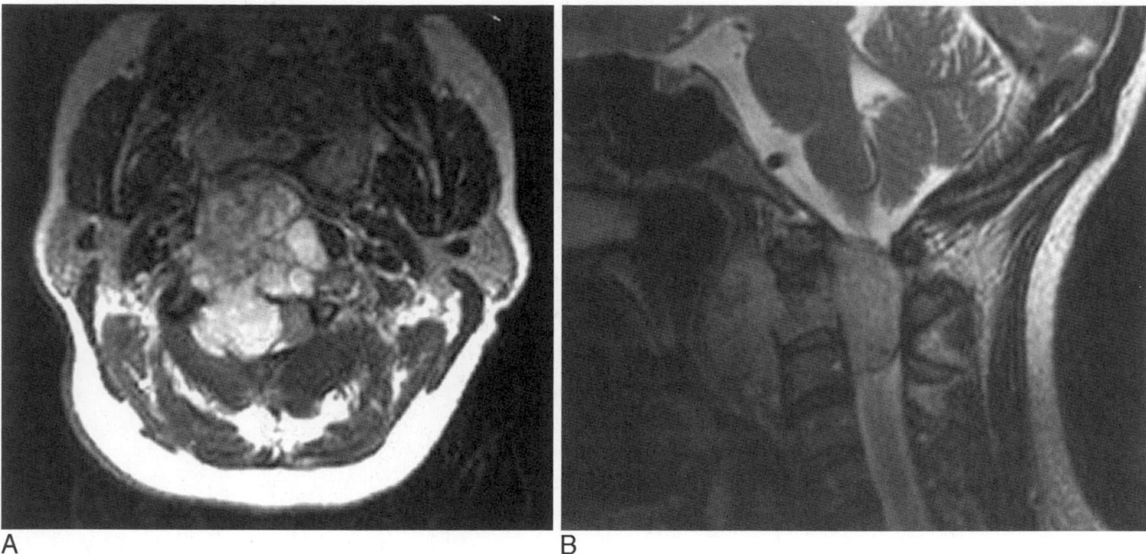

Figure 60.34 Chordoma. Axial and sagittal MR showing the typical soft-tissue mass and bone destruction. The cord is markedly displaced to the left. (Courtesy of Dr Justin Cross.)

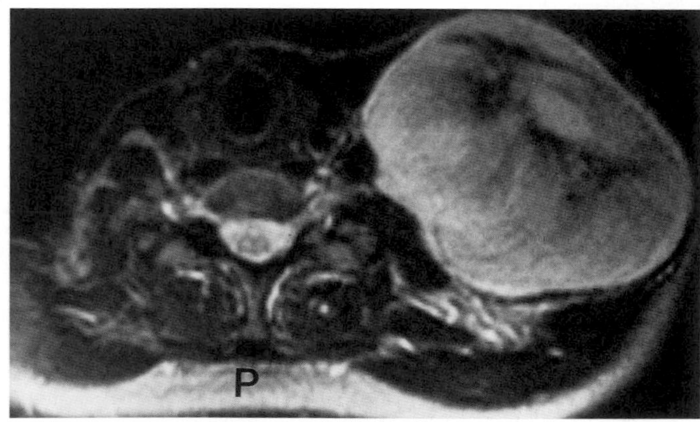

Figure 60.35 Extraspinal neurofibroma. Axial T2W gradient-recalled echo MRI showing a huge neurofibroma in the left posterior triangle without spinal involvement. (P = posterior.)

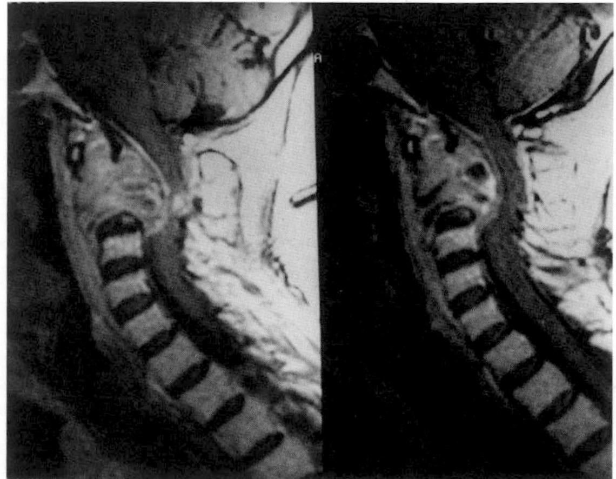

Figure 60.36 Osteoclastoma (giant cell tumour) of C2. Sagittal T1W MRIs made after IV gadolinium. C2 is replaced by tumour and the large extraosseous mass is compressing the spinal cord. Note similarity in appearances to the chordoma in Figure 60.34.

aged women and are very rare in the lumbar spine, whereas neurinomas occur at any level, at almost any age and are approximately equal in men and women[85]. Tumoural calcification may occur in both, but marked calcification is uncommon. Meningiomas may be associated with hyperostosis, but this is seldom conspicuous. Sometimes only diffuse thickening of the spinal roots occurs in neurofibromatosis. However, diffuse enlargement of the spinal roots may also occur in non-neoplastic processes, such as some of the hereditary sensory motor neuropathies.

Malignant tumours may disseminate in the subarachnoid space. Cerebral involvement is commonly present as well, and spinal lesions are most often found in the lumbar theca, but can occur anywhere. They are frequently multiple and in some cases there is diffuse pial spread with encasement of the spinal cord or cauda equina.

Plain radiographs may reveal expansion of the spinal canal or of one or more intervertebral foramina; this is shown in about 30 per cent of neurinomas, and very rarely with meningiomas. An associated paravertebral mass is far more suggestive of a neurinoma or other neurogenic tumour (see Fig. 60.37). Hyperostosis is uncommon with meningiomas of the spine because the bone is rarely infiltrated. Plain CT will demonstrate bone erosion, sclerosis and extradural extension is good, but purely intradural lesions may not be shown. IV contrast enhancement may be helpful if the level is known. Heavy calcification is rare in meningiomas and neurofibromas; a heavily calcified intraspinal mass is usually found to be extruded disc material and is often seen to be clearly extradural. MRI elegantly demonstrates the intraspinal as well as the extraspinal extent, spinal cord compression and displacement. The signal from spinal meningiomas is usually similar to that from the spinal cord in both T1W and T2W images, whereas that from neurinomas is usually conspicuously higher on T2W images. Even small intradural

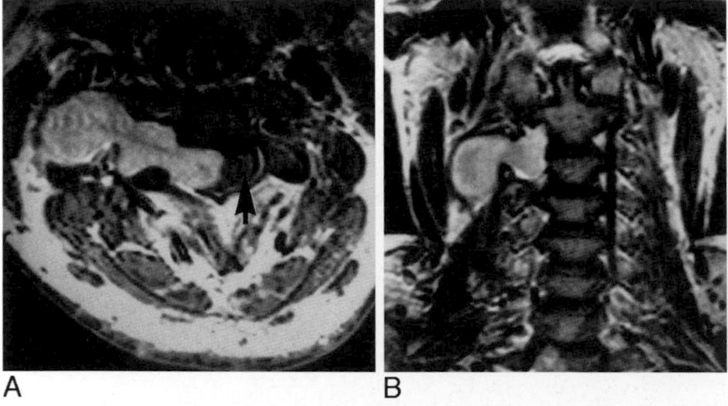

Figure 60.37 Partly intradural and partly extradural right C3 schwannoma. Axial (A) and coronal (B) T1W MRIs of the cervical spine made after the injection of IV gadolinium showing the large lobular schwannoma extending into the spinal canal and compressing the spinal cord (arrow).

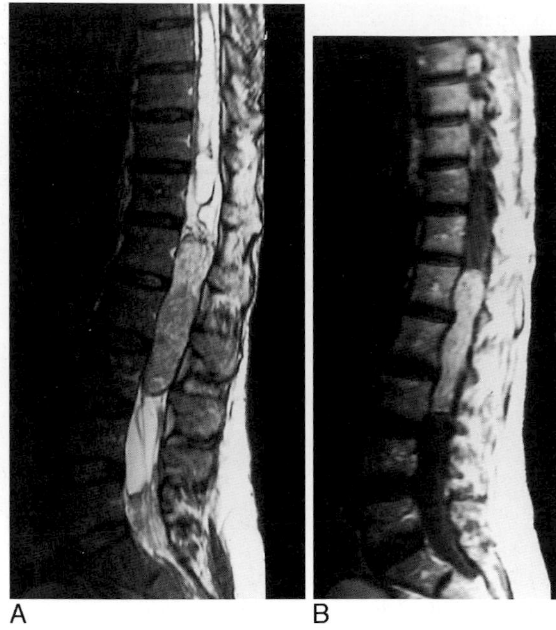

Figure 60.38 Ependymoma of the filum terminate and conus medullaris. Sagittal T2W (A) and (B) T1W post gadolinium-enhanced MRIs of the lumbar spine showing an expansile enhancing intraspinal mass and central signal change in the spinal cord above.

lesions are well shown by MRI on the high-resolution MRI techniques now available. IV contrast enhancement may be necessary to demonstrate diffuse pial spread in metastatic disease. However, CSF cytology remains considerably more sensitive in detecting diffuse leptomeningeal involvement[86]. Myelography, rarely performed nowadays, showed an intradural extramedullary lesion as a rounded, smooth contour mass, expanding rather than compressing the thecal sac and displacing the spinal cord. A plane of cleavage was usually visible between the tumour and the spinal cord.

INTRAMEDULLARY TUMOURS

Most of these are gliomas; ependymomas (Fig. 60.38) and astrocytomas occur with about equal frequency in the spinal cord, but ependymomas greatly predominate in the filum terminale, especially in children, where they are usually of the myxopapillary type[87]. Rarely, ependymomas may arise from the extradural part of the filum terminale and present as a destructive lesion of the sacrum, or a presacral mass, which is prone to metastasize especially to lung.

Spinal capillary haemangioblastomas nearly always involve the posterior columns of the spinal cord and abut against a pial surface[88]. Most are solitary, but up to 30 per cent are associated with similar lesions elsewhere in the central nervous system. Extramedullary and even extradural haemangioblastomas are encountered occasionally in the spine.

Metastases may occur within the substance of the spinal cord, and other rare intramedullary neoplasms including primary lymphoma.

About 70 per cent of intramedullary tumours are associated with cysts, and three types are described: (A) intratumoral cysts, in which the wall consists of tumour; (B) peritumoral or capping cysts, in which cone-shaped glial-lined cavities extend above and below the tumour for a limited number of spinal segments; (C) syringomyelia, in which extensive cavitation of the spinal cord is present and indistinguishable from other forms of syringomyelia in regions not involved by tumour. The latter cystic form occurs in approaching 50 per cent of all intramedullary tumours including metastases, but is probably most frequent with haemangioblastoma[87,89].

Plain radiographs only show expansion of the spinal canal in about 10 per cent of adults, 30 per cent of childhood cases overall, and is most frequent with giant myxopapillary ependymoma of the cauda equina[90]. MRI is the preferred investigation and intramedullary tumours and associated cysts are usually shown well. Signal from the tumour may be similar to cord substance, though sometimes it is lower on T1W images and frequently somewhat higher on T2W images. They may appear sharply demarcated from normal cord tissue and sometimes seem enclosed in a hypointense capsule. Astrocytoma and ependymoma cannot be distinguished reliably, nor can they be distinguished reliably from many inflammatory processes. Tumour-associated cysts are well-circumscribed tubular or cone-shaped structures of homogeneous signal intensity, low on T1W and usually high on T2W images, but about 15 per cent of apparently cystic regions are found to be solid at surgery[91]. Syringomyelia secondary to intramedullary tumour is suggested by enlargement or signal change in noncystic regions of the cord and by the appearances after administration of IV gadolinium (Gd-DTPA). Unlike the brain, the great majority of spinal cord gliomas enhance at least partially[87]. IV contrast enhancement will also help to identify solid tumours, including metastases. The spinal cord appears enlarged, the enlargement usually smooth and uniform as in syringomyelia; however the site of enlargement may be unusual for syringomyelia, and any lobulation, or focal or eccentric expansion, are valuable clues. Spinal angiography often provides definitive diagnosis of spinal haemangioblastoma, but usually is not a necessary preliminary to operative treatment. The appearance is characteristic, consisting of a usually small, relatively homogeneous, well-circumscribed dense capillary blush; the one or two arteries commonly supplying the lesion are usually slightly enlarged, and enlarged or normal-sized draining veins opacify only a little earlier than normal. Intra-operative US can distinguish cysts from solid tumour, cysts appearing as circumscribed anechoic areas. US may also assist in identifying the tumour boundary but it is not infallible[92].

TRAUMA

Clinical aspects

Acute post-traumatic myelopathy usually results from burst fractures and fracture-dislocations. If loss of cord function is complete, and remains so for 24 h, functional recovery is unlikely. Management is frequently conservative, and imaging other than CT for diagnosis usually is not indicated. When fracture is absent, pre-existing abnormalities are often present, such as cervical spondylosis or instability such as at the atlanto-axial junction. Also acute, mainly soft-tissue injury occasionally may result in sudden severe cord compression from acute disc herniation or epidural haematoma. In these situations the myelopathy is more often incomplete, and prospects for recovery can be much better. Therefore, early imaging of the spinal canal may be indicated. Many workers also believe that early stabilization and correction in spinal deformity is mandatory to optimize conditions for recovery.

In delayed post-traumatic myelopathy, the neurological impairment appears only a few hours after injury, often no explanation is found, but imaging is indicated to exclude compressive lesions such as epidural haematoma or acute disc herniations. When it appears months or years after injury, it can be due to delayed spinal instability, which recent work has shown is most likely to occur with fracture-dislocations that might have been reduced by traction in the early postinjury period; however evidence also is now substantial that post-traumatic deformity, such as angular kyphoses at the fracture site, may result in progressive cord damage manifesting clinically only after many years[72].

Progressive post-traumatic myelopathy results in worsening of existing disability or ascending functional loss. In such cases, the spinal cord usually is extensively damaged well beyond the site of injury. The entire spinal cord may be involved[93,94]. This damage manifests as diffuse atrophy with necrosis, cell loss and gliosis, and most frequently the cord is extensively cavitated. Imaging may be indicated because some workers believe it advisable to drain intramedullary cysts or correct spinal deformities and divide adhesions in such cases, in the hope that this may arrest the process. Post-traumatic pseudo-meningoceles have occasionally caused a delayed compression myelopathy or neuropathy, but usually they do not, even when large.

Acute brachial and lumbar plexus injuries resulting in a flaccid monoplegia in the cervical region are commonly due to avulsion of the spinal roots from the cord, and in the lumbar region to tearing of the nerves at the level of the root sheaths. This is usually associated with rupture of the root sheaths of the affected spinal nerves resulting in pseudo-meningoceles, or less commonly simply in irregular occlusion of the sheaths. Associated fractures may be present, especially in lumbar plexus avulsion injuries, which are seen mainly in children.

IMAGING

CT is superior to plain radiographs at detecting fractures and defining the degree of distortion of the spinal canal (Fig. 60.39). More accurate depiction of the true extent of injury will better enable instability to be predicted: fractures involving only the anterior part of the vertebral body are stable, those involving the posterior part of the body and neural arches are potentially unstable. Thin contiguous slices as on modern multidetector systems will demonstrate subtle fractures and provide multiplanar reformatted images, which are essential in assessing vertebral alignment, facet joint integrity and the craniovertebral junction. With mainly ligamentous injuries, such as complete disc rupture or avulsion of the transverse ligament of the atlas, carefully performed CT usually will reveal avulsion fractures.

Unlike CT, MRI accurately demonstrates the state of the spinal cord. The spinal cord is abnormal in most patients with acute post-traumatic myelopathy, whether or not a bony injury has occurred[95,96]. The abnormality may consist of:

1 Diffuse signal increase on T2W images, usually at the site of injury or only for one or two segments beyond
2 Cord swelling, not always present and usually only slight
3 A circumscribed area of low signal within a more extensive area of high signal on T2W images, associated with focal cord swelling, and probably representing intramedullary haematoma.

High signal on T1W images may appear, but is infrequent. It is notable that although cord contusions are always haemorrhagic pathologically, this is evident on MRI in only 50 per

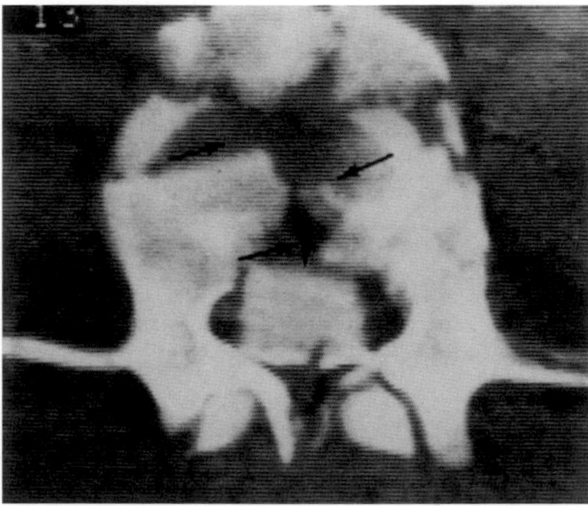

Figure 60.39 Burst fracture. Axial CT through L3 showing a comminuted fracture of the body of L3 (arrows) and a large retropulsed square bone fragment (arrowhead) occupying most of the spinal canal. Flaccid paraplegia.

cent or less. Major fractures, abnormalities of vertebral alignment and the state of the spinal canal are usually well shown. Acute disc herniations, and other lesions that may acutely compress the spinal cord such as bone fragments or epidural haematoma, also should be shown. However, MRI shows that the spinal cord is not usually significantly compressed after the injury.

Animal models that have established the extent of signal change on MRI in the acutely damaged spinal cord is related to the severity of injury. Clinical studies suggest that the extent of signal change has prognostic significance also, and mild or transient loss of function after injury usually is not accompanied by any signal change in the cord. Evidence of haematomyelia has been indicative of poor prognosis. Progression from acute injury to a localized cystic myelopathy has been followed on serial imaging[97], and in most cases, this does not lead to further functional loss. Cases with progressive myelopathy usually show extensive signal change throughout the cord on both T1W and T2W images. Cavities generally resemble syringomyelia in such cases, but often are multiple or multilocular.

Spinal cord injuries in children have been noted to differ somewhat from adults: children may develop extensive signal change in the cord with minor, remote or no spinal fracture, and any signal change usually is followed by persistent functional loss[98].

Myelography rarely needs to be performed nowadays, but it may be needed if MR is equivocal for brachial plexus avulsion injuries. The most reliable sign is failure to visualize the intradural rootlets of the avulsed spinal nerves in the cervical region when uninvolved rootlets are clearly visible.

INFLAMMATORY ARTHROPATHIES

Erosive arthropathies

Rheumatoid arthritis

The prevalence of radiological evidence of spine involvement usually has been found to be up to about 15 per cent, over 70 per cent of these cases involving the craniovertebral junction. However, autopsy studies have indicated an incidence of atlanto-axial involvement in over 80 per cent of rheumatoid arthritics. Subaxial subluxations, usually of multiple levels, are a major feature in 10 per cent. Only 2–6 per cent of cases develop a clinical myelopathy, which almost invariably is due to spinal cord compression, caused by the subluxations (especially the vertical and subaxial). In up to 40 per cent, granulomatous soft-tissue masses contribute to spinal cord compression, and in as many as 30 per cent of cases with myelopathy the subluxation is not reducible[99].

Ankylosing spondylitis and other seronegative arthritides

Ankylosing spondylitis characteristically involves mainly the spine, but the other syndromes, which include Reiter's, psoriatic, intestinal or lupus arthritis, rarely do. Even in ankylosing spondylitis, neurological complications are uncommon. They may arise from cord or root compression caused by fractures, atlanto-axial subluxation, discovertebral destructive lesions that are either inflammatory or degenerative in type, and occasionally from focal degenerative or granulomatous soft-tissue masses. The cauda equina syndrome of ankylosing spondylitis probably is an inflammatory radiculopathy, and associations with adhesions between roots and the walls of the thecal sac, and with dural ectasia have been described in some cases. Dural ectasia is rare, and may be either diffuse or saccular, the latter sometimes causing marked focal bony erosions invaginating into neural arches or vertebral bodies[37].

Imaging

In atlanto-axial subluxation due to rheumatoid arthritis, the decision to operate, and which operative strategy to employ, are influenced by:

1. Presence and severity of the spinal cord involvement
2. Whether the cord compression would be adequately diminished by regression of the inflammatory soft-tissue masses that often follow arthrodesis
3. Whether the subluxation can be reduced, and the prospect of maintaining that reduction, which in turn is influenced by:
    a. The integrity of the neural arches, especially of C1
    b. The integrity of the lateral masses of C1 and C2.

Plain CT with sagittal reconstructions is better than plain radiographs at demonstrating erosions and the integrity of structural elements. MRI shows all these features, including the soft-tissue masses and state of the spinal cord. High-resolution multiplanar MRI also usually demonstrates the bone adequately, but in some cases the addition of CT may be desirable. Subluxation is best demonstrated by plain radiographs and flexion/extension views are used as a pre-operative investigation.

INFECTIVE DISORDERS OF THE SPINE

VERTEBRAL OSTEOMYELITIS

This is usually based on a destructive discovertebral lesion. However central and subligamentous types are also occasionally encountered involving only the vertebral bodies. Rarely the neural arches are affected. Neurological involvement results from intraspinal extension of infection or more rarely instability, and occurs in less than 1 per cent of cases caused by pyogenic organisms, but in up to 40 per cent of cases caused by nonpyogenic organisms, of which the commonest is tuberculosis[100].

EPIDURAL ABSCESS

This may occur from haematogenous dissemination, or has spread from an infected disc or posterior joint, involvement of which may only be noted secondarily or in retrospect. Lesions are commonly extensive, particularly in children. Acute pain and early onset of paraplegia are characteristic.

PARAVERTEBRAL INFECTIONS

Various types of infections near the spine may be associated with subluxations. One of the most notable is atlanto-axial subluxation in the presence of retropharyngeal sepsis.

Imaging

MRI is the preferred technique and allows a firm diagnosis of pyogenic discovertebral osteomyelitis at least 2–3 weeks earlier than plain radiographs or CT. The characteristic early signs are: low signal throughout the disc and in adjacent parts of the vertebral bodies on T1W images (Fig. 60.40), and corresponding high signal on T2W images; and thinning, fragmentation and eventual loss of the dark line of the vertebral end-plates above and below the disc. This may need to be distinguished from severe disc degeneration, with high signal clefts in the disc and marked reactive changes in the adjacent vertebrae with irregular end-plates; in degeneration the changes are less uniform, both in disc and vertebral bodies, and actual bone destruction should be absent. Other features, which may be seen in infection, are perispinal extension including paraspinal abscesses (Fig. 60.41) and involvement of the anterior epidural space. Nondiscogenic forms of infective spondylitis present as localized processes, which can be difficult to distinguish from neoplasia, especially metastases. Multiple adjacent vertebrae may be involved in the subligamentous type, which would be unusual for metastases. IV Gd-DTPA results in diffuse enhancement in areas of active infection, often surrounding unenhancing foci of pus.

CT characteristically shows punched-out erosions of bone adjacent to the involved disc, giving a moth-eaten appearance, and the lesions may be associated with usually small dense sequestra. Sclerosis is often prominent. Progressive loss of disc space, and thinning progressing to loss of vertebral end-plates, followed by bone loss, wedging of adjacent vertebrae, sclerosis and regional subluxations or kyphosis, are the plain radiographic features of infective discovertebral osteomyelitis.

SPINAL MENINGITIS (ARACHNOIDITIS)

Inflammation in the subarachnoid space may lead to organizing exudates and permanent intradural adhesions[101]. The commonest causes of arachnoiditis are iatrogenic, in particular due to previous myelography using iophendylate (Myodil), but this is now becoming a rarity. It usually involves the caudal sac, rarely ascending above the L3/4 disc[102]. It also may follow other intrathecal injections such as some of the earlier ionic water-soluble agents, steroids or anaesthetic agents. Lumbar disc surgery itself is rarely a cause[83].

Arachnoiditis also may follow accidental trauma, spinal subarachnoid haemorrhage and is rarely encountered with

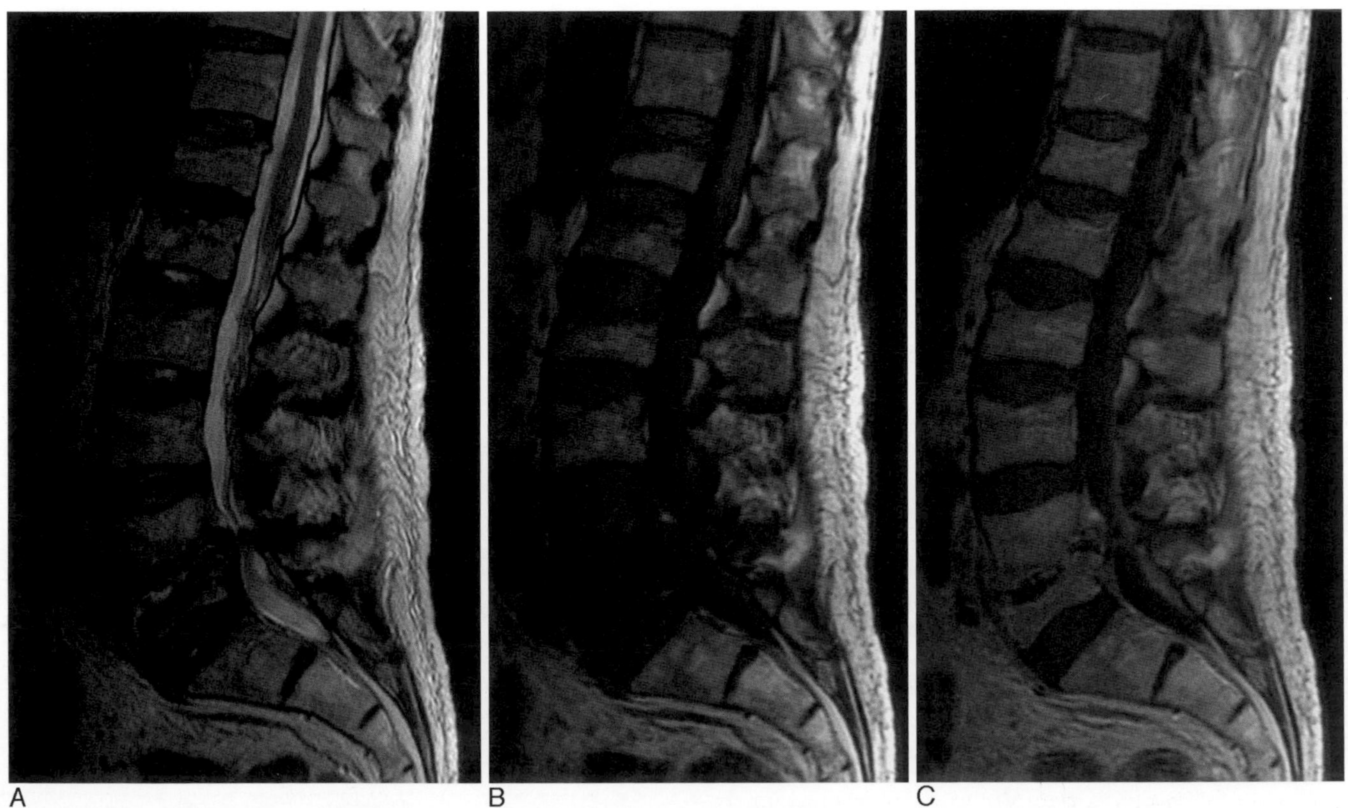

Figure 60.40 Discovertebral osteomyelitis. The L4/5 disc space is narrowed and on sagittal T2W MRI there is high signal intensity (pus) within and abnormal signal intensity in the adjacent vertebrae and destruction of the superior surface of L5. On T1W sagittal MR (B) it is difficult to distinguish the infected disc from the infected adjacent vertebrae, both of which are of intermediate signal intensity. On T1W sagittal MR after IV gadolinium (C), there is no enhancement of the pus within the infected disc but the margins of the disc and the infected adjacent vertebrae enhance avidly.

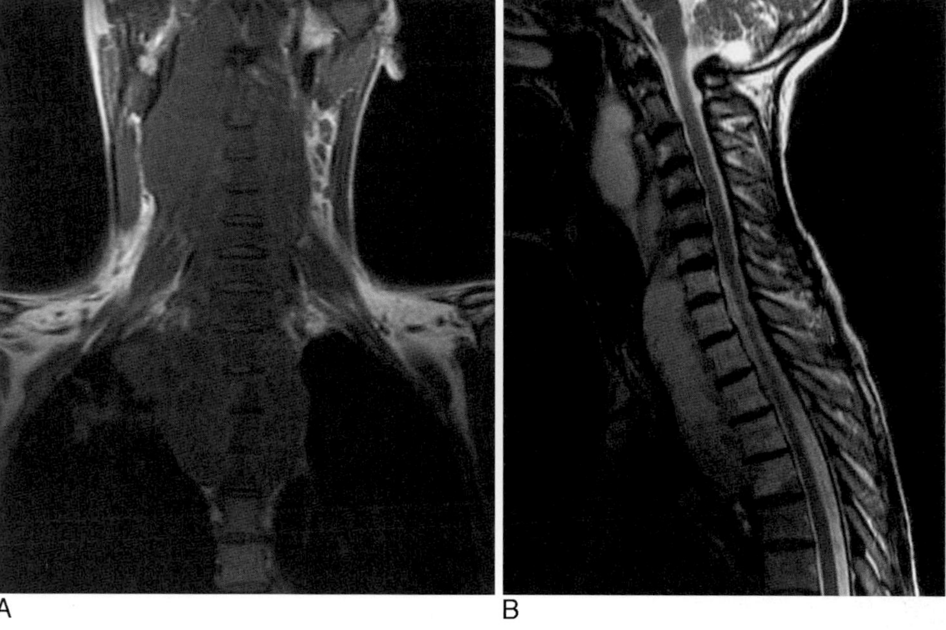

Figure 60.41 Tuberculosis and osteomyelitis. (A) Coronal T1W and (B) sagittal T2W MR images show a huge prevertebral collection and abnormal vertebrae and abnormal material in the epidural space surrounding and narrowing the cord. There is also an extensive retropharyngeal collection. (Courtesy of Dr Justin Cross.)

intraspinal tumours. Intradural infections, which include spinal tuberculosis and a variety of fungal and parasitic (especially cysticercosis) agents, characteristically cause severe generalized arachnoiditis, as can spinal sarcoidosis. Some cases are unexplained.

On rare occasions, the organized exudates become calcified and even ossified (arachnoiditis ossificans). Myelomalacia and syringomyelia often develop in extensive cases.

Imaging

MRI is the optimal investigation for demonstrating arachnoiditis and its complications (Fig. 60.42). The signs are tapering or obstruction of the lower end of the subarachnoid space, central clumping and/or peripheral adhesion of roots of the cauda equina, the latter often resulting in the appearance of an empty thecal sac though the walls of the sac commonly appear thickened. Loculation and deformity of the subarachnoid spaces, and irregular deformity of the spinal cord may be shown with central signal change in severe cases. Care may need to be exercised to distinguish crowding of roots due to intradural adhesions from that due to extradural compression, such as from degenerative spinal disease. Some infectious agents cause diffuse intradural enhancement (Fig. 60.43).

MYELITIS

Myelitis usually is due to demyelinating disease, especially multiple sclerosis. About 70 per cent of such patients also have brain lesions. Acute transverse myelitis may be the presentation of other demyelinating diseases such as neuromyelitis optica and acute disseminated encephalomyelitis (ADEM). Sarcoidosis and infections of the spinal cord are uncommon, but a wide range of organisms are documented, which include many of the enteroviruses and recently the T-cell lymphotrophic viruses, especially HTLV-1.

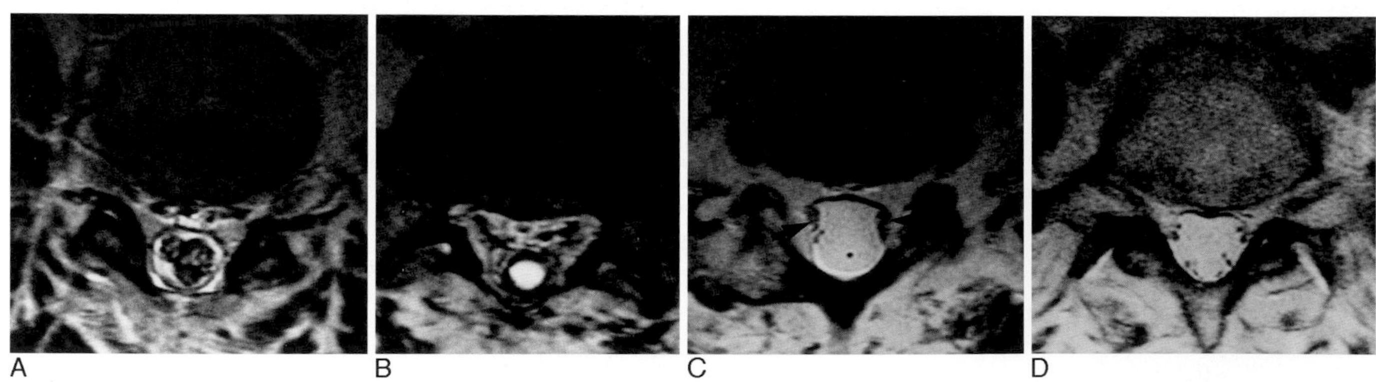

Figure 60.42 Spinal adhesive arachnoiditis. Axial high resolution (fast spin-echo) T2W MRIs of the lumbar spine showing the three main diagnostic features of this condition on MRI. (A) Central clumping of nerve roots. (B) Peripheral adhesion of roots leaving a clear central subarchnoid space. (C) Adhesion of the margins of the thecal sac near the point of exit of the root sheaths (arrows). Compare this with (D), which is normal; here rootlets are clearly seen as they enter the spinal root sheaths on each side.

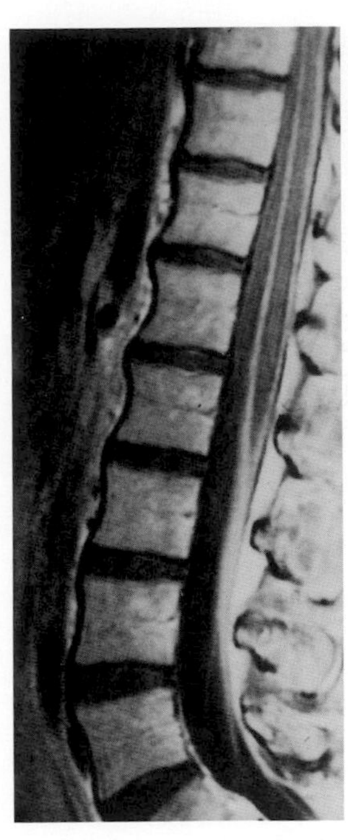

Figure 60.43 Spinal meningitis, due to Lyme disease. Sagittal T1W MRI of the lumbar spine after IV gadolinium showing diffuse enhancement of the outer surface of the cord and spinal roots.

The pathological picture is usually of inflammatory demyelination that involves several segments. In severe cases, this progresses to necrosis and cavitation. Necrosis is more common with infective causes. Granulomas or abscesses may develop with bacterial and fungal agents. Pyogenic abscesses (pyomyelia) usually arise as complications of spinal dysraphism, such as dorsal dermal sinus. Parasites such as cysticercosis may cause arachnoiditis, but intramedullary cysts sometimes occur, and may be associated with syringomyelia. Granulomas and meningeal inflammation occur in spinal sarcoidosis, which also may result in cord cavitation[70].

In acute myelitis MRI shows diffuse swelling of the spinal cord and increased signal on T2W images (Fig. 60.44). It commonly extends over multiple segments. In demyelination, over 80 per cent of acute symptomatic cord lesions are shown. Major cord swelling is present in about 30 per cent of acute lesions with extensive diffuse signal changes shrinking over 2–3 months, to leave smaller residual lesions (mainly in the cord white matter); enhancement occurs after IV Gd-DTPA within the area of more extensive signal change for up to 8 weeks, but does not persist, which may help distinguish primary demyelinating processes from other forms of inflammation such as sarcoidosis. The changes in ADEM often resolve completely. Infections usually produce similar though more florid changes to those seen in acute demyelination, but usually follow a different course on interval imaging and more often result in cavitation and focal atrophy (cysts and arachnoiditis also seen in cysticercosis). MRI of the brain often shows clinically unsuspected lesions, which may help confirm a suspected diagnosis especially of multiple sclerosis, but unsuspected brain lesions may be present in many other conditions, including HTLV-1-associated myelopathy and sarcoidosis.

VASCULAR LESIONS

Over 80 per cent of spinal arteriovenous malformations represent arteriovenous fistulas located in the spinal dura mater, usually close to a root sleeve[103] (Fig. 60.45). Such fistulae most commonly are located in the thoracic region, but can occur at any level, though in the cervical spine only around the foramen magnum. A fistula usually is supplied by one or two dural branches of a nearby spinal artery, and shunts often via a single vein into intradural veins. In symptomatic lesions, venous drainage usually is both very slow and anomalous, remaining intradural through a greater part of the spinal canal than normal. Venous stagnation is an important cause of the clinical

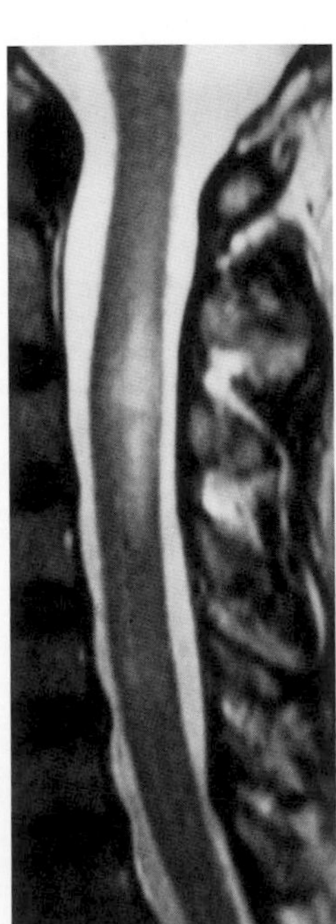

Figure 60.44 Acute myelitis, due to multiple sclerosis. Sagittal T2W MRI showing mild expansion of the upper spinal cord (low signal) and signal change (white) within.

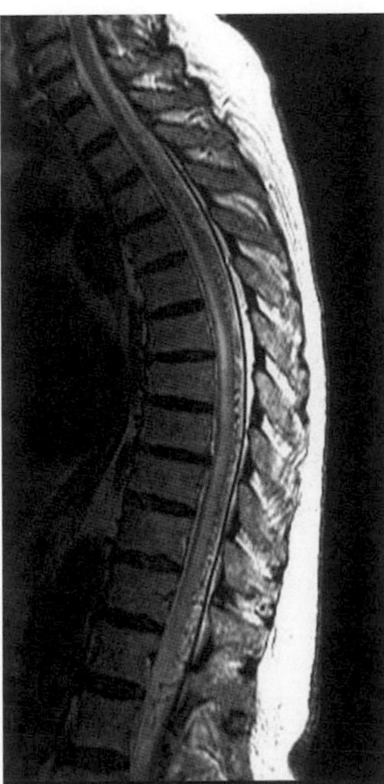

Figure 60.45 Dural arteriovenous fistula. T2W MRI showing multiple enlarged vessels on the posterior surface of the spinal cord. (Courtesy of Dr Justin Cross.)

myelopathy, and in rare cases has resulted in extensive thrombosis of the intraspinal veins with haemorrhagic infarction of the cord: the Foix–Alajouanine syndrome (subacute necrotizing myelitis)[104].

Intramedullary arteriovenous malformations

Lesions involving multiple small, thin-walled vessels in the form of a poorly circumscribed mass may occur in the spinal cord, as they do in the brain. Sometimes, mainly only in children, a pial arteriovenous fistula is present.

These lesions are supplied by radiculomedullary arteries, usually mainly by the sulco-commissural branches of the anterior spinal artery. Very occasionally there are associated vascular malformations in adjacent structures in the same body segment (Cobb's syndrome). Capillary and cavernous angiomas also occur, and sometimes are multiple, but are less common than in the brain.

MRI may demonstrate the following abnormalities in spinal dural fistulae: (A) large intrathecal and extrathecal vessels, which sometimes may be large enough to compress the spinal cord or give its surface a scalloped appearance; (B) thrombosis of intrathecal veins, either spontaneous or as a result of therapeutic embolization; (C) signal changes in the spinal cord are nearly always present in cases with persistent clinical myelopathy, which may diminish or resolve after obliteration of the shunt. Old and recent haemorrhage is seen mainly only with intramedullary malformations. The nidus may be identifiable in some intramedullary lesions and the site of a dural fistula may be shown by dynamic contrast-enhanced MRI[105]. It should be noted that normal pial veins can be prominent at the level of the lumbar enlargement of the spinal cord. The distribution of abnormally enlarged veins is a poor guide to the location of a dural fistula. Myelography was a sensitive test for detecting enlarged intrathecal veins but is rarely indicated now that MRI can provide high-resolution images of the vessels. However, these lesions are an absolute indication for spinal angiography; no other technique so precisely defines the relevant anatomy (Fig. 60.46). When searching for a dural fistula, imaging should be slow, say one frame every 2 s. A large number of spinal arteries may have to be injected before the lesion is found, and preliminary evaluation by dynamic MRI can be helpful in targeting the search and reducing its extent[105].

The study should not be regarded as negative unless: (A) all the spinal arteries from the foramen magnum to the coccyx have been opacified *adequately*, or (B) the veins thought to be abnormal have been opacified and shown to drain normally[106]. If a lesion is found, adjacent levels also should be injected, and it is advisable to identify the major radiculomedullary arteries in the same spinal region. Flush aortography does not result in adequate opacification of the relevant vessels, and often will not show these fistulae.

Embolization of arteries supplying a dural fistula may be feasible, provided the vessel to be embolized can be also shown *not* to supply the spinal cord. Embolization and surgical excision of intramedullary arteriovenous malformations may also be possible in some cases without precipitating paraplegia.

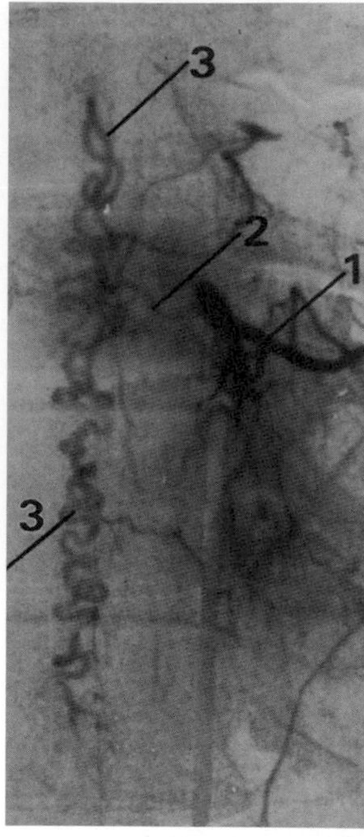

Figure 60.46 Angiogram showing dural arteriovenous fistula. 1 = intercostal artery; 2 = site of malformation, close to the intervertebral foramen, i.e. lateral to the spinal cord; 3 = draining veins on spinal cord. Frontal projection.

Other vascular malformations

Vertebral haemangiomas occur in 10 per cent of the otherwise normal population and are usually asymptomatic. They are not found in children younger than 10 years and occur rarely in the cervical spine. Occasionally, they cause back pain and very occasionally, compression of the spinal cord. Symptomatic lesions usually are associated with vertebral collapse or paraspinal extension.

Extraosseous angiomas are rare, but often are associated with nerve roots, and present with radicular pain or dysfunction.

Imaging

CT is more capable of demonstrating smaller lesions than plain radiographs. The vertebrae have a characteristic polka dot or stippled appearance. The matrix of the malformation often contains fat, so that the CT numbers are frequently in the negative range. Paraspinal extensions are well shown, especially in symptomatic cases. IV enhancement may show a soft-tissue extension as well, including intraspinal involvement. Extraosseous forms are similar to other extradural lesions. MRI commonly identifies these incidental findings. They often yield high signal because of the fat content. Lesions may be confused with metastases, when multiple or only parts of a vertebra are involved. However, the high signal on T1W images should distinguish them from nonhaemorrhagic metastases, the latter having a signal which is similar to or lower than haematopoietic marrow. MRI also shows soft-tissue extension and spinal cord compression, when present. Negative skeletal scintigraphy may help differentiate from metastases. Only rarely will spinal angiography be indicated to establish a diagnosis. Injection of the relevant intercostal or lumbar arteries shows an intense homogeneous capillary blush which, unlike a normal vertebra, typically does not respect the midline. Therapeutic embolization of symptomatic cases may result in regression, and has been used to treat both back pain and neural compression.

Spinal cord infarction

Spinal cord infarction is a rare complication of arteriosclerotic vascular disease. It may complicate aortic dissection and surgery for aortic aneurysms. The cause usually is occlusion of the sulco-commissural branches of the anterior spinal artery, the latter remaining patent. Infarction of the adjacent vertebral body may be associated[107]. Venous infarction seems to occur even less frequently, and has been due to extensive thrombosis of local pial veins in documented cases[108].

Only MRI demonstrates the pathological changes: signal change, focal or diffuse, associated only with mild swelling is seen, with enhancement in early stages. Rapid evolution over days results in contraction of the area of signal change and thinning of the involved region of the cord. Venous infarction may involve only one side of the spinal cord, such a pattern not being expected from arterial infarction.

Spontaneous epidural haematoma

This is a rare, but devastating condition in which the time to act surgically, if appropriate, is short if spinal cord function is to be restored. Acute back pain and progressive flaccid paraplegia over hours is the usual clinical picture, sometimes mistakenly diagnosed as Guillan–Barré syndrome. A cause is rarely, if ever, found even with spinal angiography (which usually is not recommended unless other indications are present); occasionally it complicates metastatic disease. These haematomas are well shown by MRI and should also be clearly visible on modern CT; they are often extensive.

MISCELLANEOUS CONDITIONS

Crystal deposition diseases

Tumour-like, paraspinal and intraspinal calcified masses sometimes occur in association with similar periarticular masses elsewhere. They may be idiopathic or part of a calcium deposition disease accompanying metabolic disorders such as renal rickets, fluorosis or osseous metaplasia in spinal ligaments, as discussed with degenerative disease. They usually consist of calcium hydroxyapatite. Similar deposits have developed rarely in the cervical spines of patients recovering from major head injuries. Calcium pyrophosphate dyhydrate crystal deposition (pseudogout) may occur in intervertebral discs, especially in the lumbar region and can be associated with discovertebral destructive lesions. Gout rarely affects the apophyseal joints, but when it does, it may produce instability and nerve root compression.

Paget's disease

The axial skeleton is one of the commonest sites of involvement, especially the lumbosacral spine. About 80 per cent of cases are polyostotic, but the cervical vertebrae are only rarely involved. The apophyseal joints usually are normal. The vertebral body is enlarged in only about 20 per cent of cases. Sometimes paraspinal or even intraspinal soft-tissue masses, consisting of poorly mineralized osteoid, develop, perhaps in response to incremental fractures. Spinal cord compression may occur. After medical treatment, the majority of cases show no radiological change, but about 20 per cent have shown increasing sclerosis; regression of paraspinal masses with improvement in neurological state can occur. Sarcomas develop in 0.15 per cent of cases of Paget's disease, but only about 3 per cent of such sarcomas involve the spine. On MRI, Pagetic bone returns an exceptionally variegated signal, and on CT an expansive mixed lytic and sclerotic appearance.

Subacute combined degeneration of the spinal cord

This is a progressive myelopathy presenting with sensory symptoms in the context of dietary deficiency of vitamin B_{12} or co-proteins. The lateral and dorsal spinal cord columns are affected, and improvement is often only partial after treatment. MRI often shows mild swelling and signal change (often subtle) in earlier stages that regress on treatment. Lesions, which are most often seen between C2 and C5, may enhance after IV contrast medium. However MRI may also remain negative[109].

REFERENCES

1. Childers J C Jr, Wilson F C 1971 Bipartite atlas. Review of the literature and report of a case. J Bone Joint Surg 53A:578–582
2. Boon D, Parsons D, Lachmann S M et al 1985 Spina bifida occulta: lesion or anomaly? Clin Radiol 36:159–161
3. McRae D L, Barman A S 1953 Occipitalization of the atlas. Am J Roentgenol 70:23–46
4. Castelliri A E, Goldstein L A, Chan D P K 1984 Lumbosacral transitional vertebrae and their relationship with lumbar extradural defects. Spine 9:493–95
5. Enzmann D R, Pele A J 1993 Cerebrospinal flow measured by phase contrast cine MR. Am J Neuroradiol 14:1301–1307
6. Mikulis D J, Wood M L, Zerdoner O A M, Poncelet B P 1994 Oscillatory motion of the normal cervical spinal cord. Radiology 192:117–121
7. Rubin J B, Enzmann D R 1987 Harmonic modulation of proton MR precessional phase by pulsable motion: origin of spinal CSF flow phenomenon. Am J Roentgenol 148:983–994
8. Youser D M, Janick P A, Atlas S W et al 1990 Pseudoatrophy of the cervical portion of the spinal cord on MR images: a manifestation of truncal artefact? Am J Neuroradiol 11:373–377
9. Yostino M T, Temeltas O M, Carter L P et al 1993 Metallic post operative artefacts on cervical MR. Am J Neuroradiol 14:747–749
10. Williams D F 1994 Editorial. Titanium: epitome of biocompatibility or cause for concern. J Bone Joint Surg 76B:348–349
11. Porter B A, Shields A F, Olson D O 1986 Magnetic resonance imaging of bone marrow disorders. Radiol Clin North Am 24:269–289
12. Dietemann J L, Dogon D, Aubin M L, Manelfe C 1992 Cervico-occipital junction: normal and pathological aspects. In: Manelfe C (ed.) Imaging of the Spine and Spinal Cord. Raven Press, New York, pp 706–715
13. Ullrick C G, Binet E F, Sanecki M G, Kieffer S A 1980 Quantitative assessment of the lumbar spinal canal by computed tomography. Radiology 134:137–143
14. Dixon A K 1986 Who has most epidural fat? Information from computed tomography. Br J Radiol 59:475–480
15. Yu S, Haughton V M, Ho P S et al 1988 Progressive and regressive changes in the nucleus pulposus. Part II. The Adult. Radiology 169:93–97
16. Czervionke L F, Daniels D L, Ho P S et al 1988 Cervical neural foramina: correlative anatomic and MR imaging study. Radiology 169:753–759
17. Raz-Fumagalli R, Haughton V M 1993 Lumbar cribriform fascia: appearance at freezing microtomy and MR imaging. Radiology 187:241–246

18. Howicki B H, Haughton V M 1992 Neural foraminal ligaments of the lumbar spine: appearance at CT and MRI. Radiology 183:257–261
19. Schellinger D, Manz H J, Vidic B et al 1990 Disc fragment migration. Radiology 175:831–836
20. Seibert C E, Barnes J, Dreisbach J N et al 1981 Accurate CT measurement of the spinal cord using metrizamide: physical factors. Am J Neuroradiol 2:75–78
21. Wilkins R H 1994 Commentary: Prevalence and percutaneous drainage of cysts of the sacral nerve root sheath (Tarlov cyst). Am J Neuroradiol 15:298–299
22. Van de Kelft E, Van Vyve M 1993 Sacral meningeal cysts and perineal pain. Lancet 341:500–501
23. Stevens J M, Kendall B E, Gedroyc W 1991 Acute epidural haematoma complicating myelography. Case Report. Br J Radiol 64:860–864
24. Johnson A J, Burrows E H 1978 Thecal deformity after lumbar myelography with iophendylate (Myodil) and meglumine iothalamate (Conray 280). Br J Radiol 51:196–202
25. Doppman J L, Di Chiro G, Ommaya A K 1969 Selective arteriography of the spinal cord. Green, St Louis
26. Rodesch G, Lasjaunas P, Berenstein A 1992 Functional vascular anatomy of the spine and spinal cord. Revista di neuroradiologiea 63–66
27. Royal College of Radiologists 2003 Making the best use of a department of clinical radiology: guidelines for doctors. Royal College of Radiologists, London. 5th edn.
28. van den Bosch M A, Hollingworth W, Kinmonth A L, Dixon A K 2004 Evidence against the use of lumbar spine radiography for low back pain. Clin Radiol 59:69–76
29. Brooks B S, Duval E R, El Hammal P et al 1993 Neuro-imaging features of neurenteric cysts: analysis of nine cases and review of the literature. Am J Neuroradiol 14:735–746
30. Rogg J M, Benzil D L, Haas R L, Knucky N W 1993 Intramedullary abscess, an unusual manifestation of a dermal sinus. Am J Neuroradiol 14:1393–1395
31. David K M, Copp A J, Stevens J M 1996 Split cervical spinal cord with Klippel–Feil syndrome: seven cases. Brain 119:1859–1872
32. Huang P P, Constantine S 1994 Acquired Chiari 1 malformations. J Neurosurg 80:1099–1102
33. Savy L, Stevens J M, Taylor D J, Kendall BE 1994 Apparent cerebellar ectopia: a reappraisal using volumetric MRI. Neuroradiology 6:360–363
34. McLone D G, Knepper P A 1989 The cause of Chiari II malformation: a unified theory. Pediatr Neurosci 15:1–12
35. Stevens J M, Serva W, Kendall B E et al 1993 Chiari malformation in adults: relation of morphological aspects to clinical features and operative outcome. J Neurol Neurosurg Psychiatry 56:1072–1077
36. Stevens J M, Kling Chong W, Barber C et al 1994 A new appraisal of abnormalities of the odontoid process associated with atlanto-axial subluxation and neurological disability. Brain 117:133–148
37. Young A, Dixon A K, Getty J, Renton P, Vacher H 1981 Cauda equina syndrome complicating ankylosing spondylitis: use of electromyography and computerised tomography in diagnosis. Ann Rheum Dis 40:317–322
38. Walters M R, Stears J C, Osborn A G 1998 Transdural spinal cord herniation: imaging and clinical spectra. Am J Neuroradiol 19:1335–1336
39. Winter R B 1983 Congenital deformities of the spine. Thiem-Stratton, New York
40. Bethem D, Winter R B, Lutter L et al 1981 Spinal disorders of dwarfism: a review of the literature and report of eighty cases. J Bone Joint Surg 63A:1412–1425
41. Crockard H A, Stevens J M 1995 Craniovertebral function anomalies in inherited disorders. Eur J Pediatr 154:504–512
42. Ulmer J L, Mathews V P, Elster A D et al 1997 Lumbar spondylolysis without spondylolisthesis. Am J Roentgenol 169:233–237
43. Stevens J M, Kendall B E, Davis C, Crockard H A 1987 Percutaneous insertion of the spinal end of a cystoperitoneal shunt as definitive treatment to relieve spinal cord compression from spinal arachnoid cyst. Neuroradiology 29:190–195
44. Potter K, Saifuddin A 2003 MRI of chronic spinal cord injury. Br J Radiol 76:347–352
45. Grant R, Hadley D M, MacPherson P 1987 Syringomyelia-cyst measurement by magnetic resonance imaging and comparison with symptoms, signs and disability. J Neurol Neurosurg Psychiatry 50: 1008–1014
46. Williams B 1972 Pathogenesis of syringomyelia. Lancet i:142–143
47. Ball M J, Dayan A D 1972 Pathogenesis of syringomyelia. Lancet ii:799–801
48. Boijsen E 1954 The cervical spinal canal in intraspinal expansive processes. Acta Radiol 42:101–115
49. Baker A S, Dove J 1983 Progressive scoliosis as the first presenting sign of syringomyelia: report of a case. J Bone Joint Surg 65B:472–473
50. Enzmann D R, O'Donohue J, Rubin J B et al 1987 CSF pulsations within non-neoplastic spinal cord cysts. Am J Neuroradiol 8:517–525
51. Quencer R M, Donovan-Post M J, Hinks R S 1990 Cine MR in the evaluation of normal and abnormal CSF flow: intracranial and intraspinal studies. Neuroradiology 32:371–391
52. Stevens J M, Olney J S, Kendall B E 1985 Post-traumatic cystic and non-cystic myelopathy. Neuroradiology 27:48–56
53. Sherman J L, Berkovich A J, Citrin C M 1986 The MR appearances of syringomyelia: new observations. Am J Neuroradiol 7:985–995
54. Vaquero J, Martinez R, Arlas A 1990 Syringomyelia-Chiari complex. Magnetic resonance imaging and clinical evaluation of surgical treatment. J Neurosurg 73:14–18
55. Milhorat T H, Johnson W D, Miller J I et al 1992 Surgical treatment of syringomyelia based on magnetic resonance imaging criteria. Neurosurgery 31:231–242
56. Vissilouthis J, Panadreon A, Anagnostasas S 1993 Theco-peritoneal shunt for syringomyelia: Report of three cases. Neurosurgery 33: 324–328
57. Yu S, Haughton V M, Ho P S et al 1988 Progressive and regressive changes in the nucleus pulposus. Part II. The adult. Radiology 169: 93–97
58. Schellinger D, Manz H J, Vidic B 1990 Disc fragment migration. Radiology 175:831–836
59. Modic M T, Steinberg P M, Ross J S et al 1988 Degenerative disc disease: assessment of changes in vertebral bone marrow with MR imaging. Radiology 166:193–199
60. Grenier N, Kressel H Y, Schiebler M L et al 1987 Normal and degenerative spinal structures: MR imaging. Radiology 165:517–525
61. Yamashita Y, Takahashi M, Matsuno Y et al 1990 Spinal cord compression due to ossification of ligaments: MR imaging. Radiology 175:843–848
62. Okada K, Oka S, Tohge K et al 1991 Thoracic myelopathy caused by ossification of the ligamentum flavum. Clinico-pathological study and surgical treatment. Spine 16:280–287
63. Jackson D E, Atlas S W, Mani J R, Norman D 1989 Intraspinal synovial cysts: MR imaging. Radiology 170:527–530
64. Crockard J M, Sett P, Geddes J F et al 1991 Damaged ligaments at the craniocervical junction presenting as an extradural tumour: a differential diagnosis in the elderly. J Neurol Neurosurg Psychiatry 54:817–821
65. Yu Y L, Du Boulay G H, Stevens J M, Kendall B E 1986 Computer-assisted tomography in cervical spondylotic myelopathy and radiculopathy. Brain 109:259–278
66. Boden S, McCowin P, Davis D, Dina T, Mark A, Wiesel S 1990 Abnormal MR scans of the cervical spine in asymptomatic patients: a prospective investigation. J Bone Joint Surg 72A:1178–1184
67. Wiesel S, Tsourmas N, Feffer H, Citrin C, Patronas N 1984 A study of the computer assisted tomography: the incidence of positive CAT scans in an asymptomatic group of patients. Spine 9:549–551
68. Stevens J M, O'Dricoll D M, Yu Y L, Ananthapavan A, Kendall B E 1987 Some dynamic factors in compressive deformity of the cervical spinal cord. Neuroradiology 29:136–142
69. Stevens J M 1993 The compressed spinal cord. Current Medical Literature. Med Imaging (R Soc Med) 5:3–8
70. Stevens J M 1995 Imaging of the spinal cord. A review. J Neurol Neurosurg Psychiatry 58:403–408
71. Al-Mefty O, Harkey H L, Marawi I 1993 Experimental compressive cervical myelopathy. J Neurosurg 79:550–561

72. Crockard H A, Heilman A E, Stevens J M 1993 Progressive myelopathy secondary to odontoid fractures: clinical, radiological and surgical features. J Neurosurg 78:579–586
73. Williams M P, Cherryman S R, Husband J E 1984 Significance of thoracic disc herniations demonstrated by MR imaging. J Comput Assist Tomogr 13:211–214
74. Bush K, Cowan N, Katz D, Gishen P 1992 The natural history of sciatica associated with disc pathology. Spine 17:1205–1212
75. Stevens J M, Clifton A G, Whitear R 1993 Appearances of posterior osteophytes after sound anterior interbody fusion in the cervical spine: a high definition computed myelographic study. Neuroradiology B5:227–228
76. Fukushima T, Takaaki I, Taoka Y, Takata S 1991 Magnetic resonance imaging study of spinal cord plasticity in patients with cervical compression myelopathy. Spine 16:534–538
77. Stockley I, Getty C J, Dixon A K et al 1988 Lumbar lateral canal entrapment: clinical, radiculographic and computed tomographic findings. Clin Radiol 39:144–149
78. Gundry C R, Heithoff K B 1993 Epidural haematoma of the lumbar spine: 18 surgically confirmed cases. Radiology 187:427–431
79. Mehali T F, Pezzuti R T, Applebaum B I 1990 Magnetic resonance imaging and cervical spondylotic myelopathy. Neurosurgery 26: 217–227
80. Jinkins J R, Osborn A G, Gerrett D, Hunt S, Story J L 1993 Spinal nerve enhancement with Gd-DTPA: MR correlation with the post-operative lumbar spine. Am J Neuroradiol 14:383–394
81. Boden S D, Davis D O, Dina T S, Parker C P, O'Malley S, Sanner J L, Wiesel S W 1992 Contrast-enhanced MR imaging performed after successful lumbar disc surgery: prospective study. Radiology 182: 59–64
82. Cavanagh S, Stevens J M, Johnson J R 1993 High resolution MRI investigation in recurrent pain after lumbar discectomy. J Bone Joint Surg 75B:524–531
83. Fitt G J, Stevens J M 1995 Post-operative arachnoiditis diagnosed by high resolution fast spin-echo MRI of the lumbar spine. Neuroradiology 37:139–145
84. Clifton A G, Stevens J M, Whitear P W, Kendall B E 1990 Identifiable causes for poor outcome in surgery for cervical spondylosis. Post-operative computed myelography and MR imaging. Neuroradiology 32:450–455
85. Levy W J Jr, Bay J, Dohn J 1982 Spinal cord meningiomas. J Neurosurg 57:804–812
86. Sze G, Krol G, Zimmerman R D, Deck M D F 1988 Malignant extra-dural spinal tumours: MR imaging with Gd-DTPA. Radiology 117:217–223
87. Balenaux D, Parizel P, Bank W O 1992 Intraspinal and intramedullary pathology. In: Manelfe C (ed.) Imaging of the Spine and Spinal Cord. Raven Press, New York, pp 513–564
88. Kaffenberger D A, Shah C P, Murtagh F R, Wilson C, Silbiger M L 1988 MR imaging of the spinal cord haemangioblastoma associated with syringomyelia. J Comput Assist Tomogr 12:495–498
89. Williams A L, Haughton V M, Pojunas K W, Daniels D L, Kilgore D P 1987 Differentiation of intramedullary neoplasms and cysts by MRI. Am J Roentgenol 149:159–164
90. Naidich T P, Doundoulakis S H, Poznanski A K 1986 Intraspinal masses: effect of plain spine radiography. Pediatr Neurosci 12:10–17
91. Rubin J M, Aisen A M, Di Pietro M A 1986 Ambiguities in MR imaging of tumoral cysts in the spinal cord. J Comput Assist Tomogr 10:395–398
92. Sosna J, Barth M M, Kruskal J B, Kane R A 2005 Intraoperative sonography for neurosurgery. J Ultrasound Med 24:1671–1682
93. Stevens J M, Olney J S, Kendall B E 1985 Post-traumatic cystic and non-cystic myelopathy. Neuroradiology 27:48–56
94. Falcone S, Quencer R M, Green B A 1994 Progressive post-traumatic myelomalacia myelopathy: imaging and clinical features. Am J Neuroradiol 15:747–754
95. Silberstein M, Nenessy O 1993 Implications of focal spinal cord lesions following trauma-evaluation with magnetic resonance imaging. Paraplegia 31:160–167
96. Kulkarni M R, McArdle C B, Kapanick D 1987 Acute spinal cord injury: MR imaging at 1.5T. Radiology 164:837–843
97. Yamashita Y, Takahiiki M, Matsumoto Y 1990 Chronic injuries of the spinal cord: assessment with MR imaging. Radiology 175:849–854
98. Davies P C, Reisner A, Hudgins P A 1993 Spinal injuries in children: role of MR. Am J Neuroradiol 14:607–617
99. Kendall B E, Stevens J M, Crockard H A 1992 The spine in rheumatoid arthritis. Rev Neuroradiol 5(Suppl 12):23–28
100. Colombo N, Berry I, Norman D 1992 Infections of the spine. In: Manelfe C (ed.) Imaging of the spine and spinal cord. Raven Press, New York
101. Kendall B E, Stevens J M, Thomas D 1991 Arachnoiditis. Curr Imaging 2:113–119
102. Johnson A J, Burrows E H 1978 Thecal deformity after lumbar myelography with iophendylale (Myodil) and meglumine iothalamate (conray 280). Br J Radiol 51:196–202
103. Kendall B E, Logue V 1977 Spinal epidural angiomatous malformations draining into intrathecal veins. Neuroradiology 13:181–189
104. Rodesch G, Berenstein A, Lasjaunias P 1992 Vascular and avascular lesions of the spine and spinal cord. In: Manelfe C (ed.) Imaging of the spine and spinal cord. Raven Press, New York, pp 565–598
105. Thorpe J W, Kendall B E, McMannus D, Millar D H 1994 Dynamic gadolinium-enhanced MRI with detection and localisation of spinal arterio-venous malformations. Neuroradiology 36:522–529
106. Willinsky R, Lasjaunias P, Terbrugge K, Hurth M 1990 Spinal angiography in the investigation of spinal arteriovenous fistula. A protocol with application to the venous phase. Neuroradiology 32:114–116
107. Yuh W T, Marsh C Y, Wang A K 1992 MR imaging of spinal cord and vertebral body infarction. Am J Neuroradiol 13:145–154
108. Henderson F C, Crockard H A, Stevens J M 1993 Spinal cord oedema due to venous stasis. Neuroradiology 35:312–315
109. Locatelli E R, Laurena R, Ballard P, Mark A S 1999 MRI in vitamin B_{12} deficiency myelopathy. Can Neurol Sci 26:60–63

CHAPTER 61

The Orbit

Tarik F. Massoud and Justin J. Cross

- Key anatomy of the orbit
- Imaging the globe
- Imaging the intraconal compartment
- Imaging the conal compartment
- Imaging the extraconal compartment
- Imaging orbital infection
- Imaging orbital trauma

The orbit and visual system is a highly complex and intricately organized region of the body, with specialized anatomical features and physiology. There are many diseases that are specific to this region, as well as many neurological diseases that afflict the sensory and motor components of the visual system. It is necessary to resort to cross-sectional and occasional angiographic imaging techniques to diagnose diseases that are not amenable to direct visual inspection and ophthalmoscopy. Computed tomography (CT) and magnetic resonance imaging (MRI) are the most useful techniques for imaging the orbit and its contents. It is usual practice in interpreting CT and MRI findings to ascribe the lesion to a certain compartment within the orbit, thus helping in anatomical interpretation and differential diagnosis. This general approach is useful when a lesion is small and/or confined to one location. However, several diseases are well known to transgress compartments as they progressively spread; the epicentre of such a process can often be assigned to a specific location.

CT remains very useful because of the inherent natural contrast provided by the presence of structures with widely different attenuation coefficients (fat, bone, fluid, muscle, adjacent air) within a confined space. A relative advantage over MRI is also the latter's sensitivity to lid and globe motion. CT is preferred over MRI for detecting small calcified optic nerve meningiomas and in a child with suspected retinoblastoma, where detection of calcification is paramount. Overall, however, MRI is gaining more acceptance because of its greater sensitivity in characterizing diseases of the orbit (especially with use of fat-suppressed T1-weighted imaging, combined head and surface coils and faster data acquisition), and the far greater ability and versatility of MRI in detecting concomitant intracranial (especially intra-axial) abnormalities.

This chapter briefly reviews key anatomical areas of the orbit, followed by discussions of the role of neuroimaging in detection and characterization of diseases of the orbit. Recently, Shields et al[1] have published a useful survey of a large number of orbital tumours and other mass lesions. The various anatomical subdivisions within the orbit that help define 'compartments' for the purpose of imaging interpretation and differential diagnosis include: the globe and the intraconal, conal and extraconal compartments. When a disease can be multicompartmental, it is discussed in the section of the compartment where it arises or is present most frequently. Only the common diseases of each compartment are discussed; the imaging findings of less common diseases are presented in Tables 61.1–61.3. The imaging findings in orbital infections and trauma are presented separately in the last two sections.

KEY ANATOMY OF THE ORBIT

The complex structures of the orbit can conveniently be clustered into several anatomical areas or compartments, including the bony orbit, globe, intraconal compartment (also containing the optic nerve), conal compartment and extraconal compartment. Gentry[2] has provided a more detailed account of the normal radiological anatomy of the orbit.

The bony orbit comprises four walls, four rims and the apex. The medial wall is formed mostly by the ethmoid bone. This is paper thin, and thus, termed the lamina papyracea. Anterior to this is the lacrimal bone and part of the horizontal portion of the frontal bone. Posterior to this is the maxillary bone and the lesser wing of the sphenoid. The lateral wall is formed mostly by the greater wing of the sphenoid. Anterior to this is the orbital surface of the zygomatic bone, and a small contribution again from part of the horizontal portion of the frontal bone. The superior wall is formed mostly by the orbital surface of the frontal bone. The inferior wall is formed mostly by the maxillary bone. The apex is where all four walls of the orbit converge. The superior orbital fissure is the space between the greater and lesser wings of the sphenoid bone. The inferior orbital fissure is formed by the space between the greater wing of the sphenoid and the posterolateral wall

Table 61.1 THE IMAGING FINDINGS OF SOME LESS COMMON DISEASES OF THE GLOBE

	Pathology	Clinical features	Key imaging findings
Congenital	PHPV (persistent hyperplastic primary vitreous)	Primary vitreous normally involutes by sixth fetal month, but occasionally persists and undergoes hyperplasia Presents with leukocoria Affects male infants more than female	Microphthalmic globe with enhancing increased density in vitreous humour on CT Soft tissue band from back of lens to posterior globe (follows Cloquet's canal) Can be unilateral or bilateral
	Retinopathy of prematurity	History of prolonged ventilation with high O_2 concentration in a premature baby Pathology shows abnormal proliferation of retinal vascular buds	Bilateral increased density in vitreous Calcification is rare
	Coat's disease	Congenital vascular malformation of retina with telangiectasia Exudation from abnormal vessels leads to retinal detachment	Increased density in all or part of vitreous Normal-sized globe No calcification
	Microphthalmia (Fig. 61.4)	Congenital underdevelopment or acquired diminution in size of the globe Associated with congenital rubella, PHPV, retinopathy of prematurity and Lowe syndrome	Congenital = small globe in a small orbit Acquired = small, calcified globe
	Macrophthalmia	Enlargement of the globe Most severe form is called buphthalmos Associated with juvenile glaucoma	Large globe in a large orbit
	Coloboma	Defect in the globe, usually near optic nerve head Involves the sclera, uvea and retina Caused by a defect in fetal optic fissure	Small globe with cystic outpouching of vitreous May be a retro-ocular cyst
Degenerative	Drusen (Fig. 61.5)	Accretion of hyaline material on optic disc May be asymptomatic or associated with headache or visual field defects	Discrete, flat calcification of optic nerve head Bilateral in 75 per cent
	Phthisis bulbi (Fig. 61.6)	End-stage injured eye	Collapsed globe May be calcified
Inflammatory	Scleritis	Anterior scleritis presents with pain, erythema, photophobia and tenderness Posterior scleritis is painless and may mimic melanoma	Thickened enhancing sclera Choroidal detachment may be present
	Sclerosing endophthalmitis	2–8-year-old child exposed to soil contaminated by dog faeces Ingestion of the ova of *Toxocara canis* results in ophthalmitis	Dense vitreous without a discrete mass No calcification
Tumour	Choroidal haemangioma	Can be isolated or associated with Sturge–Weber syndrome Benign vascular lesion	Lenticular or flat densely enhancing eye wall mass
	Medulloepithelioma	Mean age of onset 4 years Presents with ciliary body mass, lens coloboma, lens subluxation, cataract, cyclitic membrane and glaucoma About 50 per cent are teratoid and 50 per cent non-teratoid forms	Involvement of ciliary body helps differentiate from retinoblastoma Only 10–15 per cent are calcified Rarely may involve optic nerve and other locations in CNS

of the maxillary sinus. The optic canal lies between the two roots of the lesser wing of the sphenoid. The superior orbital rim is formed by the frontal bone; the lateral rim by the zygomatic and frontal bones; the inferior rim by the zygomatic and maxillary bones; and the medial rim by the frontal and maxillary bones.

The globe is mostly fluid filled and is surrounded by three major tissue layers: (A) the sclera and cornea, (B) the uveal tract (choroid, iris and ciliary body) and (C) the retina. The lens and iris divide the globe cavity into an anterior chamber filled with aqueous humor, and a posterior chamber filled with vitreous humor.

Table 61.2 THE IMAGING FINDINGS OF SOME LESS COMMON DISEASES OF THE CONAL AND INTRACONAL COMPARTMENTS

	Pathology	Clinical features	Key imaging findings
Congenital	Optic nerve hypoplasia	Can be isolated or part of a syndrome (e.g. septo-optic dysplasia)	Decreased size of optic nerve
Inflammatory	Optic neuritis (Fig. 61.13)	About 50 per cent of patients with idiopathic optic neuritis develop multiple sclerosis	Best seen on gadolinium-enhanced T1W imaging If present, look for brain demyelination using T2W imaging
		Other causes include sarcoid, radiation, pseudotumour, toxoplasmosis, TB, syphilis, virus infection	
Tumour	Leukaemia	Reported in 13–16 per cent of cases of leukaemia	Diffuse enlargement of the optic nerve with variable enhancement
		More commonly acute lymphoblastic leukaemia but described in AML and adult leukaemias	
		Presents with papilloedema and variable loss of acuity	
	Haemangioblastoma	Associated with von-Hippel Lindau (VHL)	Rarely affects orbit or optic nerve
		Progressive loss of vision	Sharply demarcated from nerve
		Retinal lesions occur in 60 per cent of patients with VHL	Densely enhancing
			Usually affect pre-chiasmatic nerve
	Haemangiopericytoma	Mean age 40–60	Superior orbital masses
		More common in women	Tend to invade locally
		Presents with proptosis, optic nerve and extra-ocular dysfunction	Marked contrast enhancement
			Florid blush on angiography
	Neurofibroma/	About 1 per cent of orbital tumours	Smooth, ovoid, solitary
	schwannoma (Fig. 61.14)	Affects young adults	Usually in the superior orbit
		Usually presents with proptosis	May be intraconal, extraconal or intramuscular
		Neurofibromatosis in 2–18 per cent	Isodense with homogeneous contrast medium enhancement on CT
			Isointense on T1 and hyperintense on T2WI
Miscellaneous	Raised intracranial pressure (Fig. 16.15)	Papilloedema, loss of venous pulsation	Dilatation of the optic nerve sheath

The optic nerve is myelinated by oligodendrocytes, and not Schwann cells like true cranial nerves. It is about 5 cm long and is divided into four segments: intra-ocular, intra-orbital, intra-canalicular and intracranial. The subarachnoid space between the dura and pia covering the optic nerve is continuous with that of the suprasellar cistern.

The six extra-ocular muscles comprise four rectus muscles and two oblique muscles. The rectus muscles originate from the annulus of Zinn and insert into the sclera of the globe. The superior oblique muscle originates from the lesser wing of the sphenoid, hooks around the trochlea (just posterior to the medial aspect of the superior orbital rim) and the trochlear tendon inserts into the sclera beneath the tendon of the superior rectus muscle. The inferior oblique muscle originates from the anteromedial aspect of the orbital floor near the lacrimal sac and inserts into the sclera after passing below the inferior rectus tendon. The lateral rectus is innervated by the abducens nerve (cranial nerve VI), the superior oblique muscle by the trochlear nerve (IV) and all other muscles by the oculomotor nerve (III). The levator palpebrae superiorus muscle originates from the lesser wing of the sphenoid and annulus of Zinn, is located above and parallel to the superior rectus muscle, and inserts into the superior lid retractor system. It is innervated by sympathetic fibres. The superior rectus and levator palpebrae superiorus muscles are difficult to separate on coronal images, and are therefore usually considered as one complex.

Thick fascial layers, collectively termed the orbital septum, situated anterior to the globe, roughly divide the more anterior skin and subcutaneous tissues (preseptal compartment) from the more posterior orbit (postseptal compartment). Infection can spread from the preseptal compartment, through an often incomplete inferior portion of the orbital septum, to the postseptal compartment. The latter comprises the globe proper (bulbar compartment) and the retrobulbar compartment, with its separate intraconal, conal and extraconal compartments.

Arterial supply to the orbit is mainly via the three large terminal branches of the ophthalmic artery, i.e. the lacrimal, nasociliary and frontal branches, in addition to smaller branches, mainly the central artery of the retina (this also supplies the inner aspect of the optic nerve) and short and long ciliary branches. Valveless veins in the orbit tend to follow arteries

Table 61.3 THE IMAGING FINDINGS OF SOME LESS COMMON DISEASES OF THE EXTRACONAL COMPARTMENT

	Pathology	Clinical features	Key imaging findings
Congenital	Cephalocele	Present soon after birth	Soft tissue and CSF continuous with the intracranial contents
		Soft mass near medial canthus	
		May be pulsatile and increase with Valsalva	
	Dermoid (Fig. 61.18)	Usually upper outer quadrant of orbit	Usually anterior, between globe and periosteum
		Fullness or small lump	Well-defined cystic masses
			Epidermoid = fluid density, dermoid = fat density on CT
			May be related to sutures
Lacrimal gland Inflammatory	Postviral	Commonest cause of acute inflammatory enlargement in younger patients	Smooth enlargement of the gland
	Sjögren's syndrome	Decreased lacrimation and dry mouth	Non-specific enlargement of the gland in acute phase
		May be primary or secondary to autoimmune connective tissue diseases	Gland may be small in chronic phase Enhancement patchy or absent
		Histology = lymphocytic infiltration of gland	
	Mikulicz disease/ syndrome	Mikulicz disease is similar to primary Sjögren's syndrome	As for Sjögren's syndrome
		Mikulicz syndrome is gland enlargement associated with sarcoid, lymphoma, leukaemia or TB	
Tumour	Benign mixed tumour (Fig. 61.19)	Same as pleomorphic adenoma Benign	Well-defined, smooth enlargement of gland
		Represents about 50 per cent of primary lacrimal gland neoplasms (rest are malignant)	Longstanding so may be bone remodelling May not enhance
		Can undergo malignant change	
	Adenoid cystic carcinoma	Most common malignant primary tumour (followed by malignant mixed tumour, adenocarcinoma and mucoepidermoid carcinoma)	Tumour is hard enough to indent globe Gland may have a serrated edge Tendency for perineural spread Enhance well
	Lymphoma (NHL)	Lacrimal gland is a common site for NHL in the orbit	Infiltrating mass Enhances well

but demonstrate greater interconnections until they form the superior ophthalmic vein, which drains through the superior orbital fissure into the cavernous sinus, and the inferior ophthalmic vein, which drains through the inferior orbital fissure to the cavernous sinus and the pterygoid plexus.

IMAGING THE GLOBE[1] (see also Table 61.1)

Retinoblastoma

Retinoblastoma is the most common tumour of the globe in children. It occurs in children less than 3 years of age presenting with leukokoria. It derives from primitive photoreceptors or neuronal retinal cells, and histologically resembles other primitive neuroectodermal tumours. Of these tumours, 75 per cent are unilateral unifocal and 25 per cent are bilateral or unilateral multifocal. When it is found bilaterally and in conjunction with a pineoblastoma, it is labelled 'trilateral retinoblastoma'; 10–40 per cent are familial (autosomal dominant, with the oncogene present on chromosome 13), and these tumours tend to be bilateral and associated with other non-ocular tumours. Retinoblastoma is highly malignant and may spread haematogenously, via lymphatics, or may spread along the optic nerve to the intracranial compartment to give drop metastases in the subarachnoid space.

Imaging is crucial for timely management and survival of patients with retinoblastoma[3]. It is imperative to perform cross-sectional imaging and not just rely on ophthalmoscopy, so as to exclude other retrobulbar tumours with globe invasion, optic nerve invasion by the retinoblastoma and intracranial metastases. CT is the preferred method to image the child with leukokoria because it is sensitive to calcification in retinoblastoma. CT demonstrates clumped or punctate calcification (in 95 per cent of cases) in the posterior part of the globe extending into the vitreous, with minimal enhancement. In advanced cases the tumour may fill the globe (Fig. 61.1). If CT shows calcification in an intra-ocular mass in a child less than 3 years of age, it should be considered a retinoblastoma until proven otherwise. Absence of calcification means this diagnosis is unlikely, since it is rare in other causes of leukokoria. On MRI, retinoblastomas are hyperintense on T1 and hypointense on T2, possibly due to calcification, or some other paramagnetic entity, or tumour protein[4]. MRI is better for detection of tumour extension both along the optic

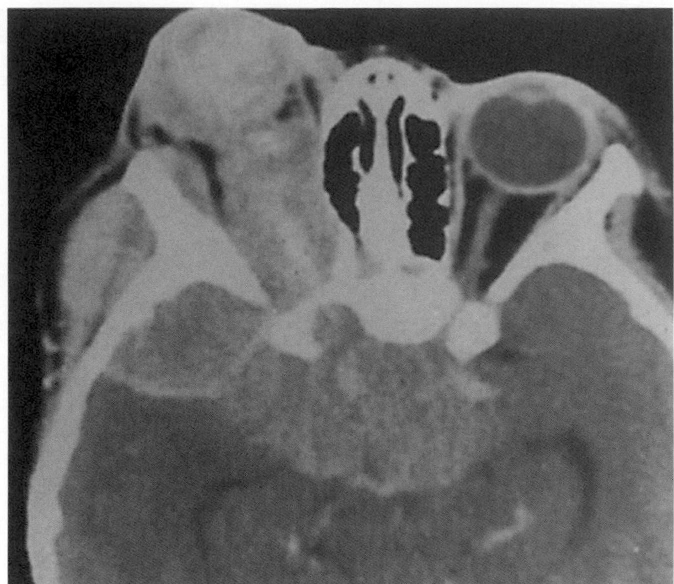

Figure 61.1 Huge retinoblastoma with orbital and intracranial involvement. Axial CT image with contrast medium. The right globe is filled by a calcified mass. The optic nerve is also calcified and surrounded by a soft tissue mass that replaces orbital fat and extends through the optic foramen. There is involvement of the suprasellar cistern, temporal lobe, greater wing of sphenoid and temporal fossa.

nerve and intracranially[5]. The tumour distribution on CT and MRI may help in differentiating recurrent tumours and second primary neoplasms[6].

Uveal melanoma

Uveal melanoma is the most common primary intra-ocular malignancy in adults. The great majority are located unilaterally in the choroid. It can metastasize to the liver and lung. Diagnosis is usually performed on ophthalmoscopy and ultrasound (US). CT and MRI are not considered in the routine workup of this disease except when it is not possible to perform adequate ophthalmoscopy, e.g. in the presence of an opaque vitreous or when there are large subendothelial effusion(s).

CT and MRI demonstrate a uveal melanoma as a soft tissue mass centred on the outer layers of the globe (Fig. 61.2). This mass bulges inward into the vitreous and may be small and flat or crescentic, or large and sharply demarcated with a 'mushroom cloud' appearance. On CT it is hyperdense and enhances after contrast medium administration. On MRI it is hyperintense on T1 and hypointense on T2 in melanotic melanomas due to the presence of paramagnetic melanin with/without haemorrhage. Metastases to the choroid from mucinous adenocarcinomas may have the same signal characteristics. Amelanotic melanomas are hypointense on T1 and hyperintense on T2, as are other tumours. Both types of melanomas enhance on MRI. MRI is better than CT for adequate differential diagnosis with choroidal haemangiomas and choroidal detachments, and for better depiction of episcleral invasion[7,8].

Ocular metastases

Only 50 per cent of patients with ocular metastases have a known primary tumour, commonly from lung or breast cancer in women and lung and the gastrointestinal tract in men. Ocular metastases occur mostly to the uveal tract (Fig. 61.3). They are seen on CT as small multiple areas of hyperdense thickening, occasionally with subretinal fluid. When found bilaterally in the posterior temporal regions near each macula, it suggests metastases rather than choroidal haemangiomas associated with Sturge–Weber syndrome.

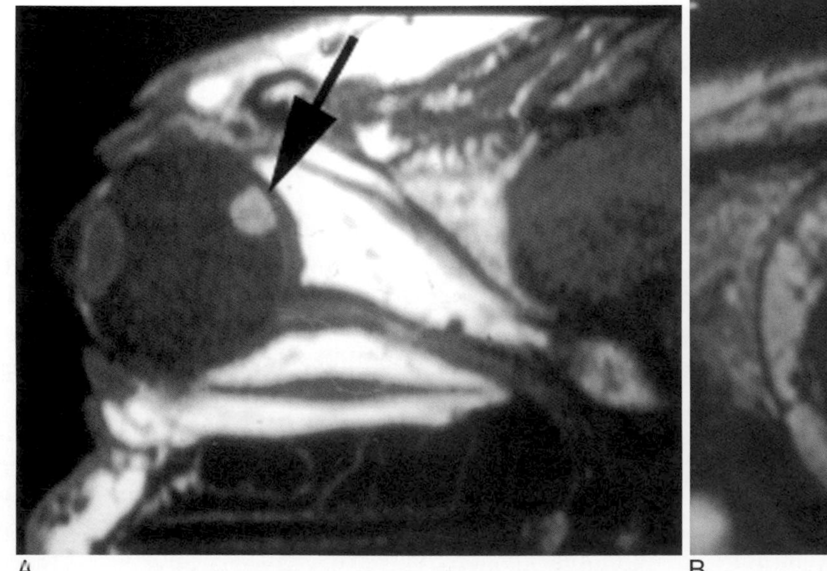

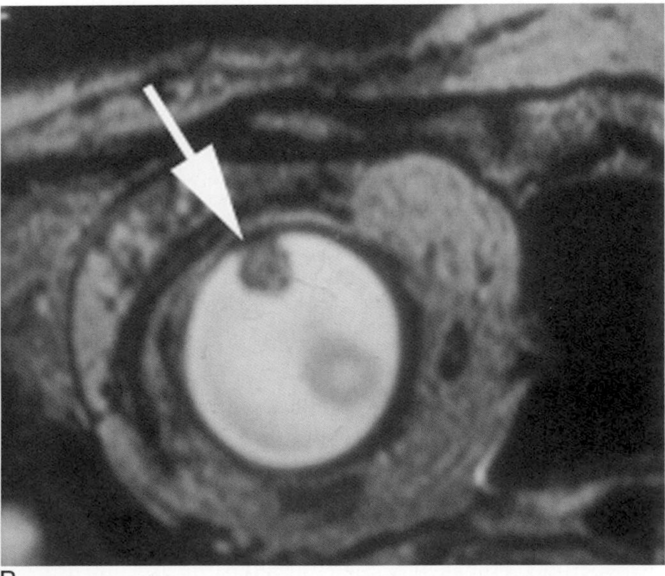

Figure 61.2 Malignant melanoma of the choroid. (A) Oblique sagittal T1-weighted MR image. (B) Oblique coronal T2*-weighted image. There is a nodule applied to the wall of the globe that is hyperintense on unenhanced T1- (black arrow) and hypointense on T2*-weighted (white arrow) images. These signal intensities are in keeping with melanin.

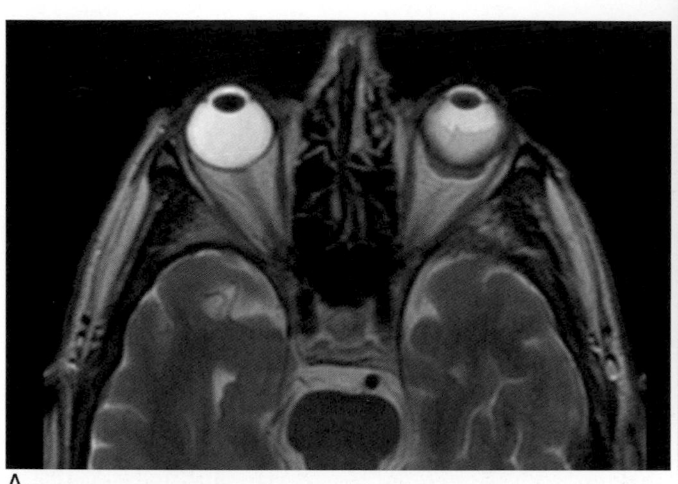

A

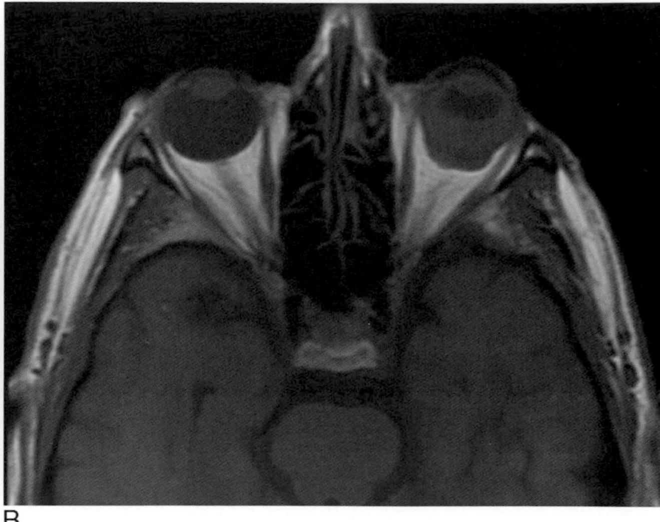

B

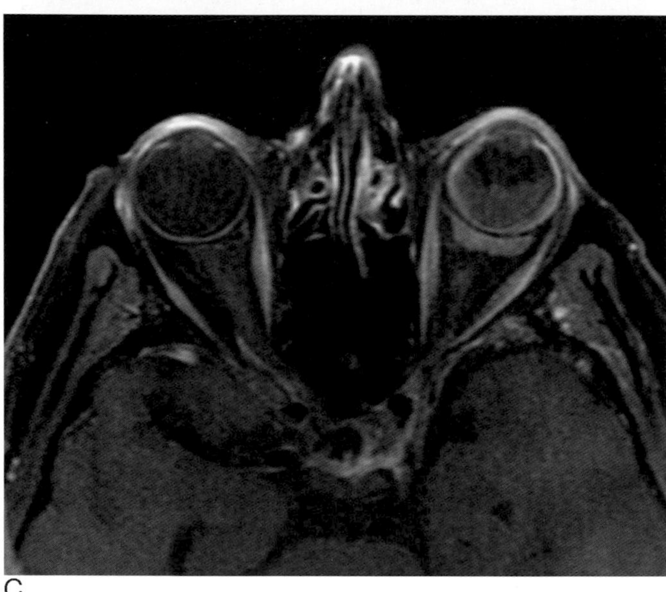

C

Figure 61.3 Ocular metastasis from systemic lymphoma. (A) Axial T2, (B) axial T1, (C) axial T1 MRI with IV gadolinium and fat suppression. There is thickening of the wall of the globe with soft tissue and enhancement extending into the vitreous and retrobulbar space.

IMAGING THE INTRACONAL COMPARTMENT[2]

Pseudotumour

Pseudotumour is the commonest cause of intra-orbital mass lesion in adults. Pseudotumour is an idiopathic inflammatory condition with rapid onset[9]. It usually presents in middle age with unilateral painful ophthalmoplegia, proptosis and chemosis. The more common acute form of the disease results in an early lymphocytic infiltrate. This has a rapid and lasting response to steroids. In the chronic form of pseudotumour there is a poor response to steroids and fibrosis sets in, requiring chemotherapy or radiotherapy as other treatment options. It is probably autoimmune, and in 10 per cent of cases is found with other systemic autoimmune conditions such as Wegener's granulomatosis, fibrosing mediastinitis, Reidel's thyroiditis, sclerosing cholangitis, retroperitoneal fibrosis, as well as polyarteritis nodosa, dermatomyositis and rheumatoid arthritis. Tolosa-Hunt syndrome is an idiopathic inflammatory condition similar to pseudotumour affecting the cavernous sinus and orbital apex, also presenting with painful ophthalmoplegia.

The morphological changes apparent on cross-sectional imaging may be found in any structure in the orbit (Fig. 61.7). In order of frequency, the retrobulbar fat, extra-ocular muscles, optic nerve, globe (uveal-scleral area) and the lacrimal gland are affected. Two patterns of the disease may be recognized: (A) the tumefactive type, where there is diffuse involvement of conal/intraconal structures, or (B) the myositic type involving extra-ocular muscles. Involvement of a unilateral single extra-ocular muscle including the tendinous insertion is highly suggestive of pseudotumour rather than thyroid ophthalmopathy. The tumefactive type of pseudotumour may be differentiated from true tumour by the history, biopsy findings and the response to steroids. Pseudotumour enhances after contrast administration, and on CT there may be subtle hyperdensity of intra-orbital fat (dirty fat). Different characteristics of attenuation change on two-phase helical CT and delayed coronal CT can be helpful in differentiating between orbital lymphoma and pseudotumour[10]. On MRI pseudotumour is hypointense to fat on T2, whereas true tumours are hyperintense to fat on T2. MRI is useful for demonstrating the presence of a variety

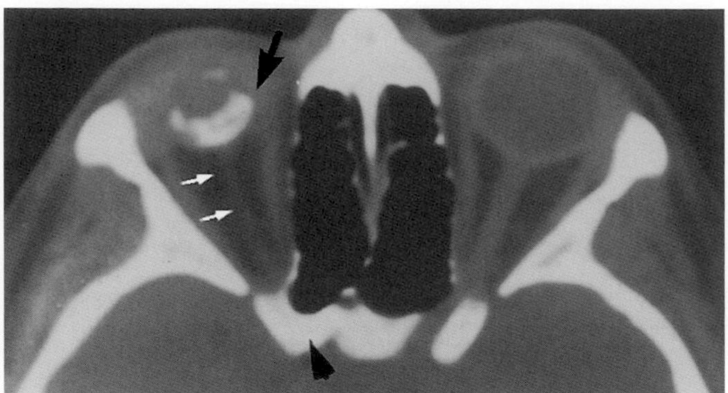

Figure 61.4 Congenital microphthalmos. Axial CT image. There is choroidal calcification (large black arrow) with a small globe, a thinned optic nerve (small white arrows) and a small orbit. Note the hypoplastic optic canal (black arrowhead).

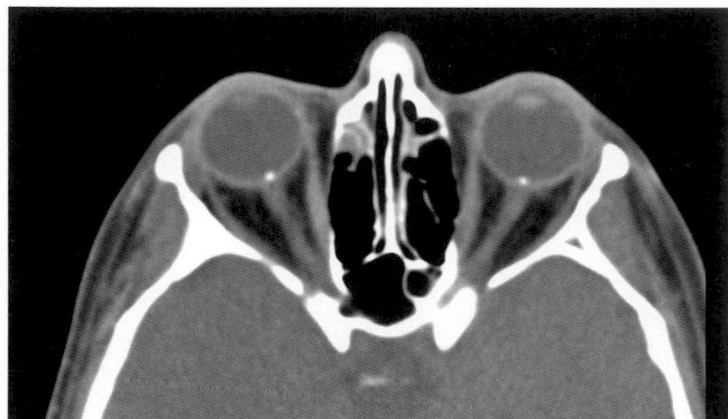

Figure 61.5 Drusen. Axial CT. There are small foci of calcification at both optic nerve heads.

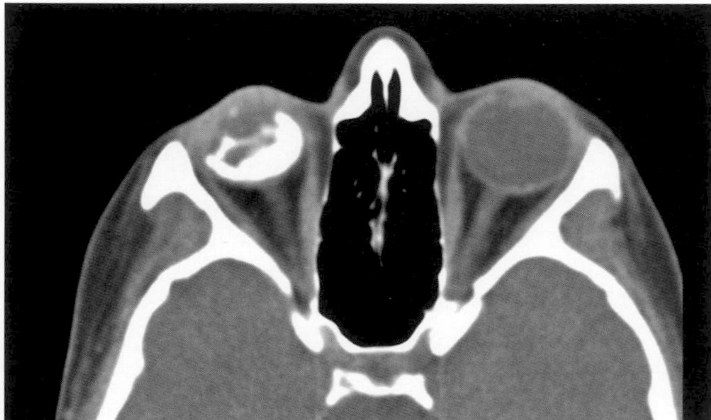

Figure 61.6 Phthisis bulbi. Axial CT. The patient had been stabbed in the right eye 2 years previously. The globe is small and densely calcified.

of extra-orbital extensions of orbital inflammatory pseudotumours[11].

Lymphoma

Orbital lymphoma presents in middle age with painless orbital swelling progressing to proptosis. There is usually no evidence of systemic disease at presentation, although this develops subsequently. Orbital lymphoma is of the B-cell variety (non-Hodgkin's lymphoma [NHL]); Hodgkins disease of the orbit is rare. Any structure in the orbit may be affected[12,13]. The lacrimal gland is involved most frequently, then the conal/intraconal compartment (the superior rectus is the commonest extra-ocular muscle involved)[14], and then the optic nerve/sheath complex, where it may simulate optic nerve meningioma or neuritis[15].

There is a wide range of radiological findings in orbital lymphoma. It may be a well-defined hyperdense enhancing mass on CT, or can produce diffuse infiltration leading to destruction of the normal anatomical architecture. It however moulds to the contour of the orbit without bone destruction, unless it is very aggressive. The combination of PET/CT may be useful in the evaluation of orbital neoplasms, especially if lymphoma is suspected[16]. On MRI lymphoma tends to be hypointense on T1, is usually hyperintense on T2, and enhances (Fig. 61.8). Bilateral orbital masses suggest the diagnosis of lymphoma. It can appear similar to pseudotumour, but lymphoma (and true tumours) tends to be superior in the orbit and the history may be of help. Moreover, comparison of lesion signal intensity to that of extra-ocular muscle appears to be a better alternative than comparison with cerebral gray matter or periorbital fat in differentiating malignant lymphoma from atypical lymphocytic infiltrates[17].

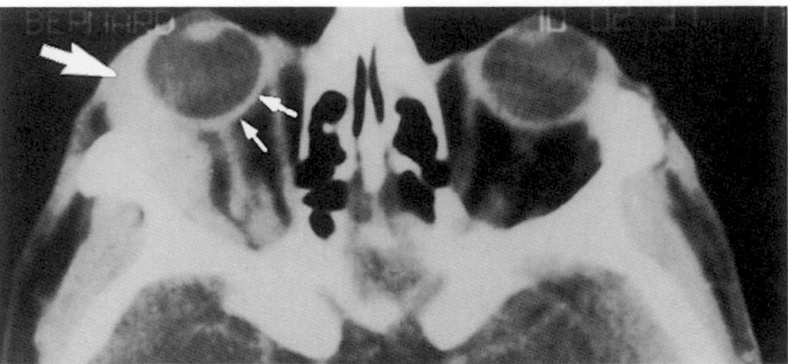

A

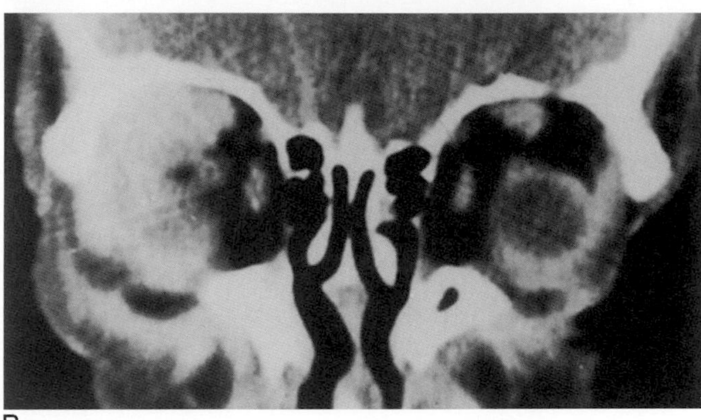

B

Figure 61.7 Orbital pseudotumour. (A) Axial and (B) coronal CT images with IV contrast medium. There is an extra- and intraconal mass with enlargement of the lacrimal gland (large arrow). There is subtle enhancement of the choroid (small arrows). The coronal image shows involvement of the extra-ocular muscles.

Cavernous haemangioma

Cavernous haemangioma is the most common orbital tumour. These lesions occur in adults 20–40 years of age and in men more than women. They present with proptosis, but vision is

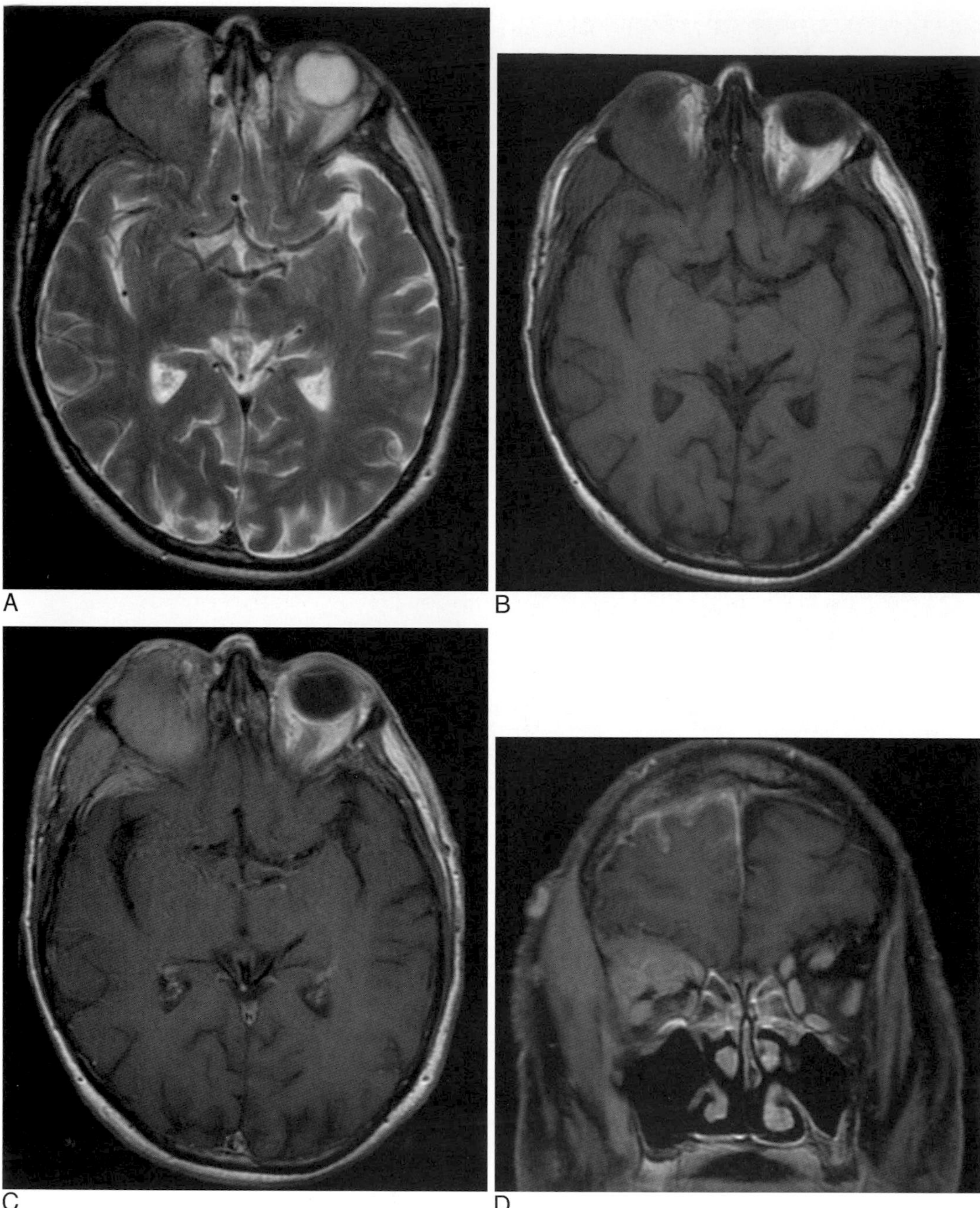

Figure 61.8 Lymphoma. (A) Axial T2, (B) axial T1, (C) axial T1 MRI with gadolinium, (D) coronal T1 with gadolinium and fat suppression. There is a diffusely infiltrating mass in the superior right orbit that is isointense to brain on T2- and slightly hypointense on the T1-weighted sequence. The mass extends outside the orbit to involve the temporal fossa. Following gadolinium, there is homogeneous signal enhancement of the mass. On coronal imaging, there is thick meningeal enhancement indicating intracranial spread of lymphoma.

usually unaffected. They are comprised of large endothelial-lined vascular spaces with a dense fibrous pseudocapsule, and are usually intraconal in location. They have no recognizable arterial feeders or draining veins, and may have phleboliths and surrounding haemosiderin/ferritin deposition, although intralesional haemorrhage is rare[18,19].

CT and MRI usually show a sharply demarcated, rounded or oval mass that spares the orbital apex[20] (Fig. 61.9). Bony deformity due to erosion may occur, but no bone destruction. CT shows these lesions to be hyperdense, and they enhance. MRI is better to show the relationship of the optic nerve and extra-ocular muscles. Cavernous haemangioma is usually isointense or hypointense on T1, hyperintense on T2, and enhances. Differences in contrast-enhancement spread patterns may be useful in distinguishing between haemangiomas and other tumours such as orbital schwannomas[21].

Capillary haemangioma

This lesion is found in infants less than 1 year of age who present with proptosis. It results from proliferation of endothelial

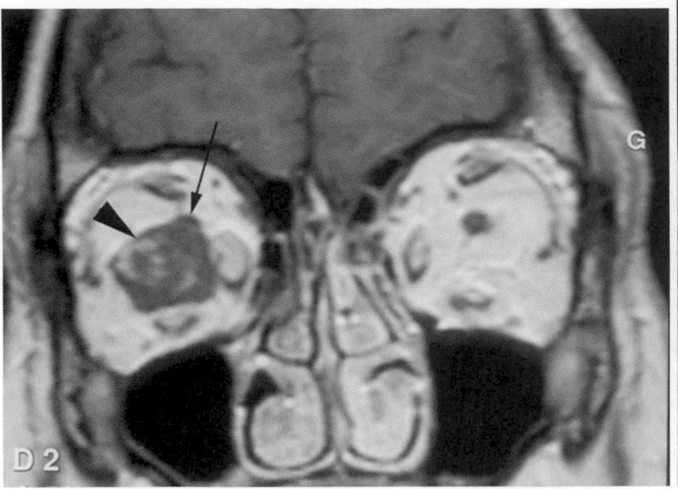

A

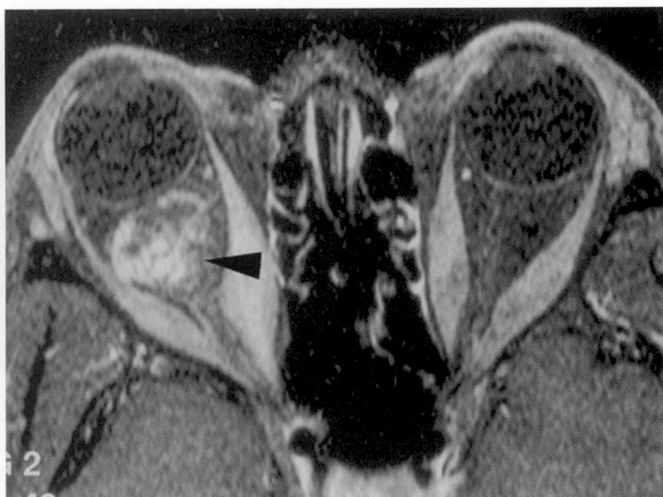
B

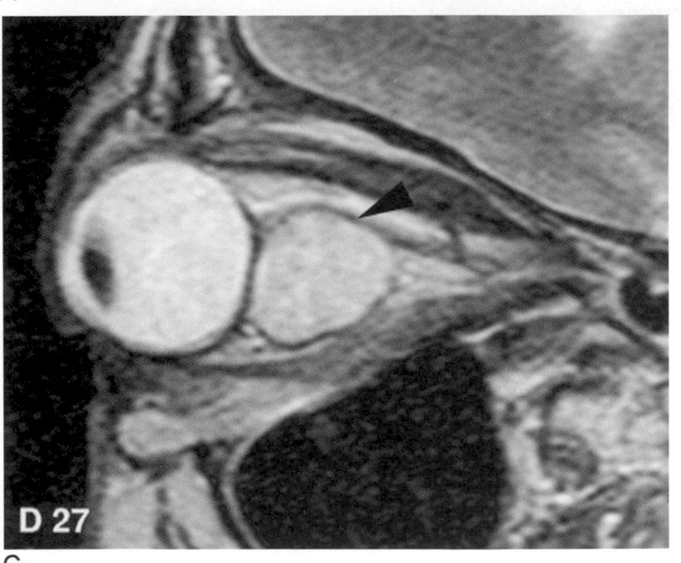

C

Figure 61.9 Cavernous haemangioma. (A) Coronal T1-weighted MR image with contrast medium. The heterogeneous mass (black arrowhead) lies inferolateral to the optic nerve (arrow). (B) Axial T1-weighted image with gadolinium and fat suppression. The heterogeneous enhancement of the mass (black arrowhead) corresponds to pooling of contrast medium within intratumoral vascular spaces. (C) Sagittal T2*-weighted image. The lesion (black arrowhead) is hyperintense and has a low intensity rim, probably because of a combination of fibrous tissue and haemosiderin/ferritin in the capsule.

cells with multiple capillaries. They regress spontaneously in the first few years of life.

CT and MRI show an enhancing mass that spans the intraconal and extraconal compartments. This mass is not usually sharply demarcated, and indeed its irregular margins may lead to confusion with malignancy. MRI is the imaging tool of choice to show the many punctate hypointense flow voids within such masses.

Optic nerve meningioma

Optic nerve meningiomas occur in middle-aged women, and more rarely in children with neurofibromatosis type 2. They are the second commonest primary tumours of the optic nerve after gliomas[22,23]. They arise from the arachnoid layer of the leptomeninges (meningoblastic rests) surrounding the optic nerve without infiltrating it, and they may be bilateral in neurofibromatosis 1 or 2. Optic nerve meningiomas may spread intracranially, but only to the prechiasmatic optic nerve sheath. Hyperostosis in a remodelled widened optic canal may be present.

Optic nerve meningiomas result usually in tubular thickening of the optic nerve/sheath complex rather than fusiform or excrescent thickening. Along with this thickening, the optic nerve tends to be seen as separate from tumour. Since these lesions are hyperdense on CT and also enhance strongly they produce a 'tram track' sign on axial images and a 'doughnut sign' on coronal images. The differential diagnosis of 'tram tracks' includes pseudotumour, sarcoid and metastasis. Calcification (psammoma bodies) is common (20–50 per cent of cases). CT may be necessary to detect the linear calcification of early lesions. On MRI, these lesions are hypointense on T1 and hyperintense on T2. They again enhance strongly, especially appreciated with fat suppression (Fig. 61.10). Early meningiomas are thus rendered more conspicuous on T1 fat-suppressed post-contrast images. Overall, MRI is better for orbital apex and intracanalicular lesions because surrounding bone makes this area difficult to outline accurately on CT. The radiological differential diagnosis of optic nerve meningiomas includes haemangioblastomas of the optic nerve in von Hippel–Lindau disease, cavernous haemangiomas and lymphoma. Meningiomas may also arise from the periostium of the orbit (the periorbita) which is in continuity with the intracranial dura mater.

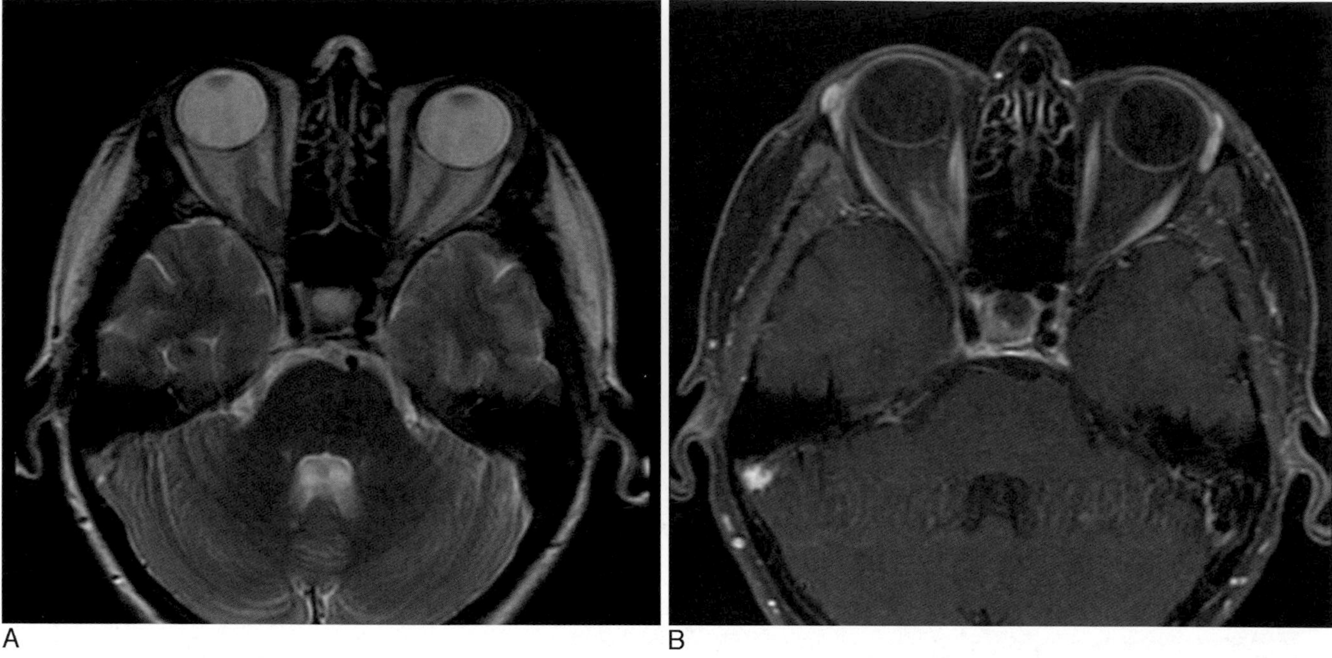

Figure 61.10 Optic nerve meningioma. (A) Axial T2, (B) axial T1 MRI with gadolinium and fat suppression. There is a mass at the right orbital apex, closely applied to the optic nerve but seen separate to it. On the contrast-enhanced image, 'tram-track' enhancement along the nerve can be seen.

Optic nerve glioma

Optic nerve gliomas are childhood slow-growing low-grade pilocytic astrocytomas, with 75 per cent of cases occurring at less than 10 years of age[22]. They cause decreased vision with minimal proptosis. Of patients with neurofibromatosis type 1, 15 per cent have optic nerve or chiasmatic gliomas that may be bilateral[24]. Bilateral tumours are virtually pathognomonic of neurofibromatosis. Optic nerve gliomas constitute 80 per cent of all primary optic nerve tumours.

These lesions result in tortuous thickening of the optic nerve/sheath complex that is most commonly tubular, but may also be fusiform or excrescent. Unlike optic nerve meningiomas, gliomas cannot be separated from the optic nerve itself (Fig. 61.11). Only half these lesions enhance, and they may contain cysts. Calcification is rare except post radiotherapy. MRI is necessary to detect involvement of the rest of the optic pathway because only 25 per cent of optic pathway gliomas are confined to the optic nerves. However, an optic nerve glioma does not itself tend to spread from the optic nerve to the intracranial compartment. MRI shows these lesions as isointense on T1 and hyperintense on T2. However, in neurofibromatosis they may be hypointense on T2 but with a hyperintense rim due to **arachnoidal gliomatosis**.

Carotid-cavernous fistulae

Carotid-cavernous fistulae (CCFs) are fistulae between the carotid siphon and the cavernous sinus. They may occur spontaneously, for example after rupture of a carotid siphon aneurysm or after trauma. Clinically they present with engorgement of the orbit and globe (sclera and conjunctiva), pulsating exophthalmos, a bruit and eventually glaucoma and visual loss in larger CCFs.

Cross-sectional imaging shows signs of orbital venous hypertension with an enlarged engorged superior ophthalmic vein and extra-ocular muscles (Fig. 61.12A). MRI shows signal void in the cavernous sinus and superior ophthalmic vein due to the presence of fast-flowing arterial blood. The enlarged cavernous sinus may be bowed convex to the middle cranial fossa. MR angiography shows filling of the cavernous sinus and superior ophthalmic vein in conjunction with the arterial anterior intracranial circulation. Conventional angiography with injections of internal and external carotid arteries can usually distinguish between 'direct' fistulae and 'indirect' ones (a dural arteriovenous malformation in the region of the cavernous sinus). Angiography may show filling of the ipsilateral or contralateral cavernous sinus via the intercavernous sinuses, and drainage into ipsilateral or bilateral superior ophthalmic veins (Fig. 61.12B), inferior petrosal sinuses, or even the cortical veins or spheno-parietal sinuses when severe.

Venous varix

A venous varix is an enormously dilated vein representing a congenital or acquired (e.g. post-traumatic) venous malformation. It may occur on its own or be associated with an intraorbital or intracranial arteriovenous malformation. Multiple varicosities may be present. Clinically they present with intermittent proptosis upon straining or coughing and retrobulbar pain.

On CT a venous varix is seen as an intraconal hyperdense lobulated mass with strong enhancement. Phleboliths and clot

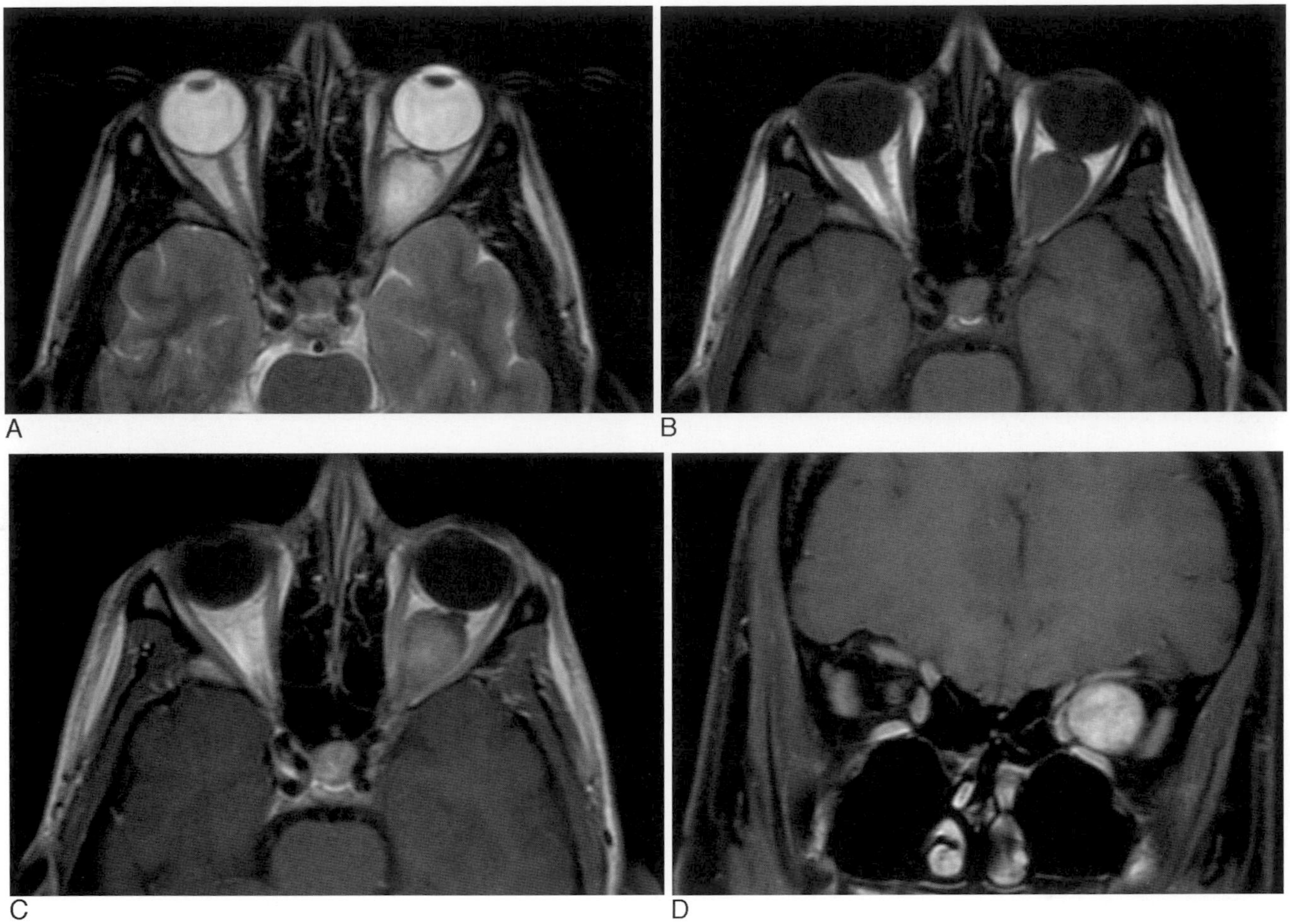

Figure 61.11 Optic nerve glioma. (A) Axial T2, (B) axial T1, (C) axial T1 MRI with gadolinium, (D) coronal T1 with gadolinium and fat suppression. There is smooth expansion of the left optic nerve extending to the orbital apex. On contrast-enhanced imaging, there is homogeneous enhancement of the mass, and the nerve cannot be distinguished from it.

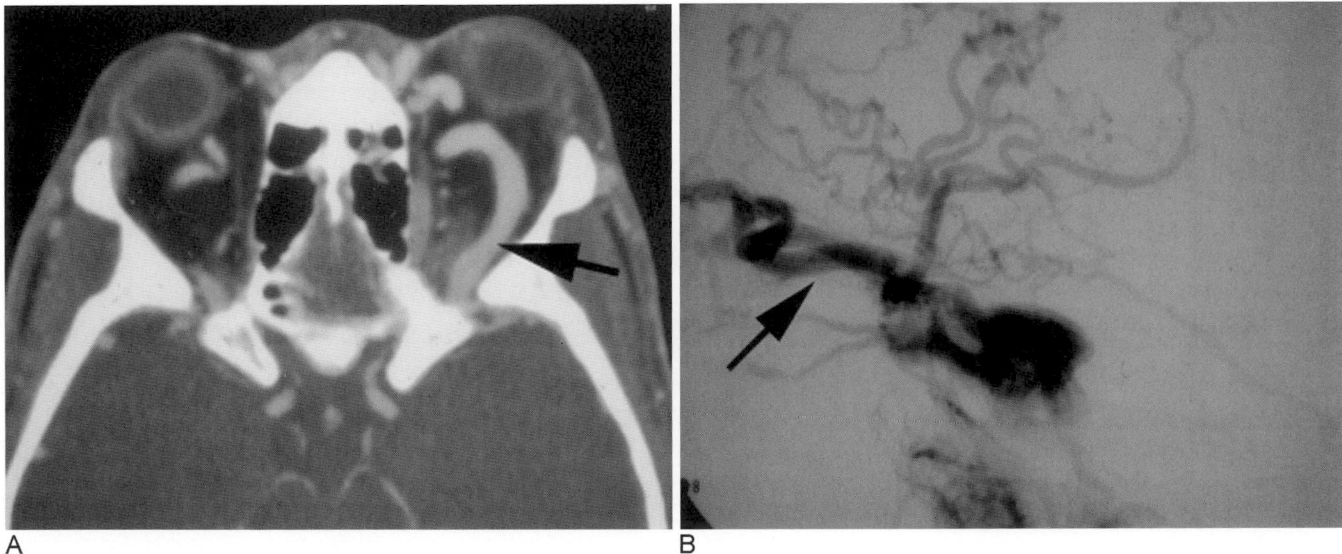

Figure 61.12 Post-traumatic high flow carotico-cavernous fistula. (A) Axial CT with contrast medium shows marked dilatation of the left superior ophthalmic vein (arrow) and moderate dilatation of the right superior ophthalmic vein. (B) Carotid angiography shows early filling of the cavernous sinus and left superior ophthalmic vein (arrow).

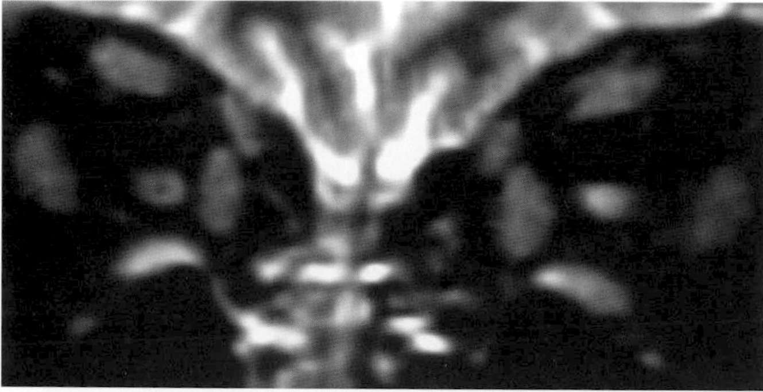

Figure 61.13 Optic neuritis. Coronal T2-weighted image with inversion recovery. There is high signal in the left optic nerve indicating optic neuritis. The patient was symptomatic and had multiple demyelinating lesions in the cerebral white matter.

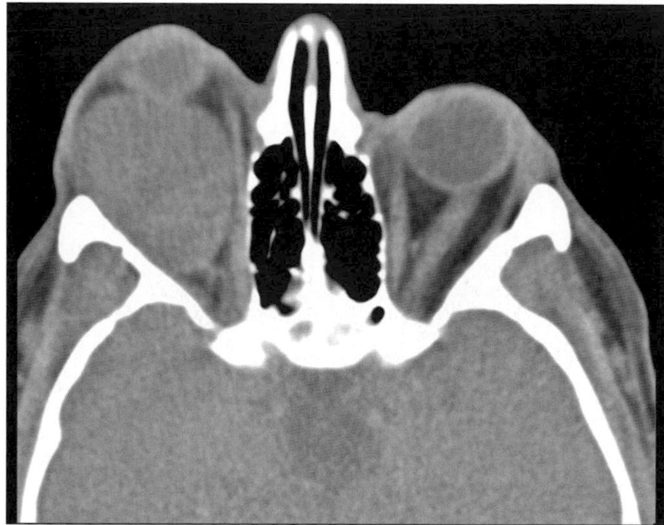

A

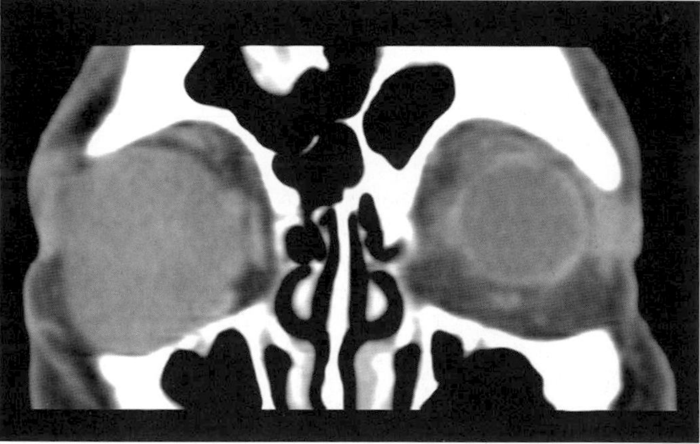

B

Figure 61.14 Intraconal schwannoma. (A) Axial and (B) coronal CT image. There is a large oval mass filling much of the orbit. It is almost isodense compared to muscle with no enhancement following IV contrast medium. The mass had not changed in size over a period of 5 years.

may be present. When small, a varix may not be seen unless it is made to enlarge with a Valsalva manoeuvre or during imaging in the prone position. Orbital phlebography is no longer required for making the diagnosis. MRI may reveal slow flow

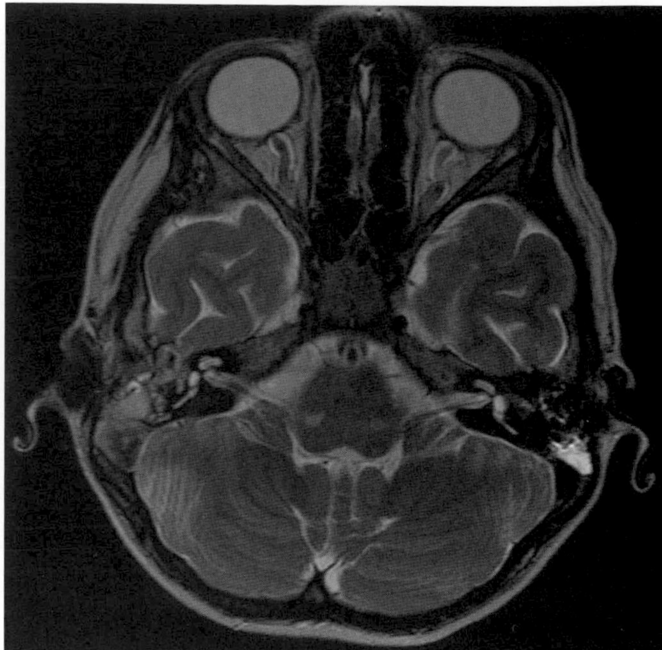

Figure 61.15 Raised intracranial pressure. Axial T2 MRI. There is dilatation of the optic nerve sheath in a patient with raised intracranial pressure secondary to right transverse sinus occlusion.

phenomena. Clot due to spontaneous thrombosis is common, which can result in variable signal intensity on MRI.

IMAGING THE CONAL COMPARTMENT[3]

Thyroid ophthalmopathy

Thyroid ophthalmopathy is the commonest cause of unilateral or bilateral exophthalmos in adults. Most patients with thyroid eye disease are hyperthyroid; only 10 per cent are euthyroid (euthyroid ophthalmopathy). It presents with insidious and painless exophthalmos and lid lag. It results from deposits of hygroscopic mucopolysaccharides and infiltration of lymphocytes, mast cells and plasma cells. Of these cases, 85 per cent are bilateral but often asymmetrical[25].

Axial CT or MRI shows fusiform enlargement and enhancement of the bellies of extra-ocular muscles, with relative sparing of the tendinous insertions (Fig. 61.16). This occurs in order of frequency in the inferior rectus, medial rectus, superior rectus, lateral rectus and oblique muscles, although most commonly all muscles are involved. Only in 10 per cent is there an isolated extra-ocular muscle involved. Importantly, if an isolated lateral rectus belly enlargement is seen, causes other than thyroid ophthalmopathy (e.g. pseudotumour) should be sought. The peak signal intensity from the most inflamed extra-ocular muscle could be the most reliable imaging correlate of clinical disease[26]. Haemodynamic information obtained by dynamic contrast-enhanced MRI may also be useful in evaluating the clinical course of thyroid ophthalmopathy[27]. For example, the mean of peak enhancement ratio values for the extra-ocular muscles in patients with Graves' disease tends to decrease according to the severity of the anatomical and clinical changes. The mean rate of enhancement also decreases according to the severity of the disease. Intra-orbital fat volume is increased, especially in the anteromedial extraconal space, although fat hypertrophy may occur also in other conditions such as following steroid therapy or in Cushing's disease. In advanced cases the lamina papyracea may show a concavity due to the raised intra-orbital pressure. Orbital apex crowding (due to the enlarged muscles and increased fat content) results in compression of the optic nerve and decreased vision (also exacerbated by the stretching of the nerve). This may require orbital decompression by removal of the medial wall or floor of the orbit. Coronal imaging with either CT or MRI is useful to assess muscle thickness and orbital apex crowding of the optic nerve.

Rhabdomyosarcoma

Rhabdomyosarcoma is one of the more common primary malignant tumours of the orbit in children aged 2–5 years. Orbital rhabdomyosarcoma is the most common site of head and neck rhabdomyosarcoma. It is highly malignant and presents with rapidly progressive exophthalmos. It originates from the extra-ocular muscles, the nasopharynx, or the paranasal sinuses. It is usually present in the superomedial orbit and may produce bone destruction.

On CT, these bulky aggressive-looking masses are isodense or slightly hyperdense, and show uniform enhancement (Fig. 61.17). On MRI they are of intermediate signal intensity on both T1 and T2 sequences. There is bone destruction in 40 per cent of cases and frequent distortion of the globe.

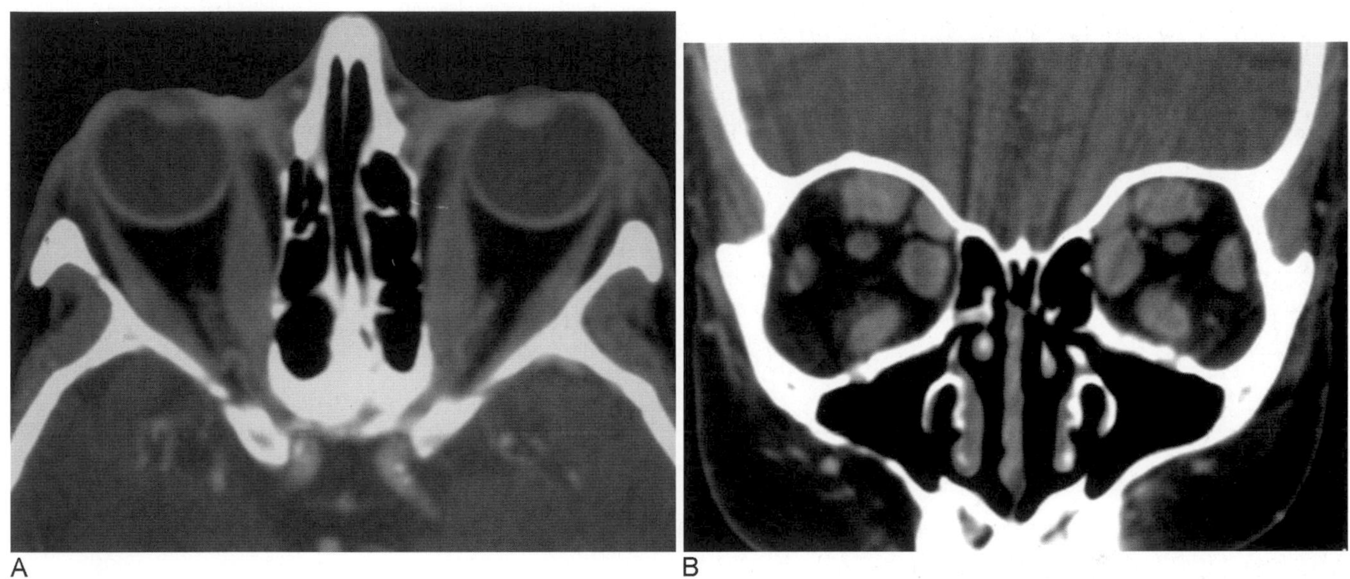

Figure 61.16 Thyroid ophthalmopathy. (A) Axial and (B) coronal CT imaging. There is generalized enlargement of the bellies of all the extra-ocular muscles, proptosis and increased intraorbital fat.

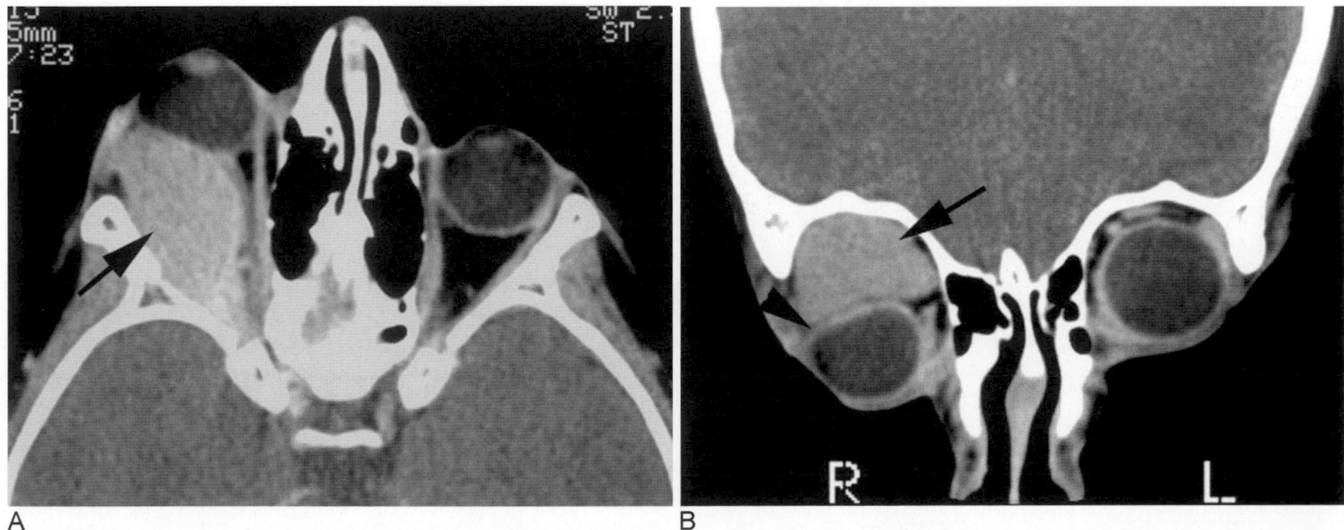

Figure 61.17 Rhabdomyosarcoma. (A) Axial and (B) coronal CT images with contrast medium. There is a large mass in the superior right orbit which is difficult to separate from the extra-ocular muscles. There is deformity of the posterior wall of the globe and marked proptosis. The mass shows uniform contrast enhancement.

IMAGING THE EXTRACONAL COMPARTMENT[4]

Retrobulbar metastases

Most retrobulbar metastases are extraconal in location, and subsequently encroach on the intraconal compartment as they increase in size to produce infiltrating poorly marginated masses. They originate mostly from the greater wing of the sphenoid, resulting in bone destruction. On CT, these lesions are isodense or hyperdense, and enhance. In children, neuroblastoma or Ewing's sarcoma produce smooth extraconal masses related to the posterior lateral wall of the orbit. They differ from rhabdomyosarcoma because of their baseline hyperdensity and lack of invasion of the preseptal compartment. In adults, an infiltrative retrobulbar mass and enophthalmos is characteristic of scirrhous carcinoma of the breast.

IMAGING ORBITAL INFECTION

Other than infection of the globe with larvae of the nematode *Toxocara canis* and the long-term development of sclerosing endophthalmitis (presented briefly in Table 61.1), both CT and MRI appearances are nonspecific for particular ocular infections. Ocular *Pseudomonas* infection may show up as a posterior scleritis cytomegalovirus (CMV) infection in human immunodeficiency virus (HIV)-positive patients and may result in arcuate enhancement of the retina.

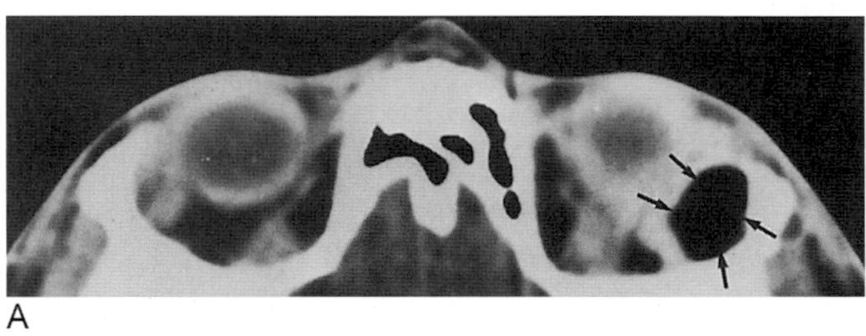

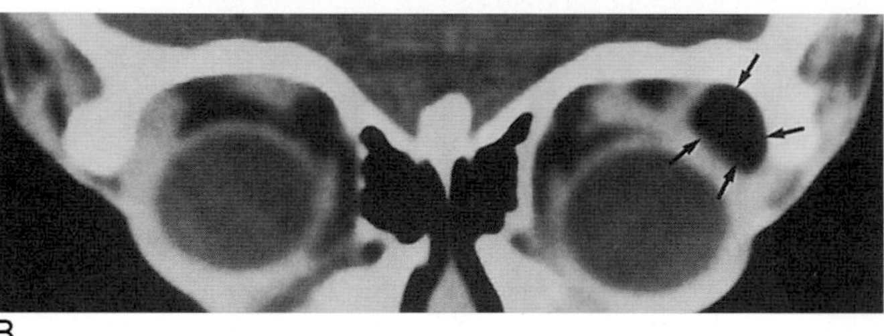

Figure 61.18 Dermoid. (A) Axial and (B) coronal CT images with contrast medium. There is a fat density mass in the superolateral left orbit with a thick enhancing capsule. Subtle deformity of the adjacent bone is noted.

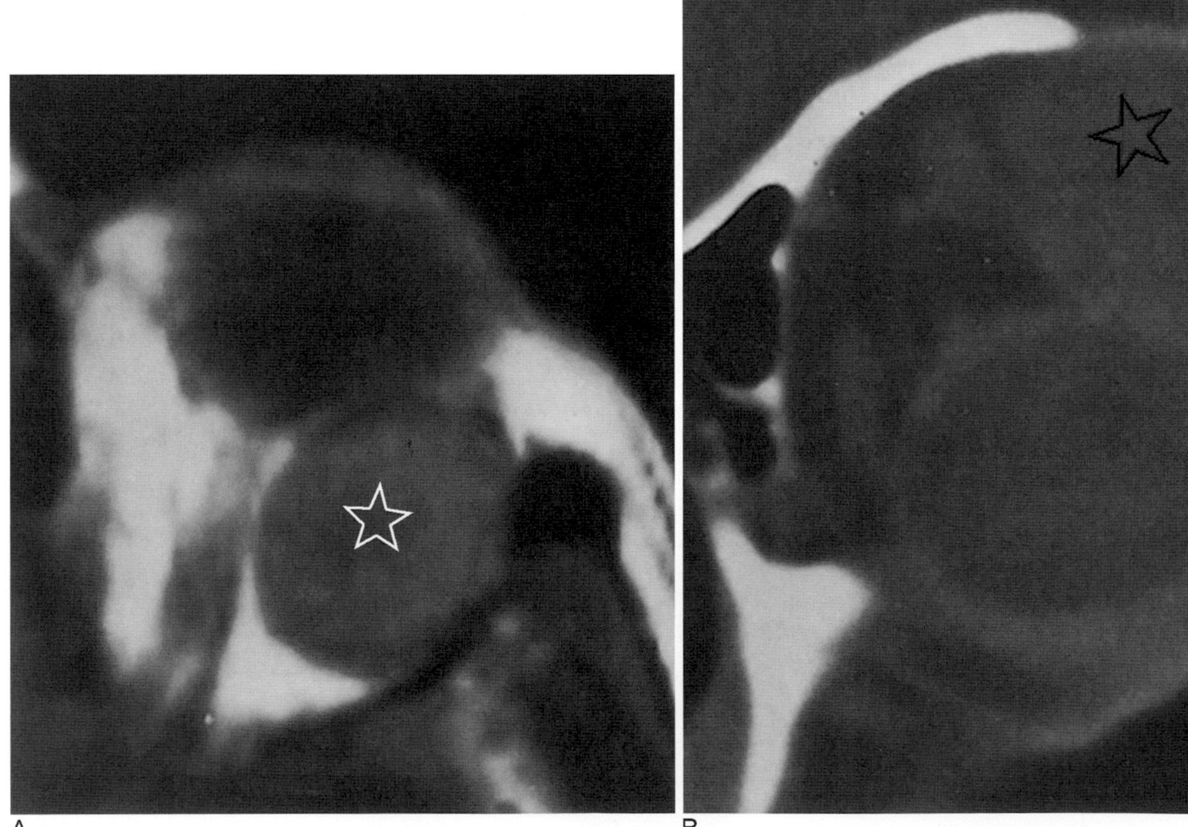

Figure 61.19 Benign mixed tumour of the lacrimal gland. (A) Axial T1-weighted MR and (B) coronal CT image with contrast medium (wide window setting). The mass (star) arises from the gland, is homogeneous and does not enhance after contrast medium. There is subtle bony remodelling.

The orbital septum acts as a mechanical barrier to spread of infection into the orbit. This is because the periorbita is reflected onto the anterior aspect of the septum and globe. Thus, preseptal cellulitis is usually confined to the eyelids. On the other hand, much more serious orbital postseptal infection can arise from sinus disease, bacteraemia, trauma, or spread of a serious infection from the skin. On CT and MRI this is seen as ill-defined tissue planes in retrobulbar structures, loss of the normal hyperintense signal of orbital fat on MRI, with or without a soft tissue mass. The latter may demonstrate ring enhancement and/or pockets of gas suggestive of abscess formation. A subperiosteal abscess may develop, especially in the presence of ethmoid sinusitis (Fig. 61.20). This can be identified as a soft tissue mass, with or without central fluid, centred on the bony (usually the medial) wall of the orbit and displacing the adjacent extra-ocular muscle whilst preserving a thin layer of extraconal fat. The lamina papyracea may or may not be destroyed. Further evaluation of the intracranial compartment using MRI is useful to exclude spread of infection in the presence of orbital cellulitis and subperiosteal infection.

IMAGING ORBITAL TRAUMA

Conventional radiography is no longer used routinely for evaluation of orbital trauma. Instead, CT is the procedure of choice, whilst MRI is reserved for examining the intracanalicular optic nerve, for detecting transection of the optic nerve, for distinguishing haematoma from any other soft tissue mass, and for examining concomitant trauma to the posterior visual pathways and intracranial contents.

There are four categories of orbital fractures to consider: zygomaticomaxillary (trimalar, tripod) fractures, LeFort fractures, orbital blowout fractures (Fig. 61.21) and orbital roof fractures.

Radiological evaluation of trauma to the globe is usually necessary in cases of suspected blunt ocular trauma or for determining the presence and location of penetrating foreign bodies.

Blunt trauma may uncommonly result in globe rupture or laceration, which is usually evident by loss of the normal globe contour on CT or MRI; dislocation of the lens may also be seen in these cases. More commonly, blunt trauma results in retinal or choroidal detachments. Retinal detachment results in a V-shaped membrane with the apex of the V at the optic disc. The associated subretinal fluid might be hyperintense on T1-weighted MRI because of proteinaceous fluid or haematoma. Choroidal detachments are distinguished by the fact that they do not extend to the optic nerve head because of the tethering effect of vortex veins.

Referrals regarding the presence and site of a penetrating intra-ocular foreign body are common. Multidetector CT is usually helpful to demonstrate glass, metal and bone fragments, whereas wood splinters and thorns are difficult to find because they are isodense to soft tissues or may resemble intraorbital air. In such cases, MRI might be useful. However, MRI is contraindicated when there is suspicion of a metallic intra-ocular foreign body because the magnetic field may cause the object to move, which may result in further trauma and intra-ocular haemorrhage.

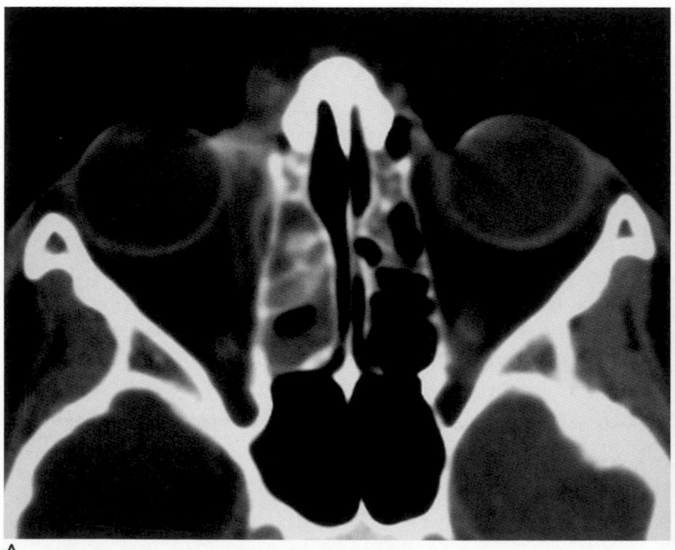

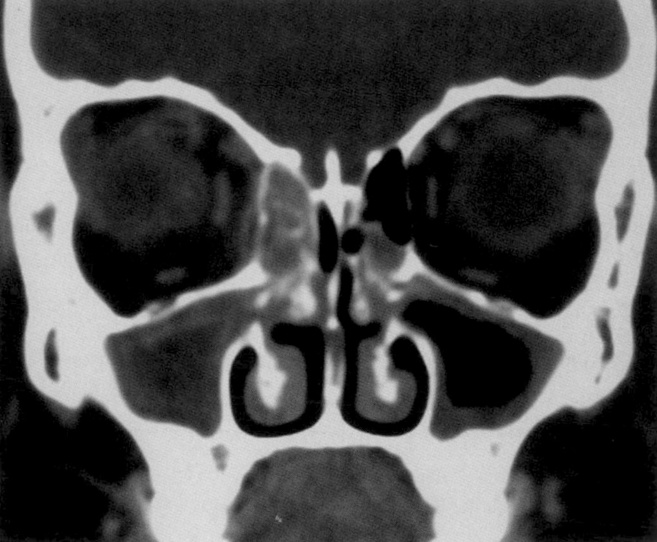

Figure 61.20 Subperiosteal abscess. (A) Axial and (B) coronal CT images with contrast medium. There is sinusitis affecting the right maxillary and ethmoid sinuses and a subtle rim enhancing fluid collection extending along the medial wall of the orbit indicating a subperiosteal abscess. Note the intact lamina papyracea despite intraorbital extension of infection.

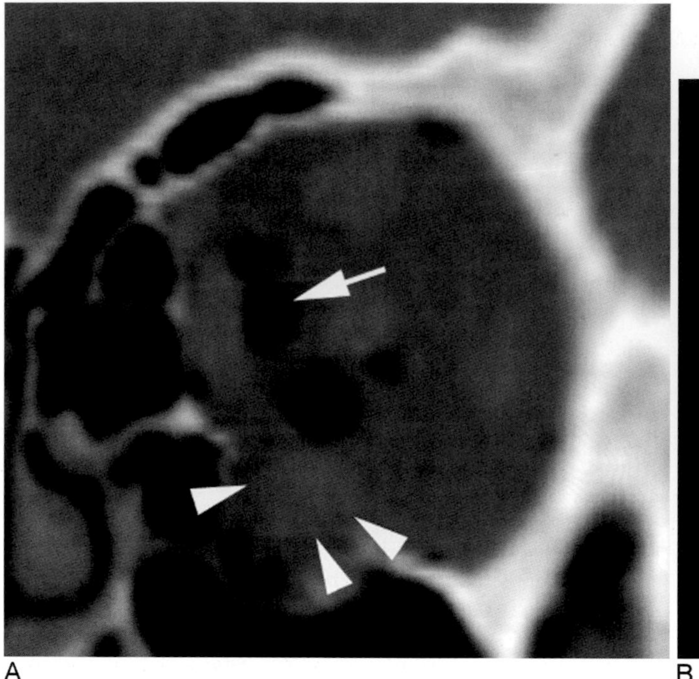

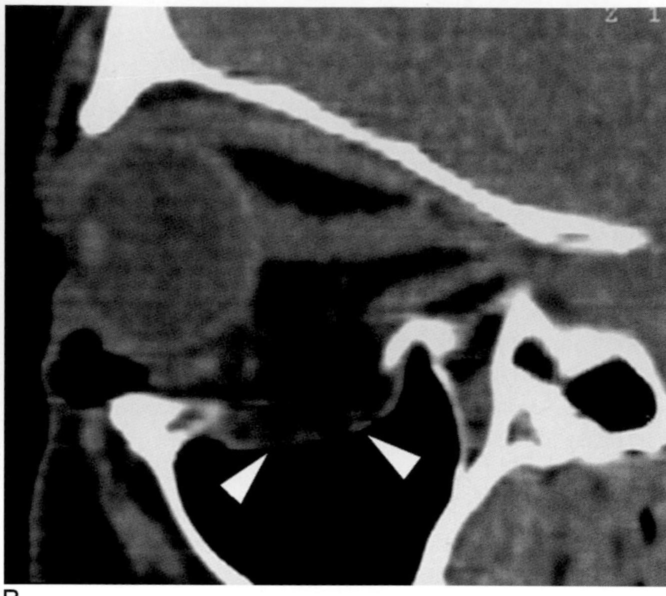

A B

Figure 61.21 Orbital blowout fracture. (A) Coronal and (B) sagittal reformatted CT images. There is intra-orbital air (arrow) and herniation of fat and inferior rectus into the maxillary sinus (arrowheads).

REFERENCES

1. Shields J A, Shields C L, Scartozzi R 2004 Survey of 1264 patients with orbital tumors and simulating lesions: The 2002 Montgomery Lecture (Pt 1) Ophthalmology 111: 997–1008
2. Gentry L R 1998 Anatomy of the orbit. Neuroimaging Clin N Am 8: 171–194
3. Apushkin M A, Apushkin M A, Shapiro M J, Mafee M F 2005 Retinoblastoma and simulating lesions: role of imaging. Neuroimaging Clin N Am 15: 49–67
4. Gizewski E R, Wanke I, Jurklies C, Gungor A R, Forsting M 2005 T1 Gd-enhanced compared with CISS sequences in retinoblastoma: superiority of T1 sequences in evaluation of tumour extension. Neuroradiology 47: 56–61
5. De Graaf P, Barkhof F, Moll A C, Imhof S M, Knol D L, van der Valk P, Castelijns J A 2005 Retinoblastoma: MR imaging parameters in detection of tumor extent. Radiology 235: 197–207
6. Tateishi U, Hasegawa T, Miyakawa K, Sumi M, Moriyama N 2003 CT and MRI features of recurrent tumors and second primary neoplasms in pediatric patients with retinoblastoma. AJR Am J Roentgenol 181: 879–884
7. Blanco G 2004 Diagnosis and treatment of orbital invasion in uveal melanoma. Can J Ophthalmol 39: 388–396
8. Recsan Z, Karlinger K, Fodor M, Zalatnai A, Papp M, Salacz G 2002 MRI for the evaluation of scleral invasion and extrascleral extension of uveal melanomas. Clin Radiol 57: 371–376
9. Jacobs D, Galetta S 2002 Diagnosis and management of orbital pseudotumor. Curr Opin Ophthalmol 13: 347–351
10. Moon W J, Na D G, Ryoo J W et al 2003 Orbital lymphoma and subacute or chronic inflammatory pseudotumor: differentiation with two-phase helical computed tomography. J Comput Assist Tomogr 27: 510–516
11. Lee E J, Jung S L, Kim B S et al 2005 MR imaging of orbital inflammatory pseudotumors with extraorbital extension. Korean J Radiol 6: 82–88
12. Fahim D K, Bucher R, Johnson M W 2005 The elusive nature of primary intraocular lymphoma. J Neuroophthalmol 25: 33–36
13. Neudorfer M, Kessler A, Anteby I, Goldenberg D, Barak A 2004 Co-existence of intraocular and orbital lymphoma. Acta Ophthalmol Scand 82: 754–761
14. Kert G, Clement C I, O'Donnell B A 2004 Orbital lymphoid tumour located within an extraocular muscle. Clin Experiment Ophthalmol 32: 651–652
15. Selva D, Rootman J, Crompton J 2004 Orbital lymphoma mimicking optic nerve meningioma. Orbit 23: 115–120
16. Chan-Kai B T, Yen M T 2005 Combined positron emission tomography/computed tomography imaging of orbital lymphoma. Am J Ophthalmol 140: 531–533
17. Akansel G, Hendrix L, Erickson B A 2005 MI patterns in orbital malignant lymphoma and atypical lymphocytic infiltrates. Eur J Radiol 53: 175–181
18. Yan J, Wu Z 2004 Cavernous hemangioma of the orbit: analysis of 214 cases. Orbit 23: 33–40
19. Scheuerle A F, Steiner H H, Kolling G, Kunze S, Aschoff A 2004 Treatment and long-term outcome of patients with orbital cavernomas. Am J Ophthalmol 138: 237–244
20. Ansari S A, Mafee M F 2005 Orbital cavernous hemangioma: role of imaging. Neuroimaging Clin N Am 15: 137–158
21. Tanaka A, Mihara F, Yoshura T et al 2004 Differentiation of cavernous hemangioma from schwannoma of the orbit: a dynamic MRI study. AJR Am J Roentgenol 183: 1799–1804
22. Miller NR 2004 Primary tumours of the optic nerve and its sheath. Eye 18: 1026–1037
23. Saeed P, Rootman J, Nugent R A, White V A, Mackenzie I R, Koornneef L 2003 Optic nerve sheath meningiomas. Ophthalmology 110: 2019–2030
24. Thiagalingam S, Flaherty M, Billson F, North K 2004 Neurofibromatosis type 1 and optic pathway gliomas: follow-up of 54 patients. Ophthalmology 111: 568–577
25. El-Kaissi S, Frauman A G, Wall J R 2004 Thyroid-associated ophthalmopathy: a practical guide to classification, natural history and management. Intern Med J 34: 482–491
26. Mayer E J, Fox D L, Herdman G et al 2005 Signal intensity, clinical activity and cross-sectional areas on MRI scans in thyroid eye disease. Eur J Radiol 56: 20–24
27. Taoka T, Sakamoto M, Nakagawa H et al 2005 Evaluation of extraocular muscles using dynamic contrast enhanced MRI in patients with chronic thyroid orbitopathy. J Comput Assist Tomogr 29: 115–120

CHAPTER 62

Ear, Nose and Throat Radiology

Philip Anslow

The introduction of cross-section imaging, notably computed tomography (CT) and magnetic resonance imaging (MRI) has hugely expanded the scope and ability of head and neck radiology to recognize and assess disease. The anatomy of the head and neck is hugely complex; pathological processes make the subject even more complex. Only advanced imaging can make a material contribution to understanding.

Imaging investigations involved in the assessment of ear, nose and throat (ENT) cases include:

- plain radiographs
- conventional tomography
- contrast medium examinations (barium swallow, etc.)
- ultrasound
- radionuclide radiology
- angiography
- CT
- MRI
- positron emission tomography (PET).

Plain radiographs and conventional tomography have virtually no place in the assessment of disease in the modern setting. Contrast medium studies still have a major role in the assessment of disorders of swallowing, particularly those where there is some sort of neuromuscular incoordination (multiple sclerosis, myasthenia, stroke). The use of ultrasound and radionuclides is discussed elsewhere in this book; ultrasound in skilled hands is fast becoming the first line investigation for many conditions. Angiography has a highly specific and limited role. This chapter concentrates on the use of CT and MRI in the assessment of disease.

In approaching this subject a number of perhaps unfamiliar clinical concepts have to be considered. The modern ENT clinic is equipped with advanced audiological and electrophysiological equipment. This allows deafness, for example, to be differentiated into *conductive*, where some problem is dampening the proper mechanical conduction of sound, and *sensorineural*, where there is a lesion in the electronic pathway – cochlea, acoustic nerve or brainstem. Microscopes for the examination of the external ear and fibre-optic endoscopes for the evaluation of the nose, postnasal space and upper airway are routinely available. In such an arena, the *detection* of disease is usually simple and pathological *characterization* has been revolutionized by the use of fine needle aspiration cytology at the time of clinic assessment. The main problem facing the ENT surgeon is then one of *extent*. The lesion is visible, its histology is known—but just how far does it go? This is the role of the radiologist.

THE EAR

THE EXTERNAL EAR

Anatomy and physiology

The external ear canal is 2–3 cm in length. While the outer one-third is lined by conventional desquamating stratified epithelium, the inner two-thirds is lined by highly specialized and unique skin directly attached to periosteum without an intervening dermal layer. This skin does not desquamate and has no hair; instead it has the unique ability of lateral migration and contains highly specialized wax to assist in toilet.

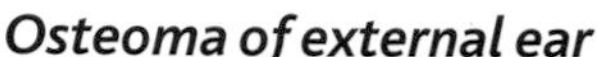

Pathology

In the ENT clinic, otitis externa, characterized by irritation and discharge, rarely requires imaging. Three conditions superficially similar to otitis externa and characterized by stenosis of the external auditory meatus (EAM) are frequently referred for imaging:

- squamous carcinoma of external ear
- 'malignant' otitis externa
- osteoma of external ear.

Squamous or basal cell carcinoma

Clinical diagnosis is easy; extent needs to be defined by cross-sectional imaging. High resolution CT (HRCT) will define the extent of bone erosion or destruction. MRI will allow better delineation of the precise extent of the soft tissue mass. Most of the information can be derived from T1- and T2-weighted images; intravenous contrast medium can add information.

Malignant otitis externa

This is a poor descriptive term. The pathology is an osteomyelitis of the outer petrous bone (Fig. 62.1). The word 'malignant' was coined because of the high mortality of the condition. A typical patient is elderly and diabetic. *Pseudomonas* is a typical organism. As the disease spreads, the facial nerve is involved, leading to palsy.

Osteoma of external ear

These benign tumours may arise spontaneously, but usually occur in those individuals fond of swimming in cold water. They enlarge slowly and usually present late with conductive deafness when the tumour fills the external meatus. CT demonstrates the typical homogeneous, well-defined dense tumour (Fig. 62.2). These tumours are surgically easy to remove but leave exposed bone in the EAM. Due to the unique nature of the skin of the EAM, it is impossible to cover or graft the bone and soft tissue re-stenosis is an almost certain consequence.

THE MIDDLE EAR

Anatomy and physiology

The tympanic membrane separates the middle ear from the external ear. The membrane is tough, normally translucent and held in tension by the action of tensor tympani. A small region, the pars flaccida in the most superior part of the drum, is less rigid than the rest of the drum (the pars tensa) and is of importance in the genesis of keratoma (see below).

The middle ear cleft is a small air-containing space (approximately 1 ml), connected to the pharynx by the Eustachian tube. Its anatomy is complex and outside the scope of this book. It contains:

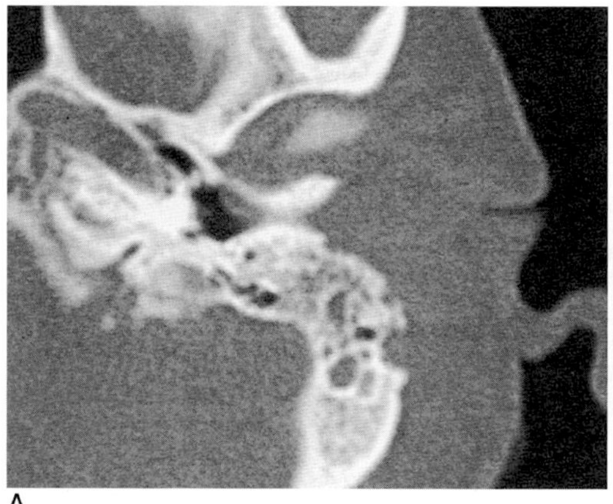

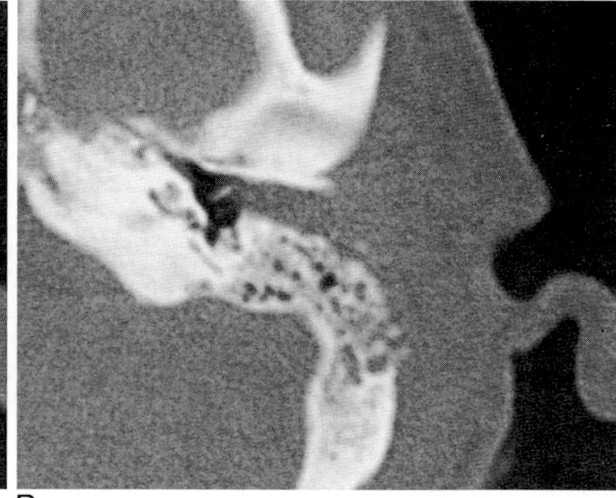

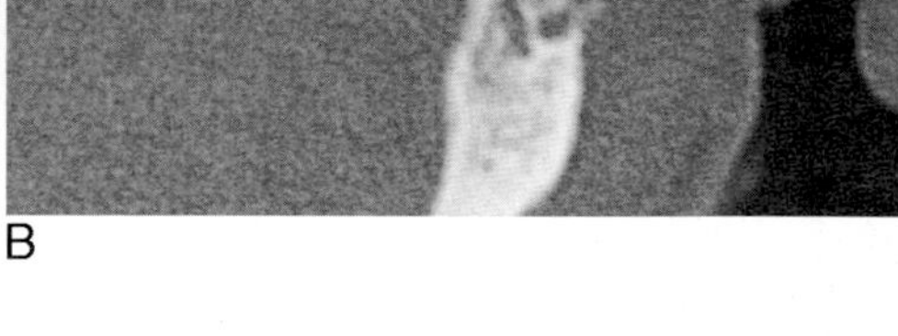

A B

Figure 62.1 Elderly diabetic man with a mass raising pinna. (A) CT: note the large and diffuse soft tissue mass, erosion of the cortical bone of the mastoid and the opacity of the mastoid air cells. (B) CT at level of external auditory meatus (EAM) shows an inflammatory mass filling the EAM but not extending into the middle ear cleft.

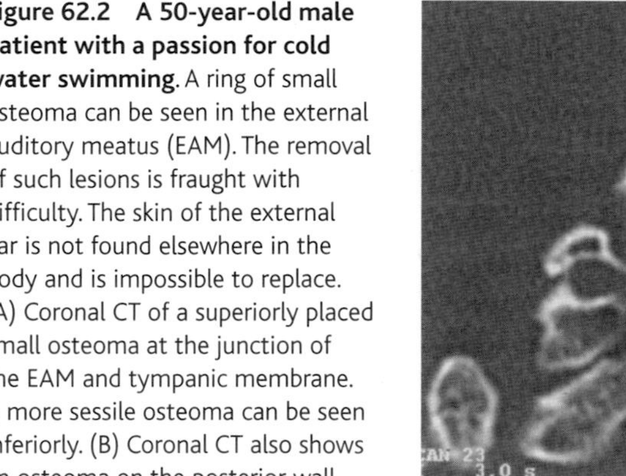

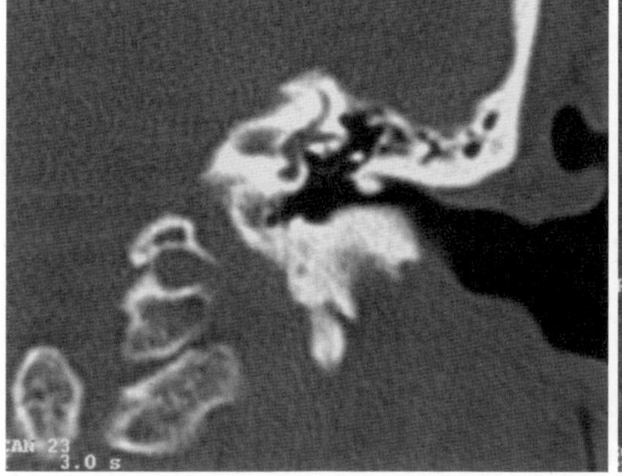

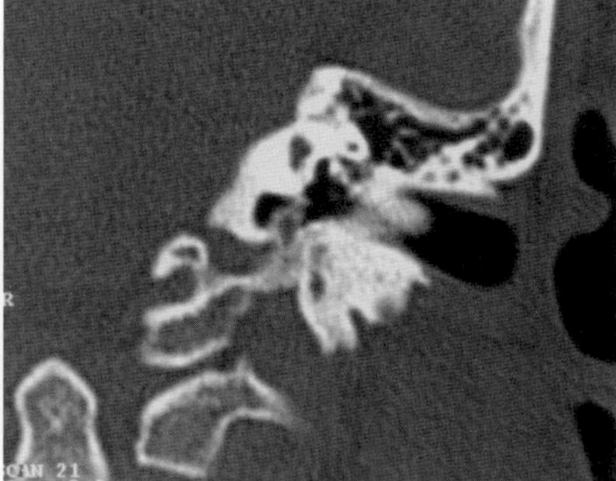

A B

Figure 62.2 A 50-year-old male patient with a passion for cold water swimming. A ring of small osteoma can be seen in the external auditory meatus (EAM). The removal of such lesions is fraught with difficulty. The skin of the external ear is not found elsewhere in the body and is impossible to replace. (A) Coronal CT of a superiorly placed small osteoma at the junction of the EAM and tympanic membrane. A more sessile osteoma can be seen inferiorly. (B) Coronal CT also shows an osteoma on the posterior wall.

- bones: malleus, incus and stapes
- muscles: tensor tympani and stapedius
- nerves: facial nerve.

Medial wall features include:
- promontory of cochlea
- promontory of horizontal semicircular canal
- round and oval windows
- facial nerve.

Important anatomical relationships include:
- mastoid air cells
- lateral venous sinus and jugular bulb
- carotid canal
- intracranial compartment and temporal lobe.

Pathology

Common pathological processes requiring imaging include:
- chronic suppurative otitis media and keratoma
- otosclerosis
- venous sinus thrombosis
- intracranial complications.

Chronic suppurtive otitis media and keratoma

This is regarded as 'safe' if there is no evidence of a bone destructive process and 'unsafe' if there is. The former requires no radiological intervention. The latter frequently requires intensive investigation using HRCT (preferably in the coronal plane; Fig. 62.3).

The primary problem lies with dysfunction of the Eustachian tube. As a consequence of negative pressure within the middle ear, the pars flaccida of the tympanic membrane is drawn inwards. When the epithelium of the pars flaccida can desquamate and be cleared by natural processes of external ear toilet, no problem arises. When this process fails, desquamated skin accumulates and forms a ball of skin—a keratoma (more frequently and incorrectly called a cholesteatoma). This can enlarge and cause bone destruction.

Otosclerosis

This is divided into two types depending on whether the hearing loss is conductive or sensorineural:

Fenestral—This is a process by which the stapes foot plate is fused to the oval window, preventing proper transmission of sound and leading to conductive hearing loss. It can be detected by HRCT (Fig. 62.4).

Retrofenestral—This is more properly an osteoporosis of the dense bone around the cochlear and labyrinth, leading to sensorineural hearing loss. Again, it can be demonstrated by HRCT.

Venous sinus thrombosis

The lateral venous sinus is an immediate relation of the posterior wall of the mastoid. Posterior extension of sepsis can cause venous thrombosis with consequent intracranial complications, e.g. haemorrhagic infarction.

Intracranial complications

These complications are mainly those of sepsis. Infection can spread to cause:

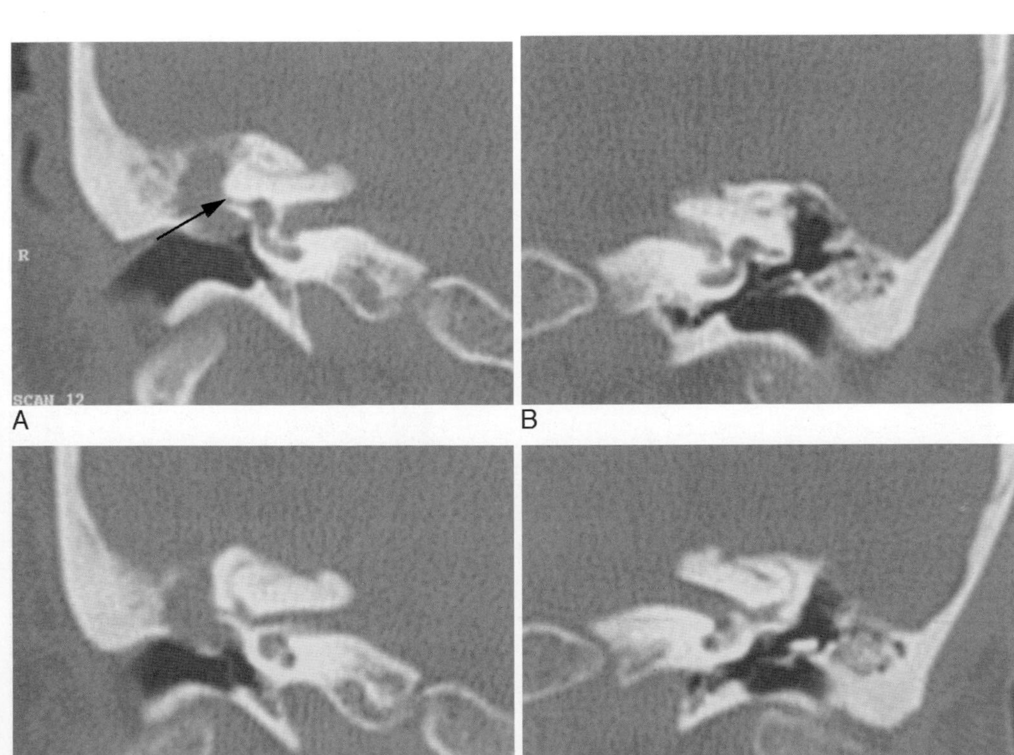

Figure 62.3 Chronic suppurative otitis media. The surgeon sees the 'tip of the iceberg' when he looks into the external auditory meatus (EAM). (A) Coronal CT showing erosion of horizontal semicircular canal (HSCC, arrow), with normal (B) for comparison. A large mass can be seen filling the attic. It has eroded into the HSCC, destroyed the ossicles and partially covers the oval window. (C) Coronal CT of erosion of the lateral wall. By comparing this with the normal side (D) the destruction of the lateral attic wall can be easily appreciated.

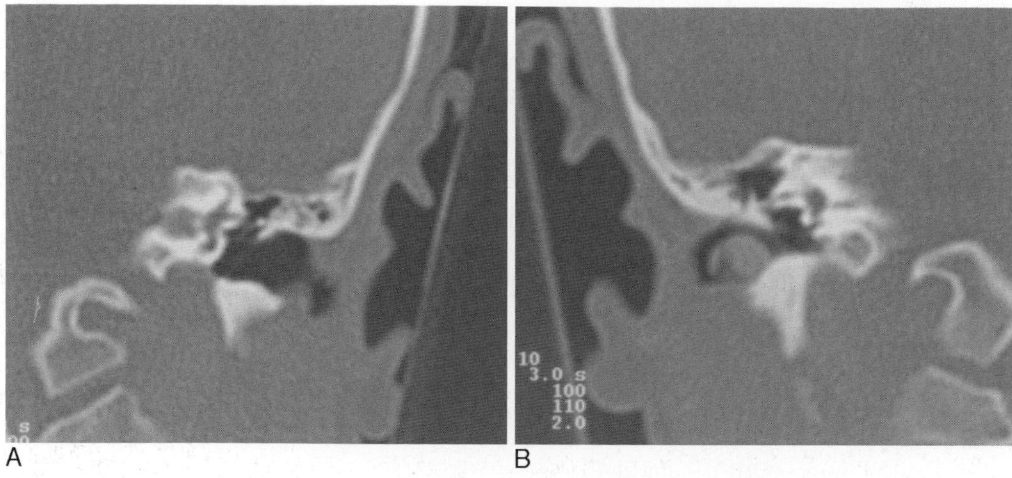

Figure 62.4 A patient with conductive hearing loss. By comparing the normal (A) and abnormal (B) sides on CT, the narrowing of the oval window can be clearly appreciated. This results in fixation of the stapes footplate and conductive hearing loss.

- extradural empyema
- subdural empyema
- cerebral abscess.

THE INNER EAR

Anatomy and physiology

Sound is transmitted from the tympanic membrane, via the ossicles, to the oval window and thence to the perilymph. Mechanical vibrations pass to the apical turn of the cochlear and return via the endolymph to the round window. As the ratio of the area of the tympanic membrane-to-oval window cross-section is 20:1, there is mechanical amplification. Hair cells in the cochlea respond to specific frequencies. Frequencies up to 20 kHz are perceived in the basal turn, down to 20 Hz in the apical turns. The range of intensity of sound perception is huge and is expressed in a logarithmic decibel scale of 0–120 dB. As an illustration, a quiet whisper is 30 dB, a lawnmower runs at 90 dB and a jet plane at takeoff is 120 dB.

The electrical output of the hair cells passes to the spiral ganglion contained in the cochlea and then in the cochlear nerves (part of the acoustic nerve) to the brainstem. Within the brainstem, nerve fibres synapse and pass in ipsi- and contralateral pathways to the medial geniculate body and then on to Heschel's gyrus in the temporal lobe.

The semicircular canal system consists of three rings at right angles to each other, and contains fluid which stimulates hair cells. These cells continue to form the superior and inferior vestibular nerves. They pass to the brainstem and are involved in reflexes involved in the control of balance via the flocculonodular lobe of the cerebellum.

Pathology

Common disease processes requiring imaging include:

- acoustic neuroma
- trauma
- glomus tumours
- facial palsy
- congenital malformations
- cochlear implantation
- bony dysplasias.

Acoustic neuroma

When these occur sporadically they are technically schwannomas. When bilateral, they indicate a diagnosis of neurofibromatosis type II.

Any patient with asymmetric sensorineural hearing loss or tinnitus could have an acoustic neuroma. However, in the vast majority the nerve has simply ceased to function. In the small minority with a tumour (perhaps 1 in 40), the size of the mass bears little relationship to the degree of deafness. Indeed a patient with a large tumour may present with signs of brainstem distortion before any features of deafness are present. This is a classical dilemma in ENT practice. A patient with asymmetrical sensorineural hearing loss *probably* has nothing, but *possibly* has a tumour which could range in diameter from a few millimetres to a few centimetres.

The wider availability of MRI has solved the clinical dilemma—high-resolution MRI can detect the smallest tumours and exclude lesions in the vast majority. The logistical and cost implications of this are, however, highly significant, especially when the yield (often < 1:40) is so small.

The choice between high resolution T2-weighted images and gadolinium-enhanced T1-weighted examinations as the optimal method of detection of small intracanalicular tumours remains a subject of much debate (Table 62.1). A contrast-enhanced study will detect tiny (1 mm) tumours missed by even the best high resolution T2 study, but their significance remains debatable (Fig. 62.5).

Trauma

Skull base fractures involving the petrous bone are uncommon, but are very important to identify because:

- there may be an associated CSF leak
- the facial nerve may be damaged
- the ossicular chain may be disrupted.

HRCT allows accurate detection and delineation of fractures. If this is performed, the classical discrimination into longitudinal and transverse subtypes becomes less common because

Table 62.1 ADVANTAGES AND DISADVANTAGES BETWEEN HIGH RESOLUTION T2-WEIGHTED AND CONTRAST-ENHANCED T1-WEIGHTED MRI

	High resolution T2	Contrast-enhanced T1
For	Inexpensive	Expensive (cost of contrast medium and additional examination time)
	Single sequence	Three sequences pre- and post-contrast and T2 weighted
Against	May miss tiny lesions	Requires injection of contrast medium
		Requires cover for possible reactions

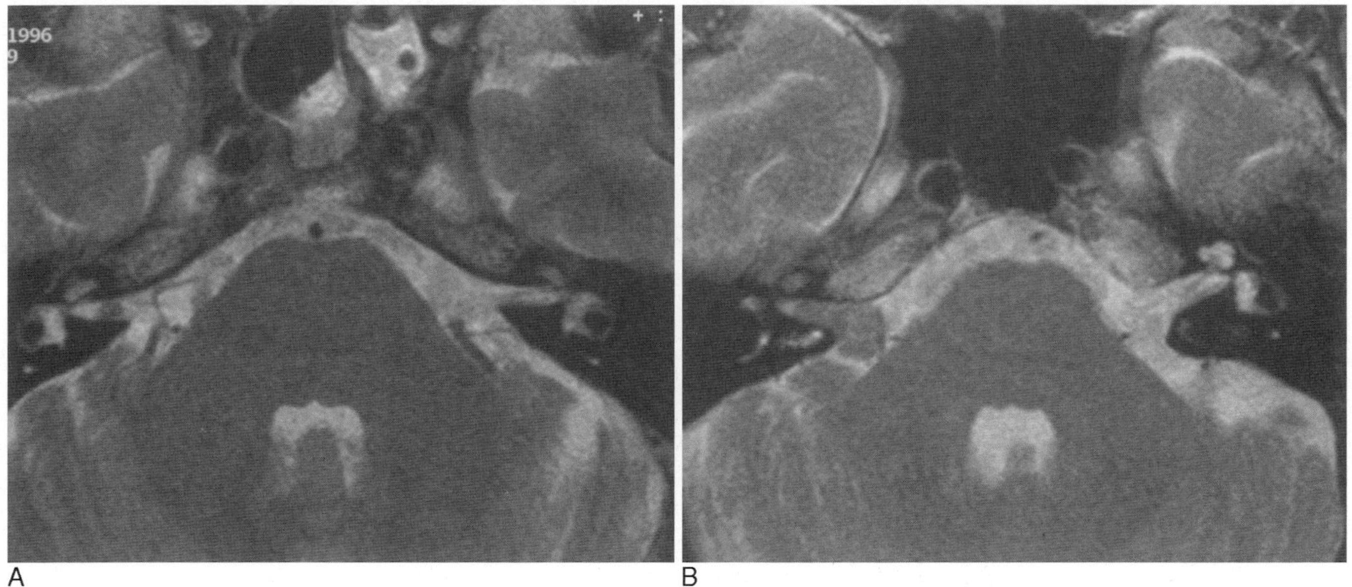

Figure 62.5 Acoustic neuromas. T2-weighted MRIs showing a small intracanalicular (A) and a larger cerebellopontine angle acoustic neuroma (B).

most are, in fact, complex. The fracture line almost inevitably takes a complex course through a complex bone!

Glomus tumours

Glomus jugulare tumours arise from chemoreceptor cells in the jugular bulb. Glomus tympanicum tumours arise close to the tympanic membrane. They both present clinically with tinnitus and as masses in the inferior aspect of the tympanic membrane. Once again, there is the classical clinical dilemma—is this tumour confined to what can be seen down an otoscope or is it the tip of a much larger tumour arising from the jugular bulb and spreading in the skull base?

CT and MRI are complementary (Fig. 62.6). CT assesses the bone destruction in the margins of the jugular bulb; fat-suppressed contrast-enhanced MRI assesses the tumour itself. Great care must be taken in the assessment of these lesions. There is a large amount of normal variation in the jugular bulb in terms of size and shape. There is complex turbulence of blood in the jugular bulb which may give rise to artefact on MRI. A glomus tumour is a vascular tumour within a vascular structure and errors of commission and omission can easily be made.

Facial palsy

Facial nerve palsy is an extremely unpleasant disorder for the patient. Apart from the problems associated with dribbling and spilling of food and drink, the loss of facial animation can lead to significant social and employment problems.

Bell's palsy is frequently seen clinically but is uncommonly imaged. A typical patient develops a sudden facial paralysis which recovers fully or incompletely after 2–3 months. If imaging is undertaken, pathological enhancement of the nerve is well described. Imaging is mandatory for atypical cases or where there is some unusual historical or clinical feature. High resolution MRI studies may reveal any number of lesions affecting the nerve from without. Intrinsic nerve lesions may demonstrate nerve swelling, signal change on T2-weighted sequences or contrast enhancement.

Congenital malformations

Malformations of the cochlea and/or labyrinth may be isolated or part of a more widespread craniofacial syndrome. There may be associated abnormalities of the middle ear, external ear, or pinna. A discussion of this extremely complex subject is outside the scope of this chapter. If a congenital malformation is suggested, it is best to go through a checklist of potential sites

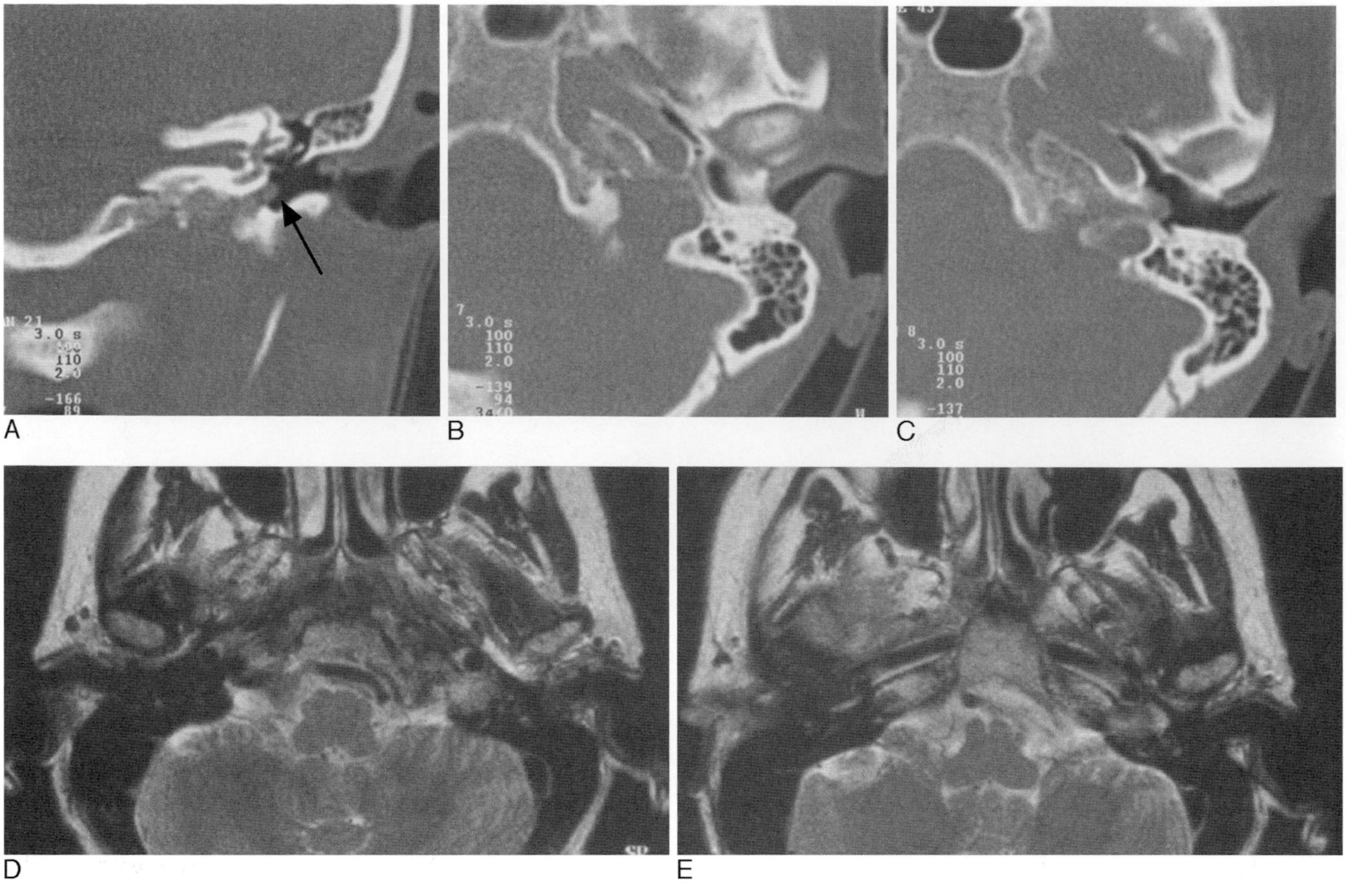

Figure 62.6 Glomus jugulare tumours. (A) Note the small soft tissue mass in contact with the inferior aspect of the tympanic membrane on coronal CT (arrow). This cannot be separated from the jugular bulb and there is loss of clarity of the bony wall of the bulb. (B) On axial CT note the lack of clarity of the bony margin of the jugular foramen. (C) The small mass projecting into the hypotympanum can be clearly seen on axial CT. (D) The high signal of the tumour can be clearly seen on axial T2-weighted MRI. Note the normal petrous bone on the other side and which is essentially black on T2-weighted images (bone, air and flowing jugular bulb blood are all black on T2-weighted images). (E) The small projection into the hypotympanum can be readily appreciated on axial T2-weighted MRI.

of abnormality—congenital malformations are rarely solitary if you look hard enough.

HRCT is the investigation of choice (Fig. 62.7) and high resolution MRI is complementary. Axial (±coronal) images allow accurate description of the abnormalities, which may include:

- cochlea: structure of basal turn; number of turns in modiolus
- vestibule: enlargement
- semicircular canal: absence; morphological abnormalities
- oval and round windows: position; orientation
- ossicles: fusion; malposition
- middle ear cleft: orientation; ventilation
- internal and external meatus: orientation; calibre
- position of jugular bulb: enlarged or absent; intact or dehiscent.

While it is possible to offer an eponymous title for some of the more common defects, it is preferable for the nonexpert to leave the description in plain English, for all to understand.

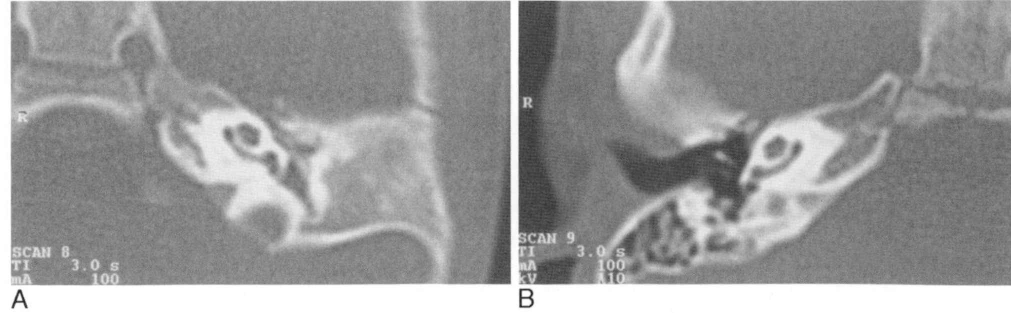

Figure 62.7 Congenital malformation of the ear. (A) Axial CT at same level as normal side. The whole of the external ear has failed to develop and is seen as a solid mass of bone. The middle ear is poorly developed and abnormally ventilated. Note also the high jugular bulb. (B) CT of normal anatomy for comparison. Note the well-developed and ventilated external auditory meatus and the cellular and ventilated mastoid.

Cochlear electrode implantation

Implantable cochlear electrodes offer a chance of hearing for some individuals, typically those whose hearing has been damaged by childhood meningitis. An array of electrodes (typically 16) is surgically introduced into the cochlea and then connected to a very complex 'black box' which is capable of spectral and volume analysis of incoming sound. After effort on behalf of the patient, good hearing can be 'learned'. Assessment of the patency of the lumen of the cochlea is an essential pre-operative requirement. HRCT will assess bony patency and high resolution MRI will then exclude fibrous adhesions within the cochlea, which might prevent passage of the electrode array.

Bony dysplasias

The petrous bone, like any other bone, may be involved in dysplasias of which the most common is fibrous dysplasia. In this disorder, the characteristic change in texture with mild expansion is easily diagnostic on HRCT. It can be mimicked by the hyperostosis induced by an intracranial meningioma.

THE NOSE AND PARANASAL SINUSES

Anatomy

The external nose consists of bone superiorly and a cartilaginous structure inferiorly. Arterial blood supply is derived from facial and ethmoidal arteries and may bleed profusely after trauma. Venous drainage into the angular vein in the medial canthus of the eye explains how nasal sepsis can spread to involve the cavernous sinus and how damage to this results in profuse subcutaneous bleeding around the eye—a 'black eye'.

The integrity of the anterior nasal cavity is maintained by the cartilaginous septum which is supported more posteriorly by the vomer. Posteriorly the cavity continues in the midline on either side of the septum. The medial nasal wall is thus the septum. The lateral nasal wall is complex and supports the three turbinates (superior, middle, inferior) and their associated airway or meatus. Thus the middle meatus lies inferior to the middle turbinate of the lateral wall of the nose.

The middle meatus is functionally the most important. It receives mucosal drainage from all the paranasal sinuses except the posterior ethmoid and sphenoid sinuses which drain into the sphenoethmoid recess. The introduction of rigid and flexible endoscopes enables these areas to be directly visualized by the ENT surgeon and has removed the need for plain radiography.

The lining of the nose is a pseudostratified ciliated columnar epithelium common to the rest of the respiratory tract. A specialized sensory epithelium lies on either side of the septum immediately beneath the cribriform plate. The neurones are specialized nonmyelinated fibres communicating with the olfactory bulbs superiorly. The most common cause of anosmia (loss of smell) is lack of ventilation of this specialized mucosa by excessive mucus.

The paranasal sinuses (frontal, ethmoid, maxillary and sphenoid) are similarly lined by a ciliated epithelium containing numerous goblet cells producing mucus. Mucus is moved from the nose and paranasal sinuses by two mechanisms:

1 *Ciliary action*—may be absent in congenital disorders such as Kartagener's syndrome, or after inhalation of toxins such as cigarette smoke.
2 *Slime trails*—mucus is swept into 'rivers of slime' by the action of cilia. Such rivers are visible by nasoendoscopy and pass into the throat. The action of swallowing 'tugs' the river of slime and assists nasal clearance of mucosa.

Physiology

The nose and nasal airway serve a number of functions:

- sense (smell)
- respiration
- air conditioner
- immune response to antigens
- sound quality.

Smell

The sense of smell adds enormously to the quality of life. Smell is a major feature of taste.

Anosmia follows when the olfactory mucosa is unventilated (common) or rarely if there is a tumour disturbing the nerves (carcinoma, esthesioneuroblastoma [Fig. 62.8], meningioma).

Respiration

The newborn baby is an obligate nasal breather. If there is choanal atresia, the baby may not be able to survive. This reliance on nasal respiration continues into adult life. In adults, mouth breathing is usually only necessary during exertion.

Air conditioning

The air conditioning function of the nose involves:

- *Heat exchange*—cold inspired air is warmed; warm expired air transfers its heat back into the nasal mucosa.
- *Humidification*—dry air is almost 100% saturated with water vapour by the time it reaches the alveoli.
- *Cleaning*—larger particles are removed; small dusts pass into the lung.

The key to these functions is the mucous blanket. Mucous production and movement is essential for proper nasal function.

Immune response

Antibodies in the nasal mucosa are in the first line of defence against air-borne pathogens. Over-reaction to allergens (as in hayfever or asthma) is uncomfortable and unpleasant and leads to mucosal thickening, oversecretion of mucus and airway obstruction.

Speech

Listening to anyone with a cold illustrates the importance of the nose in the quality of speech. The nose and sinuses act as a resonant chamber.

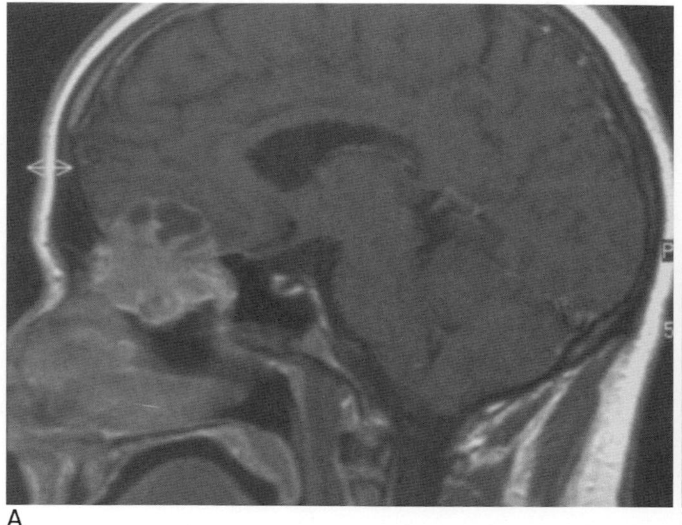
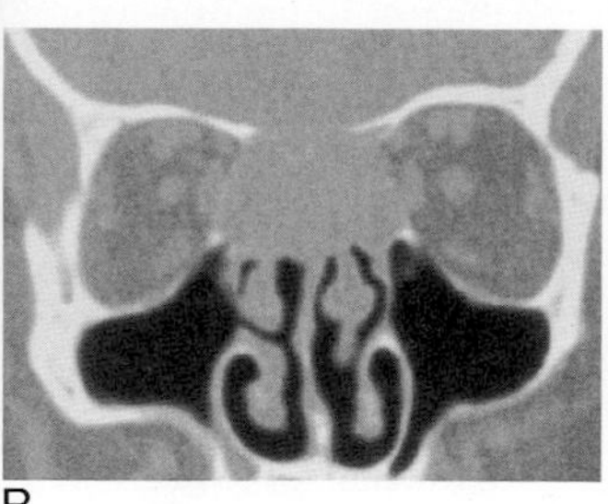

Figure 62.8 Esthesioneuroblastoma. (A) Contrast-enhanced sagittal T1-weighted MRI of mass based on cribriform plate. Note the extension inferiorly into the nose and superiorly into the brain. (B) Coronal CT shows the bony destruction of the cribriform plate and a soft tissue mass in the ethmoid. The differential diagnosis would include an ethmoid carcinoma.

Radiology and pathology

Plain radiographs are of assistance in the detection of gross disease, but interpretation is fraught with difficulty due to the great variation in normal appearance of the paranasal sinuses, and the presence of so many complex overlapping three-dimensional structures in a two-dimensional image. This is a classical example of a simple and widely available investigation which requires major expertise for correct interpretation. In any event, the advent of nasoendoscopy has allowed the surgeon direct visual access to structures hitherto invisible and has further reduced the need for plain radiographs. CT and MRI make a large and complementary contribution to the determination of the extent of disease.

Rhinosinusitis

This is an extremely common condition which is usually treated medically. Radiological investigation is rarely required unless surgical intervention is contemplated. There are a number of common causes:

- allergic—very common. Specific allergens such as pollen precipitate an immune response resulting in mucosal swelling. This may develop into allergic polyposis
- vasomotor—a disorder of autonomic regulation of nasal mucus production
- infective—all will be aware of the symptoms of the common cold
- mechanical—as in deviation of the nasal septum
- ciliary disorders—Kartagener's syndrome
- iatrogenic—overuse of nasal decongestants can result in rebound hyperaemia and finally atrophic rhinitis.

A proper understanding of nasal physiology and the development of minimally invasive surgery has changed the surgical approach away from invasive and destructive treatments (e.g. radical antrostomy—Caldwell Luc) towards logical approaches to the osteomeatal complex, such as uncinectomy to widen the ostium of the maxillary antrum. Pre-operative assessment of the bony anatomy of the nose is an essential prerequisite, best performed with coronal CT. This assessment should include:

- Identification of congenital variation: deviated nasal septum; hypoplasia and enlargement of normal structures; anomalous air cells, e.g. Haller, Ager nasi.
- Identification of extent of disease: which sinuses are involved, which spared; is the osteomeatal complex involved?; is the sphenoethmoidal recess involved?; does disease extend into orbit or cranium?
- Identification of bone destruction—this may indicate malignancy
- Identification of complications: orbital or intracranial abscess.

Almost all this information can be obtained from CT. Given the high inherent contrast in the paranasal sinus system, a low dose technique may be employed and, following the introduction of spiral CT, this investigation is commonly performed at an axial volume acquisition, subsequently reconstructed to give coronal images. However, the sphenoethmoidal recess and the posterior wall of the frontal sinus are best examined in the axial plane. Complications or suspected malignant disease may well require further contrast-enhanced studies employing higher radiographic dose rates to improve soft tissue contrast.

Common problems requiring imaging include:

- nasal polyposis
- antrochoanal polyp
- mucocoeles
- fractures
- epistaxis
- nasal and paranasal tumours.

Nasal polyposis (Fig. 62.9)

This is a common condition in adults. If it is seen in children, cystic fibrosis is a possible cause, and midline congenital anomalies such as meningocoele or encephalocoele need to be considered and excluded.

The aetiology of polyposis is uncertain, but allergy is important. Polyps can be controlled by steroids, but surgery is frequently required. Such polyps can usually be resected using an endoscope, in which case pre-operative assessment as above is sufficient.

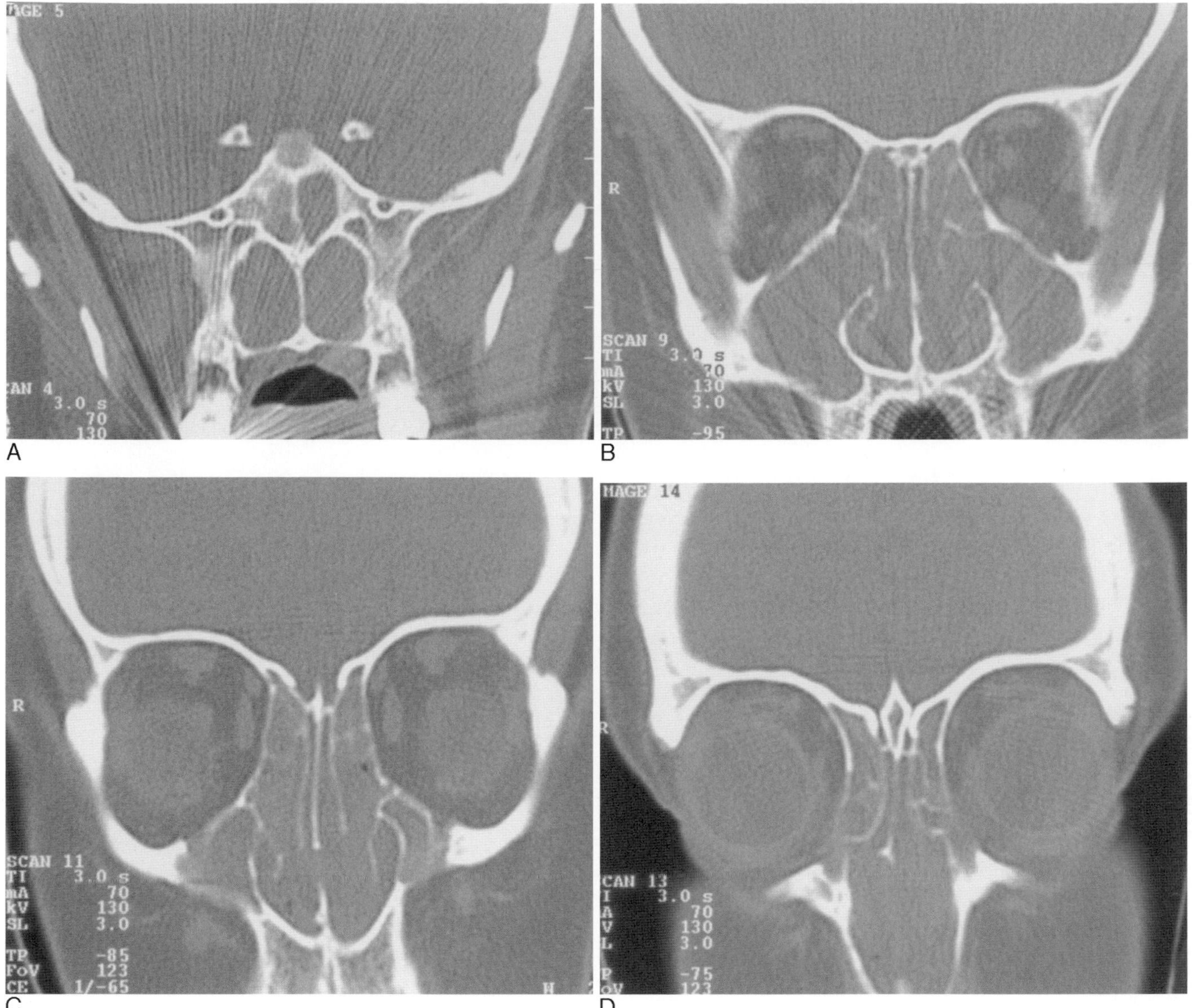

Figure 62.9 Severe nasal polyposis and airway obstruction. Four consecutive CT images, running posterior to anterior. (A) Level of posterior choana. Note the complete opacity of the normal airway. Note also marked streak artefacts from dental fillings. (B) Level of the ostia of the maxillary antra. Note again the complete opacity of the nasal airway. The ostea are widened by benign polyps and the nasal turbinates are partially eroded. (C) Level of the anterior nasal airway. Again there is complete obliteration of the airway by polyps. Note the thinning of the bone of the ethmoids. (D) Anterior nose. The polyps protrude from the sinuses into the anterior nose.

Antrochoanal polyp

This is a special unilateral polyp which arises in the maxillary antrum, passes out through the ostium which it enlarges, and then projects backwards into the postnasal space. It causes unilateral nasal obstruction. The radiological hallmark is the enlarged ostium (Fig. 62.10).

Mucocoeles

A normal sinus produces mucus, which clears by gravitational drainage and ciliary action. If the sinus ostium becomes blocked and infection does not supervene, the sinus fills with mucus. The mucus acts then as a slow-growing mass lesion, expanding the sinus and thinning the sinus wall—a mucocoele. These lesions are painless and give rise to little or no symptoms until the mass effect becomes a critical issue. Posterior ethmoid mucocoeles may encroach upon the optic nerve and lead to visual failure. Frontal or anterior ethmoid mucocoeles may extend into the orbit and give rise to proptosis.

Diagnosis is best made with CT, which will show the characteristic sinus expansion with a very thin membrane of bone surrounding it.

Mucocoeles are usually sterile, but can become infected. This is frequently a dramatic clinical presentation with rapid onset of pain and fever. Clearly an infection can rapidly spread to adjacent tissues and urgent surgical drainage is essential.

Fractures

Nasal bones Fractures of the nasal bones are common sequelae of fights. Plain radiographs are sufficient to document the injury, although they are frequently not required in simple fractures.

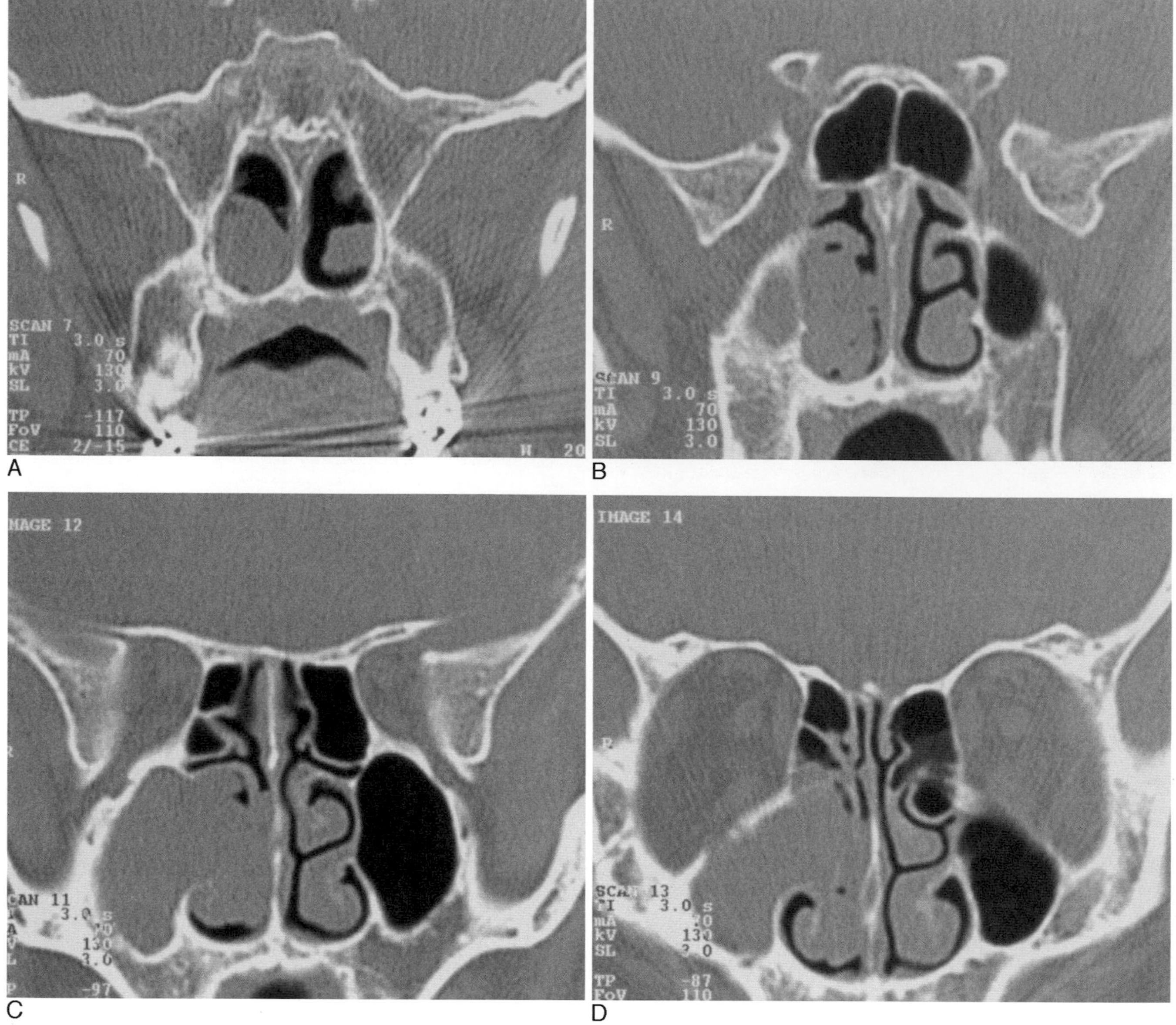

Figure 62.10 Antrochoanal polyp. Four consecutive CT images, running posterior to anterior. These benign lesions arise in the maxillary antrum close to the osteum, pass through the osteum into the middle meatus then turn 90 degrees to run posteriorly along the middle turbinate to the posterior choana. (A) Level of posterior choanal shows the posterior extent of the normal turbinates on the left side and the polyp on the right side. (B) More anterior image showing polyp intimately related to turbinates. (C) Polyp in the maxillary antrum, widening osteum, lying between middle and inferior turbinates. (D) More anterior image showing polyp traversing antrum and nasal airway.

Zygoma, orbit and middle face fractures These are beyond the scope of this chapter. Such fractures are best assessed by HRCT. Three-dimensional CT is of great value to the surgeon planning reconstruction of complex facial fractures.

'Blow-out' fractures Fist or small high velocity (e.g. squash) ball injuries to the orbit raise the intra-orbital pressure and lead to fracture of the orbital floor. The orbital fat, inferior oblique and inferior rectus muscles will prolapse into the maxillary sinus and become trapped (Fig. 62.11).

Epistaxis does not usually require radiological assessment. If the bleeding is profuse or recurrent, then a source for the bleeding may require investigation. Causes include:

- bleeding polyps.
- juvenile angiofibroma (male preponderance).
- carcinoma or other malignancy: nose, sinuses, nasopharynx.
- Wegener's granuloma.

Severe uncontrolled epistaxis may be life-threatening and requires drastic intervention. Contrast angiography and selective embolization of bleeding vessels may be life-saving. If such a service is available, the old-fashioned ligation of the external carotid artery will not be required.

Nasal and paranasal tumours

Clinical presentations include facial deformity (with or without pain), nerve involvement leading to pain, dysaesthesia and

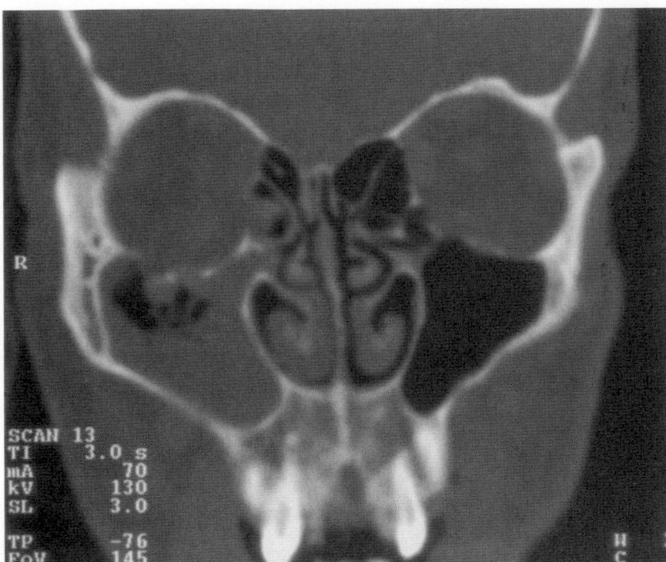

Figure 62.11 'Blow-out' fracture. Coronal CT shows normal orbital floor and ventilated antrum on left, depressed floor and blood in antrum on right. The orbit shows some opacity of the fat adjacent to the fracture due to oedema and haemorrhage. The inferior rectus is swollen but remains in the orbit. Untreated, this patient is at risk from disfiguring enophthalmos.

anaesthesia and loss of function (e.g. airway obstruction). The pathological processes include a number of very uncommon disorders which may confuse a pathologist, let alone a radiologist. The radiologist's job is one of defining extent rather than predicting histological diagnosis. Tumours vary from indolent through to very malignant.

Common indications for radiological imaging include:

- osteoma
- fibro-osseous lesions
- inverting papilloma
- juvenile angiofibroma
- granulomatous conditions
- malignant tumours.

Osteoma (Fig. 62.12) These are the most common benign tumour. They can arise anywhere but are most frequent in the frontal sinus. They are frequently incidental findings and are usually isolated. They can be part of a genetic disorder such as Gardner's syndrome.

Fibro-osseous lesions (Fig. 62.13) This is a spectrum of pathology with a purely fibrotic lesion at one end and a dysplastic bony lesion at the other. These lesions may produce considerable facial deformity and be very difficult to treat.

Inverting papilloma These frequently present as a unilateral nasal polyp causing obstruction and epistaxis. They are locally invasive tumours and require full surgical excision. Pre-operative assessment is usually satisfactory with CT, although MRI can provide additional information.

Juvenile angiofibroma Adolescent boys with heavy epistaxis characterize the disease. The tumour may be very fibrous in some individuals, more angiomatous in others. HRCT allows accurate diagnosis since these tumours start in the pterygopalatine fissure and enlarge this before they extend. The presence of a nasal mass and a widened fissure is therefore pathognomonic of the condition.

It is important to stress that these tumours may spread across the skull base and a combination of CT (to assess bone destruction; Fig. 62.14A) and contrast-enhanced MRI (to assess soft tissue extent; Fig. 62.14B–E) may be required to provide accurate pre-operative assessment. Angiography is not required to establish the diagnosis, but has a valuable role in pre-operative therapeutic embolization to reduce blood loss (Fig.62.14F).

Nasal and paranasal sinus granulomas The precise nature of the various granulomas is a matter for a pathologist. These lesions behave in a similar fashion to malignant tumours, but are characterized by small volume destructive processes leading to loss of much of the nasal bony architecture. There may, of course, be considerable coincident systemic disturbance.

Malignant tumours The types of tumour are listed above in Table 62.2. It is rarely possible to differentiate between the histological types on imaging. The most common type is squamous carcinoma, followed by adenocarcinoma, adenoid cystic carcinoma and melanoma. Lymphoma can occur as a primary tumour or can occur as a metastasis from a primary lesion elsewhere.

As always, the role of radiology is that of defining the *extent* of disease. Radiological reports should deal obsessively with detail of spread in all planes and with structures involved or destroyed. This level of detail is absolutely necessary if the correct decisions are to be taken about whether a surgical approach is appropriate and, if it is appropriate, exactly which approach is required. The radiological report forms the basis for proper planning and informed consent to proposed surgery.

CT and MRI are complementary. CT assesses bone destruction. Multiplanar MRI assesses the soft tissue component more comprehensively and has a major value to the surgeon planning an operation or the radiotherapist planning a portal (Fig. 62.15). Contrast enhancement may be of little help with the definition of the extent of the tumour mass, which is usually easily detected by standard T1 and T2 sequences, but is of enormous value in the detection of spread along nerves.

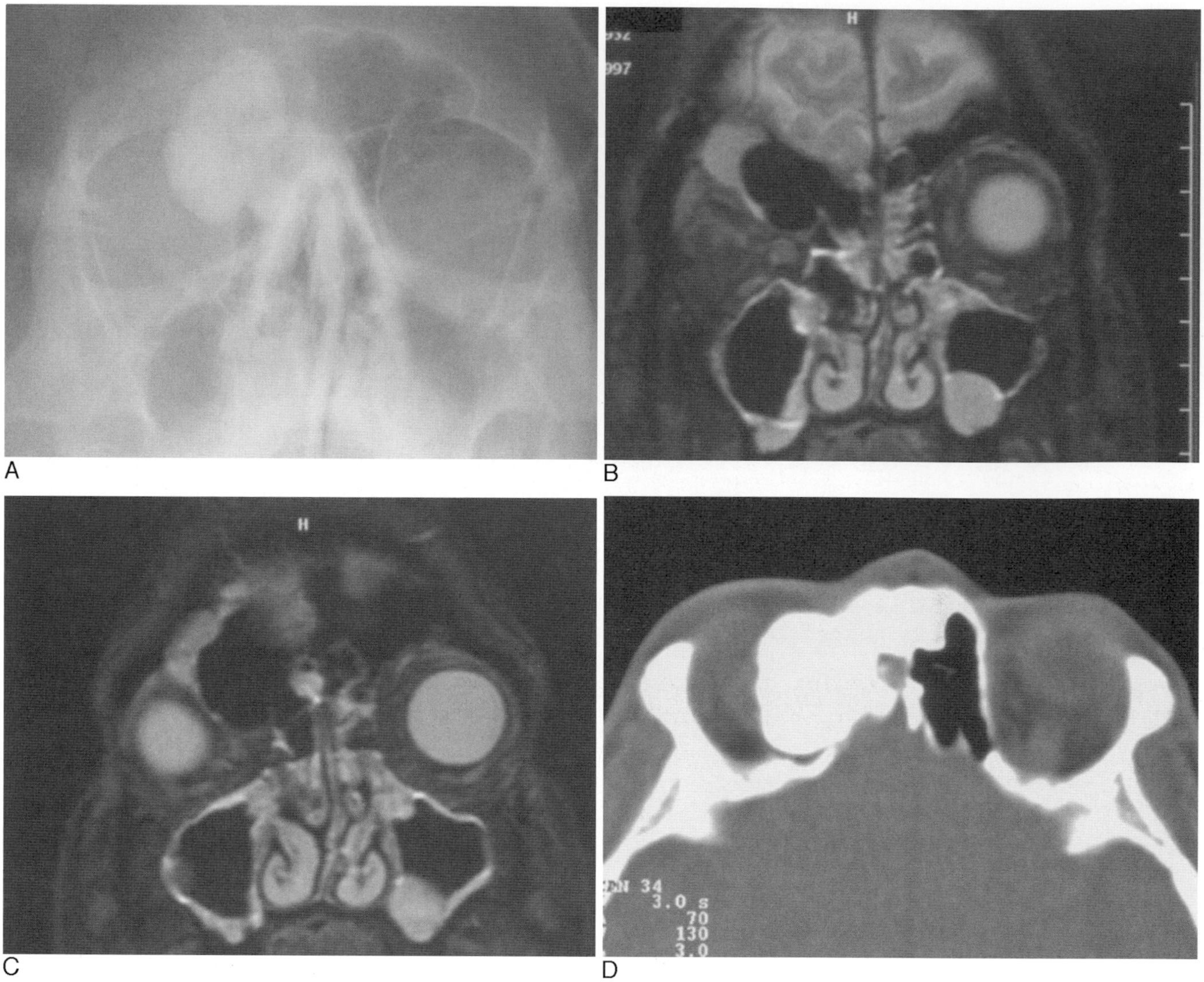

A B C D

Figure 62.12 Osteoma. (A) A rare use for a plain radiograph. The osteoma can be clearly appreciated, but the image gives no details of its involvement with the intracranial space or orbit. (B,C) The coronal STIR images underestimate the lesion since bone and air are both black on T2-weighted MRI. (D) The axial CT shows extension into the orbit.

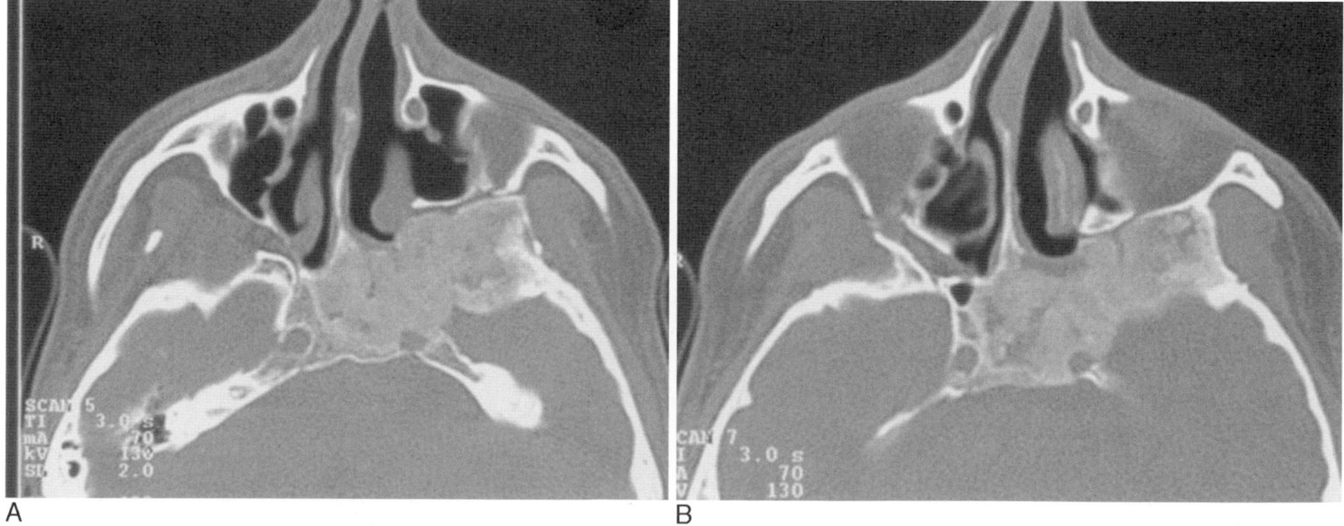

Figure 62.13 Fibro-osseous lesions. (A) The milky texture of bone typical of fibrous dysplasia is seen in this CT. (B) Fibrous dysplasia is a lesion which expands bone—note the compression of the pterygopalatine fissure.

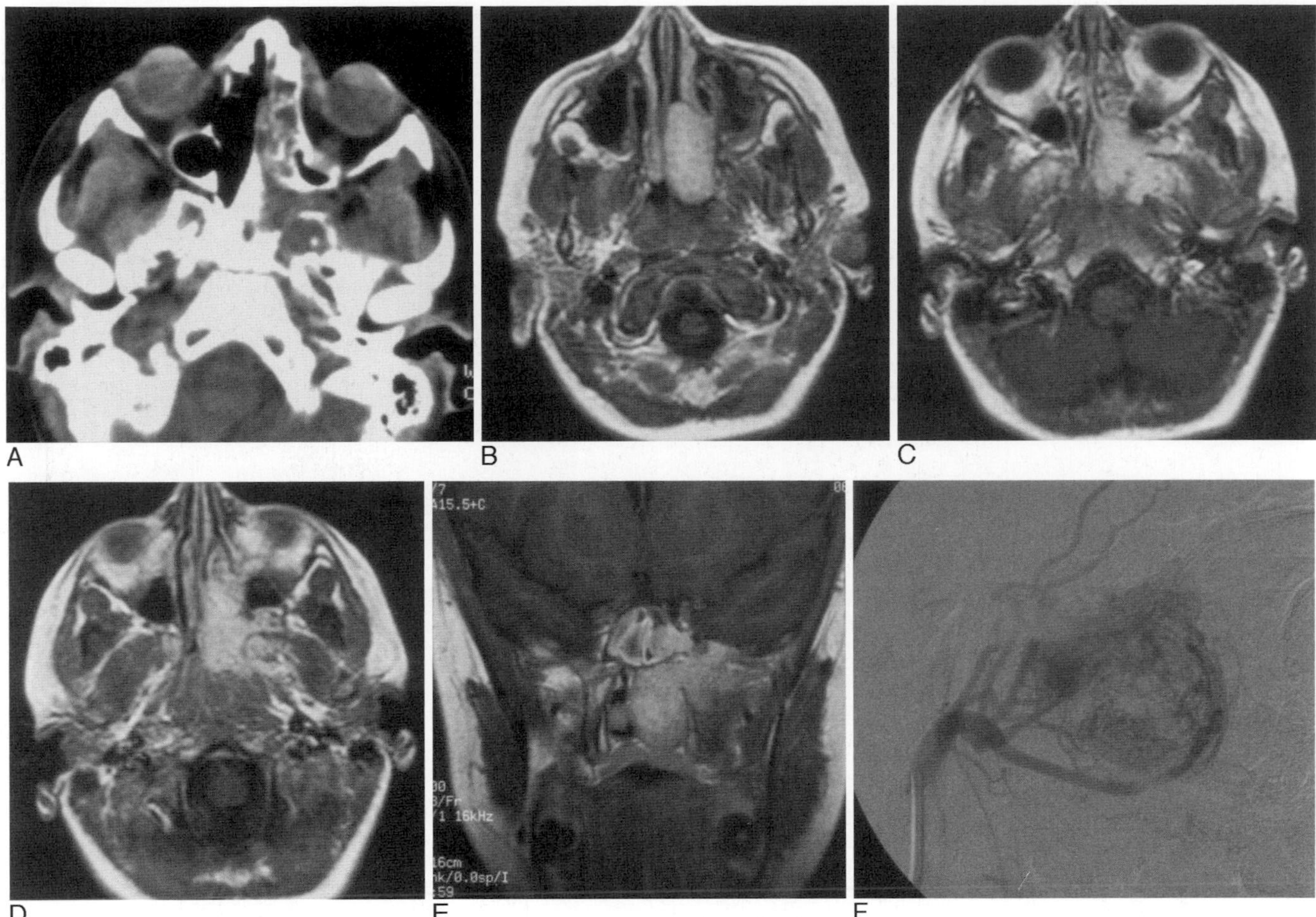

Figure 62.14 Juvenile angiofibroma in a teenager with epistaxis. (A) This axial CT was the first study performed in this patient. The critical finding is widening of the pterygopalatine fissure on the left side. This is virtually diagnostic of an angiofibroma. (B–E) Contrast-enhanced (gadolinium) T1-weighted MRIs. (B) Axial image revealing an enhancing, well-defined mass in the nose. Clinically this was visible from an anterior view through the nose and a posterior view with a mirror in the nasopharynx. (C) Axial image. Note the lateral extension of the tumour towards the infratemporal fossa. (D) Axial image. More superiorly the tumour is less well defined and more infiltrative. Note the extension into the pterygopalatine fissure is visible but more easily seen on CT. (E) Coronal image revealing the mass at the level of the posterior choana with its lateral extension. This is an essential observation for surgical planning. (F) Angiography. Lateral superselective injection into the maxillary artery shows the highly vascular nature of the tumour. This investigation was performed before therapeutic embolization and subsequent surgical resection.

Table 62.2 BENIGN AND MALIGNANT NASAL AND PARANASAL SINUS TUMOURS

	Benign	Malignant
Epithelial tumours	Papilloma	Squamous carcinoma
	Adenoma	Adenocarcinoma
	Inverting papilloma	Melanoma
		Adenoid cystic carcinoma
		Malignant salivary tumours
Mesenchymal tumours	Osteoma	Osteogenic sarcoma
	Ossifying fibroma complex	Fibrosarcoma Angiosarcoma
	Angiofibroma	Chondrosarcoma
	Chondroma	Lymphoma
		Rhabdomyosarcoma

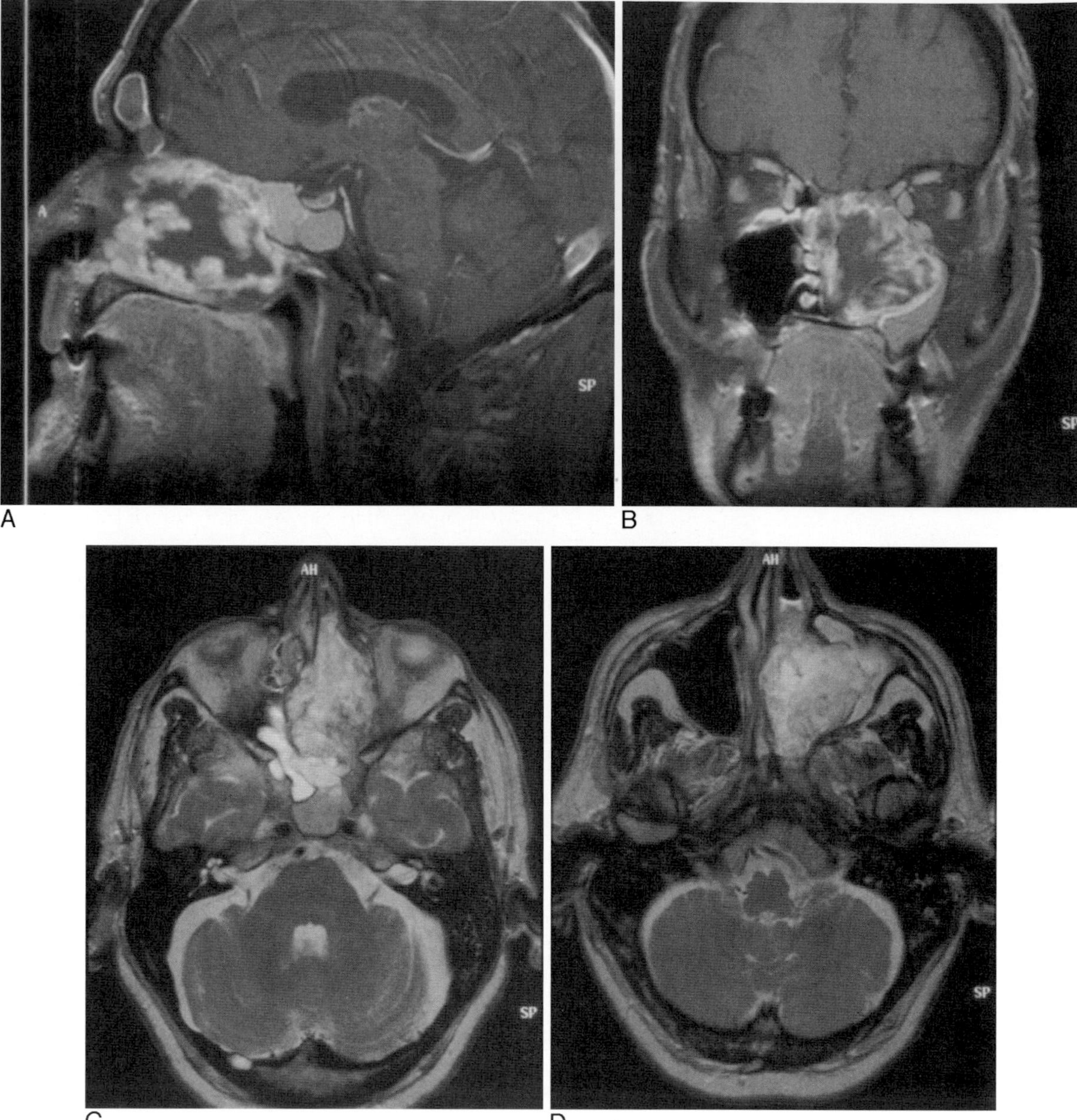

Figure 62.15 Delineation of tumour extent. The patient complained only of a blocked nose. It is the role of radiology to define extent; consequently sagittal, axial and coronal imaging all have a role to play. If contrast medium is given, it is best to employ a fat-saturation T1-weighted MR technique. (A) Sagittal T1-weighted gadolinium-enhanced MRI. This demonstrates the anterior–posterior extent of the tumour which can be seen obstructing the frontal air sinus anteriorly and the sphenoid sinus posteriorly. (B) Coronal T1-weighted gadolinium-enhanced MRI. Tumour extends laterally to bulge into the maxillary antrum. Superiorly it has invaded into the anterior cranial fossa, but not through dura. Superolaterally, the lamina papyracea of the orbit is breeched. Inferiorly the tumour is in contact with the palate. Medially the tumour has not extended far across the midline. (C) Axial T2-weighted MRI. The complex cystic and solid nature of this tumour can be clearly seen and can be easily differentiated from oedematous mucosa and obstructed sinus. (D) Axial T2-weighted MRI. The extension through the medial wall of the maxillary antrum can be clearly appreciated.

NASOPHARYNX, OROPHARYNX AND LARYNX

The 'head and neck' is a loose term to describe a specialty dealing with malignant disease of the nasopharynx, oropharynx and larynx. A multidisciplinary team approach including resective and reconstructive surgeons, oncologists, radiologists and radiotherapists is essential. Benign disorders usually fall into the remit of the ENT surgeon but are conveniently included here for completeness sake and to stress that there is frequently a benign differential diagnosis even when malignant disease is suspected.

THE NASOPHARYNX

This is a convenient anatomical description of that area of the neck bounded by the skull base superiorly and the palate inferiorly, containing the nasopharyngeal airway in its centre.

It is usefully divided into a number of compartments by very complex fascial planes. Each compartment initially contains pathological processes but eventually spread beyond the fascial plane will occur.

It is beyond the scope of this chapter to address the issue of the anatomy (and some of the relevant pathology) of the compartments precisely, but it is convenient to list them and their contents:

- mucosal: stratified squamous epithelium; small salivary glands; pharyngeal constrictor muscles; levator palatini muscle
- parapharyngeal: parapharyngeal fat
- retropharyngeal
- prevertebral
- masticator: muscles of mastication; mandible and teeth
- carotid: carotid artery; jugular vein; vagus and glossopharyngeal nerves; sympathetic trunk
- parotid: parotid gland; retromandibular vein; facial nerve.

Pathology

Mucosal and parapharyngeal spaces—nasopharyngeal carcinoma

Although this is easily the most important of the 'head and neck' cancers, it is sadly usually a large tumour at the time of diagnosis. The tumour is able to infiltrate the parapharyngeal fat 'silently' and reach large size without symptoms. Both CT and MRI demonstrate the lesion well (Fig. 62.16).

Surgery is usually not an option for these tumours and the main thrust of treatment is therefore radiotherapy. As ever, the main role of radiology is in the definition of extent for radiotherapy planning.

Masticator space

Asymmetry The development of an asymmetrical face is usually consequent upon growth of a tumour or hypertrophy of muscle. Occasionally atrophy of one side is misinterpreted as overgrowth of the other. Atrophy of muscles of mastication is consequent upon disturbance of their motor innervation—the trigeminal nerve.

Sepsis Most sepsis arises around the teeth and is clinically very easy to identify and treat. Occasionally a patient may present with trismus and little other symptomatology, when imaging may be diagnostic (Fig. 62.17).

Tumours of the muscles of mastication are rare, but are most frequently rhabdomyosarcomas.

Carotid space

Vagal neuroma Tumours of the vagus nerve are usually schwannomas and are benign. They may reach a large size due to their very slow rate of growth.

These tumours can be identified from their origin within the carotid sheath—they spread the carotid and jugular vessels apart. These tumours are characteristically of high signal on T2-weighted MRI (Fig. 62.18) and enhance avidly after intravenous contrast medium on both CT and MRI.

Paraganglionoma Tumours of the chemoreceptor cells have been mentioned above with respect to glomus jugulare tumours. Such tumours can also arise in the carotid body—carotid bulb tumours. In 10% of cases, paraganglionomas are multiple and the neck should always be examined when a glomus jugulare tumour is discovered and the skull base if a carotid bulb tumour is discovered.

Vascular anomaly The carotid artery is a common site for atheroma. Occasionally carotid aneurysms may develop spontaneously or as consequence of disease. Large aneurysms may develop layered thrombus and appear very complex on cross-sectional imaging (Fig 62.19), leading to misinterpretation as neoplasms.

Lymph node enlargement The carotid sheath is invested with a double layer of fascia and is resistant to invasion by local disease. Lymph nodes within the sheath can enlarge as part of systemic disease (e.g. lymphoma) or when the sheath is directly invaded by tumour.

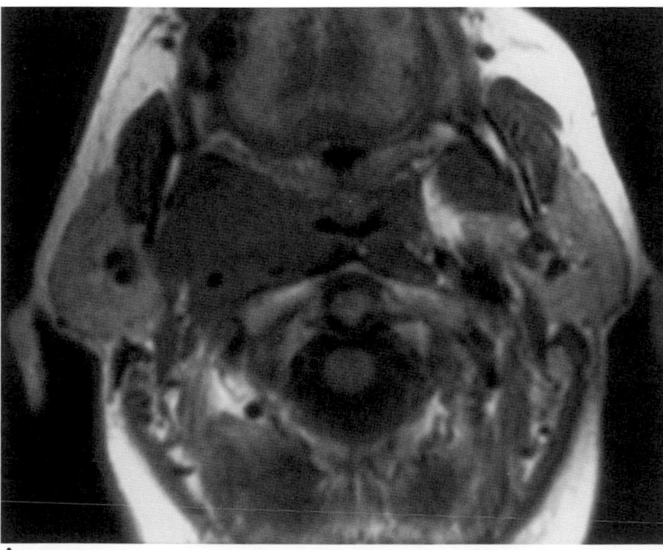
A

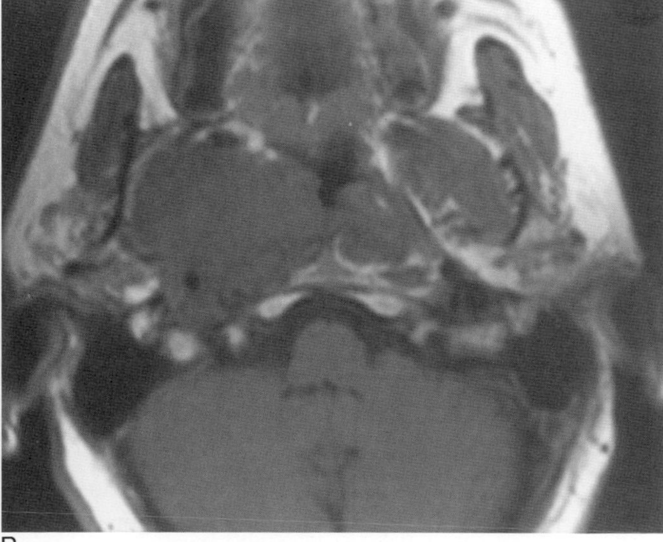
B

Figure 62.16 Nasopharyngeal carcinoma. (A,B) Axial T1-weighted MRIs show a large parapharyngeal mass in contact with the deep lobe of the parotid laterally and partially encasing the carotid.

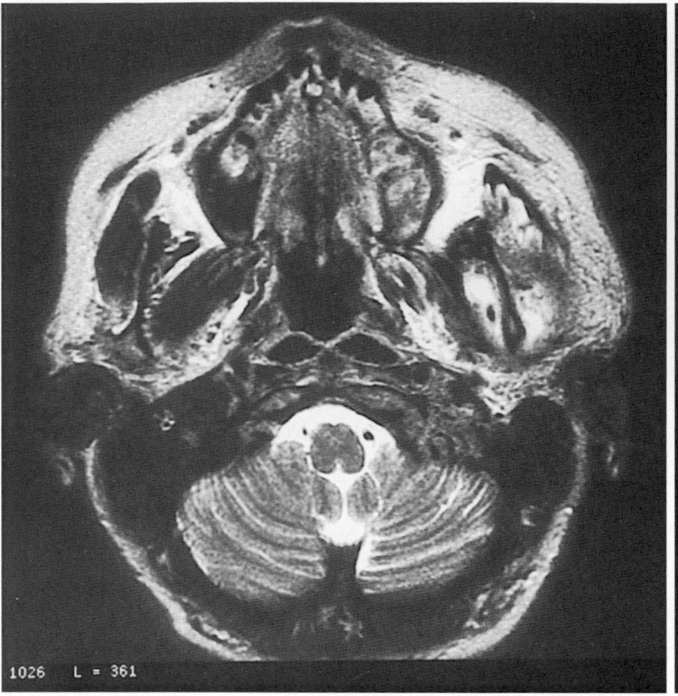

A

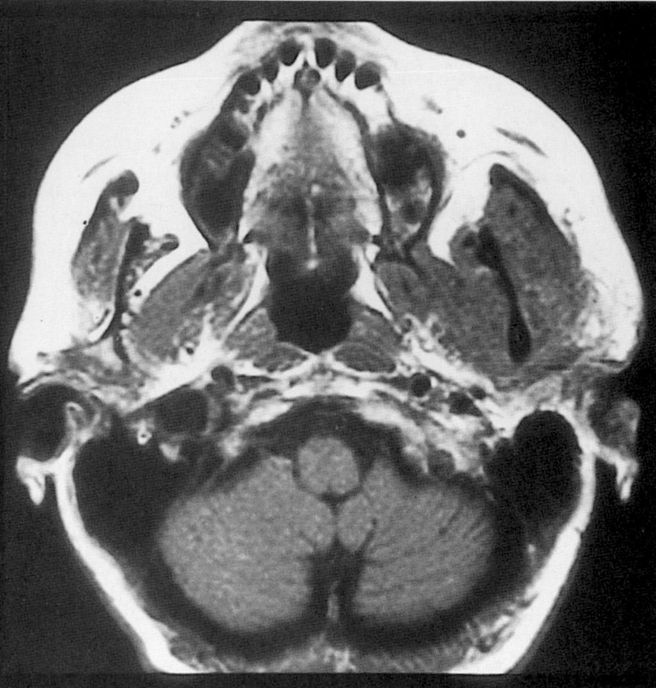
B

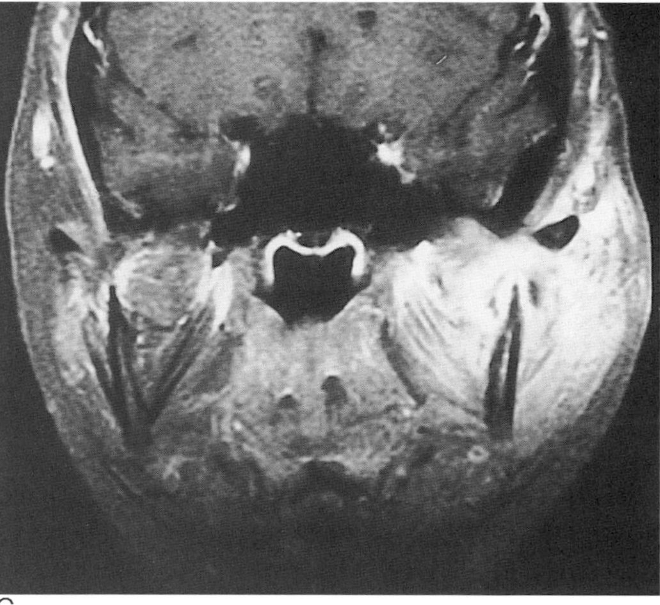
C

Figure 62.17 Sepsis. (A,B) Young woman with severe trismus. (A) Axial T2-weighted MRI shows major asymmetry between the masticator space contents on the two sides. The masseter and pterygoid on the right are normal, but on the left there is increased signal reflecting oedema of the muscles. (B) Axial T1-weighted MRI at the same level shows enlargement and reduced density of the muscles on the left side reflecting increased tissue water and muscle swelling. (C) Sepsis following incomplete treatment of a tooth infection. Coronal T1-weighted MRI after gadolinium administration. The whole of the muscle complex on the left side enhances profoundly after administration of contrast medium.

Parotid space—tumours

The majority of parotid tumours are benign and are pleomorphic adenomas. Twenty per cent are malignant and are a heterogeneous group of carcinomas, lymphomas, adenolymphomas, etc. As always the role of radiology is in the definition of extent, not histology.

Tumours of the deep lobe of the parotid deserve special mention. As they enlarge they spread medially into the parapharyngeal fat, and then are sometimes difficult to differentiate from laterally spreading parapharyngeal tumours.

The most crucial structure for the surgeon is the facial nerve which branches within the parotid before innervating the muscles of the face. The relationship of pathology to nerve is of prime importance if the nerve is to be identified and preserved. Unfortunately, it is rarely possible to identify the nerve using current imaging techniques.

ORAL CAVITY AND PHARYNX

The oral cavity includes:

- teeth (upper and lower jaw)
- bucco-alveolar sulcus (between teeth and cheek)
- tongue
- floor of mouth
- hard palate
- salivary gland openings.

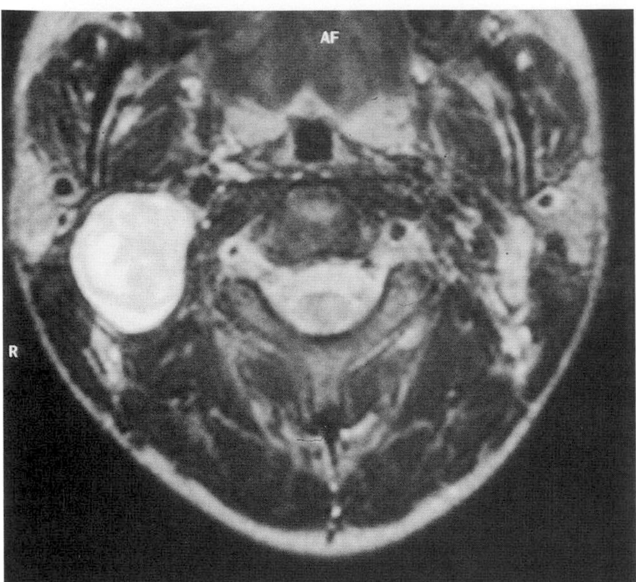

Figure 62.18 Vagal neuroma. Axial T2-weighted MRI shows a well-defined mass of high signal intensity on the right side just posterior and lateral to the flow void of the carotid artery. This is a classical appearance for a vagal neuroma.

The anterior aspect of the tonsil marks the start of the pharynx. The epithelium is a stratified squamous epithelium containing numerous minor salivary glands.

Lymphatic drainage is to the ipsilateral nodes of the internal jugular chain with the exception of the anterior mouth which can drain bilaterally. At the junction of the oral cavity and pharynx there is a complete ring of specialized lymphoid tissue—Waldeyer's ring—which includes:

- palatine tonsils (the tonsil) which lie adjacent to the posterior one third of the tongue
- adenoids (pharyngeal tonsils)
- lingual tonsils.

Sensation is derived from the mandibular branch of the trigeminal nerve anteriorly and the glossopharyngeal nerve posteriorly. Motor supply to the tongue is via the hypoglossal nerve.

The oral cavity and pharynx have obvious roles in respiration, phonation and mastication. Special function resides in taste (posterior tongue via the glossopharyngeal nerve) and swallowing.

Swallowing

This is a complex process involving mastication and preparation of food in the mouth under volitional control, followed by a very rapid nonvolitional reflex phase initiated by the elevation of the tongue forcing the food bolus to the pharynx. The reflex includes:

- switch from respiration to swallowing: stop breathing; closure of nasopharynx by elevation of soft palate; closure of airway by action of epiglottis
- elevation of larynx
- constriction of pharyngeal constrictor muscles projecting bolus into the region of the pyriform fossa
- relaxation of the cricopharyngeus muscle
- oesophageal peristalsis.

Pathology of the oral cavity

Peritonsillar abscess—quinsy

Usually secondary to streptococcal infection, an abscess here leads to severe pain and trismus. Clinical inspection and needle aspiration/formal drainage usually settles diagnosis and imaging is not required. Imaging with CT or MRI defines the extent and degree of loculation if required.

Carcinoma of the tongue

Lesions may be so small that they merely represent enlarged aphthous ulcers, or so large that they infiltrate the tongue widely. They are readily diagnosed by direct inspection and biopsy. The extent is best defined by MRI. Small lesions are simply resected or ablated. Large lesions will require full glossectomy or hemiglossectomy. The latter is a much less disruptive surgical intervention. The tongue can function well from muscular action on one side against a myocutaneous flap replacement. Critical observations include:

- Has the midline been crossed?
- Does the tumour erode or infiltrate the mandible?

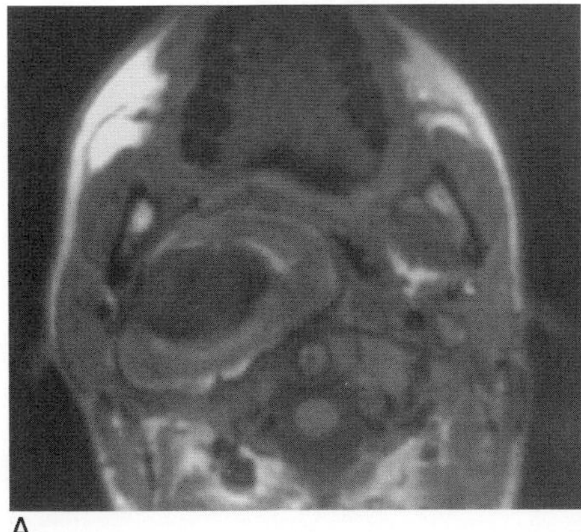
A

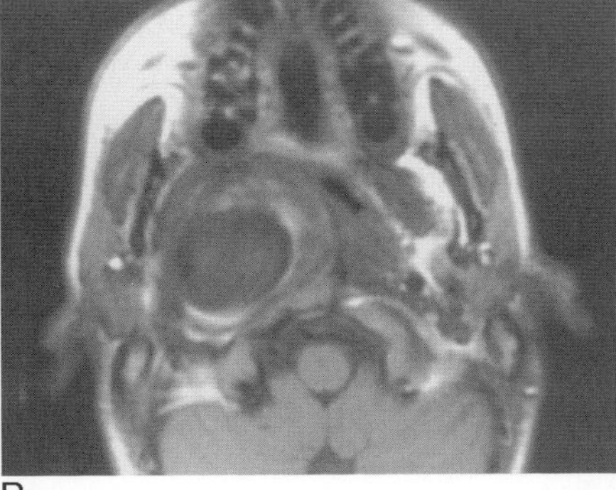
B

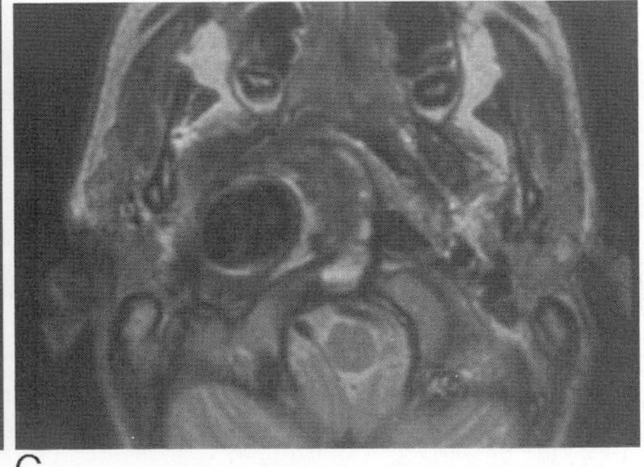
C

Figure 62.19 Carotid aneurysm. (A) Axial T1-weighted MRI in this patient who presented with a mass in his neck and had two percutaneous biopsies before the true nature of the pathology was realized! (B) Axial T1-weighted MRI at nasopharynx level shows a low signal intensity aneurysm in the lumen and organized thrombus in the wall. (C) Axial T2-weighted MRI close to the skull base shows the lumen reducing as aneurysm approaches the carotid canal.

- Does the posterior aspect of the tumour involve the root of the epiglottis and prevent its proper function?

A positive answer to these questions will result in radical surgery or radiotherapy.

Pathology of the pharynx

Carcinoma of the pharynx

These tumours are divided by their anatomical origin, e.g. pyriform fossa carcinoma or supraglottic carcinoma. All tumours infiltrate adjacent structures and along epithelial surfaces. The anatomy of the space between larynx and posterior tongue is difficult and surgical resection and reconstruction may be impossible. The integrity of the epiglottis mechanism is of paramount importance if food or fluid aspiration is to be avoided. This region requires particularly careful assessment so that the correct surgical and oncological decisions can be made.

THE LARYNX

Anatomy and physiology

The posterior walls of the pharynx are continuous with the larynx. It has two critical functions:

1 *Airway protection*—the action of the anteriorly situated epiglottis closes the tracheal airway and prevents aspiration of food and fluid.
2 *Sound generation*—the vocal cords act in a way similar to a 'reed' in a wind instrument, generating vibrations (subsequently modified by the action of tongue, palate, mouth, etc.).

The cricoid cartilage is the core structure. It resembles a signet ring with its face situated posteriorly. Attached to this, the V-shaped thyroid cartilage sits with its spine anteriorly and its open face posteriorly. The arytenoid cartilages sit within this structure, and superiorly lies the semicircular hyoid bone which links with the tongue.

The vocal cords meet in the midline anteriorly and are controlled by the intrinsic muscles of the larynx—cricoarytenoid abductors and thyroarytenoid adductors.

The superior laryngeal nerve—a branch of the vagus—conveys sensation and cricothyroid motor function. All other cord function is conveyed by the recurrent laryngeal nerve, also a branch of the vagus.

Lymphatic drainage of the supraglottis is to the upper deep cervical nodes and that of the infraglottis is to the internal jugular, peritracheal and mediastinal nodes.

Pathology

Carcinoma of the larynx (Fig. 62.20)

Tumours arising on the opposing surface of the vocal cords present early due to the effect on the voice. They are small and can be completely removed. More anterior or lateral tumours

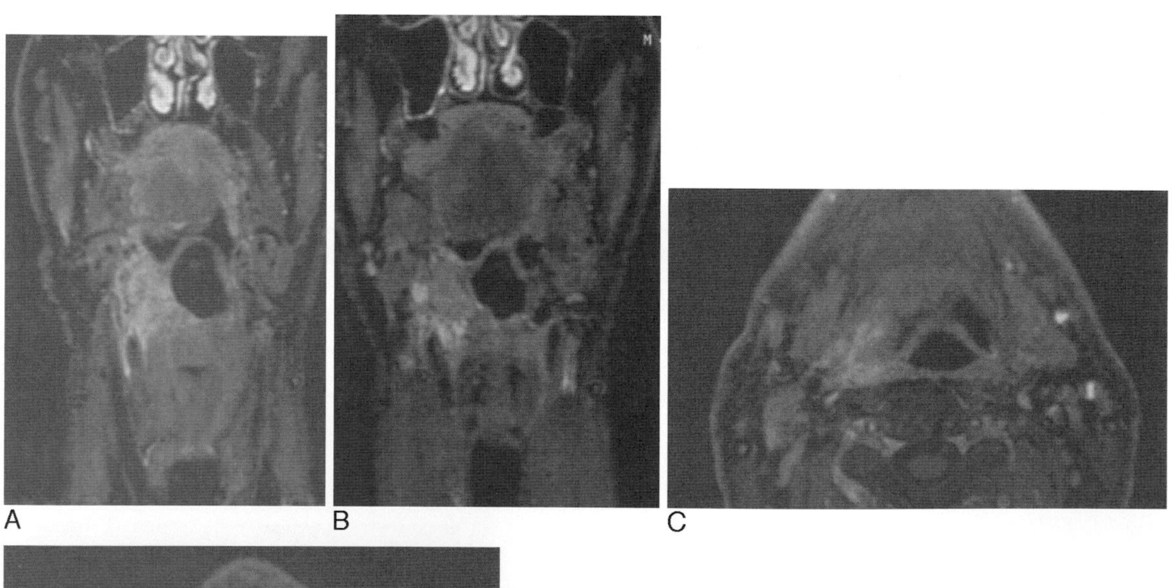

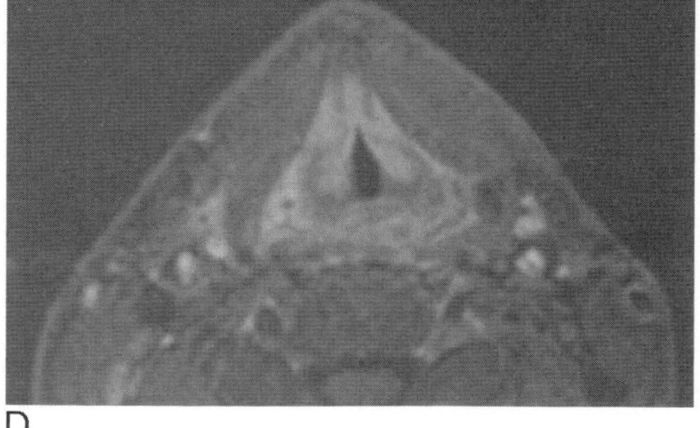

Figure 62.20 Laryngeal carcinoma in a 40 year old male smoker. (A,B) Coronal STIR MRI and (C,D) axial T1-weighted fat-saturated MRI after intravenous gadolinium. The coronal images demonstrate the superior and inferior extents while the axial images define the extent more accurately.

may present late and total laryngectomy or radical radiotherapy may be the only option. Critical observations include:

- Has the tumour spread anteriorly and escaped through the notch in the thyroid cartilage?
- Has the tumour crossed the midline?
- Does the tumour extend into the supraglottis?
- Does the tumour extend into the upper oesophagus?
- Is there invasion of the cartilage structure of the larynx (thyroid, cricoid, arytenoids)?

THE NECK

Anatomy and physiology

The neck can be divided into two triangles by the sternomastoid muscle:

- anterior triangle: sternomastoid posteriorly to mandible superiorly; midline anteriorly
- posterior triangle: sternomastoid anteriorly to trapezius posteriorly; clavicle inferiorly.

Pathology

The specific regions of the neck have been covered under the various sections of this chapter. The major subject remaining is that of lymphadenopathy.

Lymphadenopathy

Generalized lymphadenopathy is a common clinical presentation and the cause is often never known. If widespread and painful, glandular fever or other viral infection can be considered. If painless, spread from head and neck malignancy or lymphoma may be the cause. If focal and painful, a bacterial lymphadenitis may be implicated. If the cause is not immediately evident from clinical inspection and history taking, then imaging frequently has a role to play.

Palpable nodes will usually be detected by MRI or CT. Coronal STIR sequences are particularly valuable in MRI and contrast-enhanced thin section CT is equally good or even better at detecting small metastatic lesions. Ultrasound (in expert hands) and fine needle aspiration cytology or core-guided biopsy pushes the detection of small metastatic lesions even further. At present, no imaging technique is able to assess micrometastases and it remains common practice to sample the lymph nodes of the cervical chain at the time of surgical resection of tumour to detect these.

SUGGESTED FURTHER READING

Swartz J D, Harnsberger H Ric Head and Neck Imaging, Thieme

Chung V F H, Tsai S W Naso-Pharyngeal Carcinoma, Amour Publishing

O'Donaghy, Bates G, Narulea A. Clinical ENT, Oxford University Press

Laing J Clinical Analtomy of the Nose, Nasal Cavity and Paranasal Sinuses. Thieme

Lenz M CT and MRI of Head and Neck Tumours. Thieme

Rao V, Flanders A, Tom B, Dunitz M MRI and CT Atlas of Correlative Imaging in Otolaryngology

Gulya J, Shucknecht H Anatomy of the Temporal Bone with Surgical Implications. Parthanon Publishing Group

CHAPTER 63

Dental and Maxillofacial Radiology

John Rout and Jackie E. Brown

Dental radiography is performed using two techniques: intra-oral and extra-oral radiography. Diagnosing disorders affecting the teeth requires high-definition images that are obtained by using direct exposure (nonscreen) intra-oral film. Bitewing films show the crowns of the upper and lower posterior teeth on one film and are used for the detection of dental caries and the assessment of periodontal disease. Periapical film shows the tooth in its entirety together with some of the apical bone. Occlusal radiographs are larger than periapical films and are mainly used in orthodontic assessment of the upper anterior teeth and for identifying stones in the submandibular duct.

A dental panoramic radiograph demonstrates all of the teeth and jaws on one film and is indicated when a wide coverage is required. The technique is based on a form of tomography with the image layer being curved and corresponding to the shape of the jaws. Accurate patient positioning is essential as otherwise the images are prone to distortion.

Cephalometric radiography is used in orthodontic assessment and orthognathic surgery planning. The technique uses a fixed true lateral or PA head position and a long tube–film distance (approximately 2 m) to reduce image magnification.

Increasingly, conventional radiographs are being replaced by digital imaging using phosphor stimuable plates or electronic chips such as charged couple devices (CCDs).

Guidelines on the most appropriate choice for dental radiographic examination can be found in 'Selection Criteria for Dental Radiography'[1].

ANATOMY OF TEETH AND SUPPORTING STRUCTURES

In the primary dentition, there are normally 20 teeth; in adult dentition there are 32. The teeth are identified using one of two systems illustrated in Table 63.1. These are the Zsigmondy system, which uses single digits for the permanent dentition and letters for the primary (deciduous) dentition, and the Federation Dentaire International (FDI) notation, which assigns double digits for each tooth (Figs. 63.1, 63.2).[2]

All teeth consist of a crown and a root, which may be single or multiple (Fig. 63.3A, B). The crown is covered with a layer of enamel with a composition of 97 per cent mineral, thus being the most radio-opaque tissue in the body. The bulk of the tooth consists of dentine, which is 70 per cent mineralized. The root is covered by a thin layer of cementum, which has a similar radiodensity to dentine and so is indistinguishable from it. Lying within the centre of the tooth is the radiolucent soft tissue of the pulp, which runs from the pulp chamber in the crown along each root canal to the root apex, through which enter the neurovascular bundles. The tooth is supported in the jaws by the periodontal ligament, which consists largely of collagen fibres and appears as a narrow radiolucent line following the contours of the root. These fibres are inserted into a thin layer of dense bone lining the tooth socket (lamina dura), which appears as a linear radio-opaque structure, and is continuous with the cortical bone of the alveolar crest.

Table 63.1 THE ZIGMONDY (SINGLE DIGIT) AND FDI (DOUBLE DIGIT) SYSTEMS OF TOOTH IDENTIFICATION

Permanent dentition

UPPER RIGHT															UPPER LEFT
(18)	(17)	(16)	(15)	(14)	(13)	(12)	(11)	(21)	(22)	(23)	(24)	(25)	(26)	(27)	(28)
8	7	6	5	4	3	2	1	1	2	3	4	5	6	7	8
8	7	6	5	4	3	2	1	1	2	3	4	5	6	7	8
(48)	(47)	(46)	(45)	(44)	(43)	(42)	(41)	(31)	(32)	(33)	(34)	(35)	(36)	(37)	(38)
LOWER RIGHT															LOWER LEFT

Primary dentition

(55)	(54)	(53)	(52)	(51)	(61)	(62)	(63)	(64)	(65)
E	D	C	B	A	A	B	C	D	E
E	D	C	B	A	A	B	C	D	E
(85)	(84)	(83)	(82)	(81)	(71)	(72)	(73)	(74)	(75)

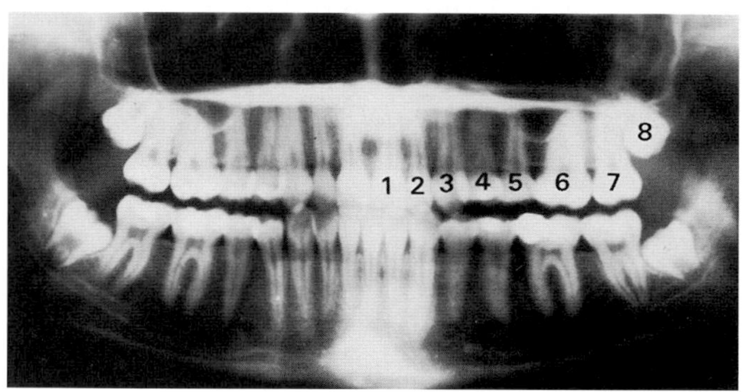

Figure 63.1 Part of a panoramic radiograph showing the permanent dentition of a normal 18-year-old. The teeth in the upper left quadrant have been numbered 1–8. The third molars are unerupted, incompletely formed and impacted.

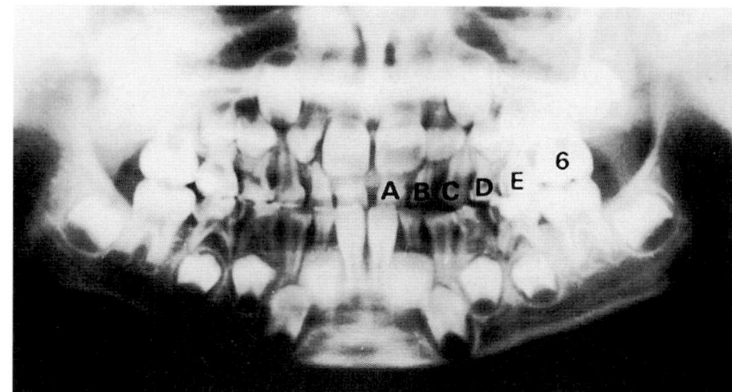

Figure 63.2 Part of a panoramic radiograph showing the dentition in a 6-year-old child. The deciduous teeth in the upper left quadrant have been labelled A–E. The first permanent molars (labelled 6) and the lower central incisors have erupted. All four primary first molars and the primary lower second molars are carious.

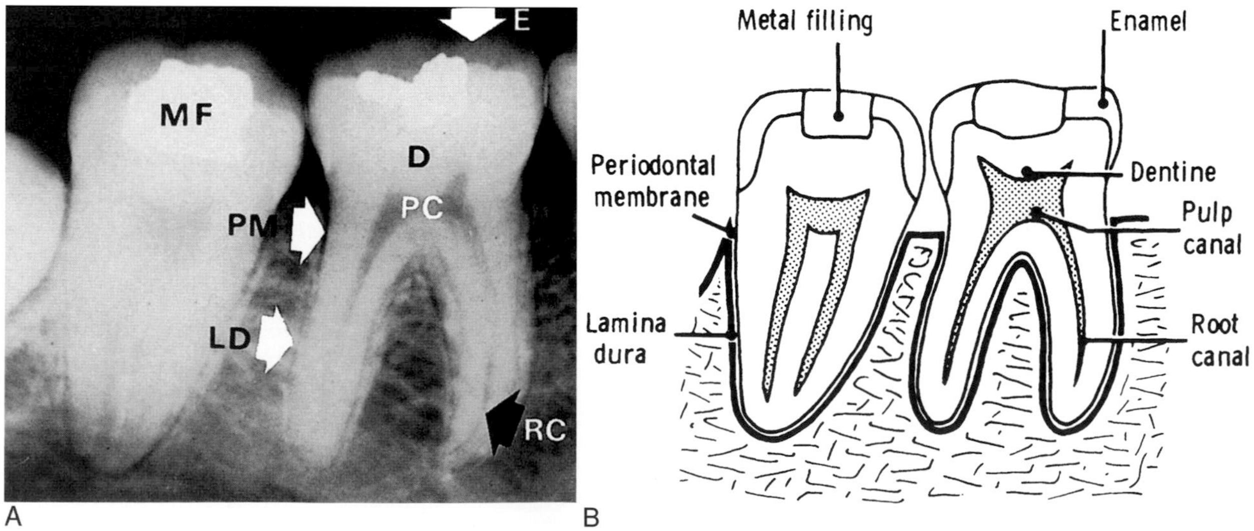

Figure 63.3 (A) Periapical radiograph labelled to show a tooth and its supporting structures. E = enamel, D = dentine, PC = pulp chamber, RC = root canal, PM = periodontal membrane (periodontal ligament space), LD = lamina dura, MF = amalgam filling. (B) Corresponding line diagram.

TOOTH ERUPTION

Normal eruption

The normal eruption times are shown in Table 63.2. The primary teeth erupt between 6–24 months and the permanent teeth between 6–21 years. Root formation is not complete until 1.5–2 years and 2–3 years after eruption for the primary and permanent teeth, respectively.

Disorders of tooth eruption

The commonest cause for failure of full eruption is insufficient room in the dental arch to accommodate the erupting tooth. This particularly affects mandibular third molars and to a lesser extent maxillary canines. Alternatively a tooth may be prevented from erupting by, for example, a tumour, cyst or supernumerary tooth. Delayed eruption occurs in certain endocrine disorders, e.g. hypothyroidism and some genetic abnormalities, e.g. Down's syndrome. Multiple failure of eruption of the permanent dentition is found in cleidocranial dysplasia (Fig. 63.4).

Disorders of tooth development

Variation in tooth number

Absence of one or more teeth is referred to as hypodontia (oligodontia) and as anodontia (rare) where there is complete absence of teeth. Hypodontia most often affects third molars, mandibular second premolars and maxillary lateral incisors (Fig. 63.5). It is seen in association with cleft lip and palate, Ellis-van Creveld (chrondo-ectodermal dysplasia) and facial-digital syndromes. Marked absence of teeth is seen in hydrotic ectodermal dysplasia.

Teeth additional to the normal series, hyperdontia, presents as either supplemental or supernumerary teeth. A supplemental tooth is an extra tooth identical in shape and form to an adjacent permanent one. The commonest supernumerary teeth are mesiodens and tuberculates, which form in the maxillary midline. Mesiodens, which are small conical teeth, form after the primary upper central incisors and occasionally erupt. Tuberculate supernumeraries develop shortly after the formation of the permanent upper central incisors and usually impede their eruption. Marked hyperdontia in the permanent dentition is seen in cleidocranial dysplasia (Fig. 63.4).

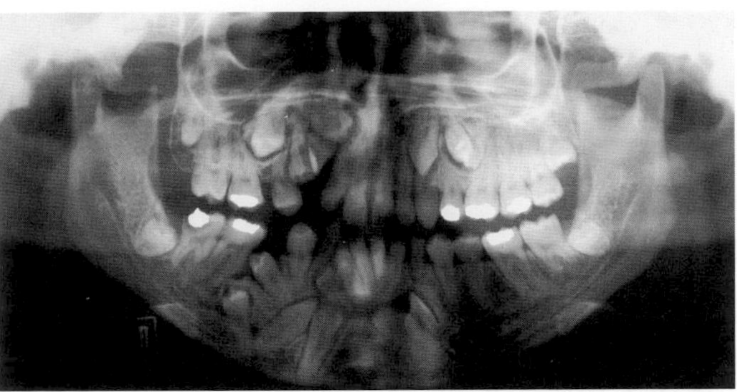

Figure 63.4 Panoramic radiograph of cleidocranial dysplasia in an adult. There are numerous unerupted teeth including several supernumeraries.

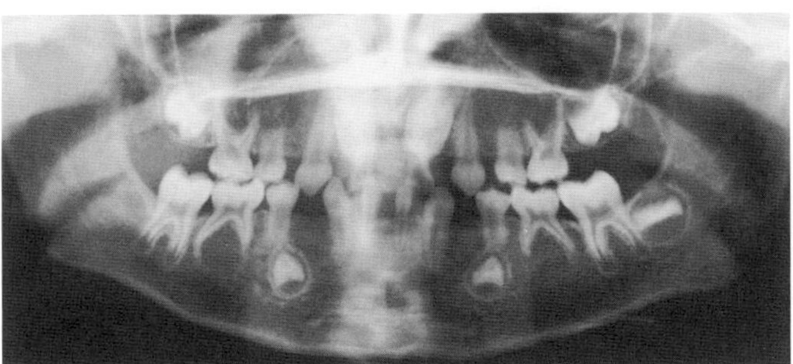

Figure 63.5 Panoramic radiograph showing a marked example of hypodontia involving both the primary deciduous and permanent dentitions in a 6-year-old child. All four lateral incisors are missing from the primary deciduous dentition and 19 permanent teeth are also absent. Note that wisdom tooth formation normally starts between 9 and 13 years of age.

Table 63.2 APPROXIMATE DATES OF ERUPTION OF THE PRIMARY AND PERMANENT TEETH

Tooth	Designation	Age(months)
Primary dentition		
Central incisors	A	6–8
Lateral incisors	B	7–10
Canines	C	16–20
First molars	D	10–14
Second molars	E	20–30
Permanent dentition		**Age (years)**
Central incisors	1	6–7
Lateral incisors	2	7–9
Canines	3	9–12
First premolars	4	10–12
Second premolars	5	10–12
First molars	6	6–7
Second molars	7	11–13
Third molars	8	17–21

Variation in tooth size

A tooth that is larger than normal is termed a macrodont and when smaller, a microdont, the latter being more common and typically affecting maxillary lateral incisors and upper wisdom teeth. Radiotherapy and/or chemotherapy can affect tooth development, resulting in arrested development such that they appear smaller than normal with short, spiculated roots (Fig. 63.6).

Variation of tooth form

Disturbance of tooth form can affect either the crown or root, or both, and may be developmental or acquired. A dens in dente is due to an infolding or invagination of the enamel into the underlying dentine towards the root, creating the appearance of a tooth within a tooth. A markedly hooked root is called dilaceration and typically affects a maxillary

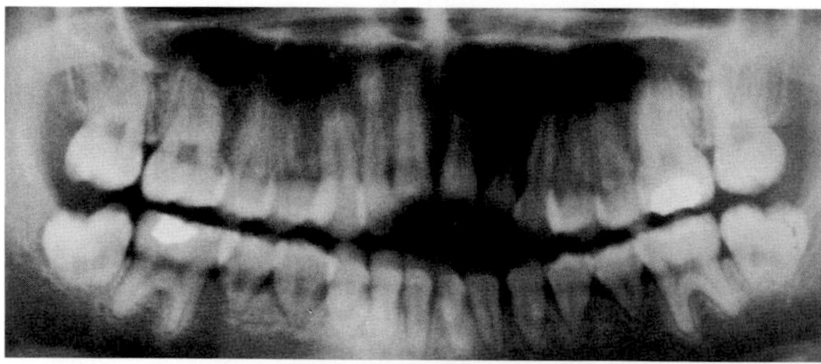

Figure 63.6 Panoramic radiograph of a child aged 12 who received radiation to the neck for lymphoma when aged 5 years. The extent to which the roots have failed to form depends on their stage of development at the time of irradiation; thus the lower incisors, which had nearly completed root formation, are relatively unharmed. The lower first molars are slightly stunted and the premolars and second molars extensively shortened. Such teeth do not suffer from excessive mobility.

central incisor usually following traumatic intrusion of the primary incisor, which displaces the developing permanent incisor. In taurodontism the pulp chamber is markedly elongated. A tooth that appears particularly enlarged may have split during its development or have become fused with an adjacent tooth.

DISTURBANCES IN STRUCTURE OF TEETH

Enamel

Enamel hypoplasia may affect a single tooth, following a localized periapical infection of its primary precursor (Turner tooth). But a more generalized form occurs as a complication of severe childhood infections or a nutritional deficiency with the manifestation depending on the time of the insult (chronological hypoplasia).

Amelogenesis imperfecta is a developmental disorder of enamel formation affecting all or most of the teeth in both dentitions. The enamel may show varying degrees of hypoplasia from being pitted (Fig. 63.7), to almost complete absence of enamel when the crown appears angular. Alternatively, the enamel may be of normal thickness but be hypomineralized such that its radiographic density is similar to that of dentine.

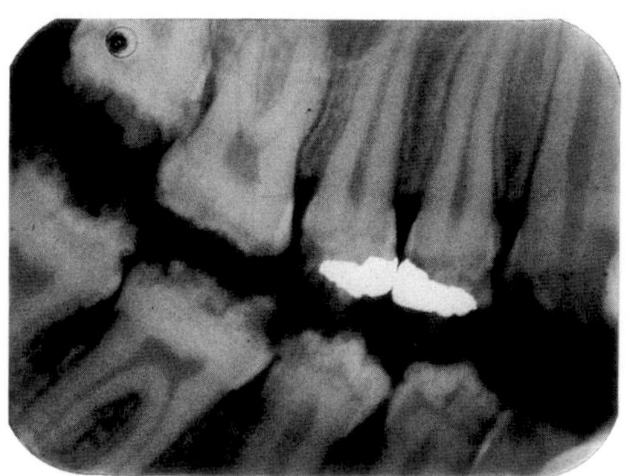
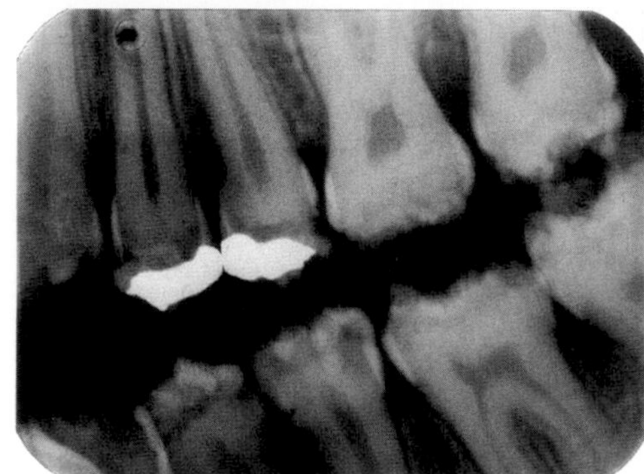

Figure 63.7 Intra-oral (bitewing) radiographs showing marked hypoplasia and pitting of the enamel, whilst the dentine appears normal. Several of the teeth are carious.

Dentine

Dentinogenesis imperfecta is a developmental anomaly of collagen formation that affects the dentine of both dentitions. The teeth are discoloured, having a brown or purple hue. The enamel chips away and the teeth rapidly wear down. The initial radiographic appearance shows bulbous crowns and large pulp chambers, which soon calcify with abnormal dentine so that little or none of the root canal is visible (Fig. 63.8). Although the teeth may appear sound, they are prone to infection resulting in pulpal necrosis and periapical radiolucencies. The appearance of the bone of the mandible and maxilla remains normal, although type IV is associated with osteogensis imperfecta.

Dentinal dysplasia resembles dentinogenesis imperfecta but is less common. In type I the crowns look normal in colour and shape but the roots of the primary and permanent teeth are short and abnormally shaped, and the pulp chambers become obliterated with dentine prior to eruption. In type II, loss of the pulp chamber and narrowing of the root canals occurs after tooth eruption. In some cases the pulp chambers may be thistle shaped.

Cementum

Hypercementosis describes the deposition of excessive amounts of cementum typically around the apical half of the root so that it appears bulbous. Usually it is localized to one or two teeth as it is caused by chronic dental infection or occlusal

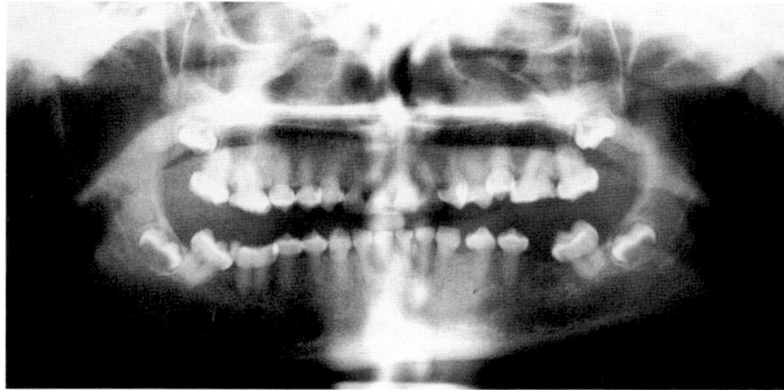

Figure 63.8 A panoramic radiograph of a young adult with dentinogenesis imperfecta. The teeth have bulbous crowns, short stumpy roots and sclerosis of the root canals.

overstress, but in Paget's disease of the jaws (Table 63.3) it is widespread.

Miscellaneous conditions

In **hypophosphataemia**, the pulps of the primary and permanent teeth are enlarged with pulp horns that extend toward the enamel/dentine junction, making the pulps susceptible to infection so that the teeth frequently become abscessed. Similar dental features are noted in hypophosphatasia but there is often premature loss of the primary teeth. In both conditions the jaws usually appear osteoporotic (osteopenic).

DENTAL CARIES

Dental caries is caused by microbial action on sugar with the formation of acid, which causes progressive demineralization

Table 63.3 DIFFERENTIAL DIAGNOSIS OF LOCALIZED RADIOLUCENT AND RADIO-OPAQUE LESIONS OF THE JAWS

Unilocular radiolucent	Multilocular radiolucent	Radio-opaque	Mixed density
Common	**Common**	**Common**	**Common**
Alveolar abscess	Odontogenic keratocyst	Root fragment	Fibrous dysplasia (early)
Apical granuloma	Central giant cell granuloma	Dense bone island	Cemento-ossifying fibroma
Radicular cyst (apical)	Ameloblastoma	Mandibular torus	Periapical cemento-osseous
Residual cyst		Periapical sclerosing osteitis	Compound odontome
Dentigerous cyst		Hypercementosis	Complex odontome
Nasopalatine duct cyst		Supernumerary tooth	Florid cemento-osseous dysplasia
Odontogenic keratocyst		Sclerosing osteitis	Benign cementoblastoma (cementoma)
Uncommon	**Uncommon**	**Uncommon**	**Uncommon**
Stafne's bone cavity	Giant cell tumour of hyperparathyroidism	Fibrous dysplasia (late)	Chronic osteomyelitis
Fibrous scar		Periapical cemento-osseous dysplasia	Osteosarcoma
Fibrous dysplasia (early)	Ameloblastic fibroma		Paget's disease
Periapical cemento-osseous dysplasia (early)	Odontogenic myxoma	Florid cemento-osseous dyplasia	
Osteomyelitis		Ossifying fibroma (late)	
Giant cell tumour of hyperparathyroidism		Complex odontome	
		Compound odontome	
Central giant cell granuloma		Paget's disease (late)	
Ameloblastoma		Osteoma/exostosis	
Lateral periodontal cyst			
Paget's disease (early)			
Brown tumour of hyperparathyroidism			
Rare	**Rare**	**Rare**	**Rare**
Carcinoma	Aneurysmal bone cyst	Metastatic carcinoma of prostate	Calcifying epithelial-odontogenic tumour (CEOT)
Metastatic carcinoma	Haemangioma		
Haemangioma	Cherubism	Cementoblastoma	Calcifying odontogenic cyst
Osteosarcoma	Glandular odontogenic cyst	Osteosarcoma	Osteoradionecrosis
Odontogenic myxoma		Chronic sclerosing osteomyelitis	Adenomatoid odontogenic tumour
Burkitt's lymphoma		Chronic osteomyelitis	Ameloblastic fibro-odontoma
Lymphoma		Osteochondroma	
Eosinophilic granuloma			
Chondroma & chondrosarcoma			
Neurofibroma			
Neurilemmoma			
Odontogenic fibroma			
Ewing's tumour			
Myeloma			

of the teeth, initially of the enamel, and then the dentine with destruction of their organic components. If left untreated it leads to the break down of the crown and bacterial infection of the pulp. It develops on the occlusal surfaces of the posterior teeth, on the approximal and cervical regions of the crown or root (if exposed), and as recurrent caries beneath restorations. The rate of mineral loss depends on a number of factors including the amount of sugar in the diet, the lack of effective oral hygiene, the presence of areas of food stagnation, and on the health of the individual. It is particularly rapid in those with reduced saliva production following radiation damage to the salivary glands.

Radiographic detection of dental decay requires images with good contrast and resolution. Despite its limitations, intra-oral radiographs are valuable in the detection and monitoring of dental decay, particularly on surfaces not easily visualized and also for occult occlusal caries, which can be extensive beneath an apparently intact enamel surface.

A carious lesion appears as a radiolucent zone, which represents an area of demineralization. An approximal lesion develops in the enamel just below the contact point with an adjacent tooth and has a triangular shape with the apex pointing towards the dentine. As the lesion progresses, its advancing surface broadens as it extends along the enamel dentine junction and penetrates into the dentine, the margin being ill defined (Fig. 63.9A, B). Adjacent carious lesions commonly develop on contiguous tooth surfaces. If left untreated, the caries reaches the pulp chamber and the weakened crown eventually crumbles away. A similar progression is seen on other tooth surfaces. The radiographic detection of dental caries can be difficult, particularly when the crown remains intact and the carious lesion is only marginally more radiolucent relative to the surrounding dentine.

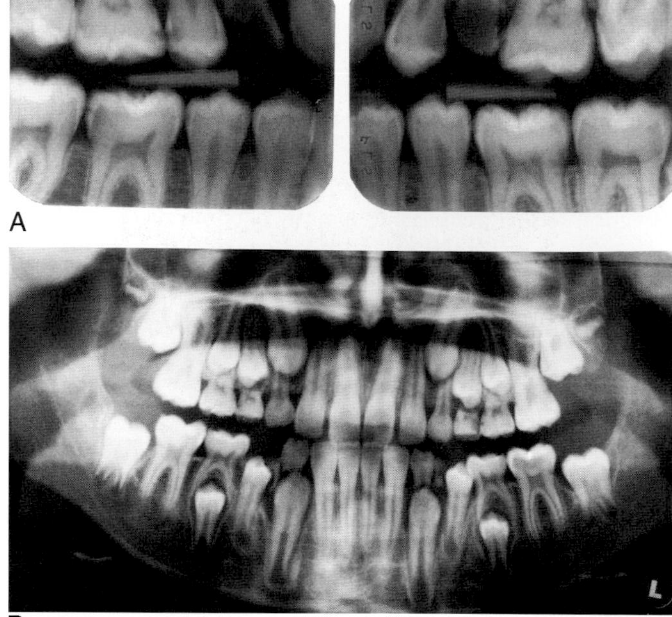

Figure 63.9 (A) Bitewing radiographs showing gross caries with crown destruction affecting the upper right first and upper left second premolars. There is approximal caries, shown as radiolucencies of the crowns, at the contact points of the other remaining upper premolars, upper and lower right first molars, and occlusal caries in the upper left first molar. (B) Panoramic radiograph of a child aged 8 in the mixed dentition. There is approximal caries in the upper right deciduous first and second molars. There is gross caries distally in the upper left deciduous first molar, which has complete root resorption by the erupting successional premolar. There are retained fragments of the roots of the deciduous first molars. The lower left permanent first molar has gross recurrent occlusal caries beneath a very small restoration. There is less extensive recurrent caries in the lower right permanent first molar. Both these teeth show periapical bone changes, most obviously the widening of the periodontal ligament space on the mesial root of the lower left permanent first molar, consistent with periapical periodontitis.

DISORDERS OF THE PULP

Dental decay that extends to the pulp results in inflammation (acute pulpitis), causing severe toothache, but has no radiological manifestations. However, regressive changes of the pulp (chronic pulpitis) due to chronic irritation can appear as calcific deposits, such as pulp stones and sclerosis (narrowing) of the root canals. Generalized pulp sclerosis is a feature of renal osteodystrophy and prolonged corticosteroid therapy. Internal resorption of the root canal or external resorption of the outer root surface may occur following pulp death.

Periapical periodontitis

Pulpal necrosis results from acute pulpitis (see earlier) or from dental trauma due to interruption of the pulp's blood supply. Bacterial action on the necrotic pulp within the root canal leads to the production of endotoxins, which exit the root apex and incite a periapical inflammatory response within the periodontal membrane (periodontitis). When this is acute, the patient suffers severe discomfort and the offending tooth is tender to touch. Apical periodontitis presents as a widened periodontal ligament space, which appears more prominent than normal. However, the condition may also be chronic and continued progression of the chronic inflammatory process eventually leads to loss of the apical lamina dura and the formation of a discrete periapical radiolucency (Fig. 63.10) due to the formation of a focal inflammatory lesion, either a granuloma, radicular cyst, or chronic abscess. All three conditions have a similar radiographic appearance, that is a periapical radiolucency that is circular or oval, usually well defined, the outline being continuous with the remaining lamina dura around the root.

Conversely, low grade stimulation from a nonvital tooth may result in reactive bone formation (sclerosing osteitis), which appears as an irregularly shaped, largely uniform area of dense bone at the root apex (Fig. 63.11).

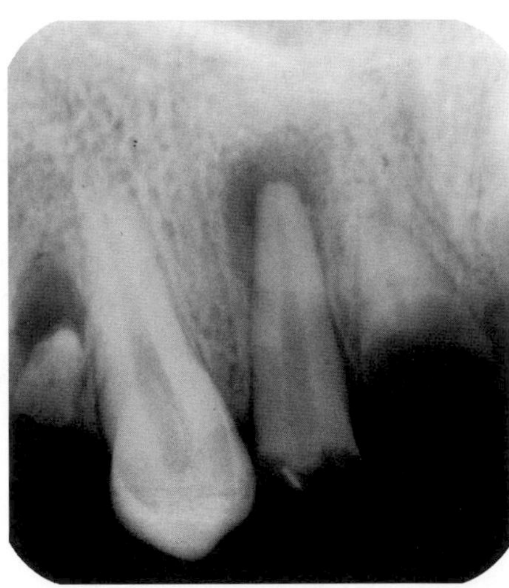

Figure 63.10 Periapical granuloma at the apex of the grossly decayed upper right lateral incisor. Although well defined, its margins are not corticated. Note the loss of the lamina dura at the tooth apex. There is a similar but smaller lesion at the apex of the exfoliating upper right first premolar root and the upper right central incisor is markedly carious.

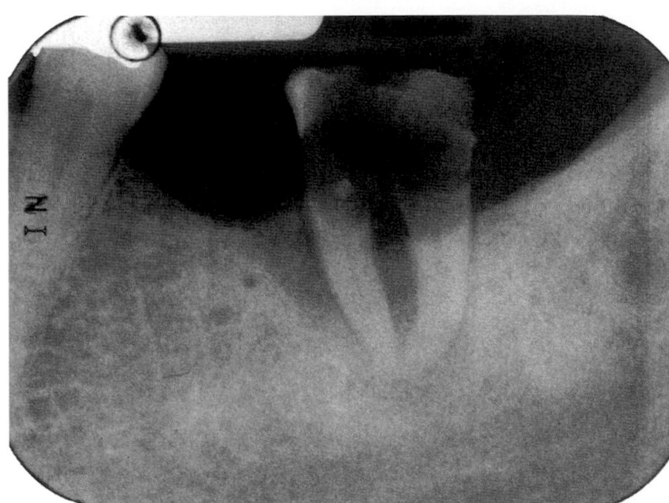

Figure 63.11 Periapical radiograph showing **sclerosing osteitis**. The lower left molar is grossly decayed and its root is surrounded by a zone of radiolucency beyond which the bone is dense as shown by the lack of trabecular spaces.

CYSTS OF THE JAWS

Cysts occur in the jaws more frequently than in any other bone because of the numerous epithelial cell residues left after tooth formation. Generally they are slow growing and painless unless infected, however some may reach a considerable size before detection.

Cysts of the jaws are divided into odontogenic when they arise from epithelial residues of the tooth-forming tissues, or non-odontogenic, these being uncommon and mainly developmental, arising from epithelium not involved with tooth formation. The four most common odontogenic cysts are the inflammatory radicular (dental) and residual cysts, and the developmental dentigerous cyst and odontogenic keratocyst.

Odontogenic and non-odontogenic cysts have a number of radiological features in common that are characteristic of slow-growing lesions, i.e. they are radiolucent, well defined and often have a cortical margin. With the exception of the odontogenic keratocyst, they have raised intracystic pressure and expand by tissue fluid transudation, and so appear as circular or oval in shape. When large, the bony cortex of the jaws becomes thinned, expanded and then perforated. Jaw cysts tend to displace structures such as tooth roots, unerupted teeth, the inferior alveolar canal, and the antral floor.

Radicular cysts are the most common (approximately 65 per cent) of the odontogenic cysts. They are derived from the cell rests of Malassez, which are epithelial remnants of root formation found in the periodontal ligament and develop at the apex of a nonvital tooth (see above periapical periodontitis). Any tooth can be affected but the majority are found on the permanent anterior teeth or first molars. When small (less than 15 mm in diameter) they resemble periapical granulomas but, unlike granulomas, can enlarge well beyond this size (Fig. 63.12). In many cases extraction of the causative tooth brings about resolution, but when this does not happen, the cyst is then termed a 'residual cyst'. Thus a residual cyst found in an edentulous part of the jaw, has a well-defined, circular radiolucency usually with a cortical margin. Many regress without treatment and some show dystrophic mineralization.

A **dentigerous cyst** (follicular cyst) arises from the reduced enamel epithelium, the tissue which surrounds the crown of an unerupted tooth. It is thus found only on teeth that are buried, particularly mandibular third molars and maxillary canines (Fig. 63.13). Cystic enlargement of the tooth follicle produces a pericoronal radiolucency, which is attached to the tooth at its neck, with the crown appearing to lie within the cyst lumen; however with large cysts this relationship may not be apparent.

Odontogenic keratocysts arise from remnants of the dental lamina, the precursor of the tooth germ. The cyst lining has a higher mitotic activity than the oral mucosa and the cyst

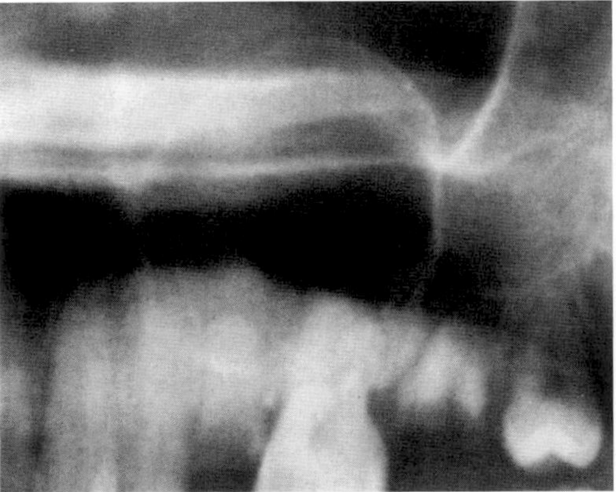

Figure 63.12 Part of a panoramic radiograph showing a corticated radiolucent lesion associated with the **carious root** of the upper left second premolar, extending into the maxillary antrum above the hard palate, consistent with a radicular cyst. Note the periapical radiolucency (granuloma/abscess) on the upper left second molar.

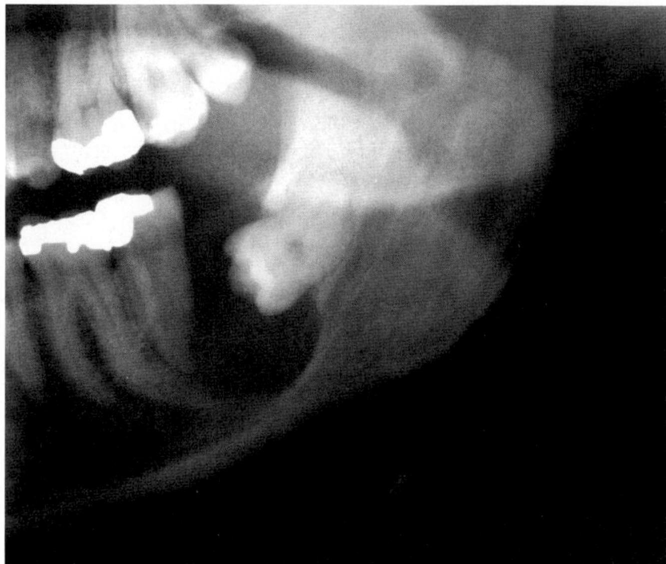

Figure 63.13 Part of a panoramic radiograph of a dentigerous cyst arising on a lower left wisdom tooth, which is unerupted and lying horizontally. It appears as a well-defined, circular radiolucency attached to the tooth at its neck. The inferior alveolar canal has been displaced inferiorly.

is thought to enlarge by mural growth and so behaves more like a benign neoplasm and is now classified as such. It appears as a unilocular or multiloculated, elongated, irregularly shaped radiolucency with a scalloped, well-defined margin (Fig. 63.14). It lacks the more ballooning characteristics of the other odontogenic cysts, which is an important diagnostic feature. Keratocysts occur most often in the lower third molar/ramus region, where they may displace, or occasionally replace an unerupted wisdom tooth and resemble a dentigerous cyst. Recurrence is common (15–20 per cent) so radiographic follow-up is necessary for several years. On CT, attenuation values of cyst fluid are higher than most other jaws cysts due to its high protein (keratin) content, ranging from 30–200 Hounsfield Units, with longstanding, multilocular cysts having the higher value[3].

Multiple odontogenic keratocysts are a feature of Gorlin-Goltz syndrome (Fig. 63.15), which also includes multiple basal cell naevi, calcification of the falx, bifid ribs, synostosis of the ribs, kyphoscoliosis, temporal and parietal bossing, hypertelorism, and shortening of the metacarpals.

There are several other less common odontogenic cysts. The lateral periodontal cyst is found on the lateral surface of a vital tooth root between two adjacent teeth, usually the lower incisor or canine teeth. The glandular odontogenic cyst mainly occurs in the anterior body of the mandible, as a multilocular or lobular, often large radiolucency that may cross the midline and has a tendency to recur.

The nasopalatine cyst is probably the commonest non-odon-togenic cyst that is believed to arise from epithelial residues in the nasopalatine canal. It appears as a round, well-defined, midline radiolucency between, but not associated with, the upper central incisor teeth.

Three lesions that may resemble jaw cysts but have no epithelial lining are sometimes considered with jaw cysts. The solitary bone cyst occurs during the first 2 decades of life,

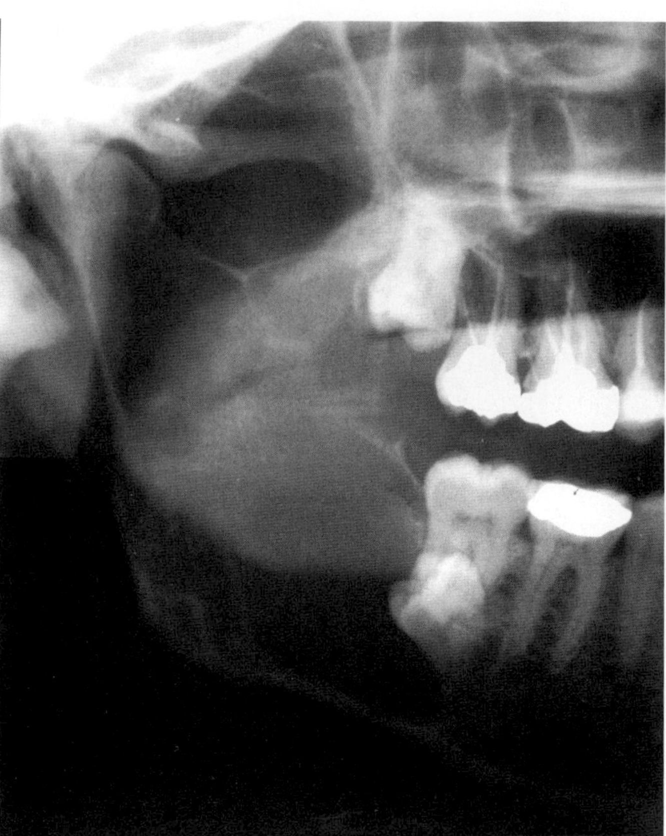

Figure 63.14 Part of a panoramic radiograph of an odontogenic keratocyst which appears as a loculated radiolucency extending from the condylar neck to the lower first molar region. There is thinning of the bony cortices but no jaw expansion, a feature associated with odontogenic keratocysts. Note the displaced lower right third molar.

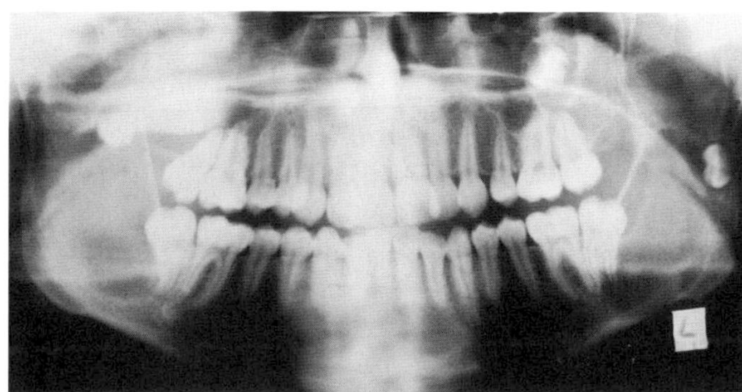

Figure 63.15 Part of a panoramic radiograph showing multiple odontogenic keratocysts consistent with **Gorlin-Goltz syndrome**. All four third molars have been extensively displaced and a lateral facial view showed the upper right one to lie posteriorly close to the orbit.

mainly in the premolar/molar regions of the mandible. Its margin is less well defined than those of odontogenic cysts and its superior border arches up between the roots of the adjacent teeth (Fig. 63.16). Tooth displacement and root resorption is uncommon. At surgery an empty cavity is found, which subsequently heals after bleeding has been induced.

The aneurysmal bone cyst is considered to be a reactive lesion of bone and is characterized by a fibrous connective tissue stroma containing many cavernous blood-filled spaces.

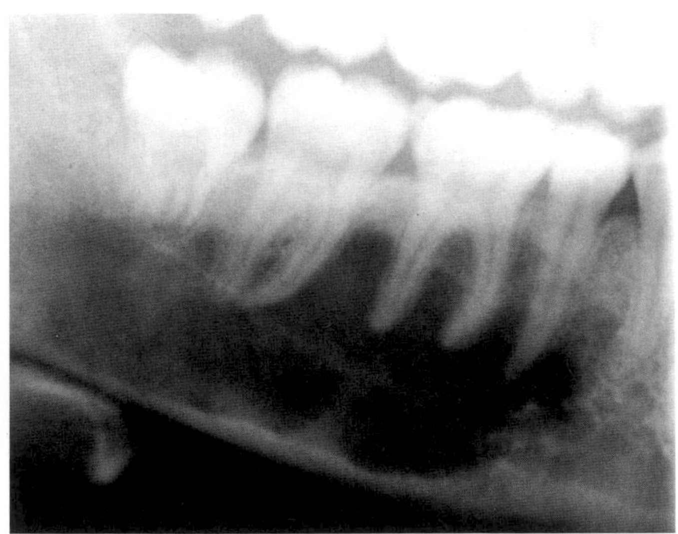

Figure 63.16 Part of a panoramic radiograph showing a partially corticated radiolucency in the right mandible involving the apices of the second premolar and first and second molars diagnosed as a solitary bone cyst. Note the characteristic scalloping between the roots of the first and second molars.

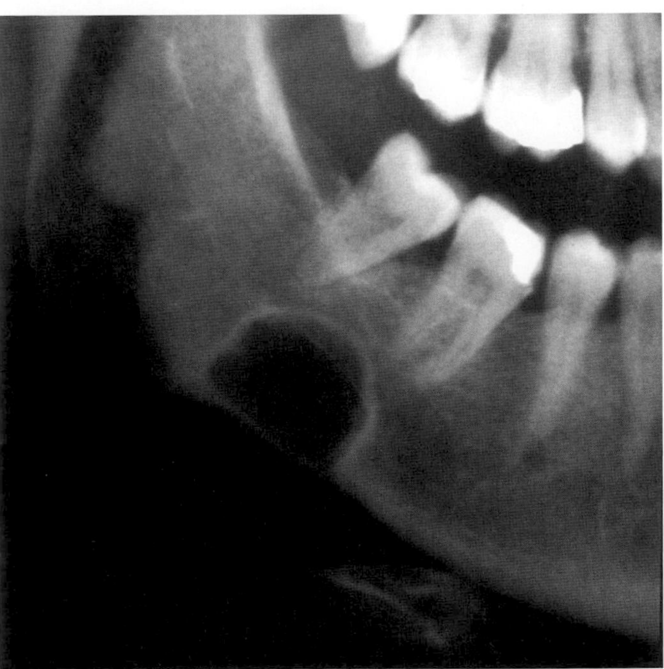

A

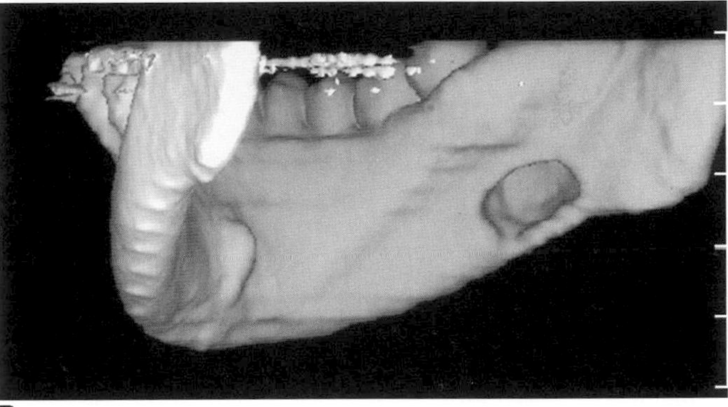

B

Figure 63.17 (A) Part of a panoramic radiograph showing a corticated radiolucency between the inferior alveolar canal and the lower border of the mandible due to the presence of a Stafne bone cavity. The 3D CT (B) shows the depression on the lingual aspect of the mandible.

It is rare and occurs mainly in the young, with over 90 per cent occurring before 30 years of age. It is typically found in the posterior region of the mandible as a well-defined, multilocular, often septated, circular radiolucency. It has a tendency to produce marked cortical expansion. Computed tomography (CT) or magnetic resonance imaging (MRI) shows the presence of fluid levels due to the presence of blood-filled cavities.

Stafne's bone cavity is asymptomatic and typically found in men over the age of 35 years. It forms a depression in the lingual cortex of the mandible just in front of the angle and below the inferior dental canal. Its origin is controversial and it has been postulated that it arises from pressure from the submandibular salivary gland, however whilst some may contain salivary gland tissue a number develop anterior to the gland. On plain radiographs, it appears as a well defined, punched out, dense radiolucency, which rarely exceeds 2 cm in diameter (Fig. 63.17A, B). Its appearance is characteristic and so does not require further imaging or biopsy. However, if CT or MRI is performed, the cavity is often found to contain fat.

DISEASE OF THE PERIODONTIUM

There are several disorders that affect the **periodontium** and these are referred to as periodontal disease. Radiographs, in particular intra-oral views (bitewings and periapical films) are helpful in the assessment of the amount of remaining bone support for the teeth, the pattern of bone loss, the detection of subgingival calculus, and local aggravating factors such as poorly contoured dental restorations.

Chronic periodontitis results from the accumulation of dental plaque on the teeth initially causing low-grade inflammation of the gingivae (gingivitis) and progresses to involve the periodontal tissues. Gingivitis has no radiological features. Chronic periodontitis is a painless condition that affects almost all adults and results in slow but gradual horizontal bone loss from the alveolar crest so that the teeth lose their support. Advanced periodontitis affects 10–15 per cent of the population, with smoking being a specific risk factor. A particularly aggressive form called rapidly progressive periodontitis occurs in young adults, where several teeth are affected by vertical bone loss resulting in angular bony defects that extend down towards the tooth apex (Fig. 63.18). Symmetrical widening of the periodontal ligament space affecting several teeth is sometimes seen in progressive systemic sclerosis or as irregular localized widening as an early feature of osteosarcoma of the jaws.

ODONTOMES AND ODONTOGENIC TUMOURS

When diagnosing odontogenic disorders, a simple rule is that they occur or are centred upon the tooth-bearing parts of

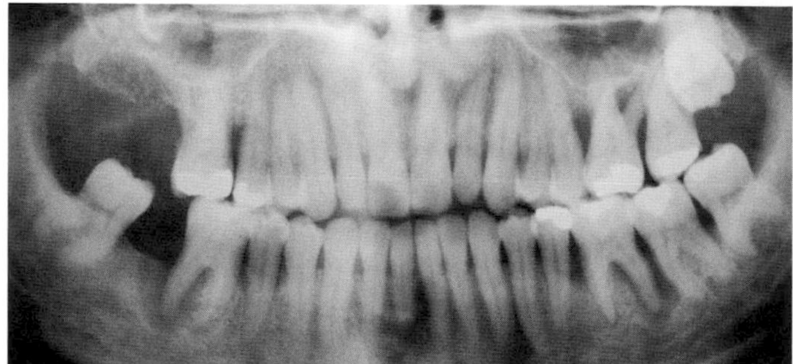

Figure 63.18 Part of a panoramic radiograph of a man aged 40 with smoking related aggressive chronic periodontal disease. There is furcation involvement of the upper left first molar and loss of up to 70 per cent of the bony attachment between the upper right first molar and second premolar and similarly on the upper left side. Combined peridontal-endodontic lesions affect both lower first molars.

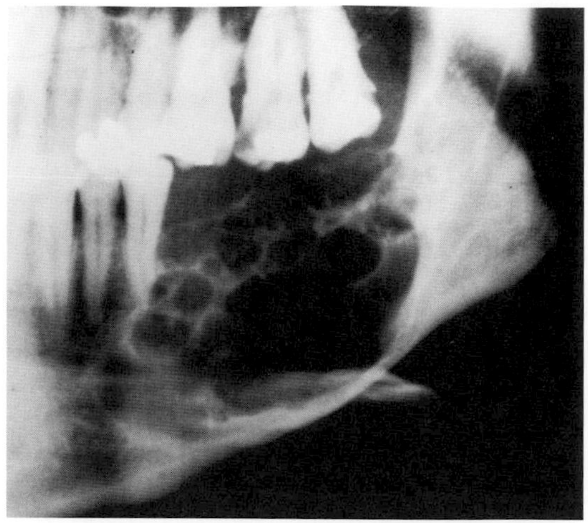

Figure 63.19 Part of a panoramic radiograph showing an ameloblastoma, which appears as an expansile, multilocular radiolucency involving the left body of the mandible.

the jaws, whereas a lesion not involving the jaw alveolus, e.g. those lying below the inferior dental canal, are unlikely to be of odontogenic origin.

Odontomes are developmental malformations or hamartomas consisting of dental hard tissues or tooth-like structures. Most are diagnosed in the second decade of life and frequently impede tooth eruption. There are two main types. The compound odontome consists of a collection of small discrete teeth called denticles and is found typically in the anterior region of the maxilla, whereas the complex odontome consists of a randomly arranged mass of enamel, dentine and cementum found predominantly in the lower premolar/molar region. Both types are densely radiopaque due to the presence of tooth enamel and are surrounded by a thin radiolucent capsular space and radio-opaque cortical margin. There are several minor developmental anomalies also classified as odontomes that can resemble teeth, but these are not described.

Odontogenic tumours are uncommon, mostly benign and arise from either the odontogenic epithelium, odontogenic epithelium and ectomesenchyme, or primarily ectomesenchyme. The commonest is the ameloblastoma, which accounts for 11 per cent of all odontogenic tumours. It occurs mainly in patients between 30–50 years of age with most (80 per cent) forming in the molar/ramus region of the mandible. When the maxilla is involved, it has the potential to spread insidiously to involve the infratemporal fossa, orbit and skull base, thus a thorough assessment is essential. The ameloblastoma has a variable radiographic appearance being a unilocular or multilocular radiolucency, but typically contains septa or locules of variable size to produce a honeycombed appearance (Fig. 63.19). The margin is well defined, often corticated but when large, produces jaw expansion with perforation of the bony cortex. A useful diagnostic feature is knife-edge resorption of the tooth roots by the tumour, which can be quite marked. The lesion is locally aggressive and requires a wide excision margin, so accurate presurgical assessment is necessary. Contrast-enhanced CT will show the tumour–bone interface but has poor soft tissue delineation. Multislice CT can be used to differentiate ameloblastoma from odontogenic keratocysts because of higher density increase during the arterial phase[4]. On T1-weighted images with gadolinium enhancement and T2-weighted images, there is good conspicuity of the tumour margin with the soft tissues, the lesion having a moderate to high signal. There is a very rare malignant variety in which the ameloblastoma probably undergoes malignant transformation with metastases most often occurring in the lungs[5]. The unicystic ameloblastoma occurs around the age of 20 years and often causes marked bony expansion (Fig. 63.20).

The odontogenic myxoma is a benign but locally aggressive tumour of odontogenic mesenchyme occurring mainly in those younger than 45 years of age. Most occur in the mandible in the premolar molar region. The lesion is usually well

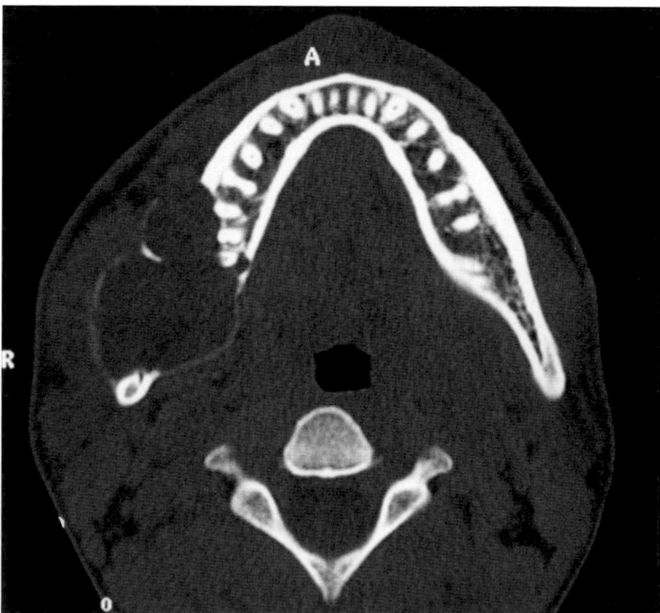

Figure 63.20 An axial CT on bone window settings of a large cystic ameloblastoma of the right side of the mandible showing marked thinning and expansion of the bone. Note the presence of root resorption.

defined, unilocular and contains a variable number of internal coarse trabeculations to produce a reticular pattern.

There are many types of odontogenic tumour, however two lesions that are well defined and contain variable amounts of focal mineral deposits are the calcifying epithelial odontogenic tumour and adenomatoid odontogenic tumour. The former is more common in men, occurs in middle life and is found mainly in the premolar/molar region of the mandible. The latter mainly affects females in the second decade of life and typically occurs anteriorly, especially in the maxilla and is associated with an unerupted tooth. The cementoblastoma is the only neoplasm of cementum; it is rare and mainly affects young males. It appears as an encapsulated radiopaque mass attached to the root, usually of a lower posterior tooth.

IMAGING IN IMPLANTOLOGY

Dental implants are placed into the jaws to replace missing teeth, giving anchorage for dental prostheses. These have gained considerable popularity since the discovery, by Branemark, that endosseous titanium implants could successfully integrate with bone. Imaging plays an essential role in pre-implant assessment, defining the volume and quality of recipient bone, identifying the location of relevant anatomical structures such as the inferior dental canal, the floor of the nose and maxillary antrum, and in assessing the status of adjacent teeth. Postoperatively, imaging is necessary to examine the degree of healing and monitor osseointegration[1].

Intra-oral periapical and dental panoramic radiography are valuable for initial pre-operative assessment but cannot identify volume of a recipient bone site or accurately localize key structures. Cross-sectional imaging is therefore indicated, particularly in complex cases, taking the form of conventional tomography, CT, MRI or Cone Beam CT (digital volume tomography). Complex tomography can be performed using dedicated multimodal maxillofacial tomography machines (Fig. 63.21) and is now available as an adjunct to conventional panoramic equipment. CT data from multiple contiguous 1–2 mm slices taken parallel to the maxillary hard palate or lower border of mandible are reformatted by dedicated multiplanar reconstruction programmes to give cross-sectional slices cross-referenced with axial plan views of the dental arch. Newly emerging cone-beam CT machines offer a similar imaging capability but with substantially lower radiation exposure, due to use of exclusively hard tissue imaging parameters. While cross-sectional tomography is used for assessment prior to placement of small numbers of implants, CT is normally reserved for complex cases involving implants in multiple quadrants. More recently MRI has been shown to be a feasible alternative to CT[6]. A stent is generally needed for any form of cross-sectional imaging to indicate chosen implant sites – this may be metallic (tomography), gutta percha or brass (CT), or gadolinium (MRI).

In the postoperative phase intraoral periapical radiographs taken perpendicular to the implant, are most useful, monitoring osseointegration and identifying peri-implant bone loss, especially at the neck, which may indicate early failure of integration.

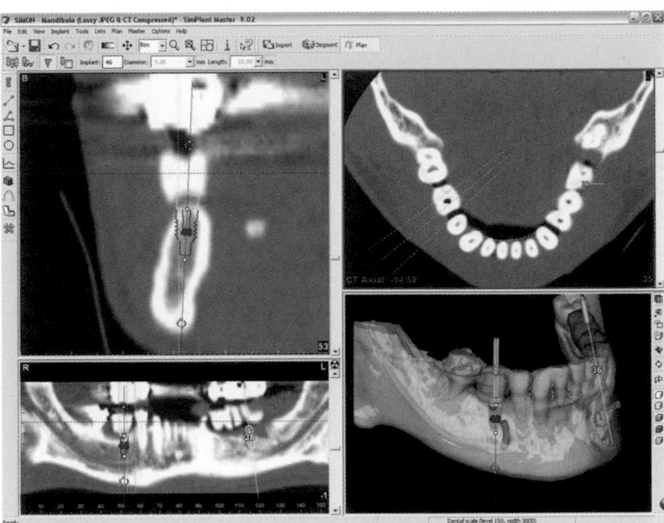

Figure 63.21 Images reconstructed from fine axial CT slices of an implant site within the mandible (SimPlant). An original axial slice is cross-referenced with a cross-sectional slice, a panoramic-like reconstruction and three-dimensional (3D) surface-rendered views. The software allows precise planning of implant placement to avoid injury to adjacent structures and helps predict the aesthetic outcome. (Courtesy of Mr Sean Goldner).

DISORDERS OF BONE

Developmental disorders

Fibrous dysplasia is a localized abnormality in which cancellous bone is replaced by fibrous tissue containing varying amounts of calcified tissue. When the jaws are affected, the maxilla is involved twice as frequently as the mandible. An immature lesion is largely radiolucent and may mimic a dental cyst, but more frequently fibrous dysplasia presents as a radiopacity, typically having an orange peel or ground-glass texture (Fig. 63.22). On radiographs the margins are usually indistinct, blending in with the normal adjacent bone. It may displace teeth or prevent their eruption. Large lesions produce jaw expansion, with thinning of the bony cortices and displacement of the antral floor. It can resemble both a cemento-ossifying fibroma, which is better defined, and an osteosarcoma, which produces destructive changes.

Cherubism is a rare dysplasia of bone that develops during the first decade of life. It occurs bilaterally in both jaws, but more commonly affects just the mandible. It develops in the posterior aspects of the jaws as a multilocular, honeycombed, expansile radiolucency. Tooth displacement is common. It regresses spontaneously after skeletal growth ceases.

Periapical cemento-osseous dysplasia and **florid cemento-osseous dysplasia** are similar conditions, with the latter being a more extravagant version of the former. They occur mainly in women, particularly of Afro-Caribbean origin, after 25 years of age. Both conditions are characterized by

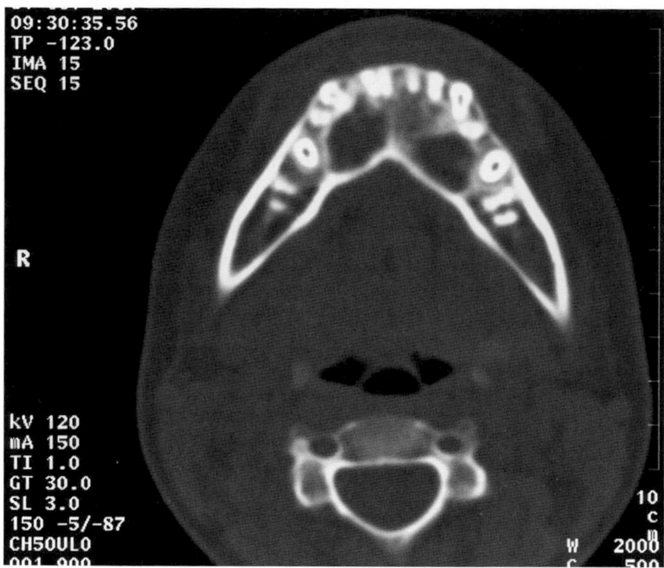

Figure 63.22 Axial CT on bone window setting of **fibrous dysplasia** of the anterior aspect of the mandible. There is thinning and expansion of the bony cortical plates. The lesion shows areas of low attenuation, lingual to the teeth, due to the presence of fibrous tissue.

the formation of multiple deposits around the tooth roots and the mandible is more frequently involved than the maxilla. In periapical cemento-osseous dysplasia, although the teeth are clinically sound, radiolucent lesions form at the apices of the teeth, which resemble periapical granulomas (see earlier). Gradually cemental-like tissue is deposited within so that it become increasingly radiopaque. When mature it becomes almost totally radiopaque but is surrounded by a thin, peripheral radiolucent zone, which helps distinguish it from sclerosing osteitis. The appearance of florid cemento-osseous dysplasia is similar to periapical cemental dysplasia but the lesions are larger, may produce jaw expansion, are more numerous, and often in both the maxilla and mandible. When extensive the condition may resemble Paget's disease of bone.

Inflammatory disorders

Osteomyelitis of the jaws is uncommon, which is surprising considering the frequency of dental sepsis. It may develop from a dental abscess or complicate tooth extraction. In acute osteomyelitis, there is thinning and discontinuity of the bony trabeculae to produce ill-defined, patchy areas of radiolucency within the cancellous and cortical bone. With time bony sequestrae form and are recognized as irregularly shaped islands of bone set against a region of radiolucency (Fig. 63.23). The features of osteomyelitis are more readily visualized on CT, which also is useful to show periosteal bone formation. On MRI, the marrow usually shows a low signal intensity on T1 and a high signal on T2 weighted images. If the disease becomes chronic, the bone becomes diffusely affected and extensively involved with sclerosis of the marrow spaces. CT will demonstrate the internal structure and the presence of sequestration.

In **diffuse sclerosing osteomyelitis**, the bone becomes increasingly dense and radio-opaque as a result of a proliferative response to low-grade infection. Bone deposition results in obliteration of the marrow spaces with gradual spread through

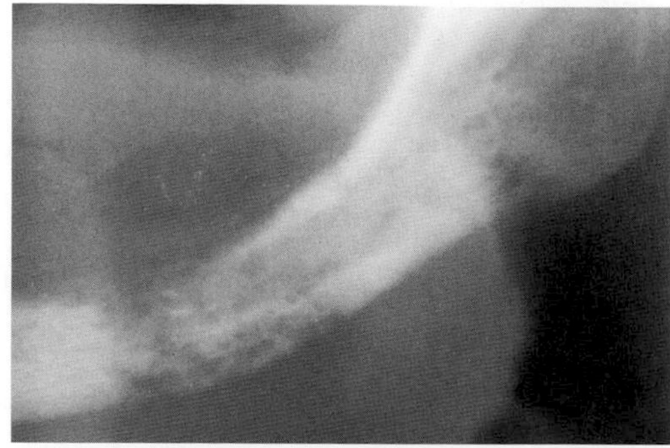

Figure 63.23 Part of a panoramic radiograph of the right mandible of a patient who developed **acute osteomyelitis** following the extraction of a premolar root 3 weeks previously. There are three sequestra in the alveolar portion of the mandible.

the mandible, however lytic areas are also seen. MRI shows a thickened cortex.

Osteoradionecrosis is an inflammatory condition that can affect the mandible if it is included in the radiation field after a dose of 45–50 Gy has been delivered. It is a clinical diagnosis and presents as areas of exposed necrotic bone. The radiographic features resemble those of chronic osteomyelitis. A similar condition called osteonecrosis may occur in the mandible in patients taking bisphosphonates.

Metabolic, endocrine, and haematological disorders of bone

Osteoporosis is found in the jaws as elsewhere in the skeleton. It affects the mandible, which becomes osteopenic, as the marrow spaces enlarge and the trabeculae thin. The cortical outline of the inferior alveolar canal becomes inconspicuous and the lower border of the mandible becomes thinner than normal.

Hyperparathyroidism of the jaws results in a general demineralization of the bone, creating a 'ground glass' appearance, loss of the lamina dura, formation of brown tumours, and subperiosteal erosions at the angle. Brown tumours develop in the facial bones, particularly in longstanding cases and appear radiolucent, with margins that are often ill defined but can also appear cystic.

Haematological replacement disorders may affect the jaws, the radiological manifestations depending on the severity of the condition. In moderate to severe thalassaemia, the jaws become radio-lucent with the presence of coarse trabeculations due to marrow hyperplasia and the maxillary antrum is reduced in size (Fig. 63.24). The skull takes on a granular appearance, with thickening of the diploic spaces and occasionally a 'hair on end' appearance.

In **sickle cell disease** similar manifestations are apparent, however several sclerotic areas are seen as a consequence of dystrophic mineralisation of small thrombi.

Paget's disease of bone is sometimes seen in the jaws, the maxilla being more commonly involved than the mandible. The radiographic disease depends on its stage of development progressing from an initial radiolucent stage to assume a more granular or 'ground glass' appearance. Later the bony trabeculae become coarse and arranged in a horizontal linear pattern

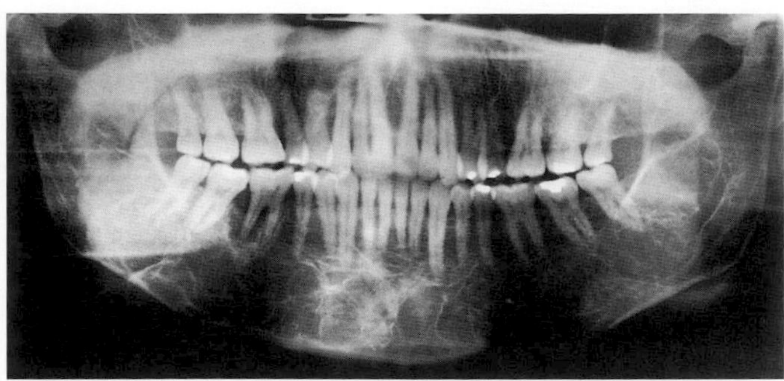

Figure 63.24 Panoramic radiograph of a case of **thalassaemia.** There is marked increase in the height of the mandible, which is composed of coarse trabeculae enclosing large marrow spaces and the small maxillary sinuses. Note the generalized loss of the lamina dura and the periodontal abscess on the distal root of the lower right first molar.

and finally the bone becomes radio-opaque with focal collections of dense bone creating a 'cotton wool' appearance.

The **central giant cell granuloma** is probably a reactive lesion and not neoplastic. It most often is detected during the first three decades of life with twice as many being discovered in the mandible as the maxilla. The lesion is usually multilocular, often well defined, lacks cortication but some have ill defined borders suggestive of a destructive lesion. Although largely radiolucent, the internal appearance varies from being almost devoid of any internal structures to those containing wispy septae (Fig. 63.25).

TUMOURS OF BONE

The **cemento-ossifying fibroma** is a tumour of bone but it can also be considered as a fibro-cemento-osseous lesion. Its behaviour varies from those showing slow growth to others being quite aggressive. It occurs mainly in young adults, mostly in the body of the mandible. The radiographic appearance depends on its degree of mineralization, and typically contains a wispy or tufted bony trabecular pattern (Fig. 63.26). The lesion is encapsulated and so appears well defined, helping to distinguish it from fibrous dysplasia.

Osteomas of the maxillofacial bones and jaws are usually slow-growing, painless and thus discovered by chance. However a large osteoma in the frontal sinuses may obstruct the drainage pathway and cause secondary infection. In the jaws, osteomas more commonly affect the mandible than the maxilla and, whilst any site can be involved, they tend to be found posteriorly on its medial aspect (Fig. 63.27). CT assists in showing the site of origin and provides three-dimensional (3D) topographic detail. Multiple osteomas are a feature of Gardner's syndrome (familial adenomatous polyposis) and precede the formation of intestinal colonic polyposis.

Osteosarcoma is uncommon in the jaws, accounting for only 7 per cent of all osteosarcomas. It tends to be slower growing and occurs about 10 years later than osteosarcoma of the long bones. The mandible is more commonly affected than the maxilla. Maxillary lesions tend to arise from the alveolar ridge, and mandibular ones in the body. It has a destructive appearance and its density varies from being radiolucent, to patchily radio-opaque or predominantly sclerotic. An important early dental radiographic sign is widening of the periodontal ligament space due to tumour spread along the periodontal ligament, however this feature is also seen in other sarcomas (e.g. fibrosarcoma Ewing's sarcoma). When the periosteum is elevated a 'hair-on-end', sunray or onion skin appearance may be visible. CT is required to demonstrate accurately tumour calcification, bone destruction, and bone reaction (Fig. 63.28),

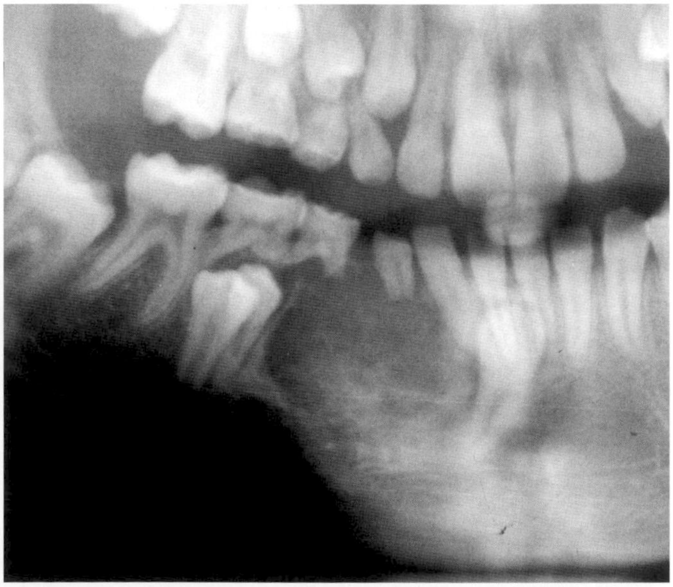

Figure 63.25 Part of a panoramic radiograph of a **central giant-cell granuloma** of the right side of the mandible, which appears as a well-defined radiolucency containing numerous coarse bony trabeculae. There has been displacement of the premolar teeth posteriorly and the canine anteriorly.

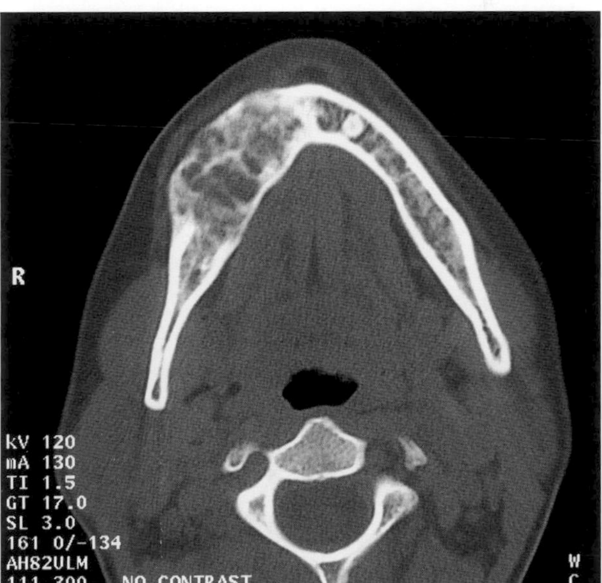

Figure 63.26 Bone window setting of an axial CT of a **cemento-ossifying fibroma** of the mandible showing mainly buccal expansion and thinning of both cortical plates, which remain intact. The lesion is of mixed attenuation as it contains areas of fibrosis, mineralization, and coarse bony trabeculations.

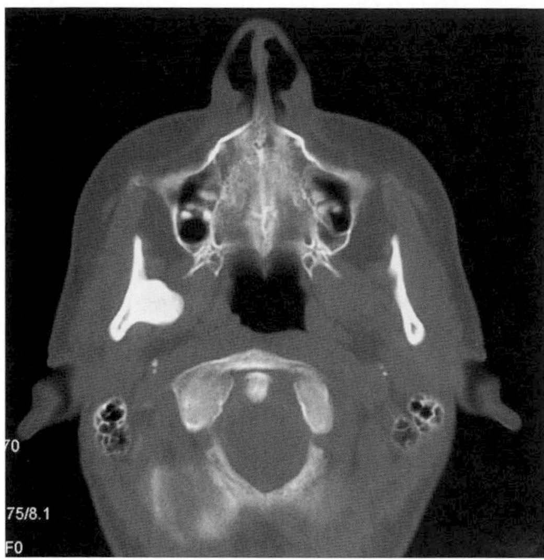

Figure 63.27 Bone window setting of an axial CT showing a dense (compact) osteoma arising from the medial aspect of the ramus of the right mandible.

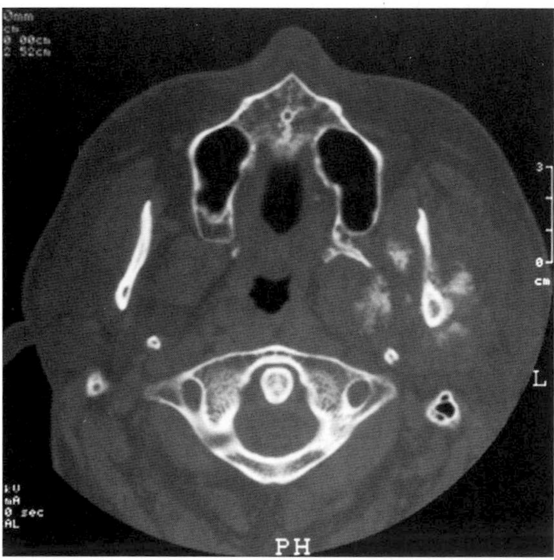

Figure 63.28 Bone window setting of an axial CT of **osteogenic sarcoma** of the left mandibular ramus. There is bone destruction in the region of the sigmoid notch. The lesion contains areas of neoplastic bone formation and extends medially towards the lateral pterygoid plate, posteriorly to the styloid process, and laterally resulting in facial swelling. (Courtesy of Mr S. Dover, Birmingham).

whilst MRI (T1- and T2-weighted images) will provide better information on the intramedullary and extraosseous components of the tumour[7].

Primary carcinoma of the overlying oral mucosa can invade the jaws to produce an ill-defined, noncorticated area of bone destruction. Bone destruction around the tooth roots gives an appearance of teeth floating in space. Very rarely, carcinoma may arise from malignant transformation of a cyst lining or epithelial residues within the jaw bone to produce an ill-defined osteolytic lesion. It affects older patients usually during in the 6th or 7th decades of life.

Metastatic tumour involvement of the jaws is uncommon, being less than 1 per cent. Primary sites include the breast, kidney, lung, colon, and prostate. They form predominantly in the posterior aspects of the mandible, resulting in loss of the outline of the inferior alveolar canal and destruction of the cortical plates. Typically their outline is moderately to poorly defined, with irregular margins that appear destructive (Fig. 63.29) without new bone formation. Some metastatic deposits are characterized by the development of several areas, often small, of bone destruction. Although most lesions that metastasize to the jaws are lytic, others, notably from the prostate, can produce bone and appear radio-opaque.

An **extranodal lymphoma** can affect the maxilla and posterior aspect of the mandible and generally appears as an ill-defined noncorticated radiolucency (Fig. 63.30). Eosino-

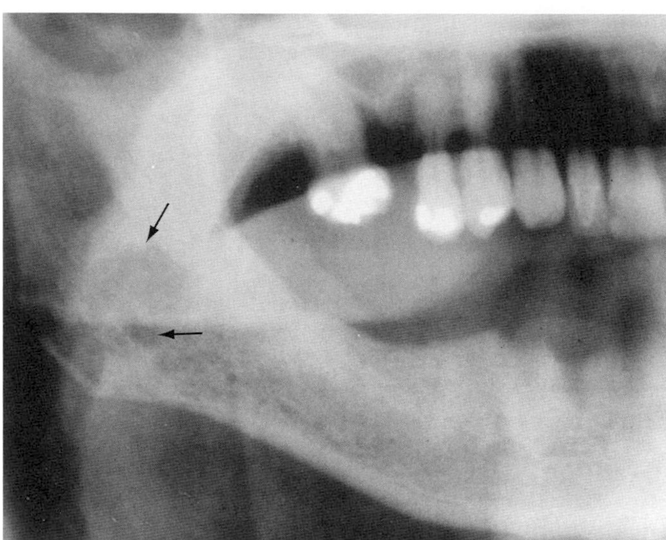

Figure 63.29 Panoramic radiograph showing metastatic carcinoma of the lung. The patient had his remaining lower teeth extracted 2 weeks previously because of toothache. Note the soft-tissue swelling in the lower right third molar region. The outline of the socket is no longer visible nor is the course of the inferior dental canal. There are multiple punched-out radiolucencies in the right angle (arrows) with erosion of the inferior cortex.

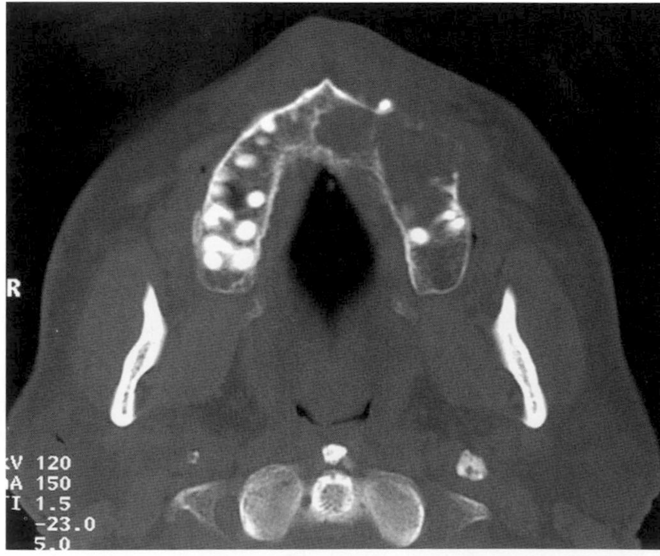

Figure 63.30 **Extranodal lymphoma** of the maxilla shown on a bone window setting axial CT at the level of the alveolus. Although a few areas of the lesion are well defined, the overall appearance is destructive with loss of much of the buccal alveolar plate.

philic granuloma and the other Langerhans' cell histiocytosis are occasionally found in the jaws, where they may mimic dental periapical or periodontal disease. Multiple myeloma is uncommon in the jaws; the mandible is more frequently affected than the maxilla, with a predilection for the posterior body and angle. Typically the lesions are well defined but lack a cortical margin and so appear punched out, but some have ragged margins.

TRAUMA

Teeth

The teeth, particularly the anterior ones, are frequently involved in traumatic injuries to the face. They may be partially or completely avulsed or the crowns or roots may be fractured. Crown fractures may just involve the enamel, or the enamel and dentine, or if at a lower level expose the pulp. Root fractures occur less frequently and if undisplaced can be difficult to detect on radiographs when two different angled views may be required. Dental trauma can be associated with a localized dento-alveolar fracture in which a block of bone becomes detached containing several teeth. Intra-oral radiographs best demonstrate traumatic injuries of the teeth.

Fractures of the facial skeleton

The facial skeleton is a complex arrangement of bones, air cavities and soft tissues attached to the skull base. Fractures in this region may be confined to the maxilla or involve other parts of the facial skeleton, such as the zygoma and nasal bones. Maxillary fractures are still classified according to the system described by Le Fort in 1900, who defined three principle types of fractures after applying blunt trauma to the faces of cadavers. The classification is contentious because fractures do not always follow the exact pattern he described (Fig. 63.31). Plain films form the initially assessment, but many of these injuries are complicated and require evaluation with axial and coronal CT or cone beam CT.

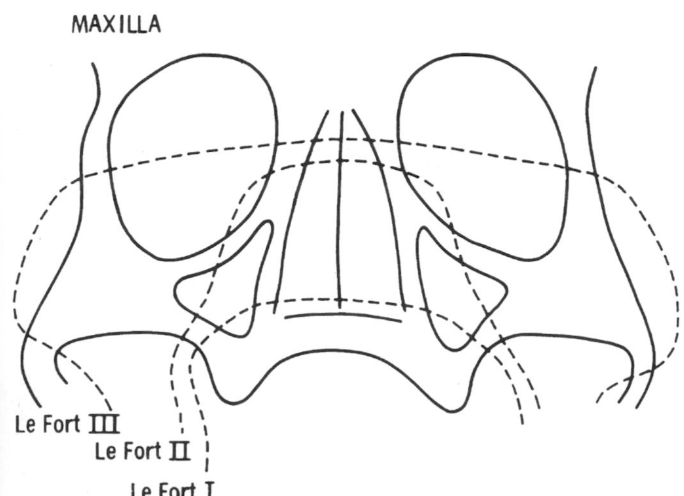

Figure 63.31 Fracture lines in Le Fort I, II, and III fractures.

In a **Le Fort I fracture** (Fig. 63.32), the tooth-bearing part of the maxilla is separated from the rest of the maxilla by trauma to the lower part of the face. The fracture line passes above the teeth but below the zygomatric buttress. It runs from the piriform fossa posteriorly to the pterygoid plates and involves the lower part of the nasal septum resulting in detachment of the dentoalveolar fragment from the remainder of the maxilla. The posterior portion may drop inferiorly, resulting in an open bite, and this is a useful diagnostic feature, as the Le Fort I fracture can often be difficult to detect on radiographs.

The **Le Fort II fracture** (Fig. 63.33) runs along the nasal bridge, through the lacrimal bones across the medial orbital walls, and orbital rims wall to involve the anterior and posterolateral wall of the maxillary sinuses and pterygoid plates. The nasal septum is fractured at a variable level.

In the **Le Fort III** or **suprazygomatic fracture** (Fig. 63.34), there is complete separation of the midface from the cranial base resulting in clinical lengthening of the face. The fracture line runs through the nasal bones, the frontal processes of the maxilla, posterolaterally through the medial and lateral orbital walls, and through the zygomatic arches. The nasal septum is fractured superiorly.

In practice, many fractures do not exactly fit these descriptions. Fractures caused by sharp-edged objects can produce comminuted fractures of the maxilla (Fig. 63.35) without affecting the tooth-bearing alveolar bone, and some fractures are not symmetrical. For instance, Le Fort I, II, and III fractures may be unilateral (Figs. 63.35, 63.36), or a Le Fort I or II may

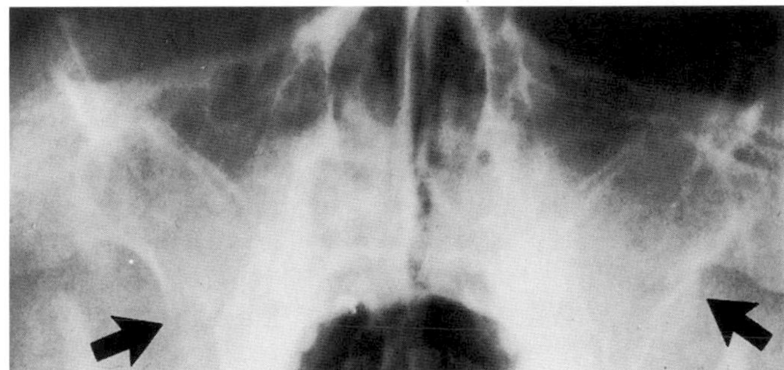

Figure 63.32 Le Fort 1 fracture. The fractures of the lateral walls of the maxillary sinuses have been arrowed. The fractures of the medial walls cannot be seen on this projection.

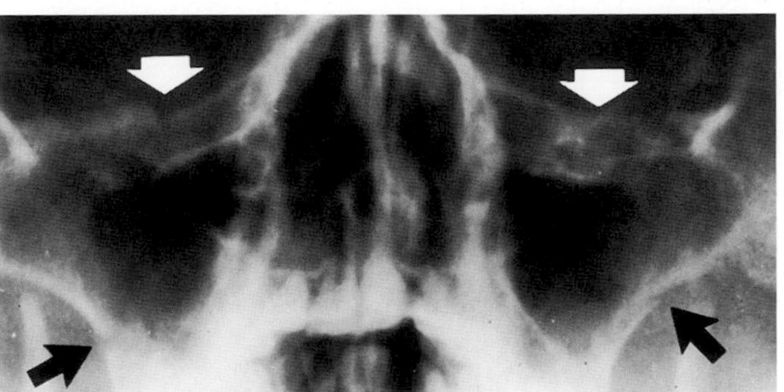

Figure 63.33 Le Fort II fracture. The fractures of the inferior margins of the orbits and of the lateral walls of the maxillary sinuses have been arrowed. The fracture of the nasal bone is not visible on this projection.

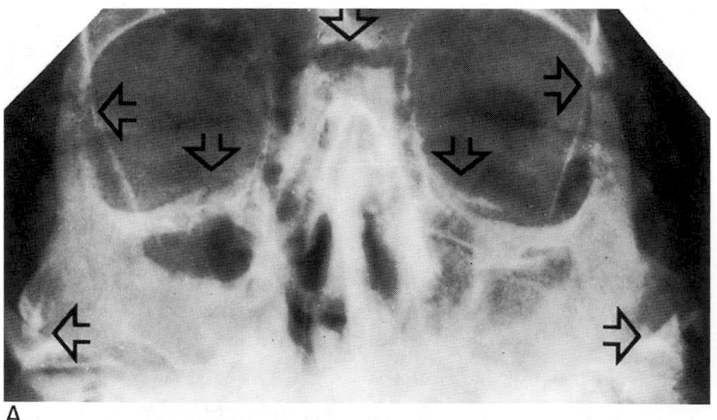

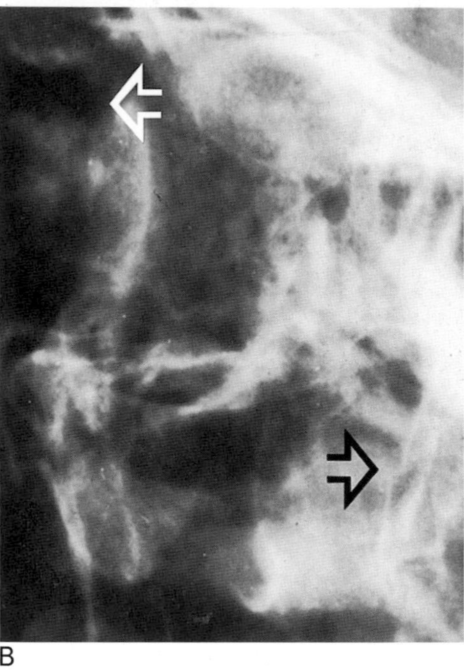

Figure 63.34 Combined Le Fort II and Le Fort III fractures. (A) There are fractures of the nasal bones, lateral orbital margins, inferior orbital margins and zygomatic arches. All have been marked with arrows. There is a fluid level in the right maxillary sinus and opacification of the left maxillary sinus. (B) Lateral view of fractures shown in A. There is a fracture of the nasal bones with wide separation (white arrow) and there are fractures of the posterior walls of the maxillary sinuses (black arrow).

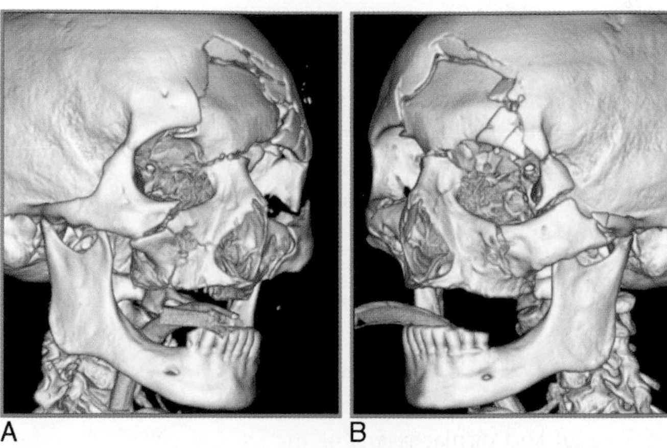

Figure 63.35 3D CT scans showing multiple fractures of the facial bones (Le Fort II and unilateral Le Fort III) and depressed fracture of frontal ethmoidal complex. Note the asymmetrical pattern of the fractures with the more severe injury involving the left side.

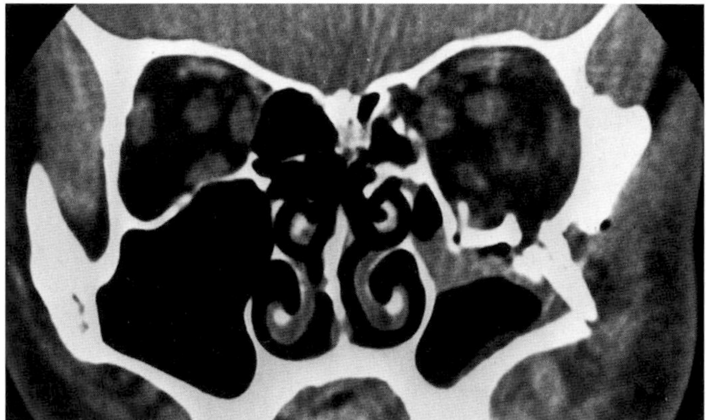

Figure 63.36 Coronal CT of a unilateral left-sided Le Fort II fracture. There are fractures of the medial wall of the orbit, the floor and inferior rim of the orbit, and the anterior wall of the maxillary sinus.

coexist with a Le Fort III (Fig. 63.34). Nevertheless the Le Fort classification is still widely used as it allows these complicated fractures to be described simply.

Fractures of the zygomatic complex

The zygomatic bone contributes to the lateral and inferior margins of the orbit, the lateral wall of the maxillary sinus, and the anterior end of the zygomatic arch, thus fractures of the zygomatic bone involve all the sites (Fig. 63.37) usually with fractures in the region of the zygomatico-frontal suture, zygomatico-temporal suture, infra-orbital rim and the lateral wall of the antrum. As not all of the fractures are always visible on a single film the presence of even one fracture should raise the suspicion that other fractures are present and, dependent

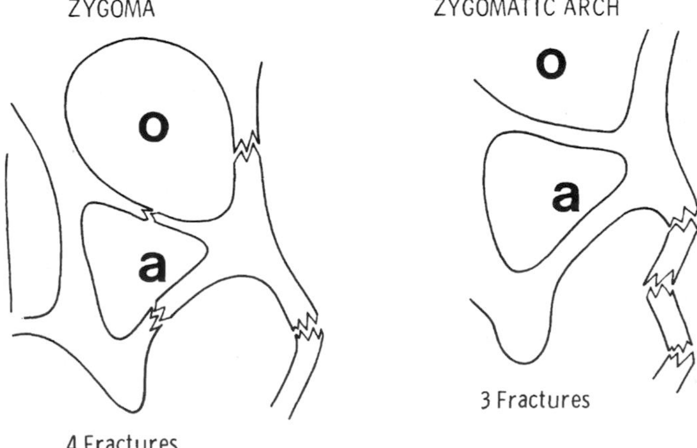

Figure 63.37 Diagram of the **usual sites of fracture of the zygoma and of the zygomatic arch.** o = orbit, a = antrum.

upon clinical findings, other imaging may be required. Severe trauma may result in a comminuted fracture of the zygomatic complex (Fig. 63.38A, B). The zygomatic arch may be fractured in association with a fracture of the zygoma as described earlier, or it may be fractured alone as a result of direct trauma to the side of the head and is seen as three points of fracture (Fig. 63.37).

Blow-out fractures of the orbit

A blow-out fracture occurs following blunt trauma to the front of the orbit. The inward force of the eyeball produces a temporary increase in pressure within the orbit, resulting in fracture and displacement of the thin bone of the orbital floor, but leaving the orbital rim intact. The orbital soft tissues herniate through the defect into the maxillary sinus. This often shows as soft tissue opacity in the upper aspect of the sinus on an occipitomental radiograph and sometimes a fluid level when blood is present. CT is helpful in defining the extent of the defect of the orbital floor and the involvement of the external ocular muscles in the fracture (Fig. 63.39). Coronal CTs demonstrate soft tissue displacement more clearly than axial. Orbital ultrasound (US) with a curved-array transducer has been shown to be useful in the detection orbital wall and orbital rim fractures[8]. Failure of recognition of a blow-out fracture or fusion of malpositioned bony fragments may lead to entrapped tissues, fibrosis, and possible diplopia. Orbital floor fractures are often accompanied by fracture of the medial wall (lamina papyracea) of the orbit.

RADIOLGICAL INVESTIGATION OF MAXILLARY FRACTURES

The initial radiographic investigation of a patient with a suspected fracture of the maxilla should be limited to a standard occipitomental, a 30-degree occipitomental (both taken postero-anterior (PA) if possible as this provides better bony detail than antero-posterior (AP) projections and with patient cooperation), and a true lateral view centred on the maxilla. These radiographs may be sufficient to diagnose and assess the fractures, but other imaging is often necessary, particularly in the more severely injured patient.

It should be remembered that recent undisplaced fractures may be not always be demonstrated on routine plain films and soft tissue oedema may obscure detail. Displaced fractures of the orbital mar-gins should show on the occipitomental views. In the Le Fort I and II fractures, there is usually a step or break in the posterior wall of the maxillary sinus on the lateral view (Fig. 63.34). Fractures of the zygomatic arches usually show on occipitomental projections, but may be better visualized on an underpenetrated submentovertical view.

Computed tomography (CT) is useful in the diagnosis and assessment of Le Fort II and Le Fort III fractures, naso-orbital fractures, orbital blow-out fractures, skull base fractures and may be helpful with Le Fort I and zygomatic complex fractures. CT demonstrates the amount of displacement or rotation of the fractured fragments, injury to the globes, optic nerve compression from bone fragments, fracture of the cribriform plate, and the possible presence of foreign bodies. Axial slices parallel to the occlusal plane are appropriate for detecting maxillary fractures allowing simple repeatability and limiting artefacts produced by metallic dental restorations. Thin slices are desirable for good bone detail and need not be contiguous unless 3D reconstruction is planned. Coronal slices at right angles to the occlusal plane demonstrate fractures of the orbital floor better than axial scans, but may not be possible in the elderly or uncooperative or recently injured patient. Thin noncontiguous slices (e.g. 2 mm at intervals of 4 or 5 mm) are adequate in most cases and should cover the orbital floors from the orbital rim to the optic foramina. Coronal slices that suffer from artefacts from dental restorations can be reduced by angling away from the true coronal position, or avoided by reconstruction from contiguous axial slices but at the cost of impaired resolution.

CT with 3D reconstruction may be used to demonstrate graphically fractures of the facial skeleton (Fig. 63.38B) and is helpful in the management of residual traumatic deformities that require reconstructive surgery. Multislice CT results

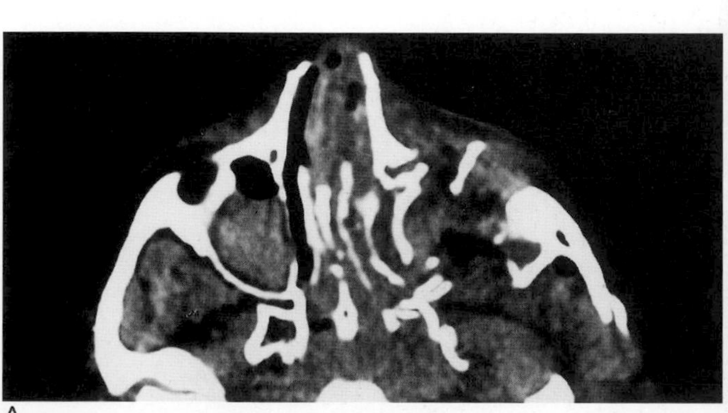

A

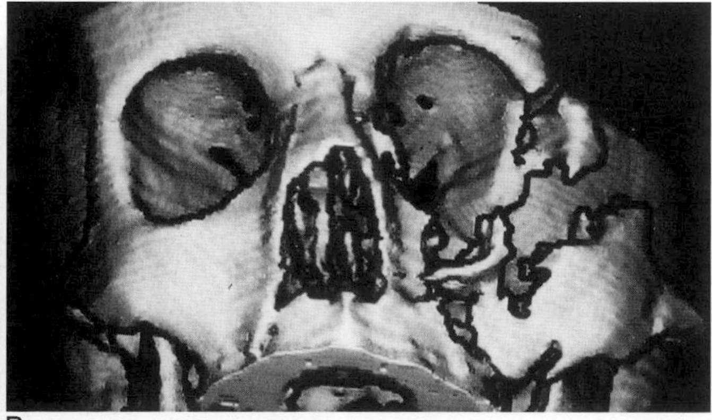

B

Figure 63.38 Comminuted fracture of the left zygoma on axial CT. (A) There are multiple fractures of the anterior, posterolateral and medial walls of the maxillary sinus. There is air in the soft tissues of the cheek and infratemporal fossa. (B) 3D CT reconstruction of a comminuted fracture of the left zygoma (same case as **A**).

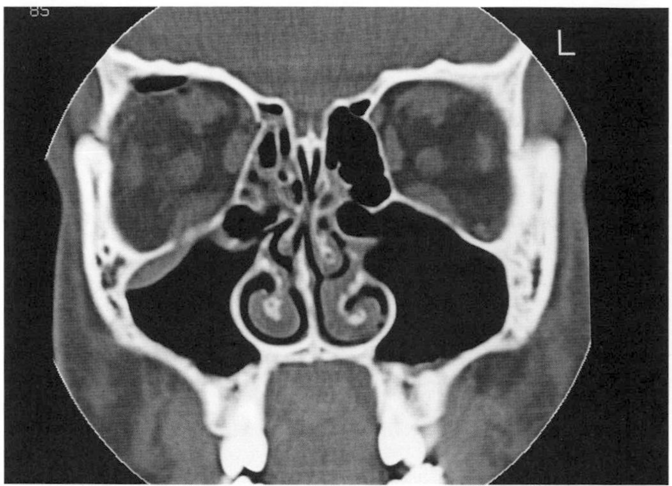

Figure 63.39 Coronal CT showing a **blow-out fracture of the floor of the right orbit.** Fractures of the lamina papyracea (with blood within the ethmoid complex) and orbital floor (with herniation of orbital contents and air within orbital cavity) are arrowed.

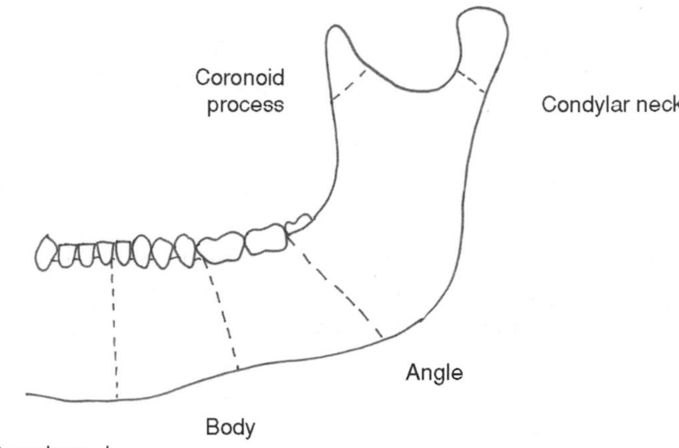

Figure 63.40 Line diagram showing **common sites of fracture** of the mandible.

in greatly increased speed of data acquisition and reconstruction so that more slices can be recorded with thinner sections than previously with spiral CT. Rapid data acquisition and multiplanar reconstructed images are relevant, particularly for severely injured patients as the result of, for example, blunt trauma from road traffic accidents who may have intracranial pathology or cervical vertebra trauma where there may be patient positioning problems.

Fractures of the mandible

Fractures of the mandible tend to occur at specific sites, as shown in Fig. 63.40. They are best demonstrated on a dental panoramic radiograph (Fig. 63.41), (or right and left oblique lateral mandibular views), together with a PA mandible radiograph. However, a fracture in the parasymphyseal region may not show on either of these films but will be demonstrated on intra-oral views, which are useful where the teeth are also thought to be fractured. A fracture on one side of the mandible is frequently accompanied by a contralateral fracture, particularly of the condylar neck.

Temporomandibular joint

The temporomandibular joint (TMJ) is a complex diarthrodial, synovial joint. It contains the mandibular condyle, which sits in the glenoid fossa when the mouth is closed. Anteriorly lies the articular eminence and posteriorly the external auditory meatus. The joint is divided into an upper and lower joint compartment by a biconcave, fibrocartilagenous disc, which acts as a cushion for the mandibular condyle. The disc lies above the condyle and is attached posteriorly by fibro-elastic tissue to the base of the skull, neck of the mandibular condyle, and elsewhere to the fibrous joint capsule. The capsule is lined by a synovial membrane and encloses the joint. Fibres of the lateral ptergyoid muscle insert into the anterior aspect of the capsule and articular disc as well as to the anterior aspect of the condylar neck.

Figure 63.41 Panoramic radiograph showing **bilateral fractures of the mandible** in the right canine region and left wisdom tooth region.

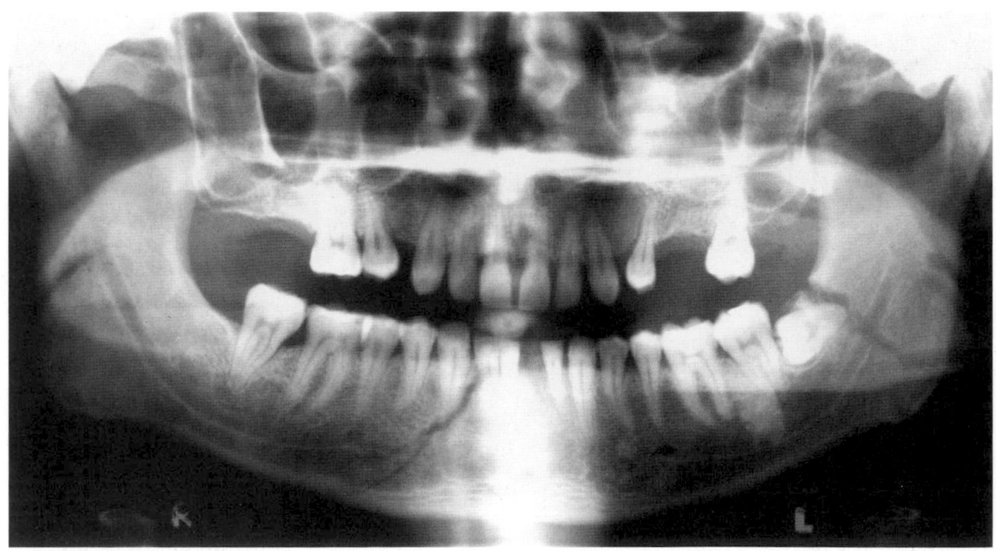

The temporomandibular joint is susceptible to conditions that affect other joints including developmental abnormalities, arthritic, traumatic, and neoplastic disease.

DEVELOPMENTAL ABNORMALITIES

These usually affect the temporal and condylar components, mainly consisting of changes in size and form, and usually result in alteration in the growth of the affected side of the mandible.

Hypoplasia of the mandibular condyle is failure of the condyle to attain full size. It may be localized to the joint or can be part of a generalized disorder, e.g. first arch syndrome. It results in underdevel-opment of the affected side of the mandible. Condylar hyperplasia causes enlargement of the mandibular condyle due to overactivity of the cartilaginous growth centre. It produces either a posterior open bite on the affected side or a centre line shift of the mandible relative to the maxilla. Radionuclide imaging may be required to demonstrate whether growth of the condylar cartilage is active prior to corrective treatment. In Hurler's syndrome (gargoylism) the articular surface of the condyle is usually concave instead of convex, an appearance thought specific for this syndrome.

A bifid condyle is believed to result from obstructed blood supply or trauma during its development. There are no clinical features and it appears as a notch or indentation on the articular surface of the condyle.

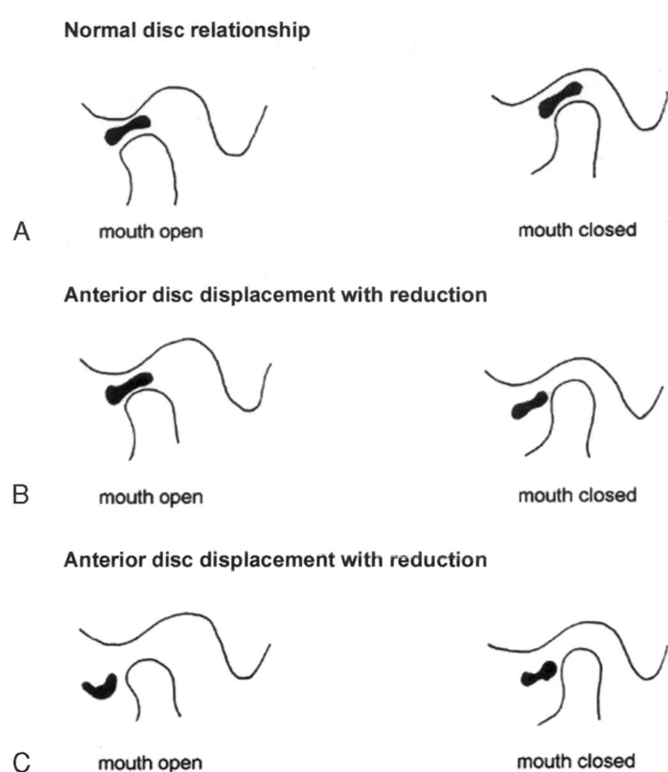

Figure 63.42 Diagrammatic representation of the **articular disc** (shaded). (A) In a normal position in relationship to condylar head, and (B) in an anteriorly displaced position with reduction on opening, and (C) with a nonreducing disc.

Temporomandibular joint dysfunction

Temporomandibular joint dysfunction is a common condition and consists of myofascial pain, resulting in muscle spasm, facial discomfort and/or internal derangement of the articular disc. Myofascial pain occurs in all age groups but is particularly common in young female patients. It presents as muscle tenderness, jaw stiffness and headaches, and is associated with stress and anxiety, tooth clenching, and occlusal disharmony. The condition is a type of fibromyalgia and as the bony tissues are not affected it has no specific radiological changes.

Internal derangement is an abnormality of the position of the articular disc, which may also show an altered morphology. The normal disc position in relation to the mandibular condyle is illustrated in Fig. 63.42. When the disc becomes displaced, it does so usually in an anteromedial, medial or sometimes lateral position relative to the condylar head. The condition may be painful and cause clicking or jaw locking, however several studies have shown displaced discs in individuals without symptoms. Discomfort is more prevalent in patients with disc displacement without reduction, particularly in combination with osteoarthrosis and bone marrow oedema.

The diagnosis is made from the clinical findings and in most cases the condition improves or resolves with conventional therapy. When this fails and more aggressive treatment is planned or when the diagnosis is uncertain, the disc position can be demonstrated using arthrography or MRI with the latter being the technique of choice[9].

The joint can be imaged using protein density or T1 and T2 sequences using 3 mm parasagittal slices, the angulation being determined by the medial angulation of the condylar head. On MRI, the disc appears as a biconcave (bow tie shaped) structure of low attenuation sandwiched between the anterior aspect of the articulating surface of the condyle and the glenoid fossa. Anterior disc displacement with reduction of the disc is shown in Fig. 63.43A and B. When the mouth is opened, the anteriorly displaced disc reduces or moves back to a normal position relative to the condylar head; this manoeuvre often results in a click, which can be apparent to the patient and palpated by the clinician. However, if the disc remains anteriorly displaced (Fig. 63.44) it may interfere with forward translation of the condyle, resulting in locking and restricted mouth opening, and pressure on the disc may cause it to become distorted.

T2-weighted images can be used to show joint effusions and inflammatory change. The significance of joint effusion is controversial as it can occur in the nonpainful joint. However, it is observed more often in joints with more advanced stages of disc displacement, i.e. nonreducing discs, and it is thought to represent the presence of synovitis[10]. Images taken in a coronal plane demonstrate disc displacement medially or laterally; this view is useful to show degenerative changes to the articular surface. The use of plain radiographs to assess joint space as a predictor of disc displacement has been shown to have a low predictive value[11].

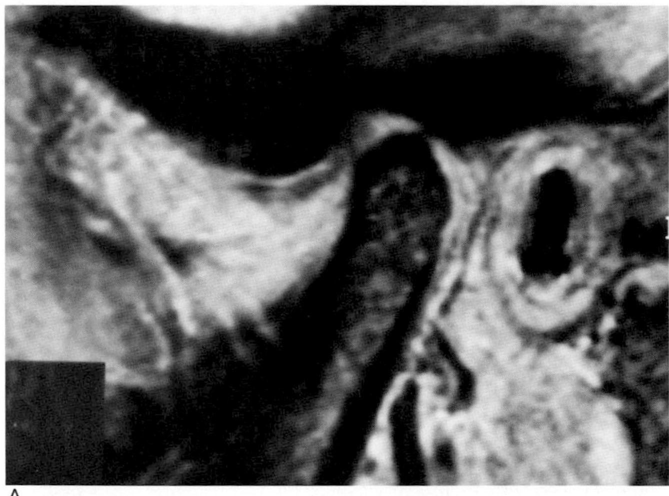
A

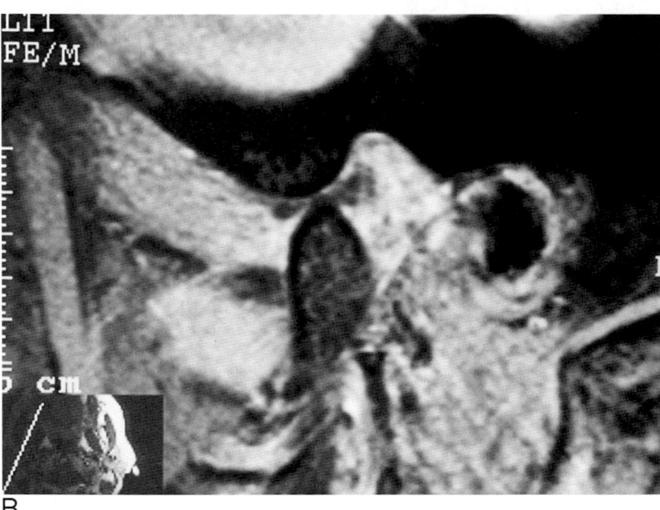

B

Figure 63.43 Anterior reducible subluxation of disc. Fast-field echo (FFE) MRI parasagittal images showing an anteriorly positioned disk (A), which reduces on opening (B) to lie over the condyle.

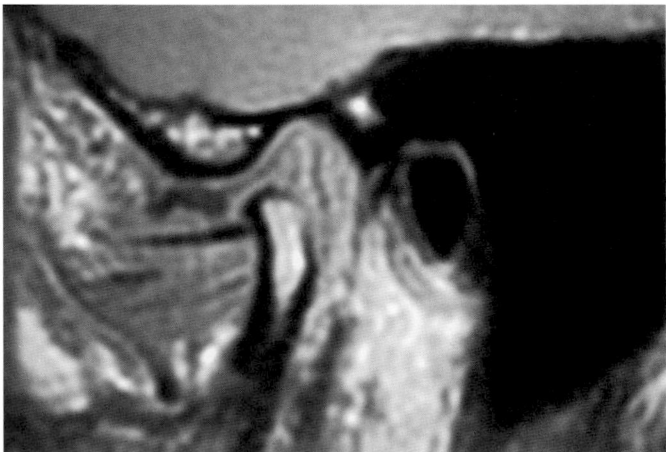

Figure 63.44 Parasagittal T1-weighted MRI image with the mouth open showing a nonreducing, anteriorly displaced disc.

Arthritides

Degenerative joint disease (osteoarthritis) can develop at any age but its incidence increases with age. It is thought to occur when the joint is unable to adapt to remodelling forces. There may be no symptoms or there may be discomfort and joint tenderness similar to temporomandibular joint dysfunction (TMJ) but crepitus is often present. The radiographic features are shown diagrammatically (Fig. 63.45), and include flattening and irregularity of the condylar surface, sclerosis, and osteophyte formation, which is seen mainly on the anterosuperior condylar surface (Fig. 63.46).

Inflammatory arthritis. Rheumatoid arthritis is a common condition in which the TMJ becomes involved in about half of cases. Symptoms include pain, swelling, and jaw stiffness. Radiographic changes consist of loss of bone density and formation of erosions leading to a somewhat pointed condylar head. T2-weighted coronal MRI images are valuable for demonstrating the presence of joint inflammation. Other

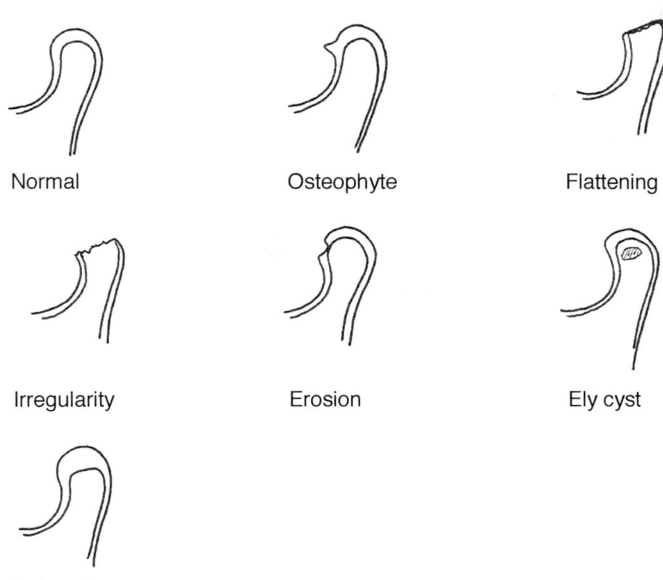

Figure 63.45 Diagrammatic representation showing various **degenerative changes that affect the mandibular condyle**.

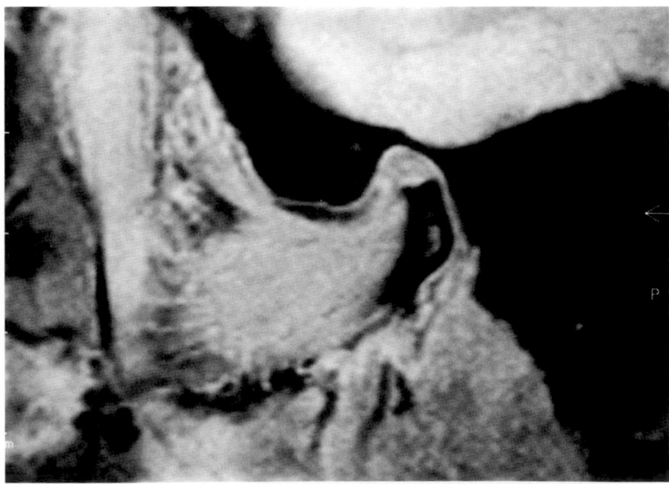

Figure 63.46 TMJ. **Degenerative arthritis**. Parasagittal MR image. Osteophytic change is present at the anterior aspect of the articular surface of the condyle; the articular disc is grossly distorted and lies immediately inferior to the articular eminence.

inflammatory arthritides may affect the joint, including systemic lupus, systemic sclerosis, psoriasis, Reiter's syndrome, juvenile chronic arthritis, and synovial osteochondromatosis, which results in joint swelling and the presence of numerous loose calcific bodies (Fig. 63.47).

Juvenile chronic arthritis occurs during the first 2 decades of life and is characterized by intermittent synovial inflammation. It causes pain and tenderness of one or both joints and if severe will affect mandibular growth. The condyle becomes radiolucent and its surface develops erosions and irregularity.

Injury

Isolated fractures of the condylar neck can occur but often accompany fractures of the mandible, especially following a blow to the chin, and are usually visible on a dental panoramic radiograph and a PA condylar view. The slender condylar neck acts as a stress breaker, reducing the likelihood of the condyle being driven up into the middle cranial fossa. Fractures of the condylar neck may be simple and undisplaced or displaced with the condyle being pulled forwards and medially by the lateral pterygoid muscle (fracture dislocation). Intracapsular fractures are difficult to demonstrate on plain films and if suspected may require evaluation with CT if symptoms persist. Haemarthrosis and ankylosis may complicate recovery.

Acute dislocation of the TMJ occurs following a blow to the mandible when the mouth is open. It is diagnosed from the clinical presentation. The role of radiology is to exclude a fracture or other contributing disease. Recurrent dislocation can develop spontaneously and may be a feature of Marfan's syndrome and Ehlers–Danlos syndrome.

Ankylosis of the TMJ may follow a traumatic haemarthrosis or infective arthritis. When this happens in childhood, many cases are complicated by hypoplasia of the condyle secondary to concurrent damage to the epiphyseal growth centre. CT is required to show the extent of the ankylosis (Fig. 63.48).

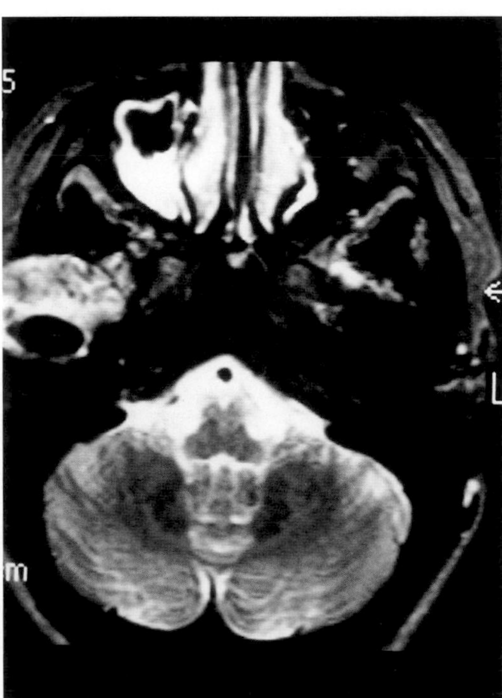

Figure 63.47 Osteochondromatosis of the TMJ. Axial T2W MR view showing mass draped around the right condyle.

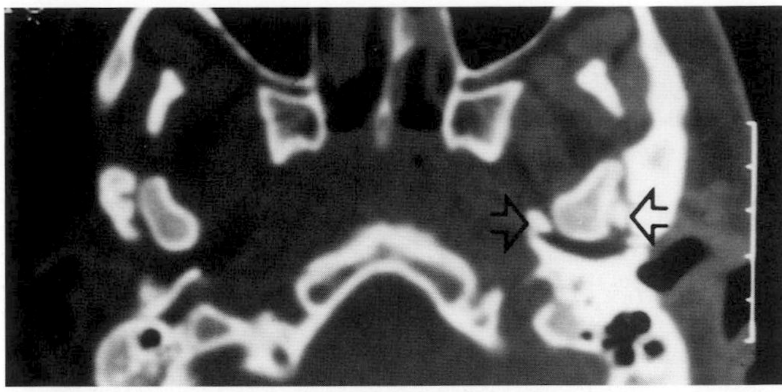

Figure 63.48 Bony ankylosis of the left TMJ on axial CT. There are two bone fragments (arrows) between the mandibular condyle and the glenoid fossa, and there is partial bone union between the lateral bone fragment, the condyle, and the glenoid fossa. Both mandibular condyles are rotated due to the fractures of the condylar necks. The patient had developed permanent trismus following an accident in childhood. (Courtesy of Dr Otto Chan).

Neoplasms of the temporomandibular joint are uncommon and include osteoma, osteochondroma, chondrosarcomas and rarely, metastatic deposits.

SALIVARY GLAND DISORDERS

There are three paired major salivary glands – the parotid, submandibular and sublingual glands – and many minor salivary glands supplying saliva to lubricate, cleanse and aid early digestion within the mouth.

The **parotid gland** lies between the posterior border of the man-dibular ramus and the sternomastoid muscle attaching to the mastoid process. It is enclosed in deep cervical fascia and traversed by the retromandibular vein, external carotid artery, and facial nerve. The retromandibular vein is easily visible on all forms of cross-sectional imaging and indicates the plane of the dividing plexus of the facial nerve lying just laterally. In this plane lies the major intraglandular ductal system, and this divides the gland into a larger superficial and smaller deep portion. While tumours are more common in the superficial lobe, surgical approach to the deep lobe involves dissection of the nerve branches, with attendant risk of nerve damage. The parotid gland drains through Stensen's duct, running horizontally forward approximately 1 cm below the zygomatic arch on the surface of masseter to turn medially, perforate the buccinator muscle, and emerge on a papilla on the buccal mucosa opposite the 1st maxillary molar tooth. The sharp sigmoid bend in the anterior portion of the parotid duct is a common site for impaction of small salivary stones and is the location of the proposed 'buccinator window anomaly', a possible obstructive phenomenon.

The **submandibular gland** wraps around the posterior free border of the mylohyoid muscle, medial to the posterior body of mandible and descends for 2–3 cm into the suprahyoid neck. The main Wharton's duct passes up from the hilum of the gland, around the posterior margin of mylohyoid, turning anteriorly in the floor of the mouth to open through a small papilla situated on either side of the lingual frenum, behind the lower incisor teeth.

The sublingual glands lie anteriorly in the floor of mouth above the mylohyoid muscle. Each gland opens by a single Bartolin's duct or by multiple ducts into the floor of mouth or terminal part of Wharton's duct.

Radiological techniques and their application

Plain radiographs are of limited value. An intra-oral true mandibular occlusal view detects radio-opaque salivary calculi in the anterior submandibular duct, of which 60–80 per cent are radio-opaque, while a PA view of the cheek may detect the 20–40 per cent of parotid stones that are radio-opaque. A negative result does not preclude obstruction.

Sialography has limitations in demonstrating parenchymal disease but remains a highly sensitive test of ductal abnormalities. Cannulation of the parotid duct is normally straightforward but the submandibular duct orifice may be very fine and difficult to identify. The sublingual duct and gland may only be incidentally demonstrated. Direct visualization of ductal filling under fluoroscopy, particularly using digital subtraction techniques (Fig. 63.49), has benefits over the traditional plain film method and water-soluble contrast media should be used to avoid the permanent foreign body reaction sometimes seen when oily media are extravasated from the ductal system. Sialography has no place in the investigation of mass lesions and is indicated primarily for symptoms directly related to the ductal system such as obstruction and sialectasis.

Interventional sialography offers a minimally invasive alternative to formal surgical sialadenectomy or sialolithectomy. Small mobile stones may be extracted from the duct system by Dormia basket or balloon catheter, and duct strictures dilated by angioplasty balloon (Figs 63.50A, B; 63.51A, B)[12,13].

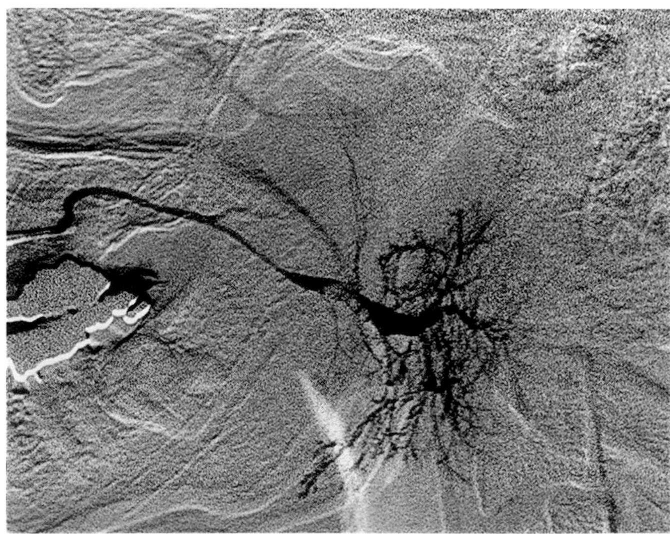

Figure 63.49 Collection of calculi at hilum of parotid gland. There is minor sialectasis (irregularity of calibre of some intraglandular ducts).

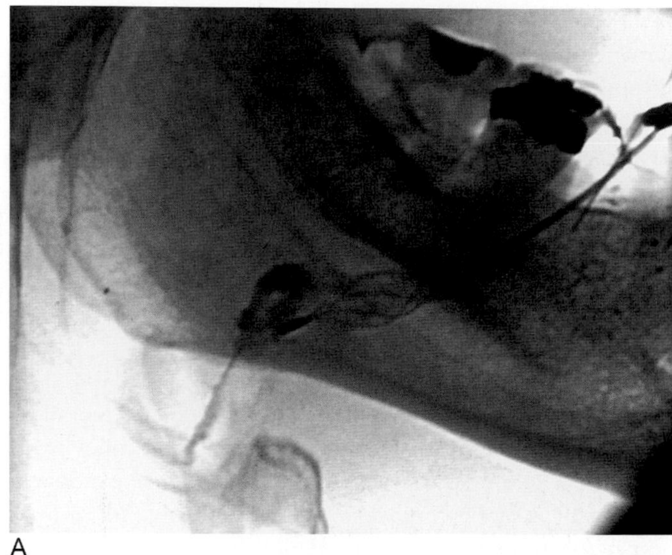

A

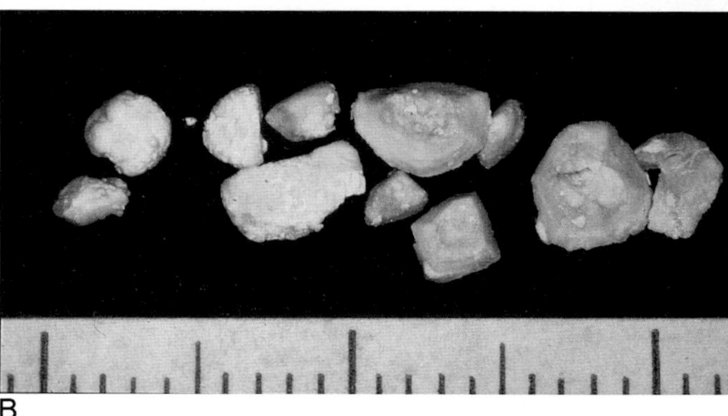

B

Figure 63.50 (A) An intraoperative sialogram showing an **open Dormia basket within the submandibular duct** during removal of a salivary stone. (B) Resultant fragmented salivary stone removed from submandibular gland shown in A.

Ultrasound (US) has increasingly become the first-line investigation for masses within the salivary glands and can readily investigate sialadenitis to detect causative stones or resultant duct dilatation, features facilitated by administering a sialogogue prior to investigation (Fig. 63.52). It is highly sensitive for the 70–80 per cent of tumours within the superficial parotid gland when compared with CT, though has limitations when imaging the deep pole.

CT is sensitive for the detection of salivary calculi though not resolving enough to show details of duct morphology in obstruction (Fig. 63.53). MRI has largely superseded it for tumour assessment though it can be useful in imaging early involvement of cortical bone. The technique of **CT sialography** has been displaced by **MR sialography**.

MRI has major advantages for salivary gland imaging, particularly related to its high soft tissue contrast and multiplanar data acquisition. Gadolinium enhancement is not required in uncomplicated cases, but can be of major importance in the assessment of recurrent tumours (Fig. 63.54).

Magnetic resonance sialography using heavily T2-weighted sequences (Fig. 63.55) (use image of grossly dilated parotid duct) allows noninvasive assessment of obstructive disease by imaging stimulated ductal saliva and correlates well

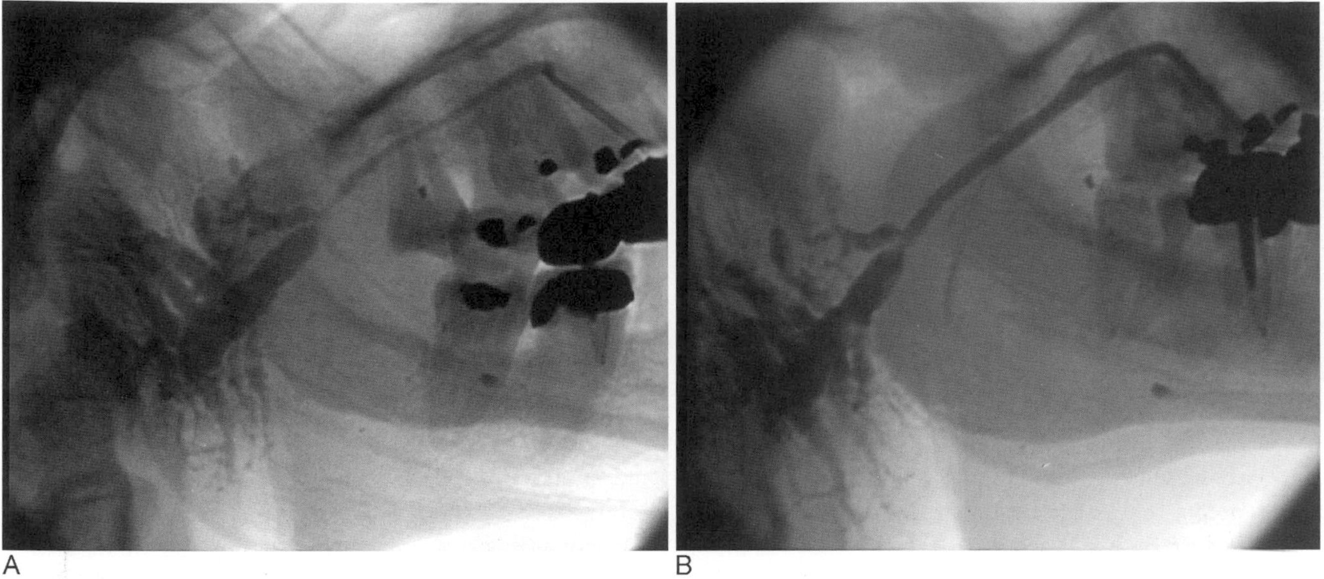

Figure 63.51 (A) Sialogram showing a **diffuse stricture at the entrance to the hilum** of the parotid gland. (B) Postoperative sialogram showing dilatation of duct stricture following balloon ductoplasty.

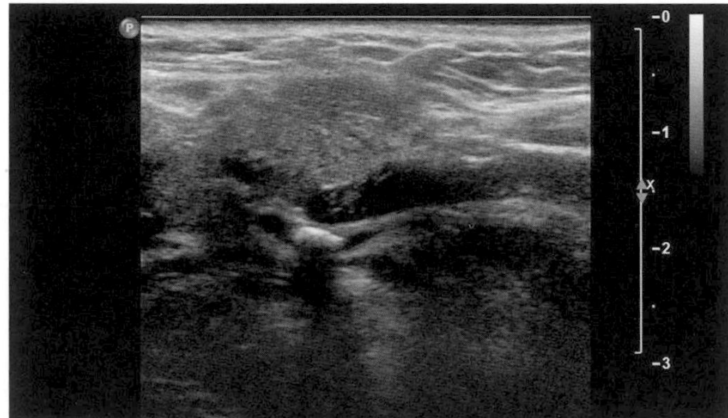

Figure 63.52 Ultrasound image of a **salivary stone** in the proximal portion of the submandibular duct.

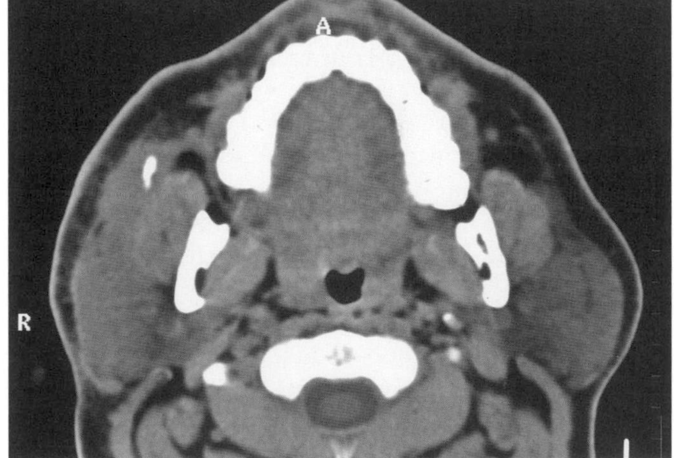

Figure 63.53 Extensive **benign pleomorphic adenoma** of the left parotid deep lobe on axial T2W MR.

with or even improves on conventional sialography in conditions such as **Sjögren's syndrome**[14,15].

Radionuclide radiology is most commonly used to assess glandular function in obstruction and inflammatory conditions. Low resolution and lack of uptake of ^{99m}Tc sodium pertechnetate in adenolymphomas (**Warthin's tumours**) limits its value in tumour imaging. **Positron emission tomography** has been used to image salivary gland tumours but, while being actively taken up by growing neoplasms, is also concentrated in lymphoid tissue and salivary glands. It has higher uptake in both malignant tumours and in the benign Warthin's tumour[16]. The most commonly used

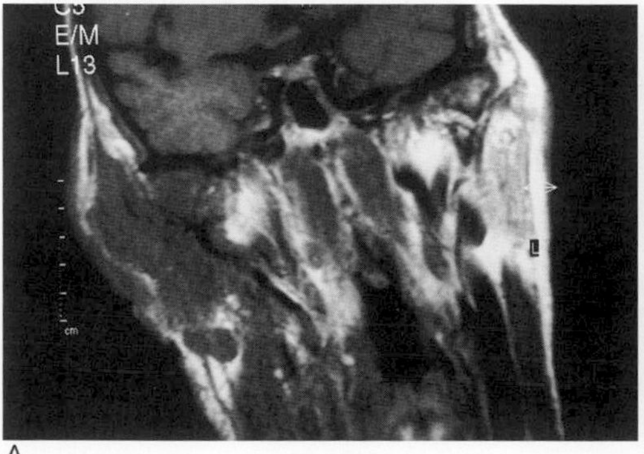

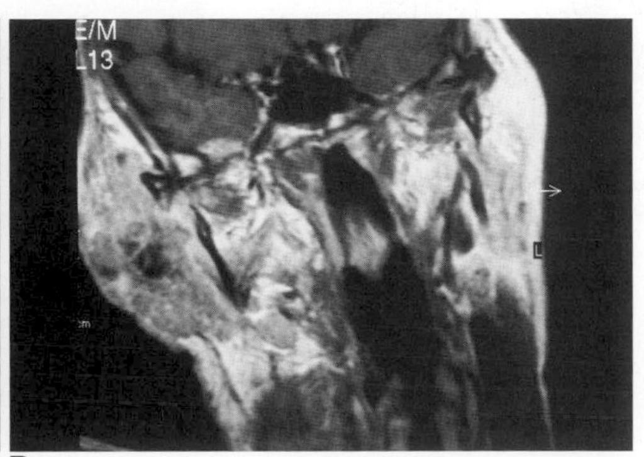

Figure 63.54 Extensive recurrent **parotid adenocarcinoma** with intra-cranial extension. Pre- (A) and post- (B) gadolinium T1W coronal MR images. Note intracranial enhancement in (B) suggesting tumour invasion via the foramen spinosum.

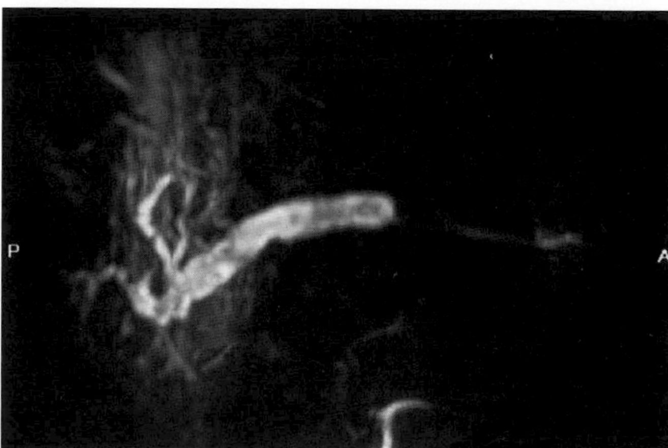

Figure 63.55 MR sialography image showing **gross dilatation of the main duct** and some of the secondary ducts. Areas of low signal in the main duct are due to the presence of several large stones. The distal part of the duct is normal. (Courtesy of Dr M. Becker, Geneva).

glucose analogue is secreted in saliva so small supraglottic, tongue base and laryngeal tumours and tumours measuring less than 1 mm may be missed. PET has strengths in assessing the post-treatment neck but may not distinguish tumour from acute infection or early wound healing[17].

Calculi and duct strictures

Calculi cause obstruction of the salivary glands typically resulting in mealtime-related swelling of the affected gland and predisposing to infection, sialectasis, and eventual gland atrophy. They are more common in the submandibular duct system (around 85 per cent) where 60–80 per cent are radio-opaque and are found particularly at the genu of the submandibular duct – that portion of the duct making an acute bend over the posterior free border of the mylohyoid muscle to enter the gland hilum. Only 20–40 per cent of parotid calculi are radio-opaque and are normally detected in the parotid hilum or main duct overlying the masseter muscle. CT is highly sensitive for small stones but US is a convenient and effective way of detecting the majority of salivary calculi (89–94 per cent sensitivity, 100 per cent specificity), except those lying in the most anterior parts of each duct. Single and multiple calculi may be found in dilated duct segments and may be associated with distally placed strictures.

Strictures of the salivary ducts result from inflammation caused by infection or calculi and are best demonstrated by sialography or MR sialography[18]. These may appear point or diffuse with proximal dilatation of the duct system. Approximately 25 per cent of salivary obstructions are due to strictures. 'Sialadochitis' describes the combination of duct dilatation and stenosis that follows obstruction complicated by infection.

Sialectasis

Sialectasis develops in sialadenitis and radiologically demonstrates degenerative changes seen within the terminal salivary ducts and acini as a result of obstruction, infection and other conditions such as Sjögren's syndrome (see later). Progression from widened and tortuous ductules to frank cavitation is seen (cavitatory sialectasis).

Inflammatory conditions

Infective sialadenitis of viral or bacterial origin causes generalized glandular enlargement on cross-sectional imaging with heterogeneous reduced echogenicity on US, increased attenuation on CT, and high signal on T2-weighted MRI (Fig. 63.56). Abscess formation is shown as an ill-defined hypoechoic area on US, with equivalent changes on CT and MR; acute inflammation is also evidenced by inflammatory stranding through the gland to the overlying tissues. Focal chronic inflammatory sialadenitis (Kuttner tumour) presents as a localized area of hypoechoic tissue in the submandibular gland on US and may be mistaken for tumour[19]. Sialography is indicated in cases of recurrent infection in order to demonstrate any underlying calculus or duct stricture.

Sjögren's syndrome causes damage to intercalated salivary duct walls allowing leakage of contrast media during sialography and creating a characteristically fine **punctate sialectasis** in approximately 70 per cent of cases. This is evenly distributed throughout salivary gland tissue – normally a parotid gland is chosen to demonstrate involvement. Similar abnormalities have been described in association with other connective tissue disorders such as rheumatoid arthritis, systemic lupus erythematosus, ankylosing spondylitis, Reiter's disease, polyarteritis nodosa and scleroderma where, in the absence of clinical features of Sjögren's syndrome, sialographic signs are estimated to exist in 5–15 per cent of cases. MR shows a speckled honeycomb appearance in moderately affected cases on both T1- and T2-weighted images, which is said to be specific and similar appearances may be found in the lacrimal glands. MR sialography has shown improved sensitivity and 100 per cent

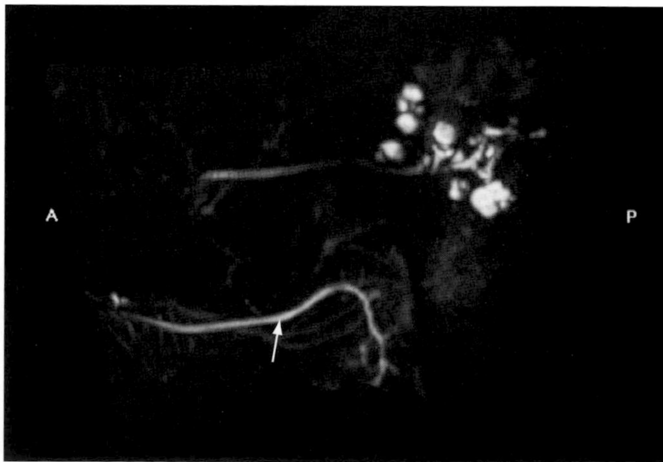

Figure 63.56 MR sialography image showing **chronic sialadenitis of the parotid gland** with focal globular high signal areas of sialectasis within the parenchyma of the gland. The main duct appears normal. The submandibular duct and gland (arrow) (seen later) appear normal. (Courtesy of Dr M. Becker, Geneva).

specificity over conventional sialography in diagnosis of Sjögren's syndrome[14]. US shows a heterogeneous reticular pattern of small low reflective foci and has a role in monitoring for lymphoma development, which may complicate late Sjögren's syndrome. Sjögren's syndrome sufferers have a 44 times greater risk of developing mucosal-associated lymphoid tissue (**MALT**) lymphoma.

Sarcoid results in generalized glandular enlargement with multiple small granulomatous areas of high attenuation on CT (Fig. 63.57), low reflectivity on US and diffuse high signal on MR. There is, in common with all inflammatory conditions, high activity on ^{67}Ga scintigraphy.

Human immunodefiency virus (HIV)-associated salivary gland disease is a spectrum of disorders that affects approximately 20 per cent of children and 0.5 per cent of adults with HIV, and includes lymphoepithelial infiltration that may progress to lymphoma. The combination of multiple intra-parotid cysts (which are otherwise rare) and cervical lymphadenopathy should alert the radiologist to this syndrome, which can occur at any stage from early post infection to full-blown acquired immune deficiency syndrome (AIDS).

Benign lymphoepithelial infiltration represents a spectrum from reactive to neoplastic change and can occur as an isolated abnormality, but is more commonly a feature of major salivary gland involvement in Sjögren's syndrome (30–50 per cent). The CT appearance in advanced disease is highly suggestive, with grossly enlarged glands containing multiple well-defined round areas of low attenuation (Fig. 63.58). Ga-citrate scintigraphy has been advocated as a method of assessing the progression of this disease, which is complicated by malignant lymphoma in 5 per cent and anaplastic carcinoma in about 1 per cent of patients. Lymphadenopathy affecting intraparotid nodes is not unusual and may mimic primary salivary tumour.

Salivary gland tumours

Most salivary gland tumours are benign and can develop at any age. Of these tumours, 80 per cent are found in the parotid glands, 5 per cent in the submandibular, 1 per cent in the sublingual, and the remaining 15 per cent in the minor salivary glands. The overall incidence of malignancy is 10–20 per cent, and the smaller the major gland the higher the rate of malignancy.

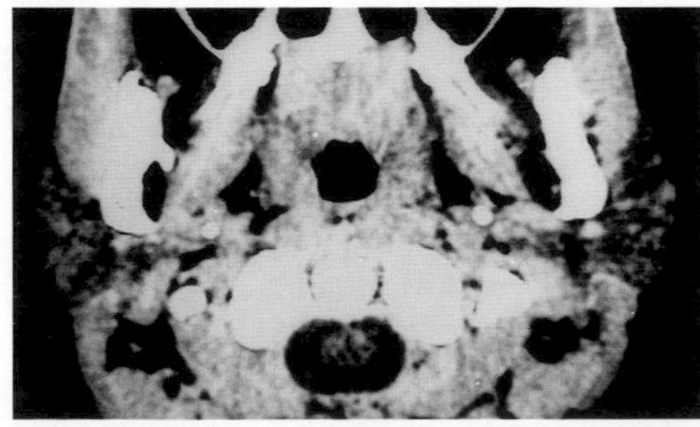

Figure 63.57 Sarcoid of the parotid glands. There is generalized glandular enlargement and multiple small areas of increased attenuation.

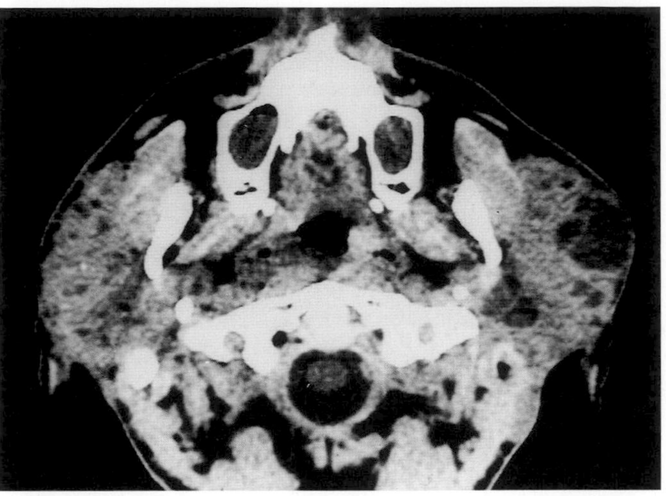

Figure 63.58 Benign lympho-epithelial infiltration of the parotids. The glands are grossly enlarged and contain multiple areas of reduced attenuation.

Benign pleomorphic adenomas (benign mixed tumours) account for around 80 per cent of salivary tumours and typically arise in the superficial portion of the parotid gland, being most common in middle-aged women. These appear uni- or mildly loculated hypoechoic lesions on US and characteristically give a low signal on T1- but high signal on T2-weighted MRI.

Adenocarcinomas are usually of distinctive histological appearance, the commonest being adenoid cystic carcinoma and muco-epidermoid carcinoma. These tumours grow slowly and are difficult to eradicate; the adenoid cystic type in particular have a propensity for insidious perineural spread. MRI can usually identify the presence, though not the extent, of perineural spread. Mucoepidermoid tumours are commonest in the minor salivary glands of the palate.

Other salivary tumours include the benign **adenolymphoma (Warthin's tumour)**, **lipoma, lymphoma**, and **tumours of the minor salivary glands.** Warthin's tumours are notably found in the parotid tail of older men, may be multiple (20 per cent) and occasionally bilateral (6.5 per cent). Lipomas give a characteristic hypoechoic appearance with numerous layered highly reflective internal strands on US and markedly low attenuation on CT.

Distinction between benign and malignant tumours is based upon criteria, some of which are common to all cross-sectional imaging, others being specific to a particular modality. Benignity is best identified by the presence of a capsule or well-defined outline, however notably many salivary malignancies are relatively low grade and are well defined in the early stages. Beyond this, CT may not be particularly discriminating, since many lesions show similarly increased attenuation, though more recently diffusion studies have allowed better differentiation.

MRI has a sensitivity of about 75% for identifying benign features; this can be improved by using gaddinium enhancement. Ultrasound normally depicts benign lesions as homogenous, hypoechoic and without regional lymphadenopathy. Additionally, colour flow Doppler indicates vascularity and may present evidence of neo-angiogenesis common in malignant tumours. Concurrent inflammatory change or haemorrhage can be confused with malignancy here. Contrast-enhanced MRI remains preferable for demonstrating recurrent tumour in areas that may be inaccessible to US and that give only nonspecific soft tissue change on CT. Whilst sialography is not recommended for the assessment of mass lesions, the incidental finding of distortion or amputation of intraglandular ducts should arouse concern as to the presence of a benign or malignant tumour, respectively.

Trauma

Laceration of the main parotid duct or of a larger intraglandular branch occasionally results from a penetrating facial injury, or is a rare complication of surgery. In recent injury, US may detect a fluid collection and sialography will show extravasation of contrast from the duct system into the soft tissues. Later, healing frequently results in duct stenosis.

Disorders of function

Salivary gland function may be quantified by time–activity curves with ^{99m}Tc-pertechnetate scintigraphy and may distinguish between the functioning, the obstructed and the nonfunctional gland. This may supplement sialography or be undertaken when sialography is not possible, and has been used to demonstrate recovery of salivary function following removal of an obstructing calculus[20].

SOFT TISSUES

Recent improvements in near-field imaging, and in colour flow and power Doppler performance, combined with its established values of high soft-tissue contrast and ease of use in guided biopsy, have increasingly led to US being seen as the first-line investigation for masses in the superficial soft tissues of the maxillofacial region. The potential for operator variability with US is one reason why axial CT remains widely used, as it demonstrates most lesions and assesses their relationship to adjacent structures, although IV contrast is often required for the accurate assessment of cervical lymphadenopathy. MRI, by virtue of its high soft-tissue contrast and multiplanar capabilities, will show most masses with similar or greater ease and has the additional advantage that different sequences may contribute information about the nature of a lesion.

US improves on clinical examination of the parotid, submandibular and cervical regions, and is a rapid and accurate means of distinguishing between cervical lymphadenopathy, salivary and other soft tissue neck lesions. Patterns suggestive of malignant involvement of cervical lymph nodes include a round shape (a short axis measurement over 1 cm becoming significant), absence of hilus, irregular outline, heterogeneous internal pattern including coagulation or cystic necrosis, disorganized peripheral colour flow pattern on Doppler US, nodal clusters, and fusion of nodes[21]. US has been found to be better than CT at detecting malignant cervical nodes but has the disadvantage of being unable to access deep nodes such as those within the retropharyngeal region. Identification of these features in combination with US-guided fine-needle aspiration cytology (FNAC) gave 100 per cent accuracy compared with CT (77–89 per cent), MR (88 per cent) and US alone (83–98 per cent)[22].

Infection in the head and neck region is characterized by spread along fascial-bound compartments (mucosal, submandibular, parapharyngeal, carotid, masticator, retropharyngeal, and prevertebral). CT or MRI are useful for the assessment of such spread (Fig. 63.59).

Malignant tumours within the oral cavity and environs are predominantly squamous cell carcinomas. MRI has become the first-choice examination for imaging both the extent of the local tumour and any regional lymphadenopathy, but may be oversensitive in the assessment of recurrent disease. MRI is also useful for the assessment of marrow involvement and is steadily encroaching on CT's superiority in demonstration of cortical bone involvement from tumours such as those in the floor of the mouth (Fig. 63.60). The imaging of

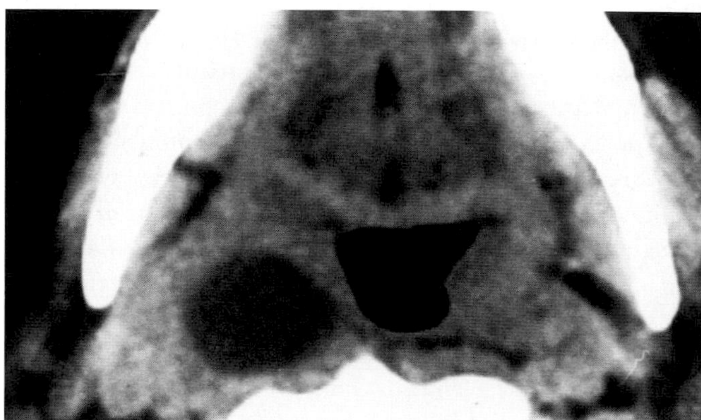

Figure 63.59 Abscess in the right oropharyngeal region on axial CT. The patient had received antibiotic treatment for recurrent throat infections and sterile pus was subsequently aspirated from the lesion.

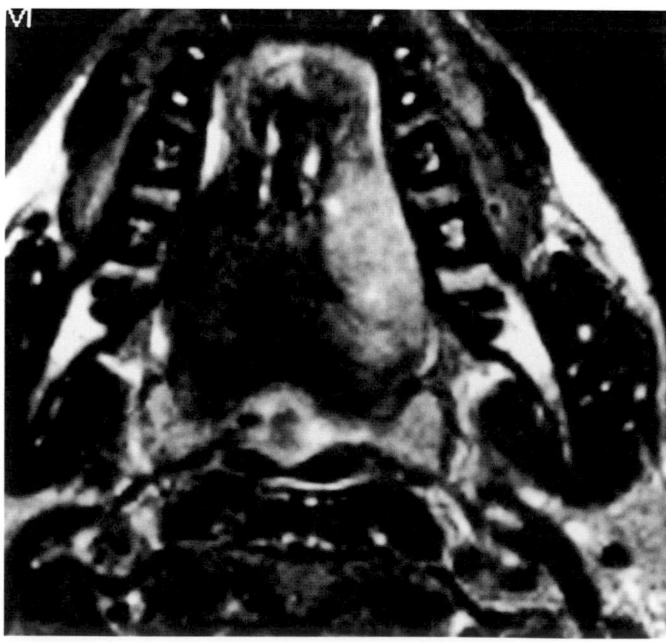

Figure 63.60 Carcinoma of the left side of the tongue, T2-weighted axial MRI. The high signal tumour extends to the midline.

primary lesions is relatively straightforward, but controversy remains surrounding the place of imaging in the assessment of lymph node involvement. Some studies state categorically that MRI lacks sufficient sensitivity and specificity to replace elective neck dissection for both staging and prognostic purposes[23], but more recently imaging has shown increased sensitivity in detecting nodal metastases using US and combinations of PET and sentinel node biopsy. MRI has successfully predicted those patients in need of neck dissection[24], and has successfully revealed micrometastases (described as intranodal tumour deposits of less than 2 mm diameter at any level of sectioning), which may be undetectable by cross-sectional imaging[23,25]. Positron emission tomography (PET), utilizing either ^{18}F-fluorodeoxyglucose (FDG-PET) or ^{11}C-tyrosine (TYR-PET) has a similar sensitivity (72 per cent) to CT (89 per cent) for the detection of lymph node metastases, but this may be improved by co-registration with PET (96 per cent sensitivity, 98.5 per cent specificity), or by supplementary sentinel node biopsy[24,26]. PET and PET/CT currently viewed as a particularly promising technique for the detection of occult primary lesions and recurrent tumours, especially in the post-radiotherapy situation. Recurrent neck disease, even when subclinical, may however be predicted with US and US-guided FNAC. The propensity for regional metastases from squamous cell carcinomas to present late after treatment of the primary lesion is an indication for prolonged follow-up (Fig. 63.61). Lymphomas may arise in Waldeyer's ring and the salivary glands, including the minor glands.

Benign tumours that require imaging in adults are relatively rare other than some **dermoids**, which present at lines of embryonic fusion; vascular abnormalities, which may grow extremely large leading to secondary growth disturbances; and salivary gland tumours, as already discussed. Colour flow Doppler US and magnetic resonance angiography may be helpful in assessment, but conventional angiography may be necessary, particularly prior to embolization. Phleboliths within such lesions may be apparent on plain films.

A wide spectrum of lesions present in the newborn, infants and children, often benign vascular abnormalities (Figs 63.62, 63.63) but other hamartomas (Fig. 63.64) and malignant tumours may be seen.

Thyroglossal and branchial cysts have characteristic positions. Thyroglossal cysts arise from epithelial tissue trapped during the embryonic descent of the thyroid gland, and present as defined midline cystic structures lying on a line between the base of the tongue and the thyroid gland (Fig. 63.65). Branchial cysts arise from epithelium trapped during incorporation of the second branchial arch, and presents as ovoid fluid-containing lesions lying deep to the sternomastoid muscle, protruding anterior to its anterior border.

Masseteric enlargement is usually secondary to muscular hypertrophy, which may be unilateral or bilateral, and often

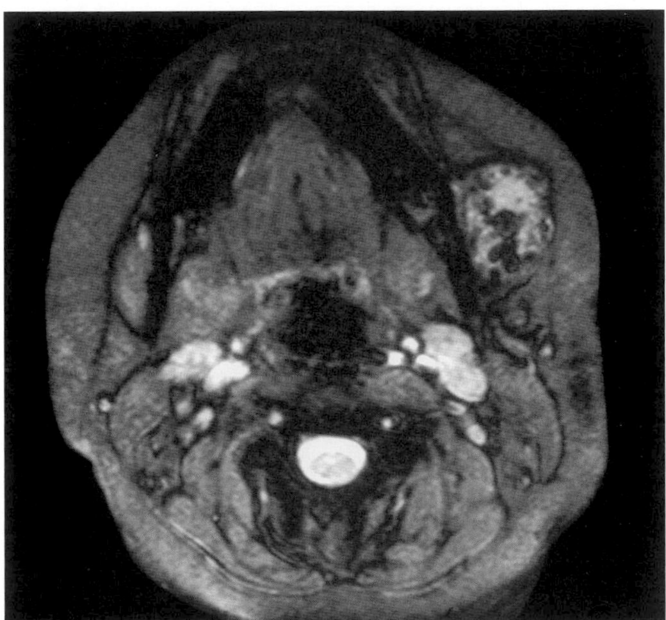

Figure 63.62 Axial MRI of an arterio-venous malformation within the masseter muscle of a 10-year-old. Low signal areas represent calcific deposits and flow voids, suggest a high flow lesion.

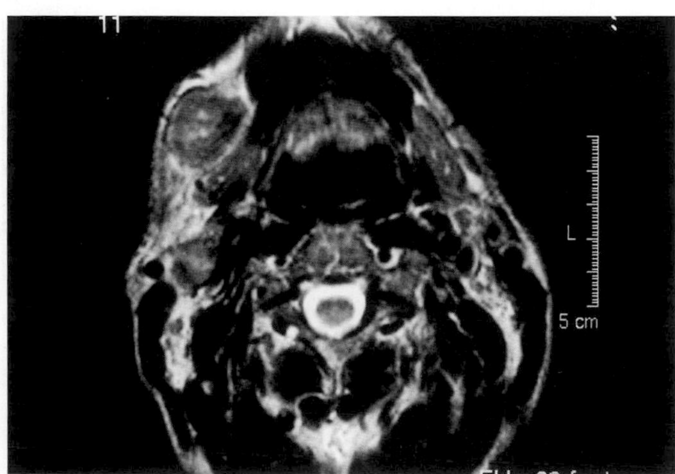

Figure 63.61 Metastatic deposit below mandible presenting 7 years post surgical excision of small ipsilateral lower lip squamous carcinoma.

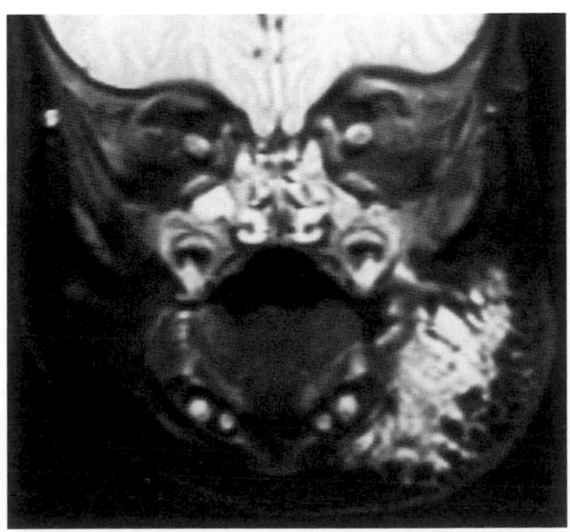

Figure 63.63 Lymphangioma in an infant. Coronal STIR MRI.

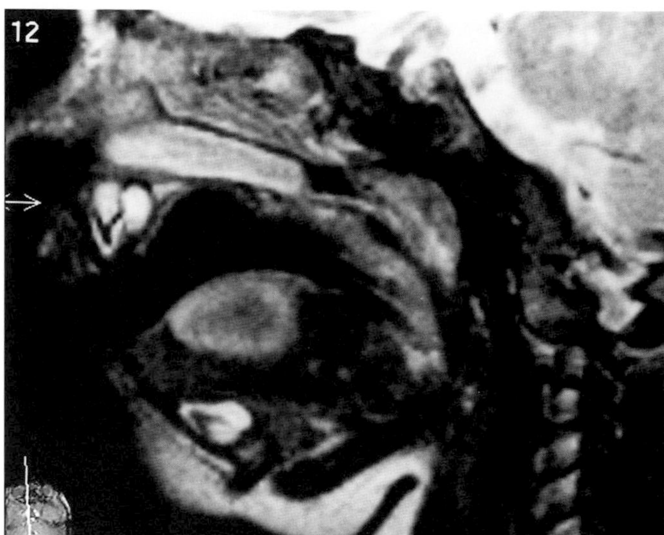

Figure 63.64 Fibroma of the tongue in an infant. Sagittal T1-weighted MRI.

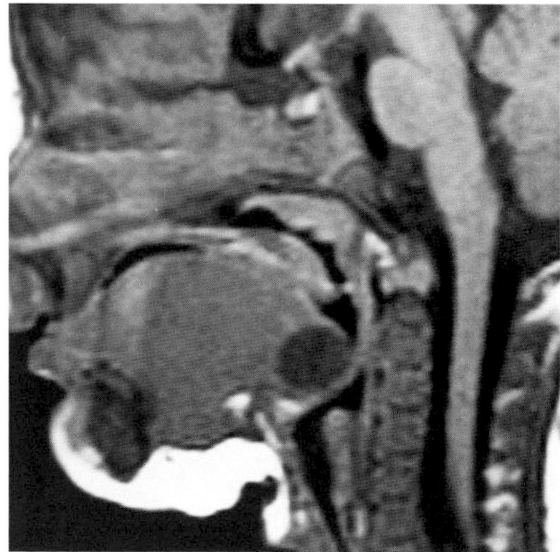

Figure 63.65 Thyroglossal cyst at base of tongue. Sagittal T1-weighted MRI.

concurrently involves the pterygoid muscles. US is valuable for diagnosis[27]. Rare causes include malignant lymphoma, leukaemic infiltration, haemangioma and rhabdomyosarcoma.

Calcification is occasionally seen in the walls of the facial and lingual arteries in patients with hypercalcaemia or renal failure. Small areas of subcutaneous calcification have been reported in Gorlin's syndrome and Ehlers–Danlos syndrome.

REFERENCES

1. Faculty of General Dental Practitioners (UK) 2004 Selection Criteria for Dental Radiography, 2nd edn. The Royal College of Surgeons of England, London
2. Browne R M, Edmondson H D, Rout P G J 1995 Atlas of Dental and Maxillofacial Radiology. Mosby-Wolfe, London
3. Yoshiura K, Higuchi Y, Ariji Y et al 1994 Increased attenuation in odontogenic keratocysts with computed tomography: a new finding. Dentomaxillofac Radiol 23: 138–142
4. Kawai T, Murakami S, Kishino M et al 1998 Diagnostic imaging in two cases of recurrent maxillary ameloblastoma: comparative evaluation of plain radiographs, CT and MR images Br J Oral Maxillofac Surg 36: 304–310
5. Verneuil A, Sapp P, Huang C et al 2002 Malignant ameloblastoma: classification, diagnostic, and therapeutic challenges. Am J Otolaryngol 23: 44–48
6. Gray C, Redpath T W, Smith F W 1998 Low-field magnetic resonance imaging for implant dentistry. Dentomaxillofacial Radiol 27: 225–229
7. Lee Y Y, van Tassel P, Nauert C et al 1988 Craniofacial osteosarcomas: plain film, CT, and MRI findings in 46 cases. Am J Roentgenol 150: 1397–1402
8. Jank S, Emshoff R, Etzelsdorfer M et al 2004 Ultrasound versus computed tomography in the imaging of orbital floor fractures. J Oral Maxillofac Surg 62: 150–154
9. Tasaki M M, Westesson P L 1993 Temporomandibular joint: diagnostic accuracy with sagittal and coronal MRI imaging. Radiology 186: 723–729
10. Segami N, Suzuki T, Sato J et al 2003 Does joint effusion on T2 magnetic resonance images reflect synovitis? Part 3. Comparison of histological findings of arthroscopically obtained synovium in internal derangements of the temporomandibular joint. Oral Surg Oral Med Oral Pathol Oral Radiol Endod 95: 761–766
11. Wilson D J 1990 Imaging. In: Norman J E de B, Bramley P (eds). A Textbook and Colour Atlas of the Temporomandibular Joint. Wolfe, London, pp 90–109
12. Brown J E, Drage N A, Escudier M P et al 2002 Minimally invasive radiologically guided intervention for the treatment of salivary calculi. Cardiovasc Intervent Radiol 25: 352–355
13. Drage N A, Brown J E, Escudier M P et al 2002 Balloon dilatation of salivary duct strictures – report on 36 treated glands. Cardiovasc Intervent Radiol 25: 356–359
14. Niemela RK, Takalo R, Paakko E et al 2004 Ultrasonography of salivary glands in primary Sjögrens syndrome. A comparison with magnetic resonance imaging and magnetic resonance sialography of parotid glands. Rheumatology 43: 875–879
15. Ohbayashi N, Yamada I, Yoshino N, Sasaki T 1998 Sjogren syndrome: comparison at assessments with MR sialography and conventional sialography. Radiology 209: 683–688.
16. Uchida Y, Minoshima S, Kawata T et al 2005 Diagnostic value of FDG PET and salivary gland scintigraphy for parotid tumors. Clin Nucl Med 30: 170–176
17. Jones J, Farag I, Hain S F, McGurk M 2005 Positron emission tomography (PET) in the management of oro-pharyngeal cancer. Eur J Surg Oncol 31: 170–176
18. Becker M, Marchal F, Becker C D et al 2000 Sialolithiasis and salivary ductal stenosis: diagnostic accuracy of MR sialography with a three-dimensional extended-phase conjugate symmetry rapid spin-echo sequence. Radiology 217: 347–358
19. Ahuja A T, Richards P S, Wong K T et al 2003 Kuttner tumour (chronic sclerosing sialadenitis) of the submandibular gland: sonographic appearances. Ultrasound Med Biol 29: 913–919
20. Makdissi J, Escudier M P, Brown J E et al 2004 Glandular function after intraoral removal of salivary calculi from the hilum of the submandibular gland. Br J Oral Maxillofac Surg 42: 538–541
21. Evans R M, Ahuja A, Rhys Williams S et al 1991 Ultrasound and ultrasound guided fine needle aspiration in cervical lymphadenopathy. Br J Radiol 64(P): 58 [Abstract]
22. Ying M, Ahuja A, Brooks F 2004 Accuracy of sonographic vascular features in differentiating different causes of cervical lymphadenopathy. Ultrasound Med Biol 30: 441–447
23. Wide J M, White D W, Woolgar J A et al 1999 Magnetic resonance imaging in the assessment of cervical nodal metastases in oral squamous cell carcinoma. Clin Radiol 54: 90–94
24. Kovacs A F, Dobert N, Gaa J et al 2004 Positron emission tomography in combination with sentinal node biopsy reduces the rate of elective neck dissections in the treatment of oral and oropharyngeal cancer. J Clin Oncol 22: 3973–3980

25. El-Sayed I H, Singer M I, Civantos F 2005 Sentinel lymph node biopsy in head and neck cancer Otolaryngol Clin North Am 38:145–160, ix–x
26. Schwartz D L, Ford E, Rajendran J et al 2005 FGD-PET/CT imaging for preradiotherapy staging of head-and-neck squamous cell carcinoma. Int J Radiat Oncol Biol Phys 61: 129–136
27. Morse M, Brown E F 1990 Ultrasonic diagnosis of masseteric hypertrophy. Dentomaxillofacial Radiol 19: 18–20

FURTHER READING

Ahuja A T, Evans R M 2000 Practical Head and Neck Ultrasound, Radionuclide Radiology, Greenwich Medical Media Limited

White S C, Pharoah M J 2004 Oral Radiology Principles and Interpretation, 5th edn Mosby

SECTION

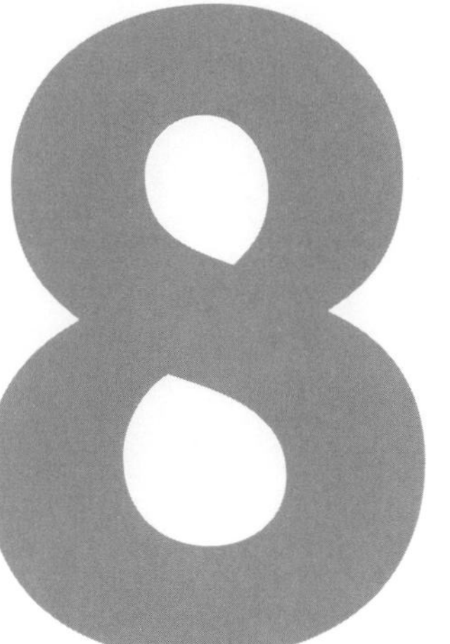

Paediatric Imaging

CHAPTER 64

The Neonatal and Paediatric Chest

Isla Lang and Alan Sprigg

The neonatal chest
- Radiation risks and radiological techniques
- The normal chest, variations and artifacts
- Normal lung development
- Neonatal respiratory distress

The older paediatric patient
- Technical factors
- The thymus
- Tachypnoea—respiratory or cardiac cause?
- Infection
- The radio-opaque chest
- Imaging the child on the intensive care unit
- The wheezy chest
- Congenital chest abnormalities
- Cystic fibrosis
- Paediatric interstitial disease
- Immunodeficiency

THE NEONATAL CHEST

Isla Lang

RADIATION RISKS AND RADIOLOGICAL TECHNIQUES

'Radiation exposure in the first 10 years of life is estimated to produce a risk of total aggregated detriment 5–7 times greater than exposure after the age of 50'[1]. Radiation in the neonate should be kept to a minimum and the radiographs performed by experienced radiographers. Routine lateral views of the chest are unnecessary. A short exposure time, high kV–low mAs technique with fast film–screen combinations should be used. Accurate collimation of the light beam and lead masking on top of the incubator should be performed. Gonad shielding should be used if an abdominal radiograph is also being performed[2].

THE NORMAL CHEST, VARIATIONS, AND ARTEFACTS

The normal appearance of the neonatal chest differs from that of older children. It is almost cylindrical in shape. Small degrees of rotation lead to considerable malprojections of the anterior ribs and sternum. On a rotated chest radiograph sternal ossification centres may simulate healing rib fractures or lung opacities (Fig. 64.1). The ribs have a more horizontal orientation with the usual level of the diaphragm at the sixth to eighth anterior rib. The normal cardiothoracic ratio can be as large as 65% due to the presence of the thymus. The size of the thymus can be highly variable. A normal thymus does not compress or displace other structures (Fig. 64.2). The thymus

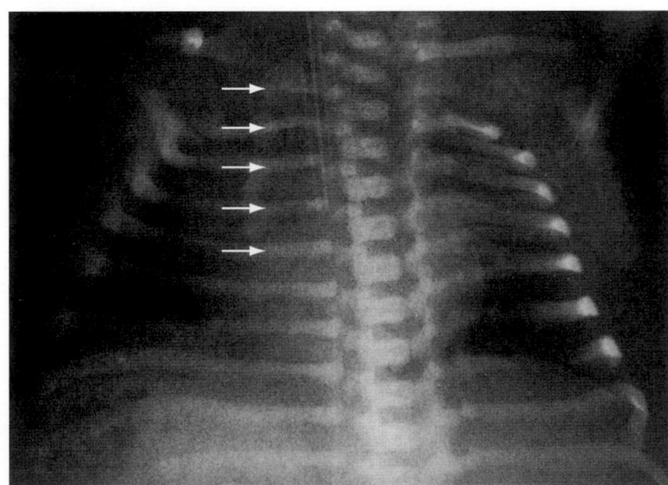

Figure 64.1 Rotated radiograph showing the **sternal ossification centres** simulating healing rib fractures (arrows).

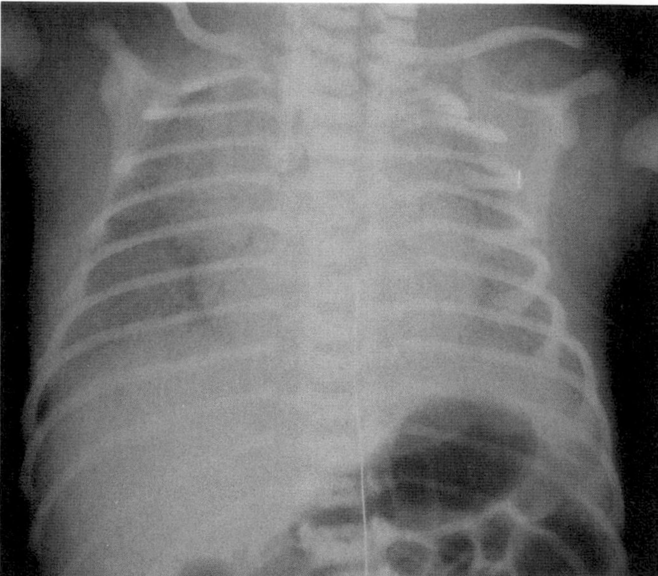

Figure 64.2 Prominent thymus in a premature baby with mild respiratory distress syndrome.

may involute rapidly in association with prenatal or postnatal stress or following the administration of exogenous steroids.

It is important to recognize certain artefacts on a neonatal radiograph. The hole in the top of the incubator may mimic a lung cyst or pneumatocele. Redundant skin, particularly in the preterm neonate, can result in a long vertical skinfold which can simulate a pneumothorax (Fig. 64.3). Deep retractions of the lower sternum in respiratory distress can produce a central radiolucency that simulates a pneumomediastinum on frontal radiographs[3].

Evaluation of tubes and lines

All tubes, catheters, and lines should be evaluated on each radiograph carried out on an infant as they are often the major reason for taking the radiograph. The trachea in the infant is often short and narrow. Optimal positioning for an endotracheal tube (ETT) is approximately 1–1.5 cm above the carina. Considerable changes in ETT position can occur because of head and neck movement. Flexion moves the ETT inferiorly, when the tube may extend into the right main bronchus. Radiographic clues of malposition of the ETT in the oesophagus, for example, are: low position, a tracheal column distinct from the ETT, pulmonary underaeration, air in the distal oesophagus, and gaseous distension of the gastrointestinal tract.

Umbilical arterial and venous lines should be differentiated from each other. This is normally possible on an antero-posterior (AP) view of the chest and abdomen but occasionally a lateral view may be required. The **umbilical arterial line** initially courses caudally through the internal and common iliac arteries to enter the aorta, and lies just lateral to the left side of the spine. The tip should ideally lie between T6 and T10 to avoid the spinal arteries, or at L3–L5 below the level of the bowel and renal arteries. The **umbilical vein catheter** courses directly cephalad on the right side of the abdomen and enters the left portal vein, at which point it may enter the ductus venosus and then the inferior vena cava. Radiographs should confirm that the tip lies above the liver and has not passed into a tributary vein (Fig. 64.4). Central lines and peripheral vascular lines extending from the periphery also need to be evaluated. These are often small and the position of

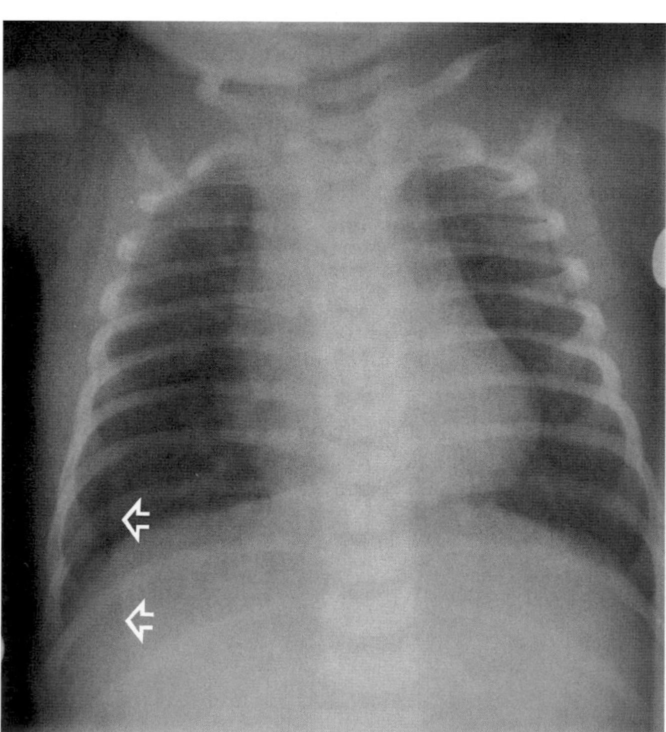

Figure 64.3 Skinfold (arrows) simulating a pneumothorax.

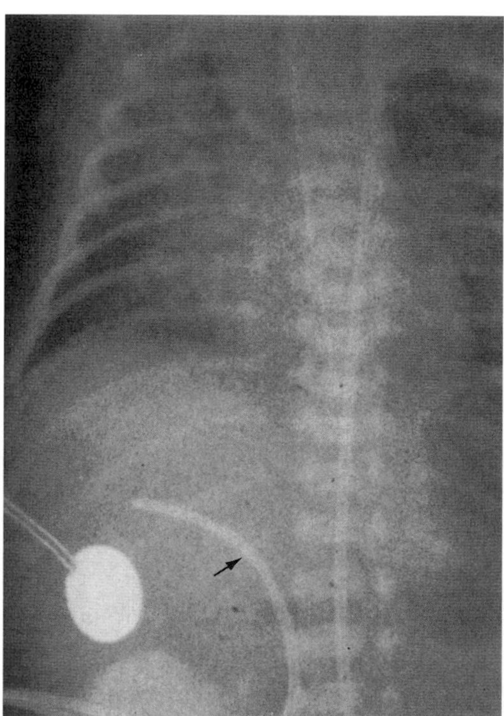

Figure 64.4 Tubes and lines. The tip of the umbilical arterial line is at T3 which is high and the top of the umbilical venous line (arrow) lies within the liver. The positions of both were altered following this radiograph.

the tip may be difficult to determine. In this situation a radiograph following contrast medium in the line may be helpful.

Feeding may be through a nasogastric or a nasojejunal tube. The position of the tips of these tubes should be recorded as infusion of enteral feeds into a malplaced tube may have serious consequences. Perforation of the oesophagus by a nasogastric tube in the neonate may cause very few symptoms[3,4].

NORMAL LUNG DEVELOPMENT

The pulmonary tract develops in the third week after conception as an outpouching from the primitive foregut. By the sixth week primitive lung buds are present. Between 6 and 16 weeks there is extensive branching of the respiratory tree. Between 16 and 28 weeks, multiple alveolar ducts arise from the respiratory bronchioles and the primitive alveoli form. True alveolar development extends from approximately 26 weeks gestation to term and continues for the first 2 years after birth, after which alveoli increase in size but not in number.

Normal respiration requires production of **surfactant**. The lamellar bodies that store surfactant appear at around 22 weeks gestation. Surfactant is produced within the endoplasmic reticulum of type 2 pneumocytes within the alveoli from about 24 weeks gestation. The pulmonary surfactant lowers alveolar surface tension. Glucocorticoids and thyroid hormones accelerate surfactant release towards term[5].

NEONATAL RESPIRATORY DISTRESS

A neonate with respiratory distress clinically presents with tachypnoea, rib recession, and grunting.

There are many causes of respiratory distress and a chest radiograph can help to differentiate between them. These include primary pulmonary disease, which can be divided into those that can be treated medically and those requiring surgery. In general, medical conditions in the newborn cause bilateral pulmonary disease, whereas surgical problems are often unilateral and frequently produce contralateral shift of the mediastinum. Cardiac disease is an important cause of respiratory symptomatology in the neonate, for which ultrasound (US) is particularly useful.

Extrapulmonary lesions are also important and should be suspected if the chest radiograph is normal or only mildly abnormal in the presence of respiratory distress. These include upper airway obstruction, musculoskeletal abnormalities of the chest, lesions of the diaphragm and abdomen, as well as distant pathology in the central nervous system or metabolic or haematological derangements[3].

Transient tachypnoea of the newborn

Before delivery, the lungs are filled with amniotic fluid. Approximately one-third of fetal lung fluid is cleared out of the airways by the thorax being squeezed in the birth canal, one-third is absorbed by the pulmonary capillaries, and one-third by the lymphatics. Within the first few breaths, it is rapidly cleared and the lungs quickly become fully aerated as normal respiration ensues. If this process is impaired, 'wet lung' or transient tachypnoea of the newborn (TTN) develops. It is commonly associated with delivery by caesarean section, prematurity, and some cases of maternal diabetes. The infant is usually tachypnoeic soon after birth and has mild to moderate hypoxia. Radiographs demonstrate prominent pulmonary interstitial markings, fluid in the interlobar fissures and intrapleural space, and slight overaeration (Fig. 64.5). In severe cases the radiographic appearance is that of alveolar oedema or a reticular granular appearance similar to that of respiratory distress syndrome of the newborn, with the only difference being that pulmonary aeration is normal to slightly increased. The changes are usually symmetrical but sometimes the right side is affected more than the left[3]. The major diagnostic feature is the mild symptomatology, with clinical and radiographic resolution occurring by 48–72 h of age.

Respiratory distress syndrome

Respiratory distress syndrome (RDS) remains the most common life-threatening respiratory disorder of newborns. Most neonates with RDS are premature. Approximately 50% of neonates born between 26 and 28 weeks and 20–30% of neonates born at 30–31 weeks of gestation develop RDS[6]. It occasionally occurs in infants older than 36 weeks gestation. Other risk factors include infants of poorly controlled diabetic mothers, fetal asphyxia, maternal or fetal haemorrhage, and multiple gestations. It is more common and more severe in boys and occurs more commonly in black than in white children.

RDS is due to a deficiency of alveolar surfactant. The initial response to a deficiency of surfactant is for the smaller alveoli to

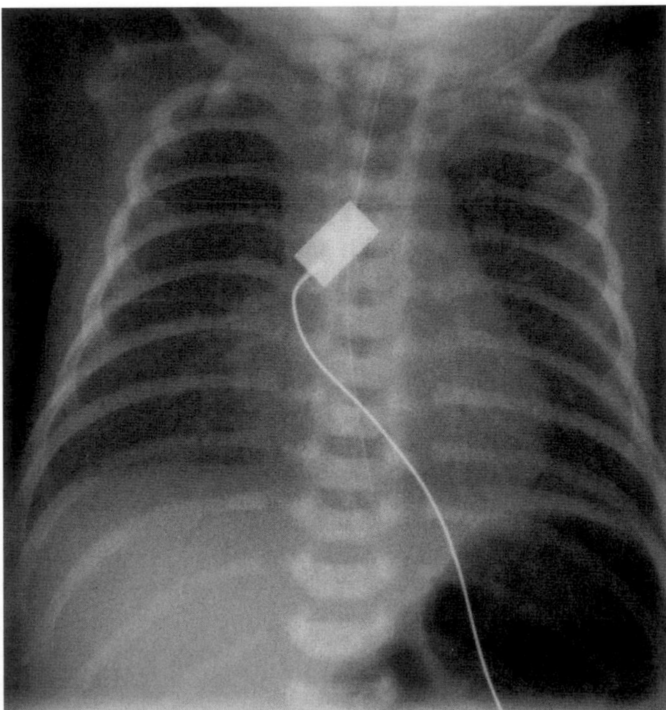

Figure 64.5 Baby with transient tachypnoea of the newborn. Chest radiograph shows hyperinflated lungs, streaky shadowing, and a little fluid in the horizontal fissure.

collapse while the larger ones hyperinflate. The lungs become stiff and increased respiratory effort is needed to inflate the lungs. The lung tissue becomes progressively traumatized and there is exudation of plasma from the pulmonary capillaries into the alveolar space. Secondary influx of white cells into the plasma exudate leads to organization of the plasma proteins with the development of a thick membrane composed of protein, white cells, and inflammatory debris. This membrane stains pink with standard histological preparations and gives rise to the alternative name for the condition—**hyaline membrane disease**.

Clinically, infants with RDS will have respiratory distress which worsens during the first 18–24 h of life, with gradual improvement generally starting by the third day. Advances in perinatal medical management that have significantly modified the natural history of RDS include antenatal corticosteroid administration, surfactant replacement therapy, and ventilatory assistance.

The chest radiograph will usually be abnormal at 6 h. There is normal to decreased aeration of the lungs as compared to TTN, where there is increased aeration. Initially the patent terminal airways are surrounded by airless alveoli, giving the characteristic fine reticular shadowing seen throughout both lungs with accentuation of the air bronchograms. As the condition progresses, influx of plasma renders the lungs more radio-opaque, the reticulogranular shadowing becomes more confluent, and there is progressive loss of clarity of the diaphragmatic and cardiac contours. Uncomplicated RDS is a bilaterally symmetrical disease: there may be some gradation in radiographic opacification between the upper and lower zones. Asymmetric changes may be seen when some areas have been differentially aerated by, for example, a misplaced ETT, asymmetric surfactant administration, and presence of localized pathology such as interstitial emphysema, pulmonary haemorrhage, or superimposed infection. Clearance of the lungs will depend on how quickly the individual baby is able to synthesize adequate amounts of endogenous surfactant and may take from 1–2 d to several weeks[3–5,7] (Fig. 64.6).

Very small infants, less than 25 weeks gestation, often do not develop typical RDS. Their lungs initially appear well aerated radiographically but they often have major problems that may involve the respiratory system, such as apnoea of prematurity, lobar atelectasis, pneumonia, patent ductus arteriosus, and intraventricular haemorrhage. The ventilatory pressures used are often low and complications such as chronic lung disease are relatively common[3].

Lung problems associated with neonatal intensive care and management of respiratory distress syndrome

Surfactant therapy

Surfactant acts synergistically with antenatal corticosteroid therapy to reduce the severity of RDS.

Post treatment, the radiographs usually show a marked uniform improvement in lung aeration. Asymmetrical or focal improvement of lung aeration may occur, usually in the central or upper regions of the right lung (Fig. 64.7). Possible explanations for asymmetrical improvement are maldistribution due to malapplication of synthetic surfactant, and focal clearing due to insufficient dose of surfactant. In asymmetric clearing, it is important to exclude a pneumothorax or pneumomediastinum. Pulmonary haemorrhage may occur following surfactant treatment[8,9].

Ventilation

Many babies receiving intensive care will require some form of positive pressure artificial ventilation. This may be in the form of a moderate elevation of airway pressure through nasal prongs or a facemask (**continuous positive airway pressure [CPAP]**) or by a cyclical inflation of the lungs through an ETT (**intermittent positive pressure ventilation [IPPV]**). Pressures in the range of 2–6 cmH_2O are used during CPAP and peak pressures between 12 and 26 cmH_2O are commonly used during IPPV.

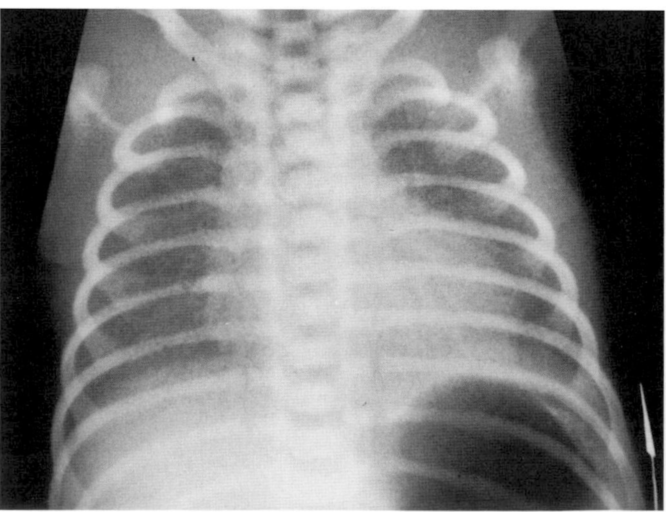

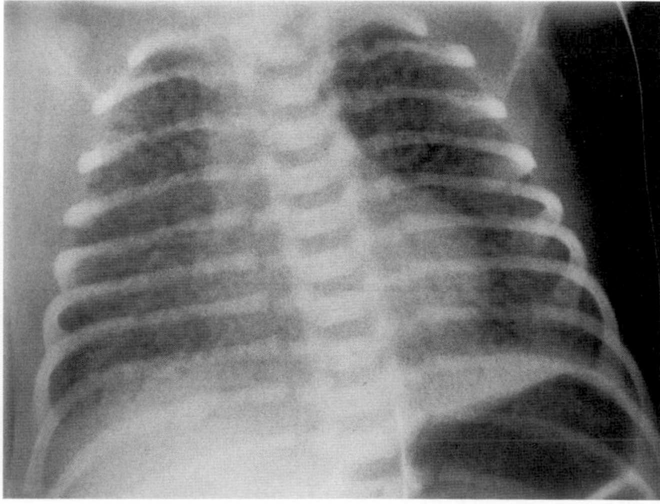

Figure 64.6 Preterm baby with respiratory distress syndrome. (A) Day 1: mild ground-glass appearance within both lungs. (B) Day 3: worsening opacification with air bronchograms.

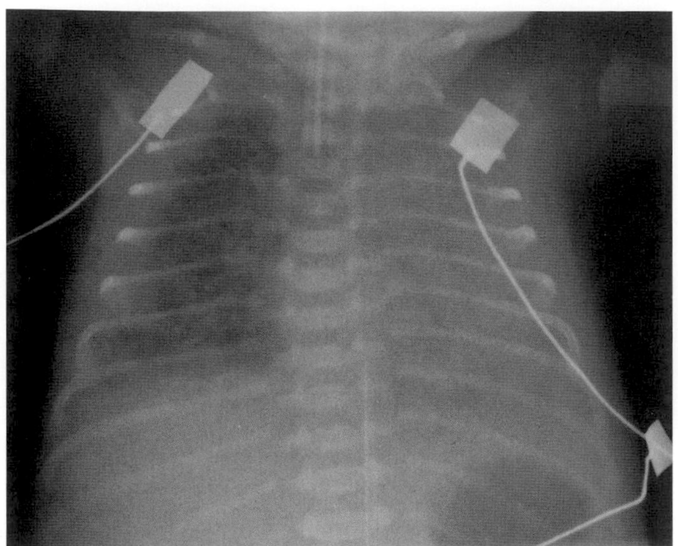

Figure 64.7 Surfactant therapy. Asymmetric improvement of lung aeration has occurred following surfactant treatment.

Normally ventilation rates approximate the normal respiratory rates of the infant (30–90 breaths min^{-1}) but on occasion, oscillatory ventilation rates of 600–900 cycles min^{-1} may be utilized. High-frequency ventilation allows adequate gas exchange at lower peak inspiratory pressures and complications of barotrauma resolve more quickly than with conventional ventilation. The efficiency of high-frequency oscillatory ventilation is normally measured by radiological assessment of the degree of lung filling. Frequent chest radiographs may therefore be required for monitoring treatment progress. The right diaphragm should be seen to lie at a level between the posterior ends of the eighth and ninth ribs[4,5].

Early effects of ventilation and respiratory distress syndrome. Mechanical ventilation is an important risk factor contributing to air leak in premature babies treated for lung disease. Leakage of air from the pulmonary parenchyma into the pleural cavity is the most common, leading to a pneumothorax (Fig. 64.8). The pneumothorax is often under tension, resulting in contralateral shift of the mediastinum. The pleural air may collect anywhere within the pleural space. Large collections are easily seen. Frequently the pleural air lies anterior and medial to the lung and is more difficult to diagnose, the only sign being increased radiolucency of the ipsilateral hemithorax. There is often increased sharpness of the mediastinal border which, unlike in a pneumomediastinum, extends from the superior extent of the lung to the diaphragm. The thymus is compressed by the pneumothorax rather than being elevated by it, as in a pneumomediastinum. Pleural air may frequently collect at the apex or base of the lung or within an interlobar fissure.

Leakage into other adjacent structures may result from a pneumomediastinum when air may dissect outside the mediastinum into the neck, or underneath the lung into an extrapleural location, or into the retroperitoneal space or peritoneal cavity. Less commonly, a pneumopericardium or diffuse vascular air embolism may occur.

Air may also leak into the interstitial space and spread throughout the lymphatics and along the perivascular sheaths, producing **pulmonary interstitial emphysema (PIE)**. The radiological appearance is of small bubbles of air radiating out from the hilum. When severe, the lungs are overinflated and cardiac compression may occur (Fig. 64.9). Treatment is difficult; high-frequency ventilation may reduce the incidence of pneumothorax but in some cases PIE may become worse due to further air trapping. Unilateral PIE may improve with decubitus positioning, with the affected side dependent: occasionally obstruction of the bronchus to the affected portion of the lung is necessary. The condition may be associated with later chronic lung disease[4,10].

Late effects of ventilation and respiratory distress syndrome Bronchopulmonary dysplasia (BPD) or **chronic lung disease of prematurity (CLD)** is a chronic lung disease that develops in infants treated with positive pressure

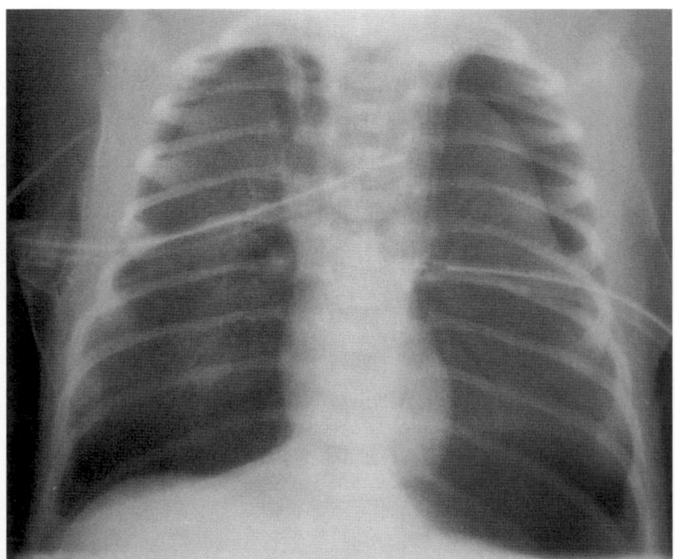

Figure 64.8 Severe respiratory distress syndrome with bilateral pneumothoraces.

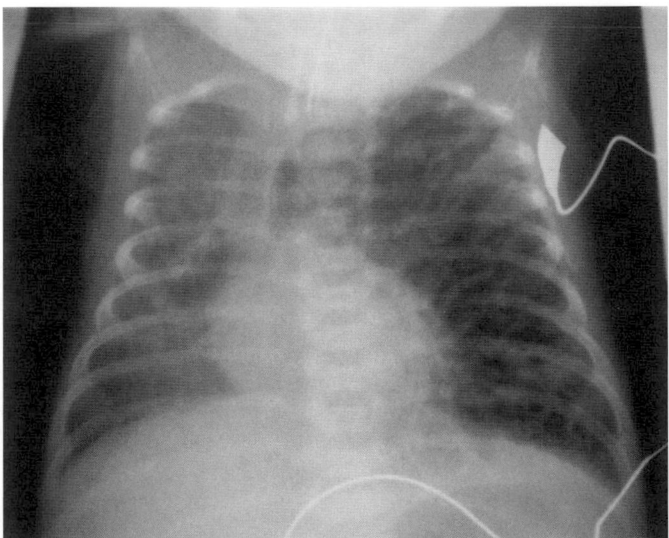

Figure 64.9 Pulmonary interstitial emphysema. Small bubbles of air radiate from the left hilum after leaking into the interstitial space. The left lung is overinflated.

mechanical ventilation and oxygen. Since the original description of BPD by Northway et al in 1967, the epidemiology has changed significantly[11]. New treatments and technologies have improved the outcome for premature infants and as a result the number of babies affected by BPD has increased and many need continuous domiciliary oxygen.

Classically BPD has been defined clinically as oxygen dependency at 28 days of age associated with an abnormal chest radiograph. However, typical histological changes of BPD may be present at autopsy in infants dying within the first week of life. The above definition also fails to account for differences in gestational age. BPD therefore represents a continuum of lung damage and repair that often begins before the diagnosis is traditionally established. Chronic lung inflammation is caused by a number of factors: barotrauma due to positive pressure ventilation, oxygen toxicity, infection, altered inflammatory response, deficiency of antioxidant defences, and many others. The contribution of different factors varies between patients and a number of less mature infants may develop BPD without ventilatory support or an initial oxygen requirement.

Pathologically the condition is characterized by areas of hyperexpansion and atelectasis interspersed with patchy areas of fibrosis. Hyperexpansion may be so severe as to result in moderate-sized pulmonary cysts, and fibrosis may vary from scattered strands of fibrous tissue to complete fibrosis and collapse of entire lobes. Characteristic radiographic appearances are patchy or linear strands of increased density with localized areas of unequal aeration and generalized hyperaeration (Fig. 64.10). Cardiomegaly may occur in severe cases and signifies pulmonary hypertension.

The chest radiograph may return to normal in babies whose disease remains mild. Severe BPD may be fatal or lead to debilitating chronic pulmonary insufficiency. Follow-up in babies with BPD shows an increased number of later respiratory infections and an increased incidence of reactive airway disease.

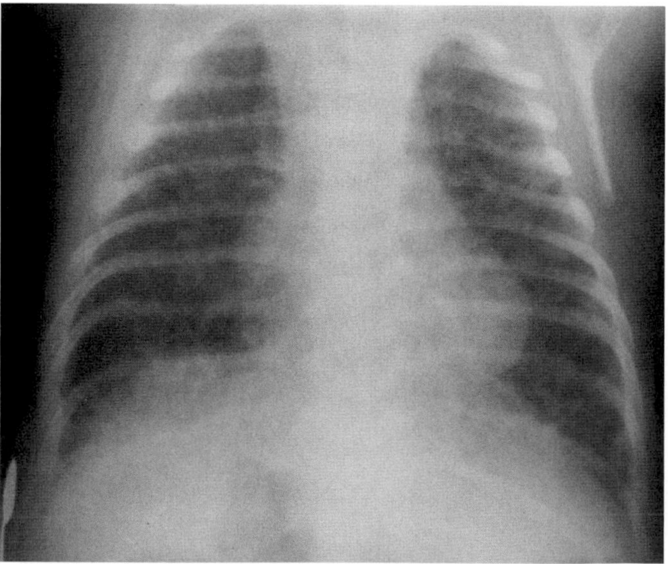

Figure 64.10 Chronic lung disease. The lungs are hyperexpanded with areas of hyperinflation interspersed with areas of fibrosis. Both lungs were equally affected.

Wilson–Mikity syndrome is described in immature infants who are initially well and do not require ventilation, but who show signs of respiratory distress in the second week[12,13]. The lungs develop streaky opacification and small cystic lucencies throughout. Respiratory failure may be progressive and symptoms may persist for many months.

Pulmonary agenesis and hypoplasia

The interaction between the branching airway and its investing lung is essential for normal lung development. Interference with this development by intrathoracic or extrathoracic compression results in pulmonary agenesis or hypoplasia. Bilateral pulmonary hypoplasia is associated with oligohydramnios which occurs in renal agenesis (Potter's syndrome) or following early rupture of membranes. Other extrathoracic causes include marked distension of the abdomen by a mass, neuromuscular disease of the chest, or skeletal dysplasias, such as asphyxiating thoracic dystrophy. Intrathoracic causes are usually unilateral, such as congenital diaphragmatic hernia, congenital cystic adenomatoid malformation, or pleural effusions. The severity of the hypoplasia depends on when the compression occurs in utero.

The diagnosis is made on the history and plain radiograph findings. It should be suspected when ventilation is much harder than expected. The plain radiograph may show an underlying lesion or the chest may be bell shaped; pneumothoraces may occur as a complication.

Pulmonary haemorrhage

Small areas of haemorrhage are frequently seen at autopsy in association with other neonatal lung problems such as RDS, congenital heart disease, aspiration pneumonia, and BPD. Radiographically it is often difficult to distinguish haemorrhage from the underlying disease. Massive pulmonary haemorrhage develops suddenly with the production of blood-stained secretions. On the radiograph there is diffuse homogeneous opacification (Fig. 64.11). In very small premature or severely asphyxiated infants, this is often a terminal event. Less severe pulmonary haemorrhage resolves over several days.

Meconium aspiration syndrome

Infants who suffer hypoxic stress in utero may pass meconium into the amniotic fluid which is then inhaled. Meconium consists of hyperosmolar, viscid intestinal secretions. Inhalation of small amounts may be innocuous, while inhalation of large amounts results in patchy widespread collapse and consolidation combined with a severe inflammatory reaction. The viscous inhaled meconium may cause complete bronchial obstruction or a partial occlusion with a 'ball valve' effect that may lead to areas of hyperinflation in the peripheral lung. The chest radiograph shows patchy areas of collapse and consolidation with areas of hyperinflation (Fig. 64.12).

Pneumothorax and pneumomediastinum are frequent complications which may result in hypoxia and lead to pulmonary artery vasoconstriction, pulmonary hypertension, and right-to-left shunting across the ductus arteriosus (persistent fetal circulation). The best treatment is immediate removal of the

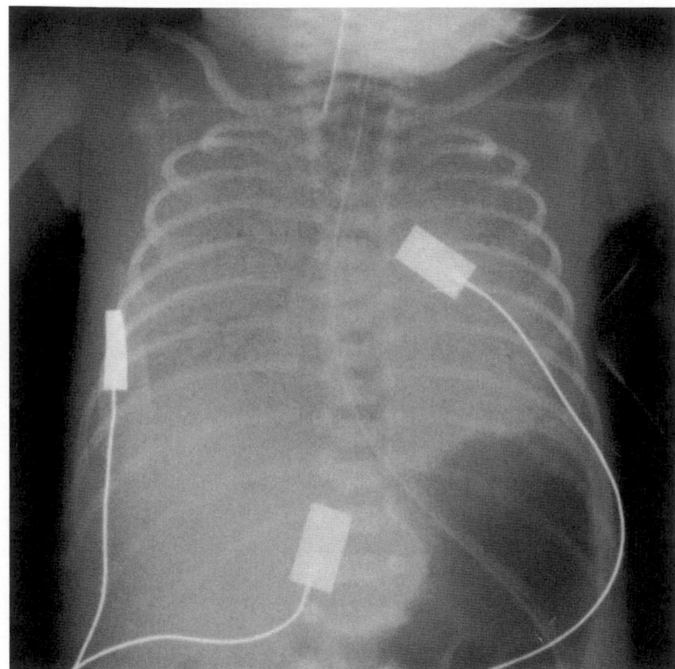

Figure 64.11 Pulmonary haemorrhage. Bilateral diffuse opacification within the lungs in a preterm infant. Both lungs were equally affected.

meconium by suction of the airways using an ETT at the time of delivery. If this is not possible, management is often difficult and recovery is often slow. Occasionally treatment with extracorporeal membrane oxygenation (ECMO) is required. The overall mortality is up to 25%.

Neonatal pulmonary infection

Infections can be acquired transplacentally, the most common organisms are TORCH (toxoplasma, rubella, cytomegalovirus, and herpes); others include listeriosis, tuberculosis, and congenital syphilis. Peripartum infection is usually by the inhalation of infected amniotic fluid or maternal tract secretions (group B streptococcus, *Esherichia coli*). Babies born following premature rupture of membranes are particularly at risk. After the first week of life, hospital infections caused by Gram-negative organisms and *Staphylococcus aureus* occur more commonly. Viral infections also may cause severe and life-threatening disease.

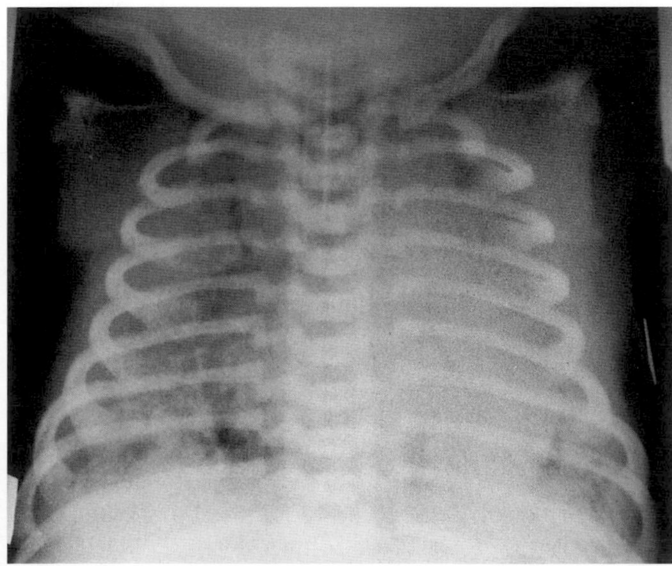

Figure 64.12 Meconium aspiration. Bilateral collapse and consolidation within the lungs in a term infant.

The diagnosis is clinical as radiographic findings vary. The spectrum includes streaky shadows resembling transient tachypnoea of the newborn, perihilar and patchy pulmonary opacities resembling aspiration, and homogeneous opacification resembling RDS. Some pneumonias have characteristic patterns. Pleural effusions frequently occur in group B streptococcal infection. Pneumatocele formation is uncommon in the neonate but may be seen in association with *E. coli*, *Haemophilus influenzae,* and now less frequently with *Staph. aureus*. Chlamydial infection is usually acquired via the birth canal but does not produce pulmonary disease until 4–6 weeks. The baby is often afebrile, may have conjunctivitis and a cough, and the radiograph shows overinflation with marked bilateral symmetric interstitial changes. Viral infections may show marked inflammatory changes with evidence of oedema.

Pleural effusions

Pleural effusions are an uncommon cause of respiratory distress. They may develop as part of a generalized oedema, as in hydrops fetalis, fetal anaemia, and fetal cardiac failure, or in response to local inflammation following perinatal infections, or due to a defect of lymphatic drainage of the pleural spaces.

Chylothorax is the most common cause of an isolated pleural effusion and predominantly affects the right hemithorax. Many different aetiologies have been implicated including congenital anomalies and birth trauma.

Congenital diaphragmatic hernia

Congenital diaphragmatic hernia occurs in 1 in 2500 live births. The most common site is posterolateral, to which the inaccurate but established term **Bochdalek hernia** is applied. It involves the left diaphragm in 70% of cases. Anterior herniation through or adjacent to the **foramina of Morgagni** usually presents later.

The diaphragm initially develops as an incomplete septum in the region of the lower cervical vertebrae and then migrates caudally to produce the pleural spaces. The diaphragmatic septum is derived from several separate elements which fuse between the sixth and seventh weeks of gestation to close the posterolateral diaphragmatic defects that are initially present. Failure of closure allows the developing intra-abdominal contents to become displaced into the thoracic cavity and results in congenital diaphragmatic hernia. In many affected infants the condition is compounded by severe respiratory difficulty secondary to pulmonary hypoplasia, persistent fetal circulation, and a degree of surfactant deficiency.

Antenatal US screening allows early diagnosis, counselling, and appropriate labour ward management. Typical postnatal radiograph findings show an opaque hemithorax with deviation of the mediastinum away from the lesion. A nasogastric tube within the stomach, as well as deflating the bowel, is a useful marker for determining the degree of mediastinal shift and the position of the stomach. Once the gastrointestinal tract starts to fill with air, radiolucencies will be seen in the affected hemithorax and there will be progressive deviation of the mediastinum (Fig. 64.13). In addition to the upper alimentary tract, parts of the colon, spleen, kidney, and pancreas can herniate into the chest and their position can be identified by US examination. Malrotation and malfixation of the small bowel are associated problems. The presence of the stomach in the thorax is usually associated with earlier herniation and more severe pulmonary hypoplasia. Radiographically, the differential diagnosis includes congenital cystic adenomatoid malformation and pneumatocele formation.

The treatment is surgical repair. The neonate normally undergoes a period of stabilization and assisted ventilation for 24–48 h before correction of the defect is performed. ECMO is occasionally required to support the neonate. Usually congenital diaphragmatic hernia is isolated. Other associated anomalies include congenital heart disease, limb deformities, extra pairs of ribs, and lung sequestration.

Congenital cystic adenomatoid malformation and bronchopulmonary sequestration

Congenital cystic adenomatoid malformation (CAM) is a rare lesion characterized by a multicystic mass of pulmonary tissue with proliferation of bronchiolar structures. CAMs are usually unilobar, usually communicate with the normal tracheobronchial tree, and receive their blood supply from a normal pulmonary artery and vein. The natural history and prognosis of these lesions are extremely variable. The prognosis depends on the size rather than the type of lesion, larger lesions having a worse prognosis. Lesions identified prenatally may involute in utero. Prenatal magnetic resonance imaging (MRI) is helpful in the diagnosis of CAM, distinguishing it from a congenital diaphragmatic hernia[14,15]. Radiographically in the first hours of life, the chest radiograph may show a shift of the mediastinum by a soft tissue mass, which represents retained lung fluid within the CAM. The fluid is absorbed and this area is replaced by an air-filled cystic lesion. If the child has severe pulmonary compromise and the contralateral lung is not hypoplastic, early surgical removal may be required.

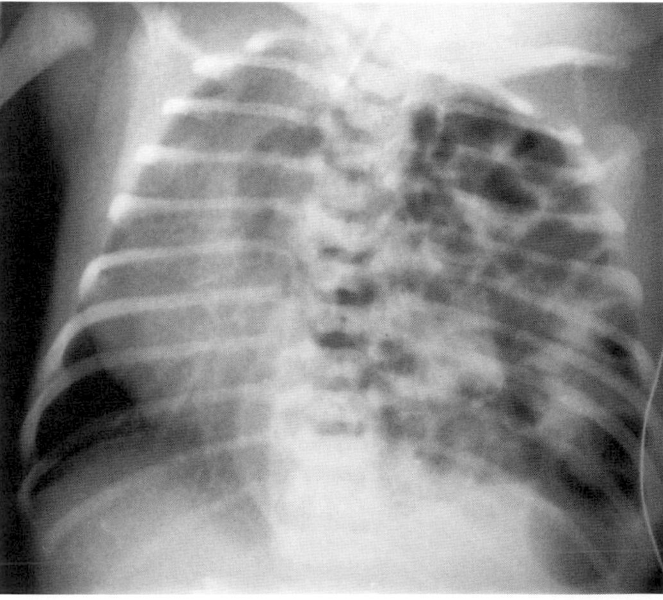

Figure 64.13 Congenital diaphragmatic hernia showing bowel extending from the abdomen in the left hemithorax and shift of the mediastinum to the right side.

Bronchopulmonary sequestration (BPS) represents a mass of nonfunctioning lung tissue that does not communicate with the normal bronchial tree and receives its vascular supply from the systemic circulation. Lesions may be intralobar or extralobar. The in utero US appearance is of a solid, well-defined highly echo-reflective mass. The anomalous systemic arterial supply is often difficult to visualize despite colour flow Doppler due to its small size and position. These lesions often appear to involute in utero. After birth these babies should be followed into childhood with chest radiographs, as the outcome of lesions seen antenatally but not detectable at birth is uncertain[16]. These lesions may not be detected antenatally or neonatally and the child presents at an older age with recurrent focal infections, bronchiectasis, haemoptysis, or an asymptomatic pulmonary mass.

Congenital lobar emphysema

Congenital lobar emphysema may be a cause of respiratory distress in the neonate. It is characterized by marked overaeration of a single pulmonary lobe, usually an upper lobe, less commonly the right middle lobe. The cause of the abnormality is unknown. Different aetiologies are suggested, including congenital absence of bronchial cartilage leading to bronchomalacia, compression of the bronchus by a vascular sling, reduplication cyst, or inflammation. A primary alveolar abnormality has also been suggested where there is an increase in the size and number of the alveoli in the affected lobe.

Immediately after birth, radiologically, the affected lobe may be opaque but will gradually become hyperlucent due to reduced pulmonary vascularity (Fig. 64.14). There will be gross overinflation with compression of the remaining lobes of the lung and contralateral mediastinal shift. Severe respiratory distress may be present and requires urgent lobectomy, but in some cases the respiratory distress is mild, surgery can be delayed, and spontaneous resolution may occur. In cases where the diagnosis is difficult, computed tomography (CT) may be helpful.

There is a well-established association between congenital heart disease and infantile lobar emphysema, particularly ventricular septal defects and tetralogy of Fallot[3,4].

Persistent fetal circulation

Persistent fetal circulation with right-to-left shunt through the patent ductus arteriosus (PDA) is often a life-threatening condition usually seen in term or post-term asphyxiated babies who have depressed respiration. It is also seen in babies with meconium aspiration syndrome, polycythaemia, pulmonary hypoplasia, and myocardial ischaemia. Chest radiographs in idiopathic cases are often normal or sometimes show mild pulmonary oligaemia, retained lung fluid, and cardiomegaly. Echocardiography is essential to demonstrate right-to-left shunting and any cardiac anomalies.

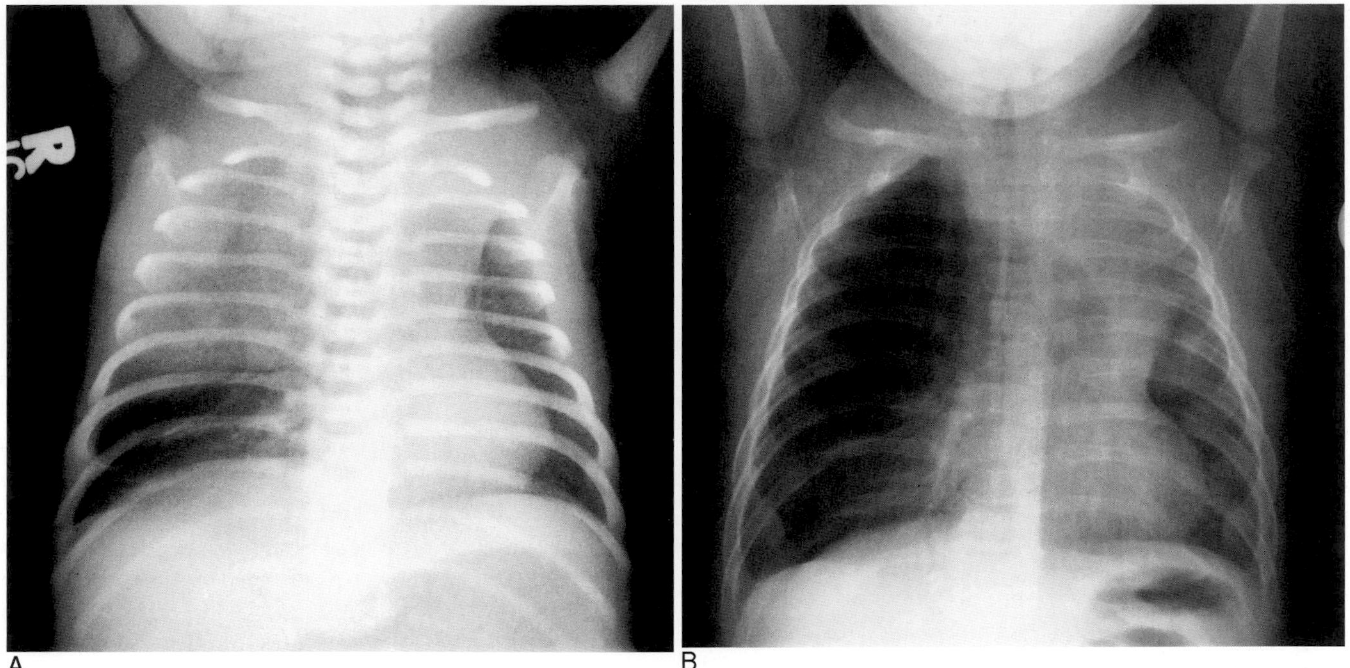

Figure 64.14 Congenital lobar emphysema. (A) Age 4 days: opacification in the right upper lobe. (B) Age 3 months: increased lucency and overinflation of the right upper lobe.

Cardiac causes of respiratory distress

The most common cardiac cause of respiratory distress is a PDA. Approximately 80% of infants will have a PDA during the first 4 d of life. The PDA only becomes pathological when there is significant right-to-left or left-to-right shunting. The diagnosis is made by echocardiography when several techniques can be used. A PDA can be seen directly with 2D or colour Doppler US and/or the left atrial-to-aortic root diameter can be measured using M-mode US, a non-specific indicator of left heart overload. A ratio greater than 1.4 on day 3 in an otherwise normal heart is indicative of a haemodynamically significant PDA[17,18]. In very premature infants, pulmonary oedema due to a PDA may form a major part of their pulmonary disease and often occurs early.

Most congenital cardiac abnormalities are suspected from the clinical presentation of the neonate and are usually diagnosed on the echocardiogram (see Ch. 23). Several cardiac conditions such as infradiaphragmatic total anomalous pulmonary venous drainage (TAPVD) causing respiratory distress are difficult to diagnose and may not be detected on the initial echocardiogram.

Late sequelae of neonatal lung disease

Radiographic changes in survivors of uncomplicated RDS are uncommon and usually consist of mild linear shadowing representing fibrosis or deep pleural fissuring. Radiographic changes occur in approximately 75% of survivors of neonatal BPD. Most commonly, linear shadowing representing pulmonary fibrosis and pleural fissuring is seen; less commonly areas of irregular aeration and distortion of the bronchovascular architecture. The plain radiograph abnormalities decrease with age. In adolescence, there may be increased bronchial lability and an increase in the AP diameter of the chest is common.

THE OLDER PAEDIATRIC PATIENT

Alan Sprigg

Respiratory tract disease is common in clinical paediatrics; frontal chest radiographs are widely performed; a lateral view is usually only performed after radiology review. Lower respiratory tract infection (LRTI) is widespread and any inflammatory change in the airways of children will produce symptoms. Whether of viral, bacterial or allergic origin, any narrowing of the small airway in children causes increased resistance to airflow, leading to noisy breathing, wheeze, tachypnoea, and 'respiratory distress'. Tenacious mucus in the airways causes lobar collapse at an earlier stage than in adults. Conducted sounds from the upper airways and crying in small children make it difficult for physicians to exclude LRTI on examination and the chest is a common source of 'sepsis'.

Patterns of consolidation or collapse are similar to those in adults and only lesions showing different appearances in paediatrics compared to adult medicine will be considered further here.

TECHNICAL FACTORS

Poor inspiration may cause significant misinterpretation of a chest radiograph. At least five anterior rib ends should be visualized above the diaphragm before a chest radiograph can be considered adequate (Fig. 64.15). Rotation of the patient causes similar problems in interpretation of mediastinal shift and air trapping as in adult practice. A postero-anterior (PA) erect radiograph taken at full inspiration is optimal, but AP supine views are often obtained in infants. Performing chest radiography on a crying, uncooperative, tachypnoeic child is challenging.

THE THYMUS

The mediastinum of infants appears abnormally wide or misshapen, due to the variable appearance of the thymus (Fig. 64.16). Enlargement of the thymus on follow-up radiography may occur after an acute illness—normal 'thymic rebound', and may simulate mediastinal mass. The normal thymus is said not to displace the trachea posteriorly unlike a true anterior mediastinal mass. The thymus is of lower attenuation than other mediastinal structures, allowing vessels to be seen through it.

US is useful to confirm that mediastinal widening is due to a normal thymus[19] before resorting to CT or MRI[20]. The normal thymus has a uniform reflectivity on US. It may extend to the right or left chest wall or anteriorly to the right or left cardiophrenic angles, simulating consolidation or a mass lesion.

TACHYPNOEA—RESPIRATORY OR CARDIAC CAUSE?

Differentiating cardiac from respiratory causes of 'respiratory distress' in an infant can be as difficult clinically as it is radiographically. In small children below the age of 1 year, the cardiothoracic ratio may be well over 50% (see above), whereas in older children it should be 50% or less, even though this is a very imprecise rule—as in adults. Significant cardiac disease may exist without a murmur and the heart size may be normal. Cardiac US is performed to exclude symptomatic cardiac disease. Dextrocardia or situs inversus may be seen on a chest radiograph.

Cardiac failure in children rarely causes pleural effusions. Mild interstitial oedema leads to peribronchial cuffing, overexpanded lungs with fluid in the horizontal fissure. Abnormal pulmonary vascularity (plethora or oligaemia) may be identifiable, but normal pulmonary vascularity does not exclude valvular stenosis or significant shunts.

INFECTION

Suspected infection is the most common reason for a paediatrician requesting a chest radiograph but radiography is seldom helpful in predicting specific bacteriology[21]. Viral infection is far more common than bacterial pneumonia in children and produces nonspecific changes. The most common finding is of overexpansion due to airway inflammatory

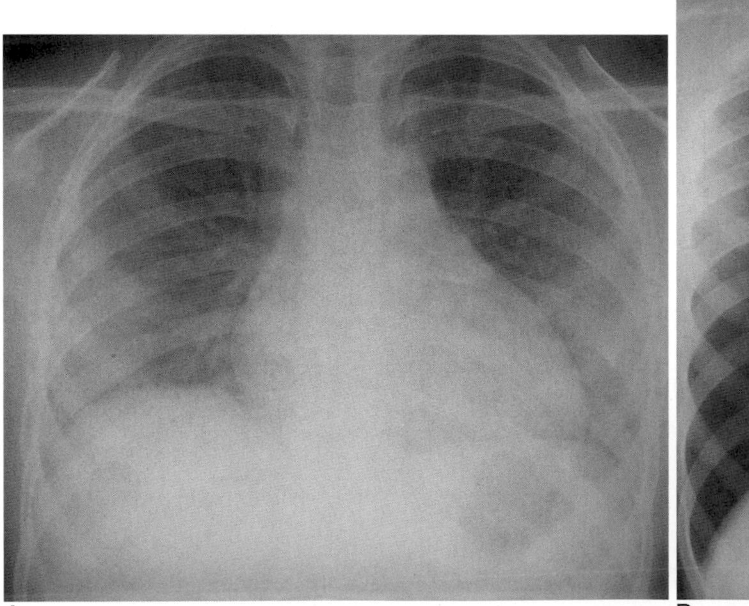

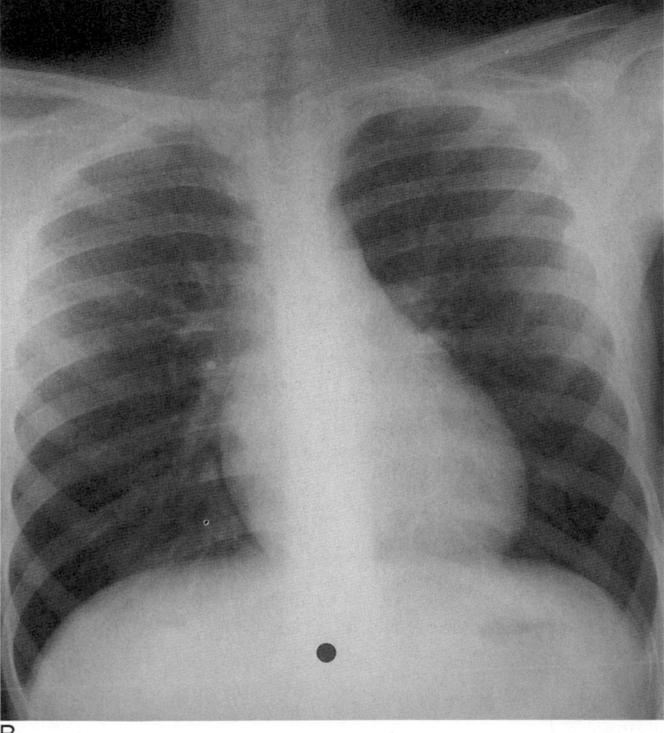

A B

Figure 64.15 Chest radiograph at different phases of respiration. (A) Four anterior rib ends above the diaphragm (expiration). (B) Six anterior rib ends (inspiration). These two radiographs on the same child at the same examination show how poor inspiration may simulate consolidation in the bases and apparent cardiomegaly.

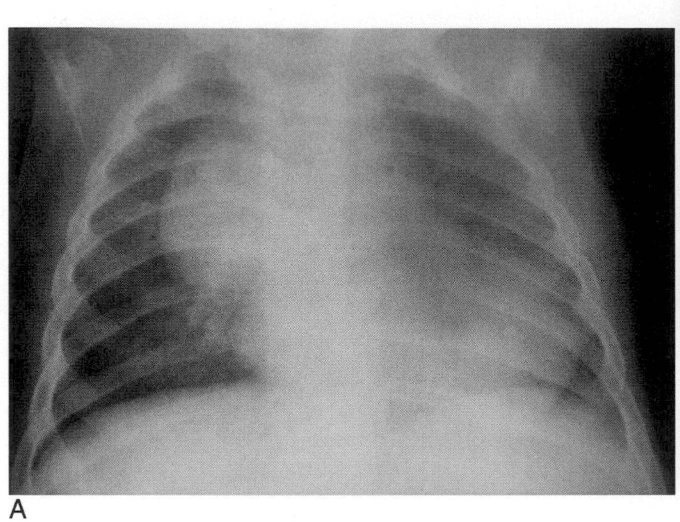
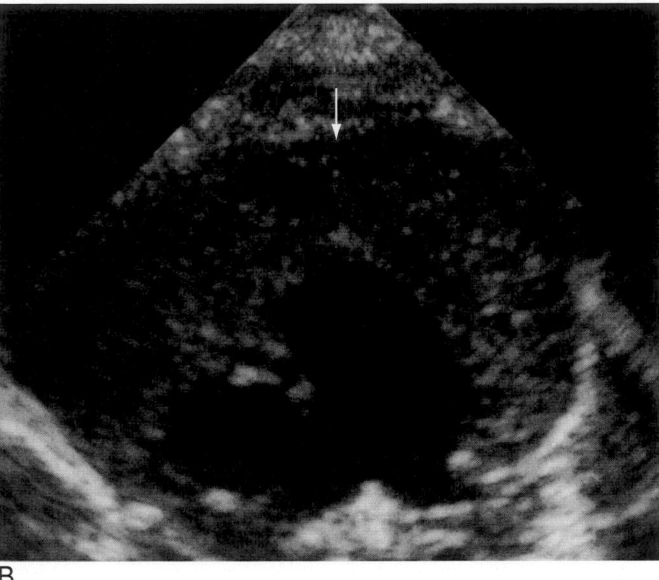

Figure 64.16 Normal thymus. (A) Chest radiograph with the thymus (sail sign) on the right mimicking right upper lobe consolidation. (B) Transverse US of the chest shows a normal thymus (arrow) around the great vessels. The normal thymus has a homogeneous reflectivity.

narrowing response, giving rise to wheeze and tachypnoea. Typical changes include peribronchial thickening, increased linear markings (interstitial infiltrates) radiating outwards from the hila, giving rise to 'perihilar flaring', and overexpansion of the lungs with flattening of the diaphragm.

Routine follow-up radiography is not necessary if the child has recovered completely clinically[22]. Radiographic changes may persist for weeks, despite clinical resolution.

A follow-up chest radiograph is useful following a complex clinical course, if there are residual clinical symptoms or after extensive lobar collapse/consolidation. The repeat chest radiograph should be delayed for several weeks.

Bronchiolitis[23]

This is the characteristic 'viral' infection of infancy, due to respiratory syncytial virus (RSV) infection, with increased incidence in spring and winter. Small children have limited energy reserves and may present with respiratory failure or respiratory arrest. Secondary bacterial infection may occur. Chest radiographs help detect the complications of bronchiolitis, rather than making the primary diagnosis. Pneumothorax occurs infrequently unless the infant is artificially ventilated. Bronchiolitis may cause a child with pre-existing pulmonary disease (e.g. BPD complicating prematurity) to go into respiratory failure. It is useful to have a 'baseline' chest radiograph on all children with chronic lung disease, before they are discharged from the neonatal nursery.

Round pneumonia[24]

Children with 'round pneumonia' present with acute pyrexia and pleuritic chest pain. The chest radiograph shows a rounded or spherical opacity with poorly defined margins, simulating a pulmonary mass (Fig. 64.17); CT may be needed for clarification. An air bronchogram is uncommon, but the clinical history and the radiographic findings are characteristic. A solitary metastasis or posterior mediastinal tumour may be considered in differential diagnosis but they usually have sharp margins. Round pneumonia resolves rapidly with treatment.

Specific infections

Pertussis[25]

The chest radiograph is usually taken to exclude complications rather than to confirm a clinical diagnosis. A poorly defined cardiac outline due to sublobar consolidation is often seen with *Bordetella pertussis* infection but it is not specific. Air trapping is seen in the acute phase.

Mycoplasma[26]

This is an atypical pneumonia and is a cause of segmental consolidation or persistent atelectasis after infancy. Small pleural effusions and a diffuse reticulonodular pattern may be seen, but these appearances are not specific for *Mycoplasma pneumoniae*.

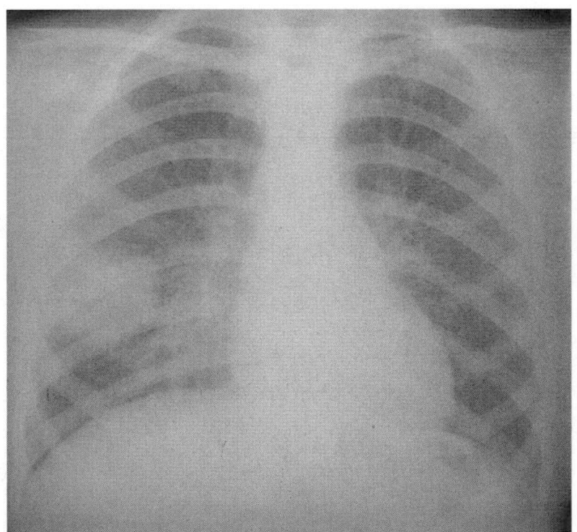

Figure 64.17 Round pneumonia. There is a rounded opacity at the right base in a pyrexial child. The shadow has ill-defined borders unlike a primary tumour or metastasis.

Staphylococcus[27]

Staphylococcus aureus infection occurs mainly in infancy or in immunocompromised children. In the acute phase it can cause a necrotic cavitating pneumonia. Following clinical resolution thin-walled 'ghost cavities' may persist for months (Fig. 64.18). They usually resolve without interference. Pyopneumothorax may occur.

Tuberculosis[28]

Infection with *Mycobacterium tuberculosis* in children may show a different pattern from that in adults. It should still be considered in the differential diagnosis of atypical pneumonia, consolidation that is slow to resolve, or persisting hilar adenopathy.

The classic pathological description is of primary and secondary tuberculosis. Primary and miliary forms are more commonly seen in young children.

In paediatric primary tuberculosis the lung focus may not be evident until it heals. It may present as consolidation with hilar nodal enlargement, persisting lobar collapse/consolidation due to endobronchial disease, or isolated nodal enlargement.

Secondary tuberculosis is similar to adults. Miliary tuberculosis can occur at any age. Chest radiography shows a miliary nodular pattern (Fig. 64.19), sometimes with coexisting nodal enlargement or consolidation (Fig. 64.20). The chest radiograph in tuberculous meningitis (TBM) is often normal.

Tuberculosis has a higher incidence in children who are malnourished or live in poor circumstances, those from areas where there is a high natural incidence of tuberculosis, and those who are immunocompromised.

Hilar adenopathy

Hilar enlargement is most commonly due to uncomplicated pulmonary infection rather than tumour or tuberculosis. Persistent hilar enlargement should be further investigated, especially if there are clinical risk factors for tuberculosis. If there is coexistent paratracheal adenopathy this must be investigated further. Sarcoidosis[29] is an uncommon cause of hilar adenopathy in children. Paediatric sarcoidosis usually presents with systemic features rather than primary pulmonary disease.

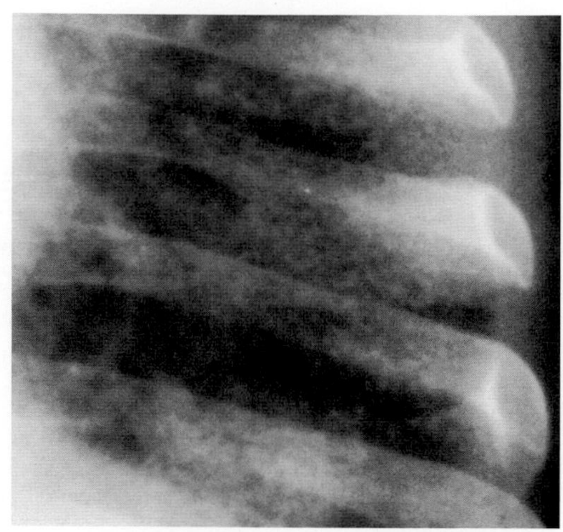

Figure 64.19 Miliary tuberculosis. Fine nodular pattern throughout the lungs.

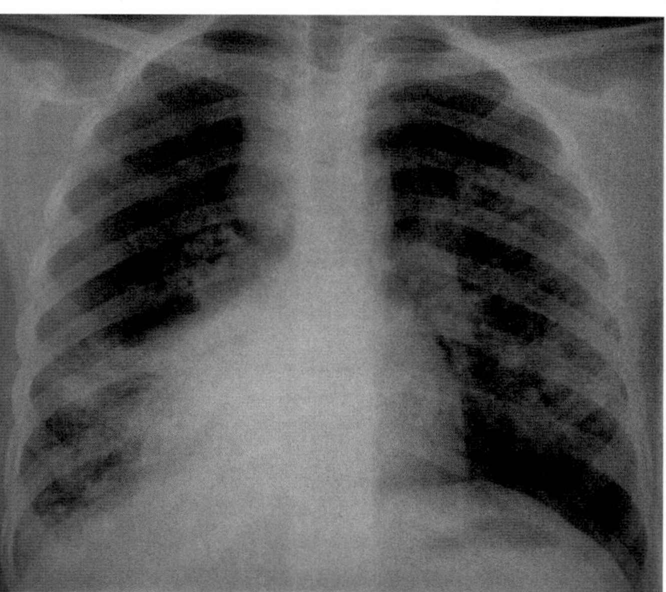

Figure 64.20 Tuberculosis in a 10 year old. A chest radiograph shows right paratracheal adenopathy, right middle lobe and lower lobe consolidation with a coarse miliary pattern throughout the lungs.

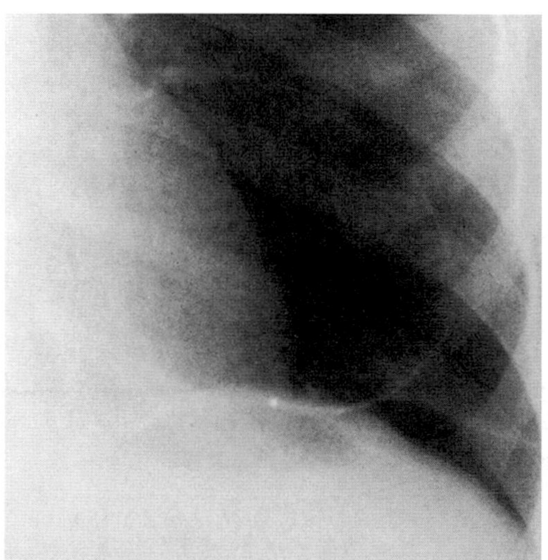

Figure 64.18 Staphylococcal infection. Following staphylococcal pneumonia, a thin-walled 'ghost cavity' may persist for several months.

Middle lobe syndrome

The right middle lobe frequently collapses due to mucus plugging, especially in asthmatic patients. It is also a common site for foreign bodies. Tuberculosis is now a less common cause of middle lobe disease.

Aspiration pneumonia[30–32]

Gastro-oesophageal reflux (GOR) is a common problem in paediatrics, especially in children with neuromuscular disorder or cerebral palsy. Nasogastric feeding tubes predispose to GOR. GOR can cause recurrent pneumonia or apnoea. The affected lobe depends on the child's posture, the upper lobes being more commonly affected in infants who spend more time supine than in the older child who sits upright.

H-shaped tracheo-oesophageal fistula

This, the rarest form of tracheo-oesophageal fistula (TOF), should be considered as a possible cause of recurrent pneumonia and can be demonstrated on a tube oesophogram. However, even good quality oesophogram tube studies may not demonstrate a narrow H-shaped fistula.

Pleural effusion

In children, pleural effusions can be due to many causes but are most often due to infection (Table 64.1)—often pneumococcal or less frequently staphylococcal, anaerobic, streptococcal, haemophilus, mycoplasma or tuberculous infection. Underlying collapse of a lung may result in elevation of the diaphragm, liver or spleen, making clinical assessment of the extent of the effusion difficult. An effusion is easily confirmed using US, and by defining extent, stranding and depth US guidance can aid the placement of a diagnostic tap or drain. It can influence a decision to perform closed drainage, thoracoscopy, or decortication if there is an empyema (Fig. 64.21).

Table 64.1 CAUSES OF PLEURAL EFFUSION
Small
Bacterial chest infection
Empyema
Tuberculosis
Subdiaphragmatic cause (sepsis or a mass)
Postoperative (sympathetic or chylothorax)
Thoracic tumour
Cardiac failure or fluid overload
Hypoproteinaemia (nutritional or nephrotic/gut)
Large (radio-opaque chest): US for assessment
As above but especially:
Empyema
Tumour—lymphoma, leukaemia
Infective—consider tuberculosis
Diaphragmatic hernia (obstructed)

THE RADIO-OPAQUE CHEST

In children infection is the most common cause of the unilaterally opaque chest radiograph. Other causes include bronchial obstruction due to intrinsic tumour (e.g. carcinoid) or extrinsic tumour (e.g. lymphoma/leukaemia nodes), pleural tumour (Askin tumour or other sarcoma), and delayed presentation of a congenital diaphragmatic hernia. A combination of US, CT, or MRI and diagnostic aspiration is used.

IMAGING THE CHILD ON THE INTENSIVE CARE UNIT

Intensive care chest imaging provides similar problems to adult practice, but respiratory arrest is much more common in paediatrics compared to cardiac arrest. Respiratory failure due to infection or septicaemia is a frequent reason for admission to the intensive care unit (ICU). The small size of the paediatric airway, tracheomalacia, or tenacious secretions cause lobar collapse, often of the right upper lobe.

Non-cuffed ETTs are used in children to minimize pressure damage to the trachea but this allows ETT movement

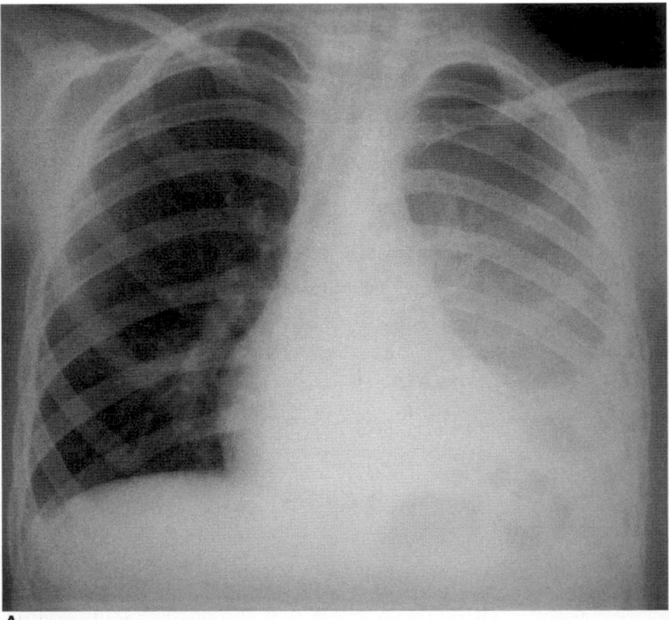

A

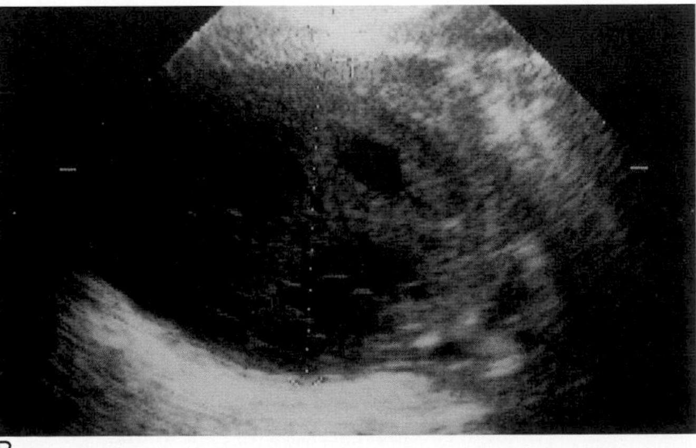

B

Figure 64.21 Ultrasound in pleural effusions. (A) Chest radiograph of left-sided pleural effusion, elevated left diaphragm and scoliosis to the left. (B) Longitudinal US shows mixed reflectivity with thick internal septa in the fluid on the right of the image, due to a loculated empyema. Thick pus was drained at thoracotomy.

with changes in the child's position—a common cause of a tube migrating from the trachea into a bronchus. Rapid re-expansion usually occurs following correction of ETT malposition (Fig. 64.22), improving gas exchange.

Misplaced central venous lines are a significant risk in paediatrics. Peripheral small bore catheters inserted for parenteral nutrition pose a significant risk for cardiac tamponade if their tip is left in the right atrium.

Rib fractures are rarely caused by cardiopulmonary resuscitation in children, because their ribs are very compliant[33,34]. The radiologist may be the first person to identify rib fractures on a chest radiograph. In infants this raises the possibility of nonaccidental injury. If there is no history of significant trauma to explain rib fractures, the findings should be discussed directly with the paediatrician who can ensure the child is protected from further injury.

THE WHEEZY CHEST

Asthma

The diagnosis of asthma is clinical, not radiographic. Asthma is common but other causes of wheezing are rare (e.g. mediastinal mass, inhaled foreign body, or congenital airway abnormality). Chest radiography may be requested if wheezing is persistent. It should only be performed to exclude complications in a known asthmatic patient, e.g. consolidation with wheeze and pyrexia, or when a child is not responding to bronchodilators. The radiographic changes of asthma are those of overexpansion (flat diaphragm, square chest shape) with bronchial wall thickening or peribronchial cuffing. Right middle lobe collapse is often due to mucus plugging. Air leaks are uncommon.

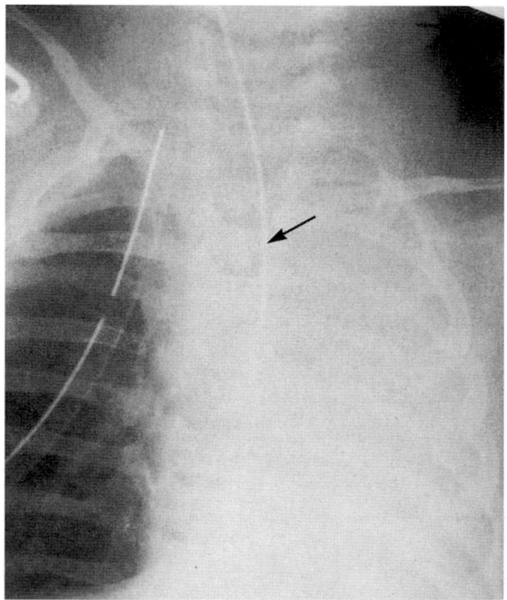

Figure 64.22 Displaced endotracheal tube (ETT) down the right main bronchus. The tip of the tube (arrow) is distal to the left main bronchus, resulting in complete collapse of the left lung and mediastinal shift to the left. Post right thoracotomy. The left lung completely re-inflated 1 h later following repositioning of the ETT.

Mediastinal shift

As in adults, mediastinal shift may be due to reduction in volume on one side (e.g. lobar collapse) or increased volume on the other side (e.g. effusion or air trapping). Chest radiography is used to define the side of abnormality and the differential diagnosis (Table 64.2). Uncomplicated asthma does not cause mediastinal shift.

Most small children will not cooperate to produce paired inspiration and expiration radiographs to look for mediastinal shift. Fluoroscopy allows assessment of diaphragmatic movement and mediastinal shift with varying phases of respiration, as most small children cry when placed on a screening table!

Functional imaging of the abnormal lung is by radionuclide radiology; perfusion (Q) and ventilation (V) scintigrams will assess V/Q mismatching. Nebulized ^{99m}Tc-DTPA may precipitate in the bronchi in children, making assessment of regional ventilation difficult. ^{81m}Krypton aerosol ventilation scintigraphy allows a continuous 'wash-in' phase assessment without precipitation in the airways, but access to ^{81m}krypton ventilation scintigraphy is limited by difficulty of supply.

Inhaled foreign bodies[35,36]

Small children frequently put objects in their mouths. A history of possible inhalation of a foreign body (FB) with the sudden onset of wheezing is an indication for further investigation. There may be no direct history of inhalation of a FB in a child presenting with wheeze or recurrent infection. Less obvious symptoms include persistent cough or recurrent pneumonia. Persisting collapse or consolidation in one lobe should alert the radiologist to the possibility of an endobronchial FB.

Bronchoscopy should be performed if there is a good history. Whilst a FB may lodge in any bronchus, the right bronchus intermedius is a common site.

The chest radiograph may identify a radio-opaque FB in the airway, air trapping, or lobar collapse, so it is important to review the whole airway with a suspicious history (Fig. 64.23). Unfortunately most inhaled FBs are radiolucent (e.g. plastic toys and peanuts). Comparison of the aeration and perfusion of the same areas of lung on both sides will show areas of air trapping or reflex oligaemia (Fig. 64.24). Fluoroscopy can be

Table 64.2 MEDIASTINAL SHIFT
Towards the abnormal side
Lobar collapse (mucus plug, foreign body)
Pulmonary agenesis or hypoplasia (primary or secondary)
Scimitar syndrome (hypogenetic lung)
Bronchopulmonary sequestration (basal)
Swyer James (MacLeod) syndrome
Away from the abnormal side
Pneumothorax
Pleural effusion (without collapse)
Air trapping: foreign body, congenital lobar emyphsema (apical), bronchial atresia
Cystic congenital adenomatoid malformation
Diaphragmatic hernia

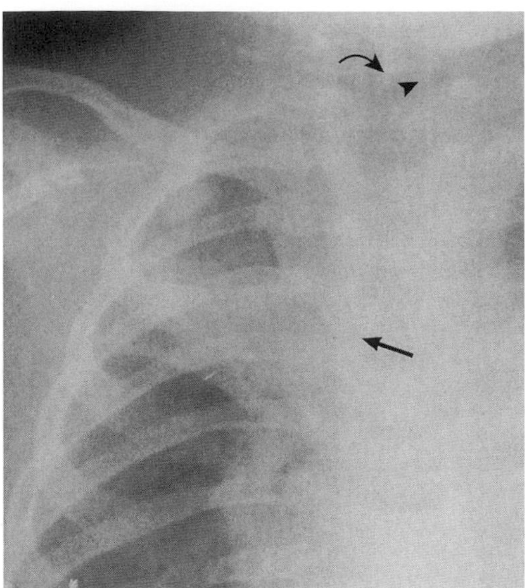

Figure 64.23 Intubated child with stridor. Endotracheal tube (ETT) and nasogastric tube in place. There is an opaque foreign body (arrow) faintly seen in the right main bronchus, right upper lobe collapse, and right middle lobe consolidation. Arrowhead = nasogastric tube; curved arrow = ETT.

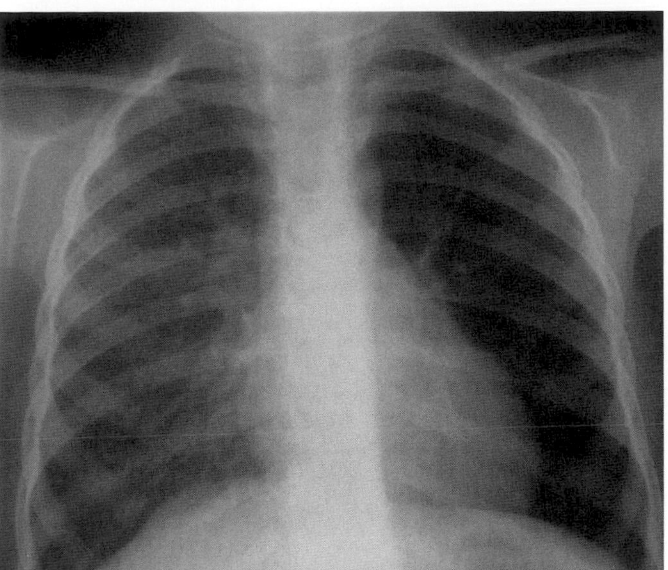

Figure 64.24 Foreign body in the left bronchus (not radio-opaque). Relative oligaemia and small blood vessels at the left lung are due to poor ventilation and reflex vasoconstriction on the left side.

used to demonstrate air trapping (ball valve effect) with mediastinal shift in an uncooperative child (Fig. 64.25).

Peanuts are common inhaled FBs that contain oil, causing endobronchial inflammation or stenosis. Peanuts often fragment during bronchoscopic removal, embolizing into smaller bronchi and causing increased consolidation on the post-bronchoscopy radiograph.

Petroleum product inhalation is usually due to inappropriate storage in 'pop' bottles. An early chest radiograph may be falsely reassuring[37]. Radiography may show pneumonitis hours later. Pneumatoceles are a late complication.

Stridor

Tracheal 'buckling' seen on a frontal chest radiograph is a normal variant due to the flexibility and movement of the infant's trachea with respiration and posture. Stridor is often due to viral or bacterial infection. Congenital stridor may be due to tracheal compression by a vascular ring (arch anomaly or pulmonary artery sling). Initial assessment is by contrast medium studies of the oesophagus with AP and lateral views.

CONGENITAL CHEST ABNORMALITIES

Congenital lobar emphysema

This most commonly presents in infancy beyond the neonatal period and involves an upper lobe. The chest radiograph shows mediastinal shift away from the side of the abnormality and reduced vascularity in the affected lobe (Fig. 64.26). CT and V/Q scintigraphy are useful in indeterminate cases, showing

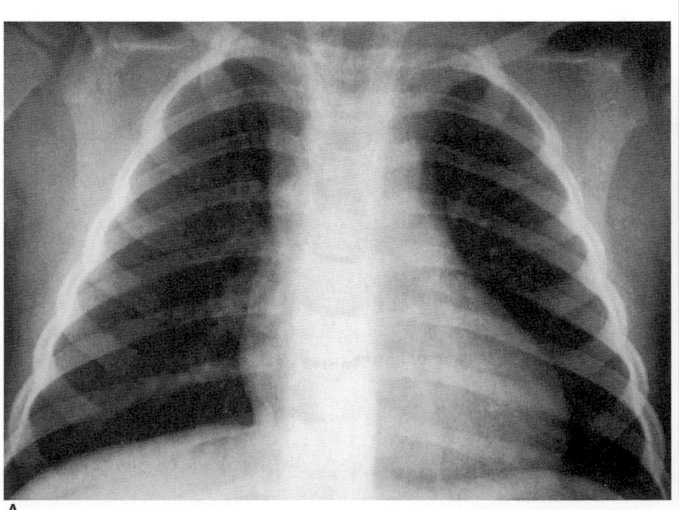

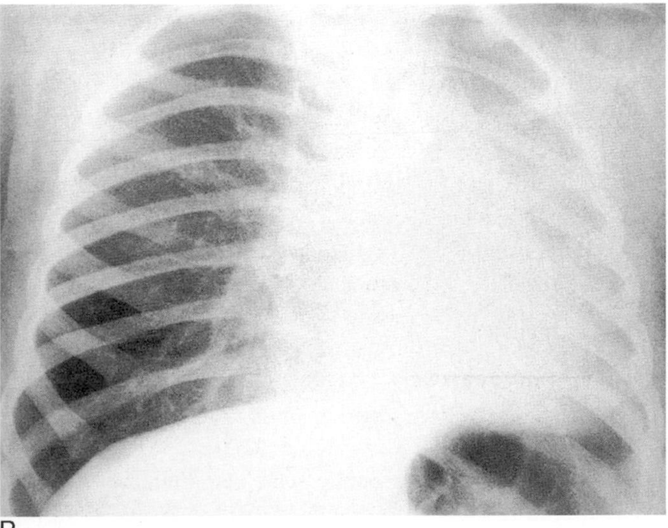

Figure 64.25 Obstructive emphysema due to foreign body. (A) The chest radiograph taken on full inspiration is normal. (B) The expiration film shows a marked mediastinal shift to the left. There was a foreign body in the right main bronchus, causing air trapping due to a 'ball valve' effect.

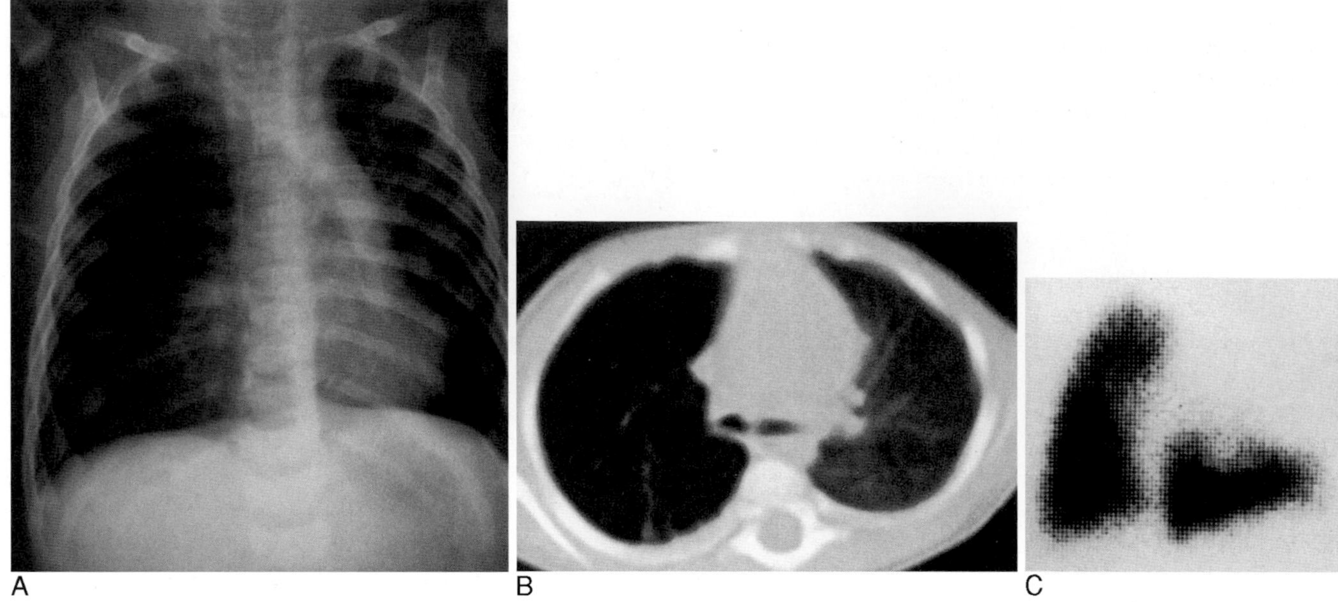

Figure 64.26 Congenital lobar emphysema. Eleven-month-old with respiratory distress. (A) Chest radiograph shows mediastinal shift to the left and oligaemia in the right upper lobe. (B) CT shows overexpansion, small pulmonary vessels and oligaemia on the right side. (C) Scintigraphy with ^{99m}Tc-macroaggregates shows poor perfusion in the right upper lobe; right posterior oblique view.

extent and reduced perfusion, with absent ventilation on the early phase, delayed entry of isotope activity in the affected lobe and retention in the late phase.

Congenital diaphragmatic anomalies[38,39]

The diaphragm originates from muscle slips from the ribs fusing into a central tendon and creating separate abdominal and chest cavities. If the central tendon of the diaphragm is abnormally lax, it causes **eventration**. If there is a diaphragmatic defect a congenital diaphragmatic hernia occurs often presenting in the neonatal period but delayed presentation does occur.

Diaphragmatic paralysis may be due to damage to the phrenic nerve during a difficult delivery. Acquired paralysis is uncommon without prior surgical intervention.

An abnormal diaphragm may be identified on a chest radiograph taken for other reasons. It may be elevated or have associated mediastinal shift. If there is unilateral diaphragmatic elevation, it is important to exclude a subdiaphragmatic cause (e.g. abdominal mass, subpulmonary effusion, or subphrenic sepsis).

US is very useful, as this may show a mass, collection, or impaired diaphragmatic excursion, and can assess paradoxical or asymmetric movement with respiration, which is best assessed on a transverse (slightly coronal) image as this can allow simultaneous visualization of both diaphragms.

Fluoroscopy is used to assess both hemidiaphragms as they move with respiration. The lateral position can assess relative movement. Older children can cooperate for the 'sniff test' and crying infants produce a rapid inspiratory excursion of the diaphragms at the end of a scream.

Unilateral diaphragmatic paralysis involves the whole hemidiaphragm but in eventration there is usually a localized hump in the diaphragm. The differentiation between diaphragmatic hernia and eventration can be difficult especially on the right side where the liver may act as a central obturator in the hernia, causing a localized hump in the diaphragm.

A hernia should be considered in the differential diagnosis of a basal cystic mass in the chest (Table 64.3) and excluded by the use of gastrointestinal contrast studies.

Anterior (midline Morgagni) hernias may present in childhood or in adult life. They can be difficult to diagnose on the chest radiograph if the omentum herniates rather than the gas-filled transverse colon. Contrast gastrointestinal studies are useful if there is apparent gut herniation (Fig. 64.27). CT or coronal MRI is useful to confirm herniation of fatty omentum in the differentiation of a paracardiac mass.

Table 64.3 CAUSES OF PAEDIATRIC LUNG CYSTS
Cystic fibrosis
Cystic bronchiectasis
Bronchopulmonary dysplasia (neonate and older)
Tuberculosis (apical thick walled)
Mycetoma (apical cyst with contents)
Pulmonary abscess (thick wall, fluid level)
Empyema (pleural)
Streptococcal pneumatocele (thin wall, post infective)
Cavitating pneumonia
Bronchopulmonary sequestration (basal)
Cystic congenital adenomatoid malformation (basal cysts of varying size)
Diaphragmatic hernia (basal cysts of similar size)
Hiatal hernia (basal posterior)
Morgagni hernia (midline anterior)
Hydatid disease (in endemic areas)
Kerosene inhalation (pneumatocele)
Histiocytosis and interstitial disease

Posterior **Bochdalek hernias** are often diagnosed antenatally or present in the neonate with a large diaphragmatic defect. In the older child the diaphragmatic defect is usually much smaller and the child may present with a loop of gut herniating into the chest through a small defect with subsequent obstruction or gut ischaemia. The clinical presentation is variable with collapse, septicaemia, a cystic chest mass, or a 'white-out' chest. A herniated stomach may simulate an isolated cavity in the left lung with a fluid level. Passage of a nasogastric tube can confirm that the stomach is in the chest (Fig. 64.28). If oral contrast studies are performed, they should be followed through until the entire colon has been demonstrated to the rectum. Confirmation that the stomach and small bowel are normally sited does not exclude a colonic hernia.

Hiatal hernias are seen in children as well as in adults. Para-oesophageal hernias may present as a cystic mass in the right or left side of the chest.

Congenital cystic adenomatoid malformation[40]

These commonly present in the neonate, often diagnosed on antenatal US. They may be found in older children on a chest radiograph taken for other reasons or who present with symptoms due to obstructive emphysema and mediastinal shift or secondary to infection. A spectrum of cystic change is found but three main forms are described: macrocystic (type 1) (Fig. 64.29), microcystic (type 3), or a mixed pattern (type 2). Congential cystic adenomatoid malformation (CCAM) is included in the differential diagnosis of cystic lesions of the paediatric chest. CCAM shares some histological features with bronchopulmonary sequestration (BPS), which is also a basal disorder.

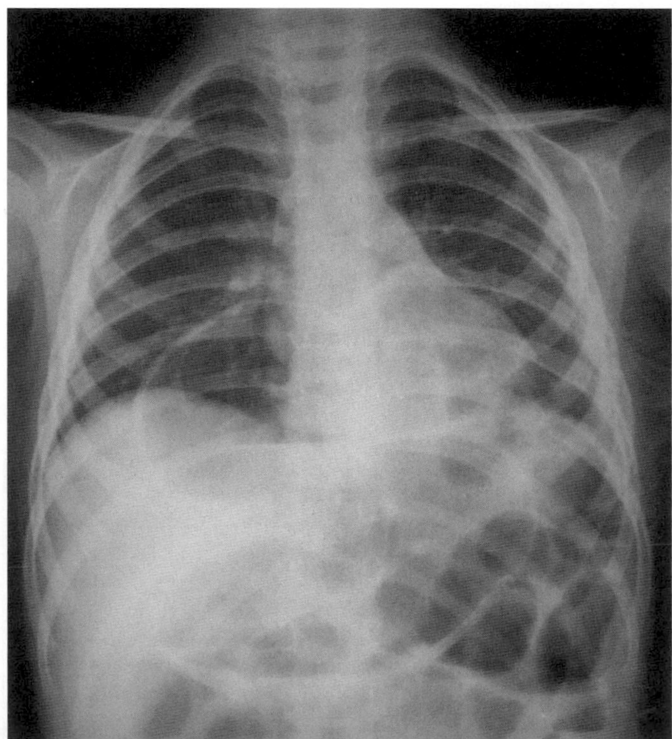

A

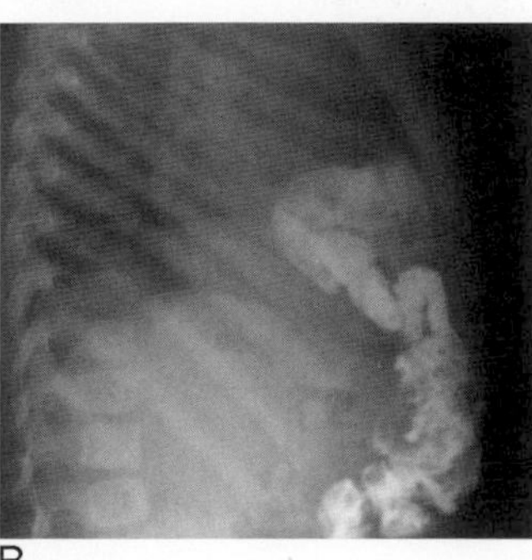

B

Figure 64.27 Morgagni diaphragmatic hernia. (A) Chest radiograph shows a cystic structure projected over the heart. (B) A barium follow-through shows the colon in the anterior hernia on the delayed lateral view.

Bronchopulmonary sequestration[41,42]

BPS is often diagnosed on obstetric US and overlaps with CCAM. It is due to a developmental abnormality of lobar formation with abnormal vascular supply. It usually presents with a persisting basal opacity on serial radiography, mimicking lower lobe collapse/consolidation or cavitation, and is frequently left sided. It is important to exclude sequestration with a persisting basal lung lesion. Its arterial supply is from the systemic circulation from the aorta above or below the diaphragm. Pre-operative colour Doppler abdominal US may demonstrate the abnormal vessel(s) if they arise from the abdominal aorta, but may miss the arterial supply from the thoracic aorta. CT angiography (CTA) or MR angiography (MRA) can define the arterial feeder(s) and may show anomalous draining veins.

Scimitar syndrome (hypogenetic lung, pulmonary venolobar syndrome)

This congenital anomaly shares some features with sequestration except that the lung is normally connected to the bronchial tree, but the vein draining the lobe (usually the right lower lobe) drains into the inferior vena cava or portal vein, rather than to the left atrium. The aberrant basal pulmonary vein may be found coincidentally on a chest radiograph or the child may present with features of a left-to-right shunt. The characteristic appearance on chest radiography is of a small ipsilateral lung with mediastinal shift towards the affected side. An abnormal vessel is usually seen draining down and enlarging towards the diaphragm in the shape of a 'scimitar' sword.

Pulmonary vascular malformations[43]

These are similar in appearance to those in adults. Pulmonary or aortic angiography is diagnostic. Radionuclide imaging is used to screen for a right-to-left shunt. Normally, ^{99m}Tc-microspheres injected intravenously do not pass through the lung capillaries. With a right-to-left shunt they can pass through into the systemic circulation and lodge in the kidneys and other organs (Fig. 64.30). Pulmonary systemic shunting may also occur with BPS, scimitar syndrome, bidirectional cardiac shunts, or other arteriovenous malformations.

Pulmonary agenesis and hypoplasia

An early insult to lung bud development or vascular supply will interfere with lung development in later pregnancy. Total agenesis of the lung is associated with absence of the pulmonary

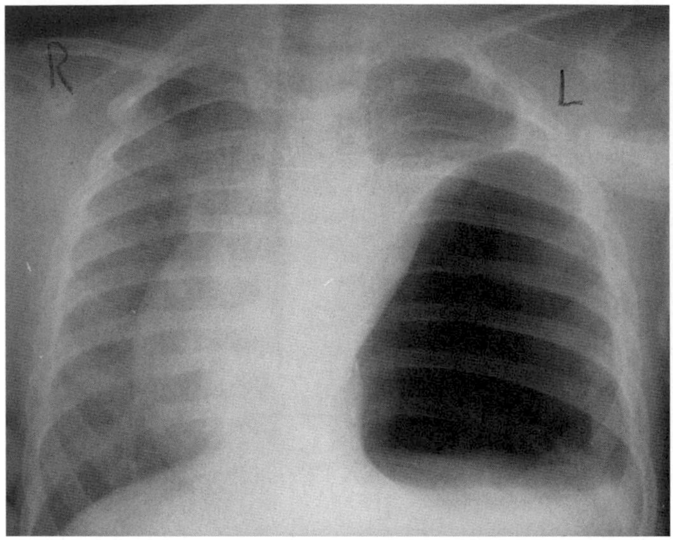

Figure 64.28 Left diaphragmatic hernia. A 2 year old child with acute dyspnoea due to gastric herniation and volvulus. Absent gastric bubble in the abdomen. A nasogastric tube was later passed into the 'pulmonary cyst', confirming gastric herniation.

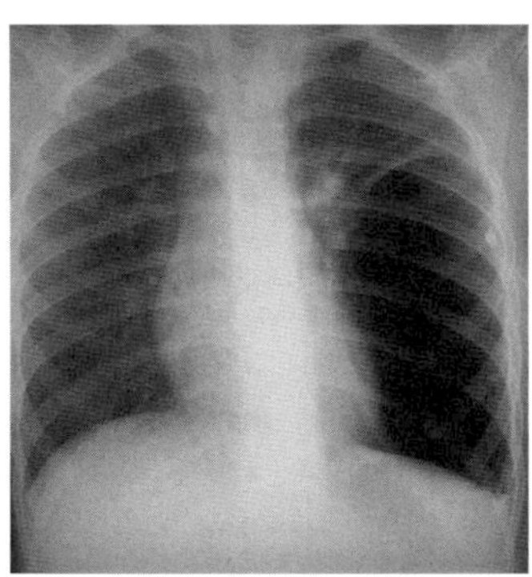

Figure 64.29 Congenital cystic adenomatoid malformation of lung (CCAM). A 4 year old child presented with acute dyspnoea. Chest radiograph shows a cystic lesion in the left lower lobe, confirmed histologically as a CCAM type 1.

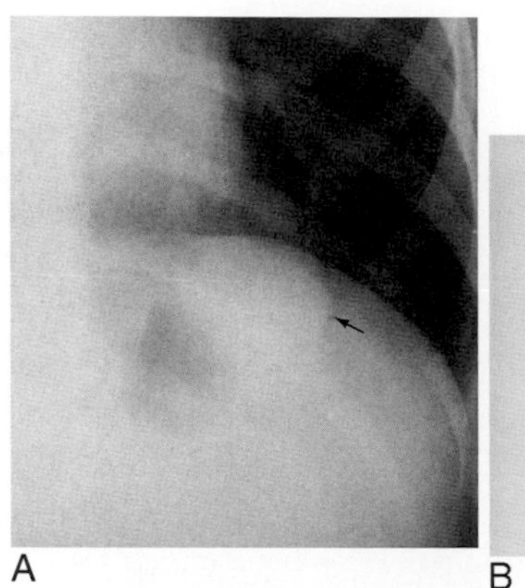

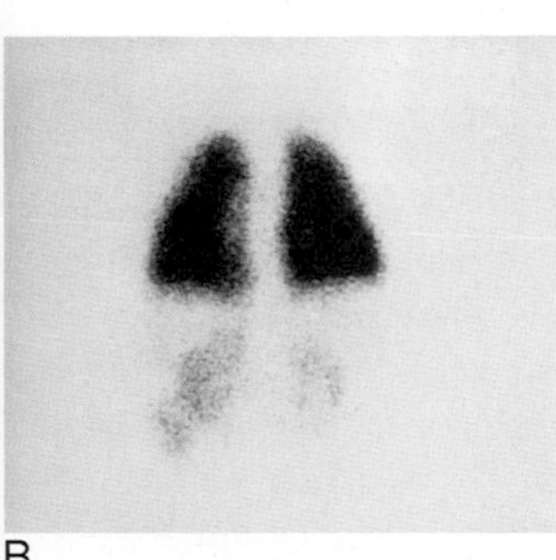

Figure 64.30 Pulmonary arteriovenous malformation (AVM). (A) Chest radiograph shows a round opacity (arrow) in the left base posterior to the diaphragm, with large lower lobe vessels. (B) ^{99m}Tc-macro-aggregate scintigraphy shows normal activity in the lungs and abnormal activity in the kidneys due to shunting from right to left across the AVM. (Courtesy of Professor H.M. Carty, Liverpool, UK.)

artery and bronchial development. Chest radiography demonstrates mediastinal shift and the absence of lung markings on the affected side. Cross-herniation of the normal lung from the opposite side may cause confusion.

CT and radionuclide imaging correlated with a recent chest radiograph are helpful. Scintigraphy shows no perfusion or ventilation in the affected lung. Angiography (or echo) confirms a small or absent pulmonary artery on the affected side (Fig. 64.31).

Pulmonary hypoplasia is a less severe form of the above and may be unilateral or bilateral. Causes include neuromuscular disease, skeletal dysplasia (e.g. asphyxiating thoracic dystrophy) or pulmonary compression due to oligohydramnios. A chest radiograph shows a 'bell-shaped' chest and slender ribs. Unilateral hypoplasia is due to a primary pulmonary embryological defect or is secondary to diaphragmatic hernia or CCAM resection. The acquired form overlaps with the Swyer James (MacLeod) syndrome, which is due to infection of the developing lung in infancy (Fig. 64.32), but unlike Swyer James syndrome, pulmonary hypoplasia shows no evidence of air trapping.

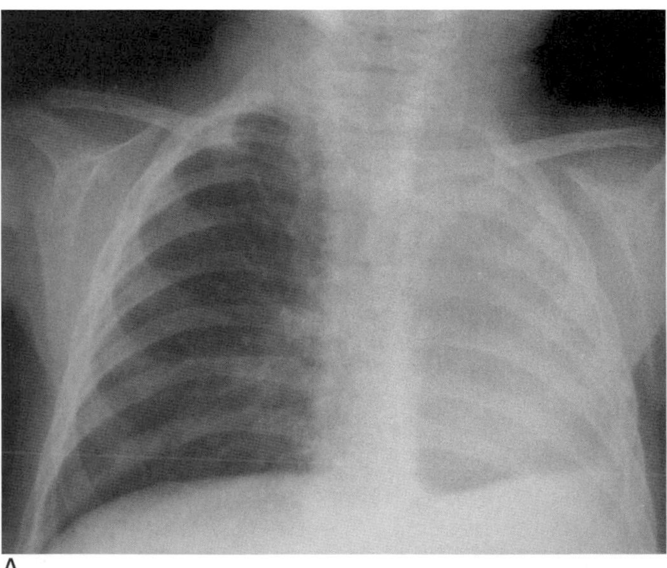

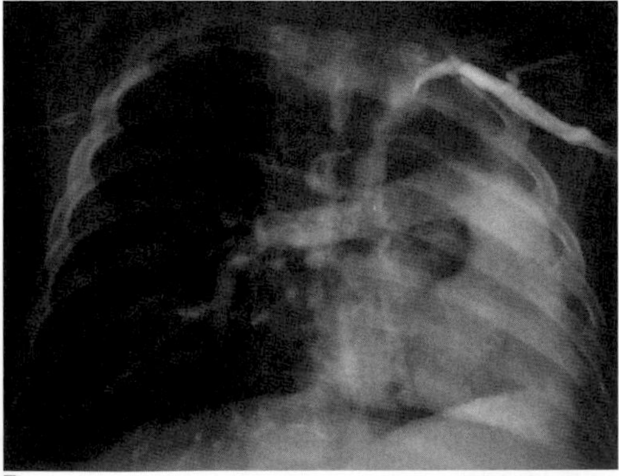

Figure 64.31 Pulmonary agenesis. (A) Chest radiograph. The heart is displaced to the left and the right lung is overexpanded into the left chest, obscuring the heart. (B) A right heart angiogram shows the large right pulmonary artery but no left pulmonary artery, confirming left pulmonary agenesis.

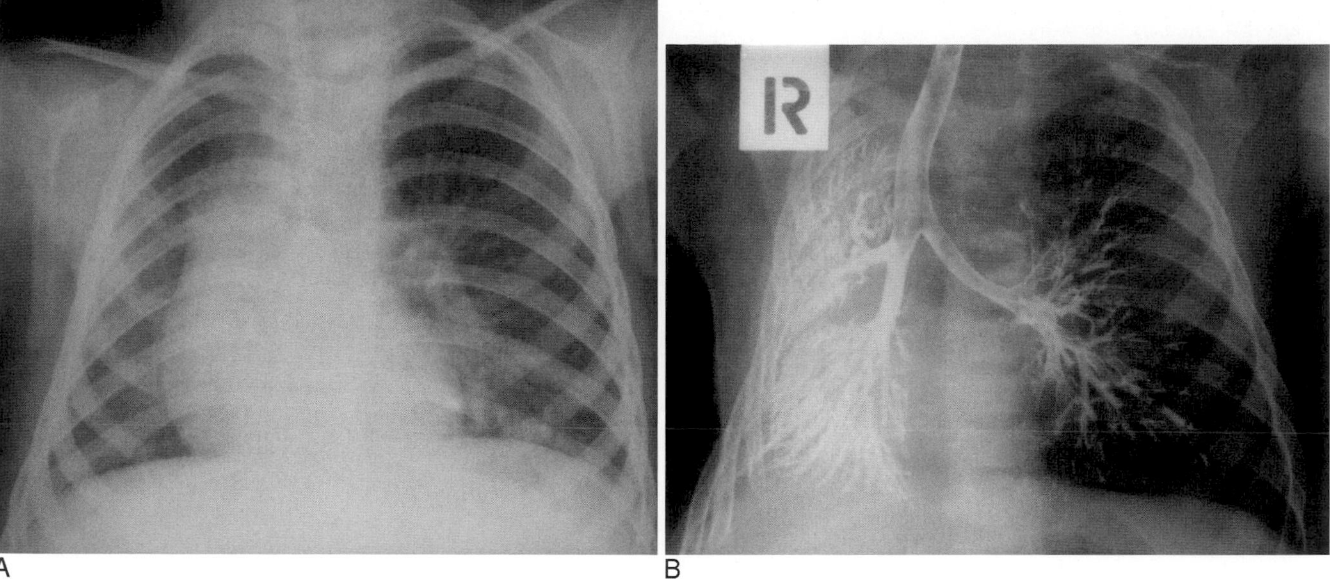

Figure 64.32 Hypoplasia of the right lung. (A) The chest radiograph shows mediastinal shift to the right and a small undervascularized right lung. (B) Bronchography shows normal right bronchial branching with attenuation. Normal left bronchi.

THE MEDIASTINUM[44–48]

The mediastinum may be divided into compartments, as in adult chest disease, but the causes of mediastinal masses are different (Table 64.4). Primary malignancy and acquired vascular disease are rare. Congenital malformations are common.

In the radiographic investigation good quality frontal and lateral chest radiographs are essential. US, CT/CTA or MRI/MRA will give further information on mediastinal masses in the assessment of vascular rings or in congenital malformation (Table 64.5). Many tumours spread across compartment boundaries—an 'anatomical' approach to mediastinal pathology is only a guide. The imaging findings must be correlated with clinical data (e.g. blood count to exclude leukaemia and clinical examination to search for other sites of nodal enlargement) before resorting to mediastinal biopsy. Imaging guides the approach of the biopsy by defining the extent of disease and its relation to major vascular and spinal structures. Involvement of pericardium, major vessels or spine may necessitate cardiac or neurosurgical assistance.

Anterior mediastinal masses are most commonly nodal (lymphoma or leukaemia) (Fig. 64.33). There may be significant compression of the trachea with an anterior mass (Fig. 64.34)—important information for the anaesthetist. A multilocular cystic mass is usually a hygroma or lymphangioma, but this may have components of haemangioma.

Calcification in a middle or anterior mediastinal mass suggests a teratoma or hamartoma, whereas a cystic mass in the middle mediastinum is most commonly a bronchogenic cyst (Fig. 64.35). Bronchogenic cysts usually have a slender connection to the carina and may occur away from the carina, but they only occasionally show air within the cyst. Foregut remnants (bronchogenic cysts, oesophageal duplication, neurenteric cyst) are due to failure of normal embryology as the primitive notocord, oesophagus, and trachea develop and separate.

Table 64.4 CAUSES OF MEDIASTINAL MASS, BY COMPARTMENT

Anterior (superior)
Normal thymus**
Thymic infiltration (leukaemia, lymphoma, histiocytosis)**
Nodal mass**
Thyroid
Cystic lymphangioma/haemangioma
Thymic cyst or thymoma
Teratoma
Plexiform neurofibroma
Anterior (inferior)
Cardiac*
Pericardial cysts, tumours, and fat pads
Morgagni hernia (gut or omentum)
Middle
Nodal mass (as above), granulomatous disease (TB)**
Vascular and aortic ring anomalies*
Bronchogenic cyst (foregut duplication, neurenteric cyst)*
Venous anomalies (left superior vena cava)
Plexiform neurofibroma
Posterior
Sympathetic chain tumours (neuroblastoma ganglioneuroma sequence)**
Hiatal and diaphragmatic hernia (intrathoracic kidney)**
Spinal related tumours (plus neuroblastoma from abdomen)*
Spinal sepsis (staphylococcal, tuberculosis)*
Bronchopulmonary sequestration*
Oesophageal duplication, neurenteric cyst
Neurofibroma
Phaeochromocytoma
Extension of abdominal pathology (e.g. pancreatitis with pseudocyst)
Extramedullary haematopoiesis (haemoglobinopathy)

** = Common; * = occasional; others are uncommon.

Table 64.5 INVESTIGATION OF A MEDIASTINAL MASS

1. **Plain radiography.** Chest PA and lateral, localized spine and rib views if posterior
2. **US if mass anterior**, pericardial or basal (solid or cystic mass, nodal or vascular/cardiac)
3. **CT.** Post intravenous contrast medium. Gives details of location and the relationship to vessels and extension. CT essential for lung detail and metastases.
4. **MRI.** Pre- and post-gadolinium. MRI is used if there is a posterior mass, associated spinal anomaly or clinical evidence of cord involvement. Axial, sagittal and coronal sections are essential.

Additional imaging

5. **Contrast studies**: Oesophogram if the mass involves the middle or posterior mediastinum or clinical symptoms of dysphagia or stridor. Late image for ? diaphragmatic hernia
6. **Radionuclide imaging**

^{99m}Tc-Pertechnetate: duplication cyst of the oesophagus

^{123}I-MIBG: neuroblastoma-like tumour, whole body

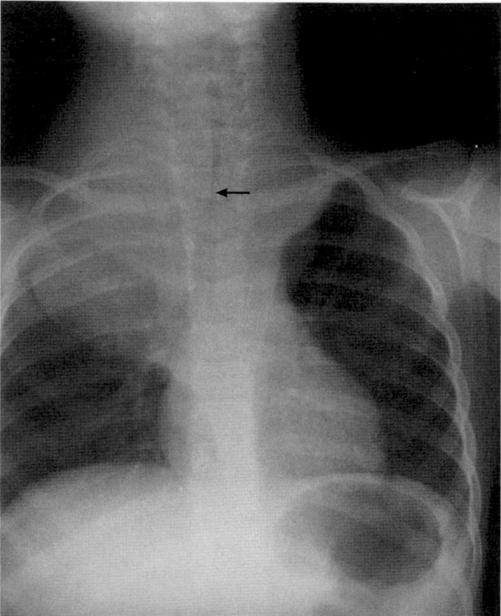

Figure 64.34 Neurofibromatosis (plexiform). There is a large mediastinalmass extending into the neck and causing tracheal compression (arrow).

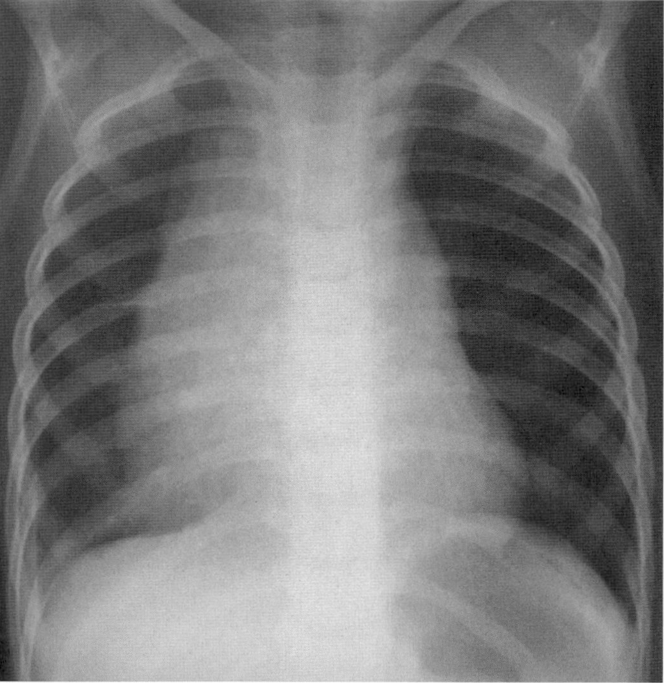
A

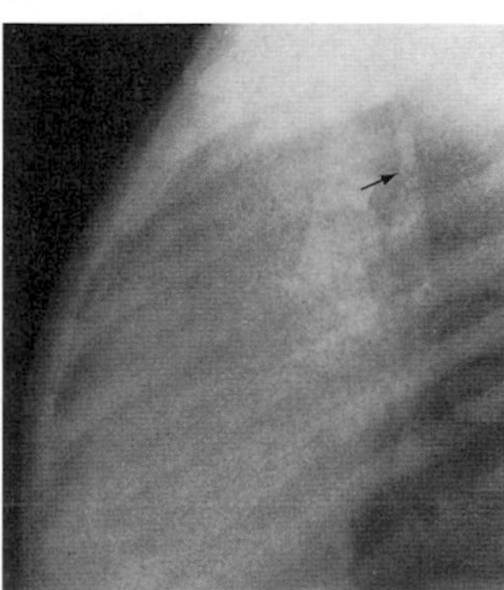
B

Figure 64.33 Anterior mediastinal mass. Chest radiograph (A) PA and (B) lateral. Large anterior mediastinal mass displacing the trachea posteriorly (arrow) due to T-cell acute lymphoblastic leukaemia. Similar appearances may be seen with lymphoma.

A middle or posterior mediastinal mass with an associated spinal anomaly may have an extra- or intra-dural extension. MRI is essential. Resection of the mediastinal component without identifying a spinal communication may result in postoperative meningitis or cord compromise.

Calcification in a posterior mass suggests a sympathetic chain tumour, commonly a neuroblastoma or ganglioneuroma (Fig. 64.36). Extradural encroachment into the spinal canal often occurs via adjacent foramina at several levels, presenting as paraparesis. Pre-operative MRI is needed to assess extent. Later ^{123}I-MIBG imaging may be needed for staging neuroblastoma. One in 10 of all neuroblastomas occur in the chest. Abdominal neuroblastoma may also extend into the chest, producing a paravertebral mass or effusion.

Vascular anomalies

Abnormal vessels seen on CT or US may indicate a primary vascular problem or represent an abnormal vascular supply to or from a congenital abnormality (e.g. scimitar syndrome, pulmonary AVM, or BPS). Abnormal embryologic development of the aortic arch leads to persistence of the primitive aortic arch or its branches. This may give an abnormal mediastinal contour but usually presents with stridor.

Tumours

Primary bronchial or pulmonary tumours are rare in paediatric practice compared to adults. Bronchial carcinoid tumour is an infrequent primary tumour occurring in adolescents. Multiple pulmonary metastases are unusually associated with an obvious primary tumour elsewhere (Table 64.6).

Chest wall tumours are more common than primary lung tumours. The Askin tumour is a sarcoma arising from the

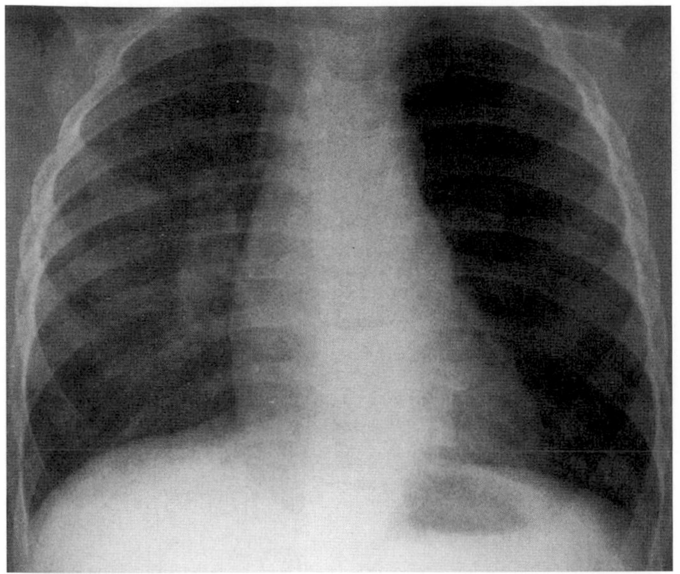

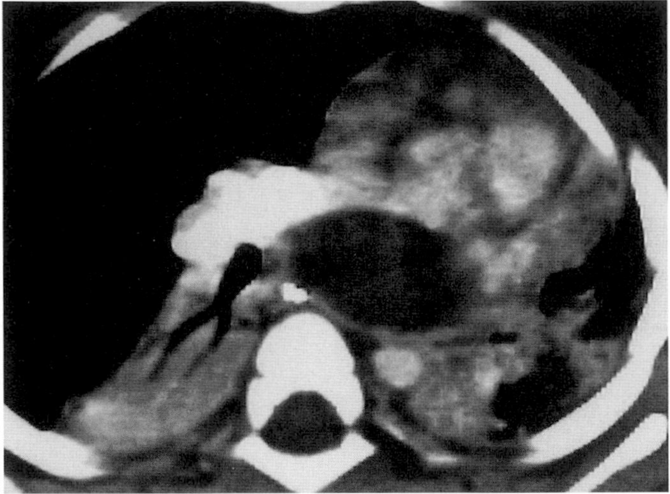

Figure 64.35 Bronchogenic cyst. (A) Chest radiograph. Obstructive emphysema in the left chest is due to a central mediastinal mass (arrow). (B) Contrast-enhanced CT (under general anaesthetic) shows a central low attenuation mass (arrow) causing compression of the carina and bilateral lower lobe collapse.

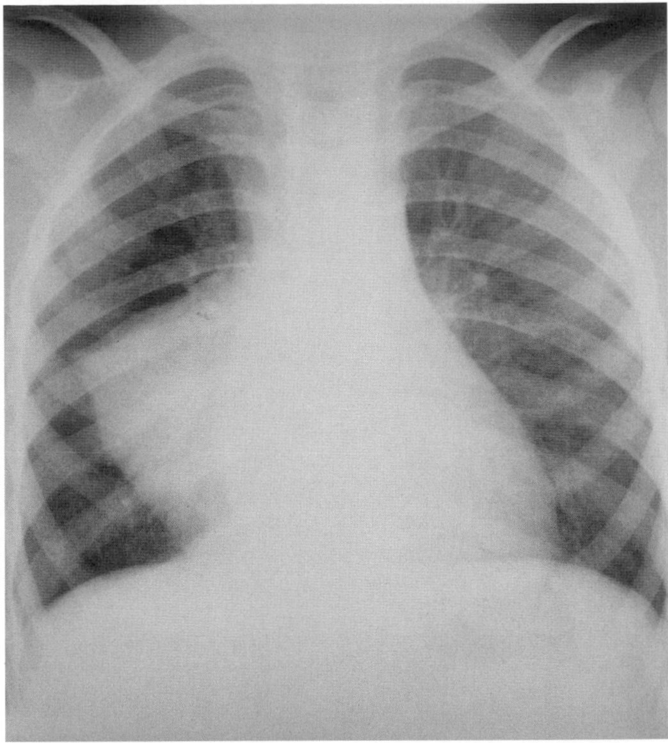

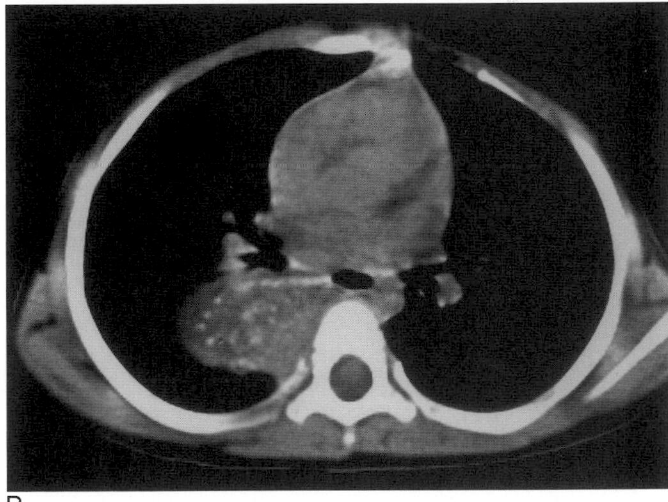

Figure 64.36 Neuroblastoma. (A) Chest radiography shows posterior mass on the right in a child with chest pain and no clinical features of infection. (B) CT chest (noncontrast) shows calcification in the mass adjacent to the spine. There was no evidence of extradural extension on MRI.

chest wall, often with rib involvement[49] and a pleural effusion. Primary sarcoma arising in the rib often presents late, with a pleural lesion with rib involvement (Fig. 64.37). Skeletal scintigraphy is used to detect multiple sites of tumour or other metastases. Bone involvement of the spine or ribs is also common in mediastinal and chest wall tumours (Table 64.7).

Initial staging of mediastinal tumours is performed with contrast-enhanced spiral CT. Percutaneous biopsy is possible for even small lesions[50]. Spiral CT should be performed before considering thoracotomy for resection of an apparently isolated metastasis or nodule seen on a chest radiograph.

Basal atelectasis is a significant problem in the young child that needs anaesthesia for chest CT. Positive end-expiratory pressure will help prevent this[51] and change in posture from supine to prone may differentiate atelectasis from disease. Peripheral pulmonary metastases are often seen in the posterior inferior recess and may be masked by atelectasis in the supine position.

Table 64.6 POTENTIAL SOURCES OF PULMONARY METASTASES
Nephroblastoma (Wilms' tumour)
Primary bone sarcoma (Ewing or osteosarcoma)
Rhabdomyosarcoma
Testicular tumour (in the adolescent)

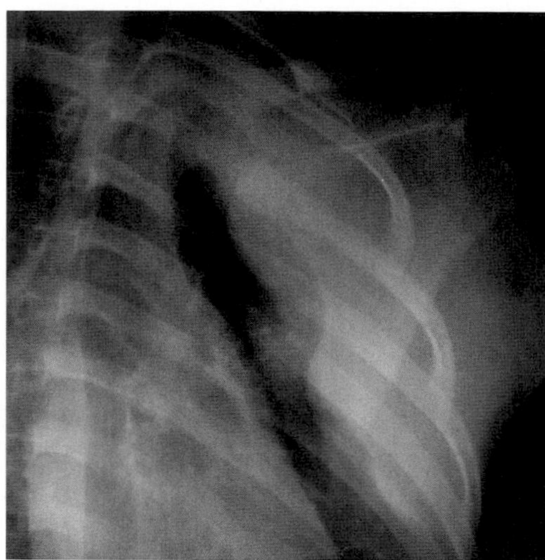

Figure 64.37 Ewing sarcoma. Oblique view of a lobulated, peripheral left chest mass and an abnormal third rib.

Table 64.7 BONE INVOLVEMENT IN THE THORAX
Spine
Direct
Primary spinal tumours (Ewing/osteosarcoma, osteoid osteoma, aneurysmal bone cyst)
Neuroblastoma-like tumour—ribs and spine
Sepsis
Neurenteric cyst
Metastatic
Leukaemia
Neuroblastoma
Histiocytosis (LCH)
Ewing/osteosarcoma
Lymphoma
Ribs
All of the above involving spine plus:
Actinomyces infection (apical)
Osteomyelitis
Askin tumour (PNET)

CYSTIC FIBROSIS

Cystic fibrosis (CF) is associated with chronic pulmonary sepsis and malabsorption (pancreatic exocrine insufficiency, cirrhosis, and gut involvement). It is an autosomal recessive disease with a carrier frequency of 1 in 25. CF may present as neonatal meconium ileus or in the older child with malabsorption or respiratory problems. The pulmonary features include chronic sepsis, mucus plugging due to abnormally thick sputum, and abnormal cilial motion that results in bronchiectasis, cavitation, and pulmonary fibrosis, and ultimately pulmonary hypertension plus episodic acute infective exacerbations. Other radiographic features include chronic sinusitis, nasal polyposis, nail clubbing, and symptoms of HPOA (hypertrophic pulmonary osteoarthropathy)[52].

Early radiographic features include air trapping and bronchial wall thickening, features that are radiographically indistinguishable from asthma or recurrent pneumonia due to other causes. Later a diffuse interstitial pattern, bronchiectasis, and cyst formation occur. The lung disease progresses at a variable rate to an 'end-stage lung' in early adult life. Late radiographic features show pulmonary hypertension with hilar enlargement and peripheral oligaemia with a background of chronic lung change (Fig. 64.38), and a barrel-shaped chest.

Serial radiography at yearly intervals is used to monitor progression of the pulmonary disease. PA and lateral radiographs are usually performed to allow radiographic 'scoring' of progression. Various scoring systems have been devised for clinical and radiographic assessment (Crispin–Norman, Shwachmann)[53]. A scoring system based on thin section CT has also been used (Bhalla)[54]. CT will show significantly more change than is detectable on a chest radiograph. The low-dose spiral CT technique minimizes radiation dose[55]. CT is especially useful when symptoms are disproportionate to chest radiograph changes[56].

Some children have a 'target lobe' where the bronchiectasis and cyst formation is maximal, and where infection seems to recur. Cysts may fill with secretions and show transient filling and clearing on serial radiography, which does not always signify acute infection. Chronic infection on sputum analysis with *Staph. aureus* is common, and in the later phase with *Pseudomonas aeruginosa*. Lobar collapse also occurs

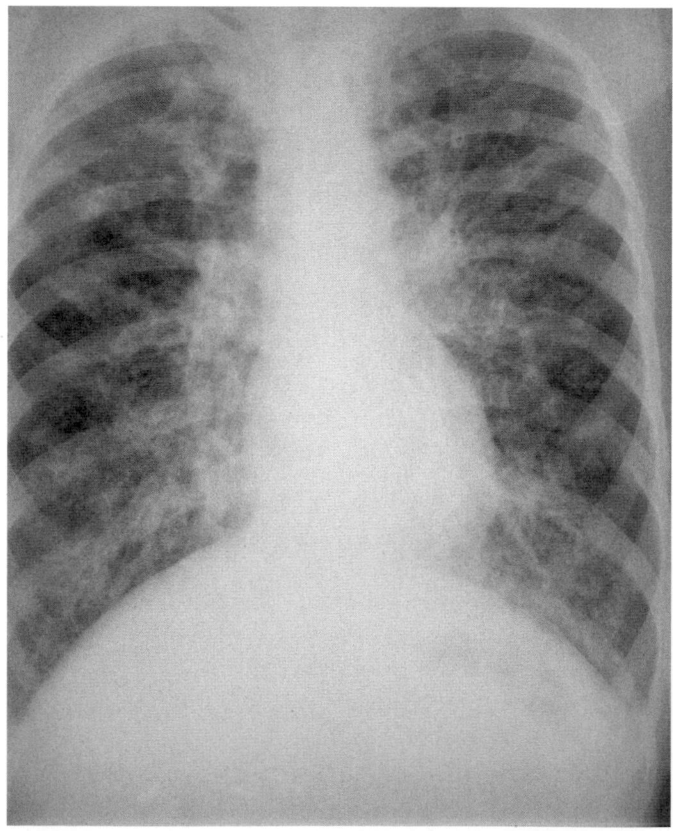

Figure 64.38 Cystic fibrosis. Chest radiograph shows thick-walled bronchi and cysts in all the lobes with increased reticular pattern. Both lungs are overexpanded with large hila indicating pulmonary hypertension.

secondary to mucus impaction, a finding that alters physiotherapy treatment.

Children with CF also have an increased risk of bronchopulmonary aspergillosis. Recurrent, transient, parenchymal opacities together with peripheral and sputum eosinophilia with specific immunology titres are diagnostic[57].

Haemoptysis may be due to bronchiectasis but occasional massive haemoptysis occurs due to arterial bleeding from an infected cavity or secondary to bronchial arterial hypertrophy due to cor pulmonale. Selective bronchial arteriography and embolization may be life saving. Pneumothorax is uncommon, but may be life threatening.

Bronchiectasis and Kartagener's syndrome

Bronchiectasis is usually idiopathic but also complicates CF, Kartagener's syndrome, and cilial dysmotility. It is a recognized complication of adenovirus, measles, and pertussis infection. High-resolution spiral CT is more sensitive and much less invasive than bronchography.

Kartagener's syndrome has additional associations with dextrocardia and facial sinusitis. The underlying problem is cilial dysmotility producing inadequate clearance of sputum. This also relates to the failure of the heart to rotate to the usual left-sided position.

PAEDIATRIC INTERSTITIAL DISEASE[58]

There is a long differential diagnosis for interstitial change in the paediatric chest. A list of common associations is given in Table 64.8. The reader is referred to further texts for details of each syndrome.

Clinical correlation is essential, including a drug history, full clinical examination (e.g. iritis, arthropathy, nodal enlargement, etc.) together with pulmonary function testing, biochemical screening (for collagen vascular disease), and then further imaging. If interstitial disease is suspected from a plain chest radiograph, clinical history, or physiological measurements, high-resolution thin-section CT helps determine the presence, extent, and distribution of disease.

Atelectasis complicates sedation due to hypostatic change. For spiral CT in small children, sedation or general anaesthesia is often needed. Controlled respiration under general anaesthesia also ensures adequate inspiration, minimizes motion artefact, and also allows scanning in expiration to assess air trapping[59]. Positive end-expiratory pressure used in anaesthesia minimizes atelectasis. Anaesthetic cooperation is important for optimal paediatric imaging, including endotracheal intubation rather than laryngeal mask airway if suspended respiration or prone positioning is needed. If chest CT is being performed as one of a series of investigations under anaesthesia (e.g. bronchoscopy or MRI), then CT should be performed first, as atelectatic changes often progress with duration of anaesthesia and medical intervention.

If the child will stay still but cannot coordinate inspiration/expiration, then selected sections can be made in both decubitus positions—the dependent lung simulating an 'expiration phase'.

CT also assists in planning the best site for lung biopsy to obtain histology, and confirms associated air trapping, bronchiectasis, and cystic disease[60]. Lung biopsy should not be obtained from an area of dense fibrosis as the pathologist may only see 'end-stage diffuse fibrosis'.

Fibrosing alveolitis is one of the more frequent causes of paediatric interstitial lung disease. It has a better outlook in children than in adults and may resolve spontaneously or after a short course of treatment. Sarcoidosis is uncommon in children prior to adolescence. 'Honeycomb lung' is rare in paediatric practice, but is more commonly seen with histiocytosis (Fig. 64.39) and tuberous sclerosis.

Table 64.8 CAUSES OF 'INTERSTITIAL' LUNG PATTERN
Cystic fibrosis
Mycoplasma pneumonia
Interstitial oedema (cardiac or fluid overload)
Histiocytosis
Sarcoidosis
Fibrosing alveolitis
Idiopathic interstitial pneumonitis
Neurofibromatosis
Tuberous sclerosis
Rheumatoid and collagen vascular disease
Drug reactions
Lymphangiectasia
Leiomyomatosis
Storage disorders (Gaucher, Neimann Pick)
Pulmonary haemosiderosis (late, following multiple bleeds)

IMMUNODEFICIENCY[61–64]

The lung is a common site of involvement in the immunocompromised child. There is easy access for inhaled pathogens and the lung is also a common site for haematogenous spread of infection from long tubes used for venous access. The paediatric lung also has a large amount of 'bronchial associated lymphoid tissue' (BALT) involved in the immune response. Over half the children dying from acquired immunodeficiency syndrome (AIDS) have pulmonary involvement.

Immunocompromise in children usually arises from one of three causes:

- congenital or combined immunodeficiency syndromes (SCIDs, etc)
- induced immunodeficiency due to steroids or chemotherapy
- acquired immunodeficiency syndrome (HIV and AIDS related).

Pulmonary infection with atypical organisms may occur or the common pathogens may exhibit an abnormal response. Common bacterial (*Streptococcus pneumoniae* and *Haemophilus influenzae*) or viral infections (chicken pox or measles) may have a devastating effect on the lung in an immunocompromised child. If virology cannot give a rapid diagnosis, then broncho-alveolar lavage (BAL), transbronchial or imaging-guided

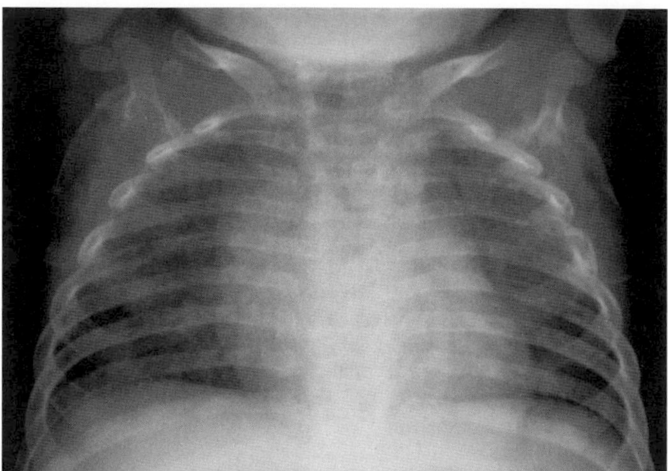

Figure 64.39 Interstitial disease—histiocytosis. There are multiple lytic bone lesions (especially of the right scapula), mediastinal adenopathy, and interstitial infiltrates.

biopsy should be performed. Alternatively a limited thoracotomy and biopsy is performed to obtain an open lung biopsy for histology and culture.

***Pneumocystis juroveci (carinii)* pneumonia (PCP)** infection is as common as in adults. The child is usually pyrexial and hypoxaemic and may progress rapidly to respiratory failure. The chest radiograph shows progressive bilateral infiltrates, evolving to bilateral diffuse airspace (alveolar) opacification.

With human immunodeficiency virus (HIV) and immunocompromise **tuberculosis** may be the first presentation, which may predate the development of 'AIDS' by several months. The chest radiograph may not show a miliary pattern even with disseminated disease. Infection with *Mycobacterium avium intracellulare* (MAI) also occurs, usually with hilar adenopathy, pulmonary infiltrates, and lobar collapse. Fungal infections are also common (Fig. 64.40).

Lymphocytic interstitial pneumonitis (LIP) is associated with immune compromise as well as Sjögren's syndrome, chronic active hepatitis, and myasthenia. The course in children is not as aggressive as in adults, as it progresses less commonly to lymphoma. The initial symptoms are mild with slowly progressive dyspnoea and hypoxia. Chest radiograph findings include hilar and paratracheal adenopathy, with reticulonodular infiltrates and patchy alveolar opacification. It progresses to cystic and cylindrical bronchiectasis, but can be treated with steroids.

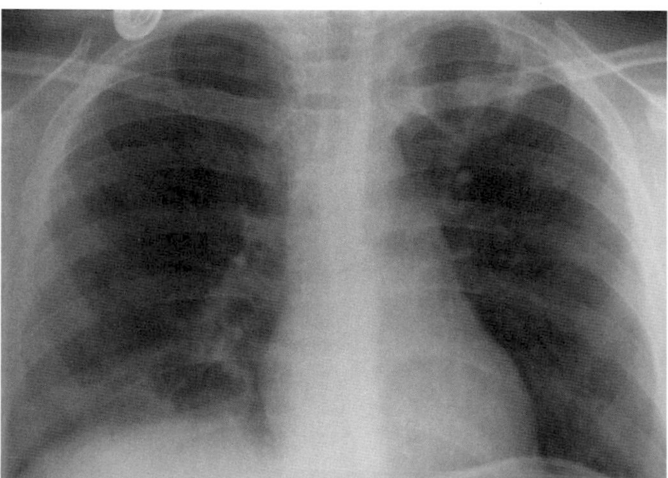

Figure 64.40 Mycetoma in an immunosuppressed patient. There are multiple cavitating lesions in the left apex and also right base with internal contents in the apical lesion.

There is considerable overlap in the appearances of the various differing infections in the immunocompromised child. The child is usually treated empirically following blood and sputum culture on the basis of the most probable infection. If there is a poor clinical response, a more invasive biopsy may have to be performed to identify the causative organism or pathological process.

REFERENCES

1. National Radiation Protection Board 1993 Occupational, public and medical exposure, vol 4, no 2. NRPB, Chilton
2. Cook J V, Shah K, Pablot S et al 1998 Guidelines on best practice in the x-ray imaging of children. AGFA, UK, pp 9–10
3. Newman B, Bowen A, Oh K S 1990 A practical approach to the newborn chest. Curr Probl Diagn Radiol 19: 41–84
4. Gibson A T, Steiner G M 1997 Imaging the neonatal chest. Clin Radiol 52: 172–186
5. Agrons G A, Harty M P 1998 Lung disease in premature infants: impact of new treatments and technologies. Semin Roentgenol 33: 101–116
6. Whitsett J A, Pryhuber G S, Rice W R et al 1994 Acute respiratory disorders. In: Avery G B, Fletcher M A, MacDonald M G (eds) Neonatology: pathophysiology and management of the newborn, 4th edn. JB Lippincott, Philadelphia, pp 429–452
7. Pilling D W, Pilling E L The neonatal chest. In: Carty H, Brunelle F, Stringer DA, Kao S C S (eds) 2005 Imaging children, 2nd edn. Churchill Livingstone, New York, pp 1023–1047
8. Dinger J, Schwarze R, Rupprecht E 1997 Radiological changes after therapeutic use of surfactant in infants with respiratory distress syndrome. Pediatr Radiol 27: 26–31
9. Slama M, Andre C, Huon C et al 1999 Radiological analysis of hyaline membrane disease after exogenous surfactant treatment. Pediatr Radiol 29: 56–60
10. Greenhough A, Dixon A K, Roberton N R C 1984 Pulmonary interstitial emphysema. Arch Dis Child 59: 1046–1051
11. Northway W H, Rosan R C, Porter D Y 1967 Pulmonary disease following respirator therapy of hyaline-membrane disease. N Engl J Med 276: 357–368
12. Wilson M G, Mikity V G 1960 A new form of respiratory disease in premature infants. Am J Dis Child 99: 489
13. Grossman H, Berdon W E, Mizaki A et al 1965 Neonatal focal hyperaeration of the lungs (Wilson Mikity syndrome). Radiology 85: 404–417
14. Hubbard A M, Crombleholme T M 1998 Anomalies and malformations affecting the fetal/neonatal chest. Semin Roentgenol 33: 117–125
15. Hubbard A M, Adzick N S, Cromblehome T M 1997 Value of prenatal MR imaging in preparation for fetal surgery of left congenital diaphragmatic hernia. Radiology 203: 636–640
16. Lacey D E, Shaw N J, Pilling D W et al 1999 Outcome of congenital lung abnormalities detected antenatally. Acta Paediatr 88: 454–458
17. Archer N 1993 Patent ductus arteriosus in the newborn. Arch Dis Child 69: 529–532
18. Evans N 1993 Diagnosis of patent ductus arteriosus in the preterm newborn. Arch Dis Child 68: 58–61
19. Carty H 1990 Ultrasound of the normal thymus in the infant: a simple method of resolving a clinical dilemma. Br J Radiol 63: 737–738
20. Siegel M J, Glazer H S, Wiener J I, Molina P L 1989 Normal and abnormal thymus in childhood: MR imaging. Radiology 172: 367–377

21. Wahlgren H, Mortensson W, Eriksson M, Finkel Y, Forsgren M 1995 Radiographic patterns and viral studies in childhood pneumonia at various ages. Pediatr Radiol 25: 627–630
22. Gibson N A, Hollman A S, Paton J Y 1993 Value of radiological follow up of childhood pneumonia. BMJ 307: 1117
23. Simpson W, Hacking P M, Court S D M, Gardner P S 1974 The radiological findings in respiratory syncytial virus infection in children. Pediatr Radiol 2: 155–160
24. Rose R W, Ward B H 1973 Spherical pneumonias in children simulating pulmonary and mediastinal masses. Radiology 106: 179–182
25. Bellamy E A, Johnston I D A, Wilson A G 1987 The chest radiograph in whooping cough. Clin Radiol 38: 39–43
26. Guckel C, Benz-Bohm G, Widemann B 1989 Mycoplasmal pneumonias in childhood. Pediatr Radiol 19: 499–503
27. Macfarlane J, Rose D 1996 Radiographic features of staphylococcal pneumonia in adults and children. Thorax 51: 539–540
28. Cremin B J 1995 Tuberculosis: the resurgence of our most lethal infectious disease—a review. Pediatr Radiol 25: 620–626
29. Lakshmana D N, Hingsbergen E A, Jones J E 1999 Adult diseases in children. Pediatr Radiol 29: 244–254
30. Simpson H, Hampton F 1991 Gastro-oesophageal reflux and the lung. Arch Dis Child 66: 277–283
31. Couriel J M, Bisset R, Miller R, Thomas A, Clarke M 1993 Assessment of feeding problems in neurodevelopmental handicap: a team approach. Arch Dis Child 69: 609–613
32. McVeagh P, Howman-Giles R, Kemp A 1987 Pulmonary aspiration studied by radionuclide milk scanning and barium swallow. Roentgenography. Am J Roentgenol 141: 917–921
33. Spevak M R, Kleinman P K, Belanger P L, Primack C P, Richmond J M 1994 Cardiopulmonary resuscitation and rib fractures in infants—a post mortem radiologic-pathologic study. JAMA 272: 617–618
34. Feldman K W, Brewer D K 1984 Child abuse, cardiopulmonary resuscitation and rib fractures. Pediatrics 73: 339–342
35. Blazer S, Naveh Y, Friedman A 1980 Foreign body in the airway—a review of 200 cases. Am J Dis Child 134: 68–71
36. Svedstrom E, Puhakka H, Kero P 1989 How accurate is chest radiography in the diagnosis of tracheobronchial foreign bodies in children? Pediatr Radiol 19: 520–522
37. Harris V J, Brown R 1975 Pneumatoceles as a complication of chemical pneumonia after hydrocarbon ingestion. Am J Roentgenol Radium Ther 125: 531–537
38. Oh K S, Newman B, Bender T M, Bowen A 1988 Radiologic evaluation of the diaphragm. Radiol Clin North Am 26: 355–364
39. Moccia W A, Kaude J V, Felman A H 1981 Congenital eventration of the diaphragm. Pediatr Radiol 10: 197–200
40. Cohen M, Sprigg A. 2005 Cystic malformations of the lung—a diagnostic approach. Cell Pathol 6: 94–99
41. Felker R E, Tonkin I L D 1990 Imaging of pulmonary sequestration. Am J Roentgenol 154: 241–249
42. Doyle A J 1992 Demonstration of blood supply to pulmonary sequestration by MR angiography. Am J Roentgenol 158: 989–990
43. Chilvers E R, Peters A M, George P, Hughes J M B, Allison D J 1988 Quantification of right to left shunt through pulmonary arteriovenous malformations using 99mTc albumin microspheres. Clin Radiol 39: 611–614
44. King R M, Telander R L, Smithson W A, Banks P M, Han M T 1982 Primary mediastinal tumors in children. J Pediatr Surg 17: 512–520
45. Merten D F 1992 Diagnostic imaging of mediastinal masses in children. Am J Roentgenol 158: 825–832
46. Carty H, Martin J 1993 Review: staging of lymphoma in childhood. Clin Radiol 48: 151–159
47. Carachi R, Burgner D P 1994 Thoracic foregut duplications. Arch Dis Child 71: 395–396
48. Kincaid P K, Stanley P, Kovanlikaya A, Mahour G H, Rowland J M 1999 Coexistent neurenteric cyst and enterogenous cyst—further support for a common embryologic error. Pediatr Radiol 29: 539–541
49. Fink I J, Kurtz D W, Cazenave L, et al 1985 Malignant thoracopulmonary small-cell (Askin) tumour. Am J Roentgenol 145: 517–520
50. Connolly B L, Chait P G, Duncan D S, Taylor G 1999 CT-guided percutaneous needle biopsy of small lung nodules in children. Pediatr Radiol 29: 342–346
51. Sargent M A, McEachern A M, Jamieson D H, Kahwaji R 1999 Atelectasis on pediatric chest CT: comparison of sedation techniques. Pediatr Radiol 29: 509–513
52. Amodio J B, Berdon W, Abramson S, Baker D 1987 Cystic fibrosis in childhood: pulmonary, paranasal sinus and skeletal manifestations. Semin Roentgenol 22: 125–135
53. Te Meerman G J, Dankert-Roelse J, Martijn A, Van Woerden H H 1985 A comparison of the Shwachmann, Crispin–Norman and Brasfield methods of scoring chest radiographs of patients with cystic fibrosis. Pediatr Radiol 15: 98–101
54. Bhalla M, Turcios N, Aponte V, et al 1991 Cystic fibrosis: scoring system with thin section CT. Radiology 179: 783–788
55. Rogalla P, Stover B, Scheer I, Juran R, Gaedicke G, Hamm B 1998 Low-dose spiral CT: applicability to paediatric chest imaging. Pediatr Radiol 28: 565–569
56. Santamaria F, Grillo G, Guidi G et al 1998 Cystic fibrosis: when should high-resolution CT of the chest be obtained? Pediatrics 101: 908–913
57. Simmonds E J, Littlewood J M, Evans E G V 1990 Cystic fibrosis and allergic bronchopulmonary aspergillosis. Arch Dis Child 65: 507–511
58. Owens C 2004 Radiology of diffuse interstitial pulmonary disease in children. Eur Radiol 14 (suppl): L2–L12
59. Arakawa H, Webb W R 1998 Air trapping on expiratory high-resolution CT scans in the absence of inspiratory scan abnormalities. Am J Roentgenol 170: 1349–1353
60. Wilkinson A G, Paton J Y, Gibson N, Howatson A G 1999 CT-guided 14-G cutting needle lung biopsy in children: safe and effective. Pediatr Radiol 29: 514–516
61. Sotomayer J L, Douglas S D, Wilmott R W 1989 Pulmonary manifestations of immune deficiency diseases. Pediatr Pulmonol 6: 275–292
62. Haller J O, Cohen H L 1994 Pediatric HIV infection: an imaging update. Pediatr Radiol 24: 224–230
63. Haller J O, Ginsberg K J 1997 Tuberculosis in children with acquired immunodeficiency syndrome. Pediatr Radiol 27: 186–188
64. Oldham S A A, Castillo M, Jacobson H L, Mones J M, Saldana M J 1989 HIV-associated lymphocytic interstitial pneumonia: radiologic manifestations and pathologic correlation. Radiology 170: 83–87

Suggested further reading

Carty H, Brunelle F, Stringer D A, Kao S C S (eds) 2005 Imaging children, 3rd edn, vol 1. Churchill Livingstone, Edinburgh, chapter 7, pp 1021–1178

A practical paediatric radiology text in two volumes.

Duncan A W 1999 Emergency chest radiology in children. In: Carty H (ed) Emergency pediatric radiology. Springer Verlag, Berlin, chapter 2, pp33–116

Kuhn S P, Slovis T L, Haller J O (eds) 2004 Caffey's pediatric diagnostic imaging, 10th edn, vol 1. Mosby, St Louis, pp 48–103, 765–1126

A paediatric reference text in two volumes.

Newman B (ed) 1993 The pediatric chest. Radiol Clin North Am 31: 453–704

An excellent 'clinics' covering the pediatric chest.

Swischuk L (ed) 1997 Imaging of the newborn infant and young child, 4th edn. William and Wilkins, Baltimore, pp 1–158

CHAPTER 65

Paediatric Abdominal Imaging

Anne Paterson, Louise E. Sweeney and Bairbre Connolly

Paediatric gastrointestinal (GI) radiology is most appropriately considered according to the age of the patient. For this reason, this chapter has been divided into two main sections. The first half of the chapter concentrates on neonatal GI disease, the latter half on GI problems in the infant and older child. Throughout the chapter, the relevant clinical features of each condition are presented, followed by the applicable imaging strategy in each case. Radiological techniques that are peculiar to paediatric radiology are discussed in more detail.

The clinical features of neonatal GI disease (Table 65.1) are varied, but may coexist in different conditions. Each problem is therefore presented under the heading of its most common physical symptoms.

The spectrum of GI disease in the infant and older child overlaps with conditions seen in adult patients. This chapter deals primarily with problems specific to paediatrics and the reader is referred to the Chapters on adult GI diseases for further information. Common complaints such as abdominal pain, constipation, abdominal trauma (including nonaccidental injury), nonbilious vomiting, abdominal distension, malabsorption, and GI bleeding are detailed. The GI manifestations of cystic fibrosis, the abdomen in the immunocompromised child, and other miscellaneous GI problems are also discussed. For completeness, this chapter has been expanded to include paediatric hepatic and biliary disease.

Table 65.1 PRESENTING FEATURES OF NEONATAL GASTROINTESTINAL DISEASE
Visible defects in the anterior abdominal wall
Respiratory distress and choking
Nonbilious vomiting
Bilious vomiting
Abdominal distension
Delayed passage of meconium
Rectal bleeding
Jaundice

THE NEONATE

CLINICAL FEATURES OF NEONATAL GASTROINTESTINAL DISEASE

Visible abnormalities of the anterior abdominal wall

The ventral wall of the embryo is formed during the fourth week of intrauterine development as the cephalic, caudal, and lateral edges of the flat, trilaminar embryonal disc fold in upon themselves. The resultant embryo is cylindrical in shape and protruding centrally from its ventral surface are the remains of the yolk sac connected to the midgut; a structure that later becomes the umbilical cord.

If this complex process is incomplete, then several types of anterior abdominal wall defect may result. Such defects may be detected and characterized by antenatal ultrasound (US). The management and planning of the remainder of the pregnancy and the subsequent delivery of the infant are all affected by the prenatal diagnosis.

Omphalocele

An omphalocele (exomphalos) is a midline anterior abdominal wall defect through which the solid abdominal viscera and/or bowel may herniate. Larger omphaloceles containing liver tissue are thought to be due to failure of fusion of the lateral body folds. Omphaloceles containing only bowel are thought to arise due to persistence of the physiological herniation of gut after the 10th week of fetal development[1]. The umbilical cord inserts at the tip of the defect. A giant omphalocele is said to be present when the liver and biliary structures are contained within the herniated membranes.

Prognosis is dependent upon associated anomalies. Chromosomal abnormalities are seen in around 50% of patients[2]. Trisomy 13 and 18 are common. The Beckwith–Wiedemann syndrome has an omphalocele (exomphalos), macroglossia, and gigantism as its primary components (the 'EMG' syndrome). Visceral abnormalities are present in up to 70% of cases[2].

Gastroschisis The term gastroschisis literally means 'split stomach'. There is a small defect or split in the ventral abdominal wall, classically to the right side of a normally positioned umbilicus. Gastroschisis typically occurs in the absence of other anomalies and is thought to be due to a localized intrauterine vascular accident, which leads to full-thickness necrosis of a portion of the anterior abdominal wall[3].

Antenatal US shows (usually only) bowel loops floating freely in the amniotic fluid. There is no covering membrane. Exposure to amniotic fluid damages the bowel; this too may be suspected antenatally if the extruded loops of bowel are dilated and thickened[1]. Postnatally, this can result in a thick, fibrous 'peel' coating the loops of bowel. Short bowel syndrome and intestinal dysmotility are serious consequences of gastroschisis. Associated intestinal atresias and stenoses are secondary to the prenatal ischaemic insult[3]. Necrotizing enterocolitis (NEC) is reported in up to 20% of patients with gastroschisis[3].

The morbidity and mortality associated with gastroschisis is mainly due to the additional GI problems, compounded by the prolonged total parenteral nutrition that some patients require; cholestatic liver disease is the major problem. The establishment of enteral feeding often takes longer in preterm infants, resulting in increased hospital stays for this group[4]. Respiratory embarrassment may occur following repair of the defect. Around one-third of male patients have cryptorchidism, which may result in the testes passing through the abdominal wall defect. Most testes descend to the scrotum after being returned to the abdominal cavity[2]. Upper GI contrast medium studies in infants with repaired gastroschisis will often demonstrate gastro-oesophageal reflux (GOR), malrotation, dilatation of small bowel loops, and a markedly prolonged transit time. GI transit times greater than 2 d are not uncommon and do not necessarily indicate intestinal obstruction.

Cloacal exstrophy is a rare, midline, infra-umbilical defect that arises due to an abnormality of the caudal body fold. Cloacal exstrophy is more common in boys and is composed of an omphalocele, imperforate anus, spinal dysrhaphism, and ambiguous genitalia. The caecum opens onto the anterior abdominal wall between two exstrophied hemibladders.

Postnatally the bladder and bowel are separated and repaired, and the anterior abdominal wall defect is closed. In the past, genetic male infants with cloacal exstrophy have commonly undergone bilateral orchidectomy and been reared as girls, as the external genitalia are frequently rudimentary. Genetic female infants usually have a double vagina and two hemi-uteri. Genital tract imaging and surgery may be delayed until later in childhood.

Early postnatal imaging includes US examination of the renal tracts, and upper GI contrast medium studies to detect malrotation and to outline the length of bowel present. Magnetic resonance imaging (MRI) will exclude an associated spinal cord abnormality and delineate the pelvic organs and pelvic floor musculature.

Choking and respiratory distress

The neonate with disease affecting the proximal GI tract often presents with respiratory symptoms. These symptoms include choking with feeds, cyanosis, and respiratory distress. Conditions that present in this way include oesophageal atresia (OA) with or without tracheo-oesophageal fistula (TOF), laryngeal clefts, swallowing disorders, diaphragmatic hernias, vascular rings, and gastro-oesophageal reflux (GOR); the latter is by far the most common. The chest radiograph may show airspace disease and atelectasis, should aspiration have occurred.

Oesophageal atresia and tracheo-oesophageal fistula

OA with or without a fistulous connection to the trachea occurs in 1 in 3000–4500 live births. It is due to abnormal partitioning of the laryngotracheal tube from the oesophagus by the tracheo-oesophageal septum during the fourth week of gestation. Five different major anomalies result (Fig. 65.1). The atretic segment of the oesophagus tends to be at the junction of its proximal and middle thirds, and a TOF, if present, is usually found proximal to the carina. Occasionally an isolated TOF occurs without OA; this is the H- (or N-) type fistula.

Half of all children with OA and TOF have associated congenital anomalies. Features of the VACTERL spectrum (vertebral anomalies, anorectal malformation, cardiovascular malformation, tracheo-oesophageal fistula with oesophageal atresia, renal anomalies, and limb defects) are commonly found, with cardiac and other GI malformations—notably duodenal atresia and stenosis, and anorectal malformations. Trisomy 18, trisomy 21, and Potter's syndrome are other recognized associations[5]. A more distal congenital oesophageal stenosis may also be present[6]. The mortality rates in patients with OA and TOF are usually no longer due to the OA itself, but to the associated malformations, especially congenital cardiac anomalies.

The diagnosis of OA may be suspected antenatally, when US demonstrates maternal polyhydramnios. A fetus with OA and no distal fistula will also have absence of the gastric bubble. With a TOF, there may be a normal or slightly small gastric bubble and associated polyhydramnios.

The remaining infants present almost immediately in the postnatal period with choking, coughing, cyanosis, and

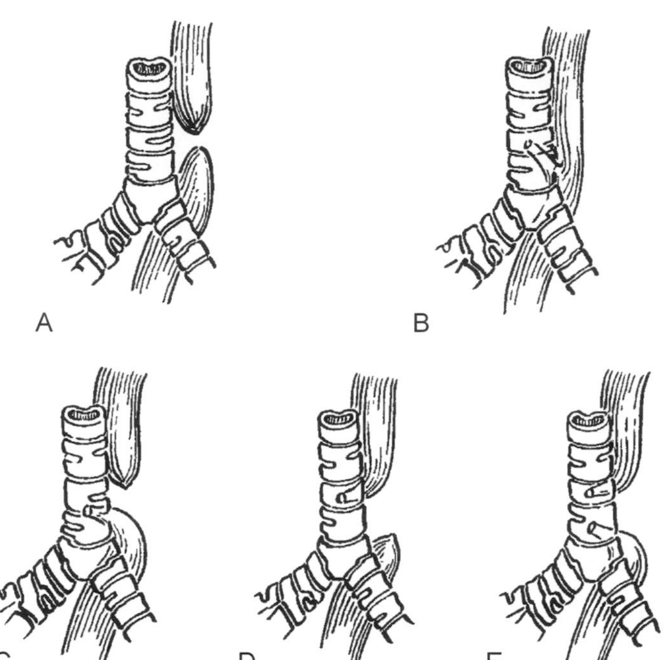

Figure 65.1 Oesophageal atresia (OA) and tracheo-oesophageal fistula. Diagrammatic representation (A) isolated OA (9%), (B) H-type fistula (6%), (C) OA with distal tracheo-oesophageal fistula (TOF) (82%), (D) OA with proximal TOF (1%), and (E) OA with TOF from both proximal and distal oesophageal remnants (2%).

drooling; these symptoms tend to be exacerbated during attempts to feed the infant. Patients with an H-type fistula are usually symptomatic from birth.

The initial radiograph will show the orogastric tube curled in the proximal oesophageal pouch (Fig. 65.2). The diagnosis can be confirmed if air is gently injected via the tube to distend the oesophageal pouch. The lungs may show features of an aspiration pneumonitis. Vertebral anomalies and an abnormal cardiac silhouette may be visible. The presence of gas in the abdomen implies a distal fistula. More recently, the ultrasound appearance of OA with or without TOF has been described in the literature and this is a promising technique for use at the bedside of a sick neonate[7].

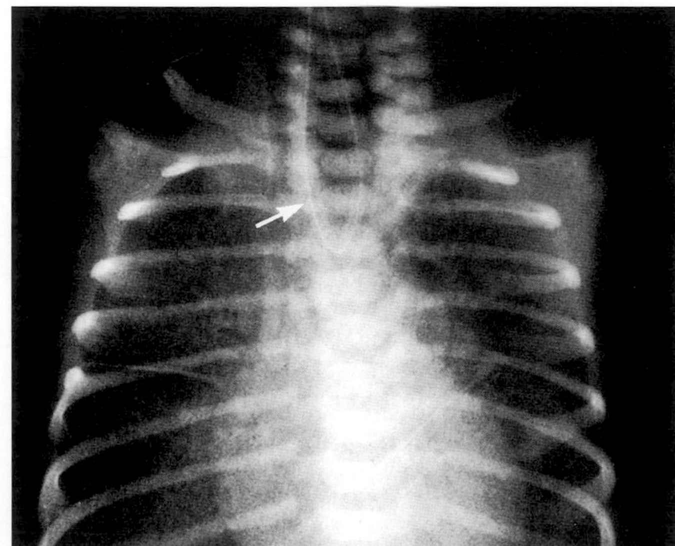

Figure 65.2 Oesophageal atresia. Supine chest radiograph shows orogastric tube curled in the proximal oesophageal pouch.

A gasless abdomen is seen with isolated OA and OA with a proximal fistula. Obstruction or atresia of the fistulous tract will also result in a gasless abdomen. In isolated OA, a long gap between the atretic segments is seen in association with 13 pairs of ribs[8]. The gap between the oesophageal pouches can be assessed following the formation of a feeding gastrostomy. Under fluoroscopic guidance, a Hegar dilator is inserted through the gastrostomy and retrogradely into the distal oesophagus. A Repogle tube is simultaneously used to delineate the superior pouch. As both tubes are radio-opaque, the degree of separation between the pouches is easily visualized. Alternatively, following simultaneous injection of air—into the upper pouch via the indwelling Repogle tube and via the gastrostomy—coronal computed tomography (CT) images can delineate the gap between the oesophageal pouches, which assists surgical management[9].

Neonates with an H-type fistula commonly have an abdomen distended by gas. The fistula is easy to miss on a routine upper GI study. An oesophogram with the patient placed prone and using a horizontal X-ray beam is recommended. The contrast medium is injected under pressure, via a nasogastric tube, with its tip in the distal oesophagus. The tube is slowly withdrawn under fluoroscopic guidance. The majority of these fistulas are seen at the level of the thoracic inlet (Fig. 65.3). Combined bronchoscopy and oesophagoscopy should be performed if there is a high clinical index of suspicion with negative imaging.

Contrast medium is rarely necessary to outline the proximal oesophageal pouch, but is occasionally required to exclude a proximal pouch fistula. Small quantities (1–2 ml) of isotonic, nonionic contrast medium should be used under fluoroscopic guidance; this will do little damage to the lungs should it be aspirated. A proximal fistula can also be demonstrated if air is injected into the Repogle tube during multidetector CT (MDCT). Multiplanar reconstructions and volume rendered images will then define the abnormal anatomy[10].

Post surgical radiology The immediate complications following OA and TOF repair are recurrence of the TOF, which occurs in up to 10% of patients, and anastomotic breakdown in a further 10–20% of patients[11,12]. A recurrent fistula may be difficult to demonstrate but is suspected radiologically if the oesophagus is gas filled on the plain radiograph and if contrast medium studies show 'beaking' of the anterior oesophageal wall[11].

Other common complications following OA and TOF repair include anastomotic strictures, disordered oesophageal and more distal GI motility, and GOR. These problems may persist into adulthood and be lifelong. The incidence of strictures is increased in those patients who have had long gap OA with a delayed primary repair; figures of up to 80% have been reported[12]. Many surgeons will request postoperative oesophograms following OA and TOF repair and before the child is fed.

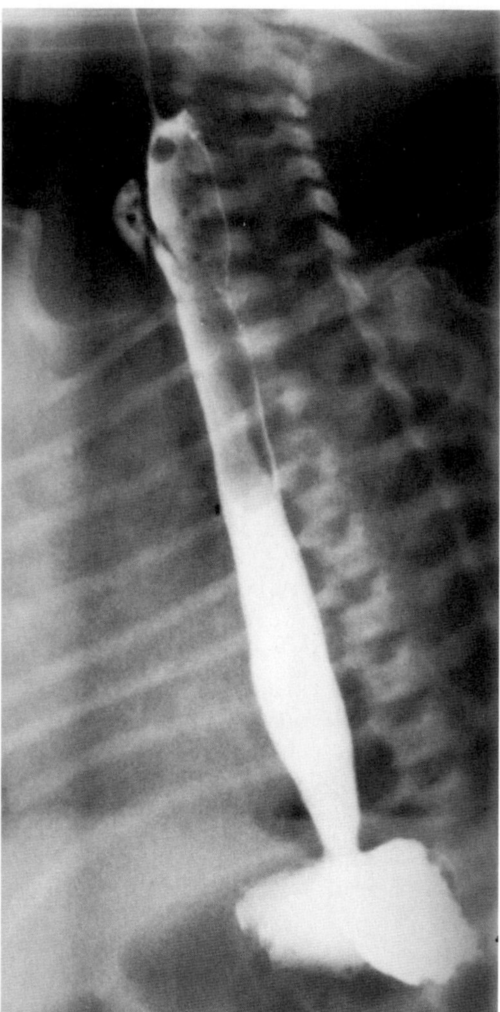

Figure 65.3 H-type tracheo-oesophageal fistula. Upper GI contrast study shows the fistula running obliquely at the level of the thoracic inlet.

Oesophageal strictures in this group of patients can easily and safely be treated by balloon catheter dilatation using fluoroscopic or endoscopic guidance[13–15].

Nonbilious vomiting

Vomiting is a common problem in children of all ages and its presence as a symptom does not necessarily indicate GI disease. Vomiting is common with infections in any body system, in metabolic disease, disorders of the central nervous system, and as a side-effect of drugs and poisons. Neonatal nonbilious vomiting due to GI causes implies a lesion proximal to the ampulla of Vater and is most frequently due to GOR. A full clinical history and physical examination are the most important factors in determining what imaging investigations (if any) are required.

Obstruction of the stomach Congenital gastric obstruction is rare. It is usually due to a web or diaphragm in the antrum or pylorus. Occasionally a true atresia is present with a fibrous cord uniting the two blind ends. Pyloric atresia is associated with epidermolysis bullosa simplex, when there are mutations in the gene PLEC 116. The diagnosis may be suspected antenatally due to maternal polyhydramnios and a large fetal gastric bubble. Postnatally upper abdominal distension and nonbilious vomiting occur. The symptoms may be intermittent and mild when the obstruction is incomplete.

With complete obstruction, a plain radiograph will show a dilated stomach with no distal air. The upper GI series will show vigorous gastric peristalsis and consistent filling defects in the antrum or pylorus at the site of the web. An antral web shows the 'pseudo double bubble', as barium outlines first the space between the antrum and pylorus, and second the duodenal bulb. At US, webs appear as persistent, linear, echogenic structures arising from the antral or pyloric walls and extending centrally[17].

Bilious vomiting

Bilious vomiting in the neonate may be the presenting symptom of both 'medical' and 'surgical' conditions. Medical conditions include functional immaturity of the colon and gastroenteritis. Surgical conditions include obstructions distal to the ampulla of Vater, of which malrotation and midgut volvulus constitute the greatest emergency. Unfortunately, the plain abdominal radiograph cannot always accurately distinguish between the conditions mentioned. If the plain radiograph demonstrates a complete high intestinal obstruction then no further imaging is required. If the radiograph shows a low intestinal obstruction (i.e. distal to the mid ileum), a contrast medium enema is preferred. Should any other plain radiographic findings be present, then an upper GI contrast medium study must be performed. Care must be taken not to overfill the stomach with contrast medium as this can obscure the position of the duodenojejunal flexure.

Malrotation and volvulus Malrotation is a serious congenital abnormality of the GI tract, as it predisposes to duodenal obstruction and midgut volvulus, which can lead to ischaemic necrosis of the small bowel. Undiagnosed midgut volvulus carries a high mortality rate.

In fetal life, the gut begins as a straight, midline tube which as it elongates and develops herniates into the base of the umbilical cord. Between the 6th and 10th weeks of fetal development, the midgut loop rotates 90 degrees anticlockwise around the axis of the superior mesenteric artery (SMA). At this stage the duodenojejunal (proximal) loop thus lies to the right, and the caecocolic (distal) loop to the left side. During the 10th week, the intestines return to the abdominal cavity; the proximal loop of bowel enters first, followed by the distal loop. Both the proximal and distal loops undergo a further 180 degrees of anticlockwise rotation as they return to the abdominal cavity; a total of 270 degrees of rotation. The duodenojejunal loop comes to lie posterior to and the caecocolic loop anterior to the SMA. The duodenojejunal junction (fixed by the ligament of Treitz) should lie in the left upper quadrant of the abdomen, and the ileocaecal junction in the right lower quadrant. The small bowel mesentery extends over the distance from the ligament of Treitz to the ileocaecal junction[18,19].

Malrotation is a generic term used to describe any variation in the position of the intestines, and is in itself not necessarily symptomatic. Malfixation of the intestines invariably accompanies malrotation in an attempt to fix the gut in place. Peritoneal (Ladd) bands stretch from the abnormally high lying caecum, across the duodenum to the region of the portahepatis and the anterior and posterior abdominal walls. The Ladd bands can cause duodenal obstruction. In addition the abnormal positions of the duodenojejunal junction and the caecum mean the base of the small bowel mesentery is short. The midgut has a propensity to twist around this narrow base, compromising its vascular supply (midgut volvulus).

Most patients have isolated malrotation of the bowel, but there is an increased incidence of associated duodenal stenosis and atresia. Patients with omphalocele, gastroschisis, and congenital diaphragmatic hernia all have malrotation and abnormal fixation of the bowel, although volvulus in these patients is rare after repair of the primary abnormality[20]. The heterotaxy syndromes, Hirschsprung's disease, and megacystis–microcolon–intestinal hypoperistalsis (Berdon) syndrome are also associated with malrotation and volvulus. Congenital short bowel without atresia is an extremely rare condition that can occur with malrotation[21].

Babies with malrotation commonly present within the first month of life, with bilious vomiting. Older children may present with non-specific symptoms of chronic or intermittent abdominal pain, nonbilious emesis, diarrhoea, or failure to thrive. Volvulus, though less common in the older child, still occurs. On physical examination the child may appear relatively well. When bowel ischaemia and necrosis have developed, symptoms of shock supervene. It is important to suspect malrotation and volvulus in a child of any age with bilious vomiting, and to perform an upper GI contrast medium study.

There are no specific plain radiographic findings in malrotation, even with volvulus. The radiograph may be completely normal if the volvulus is intermittent or if there is incomplete duodenal obstruction due to a loose twisting of the bowel. If the volvulus is tight, then complete duodenal obstruction results, with gaseous distension of the stomach and proximal duodenum, mimicking the 'double bubble' of duodenal atresia. The classical picture is of a partial duodenal obstruction, with mild distension of the stomach and proximal duodenum, with some distal gas (Fig. 65.4).

A pattern of distal small bowel obstruction is seen in a closed loop obstruction and represents a more ominous finding. The small bowel loops may be thick walled and oedematous, with pneumatosis sometimes evident. These findings represent small bowel necrosis; the volvulus is so tight that venous occlusion has occurred and the gas cannot be re-absorbed from the bowel lumen. A gasless abdomen is seen if vomiting has been prolonged, and in closed loop obstruction with viable small bowel or massive midgut necrosis. Radiographic examination should cease after the plain radiograph in the neonate with bilious vomiting and a complete duodenal obstruction, or a seriously ill child with obvious signs of peritonism; surgery is indicated. In all other children with bilious vomiting an upper GI contrast medium study is required. The examination is usually performed with barium.

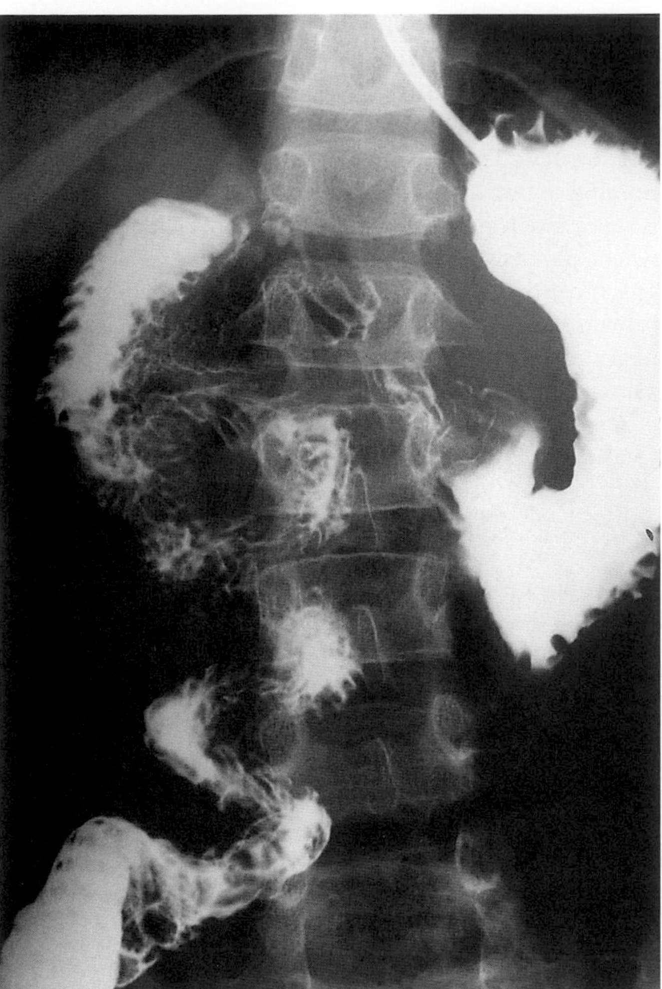

Figure 65.4 Malrotation and volvulus. Upper GI contrast medium study demonstrates the classical 'corkscrew' pattern of the duodenum and jejunum spiralling around the mesenteric vessels.

The intestines in malrotation are malfixed, and the purpose of the upper GI study is to locate the position of the duodenojejunal junction. On a supine radiograph the normal duodenojejunal junction lies to the left of the left-sided pedicles at the height of the duodenal bulb. When malrotation is present, the duodenojejunal junction is usually displaced inferiorly and to the right side. On a lateral view, the junction of the second and third parts of the duodenum is normally retroperitoneal, but it turns sharply anterior in malrotation. The more distal jejunal loops lie to the right of the midline. The caecal pole may lie high, and more to the left side than normal in patients with malrotation. Given that the caecal position is normal in a significant number of patients with malrotation, a barium meal is preferable to a barium enema in this situation. In cases of doubt over the position of the duodenojejunal junction, a delayed radiograph to demonstrate the position of the ileocaecal junction is useful. The normal duodenojejunal junction may be mobile, especially in children younger than 4 months of age. The duodenojejunal junction can be displaced temporarily by a distended colon or stomach, an enlarged spleen, an indwelling naso-enteric tube, or manual palpation.

The 'corkscrew' pattern of the duodenum and jejunum spiralling around the mesenteric vessels is pathognomonic for midgut volvulus on the upper GI study. When Ladd bands are causing duodenal obstruction rather than volvulus, the duodenojejunal course has been described as 'Z-shaped' rather than spiral[22,23].

US may demonstrate the dilated, fluid-filled stomach and proximal duodenum when obstruction is present. The relationship of the superior mesenteric vein (SMV) to the SMA is abnormal in about two-thirds of patients with malrotation, when the vein lies ventral or to the left of the artery. This sign is neither sensitive nor specific for malrotation, as some patients have abnormally related superior mesenteric vessels in the absence of malrotation[24,25]. The volvulus itself may be demonstrated with US as the 'whirlpool sign'. Colour Doppler studies show the SMV spiralling clockwise around the SMA. US is a useful screening tool in the infant with bilious vomiting, but the upper GI study remains the standard technique for the diagnosis of midgut malrotation and volvulus.

Duodenal atresia and stenosis Duodenal atresia is much more common than duodenal stenosis. Both atresia and stenosis are caused by failure of recanalization of the duodenal lumen after the sixth week of fetal life. Duodenal obstruction may also be caused by partial or complete webs or diaphragms. Extrinsic duodenal compression by an annular pancreas or preduodenal portal vein may contribute to the obstruction in some patients. Regardless of the cause, in 80% of cases, the level of the obstruction is just distal to the ampulla of Vater.

Associated anomalies occur in the majority of patients with duodenal atresia or stenosis. Down's syndrome is present in 30% of patients and congenital heart disease in 20%. Malrotation is present in 20–30% of patients and can only be diagnosed before surgery if the duodenal obstruction is partial. Components of the VACTERL association may also be present.

Duodenal atresia may be diagnosed antenatally when the dilated stomach and duodenal cap are seen with US in late pregnancy. Maternal polyhydramnios and consequent prematurity are common. Infants otherwise present early in the postnatal period with bilious vomiting and upper abdominal distension. Nonbilious emesis occurs in those infants with a pre-ampullary obstruction.

Radiographs show a gas-filled 'double bubble' of the stomach and duodenal cap (Fig. 65.5). If the stomach has been decompressed by vomiting or an orogastric tube, then air can be injected via the tube to confirm the diagnosis. With a complete obstruction, no distal gas is seen. If the obstruction is partial or, in the rare cases of a bifid pancreatic duct, straddling the atretic segment, then distal gas will be present.

In an upper GI study, duodenal stenosis is seen as a narrowed area in the second part of the duodenum. A duodenal web may be seen as a thin, filling defect extending across the duodenal lumen. If the study is performed via a nasogastric tube, then the pressure of the tube on the obstructing web causes indrawing of the duodenal wall at the site of the web's attachment (the 'duodenal dimple')[26]. A duodenal web may also be diagnosed using US[27].

Small bowel atresia and stenosis Jejunal and ilealatresias have a common aetiology and are due to intrauterine vascular problems. The vascular insult may be a primary or secondary event (e.g. due to antenatal volvulus or intussusception). As with the duodenum, atresia is more common than stenosis, and the proximal jejunum and distal ileum are more frequently affected.

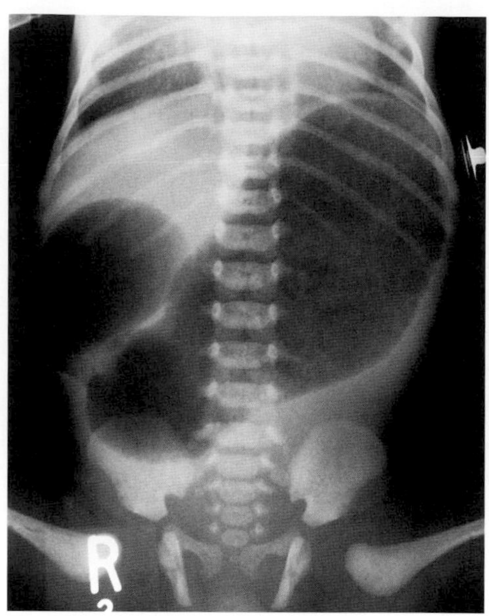

Figure 65.5 Duodenal atresia. Supine radiograph shows the classical 'double bubble' appearance.

The 'apple peel' syndrome is thought to follow intrauterine occlusion of the distal SMA. There is a proximal jejunal atresia, with agenesis of the mesentery and absence of the mid small bowel. The distal ileum spirals around its narrow vascular pedicle; an appearance that gives the syndrome its name. A malrotated microcolon is also usually present[28,29]. A second, more complex type of intestinal atresia is the syndrome of multiple intestinal atresias with intraluminal calcifications[30,31].

The majority of infants with a small bowel atresia present with bilious vomiting in the immediate postnatal period. With more distal atresias abdominal distension is also present.

On the plain radiograph, there are dilated loops of small bowel down to the level of the atresia. The loop of bowel immediately proximal to the atresia may be disproportionately dilated and have a bulbous contour. With stenosis rather than atresia, bubbles of distal gas are present. Occasionally fine intraluminal calcifications will be seen with a more distal atresia, though these are not as dense as in the familial multiple atresia syndrome. A meconium peritonitis with calcification of the peritoneum will be present if an intrauterine perforation has occurred.

Abdominal distension

Abdominal distension in the neonate may be due to mechanical or functional bowel obstruction, an abdominal mass lesion (Table 65.2), ascites, or a pneumoperitoneum. A supine abdominal radiograph will show the distribution and calibre of the bowel loops, intra-abdominal calcifications (Table 65.3), the presence of pneumatosis or portal venous gas, and possibly a soft tissue mass. A pneumoperitoneum may be detected on

Table 65.2 CAUSES OF A NEONATAL INTRA-ABDOMINAL MASS LESION
Complicated meconium ileus
Dilated bowel proximal to an obstruction
Mesenteric or duplication cyst
Abscess
Genitourinary causes
Hydronephrosis
Renal cystic disease
Mesoblastic nephroma
Wilms' tumour
Adrenal haemorrhage
Neuroblastoma
Retroperitoneal teratoma
Ovarian cyst
Hydrometrocolpos
Haemangio-endothelioma
Hepatoblastoma
Choledochal, hepatic, or splenic cysts

Table 65.3 CAUSES OF NEONATAL INTRA-ABDOMINAL CALCIFICATIONS
Complicated meconium ileus
Intraluminal calcifications
Low obstruction
Anorectal malformations with a fistula to the urinary tract
Adrenal
Haemorrhage
Neuroblastoma
Wolman's disease
Hepatobiliary disease
Haemangio-endothelioma
Hepatoblastoma
TORCH infections
Duplication and mesenteric cysts
Nephrocalcinosis
Intravascular thrombus
Teratomas

a supine radiograph, but if small is more likely to be seen on a (preferably left-side down) lateral decubitus or a lateral 'shoot through' radiograph with a horizontal beam.

US will identify free fluid or the presence of a mass lesion, and is able to confirm the origin of the latter. The majority of neonatal abdominal masses are benign and arise in relation to the genitourinary (GU) tract or are hepatobiliary in origin. Contrast medium studies, scintigraphy, CT, or MRI may follow depending upon the US findings.

Necrotizing enterocolitis (NEC) is the term used to describe the often severe enterocolitis that affects primarily premature infants. The increased survival rates of these very low birth weight infants of younger gestational age has led to an increased incidence of NEC in recent years[32]. The precise aetiology of the condition remains unknown, but immaturity of the gut mucosa and immune response, coupled with ischaemia/hypoxia, are felt to contribute[32]. Sepsis, early enteral feeding, umbilical arterial and venous cannulation, and maternal cocaine abuse are implicated as additional risk factors,[32–34] whilst breastfeeding is associated with a decreased risk of NEC developing[32]. Mini-epidemics of NEC are known to occur in neonatal intensive care units, suggesting a possible infectious cause. Aside from premature infants and those with low birth weight, NEC is also seen in term infants, particularly those with polycythaemia, cyanotic congenital heart disease, and gastroschisis. In the latter subgroups the condition often develops several weeks after surgery.

Initially superficial, the inflammatory process in NEC can extend to become transmural. Diffuse or discrete involvement of the bowel can occur, with the most commonly affected sites being the terminal ileum and colon. Almost half of all cases involve both small and large bowel. The overall mortality rate from NEC is approximately 30%, though this figure is higher in low birth weight infants. The initial clinical symptoms and signs are non-specific and include lethargy, hypoglycaemia, temperature instability, bradycardia, feeding intolerance, increased gastric aspirates, and gastric distension. Disease progression leads to vomiting and diarrhoea (often with the passage of blood or mucus in the stool), and eventually to shock. Severely affected infants may have visibly erythematous anterior abdominal walls, with palpable distended loops of bowel.

The initial radiographic features of NEC are non-specific. One of the earliest findings is diffuse gaseous distension of both small and large bowel or isolated gastric distension. If the diameter of a loop of bowel is greater than the width of the L1 vertebral body, then it is likely to be dilated[35]. Serial radiographs (usually taken every 6–12 h, depending upon the level of clinical suspicion) will demonstrate fixed dilatation of one or more bowel loops, and thickening (oedema) and loss of distinction of the bowel walls as the disease progresses. The use of the contrast medium enema in the acute situation to exclude NEC, when both the clinical and plain radiographic signs are ambiguous, has been suggested by some authors[36,37]. The risks of sepsis and perforation mean this practice is controversial.

A more specific sign of NEC on the plain radiograph is intramural gas (pneumatosis intestinalis), which may be submucosal when it appears as 'bubbly' lucencies in the bowel wall or subserosal when linear lucencies are visualized. Not all infants with NEC will have pneumatosis (Table 65.4). More extensive pneumatosis correlates with an increased severity of NEC. Portal venous gas is seen in approximately 10% of cases and is associated with severe NEC, but its presence does not necessarily imply a fatal outcome (Fig. 65.6). The disappearance of intramural or portal venous gas may herald imminent perforation rather than recovery[38]. There are no definite radiographic signs to help identify those infants most at risk of perforation. Indicators include a solitary, dilated loop of

Table 65.4 CAUSES OF PNEUMATOSIS INTESTINALIS IN THE NEONATE AND OLDER CHILD
Necrotizing enterocolitis
Bowel ischaemia, inflammation, and obstruction
Cyanotic congenital heart disease
Hirschprung's disease
Gastroschisis
Anorectal atresia
Inflammatory bowel disease
Lymphoma
Leukaemia
Cytomegalovirus and rotavirus gastroenteritis
Colonoscopy
Caustic ingestion
Short bowel syndrome
Congenital immune deficiency states
Clostridium infection
Chronic granulomatous disease of childhood
Chronic steroid use
Post hepatic, renal, or bone marrow transplant
Collagen vascular disease
Graft versus host disease
AIDS

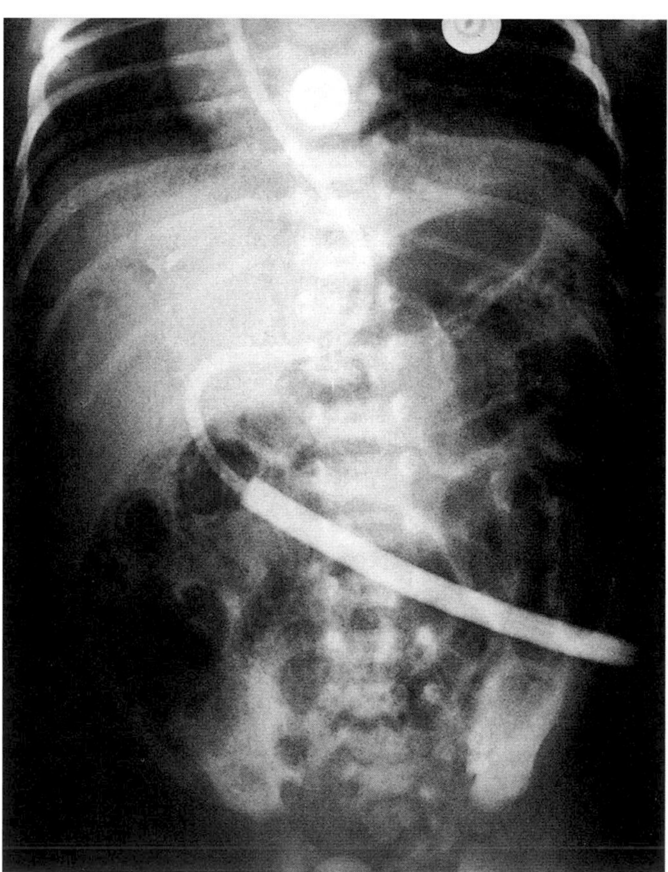

Figure 65.6 Necrotizing enterocolitis. Supine radiograph demonstrates multiple dilated loops of bowel, extensive submucosal and subserosal pneumatosis, and portal vein gas.

bowel present over 24–36 h (the 'persistent loop sign')[39] and the presence of free intraperitoneal fluid[38].

US is more sensitive than a plain radiograph in the detection of ascites and portal venous gas. The latter is seen as echogenic particles flowing within the portal vein or focal areas of intrahepatic increased echogenicity. Pneumatosis intestinalis may be recognized with US. The 'circle sign' is indicative of bubbles of gas circumferentially in the bowel wall and is seen as a continuous, echogenic ring in cross-section[40].

Perforation will occur in one-third of children with NEC, most commonly in the ileocaecal region (60% of cases)[41]. Less than two-thirds of patients with a perforation will have free air visible on a plain radiograph. The supine, cross-table lateral or decubitus view is useful to detect small amounts of free intraperitoneal air, which collects between loops of bowel and is seen as the 'telltale triangle'[42]. Almost all patients with NEC who perforate do so within 30 h of diagnosis[41] and after this time supine radiographs alone probably suffice for radiographic follow-up. The presence of free intraperitoneal fluid may also be an indicator of perforation but this is seen in only a further 20% of patients[38,41].

Perforation in infants with NEC is not an absolute indication for surgical intervention. Peritoneal drains are used in the initial resuscitation of these critically ill infants, delaying the need for surgery and allowing time for systemic recovery. In some instances, a peritoneal drain may provide definitive treatment[43].

A late complication of NEC is stricturing, which can be single or multiple, and occurs in up to a third of patients. The majority of strictures are short, are found in the colon, and are diagnosed up to 3 months following the acute illness[44]. Contrast medium studies are indicated in infants following surgery, before re-anastomosis of the defunctioned bowel. In rare instances, an acquired intestinal atresia may develop following NEC. Other reported late complications of NEC include abscess formation, enteric fistulas, enterocyst formation, obstruction secondary to adhesions, malabsorption, and short bowel syndrome following surgical resection[45–47].

Delayed passage of meconium

All infants should pass meconium in the first 24–48 h of life. Failure to do so may be due to an underlying bowel atresia or obstruction (Table 65.5) and leads to progressive abdominal distension. The more common problems encountered include Hirschsprung's disease, functional immaturity of the colon (meconium plug syndrome, small left colon), meconium ileus and peritonitis, and ileal atresia.

In all cases, a supine abdominal radiograph will show the features of a low intestinal obstruction; there will be multiple dilated loops of bowel down to the level of the obstruction. Differentiation between small and large bowel to determine the precise level of the obstruction is virtually impossible in the neonate, given that both may be of similar calibre and that the haustra are poorly developed. A horizontal beam or lateral decubitus view demonstrates fluid levels or confirms perforation and is not always necessary.

Table 65.5 CAUSES OF DELAYED PASSAGE OF MECONIUM IN INFANTS
Ileal atresia
Meconium ileus
Functional immaturity of the colon
Colon atresia
Anorectal malformations
Hirschprung's disease
Megacystis–microcolon–intestinal hypoperistalsis syndrome
Extrinsic compression of the distal bowel by a mass lesion
Mesenteric cyst
Enteric duplication cyst
Paralytic ileus, sepsis, drugs, and metabolic upset

Hirschsprung's disease is a form of functional low bowel obstruction, which is due to failure of caudal migration of neuroblasts in the developing bowel. There is thus an absence of parasympathetic intrinsic ganglion cells in both Auerbach's and Meissner's plexuses in the bowel wall. The distal large bowel from the point of neuronal arrest to the anus is aganglionic. The existence of 'skip lesions' in Hirschsprung's disease is extremely unusual48. In about 75% of cases, the aganglionic segment extends only to the rectosigmoid region (short segment disease). Long segment disease involves a portion of the colon proximal to the sigmoid. Variants of Hirschsprung's disease include total aganglionosis coli and total intestinal Hirschsprung's disease. Ultrashort segment disease is rare and involves only the anus at the level of the internal sphincter.

In short segment disease there is a male preponderance but the sex ratio is equal in long segment disease[49]. The latter has a strong familial incidence; short segment disease is sporadic. Approximately 5% of children with Hirschsprung's disease have Down's syndrome. Other associations with Hirschsprung's disease include ileal and colonic atresias, cleft palate, polydactyly, craniofacial anomalies, cardiac septal defects and other neurocristopathies[50–53].

Neonates present with abdominal distension, vomiting (which may be bilious) and failure to pass meconium. Stooling may follow a digital rectal examination or the insertion of a rectal thermometer, before the symptoms recur. Children who present later in childhood are unusual but may do so with a history of chronic constipation and failure to thrive, or rarely with an acute abdomen secondary to colonic volvulus[54].

Severe bloody diarrhoea, sepsis, and shock are associated with Hirschsprung's enterocolitis, which occurs in up to 30% of patients in both the pre- and post-operative periods. Enterocolitis is the leading cause of death in Hirschsprung's disease and has an increased frequency in long segment disease. Other postoperative complications of Hirschsprung's disease include fistulas and stenoses at the anastomotic site. In the longer term, chronic constipation, soiling, and incontinence are recognized. A suction or full thickness rectal biopsy is required for the definitive diagnosis of Hirschsprung's disease.

The abdominal radiograph will typically show a low bowel obstruction, commonly with colonic dilatation out of proportion to the small bowel. The absence of rectal gas is one of the plain radiographic findings in Hirschsprung's disease but the sign is not specific, being more commonly seen in infants with sepsis and NEC[55]. About 5% of infants will have a pneumoperitoneum; the perforation occurs most commonly in the ascending colon and may be appendiceal. Perforation is more common in long segment disease. Intraluminal small bowel calcifications may also be present in long segment disease[56,57].

A water-soluble contrast medium enema should be performed and has a diagnostic accuracy equivalent to barium[58]. The catheter tip is placed just inside the rectum. It is important that a balloon catheter is *not* used. A balloon can obscure the diagnostic features or worse, perforate the stiff, aganglionic bowel. The most important radiograph is a lateral view of the rectum during slow filling (Fig. 65.7). In short segment disease the rectum will be narrow and there will be a cone-shaped transition zone to the more proximal, dilated, ganglionated bowel. The radiological transition zone is commonly found to be distal to the pathological transition zone. Irregular contractions may be seen in the denervated rectum. The transition zone may not be present in the neonate, as it takes time for the proximal bowel to dilate. A useful calculation is the recto:sigmoid ratio; the rectum should always be the most distensible portion of the bowel and have a diameter greater than that of the sigmoid colon (recto:sigmoid ratio > 1). In short segment disease this ratio is reversed.

Retention of contrast medium above the sigmoid colon on a delayed radiograph after 24 h is a non-specific sign of Hirschsprung's disease. With coexistent enterocolitis, mucosal oedema, ulceration, and spasm are seen, although an enema would obviously be contraindicated in the infant with fulminant colitis (Fig. 65.8). Giant stercoral ulcers may also be

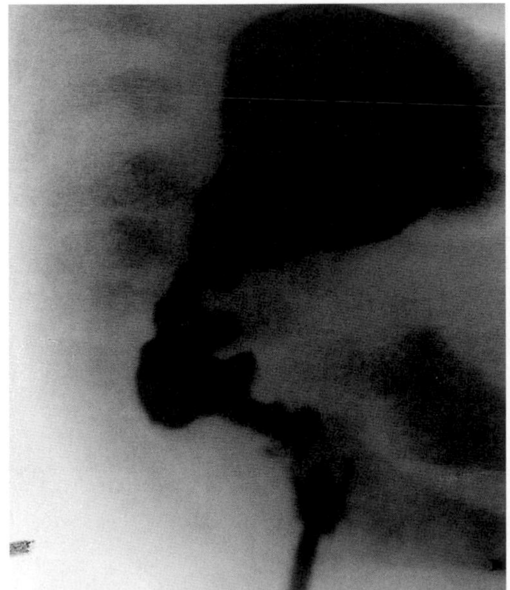

Figure 65.7 Rectosigmoid Hirschsprung's disease. Lateral view, contrast medium enema. The cone-shaped transition zone, abnormal rectosigmoid ratio, and tertiary rectal contractions are demonstrated.

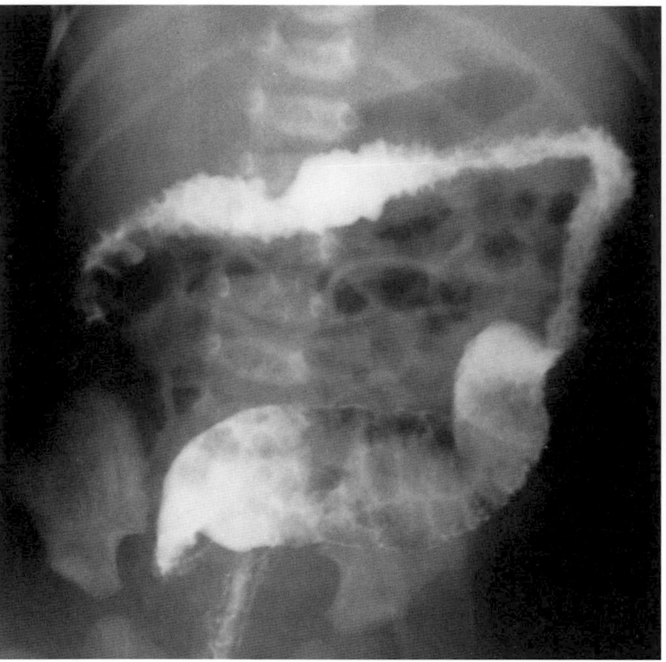

Figure 65.8 Hirschsprung's enterocolitis. Contrast medium enema shows extensive ulceration of the entire colon.

seen in older children with a delayed presentation[49]. The radiological features of Hirschsprung's disease may be absent in the neonate and overall the contrast medium enema has a false-negative rate of 20–30%[58].

In total aganglionosis coli the findings are notoriously unreliable but include shortening of a normal calibre colon, with loss of the normal redundancy of the flexures. Muscle spasm, a pseudo-transition zone, and easy reflux of contrast medium into the terminal ileum are also reported. Occasionally a microcolon is seen[49].

Functional immaturity of the colon Immature left colon (meconium plug syndrome or small left colon) is a relatively common cause of neonatal bowel obstruction.

Prematurity, birth by caesarean section, maternal diabetes and drug ingestion, and treatment of mothers with magnesium sulphate during labour have all been reported as risk factors to infants.[33,59,60] The condition is *not* associated with cystic fibrosis. The exact cause of the syndrome remains unknown, but immaturity of the myenteric plexus had been postulated as a theory[61].

The affected infants present with symptoms and signs of bowel obstruction, though they tend to be less ill than those with mechanical obstruction; the abdomen is less distended and vomiting is not necessarily a prominent feature. There is delayed passage of meconium.

The plain radiograph shows distension of both small and large bowel loops to the level of the inspissated meconium plugs. Few fluid levels are seen. The contrast medium enema typically shows a microcolon distal to the splenic flexure, at which point there is an abrupt transition to a mildly dilated proximal colon (this differs from Hirschsprung's disease in which the transition zone is more gradual and which is uncommon at the level of the splenic flexure) (Fig. 65.9). The rectum is usually distensible in the patient with functional immaturity of the colon and consequently the rectosigmoid

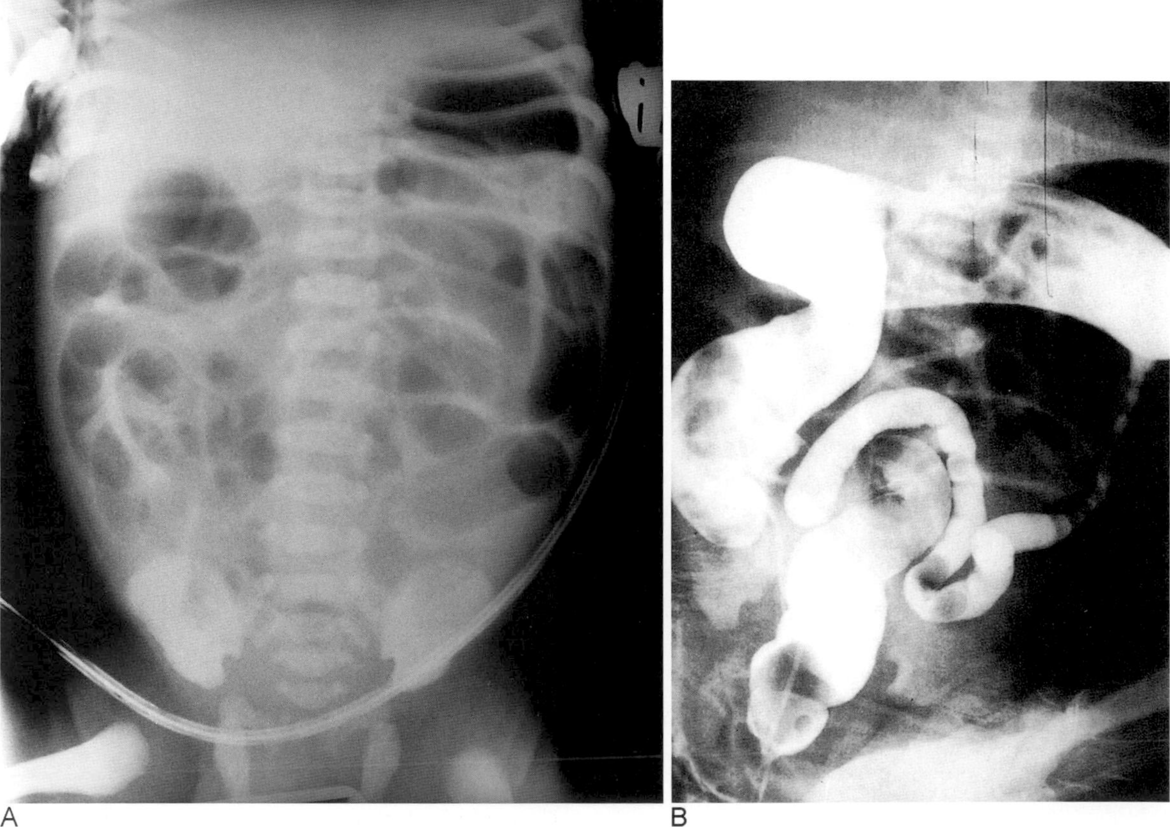

Figure 65.9 Small left colon syndrome. (A) Supine radiograph shows a low obstruction with multiple dilated loops of bowel. (B) Contrast medium enema shows a microcolon distal to the splenic flexure. The transition point is abrupt.

ratio is normal. Discrete plugs of meconium are seen as filling defects in the dilated colon. In the premature infant, the whole colon may be small[59]. When performed with water-soluble contrast medium, the enema is not only diagnostic, but therapeutic. A variable amount of meconium is typically passed soon after the examination, with a gradual recovery of the infant over the next few hours or days. Bowel perforation has occasionally been reported[59].

The main differential diagnosis is Hirschsprung's disease. If there remains doubt as to the diagnosis following the enema, then a suction rectal biopsy is recommended.

Colon atresia is rare when compared with other intestinal atresias, and colonic stenosis is rarer still. The right colon is most commonly affected. As with small bowel atresias, the atresia may take the form of a diaphragm or web, fibrous cord or mesenteric gap defect, with the latter occurring most frequently. Colon atresia is thought to be due to an in utero vascular accident[62]. More proximal atresias, gastroschisis, and Hirschsprung's disease may be found in association[52,62,63].

The abdominal radiograph will show the features of a low intestinal obstruction. If multiple atresias are present, then the bowel will be distended only to the level of the most proximal atresia, giving a misleading initial abdominal radiograph. A contrast medium enema usually demonstrates a distal microcolon, with obstruction to the retrograde flow of contrast medium at the point of the atresia. If a colonic diaphragm or web is present, then the column of barium may terminate in a 'wind sock' configuration, as the obstructing membrane balloons into the proximal air-filled colon.

Meconium ileus is a form of distal intestinal obstruction caused by inspissated pellets of meconium in the terminal ileum. Over 90% of infants with meconium ileus have cystic fibrosis and meconium ileus is the presenting feature of cystic fibrosis in 10–15% of affected patients. Of patients with cystic fibrosis, those with the ΔF508 mutation have a higher incidence of meconium ileus64. Black patients with cystic fibrosis have a lower incidence of meconium ileus than white patients[64]. Children who present with meconium ileus as neonates go on to develop more severe respiratory disease than those without meconium ileus[65,66].

Over half of the affected infants have uncomplicated meconium ileus. In utero these babies produce meconium which is thick and tenacious, and which fills and distends the small bowel loops. The meconium desiccates in the terminal ileum and becomes impacted, causing a high grade obstruction. A functional microcolon results. Meconium ileus is described as complicated when intra-uterine volvulus, atresia, gangrene, perforation or meconium peritonitis supervene.

The presenting clinical symptoms and signs of noncomplicated meconium ileus are vomiting, abdominal distension, and failure to pass meconium.

The plain abdominal radiograph will show dilatation of small bowel loops, which are of varying calibre. Fluid levels are scant. Often a 'soap bubble' appearance is visible (classically in the right iliac fossa), which is caused by the admixture of meconium with gas (Fig. 65.10). This sign is suggestive of, but not diagnostic for, meconium ileus, as it may be seen in other forms of low bowel obstruction.

US may be useful in differentiating between meconium ileus and ileal atresia. In meconium ileus, the dilated bowel loops are filled with echogenic material, whereas in ileal atresia the bowel contents are echo poor[67].

The contrast medium enema in meconium ileus demonstrates a virtually empty microcolon. Reflux of contrast medium into the terminal ileum will show that it too is small in calibre and numerous pellets of meconium are outlined (Fig. 65.11). A spiral appearance of the small bowel loops has been described secondary to intrauterine volvulus in more complicated cases[68]. More proximal reflux of contrast medium will show the dilated mid ileal loops. The contrast medium enema in uncomplicated meconium ileus may be therapeutic as well as diagnostic. In 1969, Noblett described the nonoperative management of uncomplicated meconium ileus using a Gastrografin enema[69]. Gastrografin is a water-soluble contrast medium that is hypertonic to plasma and draws water into the bowel lumen by osmosis, softening the viscous meconium and allowing it to be passed. The detergents contained within Gastrografin may also aid in relieving the obstruction. The success rate of Gastrografin enemas in relieving the obstruction in meconium ileus is approximately 60%[67,70]. The enema can be complicated by perforation in up to 5% of patients[70]. Due to the hypertonicity of Gastrografin, there is a risk of fluid and electrolyte imbalance in the infant, and the enema should not be performed unless the baby is well hydrated and intravenous fluids are running. Serum electrolytes need to be monitored.

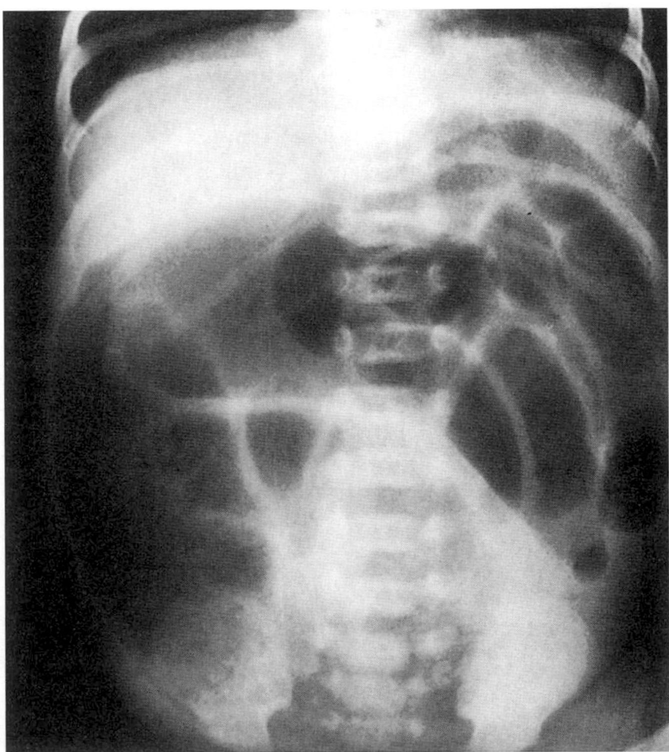

Figure 65.10 Meconium ileus. Supine radiograph shows a low obstruction with multiple, dilated loops of bowel and a 'soap bubble' appearance in the right lower quadrant.

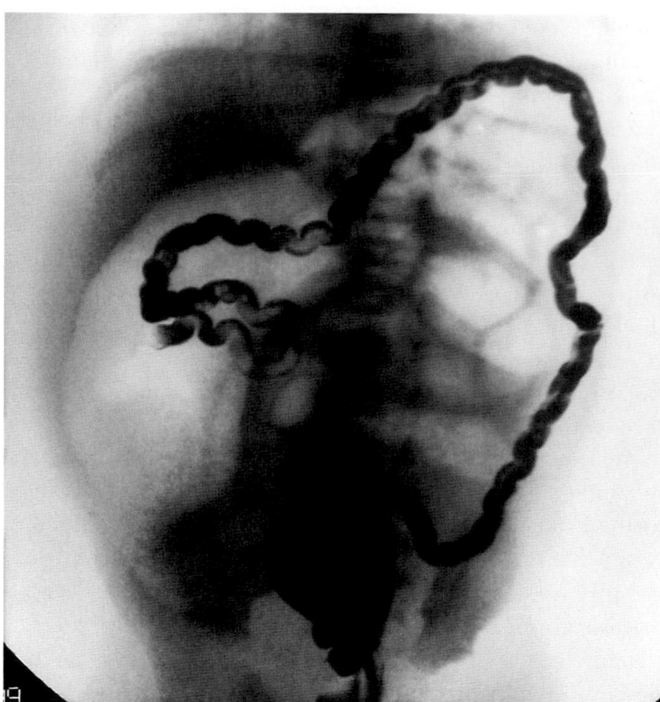

Figure 65.11 Meconium ileus. Contrast enema demonstrates the empty microcolon. Contrast refluxes into the narrow terminal ileum, where pellets of meconium are outlined.

Full strength Gastrografin is no longer commonly employed in the management of meconium ileus, rather it is diluted to half strength with saline or water, or another water-soluble contrast medium is substituted[70]. If the infant's clinical condition remains stable, then the enema can be repeated as necessary until the obstruction is relieved. Enemas in infants with suspected meconium ileus should only be performed in specialist paediatric centres. If nonoperative treatment fails or complications occur during the enema, then the infant needs surgery.

The presence of complicated meconium ileus may be suggested by the plain radiographic findings; intra-abdominal or scrotal calcifications, bowel wall calcification, prominent air–fluid levels, and soft tissue masses.

Volvulus of a heavy, meconium-laden loop of bowel is common[71]. Volvulus can lead to intestinal stenoses, atresias, gangrene and perforation. Perforation of bowel in utero leads to chemical meconium peritonitis. The extruded bowel contents cause an intense inflammatory reaction, with fibrosis and calcification to follow—the characteristic 'snow storm' ascites picture on US examinations[60]. Not all meconium peritonitis is due to meconium ileus, and the associated calcifications are seen more commonly from other causes (e.g. small bowel atresia or intrauterine intussusception)[72,73]. A meconium pseudocyst is formed in meconium ileus when there is vascular compromise in association with an intra-uterine volvulus. The ischaemic bowel loops become adherent and necrotic, and a fibrous wall develops around them. The wall may calcify and the cyst can have a secondary mass effect upon the adjacent loops of bowel[71].

Distal ileal atresia Ileal atresia is due to a prenatal vascular insult. If the atresia is in the distal ileum, then the infant will present with abdominal distension and delayed passage of meconium.

The plain radiograph will show a low obstruction with multiple dilated loops of bowel, one loop of which characteristically has a long air–fluid level. The radiographic findings are similar to those of meconium ileus. The contrast medium enema will outline a microcolon and contrast medium cannot be refluxed into the dilated small bowel. If the atresia has occurred secondary to an ischaemic insult late in the pregnancy, then the colon calibre may be near normal due to the already accumulated succus entericus in its lumen.

Anorectal malformations The incidence of anorectal malformations (imperforate anus or anorectal atresia) is 1 in 1500–5000 live births[74]. The precise aetiology is unknown, but the condition results from failure of descent and separation of the hindgut and the GU tract during the second trimester. The abnormality consists of anorectal atresia, with or without an anomalous connection between the atretic anorectum and the GU tract.

Associated congenital anomalies are common. The VACTERL sequence occurs in around 45% of patients, the OEIS complex (omphalocele, bladder exstrophy, imperforate anus and sacral anomalies) in up to 5% of patients[74]. Between 2 and 8% of patients have Down's syndrome and these patients tend to have imperforate anus without fistulas[74,75]. Currarino's triad is the association between an anorectal malformation (commonly anorectal stenosis), bony sacral anomalies (classically a 'scimitar sacrum' with unilateral hypoplasia of the lateral aspect of the vertebral bodies) and a presacral mass lesion (which may be an enteric cyst, teratoma, anterior meningocele or dermoid).

Anorectal atresias are classified into high or low lesions depending upon whether the rectum ends above or below the puborectalis sling. The distinction between high and low lesions is clinical rather than radiological, and has important therapeutic and prognostic consequences. In both male and female patients with low lesions, there is usually a visible perineal opening. The orifice may be located more anteriorly than normal (an ectopic anus) and it may be stenotic or covered with a membrane[76]. Low lesions do not have a communication with the GU tract. Female patients with low lesions will have separate urethral and vaginal orifices with an intact hymen[76]. Low lesions also include isolated rectal atresia or stenosis. This type of lesion is treated surgically with an anoplasty or dilatation soon after birth.

In both male and female patients with high lesions, no visible perineal fistula is present. Male patients will usually have a fistulous tract between the atretic anorectum and the posterior urethra. Less commonly there is a fistula to the bladder or anterior urethra. Female patients have fistulas from the atretic anorectum to the vagina or vestibule. Rarely, in both male and female patients, the rectum ends blindly. High lesions are initially managed with a colostomy, with definitive repair being performed at a later stage.

The traditional radiological approach to the baby with imperforate anus is the inverted lateral radiograph. A radio-opaque marker is placed over the anal dimple and the distance between the pouch of rectal gas and the marker is measured. False interpretation may occur within the first 24 h of life when gas may not have reached the rectum, if the infant had not been held prone for long enough, or when meconium is impacted in the distal rectum. Similarly, if the infant is crying or straining, the rectal pouch descends through the levator sling and a high lesion may be misinterpreted as a low one. Transperineal US has been used to measure the distance of the rectal pouch from the perineum[77] but interpretation suffers from similar problems to the inverted lateral radiograph. For these reasons, neither of these techniques is recommended. Instead the infant should be clinically assessed to determine whether the lesion is a low or high one (as outlined above).

Plain radiographs are more useful if they demonstrate intravesical air (implying a high lesion with a rectovesical or recto-urethral fistula in a boy) (Fig. 65.12) or calcified intraluminal meconium (again implying a high lesion in a boy; meconium calcifies when it comes into contact with urine)[78]. The plain abdominal radiograph is useful in the identification of any associated bony anomalies of the spine.

An augmented pressure colostogram[79] is performed in infants with high lesions following the initial formation of a colostomy (Fig. 65.13). A Foley catheter is inserted into the distal segment of colon and its balloon gently inflated to 5 ml. Retrograde traction is then applied to the catheter, so that the balloon seals the stoma. Water-soluble contrast is then hand injected under mild pressure to distend the distal colon and define the fistulous tract. The level of the fistula determines the surgical approach at the time of the definitive repair.

Renal US is mandatory as an ancillary investigation in all infants with anorectal atresia. Spinal US should also be performed as spinal cord lesions (e.g. cord tethering) are not uncommon[80]. Both pre- and post-operative MRI studies may be used to study the pelvic floor musculature and can also reveal any associated renal and spinal malformations.

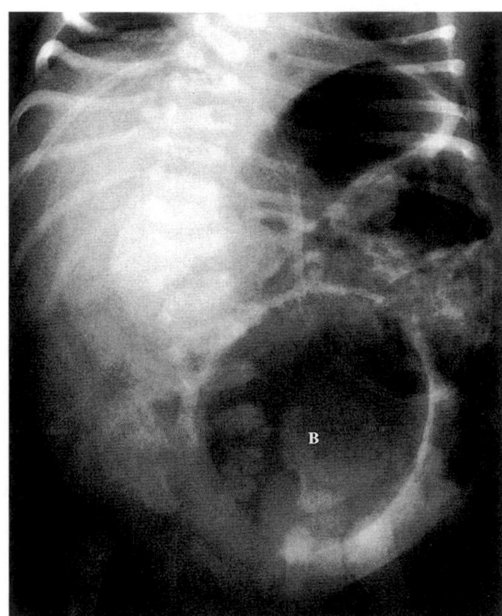

Figure 65.12 Colovesical fistula. Supine abdominal radiograph shows intravesical air and vertebral segmentation anomalies in a male infant with a high anorectal malformation. B = bladder.

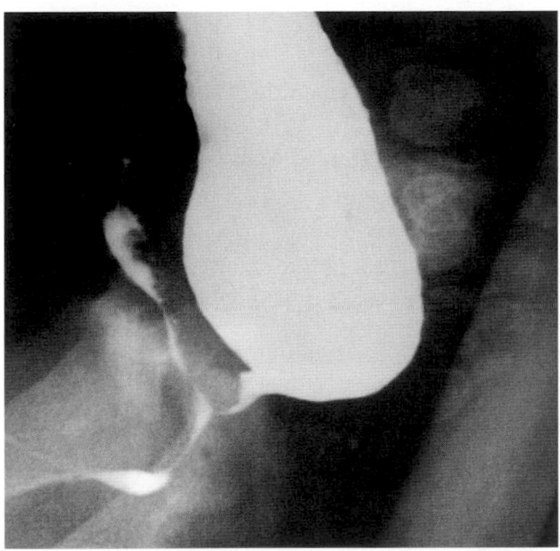

Figure 65.13 Recto-urethral fistula. Augmented pressure colostogram in a male infant with a high anorectal malformation.

THE INFANT AND OLDER CHILD

ABDOMINAL PAIN

Abdominal pain in infants and children is common and is caused by a variety of disorders (Table 65.6). It is better localized in older children than in infants. Plain radiographs of the abdomen are required for suspected mechanical obstruction, perforation and trauma, location of foreign bodies and calculi, and basal pneumonia

In non-specific abdominal pain the plain radiographs are frequently unhelpful. US is useful in the diagnosis of a number of GI disorders, including acute appendicitis, intussusception, Henoch-Schönlein purpura (HSP), and mesenteric adenitis, and in excluding other pathology as a cause of abdominal pain. CT is the best investigation for abdominal trauma and is also used in the diagnosis of acute appendicitis in clinically difficult cases.

Intussusception

Intussusception is a common surgical emergency in infants and young children. It consists of a telescoping of a segment of bowel (intussusceptum) into a more distal segment (intussuscipiens). The majority of children are under 1 year of age, with a peak incidence between 5 and 9 months of age. Ileocolic intussusceptions are the most common type. Ileo-ileocolic, ileo-ileal, and colocolic are much less common. Most (over 90%) have no lead point and are due to lymphoid hypertrophy, usually following a viral infection. Pathological lead points (which include Meckel's diverticulum, intestinal polyp, duplication cyst, and lymphoma) occur in 5–10% of patients.

The clinical presentation is characterized by episodes of intermittent colicky pain. Other common findings include vomiting, 'red currant jelly' stools (containing blood and

Table 65.6 CAUSES OF ABDOMINAL PAIN IN INFANTS AND CHILDREN
Constipation
Acute appendicitis
Gastroenteritis
Intussusception
Bowel obstruction
Mesenteric adenitis
Trauma
Perforated Meckel's diverticulum
Cholelithiasis (biliary colic/acute cholecystitis)
Henoch–Schönlein purpura
Inflammatory bowel disease
Acute or chronic pancreatitis
Ingested foreign body
Peptic ulcer

mucus), and a palpable abdominal mass. Later drowsiness and lethargy develop.

A supine abdominal radiograph may detect the intussusception and its complications, or suggest alternative diagnoses (Fig. 65.14). Findings include the presence of a soft tissue mass, distal small bowel obstruction, absence of gas from the colon, difficulty in assessing the position of the caecum, or pneumoperitoneum. Abnormal radiolucencies in the soft tissue mass are due to mesenteric fat trapped in the intussusception. The abdominal radiograph may be normal in over 50% of cases of intussusception.

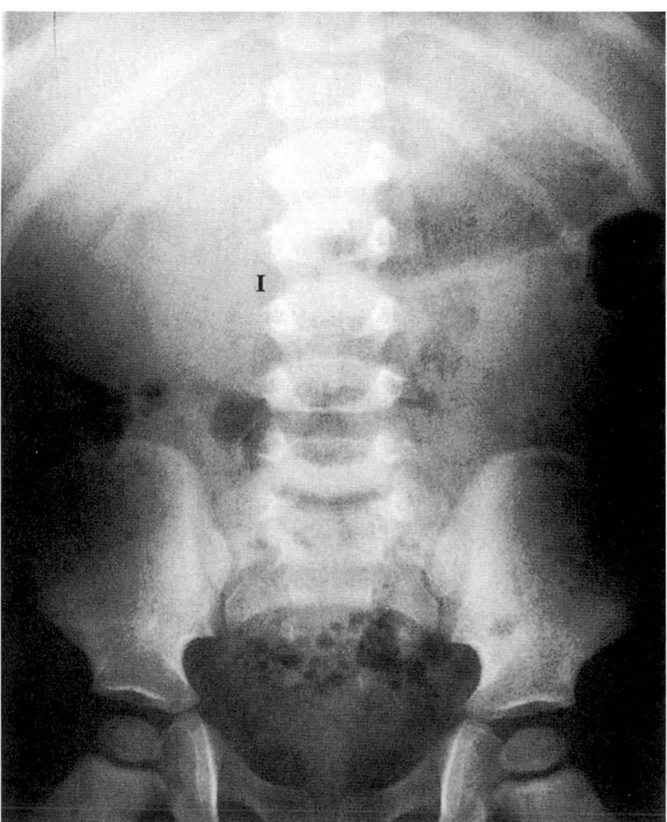

Figure 65.14 Intussusception. Supine radiograph of the abdomen shows the intussusception as a round soft tissue mass in the right upper quadrant outlined by a faint curvilinear rim of bowel gas. I = intussusceptum.

Ultrasonography is an accurate method for the diagnosis of intussusception, the assessment of bowel viability, and reducibility[81]. It has also been used to monitor hydrostatic reduction and to avoid the need for a diagnostic enema. A high-frequency linear array transducer should be used. Spontaneous reduction of intussusception has also been documented by US, which shows intussusception as a mass of 3–5 cm in diameter, with a 'target' appearance on transverse images creating a 'sandwich' longitudinal appearance. Similar findings may occur with bowel wall thickening due to oedema, inflammation, or haematoma (Table 65.7). The presence of a small amount of free intraperitoneal fluid is common. A 'crescent in doughnut' appearance on the transverse image represents the apex of the intussusception and its trailing mesentery, which causes a crescentric echogenicity (Fig. 65.15). Enlarged lymph nodes may be seen in the intussusception. Fluid can become trapped between the intussusceptum and intussuscipiens and is associated with vascular compromise[82]. Doppler interrogation can be used to assess blood flow in the intussusceptum, although nonvisualization of blood flow by colour Doppler ultrasound is not a contraindication to air enema reduction[83].

US may demonstrate lead points such as a duplication cyst, Meckel's diverticulum, or lymphoma, which may be missed on fluoroscopy[84]. Following reduction by contrast medium enema, US is also useful to confirm complete reduction or to show a residual ileocolic or ileo-ileal intussusception in difficult cases. The post-reduction 'doughnut' sign may be seen after a successful reduction and represents oedema at the ileocaecal valve.

Reduction of the intussusception should only be attempted after surgical consultation. Absolute contraindications to enema reduction include signs of bowel perforation with free intraperitoneal gas on the abdominal radiograph and the presence of septicaemic shock or peritonitis. Pneumatic reduction of intussusception using air under fluoroscopic guidance is the preferred method (Fig. 65.16)[85,86]. It has been shown to be safe, with a lower absorbed radiation dose compared with barium enema and has largely replaced hydrostatic reduction by barium enema. Pneumatic reduction of intussusception using carbon dioxide has also been described. Hydrostatic reduction with water-soluble contrast medium under US control has the advantage of avoiding radiation exposure and gives a more detailed view of the

Table 65.7 CAUSES OF BOWEL WALL THICKENING ON ULTRASOUND
Intussusception
Sepsis
Typhlitis
Trauma
Henoch–Schönlein purpura
Lymphoma
Fibrosing colonopathy of cystic fibrosis
Meckel's diverticulum

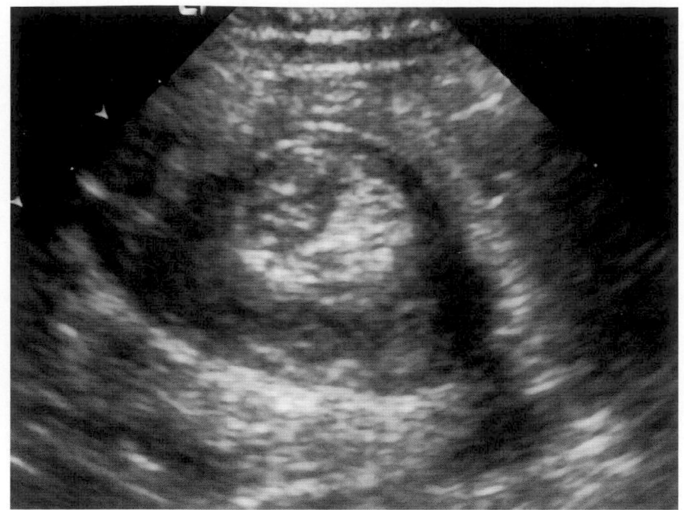
A

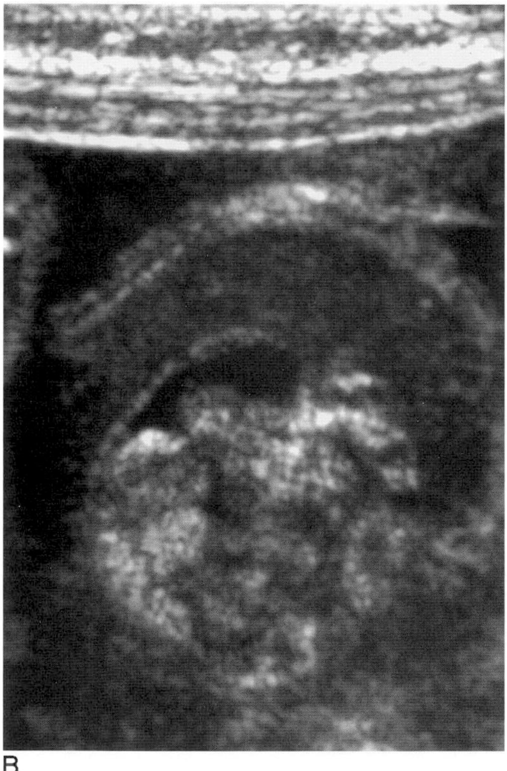
B

Figure 65.15 Intussusception. Ultrasound showing (A) crescent in doughnut appearance and (B) fluid trapped between the intussusceptum and intussuscipiens, and some free intraperitoneal fluid.

intussusception[87,88]. Success rates of 85% or higher have been reported with air and hydrostatic reduction. Delayed attempts at reduction by air enema have been used successfully where the initial air enema has failed[89].

The main complication of the contrast medium enema is perforation. This complication rate can be kept low when the enema is performed by an experienced radiologist using a pump which can limit the pressure and has a safety release valve. Perforation occurring with an air enema is safer than with liquid enemas. The perforation tends to be smaller and is associated with less faecal spillage and less peritoneal contamination.

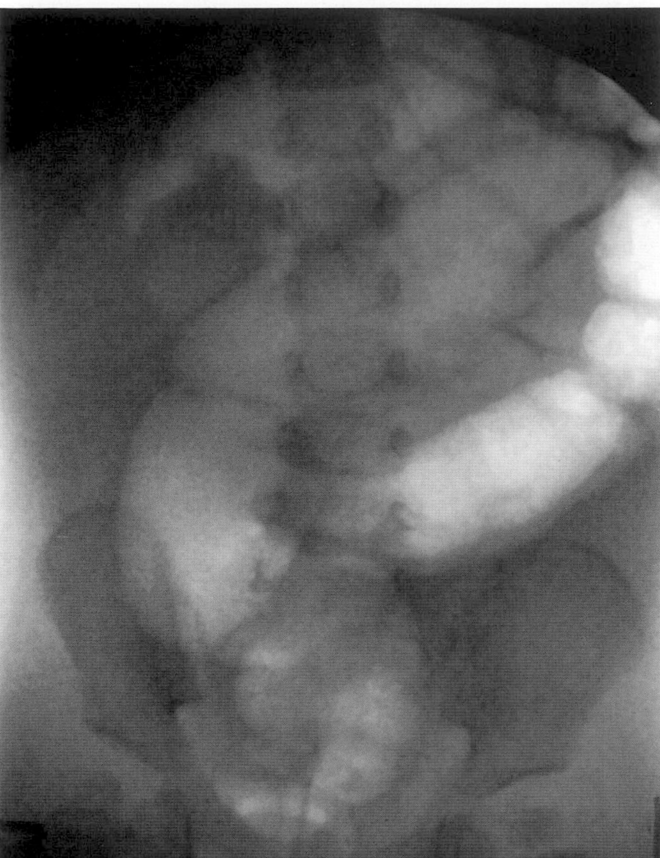

Figure 65.16 Intussusception. Air outlines the intussusception in the transverse colon during an air enema.

Acute appendicitis

Acute appendicitis is the most common indication for emergency abdominal surgery in children. Most children with acute appendicitis who present with typical clinical findings do not require imaging. Approximately 30–40% have atypical findings. Accurate clinical diagnosis can be particularly difficult in very young children and infants. Imaging can help to diagnose or exclude acute appendicitis as a cause of their acute abdominal pain or suggest alternative diagnoses[90].

Plain radiographs of the abdomen are usually normal in nonperforated appendicitis or demonstrate non-specific findings. US is helpful if the diagnosis is equivocal. This is performed using a linear array high-frequency transducer. The swollen appendix is usually a tubular, fluid-filled structure, which is noncompressible and measures 6 mm or more in diameter (Fig. 65.17). The echogenic mucosal lining may be intact or poorly defined, indicating perforation is imminent. A faecolith can sometimes be present at its tip; this may be detected on an abdominal radiograph (15% of cases; Fig. 65.18) or ultrasonography. A peri-appendicular fluid collection occurs with early perforation. Increased peri-appendiceal echogenicity represents inflammation of the surrounding fat. Colour Doppler usually shows hyperaemia of the appendiceal wall but may be limited if the inflammation is confined to the appendiceal tip[91,92]. Enlarged reactive lymph nodes are commonly seen. A perforated appendix is indistinguishable on ultrasound from other forms of intraperitoneal abscess.

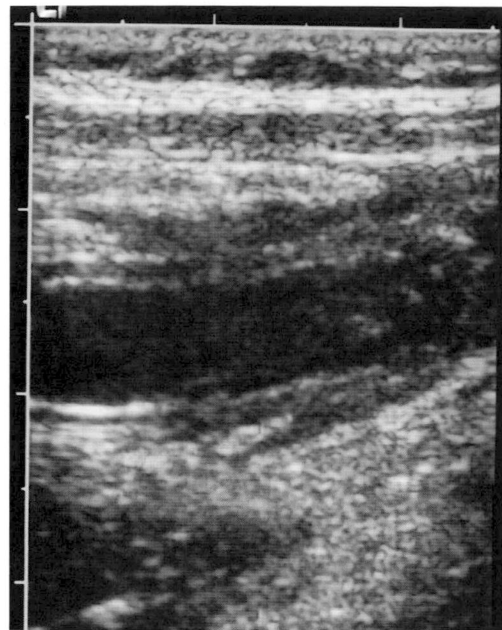

Figure 65.17 Acute appendicitis. Ultrasound shows an enlarged appendix with a fluid-filled lumen.

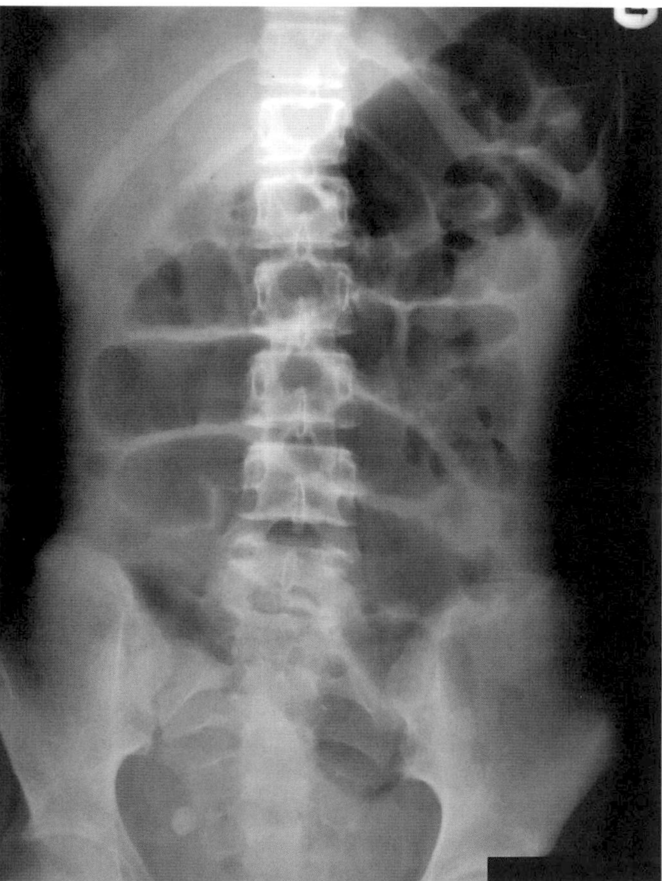

Figure 65.18 Appendicolith and small bowel dilatation in a child with acute appendicitis.

CT has a role in the diagnosis of acute appendicitis[93–95] in those patients where US has been difficult because of bowel gas or a retrocaecal appendix. US and CT are both sensitive and specific for the diagnosis of acute appendicitis but they should be reserved for those cases where the clinical diagnosis is difficult[96,97]. In the postoperative period both US and CT demonstrate a phlegmon or abscess (Fig. 65.19). The CT appearances of acute appendicitis in children are similar to those in adults[98].

Mesenteric lymphadenopathy

Mesenteric lymphadenopathy can occur in association with intra-abdominal or pelvic infection, inflammation, or malignancy, and can mimic an acute abdomen. It is a common cause of abdominal pain in children. In most cases the cause is never found. Mesenteric lymphadenitis is a diagnosis made by exclusion. Enlarged lymph nodes in the root of the mesentery may be seen on US in children with acute and chronic recurrent abdominal pain[99–102]. US is useful in establishing a primary diagnosis in these children.

Henoch–Schönlein purpura (HSP)

Henoch–Schönlein purpura (HSP) is an idiopathic, systemic vasculitis of unknown aetiology, which is characterized by a purpuric skin rash, abdominal pain, arthralgia, and nephritis. GI involvement occurs in 50–75% of patients who have abdominal pain, vomiting, and bleeding. The vasculitis can involve the bowel wall leading to GI bleeding. The duodenum and upper jejunum are the most common sites of the GI tract to be involved.

Plain radiographs of the abdomen may show bowel wall thickening due to haemorrhage and oedema, or small bowel obstruction or perforation. US features include bowel wall thickening, haematoma, ileus, peritoneal fluid, pneumatosis coli, gallbladder wall thickening, and intussusception (Fig. 65.20)[103]. The majority of intussusceptions in HSP are ileoileal, may be transient, and are not amenable to pneumatic or hydrostatic reduction. Contrast studies may show mucosal thickening, 'thumb printing', and separation of bowel loops. In most cases the changes of HSP are completely reversible and healing takes place in 3–4 weeks.

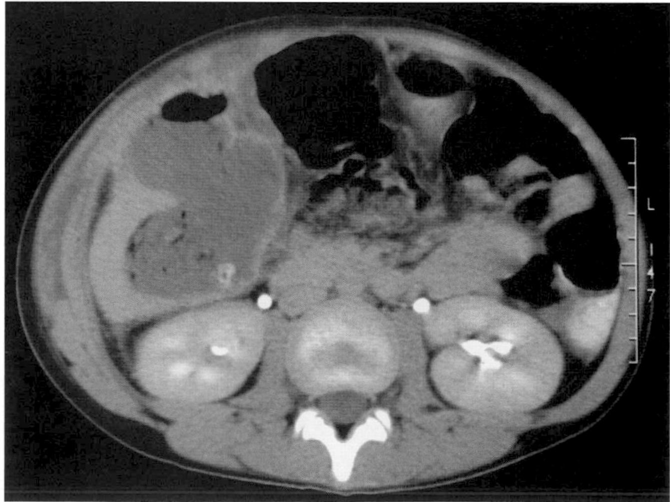

Figure 65.19 Acute appendicitis. CT showing an appendix abscess extending to the anterior abdominal wall. The abscess contains gas and an appendicolith.

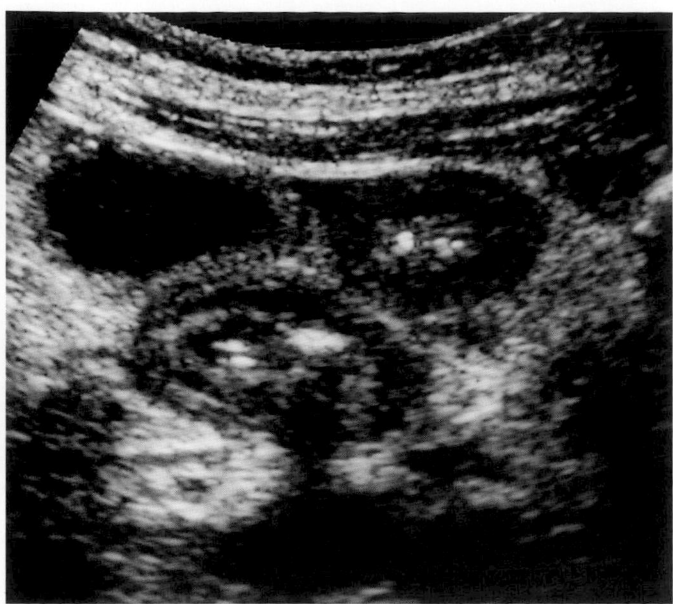

Figure 65.20 Henoch–Schönlein purpura. Transverse ultrasound shows the hypo-echoic thickened bowel wall and echogenic areas in the mucosa representing pneumatosis coli.

Constipation

Constipation is a common problem in infants and children and has been defined clinizcally as an alteration in the frequency, consistency, or ease of passage of stool[104]. This can lead to encopresis or faecal soiling, and occasionally can cause acute, severe abdominal pain. There is also an association with bedwetting, daytime urinary incontinence, and recurrent urinary tract infection. Causes of constipation are listed in Table 65.8. Chronic constipation often follows an inadequately managed acute episode. The majority of constipated children have functional constipation, which is not associated with organic abnormalities or drugs. These children have normal ganglion cells; many have emotional problems.

Table 65.8 CAUSES OF CONSTIPATION
Functional
Neurogenic
Aganglionosis
Hypoganglionosis
Neuronal intestinal dysplasia
Chronic intestinal pseudo-obstruction
Disorders of the spinal cord
Cerebral palsy
Dietary
Anal fissures
Strictures
Endocrine disorders
Metabolic disorders
Cystic fibrosis
Tumours
Lymphoma of bowel
Pelvic rhabdomyosarcoma
Presacral teratoma
Drugs
Opiates
Anticholinergics

The diagnosis of constipation in children is essentially clinical, and imaging is not usually required. The plain abdominal radiograph will demonstrate the degree of faecal loading and dilatation of the large bowel; its routine use in the diagnosis of constipation is not recommended. The presence of faecal loading on the plain radiograph does not necessarily indicate constipation. US can help differentiate a faecal mass from a true mass. Other imaging techniques described for the evaluation of constipation include the measurement of colonic transit time using radio-opaque markers, fluoroscopy, and MRI defaecography, or a scoring system for the evaluation of faecal loading on the plain abdominal radiograph[105–107]. These are only indicated in a highly selected group of children.

Intestinal motility disorders Intestinal motility disorder is a term used to describe a variety of abnormalities that have in common reduced motility of the bowel and no organic occlusion of the bowel lumen. They can be divided into acute and chronic disorders (Table 65.9)[105].

Acute dysmotility includes paralytic ileus in which there is temporary cessation of peristalsis in the gut. This simulates intestinal obstruction, as there is failure of propagation of intestinal contents. Acute gastro-enteritis can simulate small bowel obstruction by causing a local paralytic ileus, with dilatation of the affected segment of bowel and multiple fluid levels on an erect plain radiograph of the abdomen.

Chronic motility disorders include primary abnormalities of the bowel—Hirschsprung's disease (aganglionosis), hypoganglionosis which is rare and mimics Hirschsprung's disease, and neuronal intestinal dysplasia, which is a defect of autonomic neurogenesis characterized by an absent or rudimentary sympathetic ganglion innervation of the gut or by hyperplasia of cholinergic nerve fibres and hyperplasia of

Table 65.9 BOWEL MOTILITY DISORDERS
Acute
Paralytic ileus
Systemic illness including shock, hypoxia, sepsis
Chemical/hormonal upset
Functional immaturity of bowel in neonate
Meconium plug syndrome
Inspissated milk syndrome
Small left colon syndrome
Chronic
Hirschprung's disease
Hypoganglionosis
Neuronal intestinal dysplasia
Chronic intestinal pseudo-obstruction
Nonfunctional
Functional
Megacystis–microcolon–intestinal hypoperistalsis syndrome

neuronal bodies in intramural nerve plexuses[108]. The majority of cases of neuronal dysplasia present with severe constipation but tend to spontaneously recover colonic motility between 6 and 12 months of age. Plain radiographs of the abdomen may show signs of obstruction of bowel and the barium enema may show dilatation of bowel. Diagnosis is by biopsy.

Chronic intestinal pseudo-obstruction (CIP) is rare and represents a spectrum of diseases that have in common clinical manifestations consisting of recurrent symptoms mimicking bowel obstruction over weeks or years. The age of presentation varies from newborn to adult. The condition is due to a visceral neuropathy or myopathy, which can be familial or nonfamilial, resulting in a lack of coordinated intestinal motility. Megacystis–microcolon–intestinal hypoperistalsis syndrome is the most severe form of CIP and is usually fatal in the first year of life. Immune deficiencies have also been reported to be linked to CIP.

Plain radiographs of the bowel will show dilated loops of bowel with air–fluid levels. A contrast medium enema can exclude mechanical obstruction in children with acute symptoms[109].

Abdominal trauma

Blunt abdominal trauma in children most often results in injury to the liver, spleen, and kidney, and management is conservative in those who are haemodynamically stable. The mechanism of injury is usually a road traffic accident, crush injury, or fall. Surgery is indicated in those who are haemodynamically unstable or have penetrating injuries or bowel rupture. The decision to operate on a child is clinical. Imaging will assist decisions about the intensity of conservative treatment or detect subtle findings in bowel injury and expedite surgical management[110].

Plain radiographs should include a supine abdominal radiograph and if possible an erect chest radiograph or decubitus abdominal radiograph, with the right side elevated if perforation is suspected. Fractures of the spine, pelvis, and ribs may be identified. CT is indicated in children with severe blunt abdominal trauma (Fig. 65.21, Table 65.10). US is less sensitive than CT

Table 65.10 CT SIGNS OF BOWEL INJURY
Free intraperitoneal fluid
Bowel wall thickening
Mesenteric haematoma
Extraluminal air
Bowel dilatation
Bowel wall enhancement
Extravasation of oral contrast

for detection of bowel and visceral injuries, but it has a role where CT is unavailable or may be delayed[111,112]. The radiological appearances in children are similar to those in adults. The detection of bowel and mesenteric injury can be more difficult. Prompt recognition is important, as surgical intervention may be required. The mechanism of injury is important. A history of bicycle handlebar injury, lap belt injuries, or suspected nonaccidental injury should arouse suspicion of bowel injury. Lap belt injuries are also often accompanied by injury to the lumbar spine due to hyperflexion, resulting in transverse fractures of L1 and L2 or a Chance fracture.

The **hypoperfusion complex** or shock bowel is due to poorly compensated hypovolaemic shock, which results in dilated, fluid-filled loops of bowel, and is a more frequent finding in children than adults. On CT there is intense contrast enhancement of the bowel wall, which may be thickened. The major abdominal blood vessels and kidneys also show intense enhancement, and the calibre of the aorta and inferior vena cava are reduced. Enhancement of the spleen and pancreas is decreased due to splanchnic vasoconstriction (Fig. 65.22).

Hepatic periportal low attenuation zones on CT are common in children who have hepatic injury, but also can be seen in children with nonhepatic visceral injury or in the absence of intra-abdominal injury[113,114]. There is high mortality associated with hypoperfusion complex. This abnormality (periportal tracking) is associated with physiological instability and a higher mortality

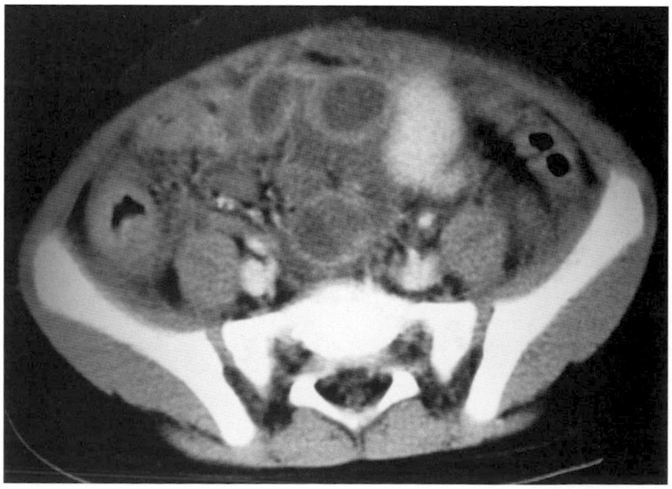

Figure 65.21 Jejunal perforation. Axial CT in a 13 year old boy following a lap belt injury to the abdomen shows subcutaneous haemorrhage, haemoperitoneum, free gas, dilatation of the small bowel, and bowel wall thickening.

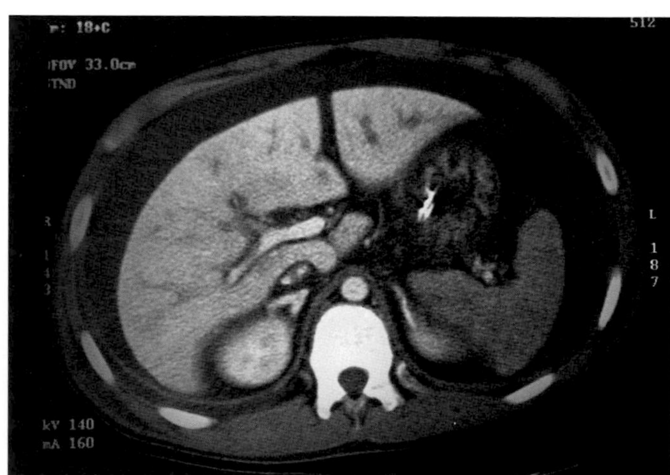

Figure 65.22 Hypoperfusion complex. Axial CT showing periportal low attenuation, small IVC, diminished and patchy enhancement of the spleen, intense enhancement of the adrenal glands and kidneys, and a haemoperitoneum.

rate. It is thought to be due to distension of the periportal lymphatics following vigorous hydration of haemodynamically unstable patients. It is not an indication for surgery.

Nonaccidental injury (NAI) Clinical presentation of NAI to the abdomen may be delayed for several days after the trauma has occurred, and is usually with abdominal pain, vomiting, signs of peritonism or obstruction. Bowel injury is more common in NAI than in accidental trauma. The duodenum and proximal jejunum are the most commonly injured parts of the bowel.

Perforation may be diagnosed on the plain radiograph. US may demonstrate a duodenal haematoma and more proximal bowel dilatation. In the acute phase, upper GI contrast medium studies will demonstrate the intramural mass, with thickening of the mucosal folds giving a 'coiled spring' appearance. Perforation of bowel, mesenteric or visceral injuries, or hypoperfusion syndrome may all be found in association with NAI and are best demonstrated by CT[115].

Nonbilious vomiting

Hypertropic pyloric stenosis (HPS) The aetiology of HPS is unknown. It presents with projectile vomiting. Associated clinical findings include weight loss, dehydration, and hypochloraemic alkalosis. The age of presentation is typically between 4 and 6 weeks. There is often a family history. It tends to occur in first born male infants (male-to-female ratio 3:1). No imaging is required if an experienced clinician can reliably palpate the hypertrophied pylorus.

US has proven to be an accurate method for the diagnosis of HPS and has replaced the barium meal in vomiting infants (Fig. 65.23, Table 65.11)[116]. Pylorospasm may mimic HPS on US. The measurements vary in pylorospasm with time, which can help distinguish it from HPS[117]. Occasionally, if US fails to confirm the diagnosis of HPS or if GOR is the likely diagnosis, a barium meal is performed. The pyloric canal is elongated ('string' sign) and indents the distal antrum to produce the 'tit' deformity (Fig. 65.24). Gastric emptying is delayed and GOR is usually present due to gastric outlet obstruction. Treatment is by pyloromyotomy.

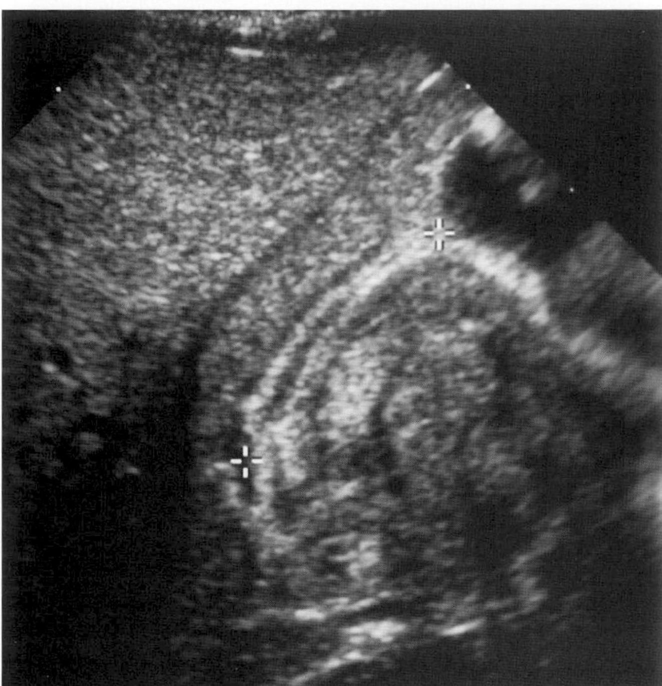

A

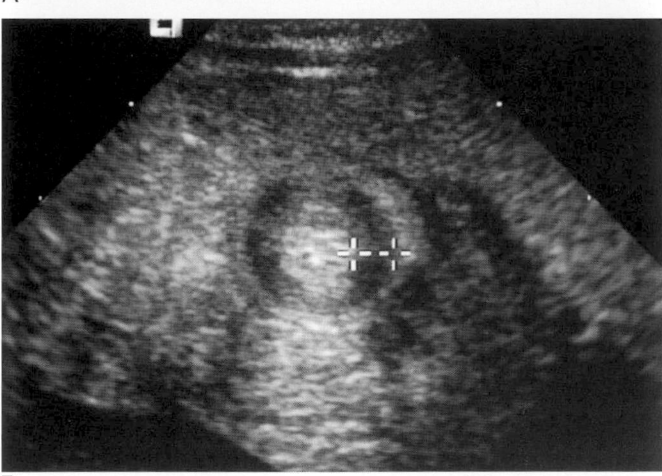

B

Figure 65.23 Hypertropic pyloric stenosis. (A) Longitudinal ultrasound shows the thickened hypo-echoic muscle. The margins of the pyloric canal appear as parallel, curvilinear echogenic lines. (B) Transverse ultrasound of the pylorus with central echogenic mucosa and surrounding hypo-echoic muscle.

Gastro-oesophageal reflux and hiatal hernia GOR is common in neonates and young children. In the majority of cases the reflux is physiological and is due to a poorly developed lower oesophageal sphincter, with a short intra-abdominal oesophageal course. As the child grows, the lower oesophageal sphincter matures and the GOR tends spontaneously to cease. Pathological reflux occurs when reflux oesophagitis or respiratory symptoms develop.

The most frequent presenting symptom of GOR is nonbilious vomiting. Other documented symptoms include failure to thrive and rectal bleeding, and in older children heartburn and dysphagia. Respiratory consequences of GOR include aspiration and pneumonia, exacerbation of reactive airways disease, and laryngospasm. GOR has also been implicated in apnoea and the sudden infant death syndrome[118,119]. Children with underlying chronic respiratory disease, neurological impairment or a history of oesophageal atresia repair have a higher incidence of reflux.

There is no agreed perfect method for detecting pathological GOR, but the current 'gold standard' is 24-h pH probe monitoring. An upper GI series is relatively insensitive for the

Table 65.11 ULTRASOUND FEATURES OF HYPERTROPIC PYLORIC STENOSIS
Canal length > 16 mm
Transverse pyloric diameter > 11 mm
Muscle wall thickness > 2.5 mm
Pyloric canal does not open
Gastric peristalsis is usually increased
Poor gastric emptying/large gastric residue

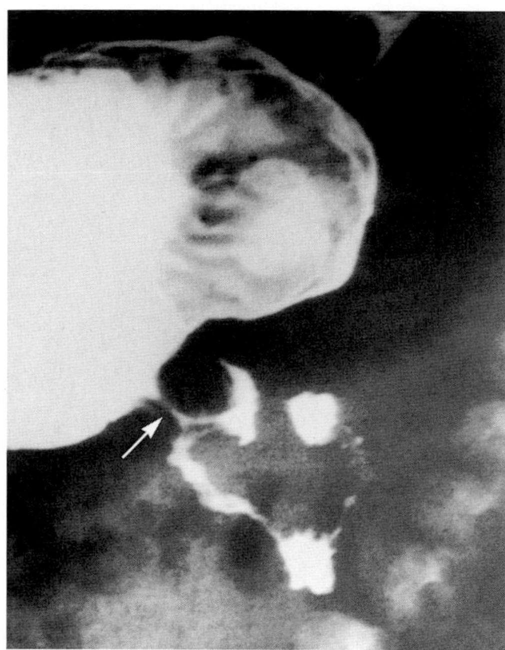

Figure 65.24 Hypertropic pyloric stenosis. Barium meal showing the narrow pyloric canal with a double track of barium. The hypertrophied pylorus indents the base of the duodenal cap.

detection of GOR, given the brief duration of the examination. Contrast medium studies are valuable to detect anatomical abnormalities which may be causing the child's symptoms, such as a hiatal hernia or an antral web, or occur consequent to the symptoms, such as a peptic oesophageal stricture. Hiatal hernias are uncommon in childhood but may be large and associated with severe GOR. A hiatal hernia is sometimes visualized as a retrocardiac mass on the frontal chest radiograph, often with an air–fluid level present. The majority of childhood hiatal hernias are of the sliding type, with the gastro-oesophageal junction seen above the level of the oesophageal diaphragmatic hiatus. The para-oesophageal ('rolling') type of hiatal hernia is rare in childhood. The stomach is displaced above the diaphragm and lies next to a normally positioned oesophagus.

Gastro-oesophageal scintigraphy, capturing images over the entire postprandial period, is more sensitive in the detection of GOR. Scintigraphy is performed using ^{99m}Tc-labelled sulphur colloid, which is mixed with formula feed or breast milk and given to the child orally. The number of episodes of GOR and the duration of each episode is documented.

US has also been used to detect reflux and to monitor gastric emptying[120,121], but is time consuming.

Surgery may be required in children who have persistent GOR and symptoms despite optimal medical therapy. The standard operation is the Nissen fundoplication; postoperative fluoroscopy can demonstrate a malpositioned fundoplication, loosening or breakdown of the wrap, oesophageal obstruction and perforation, and gastric volvulus[122].

Abdominal distension

Enteric duplication cysts are uncommon congenital anomalies and are due to abnormal canalization of the GI tract. They can occur anywhere along the length of the gut but are most frequent in the ileum where they lie along the mesenteric border and share a common muscle wall blood supply. They have a mucosal lining and 43% contain ectopic gastric mucosa. The majority of duplication cysts do not communicate with the GI tract. Duplication cysts may be diagnosed antenatally. Clinically they usually present in the first year of life with vomiting or abdominal pain. Less often presentation is with an asymptomatic palpable abdominal mass or melaena. Infection or haemorrhage into the cyst can cause it to enlarge and suddenly cause pain. A duplication cyst may act as a lead point of an intussusception. An oesophageal duplication can cause stridor.

Plain radiographs may show a mediastinal soft tissue mass in the case of an oesophageal duplication cyst or associated vertebral anomalies. An abdominal radiograph may show displacement of bowel loops by a mass or rarely gas might be seen in the cyst if there is communication with the GI tract. US will demonstrate the cyst, which is usually spherical in shape and less often tubular. It will have an inner echogenic mucosal layer and an outer hypo-echoic muscular layer (Fig. 65.25)[123]. Contrast medium studies may show displaced or obstructed loops of bowel. ^{99m}Tc-pertechnetate is taken up by ectopic gastric mucosa and is helpful in diagnosing duplication cysts which present with gastrointestinal bleeding[124].

Mesenteric cyst (lymphangioma) Intra-abdominal lymphangiomas are relatively rare and may be found in the mesentery, omentum, or retroperitoneum; the most common site is in the ileal mesentery. The cysts are true congenital abnormalities and arise due to sequestration of the mesenteric lymphatic vessels[125]. The cysts are lined by endothelial cells. Children usually present in the first decade, with increasing abdominal girth or a palpable abdominal mass. A more acute presentation can occur, with vomiting and abdominal pain following haemorrhage into the cyst, infection, or torsion. The cysts can grow large enough to cause intestinal or ureteric compression.

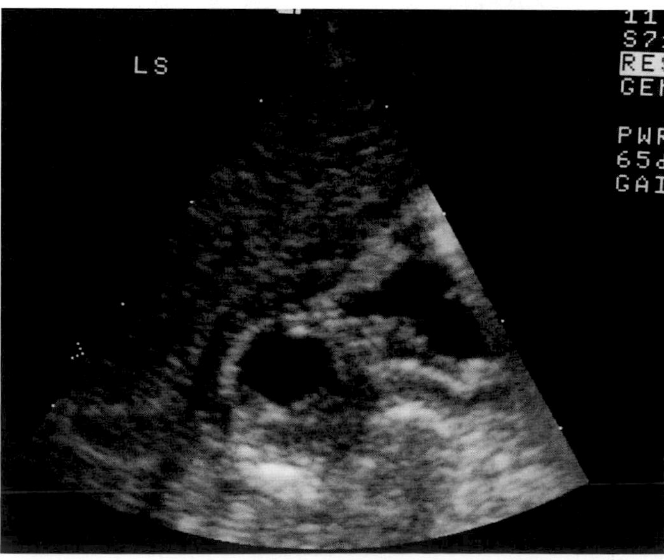

Figure 65.25 Duplication cyst of pylorus. Ultrasound showing echogenic mucosal layer and hypo-echoic outer muscular layer.

Plain abdominal radiographs show a soft tissue mass which displaces adjacent bowel loops. Occasionally the cyst wall is calcified. US examination demonstrates a thin-walled, uni- or multi-locular cystic mass that may be adherent to the solid organs and bowel. The cyst wall consists of a single layer, which contrasts with the double layered wall seen with enteric duplication cysts. If the intracystic fluid is chylous, infected, or haemorrhagic, then echogenic debris will be present. CT and MRI more precisely define the anatomical margins of the cyst (Fig. 65.26). The thin septae are more difficult to visualize with CT than US, but may enhance following the administration of intravenous contrast material. The attenuation values of the cyst contents vary; an uncomplicated lesion will have attenuation values similar to those of water. Negative attenuation values may be recorded if the fluid is chylous, and haemorrhagic and infected cysts have increased attenuation values. The MRI characteristics will similarly vary, depending upon the cyst contents.

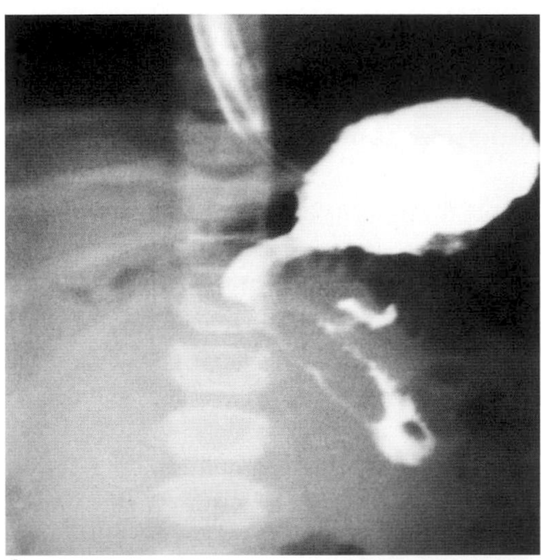

A

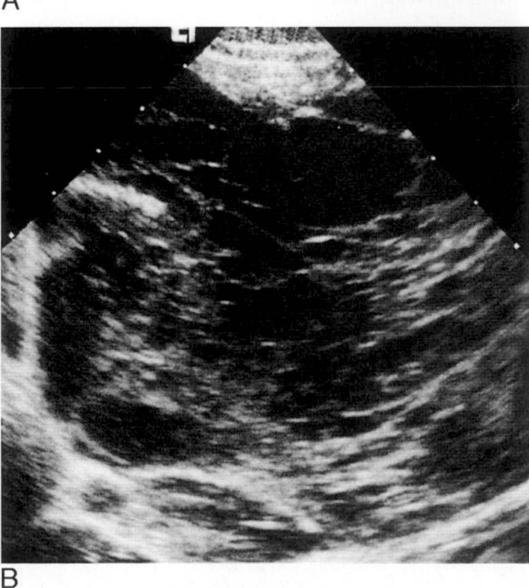

B

Figure 65.26 Mesenteric cyst. (A) Upper GI contrast medium study performed in a patient with bilious vomiting shows extrinsic duodenal compression and displacement by a central abdominal mass. (B) The mass is confirmed to be a septated cyst at ultrasound.

Malabsorption

Malabsorption is a non-specific finding occurring in many childhood diseases (Table 65.12). When clinically suspected, the diagnosis is made by jejunal biopsy. Only a few of these conditions are important to the paediatric radiologist. Structural abnormalities causing malabsorption include malrotation, blind loop syndrome, or short gut syndrome. Malabsorption secondary to short gut syndrome can occur in a neonate who has had a large length of small bowel surgically excised, e.g. for multiple small bowel atresia. Flocculation, fragmentation, and segmentation of barium are non-specific signs of malabsorption (Fig. 65.27).

Gastrointestinal bleeding

GI bleeding in infancy and childhood can involve any part of the intestinal tract. The causes are varied (Table 65.13). The age of the child and clinical presentation may enable a diagnosis to be made or narrow the differential diagnosis and then appropriate imaging will allow a specific diagnosis to be made, e.g. intussusception, HSP, and NEC. In many other cases fibre-optic endoscopy and biopsy can identify the sources of the bleeding. Other techniques that may be required include ^{99m}Tc-sulphur colloid or labelled red blood cell scintigraphy and occasionally angiography if there is continued or recurrent haemorrhage[126].

Inflammatory bowel disease

Inflammatory bowel disease (IBD) presents in childhood in approximately 25% of cases. The radiology is described in more detail in Chapter 33. The aetiology of IBD in children includes ulcerative colitis, Crohn's disease, infective colitis, typhlitis, radiation enteritis, graft versus host disease, and Kawasaki syndrome. Often the cause is clinically obvious, e.g. neutropenic colitis. Investigation is similar to adults. US has a greater role in children as bowel imaging is easier[127,128]. Thickened bowel

Table 65.12 CAUSES OF MALABSORPTION
Cystic fibrosis
Coeliac disease
Cows' milk protein sensitivity
Disaccharidase deficiency
Malrotation
Previous gut resection
Blind loop syndrome
Eosinophilic gastroenteritis
Graft versus host disease
Immunoglobulin A deficiency syndrome
Schwachman–Diamond syndrome
Hereditary angioneurotic oedema
Intestinal lymphangiectasia
Tropical sprue
Microvillus inclusion disease
Zollinger–Ellison syndrome
Abetalipoproteinaemia

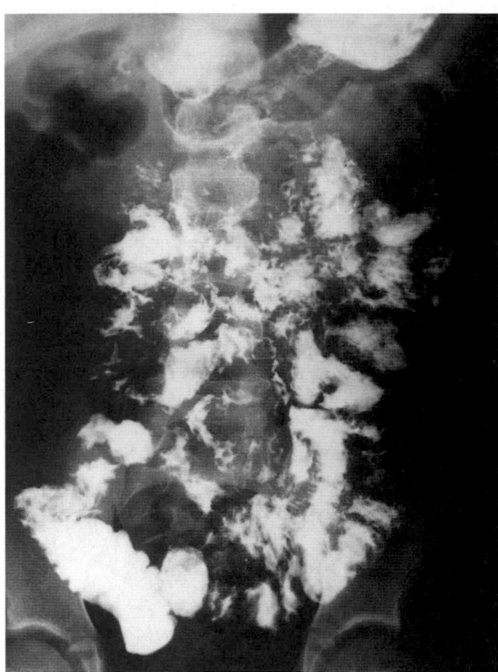

Figure 65.27 Malabsorption. Small bowel series showing segmentation and flocculation of barium, and mild dilatation of the bowel in a child with coeliac disease.

is the typical finding, but is non-specific. Most children with IBD present with weight loss and diarrhoea. Crohn's disease may present at any age, often with failure to thrive, abdominal pain, and chronic low grade fever, in addition to the usual symptoms. Endoscopy and barium studies will diagnose most cases of childhood Crohn's disease. Further imaging with US and radionuclide studies with labelled white cells may be required if endoscopy and barium studies are negative and there is strong clinical suspicion, although CT can be unreliable in the proximal bowel[129]. CT is useful for demonstrating abdominal abscesses. Gadolinuim-enhanced MRI has also been described in the diagnosis of IBD, though it is not used routinely[130].

Table 65.13 CAUSES OF GASTROINTESTINAL BLEEDING
Necrotizing enterocolitis
Intussusception
Midgut volvulus
Anal fissure
Gastroenteritis
Typhilitis
Henoch–Schönlein purpura
Meckel's diverticulum
Polyposis syndromes
Inflammatory bowel disease
Haemolytic uraemic syndrome
Foreign body
Peptic ulceration
Vascular malformation

Polyposis syndromes

Intestinal polyposis syndromes are rare in children. They are more commonly found in adult life and are described in Chapter 33. They include familial polyposis coli, Gardner syndrome, Turcot syndrome, juvenile polyposis coli, Peutz–Jegher's syndrome, and generalized polyposis coli[131,132]. Most have an autosomal dominant mode of inheritance and many have a significant risk of malignancy. The colon is predominantly affected in polyposis syndromes, with the exception of Peutz–Jegher's syndrome, which mainly affects the small bowel[133].

Juvenile polyposis coli is a rare condition in which multiple polyps occur in the colon. The polyps do not have malignant potential but there is an association with a family history of large bowel malignancy. Presentation is in the first decade of life, most often between 4 and 6 years of age. Rectal bleeding is the usual presenting complaint; anaemia, intussusception, and rectal prolapse can occur. The polyps are thought to be mucous retention cysts occurring secondary to inflammation.

Double contrast medium GI studies are the gold standard radiological methods for diagnosis. US and MRI can demonstrate polyps and could be used for follow-up, but polyps less than 1.5 cm in diameter may be missed on MRI and clusters of polyps may be seen as a mass lesion[132].

Gastrointestinal tumours

Gastrointestinal tumours are rare in children. Endoscopy may diagnose tumours in the upper GI tract and large bowel. Benign tumours may occur as part of a syndrome, e.g. polyposis syndromes. They may all present in childhood but are more common in adults. Presentation may be with gastrointestinal bleeding, anaemia, and abdominal pain. The neoplasm can act as a lead point for intussusception. Imaging is by double contrast medium barium enema, small bowel series, and/or CT.

Lymphoma is the most common primary malignant intestinal tumour in childhood. Involvement of the bowel and mesentery is almost always caused by non-Hodgkin's lymphoma and is rare in Hodgkin's disease. It is usually found in the ileocaecal region and may present with abdominal pain, mass, bowel obstruction, weight loss, or intussusception. Bowel involvement with Hodgkin's disease is usually caused by direct invasion from adjacent involved lymph nodes. US is useful for initial imaging. CT is required for staging; it can identify tumour in the bowel wall and may show additional disease in the abdominal lymph nodes, liver, spleen, or kidneys. Barium studies may show strictures, obstruction, mass lesions, or ulceration (Fig. 65.28)[134]. Positron emission tomography (PET)–CT has a role in staging and evaluating tumour response to therapy[135,136].

Omphalomesenteric (vitelline) duct remnants

The omphalomesenteric (vitelline) duct is a normal fetal structure that connects the midgut to the extra-embryonic yolk sac. It runs alongside the allantois (later the urachus/median umbilical ligament) within the umbilical cord. The omphalomesenteric duct usually involutes in the mid first trimester. Its persistence can give rise to a variety of congenital malformations.

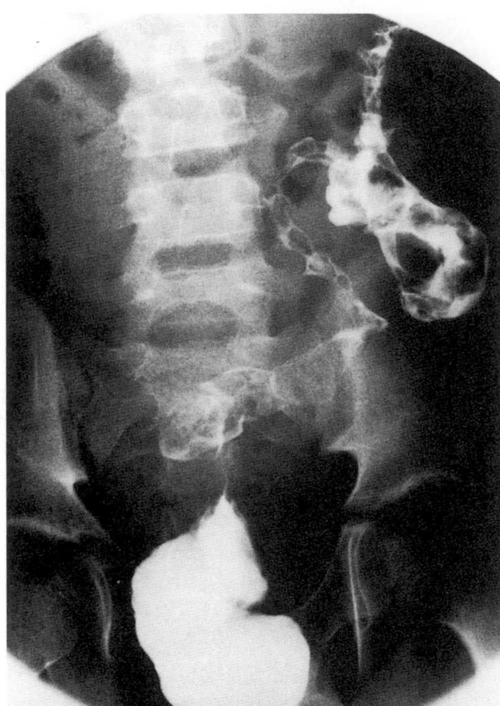

Figure 65.28 Lymphoma of the large bowel in a 9 year old boy who presented with constipation. Barium enema shows narrow, irregular descending and sigmoid colons.

Table 65.14 COMPLICATIONS OF OMPHALOMESENTERIC DUCT REMNANTS
Diverticulitis ± perforation
Bleeding (ectopic gastric mucosa)
Enterolith formation
Nonhaemorrhagic inflammation and ulceration secondary to the presence of ectopic mucosa
Gastric
Pancreatic
Duodenal
Colonic
Biliary
Intussusception
Fibrous bands
Obstruction
Volvulus
Internal hernias
Littre's hernias (prolapse of the diverticulum into an inguinal hernia sac)
Impacted foreign bodies
Wall inflammation
Perforation
Ileal prolapse onto the anterior abdominal wall
Omphalomesenteric fistula
Umbilical sinus
Mucosal polyp, granulation tissue, or cyst at the umbilicus

The majority of symptomatic omphalomesenteric ducts occur in boys and patients most commonly present before the age of 2 years. The clinical symptoms and signs depend upon the underlying abnormality (Table 65.14). If the entire duct remains patent, then there is a discharge of faeces from the umbilicus or the ileum can prolapse onto the anterior abdominal wall. Injection of contrast medium into a discharging umbilical fistula will outline loops of ileum when the omphalomesenteric duct is wholly patent.

Meckel's diverticulum The most common type of omphalomesenteric duct remnant is the Meckel's diverticulum, which arises on the antimesenteric border of the ileum. The diverticulum is present in 2–4% of V population. The size of Meckel's diverticula varies with those greater than 5 cm in length being considered 'giant'. Most are located within 60 cm of the ileocaecal junction. All the layers of the intestine are contained within their walls and frequently islands of gastric and/or pancreatic mucosa are seen within them. The typical clinical presentation of a child with a Meckel's diverticulum is with melaena or abdominal pain. Intussusception or a volvulus around a Meckel's diverticulum presents with symptoms and signs of a small bowel obstruction. Peritonitis may follow perforation of a Meckel's diverticulum.

Meckel's diverticula which haemorrhage contain ectopic gastric mucosa in 95% of cases[137] and ^{99m}Tc-pertechnetate scintigraphy can be diagnostic. The sensitivity of this investigation is increased when the patient receives premedication with ranitidine[138]. Differential diagnoses of a positive result include ectopic mucosa in an enteric duplication cyst, haemangiomata and IBD.

ABDOMINAL MANIFESTATIONS OF CYSTIC FIBROSIS

Cystic fibrosis is an inherited autosomal recessive disease. Pulmonary disease is the predominant cause of mortality. The GI complications of cystic fibrosis result from abnormally viscid secretions within hollow viscera and ducts of solid organs. Bowel obstruction due to meconium ileus or meconium plug syndrome may be present at birth (see above).

Distal intestinal obstruction syndrome

Distal intestinal obstruction syndrome (DIOS) presents in 10–15% of older children with cystic fibrosis as colicky abdominal pain, constipation, and a palpable mass in the right iliac fossa due to impaction of mucofaeculent material in the terminal ileum and right colon[139]. Abdominal distension, nausea, and vomiting are common. DIOS is potentially fatal and can mimic other causes of abdominal pain, e.g. acute appendicitis, intussusception, or subacute obstruction of small bowel due to stricture or adhesions.

Radiographs of the abdomen will show faecal loading of the colon, a bubbly appearance or mass in the right side of the abdomen, and dilated loops of small bowel (Fig. 65.29). Treatment is with oral Gastrografin and, if required, a Gastrografin enema to soften and mobilize the stool.

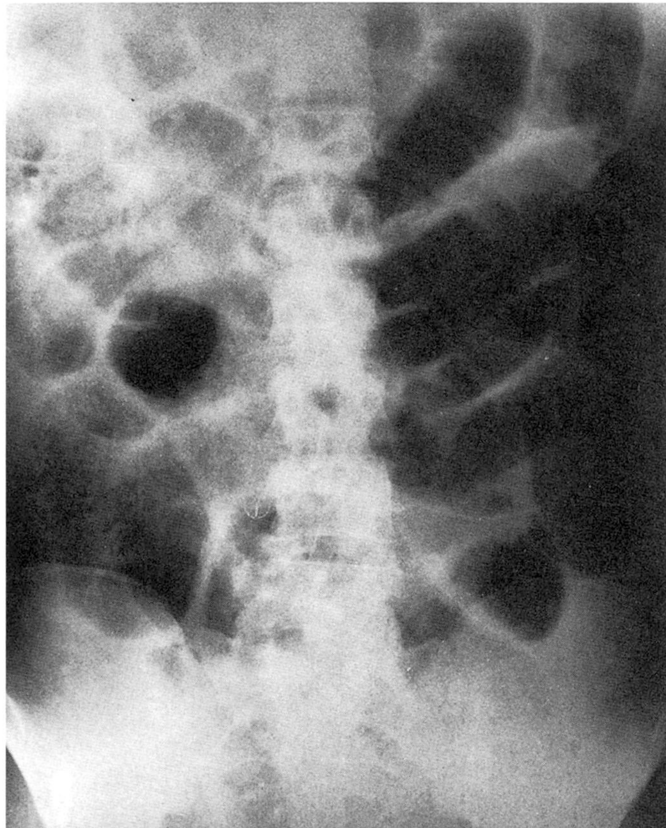

Figure 65.29 Distal intestinal obstruction syndrome. Supine abdominal radiograph shows faecal loading, with a bubbly appearance in the right side of the abdomen and dilated loops of small bowel.

Intussusception

Intussusception occurs as a complication of cystic fibrosis in 1% of patients. The average age of presentation is 9–12 years, much older than in idiopathic intussusception. It is thought that the thick, putty-like faeces act as a lead point. The intussusceptions are usually ileocolic, although transient ileo-ileal intussusception can also occur. Common presenting symptoms include colicky abdominal pain and vomiting. It can present in a similar way to DIOS and delay the diagnosis. The passage of bloody stool is less common. Clinical examination can be normal.

The imaging findings of intussusception in cystic fibrosis are the same as those seen in idiopathic intussusception.

Fibrosing colonopathy

Colonic stricture is a recognized complication in children and can lead to intestinal obstruction[140]. It is due to irreversible and sometimes progressive narrowing of the bowel lumen. High strength pancreatic enzyme supplements have been implicated in the aetiology. The right side of the colon is most frequently affected. Presentation is with signs and symptoms of distal intestinal obstruction.

Plain radiographs occasionally can be helpful by demonstrating thickening of the colon wall. MRI can also be used to evaluate patients with fibrosing colonopathy[141]. US has been shown to be useful in assessing the thickness of the colonic wall[142,143]. Contrast medium enema findings include loss of haustration, shortening of the colon, narrowing of the colonic lumen, and nodular thickening of the colonic wall. Treatment is by surgical resection of the affected segment. Histological findings include submucosal fibrosis and fatty infiltration.

Other bowel manifestations

The duodenum and small bowel are frequently abnormal in older children with cystic fibrosis. Thickened nodular mucosal folds can be demonstrated on the upper gastrointestinal series. Peptic ulcer, GOR, and associated complications of oesophagitis and oesophageal stricture are well recognized in cystic fibrosis. The US criteria for acute appendicitis are not reliable in children with cystic fibrosis as the appendix in asymptomatic children is often larger than normal[144].

Pancreatic abnormalities

Pancreatic insufficiency occurs in 80–85% of children with cystic fibrosis and manifests as malabsorption, chiefly of fat and protein. Approximately 30–50% of patients have glucose intolerance and 1–2% require insulin therapy[140].

Plain radiography of the abdomen may show punctate calcification in the distribution of the pancreas. US may show a small echogenic pancreas. The CT and MRI appearance depends on the amount of fatty replacement and degree of pancreatic fibrosis (Fig. 65.30).

Hepatobiliary disease

In children with cystic fibrosis, cirrhosis of the liver may result from impaired bile drainage due to inspissated bile or fibrosis, and the prevalence increases with age. US abnormalities of the liver include a heterogeneous echo pattern, parenchymal nodularity, and periportal increased echogenicity due to fibrosis. The gallbladder may be small and the wall thickened due to chronic cholecystitis. Gallstones are found in up to 10% of children with cystic fibrosis. US findings in portal hypertension include splenic enlargement and gastric varices at the porta hepatitis. Clinical signs of cirrhosis in children

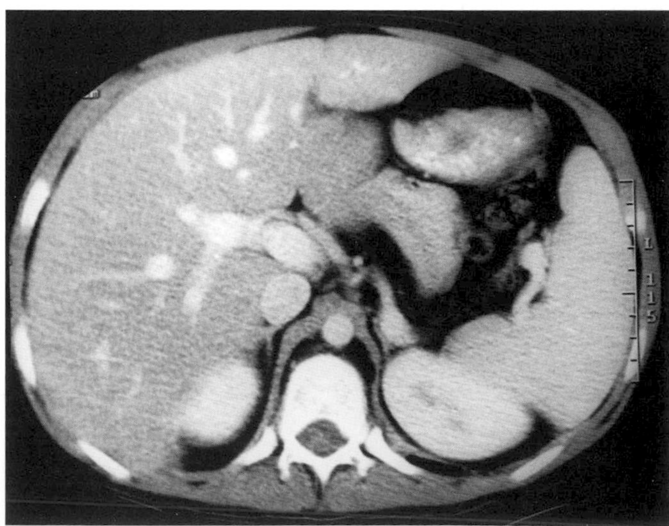

Figure 65.30 Axial CT of the pancreas in child with cystic fibrosis, showing fatty replacement of the pancreas.

may occur late, by which time the disease is advanced. US can detect liver disease before it manifests itself clinically and biochemically[145–147].

Intra-abdominal malignancy

There have been several reports of GI malignancy occurring in patients with cystic fibrosis, the frequency increasing as the survival of these children improves. The lesions include cancers of the oesophagus, stomach, small bowel, colon, liver, biliary tract, pancreas, and rectum[148].

THE IMMUNOCOMPROMISED CHILD

Gastrointestinal manifestations of acquired immune deficiency syndrome

Opportunistic infections account for most of the GI tract manifestations of acquired immune deficiency syndrome (AIDS) in children[149]. Primary lymphoma and Kaposi's sarcoma occur in the adult GI tract but are rare in human immunodeficiency virus (HIV) infected children. The most common symptoms include acute or chronic diarrhoea, failure to thrive, oesophagitis due to candida, and less often cytomegalovirus (CMV) or herpes simplex virus. Imaging with double-contrast medium upper GI studies will accurately diagnose oesophageal lesions of candidiasis.

Persistent chronic or recurrent diarrhoea can be caused by a number of organisms, including cryptosporidium, giardia, and *Mycobacterium avium–intracellulare* complex. Imaging is not usually required. Small bowel obstruction secondary to intussusception can occur in AIDS; a lead point such as lymphoma should be sought. Colitis in children with AIDS is also common and is caused by a number of organisms including shigella, salmonella, abdominal tuberculosis, and CMV. Presentation is usually with crampy abdominal pain and fever. Plain abdominal radiographs may show colonic dilatation, oedema, and thumbprinting of the bowel wall, and sometimes pneumatosis intestinalis.

Abdominal lymphadenopathy is common in paediatric AIDS. It can be caused by infection, idiopathic lymph node enlargement where no cause is found, or Kaposi's sarcoma and lymphoma[150]. US is useful in the evaluation of the abdomen for lymphadenopathy. CT has the advantage that other intra-abdominal organs, the bowel, and mesentery can also be assessed.

Section 3 contains further descriptions of the GI tract manifestations of AIDS.

Typhlitis

Typhlitis or neutropenic colitis is a complication of treatment of childhood malignancy or bone marrow transplantation. Presentation is with severe abdominal pain, often in the right iliac fossa, diarrhoea and fever. The caecum and ascending colon are most often involved. Bacterial and fungal infection of the bowel wall leads to inflammation and oedema, and occasionally haemorrhage and necrosis.

The findings on the plain abdominal radiograph are non-specific and include thickening of the colonic wall causing thumbprinting, small bowel dilatation, a mass in the right iliac fossa, and occasionally pneumatosis coli. US and CT will show colonic wall thickening, ascites, pericaecal fluid, and an inflammatory mass if present. In children, US is usually preferred because of its portability and lack of ionizing radiation (Fig. 65.31)[151–153].

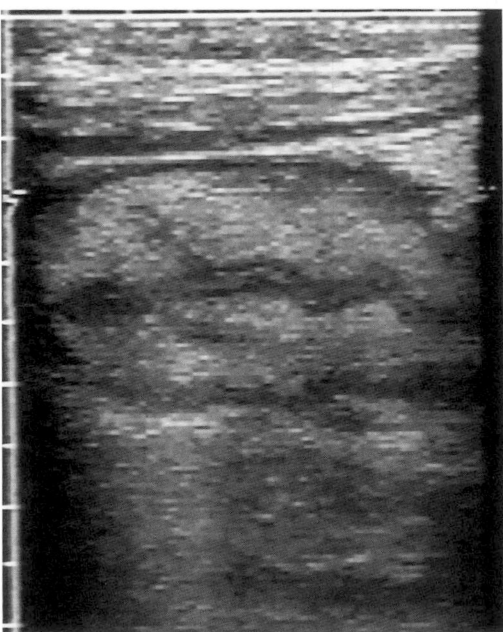

A

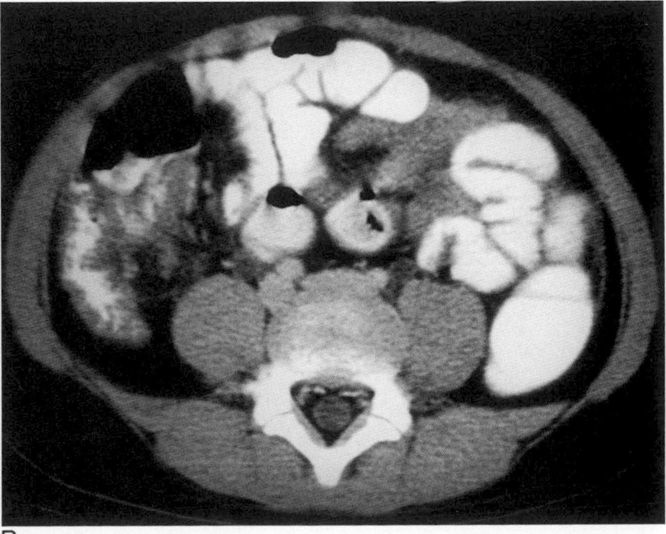

B

Figure 65.31 Typhlitis. (A) Ultrasound showing thickened bowel wall. (B) Axial CT showing thickening of the wall of the ascending colon.

MISCELLANEOUS GASTROINTESTINAL PROBLEMS

Foreign body ingestion

Ingestion of foreign bodies is common in children. The majority will pass uneventfully through the GI tract. The most common site of hold up in the oesophagus is at the level of the cricopharyngeus (80%). Oesophageal foreign bodies may rarely become embedded in the oesophageal wall causing oedema and compression of the trachea. Perforation of the oesophagus is rare. There is usually a history of choking, coughing, excessive salivation, dysphagia, or vomiting. Some children with impacted coins are asymptomatic. Infants may present with stridor and airway obstruction.

A lateral radiograph of the soft tissues of the neck and a frontal radiograph of the chest and abdomen will readily demonstrate the majority of opaque foreign bodies (Fig. 65.32)[154]. If the type of foreign body ingested is known it can be helpful to X-ray the object to assess its density. A barium swallow will be required to make the diagnosis of an impacted nonopaque foreign body[155,156]. Batteries are important to recognize because if not removed they can corrode and leak causing caustic burns in the stomach[157]. Ingestion of multiple magnets can cause necrosis, ulceration, and even perforation of bowel when two magnets in separate loops of bowel are attracted together[158,159]. Removal of foreign bodies from the oesophagus is by oesophagoscopy. Extraction of foreign bodies using a Foley catheter under fluoroscopy has been described, but it is a potentially hazardous procedure and oesophagoscopy is considered the safest technique for removal of oesophageal foreign bodies[160].

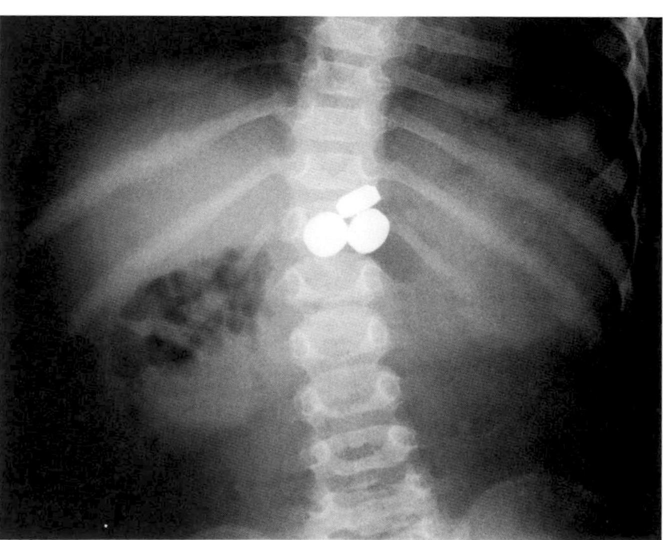

Figure 65.32 Ingested batteries in the stomach.

Caustic ingestion

The substances most often swallowed include household cleaning products, alkaline caustics, and acids. Caustic substances can cause burns to the mouth, ulceration, necrosis, and perforation of the oesophagus, and later stricture formation is common. Acid gastric secretions tend to neutralize the ingested alkalis and reduce damage to the stomach.

In the acute phase in severe cases the chest radiograph may show a dilated air-filled atonic oesophagus. Oesophagoscopy will demonstrate the extent and severity of the oesophageal involvement and imaging is not usually required. If the endoscopic examination was limited because of the risk of oesophageal perforation, upper GI contrast medium studies using water-soluble contrast medium may be required to show the extent of the oesophagitis in the acute phase (Fig. 65.33)[161,162]. In the healing phase contrast medium studies will demonstrate oesophageal strictures. These may require serial dilatation. Carcinoma arising in caustic strictures can occur many years after the initial injury[163].

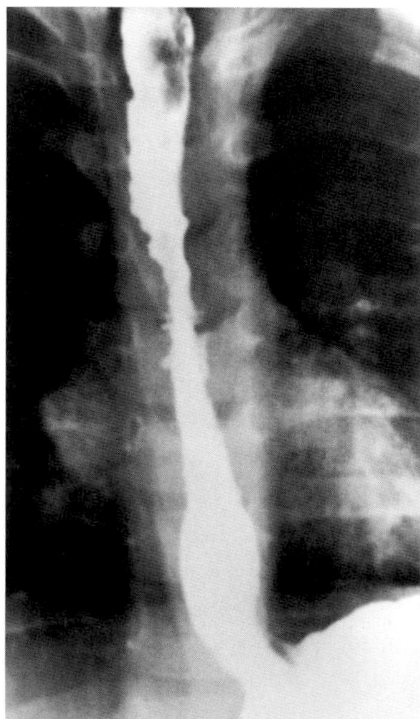

Figure 65.33 Corrosive oesophagitis. Upper GI contrast medium study showing oesophageal ulceration and narrowing of the middle third, due to oedema.

THE PAEDIATRIC LIVER, BILIARY SYSTEM AND SPLEEN

LIVER DISORDERS

Imaging techniques

Paediatric hepatic and splenic imaging employs many useful and complementary techniques[164–167]. US is the optimal technique for most paediatric and neonatal conditions of the liver and spleen. New high-resolution US equipment enables exquisite detail of liver anatomy, parenchymal information, as well as vascular/perfusion information with colour, pulse wave, and power Doppler imaging. Choice of probe is age and size dependent (vector 3.5–8 MHz; linear 7–10 MHz for parenchymal abnormalities). Other cross-sectional imaging techniques (CT, MRI) have many advantages for the display of anatomy and disease, but have inherent limitations of radiation, spatial resolution, lack of body fat in neonates, need for sedation and/or availability. Experience with MR venography (MRV), MR angiography (MRA), and MR cholangiography (MRC) in children is still growing[167–170]. Physiology, anatomy, and functional information is available with radionuclide imaging[171–173]. The role for PET/CT is still being established. Percutaneous transhepatic (transcholecystic) cholangiography (PTC or PTTC) maintains a role in therapeutic procedures. Since the development of the paediatric duodenoscope, endoscopic retrograde cholangiopancreatography (ERCP) plays a complementary diagnostic and therapeutic role even in the young child[174]. The diagnostic role of angiography is limited; however, it is essential in select therapeutic interventions. Percutaneous image guided procedures such as biopsy, drainages, biliary stenting, and embolizations are performed with accuracy, safety, and increasing frequency in children.

Diagnostic approach

Newborn infants or children require evaluation for a wide variety of congenital and acquired abnormalities, anatomical and functional disorders, infections, and inherited inborn errors of metabolism. The various associations between congenital abnormalities and syndromes must be remembered, e.g. renal cystic disease with hepatic fibrosis, congenital cardiac lesions with left- and right-sided isomerism, and TORCH (toxoplasma, orphan virus, rubella, CMV, and herpes virus) infections with liver, spleen, and brain involvement[175].

Clear communication and multidisciplinary teamwork with the referring physicians are essential to evaluate appropriately the clinical question. Clinically relevant and timely reports must be provided. In interventional cases, communication regarding preprocedural correction of coagulation abnormalities, diagnostic and therapeutic aims of the procedure, and alternatives is imperative.

Anatomy and normal variants

At about 4 weeks of gestation, the caudal portion of the foregut develops as a ventral outgrowth into the liver and biliary tree. The liver develops from the larger cranial portion of the hepatic diverticulum, and the smaller caudal portion develops into the gallbladder and cystic duct[176].

The newborn liver is less reflective on US than the echogenic newborn kidney. Commonly by 3–4 months of age this has reverted to the reverse adult pattern. The liver is normally right sided, but may be transverse and symmetric in the midline (bridging) as in polysplenia or asplenia, or left sided as in situs inversus. It is distinguished from the spleen in these situations by its internal portal and hepatic venous anatomy, echogenic portal vein walls, and the location of the gallbladder if present. Congenital agenesis or hypoplasia of a lobe is unusual, but is more common on the left than the right. Acquired atrophy may be due to left portal vein occlusion.

The newborn extrahepatic biliary tree is difficult to see without new high-resolution US equipment. The proximal intrahepatic ducts should not exceed 2 mm in diameter. There is a normogram available for normal sized biliary structures according to age. The upper limit of normal for the common bile duct is 2 mm (<1.27 mm) for the first year, 4 mm (<3.3 mm) for older children, and less than 7 mm for adolescents/adults[177]. The normal gallbladder is at least 1.5 cm in neonates, reaching a maximum in children of 7.5 cm in length and 3.5 cm in diameter[178].

In the neonate, the umbilical vein runs in the falciform ligament from the umbilicus to the anterior surface of the liver, where it divides the medial and lateral segments of the left lobe; it intersects the left portal vein and runs from there via the ductus venosis into the inferior vena cava (IVC) (Fig. 65.34)[179]. The ductus venosis and umbilical vein are patent in the premature or early newborn (<48 h) and in two-thirds of those up to 1 week of age; they obliterate within 2–3 weeks and become highly reflective and may calcify. Patency beyond this period or recanalization of a previously obliterated umbilical vein (+ collaterals) is associated with portal hypertension or abnormalities in the venous drainage of the liver. Variations in

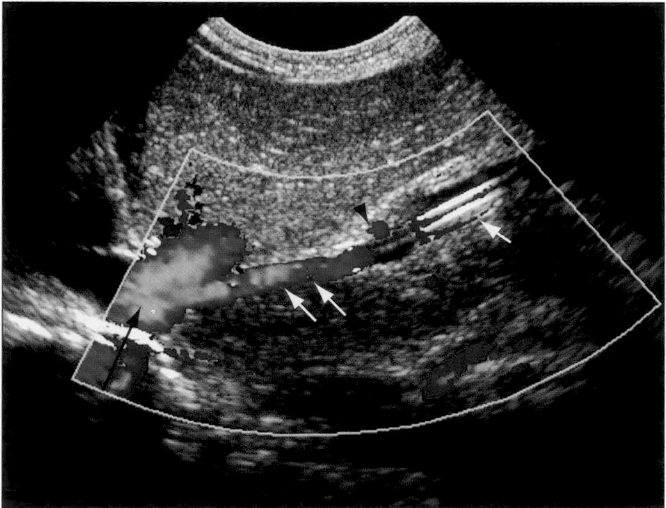

Figure 65.34 Liver. Venous anatomy in newborn. Ultrasound sagittal view through the liver showing an umbilical vein catheter in the umbilical vein (single white arrow) approaching the left portal vein (arrowhead). Blood flow is seen by colour Doppler in the ductus venosus (double arrows) as it enters the inferior vena cava (single black arrow).

venous anatomy of the liver are common. Preduodenal portal vein (seen on US or CT uncommonly) may be associated with biliary atresia.

The normal size of the spleen increases with age, the long axis approximately 6 cm at 3 months, 7 cm at 1 year, 8 cm at 2 years, 9 cm at 4 years, 10 cm at 8 years, and 12–13 cm at 15 years[180]. Anomalies of splenic size, number, and position are common. The spleen may vary in position, 'a wandering spleen'. When the spleen has a long mesenteric pedicle it may tort and infarct. Accessory spleens occur in 10% of the normal population: 90% are solitary, 9% are double, and less than 3% are multiple (Fig. 65.35). Accessory spleens, remaining following splenectomy for haematological problems, may hypertrophy and cause recurrent disease. Multiple functional peritoneal deposits of splenic tissue 'splenosis' may occur post traumatic rupture of the spleen or surgical splenectomy. Splenogonadal fusion is a rare variant occurring as a fibrous band or a tongue of ectopic splenic tissue (usually left sided and in boys).

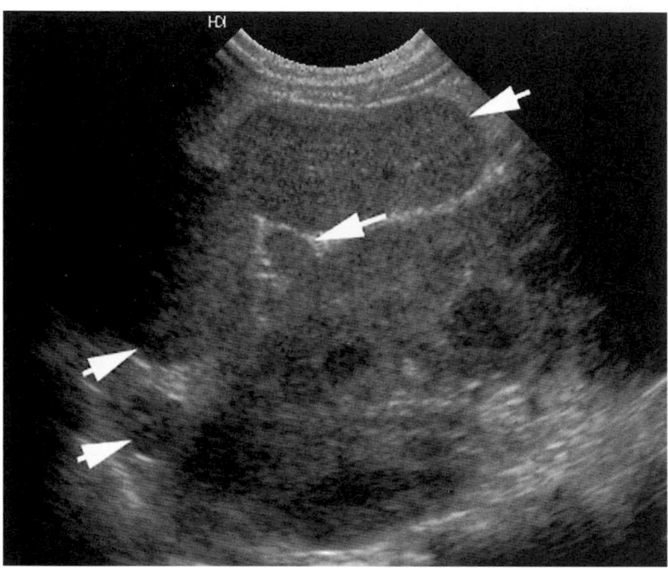

Figure 65.35 Accessory spleens. Patient with left atrial isomerism and numerous splenunculi seen on ultrasound adjacent to the left kidney. This patient also had a midline liver, interruption of the inferior vena cava with hemi-azygos continuation, as well as polysplenia.

The normal spleen on CT has a higher attenuation than liver and enhances heterogeneously in the early phase of enhancement. On MRI, the spleen has lower signal intensity on T1-weighted imaging than liver and slightly greater signal intensity than muscle. On T2-weighted images, the spleen has higher signal intensity than the liver.

Liver and spleen abnormalities are associated with cardiac isomerisms (right isomerisms with asplenia, midline gallbladder, two right lobes of liver, GI malrotation; left isomerism with polysplenia, midline liver, interruption of the IVC with azygos continuation of the IVC and preduodenal portal vein, biliary atresia, and may be splenogonadal fusion)[175]. Once one anomaly has been identified, the radiologist should search for other anomalies (Fig. 65.36).

Jaundice

Prolonged neonatal jaundice (>10 d) is common. Causes of neonatal jaundice include physiological jaundice of prematurity, breast milk jaundice, ABO incompatibility, and other haemolytic jaundice, and sepsis of any cause. If the cause is clear, the infant does not require liver imaging. Metabolic causes, though uncommon, are an important group in the newborn period (galactosaemia, α_1-antitypsin deficiency, cystic fibrosis, etc.). Clinical information regarding the gestational age of the infant, perinatal history, age of onset of jaundice, and the distinction between unconjugated and conjugated hyperbilirubinaemia is required. Unconjugated hyperbilirubinaemia is caused by prehepatic and hepatic forms of liver disease. Conjugated hyperbilirubinaemia (almost always pathological)

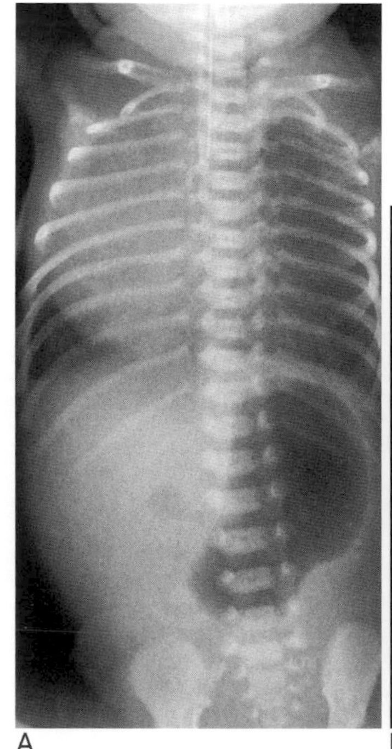

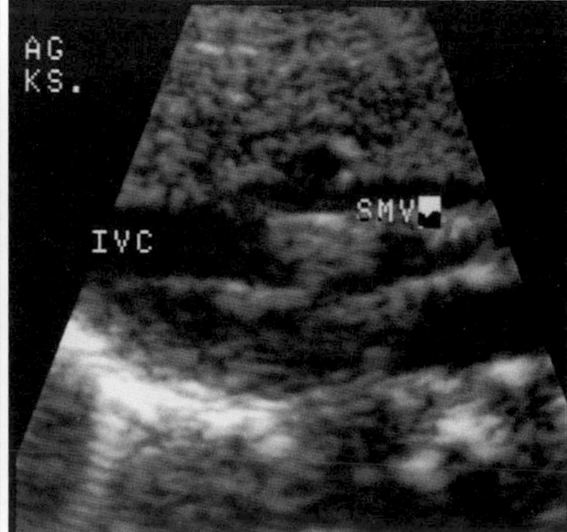

A B

Figure 65.36 Congenital abnormalities. (A) Neonate with multiple congenital abnormalities. Note the duodenal atresia with 'double bubble' sign, the dextrocardia, the nasogastric tube arrested at the T3 level suggestive of oesophageal atresia, and because of the gas in the stomach it therefore represents a tracheo-oesophageal fistula. (B) This child was found to have an absent portal vein with the superior mesenteric vein draining into the inferior vena cava as seen on the longitudinal ultrasound view.

can be divided into the extrahepatic obstructive forms—biliary atresia, Alagille syndrome, biliary hypoplasia, choledocal cyst, etc, and the hepatic forms—total parental nutrition (TPN), cholestasis, etc.[181,182]. Up to 80% of infants referred with persistent jaundice have biliary atresia or neonatal hepatitis. A multidisciplinary approach to the evaluation of neonatal jaundice up to and including liver biopsy is necessary. Jaundice in later life may result from a myriad of congenital, inherited, and acquired causes, which overlap with those seen in adults.

Biliary atresia In the infant with prolonged neonatal jaundice (defined as longer than 10 d), the diagnosis of biliary atresia is urgent, as outcome depends on early diagnosis and surgical establishment of biliary drainage before the onset of cirrhosis[183]. The distinction between biliary atresia and biliary hypoplasia and neonatal hepatitis can be difficult as imaging features may overlap[181]. The role for MRI and PTC/PTTC is still evolving.

In biliary atresia, the infant presents in the neonatal period with persisting (slightly fluctuating) jaundice, pale stools, and hepatomegaly. It is slightly more common in girls. The aetiology is uncertain (perinatal/embryonic; environmental, infectious, immune and genetic aetiologies have been suggested) but the result is a progressive obliterative inflammatory process, affecting the extrahepatic biliary tree and progressing centrally towards the intrahepatic interlobar ducts[184–186]. It is classified into different types (Fig. 65.37).

On US, the liver becomes large and coarse, with increased periportal reflectivity. Unlike obstructive jaundice in the older child or adult, the biliary tree in biliary atresia does not usually distend or dilate, due to the obliterative inflammatory process. The gallbladder is usually absent or rudimentary; it is visible but small in 20%. The presence of a normal-sized gallbladder, which distends with fasting and contracts with feeding, suggests a diagnosis other than biliary atresia[187]. The presence of the 'triangular cord sign' and absent or small gallbladder are high predictors of biliary atresia. The triangular cord is a highly reflective focus at the hilum of the liver cranial to the portal vein, likely representing the obliterated fibrosed biliary tree. Associated abnormalities occur in 10%: preduodenal portal vein, choledochal cyst, absent IVC, polysplenia, asplenia, trisomy 13, and situs inversus.

To distinguish biliary atresia from severe cholestasis, a ^{99m}Tc-DISIDA scintigram should be performed in conjunction with US. Preparation with phenobarbital (5 mg kg^{-1} d^{-1}) for 5 d before data acquisition is optimal. ^{99m}Tc-DISIDA is injected intravenously, extracted by the hepatocytes, secreted into bile canaliculi, and excreted into bowel. Sequential imaging during the first 60 min with delayed images at 2, 4, 6, and 24 h is performed. In biliary atresia, the extraction is often normal with hepatic activity seen by 5 min. Failure to show radiopharmaceutical excretion at 24 h, despite good parenchymal extraction, is suggestive of biliary atresia (Fig. 65.38). Radiopharmaceutical within the bowel by 24 h excludes the diagnosis of biliary atresia. The differential diagnosis includes severe hepatocellular dysfunction. Percutaneous liver biopsy is required for definitive diagnosis showing bile duct proliferation, periportal fibrosis, bile plugs, and cholestasis.

Traditionally at laparotomy a cholangiogram was performed through a needle placed in the gallbladder or its remnant. Preoperative PTC/PTTC and MRI may play a role in difficult cases.

The treatment for biliary atresia is usually a porto-enterostomy (Kasai procedure), whereby a jejunal loop is brought as a Roux-en-Y up to the excavated porta hepatus to allow bile to drain through minute bile remnants or canaliculi into the bowel. The alternative is liver transplantation, which carries significant morbidity and long-term immunosuppression. Although the results of the Kasai procedure are suboptimal long term (at 10 years, >50% failure, <20% jaundice free), it remains the primary treatment in patients who present before 60 d[188]. In late stages of biliary atresia (even post successful Kasai), the liver becomes large and firm with a coarse parenchymal pattern; ultimately cirrhosis, portal hypertension ± varices, splenomegaly, and ascites develop. Persistence of the triangular cord sign on US post Kasai may be a poor prognosticator. Generally, the biliary tree does not dilate; however, epithelial lined bile cysts and lakes may be seen as irregular areas of low reflectivity on US. Ultimately 70–80% of patients with biliary atresia will require liver transplantation.

Biliary hypoplasia (Alagille syndrome)

The clinical presentation of biliary hypoplasia is similar to that of biliary atresia but may present later and is of variable severity. It can be an isolated finding, i.e. 'non-syndromic' or 'syndromic' (previously known as arteriohepatic dysplasia/Alagille

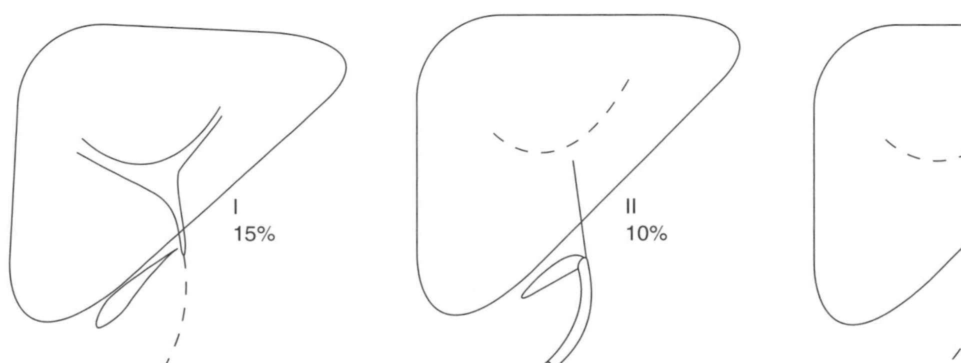

Figure 65.37 Types of biliary atresia.

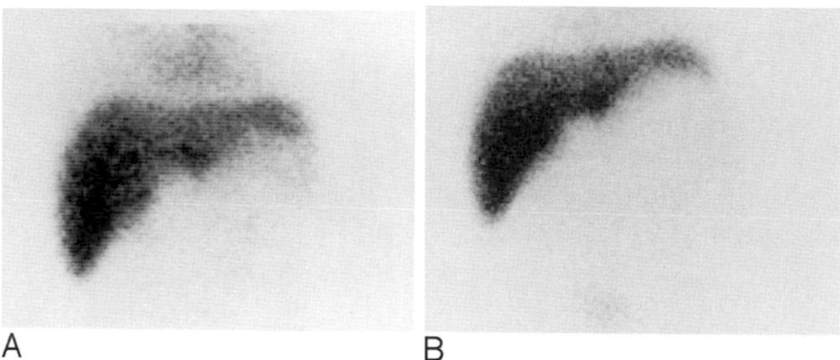

Figure 65.38 Biliary atresia. Radionuclide study of a 2 month old baby boy. ^{99m}Tc-DISIDA scintigram. Following preparation with phenobarbital for 5 d, this radionuclide scintigram using ^{99m}Tc-DISIDA shows good extraction of the tracer by the liver at 2 min, and no excretion by the biliary tree into the bowel by 6 h (A) or 24 h (B). Biopsy confirmed biliary atresia. Ultrasound showed no gallbladder present.

syndrome), which is associated with forehead bossing, pointed chin, posterior embryotoxin of the eye, butterfly vertebrae, renal anomalies (hypoplastic/dysplastic kidneys and cystic disease), and peripheral pulmonary branch stenosis (Fig. 65.39A). US shows a normal liver, a normal or small gallbladder, and no triangular cord sign (Fig. 65.39B). Radionuclide imaging (using DISIDA) may fail to show excretion into the bowel in about 50% of biliary hypoplasias (Fig. 65.39C). Liver biopsy reveals a paucity in number of intralobular bile ducts per high power field. Cholangiography, intra-operative or by PTC/PTTC, shows patency of the thin spidery ducts (Fig. 65.39D). Management is conservative. A Kasai procedure is not indicated.

Late presentation is associated with complications of the disease, e.g. cirrhosis and portal hypertension (PHT) or carcinoma, and may require treatment by liver transplantation.

Choledochal cyst

Choledochal cyst is a congenital segmental dilatation of bile ducts which may be detected antenatally. The classic triad (obstructive jaundice, pain, right upper quadrant mass) are the presenting features in one-third of children. Thirty per cent of patients present in the newborn period or infancy with a mass or obstructive jaundice, 50% present by 10 years, and 80% by young adulthood. Presentation with abdominal pain, pale stools, obstructive jaundice, and fever can mimic hepatitis unless a mass is found. The male-to-female ratio is 1:3. Different types of choledochal cyst occur (Type I–V) (Fig. 65.40). The aetiology is unclear; it may relate to the 'common

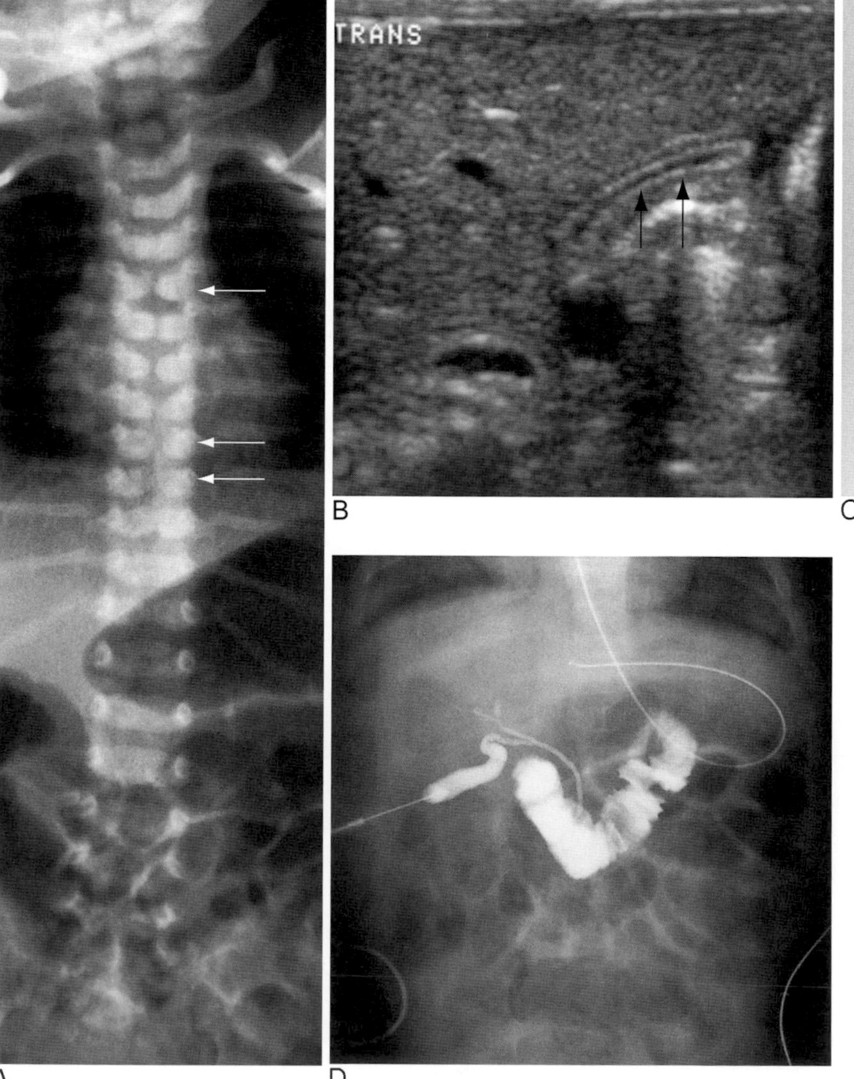

Figure 65.39 Alagille syndrome. Biliary hypoplasia. (A) Plain AP radiograph of the spine in a neonate with Alagille syndrome showing numerous hemivertebrae (arrows). (B) Ultrasound of the liver in a 2 month old boy with Alagille syndrome showing a small gallbladder (arrows). (C) Radionuclide scintigraphy in another child shows good extraction of the ^{99m}Tc-DISIDA by the liver, and excretion of some tracer into the bowel at 24 h. Both infants had biopsy-proven biliary hypoplasia. (D) Second image of a 2 month old boy with prolonged neonatal jaundice. Pre-operative cholangiogram shows a diminutive or hypoplastic but patent biliary tree consistent with biliary hypoplasia (nonsyndromic). This was confirmed on biopsy.

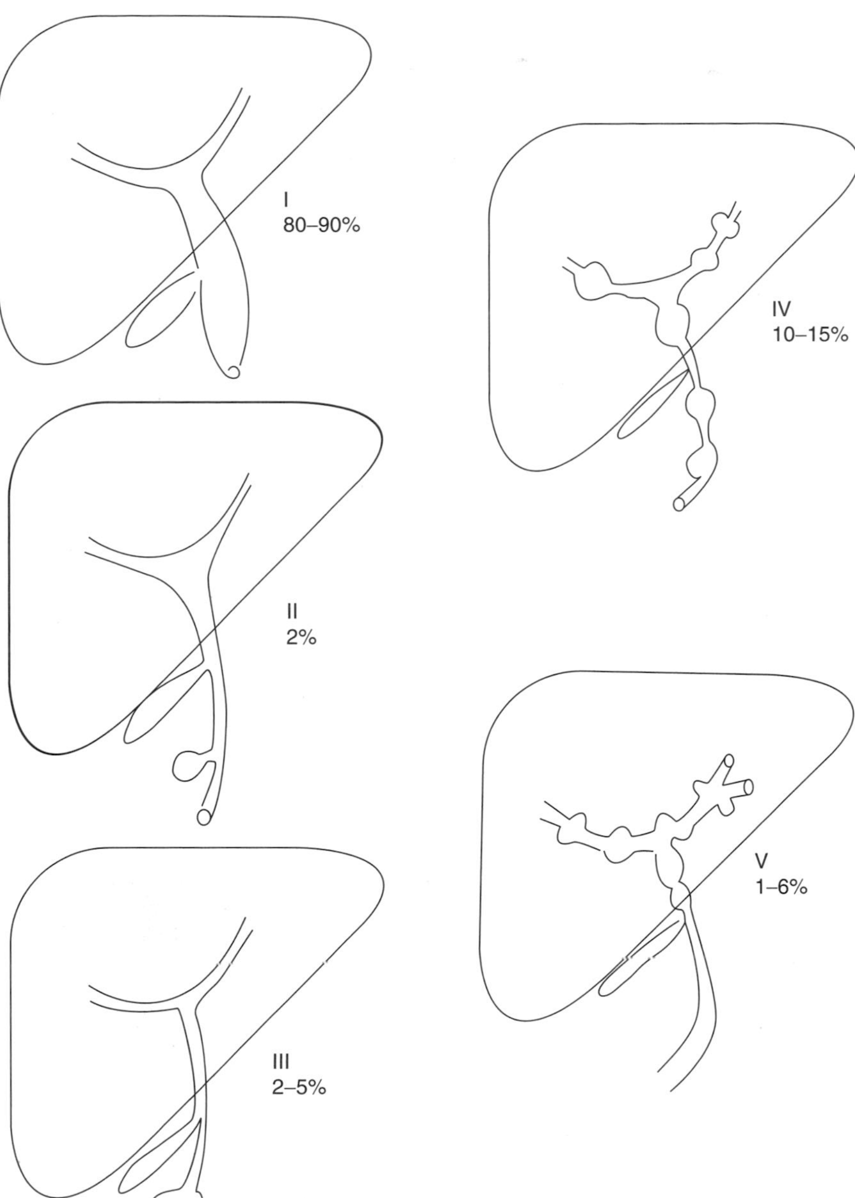

Figure 65.40 Types of choledocal cyst.

channel' theory (common insertion of pancreatic and common bile duct) (Fig. 65.41) or part of the spectrum of biliary atresia and Type V (Caroli's), due to a developmental defect during fetal hepatogenesis[184,189].

On US the biliary tree shows a fusiform or saccular dilatation of varying size involving the common hepatic duct or common bile duct, with or without dilatation of the proximal intrahepatic portions of the bile ducts, with an abrupt transition to normal (Fig. 65.42). The peripheral ducts are not dilated. The gallbladder is usually normal but may be hypoplastic or duplicated. Distinguishing a small fusiform choledochal cyst (Type IV) from a dilated common bile duct due to other causes may be difficult. An abrupt transition between the dilated and nondilated portion of the bile duct favours a choledochal cyst (Fig. 65.41). Sludge or stones may develop within it.

Biliary scintigrams (^{99m}Tc-DISIDA) may show accumulation of tracer in the choledochal cyst. MRC (fasting) may satisfactorily demonstrate the bile and pancreatic duct anatomy[170]. ERCP shows the distal common connection, the cystic dilatation and the abrupt transition to nondilated ducts (Fig. 65.41), whilst PTC and PTTC outline the intrahepatic duct anatomy optimally[174]. Both, however, are invasive with risks of cholangitis and pancreatis (ERCP), bleeding, and bile leak (PTC + PTTC). Treatment is by surgical excision of the choledochal cyst and porto-enterostomy. Complications of choledochal cyst include ascending cholangitis, bleeding, cirrhosis, stone formation, portal hypertension, and malignancy (incidence increasing with age, up to 40% in adults). The differential diagnosis includes any right upper quadrant cystic mass/obstruction of the biliary tree.

Caroli's disease (Type V choledochal cyst) is rare, characterized by segmental nonobstructive dilatation or ectasia of the intrahepatic bile ducts, probably equivalent to Type V choledochal cyst. The aetiology is uncertain, may be developmental,

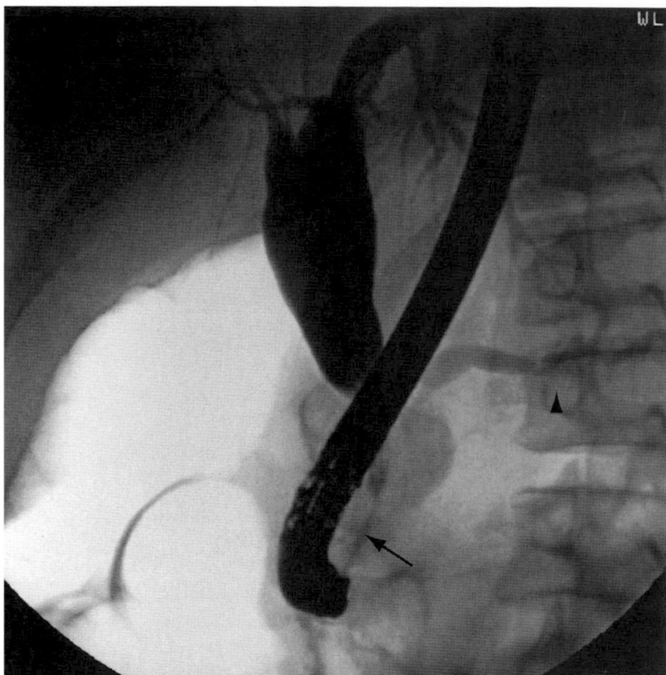

Figure 65.41 ERCP in choledochal cyst. Radiograph of an ERCP examination showing a moderate sized fusiform choledochal cyst in this 16 year old boy. Contrast medium fills the pancreatic duct (arrowhead) and the common channel is seen (arrow).

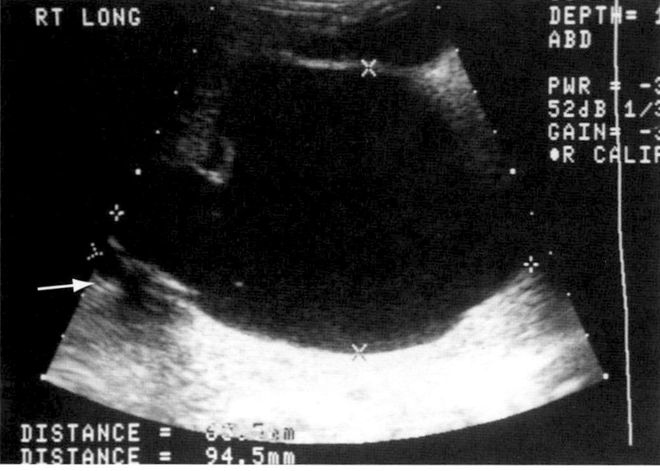

Figure 65.42 Choledochal cyst. Ultrasound through the upper abdomen in this 2½ year old girl showing a large choledochal cyst (6.3 cm × 9.4 cm) in longitudinal section and seen in transverse view anterior to the right kidney (arrow) and situated at the portal hepatis.

possibly autosomal recessive, or part of a syndrome with congenital hepatic fibrosis and autosomal recessive polycystic kidney disease[190]. Patients present in late childhood or early adulthood with cholangitis. Biliary involvement may be diffuse or focal or involve only one lobe (usually left). US shows multiple low reflective cystic areas with a central dot of high reflectivity representing the portal vein branch surrounded by an ectatic bile duct, and sacular or beaded biliary ducts (Fig. 65.43). Heterogeneous areas of high reflectivity in these biliary dilatations may represent stone, sludge, or infection presenting as cholangitis or abscess. ERCP and MRI demonstrate the saccular biliary tree. Cholangiocarcinoma can develop late.

Total parenteral nutrition cholestasis Although TPN may be life-saving, its use is associated with liver disease. Conjugated hyperbilirubinaemia may occur within 2 weeks of starting TPN, especially in low birth weight infants, infants after extensive bowel resection, and according to the composition of the TPN[191]. Imaging excludes other causes of jaundice. Ultrasound shows biliary sludge or enlargement of the gallbladder. Cholestasis may resolve if enteral feeding is started; failure to achieve enteral nutrition leads to progressive liver failure and portal hypertension, with some patients ultimately requiring liver transplantation[181,182].

Neonatal hepatitis The term neonatal hepatitis includes a large group of disorders, the majority of whom are idiopathic. Definitive diagnoses include antenatal infections such as CMV, rubella, enteroviruses, toxoplasmosis, herpes simplex, and spirochaete, as well as metabolic disorders, e.g. cystic fibrosis, α_1-antitrypsin deficiency, tyrosinaemia, and galactosaemia[182]. US features are non-specific and include hepatomegaly, heterogeneous coarse liver parenchyma, and a visible gallbladder (> 1.5 cm) without the triangular cord sign. Cranial ultrasound may identify structural abnormalities or calcification within the brain. Extraction of ^{99m}Tc-DISIDA into the liver is often reduced and excretion into the bowel may be reduced proportional to the degree of cholestasis and hepatocellular dysfunction (and excludes biliary atresia). In severe neonatal hepatitis, the cholestasis is so severe that the reduced extraction and excretion make it difficult to distinguish from biliary atresia[173]. MRC may help. Percutaneous needle biopsy of the

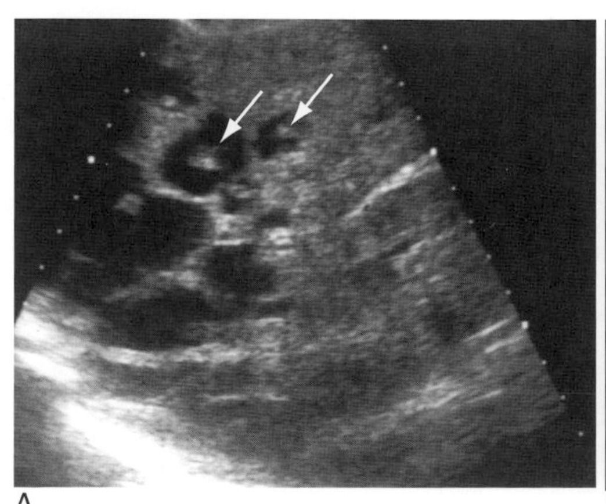

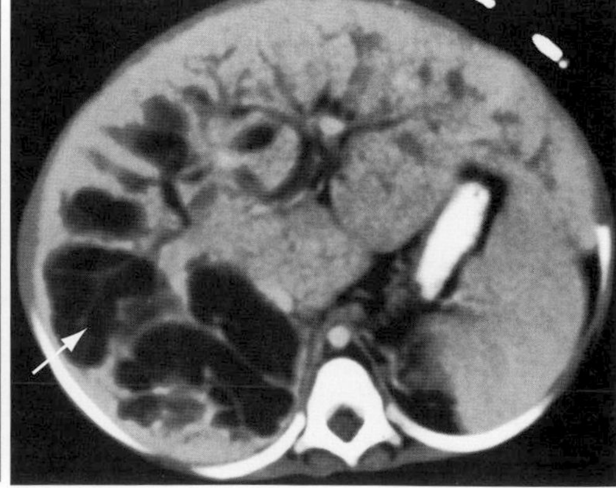

A B

Figure 65.43 Caroli's disease. (A) Transverse ultrasound image through the liver showing fluid-filled spaces with a central hyperreflective centre or dot (arrows), consistent with bile lakes of Caroli's disease surrounding a portal vein branch. (B) CT of the same patient showing the low attenuation areas surrounding the portal vein branches (arrow). The whole liver is involved, the right lobe more than the left.

liver is frequently needed to reach a definite diagnosis. Five to 10% develop persistent fibrosis.

Spontaneous perforation of the bile ducts This is an uncommon disorder, which presents in the first three months of life with jaundice, ascites, and pale stools[192]. The cause is uncertain, and the perforation occurs at the junction of the cystic duct and common hepatic duct, or the cystic duct and gallbladder. Jaundice results from reabsorption of bile from the peritoneum. Liver function tests are usually normal. US shows ascites generalized or localized to the right upper quadrant which may contain debris. Radionuclide scintigrams using ^{99m}Tc-DISIDA are very sensitive at identifying the presence of radionuclide in the peritoneum and occasionally the site of a leak. Aspiration confirms the diagnosis. Surgical or percutaneous drainage is required with spontaneous healing occurring in about 1 month.

Haemolytic anaemia

Haemolytic anaemia as a cause of jaundice is not confined to the neonatal period. US shows a normal liver, possibly pigment stones in the gallbladder, and splenomegaly. The common causes in infants are haemolytic anaemia of the newborn, Rhesus disease, and autoimmune haemolytic anaemia, and in the older child, the haemoglobinopathies and enzyme deficiencies.

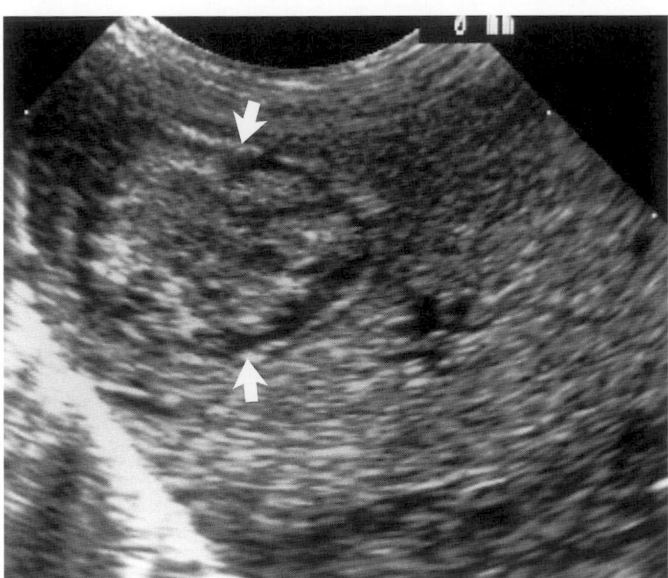

Figure 65.44 Liver abscess. Premature male infant (860 g) with sepsis secondary to an umbilical line. A 4 × 2 cm ovoid area high in the liver towards the diaphragm showing a rim of increased reflectivity (arrows) and central heterogeneous mixed reflections, and a thin surrounding low reflective rim. This was percutaneously aspirated and drained under ultrasound guidance and pus obtained (*Staph. aureus*). The child did well following drainage.

Infectious disorders

The majority of viral infections of the liver are diagnosed clinically with serology. Imaging is supportive (US ± CT ± confirmation with biopsy [targeted, percutaneous or transjugular]).

In children bacterial liver abscesses occur from (A) bacterial seeding from portal venous drainage of an area of sepsis; (B) direct spread of sepsis from a contiguous focus; or (C) infected traumatic lacerations[193,194]. Chronic granulomatous disease of childhood (an X-linked recessive disorder with inability of leukocytes to lyse bacteria) may be complicated by liver abscess, as can other immune deficiency states[195]. In the neonatal period, liver abscesses may occur secondary to necrotizing entercolitis and from extravasation from umbilical vein lines (Fig. 65.44). Many are cryptogenic. The common organisms in liver abscesses include Klebsiella, *Staphylococcus aureus*, *Escherichia coli*, aerobic streptococci, and anaerobes.

Percutaneous therapy (aspiration + drainage by US or CT, going through a seal of normal liver) has reduced morbidity and mortality from liver abscesses. The lesions may calcify when healed.

Nonbacterial abscesses such as amoebiasis and hydatid echinococcus disease are endemic to certain areas and have specific imaging characteristics (see Ch. 35).

In children the incidence of opportunistic infections in the liver has increased commensurate with transplantation, chemotherapy, immunosuppression, and HIV. Fungal infections most commonly present as microabscesses or target lesions, and must be differentiated from lymphoproliferative disease (Fig. 65.45). HIV infection in children most commonly causes hepatomegaly, with increased or decreased reflectivity of hepatic parenchymal texture, splenomegaly, and focal hypo-echoic lesions representing opportunistic infection or granulomatous foci. Gallbladder wall thickening, gallstones, and sludge are also seen.

Liver tumours

Tumours of the liver are uncommon in children, primary hepatic neoplasms accounting for just 0.5–2% of all paediatric

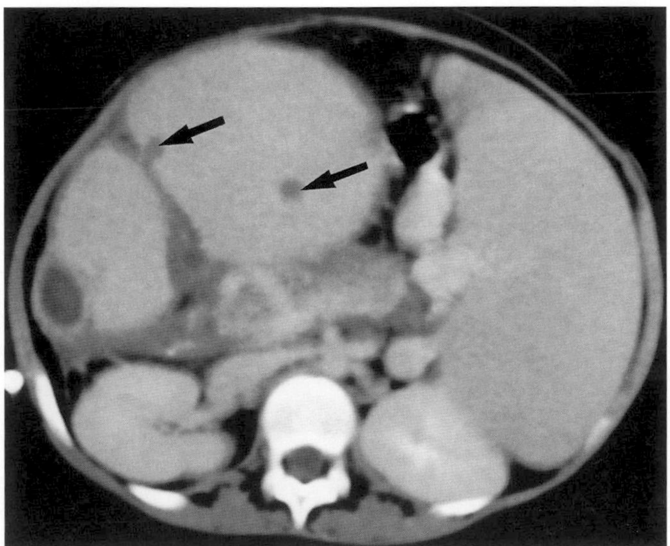

Figure 65.45 Liver graft. Lymphoproliferative disease. Axial CT images through the liver of a reduced liver graft showing several low attenuation small nodules (arrows) scattered throughout the parenchyma. Histology obtained by ultrasound-guided biopsy proved these to be post-transplant lymphoproliferative disease. Fungal infection could look similar.

malignancies (solid/nonsolid). They usually present with an incidental lump or mass felt by a parent, or as an incidental finding on ultrasound performed for another reason. They may be benign (one-third) or malignant (two-thirds)[196,197]. The latter may be primary or secondary. Therapies currently involve combinations of surgery, chemotherapy, and transplant.

Categorized by age, haemangiomas, hepatoblastoma, and mesenchymal hamartomas occur in the neonatal period. In the young child, hepatoblastoma, metastases, haemangiomas, and rhabdomyosarcoma occur. In the older child hepatocellular carcinoma, lymphoma, metastases, undifferentiated sarcomas, and adenomas are more common.

The benign tumours are commonly vascular in origin, e.g. haemangioma. Although most are asymptomatic, they may present with cardiac failure or thrombocytopenia. Imaging characteristics of many tumours have been described using ultrasound, Doppler, CT, radionuclide radiology, and MRI[164,167,197–199]. Plain radiographs are usually non-specific but may show calcification ± soft tissue enlargement.

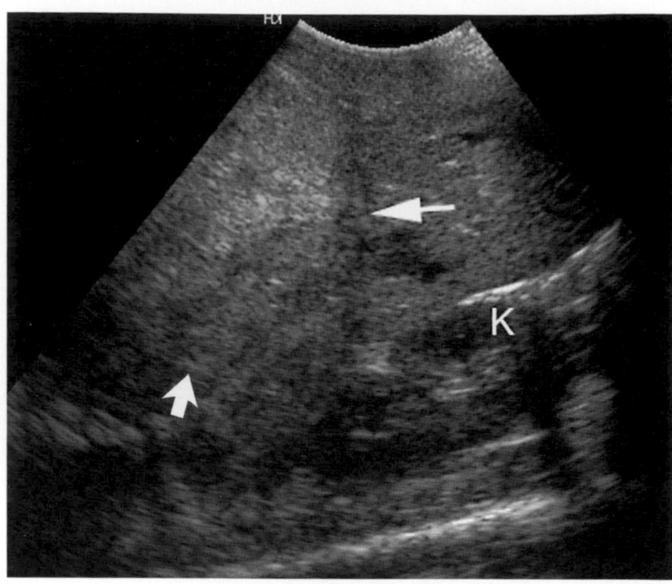

Figure 65.46 Hepatoblastoma. Parasagittal view through the upper abdomen on the right through the right lobe of the liver showing a solid mass (arrow) of increased reflectivity when compared to the adjacent normal liver and adjacent posteriorly placed kidney (K). The mass shows compression on the inferior vena cava (thick arrow).

Malignant tumours

Hepatoblastoma is the third most common abdominal tumour in infancy (second to Wilms' tumour and neuroblastoma) with a peak incidence at under 2 years of age and a male preponderance (2:1). It is associated with Beckwith–Wiedemann syndrome (chromosome 11) and familial adenomatus polyposis (chromosome 5). Many are detected as asymptomatic masses; advanced tumours are associated with anorexia, weight loss, pallor, anaemia, and abdominal pain. Twenty per cent have metastases at presentation. Serum α-fetoprotein (AFP) levels are elevated in over three-quarters of cases.

Calcification is seen in about 50% on abdominal radiography. Ultrasound shows a heterogeneous mass of mixed high and low reflectivity, which may have calcification, cystic areas of necrosis, and a pseudocapsule (Fig. 65.46). Size varies from small to very large. They may be single, multifocal, or exophytic. The tumour may show pressure on, splaying or infiltration of, hepatic or portal veins and IVC. Increased activity on the angiographic phase and a photopenic area on delayed ^{99m}Tc-sulphur colloid scintigraphy are seen. A mixed low attenuating lesion ± calcification with peripheral rim enhancement is seen on CT (Fig. 65.47). When large it is difficult to determine the organ of origin, e.g. arising from the liver, kidney, or adrenal. MRI (spin echo, MRA, MRV) assesses the extent of the tumour, its relation to the vascular and liver segmental anatomy, its blood supply, and its resectability. In general, the tumour has heterogeneous low signal on T1-weighted imaging (haemorrhage may be bright), and high signal on T2-weighted imaging with hypo-intense fibrous septae (Fig. 65.47). Angiography and venography are now largely obsolete. The diagnosis is confirmed by percutaneous needle biopsy taking numerous cores from the least necrotic areas (most solid on US) for histology, immunohistochemistry, and molecular studies. The differential diagnosis includes haemangioma, metastatic neuroblastoma, mesenchymal hamartoma, and hepatocellular carcinoma.

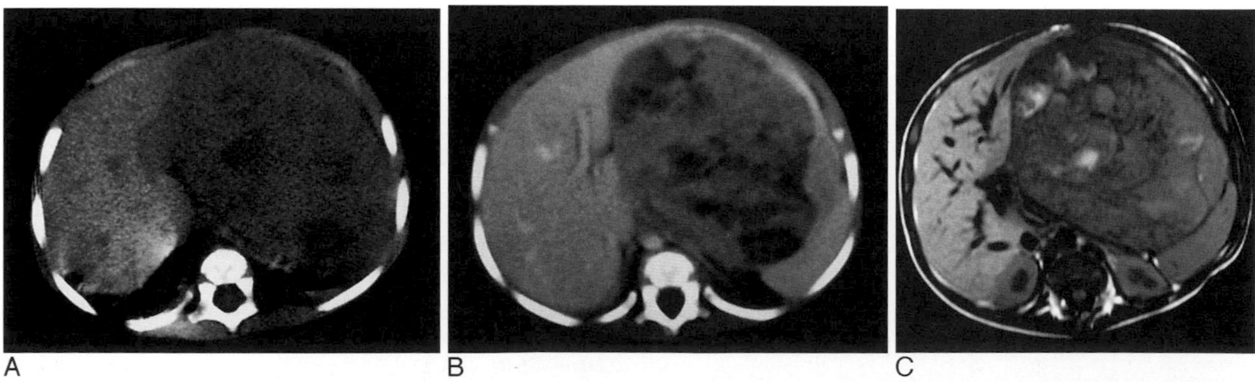

Figure 65.47 Hepatoblastoma. (A,B) A 17 month old boy with abdominal distension. A large, low attenuation, solid heterogeneous mass is seen on CT, without calcification, and with patchy enhancement. This mass was histologically shown to be a hepatoblastoma. (C) MRI T1-weighted image shows a low signal, discrete large mass with areas of increased signal consistent with blood. The portal structures are displaced to the right. Low signal septae are seen though the lesion.

Hepatocellular carcinoma This uncommon paediatric tumour may present in the older child (usually older than 4 years) de novo or in the presence of underlying liver disease—previous adenoma, chronic hepatitis, biliary atresia, inborn errors of metabolism (e.g. α_1-antitrypsin deficiency), etc. It is the second most common primary malignant hepatic tumour in childhood. Over half of the children will have elevated AFP. The imaging characteristics are detailed in Chapter 35.

Other malignant tumours Rare hepatic malignant tumours include fibrolamellar hepatocellular carcinomas occurring in adolescents, a solitary lobulated mass with a central fibrous scar, described fully in the Chapter 35. Undifferentiated embryonal sarcomas occur in older children (6–10 years), and may be solid, cystic, or mixed. They present with pain and swelling. US demonstrates a large solid mass with hypo-echoic areas. CT shows low attenuation mass with septae and fibrous pseudocapsule. Hepatic angiosarcomas, also very rare, are highly malignant, present around 3–4 years of age predominantly in girls with systemic symptoms. US and CT show multiple heterogeneous foci; they enhance centripetally. Survival is poor.

Rhadomyosarcoma, a mesenchymal tumour, rarely involves the biliary tree. It presents in children between 2 and 5 years of age with malaise, fever, pain, obstruction, jaundice, and ductal dilatation, with or without haemobilia when it involves a large bile duct. A focal irregularity or large lobulated mass of increased reflectivity arising in the region of the porta hepatis, gallbladder, or biliary tree is detected by US, CT, or MRI. When arising in more peripheral ducts, it may not be considered until a needle biopsy yields the correct diagnosis. The tumour is photopenic on ^{99m}Tc-sulphur colloid. Cholangiocarcinoma rarely occurs in children and is described in Chapter 36.

Hepatic or splenic involvement with leukaemia and lymphoma is more commonly detected at autopsy than by imaging; it may present as diffuse hepatomegaly or as focal nodules or masses (usually hypo-attenuating and hypo-echoeic).

In a child with a known tumour, the differential diagnosis of focal liver or spleen lesions includes metastases, focal infection, or pre-existing incidental focal lesions. The imaging characteristics are similar to those in adults.

Wilms' tumour and neuroblastoma are the most common tumours to metastasize to the liver in children; 60% of neuroblastomas present with metastatic disease. Metastatic neuroblastoma to the liver may be seen as discrete focal lesions, simulating a primary liver tumour or as a diffuse infiltrative multifocal tumour, with areas of low reflectivity ± calcification, giving it an extremely coarse speckled appearance (Fig. 65.48).

Benign tumours Haemangiomas are the most common liver tumours of infancy. The classification of vascular anomalies by Mulliken et al divides lesions into vascular tumours and vascular malformations. Haemangiomas have abnormal parenchyma and fall into the former category. They form a heterogeneous group of benign mesenchymal tumours which present before 6 months of age. They may be focal, multifocal, or disseminated haemangiomatosis (three or more organs involved). Haemangiomas may show hypervascularity of the mass associated with (A) slow flow without shunting; (B) high flow without shunting; (C) arterial-to-venous shunting; (C) venous-to-venous shunting; or (E) mixed shunting[200]. Most are asymptomatic; others may be associated with high output failure, thrombocytopaenia, and hypothyroidism, and are difficult to treat.

US shows single focal or multiple discrete solid hyperechoic masses. When multiple, it is difficult to identify normal liver parenchyma (Fig. 65.49). Vascular spaces with shunting in the lesions may be visible in addition to enlarged hepatic veins. Aortic narrowing below the coeliac artery in the high flow lesions is seen. On unenhanced CT the low attenuation lesions are seen—often of similar attenuation to blood in vessels; following intravenous enhancement, the periphery of the lesions takes up contrast medium first (Figs 65.50, 65.51) Red blood cell scintigraphy may be a useful technique in identifying haemangiomas. MRI shows lesions that are low signal on T1-weighted imaging and high on T2-weighted imaging with or without flow voids near or inside the lesions[201].

Angiography only plays a role in those patients who have failed medical therapy (steroids, vincristine, interferon) and require therapy for their high output failure. Embolization is challenging; its role is to temporize until involution occurs naturally (after a year or so). Multiple approaches may be needed via the hepatic artery, branches of the superior

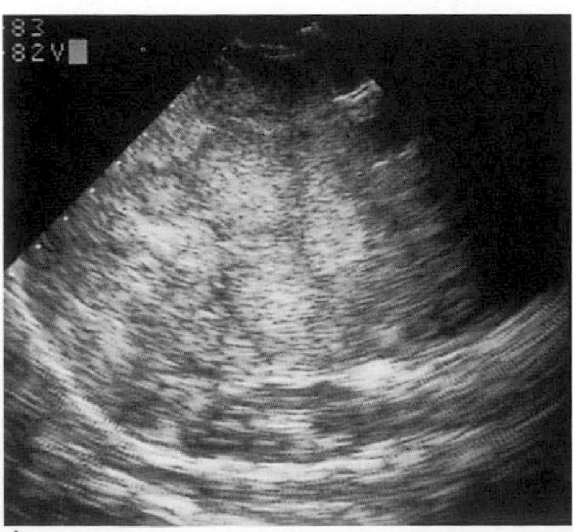

A

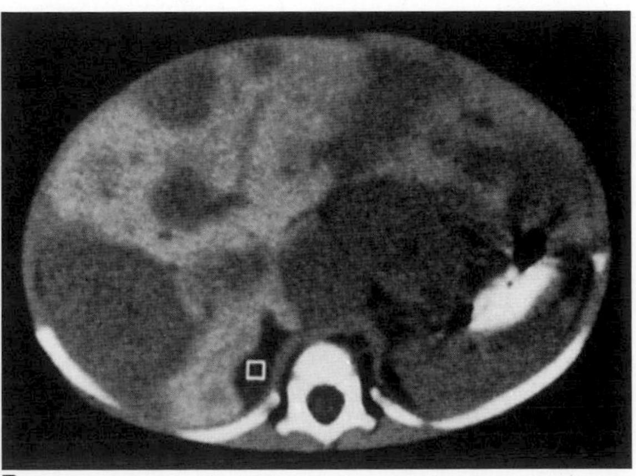
B

Figure 65.48 Metastatic neuroblastoma. (A) A 3 month old boy with abdominal distension and anaemia. Sagittal ultrasound through the right lobe of the liver shows numerous solid foci of high reflectivity throughout the parenchyma. (B) Axial CT image through the liver (without intravenous contrast medium) shows low attenuating rounded lesions in the liver, becoming confluent in some areas. Biopsy confirmed metastatic neuroblastoma.

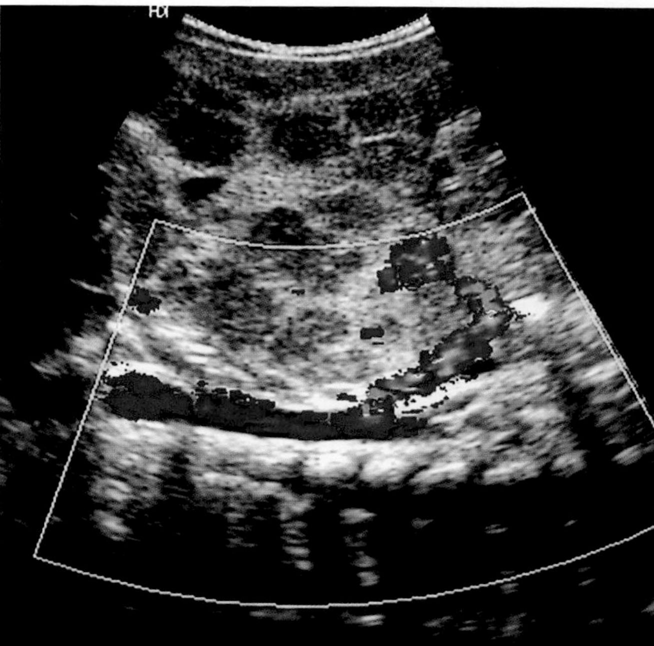

Figure 65.49 Haemangioma. Midline sagittal view of the upper abdomen in a 6 month old girl in severe congestive cardiac failure. The liver shows numerous rounded lesions of low reflectivity scattered throughout the liver parenchyma. On longitudinal views, the aorta is seen to give off a large coeliac artery to the liver and the aorta below this is significantly smaller. Note the nodules of the liver tumour do not show vascularity on colour Doppler, except for one area adjacent to the coeliac artery which most likely represents volume averaging of a feeding vessel.

mesenteric artery, the portal vein, and hepatic veins. Overaggressive embolization risks hepatic infarction (Fig. 65.52).

Mesenchymal hamartoma is rare but is said to be the second most common benign liver tumour or developmental lesion presenting in children, usually younger than 2 years of age (peak 15–22 months). Hamartomas are usually large (5–29 cm, mean 16 cm) and mixed solid cystic, containing a mixture of bile ducts and mesenchyme, multiseptated with a cystic/gelatinous composition[202,203]. When small they appear more solid (Fig. 65.53). On CT, they are of low attenuation with variable septation and fluid loculation. The tumour is hypovascular, but atrioventricular shunting can occur through enlarged irregular tortuous feeding vessels. MRI shows the multiseptated fluid areas (low on T1- and high on T2-weighted imaging) displacing major vessels. Excision of the tumour is usually therapeutic.

Focal fatty infiltration, focal nodular hyperplasia (FNH; benign tumour of epithelial origin), and adenomas are seen far more commonly in adults than children; as a result they may pose a diagnostic dilemma when they do occur (Fig. 65.54). Adenomas occur in children with metabolic disorders (e.g. glycogen storage disorders) or adolescents on the contraceptive pill, and may undergo malignant change.

BILIARY DISEASE

In children gallstones are being detected with increased frequency with the widespread application of US. Gallstones are

Figure 65.50 Haemangioma. A 3 month old boy with congestive cardiac failure. (A) Unenhanced CT image shows numerous low attenuation nodules throughout the liver parenchyma, with very little normal parenchyma. (B) Following intravenous contrast medium these nodules enhance intensely from the periphery. The aorta is seen to be of adequate size; below this and distal to the take off of the coeliac axis the aorta became significantly smaller in size (< 50%) (not shown).

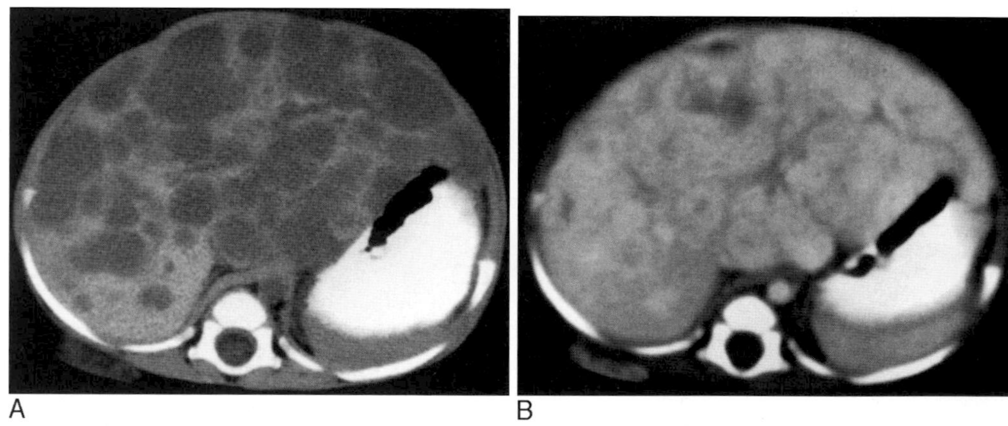

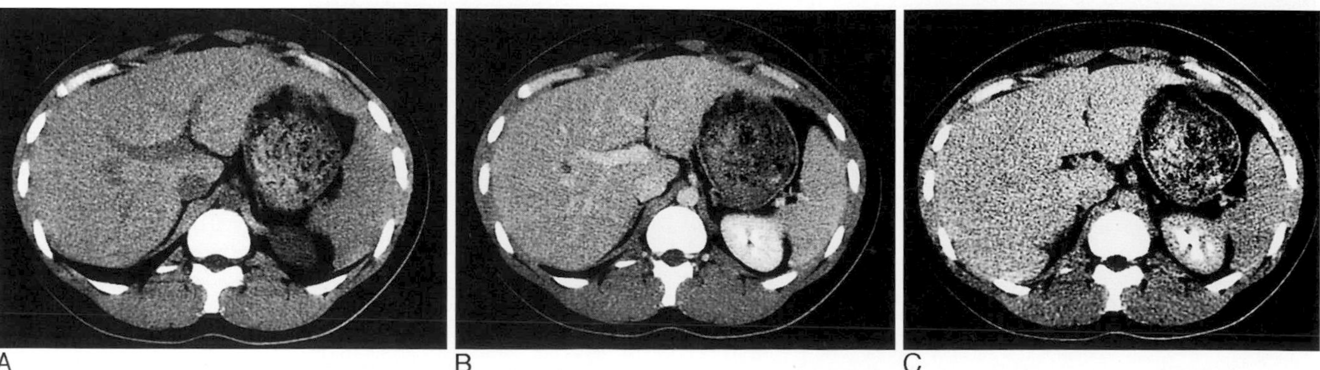

Figure 65.51 Haemangioma. Three-phase axial CT through the liver shows the small, low attenuation area posterior to the right portal vein on the enhanced CT (A), which has peripheral to central filling following administration of contrast medium (B,C).

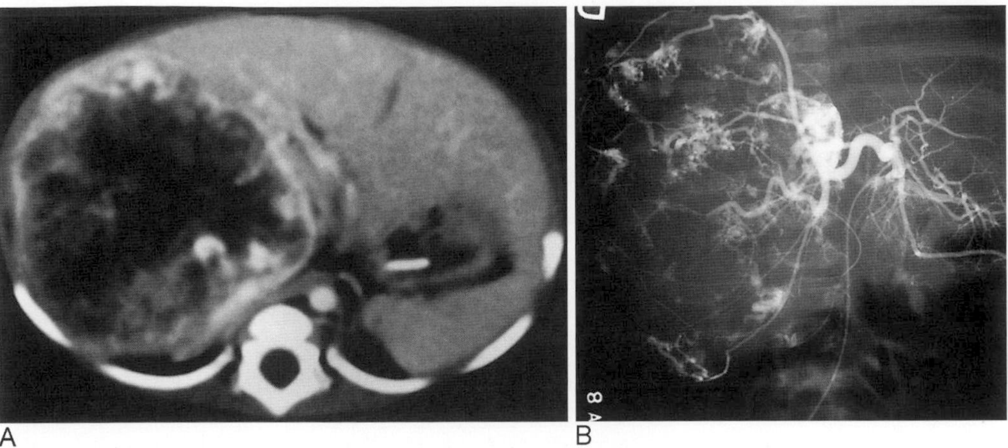

Figure 65.52 Haemangioma. A 3 month old boy with an asymptomatic mass in the right upper quadrant. (A) Axial CT image shows a large focal low attenuation mass in the right lobe with enhancing peripheral vessels. The mass is largely avascular centrally. (B) Selective coeliac axis angiogram into the hepatic artery shows the large hepatic artery feeding irregular tumour vessels with mass effect. Surgical excision proved this to be a cavernous haemangioma. The patient also had a small cutaneous haemangioma on his neck.

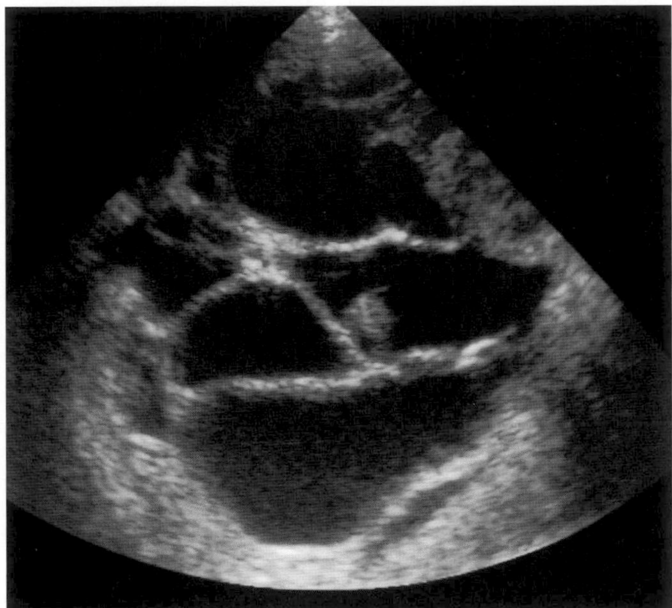

Figure 65.53 Mesenchymal hamartoma. Ultrasound through the right lobe of the liver showing a round septated partly solid, partly cystic mass.

associated with TPN, diuretics, haemolytic anaemias, cystic fibrosis, metabolic disorders, inflammatory bowel disease, short gut syndrome, structural abnormalities of the biliary tree, prematurity, and dehydration. Many children are asymptomatic; the stones resolve or pass spontaneously so treatment is controversial[204]. Imaging appearances are similar to those in adults (see Ch. 36, The Biliary System).

Calculous cholecystitis is rare in children; 50% of those with acute cholecystitis will have no stones evident. Biliary sludge is commonly seen. Kawasaki disease and systemic vasculitis may cause cholecystitis, but more commonly an acute hydrops of the gallbladder. The biliary tree in children may be involved in sclerosing cholangitits and in cystic fibrosis (see above)[170].

VASCULAR DISEASES OF THE LIVER

Vascular lesions of the liver are uncommon in children. They may be congenital or acquired—haemangiomas, vascular malformations, portal vein thrombosis, Budd–Chiari syndrome, etc.[200,201,205,206].

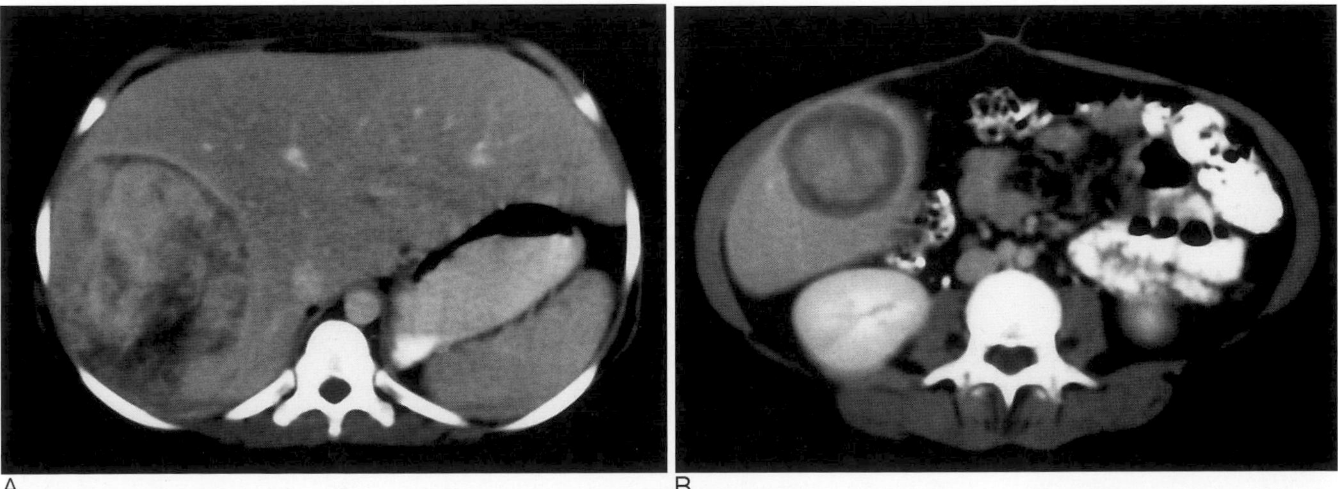

Figure 65.54 Hepatic adenoma. A 16 year old girl with glycogen storage disease, type I. Axial CT images through the liver in this teenage girl show (A) a large heterogeneous adenoma in the right lobe and (B) a smaller adenoma in the lower aspect of the right lobe (B). This girl underwent successful liver transplantation, and histology of the explanted liver showed both to be adenomas.

Portal hypertension

Portal hypertension (PHT) is categorized into prehepatic, hepatic, and post-hepatic causes. Prehepatic (extrahepatic) PHT results from portal vein thrombosis and extrinsic occlusion of the portal vein; liver function is normal. Hepatic causes include cystic fibrosis, metabolic liver disease, and numerous causes of cirrhosis, including drug induced. Post-hepatic causes in children include IVC webs, Budd–Chiari syndrome, cardiac causes, and veno-occlusive disease. US (colour and pulsed Doppler) detecting flow and its direction may distinguish the three. MR/MRA/MRV are complementary investigations[207].

Portal vein thrombosis

Portal vein thrombosis used to be a common sequela of umbilical venous catheterization and umbilical sepsis. In the older child, trauma, pancreatitis, splenectomy, tumours, inflammatory masses, and dehydration are recognized as causes. Late sequelae of portal vein thrombosis include PHT, splenomegaly, ascites, and varices. With US, occlusion of the portal vein may be seen early in its course as a swollen vein containing highly reflective thrombus. Later a leash of collateral vessels is seen surrounding the thrombosed/obliterated/partly recanalized main portal vein, 'cavernous transformation'. These collateral vessels permit ongoing hepatopetal flow as the liver parenchyma and the sinusoidal pressures are normal. When large, collaterals in cavernous transformation may have mass effect on the biliary tree, pancreatic duct, and the region of the pancreatic head. As PHT develops oesophageal, gastric, or duodenal varices may be seen. Natural collaterals and shunting develop—splenorenal, umbilical, etc. On CT, the portal vein appears of low density, enhances poorly and is surrounded by peripheral enhancing collaterals. Focal intrahepatic portal vein thrombosis can also occur with thrombosis of the left portal vein leading to focal areas of infarction in the left lobe of the liver, which may become secondarily infected.

Hepatic causes

Hepatic causes of PHT, arising from the myriad of causes of fibrosis or cirrhosis, lead to similar sequelae in terms of collaterals, varices (Fig. 65.55), and splenomegaly. Because liver synthetic function may be affected, the prognosis is poorer than with portal vein thrombosis. The imaging features of coarse liver parenchyma, mixed size nodularity, and shrunken liver are similar to the findings in adults.

Budd–Chiari syndrome

Budd–Chiari syndrome is rare in children. It presents as an acute, subacute or chronic phenomenon, from a congenital or acquired aetiology, and is due to occlusion of the small centrilobular veins, major hepatic veins, or IVC[208]. Uncommon causes are a congenital IVC web or membrane, or interruption with agenesis. Acquired causes include thrombosis secondary to hypercoaguable states, vessel wall injury, right heart pathology, tumours, postoperatively or idiopathic. Hepatomegaly, splenomegaly, retrograde portal venous flow, ascites, and large venous collaterals result.

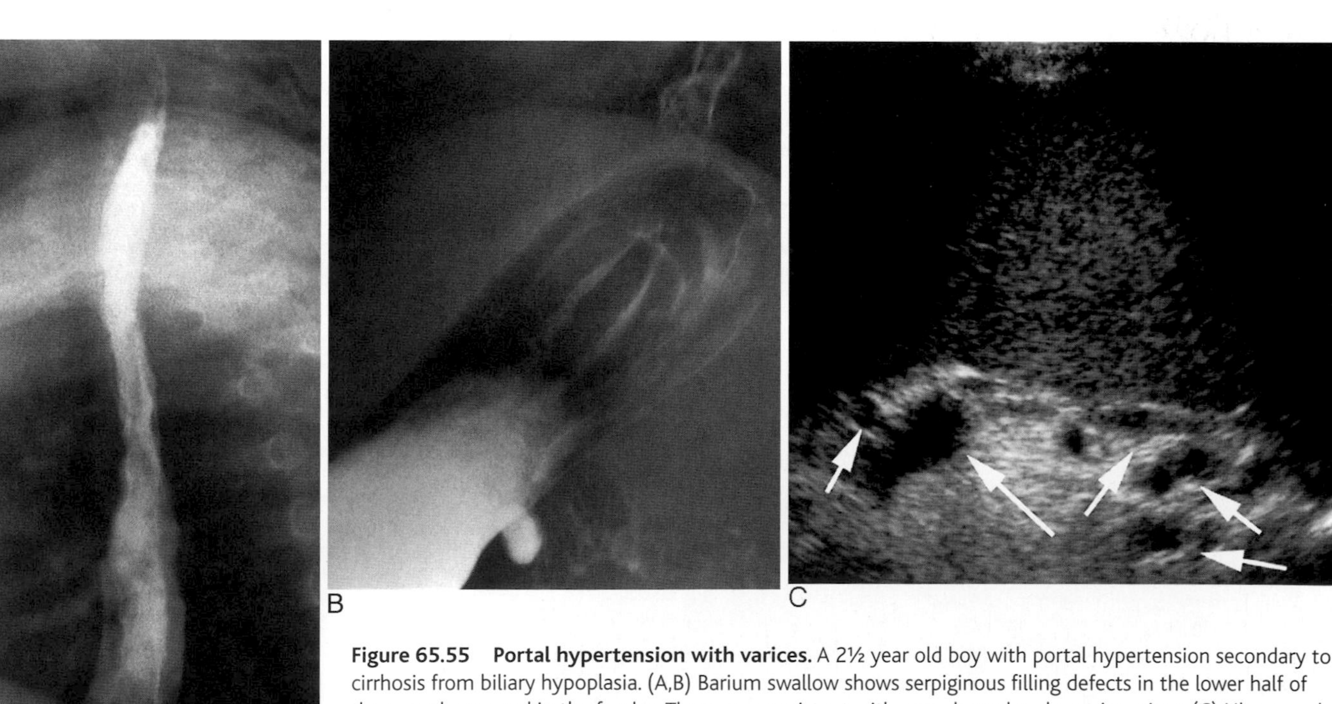

Figure 65.55 Portal hypertension with varices. A 2½ year old boy with portal hypertension secondary to cirrhosis from biliary hypoplasia. (A,B) Barium swallow shows serpiginous filling defects in the lower half of the oesophagus and in the fundus. These are consistent with oesophageal and gastric varices. (C) Ultrasound of the splenic hilum shows numerous rounded vessels of low reflectivity which filled with colour on Doppler interrogation, consistent with splenic varices (arrows).

Veno-occlusive disease (VOD) is allied to classic Budd–Chiari but is an acquired phenomenon, seen in the immunosuppressed child secondary to chemotherapy or bone marrow transplantation. This obstruction occurs at the microscopic level of the central and sublobular veins. A definitive diagnosis requires biopsy, frequently via a transjugular route because of coagulopathy during which hepatic venography, free and wedged pressures are performed (Figs 65.56–65.58). Occasionally, hepatic venography confirms the presence of a web or obstruction to the IVC which may be managed by dilatation preferably without stenting.

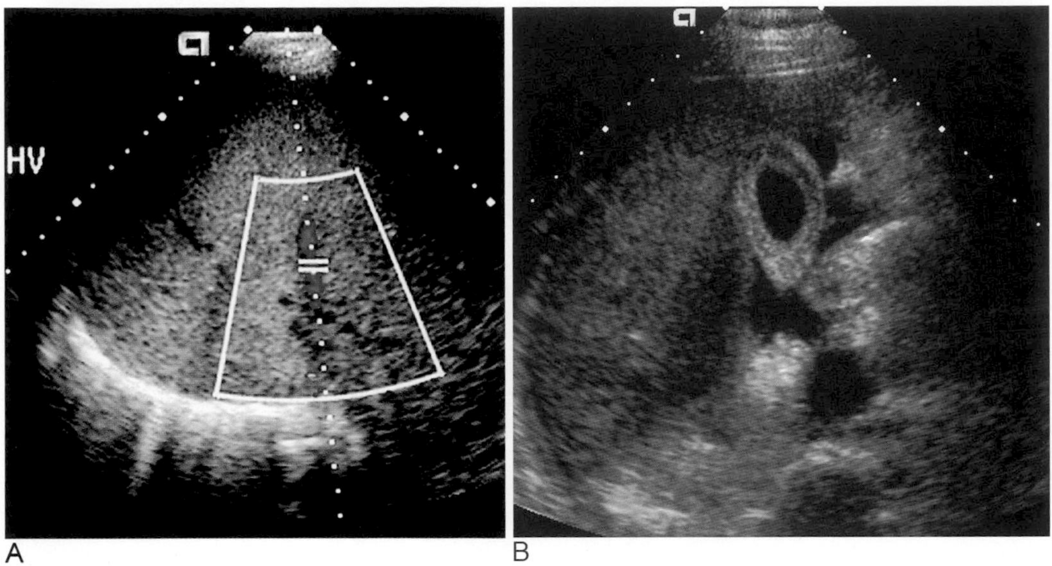

Figure 65.56 Budd–Chiari syndrome. Ultrasound. (A) Ultrasound images of a teenage girl's liver with a 2 week history of abdominal distension, on a background history of sagittal sinus thrombosis and lassitude. One hepatic vein is visible with dampened hepatic venous flow. The other hepatic veins are only faintly seen and show no flow on colour or pulse Doppler. (B) Image shows ascites and apparent thickening of the gallbladder wall secondary to the ascites.

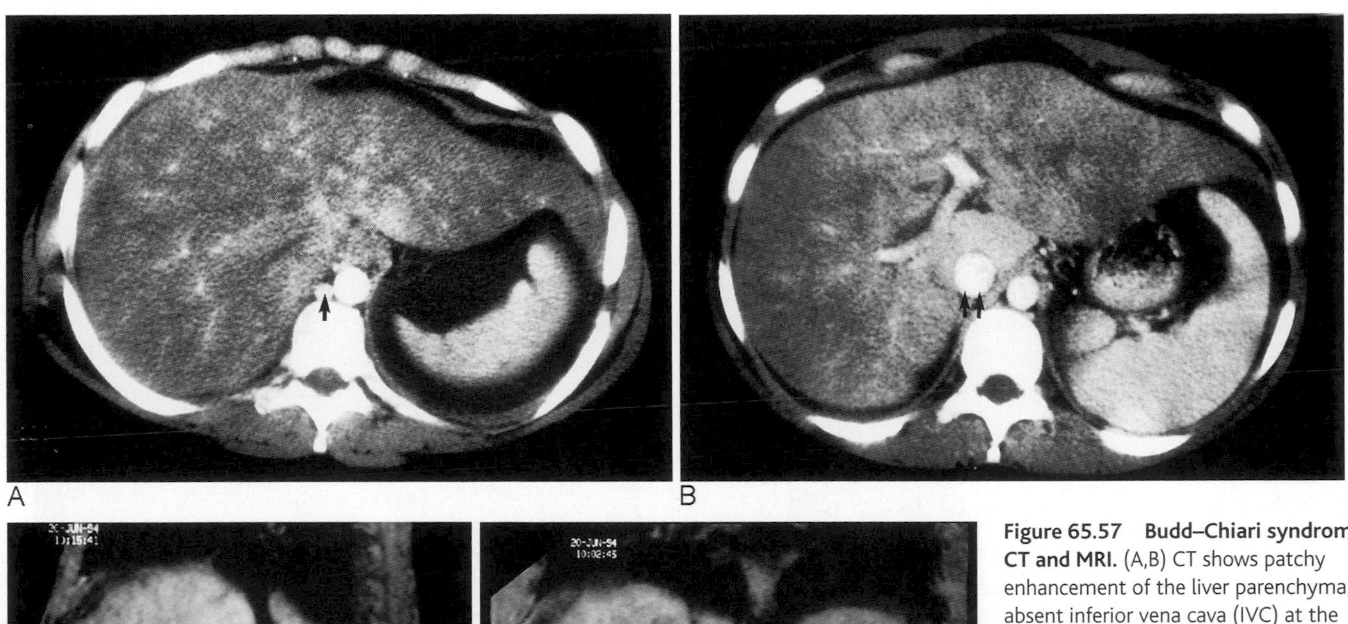

Figure 65.57 Budd–Chiari syndrome. CT and MRI. (A,B) CT shows patchy enhancement of the liver parenchyma, absent inferior vena cava (IVC) at the level of the liver, with prominence of the azygos vein (A) (arrow); and more inferiorly enhancement of the caudate lobe with distension of the obstructed IVC (two small arrows) (B). (C,D) Compared with the previous patient, these sagittal (C) and coronal (D) MRI T1-weighted images show a patent IVC (arrow) but absence of any recognizable hepatic veins in this child with more chronic features of Budd–Chiari syndrome.

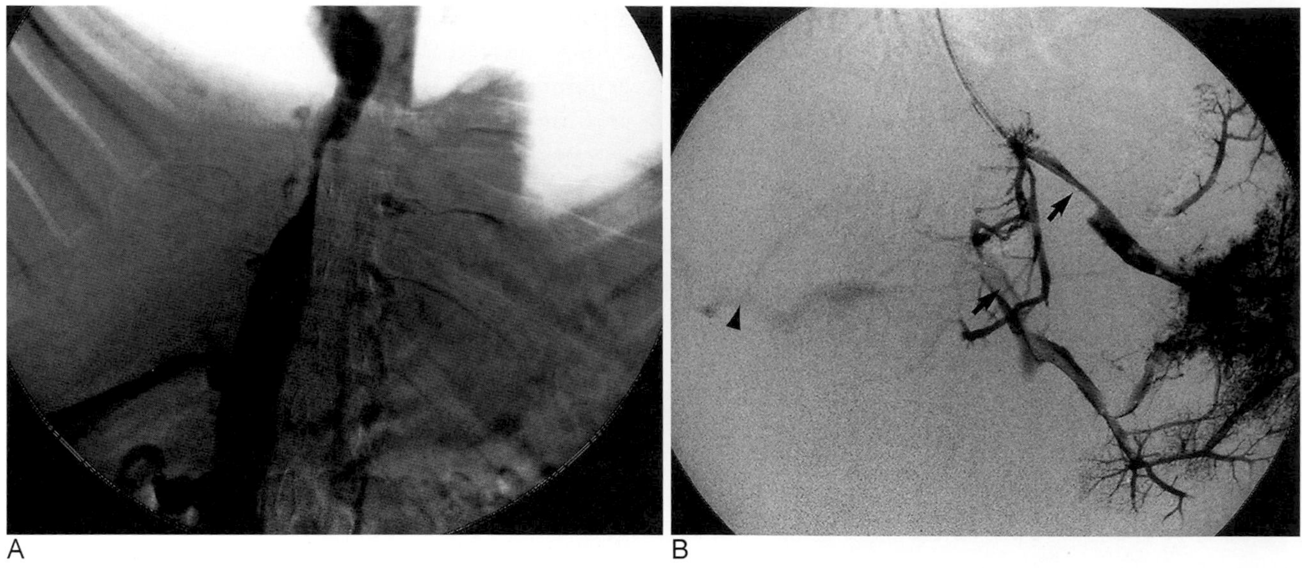

Figure 65.58 Venacavogram and hepatic venogram. (A) Cavogram in a 12 year old girl with jaundice and abdominal distension. There is compression of the inferior vena cava and its anterior and lateral dimensions, with collateral filling in a retrohepatic and inferohepatic direction and into the caudate lobe. (B) Attempts at cannulation from above, via the jugular vein, into the right or middle hepatic veins was not possible. Canulation into a small left hepatic vein branch shows extensive intraluminal filling defects consistent with clot (arrows) and abnormal staining pattern due to the high pressures, despite the catheter not being wedged. Faint filling of the portal vein is seen (arrowhead).

Interrupted inferior vena cava

During embryology, if the right subcardinal vein does not connect appropriately with the liver, the blood from the lower part of the body flows up the azygos vein with interruption of the retrohepatic IVC. US recognition is important in children before future surgery. The IVC is seen to run in a straight posterior direction into the chest, with loss of the normal anterior curve as is usually seen behind the liver where it enters the right atrium in the normal fashion. This is referred to as azygos continuation of the IVC (Fig. 65.59).

Portal vein gas

Portal vein gas is not uncommon in children, occurring usually in the context of necrotizing entercolitis, infectious and inflammatory bowel disorders, uncommonly in severe bowel gangrene or infarction, and occasionally as a benign incidental finding. US, more sensitive than plain radiography, demonstrates gas as bright echogenic foci in the main portal vein extending out to the periphery of the liver, with audible high pitched sounds on Doppler (Fig. 65.60).

Congenital and acquired vascular malformations

Congenital malformations usually present in infancy as an incidental finding on US or with cardiac failure. The acquired types may follow trauma. Intrahepatic shunts are of three varieties: arteriovenous (acquired vascular malformations [AVMs], associated with hereditary haemorrhagic telangiectasia), arterioportal (associated with Ehlers–Danlos, cirrhosis, and traumatic), or venovenous (portcaval or portohepatic), or mixed[205,206]. Although diagnosed by US and/or MRI, accurate delineation before any embolization requires angiography. Direct percutanous transhepatic coil deposition may be indicated in difficult cases of portal-to-hepatic venous shunting, either in isolation or with haemangiomas. Embolization

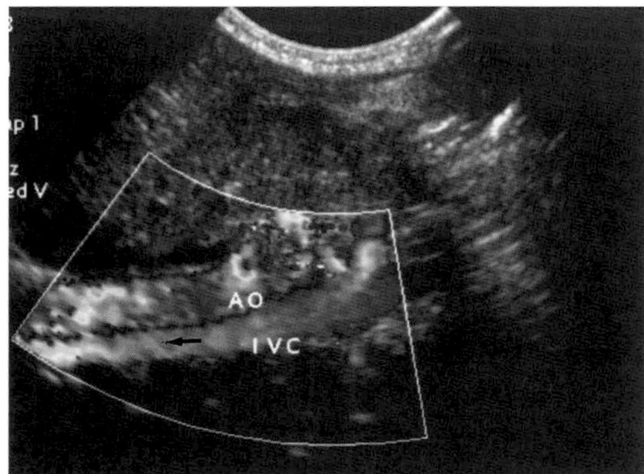

Figure 65.59 Interrupted inferior vena cava (IVC). Azygos continuation. Ultrasound of the neonate with colour Doppler shows the straight aorta in the upper abdomen running into the chest, and the IVC continuing in a posterior position as the azygos vein (arrow).

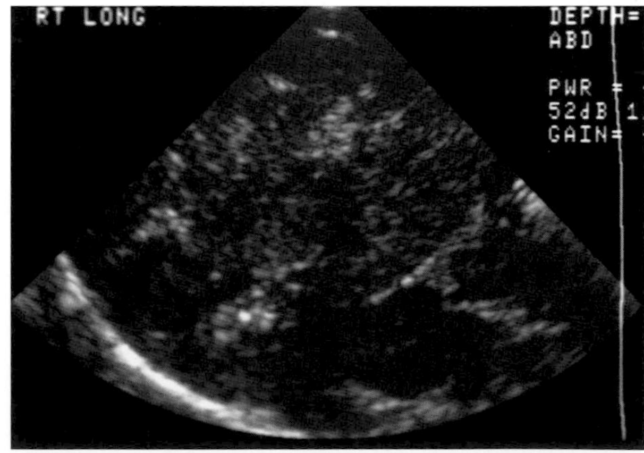

Figure 65.60 Portal venous gas. Ultrasound image of the liver in a newborn with scattered bright reflections throughout the liver parenchyma consistent with gas in the portal venous system.

in AVMs may risk arterial ischaemia. Pure venous or venolymphatic malformations are uncommon in the liver.

LIVER TRANSPLANTATION

Whole livers (cadaveric) or reduced liver grafts (living or cadaveric donors), in the form of a left lateral segment (II and III or II, III, IV) are used in children[209]. Imaging of the reduced liver graft requires an understanding of its anatomy: the liver is divided along the division of the segments above, preserving the left portal vein, the left hepatic duct, and an arterial supply to the left lobe. The raw surface of the liver is sealed by various methods (coagulation, cautery, ties, etc.) and transplanted in its orthotopic position with the raw surface facing a right lateral position. Early postoperatively complex collections seen on US may develop posterolaterally along the raw surface, e.g. haematomas and bilomas. Early hepatic artery thrombosis, before any potential for arterial collaterals, is an emergency with probable loss of the graft from acute hepatic necrosis. Careful Doppler study is necessary and possibly angiography. For a full description of complications, see Chapter 35[210–213].

In the child, the delicate balance of immunosuppression and immune competency has led to the appearance of post-transplant lymphoproliferative disease (PTLD). PTLD may occur in the transplanted organ itself or in a remote organ. The appearance of masses in the liver, spleen, nodes, brain, tonsils, mesentery, or chest raises the suspicion of PTLD. Combined with Epstein–Barr virus serology, biopsy is usually recommended to diagnose PTLD. For a full discussion of imaging of PTLD, see Chapter 72.

THE SPLEEN

US is the method of choice for evaluation of spleen size and parenchymal texture. Radiolabelled sulphur colloid is useful in detection of ectopic spleen or asplenia. Coronal MRI is useful when the spleen is very large. The parenchymal texture should be homogeneous. Focal abnormalities suggest neoplasm, cyst, abscesses, or infection[214–217]. A linear high-frequency probe will help detect subtle abnormalities of parenchymal texture. Homogeneous splenomegaly is associated with portal hypertension, leukaemia, lymphoma, or various haematological disorders, infections, and tumours. MRI enables a full evaluation of focal lesions, as well as an accurate extent of massive splenomegaly (e.g. infiltrative disorders such as Gaucher's disease)[218].

Infections

In immunocompromised children, small microabscesses, most notably fungal in origin, appear as lesions of low reflectivity with or without a central focus of high reflectivity (target lesion)[193]. On enhanced CT, these lesions are of low attenuation. US-guided biopsy provides microbial confirmation. Infectious mononucleosis, common in children, normally presents with diffuse splenomegaly. Splenic granulomas can be seen in tuberculosis, histoplasmosis, and coccidioidomycosis, as well as in those children suffering from chronic granulomatous disease of childhood. These areas may calcify. Multiple lesions in the spleen are seen in HIV infection, cat scratch disease (Fig. 65.61), and histiocytosis. A snowstorm appearance on ultrasound is due to small foci of high reflectivity in *Pneumocystis jiroveci (carinii)*.

Calcification

Calcification of the spleen may be seen on plain radiography, CT, or US. Diffuse patchy calcification is seen in the haematological disorders of sickle cell disease and represents splenic infarctions. Calcification of cyst walls occurs in infections such as echinococcal disease. Calcified granulomas also occur in tuberculosis, histoplasmosis, and chronic granulomatous disease, or in opportunistic infections.

Tumours

Tumours of the spleen are benign or malignant[215–217,219]. The benign group includes splenic cysts which are epithelial in nature (e.g. epidermoid, dermoid, transitional cell) or endothelial in nature (e.g. lymphangiomas, haemangiomas, hamartomas). These lesions may reach huge proportions and become symptomatic from capsular distension and pressure. Cholesterol-containing cysts have low level shimmering reflections within them on US (Fig. 65.62). Lymphangiomatous cysts show fine septations within the cyst. A hamartoma is an uncommon solid benign tumour in the spleen in children (Fig. 65.63). Malignant neoplasms of the spleen are usually metastatic or haematogenous in aetiology, e.g. leukaemia and lymphoma. In leukaemia and lymphoma, the spleen can be grossly enlarged homogeneously or heterogeneously with multifocal deposits of reduced reflectivity. Angiosarcoma is the most common malignant tumour of the spleen and presents as a solid heterogeneous mass within the spleen. US-guided needle biopsy of a splenic lesion may be indicated for diagnosis (Fig. 65.63) as the differential diagnosis is wide and more than one pathology can coexist.

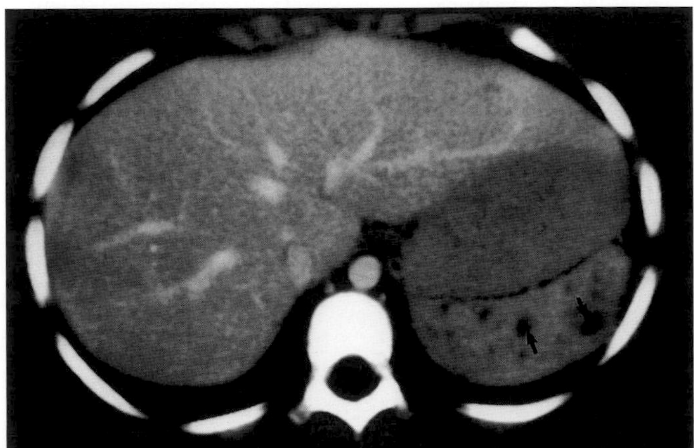

Figure 65.61 Cat scratch disease. Axial CT through the upper abdomen of a 5 year old girl with fever for 4 weeks shows multiple low attenuating lesions in the spleen. Ultrasound-guided biopsy of these lesions showed cat scratch disease. She improved following treatment with clarithromycin.

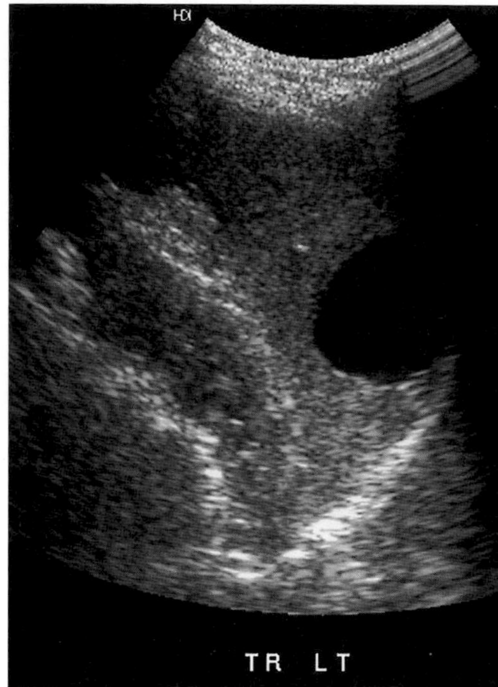

Figure 65.62 Splenic cyst. Incidental splenic cyst seen in a 5 year old girl with smooth walls, no internal reflections and no flow on colour Doppler. A cholesterol containing cyst looks similar but with low level reflections within it.

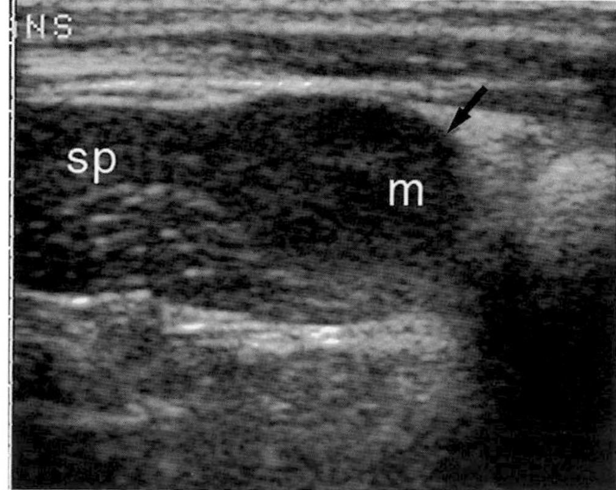

Figure 65.63 Leiomyosarcoma secondary to immunosuppression. Ultrasound of spleen showing a rounded lesion of low reflectivity towards the splenic edge (arrow) in a patient after liver transplantation. m = mass, sp = spleen.

Acknowledgements

We wish to acknowledge the advice and assistance given by Dr Martin Charron and Dr Philip John.

REFERENCES

1. Emanuel P G, Garcia G I, Angtuaco T L 1995 Prenatal detection of anterior abdominal wall defects with US. RadioGraphics 15: 517–530
2. Weber T R, Au-Fliegner M, Downard C D et al 2002 Abdominal wall defects. Curr Opin Pediatr 14: 491–497
3. Howell K K 1998 Understanding gastroschisis: an abdominal wall defect. Neonatal Netw 17: 17–25
4. Ergün O, Barksdale E, Ergün F S et al 2005 The timing of delivery of infants with gastroschisis influences outcome. J Pediatr Surg 40: 424–428
5. Chittmittrapap S, Spitz L, Kiely E M et al 1989 Oesophageal atresia and associated anomalies. Arch Dis Child 64: 364–368
6. Newman B, Bender T M 1997 Esophageal atresia/tracheoesophageal fistula and associated congenital esophageal stenosis. Pediatr Radiol 27: 530–534
7. Gassner I, Geley T E 2005 Sonographic evaluation of oesophageal atresia and tracheo-oesophageal fistula. Pediatr Radiol 35: 159–164
8. Kulkarni B, Rao R S, Oak S et al 1997 13 pairs of ribs—a predictor of long gap atresia in tracheoesophageal fistula. J Pediatr Surg 32: 1453–1454
9. Luo C-C, Lin J-N, Wang C-R 2002 Evaluation of oesophageal atresia without fistula by three-dimensional computed tomography. Eur J Pediatr 161: 578–580
10. Soye J A, Yarr J, Dick A C et al 2005 Multidetector row computed tomography three-dimensional volume reformatted 'transparency' images to define an upper pouch fistula in oesophageal atresia. Pediatr Radiol 35: 624–626
11. Stringer D A, Ein S H 1984 Recurrent tracheo-esophageal fistula: a protocol for investigation. Radiology 151: 637–641
12. Nambirajan L, Rintala R J, Losty P D et al 1998 The value of early postoperative oesophagography following repair of oesophageal atresia. Pediatr Surg Int 13: 76–78
13. Lang T, Hümmer H P, Behrens R 2001 Balloon dilation is preferable to bougienage in children with esophageal atresia. Endoscopy 33: 329–335
14. Yeming W, Somme S, Chenren S et al 2002 Balloon catheter dilatation in children with congenital and acquired esophageal anomalies. J Pediatr Surg 37: 398–402
15. Lan L C L, Wong K K Y, Lin S C L et al 2003 Endoscopic balloon dilatation of esophageal strictures in infants and children: 17 years' experience and a literature review. J Pediatr Surg 38: 1712–1715
16. Nakamura H, Sawamura D, Goto M et al 2005 Epidermolysis bullosa simplex associated with pyloric atresia is a novel clinical subtype caused by mutations in the Plectin gene (PLEC1). J Mol Diagn 7: 28–35
17. Chew A L, Friedwald J P, Donovan C 1992 Diagnosis of congenital antral web by ultrasound. Pediatr Radiol 22: 342–343
18. Snyder W H Jr, Chaffin L 1954 Embryology and pathology of the intestinal tract: presentation of 40 cases of malrotation. Ann Surg 140: 368–379
19. Filston H C, Kirks D R 1981 Malrotation the ubiquitous anomaly. J Pediatr Surg 16 (Suppl 1): 614–620
20. Levin T L, Liebling M S, Ruzal-Shapiro C et al 1995 Midgut malfixation in patients with congenital diaphragmatic hernia: what is the risk of midgut volvulus? Pediatr Radiol 25: 259–261
21. Tiu C M, Chou Y H, Pan H B et al 1984 Congenital short bowel. Pediatr Radiol 14: 343–345
22. Ablow R C, Hoffer F A, Seashore J H et al 1983 Z-shaped duodenojejunal loop: sign of mesenteric fixation anomaly and congenital bands. Am J Roentgenol 141: 461–464
23. Long F R, Kramer S S, Markowitz R I et al 1996 Radiographic patterns of intestinal malrotation in children. RadioGraphics 16: 547–556
24. Dufour D, Delaet M H, Dassonville M et al 1992 Midgut malrotation, the reliability of sonographic diagnosis. Pediatr Radiol 22: 21–23
25. Zerin J M, Polley T Z Jr 1994 Malrotation in patients with duodenal atresia: a true association or an expected finding on postoperative upper gastrointestinal barium study? Pediatr Radiol 24: 170–172
26. Dwek J R, Teich S 1999 The duodenal dimple: a specific fluoroscopic correlate to the duodenal web. Pediatr Radiol 29: 467–468
27. Yoon C H, Goo H W, Kim E A-R et al 2001 Sonographic windsock sign of a duodenal web. Pediatr Radiol 31: 856–857
28. Schiavetti E, Massotti G, Torricelli M et al 1984 "Apple peel" syndrome. A radiological study. Pediatr Radiol 14: 380–383
29. Seashore J H, Collins F S, Markowitz R I et al 1987 Familial apple peel jejunal atresia: surgical, genetic, and radiographic aspects. Pediatrics 80: 540–544

30. Guttman FM, Braun P, Garance PH et al 1973 Multiple atresias and a new syndrome of hereditary multiple atresias involving the gastrointestinal tract from stomach to rectum. J Pediatr Surg 8:633–640
31. Lambrecht W, Kluth D 1998 Hereditary multiple atresias of the gastrointestinal tract: report of a case and review of the literature. J Pediatr Surg 33: 794–797
32. Noerr B 2003 Part 1. Current controversies in the understanding of necrotizing enterocolitis. Adv Neonatal Care 3: 107–120
33. Carty H, Brereton R J 1983 The distended neonate. Clin Radiol 34: 367–380
34. Albanese C T, Rowe M I 1995 Necrotizing enterocolitis. Semin Pediatr Surg 4: 200–206
35. Edwards D K 1980 Size of gas-filled bowel loops in infants. Am J Roentgenol 135: 331–334
36. Uken P, Smith W, Franken E A et al 1988 Use of the barium enema in the diagnosis of necrotizing enterocolitis. Pediatr Radiol 18: 24–27
37. Kao S C, Smith W L, Franken E A Jr et al 1992 Contrast enema diagnosis of necrotizing enterocolitis. Pediatr Radiol 22: 115–117
38. Leonidas J C, Krasna I H, Fox H A et al 1973 Peritoneal fluid in necrotizing enterocolitis: a radiologic sign of clinical deterioration. J Pediatr 82: 672–675
39. Leonard T Jr, Johnson J F, Pettett P G 1982 Critical evaluation of the persistent loop sign in necrotizing enterocolitis. Radiology 142: 385–386
40. Goske M J, Goldblum J R, Applegate K E et al 1999 The "circle sign": a new sonographic sign of pneumatosis intestinalis—clinical, pathologic and experimental findings. Pediatr Radiol 29: 530–535
41. Frey E E, Smith W, Franken E A Jr et al 1987 Analysis of bowel perforation in necrotizing enterocolitis. Pediatr Radiol 17: 380–382
42. Seibert J J, Parvey L S 1977 The telltale triangle: use of the supine cross table lateral radiograph of the abdomen in early detection of pneumoperitoneum. Pediatr Radiol 5: 209–210
43. Rovin J D, Rodgers B M, Burns R C et al 1999 The role of peritoneal drainage for intestinal perforation in infants with and without necrotizing enterocolitis. J Pediatr Surg 34: 143–147
44. Daneman A, Woodward S, de Silva M 1978 The radiology of neonatal necrotizing enterocolitis (NEC). A review of 47 cases and the literature. Pediatr Radiol 7: 70–77
45. Paley R H, McCarten K M, Cleveland R H 1979 Enterocolonic fistula as a late complication of necrotizing enterocolitis. Am J Roentgenol 132: 989–990
46. Virjee J P, Gill G J, Desa D et al 1979 Strictures and other late complications of neonatal necrotising enterocolitis. Clin Radiol 30: 25–31
47. Ball T I, Wyly J B 1986 Enterocyst formation: a late complication of neonatal necrotizing enterocolitis. Am J Roentgenol 147: 806–808
48. Haney P J, Hill J L, Sun C C 1982 Zonal colonic aganglionosis. Pediatr Radiol 12: 258–261
49. De Campo J F, Mayne V, Boldt D W et al 1984 Radiological findings in total aganglionosis coli. Pediatr Radiol 14: 205–209
50. Roshkow J E, Haller J O, Berdon W E et al 1988 Hirschsprung's disease, Ondine's curse, and neuroblastoma—manifestations of neurocristopathy. Pediatr Radiol 19: 45–49
51. Janik J P, Wayne E R, Janik J S et al 1997 Ileal atresia with total colonic aganglionosis. J Pediatr Surg 32: 1502–1503
52. Siu K L, Kwok W K, Lee W Y et al 1999 A male newborn with colonic atresia and total colonic aganglionosis. Pediatr Surg Int 15: 141–142
53. Amiel J, Lyonnet S 2001 Hirschsprung disease, associated syndromes, and genetics: a review. J Med Genet 38: 729–739
54. Sarioglu A, Tanyel F C, Buyukpamukcu N et al 1997 Colonic volvulus: a rare presentation of Hirschsprung's disease. J Pediatr Surg 32: 117–118
55. Bradley M J, Pilling D 1991 The empty rectum on plain X-ray. Does it have any significance in the neonate? Clin Radiol 43: 265–267
56. Fletcher B D, Yullish B S 1978 Intraluminal calcifications in the small bowel of newborn infants with total colonic aganglionosis. Radiology 126: 451–455
57. Rosenfield N S, Ablow R C, Markowitz R I et al 1984 Hirschsprung disease: accuracy of the barium enema examination. Radiology 150: 393–400
58. O'Donovan A N, Habra G, Somers S et al 1996 Diagnosis of Hirschsprung's disease. Am J Roentgenol 167: 517–520
59. Amodio J, Berdon W, Abramson S et al 1986 Microcolon of prematurity: a form of functional obstruction. Am J Roentgenol 146: 239–244
60. Berrocal T, Lamas M, Gutierrez J et al 1999 Congenital anomalies of the small intestine, colon, and rectum. RadioGraphics 19: 1219–1236
61. Heaton N D, Howard E R, Garrett J R 1991 Small left colon syndrome: an immature enteric plexus. J R Soc Med 84: 113–114
62. Winters W D, Weinberger E, Hatch E I 1992 Atresia of the colon in neonates: radiographic findings. Am J Roentgenol 159: 1273–1276
63. Landes A, Shuckett B, Skarsgard E 1994 Non-fixation of the colon in colonic atresia: a new finding. Pediatr Radiol 24: 167–169
64. Hamosh A, Fitz-Simmons S C, Macek M Jr et al 1998 Comparison of the clinical manifestations of cystic fibrosis in black and white patients. J Pediatr 132: 255–259
65. Evans A K C, Fitzgerald D A, McKay K O 2001 The impact of meconium ileus on the clinical course of children with cystic fibrosis. Eur Respir J 18: 784–789
66. Li Z, Lai H J, Kosorok M R et al 2004 Longitudinal pulmonary status of cystic fibrosis children with meconium ileus. Pediatr Pulmonol 38: 277–284
67. Neal M R, Seibert J J, Vanderzalm T et al 1997 Neonatal ultrasonography to distinguish between meconium ileus and ileal atresia. J Ultrasound Med 16: 263–266
68. Navarro O M, Daneman A, Miller S F 2004 Contrast enema depiction of small-bowel volvulus in complicated neonatal bowel obstruction. Pediatr Radiol 34: 1020–1023
69. Noblett H R 1969 Treatment of uncomplicated meconium ileus by Gastrografin enema: a preliminary report. J Pediatr Surg 4: 190–197
70. Kao S C, Franken E A Jr 1995 Nonoperative treatment of simple meconium ileus: a survey of the Society for Pediatric Radiology. Pediatr Radiol 25: 97–100
71. Leonidas J C, Berdon W E, Baker D H et al 1970 Meconium ileus and its complications. A reappraisal of plain film roentgen diagnostic criteria. Am J Roentgenol Radium Ther Nucl Med 108: 598–609
72. Finkel L I, Slovis T L 1982 Meconium peritonitis, intraperitoneal calcifications and cystic fibrosis. Pediatr Radiol 12: 92–93
73. Lang I, Daneman A, Cutz E et al 1997 Abdominal calcification in cystic fibrosis with meconium ileus: radiologic–pathologic correlation. Pediatr Radiol 27: 523–527
74. Hassink E A, Rieu P N, Hamel B C et al 1996 Additional congenital defects in anorectal malformations. Eur J Pediatr 155: 477–482
75. Torres R, Levitt M A, Tovilla J M et al 1998 Anorectal malformations and Down's syndrome. J Pediatr Surg 33: 194–197
76. Seibert J J, Golladay E S 1979 Clinical evaluation of imperforate anus: clue to type of anal-rectal anomaly. Am J Roentgenol 133: 289–292
77. Donaldson J S, Black C T, Reynolds M et al 1989 Ultrasound of the distal pouch in infants with imperforate anus. J Pediatr Surg 24: 465–468
78. Berdon W E, Baker D H, Wigger H J et al 1975 Calcified intraluminal meconium in newborn males with imperforate anus. Enterolithiasis in the newborn. Am J Roentgenol Radium Ther Nucl Med 125: 449–455
79. Gross G W, Wolfson P J, Pena A 1991 Augmented-pressure colostogram in imperforate anus with fistula. Pediatr Radiol 21: 560–562
80. Metts J C, III, Kotkin L, Kasper S et al 1997 Genital malformations and coexistent urinary tract or spinal anomalies in patients with imperforate anus. J Urol 158: 1298–1300
81. Daneman A, Navarro O 2003 Intussusception part 1: a review of diagnostic approaches. Pediatr Radiol 33: 79–85
82. Harrington L, Connolly B, Hu X et al 1998 Ultrasonographic and clinical predictors of intussusception. J Pediatr 132: 836–839
83. Harquinet S, Aniishiravani M, Vunda A et al 1998 Reliability of color Doppler and power Doppler sonography in the evaluation of intussuscepted bowel viability. Pediatr Surg Int 13: 360–362
84. Navarro O, Daneman A 2004 Intussusception part 3: diagnosis and management of those with an identifiable or predisposing cause and those that reduce spontaneously. Pediatr Radiol 34: 305–312
85. Gu L, Alton D J, Daneman A et al 1988 Intussusception reduction in children by re-insufflation of air. Am J Roentgenol 150: 1345–1348

86. Daneman A, Navarro O 2004 Intussusception part 2: an update on the evolution of management. Pediatr Radiol 34: 97–108
87. Crystal P, Hertzanu Y, Farber B et al 2002 Sonographically guided hydrostatic reduction of intussusception in children. J Clin Ultrasound 30: 343–348
88. Rohrschneider W K, Troger J 1994 Hydrostatic reduction under US guidance. Pediatr Radiol 25: 530–534
89. Navarro O, Daneman A, Chae A 2004 Intussusception: the use of delayed repeated attempts and the management of intussusceptions due to pathologic lead points in pediatric patients. Am J Roentgenol 182: 1169–1176
90. Patriquin H B, Garcier J M, Lafortune M et al 1995 Appendicitis in children and young adults: Doppler sonographic-pathologic correlation. Am J Roentgenol 166: 629–633
91. Kessler N, Cyteval C, Gallix B et al 2004 Appendicitis: Evaluation of, sensitivity, specificity, and predictive values of US, Doppler US and laboratory findings. Radiology 230: 472–478
92. Sivit C, Siegel M, Applegate K et al 2001 When appendicitis is suspected in children. RadioGraphics 21: 247–262
93. Sivit C, Applegate K 2003 Imaging of acute appendicitis in children. Semin Ultrasound CT MR 24: 74–82
94. Sivit C 2004 Imaging the child with right lower quadrant pain and suspected appendicitis: current concepts. Pediatr Radiol 34: 447–453
95. Carty H 2002 Paediatric emergencies: non-traumatic abdominal emergencies. Eur Radiol 12: 2835–2848
96. Taylor G 2004 Suspected acute appendicitis in children: in search of the single best diagnostic test. Radiology 231: 293–295
97. Garcia Pena B M, Cook E F, Mandl K D 2004 Selective imaging strategies for the diagnosis of appendicitis in children. Pediatrics 113: 24–28
98. Fefferman N, Roche K, Pinkney L et al 2001 Suspected appendicitis in children: focused CT technique for evaluation. Radiology 220: 691–695
99. Sivit C J, Newman K D, Chandra R S 1993 Visualization of enlarged mesenteric lymph nodes at US examination. Pediatr Radiol 23: 471–475
100. Karmazyn B, Werner E, Rejaie B et al 2005 Mesenteric lymph nodes in children: what is normal? Pediatr Radiol 35: 774–777
101. Vayner N, Coret A, Polliack G et al 2003 Mesenteric lymphadenopathy in children examined by US for chronic and /or recurrent abdominal pain. Pediatr Radiol 33: 864–867
102. Rathaus V, Shapiro M, Grunebaum M et al 2005 Enlarged mesenteric lymph nodes in asymptomatic children: the value of the finding in various imaging modalities. Br J Radiol 78:30–33
103. Connolly B, O`Halpin D 1994 Sonographic evaluation of the abdomen in Henoch-Schönlein purpura. Clin Radiol 49: 320–323
104. Fotter R 1998 Imaging of constipation in infants and children. Eur J Radiol 8: 248–258
105. Wagener S, Shankar K, Turnock R et al 2004 Colonic transit time—what is normal? J Pediatr Surg 39: 166–169
106. Blethyn A J, Verrier Jones K, Newcombe R et al 1995 Radiological assessment of constipation. Arch Dis Child 73: 255–258
107. Roos J, Weishaupt D, Wildermuth S et al 2002 Experience of 4 years with open MR defaecography: pictoral review of anorectal anatomy and disease. RadioGraphics 22: 817–832
108. Franken E A, Smith W L, Frey E E et al 1987 Intestinal motility disorders of infants and children: classification, clinical manifestations and roentgenology. Crit Rev Diagn Radiol 27: 203–236
109. Goulet O, Jobert-Giraud A, Michel J-L et al 1997 Chronic intestinal pseudo-obstruction syndrome in pediatric patients. Eur J Pediatr Surg 9: 83–90
110. Rance C H, Singh S J, Kimble R 2000 Blunt abdominal trauma in children. J Paediatr Child Health 36: 2–6
111. Emery K, McAneney C, Racadio J et al 2001 Absent peritoneal fluid on screening trauma ultrasonography in children: a prospective comparison with computed tomography. J Pediatr Surg 36: 565–569
112. Strouse P J, Close B J, Marshall K W et al 1999 CT of abdominal and mesenteric trauma in children. RadioGraphics 19: 1237–1250
113. Sivit C J, Taylor G A, Eichelberger M R et al 1993 Significance of periportal low attenuation zones following blunt abdominal trauma in children. Pediatr Radiol 23: 388–390
114. Sivit C J, Eichelberger M R, Taylor G A 1994 CT in children with rupture of the bowel caused by blunt trauma: diagnostic efficacy and comparison with hypoperfusion complex. Am J Roentgenol 163: 1196–1198
115. Rao P 1999 Emergency imaging in non-accidental injury. In: Carty H (ed) Emergency paediatric radiology. Springer, Berlin, pp 348–380
116. Hernanz-Schulzman M 2003 Infantile hypertrophic pyloric stenosis. Radiology 227: 319–331
117. Cohen H L, Zinn H L, Haller J O et al 1998 Ultrasonography of pylorospasm: findings may simulate hypertrophic pyloric stenosis. J Ultrasound Med 17: 705–711
118. Orenstein S R, Orenstein D M 1988 Gastroesophageal reflux and respiratory disease in children. J Pediatr 112: 847–858 [published erratum appears in J Pediatr 1988; 113: 578].
119. Yulish B S, Rothstein F C, Halpin T C Jr 1987 Radiographic findings in children and young adults with Barrett's esophagus. Am J Roentgenol 148: 353–357
120. Westra S J, Wolf B H, Staalman C R 1990 Ultrasound diagnosis of gastroesophageal reflux and hiatal hernia in infants and young children. J Clin Ultrasound 18: 477–485
121. Newell S J, Chapman S, Booth I W 1993 Ultrasonic assessment of gastric emptying in the preterm infant. Arch Dis Child 69(1 Spec No): 32–36
122. Trinh T D, Benson J E 1997 Fluoroscopic diagnosis of complications after Nissen antireflux fundoplication in children. Am J Roentgenol 169: 1023–1028
123. Segal S R, Sherman N M, Rosenberg H K et al 1994 Ultrasonographic features of gastrointestinal duplications. J Ultrasound Med 13: 863–870
124. Macpherson R I 1993 Gastrointestinal tract duplications: Clinical, pathologic, and radiologic considerations. RadioGraphics 13: 1063–1080
125. Stoupis C, Ros P R, Abbitt P L et al 1994 Bubbles in the belly: imaging of cystic mesenteric or omental masses. RadioGraphics 14: 729–737
126. Vinton N E 1994 Gastrointestinal bleeding in infancy and childhood. Gastroenterol Clin North Am 23: 93–122
127. Baud C, Saguintaah M, Veyrac C et al 2004 Sonographic diagnosis of colitis in children. Eur Radiol 14: 2105–2119
128. Ali S I, Carty H M L 2000 Paediatric Crohn's disease. Eur Radiol 10: 1085–1094
129. Grahnquist L, Chapman S C, Hvidsten S et al 2003 Evaluation of ^{99m}Tc-HMPAO leucocyte scintography in the investigation of pediatric inflammatory bowel disease. J Pediatr 143: 48–53
130. Darbari A, Sena L, Argani P et al 2004 Gadolinium-enhanced magnetic resonance imaging: a useful radiological tool in diagnosing pediatric IBD. Inflam Bowel Dis 10: 67–72
131. Hyer W 2001 Polyposis syndromes: pediatric implications. Gastrointest Endosc Clin North Am 11: 659–682
132. Corredor J, Wambach J, Barnard J 2001 Gastrointestinal polyps in children: advances in molecular genetics, diagnosis, and management. J Pediatr 138: 621–628
133. Kurugoglu S, Aksoy H, Kantarci F et al 2003 Radiological work-up in Peutz–Jeghers syndrome. Pediatr Radiol 33: 766–771
134. Cohen M D 1992 Reticulo-endothelial tumours. In: Imaging of children with cancer. Mosby, St Louis, pp 89–126
135. Hudson M M, Krasin M J, Kaste S C 2004 PET imaging in pediatric Hodgkin's lymphoma. Pediatr Radiol 34: 190–198
136. Wegner E A, Barrington S F, Kingston J E et al 2005 The impact of PET scanning on management of paediatric oncology patients. Eur J Nucl Med Mol Imaging 32: 23–30
137. Khati N J, Enquist E G, Javitt M C 1998 Imaging of the umbilicus and periumbilical region. RadioGraphics 18: 413–431
138. Rerksuppaphol S, Hutson J M, Oliver M R 2004 Ranitidine-enhanced 99m technetium pertechnetate imaging in children improves the sensitivity of identifying heterotopic gastric mucosa in Meckel's diverticulum. Pediatr Surg Int 20: 323–325

139. Agrons G A, Corse W R, Markowitz R I et al 1996 Gastrointestinal manifestations of cystic fibrosis: Radiologic–pathologic correlation. RadioGraphics 16: 871–893
140. Smyth R L, van Vetzen D, Smyth A R et al 1994 Strictures of the ascending colon in cystic fibrosis and high strength pancreatic enzymes. Lancet 342: 85–86
141. Almberger M, Iannicelli E, Antonelli M et al 2001 The role of MRI in the intestinal complications in cystic fibrosis. J Clin Imaging 25: 344–348
142. Zerin J M, Kuhn-Fulton J, White S J et al 1995 Colonic strictures in children with cystic fibrosis. Radiology 194: 223–226
143. Dialer I, Hundt C, Bertele-Harms R M et al 2003 Sonographic evaluation of bowel wall thickness in patients with cystic fibrosis. J Clin Gastroenterol 37: 55–60
144. Lardenoye S W, Puylaert J B, Smit M J et al 2004 Appendix in children with cystic fibrosis: US features. Radiology 232: 187–189
145. Patriquin H, Lenaerts C, Smith L et al 1999 Liver disease in children with cystic fibrosis: US-biochemical comparison in 195 patients. Radiology 211: 229–232
146. Lenaerts C, Lapierre C, Patriquin H et al 2003 Surveillance for cystic fibrosis-associated hepatobiliary disease: Early changes and predisposing factors. J Pediatr 143: 343–350
147. Williams S M, Goodman R, Thompson A et al 2002 Ultrasound evaluation of liver disease in cystic fibrosis as part of an annual assessment clinic: a nine year review. Clin Radiol 57: 365–370
148. Neglia J P, Fitzsimmons S C, Maisonneuve P et al 1995 The risk of cancer among patients with cystic fibrosis. N Engl J Med 332: 494–499
149. Haller J O, Cohen H L 1994 Gastrointestinal manifestations of AIDS in children. Am J Roentgenol 162: 387–393
150. Andronikou S, Welman C J, Kader E 2002 The CT features of abdominal tuberculosis in children. Pediatr Radiol 32: 75–81
151. McCarville B, Adelman C S, Li C 2005 Typhlitis in childhood cancer. Cancer 104: 380–387
152. Cartoni C, Dragoni F, Micozzi A et al 2001 Neutropenic enterocolitis in patients with acute leukaemia: prognostic significance of bowel wall thickening detected by ultrasonography. J Clin Oncol 19; 756–761
153. Kirkpatrick I D C, Greenberg H M 2003 Gastrointestinal complications in the neutropenic patient : Characterization and differentiation with abdominal CT. Radiology 226: 668–674
154. McGahen E D 1999 Esophageal foreign bodies. Pediatr Rev 20: 129–133
155. Eggli K D, Potter B M, Garcia V et al 1986 Delayed diagnosis of oesophageal perforation by aluminium foreign bodies. Pediatr Radiol 16: 511–513
156. O'Hara S, Donnelly L F, Chuang E et al 1999 Gastric retention of zinc-based pennies: radiographic appearance and hazards. Pediatr Imaging 213: 113–117
157. Neilson I R 1995 Ingestion of coins and batteries. Pediatr Rev 16: 35–36
158. Tay E T, Weinberg G, Levin T L 2004 Ingested magnets: the force within. Pediatr Emerg Care 20: 466–467
159. Cauchi J A, Shawis R N 2002 Multiple magnet ingestion and gastrointestinal morbidity. Arch Dis Child 87: 539–540
160. Macpherson R I, Hill J G, Othersen H B et al 1996 Esophageal foreign bodies in children: diagnosis, treatment and complications. Am J Roentgenol 166: 919–924
161. Nagi B, Kochhar R, Thapa B R et al 2004 Radiological spectrum of late sequelae of corrosive injury to upper gastrointestinal tract. A pictorial review. Acta Radiol 45: 7–12
162. Nuutinen M, Uhari M, Karvali T et al 1994 Consequences of caustic ingestions in children. Acta Pediatr 83: 1200–1205
163. Fasulakis S, Andronikou S 2003 Balloon dilatation in children for oesophageal strictures other than those due to primary repair of oesophageal atresia, interposition or restrictive fundoplication. Pediatr Radiol 33: 682–687
164. Donnelly L F, Bisset G S 3rd 1998 Pediatric hepatic imaging. Radiol Clin North Am 36: 413–427
165. Siegel M J 2001 Pediatric liver imaging. Semin Liver Dis 21: 251–269
166. Hudson-Dixon C M, Long B W, Cox L A 1999 Power Doppler imaging: principles and applications. Radiol Technol 70: 235–243
167. Siegel M J 1995 MR imaging of the pediatric abdomen. Magn Reson Imaging Clin North Am 3: 161–182
168. Guibaud L, Lachaud A, Touraine R et al 1998 MR cholangiography in neonates and infants: feasibility and preliminary applications. Am J Roentgenol 170: 27–31
169. Miyazaki T, Yamashita Y, Tang Y, Tsuchigame T, Takahashi M, Sera Y 1998 Single-shot MR cholangiopancreatography of neonates, infants, and young children. Am J Roentgenol 170: 33–37
170. Chan Y L, Yeung C K, Lam W W, Fok T F, Metreweli C 1998 Magnetic resonance cholangiography–feasibility and application in the paediatric population. Pediatr Radiol 28: 307–311
171. Roca I, Ciofetta G 1998 Hepatobiliary scintigraphy in current pediatric practice. Q J Nucl Med 42: 113–118
172. Nadel H R 1996 Hepatobiliary scintigraphy in children. Semin Nucl Med 26: 25–42
173. Gilmour S M, Hershkop M, Reifen R, Gilday D, Roberts E A 1997 Outcome of hepatobiliary scanning in neonatal hepatitis syndrome. J Nucl Med 38: 1279–1282
174. Cheng C L, Fogel E L, Sherman S et al 2005 Diagnostic and therapeutic endoscopic retrograde cholangiopancreatography in children: a large series report. J Pediatr Gastroenterol Nutr 41: 445–453
175. Applegate K E, Goske M J, Pierce G, Murphy D 1999 Situs revisited: imaging of the heterotaxy syndrome. RadioGraphics 19: 837–852; discussion 853–834
176. Moore K P, Persaud T V N 2002 The developing human, clinically oriented embryology, 6th edn. W B Saunders, Philadelphia
177. McGahan J P, Phillips H E, Cox K L 1982 Sonography of the normal pediatric gallbladder and biliary tract. Radiology 144: 873–875
178. Hernanz-Schulman M, Ambrosino M M, Freeman P C, Quinn C B 1995 Common bile duct in children: sonographic dimensions. Radiology 195: 193–195
179. Schlesinger A E, Braverman R M, DiPietro M A 2003 Pictorial essay. Neonates and umbilical venous catheters: normal appearance, anomalous positions, complications, and potential aid to diagnosis. Am J Roentgenol 180: 1147–1153
180. Rosenberg H K, Markowitz R I, Kolberg H, Park C, Hubbard A, Bellah R D 1991 Normal splenic size in infants and children: sonographic measurements. Am J Roentgenol 157: 119–121
181. Shah H A, Spivak W 1994 Neonatal cholestasis. New approaches to diagnostic evaluation and therapy. Pediatr Clin North Am 41: 943–966
182. Venigalla S, Gourley G R 2004 Neonatal cholestasis. Semin Perinatol 28: 348–355
183. Davenport M 2005 Biliary atresia. Semin Pediatr Surg 14: 42–48
184. Torrisi J M, Haller J O, Velcek F T 1990 Choledochal cyst and biliary atresia in the neonate: imaging findings in five cases. Am J Roentgenol 155: 1273–1276
185. Mack C L, Sokol R J 2005 Unraveling the pathogenesis and etiology of biliary atresia. Pediatr Res 57: 87R–94R
186. Bezerra J A 2005 Potential etiologies of biliary atresia. Pediatr Transplant 9: 646–651
187. Park W H, Choi S O, Lee H J, Kim S P, Zeon S K, Lee S L 1997 A new diagnostic approach to biliary atresia with emphasis on the ultrasonographic triangular cord sign: comparison of ultrasonography, hepatobiliary scintigraphy, and liver needle biopsy in the evaluation of infantile cholestasis. J Pediatr Surg 32: 1555–1559
188. Petersen C 2004 Surgery in biliary atresia—futile or futuristic? Eur J Pediatr Surg 14: 226–229
189. Sherman P, Kolster E, Davies C, Stringer D, Weber J 1986 Choledochal cysts: heterogeneity of clinical presentation. J Pediatr Gastroenterol Nutr 5: 867–872
190. Brancatelli G, Federle M P, Vilgrain V, Vullierme M P, Marin D, Lagalla R 2005 Fibropolycystic liver disease: CT and MR imaging findings. RadioGraphics 25: 659–670
191. Krawinkel M B 2004 Parenteral nutrition-associated cholestasis—what do we know, what can we do? Eur J Pediatr Surg 14: 230–234

192. Chardot C, Iskandarani F, De Dreuzy O et al 1996 Spontaneous perforation of the biliary tract in infancy: a series of 11 cases. Eur J Pediatr Surg 6: 341–346
193. Brook I 2004 Intra-abdominal, retroperitoneal, and visceral abscesses in children. Eur J Pediatr Surg 14: 265–273
194. Seeto R K, Rockey D C 1996 Pyogenic liver abscess. Changes in etiology, management, and outcome. Medicine (Baltimore) 75: 99–113
195. Khanna G, Kao S C, Kirby P, Sato Y 2005 Imaging of chronic granulomatous disease in children. RadioGraphics 25: 1183–1195
196. Emre S, McKenna G J 2004 Liver tumors in children. Pediatr Transplant 8: 632–638
197. von Schweinitz D, Gluer S, Mildenberger H 1995 Liver tumors in neonates and very young infants: diagnostic pitfalls and therapeutic problems. Eur J Pediatr Surg 5: 72–76
198. Pobiel R S, Bisset G S, 3rd 1995 Pictorial essay: imaging of liver tumors in the infant and child. Pediatr Radiol 25: 495–506
199. Donnelly L F, Bisset G S 3rd 2002 Unique imaging issues in pediatric liver disease. Clin Liver Dis 6: 227–246, viii
200. Kassarjian A, Dubois J, Burrows P E 2002 Angiographic classification of hepatic hemangiomas in infants. Radiology 222: 693–698
201. Teo E L, Strouse P J, Prince M R 1999 Applications of magnetic resonance imaging and magnetic resonance angiography to evaluate the hepatic vasculature in the pediatric patient. Pediatr Radiol 29: 238–243
202. Koumanidou C, Vakaki M, Papadaki M, Pitsoulakis G, Savvidou D, Kakavakis K 1999 New sonographic appearance of hepatic mesenchymal hamartoma in childhood. J Clin Ultrasound 27: 164–167
203. Murray J D, Ricketts R R 1998 Mesenchymal hamartoma of the liver. Am Surg 64: 1097–1103
204. Keller M S, Markle B M, Laffey P A, Chawla H S, Jacir N, Frank J L 1985 Spontaneous resolution of cholelithiasis in infants. Radiology 157: 345–348
205. Burrows P E, Dubois J, Kassarjian A 2001 Pediatric hepatic vascular anomalies. Pediatr Radiol 31: 533–545
206. Gallego C, Miralles M, Marin C, Muyor P, Gonzalez G, Garcia-Hidalgo E 2004 Congenital hepatic shunts. RadioGraphics 24: 755–772
207. Ohta M, Hashizume M, Tomikawa M, Ueno K, Tanoue K, Sugimachi K 1994 Analysis of hepatic vein waveform by Doppler ultrasonography in 100 patients with portal hypertension. Am J Gastroenterol 89: 170–175
208. Okuda K, Kage M, Shrestha S M 1998 Proposal of a new nomenclature for Budd–Chiari syndrome: hepatic vein thrombosis versus thrombosis of the inferior vena cava at its hepatic portion. Hepatology 28: 1191–1198
209. Kelly D A 1998 Pediatric liver transplantation. Curr Opin Pediatr 10: 493–498
210. Patenaude Y G, Dubois J, Sinsky A B et al 1997 Liver transplantation: review of the literature. Part 3: Medical complications. Can Assoc Radiol J 48: 333–339
211. Patenaude Y G, Dubois J, Sinsky A B et al 1997 Liver transplantation: review of the literature. Part 2: Vascular and biliary complications. Can Assoc Radiol J 48: 231–242
212. Patenaude Y G, Dubois J, Sinsky A B et al 1997 Liver transplantation: review of the literature. Part 1: Anatomic features and current concepts. Can Assoc Radiol J 48: 171–178
213. Westra S J, Zaninovic A C, Hall T R, Busuttil R W, Kangarloo H, Boechat M I 1993 Imaging in pediatric liver transplantation. RadioGraphics 13: 1081–1099
214. Vural M, Kacar S, Kosar U, Altin L 1999 Symptomatic wandering accessory spleen in the pelvis: sonographic findings. J Clin Ultrasound 27: 534–536
215. Paterson A, Frush D P, Donnelly L F, Foss J N, O'Hara S M, Bisset G S 3rd 1999 A pattern-oriented approach to splenic imaging in infants and children. RadioGraphics 19: 1465–1485
216. Karakas H M, Tuncbilek N, Okten O O 2005 Splenic abnormalities: an overview on sectional images. Diagn Interv Radiol 11: 152–158
217. Freeman J L, Jafri S Z, Roberts J L, Mezwa D G, Shirkhoda A 1993 CT of congenital and acquired abnormalities of the spleen. RadioGraphics 13: 597–610
218. Elsayes K M, Narra V R, Mukundan G, Lewis J S Jr, Menias C O, Heiken J P 2005 MR imaging of the spleen: spectrum of abnormalities. RadioGraphics 25: 967–982
219. Thompson S E, Walsh E A, Cramer B C et al 1996 Radiological features of a symptomatic splenic hamartoma. Pediatr Radiol 26: 657–660

SUGGESTED FURTHER READING

Carty H, Brunelle F, Stringer D A, Kao S C S (eds) 2005 Imaging children. Churchill Livingstone, Edinburgh

Kuhn J P, Slovis T L and Haller J O (eds) 2004 Caffey's pediatric diagnostic imaging. Mosby, Philadelphia

Stringer D A 1989 Pediatric gastrointestinal imaging. BC Decker, Toronto

CHAPTER 66

Imaging of the Kidneys, Urinary Tract and Pelvis in Children

Rose de Bruyn, Isky Gordon and Kieran McHugh

Congenital anomalies
- Renal anomalies
- Uterus and vagina
- Undescended testis

Imaging techniques
- Ultrasound
- Cystography
- Nuclear medicine
- Urography (plain radiograph and intravenous urogram)
- Computed tomography
- Magnetic resonance imaging
- Interventional procedures

Integrated imaging
- The neonate
- Bladder anomalies
- Urethral anomalies
- Duplex kidney
- Urinary tract infection and vesico-ureteric reflux
- Hypertension
- Renal cystic disease
- Renal transplantation
- Tumours
- Scrotal masses
- Ovarian masses
- Presacral masses
- Nephrocalcinosis (renal calculus)
- Inflammatory diseases of the scrotum

Advances in imaging in infants and children relies heavily on real-time ultrasound (US) for anatomy, and nuclear medicine studies for functional assessment using either dynamic or static agents such as ^{99m}technetium-dimercapto-succinic acid (^{99m}Tc-DMSA). Intravenous urography (IVU) is now only used to outline calyceal anatomy. Micturating cystourethrography (MCUG) remains crucial for the male urethra. Assessment of vesico-ureteric reflux (VUR) can be done using either radionuclide cystography, MCUG, or US. The use of magnetic resonance imaging (MRI) is developing and its role will become clearer in the future. In tumours computed tomography (CT) and MRI have a crucial role. Angiography is reserved for special clinical situations and, although invasive with a high radiation burden, it still remains the gold standard. CT and MR angiography (MRA), however, are emerging as possible replacements for angiography for diagnostic purposes in the main renal artery. Angioplasty, embolization, antegrade studies, and drainage procedures are becoming more common. It should be borne in mind that each imaging technique has its strengths and weaknesses.

A guiding principle in paediatrics is to choose the least invasive but most appropriate imaging technique with the lowest radiation dose whenever possible. Consequently, almost all genitourinary studies in children should start with US, with the probable exception of severe abdominal trauma. The attitude of every member of the radiology department should be positive, reassuring, and sympathetic. Explanations to allay anxiety must be offered to the child and parent/carer at all stages of the referral for imaging. Ideally we wish for a cooperative child who can also express his/her fears and anxieties. With sufficient information, the parent/carer can frequently help the child overcome anxiety, especially if he/she remains with the child throughout the examination. With this approach, sedation is rarely used in most examinations of the urinary tract (exceptions being CT and MRI in the young or uncooperative). Sedation is positively discouraged for cystography as the child may be too sleepy to void. No special equipment is required for genitourinary examinations in children. All staff must be appropriately trained.

CONGENITAL ANOMALIES

RENAL ANOMALIES

Unilateral renal agenesis occurs in around 1 in 1250 live births. Antenatal diagnosis is uncommon, suggesting that agenesis may be an involuted multicystic kidney. It is difficult to differentiate between unilateral agenesis and a small nonfunctioning kidney, especially if it is ectopically located. This is of clinical importance in a girl who is constantly wet and in whom the small kidney drains via an ectopic ureter, and in a child with hypertension, where the small kidney may be the source of excess renin. To exclude a small ectopic kidney requires ^{99m}Tc-DMSA imaging with anterior views. MRI is useful if there is a dilated ureter but the IVU has no role. Bilateral renal agenesis is incompatible with life. Newborns who die from chronic renal failure do so towards the end of the first weeks of life and those who die in the first hours or day of life usually do so from respiratory causes.

Abnormalities of position

An ectopically placed kidney is of little clinical significance, but a malrotated kidney may develop urological complications, be more susceptible to trauma, or indicate that pathology in an adjacent organ is displacing the kidney. In malrotation, the upper pole of the kidney is located more laterally than the lower pole, and the upper pole calyces are therefore lateral to the lower pole calyces. US will ensure that there is no suprarenal mass lesion causing the malrotation. The ectopic kidney may lie within the bony pelvis and present as a mass; its surgical removal owing to the mistaken diagnosis of tumour is well recorded. Occasionally the kidney continues to migrate beyond the normal renal fossa and ends up in the thorax. This anomaly is associated with eventration of the diaphragm so that in some cases the kidney migrates upwards to lie behind the heart in the thorax and may resemble a posterior mediastinal mass on the chest radiograph.

Abnormalities of fusion

The duplex kidney is common and can have varied manifestations (see below). The most common fusion abnormality is that of the horseshoe kidney with fusion of the lower poles; this is always associated with malrotation so that the pelves and ureters pass anteriorly over the fused lower poles. The two well-recognized complications are renal pelvis dilatation (with or without obstruction) and renal calculi. The abnormal position also leaves the kidney more susceptible to injury. There is a slightly increased risk of Wilms' tumour in a horseshoe kidney. In the uncomplicated horseshoe anomaly US may not detect the abnormal axes of the kidneys, and is therefore not reliable to exclude a horseshoe kidney. When a child presents with intermittent pain and/or haematuria and the US diagnosis is that of a horseshoe kidney, calculi may be missed and plain radiographs or, rarely, nonenhanced CT may be useful. Radionuclide imaging (^{99m}Tc-DMSA) with an anterior view is useful to show all functioning renal tissue, especially over the spine. MRI can easily demonstrate a horseshoe kidney but usually requires anaesthesia in younger patients.

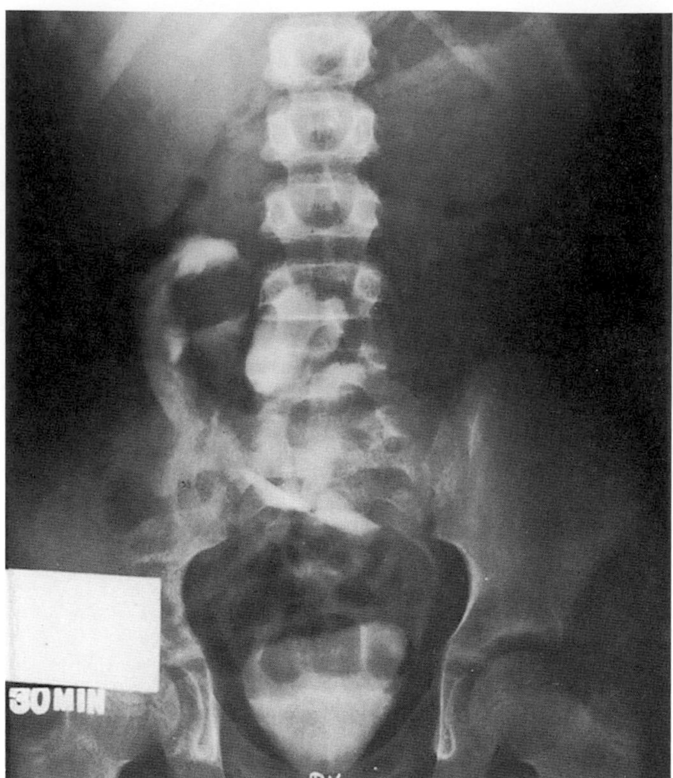

Figure 66.1 Renal ectopia. Crossed fused renal ectopy demonstrated on an intravenous urogram.

Crossed fused renal ectopia occurs when one kidney is displaced across the midline and is fused inferiorly to the other relatively normally positioned kidney. Both ureters enter the bladder in a normal position (Fig. 66.1). The importance of this condition is that it may present as an abdominal mass or as an obstructive uropathy with a pelvi-ureteric junction (PUJ) obstruction. US reveals an unusually large kidney on the affected side and an absent kidney on the opposite side. A dynamic renogram, such as a ^{99m}Tc-mercaptoacetyltriglycine MAG3 study, is required and especially if surgery is being considered for PUJ obstruction. There is an increased incidence ofVUR into the crossed kidney and if further anatomical information concerning the ureter and pelves is required an MCUG may prove helpful. The ^{99m}Tc-DMSA scintigram shows patchy uptake of the isotope owing to the anatomical abnormality and dysplasia that exists to some degree. A rare fusion anomaly is seen when both kidneys have failed to ascend from the pelvis, which is referred to as a pancake kidney (Fig. 66.2).

UTERUS AND VAGINA

In the absence of anti-Müllerian hormone secretion by a fetal testis, the Müllerian ducts meet in the midline by 8 weeks' gestation and subsequently differentiate into the uterus, cervix, Fallopian tubes, and proximal two-thirds of the vagina. The distal third of the vagina is formed by the urogenital sinus.

Müllerian duct development into the uterus depends on the formation of the Wolffian (mesonephric) duct.

Congenital anomalies of the uterus and vagina are uncommon; there is a high incidence of associated renal (50%) and skeletal anomalies (12%). The anomalies usually present as an abdominal or pelvic mass, secondary to obstruction; later they may cause serious complications of sexual function, pregnancy, and labour. The main role of imaging is to document the presence or absence of the uterus and to identify the gonads (Figs 66.3, 66.4). US and sometimes genitography are used routinely, MRI being reserved for cases in which the previous studies were inconclusive. Congenital anomalies of the vagina include complete or partial agenesis, stenosis, septation, and imperforate membrane, all of which cause obstruction (Fig. 66.5). Clinically, the older girl presents with symptoms of menstruation but no bleeding; a palpable mass with haematometrocolpos is found at US (Fig. 66.6). The Mayer–Rokitansky–Kuster–Hauser syndrome is the second most common cause of primary amenorrhoea and includes vaginal atresia, a spectrum of uterine anomalies (hypoplasia or

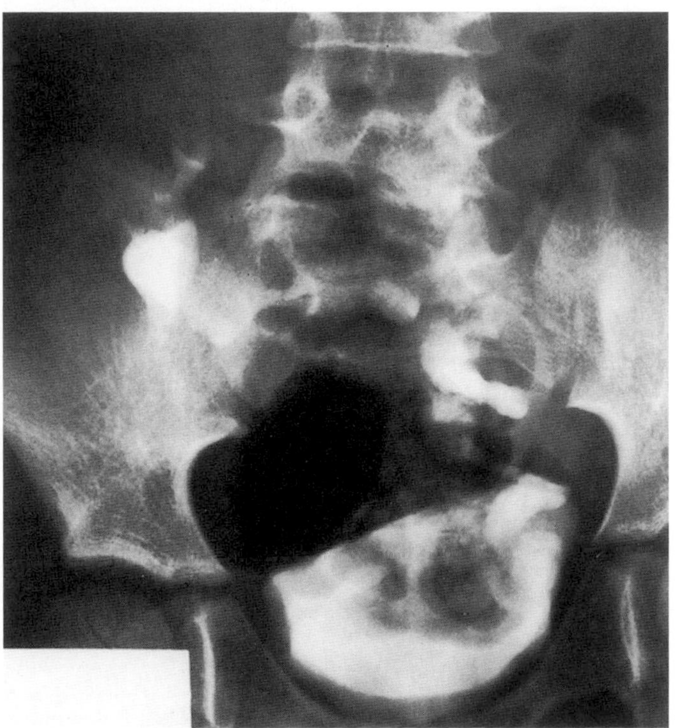

Figure 66.2 Pancake kidney demonstrated on an intravenous urogram. Note the patient also has a hypoplastic sacrum.

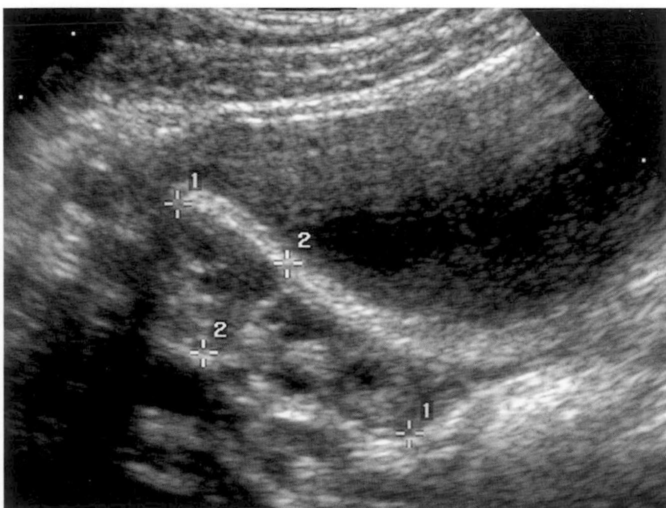

Figure 66.3 Normal ovaries. Oblique US of the right ovary in an 8 year old girl. This shows the normal appearance of multiple follicles in the ovary.

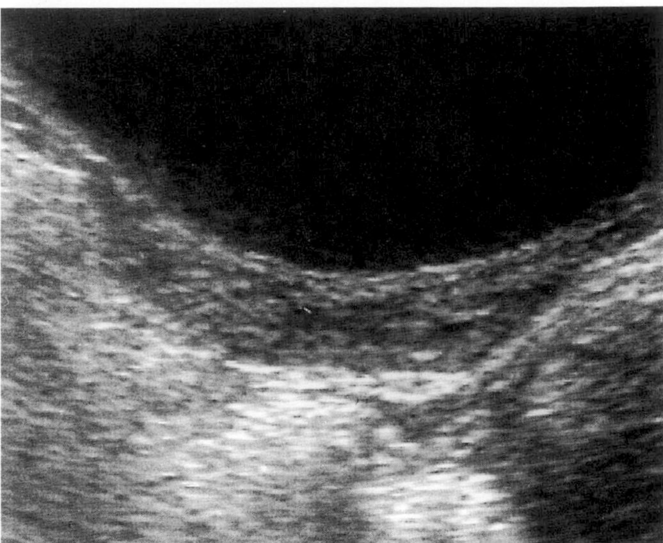

Figure 66.4 Normal uterus. Sagittal US of a prepubertal uterus in a 6 year old girl. The fundus and cervix are of equal size; there are no endometrial echoes.

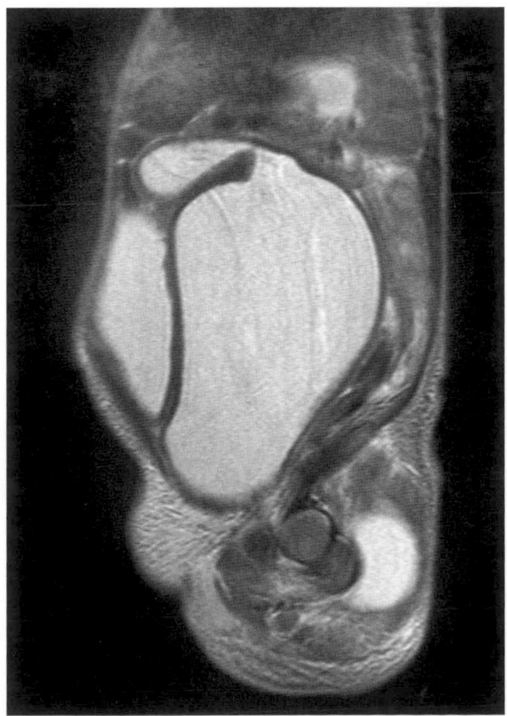

Figure 66.5 Hydrocolpos. T2-weighted parasagittal MRI showing a markedly distended vagina in a neonate with fluid also seen superiorly in a less distended uterine cavity, seen posterior to the bladder.

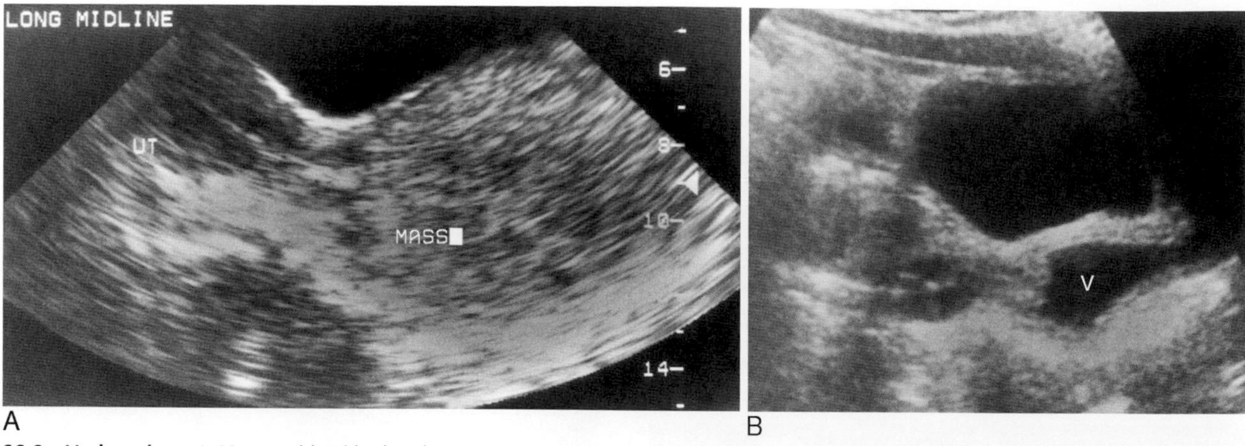

Figure 66.6 Hydrocolpos. A 10 year old girl had undergone menarche and presented with a 10 d history of spotty vaginal bleeding. (A) A longitudinal midline US image of the pelvis shows a heterogeneous mass in the region of the vagina, clearly separated from the uterus. On physical examination, there was an imperforate hymen which was punctured, releasing 500 ml of blood from the vagina. (B) A follow-up study on the following day showed resolution of the echogenic material, with only a small amount of fluid present within the vagina (v), outlining the uterine cervix.

duplication), and normal Fallopian tubes and ovaries. Imaging assists in the demonstration of uterus didelphys, unilateral hydrometrocolpos, and ipsilateral renal agenesis.

UNDESCENDED TESTIS

Cryptorchidism is present in 4% of full-term newborns, but the rate decreases to 0.8% by the first year as many testes descend spontaneously to the scrotal sac. As there is a risk of infertility and malignancy in the undescended testis, early diagnosis and treatment are important. The ectopic testis may be located anywhere from the retroperitoneum to the scrotum. Most ectopic testes are positioned within the inguinal canal and are easily visualized by US. Ipsilateral renal agenesis is associated with an absent testis so the examination should include renal US. The normal testis has high T2 signal but, contrary to early reports, MRI is poor at locating the undescended testis. Laparoscopy is increasingly used as the definitive investigation for an undescended testis.

IMAGING TECHNIQUES

ULTRASOUND

US is noninvasive and provides anatomical information of the retroperitoneal, intra-abdominal, and pelvic structures. It is independent of function. In the young child, US should always start with views of the bladder, since the child may micturate at any moment and the distended bladder provides an acoustic window for the lower urinary tract, uterus, adnexae, prostate gland, seminal vesicles, and pelvic musculature and vessels. Following micturition, the residual bladder volume should be estimated. Measurements of bipolar renal lengths should form part of the routine examination and be recorded[1,2] (Fig. 66.7). Normative graphs for age, weight, and height, and for the single kidney should be referred to in all reports (Fig. 66.8). In the normal neonatal kidney the renal cortex is more reflective than the adjacent normal liver, the medullary pyramids are hypoechoic and thus appear prominent, and there is an absence of renal sinus fat. These neonatal US appearances tend to become less prominent during the first 6 months of age. US is sensitive in the detection of hydronephrosis, nephrocalcinosis, and renal calculi. Doppler US is important in many conditions, e.g. suspected renal vein thrombosis or immediately following renal transplantation.

Visualization of the ovaries by US in girls depends on their location and size, and the age of the child. Ovarian volume is calculated using the formula according to a prolate ellipse: length × depth × width × 0.523. The mean ovarian volume before 6 years of age is usually 1 cm^3. After the age of 6, the ovaries gradually begin to enlarge and there is a marked increase after puberty[3]. Menstruating adolescents have a mean ovarian volume of 9.8 cm^3. In neonates the ovaries can be found anywhere in the abdomen and the pelvis. In childhood and adolescence, the ovaries move posterolaterally to the uterus, but due to the mobile ligamentous attachments may be elsewhere in the pelvis[4]. The appearance of the ovaries is heterogeneous, secondary to the presence of normal small follicles. Ovarian cysts are seen at all ages. Primordial (nonstimulated follicles) measure less than 9 mm in diameter, while stimulated follicles range between 9 mm and 3 cm in diameter, and these are asymptomatic.

The uterus in the neonatal period is quite large (2.3–4.6 cm in length) and thickened with clearly visible endometrial lining caused by the circulating maternal oestrogens. By 2–3 months of age it has changed to a prepubertal configuration with a tubular appearance; the fundus and cervix are the same size and endometrial echoes are no longer present. At puberty, the fundus starts to enlarge and becomes up to three times the size of the cervix. The total uterine length increases to 5–7 cm and the appearance of the endometrial lining will vary with the phase of the menstrual cycle.

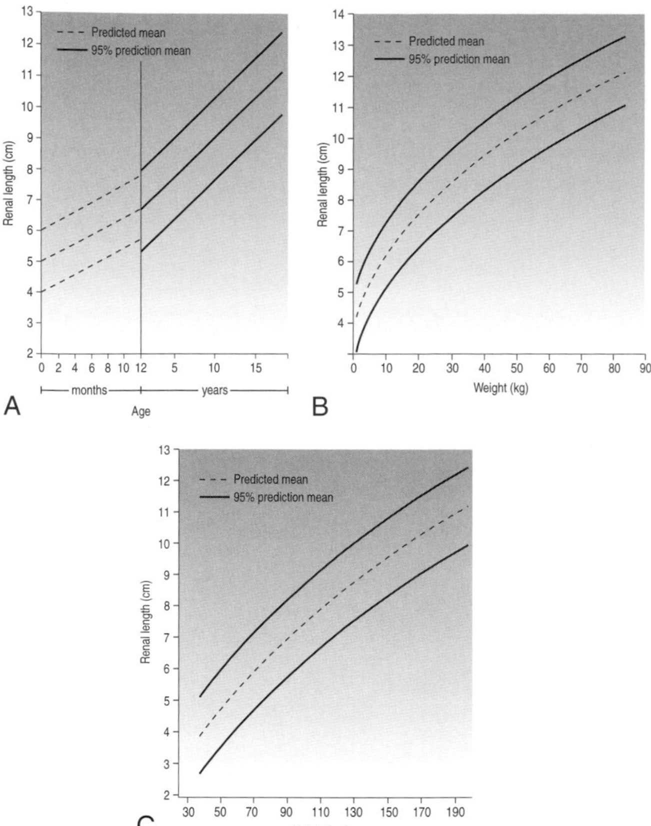

Figure 66.7 Renal growth chart. Normal renal growth charts for age, weight and height in normal children. Renal patients are often poorly grown so it is best to use charts with all the growth parameters recorded. (Reproduced with permission from Han B K, Babcock D S 1985 Am J Roentgenol 145: 611–616.)

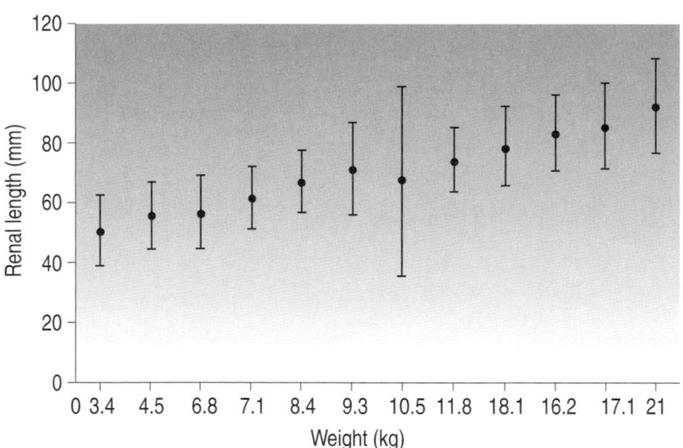

Figure 66.8 Standards for a single functioning kidney. Plot of mean renal length measurements against weight together with values for 2 SDs above and below mean for a single functioning kidney in children.

The vagina is identified on US by internal linear bright echoes. Commonly a urine-filled vagina is seen after a girl has voided. On MRI the vagina is best seen on thin axial or sagittal T2-weighted MRI. As with the uterus, the appearance and the thickness of the vaginal epithelium and the signal from the vaginal wall change with the phases of the menstrual cycle.

The prostate has an ellipsoid configuration in boys. Its texture is more homogeneous than in adults. The seminal vesicles can be identified in older boys and adolescents, but are difficult to visualize in infants and young boys. The normal testis changes in appearance during childhood. It has a homogeneous texture and is spherical or oval in shape during the neonatal period, measuring 7–10 mm in diameter. The epididymis and mediastinum testis are usually not seen at this point, but are clearly identified by puberty. Testicular size in adolescence ranges from 3 to 5 cm in length and from 2 to 3 cm in depth and width. Testicular flow, as measured by Doppler US, also changes with age. The testis in infants seldom shows colour flow, in spite of optimized slow flow settings. Power-mode Doppler US improves depiction of intratesticular flow in normal pre- and post-pubertal testes, but there are several cases of normal prepubertal testes that show no flow with this technique.

The ability to delineate normal and abnormal anatomy is directly related to the skill of the ultrasonographer who must be experienced in examining children and fully conversant with the spectrum of diseases in childhood. A quiet environment, appropriate to the needs of children, leads to better results. One important limitation of US is in the detection of renal scars.

CYSTOGRAPHY

There are four different methods for undertaking cystography in children. The ideal principle of using the lowest radiation burden and the least invasive technique must be borne in mind, remembering that the MCUG generally has a high radiation dose. All techniques except indirect radio-isotope cystography (IRC) require a bladder catheter. The MCUG, however, is the only technique that can visualize the male urethra adequately. The least invasive method is the IRC and it has a low radiation burden using ^{99m}Tc-MAG3; it is also the only physiological examination. However, it requires a toilet-trained child. US cystography involving bladder catheterization and the use of US contrast agents is not widely available. Intermittent or transitory VUR may be missed whatever technique is used.

Micturating cystourethrogram

This is the definitive method of assessing the lower urinary tract but may reveal upper tract detail if VUR is present. It is necessary in all boys in whom there is any suspicion of urethral pathology; images of the urethra are best achieved during voiding in an oblique projection.

Indications An MCUG is indicated in all boys with suspected urethral pathology. It is often also done in those under 3 years of age with a urinary tract infection (UTI) who have an abnormal US or DMSA scintigram; when ureteric dilatation is found; for terminal haematuria accompanied by lower urinary tract symptomatology; and also possibly in renal failure of undetermined cause with an abnormal US; in certain voiding problems, particularly when a thick-walled bladder is seen on US; and for infant screening in those who have an older sibling with VUR.

Method A small (6F) feeding tube, rather than a balloon catheter, is inserted via the urethra under strict aseptic conditions. If a balloon catheter is already in place, the balloon should be deflated for the cystogram. Oblique voiding images of the male urethra are mandatory without the catheter in situ. An adequate voiding image of the male urethra can be difficult to achieve and so simultaneous videotape recording is useful for review.

Dilute contrast medium, ideally warmed to body temperature, is administered either via drip infusion or careful injection; slow filling is ideal. With good urethral distension during voiding, posterior urethral valves will not be obscured by a 6F feeding catheter. If posterior urethral valves are discovered, then the bladder should be left on open catheter drainage so as not to leave a closed system that may become infected. Cyclic or double voiding leads to higher sensitivity in the detection of reflux.

Contraindications For the follow-up of known VUR, a radio-isotope cystogram should be carried out. A direct radio-isotope cystogram (DIC) is adequate for diagnosing VUR in girls who are not toilet trained, and have a UTI and abnormal ^{99m}Tc-DMSA findings.

Direct radio-isotope cystogram

Indications

A DIC is indicated **w**henever renal reflux must be excluded. This group of patients mainly includes young girls with a history of UTI and boys who require follow-up cystography (having previously had an MCUG).

There are no contraindications.

Method

This is similar to MCUG—instilling ^{99m}Tc-pertechnetate (20 MBq) and warm normal saline until the bladder is full, when micturition should occur. The entire procedure is carried out on top of the gamma camera linked to a computer system with a double disposable nappy on the infant. Both renal areas and the bladder are kept in the field of view. Sedation is never required.

Ultrasound cystogram

Although described some time ago, this technique is not used frequently as the US contrast agents are not licensed for intravesical or paediatric use in many countries. A bladder catheter is required and it follows the concept of the MCUG. The advantage is lack of irradiation; the disadvantages include the need for catheterization and the logistic difficulty of doing bilateral renal US during voiding.

Indirect radio-isotope cystogram

The IRC is physiological, will assess renal and bladder function, does not require a bladder catheter, and will detect reflux under normal voiding conditions. IRC is undertaken following the intravenous injection of diethylene triamine penta-acetate (^{99m}Tc-DTPA), ^{123}I-hippuran or, commonly, ^{99m}Tc-MAG3. Once the majority of the isotope is in the bladder, the child is asked to void in front of the gamma camera.

Indications

The indications are:

- whenever renal reflux must be excluded in the older toilet-trained child
- ureteric dilatation in the toilet-trained child
- children with bladder dysfunction, including posterior urethral valves, where the entire nephro-urological system can be evaluated.

Method

Following a routine ^{99m}Tc-MAG3 scintigram, the child returns to the gamma camera, which has been turned horizontal, when he/she wishes to void. The child sits with the camera at his/her back; often the boys stand. Acquisition starts 30 s before micturition and continues for 30 s afterwards with continuous data acquisition. Processing includes viewing the data in cine mode, drawing regions of interest (ROI) over the bladder and kidneys, as well as creating a compressed image of the entire procedure.

NUCLEAR MEDICINE

Dynamic renogram

The isotopes used are either ^{99m}Tc-DTPA, ^{123}I-hippuran or, commonly, ^{99m}Tc-MAG3. Analysis includes renal perfusion, divided renal function (DRF), and drainage of the collecting systems. (A diuretic is required in the presence of a dilated collecting system.) ^{99m}Tc-DTPA uptake reflects glomerular function while ^{99m}Tc-MAG3 uptake reflects tubular function. In most clinical situations this difference is unimportant.

Indications

The indications are:

- to assess DRF and drainage in suspected obstruction or before surgery on the collecting system
- postoperative evaluation of the collecting system
- for IRC
- following renal transplantation
- renography with captopril stimulation for renovascular hypertension.

Method

Hydration The child should be encouraged to drink from the time of arrival in the department until the actual injection. Voiding before the injection is recommended. An anaesthetic cream should be applied 45 min before the injection.

The administered dose is scaled on a body surface basis, with a maximum dose of 80 MBq for ^{99m}Tc-MAG3 and 200 MBq for ^{99m}Tc-DTPA, and a minimum dose of 20 MBq for both tracers. The effective dose equivalent (EDE) for a 5 year old child using ^{99m}Tc-DTPA is 0.63 mSv while for ^{99m}Tc-MAG3 it is 0.40 mSv.

The gamma camera is face up using a low energy, general purpose collimator with the child supine. To reduce movement, sandbags are placed on either side of the child with Velcro straps around the child and the sandbags. The heart, kidneys, and bladder should all be included in the field of view. A frame rate of 10 or 20 s per frame is required and the study should continue for 20 min.

In the presence of a full bladder, drainage from the kidney may be delayed. The use of a diuretic usually causes the child to void, often within 15–20 min; additional data should be routinely acquired after micturition and a change in posture so that analysis of the kidneys can be undertaken when the bladder is empty. The change in posture should be for approximately 5 min before the 1-min late series dynamic data are acquired.

Diuretic administration 1 mg kg^{-1} of frusemide with a maximum dose of 20 mg can be given at appropriate times.

Differential renal function estimation The relative function of each kidney is expressed as a percentage of the sum of the right and left kidneys. It is computed from the renogram, during the period 60–120 s from the peak of the vascular curve. The integral and the Patlak–Rutland plot method are the only two internationally recommended techniques.

Interpretation of diuretic challenge Simple analysis of the post-frusemide curve only is strongly discouraged since this curve fails to take into consideration the effect of gravity, the bladder status, and the function of that particular kidney. The routine use of the post-micturition image plus assessment of washout relative to the uptake function of the kidney will overcome all these difficulties. Good drainage is easy to define, since the images, curves, and numerical data all reveal little tracer in the kidney and dilated collecting system at the end of the study. However, when drainage is reduced then there is little agreement as to what constitutes moderate drainage or poor drainage. The significance of impaired drainage is also strongly debated and the relationship between impaired drainage and different treatment modalities is not clear. Using pelvic excretion efficiency (PEE), good drainage is defined as a kidney and renal pelvis clearing 84% or more of the isotope which has been taken up by the kidney at the end of the study.

Static renal scintigraphy

^{99m}Tc-DMSA binds to the proximal convoluted tubules, resulting in fixation of the isotope and an unchanging image over many hours with only 10% of the injected dose excreted in the urine. It provides an accurate image of renal parenchymal function and DRF.

Indications

All indications are to detect a focal renal parenchymal abnormality:

- in UTI, renal involvement in the acute phase can be diagnosed by ^{99m}Tc-DMSA
- exclusion of a scar requires a normal ^{99m}Tc-DMSA study
- when only one kidney has been identified and doubt exists about the presence of a second kidney
- in the follow-up of pyelonephritis
- assessment of focal parenchymal abnormalities in the presence of hypertension
- in children with urinary incontinence and a suspected duplex kidney with ectopic drainage of the upper moiety (this may be a difficult diagnosis)
- in children with gross dilatation (e.g. prune belly syndrome) where assessment of drainage is not possible but DRF is required.

There are no contraindications.

Method

Posterior and both posterior oblique projections are routine. Anterior views including the empty bladder are essential when an ectopic kidney is to be excluded. The child is kept still with sandbags and Velcro straps. Sedation is almost never used.

UROGRAPHY (PLAIN RADIOGRAPH AND INTRAVENOUS UROGRAM)

A plain abdominal radiograph is essential before every IVU, especially in the presence of renal calculi. In the presence of chronic renal failure the femoral epiphyses may slip and renal osteodystrophy should be sought. IVU is now an infrequent examination and may be replaced by MRI in time.

Indications

The indications are:

- for suspected renal calculi
- in suspected autosomal recessive polycystic kidney disease
- when an occult duplex kidney is considered, especially if US and ^{99m}Tc-DMSA imaging are normal
- to define ureteric anatomy in the context of primary enuresis
- to define ureteric anatomy in known duplex kidneys
- if a small kidney is discovered on US or isotope examination and no VUR is found, then an IVU to show the calyceal anatomy may prove helpful in establishing the cause, e.g. previous ischaemia
- occasionally in the post-transplant setting to demonstrate ureteric anatomy.

Method

The IVU should be individualized to answer specific clinical questions. To evaluate calyceal anatomy, images approximately 5 min after the injection of contrast medium should be obtained in the coned AP as well as the AP supine renal window view (caudal angle 34 degrees approximately centred on the xiphisternum) as a routine. The latter view will project the bowel gas over the lower abdomen. A US study rather than a post-micturition radiograph is recommended to assess bladder emptying.

COMPUTED TOMOGRAPHY

CT generally has a limited but specific role in the evaluation of the paediatric genitourinary tract. The recommended dose of standard nonionic contrast medium, e.g. iohexol 300, for most abdominal studies is 2 ml kg^{-1}.

Indications

The indications are:

- all patients with a suspected malignant renal or pelvic lesion or suspected abscess after intravenous contrast enhancement

- follow-up of known malignant tumours, although MRI is now regarded as equally reliable in assessing abdominal masses
- major abdominal trauma with suspicion of serious pelvic injury or fracture, or if haematuria is present or bladder rupture is suspected
- less common indications may include a suspicion of chronic renal infection or tuberculosis, or of nephrocalcinosis when a US study is inconclusive
- CT angiography (CTA) may replace conventional angiography in certain circumstances, e.g. assessment of post-transplant arterial complications or in the evaluation of a suspected large vessel aneurysm.

Method

For the majority of studies intravenous contrast enhancement is so crucial that nonenhanced images are often noncontributory, unless calcification or calculi specifically are being sought. With the new multidetector systems, a low milliampere setting, ideally based on weight, to reduce dose is essential in small patients. In cases of abdominal trauma, delayed imaging after an interval of 10–15 min can be a useful method of detecting extravasation of contrast medium from the genitourinary tract.

MAGNETIC RESONANCE IMAGING

All pelvic masses are best assessed with MRI. Spinal MRI is warranted in patients with a suspected spinal cord tethering or a neuropathic bladder. Fat-suppressed gadolinium-enhanced sequences may be as sensitive as ^{99m}Tc-DMSA scintigraphy in the detection of acute pyelonephritis. The normal renal medulla on MRI has a longer T1 relaxation time than the cortex such that T1-weighted imaging yields good corticomedullary differentiation. Heavily T2-weighted sequences, e.g. rapid acquisition relaxation enhancement (RARE), can yield an MR urogram (MRU) that is comparable to the standard IVU in terms of anatomical detail. MRU can be performed rapidly, independent of renal function. There is as yet little literature regarding the accuracy of MRA in the assessment of the renal vasculature in children, but it is likely to have a role to play in assessing the first- and second-order branches. Simple and complicated cysts, and haemorrhagic or fat-containing lesions, can be accurately diagnosed with MRI. MRI can replace CT in the assessment of a Wilms' tumour; however, thoracic CT is needed to exclude pulmonary metastases.

Indications

The indications are:

- children with a neuropathic bladder or an abnormal spinal radiograph require exclusion of spinal cord pathology, which is best achieved with MRI
- to stage the intra-abdominal extent of Wilms' tumours
- evaluation of pelvic tumours
- gadolinium-enhanced MRA may have a future role in the assessment of hypertension but conventional arteriography currently remains the reference technique
- future indications may include confirmation of renal involvement in acute pyelonephritis.

Method

Coronal imaging produces images akin to an IVU. Contrast enhancement is necessary to detect acute pyelonephritis and roughly to predict tumour vascularity. MRU with heavily T2-weighted techniques can be performed as a single-shot, fast spin-echo sequence. If upper tract obstruction is suspected, a prolonged dynamic series with intravenous frusemide after gadolinium injection may eventually replace dynamic renography. During post-processing, signal intensity versus time, similar to a renogram curve, can be plotted utilizing a ROI over the renal pelvis. Additional anatomical information, such as renal pelvis diameter in response to frusemide administration, can be measured simultaneously. MRA techniques employing gadolinium enhancement, rather than nonenhanced time-of-flight or phase-contrast sequences, are more robust and reproducible in the evaluation of the renal vasculature.

INTERVENTIONAL PROCEDURES

Angiography

Angiography with its high radiation dose and invasiveness is reserved for special clinical situations. It is best undertaken by an experienced operator.

Indications

The indications are:

- hypertension with a high suspicion of renovascular disease, including suspected vasculitis, especially polyarteritis nodosa. Renal vein sampling for renin values is useful in some cases to evaluate which kidney is causing the hypertension
- before interventional procedures, e.g. embolization for arteriovenous malformations or balloon dilatation for renal artery stenosis
- rarely now in bilateral Wilms' tumours before surgery
- testicular vein embolization for varicocele obliteration.

Method

Angiography should use the smallest catheter compatible with good results. Selective arteriography with magnification and oblique views is essential to look for lesions in small renal vessels.

Antegrade pyelogram

This investigation should be carried out by an experienced operator in the radiology department or in theatre, usually before surgery, to provide anatomical detail of the renal pelvis and/or ureter unavailable from US or IVU. Occasionally antegrade studies are combined with pressure flow measurements with or without urodynamic studies to determine the physiological significance of a dilated upper urinary tract.

Nephrostomy

The placement of a pigtail catheter in a dilated renal pelvis or ureter should be undertaken by an experienced operator under US guidance. The technique in children is similar to that in adults. US guides the needle insertion into, preferably, a lower pole calyx for contrast delineation of the collecting system. The nephrostomy tube is then placed appropriately. Different sized drainage catheters are used depending on the child's size and need for drainage. The complications of placing a nephrostomy tube are generally those of catheter placement, extravasation of contrast medium, and leakage of urine.

Retrograde pyelogram

The instillation of dilute contrast medium into a ureter via a catheter inserted into the distal ureteric orifice is usually undertaken by a urologist in the operating theatre. With modern flexible ureteroscopes, the contrast medium may be instilled into the upper ureter or even the renal pelvis. This is done to outline the ureter and its drainage.

INTEGRATED IMAGING

THE NEONATE

The immature kidney of the neonate is different from that in the older child, both in its US appearance and also in the handling of radio-isotopes or contrast medium. There is difficulty in disposing of an osmotic and/or a sodium load and consequently a greater risk of volume overload with excess intravenous contrast medium. In the neonate and infant there is a relatively large extracellular fluid space so that readily diffusible substances injected intravenously (^{99m}Tc-DTPA or iodinated agents for IVU or CT, or gadolinium for MRI) have a large volume of distribution and therefore a relatively low plasma concentration.

Normal imaging

High-quality dynamic isotope studies are generally best achieved when some renal maturity has occurred (at about 4 weeks of age). Renal immaturity dictates the use of ^{99m}Tc-MAG3 since this isotope remains in the blood pool rather than DTPA. Renal immaturity precludes the exclusion of a minor parenchymal abnormality in the first months of life. However, in the presence of renal failure and/or bilateral dilatation, ^{99m}Tc-DMSA imaging has proved very helpful in deciding whether both kidneys are equally involved in the disease processes or if all the function is from only one kidney. There is no minimum age in such a clinical situation to undertake ^{99m}Tc-DMSA scintigraphy.

There is no indication for an IVU in the neonatal period. An IVU in the neonatal period may aggravate renal venous thrombosis (RVT) or medullary necrosis. Even in normal neonates, an IVU may fail to outline the kidneys, especially in the first 48 h of life. MRU has not been fully explored in the newborn.

Prenatal diagnosis of renal/urological abnormality

Newborns with a prenatal US diagnosis of a renal tract abnormality do not form a homogeneous group. Postnatal US in the neonatal period guides further imaging following an abnormal prenatal US. A fetus at 18–20 weeks' gestation with a renal pelvis of 5 mm or greater, which enlarges or remains static, is generally referred for investigation postnatally. In many situations the natural history is unclear and therefore the question arises in many asymptomatic infants whether any surgical correction should be undertaken. Management is complex so a simple attitude cannot be adopted from the data in the literature. An absolute indication for surgery is unequivocal obstruction, e.g. complicated ureterocele, posterior urethral valve, or major infection complicating a hydronephrosis.

Differential diagnosis

The infant with one normal kidney and contralateral hydronephrosis must be distinguished from the infant with bilateral hydronephrosis with or without a normal bladder. Postnatal imaging is heavily dependent on the prenatal US assessment of the urinary tract in respect of how quickly postnatal imaging should be undertaken. The full differential diagnosis is listed in Table 66.1.

The most common referral is that of mild pelvic dilatation seen in early pregnancy at around 18 weeks' gestation: postnatal US is usually normal in these cases. In more specialized centres, isolated unilateral renal pelvic dilatation (RPD) is a more common referral (see section on cystic disorders below for a description of multicystic dysplastic kidney).

Unilateral renal pelvic dilatation

RPD or hydronephrosis may be defined as calyceal dilatation plus RPD of greater than 10–15 mm in its AP diameter with no US evidence of a dilated ureter[5]. This was referred to loosely in the past as PUJ obstruction or PUJ stenosis. On antenatal US the AP renal pelvis is greater than 50% of the longitudinal length of the kidney. This equates to approximately a 5-mm

Table 66.1 DIFFERENTIAL DIAGNOSIS OF PRENATAL HYDRONEPHROSIS
Unilateral pathology
Renal pelvic dilatation (RPD)
Vesico ureteric reflux (VUR)
Megaureter (with or without reflux)
Multicystic dysplastic kidney
Complicated duplex kidney
Upper moiety dilatation—either ureterocele or ectopic drainage
Lower moiety dilatation—usually VUR but rarely RPD only
Bilateral pathology
Bilateral renal pelvic dilatation
Bilateral VUR
Bilateral megaureter (with or without reflux)
Bladder pathology, e.g. neurogenic bladder
Bladder outlet pathology (posterior urethral valves)
Bilateral complicated duplex kidneys
Multicystic kidney on one side and cystic dysplastic kidney on opposite side

pelvis at 20 weeks' gestation and a 10-mm pelvis in the third trimester. RPD is commonly unilateral but may be bilateral; the importance of this distinction is that if it is unilateral then there is no urgency in terms of investigation.

All these infants are asymptomatic. Only about 25% now undergo surgery. Natural history studies suggest that RPD is a relatively benign condition and help define how to investigate and manage these children.

Obstruction is not easily defined. The effects of obstruction are hydronephrosis, parenchymal atrophy, and impaired renal function. These changes do not define or predict the potential for progressive renal deterioration. The only accepted diagnosis of obstruction is that if nothing is done either function deteriorates or dilatation increases. If the function and dilatation remain unchanged then that kidney is not obstructed and is in equilibrium. These children with RPD should not be confused with those who have symptoms of loin pain and intermittent PUJ obstruction.

Imaging protocol

There is no available test that will predict which kidney with a prenatal RPD will deteriorate if left alone. A US examination should be undertaken 48–72 h after birth to assess calyceal and pelvic dilatation, measure the transverse diameter of the pelvis, and confirm the structural normality of the bladder and opposite kidney. With a secure diagnosis of unilateral calyceal and RPD dilatation, a diuretic MAG3 renogram and follow-up US are required. The exact timing of follow-up will depend on the size of the RPD and DRF. Marked RPD or poor function require closer follow-up than 15–20-mm RPD and/or normal DRF. With stable imaging follow-up is less frequent. Long-term follow-up is recommended until at least 15–20 years of age. There is no role for an MCUG in these children.

Bilateral renal pelvic dilatation

There is uncertainty about the management of bilateral RPD. When and on which side to operate is uncertain and how to judge the results of US and diuretic ^{99m}Tc-MAG3 is very difficult.

The investigative protocol in this situation should be as for the unilateral RPD dilatation, but here includes an MCUG as well as formal sequential glomerular filtration rate (GFR) estimation. Some surgeons will opt for a non-surgical approach as long as the degree of dilatation and differential function are stable, while others prefer to operate on the better functioning kidney, and yet others will operate on the worse kidney or the one with the greater dilatation. Until more data become available, no rigid approach can be recommended.

Normal postnatal ultrasound or mild dilatation

This is the largest group of children seen with a prenatal US diagnosis of hydronephrosis. Early studies show that the MCUG revealed no bladder obstruction and a normal bladder wall thickness, but VUR may be present with a marked male preponderance[6]. Grade IV or V (see Fig. 66.20 for grading) reflux stops spontaneously within 2 years in 20%. Postnatal US is normal in the vast majority. Between 30% and 50% of these children had reduced function on isotope renography; however, following UTI this increased to 71% (Fig. 66.9)[7]. This is the rationale for the use of prophylactic antibiotics in this group of infants. These data suggest that there is a developmental abnormality resulting in both VUR and an abnormal kidney.

If the initial US is normal and the child is on chemoprophylaxis then it may be argued that nothing more need be done from an imaging aspect. If the US is abnormal, then further imaging is guided by the abnormality seen.

Megaureter

Hydronephrosis with a dilated ureter is dealt with in the same way as pelvic dilatation above (Fig. 66.10). The investigative protocol is similar to that of RPD plus a MCUG to document or exclude VUR. The US must in addition focus on the bladder and vesico-ureteric junction since it is imperative to exclude a small ureterocele or other bladder abnormality. Usually the bladder appears normal on both US and MCUG, in which case there may be a functional abnormality. Management is also complex as some surgeons believe that re-implantation of a ureter into the bladder in a child younger than 1 year of age may result in abnormal bladder function in later life. The role of urodynamics remains uncertain. With a suspected neuropathic bladder, a spinal US in early infancy can exclude spinal cord pathology.

With increasing dilatation or fall in function on diuretic ^{99m}Tc-MAG3 studies, the insertion of a double J stent from the ureter into the bladder requires an antegrade study. Follow-up imaging is with US and diuretic ^{99m}Tc-MAG3 studies post stent insertion, as well as after stent removal.

Renal failure

The neonate may be in acute renal failure due to an episode around the time of labour or acquired sepsis resulting in RVT, medullary or acute tubular necrosis (ATN), or any combination of these conditions. The US should identify the size of each kidney, and the echogenecity of the cortex and medulla compared to the liver and spleen. All these disorders result in an echogenic kidney with loss of the normal corticomedullary differentiation. In ATN the kidneys are usually symmetrically abnormal. In RVT they are asymmetrically involved, swollen, with poor corticomedullary differentiation; the interlobular arteries are prominent and often no venous flow can be seen at the renal hilum or in parts of the swollen kidney on Doppler interrogation (Fig. 66.11). Thrombus in the inferior vena cava (IVC) is well recognized. There may be adrenal haemorrhage in this clinical setting, readily seen on US (typically left-sided as the left adrenal vein drains into the left renal vein). The pathogenesis in RVT is dynamic so the US findings change depending on the stage of the pathology. RVT can ultimately result in a small scarred kidney. To assess the long-term damage ^{99m}Tc-DMSA scintigraphy (between 4 and 12 months of age) should be performed.

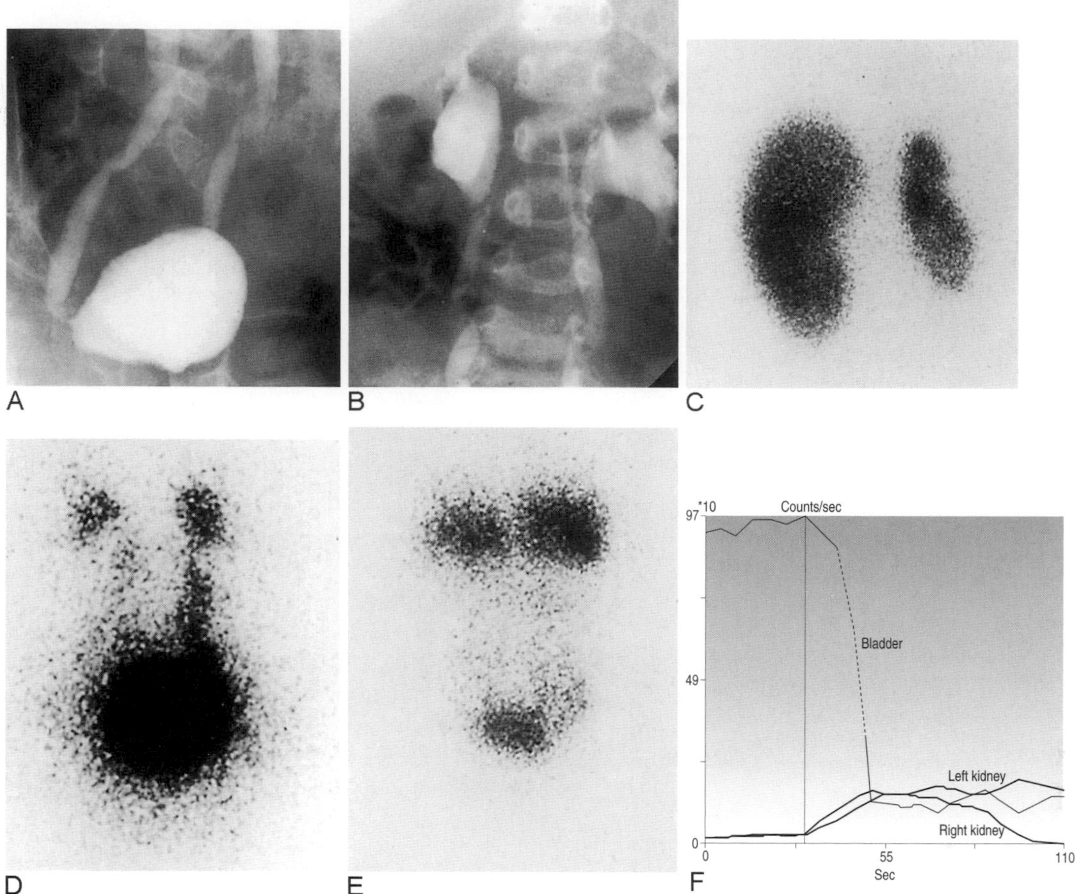

Figure 66.9 Antenatal diagnosis of bilateral hydronephrosis. Due to vesico-ureteric reflux (VUR). This diagnosis was confirmed postnatally. (A) The micturating cystourethrogram (MCUG) shows bilateral VUR with a normal bladder. (B) The calices and pelves on the MCUG appear normal. There was no evidence of bladder outflow obstruction. (C) ^{99m}Tc-DMSA scintigram shows a normal left kidney with a small scarred right kidney. The left kidney contributed 76% to overall function and the right kidney 24%. The left kidney took up 34.6% of the injected dose and the right kidney 9.3%. (D) Indirect radio-isotope cystogram (IRC) with ^{99m}Tc-MAG3 at age 3 years. The radionuclide may be noted in the bladder and there is still some in both kidneys as well as in the right ureter. This image was obtained 1 h after the intravenous injection of ^{99m}Tc-MAG3. (E) IRC at the end of micturition shows the bladder to be almost empty and the ureters empty, but marked activity is noted in both kidneys. (F) The curves show prompt bladder emptying with a bilateral renal reflux of 5 ml into the right kidney and 4 ml into the left kidney. The bladder volume was 55 ml with a voided volume of 40 ml and a urine flow rate of 2 ml s^{-1}.

Associated congenital abnormalities

Children with anorectal anomaly, tracheo-oesophageal fistula, or VACTERL association have a high incidence of renal abnormalities such as crossed fused ectopia and a single kidney. All require US, with further imaging dictated by the US findings.

BLADDER ANOMALIES

Exstrophy/epispadias

Exstrophy and epispadias represent a spectrum of anomalies. Boys are affected three times as frequently as girls. The diagnosis is clinically apparent in cases of exstrophy and in epispadias in the male infant. Female epispadias is rare and may present as an occult cause of enuresis. A measurement of pubic symphysis diastasis can be used as a radiological criterion to estimate the degree of abnormality present in this spectrum. Diastasis of only several millimetres more than the normal 10 mm suggests epispadias, whereas separation of the pubic bones by more than 25 mm is characteristic of exstrophy (Fig. 66.12). The genital structures are normal, as are the upper urinary tracts initially, though minimal distal ureteric dilatation may be present at birth. Subsequently, following surgery, complications such as VUR or obstruction (which may be silent) must be sought, particularly with any type of diversion. Additionally, the incidence of adenoma or adenocarcinoma at such anastomoses is higher than would be expected, so regular evaluation is important and this is best done using a combination of US and MAG3 to assess the ureters and bladder. Loopograms may also be required following diversion.

Prune belly syndrome (prune belly triad syndrome; abdominal musculature deficiency syndrome)

The prune belly syndrome (PBS) is generally readily apparent clinically and consists of absent abdominal wall muscles, undescended testes, and renal dysplasia associated with gross dilatation of the collecting systems. The incidence of the condition

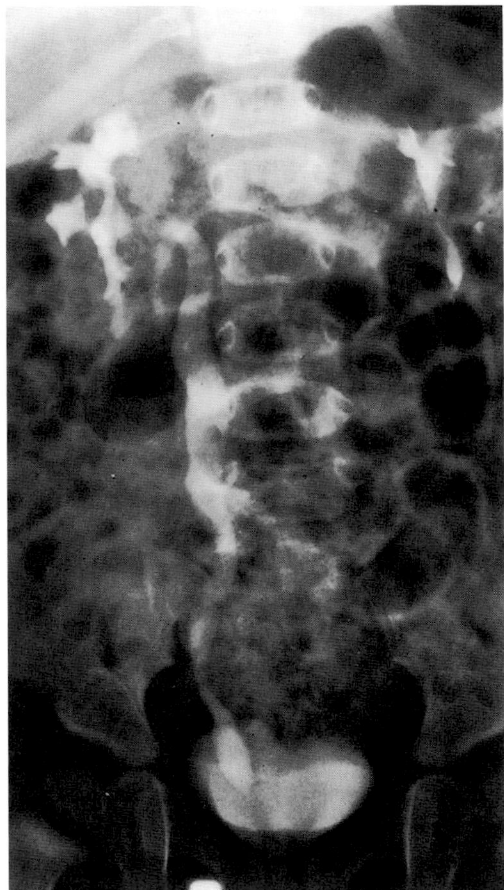

Figure 66.10 Primary megaureter demonstrated on an intravenous urogram. The entire right ureter is dilated, particularly the distal ureter. There is little dilatation of the upper collecting system.

has fallen due to antenatal diagnosis with subsequent termination of pregnancy. Both the pathogenesis and optimal therapy in management are debated.

All affected children have a universal mesentery with a mobile bowel. Plain abdominal radiographs show a protuberant abdomen resulting from the lack of abdominal musculature. In the most severely affected patients, there may be urethral obstruction with severe renal dysplasia, while less severely affected individuals demonstrate an array of urinary tract abnormalities. The characteristic features are small kidneys with abnormal minimally dilated calyces and upper ureters, while the lower ureters are tortuous and show disproportionate dilatation. The bladder is thin walled, of large capacity without trabeculation, and has a wide neck. A patent urachus or a urachal diverticulum may be present. The posterior urethra is dilated proximally with a typical conical narrowing and a poor stream in the distal urethra (Fig. 66.13). Occasionally, generalized or focal anterior urethral dilatation is present. Prognosis depends on the degree of renal dysplasia.

Imaging

US demonstrates the small lobulated kidneys and upper tracts, but with marked lower ureteric dilatation and a full bladder it may not be able to 'sort out' the lower urinary anatomy. ^{99m}Tc-DMSA is valuable for DRF. IVU is rarely indicated

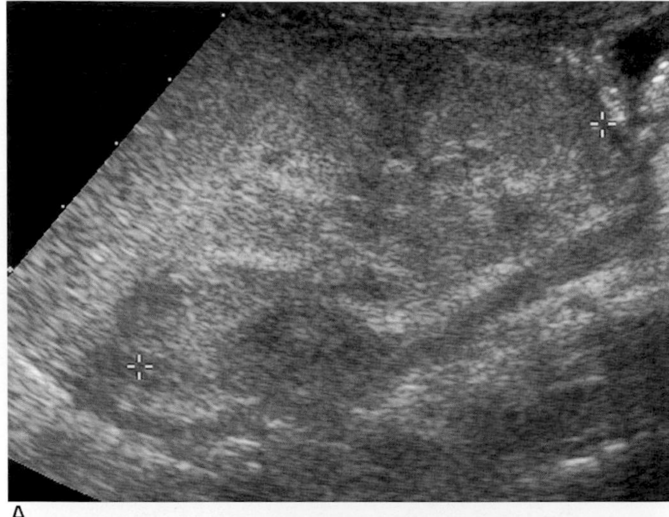

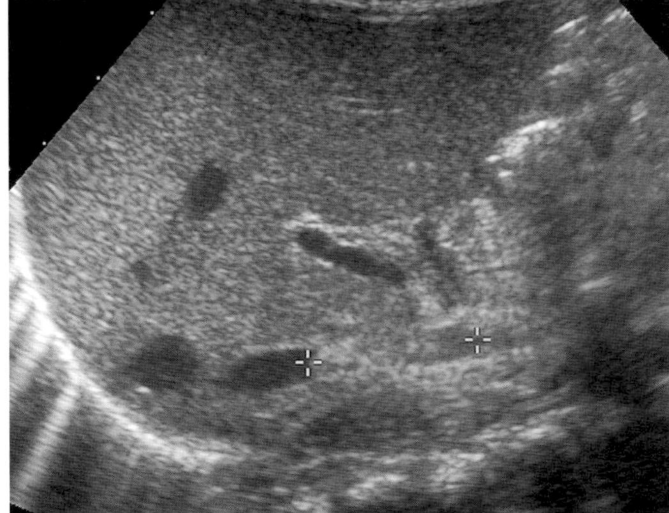

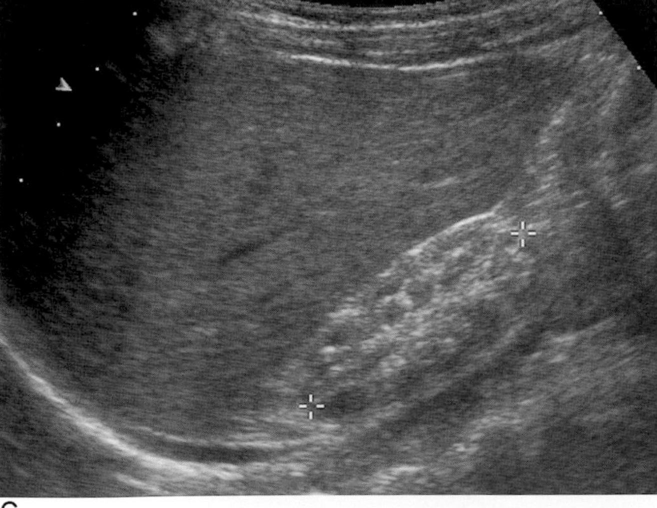

Figure 66.11 Renal vein thrombosis. (A) Longitudinal US of the right kidney in a neonate with haematuria and a palpable kidney. The kidney is large and swollen with an overall increase in the echogenicity and some prominent interlobular vessels. (B) Longitudinal US of the inferior vena cava (IVC). This shows thrombus in the IVC (between calipers). (C) Longitudinal US of the right kidney 6 months later. The kidney is small and echogenic with bright calcified intrarenal vessels.

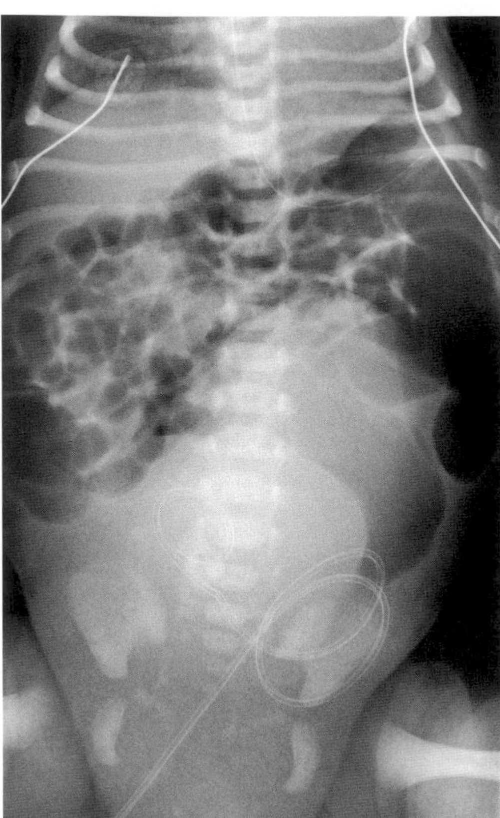

Figure 66.12 Pubic symphysis diastasis. A neonate with a cloacal anomaly. The apparent mass arising out of the pelvis was a hydrocolpos.

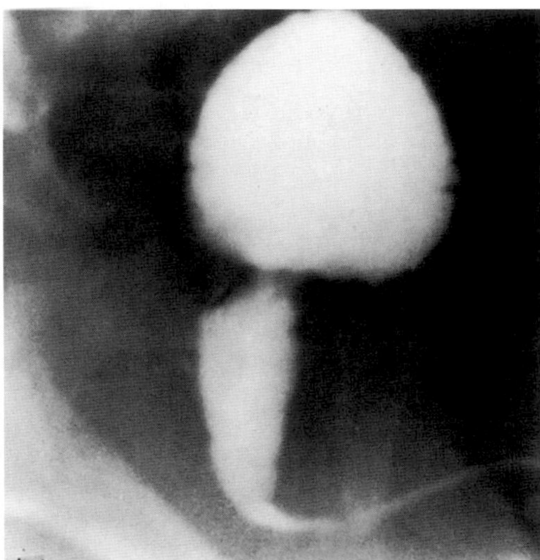

Figure 66.13 Prune belly syndrome. Image exposed near the end of micturition on a voiding cystourethrogram. The posterior urethra is dilated proximal to the membranous urethra and the calibre of the latter is normal. Posterior urethral valves are not present.

and dynamic renal scintigraphy fails to show adequate drainage due to the gross dilation. MCUG is valuable for urethral anatomy but is dangerous if sepsis arises. VUR occurs in about two-thirds of cases. The long-term follow-up is a combination of US and ^{99m}Tc-DMSA imaging at intervals, with MCUG being required if bladder outlet symptoms develop.

Neurogenic bladder

Children with this disorder commonly have a deficiency of appropriate detrusor muscle contraction and external sphincter relaxation, resulting in an uncontrolled voiding pattern with incomplete bladder emptying. Meningomyelocele is the most common associated abnormality with significant secondary musculoskeletal and bowel consequences. Defects in the sacrum can also result in a neurogenic bladder. Other abnormalities included under the broad term 'myelodysplasia' (including sacral agenesis) may have similar urological implications without obvious musculoskeletal abnormalities. When no spinal abnormality is found, the term non-neurogenic neurogenic bladder is used. Minor degrees of spinal dysraphism, such as spina bifida occulta at the lumbosacral junction, are not associated with neurological defects. The goals in the management of neurogenic bladder are preservation of renal function and attainment of continence. Initially the upper tracts are normal and deterioration of function results from poor bladder emptying with complications of infection, reflux, and hydronephrosis. Current management focuses on regular clean intermittent catheterization, the use of pharmacological agents, and occasionally the use of an artificial urinary sphincter. US, MCUG, and MAG3 scintigraphy are indicated at diagnosis and follow-up.

Classification of neurogenic bladder is mainly based on urodynamic results, which have also contributed significantly to the management of the condition. On MCUG the neurogenic bladder may be vertically orientated, thick-walled, and trabeculated with diverticular formation, but mild changes may also be seen early on. Narrowing of the urethra at the external sphincter may be shown and the remainder of the urethra is normal. Spinal US should be done in infants younger than 6 months of age. On plain radiographs it may be difficult to identify a spinal abnormality in the infant. MRI is the best technique to ensure a small mass lesion is not overlooked.

URETHRAL ANOMALIES

Delineation of the bladder neck and urethra is best achieved on the MCUG in the oblique projection. In the presence of bladder neck hypertrophy due to urethral obstruction, the posterior aspect of the bladder neck is easy to identify but the anterior boundaries of the bladder neck have no readily demonstrable landmark. When the bladder empties, a contraction ring may be seen, which looks like the bladder neck to the unwary. For these reasons it is often difficult to be certain where the bladder neck finishes and the posterior urethra begins.

Obstruction to bladder outlet

Anatomical causes of outlet obstruction include posterior urethral valve, urethral dysplasia as seen in certain syndromes (e.g. PBS), anterior urethral valve/diverticulum, and meatal stenosis, as well as post-traumatic strictures of the urethra at any level. *Functional* obstruction may be secondary to a spinal abnormality and the occult neuropathic bladder.

Intrinsic masses obstructing bladder outflow

These include rhabdomyosarcoma of the bladder, vagina, or prostate, and benign tumours such as neurofibroma, hamartoma, and haemangioma. Occasionally, a polyp on a stalk originating in either the posterior urethra or the bladder may cause an obstruction. All these mass lesions may prolapse into the urethra and so cause obstruction. The larger lesions will all be readily identified on US while smaller lesions require an MCUG using dilute contrast medium.

Male urethra

Congenital abnormalities affect both the anterior and posterior portion of the urethra, the most common abnormality being hypospadias, which has little radiological importance.

Posterior urethral valves (Fig. 66.14)

Rarely these children present with severe UTI and the diagnosis of septicaemia is now more commonly made in early infancy or during fetal development. The presence of bilateral hydronephrosis, a full bladder, and progressive oligohydramnios during pregnancy may be an indication for drainage of the bladder during pregnancy. This needs to be done early if the complications of oligohydramnios, such as pulmonary hypoplasia, are to be prevented.

Posterior urethral valves (PUVs) are categorized into either three or four types, depending on the classification used. Detailed descriptions are inappropriate in context, but Types 1 and 3 merit brief mention. Type 1 is the most common, where two folds at the level of the verumontanum have a ventral central slit-like orifice. Type 3 has a pin-point, eccentric orifice which results in forward ballooning of the valve giving a 'wind in the sail' appearance on the oblique projection during MCUG. With Type 3 valves there is a high association of renal dysplasia with minimal upper tract dilatation and there may be little improvement in renal function following ablation of this type of valve. The mild degree of dilatation of the collecting systems throughout the natural history of the condition is out of keeping with the degree of chronic renal failure.

A rare complication of PUV in the neonatal period is rupture of a calyceal fornix, leading to accumulation of urine (urinoma) around the kidney limited by fascial planes. This urinary leak may result in urinary ascites which has a significant generalized metabolic effect.

In male infants the presence of dilated ureters with or without a thick-walled bladder dictates the need for an MCUG to exclude the diagnosis of PUV. US may detect the bladder neck hypertrophy, which is a constant feature of the PUV. On MCUG the visualization of the valve may be difficult unless the correct oblique projection is obtained during micturition. Other signs include dilatation of the posterior urethra proximal to the valve, with a disparity between the respective calibres of the proximal and distal urethra. Bladder neck hypertrophy is invariable, the bladder is usually thick walled and of variable capacity (small or large), and trabeculation may be an early feature. VUR may be seen and is generally associated with poor

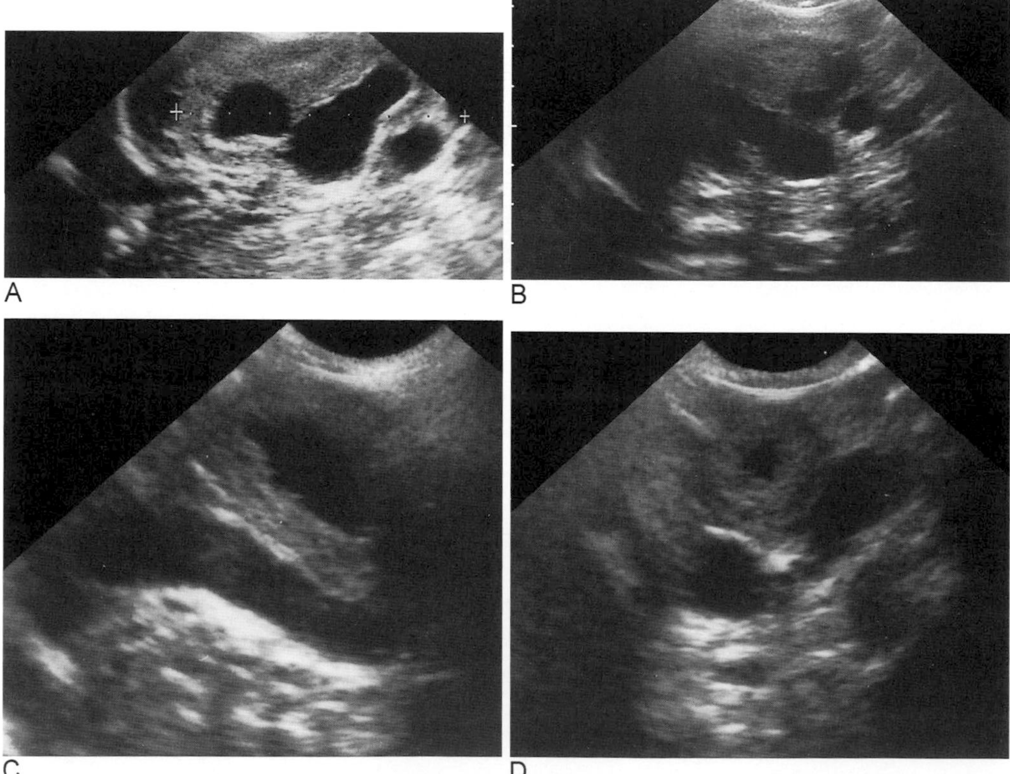

Figure 66.14 Bilateral hydronephrosis secondary to posterior urethral valves. (A) Longitudinal US of the left kidney shows hydronephrosis with a bright renal parenchyma. (B) Longitudinal US of the right kidney reveals a similar hydronephrosis to that seen on the left. (C) Longitudinal US of the bladder reveals a thick-walled bladder with a dilated ureter behind the bladder. (D) Transverse US of the bladder once again shows the thick-walled bladder with dilated ureters behind the bladder.

Continued

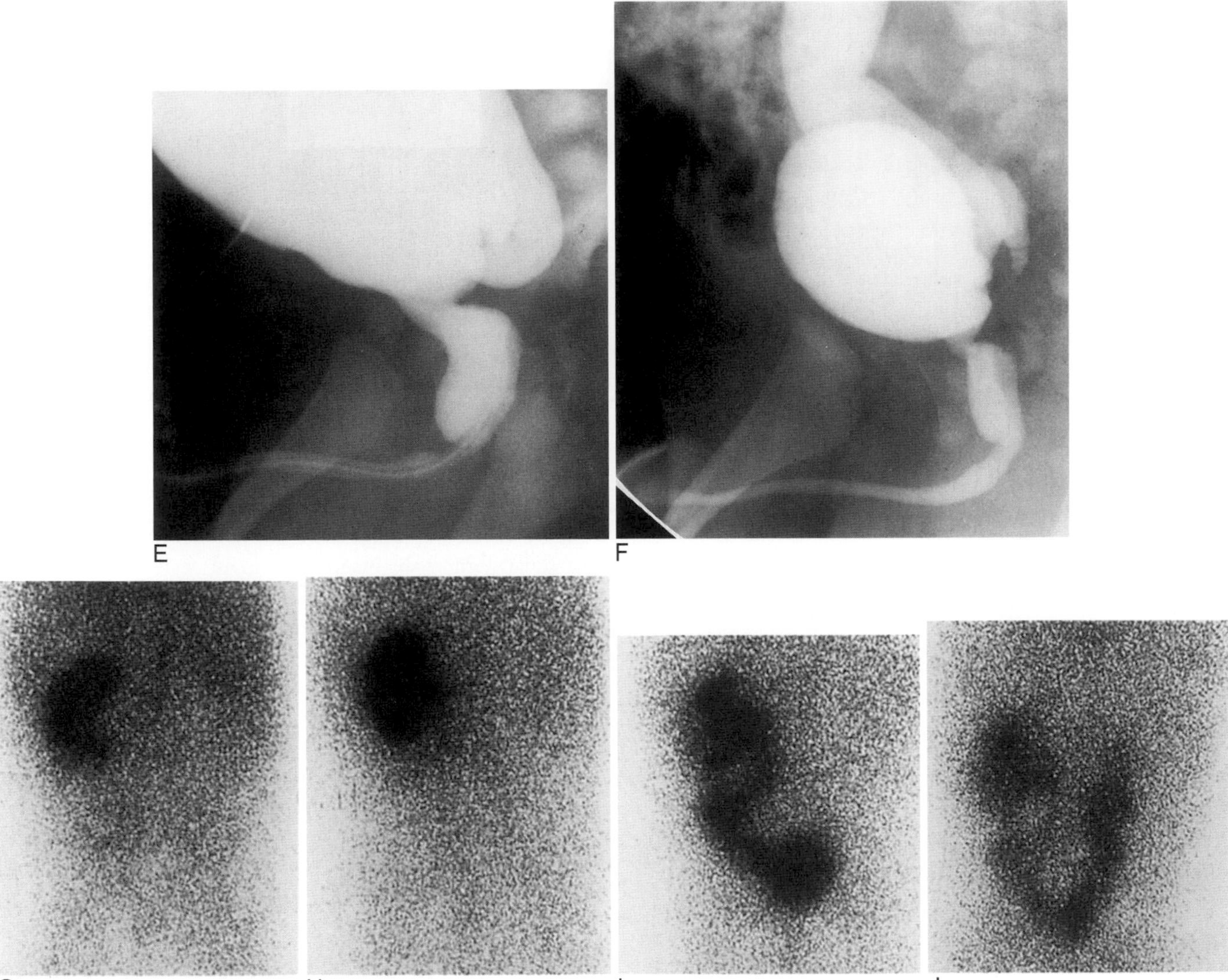

Figure 66.14 Cont'd (E) Micturating cystourethrogram (MCUG) done on the first day of life reveals bladder neck hypertrophy with a dilated posterior urethra. There is an abrupt change in calibre of the urethra, although the exact outline of the posterior urethral valve cannot be seen. Note that with a 6F feeding tube in the urethra the possibility of obscuring a posterior urethral valve was very small. Reflux into a ureter was also clearly seen. (F) MCUG 3 months after valve resection shows that the bladder neck hypertrophy is less marked and that the differential calibre of the urethra is minimal. Reflux persists; this is on the left. (G) ^{99m}Tc-DTPA scintigram. The 1-min image reveals function only in the left kidney. (H) The 20-min image shows progressive accumulation of radionuclide in the left kidney with no function in the right kidney. (I) 10 min after intravenous furosemide. The radionuclide has moved from the dilated left renal pelvis down the ureter into the bladder. (J) Following micturition the bladder has emptied and reflux is clearly seen into the nonfunctioning right kidney. The left kidney as well as the ureter have cleared the radionuclide, suggesting that no obstruction exists.

renal function on the affected side; VUR may cease following valve ablation.

Imaging

US usually suggests the diagnosis, typically showing bladder wall thickening with or without hydroureters and echogenic kidneys. US may show a urinoma. The MCUG is definitive. These two examinations allow comprehensive immediate management. A baseline, ^{99m}Tc-MAG3 scintigram should be carried out around 12 weeks following valve ablation. Long-term follow-up includes revisualization of the urethra on MCUG after the last instrumentation, as well as US and dynamic diuresis renography at regular intervals. After the age of 3 years the dynamic MAG3 renogram should be completed with an IRC so that the effect may be judged of a full bladder and bladder emptying on the upper tract.

Urethral dysplasia

The entire urethra may be dysplastic and this feature is generally associated with dysplasia of the kidneys and consequent renal failure within the first year of life. The urethra may be difficult to catheterize, even using a 6F catheter, and suprapubic cystography may be required to outline the urethra on MCUG. On fluoroscopy, a thin line of contrast medium is seen where the urethra should be, without the normal anatomical landmarks. The entire urethra is of the same calibre. The prognosis depends on the degree of renal dysplasia.

In Down's syndrome narrowing of the distal posterior urethra, not dissimilar to that seen in PBS, is seen. However there is a good stream. The narrowing is concentric and does not act as an obstructive lesion since the children can empty their bladder completely and there is no bladder neck hypertrophy.

In the presence of a single ectopic ureter, the ureter enters below the bladder base and drains a simple (i.e. nonduplex) kidney. There is elongation and narrowing of the posterior urethra between the bladder neck and verumontanum. The ureter is not usually obstructed and may be of normal calibre. The effect on the urethra is variable but is usually obstructive to some degree.

Recto-urethral fistula

This abnormality is usually associated with an imperforate anus. A high-pressure loopogram via a colostomy is the best method of demonstrating the passage of contrast medium from the bowel to the posterior urethra (close to the verumontanum). The presence of air in the bladder as shown on plain images confirms the diagnosis of a fistula. Direct rectovesical fistulas are exceedingly uncommon.

Duplication of the urethra

This is a rare abnormality in which there is usually complete duplication, with one of the urethras ending as a hypospadias (Fig. 66.15). Pathology within one of the urethras, e.g. a posterior urethral valve, must also be excluded.

Anterior urethral abnormalities

This area has been neglected by both radiologists and urologists. High-quality images are essential to exclude a syringocoele or meatal abnormalities.

Traumatic strictures

Strictures may be found at any level in the urethra following either instrumentation or external trauma.

DUPLEX KIDNEY

An uncomplicated duplex kidney is a variation of normality. A complicated duplex may be a complete or incomplete duplex. Both moieties may show equal function, and here the duplex kidney is typically longer than normal in bipolar length on US and has divided renal function of over 55% of global function. Reduced function of the upper moiety may be due to dysplasia and/or obstruction due to a ureterocele (Fig. 66.16). The lower moiety may have reduced function in association with reflux into this moiety or due to obstruction at the PUJ level.

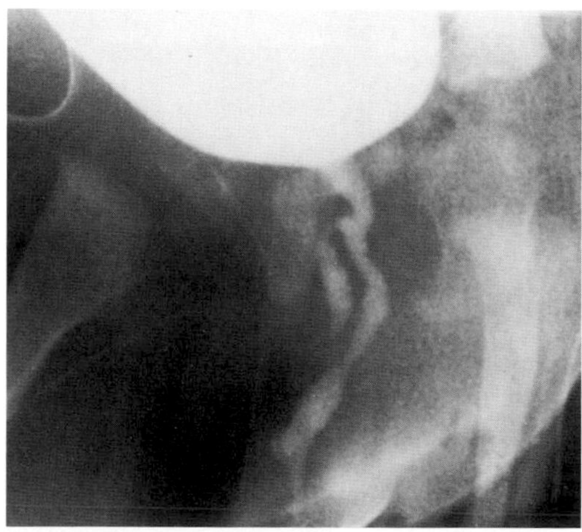

Figure 66.15 Infant with hypospadias. The urethral views of the micturating cystourethrogram demonstrate a double urethra; the dorsal urethra is severely dysplastic and the main channel is through the ventral urethra terminating in the hypospadias.

Drainage

Incomplete duplication

Drainage of the duplex kidney is by definition via two collecting systems. However, the two systems have many possible formations. There may be incomplete duplex, in which the two ureters join at any level above the bladder. This is when 'yo–yo' reflux may occur, i.e. when urine refluxes from one moiety down the ureter and then up into the other moiety, rather than going down into the bladder. It is only by using dynamic radionuclide studies that this diagnosis can be made with certainty.

Complete duplication

Here the ureters draining the two moieties never join. When both ureters drain into the bladder, the ureter draining the lower moiety is prone to reflux. The ureter draining the upper moiety usually enters the bladder as a ureterocele and is frequently obstructed. The ureterocele may vary in size from being so large that the inexperienced may mistake it for the bladder or it may be collapsed such that it is not recognizable even on a careful US examination. When one moiety drains outside the bladder, it is usually the upper moiety and this ureter can terminate in the urethra or in the vagina in girls. Such ectopic drainage of the ureter is almost always associated with dysplastic function of the upper moiety of the kidney (Fig. 66.17).

Clinical presentation

- Asymptomatic as an incidental finding
- UTI
- Pain which can be secondary to an intermittent obstruction at the PUJ level of the lower moiety or due to 'yo–yo' reflux with incomplete duplication
- Continuous wetting in the girl who has never been dry due to an ectopic insertion of the upper moiety into the vagina
- Vaginal prolapse may occur when the ureterocele prolapses out of the bladder. Prolapse of a ureterocele may also result in bladder neck obstruction and may mimic PUV in boys.

Imaging

One of the cardinal signs of a duplex system is a change in the axis of the lower moiety. This is best seen in that the calyces of the lower moiety show the lower group medial to the upper group of calyces, giving the lower moiety of the kidney a longitudinal axis pointing to the shoulder on the same side.

Ultrasound

The US findings are protean depending on the abnormalities present. The upper moiety may be normal, small, and dysplastic, or may be anechoic resembling a 'cyst' which is an obstructed ureterocoele. The latter two conditions are generally associated with a dilated ureter. The appearances of a lower moiety in complete duplication may be normal and difficult to recognize or the kidney may simply show two distinct renal pelves. The calyces and pelvis of a lower moiety may be dilated with no ureteric dilatation, which would suggest a PUJ stenosis. Reflux is likely when a dilated ureter is seen.

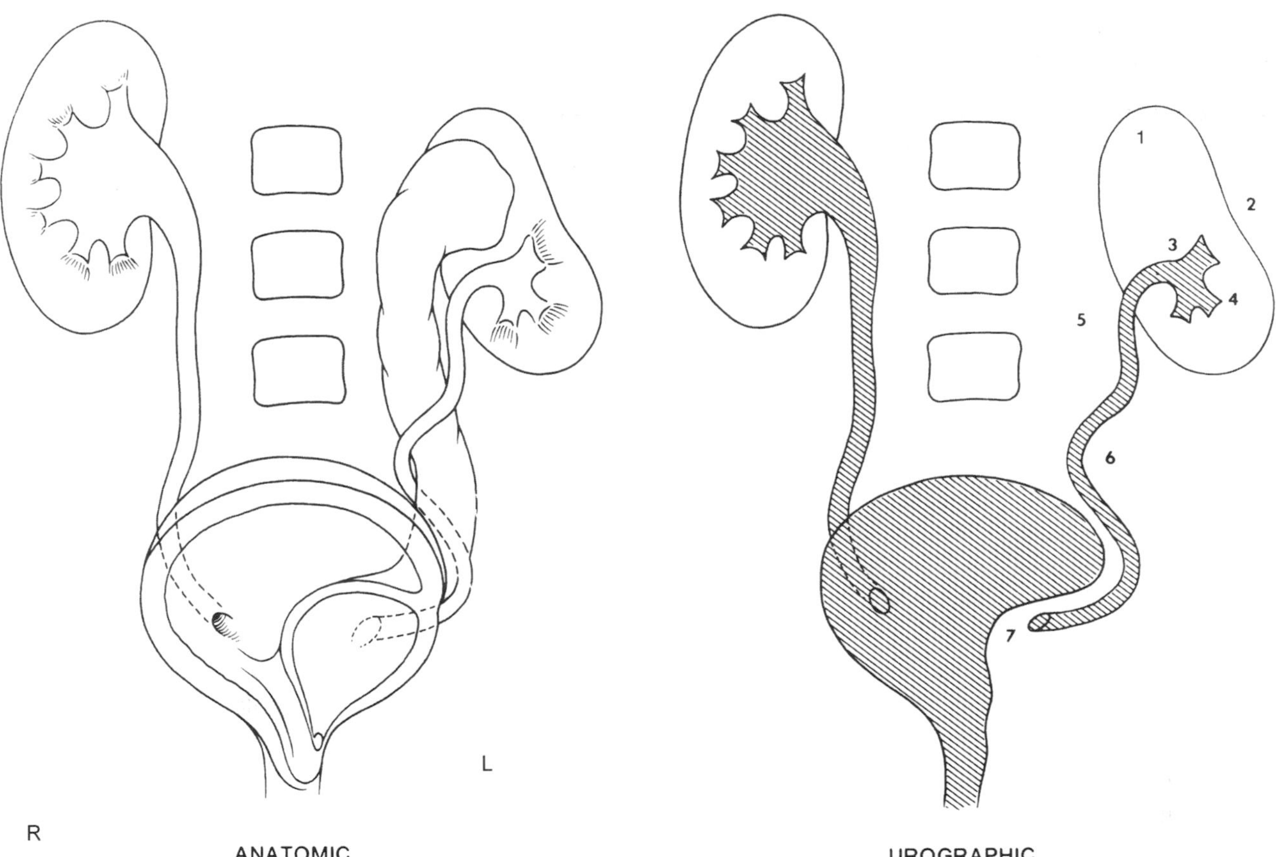

Figure 66.16 Ectopic ureterocele. Diagrammatic representation of the anatomical and urographic appearances of an ectopic ureterocele of the left upper moiety without function. Diagnosis of this entity on the urogram depends on recognition of indirect signs: 1 = increased distance from the top of the visualized collecting system to the upper border of the nephrogram; 2 = abnormal axis of the collecting system; 3 = impression upon the upper border of the renal pelvis; 4 = decreased number of calyces compared to the contralateral kidney; 5 = lateral displacement of the kidney and ureter; 6 = lateral course of the visualized ureter; and 7 = filling defect in the bladder. (Redrawn from Lebowitz R L, Avni F E 1980 Misleading appearances in pediatric uroradiology. Pediatr Radiol 10: 15–31.)

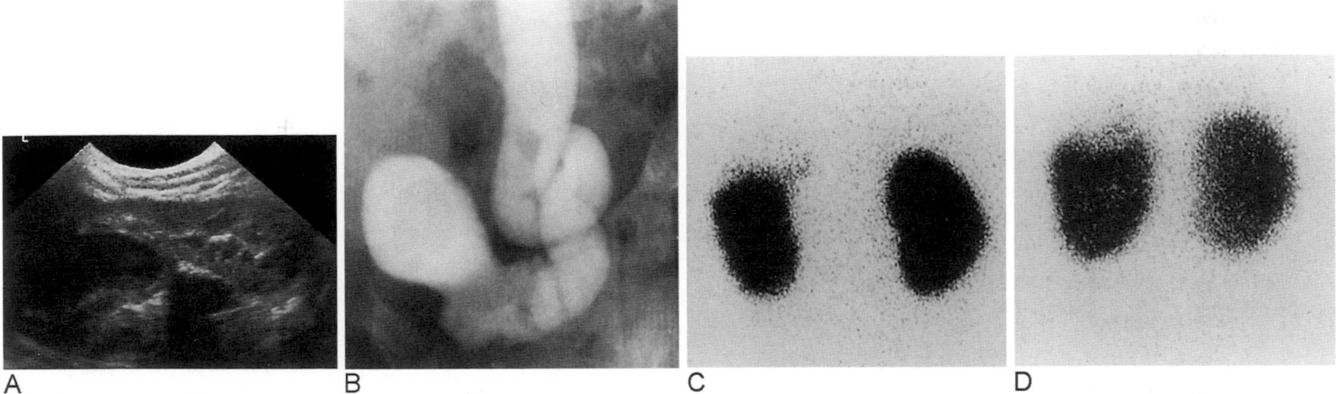

Figure 66.17 Duplex anomaly. Anomaly in a 1 year old girl with urinary tract infections. (A) Longitudinal US of the left kidney showing a dilated collecting system in the upper portion, with a normal lower pole. (B) The micturating cystourethrogram shows vesico-ureteric reflux (VUR) into a dilated ureter, which is draining the lower moiety of the left kidney; a small amount of contrast medium is seen in the bladder but no ureterocele is evident. (C) ^{99m}Tc-DMSA scintigram in the posterior (prone) projection shows a normal right kidney; the left kidney shows decreased activity in the upper pole with a little abnormal activity on the superomedial aspect. The left kidney contributed 38% to overall function and the right kidney 62%. (D) Left posterior oblique projection of the ^{99m}Tc-DMSA scintigram showing to better advantage the defect in the upper pole of the left kidney. This infant had a duplex left kidney with a ureterocele draining the obstructed upper moiety. VUR into the lower moiety had not caused any scarring.

Nuclear medicine

The appearances of a duplex kidney vary with the pathology of each moiety. ^{99m}Tc-MAG3 will assess function, drainage, and/or reflux, especially with late images. If a moiety is non-functional it will not be visualized; this is important when there is a small severely dysplastic upper moiety. A high index of suspicion when reporting on functional imaging allows the duplex kidney to be recognized easily. With incomplete duplication the upper and lower moieties may be normal or there may be reduced function of either element. With

^{99m}Tc-MAG3 the drainage from each moiety can be evaluated as well as looking for 'yo–yo' reflux.

Micturating cystourethrogrophy

If a duplex is suspected the technique must be modified; fluoroscopy begins when a small volume of contrast medium has been instilled into the bladder to allow detection of the ureterocele as a filling defect; this will be obliterated once the bladder is full of contrast medium. US, however, is the preferred method for detecting and measuring ureteroceles. VUR may be detected, usually into the lower moiety. A nonrotated frontal image centred on the kidneys is essential. Reflux into the upper moiety is rarely detected.

Intravenous urogram

This is only indicated when there is a strong clinical suspicion of a duplex as, e.g. in the girl who is always wet, yet the US and ^{99m}Tc-DMSA studies are normal. Since the ureter drains below the bladder base in this situation, there is no point in doing an MCUG. An IVU with special emphasis on the upper poles of the kidneys, including delayed images, may be useful. The only sign of a duplex system may be a little contrast on a late radiograph medial to the upper pole of one of the kidneys. MRU may now be superior in this context.

URINARY TRACT INFECTION AND VESICO-URETERIC REFLUX

UTI is common and the imaging that children undergo is important in terms of discomfort, radiation exposure, and resource utilization. An effort must be made not to overburden the radiology department or over investigate the child but at the same time not to overlook treatable pathology or long-term complications. Imaging should therefore be limited to those children with a bacteriologically proven UTI.

Clinical setting

Four per cent of all children under 8 years of age will present with a UTI each year, yet the incidence of children requiring dialysis secondary to pyelonephritis is one child per million age-related population. There are little data to support the belief that hypertension is a complication of mild renal scarring. For these reasons the 'susceptible child' who has a UTI and requires imaging needs to be identified. These children include those with: febrile infection; recurrent infections; clinical signs (poor urinary stream, palpable kidneys); unusual organisms (non-*Escherichia coli*) infections; bacteraemia; slow response to antibiotics; or unusual clinical presentation (older boy).

VUR is a sign detected in the radiology/nuclear medicine department; it is not a disease. The relationship between VUR and renal damage has been questioned[8]. A systematic review of the literature in children with UTI showed that only 20% of those with VUR showed renal damage on DMSA, while scarred kidneys were seen in children where no VUR could be demonstrated[9,10]. Further, 30% of children with a prenatal diagnosis of hydronephrosis already have an abnormal kidney at birth, thus recognizing that a child may have VUR and a maldeveloped kidney which previously was considered to be 'reflux nephropathy' (Fig. 66.18).

Imaging

The aim of imaging is to detect an obstructive uropathy or calculi, and to prevent further infections. A full US examination as soon as possible after diagnosis in the susceptible group is recommended. If the US is normal or abnormal but without dilatation, then a ^{99m}Tc-DMSA scintigram is required. If the US shows hydronephrosis a MAG3 diuretic renogram is required. When US shows a dilated ureter or an abnormal bladder then

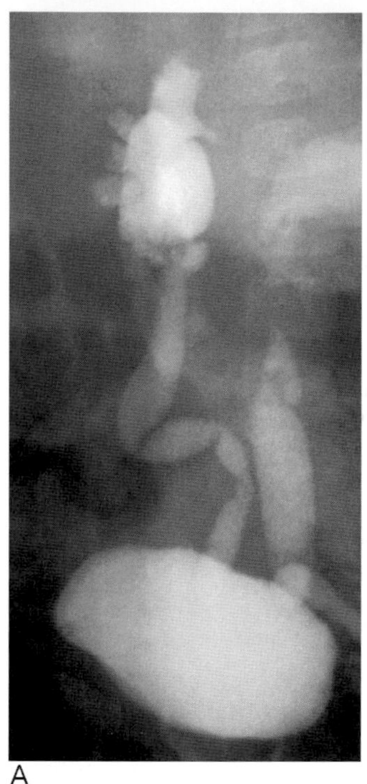

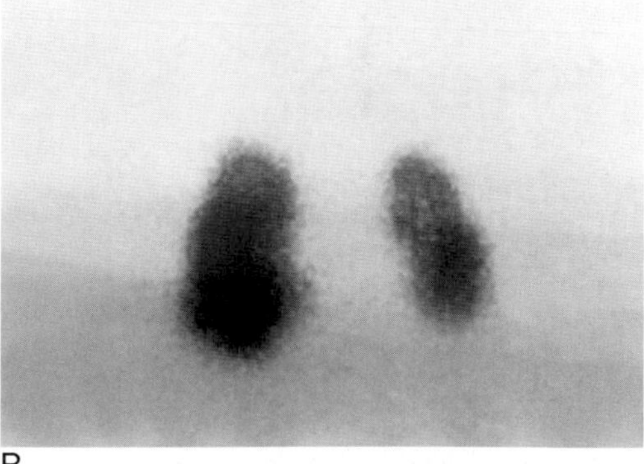

Figure 66.18 Antenatal detection of renal pelvic dilatation (RPD). This baby had antenatal US detection of RPD and this is the postnatal imaging. Longitudinal US showed that the right kidney is larger than the left. Both kidneys had irregular outlines with areas of cortical thinning. (A) Micturating cystogram on the same child showing bilateral reflux into tortuous dilated ureters and pelvicalyceal systems. (B) DMSA scintigram on the same child showing bilateral focal defects in the cortex of both kidneys with the right kidney functionally smaller than the left as seen on the US. This child had never had a urinary tract infection and the defects on DMSA are thought to be related to dysplasia during intrauterine development, which may be associated with vesico-ureteric reflux.

a MCUG plus DMSA imaging is required. If US detects a calculus an abdominal radiograph is indicated (Fig. 66.19). There is growing evidence that gadolinium-enhanced fat-suppressed T1-weighted or inversion recovery (STIR) MRI sequences may be sensitive in the detection of acute pyelonephritic lesions; comparison with ^{99m}Tc-DMSA is being undertaken[11]. In children with recurrent UTI, emphasis must be on the bladder. Frequency void charts and the physiological IRC may help identify the unstable bladder.

The follow-up of children with a damaged kidney and VUR who are on long-term antibiotic prophylaxis is unclear[10]. Imaging should be infrequent and as these children are older they should not have repeat MCUGs. One approach is to only undertake imaging if it will affect treatment, i.e. if a negative isotope cystogram will be the indication to stop long-term prophylaxis. If surgical intervention has been undertaken to stop VUR (Fig. 66.20), then a US and dynamic scintigraphy are essential to ensure that no obstruction has resulted. Current recommendations on this topic from the Royal Colleges of Physicians and Paediatrics and Child Health, and the American Academy of Pediatrics are being seriously questioned[10,12,13].

Renal abscess

This complication follows acute pyelonephritis and may be first suspected when the child develops a swinging fever with a poor response to antibiotics. Usually the abscess also has a thick wall with heterogeneous internal echogenicity. A ^{99m}Tc-DMSA scintigram will show a focal defect in a kidney which

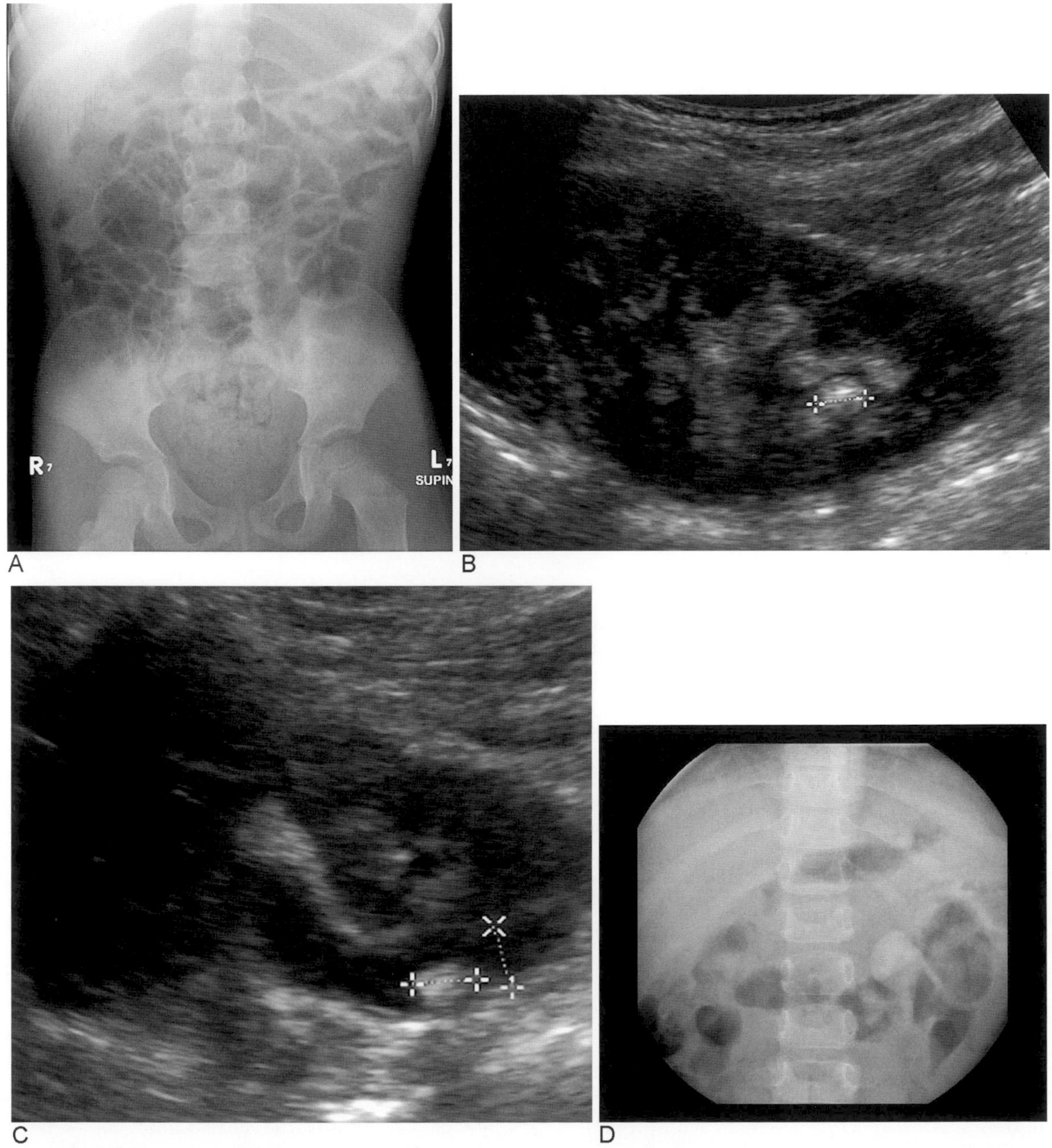

Figure 66.19 Renal calculi. (A) Plain abdominal radiograph showing small opacities overlying the left kidney. (B,C) Longitudinal US of the left kidney showing the echogenic foci of the renal calculi casting an acoustic shadow in (B) a calyx and (C) also in the upper ureter. (D) Plain abdominal radiograph showing a left staghorn calculus in a different 4 year old boy.

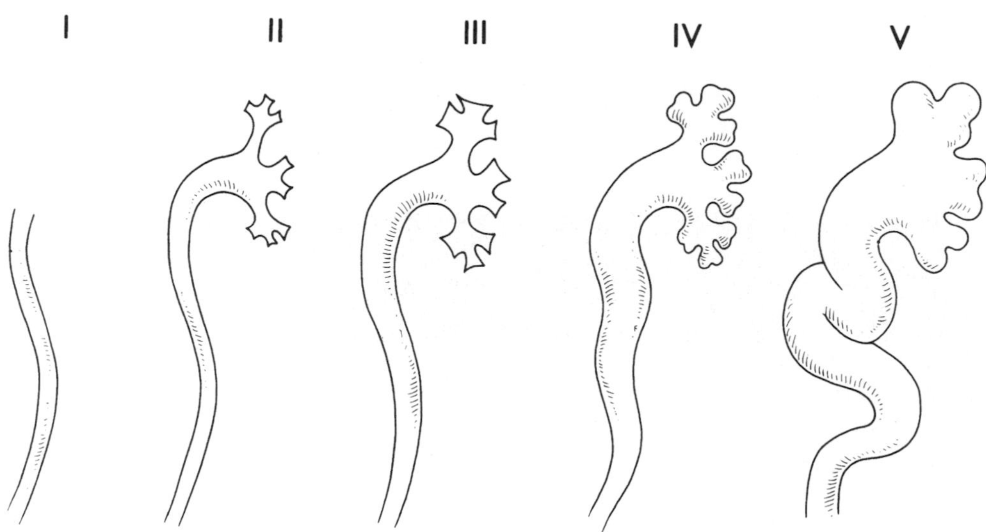

Figure 66.20 Radiographic grades of reflux. (I) Ureter and upper collecting system without dilatation; (II) mild or (III) moderate dilatation of the ureter and mild or moderate dilatation of the renal pelvis, but no, or only slight, blunting of the fornices; (IV) moderate dilatation and/or tortuosity of the ureter with moderate dilatation of the renal pelvis and calyces and complete obliteration of the sharp angle of the fornices but maintenance of papillary impression in the majority of calyces; (V) gross dilatation and tortuosity of ureters, renal pelvis, and calyces; papillary impressions are not visible in the majority of calyces. (From Levitt S B, Duckert J, Spitzer A, Walker D 1981 Report of the International Reflux Study Committee. Medical versus surgical treatment of primary vesico-ureteral reflux. Reproduced with permission from Pediatrics 67: 392–400© 1981 by the American Academy of Pediatrics.)

generally shows reduced overall uptake of isotope. CT is helpful especially if aspiration or drainage is being considered.

Xanthogranulomatous pyelonephritis

Xanthogranulomatous pyelonephritis (XPN) is a rare chronic inflammatory disease of the kidney in childhood. The clinical presentation is with weight loss, failure to thrive, malaise, anaemia, and often an abdominal mass. Urine cultures are positive in around 70% of cases with Proteus species and *E. coli* being the most common pathogens.

Frequently a calculus is evident but XPN is not generally considered to be an infected obstructed kidney but rather a kidney in which there has been an abnormal inflammatory response to infection in the presence of a stone. The imaging findings are usually sufficiently characteristic to allow pre-operative diagnosis and to avoid confusion with a Wilms' tumour. The diffuse type of XPN, affecting the entire kidney, is more common in childhood. Rarely focal involvement of only part of a kidney is seen. Focal XPN has a female predominance but the diffuse type has an equal sex distribution.

The focal type of XPN tends to manifest with a localized intrarenal mass in an otherwise normal kidney. Plain radiographs reveal an abdominal mass with calculi. US demonstrates general renal enlargement in the diffuse form with hypoechoic areas corresponding to inflammatory masses within the kidney. Calcification, particularly at the contracted renal pelvis, is usually prominent. Ureteric calculi may also be visualized. ^{99m}Tc-DMSA scintigraphy shows a nonfunctioning kidney in the diffuse form or a photon-deficient area in the focal form. CT after intravenous contrast medium characteristically shows global renal enlargement with prominent low-attenuating abscess cavities. The remaining renal parenchyma can often show some rim enhancement due to the perfusion of the inflamed, nonfunctioning kidney (Fig. 66.21).

The necrotic areas tend to be hyperintense on T2-weighted MRI, with medium signal on T1-weighted sequences, which probably represents the high protein content of the cavities. Perinephric extension is common with hilar or para-aortic adenopathy. The treatment for both types is nephrectomy but this may be difficult due to the surrounding chronic inflammation. There may be a role for pre-operative embolization to reduce peri-operative haemorrhage.

HYPERTENSION

The more severe the hypertension and the younger the child, then the more likely it is to be secondary hypertension. Renal disease is the cause of hypertension in over 90% of children after 1 year of age[14]. Any abnormal kidney may produce renin and so generate hypertension. Renal scarring and glomerular disease are the most common causes, and occasionally PUJ obstruction, neuroblastoma, or Wilms' tumours present with hypertension. Renovascular disease accounts for approximately 10% of cases, with fibromuscular dysplasia being the most common cause. Other associations are neurofibromatosis, idiopathic hypercalcaemia of infancy, an arteritic illness, or middle aortic syndrome. Phaeochromocytomas, albeit uncommon in childhood, are seen and are often both multiple and extra-adrenal in origin. Essential hypertension is also encountered, usually in milder cases, often with a positive family history of hypertension.

Imaging

US will demonstrate the small kidney, the severely scarred kidney, significant hydronephrosis, and both renal and most adrenal tumours. Doppler US of the aorta and renal arteries may reveal aortic narrowing or renal artery stenosis. Further

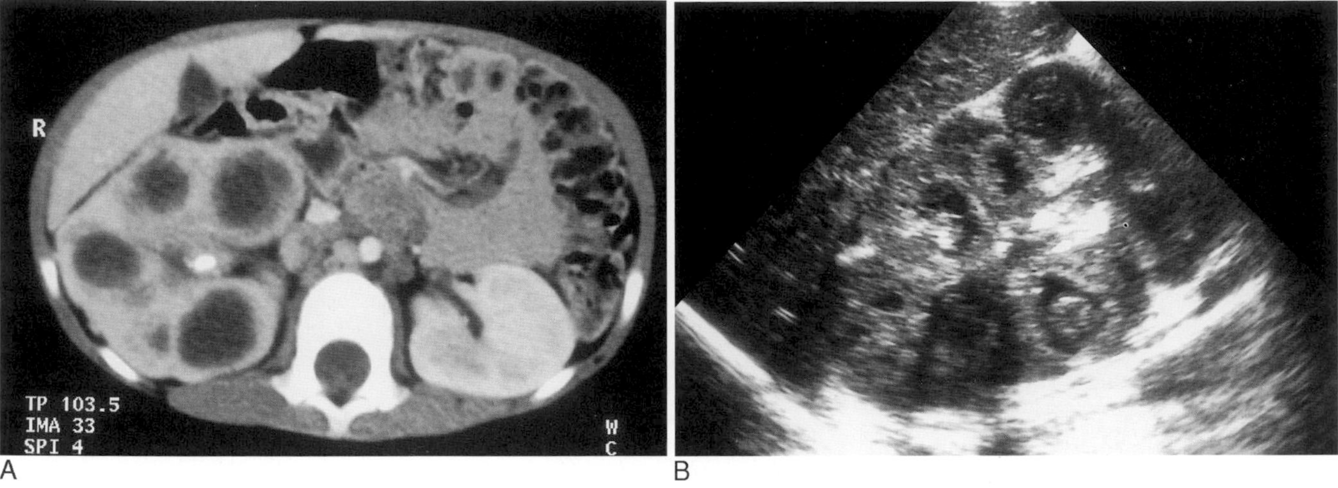

Figure 66.21 Xanthogranulomatous pyelonephritis. (A) Longitudinal US of the right kidney in a 2 year old boy showing heterogeneous reflectivity due to xanthogranulomatous pyelonephritis. (B) Axial-enhanced CT study showing calcification at the right renal hilum, renal enlargement, and low-density fluid collections within the renal substance. Although there appears to be some enhancement of the renal parenchyma, there was no renal function on isotope studies.

investigation depends upon the abnormal US findings. Doppler US, however, has proved disappointing in the detection of renovascular disease in native renal arteries. A normal US does not exclude renal scarring, renovascular pathology, or a phaeochromocytoma. The differential diagnosis of a small kidney includes renal venous thrombosis, dysplasia, reflux nephropathy, postobstructive atrophy, and arterial pathology.

With a normal US examination, a ^{99m}Tc-DMSA scintigram is the next recommended investigation. This can detect a focal parenchymal abnormality such as renal scarring. The major limitation of US and ^{99m}Tc-DMSA imaging is the possibility of unidentified renovascular disease or phaeochromocytoma. With biochemical evidence of a phaeochromocytoma imaging should be undertaken with a [^{123}I]meta-iodobenzylguanidine ([^{123}I]MIBG) scintigram followed by cross-sectional imaging, either CT or MRI, with specific attention focused on the areas of abnormal [^{123}I]MIBG uptake. With MRI there is no risk of a hypertensive crisis as no iodinated contrast medium is used.

To exclude renovascular disease, pre- and post-captopril MAG3 renography is recommended: this will exclude all surgical/angioplasty treatable causes. A negative study will not exclude middle aortic syndrome which requires angiography. Conventional arteriography demands a free flush aortic injection as well as selective renal injections in both AP and oblique projections in order to diagnose both intra- and extra-renal renovascular disease. While digital subtraction angiography is the current reference method, renal MRA with gadolinium-enhanced sequences is promising. However, CT and MRA cannot demonstrate the intrarenal vasculature adequately. It is noteworthy here that intrarenal vascular disease is more common in childhood renovascular hypertension than in adults, underscoring the need to examine the intrarenal vessels in children suspected of renovascular hypertension.

Role of angioplasty

Angioplasty is feasible in children with disease of the main or major intrarenal arteries but requires expertise in paediatric angioplasty to minimize complications. The selection of cases is possibly the most important aspect of angioplasty and this is why some institutions prefer to undertake a diagnostic study first, together with renal vein renin sampling, review of the results of all the imaging, degree of hypertension, and current drug regimen of the child, before undertaking an angioplasty. As angioplasty can cause renal arterial thrombosis, a follow-up DMSA scintigram soon after the procedure is important (Fig. 66.22).

RENAL CYSTIC DISEASE

Cystic disease of the kidney is a wide spectrum of different diseases with variable kidney involvement. Although seen at any age, antenatal US allows many now to be detected in utero.

Clinical information

No single classification of cystic kidney disease is entirely satisfactory but the most widely acceptable is based on genetics. The genetic disorders are often systemic and there may be more than one abnormal chromosome causing the disorder (Table 66.2). They present at any age, e.g. autosomal dominant polycystic kidney disease (ADPKD). Important factors include family history of renal disease, pedigree, and histopathology (if available) of affected members and consanguinity. US of parents and siblings; renal function; clinical presentation of the child; and evidence of a syndrome together with any abnormalities of the skin, eyes, lungs, cardiac, cerebral, and/or musculoskeletal systems are all important. Nongenetic conditions include both congenital and acquired disorders.

Nongenetic 'cystic kidney' (Table 66.3)

Dysplasia/cystic dysplasia

These terms used by nephrologists, radiologists, pathologists, and urologists have different meanings. Dysplasia is a histological diagnosis based on abnormal metanephric differentiation, with persistence of fetal kidney tissue in the form of nests of metaplastic cartilage associated with primitive ducts. However, most clinicians use the term when US shows a small kidney

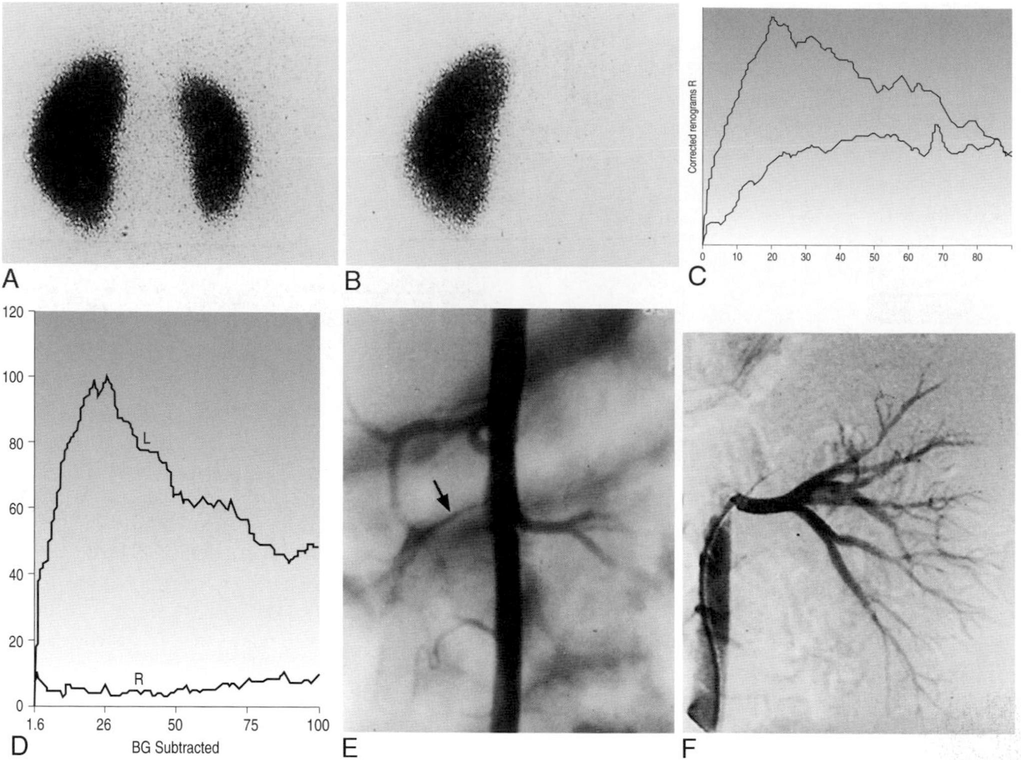

Figure 66.22 Hypertension in a 7 year old boy who presented with left facial nerve palsy, a well-recognized presenting feature of hypertension in paediatrics. (A) A ^{99m}Tc-DMSA scintigram in February 1987 shows a normal left kidney contributing 69% to overall function and a small unscarred right kidney contributing 31% to overall function. Results of US examination of this boy were normal. (B) Repeat ^{99m}Tc-DMSA scintigraphy in March 1987 following oral captopril 90 min before injection of DMSA shows absent function in the right kidney while the left kidney remains normal. (C) The ^{99m}Tc-DTPA renogram curves after background subtraction show a normal left kidney (L); the right kidney (R) shows a decreased uptake of radionuclide with a poor renogram. (D) Following oral captopril the ^{99m}Tc-DTPA renal curves reveal no change on the left but that for the right kidney is no longer normal. (E) Free-flush aortic angiogram using DMSA. The aorta is normal; the right renal artery shows narrowing from its origin all the way to the renal hilum (arrow). The left renal artery looks normal apart from narrowing at the origin of the artery inferiorly. (F) Selective left renal arteriogram reveals a normal intra-arterial supply within the left kidney.

Table 66.2 GENETIC CONDITIONS
Autosomal dominant
Autosomal dominant polycystic kidney disease
Tuberous sclerosis
Medullary cystic disease
Glomerulocystic disease
Autosomal recessive
Autosomal recessive polycystic kidney disease
Juvenile nephronophthisis
Cysts associated with syndromes
Chromosomal disorders
Autosomal recessive syndromes
X-linked syndromes

Table 66.3 NONGENETIC CONDITIONS
Cystic dysplasia or dysplasia
Multicystic dysplastic kidney
Multilocular cyst
Multilocular cystic Wilms' tumour
Localized cystic disease of the kidney
Parapelvic cyst
Simple cysts
Calyceal cyst (calyceal diverticulum)
Medullary sponge kidney
Acquired cystic kidney disease (in chronic renal failure)

with loss of the normal corticomedullary differentiation and hyper-reflectivity with a variable number and size of cysts (Figs 66.23, 66.24). Dilatation is not a common feature unless associated with VUR. There is poor function to a varying degree on ^{99m}Tc-DMSA scintigraphy which may also show focal defects that should not be interpreted as a scar since such appearances are seen in children with dysplasia who have never had a UTI. The calyces if outlined by contrast medium at the time of MCUG show loss of the fornices with resulting blunting. The calyces may be few in number and the renal pelvis may be dilated and rather perpendicular with a tortuous and dilated ureter.

If bilateral, the child will go into renal failure but end-stage renal failure is variable and may not come about until late in the second decade of life. Dysplasia is often seen in association with other congenital malformations of the kidney. The most common are the upper moiety of a duplex, posterior urethral valves, and malpositioned kidneys, as in crossed fused renal ectopia, horseshoe kidney, or the pelvic kidney. In many syndromes and genetic disorders the kidneys are affected and are called

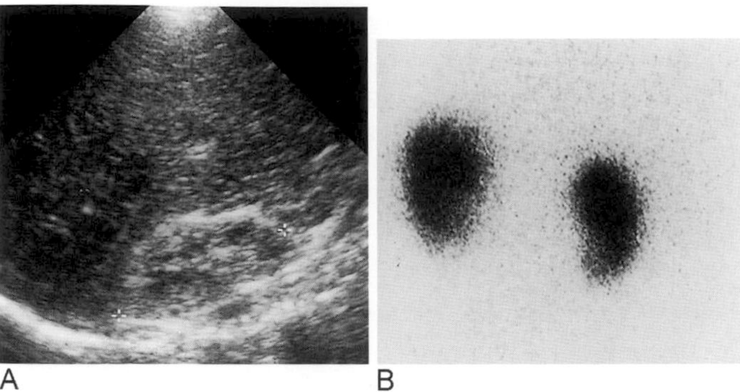

Figure 66.23 Renal dysplasia in a boy who presented at birth with rectal atresia. (A) The longitudinal US of the right kidney shows a small (32 mm) bright kidney with some differentiation between the cortex and medulla. A micturating cystourethrogram was carried out (not shown) but no vesico-ureteric reflux was seen. (B) ^{99m}Tc-DMSA scintigram reveals two equally functioning kidneys with no focal defects. Differential function: left = 50%, right = 50%. Each kidney, however, only took up 8.7% of the injected dose and the child was noted to be in chronic renal failure. He was classified as having renal dysplasia.

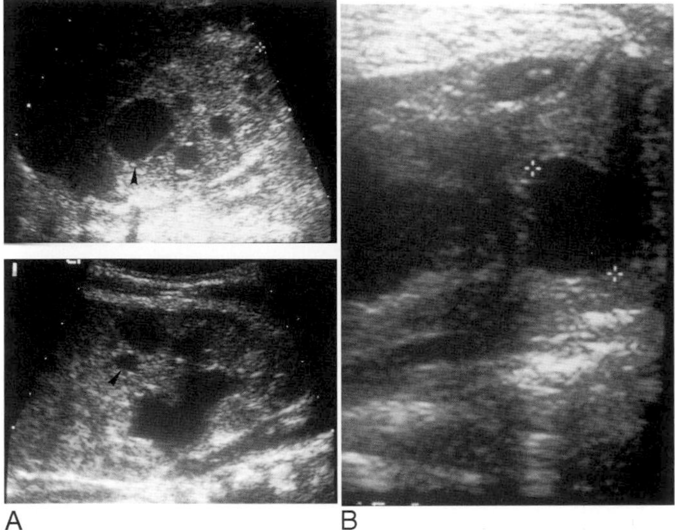

Figure 66.24 Cystic dysplasia. (A) Longitudinal US of the right (top) and left (bottom) kidneys. This shows that both kidneys are hyperechoic and contain small cysts (arrowheads). In addition, there is some dilatation of the collecting system on the left. This male infant also had dilated ureters. (B) Longitudinal US of the posterior urethra during voiding shows the dilatation of the posterior urethra. This infant had posterior urethral valves.

dysplastic with or without cysts. Some of the more common syndromes include Meckel's, Beckwith–Weidemann, Laurence–Moon–Beidl, Opitz Lemi, and oto-brachial-digital syndrome.

Multicystic dysplastic kidney

In the multicystic kidney or multicystic dysplastic kidney (MCDK) there is *no* normal overall structural pattern to the kidney, which is always nonfunctioning and the ureter is atretic. On US, there is a spectrum of appearances from a small single cyst to a large mass containing multiple, usually anechoic, cysts of varying sizes, often with a dominant large cyst situated peripherally (Fig. 66.25). There is no identifiable

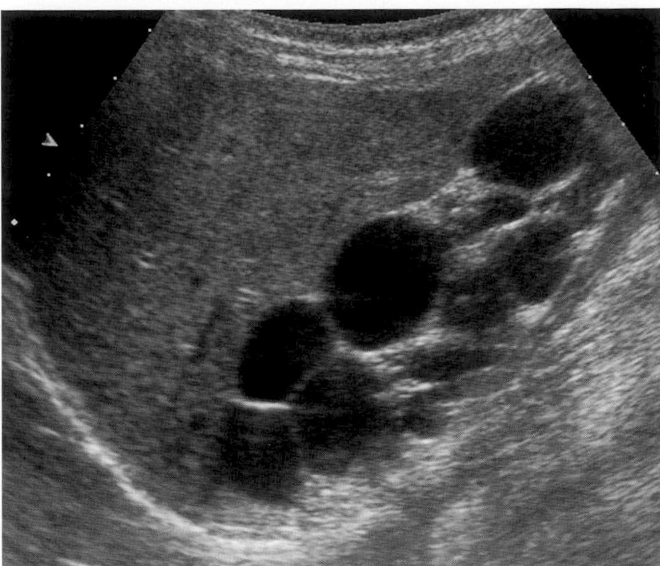

Figure 66.25 Multicystic dysplastic kidney. Longitudinal US of the right renal area. This shows the right renal fossa filled with multiple cysts of varying sizes and no normal renal parenchyma.

renal parenchyma. Histologically primitive cartilage and ductules are present. There is no increased incidence of VUR.

MCDK most commonly presents on antenatal US, is more common in boys, and the natural history is for involution. Uncommonly some persist, particularly those over 5 cm in diameter at diagnosis. A few cases complicated by either hypertension or malignancy are recorded but this is not yet accepted as a true association. Indications for surgery include a mass so large as to impede breathing or feeding, an enlarging mass, or one that by the age of 1 year remains over 5 cm in diameter. MCDK, if bilateral, is incompatible with life. The prognosis depends on the function of the contralateral kidney in which there is a 30% association of PUJ obstruction or ureteric stenosis. A MAG3 scintigram should be undertaken to assess drainage of the opposite kidney if hydronephrosis or a hydroureter is seen. MCUG is not routinely required unless the US examination reveals a contralateral dilated ureter or an abnormal bladder.

Calyceal cysts

This is not a true cystic condition but rather an observation made on US. The importance of a calyceal cyst or diverticulum is the possibility of a calculus developing within it or the theoretical existence of tuberculosis as the cause due to infundibular cicatrization. Further imaging, if any, will depend on the clinical setting.

Simple cysts

Simple renal cysts in children are extremely rare with a frequency of 0.22% and are usually detected incidentally[15]. The incidence of cysts is not related to age in this population. Simple cysts are more common following chemotherapy or abdominal radiotherapy in oncology patients. The important differential diagnosis is an abnormal upper moiety of a duplex kidney. US cannot differentiate a simple cyst from a calyceal cyst.

Localized cystic disease of the kidney

This condition is recognized as genetically, radiologically, and morphologically distinct from ADPKD. The involved segment of the kidney is usually enlarged, containing multiple, anechoic small cysts which gradually merge into normal renal parenchyma and are not sharply demarcated from the adjacent normal parenchyma. The cardinal feature which helps differentiate this condition from the multilocular cystic Wilms' tumour is the absence of a surrounding capsule on imaging and histology.

The cystic abnormality differs from ADPKD in regard to its localization into one part of the kidney and the absence of cysts in the contralateral kidney. No family history or pattern of inheritance has been reported. The lesions do not appear to be progressive in the few cases that have been reported and left in situ. Hypertension has been documented but the natural history is unclear.

Medullary sponge kidney

Medullary sponge kidney is not usually seen in childhood, but when it is the changes are the same as those seen in adults. The US appearances of renal tubular ectasia without calculi are simply an increased echogenicity of the medullae in normal sized kidneys.

Acquired cystic renal disease

In patients in chronic renal failure, cysts commonly develop (22%) without any underlying cystic renal disorder. The frequency increases with duration of dialysis with 90% developing cysts if on dialysis for over 10 years. After successful transplantation, the cysts tend to regress in size. Complications include renal cell carcinoma, haemorrhage, or infection in the cysts.

Genetic cystic disease

Table 66.4 compares some of the findings in the more common cystic renal disorders in children.

Autosomal dominant polycystic kidney disease (ADPKD)

This is rarely seen in childhood and commonly presents after the third decade of life. However, there is considerable phenotypic variability in the severity of the renal disease with some affected individuals presenting in childhood or being detected antenatally. Prevalence is approximately 1 in 1000 with two or three genetic loci identified; 90% of families have the gene located on the short arm of chromosome 16 (PKD1). The second gene is on chromosome 4 (PKD2). The location of PKD3 has not yet been found. In PKD1 families, 64% of children affected under the age of 10 years will have cysts and 90% between the ages of 10 and 19 years. There may be no family history as spontaneous mutation accounts for many cases.

The extrarenal manifestations of ADPKD include cysts in the liver, pancreas, or spleen, again rarely seen in paediatric patients. Subarachnoid haemorrhage due to intracranial aneurysm is also rare in childhood. The occurrence of subarachnoid haemorrhage tends to cluster in families. Congenital hepatic fibrosis is generally associated with autosomal recessive PKD (ARPKD; see below) but some rare cases have been described in association with ADPKD.

Ultrasound In the prenatal period, US may demonstrate highly reflective kidneys similar to ARPKD. In infancy the ultrasonic appearances vary, from a normal kidney to a few isolated cysts to a kidney packed full of cysts (Fig. 66.26). Typically the cysts are scattered throughout both the cortex and medulla with unequal involvement of the two kidneys. The intervening renal parenchyma appears normal. When found in the young child (younger than 5 years of age) with no family history, a diagnosis of tuberous sclerosis (TS) must also be considered and actively excluded (Fig. 66.27).

Intravenous urogram This probably has little role. MRI may be the examination of choice, especially when tuberous sclerosis is suspected to identify fatty tissue in an angiomyolipoma.

Tuberous sclerosis

TS is an autosomal dominant condition with a prevalence of 1 in 10 000. TS is characterized by multiple hamartomas in the brain, skin, heart, kidneys, liver, lung, and bone, and cysts are also seen in the kidneys. Genetic linkage to chromosome 9 is seen in about one-third of families, and to chromosome 16 in the same region as the ADPKD1 gene.

Table 66.4 COMPARISON OF RENAL CYSTIC DISEASES

	ADPKD	Tuberose sclerosis	ARPKD	MCDK	Simple cyst
Inheritance	D	D	R	None	None
Uni- or bi-lateral	Bilateral unequal	Bilateral	Bilateral equal	Uni- or bi-lateral	Unilateral
Kidney size	Normal or large	Normal or large	Very large > 90th centile	Small or large	Normal
Extrarenal manifestations	Cysts in liver spleen pancreas	Cardiac rhabdomyomas, intracranial tubers	Congenital hepatic fibrosis	None	None
Age at presentation	Third decade	Often < 18 months	Neonate and childhood	Antenatal, rare in childhood	Onset in adult life
Cyst size	Visible cysts of variable size	Similar to ADPKD, ± angiomyolipomas	Generally small	Large then often involute	Variable
Diagnosis	US, genetic	US, cardiac echo, cranial MRI	US, IVU, liver biopsy	US, MAG3	US, IVU
Malignancy risk	No	Yes	No	Rare	No

ADPKD = autosomal dominant polycystic kidney disease; ARPKD = autosomal recessive polycystic kidney disease, D = autosomal dominant; MCDK = multicystic dysplastic kidney; R = autosomal recessive

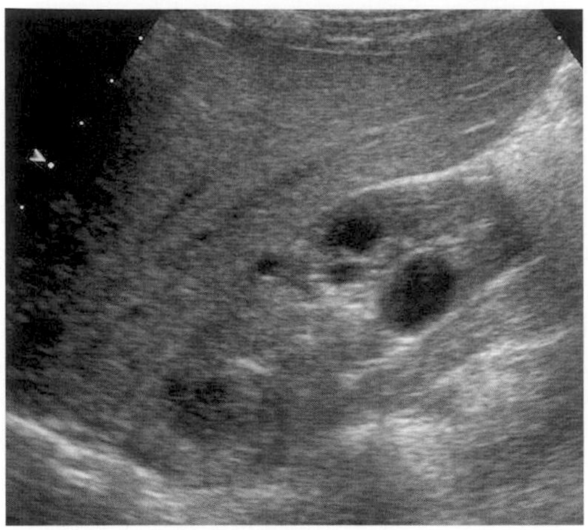

Figure 66.26 Autosomal dominant polycystic kidney disease (ADPKD). Longitudinal US of the right kidney in a child with a strong family history of ADPKD. The kidney contains a number of visible cysts in an otherwise normal looking kidney. The left kidney had very similar appearances.

The incidence of renal manifestations on imaging varies in the reported literature but is estimated to be between 47% and 73%. Angiomyolipomas are the most common lesions found in older patients and they may occur with or without cysts. Renal cysts are found less frequently (18–53%) and occur in younger patients. No imaging modality can currently differentiate cysts in TS from ADPKD. When cysts are found in the young child (younger than 5 years of age) with no family history, a diagnosis of TS must also be considered and actively excluded. Echocardiography and cranial MRI should form part of the diagnostic work-up.

Ultrasound On US (Fig. 66.27) the kidneys may have multiple cysts, resembling ADPKD. In later childhood US may demonstrate multiple small rounded echogenic foci throughout the renal parenchyma due to multiple angiomyolipomas. Complications of an angiolipoma when greater than 4 cm in diameter in particular include haemorrhage as renal vascularity is grossly abnormal. Renal cell carcinoma may also occur, although not usually in the paediatric age range. Up to 50% of patients with cardiac rhabdomyomas have TS.

Autosomal recessive polycystic kidney disease

ARPKD is a rare genetic disorder with an incidence of approximately 1 in 55 000 live births. The parents are always unaffected. The gene for ARPKD has been located on chromosome 6. Younger children tend to have the more severe renal involvement while in older children hepatic involvement predominates. Less severely affected children may present in later childhood or even in adolescence.

Ultrasound Prenatal diagnosis with US has been reported as early as 14–17 weeks' gestation but as the appearance of bilateral highly reflective kidneys during the fetal period is not specific to ARPKD, caution is necessary before suggesting this diagnosis on prenatal US. Both kidneys are always equally involved and markedly enlarged, measuring over the 95th centile for age in early infancy. As the infant grows, so the kidneys appear relatively less enlarged. The characteristic appearance is a hyper-reflective cortex and medulla, although variations, with the medulla much brighter than the cortex, may be seen. Using high-frequency probes, small 1–2-mm cysts may be detected in the medulla. Occasionally cysts of less than 2 cm may be found, especially as the child grows. In a small proportion of cases there is an evolving appearance of the kidneys such that in later childhood the kidneys contain large cysts of different sizes with an appearance indistinguishable from ADPKD (see Table 66.4).

Most children after the first year of life have some degree of hepatosplenomegaly. The spectrum of hepatic abnormalities may be subtle in the neonate. In the young child the liver is enlarged with increased echogenicity in the periportal region from bile duct proliferation and fibrosis. Single or multiple cysts communicating and closely related to the biliary tree, together with biliary ectasia, may be present. A large spleen and evidence of portal hypertension and varices may be demonstrated with US and Doppler examination, although this is not usually present in the first decade of life.

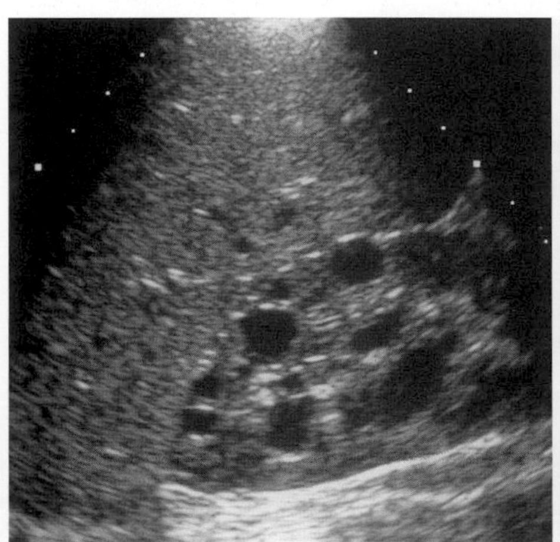

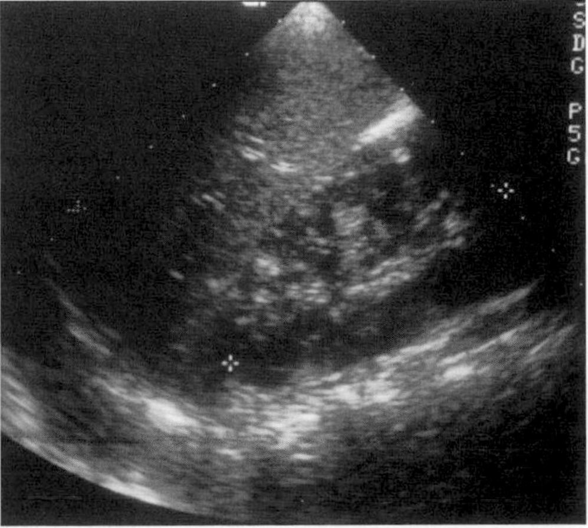

Figure 66.27 Tuberous sclerosis. (A) Longitudinal US of the right kidney. The left kidney had similar appearances. Both kidneys contain multiple cysts of varying sizes. The appearances on US are indistinguishable from autosomal dominant polycystic kidney disease. This child had the skin stigmata of tuberous sclerosis. (B) Longitudinal US of the right kidney of another patient. There were similar appearances in the left kidney. This shows the more usual appearances of tuberous sclerosis in the kidney with the small echogenic foci of angiomyolipomas.

Intravenous urogram The US appearances are not specific and some conditions may masquerade as ARPKD, such as ADPKD and glomerulocystic disease. The IVU may help differentiate these conditions by demonstrating a streaky nephrogram as contrast medium pools in the ectatic collecting ducts. The calyces may be distorted with full collecting systems. The IVU should be undertaken after 6 months of age since renal immaturity with or without associated renal impairment before this age may result in nonvisualization of the kidneys (Fig. 66.28).

^{99m}Tc-DMSA scintigraphy shows bilateral focal defects in enlarged kidneys with a high background activity. This combination of appearances on US and DMSA are characteristic of ARPKD.

The liver has a characteristic appearance. Using HIDA, a hepatobiliary agent which undergoes hepatocyte uptake, transport, and secretion into the bile, the early images reveal an enlarged left lobe of the liver in children over 1 year of age. There may be delayed passage of isotope through the liver, with areas of pooling and prominence of the duct system. This provides a valuable noninvasive method for the demonstration of subclinical biliary ectasia. This appearance has been described in Caroli's disease. US may fail to show dilatation of the bile ducts.

Juvenile nephronophthisis/medullary cystic disease

These are two different terms for conditions that have a different inheritance, different age of onset, and different associations, but a similar renal morphology and imaging. Both present with slowly progressive renal failure. Juvenile nephronophthisis (JN) has an autosomal recessive inheritance, presenting in childhood as chronic renal failure. It is characterized by an early concentrating defect, polyuria, polydipsia with growth retardation, and anaemia. The patients are in end-stage renal disease before the age of 25 years. Medullary cystic disease (MCD) shows an autosomal dominant inheritance and presents up to the fourth decade of life.

Imaging US reveals two normal-sized kidneys with a globally hyper-reflective appearance. Cysts are not a feature until late in the disease and are then typically corticomedullary. An IVU has no role. In the early stages of the disease when the tubules are affected to a greater degree than the glomeruli, the DMSA scinitigram may fail to show the kidneys yet the ^{99m}Tc-DTPA scintigram may be almost normal. The ultimate diagnosis can only be made on biopsy. Extrarenal manifestations reported in JN include skeletal abnormalities, congenital hepatic fibrosis, and mental retardation. None has been reported in MCD. In Jeune syndrome (asphyxiating thoracic dystrophy) children develop renal failure in adolescence similar to that seen in JN.

RENAL TRANSPLANTATION

Renal transplantation in very young children is now a well-established treatment, giving a significantly improved quality of life. The three most common causes of end-stage renal disease leading to transplantation are renal dysplasia, glomerular disease and pyelonephritis.

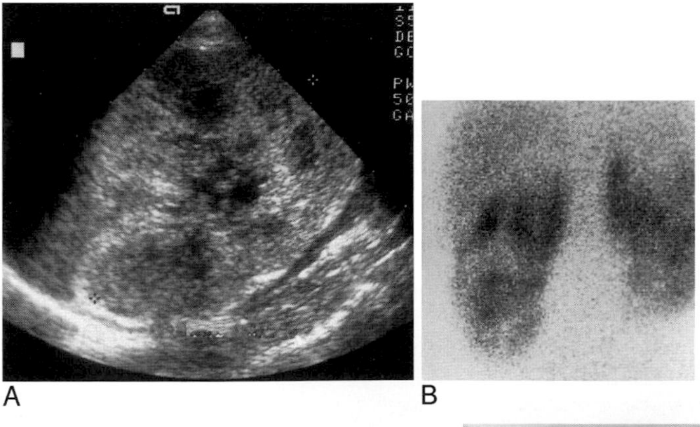

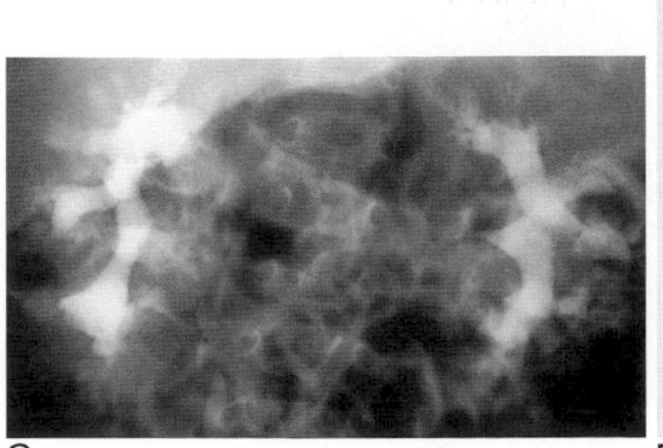

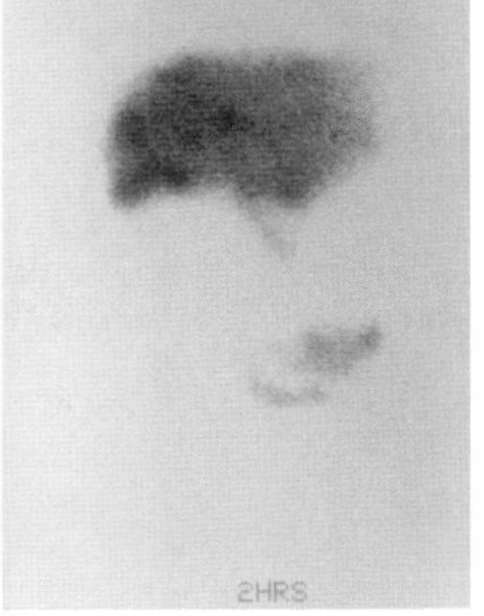

Figure 66.28 Autosomal recessive polycystic kidney disease (ARPKD). (A) Longitudinal US of the right kidney and (B) DMSA scintigram on a patient with ARPKD. US shows the typical appearances of a large hyperechoic kidney. The left kidney appeared similar. The DMSA scintigram shows photon-deficient areas in both the kidneys, particularly in the polar regions. These defects do not correspond to visible cysts on US. The child had no history of urinary tract infection. (C) Intravenous urogram on a patient with ARPKD showing the streaky radiation of contrast medium as it passes through the ectatic tubules. (D) HIDA scintigram: delayed image after 2 h showing retention of tracer within the liver, an enlarged left lobe, and a 'patchy' appearance as the tracer has accumulated in the ducts. Similar appearances have been reported in Caroli's syndrome with congenital hepatic fibrosis.

Pre-transplantation

In children with multiple congenital anomalies, anatomical variations of the aorta and IVC, e.g. high bifurcation, are common. Identification of such anomalies may be achieved using US, but MRI or CT may be required.

Post-transplantation

The major imaging techniques used are US and nuclear medicine studies with the occasional need for cross-sectional imaging or interventional techniques. The principles of imaging children post-transplantation are broadly similar to those in adults, with a few exceptions[16]. The renal artery and vein are often anastomosed to the aorta and IVC rather than to the iliac vessels.

US will identify complications, e.g. calyceal, pelvic, or ureteric dilatation, and bladder abnormalities. Colour Doppler examination is useful in the immediate post-transplant phase, especially if the child is anuric; in later follow-up, the results are disappointing with an inability to differentiate between ATN, rejection, and cyclosporin toxicity (Table 66.5). Early reports of the value of the resistive index have not been confirmed and this institution no longer reports any index of flow. ^{99m}Tc-DTPA scintigraphy will assess blood flow in the perfusion phase (0–20 s post-injection); the filtration of the kidney (1–2 min post-injection); and then transit through the kidney over 20 min with an additional image following a change in posture and micturition to assess drainage from the calyces to the bladder.

The integration of the results of different imaging techniques with clinical data will provide the best results as no single technique allows specific diagnosis of graft dysfunction. The role of MRI has not been fully evaluated. It may well replace the IVU, which is only indicated if a dilated ureter is seen and the creatinine is rising, to assess the exact level of the partial hold-up.

Late dysfunction

A late decrease in renal function may be due to rejection or drug toxicity. ^{99m}Tc-DTPA scintigraphy may suggest the diagnosis but ultimately all patients have renal biopsies. US will detect hydronephrosis/hydroureter, which if new, requires surgery. Table 66.6 gives the relevant imaging findings in some of the relevant conditions. When children develop hypertension, arterial stenosis must be considered and arteriography is required. This is uncommon with cadaveric donor kidneys as there is a patch of aorta included, but it is more likely with living donor transplant. Catheter angiography remains the reference technique in children, but the results of MRI are promising. The preferred method of treatment is angioplasty.

Lymphoceles are readily detected by US as large cystic septated collections but cannot be reliably differentiated from urinomas or large haematomas. A ^{99m}Tc-MAG3 scintigram will show whether urine enters the collection (a urinoma).

Lymphoproliferative disorder is a well-recognized complication of all transplantation with concomitant immunosuppression. The children may present with local or generalized lymphadenopathy and simply curtailing the immunotherapy may resolve the enlarged lymph nodes. There is a well-recognized association with Epstein–Barr virus. Occasionally children may present with an aggressive lymphoma requiring full chemotherapy.

TUMOURS

BENIGN TUMOURS

Nephroblastomatosis

The term 'nephrogenic rest' describes persistence of embryonic renal parenchyma (metanephric blastema) beyond 36 weeks' gestation when renal development is normally complete. Nephroblastomatosis is the presence of multiple nephrogenic rests. The abnormal foci of persistent nephrogenic cells are regarded as precursor lesions. There is an increased incidence of Wilms' tumour ('nephroblastoma') in children with nephroblastomatosis[17]. The lesions are found in association with 41% of unilateral Wilms' tumours, with 94% of metachronous bilateral Wilms' tumours and in 99%

Table 66.5 IMAGING FINDINGS IN PRIMARY NONFUNCTION

Imaging technique	ATN	RVT	RAT
US	Good arterial and venous flow	No venous flow	No venous flow, no arterial flow
US Doppler	Normal arterial and venous flow or damped due to swollen kidney	Damped systolic peak with reverse arterial flow in diastole.	Very late—no flow
^{99m}Tc-DTPA blood flow	Good	Photon-deficient area	Photon-deficient area
^{99m}Tc-DTPA filtration	Moderate	Very poor	Nil
^{99m}Tc-DTPA transit	Very slow and progressive	Often normal	Nil

ATN = acute tubular necrosis; RAT = renal artery thrombosis; RVT = renal vein thrombosis.

Table 66.6 IMAGING FINDINGS WITH A RISING CREATININE IN RENAL TRANSPLANTS

Imaging technique	Rejection	Cyclosporin toxicity	Obstruction
US	Good arterial and venous flow	Good arterial and venous flow	Dilatation of the calyces, pelvis and ureter
^{99m}Tc-DTPA blood flow	Reduced markedly	Moderate reduction	Normal
^{99m}Tc-DTPA filtration	Moderate reduction	Reduced markedly	Normal or reduced
^{99m}Tc-DTPA transit	Slow, but isotope seen	Slow with retention	Slow and progressively rising in bladder and parenchyma

of multicentric or bilateral Wilms' tumours. The malignant potential of individual lesions is uncertain; however, as only a minority of nephrogenic rests develop into Wilms' tumours and spontaneous regression may occur.

Nephroblastomatosis may either be diffuse or multifocal (Fig. 66.29), although a unifocal form may be found. The diffuse form demonstrates a thick band of reduced reflectivity on US. This abnormal tissue surrounds the renal periphery and is nonenhancing on CT and MRI. In the more common multifocal type, the nephrogenic rests resemble normal renal cortex on all modalities and can be scattered throughout the kidneys; they may be nodular or plaque-like and after contrast medium administration they become hypodense on CT and hypointense on MRI due to poor perfusion in relation to the highly vascular renal cortex.

Nephroblastomatosis yields variable signal intensity depending on cellularity and histological characteristics on T2-weighted MRI. In general, the signal intensity of nephroblastomatosis on all sequences, including gadolinium-enhanced images, tends to be relatively homogeneous in contrast to Wilms' masses which are always heterogeneous in appearance. With enhancement on either CT or MRI, the lesions are more conspicuous, which is important for the detection of small lesions. Despite characteristic imaging appearances, early histological evaluation and serial assessments are warranted because of the known malignant risk. The differential diagnosis of diffuse nephroblastomatosis on US mainly includes renal lymphoma or leukaemia.

Mesoblastic nephroma

Mesoblastic nephroma is the most common renal neoplasm in the first 3 months of life. Commonly it presents as an abdominal mass in a neonate. On US there are areas of heterogeneous reflectivity; the mass is solid but there may be hypoechoic areas due to cystic change or necrosis. Neither US nor CT can reliably distinguish mesoblastic nephroma from Wilms' tumour. The former tumours show uptake of ^{99m}Tc-DMSA. Mesoblastic nephroma does not invade the vascular pedicle nor does it metastasize. Local recurrence may result from incomplete removal or capsular penetration. With complete removal there is an excellent prognosis.

Multilocular cystic nephroma

Multilocular cystic nephroma is an uncommon cystic renal mass, derived from metanephric blastema, occasionally seen in children. It is bimodal, seen more commonly in boys under 4 years and in women in the fifth or sixth decades. It reflects a wide spectrum of histology from the completely benign on the one hand (multilocular renal cyst) to the malignant on the other (multilocular cystic Wilms' tumour). The imaging is indistinguishable between the different spectrum of histology. There are no associated anomalies. Clinically, the child presents with an abdominal mass. US will show a multilocular renal mass with multiple cysts and septations. A similar appearance is seen on CT and the lesion is nonfunctioning on isotope imaging. The hallmark on imaging is the presence of a capsule. Nephrectomy is curative and is recommended because of the malignant potential.

Angiomyolipoma

Angiomyolipoma (see section above on TS) is rarely encountered as an isolated phenomenon in children but more usually represents one of the renal manifestations of tuberous sclerosis.

MALIGNANT TUMOURS

Wilms' tumour

Wilms' tumour or nephroblastoma accounts for up to 12% of all childhood cancers with a peak incidence at around 3 years of age[18]. The most common presentation is with an asymptomatic abdominal mass. Haematuria, particularly after minor trauma, is another typical clinical manifestation while pain, fever, or hypertension (in up to one-quarter of cases) are unusual but recognized presenting features. Microscopic haematuria is present in 25% of cases. There is equal distribution between the sexes with the highest incidence being in the black population in the USA and Africa. Around 10% of Wilms' tumours are

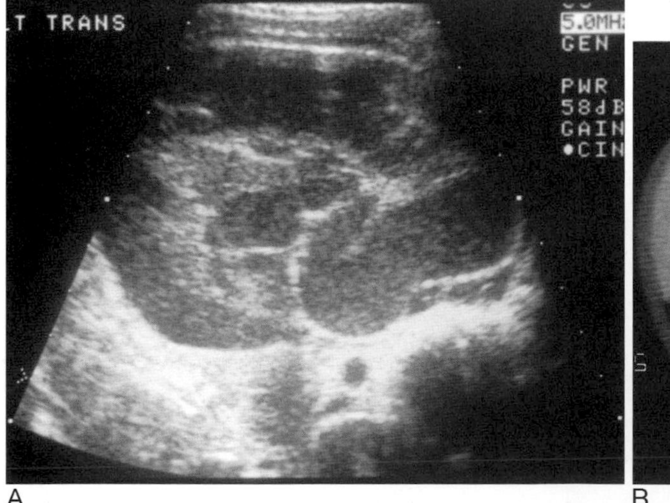

A

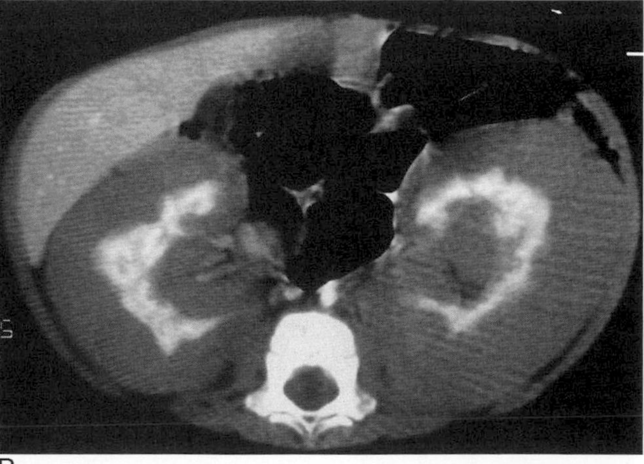

B

Figure 66.29 Nephroblastomatosis. (A) US demonstrating uniformly hypoechoic lesions surrounding the periphery of an enlarged kidney in a diffuse type of nephroblastomatosis. (B) Delayed post-contrast CT sections demonstrate these lesions, typically showing reduced vascularity in a fairly homogeneous pattern. Dense contrast medium is seen within the normal renal parenchyma.

bilateral, of which two-thirds are synchronous and one-third metachronous.

Associated congenital anomalies occur in 15% of children and include cryptorchidism and horseshoe kidney. Certain syndromes have a predisposition to Wilms' tumour. These include aniridia (absence of ophthalmic iris), Beckwith–Wiedemann (macroglossia, exomphalos, gigantism), hemihypertrophy, Denys–Drash (pseudohermaphroditism), Soto's (cerebral gigantism), Bloom's (immunodeficiency and facial telangiectasia) and Perlman's syndromes. In Denys–Drash syndrome, for example, most but not all patients will develop a Wilms' tumour, the median age at presentation being 18 months and 20% of cases are bilateral. Routine US screening to detect tumours at an early stage is controversial, because despite 3-monthly US studies large interval tumours may occur.

Nephroblastomatosis is commonly found in cases of bilateral masses. A small group of Wilms' cases are familial. Intralobar nephrogenic rests are also commonly found in such patients but there is no association of familial tumours with bilaterality. Extrarenal Wilms' tumours are rare, the most common locations are the retroperitoneum, inguinal region and pelvis. Their histology and outlook are identical to those of renal Wilms' tumours.

Wilms' tumours are solid lesions with a fibrous pseudocapsule and they have variable areas of haemorrhage and necrosis. The tumour may invade the renal vein and IVC with caval extension, often to the right atrium, seen in 4% of patients (Fig. 66.30). Metastases to local para-aortic lymph nodes and haematogenous spread to the lungs and less commonly the liver or skeleton are seen.

Epithelial (tubular, glomerular), stromal (spindle, myxoid) and blastemal (small round cells) cell lines are the histological components of nephrogenic rests, fetal kidneys and Wilms' tumours. When all three are present in malignant masses, the lesions are described as triphasic Wilms' tumours and are regarded as favourable histology. These lesions lack anaplastic changes. Unfavourable tumours comprise 6% of lesions and typically have hyperchromatic cells with large nuclei. The degree of anaplasia correlates with patient outcome. Minimally anaplastic tumours have a prognosis similar to favourable histology lesions. Clear cell sarcoma (bone metastasizing tumour) and rhabdoid tumour are no longer regarded as Wilms' variants but as biologically different entities.

The (post-surgical) staging of Wilms' tumour according to the North American National Wilms' Tumor Study Group is summarized below:

- Stage I—tumour confined to the kidney without capsular or vascular invasion.
- Stage II—tumour beyond renal capsule, vessel infiltration, biopsy performed before resection or intra-operative tumour rupture.
- Stage III—positive lymph nodes in the abdomen or pelvis, peritoneal invasion, or residual tumour at surgical margins.
- Stage IV—metastatic disease outside the abdomen or pelvis.
- Stage V—bilateral tumours at original diagnosis.

The International Society of Paediatric Oncology (SIOP) in Europe generally utilizes the same staging system with one common exception, namely masses that have been biopsied may be regarded as Stage I disease when later excised.

As with all abdominal masses, US must be the first radiological method of assessment. The tumour typically is large with a mixture of solid hyperechoic masses and relatively cystic areas; often the cystic components predominate. Normal native renal tissue can be difficult to detect and is typically stretched at the periphery of the lesion. Movement of the mass separate from adjacent organs such as the liver, indicating a lack of direct invasion, can be optimally assessed with US, a phenomenon that is difficult to evaluate on CT or MRI. The renal vein, IVC, liver and opposite kidney should be carefully assessed for spread of disease. US is also the most reliable method of excluding renal vein and IVC thrombus.

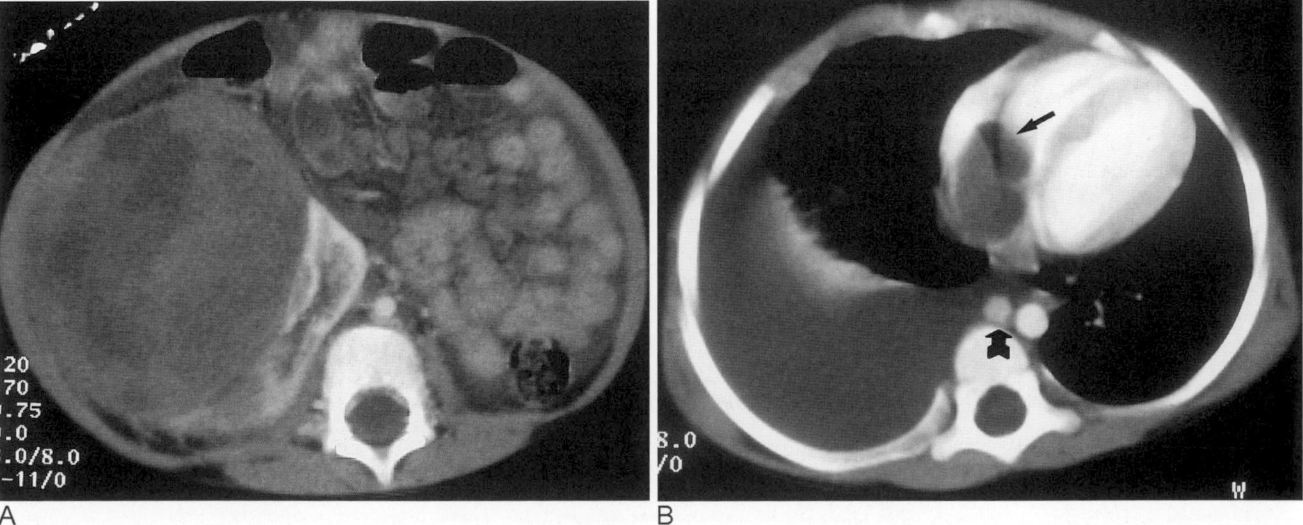

Figure 66.30 Wilms' tumour. (A) Axial CT of the abdomen after intravenous contrast medium enhancement in a 2½ year old boy showing a large mass arising from the right kidney which is of heterogeneous attenuation. The mass is seen to displace the normal enhancing renal parenchyma to the left. (B) Thoracic CT tumour thrombus was seen to extend from the inferior vena cava into the right atrium, causing a filling defect within the heart (thin arrow). Note the enlarged azygos vein (wide arrow) adjacent to the aorta and the large right pleural effusion.

Contrast-enhanced CT or MRI is necessary for further delineation of tumour extent and associated changes. CT is widely available, does not require sedation or anaesthesia, is preferred by surgeons, and is needed anyway to exclude pulmonary metastases. Wilms' tumours have a heterogeneous appearance with areas of low attenuation. Calcification is unusual, seen in less than 10% of patients. The tumour enhances to a lesser degree than normal renal parenchyma. A so-called claw or beak of normal renal tissue may be seen to be displaced by the tumour. Exclusion of adenopathy, liver abnormalities, peritoneal invasion and contralateral kidney changes should be undertaken. Small superficial or intrarenal nephroblastomatosis lesions are often not identified even with a high quality CT study.

Wilms' masses on MRI are generally hypointense on T1, variably hyperintense on T2, and enhance heterogeneously, and often poorly, with gadolinium administration (Fig. 66.31). Gadolinium is required to assess the contralateral kidney for nephroblastomatosis or another Wilms' mass. Cross-sectional imaging is playing an increasing role in needle biopsy (14G or 16G cutting needle) planning.

A controversy exists with regard to the current role of chest CT in patients at initial diagnosis. The commonly used staging systems are based on frontal and lateral chest radiographs. Although most centres perform chest CT, positive findings are ignored if no lesions can be visualized on a chest radiograph. It is argued that a pre-operative imaging protocol relying on chest radiography alone does not reduce survival and therefore chest CT is not needed. However, in a number of cases, review of a 'negative initial' chest radiograph following a positive CT revealed metastasis. For most cancers staging is based on disease distribution and on the presence or absence of disease, not on the imaging modality (chest radiography or CT) by which it is detected. Wilms' staging, however, still relies solely on plain chest radiographic findings.

The typical North American practice is initial surgical removal followed by adjuvant chemotherapy as dictated by the staging at surgery. European oncologists favour initial chemotherapy after biopsy confirmation with later resection. It is not surprising, therefore, as tumour shrinkage is often quite marked, that the percentage of Stage I and II patients is higher when pre-operative chemotherapy is used. The prognosis for Wilms' tumour patients is excellent and there is little evidence to suggest that the overall relapse-free survival is adversely affected by either approach. The 4-year overall survival rate, and presumed cure, ranges between 86% and 96% for Stages I–III disease, is up to 83% for Stage IV and 70% for Stage V disease. Patients with the much less common diffuse anaplastic Wilms' tumours have a much poorer outcome, however. Their 4-year survival rates are 45% for Stage III and only 7% for Stage IV disease.

Clear cell sarcoma of the kidney

Clear cell sarcoma of the kidney is a distinct entity accounting for 4% of all childhood renal neoplasms with a marked male preponderance. There are no known genetic associations and no reports of bilateral tumours. The peak age of incidence is similar to that of Wilms' tumour.

There are no specific radiological features to help distinguish clear cell sarcoma of the kidney from a Wilms' tumour; the distinction is histological. Although this neoplasm can metastasize to the lungs, there is a particular predilection for skeletal metastases (over 20%), hence the other known term, bone metastasizing tumour. Once diagnosed, ^{99m}Tc-MDP bone scintigraphy is indicated for staging purposes. The discovery of a secondary in the skeleton in a child with a presumed diagnosis of Wilms' tumour and no evidence of deposits in the lungs should suggest that the primary diagnosis is incorrect and that the tumour is likely to be a clear cell sarcoma of the kidney.

Rhabdoid tumour of the kidney

Rhabdoid tumour of the kidney is the most aggressive malignant renal tumour in childhood and accounts for 2% of paediatric renal neoplasms. Most cases are diagnosed in the first year of life. The mass is indistinguishable from a Wilms' tumour on imaging. A peripheral fluid crescent sign on CT has been described but it is not pathognomic and the relative rarity of the tumour diminishes the positive predictive value of this finding in an individual case. Invasion of the renal vein is common. Metastases to the lungs, liver and brain have been reported. There is also an association with simultaneous primitive neuroectodermal tumours, usually in the posterior fossa. Hypercalcaemia is a recognized finding in rhabdoid tumour but it is not specific as it is also found occasionally in mesoblastic nephroma.

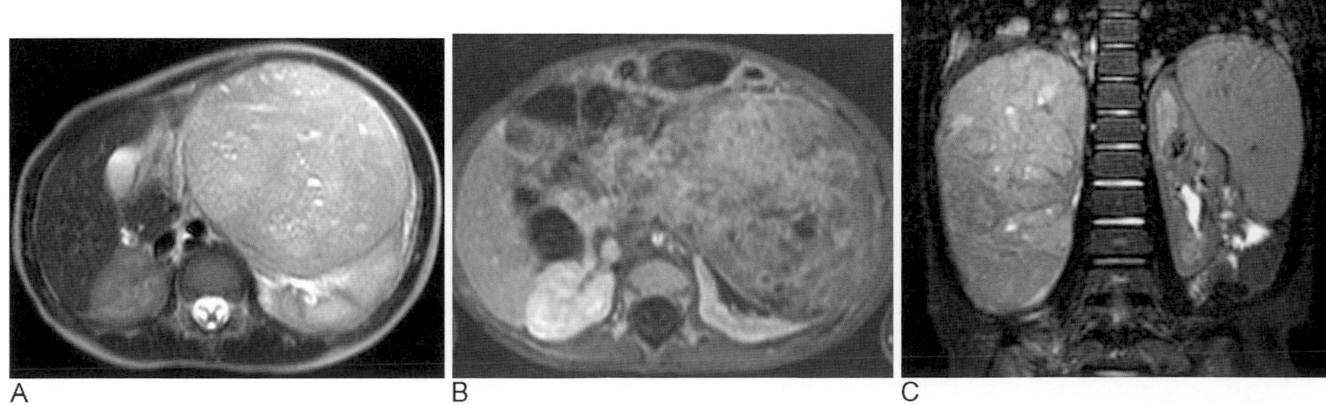

Figure 66.31 Wilms' tumours. MRI. (A) Axial T2-weighted and (B) axial T1-weighted images, post-gadolinium administration, show a large tumour growing exophytically anterior to the left kidney in a 2 year old girl. (C) Coronal T2-weighted image in another 2 year old showing a heterogeneously hyperintense, large right-sided mass.

Renal cell carcinoma

Renal cell carcinoma rarely presents in the first two decades of life, with less than 1% of all cases in children. A mass or flank pain are more common presenting features than haematuria. The mean age at paediatric presentation is 9 years. A typically solid intrarenal mass cannot be distinguished from a Wilms' tumour. Occasionally ring-like calcifications are present within the mass but the usual discriminating feature from a possible Wilms' tumour is the older age of the patient. Metastases to the lungs, liver, skeleton or brain are present in 20% of patients at diagnosis.

Lymphoma and leukaemia

Renal involvement with or without retroperitoneal adenopathy is seen in 12% of children with non-Hodgkin's lymphoma, most commonly B-cell Burkitt lymphoma. Multiple, usually bilateral, nodules are typical, although diffuse infiltration may be seen. There is generally widespread disease elsewhere. Renal enlargement on US with altered echo texture is characteristic of both renal lymphoma and leukaemia. The changes in the kidneys can be quite subtle on CT and may be more conspicuous on MRI, particularly T1-weighted images after gadolinium enhancement.

US is recommended in all children with leukaemia/lymphoma before the commencement of chemotherapy to detect tumour infiltration or calyceal dilatation. Before and during initial chemotherapy, a large fluid load is administered which in addition to the excretion of tumour metabolites may result in renal obstruction or uric acid nephropathy; those children with leukaemic or lymphomatous involvement of the kidneys need careful nephrological monitoring.

Rhabdomyosarcoma

Rhabdomyosarcoma is the most common malignant neoplasm of the pelvis in children. The genitourinary tract is the second most common site of rhabdomyosarcoma in children after head and neck locations (Fig. 66.32). Although the term suggests a mesenchymal tumour derived from striated muscle, the tumour frequently arises in sites lacking striated muscle. The two major cell types are embryonal and alveolar, of which embryonal is the more common and has a better prognosis. A botryoid subtype of embryonal rhabdomyosarcoma is characterized macroscopically by the presence of grape-like polypoid masses and accounts for 5% of cases. Botryoid tumours classically occur in the vagina, rarely metastasize and respond well to current treatment regimens.

In general, pelvic tumours may be very large at presentation and present as abdominal masses (Fig. 66.33). Prostate tumours may cause urinary obstruction and manifest with marked bladder distension or acute retention. The mass is typically solid but heterogeneous on US. Vascularity of the mass lesions can be quite variable, but some tumours are seen to enhance vividly after contrast medium administration on both CT and MRI. In addition to assessment of the primary site, the regional lymph nodes must be evaluated. Although MRI is recommended in general for all pelvic tumours, it does have some pitfalls. Oedema and later non-specific soft tissue thickening after radiotherapy may suggest an increase in tumour size or persisting tumour which can lead to discrepancies between the MRI (and CT) findings and surgical or biopsy results. Coronal or sagittal T1-weighted imaging without contrast can often be the most useful sequences for follow-up. Routine chest CT is also recommended as up to 10% of rhabdomyosarcomas have pulmonary metastases at diagnosis. ^{99m}Tc-MDP skeletal scintigraphy is performed in all cases to detect the smaller percentage of patients who have skeletal metastases.

Rhabdomyosarcomas in favourable sites such as the vagina have up to 94% 3-year survival. Tumours in the prostate and bladder, however, have a worse prognosis with a 3-year survival of approximately 70%. Prostatic tumours commonly infiltrate locally into the perivesical tissues and into the bladder base and anterosuperior spread into the space of Retzius is also recognized. The goal of therapy for bladder or bladder/prostate tumours (as it is frequently very difficult to tell the exact organ of origin) is survival with an intact bladder.

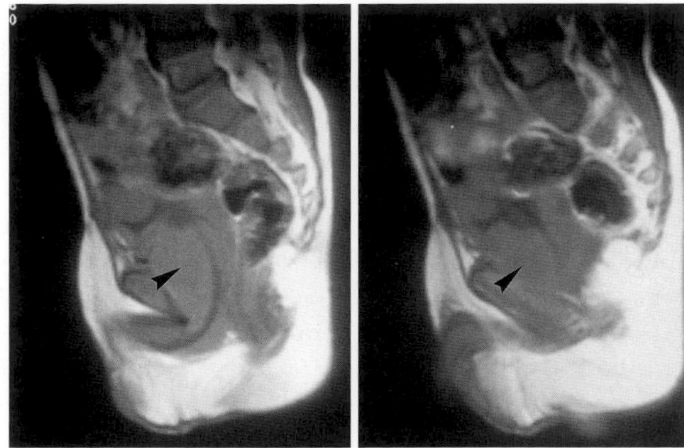

Figure 66.32 Prostatic rhabdomyosarcoma. MRI sagittal T1-weighted images through the pelvis in a 10 year old boy showing a large mass of intermediate signal intensity centred on the prostate (arrowheads). A catheter is seen to traverse the urethra with the balloon in a collapsed bladder. The appearances are those of the bladder/prostate rhabdomyosarcoma.

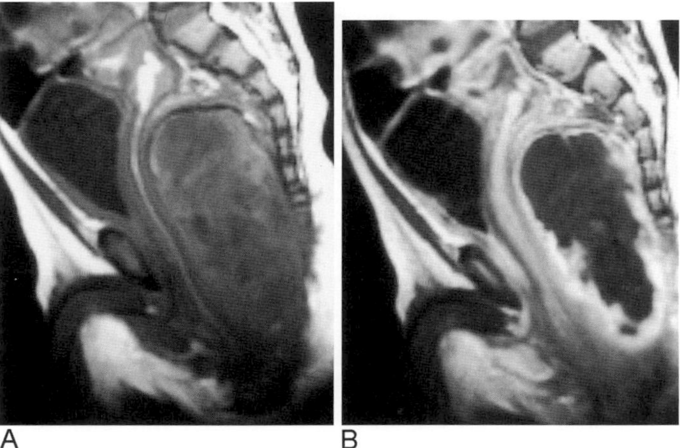

Figure 66.33 Rhabdomyosarcoma. (A) Sagittal nonenhanced T1-weighted images. (B) Sagittal T1-weighted images after gadolinium enhancement showing a large cystic mass lesion due to an embryonal rhabdomyosarcoma in the presacral region extending to the perineum. The mass demonstrates vivid peripheral enhancement after contrast medium administration, but no obvious central enhancement was seen. Note that the bladder and bowel are displaced anteriorly. No intraspinal extension was evident.

SCROTAL MASSES

Intratesticular benign and malignant tumours are relatively common neoplasms in children. Primary testicular neoplasms include germ cell tumours (most common and often with calcifications), endodermal sinus tumour and embryonal carcinoma. Paratesticular rhabdomyosarcoma accounts for 12% of scrotal tumours in boys. The testes are also secondary sites of disease in children with leukaemia, lymphoma and neuroblastoma, although much less frequently than in adults.

Paratesticular rhabdomyosarcoma includes tumours arising in the spermatic cord, testis, epididymis and penis. US is recommended to evaluate scrotal disease. A heterogeneous appearance within the testis with increased flow on Doppler may mimic infection, but clinical presentation is usually with a suspected or palpable mass rather than with signs suggesting infection. The regional lymph nodes, including the para-aortic nodes, require evaluation by both US and CT/MRI. CT studies with oral contrast medium administration are mandatory as retroperitoneal lymph node dissection may depend on the results. Paratesticular rhabdomyosarcoma has a good outlook in children younger than 10 years with a greater than 90% 5-year survival.

OVARIAN MASSES

Ovarian cysts

Simple ovarian cysts represent the majority of ovarian masses. In the neonate they usually present as abdominal masses because of the small size of the bony pelvis. When very large, they must be differentiated from other lesions such as mesenteric cysts, intestinal duplication and urachal cysts. Spontaneous resolution of some cysts has been reported. The treatment of choice is observation or aspiration if the cyst is very large. In pubertal girls, ovarian cysts result from continuous growth of a follicle after failed ovulation or when it does not involute after ovulation. Most follicular cysts are not loculated, contain clear fluid, and measure between 3 and 10 cm. Corpus luteum cysts contain serous or haemorrhagic fluid, and as with follicular cysts, usually involute spontaneously. Most ovarian cysts are asymptomatic, but when complications such as torsion, haemorrhage or rupture occur, patients present with acute abdominal pain, nausea, vomiting and leukocytosis. Torsion of the ovaries and Fallopian tubes results from partial or complete rotation of the ovary on its vascular pedicle. US is helpful in the evaluation of these patients, showing ovarian enlargement and fluid in the cul-de-sac. The presence of a fluid–debris level or septa may be an indication of bleeding or infarction. A more specific sign of torsion is the presence of multiple follicles in the cortical portion of a unilaterally enlarged ovary and a lack of Doppler signal. Physiological or pathological cysts may be found coincidentally in patients with lower abdominal or pelvic pain. Repeating the US study at a different phase of the menstrual cycle is useful.

Ovarian tumours

Ovarian neoplasms account for 10% of all childhood tumours, and 10–30% of these are malignant (the most common is malignant germ cell tumours). Tumours include dysgerminoma, immature teratoma, embryonal carcinoma, endodermal sinus tumour and choriocarcinoma. The differentiation between ovarian torsion and a tumour may be difficult. Tumour markers are helpful. Tumours are more common after puberty but can occur at any age, presenting with abdominal pain or as a palpable mass. Mature teratomas and dermoid cysts account for two-thirds of paediatric ovarian tumours and have a wide spectrum of imaging characteristics (Fig. 66.34). The most characteristic appearance on US is that of a mass of low reflectivity with an echogenic mural nodule. Calcifications and fat–fluid levels also assist in the diagnosis. Cystadenomas represent 20% of ovarian tumours in children and are of epithelial origin; they are large tumours, with loculations. Imaging cannot differentiate between malignant and benign cystadenomas. Leukaemia, lymphoma and neuroblastoma are among the primary tumours that metastasize to the ovaries in children.

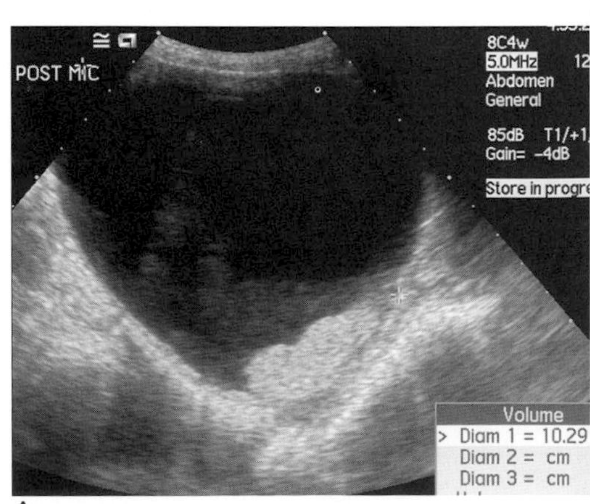

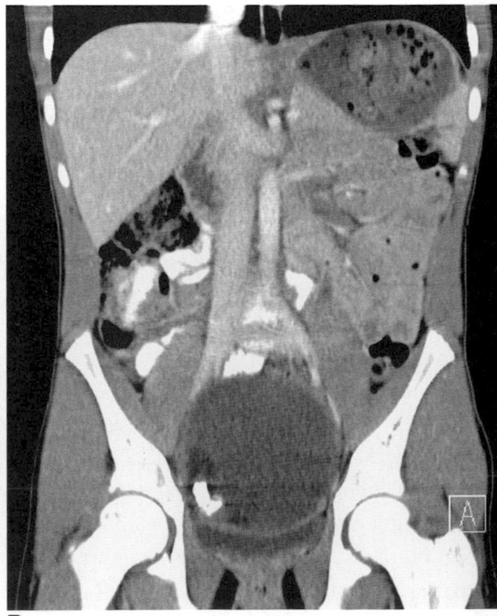

Figure 66.34 Ovarian teratomas. (A) Pelvic US in an 8 year old girl showing a mainly anechoic cystic mass, over 10 cm in diameter, with a more solid component posteriorly. (B) Coronal CT reformatted image in a 10 year old girl showing a cystic mass lesion superior to the bladder with (possibly tooth-like) calcification seen peripherally on the right side of the mass.

PRESACRAL MASSES

Sacrococcygeal teratoma is the most common presacral tumour and is a congenital lesion containing derivatives of the three germinal layers. These lesions occur more frequently in girls, are mostly nonfamilial, and are classified into four types, according to location. Type I is predominantly external and Type IV entirely presacral with no external component. The lesion may be evident at birth or present later (Type IV). Sacrococcygeal teratomas are attached to the sacrum, with the internal component best depicted on MRI (Fig. 66.35). This finding in addition to solid components allows differentiation from anterior sacral meningocoele.

Benign teratomas are usually cystic, with calcification and fat. Malignant teratomas are predominantly solid and may invade adjacent structures. All sacrococcygeal teratomas have the potential for later malignant transformation and hence require surgical removal. They can metastasize to the chest. The tumour marker for sacrococcygeal teratoma is α-fetoprotein. Other presacral lesions include anterior myelomeningocoele and neuroenteric cyst, and forms of spinal dysraphism associated with a sacral defect which are well imaged by MRI of the spine. Neuroblastoma and lymphoma are masses less commonly seen in the presacral region.

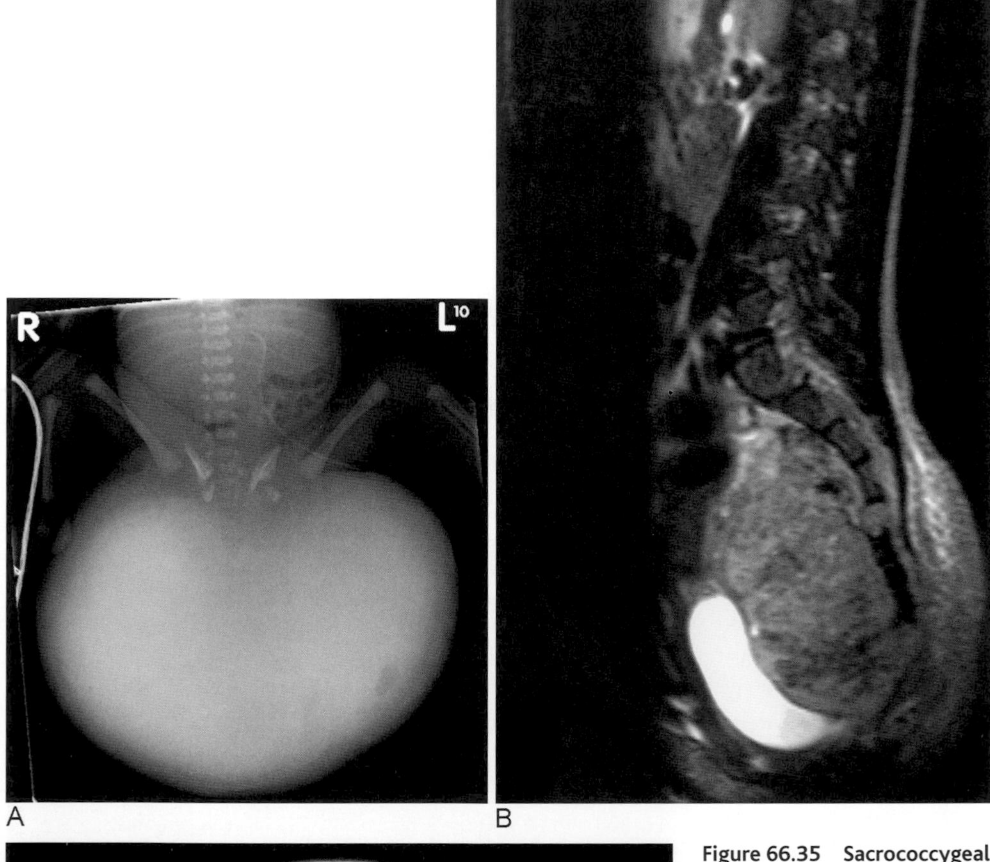

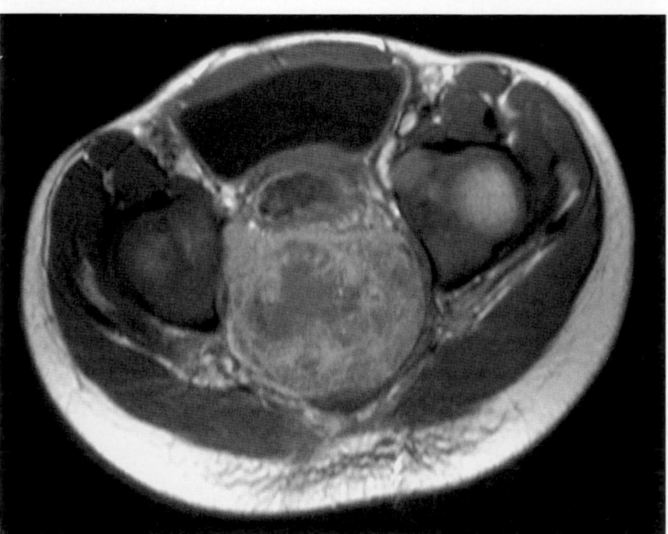

Figure 66.35 Sacrococcygeal teratomas. (A) Plain abdominal radiograph showing a very large external component to a sacrococcygeal teratoma in a newborn. (B) Sagittal T2-weighted image in another infant showing a large intrapelvic component to the sacrococcygeal teratoma. Note the teratoma, posterior to the uniformly hyperintense bladder, is of intermediate heterogeneous signal, and is invading the sacrum. (C) Axial T1-weighted image in the same patient showing the heterogeneous mass in a presacral location.

NEPHROCALCINOSIS (RENAL CALCULUS)

US is more sensitive in the early stages of calcium deposition in the kidneys than plain abdominal radiography. Increased medullary echogenicity of the kidneys in children, while nonspecific on US, may be an unexpected finding and indicative of underlying metabolic disease. It always requires a clinical explanation. Iatrogenic nephrocalcinosis (diuretics, vitamin D) is the most common cause in children for an increased echogenicity of the medullary pyramids. If this diagnosis can be excluded a large differential diagnosis remains (Table 66.7).

Renal calculi may present with pain, haematuria, or UTI, or they can be asymptomatic. US, a plain abdominal radiograph (for ureteric stones) and a ^{99m}Tc-DMSA scintigram to assess the effect in renal function are essential.

INFLAMMATORY DISEASES OF THE SCROTUM

The more common causes of acute pain and/or swelling in the scrotum include torsion of the testicular appendages, testicular torsion, epididymitis with or without orchitis, trauma, acute hydrocoele, incarcerated hernia and acute scrotal oedema. US is the optimal initial imaging investigation. Doppler examination of the testis in young children however is limited, because even modern high-resolution linear array transducers may not be able to detect slow flow in small testes. Testicular torsion shows alteration in echogenicity compared with the contralateral organ and is a surgical emergency. There is absence of flow on the Doppler studies. There may be some surrounding fluid. Epididymitis presents ultrasonically as a swollen hyperechoic epididymis with normal or increased testicular colour flow. If there is doubt about the US findings, then surgical exploration is required. Acute scrotal oedema presents clinically with abrupt onset of a swollen, painful, red scrotal sac. US confirms the thickening of the scrotal wall but shows normal underlying organs.

Table 66.7 CAUSES OF INCREASED MEDULLARY ECHOGENICITY IN CHILDREN
Nephrocalcinosis • Noniatrogenic, e.g. idiopathic hypercalcaemia in Williams' syndrome, absorptive hypercalciuria • Iatrogenic, e.g. treatment for hypophosphataemic rickets or frusemide for bronchopulmonary dysplasia or cardiac failure in a premature infant
Tubulopathies, e.g. renal tubular acidosis
Protein deposits giving transient increased medullary echogenicity in newborns
Vascular congestion, e.g. sickle cell anaemia
Infection, e.g. candidiasis and cytomegalovirus
Metabolic disease, e.g. urate deposits as in Lesch–Nyhan syndrome. Also seen in tyrosinaemia and glycogen storage disease
Oxalosis
Cystic medullary renal disease, e.g. autosomal recessive polycystic kidney disease

REFERENCES

1. Dinkel E, Ertel M, Dittrich M et al 1985 Kidney size in childhood. Sonographical growth charts for kidney length and volume. Pediatr Radiol 15: 38
2. Rottenberg G T, de Bruyn R, Gordon I 1996 Sonographic standards for single functioning kidney in children. Am J Roentgenol 167: 1255–1259
3. Bridges N A, Cooke A, Healy M J R et al 1993 Standards for ovarian volume in childhood and puberty. Fertil Steril 60: 456–460
4. Cohen H L, Ticc H M, Mandel F S 1990 Ovarian volumes measures by ultrasound: Bigger than we think. Radiology 177: 189
5. Fernbach S K, Maizels M, Conway J J 1993 Ultrasound grading of hydronephrosis: introduction to the system used by the Society for Fetal Urology. Pediatr Radiol 23: 478–480
6. Dudley J A, Haworth J M, McGraw M E, Frank J D, Tizard E J 1997 Clinical relevance and implications of antenatal hydronephrosis. Arch Dis Child Fetal Neonatal Edn 76: F31–F34
7. Yeung C K, Godley M L, Dhillon H K, Duffy P G, Ransley P G 1998 Urodynamic patterns of infants with normal lower urinary tracts or primary vesico-ureteric reflux. Br J Urol 81: 461–467
8. Moorthy I, Easty M, McHugh K, Ridout D, Biassoni L, Gordon I 2005 The presence of vesicoureteric reflux does not identify a population at risk for renal scarring following a first urinary tract infection. Arch Dis Child 90: 733–736
9. Gordon I, Barkovic M, Pinderia S, Cole T J, Woolf A S 2003 Primary vesicoureteric reflux as a predictor of renal damage in children hospitalized with urinary tract infection: a systematic review and meta-analysis. J Am Soc Nephrol 14: 739–744
10. Verrier Jones K 2005 Time to review the value of imaging after urinary tract infection in infants. Arch Dis Child 90: 663–664
11. Lonergan G J, Pennington D J, Morrison J C et al 1998 Childhood pyelonephritis: comparison of gadolinium-enhanced MR imaging and renal cortical scintigraphy for diagnosis. Radiology 207: 377–384
12. Centre for Reviews and Dissemination, University of York 2004 Diagnosing urinary tract infection (UTI) in the under fives. Effective Health Care, vol 8. London, RSM Press
13. National Institute for Clinical Evidence 2007 Urinary tract infection: diagnosis, treatment and long term management of urinary tract infection in children. Department of Health, London
14. Deal J E, Snell M F, Barratt T M et al 1992 Renovascular disease in childhood. J Pediatr 121: 378–384
15. McHugh K, Stringer D A, Hebert D et al 1991 Simple renal cysts in children: diagnosis and follow-up with ultrasound. Radiology 178: 383–385
16. Baxter G M 2001 Ultrasound of renal transplantation. Clin Radiol 56: 802–818
17. Beckwith J B, Kiviat N B, Bonadio J F 1990 Nephrogenic rests, nephroblastomatosis, and the pathogenesis of Wilms' tumor. Pediatr Pathol 10: 1–36
18. Strouse P J Pediatric renal neoplasms. Radiol Clin North Am 34: 1081–1100

SUGGESTIONS FOR FURTHER READING

Carty H, Brunelle F, Stringer D A, Kao S C S (eds) 2005 Imaging children, 2nd edn. Churchill Livingstone, Edinburgh

Kuhn J P, Slovis T, Haller J (eds) 2004 Caffey's pediatric X-ray diagnosis, 10th edn. Mosby, Philadelphia.

Gearhart J P, Garrett R A, Rink R, Mouriquant P 2001 Pediatric urology. WB Saunders, Philadelphia

CHAPTER 67

Skeletal Radiology in Children: Non-traumatic and Non-malignant

Amaka C. Offiah and Christine M. Hall

- Constitutional disorders of bone
- Localized disorders of the skeleton
- Neurocutaneous syndromes
- Non-inflammatory disorders
- Metabolic and endocrine disorders
- Toxic disorders
- Haemoglobinopathies
- Infection of the bones and joints

CONSITUTIONAL DISORDERS OF BONE

Nomenclature

The constitutional disorders of bone include osteochondrodysplasias and dysostoses.

Osteochondrodysplasias consist of dysplasias (abnormalities of bone and/or cartilage growth) and osteodystrophies (abnormalities of bone and/or cartilage texture). Abnormalities in the osteochondrodysplasias are intrinsic to bone and cartilage[1], and because of gene expression will continue to evolve throughout the lifespan of the individual.

Dysostoses occur as a result of altered blastogenesis in the first 6 weeks of intrauterine life. In contrast to the osteochondrodysplasias, the phenotype is fixed, and previously normal bones will remain so. However, more than one bone may be involved.

Inevitably there is some overlap between these groups and, from the radiological point of view, when establishing a diagnosis it is useful to consider them together. Most are genetically determined but some malformation syndromes are the result of environmental effects.

The most recent International Classification of Osteochondrodysplasias, published in 2002[1], expanded on the previous classification. The osteochondrodysplasias have been classified into 33 groups (Groups 1–33), and the dysostoses into three (Groups A–C).

Currently more than 2000 malformation syndromes are recognized and many of these will have skeletal abnormalities. In this chapter, only an approach to diagnosis can be given and only the more common conditions will be used as illustrative examples.

Prevalence

Although these conditions individually are rare, collectively they form a large group, which is expensive in both medical resources and human care and commitment. An accurate assessment of the prevalence of patients with malformation syndromes and skeletal dysplasias is difficult to achieve. As a rough estimate, approximately 1% of live births have clinically apparent skeletal abnormalities. This figure does not take into account the large numbers of spontaneous abortions or elective terminations, many of which have significant skeletal abnormalities. Nor does it detect those dysplasias presenting only in childhood, or those relatively common conditions that may never present for diagnosis because they are mild, e.g. hypochondroplasia and dyschondrosteosis, both of which merge with normality in individual cases. At orthopaedic skeletal dysplasia clinics in England and Scotland, approximately 10 000 patients are seen; 6000 of whom will require repeated hospitalization for surgical procedures and some will require more prolonged stays in institutions.

Diagnosis

Arriving at an accurate diagnosis of these conditions requires a multidisciplinary approach, i.e. combined clinical, paediatric, genetic, biochemical, radiological and pathological (molecular, cellular and histopathological) input.

Rapid advances are being made in the field of gene mapping with many conditions being localized to abnormalities at specific loci on individual chromosomes. Also, 'families' of conditions are being recognized with many common clinical and radiological features. One example of this is seen in collagen synthesis. For example, about 90% of cases of osteogenesis imperfecta are due to mutations in genes responsible for Type I collagen. Classification from genetic mutations has proved of value in determining an underlying causative defect. However, this diagnostic approach does not necessarily arrive at a precise clinical diagnosis, with prediction of natural history, morbidity, and mortality and in individual cases this form of classification is conflicting and indeterminate.

The most recent classification of skeletal dysplasias recognizes the radiological features as being paramount in accurate diagnosis. Whilst clinical features, such as cleft palate, deafness and myopia, are of diagnostic importance, the onus is still on the radiologist to evaluate the wealth of findings on the radiographic skeletal survey by careful observation and accurate interpretation, and thereby arrive at an accurate diagnosis. An approach to the radiological interpretation of skeletal surveys performed in the clinical context of a suspected dysplasia is available[2].

Because of the large number of relatively rare conditions, it is difficult or impossible for an individual radiologist to be familiar with every feature of each disorder. In addition, the radiological features of individual conditions will change with time, from infancy to childhood to adulthood, so that each of these conditions may have many age-dependent features.

Examples of this temporal change can be seen in spondylo-epiphyseal dysplasia congenita (SEDC). Radiological features in the neonate include absent ossification of the pubic rami and short femoral necks (see Fig. 67.6A). However, at the age of 12 years, the pubic rami are present and there is severe coxa vara (see Fig. 67.6C). Another example is seen in Morquio disease (mucopolysaccharidosis, MPS Type IV) in which the capital femoral epiphyses are well ossified at the age of 2 years, but at 8 years are small and flattened, and by 10 years have typically disappeared.

Each radiologist's personal experience of the individual conditions will be limited because of the vast numbers of conditions involved. Textbooks are also of limited value because of the necessarily restricted number of illustrations and obsolescence. For these reasons, skeletal dysplasias and malformation syndromes as a group lend themselves to computer-based applications and in particular to computer-assisted diagnosis. These tools should be used to help improve our diagnostic abilities.

Computer assistance may take the form of menu-driven databases of clinical and radiological features. A number of findings in a particular case can be matched and a group of conditions selected from the database for further consideration before arriving at a diagnosis, e.g. the Radiological Electronic Atlas for Malformation Syndromes (REAMS)[3]. This approach is really an automated method for cross-referencing gamuts. An alternative method is by means of a knowledge-based expert system in which experts in the field lead the user (the general radiologist) with a series of questions through a differentiation strategy to arrive at a diagnosis. Either system can be linked to a computerized image database capable of illustrating many thousands of images.

A specific diagnostic label should only be attached to a patient when it is secure. An inaccurate diagnosis may have a profound effect upon the family in terms of genetic counselling, and upon the patient in terms of management and outcome. There may be a need to monitor and re-evaluate the evolution of radiological findings over time before establishing a diagnosis. A significant proportion of cases (approximately 30%) are unclassifiable because the combination of findings does not conform to any recognized condition. It is important that data, both clinical (Table 67.1) and radiological and specimens, such as bone, tissue and blood, are stored and that the information can be widely disseminated. Only in this way will it be possible to 'match' conditions and to establish the natural history of a disorder.

Prenatal diagnosis

In the USA prenatal ultrasound (US) is less formal than in Europe; however, its use has been steadily increasing over the past two decades. By comparison, most pregnant women in the UK undergo prenatal US screening at between 14 and 18 weeks' gestation. All neonatally lethal skeletal dysplasias may be diagnosed at this stage by demonstrating short limbs, bowed limbs, or a narrow thorax. Where there has been a previously affected sibling, specific malformations such as polydactyly, polycystic kidneys, or micrognathia may be assessed. Skeletal US findings are highly significant but are not very specific, and in general it is unwise to offer a precise diagnosis on the basis of US findings alone. Pregnancy terminations offered on the grounds of such US findings should also have subsequent radiological evaluation to determine the precise diagnosis, and before genetic counselling is offered.

Many nonlethal conditions which may present at birth can also be ascertained on prenatal US. Fetal anomaly US examinations are offered to parents of previous babies who have had congenital dysplasias or malformation syndromes, and to at-risk parents with high maternal or paternal ages, or with specific environmental exposures.

Occasionally, other imaging techniques may help to confirm a suspected diagnosis prenatally. Maternal abdominal radiographs are not recommended. Too often the fetus is in such a position that diagnostic radiographic details are obscured and misdiagnosis is possible. Nor is the radiation risk to the fetus and mother justified, especially if the fetus is normal or is a potential survivor with a good quality of life.

Magnetic resonance imaging (MRI) is being used occasionally for in utero evaluation of specific anomalies when a sibling has suffered from a particular syndrome.

Chorionic villus sampling can be used for biochemical evaluation of fetuses at risk from storage disorders in those parents with a previously affected infant. Fetal chromosomal

Table 67.1 CLINICAL DATA USED IN THE DIAGNOSIS OF SKELETAL DYSPLASIAS AND MALFORMATION SYNDROMES

Stature—proportionate, disproportionate
Abnormal body proportion—short trunk, short limbs
Abnormal limb segments—rhizomelic, mesomelic, acromelic
Local anomalies and deformities—cleft palate, polydactyly
Facies—dysmorphology
Other—hearing, sight, mental retardation
Temporal changes
Pedigree

analysis from skin biopsy can be assessed when a sibling or carrier parent is affected.

Imaging

Making the diagnosis

In addition to prenatal US, a skeletal survey should be performed on any pregnancy termination resulting from a US diagnosis of short-limbed dwarfism or significant malformation. Also, a skeletal survey should be performed on any stillbirth. Although this may involve antero-posterior (AP) and lateral 'babygrams' of the entire infant, ideally additional views of the extremities should be performed. Spontaneous abortions should also have a radiographic skeletal survey. However, this can rarely be achieved.

After birth, a standard full skeletal survey is indicated when attempting to establish a diagnosis for short stature or for a dysmorphic syndrome. This should include:

- AP and lateral skull to include the atlas and axis
- AP chest
- AP pelvis
- AP lumbar spine
- lateral thoracolumbar spine
- AP one lower limb
- AP one upper limb
- postero-anterior (PA) one hand (usually the left; allows bone age assessment).

Occasionally, additional views will be required, particularly with specific clinical abnormalities, and these may include views of the feet, e.g. if polydactyly is present, or views of the cervical spine if cervical instability is suspected with specific diagnoses, or both upper and lower limbs if asymmetry or deformity is a clinical feature.

If a diagnosis cannot be established, then (limited) follow-up skeletal surveys are indicated, e.g. at 1 and 3 years, to evaluate progression and evolution of radiographic appearances.

Occasionally a technetium radionuclide skeletal scintigram showing the photon-deficient area of avascular necrosis (AVN) may be of value in differentiating bilateral Perthes disease from the small fragmented capital femoral epiphyses of multiple epiphyseal dysplasias. In this regard, contrast-enhanced MRI is also useful.

Conditions with decreased bone density may be assessed and monitored by means of bone densitometry.

Assessing complications

When a confident diagnosis is established, further imaging is essential to monitor the progress of potential complications. Complications may result as part of the natural evolution of the condition, but also may occur secondary to medical intervention.

Radiography and MRI of the cervical spine in flexion and extension will monitor instability; AP and lateral views of the spine will monitor kyphosis and scoliosis. In some conditions, progressive hip subluxation, genu varum or genu valgum may be problematic. Long limb radiographic views are sometimes used to assess asymmetry, genu varum, and genu valgum, and to monitor progression. Computed tomography (CT) is also of value in the measurement of limb asymmetry.

CT or MRI may monitor the development of hydrocephalus or the presence of neuronal migration defects and structural defects, such as the absence of the corpus callosum. CT may also demonstrate encroachment on the cranial nerve foramina and both CT and MRI are of value in assessing spinal cord compression.

US can demonstrate associated organ anomalies, e.g. cystic disease of the kidneys or hepatosplenomegaly and echocardiography may reveal associated intracardiac abnormalities.

Arthrography, US, CT and MRI are of value in the assessment of joint problems, particularly when surgical intervention is proposed.

Technetium skeletal scintigrams are occasionally used to determine the extent of bony involvement in specific disorders, e.g. the number of exostoses can be demonstrated in diaphyseal aclasis. However, it has been shown that in other patchy disorders, such as fibrous dysplasia, radiographically affected areas may not demonstrate abnormal uptake of radionuclide.

Postoperative imaging

US has a place in assessing the development of new bone formation following osteotomies and limb-lengthening procedures and plain radiography and CT in confirming the correct alignment in this situation. All imaging investigations are brought into play in the assessment of a patient following bone marrow transplantation.

Management

Only when an accurate diagnosis has been established can the prognosis and natural history of the disorder be given. For example, myopia can be corrected and retinal detachment prevented in Stickler syndrome (hereditary arthro-ophthalmopathy); cord compression can be prevented in conditions with instability in the cervical spine (Table 67.2) or with progressive thoracolumbar kyphosis and spinal stenosis, as seen in achondroplasia.

In some conditions, cure may be achieved, e.g. in the severe form of osteopetrosis (which is lethal in childhood and results in cranial nerve compressions leading to blindness in the first year of life), by means of a compatible bone marrow transplant. This not only improves life expectancy and arrests cranial nerve compression, but the radiographic changes revert to normal and the predisposition to fractures resolves. In this condition, the diagnosis needs to be established within the first 6 months of life if most complications are to be prevented.

Bone marrow transplantation has also been used with some success in treating selected patients with the mucopolysaccharidoses. The skeletal abnormalities persist but quality of life and life expectancy are improved. This treatment has resulted in iatrogenic manipulation of the natural history of the mucopolysaccharidoses and, with increased life expectancy, later complications, often the result of spinal cord compression, are now being recognized.

In many conditions, orthopaedic procedures are invaluable in maintaining or improving mobility. For example, osteotomies prevent or correct dislocations or long bone bowing deformities. Patients with osteogenesis imperfecta may require multiple osteotomies to correct severe deformities, as well as intramedullary

Table 67.2 DISORDERS WITH INSTABILITY IN THE CERVICAL SPINE

Cervical spine instability with odontoid peg absence or hypoplasia
Morquio disease (MPS Type IV)
Other mucopolysaccharidoses (MPS)
Mucolipidoses (MLS)
Achondroplasia
Down's syndrome
Metatropic dysplasia
Kniest dysplasia
Diastrophic dysplasia
Dyggve–Melchior–Clausen disease
Metaphyseal chondrodysplasia, Type McKusick
Spondyloepiphyseal dysplasia congenital (SEDC)
Multiple epiphyseal dysplasia
Pseudochondroplasia
Chondrodysplasia punctata
Cervical spine instability with cervical kyphosis (C2C3)
Diastrophic dysplasia
SEDC
Lethal
Atelosteogenesis
Campomelic dysplasia

rodding to reduce fractures, maintain alignment and provide support and stability. These patients suffer from basilar invagination resulting in compression of the brain stem. Surgical intervention may prevent severe neurological impairment (see Fig. 67.19D). Spinal deformities, kyphosis and scoliosis are common in the constitutional disorders of bone. Prevention and treatment consists of spinal bracing and timely arthrodeses or laminectomies for cord compression. Joint replacements may be necessary, especially in those dysplasias, such as multiple epiphyseal dysplasia, in which major involvement of the epiphyses may result in premature osteoarthritis. In some conditions, limb-lengthening procedures may be appropriate to improve mobility. This is usually offered in disorders with asymmetric shortening (Table 67.3; Fig. 67.1), but is sometimes offered to selected patients with achondroplasia (Fig. 67.2) or other short-limbed dysplasias for cosmetic reasons. Achondroplasia has proved particularly amenable to limb-lengthening procedures because redundant soft tissues are a feature of this dysplasia and insufficient soft tissue has proved to be a limiting factor in lengthening procedures in other conditions. An increase of approximately 30% in the length of the long bones may be achieved in achondroplasia, compared with 15% in other disorders.

Only with an accurate diagnosis in those conditions presenting at birth can those that are likely to be lethal be predicted. The diagnosis of a lethal dysplasia can prevent unnecessary and distressing prolongation of life, help to reduce parental expectations and anguish and help save on economic resources.

Termination of pregnancy may be offered with prenatally diagnosed lethal conditions, or where there is intrauterine evidence of short limbs. When a sibling has suffered from a

Table 67.3 ASYMMETRIC SHORTENING (OR OVERGROWTH)

Ollier's disease (multiple enchondromatosis)
Maffucci syndrome
Polyostotic fibrous dysplasia
McCune–Albright syndrome
Melorheostosis
Neurofibromatosis
Diaphyseal aclasis (multiple exostoses)
Chondrodysplasia punctata
Beckwith–Wiedemann syndrome
Klippel–Trenaunay syndrome
Silver–Russell syndrome
Dysplasia epiphysealis hemimelica
Sturge–Weber syndrome
Proteus syndrome
Hypomelanosis of Ito
Epidermoid nevus syndrome

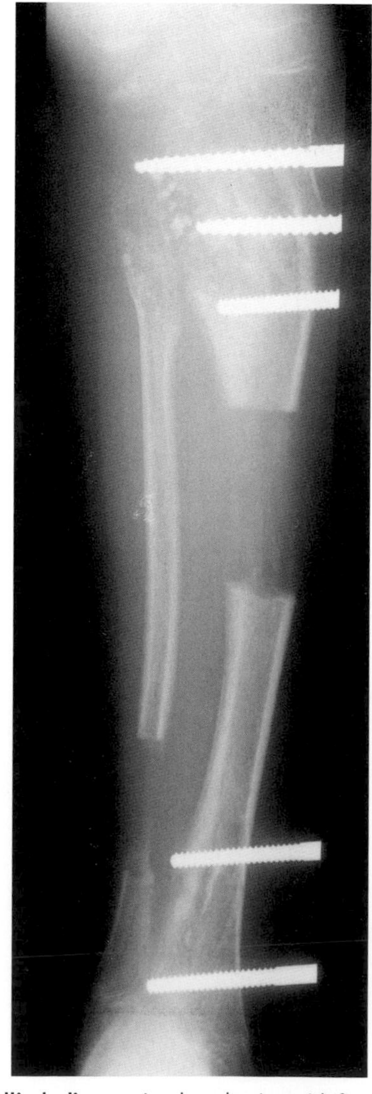

Figure 67.1 Ollier's disease. Leg lengthening with fixator in position.

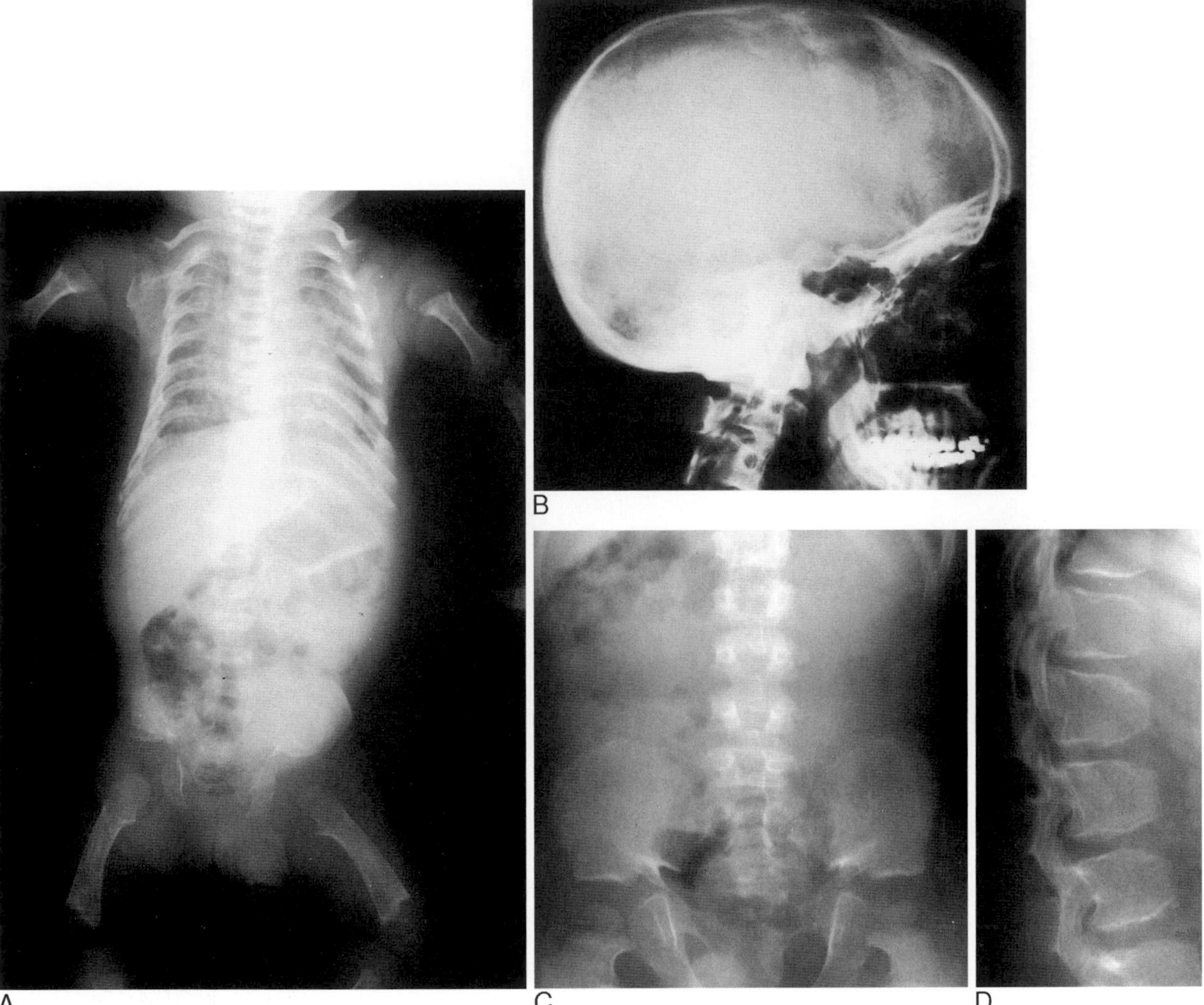

Figure 67.2 **Achondroplasia** in a neonate. (A) Sloping metaphyses, oval transradiant proximal femora, small square iliac wings with horizontal acetabular roofs, and a narrow thorax with short ribs. (B) Short skull base with prominent frontal bone and narrow cervical canal. (C) Small square iliac wings, horizontal acetabular roofs, short sacrosciatic notches, progressive caudal narrowing of the lumbar interpedicular distances and low set sacrum. (D) Mild kyphosis, posterior scalloping of the vertebral bodies and short pedicles with spinal stenosis.

disabling condition associated with particular malformations, these may be specifically looked for prenatally in subsequent pregnancies. This practice is leading to a change in the incidence of certain conditions formerly presenting at birth.

With the identification and localization of specific chromosomal abnormalities associated with particular disorders, the development of gene therapy for clinical use poses many challenges and offers great potential for the future.

Growth hormone therapy is used in selected disorders to influence final height. Growth hormone stimulates Type I collagen production and is being used, in particular, to augment growth rate in children with osteogenesis imperfecta.

Bisphosphonates are pyrophosphate analogues that inhibit osteoclast function. They have been used in osteogenesis imperfecta to improve bone density, and have also been used to treat bone pain and osteopaenia in a variety of rheumatological and dermatological conditions.

Genetic counselling

When an accurate diagnosis has been made, meaningful genetic counselling can be given, both to the parents and to the affected individual. Most conditions are inherited in an autosomal dominant or autosomal recessive manner. In conditions with an autosomal dominant inheritance, the affected individual has a one in two chance of passing the same abnormality on to his/her offspring. However, many of these conditions arise as a spontaneous mutation, which means that the parents of the affected individual, who are themselves normal, have an extremely low risk of having another affected child. In autosomal recessive conditions, both the parents are carriers of the disorder, but are not affected themselves, and they have a one in four chance of having another affected child.

Other important, although uncommon, modes of inheritance are the result of somatic or gonadal mosaicism. Mosaicism is the presence of at least two cell lines in a single individual or tissue that derive from a single zygote. Somatic mosaicism for autosomal dominant conditions results in asymmetric or patchy disorders (see Table 67.3). It is thought that when not a mosaic, these disorders are lethal. Clinical evidence of somatic mosaicism includes asymmetry, localized overgrowth, pigmentation and haemangiomas.

Osteochondrodysplasias

The clinical and radiographic features of selected osteochondrodysplasias are described in Table 67.4.

Table 67.4 CLINICAL AND RADIOGRAPHIC FEATURES OF SELECTED OSTEOCHONDRODYSPLASIAS

	Clinical features	Radiological features
Group 1 (achondroplasia group)		
Achondroplasia	Common Short limbs, short trunk Narrow thorax with respiratory distress in infancy Bowed legs Prominent forehead with depressed nasal bridge Hydrocephalus and brainstem and spinal cord compression Inheritance: autosomal dominant	'Bullet-shaped' vertebral bodies Decrease in interpedicular distance in lumbar spine caudally Short vertebral pedicles Posterior vertebral body scalloping Squared iliac wings with small sciatic notch Flat acetabular roofs Short ribs Short wide tubular bones Relative overgrowth of fibula Large skull vault, relatively short base Small foramen magnum Dilatation of lateral cerebral ventricles V-shaped notches in growth plates (chevron deformity)
Hypochondroplasia	Variable short stature Prominent forehead Inheritance: autosomal dominant	No normal widening in the interpedicular distance in the lumbar spine caudally Short relatively broad long bones Elongation of the distal fibula and ulnar styloid process Variable brachydactyly
Thanatophoric dysplasia	Most common lethal neonatal skeletal dysplasia Short markedly curved limbs Respiratory distress, small thoracic cage Inheritance: sporadic, autosomal dominant mutation	Short ribs with wide costochondral junctions Severe platyspondyly Horizontal acetabular roofs with medial spikes Small sacroiliac notches Marked shortness and bowing of the long bones, 'telephone receiver femora' Irregular metaphyses Short broad tubular bones in the hands and feet Small scapulae May be associated with 'clover leaf skull'
Group 3 (metatropic dysplasia group)		
Metatropic dysplasia (Fig. 67.3)	Short limbs Relatively narrow chest Small appendage in coccygeal region (tail) Progressive kyphoscoliosis Progressive change to a relatively short trunk Inheritance: variable, autosomal dominant or recessive	Short tubular bones with marked metaphyseal widening (dumb-bell) Platyspondyly Relatively large intervertebral discs Flat acetabular roofs Short iliac bones Short ribs with anterior widening Progressive kyphoscoliosis Hypoplastic odontoid process
Group 4 (short rib dysplasias, with or without polydactyly)		
Asphyxiating thoracic dysplasia (Jeune's; Fig. 67.4)	Often lethal Respiratory problems with long narrow thorax Short hands and feet Nephronophthisis in later life in survivors Inheritance: autosomal recessive	Small thorax with short ribs, horizontally orientated Widened costochondral junctions High clavicles Iliac bones short Horizontal acetabula with medial and lateral 'spurs' (trident) Premature appearance of the proximal femoral ossification centres Cone-shaped epiphyses in phalanges May have polydactyly
Ellis–van Creveld (chondroectodermal dysplasia; Fig. 67.5)	Short stature Short limbs, more marked distally Polydactyly	Short ribs in infancy Short iliac wings; horizontal acetabulum with medial and lateral spurs (trident)

Continued

Table 67.4 cont'd CLINICAL AND RADIOGRAPHIC FEATURES OF SELECTED OSTEOCHONDRODYSPLASIAS

	Clinical features	Radiological features
	Hypoplasia of the nails and teeth Ectodermal dysplasia with sparse hair Congenital cardiac defects, atrial septal defect, single atrium Fusion between upper lip and gum Inheritance: autosomal recessive	Premature ossification of the femoral capital epiphyses Pelvis becomes more normal in childhood Laterally sloping proximal tibial metaphysis Exostosis of the medial upper tibial shaft Carpal fusions Cone-shaped epiphyses, middle phalanges Polydactyly of hands and feet
Group 8 (Type II collagenopathies)		
Spondyloepiphyseal dysplasia congenita (SEDC) (Fig. 67.6)	Short stature with short trunk at birth Cleft palate Myopia Maxillary hypoplasia Thoracic kyphosis and lumbar lordosis Barrel-shaped chest Inheritance: autosomal dominant	Ovoid, pear-shaped irregular-sized vertebral bodies in infancy Irregular platyspondyly in later life Odontoid hypoplasia and cervical spine instability Short long bones Absent ossification of epiphyses of knees, talus, calcaneus at birth Pubic and ischial hypoplasia Hands relatively normal Severe coxa vara developing in early childhood Horizontal acetabulum
Spondyloepiphyseal dysplasia tarda (Fig. 67.7). Several types with different modes of inheritance are recognized	Usually presents in adolescence with short stature due to short trunk Joint limitation	Platyspondyly Characteristic mound of bone in central and posterior part of the vertebral end plates in the X-linked dominant type Narrow intervertebral discs Mild to moderate generalized epiphyseal dysplasia Early osteoarthritis
Group 11 (multiple epiphyseal dysplasias and pseudoachondroplasia)		
Pseudoachondroplasia (Fig. 67.8)	Short limbs with normal head and face Accentuated lumbar lordosis Genu valgum (knock knees) or genu varum (bow legs) Joint hypomobility Inheritance: autosomal dominant	Platyspondyly with tongue-like anterior protrusion of the vertebral bodies Biconvex configuration of upper and lower vertebral end plates Atlantoaxial dislocation Small femoral capital epiphyses Short iliac bones Wide Y-shaped cartilage Irregular acetabulum Small pubis and ischium Pointed proximal metacarpals Shortening of the tubular bones with expanded, markedly irregular metaphyses Small irregular epiphyses Wide costovertebral joints Relatively long distal fibula
Multiple epiphyseal dysplasia (Fig. 67.9)	Stiffness in joints with limp Early osteoarthritis Mild shortening of limbs Inheritance: autosomal dominant	Delayed ossification and irregularity of the epiphyses of the tubular bones Delayed ossification of carpus and tarsus Short tubular bones of the hands and feet Double-layered patella Only mild irregularity of the vertebral end plates Mild wedging of the vertebral bodies Mild acetabular hypoplasia Early joint degenerative changes
Group 12 (chondrodysplasia punctata/stippled epiphyses)		
Chondrodysplasia punctata (CDP) (Fig. 67.10)	Flat nasal bridge, high arched palate Cutaneous lesions such as ichthyosis Asymmetrical or symmetrical shortening of the limbs Joint contractures Cataracts Inheritance: autosomal dominant, autosomal recessive, X-linked	Stippled calcification in cartilage, particularly around the joints and in laryngeal and tracheal cartilages Shortening, symmetrical or asymmetrical, of the long bones Short digits in some types Vertebral bodies show coronal clefting Eventual disappearance of the stippled calcification in later life Punctate calcification may also be seen in Pacman dysplasia, Zellweger syndrome, fetal alcohol and warfarin embryopathies, and in some chromosomal abnormalities and mucolipidoses (Fig. 67.11)

Continued

Table 67.4 cont'd CLINICAL AND RADIOGRAPHIC FEATURES OF SELECTED OSTEOCHONDRODYSPLASIAS		
	Clinical features	**Radiological features**
Group 13 (metaphyseal dysplasias) (Figs 67.12–67.14)		
Metaphyseal chondrodysplasia (Schmid) (Fig. 67.13)	Short limbs, short stature, presenting in early childhood Genu varum (bow legs) Inheritance: autosomal dominant	Metaphyseal flaring Irregular widened growth plates, most marked at the hips Increased density and unevenness of metaphyses, particularly of upper femora and around knees Large femoral capital epiphyses Coxa vara Femoral bowing Anterior cupping of the ribs Spine normal
Group 19 (dysplasias with predominant membranous bone involvement)		
Cleidocranial dysplasia (Fig. 67.15)	Large head Large fontanelles with delay in closure Multiple supernumerary teeth Excessive mobility of the shoulders Narrow chest Inheritance: autosomal dominant	Frontal bossing Wide sutures of the skull Multiple wormian bones Persistently open anterior fontanelle Prominent jaw with multiple supernumerary teeth Variable hypoplasia or pseudoarthrosis of the clavicles Small scapulae Absent or delayed ossification of the pubic bones Hypoplastic iliac wings Short middle phalanges with cone-shaped epiphyses and tapering terminal phalanges Undermodelling of the shafts of the long bones Pseudarthrosis of long bones (rare)
Group 20 (bent bone dysplasias)		
Campomelic dysplasia	*Neonatal* Respiratory distress Cleft palate Prenatal bowing of lower limbs Pretibial dimpling *Survivors* Short stature Learning difficulties Recurrent respiratory infections Inheritance: autosomal dominant (sex reversal has been reported)	11 pairs of ribs Hypoplastic scapulae Angulation of femora at junction of proximal third and distal two-thirds Angulation of tibiae at junction of proximal two-thirds and distal third Short fibulae Progressive kyphoscoliosis Dislocated hips Deficient ossification of the ischium and pubis Hypoplastic patellae
Group 22 (dysostosis multiplex)		
Mucopolysaccharidoses (Figs 67.16, 67.17). This group of conditions is characterized by an abnormality of mucopolysaccharid and glycoprotein metabolism. Differentiation between the types is dependent upon laboratory analysis particularly of urine, leukocytes and fibroblastic cultures	Presenting typically in early childhood, the clinical manifestations are variable Short stature isassociated with a distinctive coarse facial appearance with mental retardation, corneal opacities, joint contractures, hepatosplenomegaly and cardiovascular problems Inheritance: autosomal recessive except Type II (Hunter) which is X-linked recessive	Macrocephaly Thick vault with 'ground-glass' opacity 'J'-shaped sella Wide ribs, short wide clavicles, poorly modelled scapulae Ovoid, hook-shaped vertebral bodies with thoracolumbar gibbus Odontoid hypoplasia Iliac wings flared with constricted bases to the iliac bones Small, irregular femoral capital epiphyses Coxa valga Lack of normal modelling of the long bones Thin cortices Coarse trabecular pattern Short wide phalanges with characteristic proximal pointing of the metacarpals Neurological changes include hydrocephalus, leptomeningeal cysts and a variety of abnormalities best demonstrated by MRI
Morquio's syndrome (MPS-IV)	Normal intelligence Joint laxity Knock knees Short stature	Absent odontoid peg with cervical instability leading to spinal cord compression Platyspondyly Anterior central 'beak' or 'tongue' of vertebral bodies Iliac wings flared with constricted bases of the iliac bones Progressive disappearance of femoral capital epiphyses Coxa valga Genu valgum Irregular ossification of metaphyses of long bone Small irregular epiphyses Proximal pointing of second to fifth metacarpals

Continued

Table 67.4 cont'd CLINICAL AND RADIOGRAPHIC FEATURES OF SELECTED OSTEOCHONDRODYSPLASIAS

	Clinical features	Radiological features
Group 24 (dysplasias with decreased bone density)		
Osteogenesis imperfecta—a group of conditions caused by an abnormality of Type 1 collagen. Several forms are recognized (Table 67.5; Fig. 67.18)	See Table 67.5. *Additional clinical findings* Hydrocephalus Large fontanelles not related to hydrocephalus Kyphoscoliosis Pseudarthrosis Ligamentous laxity Easy bruising Thin skin	See Table 67.5. *Additional radiological findings* Wormian bones Basilar invagination Tam O'Shanter skull Irregular calcific 'popcorn' lesions in metaphyses Hyperplastic callus Severe protrusio acetabuli Lumbar pedicles elongated 'Codfish' vertebral bodies Generalized osteoporosis
Group 26 (increased bone density without modification of bone shape)		
Osteopetrosis (Fig. 67.19). There are several types	Enlargement of the liver and spleen Bone fragility with fracture Cranial nerve palsies Blindness Osteomyelitis Anaemia Inheritance: more severe types are autosomal recessive, although a milder delayed form shows autosomal dominant inheritance	Generalized increase in skeletal density Abnormal modelling of the metaphyses, which are widened with alternating bands of radiolucency and sclerosis Bone within bone appearance Rickets and basal ganglia calcification in a recessive form with carbonic anhydrase deficiency
Pyknodysostosis (Fig. 67.20)	Short limbs Propensity to fracture Respiratory problems Irregular dentition Inheritance: autosomal recessive	Wormian bones Delayed closure of the fontanelles Generalized increase in density of the skeleton Straight mandible Prognathism Deficient ossification of distal phalanges Re-absorption of lateral end of clavicle Pathological fractures
Osteopoikilosis (Fig. 67.21)	Often asymptomatic May present with cutaneous/subcutaneous nodules	Sclerotic foci (islands), especially around the pelvis and metaphyses of long bones
Melorheostosis (Fig. 67.22)	Sclerodermatous lesions over the bony lesions Asymmetry of the affected limbs Vascular anomalies Abnormal pigmentation Muscle contractures and wasting Inheritance: nongenetic	Dense cortical longitudinal hyperostosis of the bones Appearances like wax running down the side of a candle Particularly involves the long bones, less commonly other bones
Group 27 (increased bone density with diaphyseal involvement)		
Diaphyseal dysplasia (Englemann disease)	Muscle weakness Pain in the extremities Gait abnormalities Exophthalmos Inheritance: autosomal dominant	Sclerotic skull base Progressive endosteal and periosteal diaphyseal sclerosis Narrowing of medullary cavity of tubular bones Bone images: increased activity
Group 30 (neonatal severe osteosclerotic dysplasias)		
Caffey disease (infantile cortical hyperostosis)	Usually appears in the first 5 months of life Hyperirritability Soft tissue swelling Inheritance: autosomal dominant suggested in some families (also a lethal recessive form)	Commonly affects mandible, clavicles, ulnas May be asymmetrical Periosteal new bone and cortical thickening When tubular bones are affected, abnormality is limited to the diaphyses
Group 31 (disorganized development of cartilaginous and fibrous components of the skeleton)		Proximal pointing of second to fifth metacarpals
Multiple cartilaginous exostoses (diaphyseal aclasis) (Fig. 67.23)	Multiple exostoses particularly at the ends of the long bones, ribs, scapulae and iliac bones Secondary deformity and joint limitation Ulnar deviation of the hands Inheritance: autosomal dominant	Multiple flat or protuberant exostoses Secondary joint deformities Exostoses of the iliac crest and scapula Vertebral involvement rare Cranial vault spared

Continued

Table 67.4 cont'd CLINICAL AND RADIOGRAPHIC FEATURES OF SELECTED OSTEOCHONDRODYSPLASIAS

	Clinical features	Radiological features
		Long bone exostoses point away from the adjacent joint Short ulna distally (reverse Madelung deformity) Sarcomatous change to be suspected if rapid increase in size, or pain
Enchondromatoses (± haemangiomas) (Fig. 67.24)	Asymmetrical limb shortening Expansion of affected bones Occasional pathological fracture Absence of haemangiomas (Ollier's disease) Presence of haemangiomas (Maffuci syndrome) Malignancy rare in Ollier's disease, 15% incidence in Maffuci syndrome Inheritance: nongenetic	Shortening of affected long bones Rounded and streaky radiolucencies, particularly in the metaphyses Expansion of the bone with cortical thinning Areas of calcification within the lesions Pathological fractures Joint deformity Typically markedly asymmetrical Short ulna distally (reverse Madelung deformity) Calcified haemangiomas (Maffuci syndrome, not usually seen until adolescence)
Fibrous dysplasia (Fig. 67.25). May involve one bone only (monostotic) or multiple bones (polyostotic). The association of polyostotic fibrous dysplasia, patchy café-au-lait skin pigmentation and sexual precocity, usually in girls, constitutes the McCune–Albright syndrome	Deformity and pain related to involved bones Pathological fracture Hypophosphataemic osteomalacia or rickets Usually presents in childhood Inheritance: nongenetic	Skull often shows asymmetrical thickening of the vault with sclerosis at the base: multiple rounded areas of radiolucency Obliteration of the paranasal air sinuses Marked facial deformity (leontiasis ossea) Disruption of dentition 'Ground-glass' or radiolucent area of trabecular alteration in the long bones associated with patchy sclerosis and expansion, with cortical thinning and endosteal scalloping Pathological fractures and deformities due to softening, e.g. 'shepherd's crook' femoral necks Localized or asymmetrical overgrowth Secondary spinal stenosis

Table 67.5 OSTEOGENESIS IMPERFECTA CLINICAL (BASED ON THE SILLENCE CLASSIFICATION) AND RADIOLOGICAL FINDINGS

	I	II	III	IV
Clinical findings				
Incidence	1:30000	1:30000	Rare	Unknown (rare)
Severity	Mild	Lethal	Severe	Mild/moderately severe
Death	Old age	Stillborn	By 30 years	Old age
Sclerae	Blue	Blue	Blue, then grey	White
Hearing impairment	Frequent	—	Rare	Rare
Teeth (dentinogenesis) imperfecta	IA Normal	—	Abnormal	IVA normal
	IB Abnormal	—		IVB abnormal
Stature	Normal	—	Short	Normal/mildly short
Inheritance	Autosomal dominant	Autosomal dominant	Autosomal dominant/ autosomal recessive	Autosomal dominant
Radiological findings				
Fractures at birth	<10%	Multiple	Frequent	Rare
Osseous fragility	Moderate/mild	Severe	Moderate/severe	Moderate/mild
Deformity	Mild	—	Severe	Variable

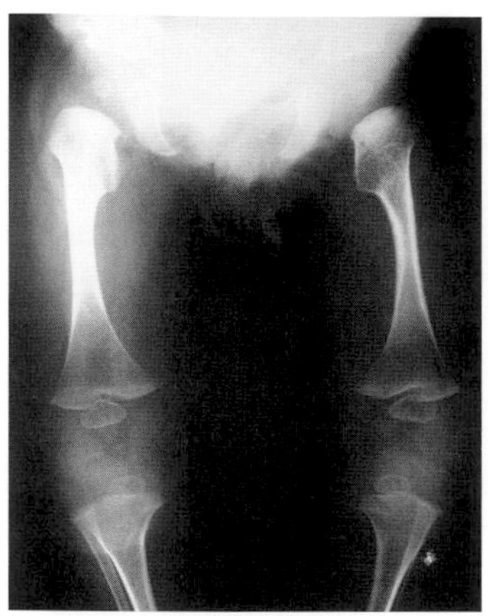

Figure 67.3 Metatropic dysplasia. 'Dumb-bell' appearance of the long bones due to wide metaphyses.

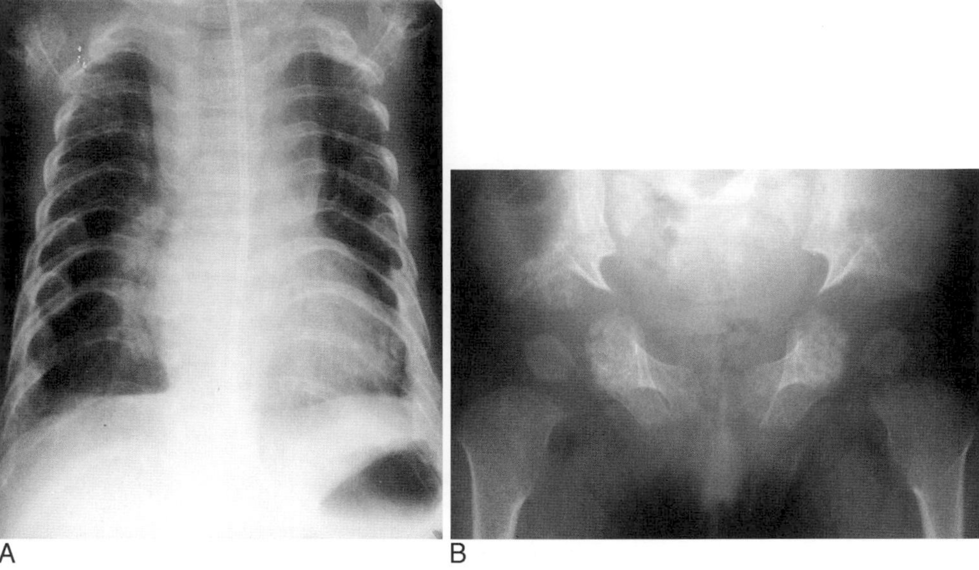

Figure 67.4 Asphyxiating thoracic dystrophy. (A) Narrow thorax and short ribs. (B) Horizontal acetabular roofs and pronounced medial spurs, less pronounced laterally ('trident' appearance).

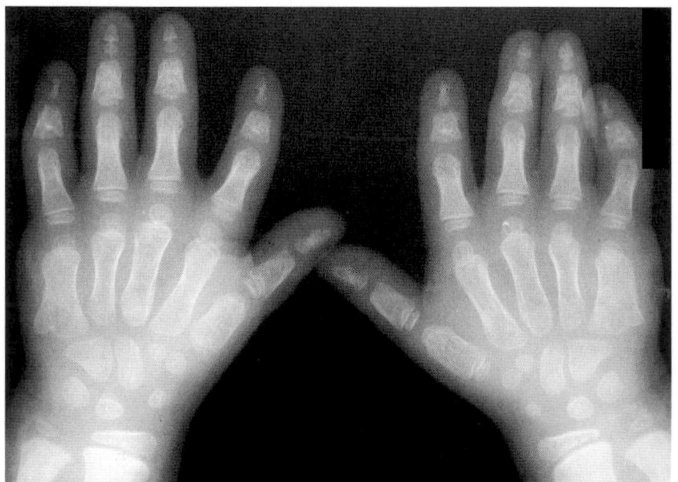

Figure 67.5 Ellis–van Creveld syndrome. Partial duplication of the fifth metacarpals (postaxial polydactyly), deformed hamate and short middle and terminal phalanges with cone-shaped epiphyses.

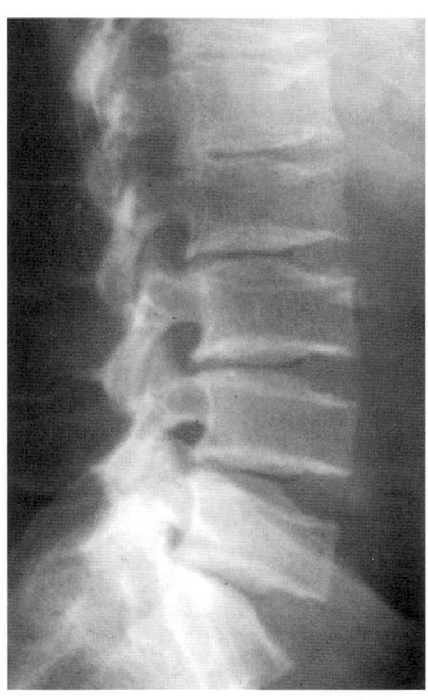

Figure 67.7 X-linked spondyloepiphyseal dysplasia tarda. Characteristic dense mounds of bone on the posterior two-thirds of the vertebral end plates are seen.

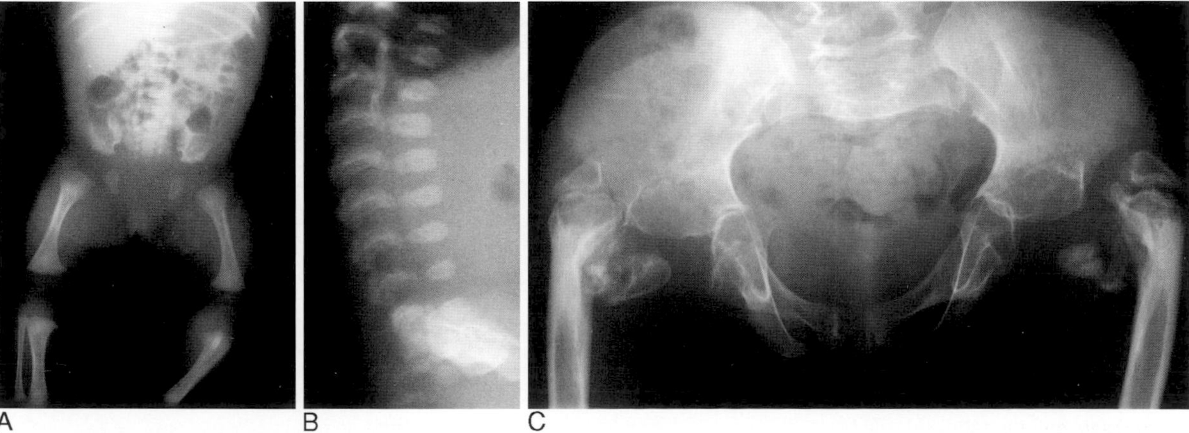

Figure 67.6 Spondyloepiphyseal dysplasia congenita in a neonate. (A) Absent ossification of the pubic rami, short femoral necks and absent ossification of the epiphyses at the knees. (B) 'Pear-shaped' vertebral bodies with posterior constriction. Note the marked variability in size between L1 and L5. (C) Severe coxa vara deformity.

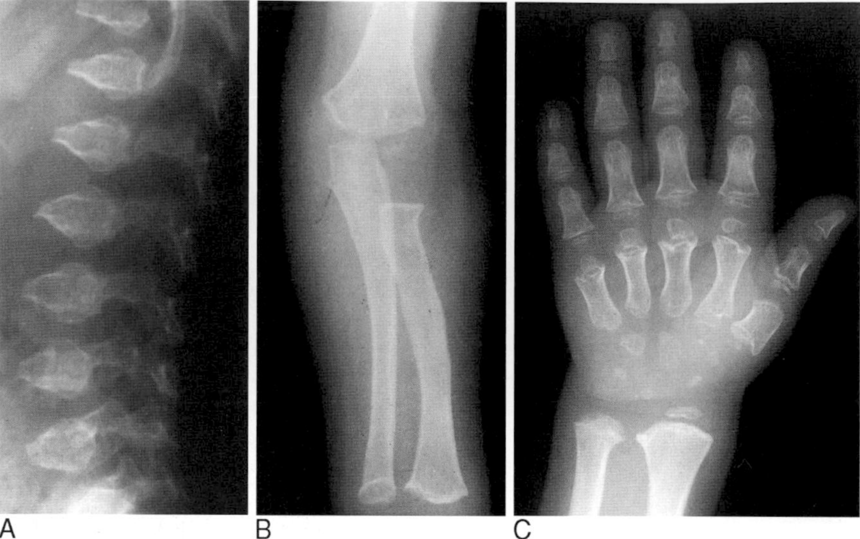

Figure 67.8 Pseudoachondroplasia. (A) Biconvex vertebral bodies with central anterior tongue and long pedicles. (B) The long bones show flared irregular metaphyses. (C) The phalanges and metacarpals are short with flared irregular metaphyses and small epiphyses. The carpal centres are small and irregular. There is proximal pointing of the second to fifth metacarpals.

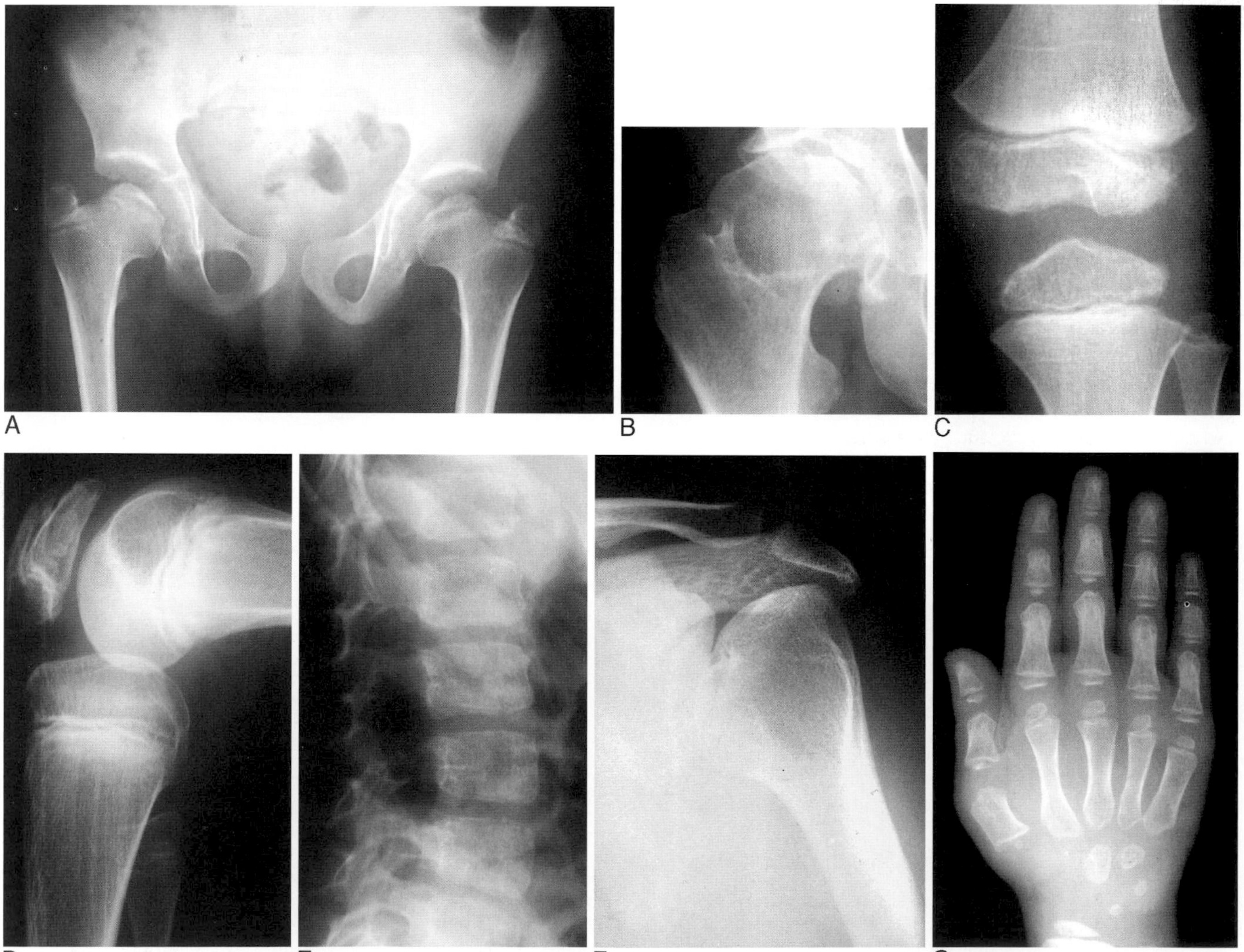

A B C

D E F G

Figure 67.9 Multiple epiphyseal dysplasia. (A) Small flattened capital femoral epiphyses with short femoral necks and coxa vara. (B) Right hip of a young adult showing premature osteoarthritis. (C) Small flattened irregularly ossified knee epiphyses. (D) Layered ossification of the patella. (E) Very mild vertebral end-plate irregularity. (F) The left shoulder shows a 'hatchet' deformity of the proximal humerus. (G) Delayed bone maturation with small carpal centres and flattened small and fragmented epiphyses.

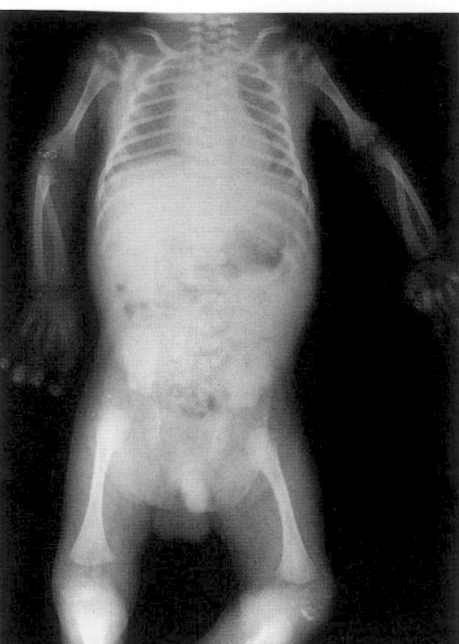

Figure 67.10 Chondrodysplasia punctata. Stippled or punctate calcification in the region of the epiphyses.

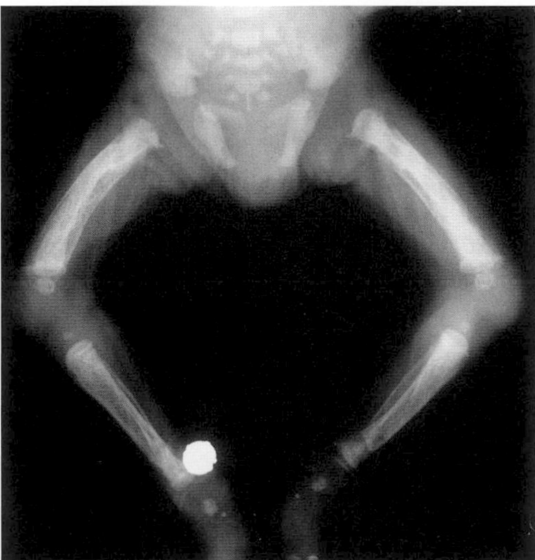

Figure 67.11 Mucolipidosis Type II. Periosteal cloaking of the long bones and some stippled ossification in the tarsus.

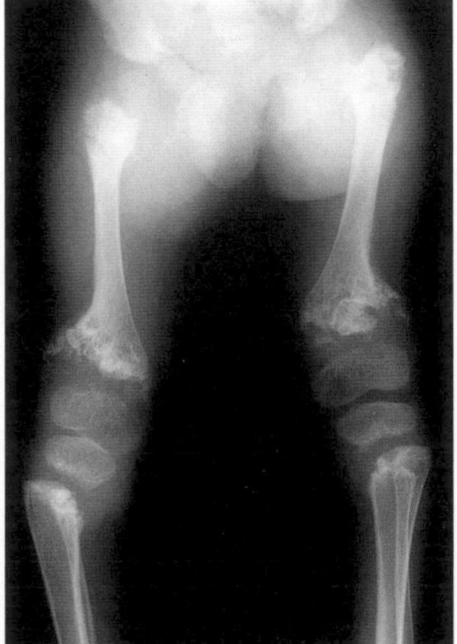

Figure 67.12 Metaphyseal chondrodysplasia, Type Jansen. Femora are short with marked expansion, irregular ossification and some sclerosis of the metaphyses. Epiphyses are large and rounded.

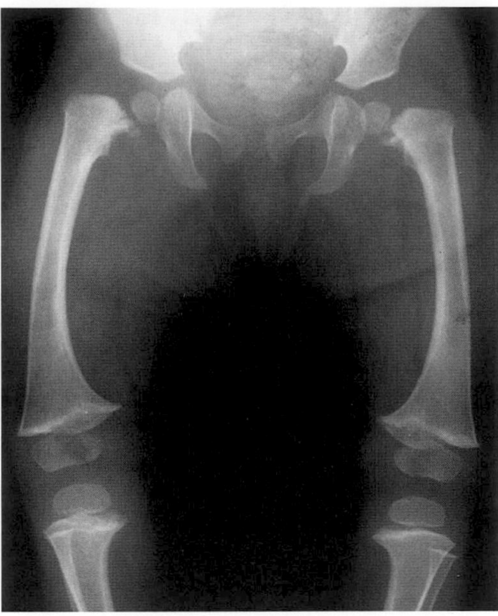

Figure 67.13 Metaphyseal chondrodysplasia, Type Schmid. There is bilateral coxa vara, the metaphyses are splayed and irregular and there is lateral bowing of the femora.

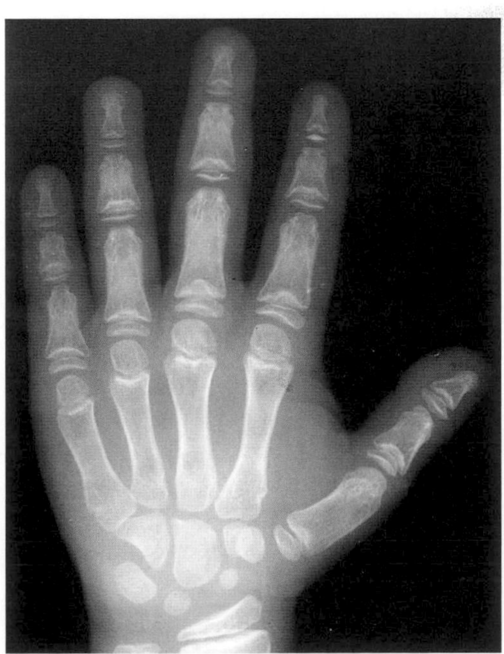

Figure 67.14 Metaphyseal chondrodysplasia, Type McKusick. The phalanges are short with multiple cone- and delta-shaped epiphyses.

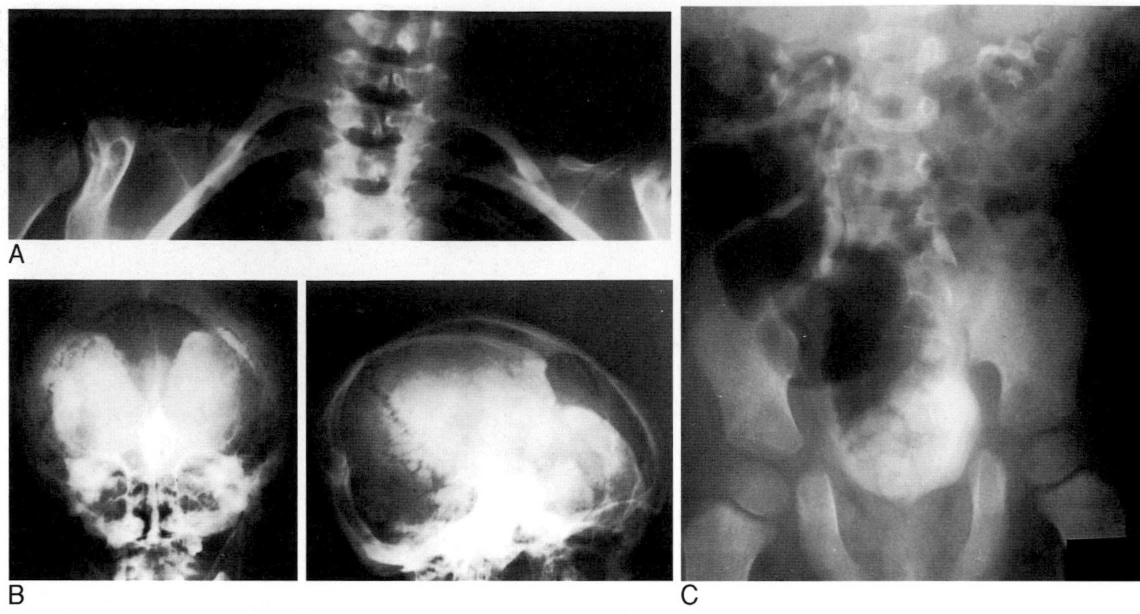

Figure 67.15 Cleidocranial dysplasia. (A) Absent ossification of the lateral portions of the clavicles, the glenoid fossae are hypoplastic, and there is dysraphism in the lower cervical spine. (B) Wide fontanelles and sagittal suture with multiple wormian bones in the lambdoid suture. (C) Mild scoliosis, narrow iliac wings, wide symphysis pubis and large rounded capital femoral epiphyses.

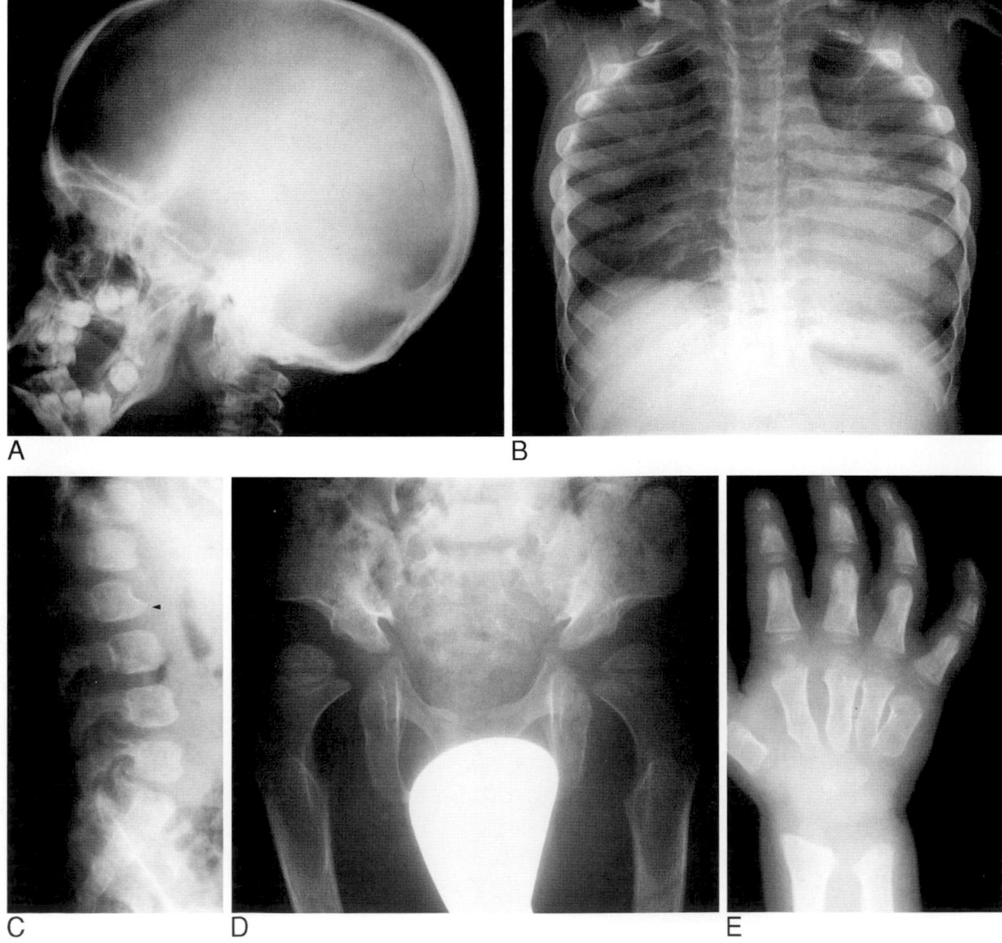

Figure 67.16 Mucopolysacch aridosis Type I–H. (A) Elongated (J-shaped) sella. The vault shows an overall ground-glass opacity and the odontoid peg is hypoplastic. (B) The ribs are broad, and the clavicles short and broad. Varus deformity of the upper humeri is seen. (C) Inferior hook (arrowhead) on the body of L2 with a mild kyphosis. (D) The iliac wings are flared laterally and the acetabular roofs are shallow. Bilateral hip subluxation with long femoral necks and coxa valga. (E) Flexion deformities of the fingers. The short bones are undermodelled, and there is proximal pointing of the second to fifth metacarpals and a V-shaped deformity of the metaphyses at the wrist.

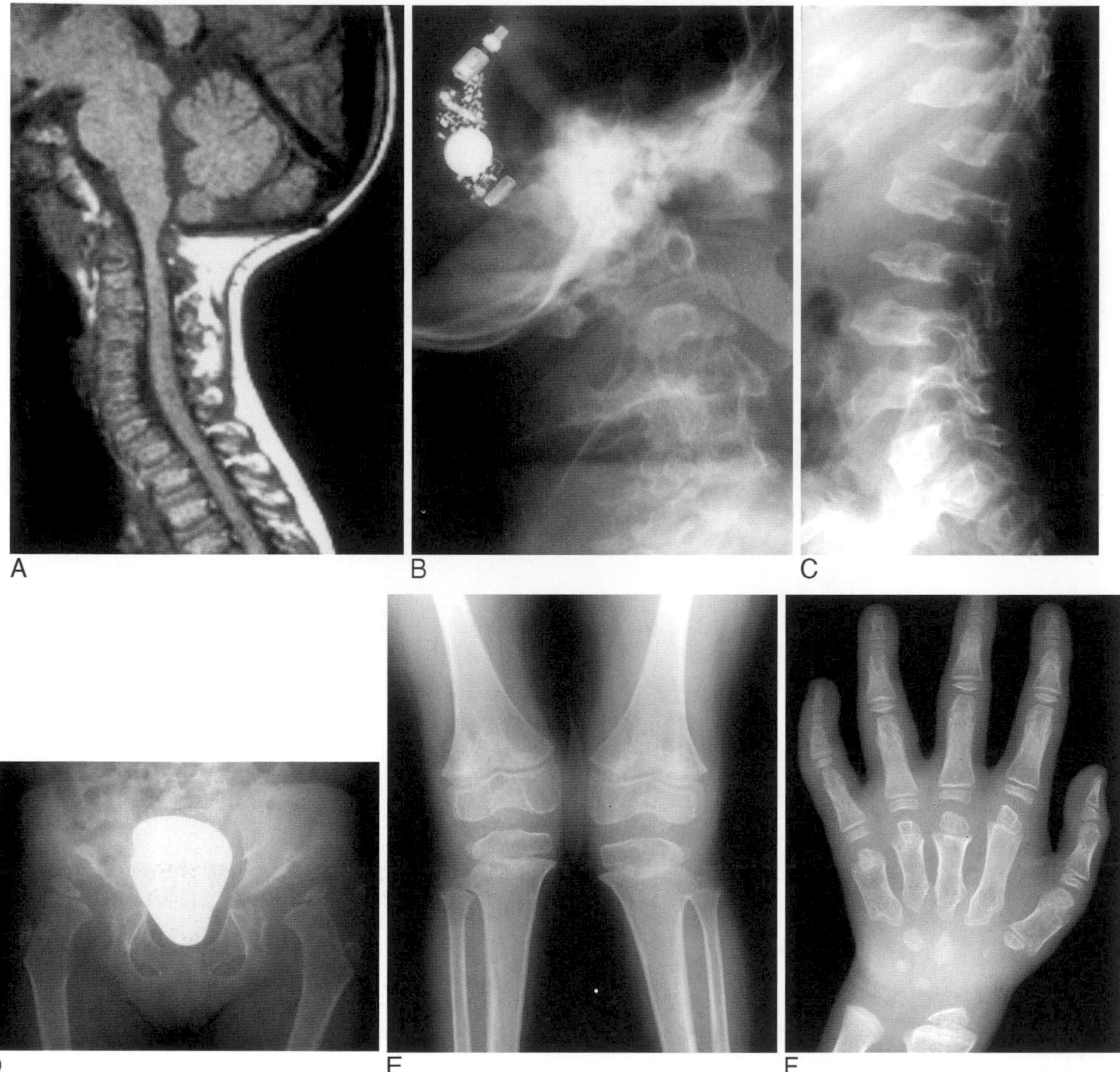

Figure 67.17 Mucopolysaccharidosis Type IV. (A) MRI showing upper cervical cord compression. (B–F) Radiographs showing (B) absent odontoid peg. A hearing aid is in position; (C) platyspondyly, posterior scalloping of the vertebral bodies and anterior 'beaks' or 'tongues', kyphosis and long pedicles; (D) flared iliac wings with sloping acetabular roofs, small and flattened capital femoral epiphyses, dislocated hips and coxa valga; (E) genu valgum, flared, irregularly ossified metaphyses and small irregular epiphyses; and (F) short metacarpals with proximal pointing of the second to fifth metacarpals, irregular epiphyses and small carpal centres.

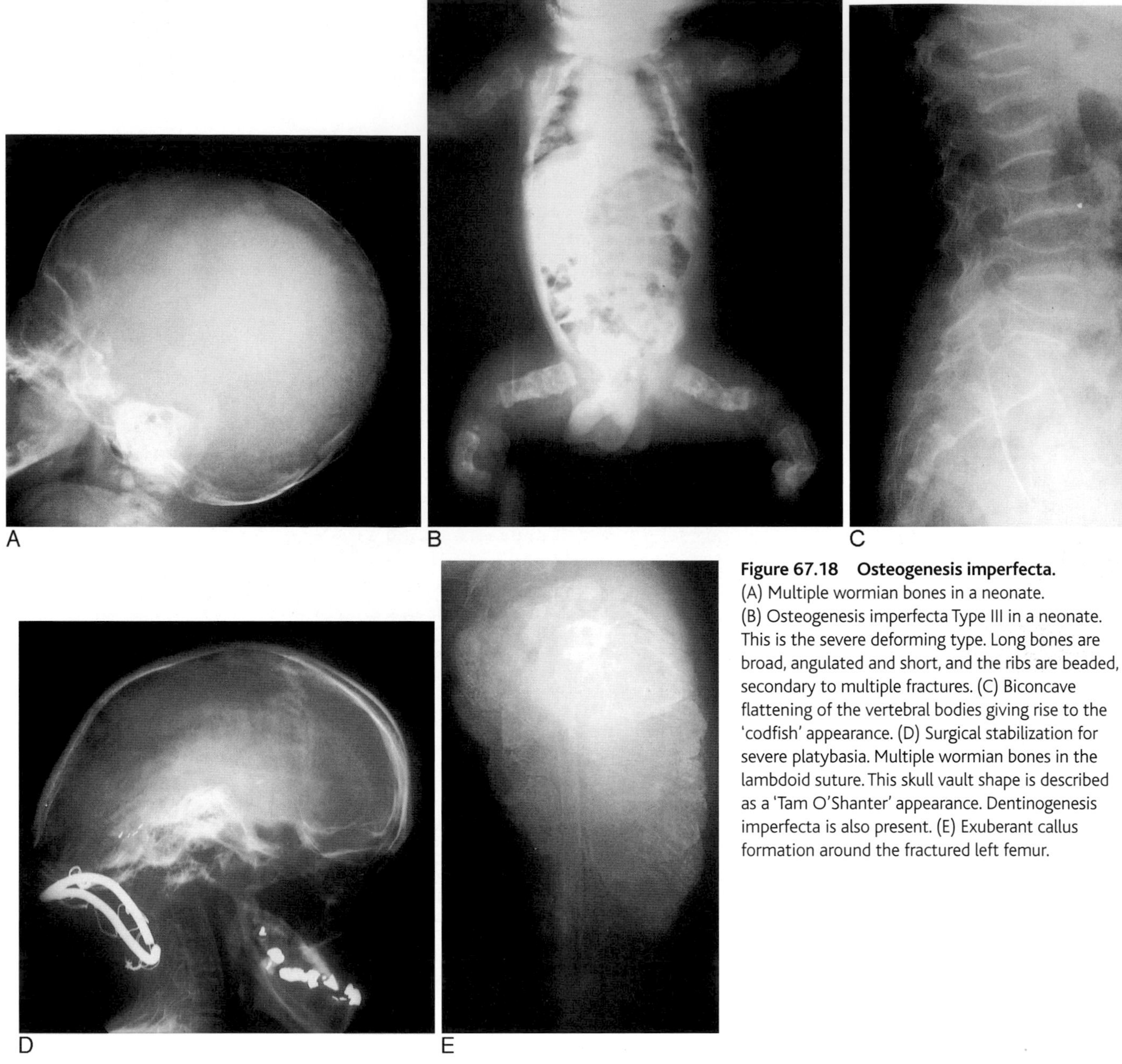

Figure 67.18 Osteogenesis imperfecta. (A) Multiple wormian bones in a neonate. (B) Osteogenesis imperfecta Type III in a neonate. This is the severe deforming type. Long bones are broad, angulated and short, and the ribs are beaded, secondary to multiple fractures. (C) Biconcave flattening of the vertebral bodies giving rise to the 'codfish' appearance. (D) Surgical stabilization for severe platybasia. Multiple wormian bones in the lambdoid suture. This skull vault shape is described as a 'Tam O'Shanter' appearance. Dentinogenesis imperfecta is also present. (E) Exuberant callus formation around the fractured left femur.

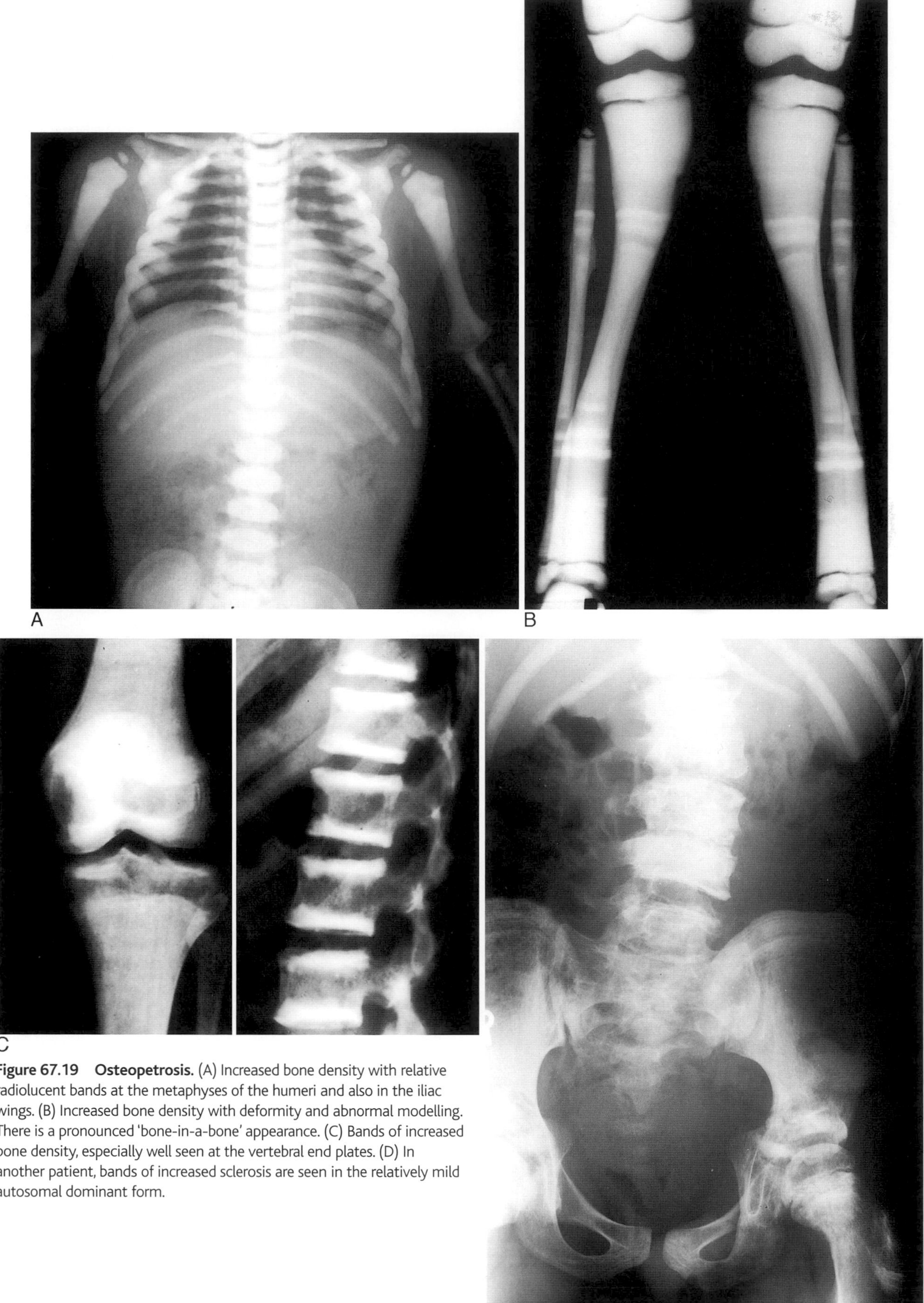

Figure 67.19 Osteopetrosis. (A) Increased bone density with relative radiolucent bands at the metaphyses of the humeri and also in the iliac wings. (B) Increased bone density with deformity and abnormal modelling. There is a pronounced 'bone-in-a-bone' appearance. (C) Bands of increased bone density, especially well seen at the vertebral end plates. (D) In another patient, bands of increased sclerosis are seen in the relatively mild autosomal dominant form.

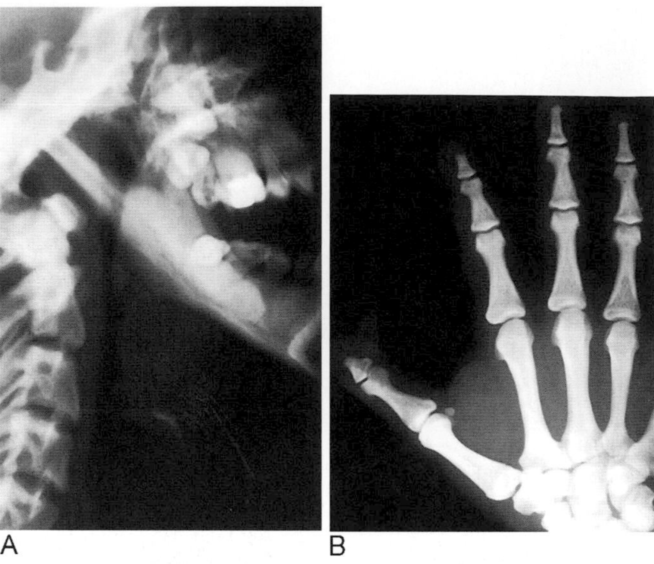

Figure 67.20 Pyknodysostosis. (A) The mandibular angle is obtuse (straight). (B) Generalized osteosclerosis. The terminal phalanges show varying degrees of hypoplasia and tapering.

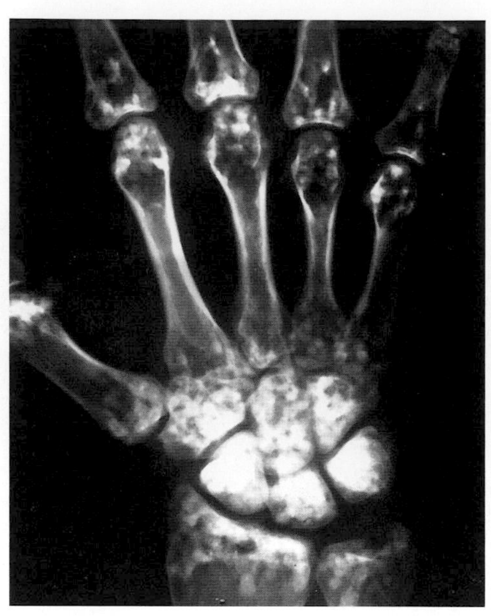

Figure 67.21 Osteopoikilosis. Multiple discrete islands of sclerosis, especially affecting the carpus, metaphyses, and epiphyses.

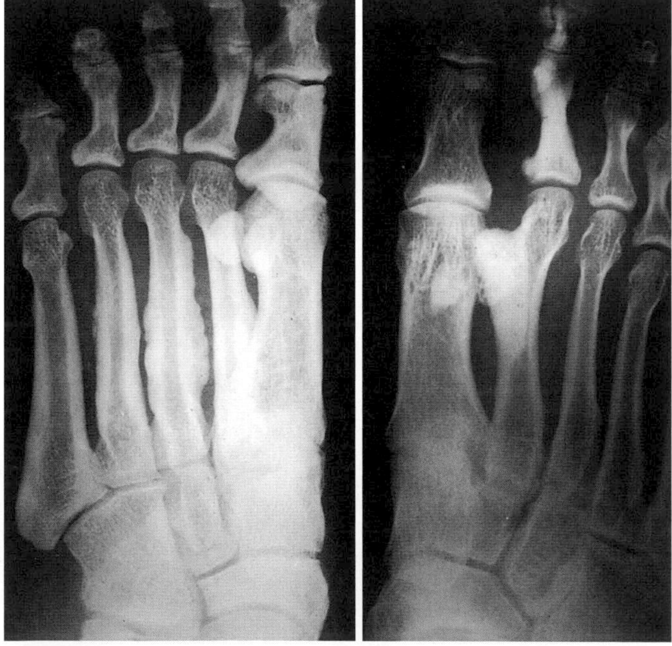

Figure 67.22 Melorheostosis (two patients). There is dense irregular cortical bone: this is sometimes described as the 'flowing candle wax' appearance. One patient demonstrates a 'ray' distribution (asymmetrical changes).

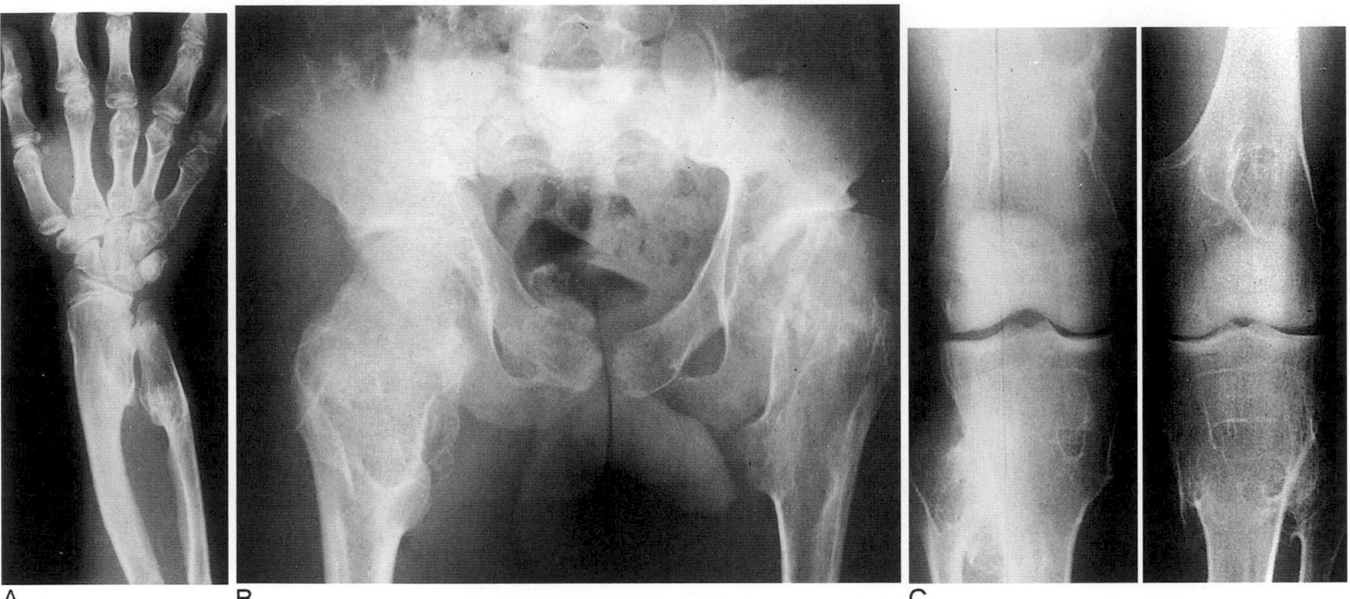

Figure 67.23 Diaphyseal aclasis. (A) Characteristic distal shortening of the ulna (reverse Madelung deformity), multiple exostoses and hypoplasia of the entire ulnar ray. (B) Multiple exostoses with deformity. (C) Multiple exostoses around the knees. They all point away from the epiphyseal plates.

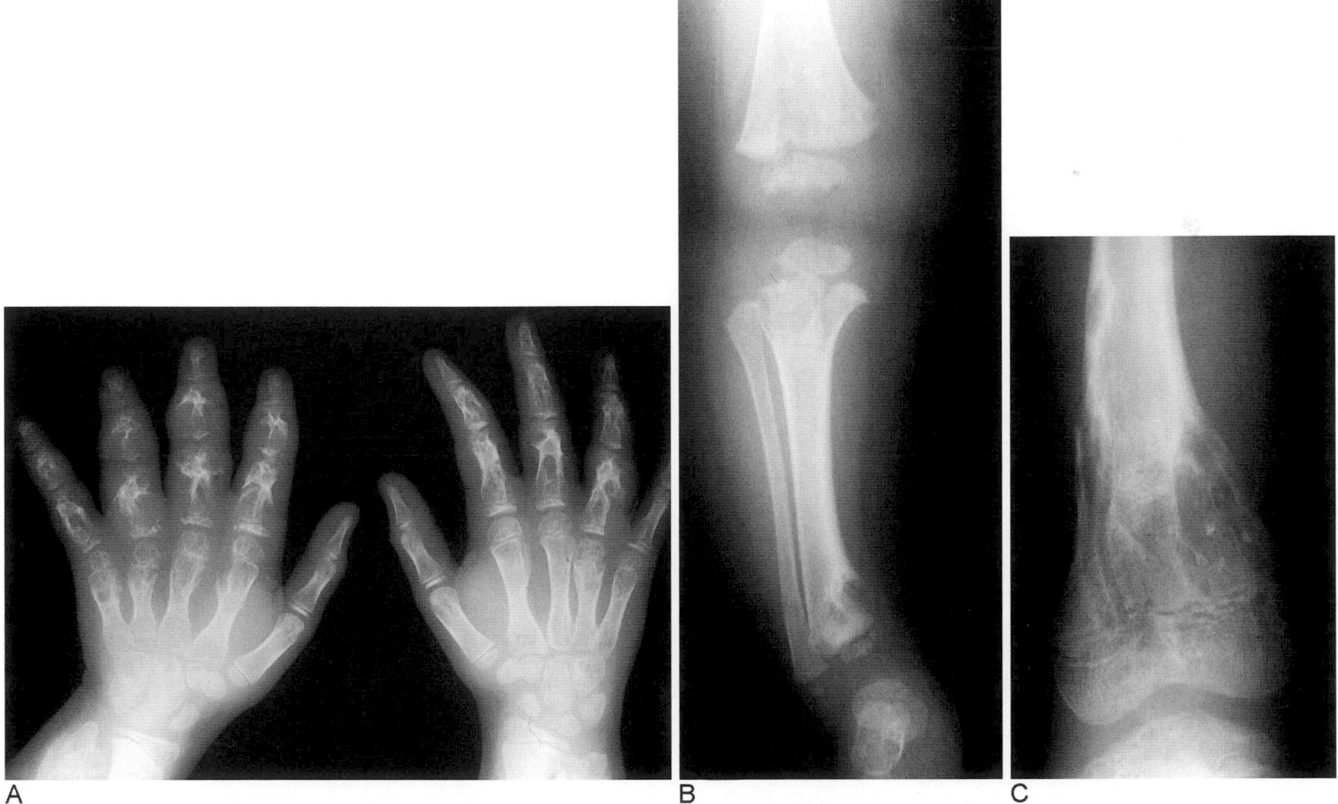

Figure 67.24 Ollier's disease. (A) Multiple enchondromas are causing clearly defined expanding lytic areas within most of the fingers. Ray distribution with sparing of the thumbs. Distal end of left ulna short (a reverse Madelung deformity). (B) The enchondromas affect predominantly the metaphyses and adjacent epiphyses with asymmetrical shortening. (C) Expanding lytic areas in distal left femur show stippled calcification indicating the chondromatous nature of the lesions.

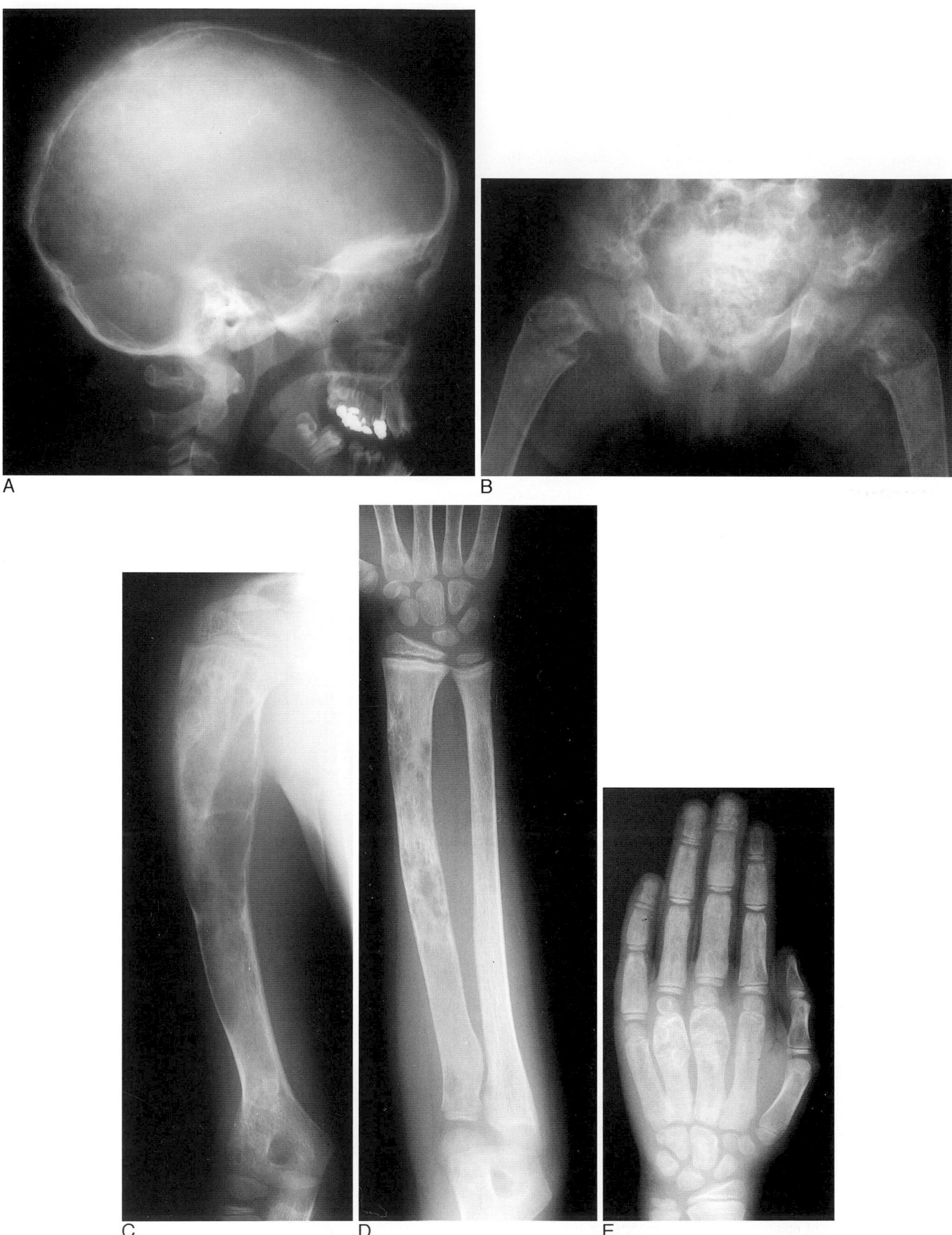

Figure 67.25 Fibrous dysplasia. (A) Patchy sclerosis affecting the vault and the base of the skull. (B) Radiolucent areas in the femoral necks and pelvic bones. Bilateral coxa vara. This is an early 'shepherd's crook' deformity. Widening of the upper femoral epiphyseal plates, due to associated hypophosphataemic rickets. (C) Multiple radiolucent areas causing expansion. The margins are sclerotic and extend over several millimetres (a 'rind' appearance). Scalloping of the cortex. (D) The radiolucent areas predominantly affect the radius in a ray distribution. (E) The metacarpals and phalanges of the second to fifth fingers show expansion and deformity. Multiple radiolucent clearly defined lesions with relative sparing of the thumb and carpus.

Group 8 (Type II collagenopathies)

Collagen forms the framework of connective tissues. At least 11 types of collagen have been identified and many of these have been mapped to specific chromosome locations. A family of disorders has been recognized in which the basic abnormality is found in Type II collagen. This gene has been localized to the long arm (q-arm) of chromosome 12 with a specific locus at 13.1–13.2. The Type II collagen fibril consists of a triple helix composed of three α-I chains. Each chain consists of long sequences of amino acids. Type II collagen forms a network with collagens Type IX and Type XI, which is crucial to the mechanical strength of articular cartilage. Type II α-I collagen, also known as cartilage collagen, is found in addition in the vitreous of the eye, in the inner ear and in the nucleus pulposus.

Conditions identified as having a Type II collagen defect are (in order of decreasing severity):

- achondrogenesis Type II
- hypochondrogenesis
- Torrence platyspondylic dysplasia
- spondyloepiphyseal dysplasia congenita (SEDC)
- spondyloepimetaphyseal dysplasia (SEMD) Type Strudwick
- Kniest dysplasia
- Stickler syndrome
- precocious osteochondrosis.

The family of dysplasias identified as having abnormalities of Type II collagen can present in a wide variety of ways, ranging from the lethal achondrogenesis Type II to the milder Stickler syndrome and premature osteoarthrosis. They have a range of epiphyseal abnormalities. The epiphyses may be small in SEDC or absent in achondrogenesis. The spine is abnormal, ranging from absent ossification of vertebral bodies in achondrogenesis Type II and hypochondrogenesis, to mild platyspondyly as seen in Stickler syndrome. In the surviving conditions, the stature may vary considerably, with severe shortening in SEDC and Kniest dysplasia and minimal shortening or even a Marfanoid appearance in Stickler syndrome.

In view of the distribution of Type II collagen within the body, the clinical findings in this family of disorders include myopia and sensorineural deafness; cleft palate is also a feature, sometimes associated with micrognathia and the Pierre–Robin sequence, and with the specific dysmorphic features of mid-face hypoplasia.

In a few patients with one of these dysplasias, the specific molecular abnormality of the Type II collagen may be identified. In achondrogenesis, at the severe end of the spectrum, the condition is often the result of a glycine substitution in the amino acid chain resulting in the formation of a mutant protein. However, in Stickler syndrome at the mild end of the spectrum, it is likely that there is a 'null' allele, a nonfunctioning mutant allele which results in a premature 'stop' code and a reduction in the amount of normal protein but not a mutant protein in the tissues.

Dysostoses

The clinical and radiographic features of Group A dysostoses are described in Table 67.6.

Chromosomal disorders

Trisomy 21 (Down's syndrome)

Craniofacial abnormalities include brachycephaly, microcephaly, hypertelorism and relatively small facial bones. The iliac wings are flared with relatively sloping acetabula. Frequently there are 11 pairs of ribs and the ribs themselves

Table 67.6 CLINICAL AND RADIOGRAPHIC FEATURES OF GROUP A DYSOSTOSES

	Clinical features	Radiographic features
Group A (localized disorders with predominant cranial and facial involvement)		
Apert's syndrome	Abnormalities present from birth Proptosis High arched/cleft palate Bifid uvula Brachyturricephaly 'Mitten'/'sock' deformities of hands/feet Inheritance: sporadic, autosomal dominant in some families	Premature fusion of coronal suture Bony and soft tissue syndactyly of the hands and feet Progressive carpal and tarsal fusions Progressive symphalangism Progressive fusion in the cervical spine (commonly C5/C6) Progressive fusion of large joints Hypoplasia of the glenoid fossae Dislocated radial heads
Mandibulofacial dysostosis (Treacher–Collins)	Symmetrical Ear deformities Deafness Downslanting eyes Lateral coloboma of the lower eyelid Hypoplastic malar bone Cleft palate Inheritance: autosomal dominant	Stenosis/atresia of the external auditory meati Maxillary hypoplasia Mandibular hypoplasia Hypoplastic paranasal sinuses

are gracile. There are often two ossification centres in the manubrium sterni. Atlanto-axial subluxation and instability with hypoplasia of the odontoid process are a frequent cause of myelopathy. There is generalized joint laxity. The vertebral bodies are relatively tall. The hands are short with clinodactyly of the little finger due to a hypoplastic middle phalanx. Congenital heart lesions include endocardial cushion defects and intra- and extra-cardiac shunts. Duodenal atresia, duodenal stenosis, Hirschsprung's disease and anorectal anomalies are associated.

45XO (Turner's syndrome)

Short stature and lymphoedema may be clinically obvious. Important radiological findings include short fourth metacarpals, a reduced angle between the distal radial and ulnar metaphyses similar to that seen in dyschondrosteosis (Madelung deformity; Fig. 67.26), flattening of the medial tibial condyle with a transitory exostosis, osteoporosis, scoliosis, coarctation of the aorta, and increased occurrence of urinary tract anomalies, such as horseshoe kidneys and delay in maturation of the skeleton.

LOCALIZED DISORDERS OF THE SKELETON

Sprengel deformity (congenital elevation of the scapula)

This is the most common congenital abnormality of the shoulder. There is a failure of the normal descent of the scapula from its initial mid cervical to its final mid thoracic position. This descent should occur between the sixth and eighth weeks of gestation. Both genders are affected equally. It may affect one or both sides. When unilateral, the left shoulder is more often involved. It may occur in isolation or in association with fusions of the cervical spine in the Klippel–Feil deformity. The scapula is elevated and rotated with the inferior edge of the glenoid pointing towards the spine. The superomedial angle is high and prominent, and the affected scapula is larger than the normal one[4]. An autosomal dominant inheritance has been suggested.

An omovertebral bone (bony or fibrous connection between the superomedial angle of the scapula and the spinous process, lamina or transverse process of a vertebral body between C4 and C7) occurs in approximately 50% of cases. Three-dimensional (3D) CT is useful for depiction both of the deformity (Fig. 67.27) and of the omovertebral bone (when present).

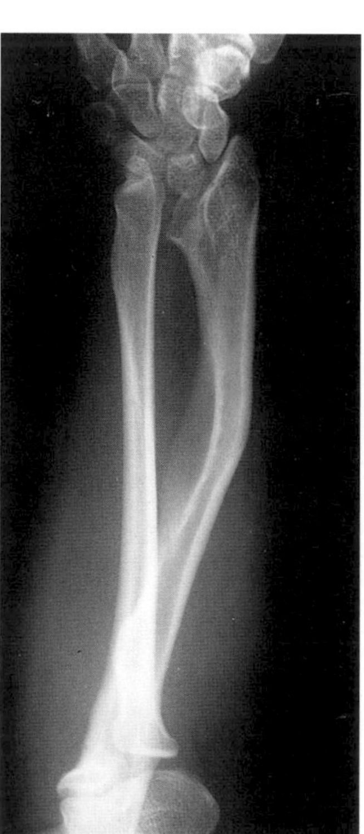

Figure 67.26 Dyschondrosteosis. Madelung deformity. The distal radial metaphysis is sloping and there is dislocation of the distal end of the ulna. The radius is bowed laterally.

Madelung deformity

This condition results from abnormality of the medial half of the distal radial epiphysis. The radii are short and bowed. There is reduction of the carpal angle, with wedging of the carpal bones between the distal radius and ulna. Madelung deformity may be inherited when it occurs as an autosomal dominant mesomelic dysplasia (dyschondro-osteosis) or it may present as an isolated disorder (Fig. 67.28A).

In reverse Madelung deformity, there is bowing of the forearm bones, in association with a short (abnormal) ulna. Causes of reverse Madelung include trauma, hereditary multiple exostoses (Fig. 67.28B) and diaphyseal aclasis.

Developmental dysplasia of the hip

This may occur as an isolated disorder (increased female incidence, breech presentation, first born children, oligohydramnios, and when there is a positive family history) or in association with other conditions (e.g. sternomastoid tumour, torticollis, talipes calcaneovalgus, arthrogryposis multiplex and trisomy 21). The incidence in the UK approaches 1 in 400 live births, while in the USA it is 3–4 in 1000.

Although guidelines may vary slightly, both in the UK and the USA, static and dynamic US examination is performed on all newborn infants with a positive Ortolani and/or Barlow test, breech presentation, or positive family history. US should

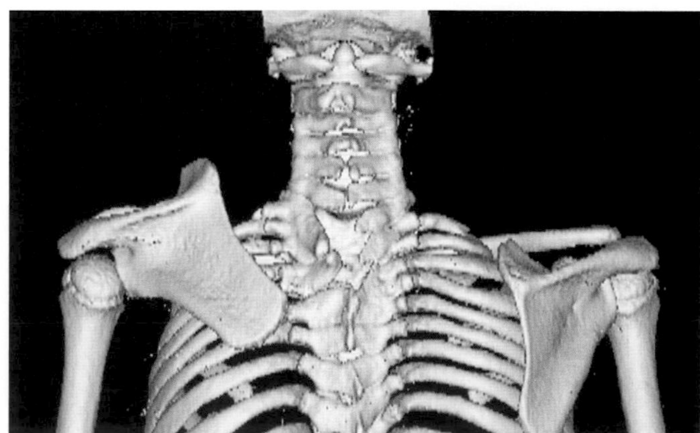

Figure 67.27 Sprengel's deformity. 3D CT of thorax on bone windows. Elevated right scapula (Sprengel's deformity). Note also the spinal dyspraphism (C5–T3) and failure of segmentation (T4/T5).

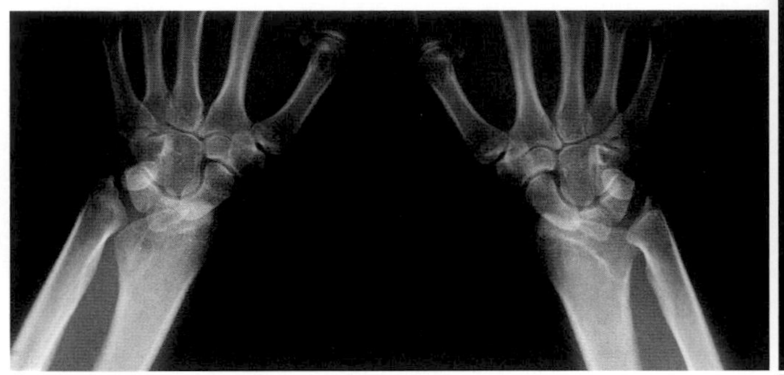

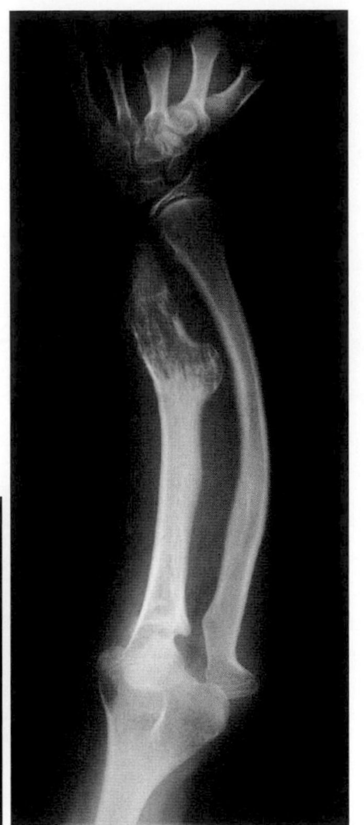

Figure 67.28 Madelung deformity. Compare (A) the bilateral Madelung deformity in dyschondrosteosis with (B) the reverse Madelung deformity in a patient with Ollier's disease—multiple enchondromatosis.

usually be performed when the infant is about 6 weeks old. A high frequency linear probe is used to obtain a coronal view of the hip joint. Measurements and their interpretation are summarized in Figure 67.29A,B and in Table 67.7. The radiographic appearances of DDH are illustrated in Figure 67.29C–E.

When ossification of the proximal femoral epiphysis renders US examination difficult, then radiographs are useful for follow-up and monitoring the response to treatment. Screening of at-risk infants has led to early detection and treatment of developmental dysplasia of the hip (DDH), and cases such as those with bilateral dislocation and formation of pseudoacetabulae (Fig. 67.29E) are now less commonly seen.

Femoral dysplasia (idiopathic coxa vara/proximal focal femoral deficiency spectrum)

The spectrum of femoral dysplasia encompasses all conditions from the mild idiopathic coxa vara (Fig. 67.30) to severe forms of proximal focal femoral deficiency in which only the distal femoral condyles develop.

Idiopathic coxa vara

In this condition, there is coxa vara (reduction of femoral neck/shaft angle). A separate fragment of bone (Fairbank's triangle)—from the inferior portion of the femoral neck—is characteristic. If the neck/shaft angle is less than 100 degrees, then without surgical intervention the varus deformity will progress.

Proximal focal femoral deficiency (PFFD)

Proximal focal femoral deficiency (PFFD) is bilateral in only 10% of cases. Varying degrees of agenesis of the proximal femur occur, and there is an association between severity of femoral dysplasia and severity of acetabular dysplasia. The lower leg may also be short, and the fibula absent or hypoplastic.

Radiography demonstrates the degree of aplasia and in younger children, MRI and/or arthrography is useful for the visualization of unossified cartilage.

Tibia vara

This refers to bowing of the legs, which may be bilateral or unilateral. Bowing may occur at the level of the knee joint or proximal tibia. Causes include physiological bowing (bilateral and self-resolving), Blount's disease, rickets, trauma, infection, neurofibromatosis, Ollier's disease, Maffucci syndrome, fibrous dysplasia and focal fibrocartilaginous dysplasia (Fig. 67.31).

Blount's disease (Fig. 67.32) affects the medial aspects of the proximal tibial epiphyses. It is unilateral in 40%. There are infantile and adolescent presentations. The infantile form of the disease occurs between the ages of 1 and 3 years. Adolescent Blount's disease has a higher post-surgical recurrence rate.

Talipes

Talipes equinovarus (congenital clubfoot) consists of varus (inversion) and equinus (fixed plantar flexion) of the hindfoot,

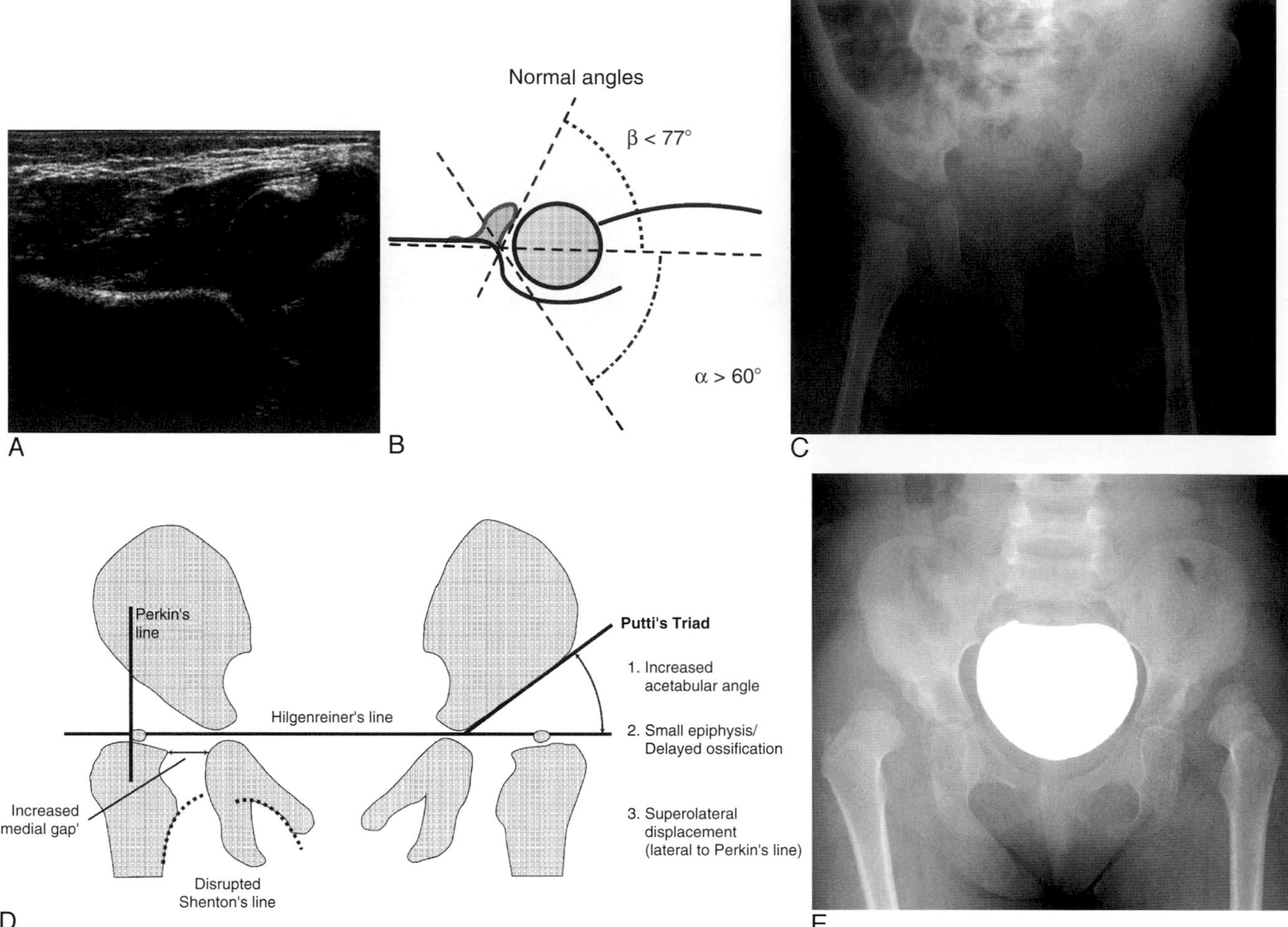

Figure 67.29 Developmental dysplasia of the hip (DDH). (A) Ultrasound of a dislocated hip. (B) Normal Graf angles. (C) AP radiograph of the pelvis with left DDH. (D) Measurements in DDH. (E) AP radiograph of the pelvis showing bilateral DDH. Note the early formation of pseudoacetabulae.

Table 67.7 GRAF ANGLES

Type	α angle (degrees)	β angle (degrees)	Bony roof	Ossific rim	Cartilage roof	Interpretation
Ia	> 60	< 55	Good	Sharp	Covers femoral head	Mature
Ib	> 60	> 55	Good	Usually blunt	Covers head	Mature
IIa	50–59	> 55	Deficient	Rounded	Covers head	Physiological ossification delay
IIb	50–59	> 55	Deficient	Rounded	Covers head	
IIc	43–49	< 77	Deficient	Rounded/flat	Covers head	
IId	43–49	> 77	Severely deficient	Rounded/flat	Compressed	On point of dislocation
IIIa	< 43	> 77	Poor	Flat	Displaced up Echo poor	Dislocated
IIIb	< 43	> 77	Poor	Flat	Displaced up Reflective	Dislocated
IV	< 43	> 77	Poor	Flat	Interposed	Dislocated

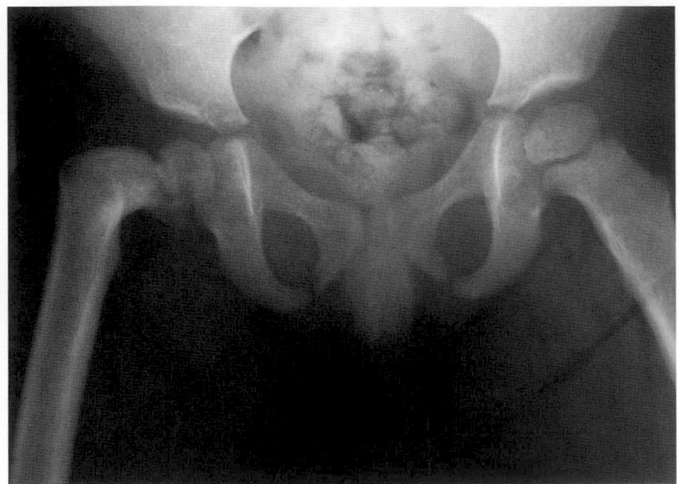

Figure 67.30 Femoral dysplasia. Right coxa vara deformity.

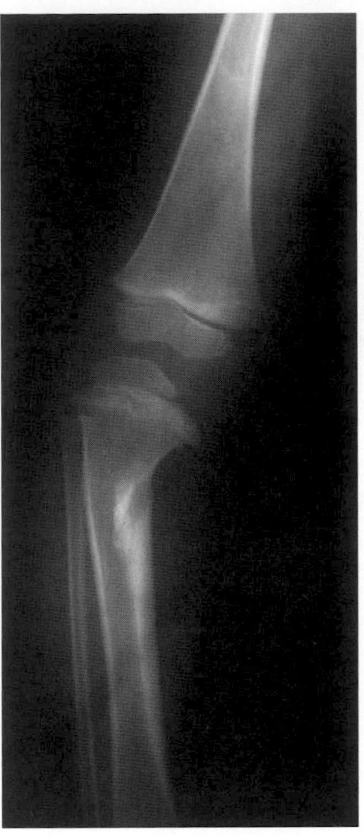

Figure 67.31 Focal fibrocartilaginous dysplasia. Note the pathognomonic appearance of the radiolucent band. This condition is usually self-resolving and in the first instance should be managed conservatively

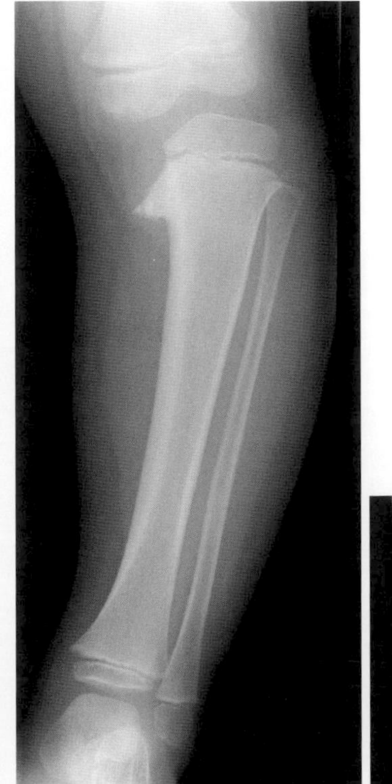

A

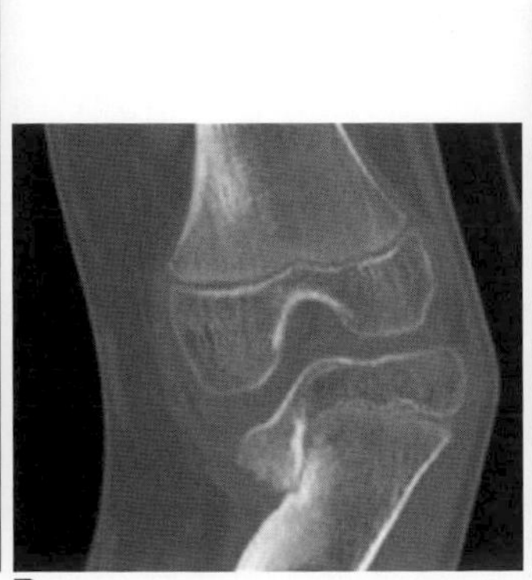

B

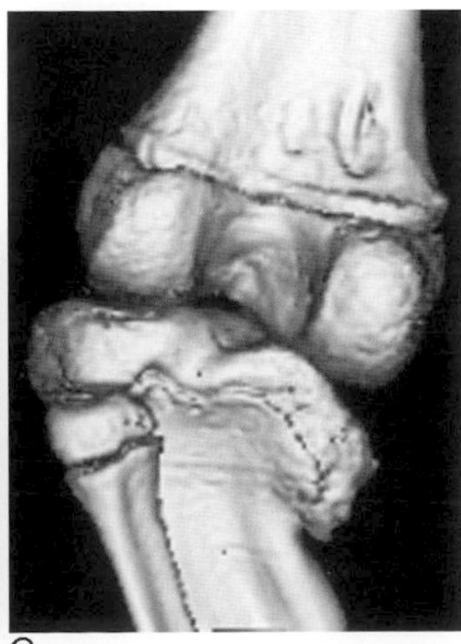

C

Figure 67.32 Blount's disease. (A) Plain radiograph, (B) coronal CT and (C) 3D CT reconstruction (posterior view).

and varus of the forefoot. It results from abnormal development around the ninth week of gestation. Aetiological considerations include genetic factors and early amniocentesis (before 11 weeks)[5,6]. It occurs two to three times more commonly in boys. Useful measurements are summarized in Table 67.8.

Idiopathic avascular necrosis of the femoral head (Perthes disease)

Osteonecrosis of the femoral head usually presents with pain or limping between 5 and 8 years of age. It is most often unilateral, but when bilateral (in 15%) it is asymmetrical, helping to distinguish it from an epiphyseal dysplasia. There are four stages of disease: devascularization; collapse and fragmentation; re-ossification; and finally the stage of remodelling.

The earliest radiographic feature is that of a radiolucent subchondral fissure—the crescent sign (Fig. 67.33A). Disease progresses with loss of height, fragmentation and sclerosis of the femoral head. A coxa magna deformity may ensue, with lateral uncovering of the capital femoral epiphysis. There may be associated irregularity of the acetabular margin. Several radiographic signs and classification systems exist to help in the diagnosis and prognosis of Perthes disease. The extent of subchondral fracture is said to be a good predictor of the final outcome[7]. More detailed classification systems include that proposed by Catterall[8] and later simplified by Salter and Thompson[9], and the more recent system proposed by Herring et al[10]. The last of these is based on the degree of resorption of the lateral femoral head pillar during the fragmentation phase. All systems have been found to be good when used by an experienced observer[11]. The centre edge angle may be used to assess the degree of femoral head coverage.

Perthes disease is occasionally bilateral and synchronous, but it is more usually metachronous (Fig. 67.33B). Synchronous disease should raise the suspicion of an epiphyseal dysplasia.

Table 67.8 DIAGNOSIS OF TALIPES

Deformity	DP radiograph	Lateral radiograph
Hind foot varus	Talocalcaneal angle: < 15 degrees Midtalar line lateral to first metatarsal base	Talocalcaneal angle: < 25 degrees
Hind foot valgus	Talocalcaneal angle: > 50 degrees in newborns; > 40 degrees in older children Midtalar angel medial to first metatarsal base	Talocalcaneal angle: > 50 degrees in newborns; > 45 degrees in older children
Hind foot equines	—	Calcaneotibial angle: > 90 degrees Plantar flexion of calcaneus
Hind foot calcaneus	—	Calcaneotibial angle: < 60 degrees Dorsiflexioun of calaneus
Forefoot varus	Narrow with increased overlap of metatarsal bases	Fifth metatarsal most plantar (normal) First metatarsal most dorsal
Forefoot valgus	Broad with reduced overlap of metatarsal bases	First metatarsal most plantar

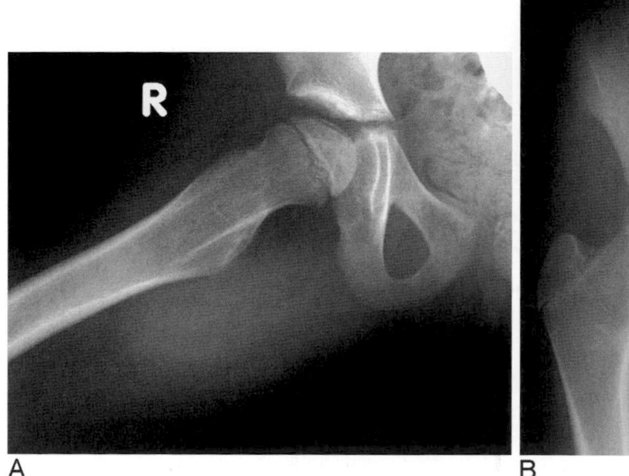

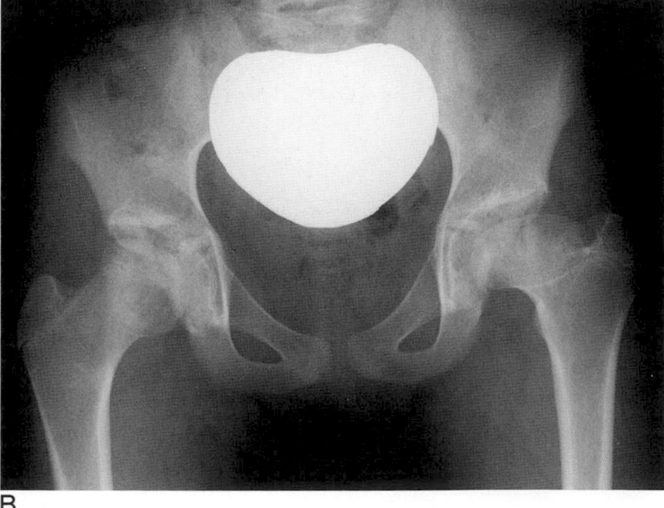

Figure 67.33 Perthes disease at (A) presentation, showing the crescent sign, and (B) 17 months later. Note the metachronous nature of the disease.

Perthes disease may be suspected from US examination. Capsular distension from a hip effusion persisting for longer than 6 weeks is associated with the development of Perthes disease[12]. Additionally, irregularity/fragmentation of the capital femoral epiphysis and poor coverage of the femoral head may be demonstrated.

While skeletal scintigraphy is highly sensitive and specific for detecting AVN, MRI has now largely replaced it (Fig. 67.34). Signal abnormalities may be detected within the first 3 months of disease onset; however, they are more clearly visualized 3–8 months after onset[13]. Six patterns of signal abnormality have been described[14]. In summary, T1-weighted images show low signal intensity, compared to high signal on T2-weighted fat-suppressed/inversion recovery (STIR) sequences. In those with normal signal intensity or complete loss of signal on both sequences (dead bone), intravenous enhancement is not necessary. In those with normal/low T1-weighted and high T2-weighted signal, intravenous contrast medium will identify areas of viable bone. The role of dynamic contrast MRI in the diagnosis of Perthes disease is under evaluation[15,16].

Slipped capital femoral epiphysis

This is the most common hip disorder of adolescence. There is no change in the relationship between the femoral head and the acetabulum–anterolateral and rotational forces of the hip muscles on the femoral shaft result in anterosuperior translation of the proximal femoral metaphysis relative to the epiphysis. By definition, it occurs through the nonrachitic physis[17].

It is more common in boys, in those of Afro-American origin, and in the obese.[18] The age range for girls is 11–12 years and for boys 12–14 years. It most commonly occurs at the time of the pubertal growth spurt at Risser grade 0, and is rarely seen in girls after menarche or in boys after Tanner stage 4. Bilateral slips occur in about 25% of Caucasian and up to 50% of Afro-American children (depending on the reported series). When unilateral, the left side is more often involved (65%). Endocrine disorders associated with SCFE include hypothyroidism, growth hormone deficiency, hypogonadism and panhypopituitarism[19,20].

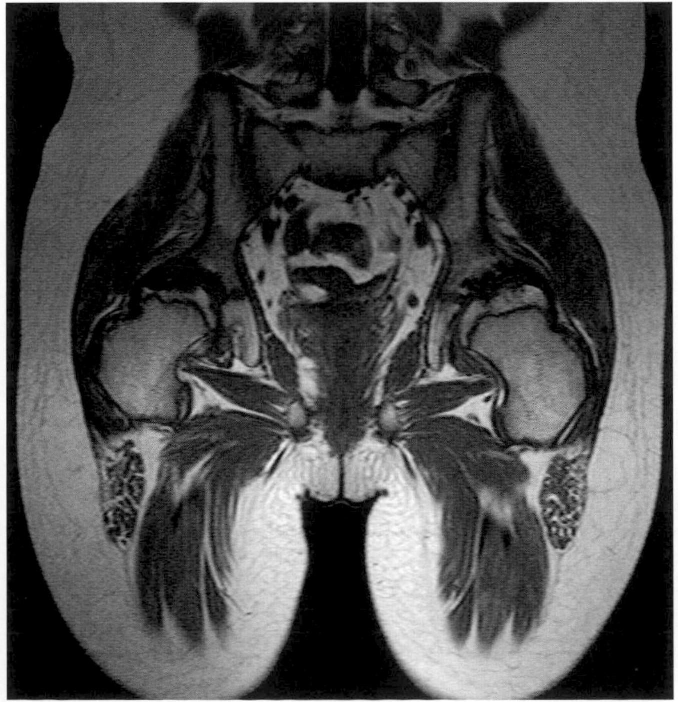

Figure 67.34 Avascular necrosis. T1 coronal MRI showing bilateral avascular necrosis.

Clinically SCFE may be classified based either on duration of symptoms—acute (symptoms for less than 3 weeks); chronic (symptoms for more than 3 weeks); or acute on chronic (symptoms for more than 3 weeks with an acute exacerbation). The second system based on patient mobility classifies SCFE as either stable (patient able to walk with or without crutches) or unstable (patient unable to walk with or without crutches)[17]. The condition is most commonly of chronic onset[18].

Radiography remains the investigation of choice. AP and frog lateral views of the pelvis are obtained. Observations include disuse osteopenia; a widened growth plate with indistinct borders; and malalignment of the epiphysis and proximal femoral metaphysis (more easily recognized on the frog lateral radiograph). On an AP radiograph malalignment may be more objectively assessed by drawing a line (Klein's line) along the outer border of the femoral neck—when extended upwards, this line should intersect approximately a sixth of the femoral epiphysis. In cases of SCFE, the Klein's line may not intersect the proximal femoral epiphysis (Fig. 67.35). The frog lateral radiograph allows an assessment of the severity of the slip according to the method outlined by Southwick[21] in which a 'slip angle' is calculated (Fig. 67.36). Based on the slip angle obtained, SCFE can be classified as mild (≤30 degrees), moderate (31–50 degrees), or severe (≥51 degrees)[22].

Some authors advocate the use of US over radiography for the diagnosis of SCFE[23]. Findings on US allow classification into stable or unstable SCFE. Absence of a joint effusion together with evidence of remodelling at the physeal–epiphyseal junction (periosteal reaction) implies a stable slip. The presence of a joint effusion with no signs of remodelling implies an unstable slip.

Complications of SCFE include chondrolysis (narrowing of the joint space), AVN and osteoarthritis.

Scoliosis

The Scoliosis Research Society has defined scoliosis as a lateral curvature of the spine greater than 10 degrees[24]. Scoliosis may

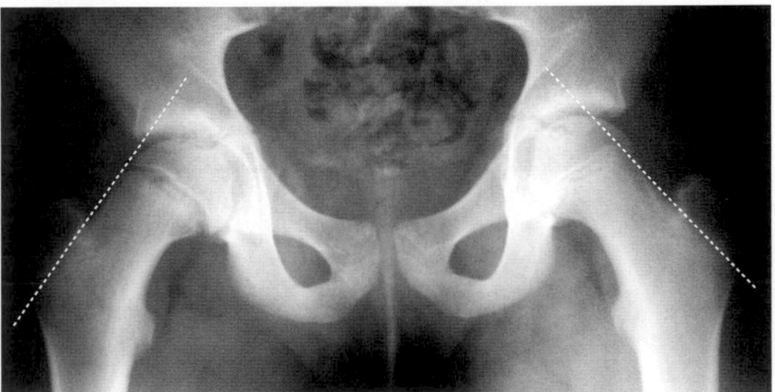

Figure 67.35 Slipped capital femoral epiphysis. Klein's line.

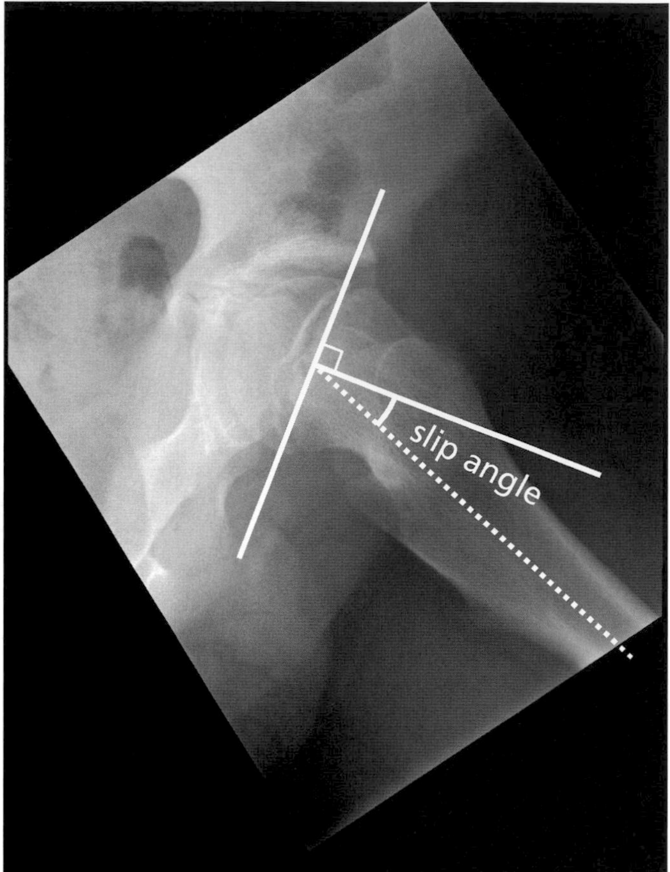

Figure 67.36 Slipped capital femoral epiphysis. Frog lateral illustrating measurement of slip angle.

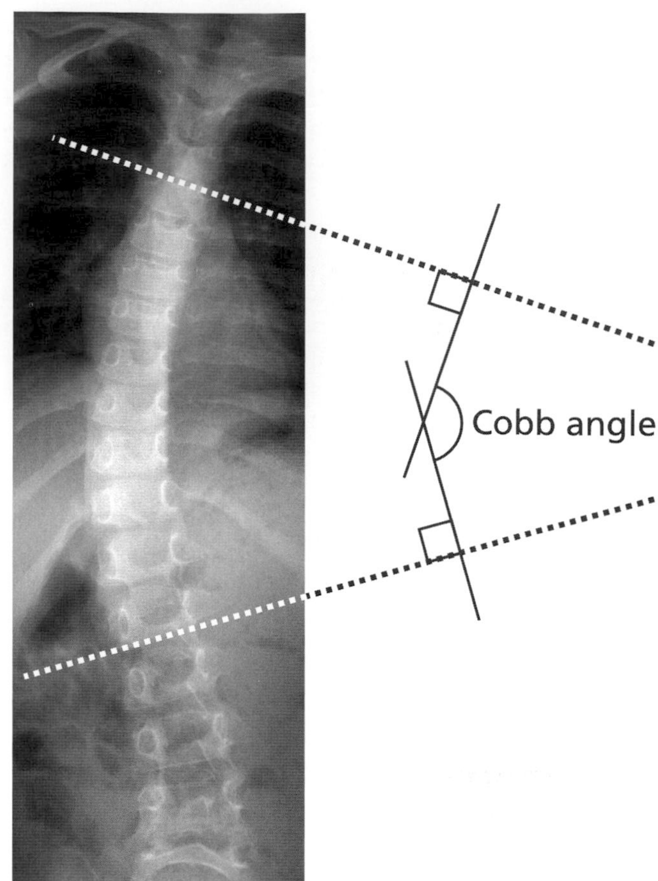

Figure 67.37 Scoliosis. AP radiograph of the spine showing measurement of the Cobb angle.

be congenital or idiopathic. In contrast to idiopathic scoliosis, congenital scoliosis is related to a developmental abnormality of the spine. Based on the age of the patient at diagnosis, idiopathic scoliosis may be further subdivided into infantile (onset before 3 years of age), juvenile (between 3 and 10 years of age) and adolescent (from 10 years to skeletal maturity). The majority of children who present with idiopathic scoliosis do so in the adolescent period[25]. There is a strong hereditary component to idiopathic scoliosis and indeed candidate regions on chromosomes 6, 9 and 16 have recently been identified[26].

Congenital scoliosis is associated with such vertebral anomalies as hemivertebrae, block vertebrae and butterfly vertebrae. It may be associated with syndromes such as Alagille, Jarcho–Levin, VACTERL, Goldenhar and Klippel–Feil. Other conditions associated with a scoliosis include connective tissue disorders (Marfan's, Ehlers–Danlos, and homocystinuria), neurological conditions (cerebral palsy, tethered cord, neurofibromatosis), and any cause of a leg length discrepancy.

The prognosis (risk of curve progression) depends on the patient's gender (worse in girls), the severity of the curve, and the child's growth potential. The latter two may be determined radiographically.

The magnitude of the curve is determined by measuring the Cobb angle (Fig. 67.37). An estimation of growth potential can be made by an assessment of the Tanner stage (clinical) and the Risser grade (radiological; Fig. 67.38). The Risser grade is based on the degree of maturation of the iliac crest apophysis, and gives an estimation of how much growth remains. It has been shown to correlate directly with the risk of curve progression[27].

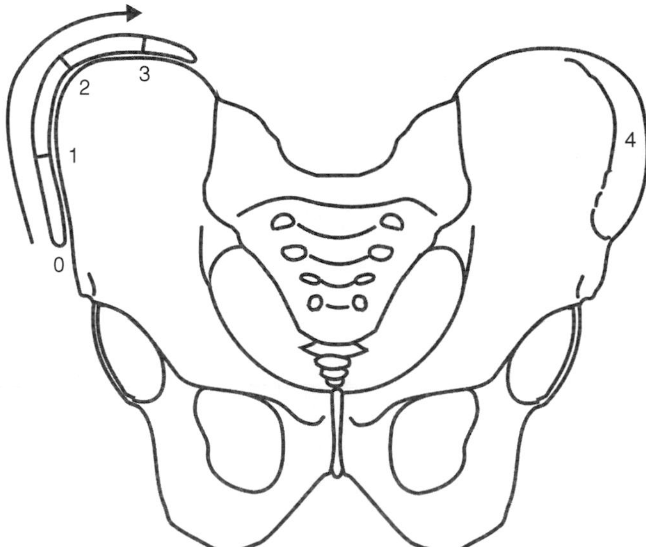

Figure 67.38 Scoliosis. Line diagram of the Risser grades (0 = iliac crest yet to ossify; 4 = full closure of apophysis).

Cross-sectional imaging (CT and MRI) is useful for the exclusion of underlying vertebral and spinal cord anomalies; indeed, MRI is advised whenever there is a left thoracic curve, pain, abnormal neurological examination, or other unexpected findings to exclude causes such as tumour, syringomyelia, or spondylolisthesis[28].

NEUROCUTANEOUS SYNDROMES

Neurofibromatosis

This is inherited as an autosomal dominant disorder. The responsible genes have been mapped to chromosomes 17q 21 (NF-I) and 22q12 (NF-II).

Clinical features include multiple neurofibromas, schwannomas, axillary freckling, café-au-lait spots and molluscum fibrosum. Up to 85% of patients with neurofibromatosis manifest musculoskeletal abnormality (Fig. 67.39 and 67.40). Other features are listed in Table 67.9.

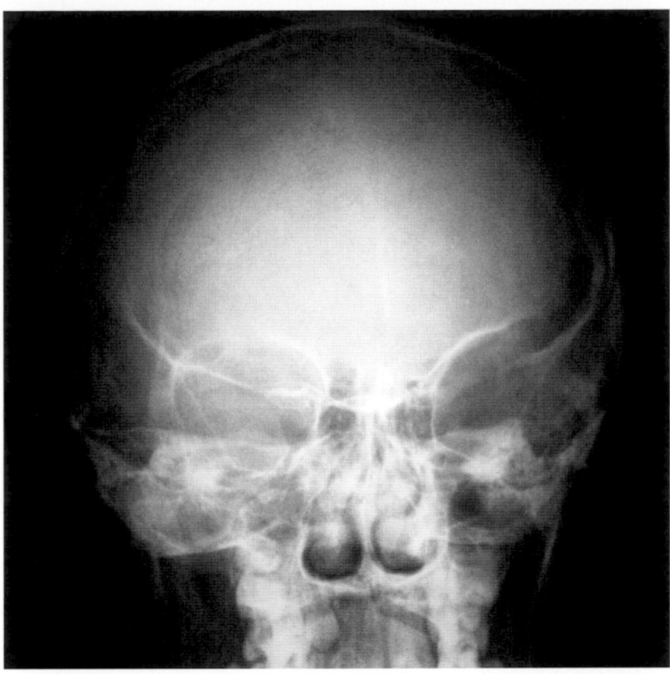

Figure 67.39 Neurofibromatosis Type 1. AP radiograph of the skull showing 'empty' left orbit.

Tuberous sclerosis

Clinical and radiographic features are listed in Table 67.10.

Juvenile idiopathic arthritis

The International League of Associations for Rheumatology (ILAR) introduced the term juvenile idiopathic arthritis (JIA) in 1997 to replace and unify the previous classifications of juvenile chronic arthritis and juvenile rheumatoid arthritis[33].

JIA is arthritis of unknown aetiology occurring before the age of 16 years. It is subdivided to include: 'oligoarthritis' (one to four joints affected in the first 6 months of the disease); 'polyarthritis' (more than four joints affected within the first 6

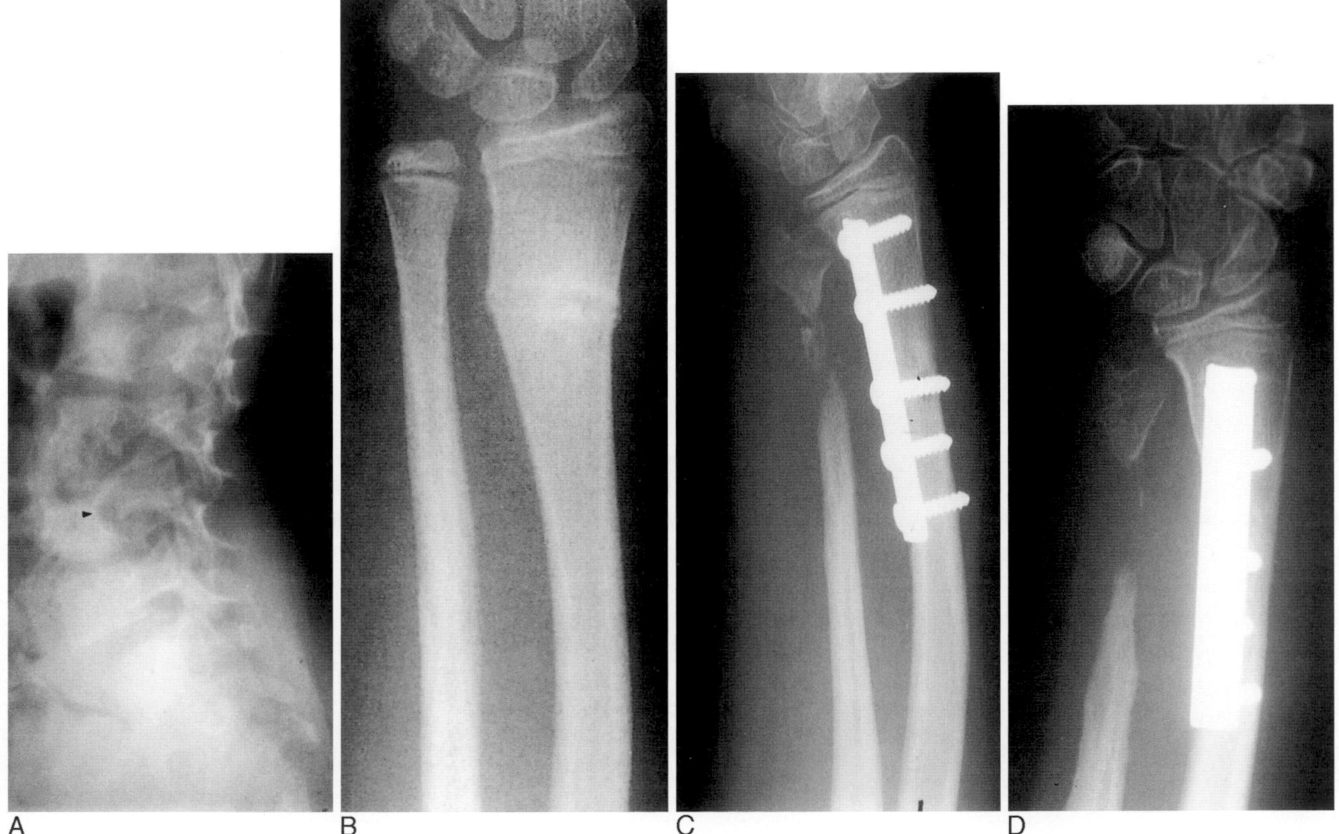

Figure 67.40 Neurofibromatosis. (A) Pronounced posterior scalloping (arrowhead) of the lumbar vertebral bodies due to dural ectasia. (B–D) Development of a pseudarthrosis in the distal shaft of the ulna following a fracture of the radius (same patient).

Table 67.9 RADIOGRAPHIC FEATURES OF NEUROFIBROMATOSIS

Soft tissues	Focal gigantism (soft tissue overgrowth or plexiform neurofibroma)
	Neurofibrosarcomas[29]
Skull	Macrocrania
	Aplasia/hypoplasia of the sphenoid wings (empty orbit; Fig. 67.39)
	Hypoplasia of posterosuperior orbital wall (pulsatile exophthalmos)
	Mesodermal dysplasia (calvarial defects)
	Neuromas and/or fibromas (with enlarged cranial foramina[30])
Spine	Angular kyphoscoliosis
	Posterior scalloping of the vertebral bodies (dural ectasia)
	Dumb-bell neurofibromas/lateral meningocoeles
Ribs	'Ribbon' ribs (mesodermal dysplasia)
	Rib notching
Tubular bones	Pseudoarthroses of the tibia, fibula, or clavicle
	Anteromedial bowing of tibia
	Fibrous cortical defects (multiple and large)
	Intraosseous cysts

Table 67.10 CLINICAL AND RADIOGRAPHIC FEATURES OF TUBEROUS SCLEROSIS

Clinical features	Radiographic features
Adenoma sebaceum	Renal angiomyofibromas[31]
Leukoderma	Cardiac myomas
Shagreen patches	Cyst-like phalangeal lesions
Subungual fibromas	Irregular undulating periosteal reaction along metacarpals and other tubular bones
Café-au-lait spots	Bone islands in the vertebral bodies and pedicles
Inflammatory arthropathy	Intracranial calcification[32]

months);'systemic arthritis' (arthritis accompanied by systemic illness); 'psoriatic arthritis'; 'enthesitis related arthritis' (often HLA B-27 positive); and 'other arthritis' (disease that does not fall into the listed groups).

The wrist is affected in 61% of patients with polyarticular JIA, being second only to the knee as the most frequently affected joint. The hip and wrist are the most vulnerable joints to radiographically visible destruction. In some children, isolated involvement of the hips with bilateral protrusio acetabuli has been documented. It has been suggested that this isolated inflammatory coxitis may represent a separate subtype of oligoarthritic JIA[34].

Joint involvement is characterized by synovial inflammation progressing to synovial hyperplasia and pannus formation. Pannus erodes cartilage and bone and leads to articular destruction and ankylosis[35]. Affected joints are swollen, stiff with reduced motion, painful, erythematous and warm.

Early prediction of the course of disease is vital in JIA in order to instigate appropriate therapy and reduce long-term disability. The best predictors of poor outcome have been shown to be severity and extent of joint involvement at onset of disease; early hip and/or wrist involvement; positive rheumatoid factor; and prolonged active disease[36].

Radiography (Fig. 67.41A–C), dual energy X-ray absorptiometry (DEXA), ultrasound, CT and MRI are all employed, both for the initial evaluation and diagnosis of patients with JIA and for monitoring response to and complications of therapy.

Radiography allows the assessment of soft tissue swelling, osteoporosis, erosions, joint destruction and ankylosis. Early in the course of the disease, the presence of effusions causes the joint spaces to appear widened. As disease progresses in severity, the joint spaces are narrowed (seen in the wrist as loss of height of the carpus) until finally there may be bony ankylosis. Inflammation causes hyperaemia with osteopaenia, relative overgrowth of the femoral condyles and patella and premature fusion of the epiphyses. Pressure from the hypertrophied synovium causes widening of the intercondylar notch. Evaluation of bone density from radiographs is subjective, and reliable detection requires that bone density be reduced to at least 30% its original value[37]. Other disadvantages of radiography include its low sensitivity for the detection of joint effusions, synovial thickening and differentiation of active from quiescent disease.

MRI (Fig. 67.41D) has the advantage of not exposing the child to radiation. Furthermore, it allows improved demonstration of articular cartilage, joint effusions, synovial hypertrophy, fibrocartilaginous structures and muscles. Contrast-enhanced MRI (Fig. 67.41E) allows assessment of the perfusion of cartilage, synovium and bone and is the most sensitive method for determining whether an arthritic condition is present[38]. Enhancement of thickened synovium suggests active disease and differentiates it from fluid.

AVN is a recognized complication of both JIA and steroid therapy. The presence of AVN may be determined using either radiography or MRI. Although it is more sensitive than radiography for the detection of early AVN, MRI is said to be less sensitive for the detection of osteochondral fractures with reported sensitivity and specificity for MRI and radiography cited as 38% and 100%, and 71% and 97%, respectively[39]. However, of particular significance is the fact that MRI may detect changes of AVN when radiographs appear normal[40]. A note of caution; standard MRI techniques do not always detect dead bone—this is because at the stage of early marrow necrosis, fat tissue is 'mummified' and preserves the same signal intensity as fat[41].

Juvenile dermatomyositis

Juvenile dermatomyositis (JDM) is a multisystem disease defined as affecting those under 18 years of age, although it more commonly affects children aged 2–15 years. It is of unknown aetiology, but both genetic and infectious agents have been implicated. The disease is characterized by a non-suppurative inflammation of skin and skeletal muscle and is associated with a typical (pathognomonic) rash.

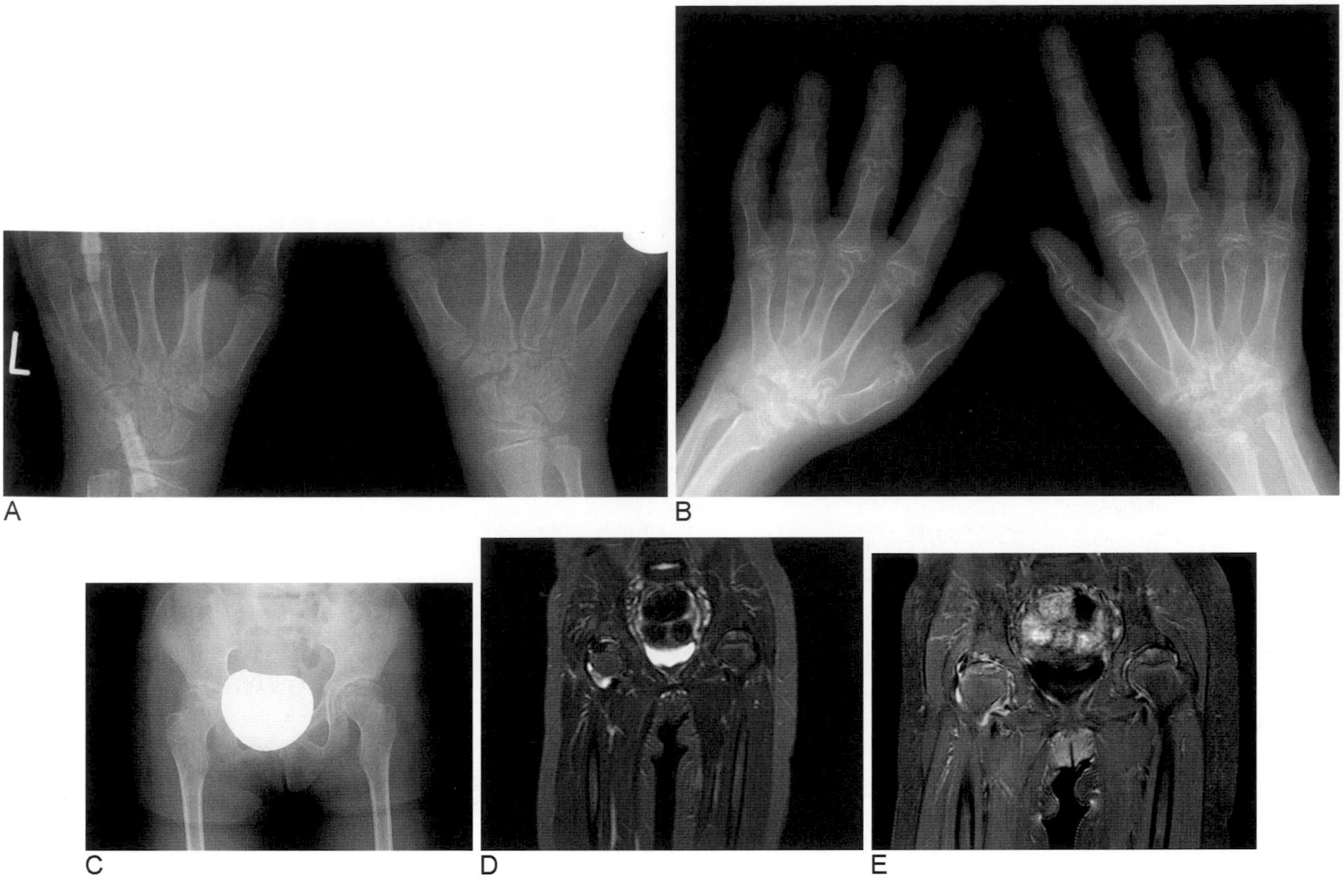

A B C D E

Figure 67.41 Juvenile idiopathic arthritis. DP radiographs of the hands showing (A) mild erosive change of carpal bones and (B) severe changes (erosions of carpal bones and phalanges, osteopaenia, loss of height of carpus). (C) AP radiograph of the pelvis with severe loss of joint space on the right. The left hip is less severely affected. (D,E) MRI in same patient as C. (D) STIR image illustrating right hip effusion and avascular necrosis of the right femoral head. (E) T1-weighted image following contrast administration demonstrates bilateral active synovitis

The diagnostic criteria (established by Bohan and Peter[42]) include this rash and any three of the four following criteria: symmetrical proximal muscle weakness, elevated muscle enzymes, diagnostic histopathology findings and characteristic features on electromyogram (EMG). The latter two are invasive procedures and with the advent of MRI the diagnosis is often based on clinical, laboratory and MRI findings.

Disease activity and response to therapy in JDM may be monitored by documenting muscle strength and function, serum muscle enzyme levels, range of joint movement, and physician's global assessment (PGA) and by MRI. The Paediatric Rheumatology International Trials Organisation (PRINTO) and the Pediatric Rheumatology Collaborative Study Group (PRCSG) have recently published preliminary core sets of measures for disease activity and damage assessment in JDM, which bring together several of the tools listed above. Despite its usefulness they do not include MRI, as it is not universally available[43].

Radiographs may be normal. Abnormal findings include loss of muscle bulk, disuse osteopaenia and soft tissue calcification (Fig. 67.42).

The MRI features of active dermatomyositis are best illustrated on T2-weighted and inversion recovery (STIR) sequences (Fig. 67.43). They include increased signal inten-

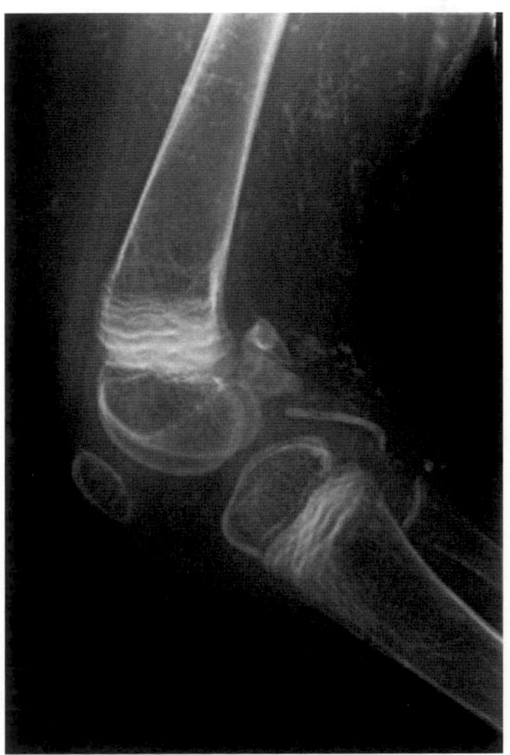

Figure 67.42 Juvenile dermatomyositis. Soft tissue calcification. Note also the pamidronate lines (see Fig. 67.44).

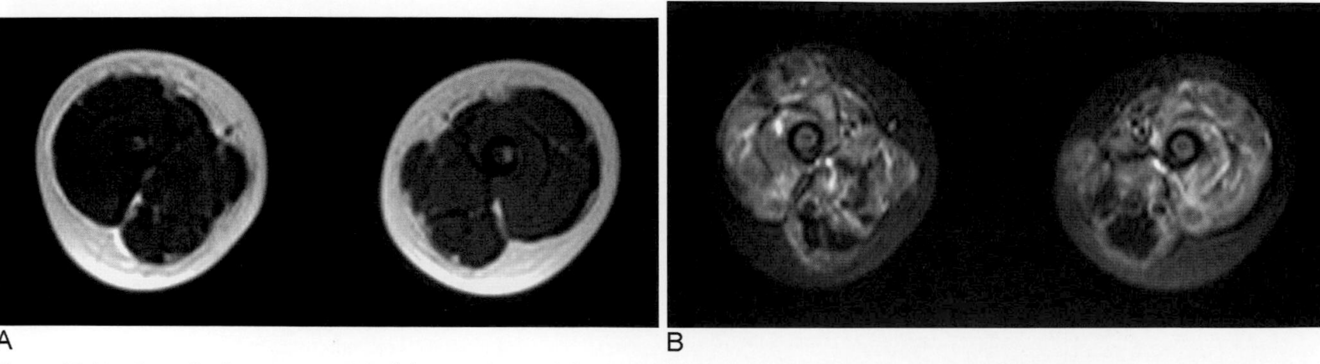

Figure 67.43 Juvenile dermatomyositis. (A) T1 axial MRI of the thighs. (B) Axial STIR of the thighs. There is bilateral active myositis with no significant loss of muscle bulk.

sity in affected muscles, perimuscular oedema, enhanced chemical-shift artefact and increased signal intensity in subcutaneous fat. More recently it has been shown that the T2 relaxation time can be used as a quantitative measure of muscle inflammation in JDM[44]. MRI will also demonstrate loss of muscle bulk with relative and absolute increases in subcutaneous fat, fatty infiltration of muscles, and occasionally soft tissue calcification. The resolution and relapse of signal abnormality during the course of JDM has been documented using serial MRI. However, there have been no controlled studies. Currently there are no recommendations for the timing of MRI in JDM, and it is not known how soon the abnormal signal intensity begins to respond to therapy or when it normalizes.

The bisphosphonates are a group of drugs that are pyrophosphate analogues. They act by reducing bone resorption through an inhibitory effect on osteoclast function. Although not yet licensed for children, they are increasingly used in this age group, most commonly to increase bone mass in osteogenesis imperfecta. However, other indications include improvement of bone pain and density in rheumatological conditions such as JIA, JDM and SAPHO (synovitis, acne, palmoplantar pustulosis, hyperostosis and osteitis) syndrome. The radiographic hallmark of bisphosphonate therapy is the presence of dense metaphyseal bands (treatment pulses) alternating with bone of normal density (periods off treatment) (Figs 67.42, 67.44).

NON-INFLAMMATORY DISORDERS

Haemophilia

In this X-linked recessive disorder, a defect in blood coagulation leads to an increased tendency to haemorrhage. Depending on the severity of the disease (and compliance with therapy), bleeding may be spontaneous or occur following relatively mild trauma. Sites of bleeding include the brain, joints, abdomen and retroperitoneal cavity.

Bleeding into the joints is common in haemophilia and usually involves the large joints of the knee (Fig. 67.45), elbow, ankle, hip and shoulder. Haemarthrosis begins in the first two decades of life, but the number of affected joints stabilizes by the age of 20.

Recurrent episodes of intra-articular bleeding cause villous synovial hypertrophy with accumulation of haemosiderin within macrophages. The arthropathy may progress to cause significant and irreversible cartilage destruction with secondary degenerative disease. Rarely (1–2% of patients) recurrent subperiosteal haemorrhage may become encapsulated and cause bony erosion, giving rise to the so-called haemophilic pseudotumour. This is more common in adult patients[45].

Based on radiography, five stages of disease may be recognized[46]; however, in any given patient, the chronology may

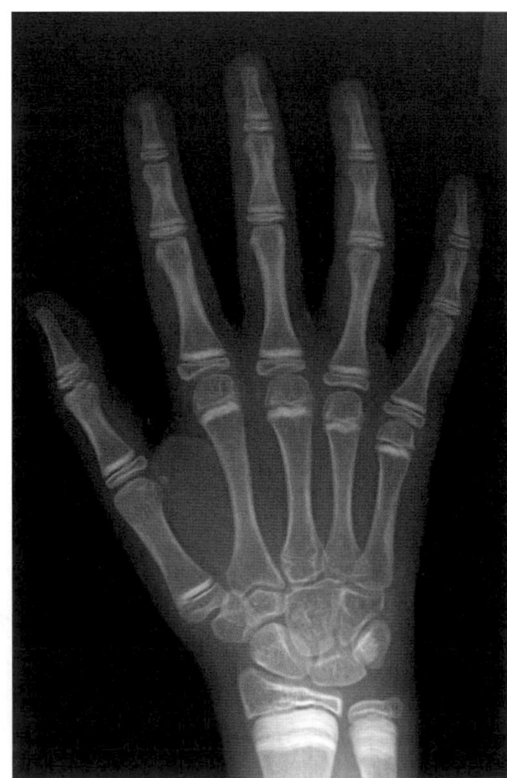

Figure 67.44 Juvenile dermatomyositis. DP radiograph of the hands showing pamidronate lines in the same patient as shown in Fig. 67.43.

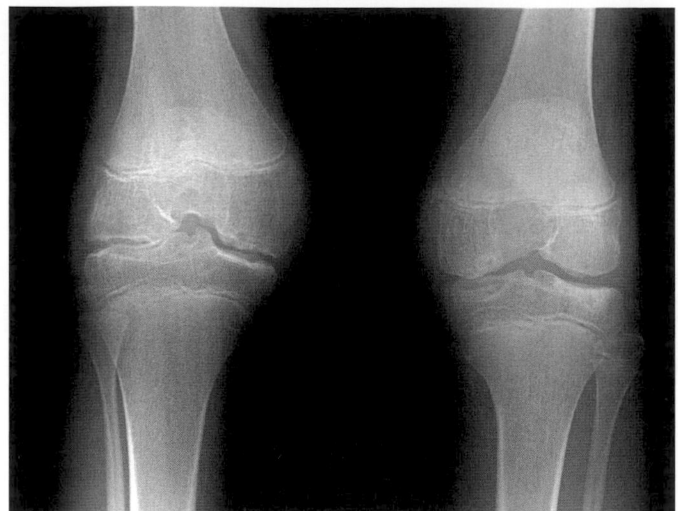

Figure 67.45 Bleeding into the joints in haemophilia. AP radiograph of the knees. There is widening of the intercondylar notches, narrow joint spaces and erosive change. The right knee is more severely affected.

not necessarily follow the stages nor is progression to the final stages inevitable in all affected joints. The stages are:

- Stage I—soft tissue swelling and/or joint effusion—normal joint surfaces
- Stage II—Stage I plus peri-articular osteoporosis—epiphyseal overgrowth
- Stage III—erosions, sclerosis and subchondral cysts—joint spaces preserved
- Stage IV—Stage III plus focal/diffuse joint space narrowing
- Stage V—stiff contracted joint with significant degenerative change.

Although CT and US may also be used in the assessment of haemophilic arthropathy, MRI (with its ability to demonstrate early disease, including synovial abnormality, ligamentous tears, peri-articular bleeding, cartilaginous and osseous bruising, erosions and joint space narrowing) is the investigation of choice and classification systems based on MRI findings are currently being developed[47–49]. Intra-articular haemorrhage will usually be evident as a joint effusion; however, fluid–fluid levels may be demonstrated. Gradient-echo sequences will more readily demonstrate deposits of haemosiderin compared to spin-echo sequences (due to magnetic susceptibility artefact). Three-dimensional spoiled gradient-echo and fast spin-echo sequences allow early identification of focal cartilage defects and thinning.

Pigmented villonodular synovitis

Pigmented villonodular synovitis (PVNS) refers to benign villous or nodular proliferation of synovium of uncertain aetiology. It most commonly affects a single joint with the knee being involved in 80%. Although most patients present in the third and fourth decades of life, the disease may also present in childhood (Fig. 67.46). Synovial joints, tendon sheaths, or bursae may be involved.

Presentation is with a slow growing painless mass that may be tender to palpation. In long-standing cases there may be destruction of cartilage, secondary degenerative change and pain.

Radiographic findings include soft tissue swelling, joint space narrowing and bony erosion (particularly in the hip where subchondral cysts with sclerotic rims are typical). Calcification is rare.

Nonenhanced CT will show high attenuation due to the haemosiderin within the mass. The synovial proliferation enhances following administration of contrast medium.

Diagnostic MRI features include a nodular lesion with areas of haemosiderin (low signal on all sequences) and haemorrhage (Fig. 67.46C). Joint effusions and bony erosions are well demonstrated. As with CT, contrast enhancement is typical.

The differential diagnosis includes haemophilia and synovial haemangioma (rare, phleboliths in soft tissue)[50].

METABOLIC AND ENDOCRINE DISORDERS

Metabolic disorders

Rickets

Rickets is osteomalacia in children. There is an excess of unmineralized osteoid. The serum alkaline phosphatase is elevated, while serum and urinary calcium and phosphate levels are low. Serum levels of calcium and phosphate are controlled in part by vitamin D.

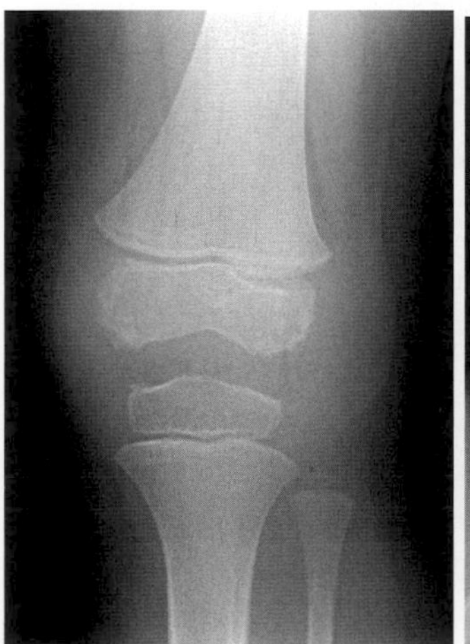
A

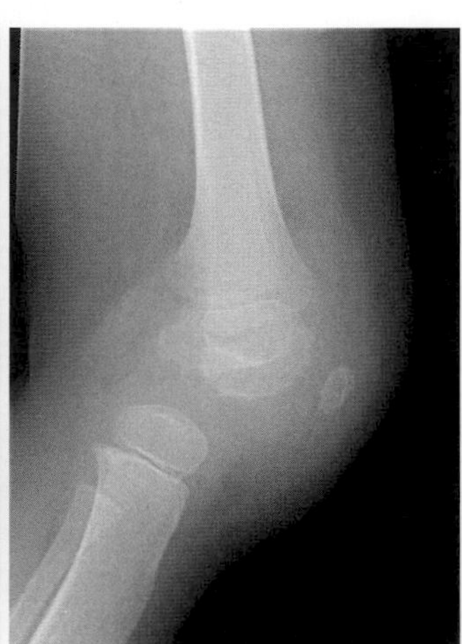
B

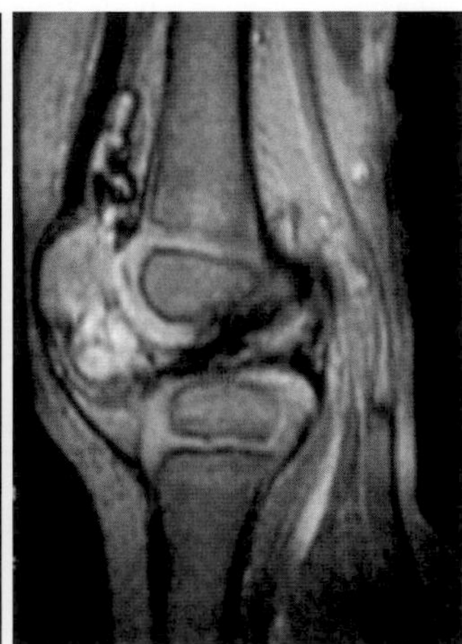
C

Figure 67.46 Pigmented villonodular synovitis. This child was unusual in that he was only 3 years of age at the time of diagnosis. (A) AP and (B) lateral radiographs of the knee showing significant soft tissue swelling. (C) Sagittal T1 MRI illustrating a mixed signal mass with areas of low haemosiderin) and high signal (haemorrhage).

The active form of vitamin D (cholecalciferol) is 1,25-dihydroxy-D3. Hydroxylation of D3 occurs first in the liver at the 25-position, and then in the kidney (regulated by parathyroid hormone) at the 1-position. It acts (with parathyroid hormone) on bone to stimulate the release of calcium and phosphate from osteoclasts; it stimulates intestinal absorption of calcium and phosphate; inhibits secretion of parathormone; and finally stimulates renal tubular re-absorption of phosphate.

The focal radiographic features of rickets are best seen at sites of rapid growth [metaphyses and epiphyses of the distal radius (Fig. 67.47A), ulna and femur and proximal humerus and tibia]. Features include widening and cupping of the metaphyses, which have irregular, frayed margins. There is apparent widening of the physis (due to the unossified zone of provisional calcification). The epiphyses have indistinct margins and are relatively osteopaenic. Looser zones may be seen, particularly at the pubic rami, medial margins of the proximal femora, posterior aspects of the proximal ulnae, axillary margins of the scapulae and the ribs. The 'rachitic rosary' occurs as a result of expansion of the costochondral junctions.

Complications include bowing of the long bones (bone softening, especially of the lower limbs), slipped capital femoral epiphysis and irregular vertebral end plates.

Renal osteodystrophy

Chronic renal failure causes rickets as a result of failure of hydroxylation of inactive 1-hydroxy-D3 to the active 1,25-dihydroxy-D3 within the renal glomeruli. In chronic renal failure there is retention of phosphate and hypocalcaemia, which leads to parathyroid hyperplasia and secondary hyperparathyroidism. In addition there is reduced gastrointestinal absorption of calcium and end-organ resistance to parathormone. Serum phosphate and alkaline phosphatase are elevated, while serum calcium is normal or low.

Radiologically, in addition to features of rickets, those of secondary hyperparathyroidism (osteosclerosis, acro-osteolysis and subperiosteal bone resorption) are also present.

Vitamin D-dependent rickets

In these autosomal recessive conditions, vitamin D levels are not reduced. Type I is due to a defect in 1-α-hydroxylase, while in Type II vitamin D-dependent rickets there is end-organ resistance to 1,25-dihydroxy-D3. Patients may have alopecia and abnormal dentition.

Vitamin D-resistant rickets

In these disorders renal tubular re-absorption of phosphate is defective. Renal excretion of calcium and phosphate is increased. Serum vitamin D levels are normal or even elevated. X-linked hypophosphatasia, vitamin D-resistant rickets with glycosuria (defective glucose and phosphate resorption), Fanconi's syndrome (Fig. 67.47B) and acquired hypophosphataemic syndrome are the four conditions in which vitamin D-resistant or -refractory rickets may be seen.

Tumour rickets

Certain tumours are thought to secrete a phosphaturic substance with consequent elevation in urine phosphate and

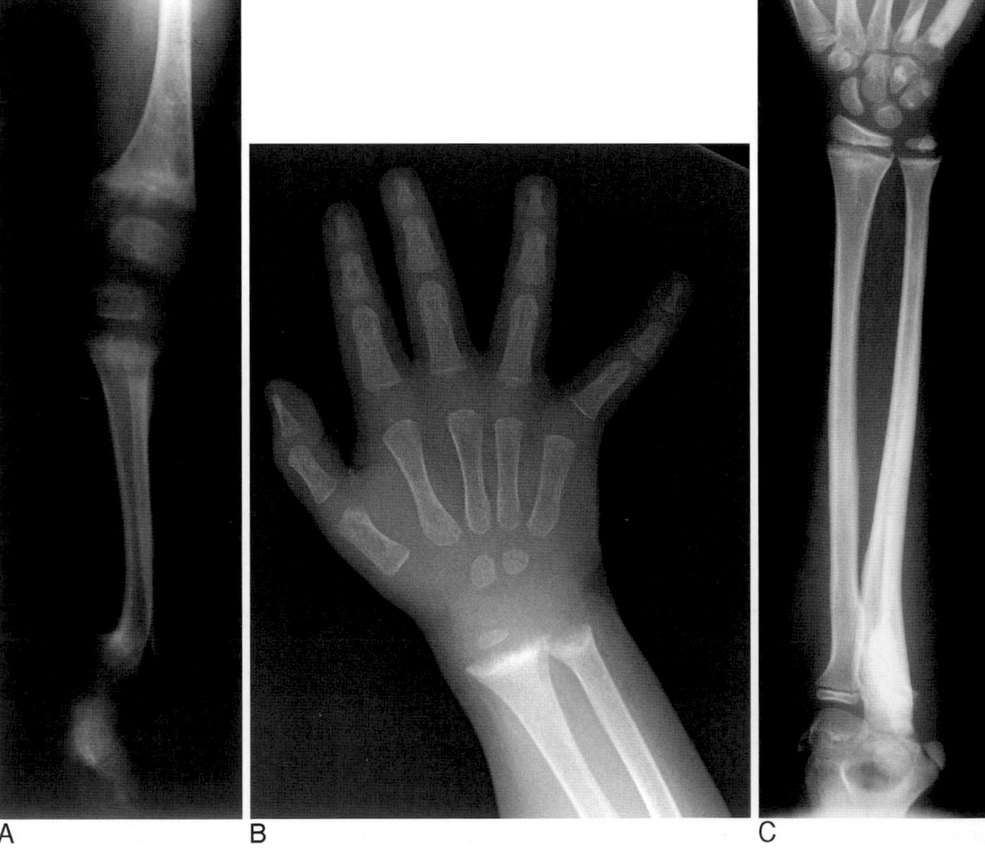

Figure 67.47 Rickets. (A) Renal osteodystrophy. (B) Child with Fanconi's disease. The dense metaphyseal band may be characteristic. (C) Linear sebaceous naevus syndrome. Note the areas of bone sclerosis.

alkaline phosphatase. Serum calcium is normal. Implicated tumours include haemangiopericytoma, linear sebaceous naevus syndrome (Fig. 67.47C), nonossifying fibroma, giant cell tumour, osteoblastoma, fibrous dysplasia and mixed sclerosing dysplasia. Resection of the tumour leads to resolution of the rickets.

Neonatal rickets

Radiographic features of neonatal rickets are not usually seen before 6 months of age. Rickets may develop in the neonate because dietary levels of calcium, phosphate, and vitamin D cannot meet the needs of a rapidly growing skeleton. Rickets occurring in preterm infants on parenteral nutrition is now relatively uncommon as a result of supplements in feeds.

Scurvy

In this condition there is deficiency (usually dietary) of vitamin C (ascorbic acid). Infants typically present between 6 and 9 months of age. There is defective osteoid production by osteoblasts with reduced endochondral bone ossification.

The bones are osteopenic with relatively dense margins (white lines of scurvy) where mineralization of osteoid continues. In the epiphyses this pencil outline is termed the 'Wimberger' sign (Fig. 67.48). Other features include metaphyseal (pelcan) spurs, which may fracture, exuberant periosteal reaction (recurrent subperiosteal bleeding), lucent metaphyseal bands and increased density of the end of the metaphyses (white line of Fraenk) (see Fig. 67.48).

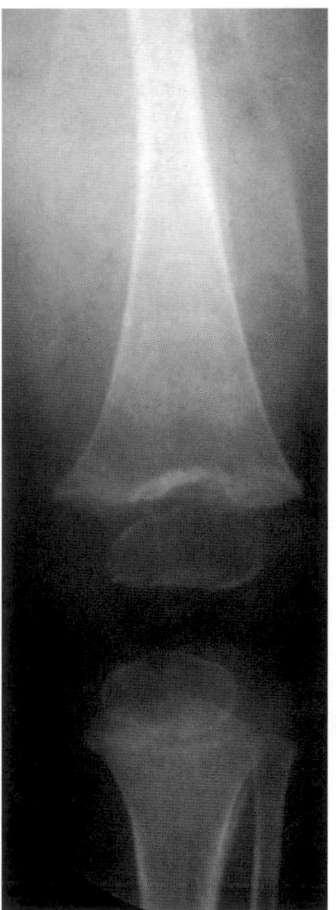

Figure 67.48 Scurvy. AP radiograph of the knee. Soft tissue calcification is seen in the walls of a large haematoma.

Gaucher's disease

This autosomal recessive storage disorder occurs most frequently in Ashkenazi Jews. The deficient enzyme is glucocerebrosidase. Glucocerebroside accumulates in the reticuloendothelial system and the bone marrow is infiltrated by lipid laden Gaucher cells. Infantile and juvenile forms are associated with mental retardation and early death. A milder adolescent form presents in childhood or early adulthood.

Radiological features include osteopenia, bone infarcts, AVN (particularly of the femoral head; Fig. 67.49A), flattening of the vertebral bodies, which may be significant (vertebra planal; Fig. 67.49B), Erlenmeyer flask deformity of the femora

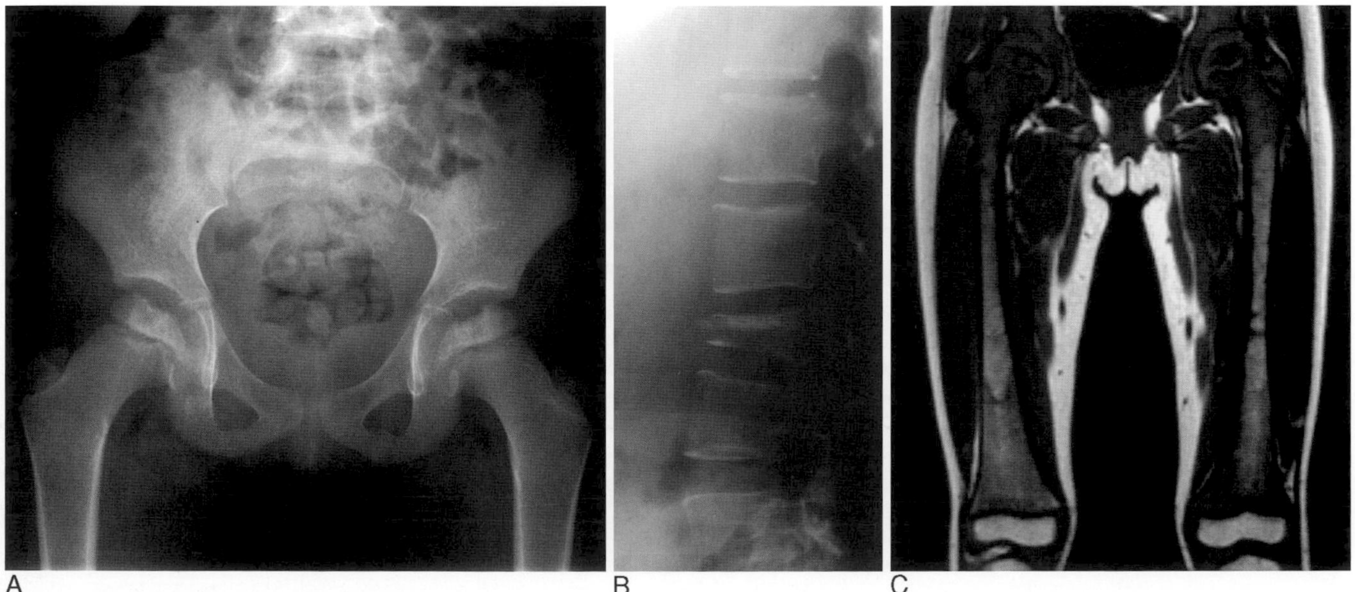

Figure 67.49 Gaucher's disease. (A) AP radiograph of the pelvis showing bilateral avascular necrosis. (B) Lateral radiograph of the spine showing vertebra plana. (C) T1-weighted coronal MRI of the femora. Note the Erlenmeyer flask deformity and marrow infiltration.

(Fig. 67.49C) and localized lytic bone lesions (focal deposition of Gaucher cells).

Radiology helps to estimate disease burden, detect skeletal complications and monitor response to treatment. In children, physiological conversion of red to yellow marrow may cause confusion when interpreting MRIs. Radiologists should be aware of the patterns of conversion of low signal red marrow to high signal fatty marrow[51,52].

ENDOCRINE DISORDERS

Hyperparathyroidism

In hyperthyroidism serum phosphate is decreased, serum calcium and alkaline phosphatase increased, and urine calcium and phosphate increased.

Primary hyperthyroidism is due to a parathyroid adenoma or may occur in multiple endocrine neoplasia and is rare in children. Secondary hyperthyroidism is seen in chronic renal failure and tertiary hyperthyroidism occurs when the parathyroid glands become resistant to the regulatory effects of serum calcium (usually in patients on haemodialysis).

Radiographs reveal features either of bone resorption and/ or bone formation. Sites of bone resorption include:

- subperiosteal (radial sides of phalanges)
- subchondral (sacroiliac joints, acromioclavicular joints, with resorption of the acromial ends of the clavicle and symphysis pubis)
- subligamentous (calcaneum at the site of insertion of the Achilles tendon)
- trabecular (diploic space causing a 'salt and pepper' skull)
- intracortical (intracortical tunnelling/striations)
- endosteal.

Additional findings include osteosclerosis (localized or diffuse), rugger-jersey spine, brown tumours, chondrocalcinosis and soft tissue and vascular calcification.

Neonatal hyperparathyroidism (Fig. 67.50) may occur as a primary disorder or as a result of poorly controlled maternal hypoparathyroidism or pseudo hypoparathyroidism. Radiological features in these infants with failure to thrive include severe osteopaenia with an increased tendency to fracture, coarse trabeculae, metaphyseal cupping and subperiosteal resorption.

Hypoparathyroidism

A reduced level of parathormone causes hypocalcaemia, hypophosphataemia and neuromuscular malfunction. It may be idiopathic or occur after surgical removal, disease, or trauma.

Radiographs demonstrate osteosclerosis, skull vault thickening, soft tissue calcification, calcification of the basal ganglia, hypoplastic dentition and thickened lamina dura. Less commonly, osteoporosis, dense metaphyseal bands, dense vertebral end plates, premature fusion of the growth plates, vertebral hyperostosis and enthesopathy may occur.

Pseudo hypoparathyroidism and pseudo pseudo hypoparathyroidism

Features in common with hypoparathyroidism include osteosclerosis, dense metaphyseal bands and calcification of the soft tissues and basal ganglia. Secondary hyperparathyroidism may be seen in 10% of patients with pseudo hypoparathyroidism (PHP), but is never seen in pseudo pseudo hypoparathyroidism (PPHP).

In PHP there is end-organ resistance to normal or increased serum levels of parathyroid hormone. Clinically there is obesity, short stature and a rounded facies. Hypocalcaemia results in muscular tetany. Radiological features include exostoses and brachydactyly [short fourth (and fifth) fingers and toes (Fig. 67.51)] with a positive metacarpal sign (a line joining the heads of the little and middle fingers fails to intersect the head of the fourth metacarpal).

Patients with PPHP have the phenotype of PHP; however, serum calcium and phosphate levels are normal. Cone-shaped epiphyses of the tubular bones of the hands and feet fuse prematurely causing brachydactyly.

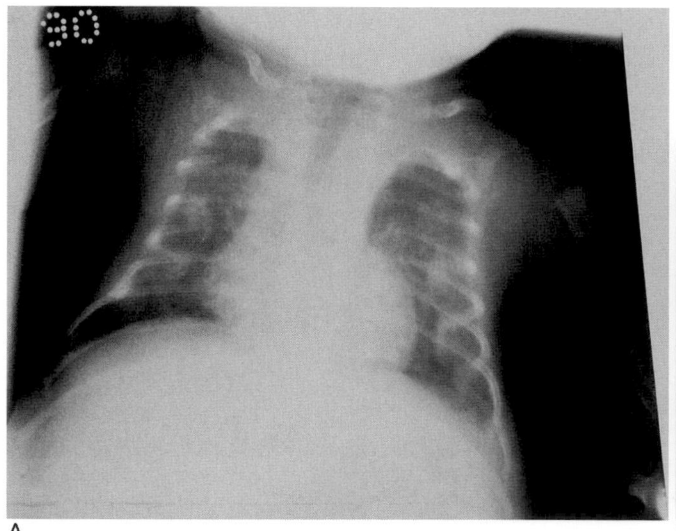

A

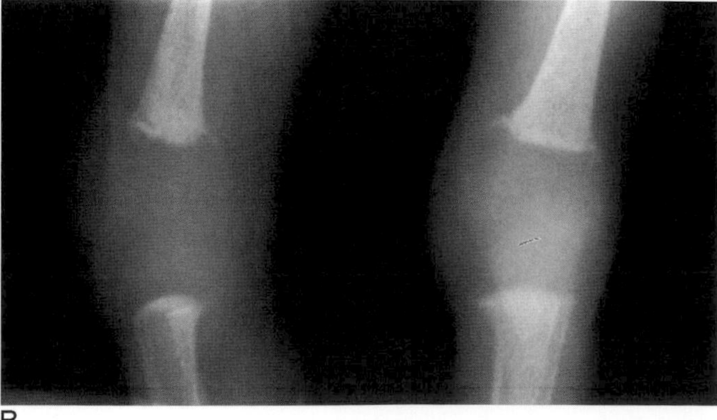

B

Figure 67.50 Neonatal hyperparathyroidism. (A) Chest radiograph showing severe osteopenia and metaphyseal spurs of both proximal humeral metaphyses. (B) AP radiograph of the knees. Note the metaphyseal spurs.

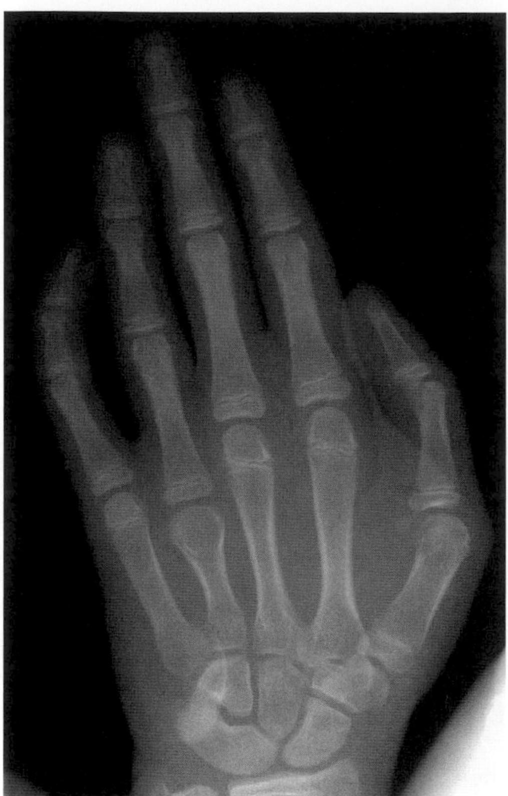

Figure 67.51 Pseudo hypoparathyroidism. AP radiograph of the hands. Note the short fourth metacarpal.

Hypothyroidism

In all types of hypothyroidism (infantile, juvenile and adult) there is either deficiency, or failure, of end-organ response to thyroxine.

Radiological features in the paediatric age group include delayed bone age, delay in appearance of secondary ossification centres, epiphyseal fragmentation, stippling and short stature. Additional findings include osteoporosis, multiple wormian bones, delay in closure of the sutures and fontanelles, delayed dentition, dense metaphyseal bands, shortened long bones, increased atlanto-axial distance, kyphosis at the thoracolumbar junction and an increased incidence of slipped capital femoral epiphysis.

TOXIC DISORDERS

Fluorosis

Although rarely seen in the UK, the incidence of all types of fluorosis in the western world is said to be increasing.

Radiologically it manifests as a generalized increase in bone density, particularly of the axial skeleton. There is periosteal proliferation, ligamentous calcification, degenerative enthesopathy and fractures. In children, exposure before the age of 8 years causes patchy opaque areas of the enamel of permanent teeth.

Lead poisoning

This manifests radiologically as dense metaphyseal bands. Other features include widened sutures (raised intracranial pressure) and radio-opacities on abdominal radiographs (ingested lead).

HAEMOGLOBINOPATHIES

Sickle cell disease

Bone pain is the most common reason for hospital admission of patients with sickle cell disease. Thromboembolic infarcts and haemolysis (with chronic anaemia and secondary marrow expansion) is the underlying pathophysiology of the skeletal complications that occur.

Acute bony involvement includes bone infarcts, osteomyelitis, stress fractures, vertebral collapse, bone marrow necrosis, orbital compression (infarction of the orbital bone) and dental complications (caries, mandibular osteomyelitis). Chronic complications include osteoporosis (secondary to marrow hyperplasia), AVN, chronic arthritis and growth failure[53].

Bone infarcts of the small bones of the hands and feet will lead to dactylitis; of the vertebral end plates to the so-called 'cod fish' or 'H-shaped' vertebrae (Fig. 67.52A); of the epiphyses will lead to joint effusions and AVN (Fig. 67.52B,C). Osteomyelitis is common, with Salmonella species being isolated in up to 70%[54]. The infection most commonly involves the diaphysis of the humerus (Fig. 67.52A), femur and tibia.

The diagnostic challenge is to differentiate acute osteomyelitis from vaso-occlusive disease. Imaging findings may be very similar. The presence of a collection or of a break in the cortex makes infection more likely than simple infarction. US-guided aspiration of subperiosteal collections is said to be useful—it not only provides a sample for laboratory examination, but decompression relieves the pain associated with both conditions[55].

Thalassaemia

Skeletal changes in thalassaemia arise from the chronic anaemia associated with the condition.

In the skull, there is widening of the diploic spaces (low signal on all MRI sequences) with thinning of the outer table of the skull vault. The trabecular markings are oriented perpendicular to the inner and outer tables and on plain radiographs this gives rise to the 'hair-on-end' appearance. There is frontal bossing and overgrowth of the facial bones with reduced pneumatization of the paranasal sinuses. The so-called 'rodent facies' arises from marrow hyperplasia in the maxillae causing lateral displacement of the orbits and ventral displacement of the central incisors[56].

In the spine there may be marked osteoporosis and cortical thinning resulting in fractures of the vertebral bodies and platyspondyly. Imaging may reveal paraspinal masses (as a result of extramedullary haematopoiesis). Cord compression can result if these masses extend into the extradural space. MRI findings are secondary to blood transfusion and chelation therapy.

There may be expansion of the head and neck of the ribs (Fig. 67.53) and osteoporosis. A rib within a rib appearance may result. Extramedullary haematopoiesis can cause erosions of the inner cortex of the ribs or manifest as a posterior mediastinal soft tissue mass.

Premature fusion of the growth plates (particularly of the proximal humerus and distal femur) is a recognized feature. Irregular sclerosis at the metaphyses and anterior rib ends is a recognized complication of treatment with desferrioxamine[57].

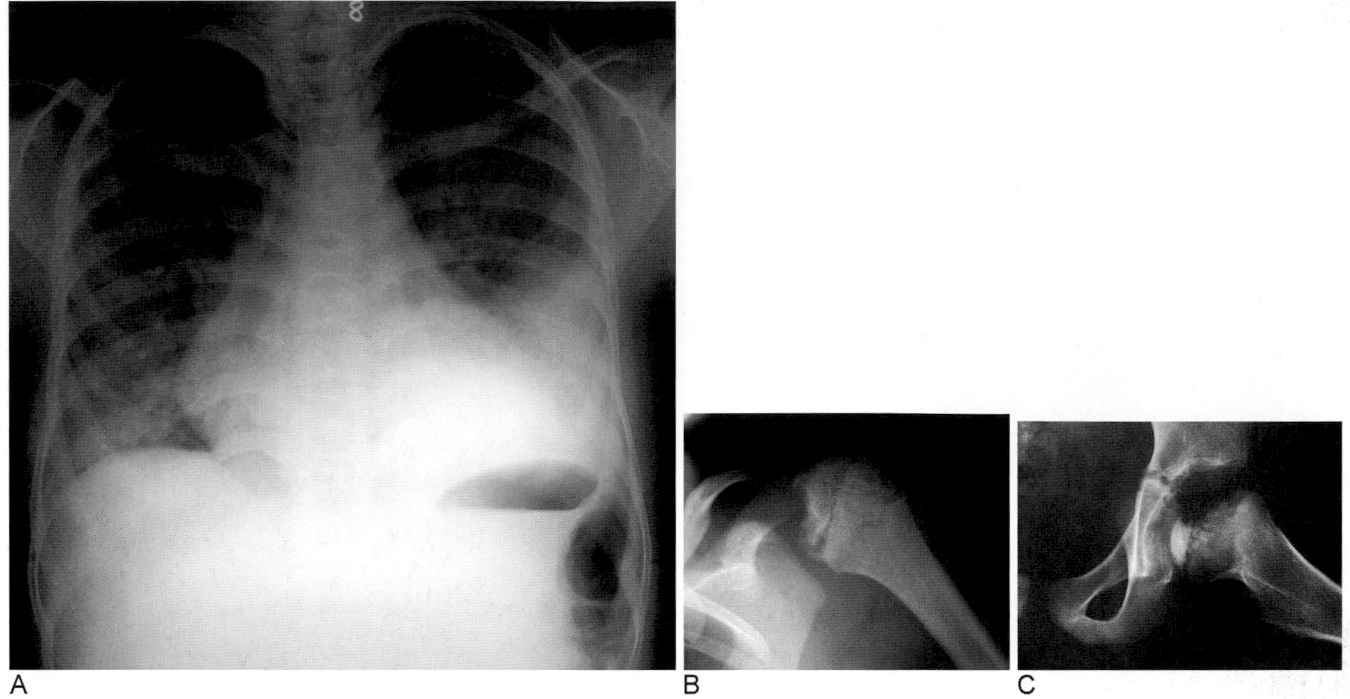

Figure 67.52 Sickle cell disease. (A) Frontal chest radiograph: heart failure, codfish vertebrae. (B,C) Radiographs of the shoulder (B) and hip (C) showing avascular necrosis.

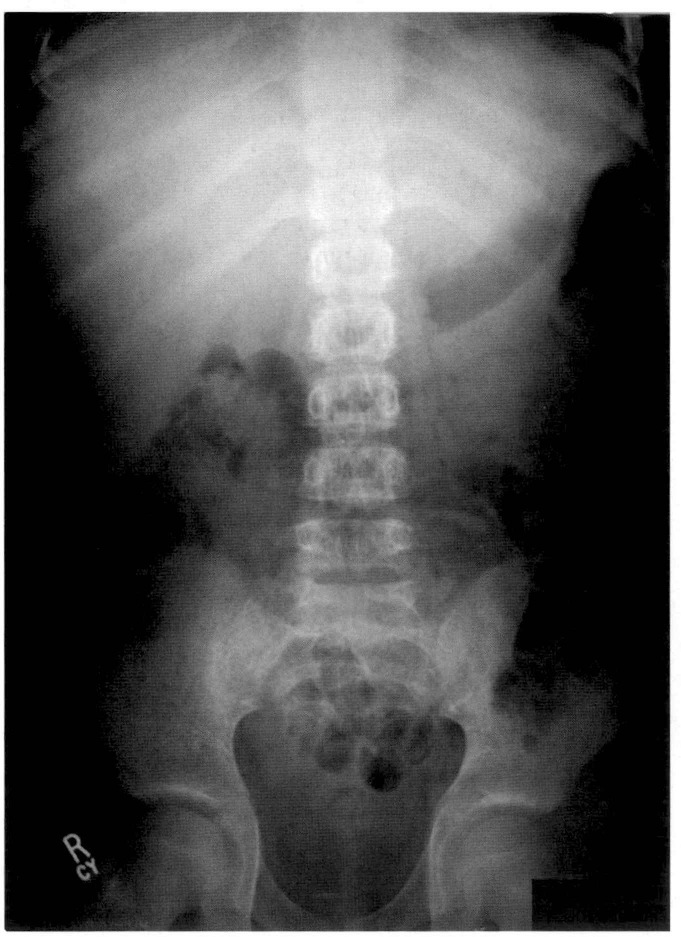

Figure 67.53 Thalassaemia. The abdomen shows coarsened trabeculae of the lumbar spine.

INFECTION OF THE BONES AND JOINTS

Osteomyelitis

Infection may reach the bone through the bloodstream (haematogenous), from direct implantation (e.g. penetrating injury, surgery), or from infection elsewhere adjacent to bone (e.g. soft tissues). Because of the rich blood supply, osteomyelitis of the long bones in children most commonly affects the metaphyses. In infants, metaphyseal vessels penetrate the growth plate, and therefore in this age group there is a higher incidence of epiphyseal and joint involvement.

Infection of the bones may be acute, subacute (Brodie's abscess), or chronic.

Acute osteomyelitis is most commonly seen in infants (*Staphylococcus aureus, Escherichia coli*) and young children (*S. aureus, Streptococcus pyogenes, Haemophilus influenzae*). Patients with sickle cell disease are more disposed to Salmonella infection. Subacute and chronic osteomyelitis result from incomplete eradication of infection following acute osteomyelitis, or from infection by less virulent organisms. Mycobacterial osteomyelitis occurs from haematogenous spread in a patient with primary tuberculosis. Fungal causes include coccidioidomycosis, bastomycosis and cryptococcosis.

In acute disease there is oedema, vascular congestion and thrombosis of small vessels. Clinical features include fever, irritability, lethargy and local signs including swelling, erythema and warmth (inflammation). If not treated promptly (or aggressively), the vascular compromise leads to areas of dead bone (sequestra), which are the hallmark of chronic infection[58]. Periosteal new bone formation is another feature of chronic osteomyelitis. This new bone (involucrum) encases areas of live bone. Pus may track from the medullary cavity through gaps in the involucrum into the soft tissues. These tracks may eventually penetrate the skin surface (sinus tracts).

Radiographic changes (Fig. 67.54A,B) may not be apparent for up to 2 weeks after the onset of disease, and therefore radiographs may appear entirely normal. More specific signs include soft tissue swelling, cortical irregularity (bony destruction) and periosteal reaction. A Brodie's abscess may be seen as a well-defined lytic lesion with a sclerotic rim. In chronic infection sequestra appear as dense foci, and soft tissue wasting and sinus tracts may be appreciated. Even on appropriate therapy, radiographic signs of improvement may lag behind clinical recovery. Spina ventosa implies tuberculous dactylitis. Radiographically there are cyst-like cavities associated with diaphyseal expansion. It more commonly affects the bones of the hands than the feet[59].

High-resolution US provides a simple and noninvasive assessment of infants and children with osteomyelitis. US helps to localize the site and extent of disease, and to confirm the presence and degree of the fluid component of the abscess, and provides guidance for interventional procedures. Chau and Griffiths[60] provide a useful review of the US appearances of musculoskeletal infection.

Skeletal scintigraphy is useful if multifocal infection is suspected.

CT helps to define the extent of cortical destruction and to exclude the presence of sequestra.

MRI (Fig. 67.54C,D) has the highest sensitivity and specificity for detecting osteomyelitis in children[61]. In subacute

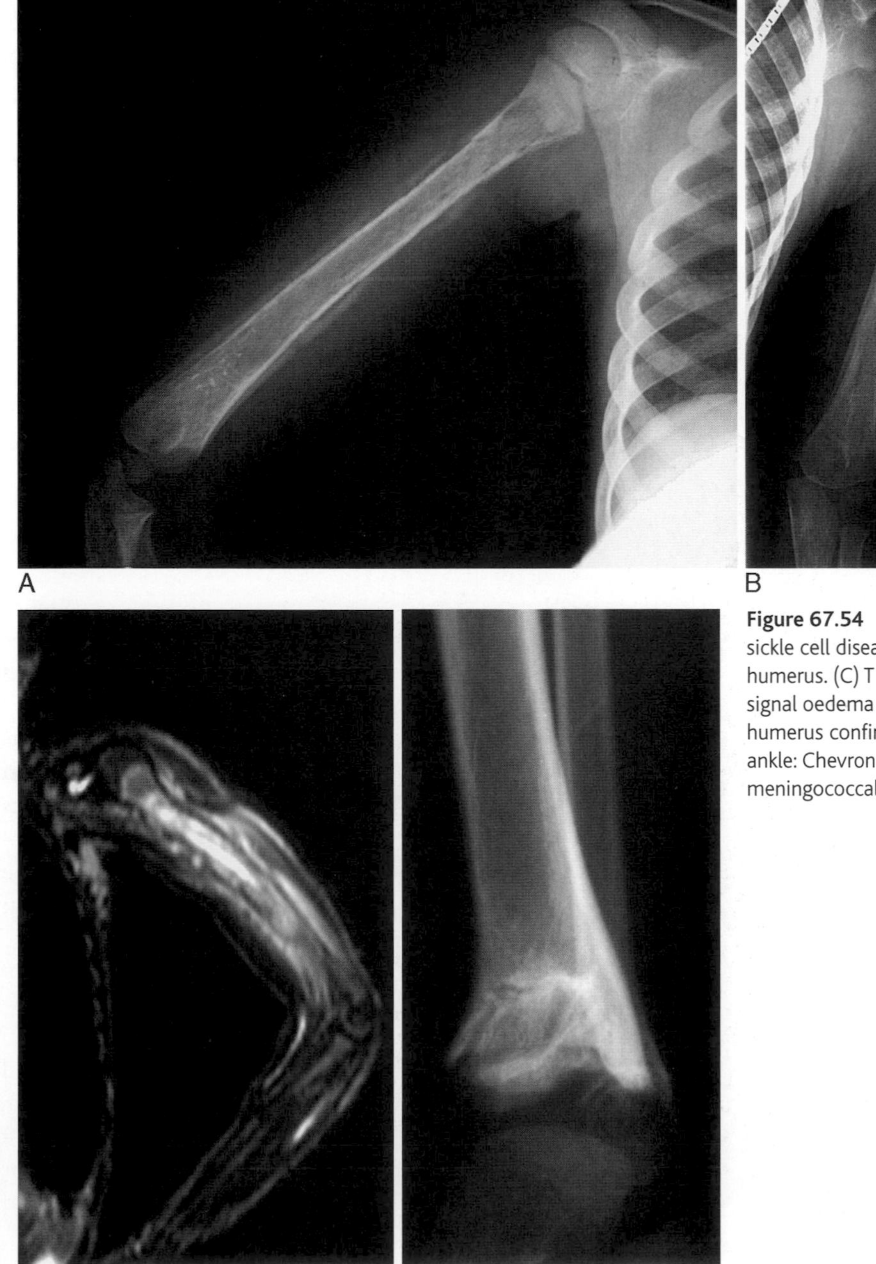

Figure 67.54 Osteomyelitis. (A) Right humerus in a patient with sickle cell disease. (B–D) Same patient. (B) Radiograph of the left humerus. (C) T1-weighted coronal MRI of the humerus showing low signal oedema in the medullary cavity. (D) Coronal STIR MRI of the humerus confirming marrow and soft tissue oedema. (E) Lateral ankle: Chevron deformity of the distal tibial metaphysis following meningococcal septicaemia.

infection a characteristic penumbra sign may be recognized[62]. This consists of a peripheral relatively high signal ring (granulation tissue) surrounding a low signal central zone (abscess cavity). Enhanced fat-suppressed sequences show avid enhancement of the granulation tissue. Contrast medium also helps to identify soft tissue abscesses. On T2-weighted sequences the high signal of reactive oedema may exaggerate the extent of infection.

Complications include joint destruction and damage to growth plates (Fig. 67.54E) resulting in limb length discrepancies, angular deformities and early osteoarthritis.

Chronic recurrent multifocal osteomyelitis

This is a condition of unknown aetiology characterized by a fluctuating clinical course of relapses and remissions. It affects multiple sites (synchronous or metachronous) and most commonly involves the long bones, clavicle, spine and pelvis. The ribs and sternum may also be affected. No causative agent is found. When associated with acne and palmoplanter pustulosis it is termed SAPHO syndrome.

Radiographic features (Fig. 67.55A,B) suggest subacute or chronic osteomyelitis; however, abscess formation, involucra, and sinus tracts are not a feature. In the tubular bones lytic

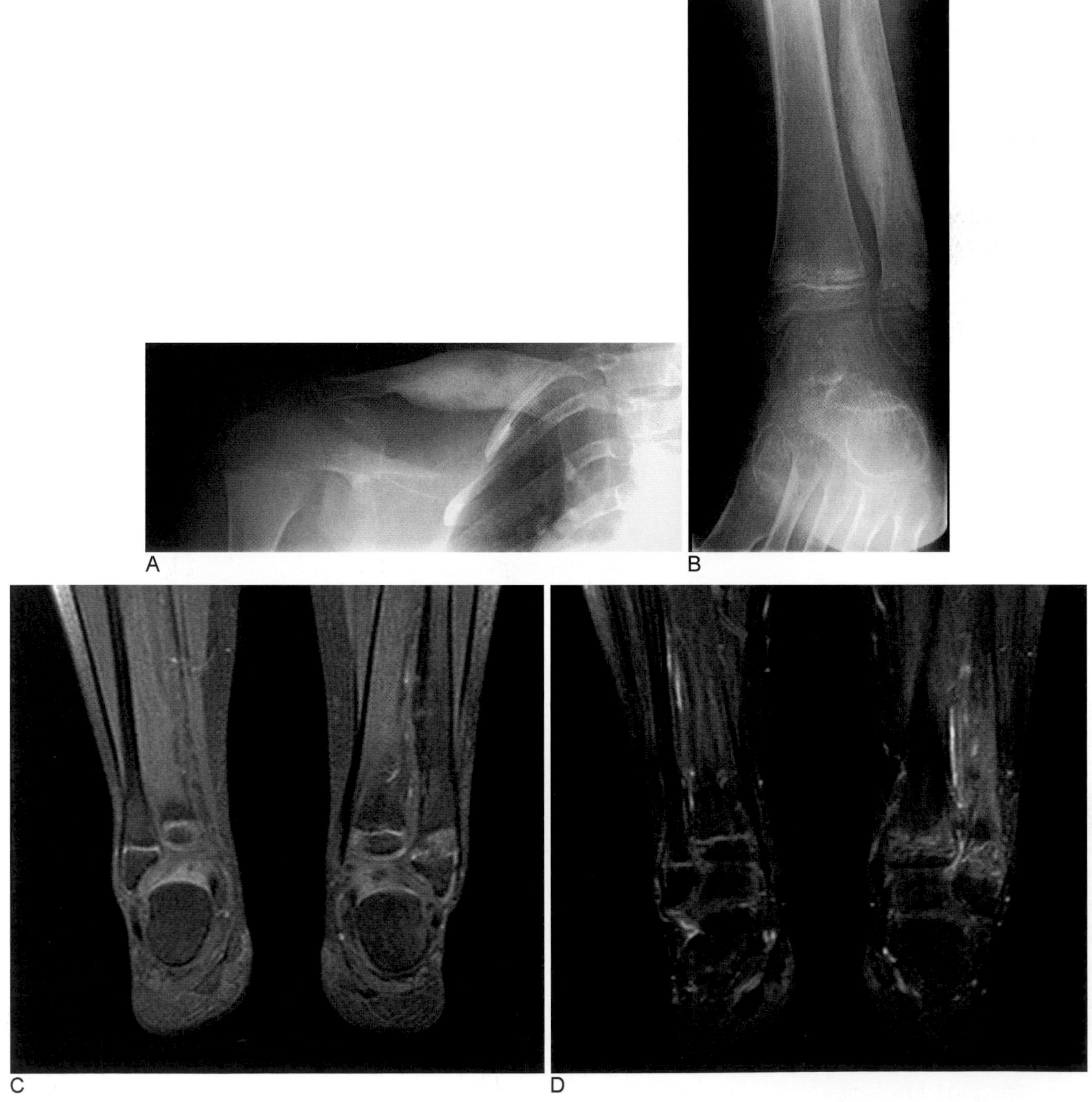

Figure 67.55 Chronic recurrent multifocal osteomyelitis. (A,B) Hyperostosis of (A) the right clavicle (the left was similarly affected) and (B) the left fibula. (C) T1-weighted coronal MRI showing hyperostosis of the left fibula. (D) Coronal STIR MRI confirming active disease in the left fibula.

metaphyseal lesions sometimes extending to the diaphysis are typical. Quiescent periods are characterized by bony expansion and sclerosis. In the clavicle, lytic medullary lesions are a feature of active disease, with expansion and sclerosis again being features of a quiescent phase. Chronic recurrent multifocal osteomyelitis (CRMO) manifests in the spine as loss of height of the affected vertebral bodies and is a differential diagnosis of vertebra plana.

Bone scintigraphy is useful for the detection of asymptomatic lesions. MRI, by failing to demonstrate abscesses and sinus tracts, excludes chronic osteomyelitis. Active disease is confirmed by the presence of high signal marrow on T2/STIR sequences (Fig. 67.55C,D).

Infective arthritis

As with osteomyelitis, infection may spread to joints via the bloodstream, direct inoculation, or spread from a contiguous site. The most common organism is *S. aureus*. Radiographic features (Fig. 67.56A,B) include soft tissue swelling, oedema and joint effusion. In infants, effusions may lead to dislocation (particularly in the hip joint). Other findings include metaphyseal irregularity and destruction. Septic arthritis in children is a clinical emergency, and early drainage is required to prevent severe bony destruction with resultant shortening and deformity. In this regard US (Fig. 67.56C) is helpful, both to exclude the presence of an effusion (a difference of 1–2 mm between the two sides is suggestive) and to assist in its drainage.

Infection of the spine (discitis and osteomyelitis)

Discitis refers to infection of the intervertebral disc space, whereas osteomyelitis of the spine implies pyogenic destruction of the vertebral body, which may then spread to involve the disc. Differentiation of the two is important, as management may differ. Discitis can involve any spinal level, but most commonly affects the lumbar region in children younger than 5 years of age[63]. Generally children with discitis are younger, and clinically less toxic than those with osteomyelitis[64]. Children with either condition will present with back pain, refusal to mobilize, or irritability depending on age at presentation. Although there is much debate as to the aetiology of discitis, a low-grade infection has been postulated. In 70% of cases, the causative organism is not identified. When an organism is cultured, it is most commonly *S. aureus*. In discitis, radiological changes are confined to the disc and adjacent vertebral end plates, in comparison to osteomyelitis, in which the disease begins in and destroys the vertebral body. Infection may then spread to an adjacent vertebral body either via the intervertebral disc or via the subligamentous spread of pus (e.g. in spinal tuberculosis).

In discitis, radiographs/CT of the spine (Fig. 67.57A) show characteristic features, including loss of disc height and irregularity of the adjacent vertebral end plates. Vertebral body height is preserved. It has been suggested that in the clinical context of suspected discitis, further imaging is not required if the radiographs demonstrate characteristic findings. However, if radiographs are normal or equivocal, or the child is toxic (suggesting spinal osteomyelitis), then further imaging is indicated[61].

MRI (with a sensitivity and specificity of 96% and 93%, respectively) is the next investigation (Fig. 67.57B) and can exclude intraspinal or other soft tissue (e.g. psoas) collections. T1 sagittal and axial and T2 sagittal views are often sufficient. In

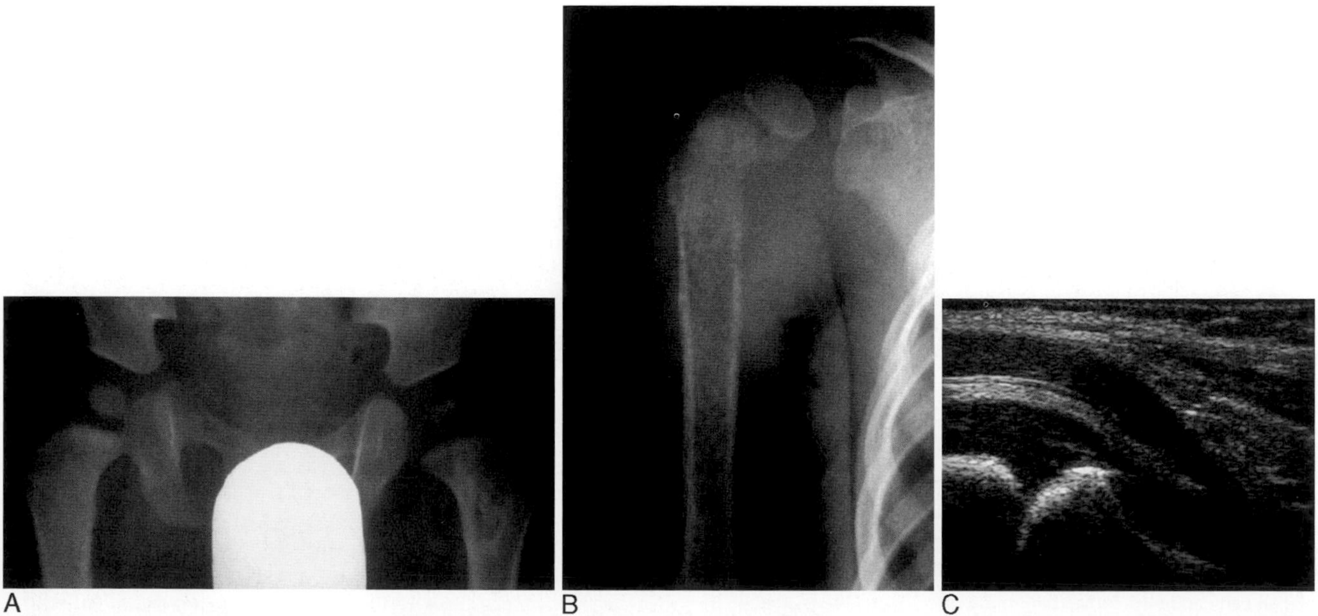

Figure 67.56 Infective arthritis. (A) AP radiograph of the pelvis. There is a lytic lesion of the left proximal metaphysis with irregularity and reduced size of the left capital femoral epiphysis. (B) Right shoulder. Osteomyelitis of the humerus is complicated by septic arthritis and a dislocated shoulder. (C) Ultrasound of the hip confirms the presence of an effusion.

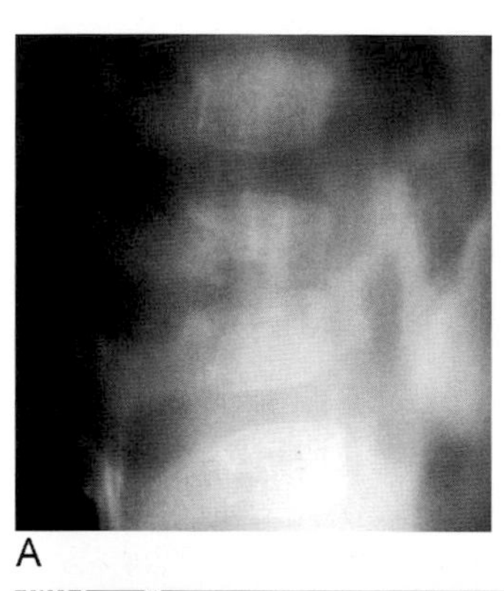

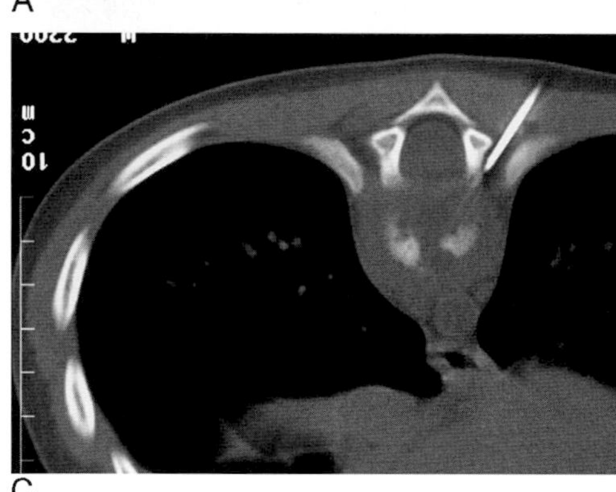

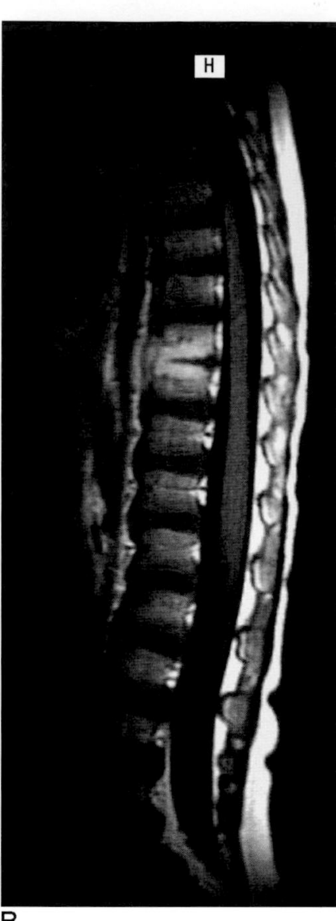

Figure 67.57 Discitis. (A) Conventional tomogram showing irregular and indistinct end plates at the affected level with narrowing of the disc space. (B) Sagittal T1-weighted MRI showing enhancement of the end plates with a small anterior collection. (C) Axial CT obtained during prone guided biopsy of the affected disc.

equivocal cases, intravenous administration of contrast medium may be helpful. The pattern of enhancement is said to aid in differentiating tuberculous spondylitis (avid, heterogeneous rim enhancement, involving several vertebral bodies) from vertebral osteomyelitis[65]. However, regardless of the pattern of enhancement, tissue should be obtained for microbiological examination, usually by CT-guided biopsy (Fig. 67.57C).

REFERENCES

1. Hall C M 2001 International nosology and classification of constitutional disorders of bone. Am J Med Genet 113: 65–77
2. Offiah A C, Hall C M 2003 Radiological diagnosis of the constitutional disorders of bone. As easy as A, B, C? Pediatr Radiol 33: 153–161
3. Radiological electronic atlas for malformation syndromes (REAMS). Oxford University Press, Oxford, 2000
4. Cho T-J, Choi H I, Chung C Y et al 2000 The Sprengel deformity: Morphometric analysis using 3D-CT and its clinical relevance. J Bone Joint Surg (Br) 82-B: 711–718
5. Kawashima T, Uhthoff H K 1990 Development of the foot in prenatal life in relation to idiopathic club foot. J Pediatr Orthop 10: 232–237
6. Farrell S A, Summers A M, Dallaire L et al 1999 Clubfoot, an adverse outcome of early amniocentesis: disruption or deformation? CEMAT, Canadian Early and Mid-Trimester Amniocentesis Trial. J Med Genet 36: 843–846
7. Wiig O, Svenningsen S, Terjesen T 2004 Evaluation of the subchondral fracture in predicting the extent of femoral head necrosis in Perthes disease: a prospective study of 92 patients. J Pediatr Orthop B 13: 293–298
8. Catterall A 1971 The natural history of Legg-Calve-Perthes disease. J Bone Joint Surg (Br) 53: 37–53
9. Salter R B, Thompson G H 1984 Legg-Calve-Perthes disease. The prognostic significance of the subchondral fracture and a two group classification of the femoral head involvement. J Bone Joint Surg Am 66: 479–489
10. Herring J A, Neustadt J B, Williams J J, Early J S, Browne R H 1992. The lateral pillar classification of Legg-Calve-Perthes disease. J Pediatr Orthop 12: 143–150
11. Wiig O, Terjesen T, Svenningsen S 2002 Interobserver reliability of radiographic classifications and measurements in the assessment of Perthes disease. Acta Orthop Scand 73: 523–530
12. Eggl H, Drekonja T, Kaiser B, Dorn U 1999 Ultrasonography in the diagnosis of transient synovitis of the hip and Legg-Calve-Perthés disease. J Pediatr Orthop B 8: 177–180
13. Lahdes-Vasama T, Lamminen A, Merikanto J, Marttinen E 1997 The value of MRI in early Perthes' disease: an MRI study with a 2-year follow-up. Pediatr Radiol 27: 517–522
14. Mahnken A H, Staatz G, Ihme N, Gunther R W 2002 MR signal intensity characteristics in Legg-Calve-Perthés disease. Value of fat-suppressed (STIR) images and contrast-enhanced T1-weighted images Acta Radiol 43: 329–335
15. Sebag G, Ducou Le Pointe H, Klein I et al 1997 Dynamic gadolinium-enhanced subtraction MR imaging—a simple technique for the early diagnosis of Legg-Calve-Perthés disease: preliminary results. Pediatr Radiol 27: 216–220
16. Lamer S, Dorgeret S, Khairouni A et al 2002 Femoral head vascularisation in Legg–Calve–Perthés disease: comparison of dynamic

gadolinium-enhanced subtraction MRI with bone scintigraphy. Pediatr Radiol 32: 580–585
17. Loder R T 2001 Unstable slipped capital femoral epiphyses. J Pediatr Orthop 21: 694–699
18. Loder R T 1996 The demographics of slipped capital femoral epiphysis: An international multicenter study. Clin Orthop Relat Res 322: 8–27
19. Loder R T, Wittenberg B, DeSilva G 1995 Slipped capital femoral epiphysis associated with endocrine disorders. J Pediatr Orthop 15: 349–356
20. Wells D, King J D, Roe T F, Kaufman F R 1993 Review of slipped capital femoral epiphysis associated with endocrine disease. J Pediatr Orthop 13: 610–614
21. Southwick W O 1967 Osteotomy through the lesser trochanter for slipped capital femoral epiphysis. J Bone Joint Surg Am 49: 807–835
22. Boyer D W, Mickelson M R, Ponsetti I V 1981 Slipped capital femoral epiphysis. Long-term follow-up study of one hundred and twenty-one patients. J Bone Joint Surg Am 63: 85–95
23. Kallio P E, Paterson D C, Foster B K et al 1993 Classification in slipped capital femoral epiphysis. Sonographic assessment of stability and remodelling. Clin Orthop 294: 196–203
24. Scoliosis Research Society 1976 A glossary of scoliosis terms. Spine 1: 57–58
25. Reamy B V, Slakey J B 2001 Adolescent idiopathic scoliosis: Review and current concepts. Am Fam Physician 64: 111–116
26. Miller N H, Justice C M, Marosy B et al 2005 Identification of candidate regions for familial idiopathic scoliosis. Spine 30: 1181–1187
27. Lonstein J E, Carlson J M 1984 The prediction of curve progression in untreated idiopathic scoliosis during growth. J Bone Joint Surg Am 66: 1061–1071
28. Oestrich A E, Young L W, Young Poussaint T 1998 Scoliosis circa 2000: radiologic imaging perspective I. Diagnosis and pre-treatment evaluation. Skeletal Radiol 27: 591–605
29. Vitale M G, Guha A, Skaggs D L 2002 Orthopaedic manifestations of neurofibromatosis in children: an update. Clin Orthop Aug: 107–118
30. Jacquemin C, Bosley T M, Liu D, et al 2002 Reassessment of sphenoid dysplasia associated with neurofibromatosis type 1. Am J Neuroradiol 23: 644–648
31. Casper K A, Donnelly L F, Chan B et al 2002 Tuberous sclerosis complex: renal imaging findings. Radiology 225: 451–456
32. Morris B S, Garg A, Jadhav P J 2002 Tuberous sclerosis: a presentation of less commonly encountered stigmata. Australas Radiol 46: 426–430
33. Petty R E, Southwood T R, Baum J et al 1998 Revision of the proposed classification criteria for juvenile idiopathic arthritis: Durban, 1997. J Rheumatol 25: 1991–1994
34. Adib N, Owers K L, Witt J D, Owens C M, Woo P, Murray K J 2005 Isolated inflammatory coxitis with protrusio acetabuli: a new form of juvenile idiopathic arthritis? Rheumatology (Oxf) 44: 219–226
35. Davidson J 2000 Juvenile idiopathic arthritis: A clinical review. Eur J Radiol 33: 128–134
36. Ravelli A, Martini A 2003 Early predictors of outcome in juvenile idiopathic arthritis. Clin Exp Rheumatol 21: S89–S93
37. Garland D E, Lewonowski K, Adkins R H, Stewart C A 1993 Visual versus quantified digital radiographic determination of bone density. Contemp Orthop 26: 591–595
38. Lamer S, Sebag G H 2000 MRI and ultrasound in children with juvenile chronic arthritis. Eur J Radiol 33: 85–93
39. Stevens K, Tao C, Lee S-U et al 2003 Subchondral fractures in osteonecrosis of the femoral head: comparison of radiography, CT and MR imaging. Am J Roentgenol 180: 363–368
40. Brody A S, Strong M, Babikian G et al 1991 Avascular necrosis: early MR imaging and histological findings in a canine model. Am J Roentgenol 157: 341–345
41. Sebag G, Ducou Le Pointe H, Klein I et al 1997 Dynamic gadolinium-enhanced subtraction MR imaging—a simple technique for the early diagnosis of Legg-Calve-Perthe's disease: preliminary results. Pediatr Radiol 27: 216–220
42. Bohan A, Peter J B 1975 Polymyositis and dermatomyositis (part 2). N Engl J Med 292: 403–407
43. Ruperto N, Ravelli A, Murray K J et al 2003 Preliminary core sets of measures for disease activity and damage assessment in juvenile systemic lupus erythematosus and juvenile dermatomyositis. Rheumatology (Oxf) 42: 1452–1459
44. Maillard S M, Jones R, Owens C et al 2004 Quantitative assessment of MRI T2 relaxation time of thigh muscles in juvenile dermatomyositis. Rheumatology 43: 603–608
45. Kerr R 2003 Imaging of the musculoskeletal complications of hemophilia. Semin Musculoskelet Radiol 7: 127–136
46. Arnold W D, Hilgartner M W 1977 Hemophilic arthropathy. Current concepts of pathogenesis and management. J Bone Joint Surg 59A: 287–305
47. Kilcoyne R F, Nuss R 2003 Radiological assessment of haemophilic arthropathy with emphasis on MRI findings. Haemophilia 9 (suppl 1): 57–63
48. Lundin B, Babyn P, Doria A S et al 2005 Compatible scales for progressive and additive MRI assessments of haemophilic arthropathy. Haemophilia 11: 109–115
49. Doria A S, Lundin B, Kilcoyne R F et al 2005 Reliability of progressive and additive MRI scoring systems for evaluation of haemophilic arthropathy in children: expert MRI Working Group of the International Prophylaxis Study Group. Haemophilia 11: 245–253
50. Masih S, Antebi A 2003 Imaging of pigmented villonodular synovitis. Semin Musculoskelet Radiol 7: 205–216
51. Maas M, Poll W L, Terk M R 2002 Imaging and quantifying skeletal involvement in Gaucher disease. Br J Radiol 75 (suppl 1): A13–A24
52. Bembi B, Ciana G, Mengel E et al 2002 Bone complications in children with Gaucher disease. Br J Radiol 75 (suppl 1): A37–A44
53. Almeida A, Roberts I 2005 Bone involvement in sickle cell disease. Br J Haematol 129: 482–490
54. Bennet O M, Namnyak S S 1990 Bone and joint manifestations of sickle cell anaemia. J Bone Joint Surg Br 72: 494–499
55. Booz M M, Hariharan V, Aradi A J, Malki A A 1999 The value of ultrasound and aspiration in differentiating vaso-occlusive crisis and osteomyelitis in sickle cell disease patients. Clin Radiol 54: 636–639
56. Tunaci M, Tunaci A, Engin G 1999 Imaging features of thalassaemia. Eur Radiol 9: 1804–1808
57. Chan Y-L, Pang L-M, Chik K-W, Cheng JCY, Li C-K 2002 Patterns of bone disease in transfusion-dependent homozygous thalassaemia major: predominance of osteoporosis and desferrioxamine-induced bone dysplasia. Pediatr Radiol 32: 492–497
58. Lazzarini L, Mader J T, Calhoun J H 2004 Osteomyelitis in long bones. J Bone Joint Surg (Am) 86: 2305–2318
59. Andronikou S, Smith B 2002 Spina ventosa—tuberculous dactylitis. Arch Dis Child 86: 206
60. Chau C L F, Griffith J F 2005 Musculoskeletal infections: ultrasound appearances. Clin Radiol 60: 149–159
61. Jorulf K S, Hirsch G 1998 Clinical value of imaging technique in childhood osteomyelitis. Acta Radiol 39: 523–531
62. Davies A M, Grimer R 2005 The penumbra sign in subacute osteomyelitis. Eur Radiol 15: 1268–1270
63. Early S D, Kay R M, Tolo V T 2003 Childhood diskitis. J Am Acad Orthop Surg 11: 413– 420
64. Fernandez M, Carrol C L, Baker C J 2000 Discitis and vertebral osteomyelitis in children: An 18-year review. Pediatrics 105: 1299–1304
65. Arizono T, Oga M, Shiota E, Honda K, Sugioka Y 1995 Differentiation of vertebral osteomyelitis and tuberculous spondylitis by magnetic resonance imaging. Int Orthop 19: 319–322

CHAPTER 68

Paediatric Musculoskeletal Trauma and the Radiology of Nonaccidental Injury

William H. Ramsden and Padma Rao

PAEDIATRIC MUSCULOSKELETAL TRAUMA

William H. Ramsden

FRACTURES

Greenstick (Fig. 68.1) and torus (Fig. 68.2) injuries are both incomplete fractures which commonly occur in children. The bone cortex and periosteum break on the convex side of a greenstick fracture, whilst a torus fracture is diagnosed when the cortex buckles on its concave side.

When a long bone bends, rather than breaks, this is known as plastic bowing (Fig. 68.3). It manifests as a subtle increase in curvature rather than a discrete fracture, but histologically multiple oblique microfractures are present at the site of greatest compression[1]. The forearm bones are most often affected and the fracture may be difficult to appreciate acutely. In addition, the 'clue' of periosteal new bone formation may not be visualized during the early healing phase[2]. It is unusual for balanced forces to cause plastic bowing of both forearm bones and the nonbowed bone may fracture or dislocate.

STRESS AND OVERUSE INJURIES

Children may develop similar stress injuries to adults, due to repeated forces acting upon a bone that are less than the force needed to fracture it acutely. In childhood the tibia is most often affected (Fig. 68.4), with significant numbers of fibular and metatarsal fractures[3].

The stresses that lead to sports-related injuries in children elicit a different response from the developing skeleton than that seen in adults. In children the main sites affected are the growth plates, muscle insertions and apophyses. Avulsion injuries are responsible for the latter two sites, and are most common around the pelvis and elbow[4].

Plain radiographs are the initial imaging investigation in both stress and avulsion injuries, and the former may be investigated by both radionuclide radiology and magnetic resonance imaging (MRI). MRI sequences that are particularly sensitive for oedema, such as inversion recovery (STIR), may show widespread changes in bone surrounding a stress injury. This should not deflect the clinician from the diagnosis if clinical circumstances and imaging appearances are otherwise appropriate.

EPIPHYSEAL INJURIES

Epiphyseal separations are often the most challenging childhood fractures to investigate. It is important to understand normal epiphyseal anatomy, so that injuries may be detected and normal growth plates correctly identified. The best example of this is at the elbow joint, where epiphyses both appear and fuse in a known sequence.

Epiphyseal injuries are grouped according to the Salter–Harris classification (Fig. 68.5), an important guide to both

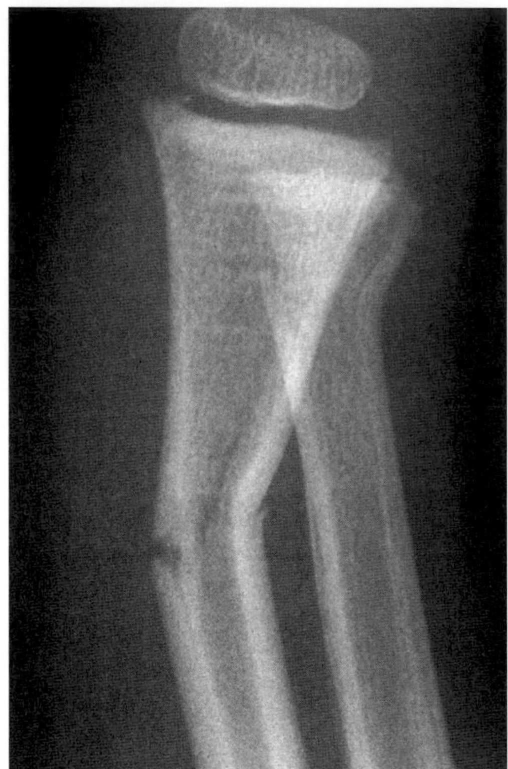

Figure 68.1 Greenstick fractures of the distal radius and ulna.

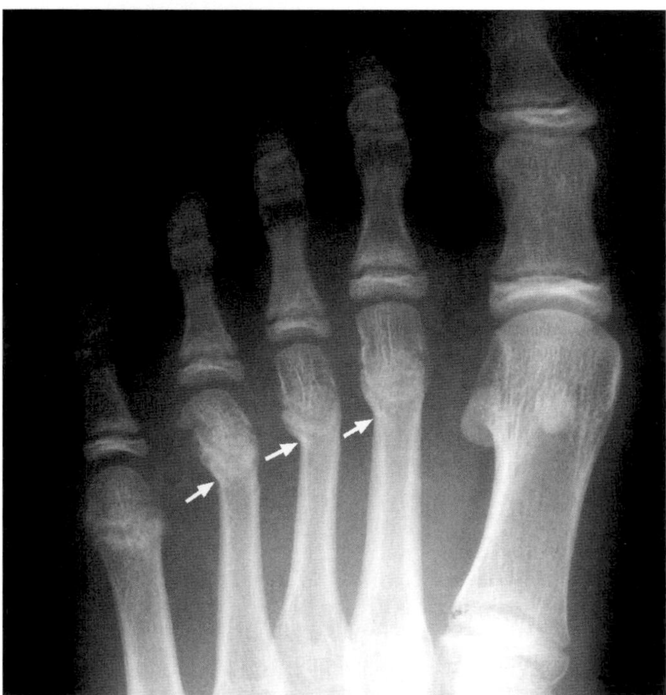

Figure 68.2 Torus fractures (arrows) of the necks of the second, third and fourth metatarsals.

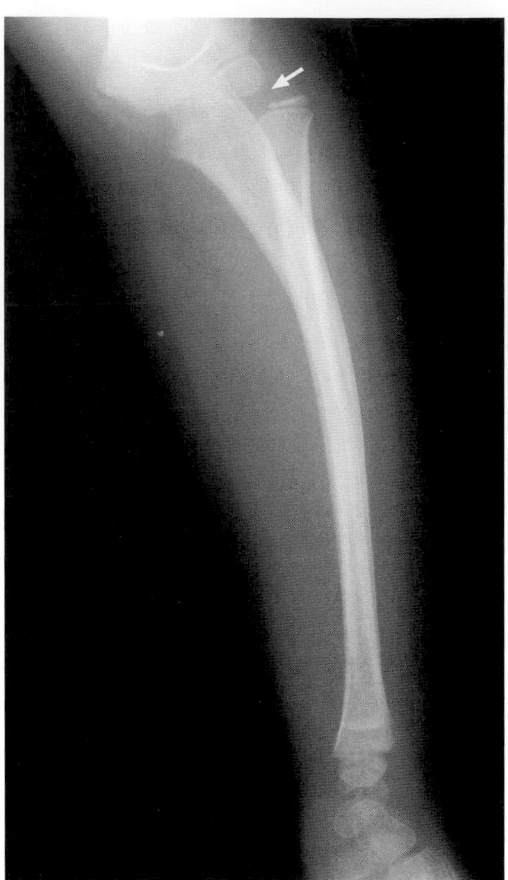

Figure 68.3 Plastic bowing of the ulna with dislocation of the radial head (arrow).

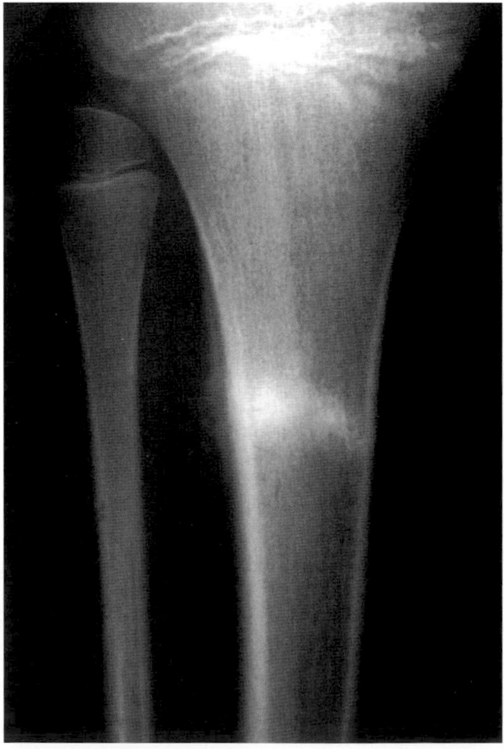

Figure 68.4 Healing stress fracture of the proximal tibia.

treatment and the prognosis of any particular fracture. The grading of injuries runs from I to V, becoming more serious as the numeral rises.

In Types I and II, the epiphysis remains intact and these injuries generally have a good prognosis. This contrasts with Types III and IV, where the epiphysis itself is fractured. The Type V fracture is a very rare crushing injury of the physeal cartilage and is more commonly seen in association with Types I–IV injuries than in isolation. Growth disturbance is the main complication that can occur and tends to be more severe with the higher grades. In spite of this classification, prognosis is worse in the lower limb for all grades.

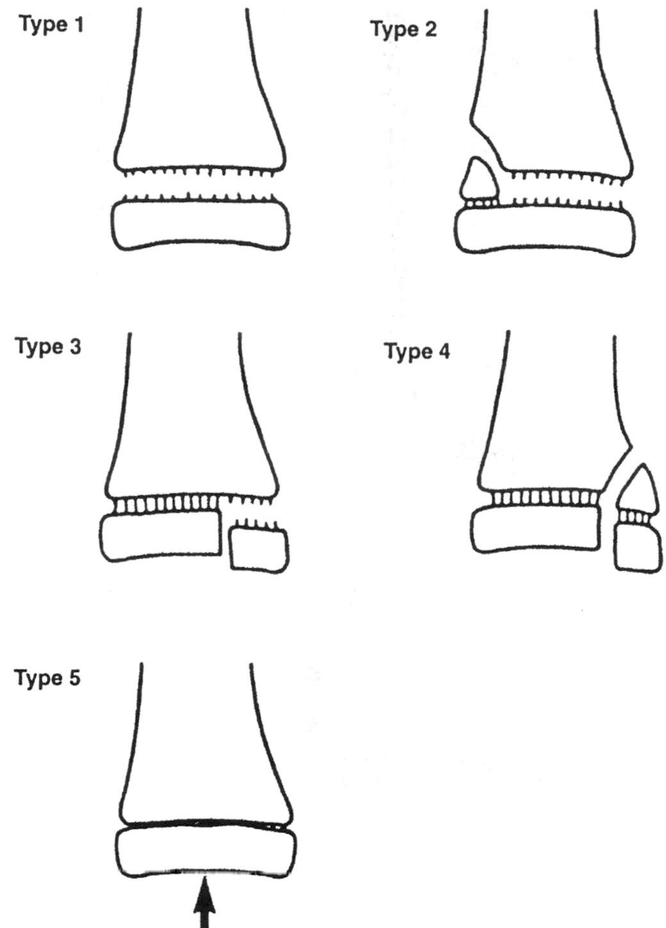

Figure 68.5 Salter–Harris classification of fractures involving the epiphyseal plate. [From Carty H (ed) 1999 Emergency pediatric radiology. Springer-Verlag, Berlin.]

Although plain radiographs are the sole imaging method required in the majority of epiphyseal injuries, computed tomography (CT) is useful in planning complex fracture treatment, and MRI is becoming increasingly important in evaluating more difficult cases.

MRI is used to visualize nonossified growth plate cartilage, and in very young children the nonossified epiphysis itself. It allows visualization of any associated soft tissue or ligamentous injury, the latter often accompanying epiphyseal injuries at the knee. Although the STIR sequence rapidly localizes injury, conventional spin-echo sequences are needed to separate bone bruises and true fractures. Gradient-echo sequences are particularly good at demonstrating the growth plate as hyperintense compared to surrounding bone.

UPPER LIMB INJURIES

Clavicle and proximal humeral fractures

The clavicle is the bone most commonly injured at birth and the main associated risk factors are heavy neonates and shoulder dystocia. There is also a risk of brachial plexus damage, although both this and the bony injury generally heal uneventfully. Clavicular fractures are common in childhood, usually due to falling onto an outstretched hand. The most common fracture type is a greenstick injury centred upon the middle third of the bone.

Acromioclavicular joint separation is uncommon in children due to the relative strength of the associated ligaments, and in young children the normal joint may often look 'wide'. In dislocation of the sternoclavicular joint the medial clavicle is usually displaced anteriorly, but it is the rarer posterior dislocation that is potentially the more serious, because of the proximity of underlying vessels. In such a situation, CT is the imaging method of choice.

Although fractures involving the proximal humeral growth plate account for a small minority of physeal injuries, they may have important consequences as this area contributes 80% to the bone's longitudinal growth. However, it needs to be noted that the normal proximal humeral growth plate has an irregular contour on a standard antero-posterior (AP) radiograph, which may be mistaken for a fracture.

Transverse and torus fractures of the proximal humeral metaphysis may also occur, most commonly around the surgical neck.

Simple bone cysts are frequently found in this area and pathological fractures often occur. Plain radiographs in the latter situation may demonstrate a characteristic 'fallen fragment sign' as cortical bone lies within a fluid-filled cavity.

Distal humeral and elbow trauma

The six epiphyses surrounding the elbow joint appear and fuse in a predictable sequence commencing with that of the capitellum, followed by the radial head, medial epicondyle of the humerus, trochlea, olecranon and finally, the lateral epicondyle. Any deviation from the above sequence following trauma should initiate efforts to locate an avulsed or malpositioned epiphysis.

Good quality frontal and lateral radiographs are the usual initial imaging investigation in elbow trauma and the latter allows detection of elbow joint effusions as they elevate fat pads. Effusions in the absence of visible bony injury may be due to occult fractures, and in children who have undergone subsequent MRI, over 50% were shown to have such injuries. However, in the largest series[5] this knowledge had little influence upon treatment or outcome.

The lateral radiograph is also particularly important in the detection of supracondylar fractures, and the diagnosis may depend upon visualization of subtle disruption of the normal relationship between the distal humeral metaphysis and capitellum. A line drawn along the anterior cortex of the humerus should pass through the middle third of the capitellum, and if it does not, a supracondylar fracture is likely to be present.

Other imaging modalities are particularly useful for demonstrating cartilaginous areas. Ultrasound (US) can demonstrate the relationship of nonossified epiphyses to the metaphyses, and CT can be used to clarify complex epiphyseal injuries before treatment. MRI combines the strengths of both modalities by its excellent demonstration of cartilaginous epiphyses in multiple planes.

Supracondylar fractures (Fig. 68.6) are usually due to falling on the outstretched hand. The usual pattern of injury is of a

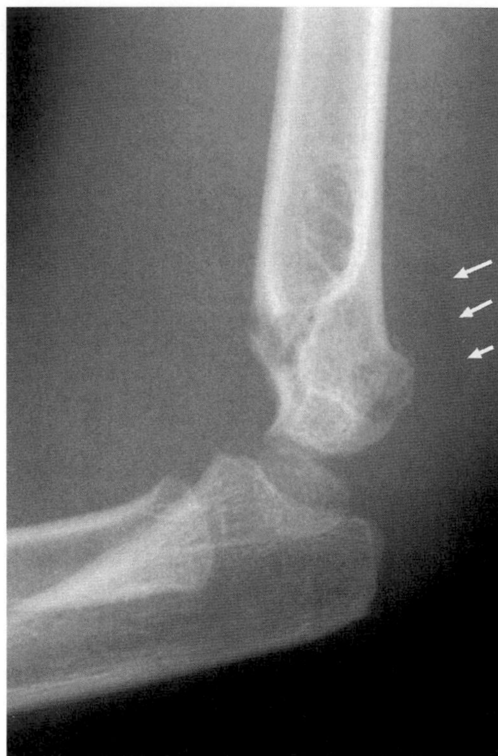

Figure 68.6 Supracondylar fracture of the distal humerus with elevation of the posterior fat pad (arrows) indicating a significant joint effusion.

transverse fracture passing just proximal to the ossified capitellum and trochlea with posterior displacement of the distal fragment. Displaced fractures may damage the brachial artery and check radiographs are essential to ensure a satisfactory position after manipulation.

Children also sustain condylar and epicondylar fractures, and avulsion of the medial epicondyle carries the significant risk of entrapment of the separated epiphysis within the elbow joint in association with dislocation. The latter may reduce spontaneously or be manipulated, but in either situation the position of the ossified epiphysis must be carefully checked on post-reduction radiographs to ensure it is not intra-articular (Fig. 68.7).

Forearm, wrist and hand fractures

The radial and ulnar shafts may fracture together or alone. In a single fracture it is most important to check for dislocation of the noninjured bone, and a line drawn along the longitudinal axis of the radius should bisect the capitellum, whatever the radiographic plane. Monteggia and Galeazzi fractures (Fig. 68.8) may both occur in childhood although the former is less common than in adults. It should also be noted these injuries can result from greenstick or bowing fractures in children (see Fig 68.3). Fractures of both forearm bones occur more commonly, but rarely even these may be associated with radial head dislocation.

Greenstick injuries of the distal forearm bones are commonly seen, as are Salter–Harris Type II epiphyseal separations of the distal radius. Distal radial fractures may or may not be accompanied by injuries to the distal ulna, but isolated ulnar fractures are uncommon.

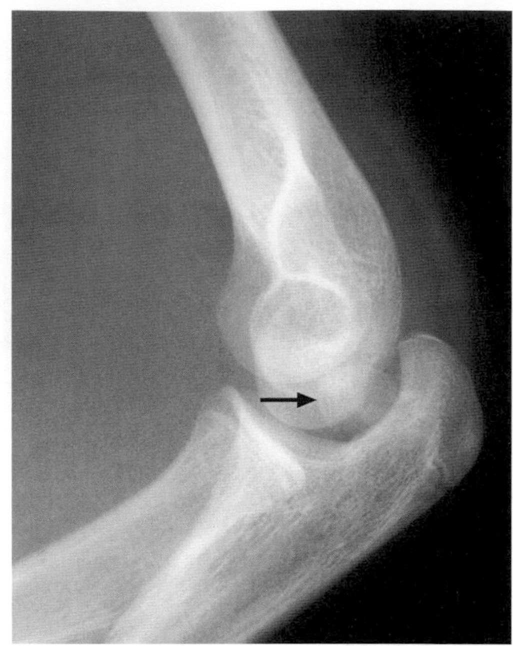

Figure 68.7 Medial epicondyle epiphysis (arrow) trapped within the elbow joint following avulsion.

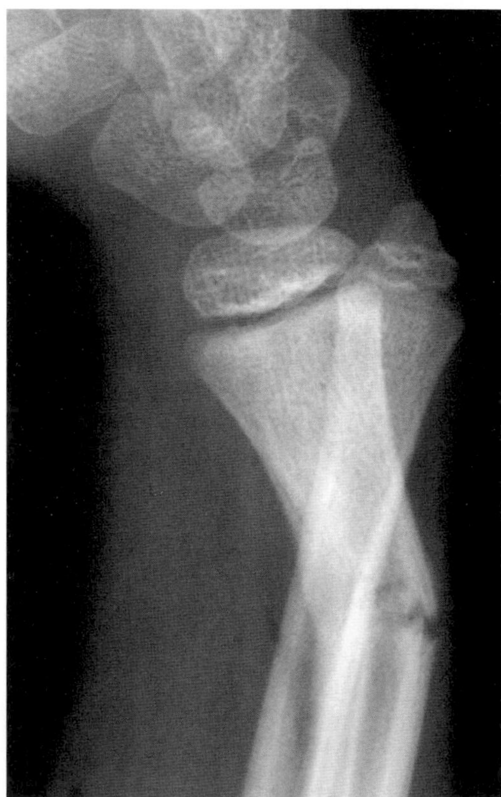

Figure 68.8 Galeazzi fracture dislocation.

Childhood carpal fractures are uncommon but when they do occur, it is the scaphoid that is most often affected. Scaphoid fractures are most commonly seen in adolescents and are extremely rare in younger children. The distal third of the scaphoid is the most common site of injury (Fig. 68.9), in contrast to the waist of the bone in adults. Thus although fracture, nonunion and avascular necrosis occasionally occur[6], their incidence is far lower than in older patients.

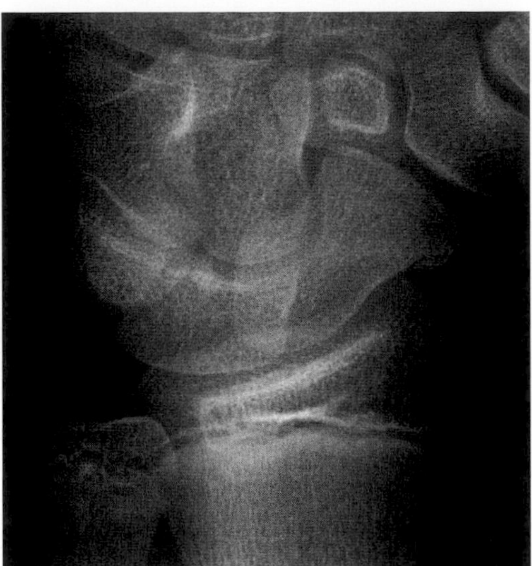

Figure 68.9 Fracture of the distal pole of the scaphoid.

Plain radiographs are used for initial evaluation. Traditionally, the patient with persistent symptoms and no demonstrable fracture has been further investigated with follow-up radiographs, and if these too are negative, bone scintigraphy. However, MRI has also been shown to be very useful in the exclusion or confirmation of scaphoid fractures, allowing appropriate management of injured patients and discharge of the remainder[7].

Metacarpal fractures are more common, with the neck of the little finger metacarpal most frequently affected. However, the most common fracture in children's hands is a Salter–Harris Type II fracture of the base of the proximal phalanx of the little finger, and this area often harbours subtle greenstick injuries.

The middle and distal phalanges are prone to avulsion of their epiphyses, and care must be taken that separated fragments are not missed on inadequate radiographs (Fig. 68.10). Injured digits require good quality AP and lateral radiographs and all the ossified phalangeal epiphyses need to be accounted for, as avulsions may travel a significant distance proximally.

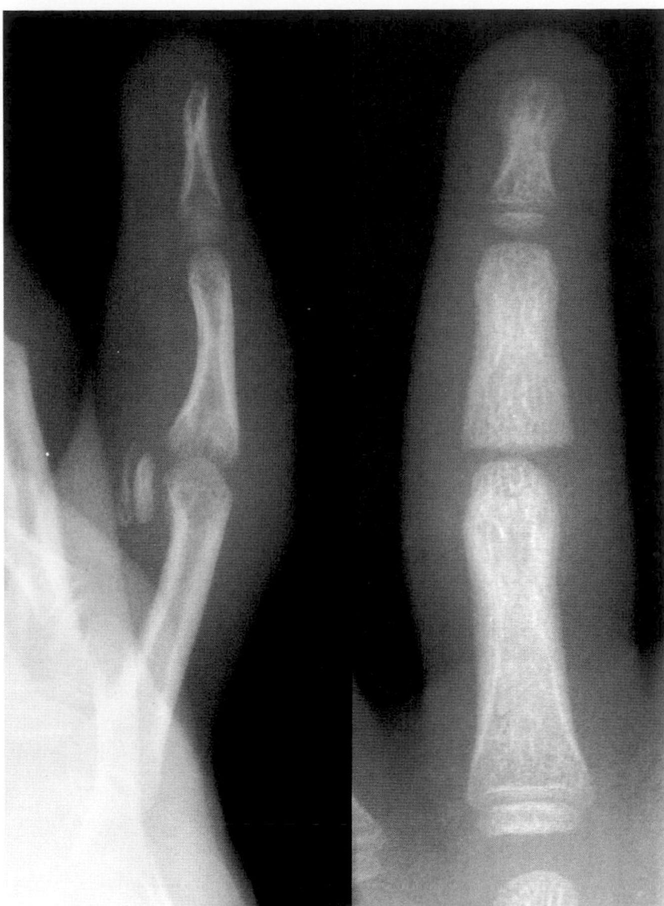

Figure 68.10 Salter–Harris Type II epiphyseal separation of the middle phalanx of the ring finger. The avulsed fragment is not visible on the AP view, but the epiphysis is missing. [From Carty H (ed) 1999 Emergency pediatric radiology. Springer-Verlag, Berlin.]

FRACTURES OF THE PELVIS AND LOWER LIMBS

Fractures of the pelvis

The system of paediatric pelvic fracture classification, proposed by Torode and Zieg in 1985[8], attempts to take account of all of a child's injuries and the associated morbidity and mortality. Pelvic fractures are divided into four types, the less severe comprising avulsion injuries (Type 1) and isolated fractures of the iliac wing (Type 2). Type 3 comprises simple ring fractures and Type 4 ring disruption, the latter having the greatest long-term morbidity[9].

Avulsion injuries are most commonly seen in adolescents and are usually due to athletic activity. These injuries may be either acute or chronic, the former being due to sudden contraction of a muscle attached to an apophysis and the latter due to repetitive traction. The ischial tuberosity is most commonly affected, as it attaches both the hamstrings and adductors. Other sites frequently affected are the anterior superior and inferior iliac spines, which attach the sartorius and straight head of the rectus femoris, respectively (Fig. 68.11).

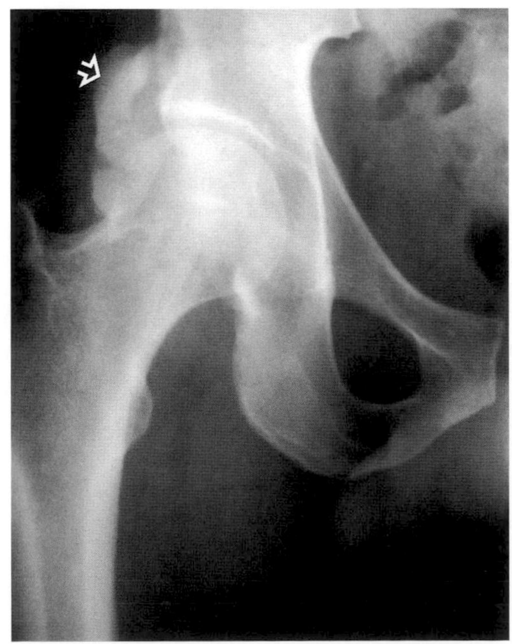

Figure 68.11 Avulsion injury. Florid new bone formation (arrow) following an avulsion injury of the reflected head of the rectus femoris muscle in a young footballer.

A standard AP pelvic radiograph will demonstrate most acute avulsion injuries, apart from those affecting the anterior inferior iliac spine, which may require an oblique view. Healing may produce much callus and subtle radiolucency, and periosteal reaction may be seen in chronic avulsion injuries, particularly in the region of the ischial tuberosity. It is important that neither is mistaken for a bone tumour.

The higher grades of fracture are usually due to road accidents. Iliac wing fractures (Type 2) are less common than in adults, associated soft tissue injury is uncommon and the overall prognosis is good.

Type 3 fractures include those involving the pubic rami and disruption of the pubic symphysis, although the elasticity of a child's pelvis means that the pubic symphysis may separate to approximately 2.5 cm without sacro-iliac joint instability. This category allows for displaced fractures providing there is no clinical instability of any other pelvic segment.

Type 4 fractures comprise those with an unstable segment due to the pelvic ring fracturing at two sites. Unsurprisingly, abdominal and genitourinary injuries are most commonly seen in association with Types 3 and 4 fractures.

Plain radiography is the usual initial investigation in suspected pelvic fractures, although it is of limited utility when used purely for screening after trauma[10]. Children suspected of having serious fractures usually proceed to CT to define better bony injury and/or associated visceral trauma.

Acetabular, hip and femoral fractures

Acetabular fractures in children are uncommon, but potentially significant because those that involve the triradiate cartilage may affect subsequent growth. A plain radiograph may be obtained initially, but CT is usually the imaging method of choice. Children who suffer hip dislocation have a lesser probability than adults of sustaining an associated acetabular injury[11]. However, in those that do, MRI is particularly useful in assessing the degree of posterior acetabular involvement (bony and cartilaginous) and consequently guiding treatment[12].

Posterior hip dislocation is the most common type and avascular necrosis of the femoral capital epiphysis is a serious complication, particularly if the hip is left unreduced for over 24 h. It is important that a careful check is made for associated fractures of the pelvis, femur and patella.

Femoral head and neck fractures are far less common in children than in adults, but complications occur more frequently and tend to be more serious. These include avascular necrosis, premature fusion of the growth plate, varus deformity and nonunion. AP and lateral radiographs are essential to check the position of the femoral capital epiphysis and the integrity of the growth plate.

Femoral diaphyseal fractures are not uncommon in children, and surrounding muscle pull may cause angulation and overlap of the opposing bone ends. Despite this, it is essential to obtain radiographs in two planes, otherwise subtle injuries may be missed.

Fractures involving the distal femoral growth plate are more likely to lead to problems with subsequent growth disturbance than those at many other locations (Fig. 68.12). This may be due to the significant force needed to disrupt the physis[13]. Although plain radiographs may reveal the physeal injury, in many cases its full extent is only revealed by MRI, and this additional information will frequently alter subsequent management[14].

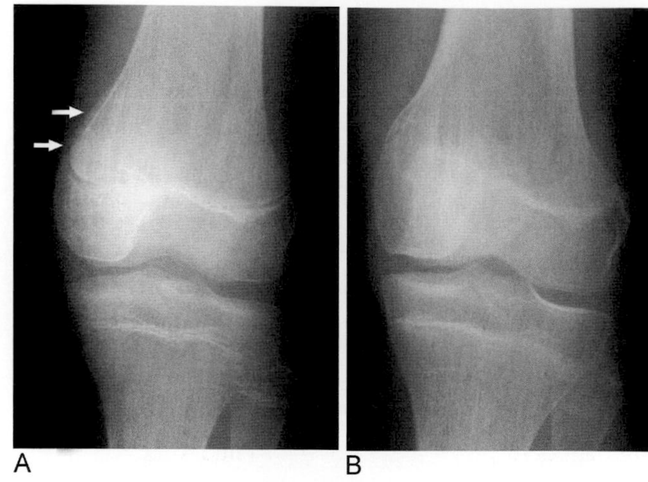

Figure 68.12 Epiphyseal injury of the distal femur. (A) Healing epiphyseal injury (arrows) of the medial aspect of the distal femur. (B) Delayed radiograph demonstrating growth arrest due to premature fusion of the medial half of the epiphysis. [From Carty H (ed) 1999 Emergency pediatric radiology. Springer-Verlag, Berlin.]

Fractures, ligamentous and cartilaginous injuries around the knee (including the tibia)

Functionally, fractures involving the anterior intercondylar eminence of the tibia (Fig. 68.13) are similar to anterior cruciate ligament disruption, and are usually due to knee hyperextension[15]. Such injuries may be subtle radiographically, the lateral view revealing a small displaced calcific fragment as the only visible sign of underlying disruption of the epiphyseal cartilage. The lesion may be missed on the AP view as the joint is flexed, and MRI provides the best means of making the

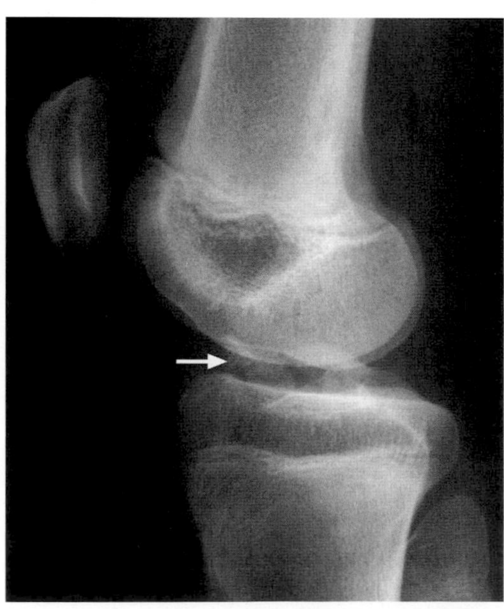

Figure 68.13 Fracture of the anterior intercondylar eminence of the tibia (arrow).

diagnosis. The injury is significant as irreducible and displaced fractures require operative fixation[13].

Hyperextension of the knee can also cause separation of the proximal tibial epiphysis (Fig. 68.14), as the adjacent metaphysis is forced backwards. The usual result is a Salter–Harris Type II fracture which may be difficult to appreciate on plain radiographs if displacement is minimal. Again, MRI provides the best means of diagnosis. Although uncommon, such injuries may be complicated by angular deformity, future leg length discrepancy and damage to the adjacent popliteal artery if displaced.

A similar mechanism of injury can cause a transverse fracture of the tibial metaphysis in young children[16]. This may result in a subtle bony injury causing a child to limp.

In children in whom ligamentous or meniscal injury is suspected, MRI is recommended, utilizing sagittal and coronal T1-weighted images, coronal T2-weighted images and sagittal T2-weighted gradient-echo images.

Uniform low signal intensity is seen in intact ligaments, whilst possible tears show as areas of increased signal, and definite tears as increased signal with disruption or deformity. Definite meniscal tears are revealed as either deformity or high signal traversing the normally low signal meniscus to reach an articular surface. When high signal within the meniscus does not reach an articular surface, appearances are regarded as equivocal.

In children medial meniscal tears are more common than injuries to the lateral meniscus, although both injuries occur significantly less frequently than in adults. A significant number of traumatized lateral menisci will be discoid. The anterior cruciate ligament is injured less frequently than the menisci and tears of the posterior cruciate ligament are uncommon. Associated injuries may also be demonstrated on MRI; examples including tears of the collateral ligaments, osteochondral fractures and bone marrow oedema[17,18].

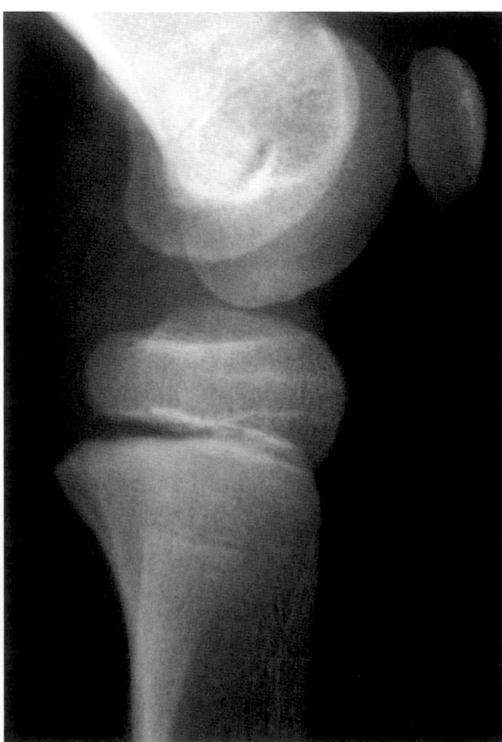

Figure 68.14 Salter–Harris Type I epiphyseal separation of the proximal tibia.

MRI is also useful in the diagnosis of osteochondritis dissecans (Fig. 68.15), which is defined as a subchondral or osteochondral defect due to necrosis of the subchondral bone, possibly following an undiagnosed injury. This may subsequently lead to separation of a subchondral fragment, resulting in an intra-articular loose body.

In the knee the condition most frequently involves the medial femoral condyle[19], and other sites classically affected include the dome of the talus and capitellum. A plain radiograph of the knee joint will reveal an oval lucency involving the articular surface of one of the femoral condyles with or without a central bony fragment. MRI can be used to predict the stability of such lesions, as unstable fragments may become intra-articular loose bodies. High signal intensity between the fragment and bone, articular fractures, focal osteochondral defects and cysts greater then 5 mm across, deep to the lesion, are all MRI predictors of instability.

The patella is infrequently fractured in children, the most common injury types being comminuted and transverse fractures following road traffic accidents. Patellar dislocation usually first occurs in adolescence and is associated with an abnormally flat sulcus between the femoral condyles and patella alta. The injury is associated with a significant number of osteochondral fractures[20], derived from either the lateral femoral condyle or the patella itself.

Full patellar dislocation will be visible on a standard plain radiographic series. If the dislocation has reduced before the child is examined, a 'skyline' view should be obtained to pursue a possible associated osteochondral fracture of the medial patella. As with other osteochondral lesions, they may be subtle or entirely chondral, in which case MRI offers the best means of detection (Fig. 68.16).

The classical toddler's fracture (Fig. 68.17) is an undisplaced, oblique fracture of the distal tibia which may not be visible on initial radiographs. It usually presents in young children as limping or refusal to weightbear. If the initial investigations are

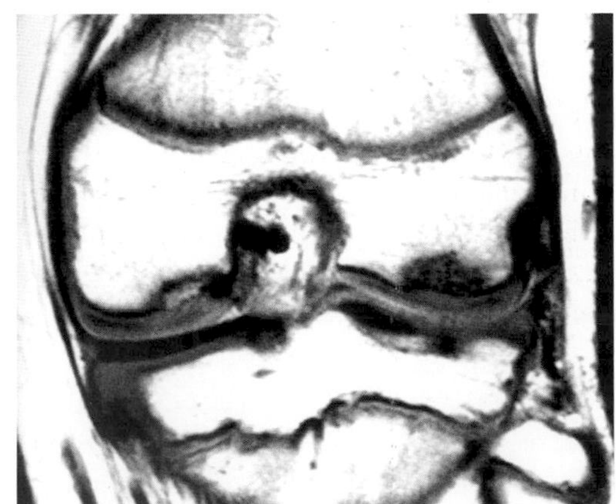

Figure 68.15 Osteochondritis dissecans. Coronal proton density MRI demonstrating characteristic defects in both femoral condyles due to osteochondritis dissecans.

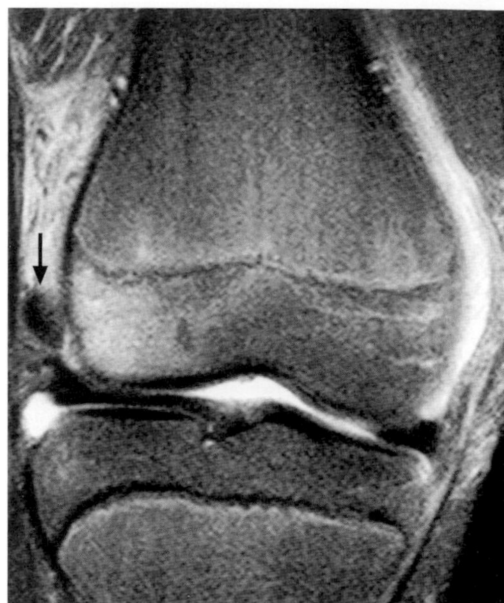

Figure 68.16 Chondral fragment. Coronal T2-weighted MRI (with fat saturation) showing a chondral fragment (arrow) avulsed following patellar dislocation with a 'bone bruise' of the adjacent distal femoral epiphysis.

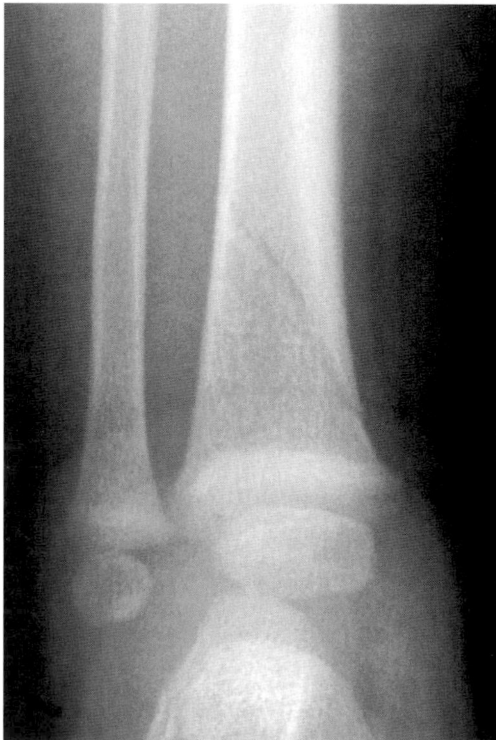

Figure 68.17 Toddler's fracture of the distal tibial metaphysis.

negative, a delayed radiograph or scintigraphy may be used to confirm the diagnosis.

Fractures around the ankle

Avulsions from the tip of the lateral malleolus and Salter–Harris Type I and II epiphyseal injuries of the distal fibula form the majority of paediatric ankle fractures. Children's physes are more likely to fail than ligaments and those of the distal tibia and fibula fuse at approximately the same time during adolescence. If only one is fused, the suspicion of an epiphyseal injury is raised.

Triplane and Tillaux fractures tend to occur in adolescence, around this time of distal tibial epiphyseal fusion. The former is a Salter–Harris Type IV epiphyseal injury comprising an oblique coronal fracture through the distal tibial metaphysis, which extends horizontally through the lateral part of the physis before running vertically through the epiphysis in the sagittal plane.

The lateral ankle radiograph suggests a Salter–Harris Type II fracture due to the extension into the metaphysis whilst the frontal view reveals a Type III injury of the epiphysis. Accurate reduction of such an injury is important and CT with multiplanar reformatting provides the best assessment of the fracture's extent before reduction (Fig. 68.18).

The Tillaux fracture occurs at a similar location and consists of a Salter–Harris Type III injury, which runs through the anterolateral aspect of the distal tibial physis until it reaches the part that has fused. It then passes downwards through the epiphysis into the joint.

The fracture is usually demonstrable on plain radiographs (Fig. 68.19), subject to the X-ray beam being parallel, which may require an oblique view. As the majority of the epiphysis has already fused the injury does not cause subsequent growth arrest, but its recognition is important so that joint congruity is restored. CT has been shown to be useful in detecting significant displacement requiring closed or open reduction[21].

Fractures of the foot

The calcaneus is the most frequently injured tarsal bone in children, but as fractures tend to involve the tuberosity and avoid the posterior facet, most are classified as extra-articular[22]. They may be very difficult to detect radiographically, and CT or scintigraphy both provide useful means of pursuing the diagnosis further.

The most common talar fracture in childhood affects the neck of the bone and displaced injuries carry the risk of subsequent avascular necrosis. However, the high cartilage-to-bone ratio of a child's talus makes it more resistant to injury than

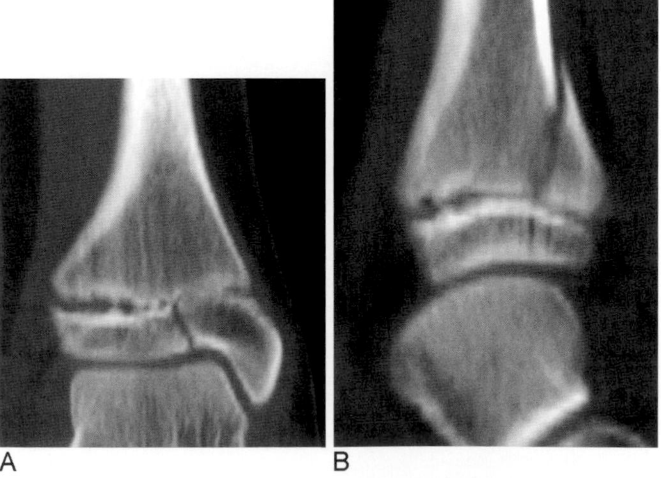

Figure 68.18 Assessment of the extent of a triplane fracture. (A) Coronal reformat of an axial CT demonstrating epiphyseal and physeal components of a triplane fracture. (B) Saggital reformat of the same case demonstrating metaphyseal extension of the fracture.

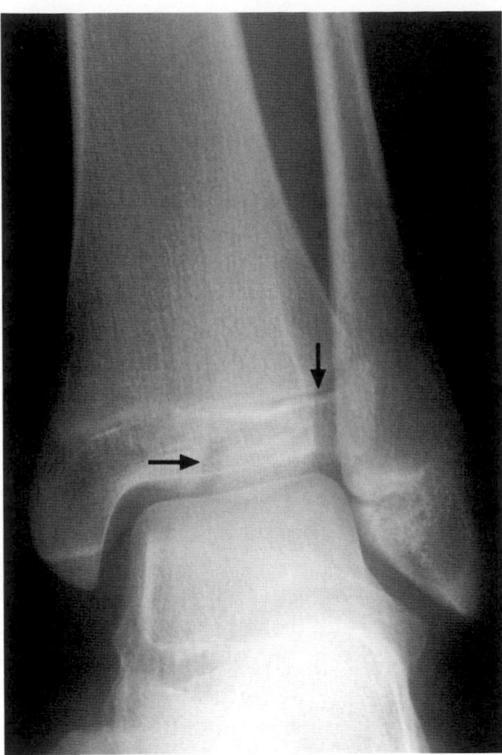

Figure 68.19 Tillaux fracture (arrows) of the distal tibial epiphysis.

that of an adult[23]. As with other tarsal bones, CT will best define the acute fracture.

The navicular may be subject to avulsion of its dorsal cortex or tuberosity. Fractures of the body of the bone may also occur, sometimes as stress injuries in young athletes. As they are usually orientated in the sagittal plane in the centre of the bone, they may be impossible to detect on plain radiography. Scintigraphy is a useful means of investigating mid foot pain in such patients (Fig. 68.20), and if increased activity is demonstrated in the navicular, CT may be used to confirm a fracture[24].

Greenstick and torus fractures are the most common types affecting the metatarsals and phalanges, and injuries to the forefoot occur more frequently than in the mid and hind foot.

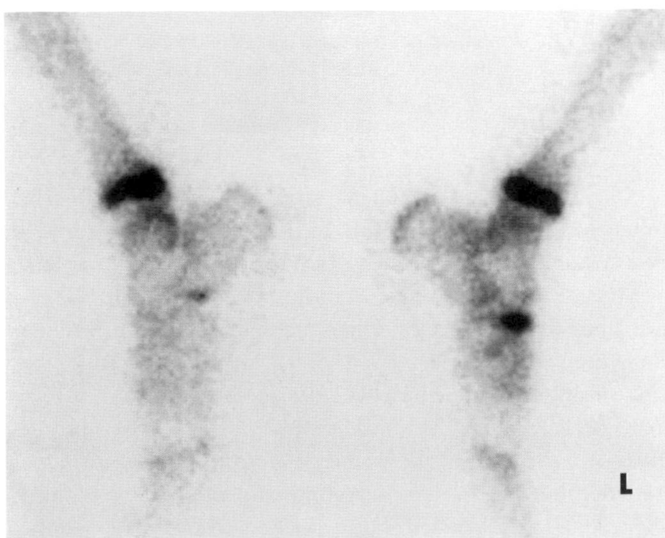

Figure 68.20 Navicular fracture. Bone scintigram showing localized increase in activity in the left navicular consistent with an occult fracture.

SPINAL INJURIES

Normal variants

There may be congenital absence of the posterior arch of the atlas and the anterior arch may not ossify until a year of age in normal children. 'Pseudospread' of the lateral masses of the atlas may also be seen on an open mouth view in young children.

Pseudosubluxation (Fig. 68.21) is the result of ligamentous laxity and horizontally orientated facet joints in young children, allied to their relatively large head size. A line connecting the anterior aspects of the spinous processes of C1 to C3 on a true lateral radiograph may help differentiate true injuries from pseudosubluxation. If this line misses the anterior aspect of the C2 spinous process by 2 mm or more, then the suspicion of a fracture or true subluxation is raised. The latter is very rare, even in severe polytrauma, whilst pseudosubluxation is relatively common in the same context[25]. Ligamentous laxity also means that the atlanto-axial distance measured on a lateral radiograph may be up to 5 mm in normal children.

Injuries to the cervical and thoracic spine

Half to two-thirds of injuries to the cervical spine in children are caused by road traffic accidents. In those under 12 years of age the majority of injuries affect the occipito-atlanto-axial segment, which partly explains the higher mortality in younger children, allied to the greater incidences of associated severe head and extraspinal trauma. Younger children (under 8 years) tend to suffer distraction and subluxation injuries whilst fractures occur more commonly in those over 8 years[26].

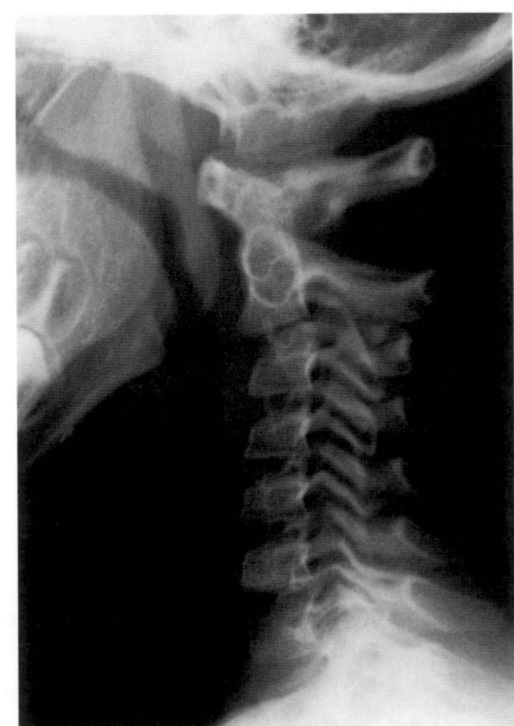

Figure 68.21 Pseudosubluxation of C2 upon C3.

In children, as in adults, the precervical soft tissues visualized on the lateral radiograph should measure 7 mm or less anterior to the second cervical vertebral body. In infants this area should measure no more than three-quarters of the AP diameter of the adjacent vertebral body. The vast majority of children with high cervical injuries will demonstrate widening of the retropharyngeal soft tissues[27], although radiographs obtained in flexion may exaggerate such thickening.

Rotary subluxation of the atlas upon the axis may or may not follow trauma in children and is a more common occurrence than in adults. The diagnosis is suspected on plain radiographs when the odontoid is positioned asymmetrically between the lateral masses of the atlas.

To differentiate this injury from transient torticollis, imaging must demonstrate lack of rotatory movement and/or locking of the lateral masses of the atlas and axis. CT is the best means to demonstrate such locking, and is performed with the head rotated both to the left and right to show that the abnormal relationship between the vertebrae does not change. It also serves to exclude an associated fracture.

Atlanto-axial dislocation in children differs from that in adults in that the child's transverse ligament usually ruptures without an associated odontoid injury, whilst adults more commonly sustain a dens fracture. Suspicion of dislocation is raised when the atlanto-axial distance exceeds 5 mm on the lateral radiograph, or if there is a large difference between flexion and extension. MRI is the method of choice for the demonstration of ligamentous injury and the cord damage that may also occur.

Older children tend to sustain injuries to the mid and lower cervical spine which correspond more to the adult pattern and distribution.

Spinal cord injury without radiographic abnormality (SCIWORA) may occur following trauma due to the disproportionate flexibility of a child's spine and spinal cord (Fig. 68.22). Either the cervical or thoracic cord may be affected, with younger children being affected more frequently[28]. Radiographs are normal, but the underlying cord injury is a significant cause of childhood paraplegia. MRI is required to delineate the cord damage, and in children with neurological signs, it must be obtained before discontinuing spinal immobilization.

In a large series of paediatric spinal fractures, the thoracic region (T2–T10) was most frequently injured[29]. The most common mechanism of trauma to the thoracic spine is hyperflexion, usually due to falls or sporting injury. This usually leads to a stable anterior wedge compression fracture, most commonly in the mid thoracic region. Multiple wedging occurs more commonly than a single fracture, and the diagnosis may be made on plain radiography.

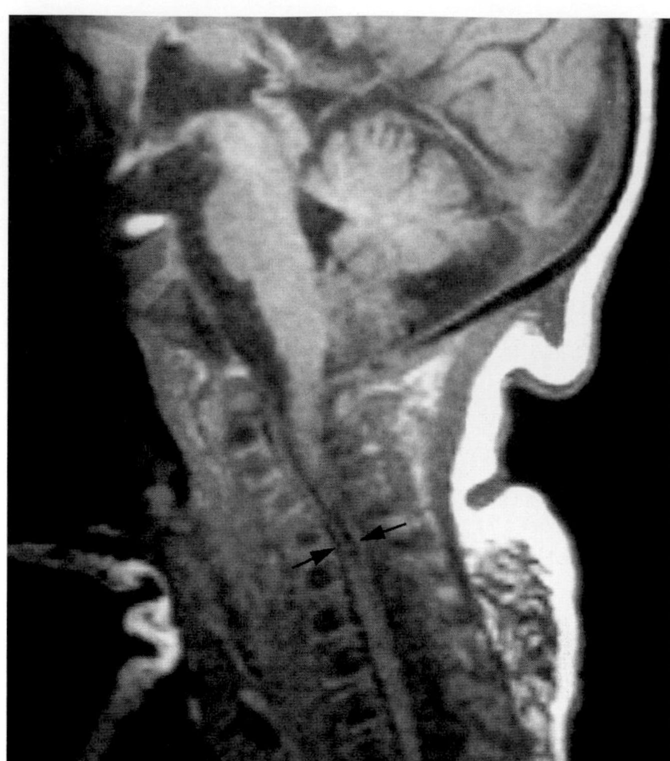

Figure 68.22 Spinal cord injury without radiographic abnormality (SCIWORA). Sagittal T1-weighted MRI demonstrating injury to the upper cervical cord (arrows) without radiographic abnormality following birth trauma.

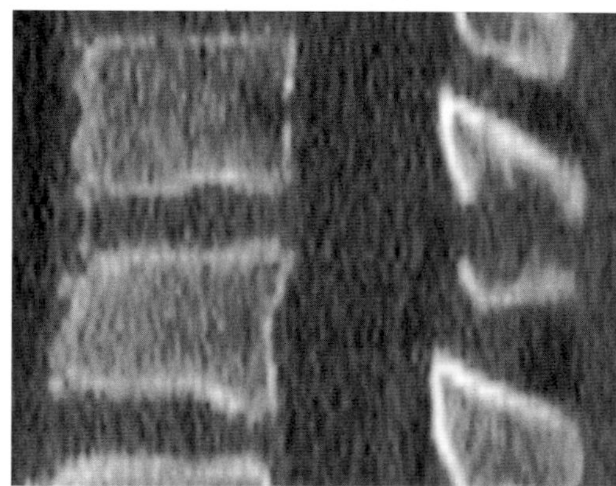

Figure 68.23 Lumbar spinal fracture. Sagittal reformat of CT showing lumbar spinal fracture following a seatbelt injury in a child. The fracture has split the spinous process posteriorly and there is a more subtle component affecting the anterior column as well.

Injuries to the lumbar spine

Hyperflexion injuries leading to wedge compression of vertebral bodies also occur in the lumbar region, but the latter area has the further association of fractures from the use of lap seatbelts as restraints in cars (Fig. 68.23). These seatbelts tend to ride up onto the anterior abdominal wall in children, leading to transmission of forces to the abdomen and spine in accidents. This leads to a high incidence of associated injury to the abdominal viscera and spinal fractures that are often more complicated than simple wedge compression.

A flexion distraction mechanism is responsible, causing ligamentous or bony disruption of the posterior column with an associated injury to the vertebral body and/or disc anteriorly. The injuries most commonly occur between the first and third lumbar vertebrae and are unstable if the posterior elements are disrupted.

Conventional abdominal CT has been shown to miss many such injuries[30], and plain radiographs of the lumbar spine, in particular the lateral view, are essential in this situation. CT has a definite role in demonstrating associated visceral trauma, and may also be utilized in a dedicated fashion to examine a known spinal fracture. Although the traumatized area may lie inferior to the conus, MRI is useful in assessing any associated damage to the cauda equina or filum terminale.

RADIOLOGY OF NONACCIDENTAL INJURY

Padma Rao

The spectrum of injuries encompassed by the terms nonaccidental injury (NAI) or child abuse range from the well-documented physical and sexual abuse to the less frequently publicized emotional abuse, neglect, deprivation and abandonment. Literature on the presentation and radiology of NAI is extensive and dates back to 1860 when Tardieu published what is thought to be the first article on the concept of the battered child[31]. Exact figures on prevalence are difficult to establish as there are cultural and geographical variations throughout different societies as to the definition of socially acceptable limits of discipline and parental control. Child abuse is not confined to any one social class or strata of society. The reported incidence of NAI has significantly increased over the past three decades, partly related to society's greater awareness and understanding of the problem, and also to the expansion in the use of diagnostic imaging in its detection and follow-up[32]. It is imperative that those involved in abuse cases remain objective in their judgement. The radiologist's role is to provide an objective assessment of the radiology and this is best carried out in the absence of any contact with the patient or his/her family.

Physical signs of abuse are not always present and radiological abnormalities alone, sometimes picked up incidentally, may provide the only evidence and confirmation of abuse. The radiologist may be the first to arouse suspicion of abuse. The radiologist's role in the management of a child can be summarized as follows:

- To document the radiological abnormalities and injuries present.
- To recognize specific injuries or patterns of injury as pathognomonic of abuse.
- To raise the suspicion of NAI and to perform a complete radiographic skeletal survey to determine the extent of bony and soft tissue injury.
- To differentiate the injuries from normal variants in the immature skeleton and to exclude underlying brittle bones or other diseases that may mimic NAI.
- To confirm a radiological diagnosis of NAI by an assessment of the number, type and differing ages of fractures with an inappropriate or incompatible history.
- To recommend further investigations as appropriate, including repeat radiography and bone scintigraphy to assist in dating fractures and confirming previously undetectable fractures, CT and MRI for intracranial and neurological abnormalities, and specific abdominal investigations to detect visceral injury.

Good communication and prompt liaison with the paediatric team, casualty department and social work team is essential in order to ensure appropriate handling of a sensitive topic. If there is any doubt as to the presence or significance of a lesion, a second opinion should be sought from a paediatric radiologist experienced in NAI cases. A wrong diagnosis of NAI can be devastating for the family. A missed diagnosis of NAI may condemn the child to continued abuse, which may ultimately lead to death.

The imaging findings must be considered together with the clinical history and presentation and be correlated with the child's age and stage of development. The radiologist must be familiar with the typical accidental injuries of childhood and have an understanding of the mechanism involved in inflicting the injuries. There is increasing reliance on multidisciplinary discussion at, for example, case conferences.

The clinical presentation is extremely variable and the child may present with the same symptoms and signs as in accidental trauma or medical illness. The initial diagnosis is often that of a medical emergency, such as meningitis or status epilepticus. Symptoms may range from minor vague symptoms (and be dismissed as insignificant) to severe life-threatening shock. The presence of skeletal injuries or typical soft tissue injuries makes a diagnosis of NAI easier but these are not always present. They are often absent in those injuries involving acceleration/deceleration forces alone. Unexplained soft tissue injury in children, especially if extensive or penetrating, should be further investigated for accompanying skeletal injury. Characteristic soft tissue injuries in abuse are bruises, a torn frenulum, cigarette burns, bite marks and scalds, usually of the lower extremities and buttocks. Retinal, subhyaloid and subconjunctival haemorrhages are associated with shaking. Retinal haemorrhage that occurs in normal neonates as a consequence of the high pressures generated during delivery resolves within a few weeks of birth.

Accidental bruising usually occurs over bony prominences. In abuse, bruising occurs frequently and multiple bruises of differing ages found in sites unlikely to be affected by accidental injury, such as the flanks or buttocks, are typical of NAI. On plain radiographs there may be swelling and disruption of the normal soft tissue planes at the site of the bruise. Calcified soft tissue haematomata may be apparent. Calcification in the soft tissues around the neck (necklace calcification), represents fat necrosis following strangulation[33]. The following circumstances should alert the physician to the possibility of NAI:

- The presence of an inappropriate, inconsistent, or conflicting history.
- The presence of unexplained soft tissue injury.
- The presence of a healing fracture or the presentation of the child in a shocked or dehydrated state resulting from a delay in seeking medical help.
- Radiological evidence of trauma exceeds that expected from the clinical history.
- The presence of skeletal injuries with a high specificity for abuse.

Other suspicious circumstances include a failure to thrive of unknown cause suggesting emotional deprivation, poor nutrition and neglect; unexplained abdominal trauma; recurrent pancreatitis; and a history of previous abuse to this child or a sibling.

SKELETAL AND SOFT TISSUE INJURY

The main determinants of the sequence of diagnostic imaging in abuse are the cardiovascular and neurological status of the child. Stability must be achieved before proceeding with further investigations.

Investigation

Skeletal survey

A recommended schedule of images is given in Table 68.1. A 'babygram' is not an adequate skeletal survey and should not be performed. In cases of sudden infant death syndrome (SIDS), the skeletal survey should be performed and ideally reported by a paediatric radiologist before the post-mortem. Questionable areas on the initial survey should be supplemented by additional views. The skeletal survey should be checked and deemed satisfactory before the child leaves the department. Repeat radiographs after 10–14 d enhance detection of occult fractures, especially of the ribs, and provide additional information on the number, type, and age of the injuries[34]. The yield from a skeletal survey decreases with increasing age and is of most value in those under 2 years of age[35]. A skeletal survey should only be performed in older children if clinically it is thought appropriate.

Scintigraphy

The role of skeletal scintigraphy in suspected or proven NAI is established. A recommended bone scintigram protocol is outlined in Table 68.2. Studies have advocated performing both scintigraphy and a skeletal survey[36,37]; an increase in sensitivity has been demonstrated of between 25% and 50% in detecting soft tissue as well as bony lesions, assuming adequate patient immobilization and positioning[38]. Pinhole collimation should be available to resolve occasional difficulties. The urinary bladder should be emptied before the delayed images of the pelvis to resolve superior and inferior rami fractures. The nuclear medicine service needs to have sufficient and specific expertise in order to interpret the studies accurately and it is therefore recommended that they are performed at a dedicated children's unit. They should *not* be performed or interpreted by the occasional practitioner.

Table 68.1 SKELETAL SURVEY

AP and lateral chest—lateral to include sternum
Upper limbs—AP both forearms, AP both humeri, PA both hands and wrists
Lower limbs—AP both femora done individually
AP both tibiae and fibulae
AP both ankles, coned, with ankle joints flexed at 90 degrees
Dorsiplantar both feet
AP abdomen and pelvis
Lateral of thoracolumbar spine
Lateral cervical spine
AP and lateral skull—add a Townes' view if there is occipital injury
Additional views at radiologist's discretion
All films to be checked by a radiologist.
It is essential to have the following:
• metal markers on all films
• correct patient identification labelling
• radiographs should ideally be done on high resolution film but there is increasing use of modern digital equipment.

Table 68.2 BONE SCINTIGRAM PROTOCOL

Patient preparation	None before injection. After injection, maintain good hydration
	Empty bladder before delayed images
	± Sedation
Radiopharmaceutical	^{99m}Tc-methyldiphosphonate
Dose	Weight adjusted percentage of adult dose
	Adult dose: 800 MBq
Images	
Radioangiogram	If there is an obvious region of interest
Blood pool	Posterior and anterior whole body passes
Delayed	3 h post injection—posterior and anterior whole body passes
	Anterior and oblique views of ribs
	Right and left lateral of skull
	Anterior lower legs: toes turned in to separate bones
	Anterior and posterior 'spot' views of torso
	Forearms (separating radius and ulna)
Pinhole images	For suspicious area or small region if magnification may assist resolution
Tomography	Rarely performed

Familiarity with the normal scintigraphic appearances in children is essential. The normal high uptake in the epiphyses should not be confused with fractures. Physiological periosteal new bone and the periosteal prominence accompanying rapid growth do not show increased isotope uptake. Scintigraphy is most sensitive in detecting rib, scapular, spinal, diaphyseal and pelvic fractures. Sensitivity is lower for flat bones, old healed fractures and metaphyseal fractures[38]. Scintigraphy is not reliable in identifying skull fractures because of the low lesion-to-background ratio and the poorer osteoblastic response in linear fractures. Scintigraphy becomes positive within hours of an injury and has been demonstrated as early as 7 h after injury[37].

Ultrasound

US is not routinely performed but may be a useful supplementary technique. It can demonstrate subperiosteal haemorrhage, fracture separation of the epiphysis, costochondral injuries and occult long bone fractures before they become evident radiographically.

Dating fractures

Precise dating of fractures is not possible. Estimates are based on the pattern of fracture healing observed in accidental trauma (Table 68.3) when both the time of injury and the interval before investigation are known. Fracture dating is easiest if the time interval between injury and the initial radiography is short. Subtle periosteal new bone may be seen as early as 4 d after a fracture. Fractures with a large amount of periosteal new bone or callus are more than 14 d old.

Table 68.3 DATING FRACTURES: RADIOGRAPHIC CHANGES IN CHILDHOOD FRACTURES (ADAPTED FROM O'CONNOR J F, COHEN J 1987 DIAGNOSTIC IMAGING OF CHILD ABUSE. WILLIAMS & WILKINS, BALTIMORE, P112)

Radiological feature	Early	Peak	Late
Soft tissue resolution	2–5 days	4–10 days	10–21 days
Periosteal new bone	4–10 days	10–14 days	14–21 days
Loss of fracture line definition	10–14 days	14–21 days	42–90 days
Soft callus	10–14 days	14–21 days	2 years to physeal closure
Hard callus	14–21 days	21–42 days	
Remodelling	3 months	1 year	

Injuries to the neck, larynx and airway

Oropharyngeal injuries

Injury to the mouth is common in abuse but radiological evidence of orophayngeal injury is uncommon. Pharyngeal perforation may occur secondary to forceful insertion of a blunt or penetrating object or orosexual abuse. The children are usually younger than 1 year old. Retropharyngeal abscess or mediastinitis may result from any cause of retropharyngeal perforation. Perforation may be further complicated by haemorrhage, interstitial emphysema and mediastinal pseudocyst formation[39–41]. Radiologically, there may be widening of the superior mediastinum on a frontal chest radiograph. A soft tissue lateral radiograph of the neck demonstrates prevertebral soft tissue thickening which may contain gas or a fluid level, or a foreign body may be evident. Oral contrast studies may demonstrate an extraluminal leak. CT and MRI are sensitive for soft tissue abnormalities.

Asphyxiation

This most frequently presents as a near miss cot death or SIDS, or recurrent apnoeic attacks. Often asphyxiation occurs in the absence of external visible signs of injury or skeletal injury. Occasionally there may be bruising. There are no specific radiological signs. A chest radiograph may demonstrate aspiration or pulmonary oedema. Both may contribute to the hypoxia. Severe or recurrent episodes of asphyxiation may result in hypoxic ischaemic brain injury.

Skeletal injuries

The frequency of skeletal trauma in NAI has been variously reported as between 11% and 55%[42]. It is most common in children under 3 years of age[43,44]. The following fractures, which occur infrequently, are considered to have a high specificity for abuse:

- metaphyseal, rib and scapular fractures
- fractures of the outer third of the clavicle
- sternal fractures
- spinous process fractures.

Other sites and patterns of injury which have moderate specificity for abuse are:

- multiple fractures, bilateral fractures and fractures of differing ages
- vertebral fractures or subluxation
- digital injuries in nonmobile children
- spiral fractures of the humerus
- epiphyseal separations
- complex skull fractures, i.e. those that are wider than 5 mm, depressed, occipital and growing fractures.

Fractures that occur frequently but have a low specificity for abuse are:

- mid-clavicular fractures
- simple linear skull fractures of the parietal bone
- single diaphyseal fractures, with the exception of spiral fractures of the humerus
- greenstick fractures.

These injuries occur commonly in young mobile children and, if isolated, should not be regarded as significant evidence for abuse. Mid-clavicular and humeral fractures are also well-known birth injuries. Again, they are isolated and there is an appropriate history.

Metaphyseal fractures

Also known as corner or bucket handle fractures (Fig. 68.24), metaphyseal fractures are highly characteristic of and specific for NAI with an incidence of between 11% and 28%[43,45]. They are most commonly seen in nonmobile abused infants under 18 months of age, and are most frequent around the knees and ankles but also occur at the shoulder, elbow, wrists and hips[45]. They may be bilateral.

Metaphyseal fractures do not usually occur in children over 2 years of age. In these children, trauma to the metaphysis results in diaphyseal or epiphyseal fracture separation. Histological changes consist of a subepiphyseal planar series of microfractures through the metaphyseal primary spongiosa, which results in separation of a part or whole of a mineralized disc and this is the portion evident radiologically[42,46]. The fractures are transmetaphyseal[46]. They may occur during shaking when acceleration/deceleration forces are applied directly to the limb, but a further well-recognized mechanism is direct wrenching or twisting of the limb using the extremities as 'handles'. At the metaphysis, the loosely attached periosteum is frequently stripped by the shearing forces, resulting in subperiosteal bleeding. During healing, this is evident as subperiosteal reaction. With small metaphyseal fractures, periosteal new bone is not seen as the fracture is entirely intracapsular and subperiosteal bleeding does not occur. The most subtle metaphyseal fracture is the metaphyseal lucent line which lies immediately adjacent to the epiphyseal plate (Fig. 68.24E)[42,47].

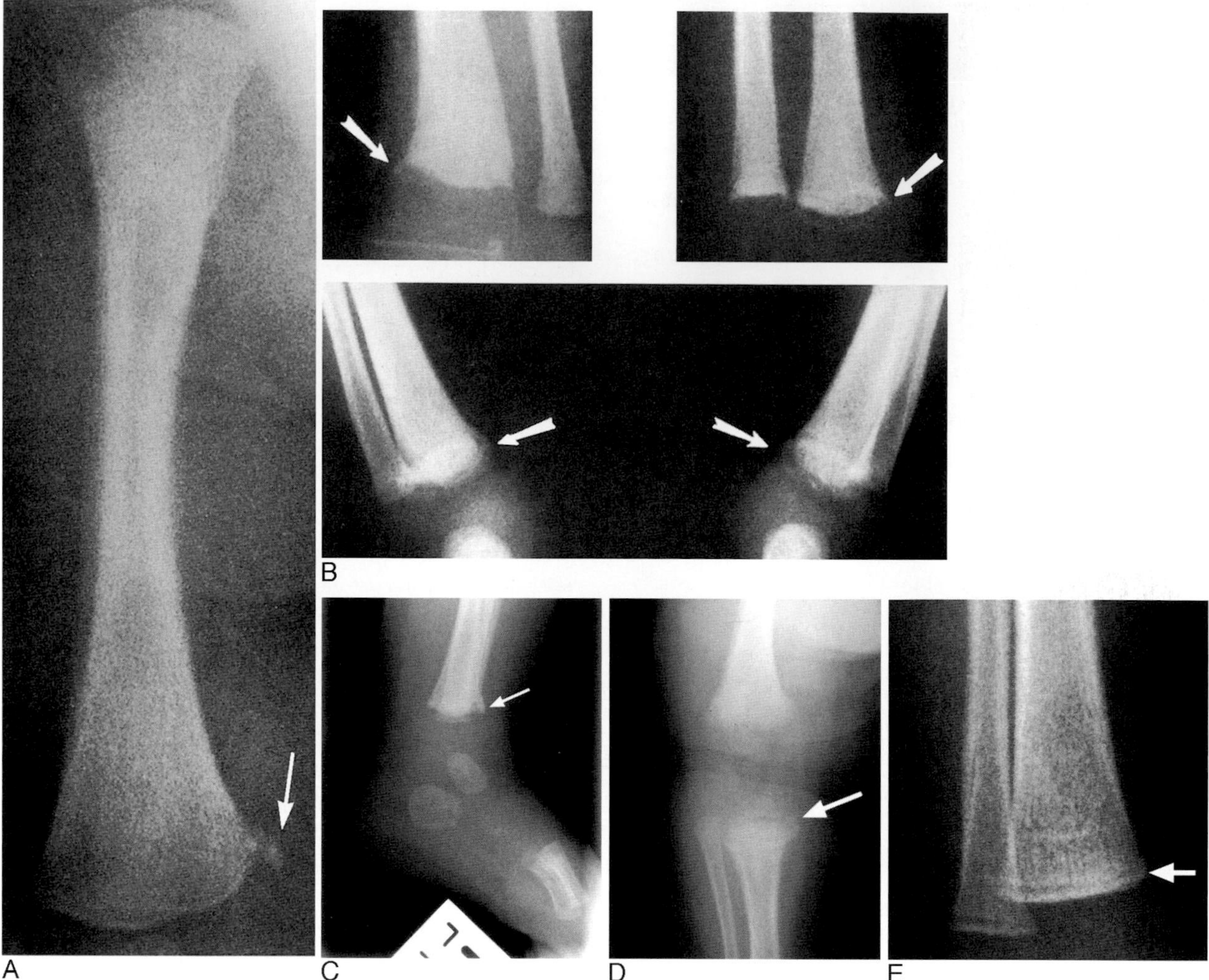

Figure 68.24 Metaphyseal fractures. (A,B) Radiographs of the right femur (A) and both ankles (B) of a 2 month old abused infant demonstrating metaphyseal corner fractures of the distal femur and both distal tibia (arrows). The angled tangential view reveals the 'bucket handle' appearance of the fracture. (C) Radiograph of the left ankle of an infant demonstrates a metaphyseal corner fracture of the distal tibia (arrow). (D) Angled tangential view of the right lower limb of an abused infant demonstrates the 'bucket handle' appearance (arrow). (E) Radiograph of the right ankle of a 6 week old abused baby with subtle metaphyseal fractures evident as a metaphyseal lucent line (arrow).

Dating metaphyseal fractures may be difficult as they do not always result in callus formation and healing occurs by gradual bone consolidation. Repeated trauma may lead to an irregular fluffy appearance. Metaphyseal fractures are usually asymptomatic and not evident clinically. They are detected incidentally when imaging for other reasons.

There are several normal variations in the appearance of the metaphyseal regions that should not be mistaken for abuse, namely, metaphyseal beaks and spurs, the metaphyseal step-off and the proximal tibial cortical irregularity[48].

Diaphyseal fractures

Diaphyseal fractures are the most common fracture in child abuse and are said to occur four times more frequently in NAI than metaphyseal fractures[43]. The femur, humerus and tibia are the most frequently injured bones (Fig. 68.25). A variety of frequencies and fracture patterns have been quoted[43,49] but no one pattern or type of diaphyseal fracture is specific to NAI.

The significance of diaphyseal fractures increases when they are multiple, bilateral, found in a state of healing, are of differing ages, when there is a fracture through the callus, and when they are associated with fractures that have a high specificity for abuse. Transverse diaphyseal fractures result from direct trauma. The infant may be pulled inappropriately by the limb and the bone fractures due to the weight of the suspended child against the fixed adult hand. Spiral fractures are more common than transverse fractures in both accidental and nonaccidental trauma. They are produced by a twisting/pulling force and are always suspicious of abuse, in particular those of the humerus.

It is important to differentiate accidental fractures and normal variants from NAI. In mobile children, the 'toddlers' fracture' (a fine spiral fracture of the tibia; see Fig. 68.17), supracondylar fractures and metaphyseal torus fractures are common accidental injuries of childhood. However, in the appropriate clinical setting, any type of fracture can occur in abuse. The importance of all humeral fractures as indicators of abuse has been emphasized[50]. Femoral fractures have been said to have a high incidence of abuse in nonmobile children,[50,51] but this has recently been debated[52]. Fractures at the subtrochanteric level are stated to be more common in NAI[51].

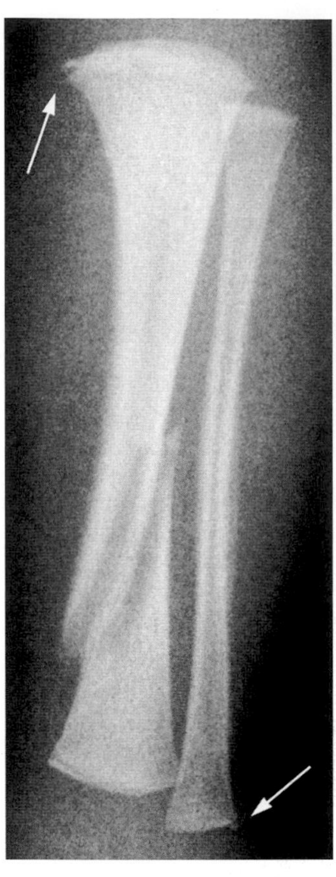

Figure 68.25 Diaphyseal fracture. Radiograph of the left lower leg of a 3 month old abused child demonstrating a mildly diastatic oblique fracture of the distal tibia. There are also metaphyseal corner fractures of the proximal tibia and distal fibula (arrows). A faint metaphyseal lucent line of the distal tibia is also noted.

Impaction fractures

Impaction buckle fractures occur most commonly at the metadiaphyseal junction of the distal femur and proximal tibia[42]. They result from impaction forces transmitted when the child is forcibly thumped down on his/her legs on a hard surface. The bone cortex buckles anteriorly and there is an incomplete crush fracture of the bone shaft. They must be differentiated from accidental torus fractures, which also occur at the metadiaphyseal junction, typically at the distal tibia. Impaction fractures also occur in the spine.

Epiphyseal fractures

Compared with accidental trauma, the frequency of epiphyseal and true Salter–Harris fractures is rare. Fracture separation of the epiphysis and dislocation is sometimes seen and can be detected by US before becoming radiologically visible[44]. In children, movement is prevented by the epiphysis being held tightly in position by the periosteum. The proximal femur and humerus are the most common sites[42]. In humeral fractures, the mechanism of injury is external rotation of the forearm. In abuse the forearm is displaced medially; in accidental injury the displacement is lateral[49]. Epiphyseal injuries are commonly complicated by orthopaedic deformity and growth disturbances.

Periosteal new bone

Physiological periosteal new bone is seen as a normal physiological phenomenon between 6 weeks and 6 months of age, and always has an organized lamellar appearance. It occurs symmetrically, is more common in the lower limbs, and is confined to the diaphysis, never extending to the metaphysis. Outside this age range the presence of periosteal new bone is abnormal. It is usually seen in fracture repair but can occur in the absence of a fracture as a consequence of a gripping or twisting force[44,53,54] or acceleration–deceleration forces alone[54,55]. In young children, the periosteum has only a loose attachment to the underlying bone and it readily separates following the formation of a subperiosteal haematoma in trauma. This results in periosteal reaction evident radiologically about 7 d post injury. Physiological periosteal new bone shows normal uptake on scintigraphy whereas uptake is increased in traumatic and other causes[37]. Repetitive injury, failure to immobilize the limb and severe twisting lead to a florid periosteal reaction which may cloak the bone and extend into the epiphysis, and this is characteristic of abuse cases. Clinically, this may present as a hot swollen limb and mimic osteomyelitis, metabolic bone disease, or dysplasia.

Digital injury

Common injuries to the hand include bruises, burns and lacerations, and rarely (0–3%) lead to fractures. These usually result from direct injury to the digits from trampling, squeezing, or forced hyperflexion[35,55]. Accidental fractures in toddlers are usually confined to the phalanges, but in abuse, involvement of the metacarpals and metatarsals is seen.

Vertebral injuries

These occur relatively rarely in NAI. The true incidence is unknown. Unless a lateral spine radiograph is performed they are frequently missed. They are due to hyperflexion and hyperextension forces arising from direct trauma or impaction against a hard surface[42], resulting in varying degrees of compression fractures of the vertebral bodies most commonly in the thoracolumbar region. Vertebral injury may be further complicated by rupture of the spinal ligament, vertebral dislocations, disc herniation, avulsion of the posterior elements which, if the injury is high enough, can lead to kyphosis, cord damage and paraplegia. Babies are susceptible to cervical spine damage because of their flexible supporting ligaments and joint capsule. MRI is indicated in the presence of abnormal neurology.

Rib fractures

The presence of rib fractures in children, whether solitary or multiple, is highly suspicious of child abuse. Accidental rib fractures are extremely rare even in the presence of major trauma. Once metabolic bone disease, rickets, prolonged parenteral nutrition, jaundice, frusemide therapy, bronchopulmonary dysplasia, osteogenesis imperfecta and bone disease of the premature have been excluded, rib fractures are considered synonymous with abuse[56]. The incidence of rib fractures in children with proven NAI varies between 5% and 27%[57]. Eighty per cent of rib fractures in NAI are clinically occult and are not associated with bruising or specific symptoms. They are discovered incidentally during the skeletal survey or when imaging for other problems. Fractures are often multiple and bilateral and affect the necks, posterior shafts and axillae[42,44], particularly medial to the costotransverse articulation (Fig. 68.26). Anterior rib fractures are also recognized but are less common.

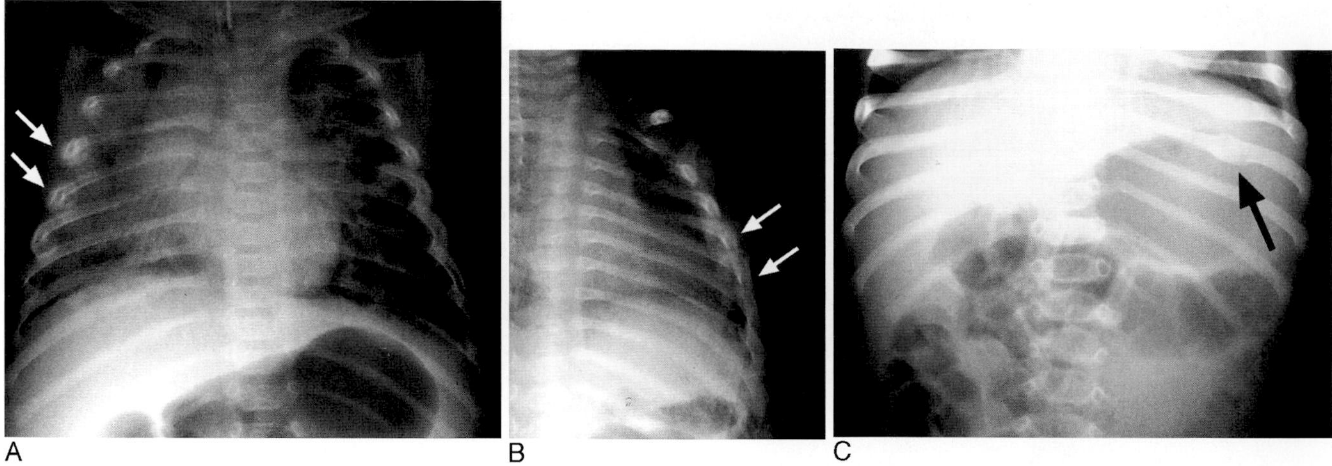

Figure 68.26 Rib fractures. (A) Chest radiograph of an intubated 3 month old abused infant demonstrating fractures of the angles of the right third, fourth and fifth ribs associated with pulmonary contusion (arrows). (B) Oblique left-sided rib views demonstrating multiple fractures of the angles of the left third to eighth ribs at different stages of healing (arrows). (C) Healing fractures of the posterior aspects of the left seventh and eighth ribs picked up as an incidental finding on a baby who presented with abdominal signs (arrow). Nonaccidental injury was later confirmed.

Rib fractures most commonly occur during episodes of violent shaking whilst the thorax is squeezed and compressed[44,45,58]. Lateral compression causes posterior fractures, and AP compression, such as from trampling, causes fractures in the mid-axillary line. Often both coexist. They can also result from direct trauma to the chest, such as trampling or kicking, which is often the cause in older children, and are rarely accompanied by underlying lung contusion, but a pleural haematoma may be seen acutely. Unlike adults, the forces sustained in cardiopulmonary resuscitation do not normally cause rib fractures in children[59,60].

Approximately 90% of rib fractures in abuse occur in children under 2 years of age and most are in those younger than 1 year old. A row of fractures involving the necks and lateral aspects may result in a flail chest. Early after injury, fractures are often difficult to detect. Rib fractures become easier to see during healing[44], and a repeat chest radiograph should be obtained 10–14 d later in suspected NAI cases.

The more subtle signs of rib fractures are often overlooked, including expansion and widening of the ribs, frequently at the neck. These fractures are pathognomonic of abuse. Fractures of the first rib are rare in both NAI and accidental trauma. If they occur, they are usually sited laterally rather than posteriorly[61]. The amount of callus formation in healing rib fractures is determined by the degree of bleeding and cortical disruption. The 'hole in the rib sign' refers to the cyst-like radiolucencies in the bones arising as sequelae to fractures.

Clavicular and scapular injury

The frequency of clavicular fractures in abuse is between 2% and 6%[45]. In mobile children, the clavicle is frequently injured in accidental trauma, usually in the midshaft, and it is the most frequently injured bone in birth trauma. Birth injuries are usually isolated and periosteal new bone is seen at around 11 d and mature callus at 1 month. In abuse, midshaft fractures also occur but the incidence of fractures to the medial and outer thirds of the clavicle increases. A fracture of the outer third of the clavicle is highly associated with abuse. Accidental clavicular fractures are rare under the age of about 3 years. They do not always present with immediate symptoms. The child later presents with persistent localized pain or swelling and a radiograph confirms a healing fracture. Scapular and sternal fractures are rare but both are highly specific for abuse. In the scapula, the acromion is the most common site of injury (Fig. 68.27). These fractures may not be evident on radiographs and are only detected on scintigraphy.

Skull fractures

Skull fractures in abuse may not necessarily differ from those occurring in accidental trauma, and no specific type of skull fracture is pathognomonic of child abuse[62]. Any type of fracture can occur (Fig. 68.28). The types of skull fracture that are rare in uncomplicated accidental trauma and may be associated with abuse are listed in Table 68.4. Skull fractures that are suspicious of abuse are those that are multiple and diastatic (Fig. 68.29); of differing ages; complex, involving both sides of the skull; depressed and nonparietal, especially those of the occiput. A depressed occipital fracture is considered specific for abuse. Skull fractures must be differentiated from normal variants and normal sutures that may mimic fractures. Growing fractures of the skull, or traumatic encephaloceles, are sometimes seen in abuse but are not specific to it.

Skull fractures are difficult to date as they do not heal by callus formation. A fracture is usually more than 2 weeks old if its edges are rounded and smooth. A scalp haematoma overlying the injury site usually develops immediately or within hours of the injury, thus indicating that an injury is likely to be recent. Most disappear after 3–4 d. A delayed appearance of a haematoma is a recognized although rare occurrence and is due to continuous slow extravasation of blood and CSF. The head injury may be complicated by a nontender swelling beneath the scalp, termed a subepicranial hygroma, which spontaneously disappears with no residual effects. It is due to a collection of CSF beneath the subepicranial aponeurosis[63], is generally

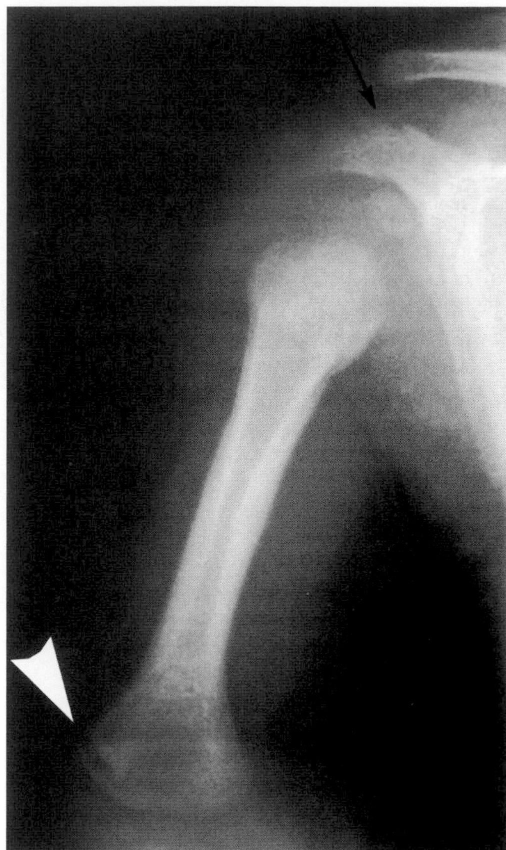

Figure 68.27 Fracture of the acromion. AP radiograph of the right shoulder and humerus of an abused child demonstrates a fracture of the right acromion process (black arrow). There is also a metaphyseal fracture of the distal humerus (white arrowhead). A thick pathological periosteal reaction of the proximal humerus extending into the metaphysis is evident. [From Rao P 1999 Emergency imaging in non-accidental injury. In: Carty (ed) Medical radiology: Emergency paediatric radiology. Springer-Verlag, Berlin.]

considered to be a benign complication of head injury, and is not associated with any significant intracranial injury.

Simple skull fractures in accidental trauma have a very low risk of intracranial sequelae[64,65]. Most head injuries in young children occur from falls from short distances which impart a predominantly translational (linear) force to the head. In one study, whilst differing fall heights were associated with some differences in the type of injury, most household falls were benign[66]. Minor accidental falls from heights of 4 feet or less are very rarely associated with serious or fatal injury[67–70]. In severe injuries or fatalities said to result from falls from heights of less than 4 feet, the putative history is likely to be inaccurate and should be viewed with a high degree of suspicion[69]. In the presence of major injury, a history of minor trauma is clearly incompatible and the reliability of the history and thus NAI must be queried. Difficulties arise in abused patients as the history is often vague and inadequate.

Medically, skull fractures become important if they are depressed, have intracranial penetration with resultant CSF leaks and risk of meningitis, or are basal and often accompanied by brainstem injury.

In the absence of a clear history of injury or bleeding disorder, an apparently spontaneous subdural haematoma on CT or MRI in an infant is caused by blood leakage from torn delicate dural veins and is usually caused by a shaking or shaking/impact injury. It is often accompanied by retinal haemorrhages but may be associated with a skull fracture. A more detailed account of the intracranial manifestations of NAI is given in the section below on brain injuries in NAI.

Differential diagnosis of abuse fractures

Several medical conditions may be associated with fractures, periosteal reactions and irregular metaphyses and these may

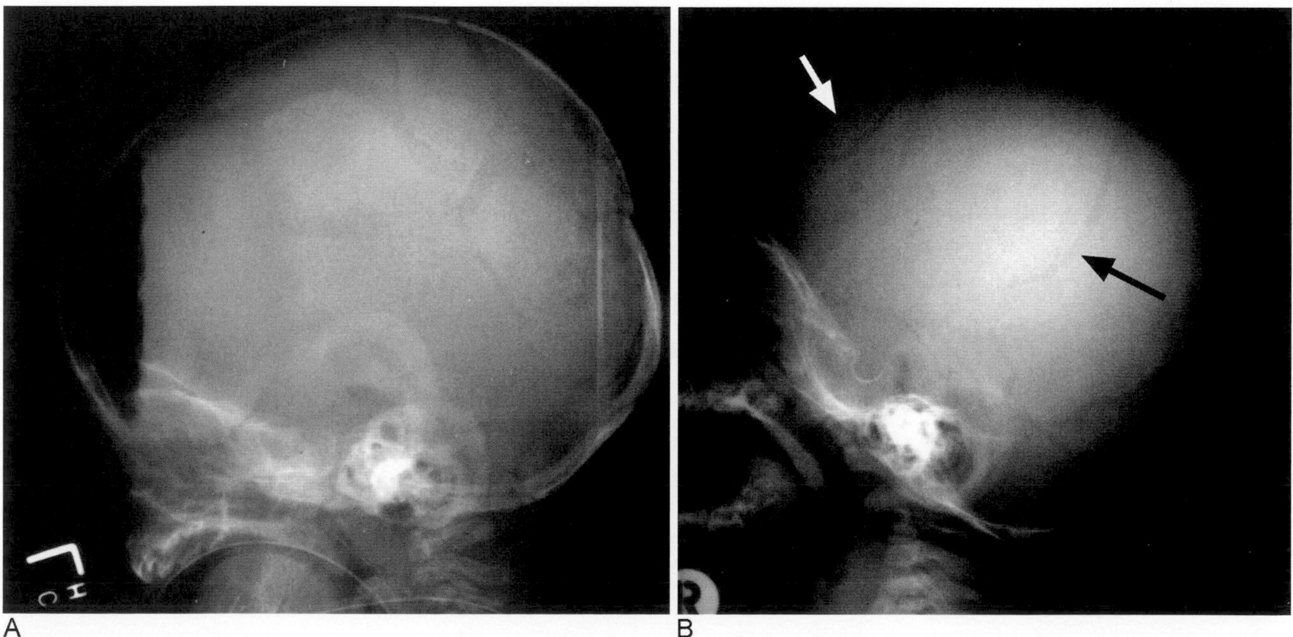

Figure 68.28 Skull fractures. (A) Lateral skull radiograph demonstrating complex, diastatic temporoparietal skull fractures associated with pneumocephalus. A linear occipital component is also present. (B) Lateral skull radiograph demonstrating multiple skull fractures in the frontal and parietal regions (arrows).

Table 68.4 FEATURES OF SKULL FRACTURES WITH A HIGHER SPECIFICITY FOR ABUSE
Complex fractures involving both sides of the skull
Multiple fractures
Diastatic fractures
Fractures of differing ages
Depressed fractures especially of the occiput

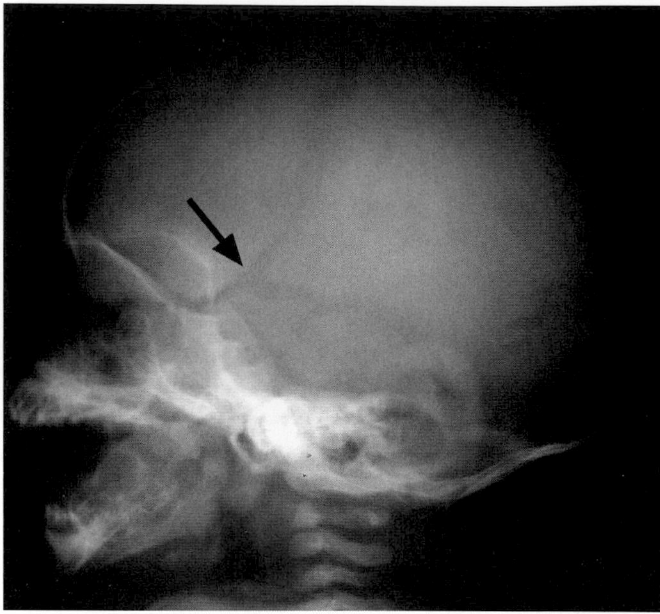

Figure 68.29 Diastatic skull fracture. Lateral projection of the skull of an 8 month old abused infant demonstrating a complex diastatic temporal fracture (arrow).

cause diagnostic confusion. In some, other associated radiological findings enable a differentiation to be made, and in others it is the nonradiological extraskeletal manifestations of the disease that aid the diagnosis (Table 68.5). Confirmation of the underlying medical condition does not automatically exclude NAI; the two may occur concurrently.

Abdominal and thoracic injury

These injuries have a lower incidence in NAI compared with skeletal and brain injuries. They are associated with significant morbidity and mortality rates in the order of 50%[71]. With increasing age, there is a clear change in the site of fatal injury from the brain to the abdomen. The average age for blunt abdominal trauma and fatal visceral injury in abuse is 2 years, i.e. after the child has become mobile.

In NAI, the duodenum, pancreas and mesentery are injured more frequently than the liver, kidneys and spleen. The reverse is true for accidental trauma[72,73]. In children younger than 5 years, in the absence of road traffic accidents, significant abdominal injuries are extremely rare. In NAI, injuries occur secondary to direct blunt trauma or to sudden deceleration after the child is thrown.

Clinical presentation varies with the severity of injury and the interval between injury and presentation. The child may present acutely with shock, hypovolaemia and peritonitis, or more insidiously with chronic weight loss, malaise,

Table 68.5 DIFFERENTIAL DIAGNOSIS OF NONACCIDENTAL INJURY IN CHILDREN (ADAPTED FROM KLEINMAN P K (ED) 1998 DIAGNOSTIC IMAGING OF CHILD ABUSE. WILLIAMS & WILKINS, P179)

Disease	Shaft fracture	Periosteal reaction	Metaphyseal abnormality
Normal bone density			
Nonaccidental injury	+	+	+
Birth trauma	+	±	±
Congenital indifference to pain	+	+	+
Myelodysplasia	+	+	+
Osteomyelitis	–	+	+
Congenital syphilis	–	+	–
Vitamin A intoxication	–	++	–
Caffey's disease	–	+	–
Prostaglandin E therapy	–		
Metaphyseal and spondylometaphyseal dysplasias	–	–	+
Osteopenic bones			
Osteogenesis imperfecta	+	–	±
Rickets	+	+	+
Scurvy	–	+	+
Leukaemia	–	+	–
Methotrexate therapy	+	–	±
Menkes' kinky hair syndrome	–	+	+

unexplained mass lesion, or functional organ impairment. The diagnosis is often delayed or missed in these late presentations and is associated with repeated admissions to casualty or visits to the general practitioner and a higher morbidity and mortality. Typical abuse injuries may be an incidental finding detected only when imaging for other reasons, e.g. lower rib fractures on an abdominal radiograph if the child presents to the surgeons with a presumed obstruction or an acute abdomen (see Fig. 68.26C). Vomiting is a nonspecific sign occurring in both acute and chronic presentations. It can be a manifestation of either abdominal or intracranial injury. If investigations fail to identify an intra-abdominal cause, an intracranial cause must be sought.

Investigation

Blood pressure is an unreliable predictor of major organ injury in children as a normal blood pressure may be maintained despite significant blood loss, and hypotension may only be apparent when the child is moribund and almost dead[72]. If the child cannot be stabilized, imaging plays no part and immediate surgery is usually required. Once stable, imaging can proceed. The abdominal radiograph is not a sensitive investigation and demonstrates pneumoperitoneum in less than 30% of patients with visceral rupture. The roles of US and CT in accidental and nonaccidental abdominal trauma in both adults and children have been extensively studied[74–76]. CT is the 'gold standard' and remains the investigation of choice for the complete assessment of the abdomen and thorax.

The advantages of US in the acute setting are that it is portable and readily available. It can give good information on solid organ injury and can detect free fluid, but overall assessment of the abdomen is limited.

The relative roles of diagnostic peritoneal lavage (DPL) and CT in the assessment of the traumatized patient have been well debated[77,78]. CT should be performed before DPL as the presence of lavage fluid masks the presence of free fluid on CT, making it difficult to interpret its significance. All CT for trauma should be performed with intravenous contrast medium. Inspection of the images on both soft tissue and wide window settings increases the sensitivity in detecting small amounts of extraluminal air.

Abdominal injury

Solid organ injury In abuse, the liver is injured more frequently than the spleen or kidneys. In accidental trauma, the spleen and kidneys are injured more frequently than the liver. The presentation and radiology of solid organ injuries are essentially the same as those in accidental trauma. Contrast-enhanced CT is the investigation of choice. A detailed account of such injuries is outside the remit of this chapter and the reader is advised to consult specialist texts.

Although the overall incidence of renal tract injuries is rare, some injuries are more specific to NAI and include bladder rupture in the absence of a pelvic fracture following a direct blow against a full bladder. Urethral injuries may be associated with sexual abuse, often with associated injuries to the rectum, perineum and genital organs. Common presentations are an inability to void and increasing bladder distension or blood at the urethral meatus[79,80]. Bruising and/or perineal haematoma and pelvic haematoma are known sequelae. Suspected urethral rupture in boys should be confirmed by retrograde urethography before passing a urinary catheter in order to prevent converting a partial tear to a full tear.

Pancreatic injuries Trauma is the most common cause of acute pancreatitis in childhood. Acute haemorrhagic pancreatitis is highly suggestive of NAI once hereditary pancreatitis and accidental injuries have been excluded. The child may present acutely with abdominal pain, vomiting and shock, or more insidiously with weight loss, anorexia and chronic abdominal pain; it is the latter group who may present repeatedly to their general practitioner or casualty and in whom the diagnosis is often missed. More rarely, vomiting and symptoms of bowel obstruction or a palpable mass due to a pancreatic pseudocyst are present[81]. Due to its retroperitoneal location, signs of pancreatitis are classically absent. The evolution of clinical signs may be slow and associated injuries often mask the few signs that are present. Hence, the diagnosis is frequently delayed, particularly as the rise in serum amylase, although a nonspecific marker, may also be delayed for 24 h or more.

In NAI the usual mechanism of injury is a direct blow over the midline where the pancreas crosses the vertebral column. The pancreas is most frequently injured at the junction of the body and tail, and acute pancreatitis, pancreatic abscess, necrosis and pseudocyst are common sequelae. Skeletal and soft tissue injuries may accompany the pancreatitis but the association with medullary fat necrosis at distant sites and lytic osseous lesions are rare. On US, approximately 50% of affected patients demonstrate diffuse/focal gland enlargement and pancreatic duct dilatation (Fig. 68.30), and a decrease in gland reflectivity occurs in the presence of interstitial oedema. Thin-section CT has the highest rate of detection of pancreatic injury although it is quoted as missing one-third of injuries[15,82]. The CT appearances of acute pancreatitis and its complications are the same

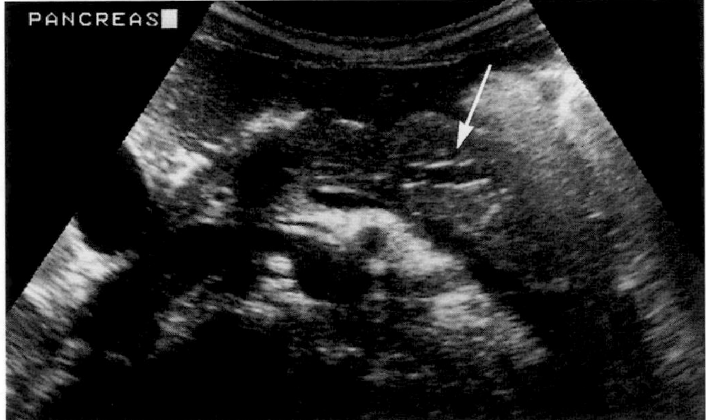

Figure 68.30 Pancreatic duct dilatation. Ultrasound of the pancreas in a young boy performed several weeks after he sustained a direct blow over the midline. In the acute stages the pancreas was enlarged and swollen. During follow-up, the pancreas demonstrates residual duct dilatation (arrow).

as those in other medical aetiologies. CT findings of peripancreatic fluid in the absence of other visceral injury are the best indicator of pancreatic injury[83,84].

Adrenal injuries These may be incidental findings detected when imaging for other abdominal trauma. Unilateral adrenal haemorrhage tends to be right sided[85] and is often clinically silent. Adrenal haemorrhage may be evident clinically when bilateral and acute adrenocortical insufficiency results[85]. On CT, haemorrhage appears as round or oval low attenuation homogeneous masses within the gland, predominantly in the medulla, but extension into the cortex is seen. There is frequently thickening of the ipsilateral diaphragmatic crus, haemorrhagic infiltration of the surrounding fat and free intraperitoneal fluid or blood. Adrenal injuries may be isolated or occur in association with injuries to the kidneys, spleen and pancreatic tail. Adrenal haemorrhages are not uncommon in the neonate and when present usually resolve within several weeks after delivery[86].

Injuries to the gastrointestinal tract These severe injuries are often diagnosed late and are thus associated with a high mortality. Bowel injuries are rare in accidental trauma but occur with a relatively high frequency in NAI due to the greater incidence of direct blows across the abdomen. The three main types of injury are mesenteric injuries, bowel disruption from partial or complete transection or perforation and haematoma formation. The mesenteric side of the bowel is more prone to vascular tears and the antimesenteric side to perforation. The duodenum, especially the second and third parts, is the area of bowel most frequently injured in abuse. Injury occurs from direct compression as the duodenum passes over the vertebral column, from shear injury or from a marked rise in intraluminal pressure when a closed loop is formed between the pylorus and ligament of Treitz[87].

Intramural haematomas of the duodenum and jejunum are the most frequent findings in bowel trauma in NAI[45,88,89]. Approximately one-third of patients sustain major vascular injuries. Vascular disruption to the small intestine is secondary to sudden deceleration or results from a compressive force of the fixed duodenum against the spine following blunt trauma. Bleeding into the submucosa and subserosa, secondary to both direct trauma and ischaemic injury, may lead to complete or partial obstruction of the lumen. Clinically, the child usually presents with abdominal pain and vomiting with signs of peritonism and obstruction. In up to 25% of patients, associated biliary and pancreatic injuries occur. The plain abdominal radiograph may demonstrate ischaemic change, proximal bowel obstruction, or free fluid. Upper gastrointestinal contrast studies are very informative. In the acute stages of a duodenal haematoma, an intramural mass with thickening of the proximal folds gives a 'coiled spring' appearance. During resolution, signs of previous haemorrhage are seen as localized masses in the duodenal wall with prominent mucosal folds[88,90] (Fig. 68.31). The haematoma may act as a lead point and result in intussusception. US may visualize the haematoma directly or demonstrate indirect signs such as proximal duodenal dilatation.

Direct trauma may result in bowel rupture and perforation[45]. The most susceptible parts are the retroperitoneal second and third parts of the duodenum, or at points of mesenteric fixation at or just distal to the ligament of Treitz and the ileocaecal junction. Perforation is the result of both compression and shearing

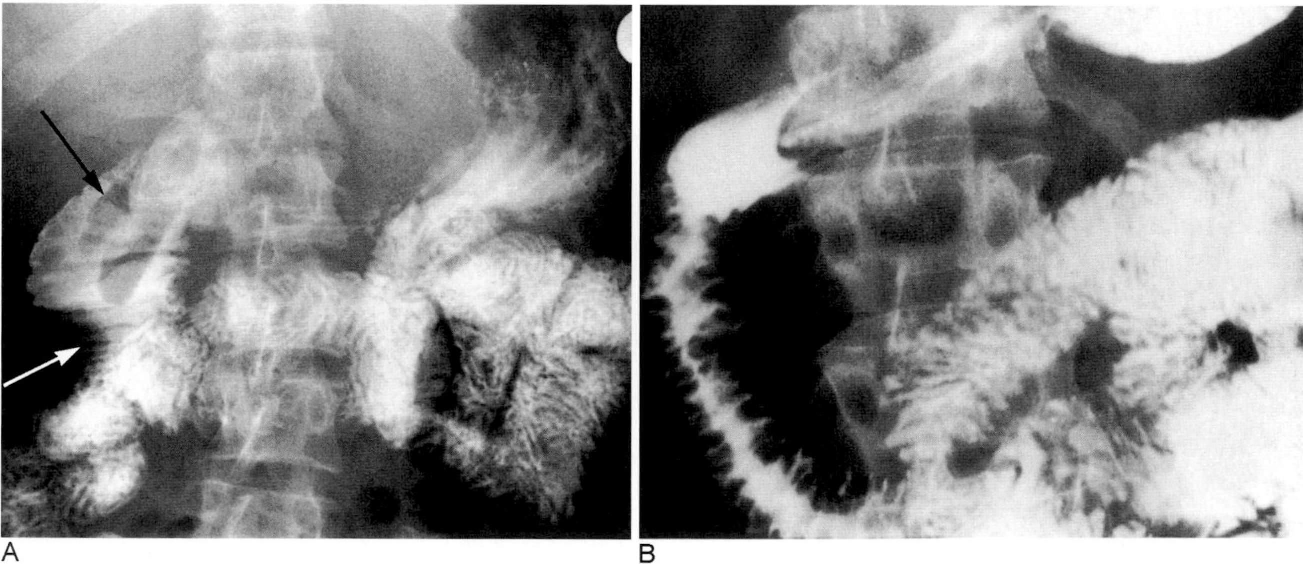

Figure 68.31 Duodenal haematoma. (A) Upper gastrointestinal contrast study following blunt trauma to the midline demonstrates the haematoma as two low density filling defects in the second part of the duodenum (black arrow) associated with prominent thickened folds giving a coiled spring appearance (white arrow). (B) Resolving duodenal haematoma of the second part of the duodenum seen as localized intramural masses associated with prominent mucosal folds. [From Rao P 1999 Emergency imaging in non-accidental injury. In: Carty (ed) Medical radiology: Emergency paediatric radiology. Springer-Verlag, Berlin.]

between opposing surfaces. A clinical presentation of perforation may be delayed and a delay of more than 24h increases the mortality rate from 5% to 60%. If sufficient free air is present, perforation is readily diagnosed on plain radiography and no other imaging is needed, surgery being the next step. An erect chest or lateral decubitus radiograph can theoretically detect as little as 1–2ml of free air, but it is not always possible to obtain these in very ill or shocked children, and a horizontal beam lateral or a supine radiograph often has to suffice. CT is again the optimal investigation. A significant amount of unexplained peritoneal fluid is the most frequent sign of bowel rupture. A very sensitive and specific sign of blunt bowel trauma is abnormally intense bowel wall enhancement on contrast-enhanced CT seen in the hypoperfusion complex/shock bowel syndrome[91–93]. The CT appearances may be confused with bowel rupture, but it is important to distinguish the two as shock bowel requires attention to haemodynamic and fluid balance while rupture requires surgery.

Mesenteric injuries include haematoma formation from trauma to small peripheral branches. Severe injuries result from complete avulsion of the superior mesenteric vessels, resulting in mesenteric ischaemia and large quantities of peritoneal blood[94]. Ischaemic strictures of the bowel are late complications[95]. On CT there is streaky infiltration of the mesentery, bowel wall thickening, haemoperitoneum and mesenteric haematoma.

The stomach is rarely injured in abuse, occurring in less than 1% of cases[96], and is usually associated with additional injury to the ribs, spleen and left kidney.

Gastric rupture after trauma usually follows a meal when the stomach is full and distended. It is also a rare consequence of failure to pass a nasogastric tube in gastric dilatation secondary to duodenal obstruction or paralysis in acute atony in neglected children. Gastric perforation and rupture are life-threatening events, potentially resulting in septic shock and death[45]. In 60% of cases, pneumoperitoneum is evident radiographically. In these children there is no need for further imaging and immediate surgery is required.

Colonic injury is rare in NAI as the colon is protected from direct trauma by the bony pelvis or by its peripheral location in the abdomen. The types of injury sustained are similar to those in the small intestine. Both the transverse colon and jejunum are subject to the same compressive force as they cross the spine. Colonic haematoma in association with jejunal haematoma has been documented[45]. Anal and rectal injuries presenting as perineal and pelvic abscesses, faecal peritonitis and rectal tears occur in association with sexual abuse. Colonic perforation may occur from direct stabbing or from forced insertion of foreign bodies.

Thoracic injury

Direct contusional injury of the lungs and pleura is rare even in the presence of rib fractures[45]. Rib fractures or bruising are not always evident and mild injuries may be undetected. In all cases of suspected abuse, if bone scintigraphy is not available, a repeat chest radiograph should be performed after 10–14d and re-assessed for fractures. Complications of direct thoracic compression, usually as a result of direct punching or stamping, are the same as those in accidental trauma. Pneumothorax and pleural effusions are not commonly seen in abusive thoracic injury, whereas they are common sequelae in accidental trauma. Contrast-enhanced CT is the investigation of choice and will also determine the presence of any associated diaphragmatic injury. In the presence of both anterior rib fractures and sternal fractures, associated myocardial injury should be suspected.

Diaphragmatic injury Rupture may be difficult to diagnose clinically as there may be few physical signs and these may be masked by other injuries. It should be considered if either hemidiaphragm is indistinct. However, the chest radiograph is normal in 10–20% of cases. In intubated patients, the positive pressure ventilation may delay herniation of abdominal contents into the thorax giving a false negative result. The true radiological diagnosis is delayed until extubation when herniation occurs leading to respiratory embarrassment.

Summary

Children may suffer from many different types of abuse. As doctors and as radiologists we are concerned with suggesting, diagnosing and confirming NAI. It is incumbent upon all of us to be aware of the possibility of abuse. There may be no skeletal manifestations or external soft tissue markers and radiology may provide the only documentation of abuse. There should be no hesitation in gaining a second opinion if uncertain or in doubtful cases. Good relationship with the paediatricians and support services is essential. Our ultimate aim is the protection of and welfare of the child.

BRAIN INJURIES

NAI is the leading cause of serious head injury and death in infants under 2 years of age[32,58]. External indicators of injury such as skull fracture (see above) or bruising may be absent[97]. The clinical presentation is often nonspecific. The child may present repeatedly to the general practitioner or casualty department with vague symptoms, such as irritability, lethargy and feeding difficulties. These symptoms are often overlooked due to their lack of specificity but they are often a precursor to more serious NAI. Acute severe presentation, such as fits, vomiting, or collapse may occur[98,99]. In the absence of bruising the initial presumed diagnosis is often meningitis.

Intracranial manifestations of head injury

Most children who suffer nonaccidental brain injury are under 2 years of age. The initial brain injury in head trauma is known as the primary injury. The two main mechanisms of intracranial trauma are impact injuries, including acceleration/deceleration and whiplash shaking injuries. Pathophysiological responses to the primary injury, such as cerebral oedema, cerebral congestion, fall in cerebral blood flow, shock and cerebral vasospasm may result in the secondary injury—hypoxic ischaemic damage[99,100]. The term 'whiplash shaken baby syndrome' describes the association of subdural and/or subarachnoid haemorrhage, massive cerebral oedema, fractured ribs and metaphyseal injury in the absence of external signs of cranial trauma[101,102].

Shaking injuries usually occur in children younger than 1 year of age but may occur up to about 2 years, the child being held by the rib cage and squeezed, resulting in fractured ribs and high central venous pressure. Retinopathy, common in NAI, is probably a consequence of high central venous pressure. In older children, who are held by the shoulders or upper arms, subperiosteal bleeding and periosteal reaction in the humeri occur. The young infant has a relatively large head in relation to his/her body, which, when associated with weak neck muscles, results in poor head support and little control. The whiplash movement causes the head to lash to and fro and rotate. Both duration and velocity of the action are important factors. The baby's brain is relatively small in relation to the size of the cranium and, as the meninges are loose, it starts to move in different directions, which generates shearing forces within the skull and brain. This action is exaggerated by the rotational element which is important in producing the brain injury and associated subdural haemorrhage[58,62,101,103–105].

Shaking alone can cause brain injury. However, many shaken children are also thrown at the end of the shake, the head impacting against a hard surface and resulting in a shaking–impact injury. The skull fracture is often the last event in the inflicted trauma.

Brain injury may be further contributed to by hypoxia sustained as the child's chest is squeezed during shaking causing impaired ventilation and respiratory embarassment[106]. Both carotid occlusion secondary to violent neck motion, or direct strangulation[106] and suffocation, such as by a hand or pillow in blocking the mouth in order to suppress crying, can contribute to hypoxia[107,108]. Innocent activity, such as playfully lifting the child above the head, does not result in brain injury. The degree of force needed is such that a neutral observer who saw a child being shaken would recognize the violence of the act and would regard it as dangerous[32].

The major complications of intracranial injury in abuse are subdural haematoma, cerebral oedema, hypoxic ischaemic encephalopathy, cortical contusions and shearing injuries. Rarer manifestations include intracerebral and intraventricular haemorrhage and extradural haematoma.

Cortical contusions occur from impact trauma and may be accompanied by a fracture. If the head is stationary, they occur at the site of impact. If the head is moving, contre coup injuries distant from the site of impact may occur. Contusions tend to occur in the temporal and frontal lobes, particularly the parasagittal cerebral cortex adjacent to the falx[100]. However, they are more common in older children and in accidental injury, and are less frequent in NAI (Figs 68.32, 68.33).

Subdural haematoma

Subdural haematoma is the most common intracranial finding in NAI. The finding of a subdural haematoma has a high specificity for abuse. It results from trauma associated with rotation between the brain and dura causing shearing of the bridging veins in the subdural space[109]. The force required to produce a subdural haematoma is severe.

Accidental causes of subdural haematoma in infants and children are rare, occurring in, for example, major road traffic accidents[65,110,111]. In these instances the incident has usually been witnessed and a history and other injuries compatible with the degree of trauma are present.

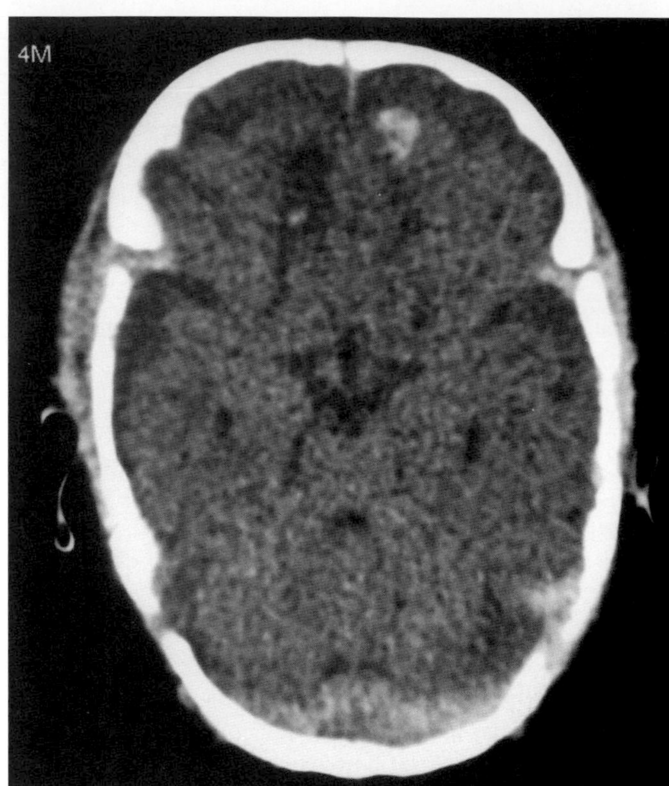

Figure 68.32 Frontal lobe contusion. Axial unenhanced CT of the brain demonstrating an area of low density in the right frontal lobe consistent with contusion. There is an area of mixed high and low density in the left frontal parasagittal region consistent with haemorrhagic contusion. Associated subdural blood is also noted.

Certain features of subdural haematoma are unusual in accidental trauma and are suspicious of NAI. These are:

- The presence of sudurals without a skull fracture, implying a shaking injury.
- Bilateral subdurals (Figs 68.33, 68.34).
- Subdurals of different ages (Fig. 68.35). The density of blood on CT and MRI varies with its age (Table 68.6).
- Subdurals in the presence of retinal haemorrhages, implying an acceleration–deceleration force.
- Acute interhemispheric fissure subdural or falx haemorrhage (Fig. 68.36). This is evident as a bright and irregularly thickened falx[112,113]. It must be distinguished from a normal falx which may appear bright against the background of an abnormally low density brain. In accidental trauma, subdural bleeds do not usually extend into the falx.

Confusion may occur in differentiating chronic bilateral subdural haemorrhage from cases of unrelated cerebral atrophy or the more common benign enlargement of the extra-axial spaces. In neither of these should blood products be present and the changes are usually symmetrical.

Brain oedema and hypoxic ischaemic encephalopathy

The 'reversal sign' describes a distinctive CT appearance in a group of children with hypoxic ischaemic cerebral injury and it carries a poor prognosis. It is highly associated with child

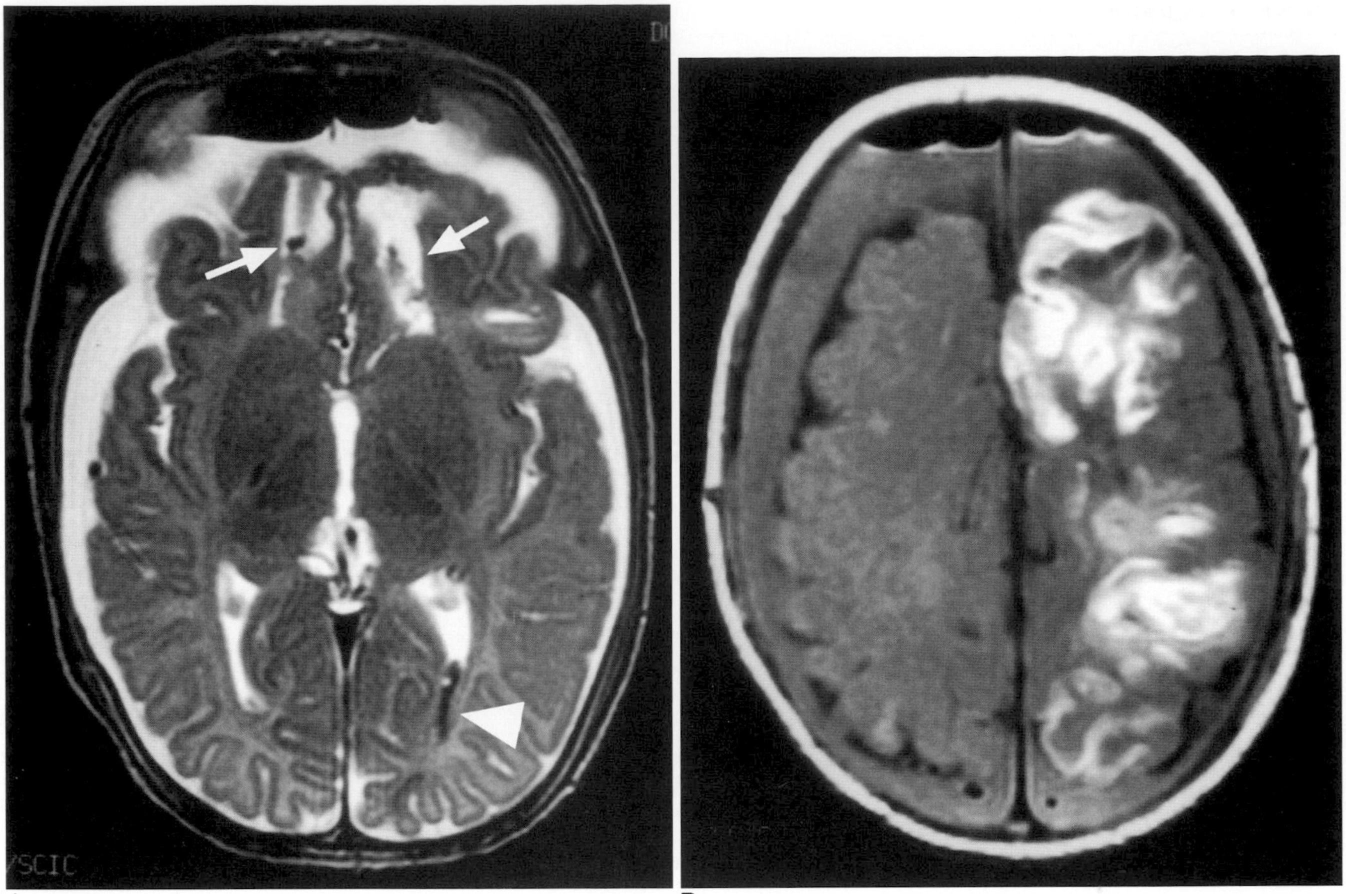

A B

Figure 68.33 Bilateral subdural haematoma. (A) Axial T2-weighted image of an abused infant after drainage of bilateral subdural collections demonstrating bilateral frontal, parasagittal haemorrhagic contusions (arrows). Intraventricular blood is also noted in the posterior horn of the left lateral ventricle (arrowhead). (B) Axial T1-weighted image demonstrating bilateral iso-intense subdural haemorrhages and pneumocephalus. There is an extensive area of high signal accompanied by punctate areas of low signal consistent with laminar cortical necrosis demonstrated in the left hemisphere.

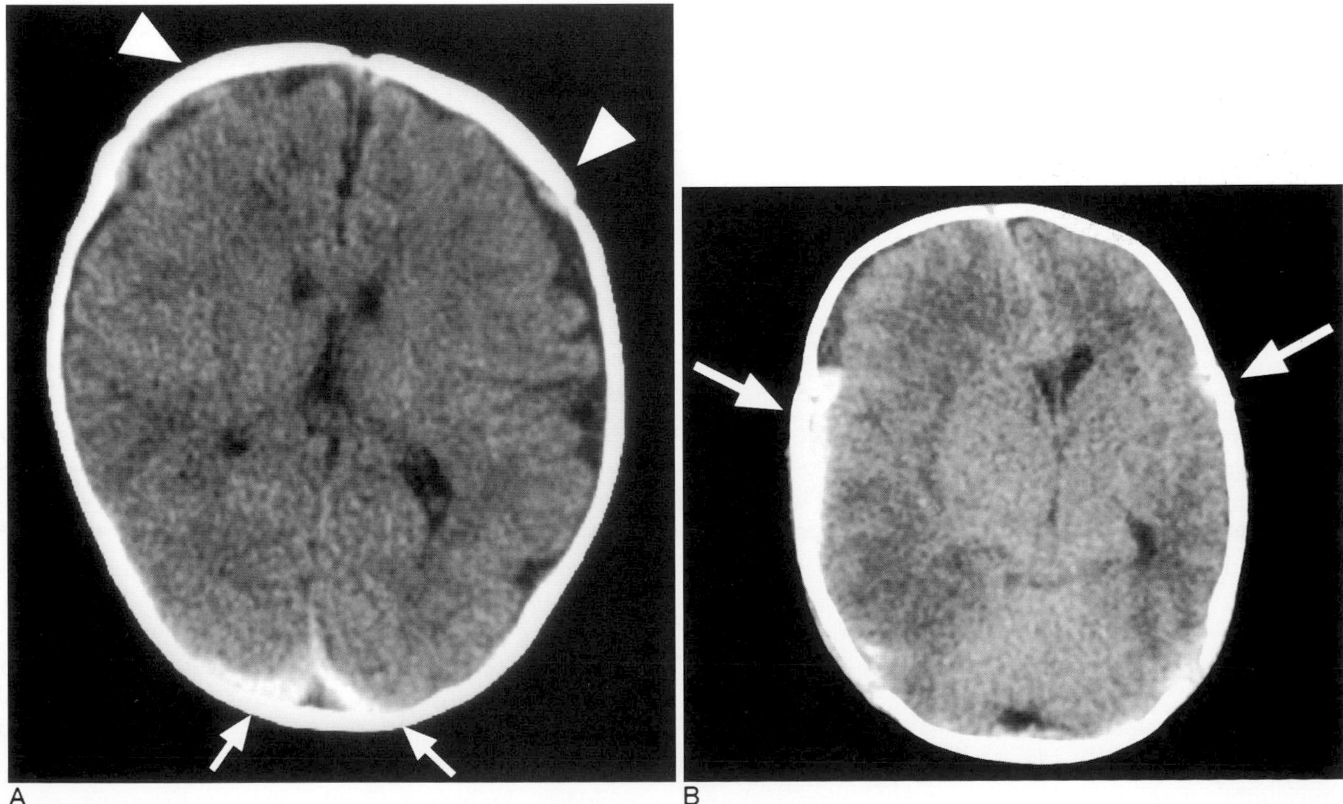

Figure 68.34 Bilateral subdural haematoma. (A) Axial unenhanced CT demonstrating a bilateral fresh high density subdural haematoma over both posterior parietal lobes (arrows) and both frontal lobes (arrowheads). (B) Axial unenhanced CT demonstrating bilateral fresh, high density subdural blood (arrows). On the right, there is associated infarction of the brain in the right middle cerebral artery territory associated with mass effect and contralateral midline shift.

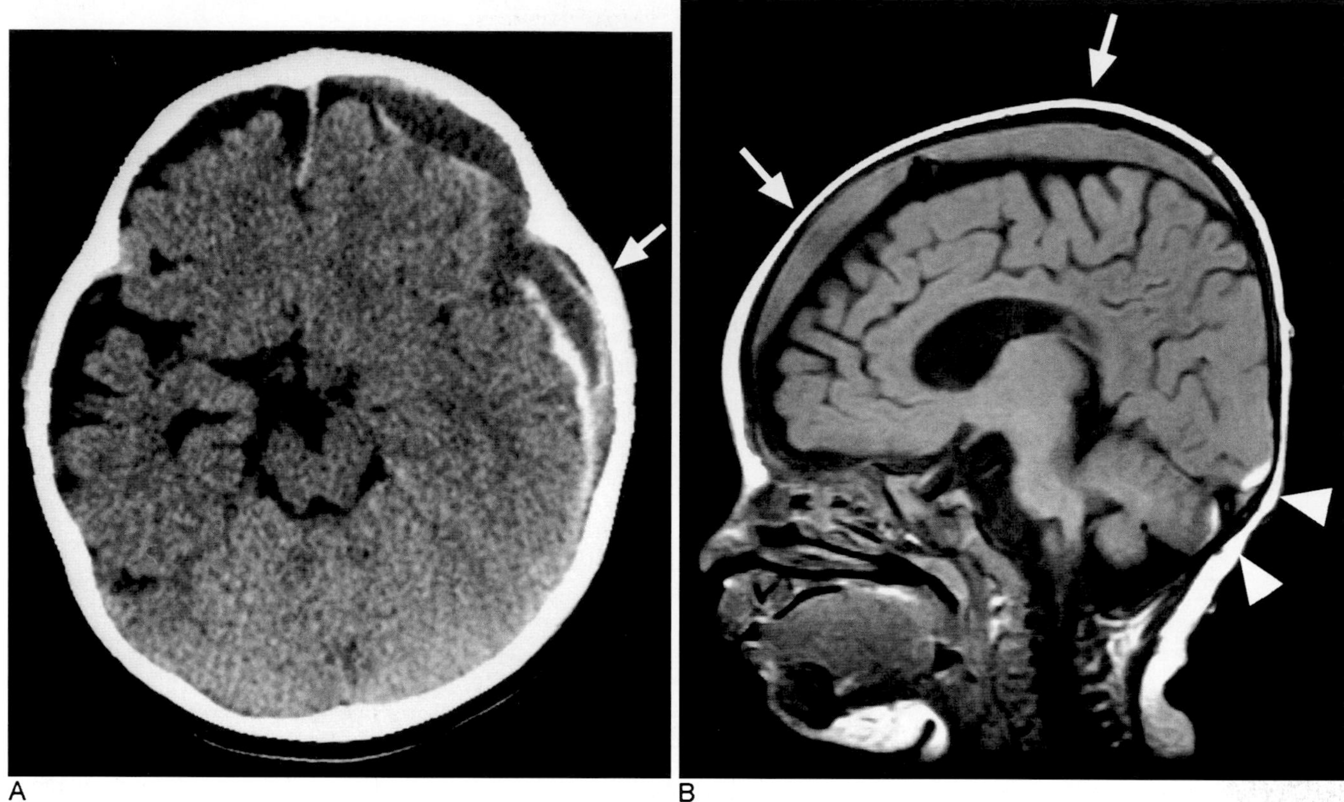

Figure 68.35 Subdural haematomas of differing ages. (A) Acute on chronic subdural haematoma. Axial unenhanced CT demonstrating subdural blood of differing ages in the left frontal and temporal regions (arrow). (B) Sagittal T1-weighted MRI slice demonstrating fresh iso-intense subdural haemorrhage over the frontal and parietal convexities (arrows). A small amount of hyperintense subdural blood is also noted in the occipital and posterior parietal region (arrowheads).

Table 68.6 CT AND MRI OF INTRACRANIAL HAEMORRHAGE: CHANGE IN DENSITY/SIGNAL WITH AGE

Time	NECT density	CECT density	T1-weighted signal	T2-weighted signal	Gradient-echo signal
4–6 h	Hyper	—	Iso-intense	Hyper	Hypo
7–72 h	Hyper	—	Iso-intense	Hypo	Very hypo
4–7 d	Hyper/iso-intese	—	Iso-intense (centre) Hyper (rim)	Hypo	Very hypo
1–4 weeks	Iso-intense/hypo	Rim enhancing	Hyper	Hyper	Hypo
Chronic	Hypo	—	Hypo	Hypo	Hypo

NECT = nonenhanced CT, CECT = contrast enhanced CT

abuse[113]. The CT features of the reversal sign are of diffusely decreased grey and white matter density with decreased or lost grey–white matter differentiation and a relative preservation in density of the thalami, basal ganglia and cerebellum (Fig. 68.37). The appearances are not unique to NAI and can result from a variety of brain insults, such as drowning, fits, status asthmaticus, cardiac arrest and accidental trauma. The evolution of the changes of hypoxic ischaemic encephalopathy is the same whatever the cause. The finding of acute interhemispheric fissure subdural haemorrhage together with the acute reversal sign should be regarded as highly suggestive of a shaking injury of NAI[114].

Complications of the brain injury include obstructive hydrocephalus from arachnoiditis, communicating hydrocephalus from alteration in the CSF dynamics, cerebral atrophy, cerebral arterial and venous infarction and multicystic encephalomalacia.

Investigations

In children, severe intracranial injury can occur in the absence of skull fracture. Skull radiography is not a reliable predictor of intracranial injury. Skull radiography is recommended in children over 2 years of age to confirm a suspected depressed fracture or penetrating injury, or where NAI is suspected, but should be performed in all children under 2 years of age with suspected injury because of the greater probability of NAI in this younger age group[66].

Any obtunded or neurologically unstable child requires cross-sectional brain imaging. Any child suspected of abuse where a skull fracture is detected, even in the absence of neurological indication, should undergo neuroimaging to confirm or exclude intracranial injury. Multiplanar CT of the brain is the initial investigation of choice. An initial series of images should be obtained without intravenous contrast

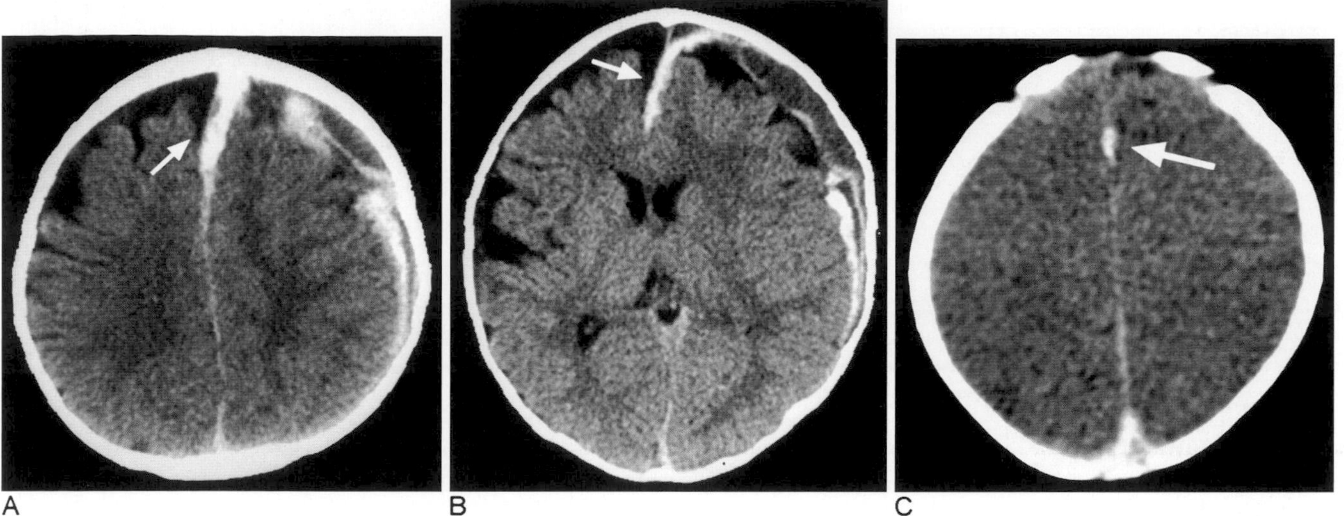

Figure 68.36 Acute interhemispheric subdural haematoma. (A) Axial unenhanced CT demonstrating acute interhemispheric fissure subdural blood (arrow). Acute on chronic subdural haemorrhage is also present over the left frontal and parietal convexity. (B) Fresh subdural blood is seen tracking along the interhemispheric fissure anteriorly (arrow). (C) Axial unenhanced CT of a different abused baby demonstrates a thickened, bright interhemispheric fissure due to the presence of fresh subdural blood (arrow). The brain is of generalized low density due to associated oedema.

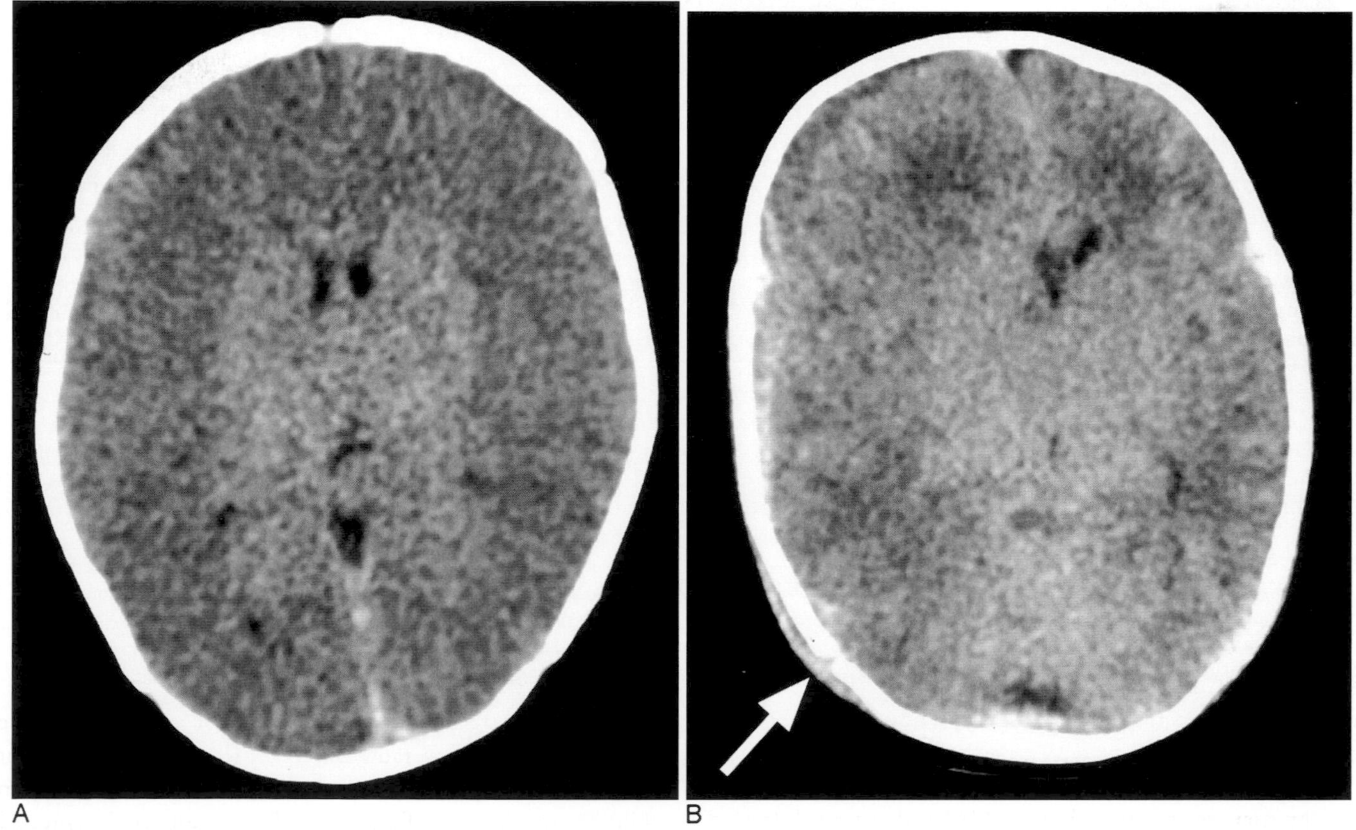

Figure 68.37 Reversal sign in hypoxic ischaemic encephalopathy. (A) Axial unenhanced CT of an abused baby who was shaken, demonstrating the 'reversal sign'. The brain is oedematous with loss of grey–white matter differentiation and reduced density. There is relative preservation in density of the thalami and basal ganglia. (B) Axial unenhanced CT demonstrating an oedematous, swollen brain with reduced grey–white matter differentiation and mass effect. Small bilateral hyperdense subdural bleeds are present. A right posterior parietal skull vault fracture is present and is associated with an overlying scalp haematoma (arrow).

medium. If an isodense subdural is suspected, intravenous contrast medium may help in its identification.

In neonates and small babies with a patent fontanelle, high resolution transfontanellar US will detect subdural collections[115] and differentiate them from subarachnoid collections. However, US lacks sufficient parenchymal definition, it is operator dependent and there are some relatively inaccessible areas of the brain. Thus US is not considered adequate as the sole investigation for the brain.

MRI is the imaging method of choice in the stable child for overall full assessment of the intracranial structures, particularly cortical contusions, shearing injuries, small haemorrhages and early ischaemia and for long-term follow-up. In the early stages, MRI may be very useful if the CT is negative when there is a strong clinical suspicion of abuse.

MRI sequence protocols for brain injury may vary between departments with different machines and field strengths. Standard T1- and T2-weighted sequences are needed and modern systems can now provide fast T2-weighted images, with or without fat suppression. There is increasing use of perfusion and diffusion imaging and spectroscopy. Depending on age, inversion recovery techniques (e.g. FLAIR) may be helpful. In the younger patient MR angiographic (MRA) techniques may be contributory when an infarct is suspected.

Acknowledgements

W Ramsden would like to thank Miss J Moran for typing the manuscript, and Professor H Carty, Dr M Elias, Dr J Foster and Mr M Hampshire for the loan of illustrations.

REFERENCES

1. Borden S IV 1975 Roentgen recognition of acute plastic bowing of the forearm in children. Am J Roentgenol 125: 524–530
2. Komara J S, Kottamasu L, Kottamasu S R 1986 Acute plastic bowing fractures in children. Ann Emerg Med 15: 585–588
3. Ohta-Fukushima M, Mutoh Y, Takasugi S, Iwata H, Ishii S 2002 Characteristics of stress fractures in young athletes under 20 years. J Sports Med Physical Fitness 42: 198–206
4. Carty H 1994 Sports injuries in children—a radiological viewpoint. Arch Dis Child 70: 457–460
5. Griffith J F, Roebuck D J, Cheng J C Y et al 2001 Acute elbow trauma in children: Spectrum of injury revealed by MR imaging not apparent on radiographs. Am J Roentgenol 176: 53–60
6. Caputo A E, Watson H K, Nissen C 1995 Scaphoid nonunion in a child: A case report. J Hand Surg 20A: 243–245
7. Johnson K J, Haigh S F, Symonds K E 2000 MRI in the management of scaphoid fractures in skeletally immature patients. Pediatr Radiol 30: 685–688
8. Torode I, Zieg D 1985 Pelvic fractures in children. J Pediatr Orthop 5: 76–84
9. Garvin K L, McCarthy R E, Barnes C L, Dodge B M 1990 Pediatric pelvic ring fractures. J Pediatr Orthop 10: 577–582
10. Rees M J, Aickin R, Kolbe A, Teele R L 2001 The screening pelvic radiograph in pediatric trauma. Pediatr Radiol 31: 497–500
11. Hamilton P R, Broughton N S 1998 Traumatic hip dislocation in childhood. J Pediatr Orthop 18: 691–694
12. Rubel I F, Kloen P, Potter H G, Helfet D L 2002 MRI assessment of the posterior acetabular wall fracture in traumatic dislocation of the hip in children. Pediatr Radiol 32: 435–439
13. Zionts L E 2002 Fractures around the knee in children. J Am Acad Orthop Surg 10: 345–355
14. Close B J, Strouse P J 2000 MR of physeal fractures of the adolescent knee. Pediatr Radiol 30: 756–762
15. Accousti W K, Willis R B 2003 Tibial eminence fractures. Orthop Clin North Am 34: 365–375
16. Swischuk L E, John S D, Tschoepe E J 1999 Upper tibial hyperextension fractures in infants: another occult toddler's fracture. Pediatr Radiol 29: 6–9
17. Zobel M S, Borrello J A, Siegel M J, Stewart N R 1994 Pediatric knee MR imaging: Pattern of injuries in the immature skeleton. Radiology 190: 397–401
18. King S J, Carty H M L, Brady O 1996 Magnetic resonance imaging of knee injuries in children. Pediatr Radiol 26: 287–290
19. Strouse P J, Koujok K 2002 Magnetic resonance imaging of the pediatric knee. Top Magn Reson Imaging 13: 277–294
20. Nietosvaara Y, Aalto K, Kallio P E 1994 Acute patellar dislocation in children: Incidence and associated osteochondral fractures. J Pediatr Orthop 14: 513–515
21. Horn B D, Crisci K, Krug M, Pizzutillo P D, MacEwen G D 2001 Radiologic evaluation of juvenile tillaux fractures of the distal tibia. J Pediatr Orthop 21: 162–164
22. Inokuchi S, Usami N, Hiraishi E, Hashimoto T 1998 Calcaneal fractures in children. J Pediatr Orthop 18: 469–474
23. Ribbans W J, Natarajan R, Alavala S 2005 Pediatric foot fractures. Clin Orthop Rel Res 432: 107–115
24. Prokuski L J, Saltzman C L 1997 Challenging fractures of the foot and ankle. Radiol Clin North Am 35: 655–670
25. Shaw M, Burnett H, Wilson A, Chan O 1999 Pseudosubluxation of C2 on C3 in polytraumatized children—prevalence and significance. Clin Radiol 54: 377–380
26. Kathol M H 1997 Cervical spine trauma. What is new? Radiol Clin North Am 35: 507–532
27. Apple J S, Kirks D R, Merten D F, Martinez S 1987 Cervical spine fractures and dislocations in children. Pediatr Radiol 17: 45–49
28. Martin B W, Dykes E, Lecky F E 2004 Patterns and risks in spinal trauma. Arch Dis Child 89: 860–865
29. Reddy S P, Junewick J J, Backstrom J W 2003 Distribution of spinal fractures in children: does age, mechanism of injury, or gender play a significant role? Pediatr Radiol 33: 776–781
30. Glass R B J, Sivit C J, Sturm P F, Bulas D I, Eichelberger M R 1994 Lumbar spine injury in a pediatric population: Difficulties with computed tomographic diagnosis. J Trauma 37: 815–819
31. Silverman F N 1972 Unrecognised trauma in infants, the battered child syndrome and the syndrome of Ambroise Tardieu. Radiology 104: 337–353
32. American Academy of Pediatrics Committee on Child Abuse and Neglect 1993 Shaken baby syndrome; inflicted cerebral trauma. Pediatrics 92: 872–875
33. Carty H 1993 Case report: Child abuse—necklace calcification—a sign of strangulation. Br J Radiol 66:1186–1188
34. Kleinman P K 1996 Follow up skeletal survey in suspected child abuse. Am J Radiol 167: 893–896
35. Nimkin K, Spevak M, Kleinman P K 1997 Fractures of the hands and feet in child abuse: Imaging and pathological features. Radiology 203: 233–236
36. Mandelstam S A, Cook D, Fitzgerald M, Ditchfield M R 2003 Complementary use of radiological skeletal survey and bone scintigraphy in detection of bony injuries in suspected child abuse. Arch Dis Child 88: 387–390
37. Sty J R, Starshak R J 1983 The role of bone scintigraphy in the evaluation of the suspected abused child. Radiology 146: 369–375
38. Conway J J, Collium M, Tanz R R et al 1993 The role of scintigraphy in detecting child abuse. Semin Nucl Med 23: 321–333
39. McDowell H P, Fielding D W 1984 Traumatic perforation of the hypopharynx—an unusual form of abuse. Arch Dis Child 59: 888–889
40. Kleinman P K, Spevak M R, Hansen M 1992 Mediastinal pseudocyst caused by pharyngeal perforation during child abuse. Case report. Am J Radiol 158: 1111–1113
41. Ablin D S, Reinhart M A 1992 Oesophageal perforation by a tooth in child abuse. Pediatr Radiol 22: 339–341
42. Carty H 1989 Skeletal manifestations of child abuse. Bone 6: 3–7
43. Loder R T, Bookout C 1991 Fracture patterns in battered children. J Orthop Trauma 5: 428–433
44. Carty H 1993 Fractures caused by child abuse. Br J Bone Joint Surg 75: 849–857
45. Kleinman P K 1990 Diagnostic imaging in child abuse. Am J Radiol 155: 703
46. Kleinman P K, Marks S C, Blackbourne B 1986 The metaphyseal lesion in abused infants: a radiological histopathological study. Am J Roentgenol 146: 895–905
47. Kleinman P K, Marks S C 1996 A regional approach to the classic metaphyseal lesion in abused infants: The proximal tibia. Am J Radiol 166: 421–426

48. Kleinman P K, Belanger P L, Karellas A et al 1991 Normal metaphyseal radiologic variants not to be confused with findings of infant abuse. Am J Roentgenol 156: 781–783
49. King J, Didendorf D, Apthorp J et al 1988 Analysis of 429 fractures in 189 battered children. J Pediatr Orthop 8: 585–589
50. Thomas S A, Rosenfield N S, Leventhal J M et al 1991 Long bone fractures in young children: distinguishing accidental injuries from child abuse. Pediatrics 88: 471
51. Beals R K, Tufts E 1983 Fractured femur in infancy: The role of child abuse. J Pediatr Orthop 3: 583
52. Schwend R M, Werth C, Johnston A 2000 Femur shaft fractures in toddlers and young children: rarely from child abuse. J Pediatr Orthop 20: 475–481
53. Caffey J 1946 Multiple fractures in the long bones of infants suffering from chronic subdural haematoma. Am J Radiol 56: 163–173
54. Chapman S 1990 Radiological aspects of non accidental injury. J R Soc Med 83: 67–71
55. Kleinman P K 1998 Skeletal trauma: general considerations. In: Kleinman P K (ed) Diagnostic imaging in child abuse. Williams and Wilkins, Baltimore, p8
56. Carty H 1995 Radiological features of child abuse. Curr Pediatr 5: 230–235
57. Kleinman P K 1998 Bony thoracic trauma. In: Kleinman P K (ed) Diagnostic imaging in child abuse. Williams and Wilkins, Baltimore, p110
58. Carty H, Ratcliffe J 1995 The shaken infant syndrome. BMJ 310: 344
59. Feldman K W, Brewer D K 1984 Child abuse, cardiopulmonary resuscitation and rib fractures. Pediatrics 73: 339
60. Spevak M R, Kleinman P K, Belanger P L et al 1990 Does cardiopulmonary resuscitation cause rib fractures in infants? Post mortem radiologic–pathologic study. Radiology 177: 162 (abstr)
61. Strouse P J, Owings C L 1995 Fractures of the first rib in child abuse. Radiology 197: 763–765
62. Carty H 1991 The non skeletal injuries of child abuse: The brain. Year Book of Pediatric Radiology, vol 3. Mosby, St Louis
63. Epstein J A, Epstein B S, Small M 1961 Subepicranial hydroma. J Paediatr 4: 562–566
64. Thornbry J R, Campbell J A, Masters S J et al 1983 Skull fracture and low risk of intracranial sequelae in minor head trauma. Am J Radiol 143: 661
65. Harwood-Nash D C, Hendrick E B, Hudson A R 1971 The significance of skull fractures in children. A study of 1187 patients. Radiology 101: 151
66. Duhaime A C, Alario A J, Lewander W J et al 1992 Head injury in very young children: mechanisms, injury types and ophthalmic findings in 100 hospitalised patients younger than two years of age. Paediatrics 90: 179–185
67. Musemeche C A, Barthel M, Cosentino C et al 1991 Paediatric falls from heights. J Trauma 31: 1347
68. Reiber G D 1993 Fatal falls in childhood. How far must children fall to sustain fatal head injury? Report of cases and review of the literature. Am J Forensic Med Pathol 14: 201
69. Chadwick D L, Chin S, Salerno C et al 1991 Deaths from falls in children. How far is fatal? J Trauma 31: 1353–1355
70. Kravitz H, Dreissen G, Gomberg R et al 1969 Accidental falls from elevated surfaces in infants from birth to one year of age. Paediatrics 44: 869–876
71. Cooper A, Floyd T, Barlow B et al 1988 Major blunt abdominal trauma due to child abuse. J Trauma 28: 1483–1487
72. Sivit C, Taylor L, Eichelberger M 1989 Visceral injury in battered children: A changing perspective. Radiology 173: 651–659
73. Filiatrault D, Garel L 1995 Paediatric blunt abdominal trauma—to sound or not to sound. Pediatr Radiol 25: 329–331
74. Turnock R R, Sprigg A, Lloyd D A 1983 CT in the management of blunt abdominal trauma in children. Br J Surg 80: 982–984
75. Sivit C J, Kaufman R A 1995 Commentary: Sonography in the evaluation of children following blunt abdominal trauma: is it to be or not to be? Pediatr Radiol 25: 326–328
76. Jamieson D H, Babyn P S, Pearl R 1996 Imaging gastrointestinal perforation in paediatric blunt abdominal trauma. Pediatr Radiol 26: 188–194
77. Alyono D, Morrow C E, Perry J F Jr 1982 Reappraisal of diagnostic peritoneal lavage criteria for operation in penetrating and blunt trauma. Surgery 92: 751–757
78. Davis J W, Hoyt D B 1990 Complications in evaluating abdominal trauma: DPL versus computerised axial tomography. J Trauma 30: 1506–1509
79. Noe H N, Jerkins G R 1992 Genitourinary trauma. In: Kelalis P P, King L R, Belman A B (eds) Clinical pediatric urology, 3rd edn. WB Saunders, Philadelphia pp1353–1378
80. Goldman S M, Sandler C M, Corriere J N Jr et al 1997 Blunt urethral trauma: A unified anatomical mechanical classification. J Urol 157: 85–89
81. Carty H 1991 The non skeletal injuries of child abuse. Part 2. The body. 1991 Year book of pediatric radiology, vol 3. Mosby, St Louis
82. Sivit C J, Eichelberger M, Taylor L 1992 Blunt pancreatic trauma in children: CT diagnosis. Am J Radiol 158: 1097–1100
83. Jeffrey R B, Federle M P, Grass R A 1983 Computed tomography of pancreatic trauma. Radiology 147: 491–494
84. King L R, Siegel M J, Balge D M 1995 Acute pancreatitis in children: CT findings of intra- and extrapancreatic fluid collections. Radiology 195: 196–200
85. Nimkin K, Teeger S, Wallach M T 1994 Adrenal hemorrhage in abuse children: Imaging and post mortem findings. Am J Radiol 162: 661–663
86. Burks D W, Mirvis S E, Shanmuganathan K 1994 Acute adrenal injury after blunt abdominal trauma: CT findings. Am J Radiol 162: 661–663
87. Cox T D, Kuhn J P 1996 CT scan of bowel trauma in the pediatric patient. Radiol Clin North Am 34: 807–818
88. Kleinman P K, Brill P W, Winchester P 1986 Resolving duodenal–jejunal hematoma in abused children. Radiology 160: 747–750
89. Fulcher A S, Das Narla L, Brewer W H 1990 Gastric hematoma and pneumatosis in child abuse. Case report. Am J Radiol 155: 1283–1284
90. Bratu M, Dower J C, Siegel B et al 1970 Jejunal hematoma, child abuse and Felson's sign. Conn Med 31: 261–264
91. Taylor G, Fallat M, Eichelberger M 1987 Hypovolaemic shock in children: Abdominal CT manifestations. Radiology 164: 479
92. Hara H, Babyn P S, Bourgeois D 1989 Significance of bowel wall enhancement on CT following blunt abdominal trauma in childhood. J Comput Assist Tomogr 13: 430–432
93. Sivit C J, Eichelberger M R, Taylor G A 1994 CT in children with rupture of the bowel caused by blunt trauma: Diagnostic efficacy and comparison with hypoperfusion complex. Am J Radiol 163: 1195–1198
94. Rizzo M J, Federle M P, Griffiths B G 1992 Bowel and mesenteric injury following blunt trauma: Diagnosis with CT. Am J Radiol 159: 1217–1221
95. Shah P, Applegate K E, Buonomo C 1997 Stricture of the duodenum and jejunum in an abused child. Pediatr Radiol 27: 281–283
96. Brunsting L, Morton J 1987 Gastric rupture from blunt abdominal trauma. J Trauma 27: 887
97. Lloyd D A, Carty H, Patterson M et al 1997 Predictive value of skull radiography for intracranial injury in children with blunt head injury. Lancet 349: 821–824
98. Ludwig S, Warman M 1984 Shaken baby syndrome. A review of twenty cases. Ann Emerg Med 13: 104
99. Brown J K, Minns R A 1993 Non accidental head injury with particular reference to whiplash shaking and medicolegal aspects. Dev Med Child Neurol 35: 849–869
100. Kleinman P K, Barnes P D 1998 Head trauma. In: Kleinman P (ed) Diagnostic imaging of child abuse, 2nd edn. Mosby, St Louis, pp 285–342
101. Caffey J 1972 On the theory and practice of shaking infants. Am J Dis Child 124: 161–169
102. Caffey J 1974 The whiplash shaken baby syndrome: manual shaking by the extremities with whiplash induced intracranial and intraocular bleedings linked with residual permanent brain damage and mental retardation. Paediatrics 54: 396–403
103. Ommaya A K, Faas F, Yamell P 1968 Whiplash injury and brain damage. An experimental study. JAMA 204: 75–79

104. Dykes L 1986 The whiplash shaken infant syndrome. What has been learned? Child Abuse Neglect 10: 211–221

105. Newton R W 1989 Intracranial haemorrhage and non accidental injury. Arch Dis Child 64: 188–190

106. Bird C R, McMahan J R, Gilles F H et al 1987 Strangulation in child abuse: CT diagnosis. Radiology 163: 373–375

107. Krugman R D 1985 Fatal child abuse: Analysis of 24 cases. Paediatrician 12: 68

108. St James-Roberts I 1991 Persistant infant crying. Arch Dis Child 66: 653

109. Guthkelch A N 1971 Subdural haematoma and its relationship to whiplash injuries. BMJ 2: 430–431

110. Boulis Z F, Barnes N R 1978 Head injuries in children—aetiology, symptoms, physical findings and X-ray wastage. Br J Radiol 51: 851–854

111. Bell W O 1995 Paediatric head trauma. In: Arensman R M (ed) Paediatric trauma. Raven Press, New York, 101–118

112. Zimmerman R A, Bilaniuk L T, Bruce D 1978 Interhemispheric acute subdural haematoma: a CT manifestation of child abuse by shaking. Neuroradiology 16: 39–40

113. Han K B, Towbin R B, De Courten-Myers G et al 1989 Reversal sign on CT: Effect of anoxic/ischaemic cerebral injury in children. Am J Neuroradiol 10: 1191–1198

114. Rao P, Carty H, Pierce A 1999 The acute reversal sign: Comparison of medical and non-accidental injury patients. Clin Radiol 54: 495–501

115. Lam A H, Cruz G B 1991 Ultrasound evaluation of subdural haematoma. Australas Radiol 35: 330

SUGGESTIONS FOR FURTHER READING

Carty H (ed) 1999 Medical radiology: Emergency pediatric radiology. Springer-Verlag, Berlin

Kuhn J P, Slovis T L, Haller J O (eds) 2003 Caffey's pediatric diagnostic imaging, 10th edn. Mosby, Philadelphia, pp 2269–2303

Rodriguez–Merchan E C, Radomisli T E (eds) 2005 Symposium: Pediatric skeletal trauma. Clin Orthop Rel Res 432: 1–131

Rogers L F 2001 Radiology of skeletal trauma, 3rd edn. Churchill Livingstone, New York, pp 111–144

Kleinman P K 1998 Diagnostic imaging of child abuse, 2nd edn. St Louis, Mosby

CHAPTER 69

Bone Tumours and Neuroblastoma in Children

Paolo Toma and Claudio Defilippi

This chapter should be read in conjunction with the descriptions of bone tumours in adults (see Chs 47, 48).

BONE TUMOURS

The most common symptom of bone neoplasms is skeletal pain and plain radiography remains the first diagnostic step. Further investigation by computed tomography (CT), magnetic resonance imaging (MRI) and radionuclide radiology may be required, depending on initial interpretation. Due to the relative rarity of bone malignancies in the paediatric age group, the diagnosis is not always appreciated by general radiologists and, in atypical cases, may be delayed due to misinterpretation. However, plain radiographic diagnosis may be impossible during asymptomatic early tumour growth and can remain extremely difficult, even when the tumour is more advanced. Unusual clinical presentation, suspected metastatic spread from an unknown primary focus, adult-type neoplasms, chemo- and radio-therapy-induced malignancies and tumours associated with genetic syndromes all lead to difficulties. Diagnostic imaging, though playing a crucial role, must be closely coordinated with clinical assessment and histology. It must be remembered that biopsy specimens are small and will only sample a portion of a lesion; thus histopathological diagnosis can be impossible without clinical and radiological data (Table 69.1)[1–7]. It is increasingly important that all potentially malignant lesions in children are referred to a centre with the necessary expertise and multidisciplinary teams so that discussion about potential biopsy

Table 69.1 ADVANTAGES AND LIMITATIONS OF DIFFERENT IMAGING TECHNIQUES IN EVALUATING MUSCULOSKELETAL NEOPLASMS (modified from ref. 2)

Characteristic	Radiography	Radionuclide radiology	CT	Contrast-enhanced CT	MRI
Cortical bone	+++	+	+++	+++	++
Bone marrow	–	+	+	+	+++
Soft tissue	+	+	++	++	+++
Intramedullary extent	+	+	++	++	+++
Extramedullary extent	+	+	++	+++	+++
Relationships to neurovascular bundle	–	–	+	++	+++
Calcifications	++	–	+++	+++	++
Skip lesions	+	++	++	++	+++
Differential diagnosis: benign vs malignant	+++	+	+	+	++
Monitoring response to therapy	+	++	++	++	+++
Tumour characterization	+++	+	++	++	++

(and the route of any biopsy) is discussed in advance with the surgeon and oncologists who will be responsible for future care. For example, a biopsy should normally be obtained through tissue planes related to subsequent surgery to avoid the risk of seeding.

The aim of initial assessment is to differentiate aggressive from chronic disease and to distinguish benign from malignant lesions.

BENIGN BONE TUMOURS

Bone-forming tumours

The bone-forming tumours are:

- osteoma
- enostosis
- osteoid osteoma
- osteoblastoma.

Osteoid osteoma

This is a painful lytic lesion (nidus) with a sclerotic host reaction. Osteoid osteoma occurs in children and adolescents but more than 80% of cases occur in the second decade of life[8]. A typical patient presents with pain, often worse at night, relieved by aspirin but not anti-inflammatory drugs.

Typically the lesions occur in the tubular bones but they may also affect the vertebral appendages. In the tubular bones the lesions are cortically based. The dense sclerotic reaction can mask the nidus on plain radiographs. Intramedullary intracapsular lesions, usually located in the proximal femur at the medial aspect of the femoral neck, may cause growth deformities and overgrowth with limb length discrepancy, muscle atrophy and associated early osteoarthritis.

Subperiosteal osteoid osteoma is less common, occurring in the tubular bones and talus[9]. Typically there is scalloping and irregular bone resorption. Another location is in the posterior elements of the spine, presenting clinically with painful scoliosis. These are seen as dense pedicles or are identified following positive scintigraphy. Very rarely, osteoid osteoma may be polyostotic.

The diagnosis (Figs 69.1, 69.2) is based on the plain radiograph, supplemented by CT with direct visualization of the nidus and the surrounding sclerotic reaction. Sometimes, calcified foci may be seen inside the nidus. CT may also reveal surrounding oedema of the soft tissues.

MRI can cause confusion; if inflammatory changes are seen near the lesion, the diagnosis may be mistaken for a more aggressive tumour or even infection. The MRI findings are extremely variable and generally non-specific. The nidus has low to intermediate signal intensity on T1-weighted images and low to high signal intensity on T2-weighted images. It may enhance with intravenous paramagnetic contrast medium. Calcification has low signal intensity on all pulse sequences. The nidus may be masked by signal changes due to associated sclerosis, bone marrow oedema and soft tissue inflammation.

Some authors[5] report a typical tumour pattern on three-phase skeletal scintigrams characterized by focal hypervascularity and high uptake[4]. A negative scintigram excludes the presence of osteoid osteoma. Scintigraphy can help to locate the lesion, especially in radiographically difficult areas such as the spine, and to confirm recurrence or incomplete removal if pain persists following surgery.

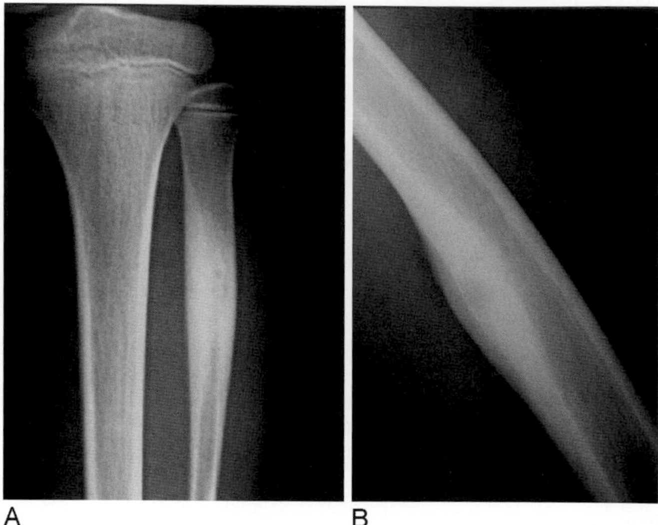

Figure 69.1 Osteoid osteoma. (A) Intracortical osteoid osteoma of the left fibular shaft: typical oval radiolucent area, representing the nidus, with calcification inside and reactive bone sclerosis. (B) Intracortical osteoid osteoma of the left femoral shaft without calcification in the radiolucent area and perifocal osteosclerosis.

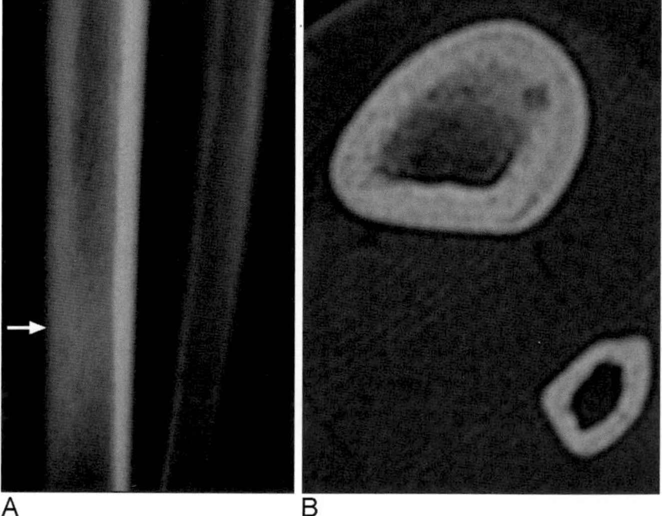

Figure 69.2 Osteoid osteoma. Intramedullary pattern. (A) Conventional radiograph shows a minimal peri-ostosis and reactive bone sclerosis (arrow). (B) CT demonstrates the nidus.

Surgery is the therapy of choice but if the nidus is excised incompletely, there is a risk of recurrence (filming of the specimen to evaluate the complete excision of the nidus is useful). Percutaneous CT-guided excision has been recently suggested with good results and rapid recovery.

Osteoblastoma

Osteoblastoma occurs mainly in children and adolescents. It is a rare benign tumour (0.5% of bone tumour biopsies) that is difficult to differentiate histologically from osteoid osteoma while, radiographically, it is quite distinct from osteoid osteoma[10,11]. Usually monostotic, the main site is the bony spongiosa of the posterior elements of the spine (Fig. 69.3); frequently the location can be either metaphyseal or diaphyseal in the long bones. Osteoblastomas are larger than osteoid osteomas and can reach 2–10 cm in diameter. Radiographically they may be lucent or sclerotic but always have a sclerotic rim, and tend to cause expansion without a large amount of reactive sclerosis. The shape can be fusiform and a real 'nidus' is usually not appreciable. Described as nonaggressive, occasionally the cortex may be broken[10].

Differential diagnosis includes osteosarcoma, if the appearance is aggressive and osteoid osteoma. Usually plain radiography, scintigraphy and CT are more than sufficient for the diagnosis.

The MRI appearance is generally non-specific, with a low to intermediate signal intensity on T1-weighted images and an intermediate to high signal intensity on T2-weighted images. MRI elegantly shows the effects on the spinal canal and cord, as well as the intra- and extra-osseous reactive changes and the possible infiltration of adjacent soft tissue[12].

Tumours of fibrous tissue origin

The tumours of fibrous tissue origin are:

- ossifying bone fibroma (OBF)
- nonossifying fibroma (NOF)
- benign fibrous histiocytoma
- metaphyseal fibrous cortical defect
- fibrous bone dysplasia (Jaffe Lichtenstein) (FBD)
- osteofibrous bone dysplasia (Campanacci) (OBD)

Nonossifying fibroma and metaphyseal fibrous cortical defects

Although histologically different, these two lesions appear radiologically similar and are conventionally treated as one process.

NOF is the most common benign tumour in children and is typically encountered during childhood and adolescence. Most lesions are discovered incidentally, often because of a pathological fracture. Radiographically these fibrous lesions appear as an osteolytic cystic defect in the metaphysis of a long bone (Fig. 69.4), usually at the site of tendon attachment to the cortical surface. It is well delineated, often multilocular, and has marginal sclerosis[1,13]. The most frequent sites are the proximal and distal tibia and proximal femur.

Eighty-two per cent of all NOFs are detected in children and they usually undergo a spontaneous resolution later in life. Although MRI is not routinely indicated for simple cases of NOF, T1-weighted MRI shows low signal intensity within the lesion compared with the skeletal muscle. On T2-weighted images, the lesion can have variable signal intensity. The lesion usually enhances avidly[14].

A metaphyseal fibrous cortical defect, which is not a true tumour, grows exclusively in the metaphyseal regions in children and adolescents, most frequently in the tibia and femur. It is a harmless proliferation of fibrous tissue in the periosteum which appears as a cortical bony defect.

On plain radiographs, there is a cortical defect separated from the inner bone by a sclerotic rim. On MRI the marginal defect presents as a hypo-intense signal on both T1- and T2-weighted sequences[15].

Cartilage-forming tumours

The cartilage-forming tumours are:

- chondroma (enchondroma) (Fig. 69.5)
- osteochondroma:
- chondroblastoma.

Osteochondroma (exostosis)

An osteochondroma is a very common benign neoplasm that results from growth plate cartilage being displaced to the

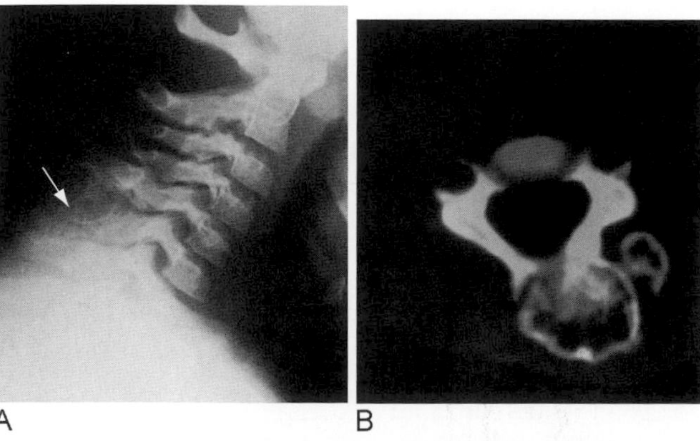

Figure 69.3 Osteoblastoma. (A) C6 posterior arch is markedly expanded by a large lucent lesion with a sclerotic rim (arrow). (B) CT confirms the lytic nature of the lesion, with lobulated regular margins and internal septa.

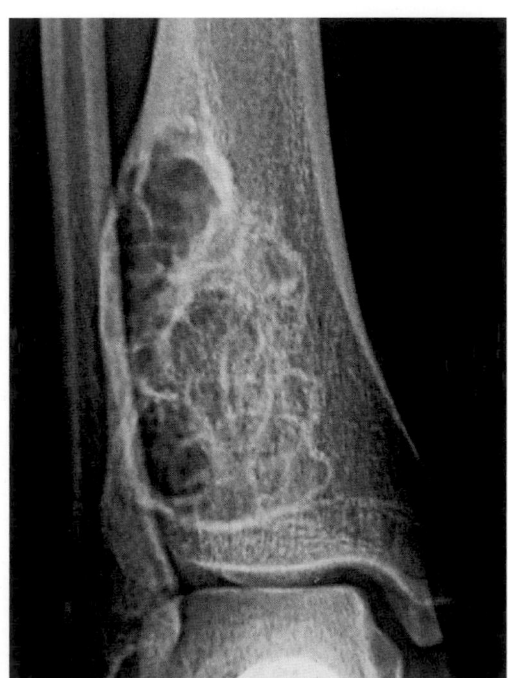

Figure 69.4 Nonossifying fibroma with a 'soap bubble' appearance eccentrically located in the right distal tibia displaying a characteristic scalloped border.

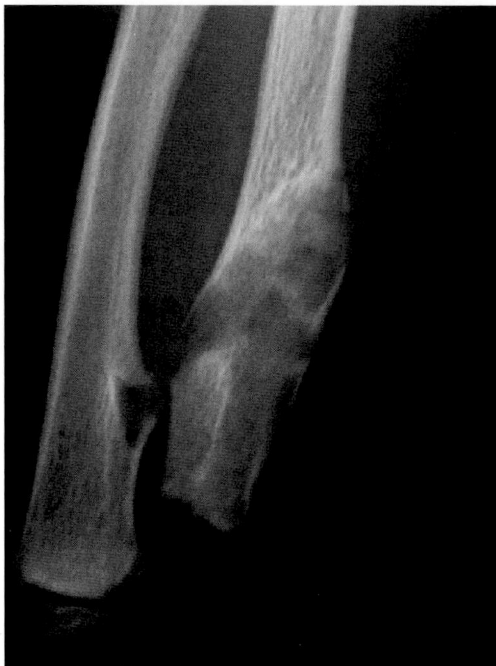

Figure 69.5 Enchondromatosis. Multiple enchondromas in the right distal forearm.

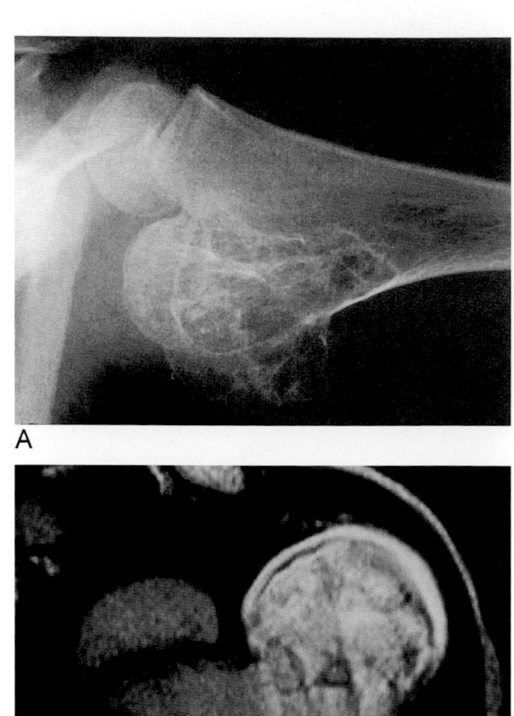

Figure 69.6 Osteochondroma. (A) 'Cauliflower' growth of a chondroma arising from the greater tuberosity of the humerus. (B) MRI (turbo T2-weighted sequence with fat saturation) shows the bright hyperintensity of the cartilaginous cap.

metaphyseal region[16]. The underlying bone is normal. The exostosis is covered by a cartilaginous cap which is the source of the growth. Osteochondromas may be flat with a broad base or sessile, referred to as a cauliflower exostosis. Clinically they feel larger than shown on the radiographs due to the unossified cartilage cap. Osteochondromas may grow until skeletal maturity. Growth after maturity suggests malignant degeneration which occurs in 1% of solitary exostoses.

Osteochondromas are usually seen as solitary lesions in the first two decades and in a monostotic form in a metaphyseal location adjacent to joints, 36% near the knee and 35% in the extremities. The base is formed of normal bone which has a cartilaginous cap, which in turn can be covered by a bursa due to chronic irritation of the overlying soft tissues which may be displaced.

The polyostotic form, called multiple hereditary exostosis or diaphyseal aclasis, is an autosomal dominant disorder. Most osteochondromas are broad based and involve a large portion of the circumference of the metaphysis with a resultant shortening of the limbs and deformity.

Plain radiography is diagnostic in the vast majority of cases. On MRI T2-weighted sequences the hyaline cartilage appears hyperintense with a good visualization of its structural layers. MRI demonstrates the cartilaginous lobulated matrix and the thickness of the cartilaginous cap of the tumour (Fig. 69.6). In children and adolescents, the cap may be as thick as 3 cm. Malignant degeneration is very rare in children.

Chondroblastoma

This is a rare benign cartilaginous tumour found almost exclusively in the epiphysis and which tends to be seen before epiphyseal closure. It is a monostotic lesion with a cartilaginous matrix, calcification in 50% and no soft tissue involvement. It is normally located in the proximal femur or proximal tibia, is usually lobulated with a sclerotic rim and can be associated with host periosteal reaction.

The diagnosis may be suggested on plain radiography by identifying a well-defined radiolucent lesion in a characteristic position. CT is useful to identify any calcified matrix. MRI appearances are non-specific with low to intermediate heterogeneous signal on T2 with a lobulated pattern. The presence of high signal on T2-weighted images depends on noncalcified chondroid matrix. Bone marrow oedema may be present and, if the location is juxtacortical, an intra-articular fluid effusion may be appreciable.

Vascular and other connective tissue tumours

These tumours are:

- bone haemangioma
- bone lymphangioma
- massive osteolysis
- myofibromatosis
- lipoma of bone.

Myofibromatosis

Myofibromatosis presents most often in infancy, but can occur even in adults. The solitary or multiple lesions involve skin, subcutaneous tissues, muscles, bones and viscera (particularly lung, heart, gastrointestinal tract and dura). Multicentric visceral involvement, especially of the lung, is considered a poor prognostic indicator associated with early death. The skeletal lesions appear lytic and sharply defined. Sclerotic margins appear later[17].

Locally aggressive tumours

These tumours are:

- desmoplastic bone fibroma
- chondromyxoid fibroma
- haemangiopericytoma
- osteoclastoma (giant cell tumour).

Chondromyxoid fibroma

This is a rare semimalignant bone tumour which accounts for only 0.5% of all bone tumours. It is mainly seen in the second decade of life but cases have been described in the first decade.

Typically, chondromyxoid fibromas are located in the metaphyseal region of the long tubular bones, near the growth plate, and can cross into the epiphysis. The lesion is well circumscribed, with an eccentric osteolytic lobulated aspect that bulges outward, thinning the cortex (Fig. 69.7). It is usually benign in character but may cause local invasion with a high recurrence rate if incompletely removed.

Haemangiopericytoma

This extremely rare soft tissue tumour may invade bone. It occurs in every age group, including children.

The tumour arises from pericytes (Zimmerman cells) and grows aggressively with local bone invasion. On a plain radiograph, osteolytic bone destruction is often mixed with sclerosis and osteolysis. The lack of clear margins indicates malignancy. MRI identifies the characteristic vascular channels, often seen in the periphery of the mass. The mass is hypervascularized, with a serpentine vascular structure which may have flow voids due to high velocity flow or T2-weighted hyperintensity because of slow flow. The main mass has an intermediate T1-weighted signal and a high T2-weighted signal. Due to its aggressive nature, there is a lack of fatty tissue, in contrast to benign haemangiomas.

Tumour-like lesions

The tumour-like lesions are:

- simple juvenile bone cyst
- aneurysmal bone cyst (ABC)
- benign fibrous cortical defect: see fibrous tissue tumours
- fibrous bone dysplasia (Jaffe Lichtenstein) (FBD)
- osteofibrous bone dysplasia (Kempson, Campanacci) (OBD)
- eosinophilic granuloma (Langerhans cell histiocytosis).

Simple bone cyst

Cystic bone lesions are relatively common in children and adults. A juvenile bone cyst or solitary or unicameral cyst is a benign lesion that develops in the centre of the metaphysis, usually of the femur or humerus near to the epiphyseal plate (Fig. 69.8). It expands the bone, thinning the cortex. With maturity, the cyst migrates down the shaft of the bone. It has smoot h margins and, if there has been haemorrhage into the cyst, is filled with clear or sanguinous fluid. The MRI signal depends on the content: usually the signal is intermediate on T1-weighted images and high on T2. It is frequently discovered by chance during incidental radiographs for other purposes. Two-thirds of patients present with a pathological fracture (Fig. 69.8) and, in other symptomatic patients, this pain is thought to be due to microfractures.

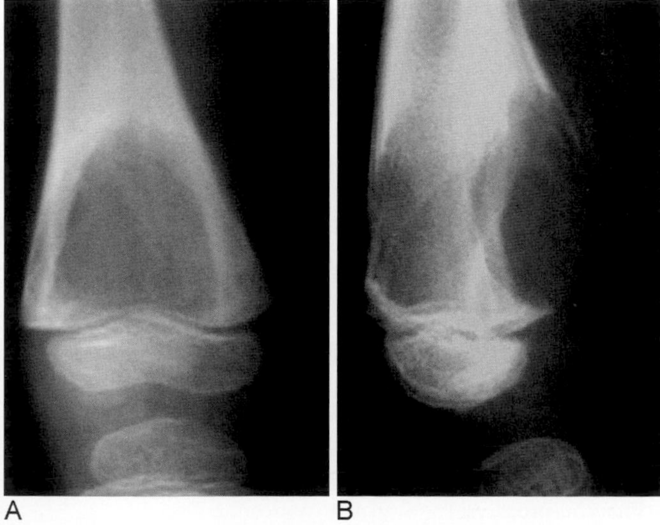

Figure 69.7 Chondromixoid fibroma of the distal femoral metaphysis. (A,B) Large osteolytic defect bulging outward.

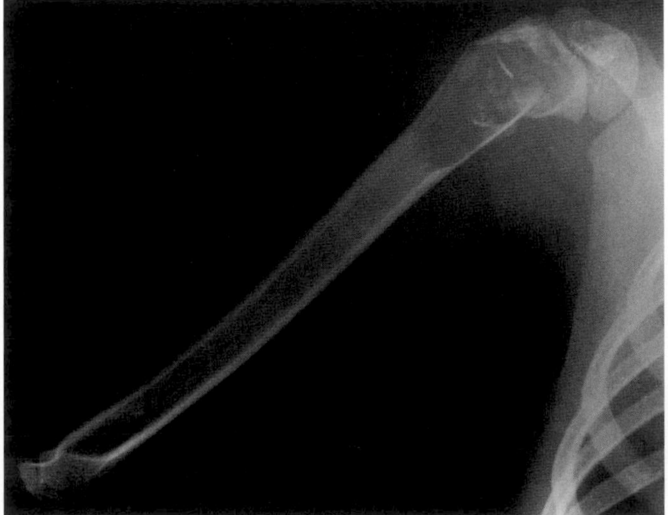

Figure 69.8 Solitary bone cyst. Large radiolucent area of the right humerus with pathological fracture, and a 'fallen' fragment.

Aneurysmal bone cyst

This is a benign, solitary expansile lesion which occurs in the vertebral appendages, the flat bones and most frequently the metaphysis of the long bones in the femur, tibia and humerus, but may also be found in the tubular bones of the hands and feet. The lesion develops eccentrically without crossing through the growth plate. It consists of a cyst, usually filled with blood. The lesion is frequently multilocular with poorly defined margins. The plain radiographic appearance is usually characteristic in the long bones. In the vertebral column, a destructive expansile lesion is seen in the appendages and may encroach on the spinal canal. Full evaluation of ABCs requires cross-sectional imaging. CT demonstrates the bone destruction and is essential before sclerotherapy. Coronal T2-weighted images, with or without fat saturation, are advantageous for visualization of the main cystic lesion, any additional cysts and fluid–fluid levels within the lesion (Fig. 69.9). Contrast-enhanced T1-weighted sequences show enhancement of cyst walls and internal septations[18,19]. Follow-up studies monitor resolution of these cysts following treatment. In selected cases percutaneous sclerotherapy under fluoroscopy guidance has been used with successful results.

Fibrous bone dysplasia (Jaffe Lichtenstein)

This is a malformation which may be mistaken for a bone tumour. FBD is a common osteolytic bone lesion in which the bone is centrally replaced by fibrous tissue[20]. Local bending or pathological fractures may occur. This is discussed more fully in the skeletal dysplasia section below. Problems with diagnosis mainly arise with the monostotic forms, which on plain radiography show widening of the medullary cavity, bony expansion and a ground-glass appearance (Fig. 69.10).

A rare condition, the McCune Albright syndrome, consists of unilateral polyostotic FBD associated with precocious puberty.

The most frequent locations for FBD are the ribs, proximal femur, skull, scapula and pelvis.

Osteofibrous bone dysplasia (Kempson, Campanacci)

This occurs in the shaft of long tubular bones. It is a multicystic lesion surrounded by a sclerotic bone, with intact cortex and no periosteal reaction. It may be multifocal. On MRI the appearances are those of all fibrous tumours. The plain radiographs are diagnostic (Fig. 69.11). This lesion is often present at birth.

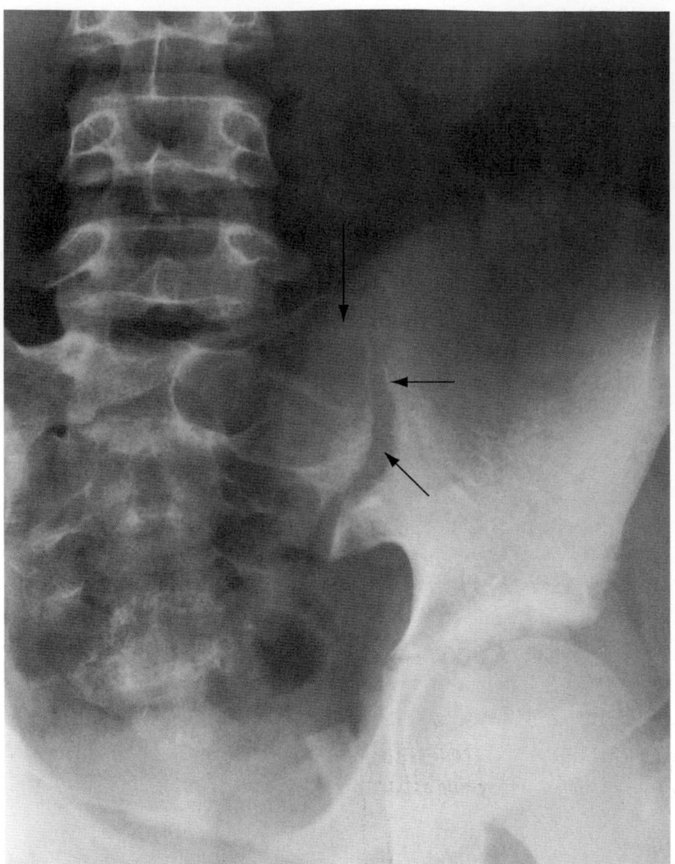

A

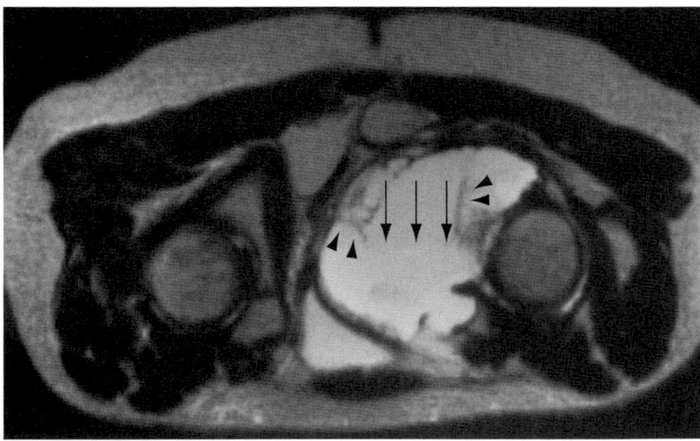

B

Figure 69.9 Aneurysmal bone cyst. (A) Large well-defined cystic lesion of the left part of the sacrum (arrows), showing the 'blow out' pattern, with septa and bridges. (B) MRI: T2-weighted sequence, axial view. Large hyperintense mass, 'soap bubble'-shaped lesion arising from the right ischiopubic region. Fluid–fluid level (arrows) and hypo-intense septa (arrowheads) are evident.

MALIGNANT BONE TUMOURS

Osteosarcoma

Osteogenic sarcoma (OS) is the most common primary malignant tumour of bone in children and accounts for 15% of all primary bone tumours[1]. Radiologically OS can be diagnosed when osteoid tissue or bone tissue formation produced by tumour cells is associated with aggressive characteristics[21]. The aetiology is unknown. The only environmental agent known to cause this tumour is ionizing radiation but radiation-induced OS only accounts for approximately 3% of all OS. The peak incidence of OS occurs in the second decade of life, a characteristic that suggests a relationship between rapid skeletal growth and the development of this neoplasm. Furthermore, OS occurs most frequently at sites where the greatest increase in length and size of bone occurs: the metaphyseal portions of the most rapidly growing bones (and parts of bones) in adolescents. Very often, patients have a history of trauma, which brings the problem to clinical attention.

The radiographic appearances of OS are variable but the most frequent is that of a destructive lesion in the metaphysis

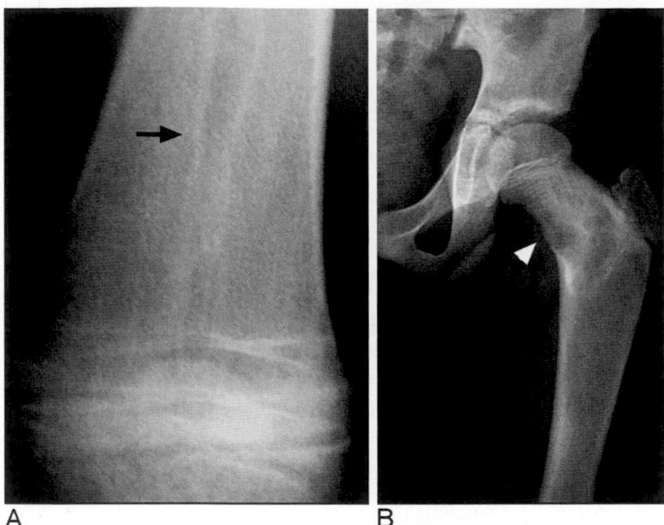

Figure 69.10 Monostotic fibrous dysplasia. (A) Initial 'candle flame' aspect (arrow). (B) Cystic-like appearance (arrowhead).

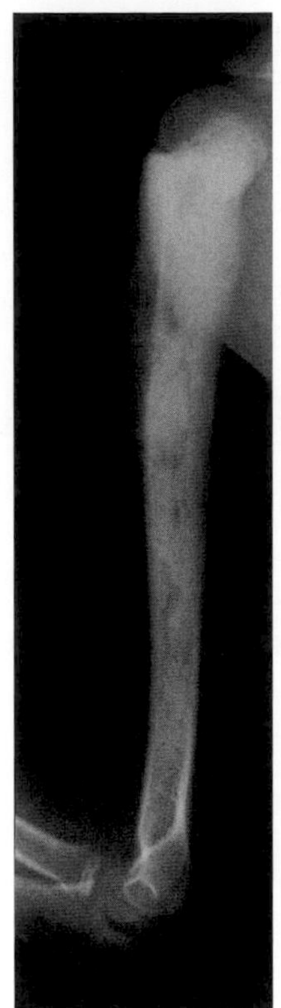

Figure 69.12 Osteosarcoma. Mixed sclerotic and lytic lesion of the right humerus, extending into the soft tissues and sparing the growth plate. A Codman triangle is visible at the upper limit of the tumour.

of a long bone, poorly demarcated margins, a Codman's triangle, aggressive periosteal reaction and a soft tissue mass[22,23]. The lesion may cross the growth plate (Fig. 69.12). CT and MRI provide the required information for staging the disease and monitoring the treatment. On MRI, tumour volume measurement and necrosis grading after chemotherapy are the main prognostic factors in monitoring OS, reflecting reduction in vascularity, peritumoural oedema and neoplastic cell mass. Because of sensitivity to oedema, MRI can overestimate tumour size if performed after biopsy. MRI is superior to CT for detecting marrow extension, relationships with vessels, transphyseal spread of tumour, soft tissue component and skip metastases because of its ability to image the tumour in axial, coronal and sagittal planes with high contrast resolution (Fig. 69.13). Thus MRI is the cross-sectional imaging method of choice. Furthermore, it can monitor the response to chemo- or radiotherapy demonstrable as changes in the intensity of the signal, in both T2- and enhanced T1-weighted sequences.

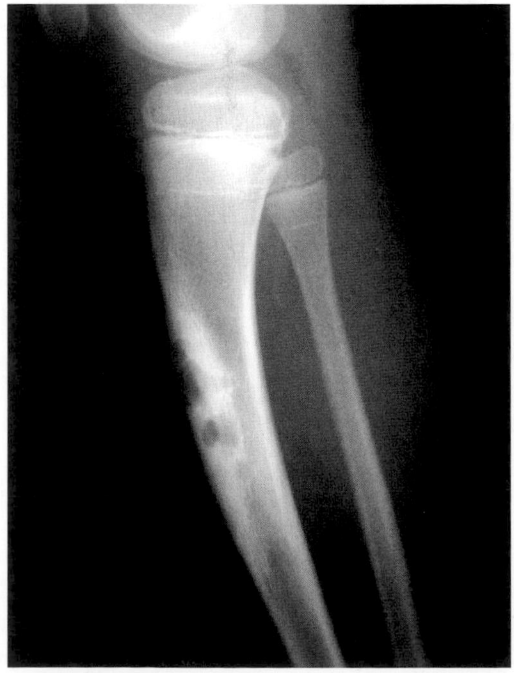

Figure 69.11 Osteofibrous dysplasia of the tibial shaft. Multicystic lesion surrounded by sclerotic bone.

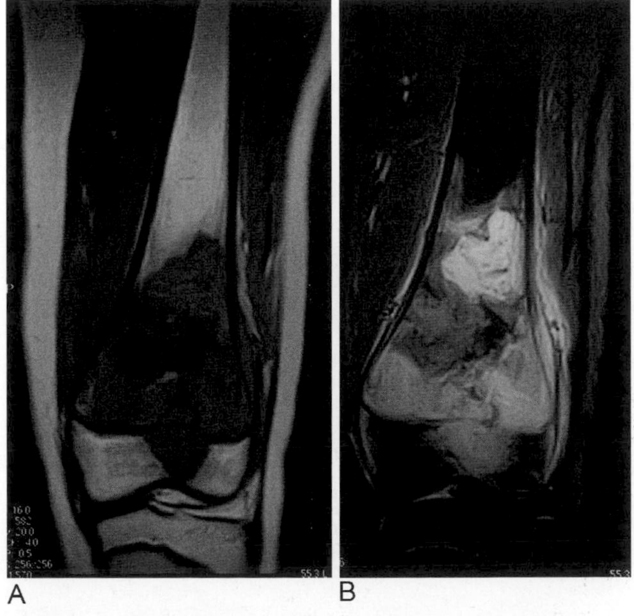

Figure 69.13 Osteosarcoma. (A) T1- and (B) T2-weighted MRI sequences of osteosarcoma in the distal femur with transphyseal extension and a small soft tissue component laterally.

Due to the cartilage cap, the rare variant osteochondroma-like parosteal osteosarcoma can be misdiagnosed as a benign lesion at MRI.

MRI staging should include T1-weighted sequences following administration of intravenous contrast medium, to differentiate between tumour and oedema. Initial staging also requires CT of the lungs. Scintigraphy is required to look for skeletal metastases. Lung secondaries may also take up the bone-seeking agents.

Successful treatment with chemotherapy leads to a decrease in tumour volume and increased signal intensity on T2-weighted images, reflecting both tumour necrosis and oedema.

Fast dynamic contrast-enhanced MRI is useful to seek recurrence of the tumour, which shows early enhancement as opposed to slow enhancement of inflammatory tissue. Following treatment, the signal intensity on T2-weighted images decreases due to the replacement of tumour cells by fibrous tissue.

Ewing's sarcoma

This tumour was originally described in 1921 by James Ewing as a radiosensitive bone neoplasm, of endothelial origin, growing in the shaft of the long bones (Fig. 69.14). It is generally accepted that the tumour is of neural origin. Ewing's sarcomas (ES) are now accepted as a group of malignant tumours, arising both from bone and extraskeletally, mostly presenting as undifferentiated neoplasms but including more differentiated forms like peripheral primitive neuro-ectodermal tumour (PNET)[24]. The term PNET includes soft tissue and bone neoplasms previously reported as peripheral neuro-epithelioma, adult neuroblastoma, small cell tumour of the chest wall (Askin tumour) and others. Extra-osseous ES, extra-osseous PNET and bone PNET account for only 13% of all these malignancies.

The aetiology and pathogenesis of ES and its variants are unknown. Association with congenital diseases is rare. ES occurs more commonly in adolescents but a second peak of incidence in very young children is well known. It is the second most common bone tumour in children and adolescents, accounting for about 10% overall, with an incidence of 0.6 per million. It is sometimes difficult at presentation to determine whether the tumour is of osseous or extra-osseous origin because of the large soft tissue component of bone tumours and the osseous involvement in soft tissue malignancies. All bones may be involved, but most of the tumours develop in the long bones and pelvis. Children with pelvic and spinal tumours often have symptoms for several months before a diagnosis is made on plain radiographs. In the pelvis the tumour arises from the iliac bone and a large soft tissue mass is usually present. This, combined with reactive bone, often causes a sclerotic appearance of the iliac blade. Signs of bone destruction are subtle initially and often overlooked. Scintigraphy is indicated in occult bone pain in children and leads to earlier diagnosis.

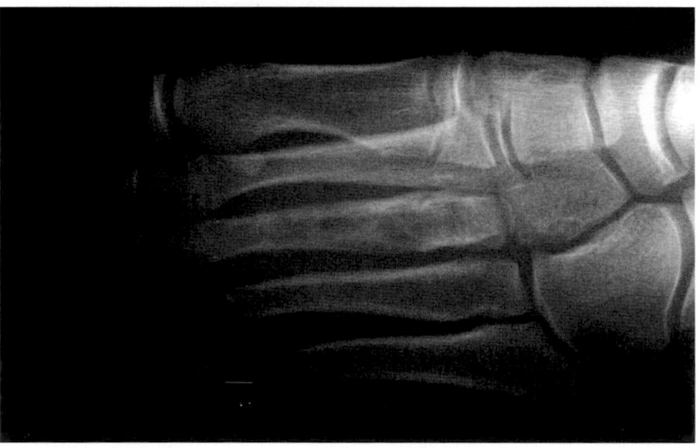

Figure 69.14 Ewing's sarcoma. Mixed lytic and sclerotic lesion of the third metatarsal bone.

The clinical presentation is non-specific: local pain and swelling can mimic an acute osteomyelitis, delaying the diagnosis. Fever and increased local temperature are often present. Children with a chest wall tumour usually present with pain. The destructive rib lesion is often initially overlooked and by the time of diagnosis there is usually a pleural effusion present.

Spread is haematogenous and metastases are found in lungs, bones and bone marrow. Lymph node, liver and skip metastases are rare.

The differential diagnosis includes osteomyelitis, other lytic bone lesions, osteosarcoma and metastases from another primary tumour. The routine imaging algorithm of these patients includes plain radiography and MRI of the primary lesion, bone scintigraphy of the skeleton looking for metastatic bone spread and plain radiography and CT for chest evaluation of metastases.

The radiographic features include both a poorly defined lytic appearance and sclerotic opacities, often accompanied by severe periosteal reaction (Fig. 69.14). The lytic pattern reflects the severe bone destruction by the neoplasm, while the sclerotic appearance should not be interpreted as tumour bone production, as documented in osteosarcoma, but is a secondary reactive phenomenon.

The extent of the disease can be defined both by CT and MRI. On MR images, the presence of high signal intensity in T2 is generally associated with tumour viability or recurrence, while the absence of high T2-weighted signal intensity has a good prognostic value. When a large soft-tissue mass is present it can still be difficult to differentiate between tumour and infection, even with Gadolinium enhancement. The diagnosis is made by biopsy. Clinical management of Ewing's sarcoma is with initial chemotherapy and then resection.

Bone metastases

Bone metastases, the most common form of malignant bone tumour in adults, are not common in children. Metastases as the first manifestation of a primary tumour are unusual as the primary is usually evident.

Bone and bone marrow are usually involved via a haematogenous pathway. The red marrow is more frequently involved than the yellow marrow and thus long bones are common metastatic sites.

Metastatic bone disease in children is most frequently due to leukaemia and neuroblastoma (Fig. 69.15), but lymphoma, ES and OS also metastasize to bone. Bone metastases are also described in rhabdomyosarcoma and medulloblastoma.

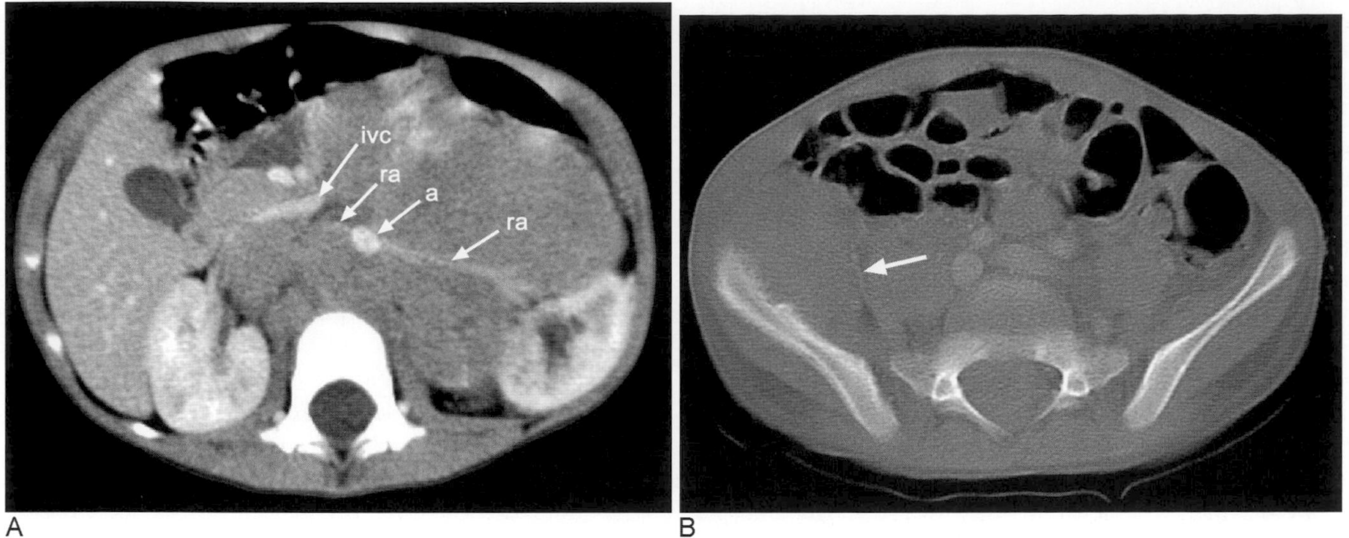

Figure 69.15 Abdominal neuroblastoma. Contrast-enhanced CT. (A) A prevertebral tumour extends across the midline in the retroperitoneum, displaces and encases the aorta (a) anteriorly and encases the renal arteries (ra). The inferior vena cava (ivc), partially encased, is displaced anterolaterally and compressed by the tumour and nodes. The mass extends to both the renal hili. (B) Infiltrative lesion to the right iliac bone with a large soft tissue component (arrow) that projects inward as a space-occupying mass.

Periosteal reaction and a lytic appearance of lesions are the most common radiographic characteristics in metastatic locations but sclerotic lesions are also reported, particularly in medulloblastoma and leukaemia. Bone changes due to metastatic spread may also include osteoporosis, radiolucent lines, cortical disruption, periosteal thickening and 'onion skin' periosteal reaction. Metaphyseal radiolucent lines are typically described in leukaemia and, less commonly, neuroblastoma. A radionuclide skeletal survey confirms secondary bone involvement but MRI is also excellent because of its great sensitivity. All procedures may have to be followed, when clinically indicated, by marrow biopsy.

Rare malignant bone tumours in children

The rare malignant tumours are:

- chondrosarcoma
- primary malignant lymphoma of bone
- haemangiosarcoma of bone.

NEUROBLASTOMA

Neuroblastoma (NB) is a malignant tumour arising from primordial neural crest cells. These cells migrate during embryogenesis to form the adrenal medulla and the sympathetic ganglia. NB occurs, therefore, in diverse but predictable locations such as the neck, thorax, abdomen and pelvis, arising from the adrenal glands or anywhere along the sympathetic chain.

NB arises in the retroperitoneum in 65% of cases and, of these, 40% of lesions occur in the adrenal glands. It is the most common extracranial solid malignancy in children and the third most common paediatric malignancy (the first is central nervous system tumours and the second leukaemia). Overall, NB represents 8–10% of all childhood cancers. Among abdominal neoplasms, NB is the second most common cancer after Wilms' tumour. The median age at diagnosis is 2 years, with 90% of diagnoses made in children younger than 5 years of age. NB is also seen in the neonatal period and may be identified in the fetus by antenatal imaging[25]. It may also be present very rarely in adolescents and adults.

Three types of neural crest tumours are known, classified according to cellular differentiation. NB is the more common and is characterized by the most primitive and malignant cells, ganglioneuroma, which is completely differentiated and benign, and ganglioneuroblastoma, which presents intermediate features between NB and ganglioneuroma.

Clinical issues

The signs and symptoms of NB reflect the tumour site and extent of disease. The tumours may manifest as an incidental mass, or may cause abdominal pain. Because metastases are so frequently present (skeleton, bone marrow, lymph nodes, liver, and, rarely, lung and brain), the clinical symptoms are often due to metastatic disease. Children may have bone and joint pain, proptosis from orbital metastases, anaemia, weight loss and fever.

Horner's syndrome may be the presenting feature of cervical or thoracic NB involving the stellate ganglion.

Children may also present with the effects of production of hormones such as catecholamines (hypertension) and vasoactive intestinal polypeptyde (VIP) (intractable watery diarrhoea). Another paraneoplastic syndrome associated with NB is myoclonic encephalopathy of infancy (MEI). The precise pathogenesis of MEI is unknown.

NB in infants younger than 1 year of age is often associated with extensive hepatic metastases. Hepatomegaly may be massive despite a small, sometimes not evident, primary lesion. These children usually have bone marrow lesions and palpable subcutaneous nodules as well (Stage IV-S). This type of NB has a better prognosis and has a tendency to spontaneous regression: the survival probability is about 79%. The very young IV-S patients are at high risk because of severe respiratory complications as a result of massive hepatomegaly.

Extradural extension (dumb-bell syndrome) is common with thoracic NB, but rare in abdominal tumours.

Approximately 95% of patients with NB have elevated levels of catecholamines [vanillylmandelic acid, homovanilic acid, norepinephrine (noradrenaline), dopamine] in the urine. A combination of a positive bone marrow aspirate and an increase of urinary catecholamine metabolites is sufficient to confirm the diagnosis.

Staging

The treatment of NB is determined by the stage of the tumour at the time of diagnosis[26]. The international NB staging system is based on radiological findings, surgical resectability, lymph node involvement and bone marrow involvement (Table 69.2)[27]. Several biological markers may also affect prognosis: serum ferritin and serum neuron-specific enolase levels, MYCN oncogene amplification, chromosome 1p deletion (loss of heterozygosity), TRK expression and histopathology (Shimada classification).

Imaging

The current evaluation of primary sites (staging and follow-up) of patients with NB consists of CT or MRI of the primary tumour and meta-iodobenzylguanidine (MIBG) scintigraphy. The evaluation of metastatic disease is based on MRI or CT of the head, orbit and neck; MRI or CT of the abdomen and pelvis; CT of the chest; skeletal scintigraphy with radiographs of abnormal sites; and MIBG scintigraphy. The diagnosis is made most frequently by ultrasound. Usually NB presents as an aggressive tumour with a tendency to invade adjacent structures: the mass surrounds and engulfs, rather than displacing, large vessels such as the aorta, coeliac artery, superior mesenteric artery and vena cava[28].

Radiographs

Chest radiographs may show a calcified mass. Paravertebral widening in the lower chest may be caused by retrocrural spread. Abdominal radiography demonstrates a nonspecific soft tissue mass with calcification in as many as 53% of patients (diffuse, mottled, finely stippled, or coalescent calcifications).

Erosion of pedicles is suggestive of intraspinal extension. Radiographs of the long bones in patients with bone metastases may be normal or may show ill-defined areas of bone destruction. A solitary lesion may appear as a lytic, moth-eaten or permeating destructive area, interspersed with sclerotic trabeculae. New periosteal bone formation, often parallel to the shaft, may be present. The radiographic features do indicate malignant growth but are not specific. The most common skeletal sites are the skull and metaphyses of long bones (humerus and femur), but they can be seen in any bone except for the hands, feet and clavicles (see Ch. 48).

Ultrasound

Performed to confirm the presence of a mass or for a routine prenatal examination, often suggests the diagnosis of abdominal NB. The mass can have varying echogenicity and is usually heterogeneous and hypervascularized on colour Doppler. Hypo-echoic areas secondary to haemorrhage and necrosis are frequent. Completely cystic NB has been described. Small echogenic foci within the mass represent calcification. The retroperitoneal location of the mass can be confirmed by demonstration of anterior displacement of the aorta and inferior vena cava (Fig. 69.16). NB classically displaces the kidney without distorting the renal collecting system.

A preliminary evaluation of intra-abdominal extension of the tumour may be performed and colour Doppler may be used in displaying vessel encasement and displacement. Hepatic metastases have a variable ultrasound appearance. Diffuse infiltration of the liver (Stage IV-S) causes hepatomegaly with heterogeneity of the parenchyma.

Computed tomography and magnetic resonance imaging

Although the primary tumour may first be detected by ultrasound, CT or MRI are required as a guide to staging, resectability, prognosis and follow-up. MRI has the advantage at diagnosis that it is excellent at assessing the bone marrow in patients with NB of the abdomen or other sites by revealing areas of abnormal signal intensity (low on T1- and high on T2-weighted images)[29].

CT of the chest, abdomen and pelvis requires a bolus intravenous administration of contrast medium. Examinations of

Table 69.2 INTERNATIONAL NEUROBLASTOMA STAGING SYSTEM

Stage 1	Localized tumour confined to the area of origin; complete gross resection, with or without microscopic residual disease; identifiable ipsilateral and contralateral lymph nodes negative microscopically
Stage 2A	Localized tumour with incomplete gross excision; identifiable ipsilateral and contralateral lymph nodes negative microscopically
Stage 2B	Unilateral tumour with complete or incomplete gross resection with positive ipsilateral regional lymph nodes; contralateral lymph nodes negative microscopically
Stage 3	Tumour infiltrating across the midline with or without regional lymph node involvement; unilateral tumour with contralateral regional lymph node involvement; or midline tumour with bilateral regional lymph node involvement
Stage 4	Dissemination of tumour to distant lymph nodes, bone, bone marrow, liver, skin or other organs (except as defined in Stage 4S)
Stage 4S	Localized primary tumour (as defined for Stages 1, 2A or 2B) with dissemination limited to skin, liver, or bone marrow (< 10% tumour cells, and meta-iodobenzylguanidine scintigram negative in the marrow). Limited to infants younger than 1 year

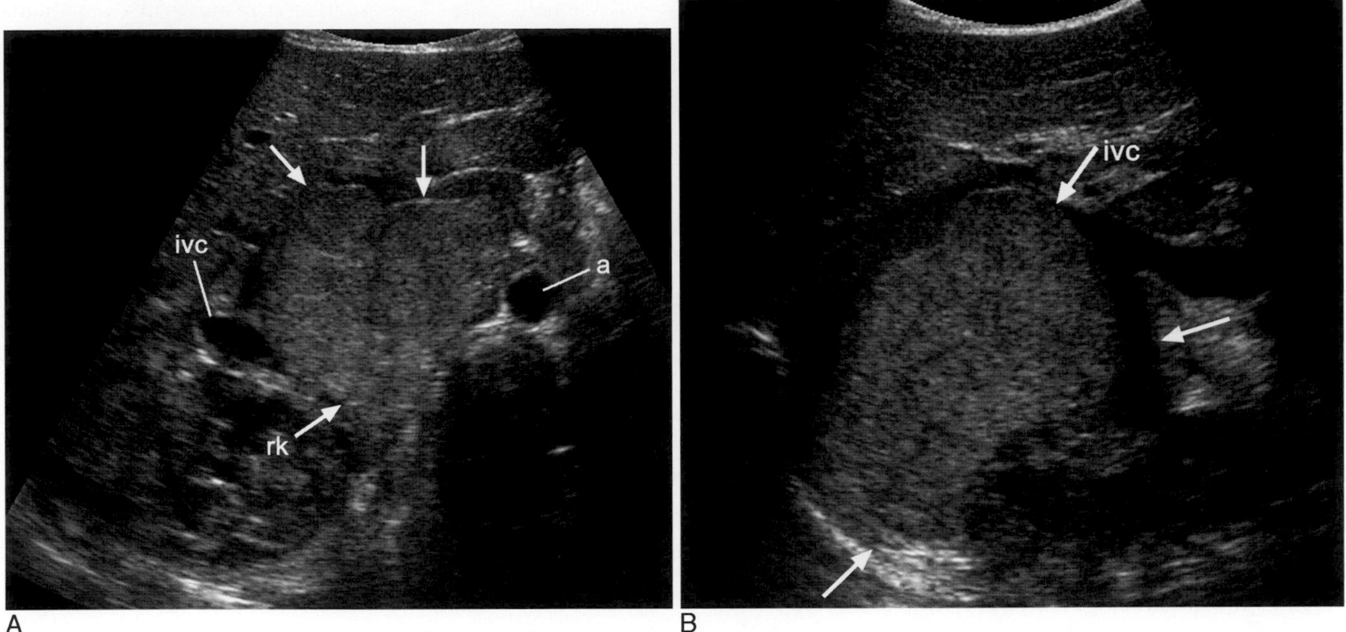

Figure 69.16 Abdominal neuroblastoma. (A) Transverse ultrasound through the right abdomen shows a solid paraspinal mass (arrows) anterior to the right kidney (rk). The aorta (a) and inferior vena cava (ivc) are displaced by the mass. (B) Longitudinal image through the right flank shows the mass (lower arrows) and the stretched inferior vena cava (ivc).

the chest should extend from the lung apices to the lower edge of the liver during relatively early enhancement; the abdominal series should cover the liver in the portal phase and extend down to the pubic symphysis.

With MRI the patient must be imaged in at least two planes by T1-weighted spin-echo and fat-saturated T2-weighted fast spin-echo sequences and transverse T1-weighted gradient-echo angiographic sequences. The T1-weighted spin-echo sequence must be repeated with fat-suppression after intravenous injection of gadolinium.

Usually the masses are large and heterogeneous. On CT, the lesions have an attenuation equal to or less than that of muscle. Tumour calcification is readily detected (calcification is seen by CT in up to 85% of cases). Low-attenuation areas represent regions of necrosis or haemorrhage. NB usually shows mild heterogeneous enhancement, reflecting areas of vascularity alternating to areas of necrosis, haemorrhage and cystic change. At MRI, NB has prolonged T1 and T2. High signal intensity on T1-weighted images represents haemorrhage. After administration of gadolinium the enhancement is heterogeneous.

With all techniques, it is essential to assess extent of tumour as clearly as possible. By definition, if the mass crosses the contralateral aspect of the vertebral body, it has crossed the midline: this determination is important in staging. Measurement of the tumour volume is crucial for prognosis and follow-up. As separation of the primary tumour from the accompanying large nodes often is not possible; measurement must include the entire mass. NB often has an invasive pattern of growth encasing the vessels, so it is crucial to define the position of the vessels and to determine the relationships of the tumour tissue to the vessels to define extent of tumour and determine operability (see Fig. 69.15).

The tumour may invade the spinal canal, kidney, or liver. Hepatic metastases and renal atrophy (ischaemia or infarction secondary to encasement or compression of the renal vessels) may be seen. Intraspinal extension may be suspected at CT but cannot be thoroughly evaluated: MRI should be performed on any paraspinal mass suspected of extending into the extradural space (Fig. 69.17).

CT or MRI allow the evaluation of skull and iliac bone metastases (see Fig. 69.15). Usually, skull metastases are located in the spheno-orbital region. They appear as an infiltrating mass causing permeative bone destruction and spiculated bony changes, which may extend into the soft tissue of the scalp or push through the inner table of the skull.

NB tends to regress in size with treatment, but the regression is frequently incomplete, leaving a small residual soft tissue mass, which is often calcified. Determining whether residual tissue is fibrosis or viable tumour usually requires an MIBG scintigram.

The ganglioneuromas have patterns similar to those of NB, mostly occurring in the posterior mediastinum.

Radionuclide radiology

CT or MRI is needed to define the local extent of disease, whereas MIBG and skeletal scintigrams are essential for determining distal spreading[30]. MIBG (^{131}I- or ^{123}I-labelled), an analogue of catecholamine precursors, is taken up by catecholamine-producing cells. In children such uptake is usually specific for NB (primary tumour and metastases). Unfortunately 30% of the primary lesions do not take up MIBG and, in other rare cases, the uptake stops despite the presence of persistent demonstrable disease. However, MIBG scintigraphy remains important in the diagnosis (characterization of

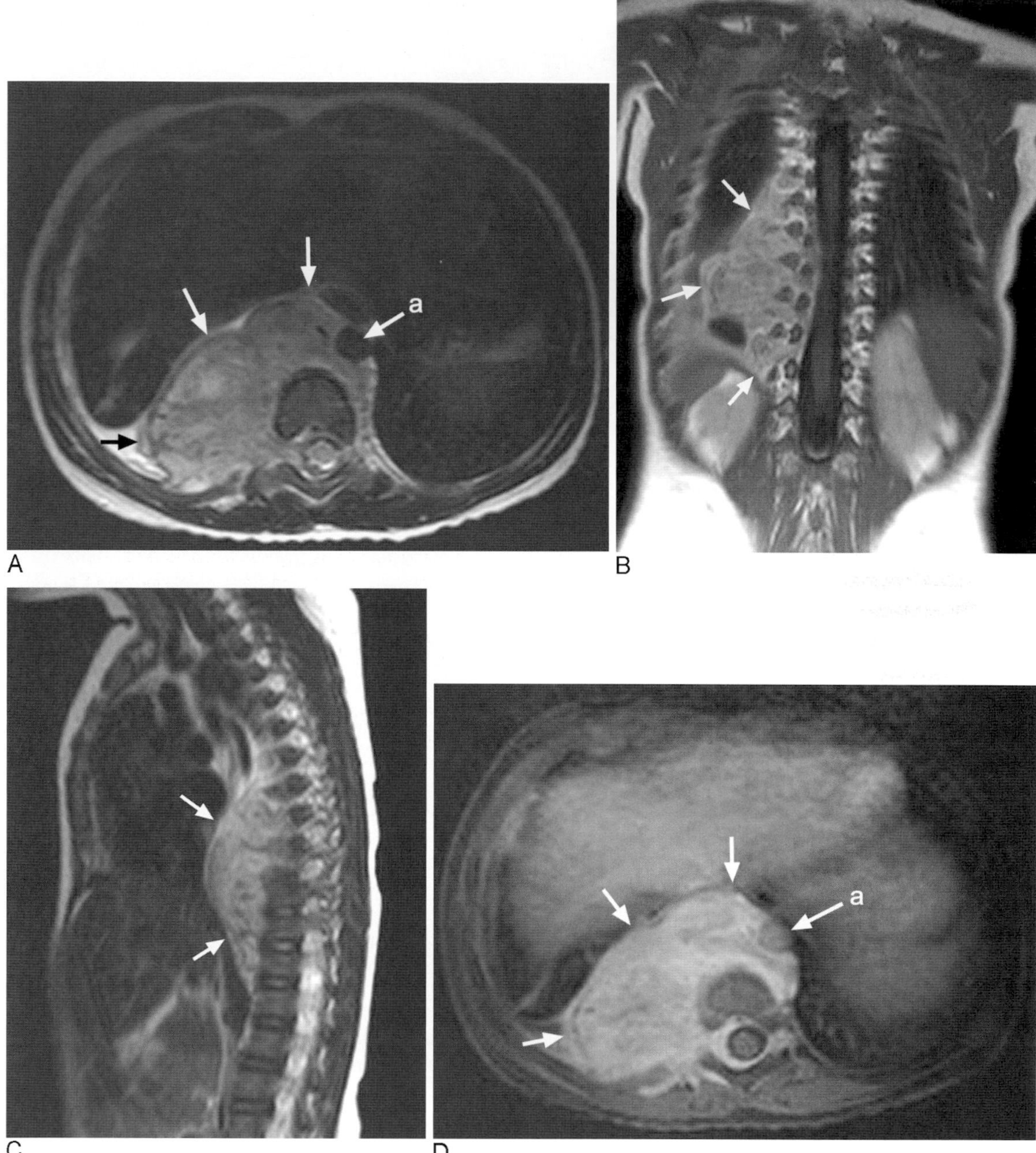

Figure 69.17 Thoracic neuroblastoma with intraspinal extension. MRI. (A–B) axial and coronal T1-weighted images with Gd-DOTA enhancement. (C) sagittal T1-weighted image with Gd-DOTA enhancement. (D) Axial T2-weighted image. Large posterior mediastinal mass (arrows) with anterior and lateral displacement of the aorta (a), which is encased. There is massive tumour extension into the canal through the right neural foramina to displace the spinal cord to the left. Extension into the right paraspinal soft tissues is evident.

the mass, localization of the primary tumour in patients with MEI, and evaluation of the intra- and extra-skeletal extent of disease), and follow-up (new areas of uptake generally indicate new active disease).

Two-thirds of patients have metastatic bone disease at diagnosis; therefore, ^{99m}Tc-MDP bone scintigraphy should be performed in all patients at diagnosis and follow-up. MIBG uptake in bone is nonspecific because cortical uptake cannot be distinguished from marrow involvement.

Positron emission tomography (PET) with [^{18}F]FDG has a major impact on the treatment of adult cancer, whereas the reported experience with tumours of childhood is limited. PET and MIBG imaging show similar patterns of diffusely abnormal skeletal findings in patients with extensive bone marrow involvement. A major drawback of PET is the lack of visualization of lesions in the cranium because of the high physiological activity in the brain.

Differential diagnosis

The differential diagnosis encompasses all paediatric abdominal masses, and particularly Wilms' tumour and neonatal adrenal haemorrhage.

Concerning Wilms' tumour, the mean age at onset is 3 years (for NB it is younger than 2 years), it grows like a ball displacing the vessels (NB surrounds vessels), and it may invade the renal vein and inferior vena cava. It arises from the kidney with the typical claw sign; calcification is uncommon. Lung metastases are present in 20% of cases (very uncommon in NB).

The diagnosis of adrenal haemorrhage is usually performed by ultrasound, which identifies the mass and shows, in sequential examinations, decreasing size and cystic evolution. Colour Doppler is useful to show avascularity of adrenal haemorrhage. MRI may show the classic signal intensity pattern of ageing blood products, but diagnostic difficulties can occur because of bleeds of different ages. Other paediatric adrenal tumours, such as phaeochromocytoma and adrenal carcinoma, are much less common.

In the neck, firm to hard masses can be cysts, ectopic thymus, abscesses, inflammatory or tumoural adenopathy, benign and malignant tumours, or parotid and thyroid lesions. The most common cancers are lymphomas, thyroid cancers, rhabdomyosarcomas and NB.

In the mediastinum, NB is located in the posterior anatomical space. Of the posterior mediastinal masses, approximately 80% are NB or ganglioneuroblastoma and ganglioneuroma. Other abnormalities can be: neurofibroma, neurenteric cyst, meningocele and paraspinal inflammation due to vertebral osteomyelitis.

REFERENCES

1. Adler C P, Kozlowski K 1993 Osteosarcoma. In: Adler C P, Kozlowski K (eds) Primary bone tumors and tumorous conditions in children. Springer Verlag, London
2. Lang P, Johnston J O, Arenal-Romero F, Gooding C A 1998 Advances in MR imaging of pediatric musculoskeletal neoplasms. MRI Clin North Am 6: 579–604
3. Brisse H, Edeline V, Neuenschwander S 2003 Imaging of malignant tumours of the long bones in children: monitoring response to neoadjuvant chemotherapy and preoperative assessment. In: Toma P (ed) Compendium 26th postgraduate ESPR course. Omicron, Genova, pp 75–82
4. Delbeke D, Habibian M R 1988 Non inflammatory entities and the differential diagnosis of positive three phase with bone scintigraphy. Clin Nucl Med 13: 844–851
5. Focacci C, Lattanzi R, Iadeluca M L, Campioni P 1998 Nuclear medicine in primary bone tumours. Eur J Radiol 27: 123–131
6. Fletcher B D 1999 Malignant bone tumors. RSNA special course in pediatric radiology: current concepts in body imaging at the millennium. RSNA Inc, Oak Brook, pp 173–182
7. Vanel D, Verstraete K L, Shapeero L G 1997 Primary tumors of the musculoskeletal system. Radiol Clin North Am 35: 213–237
8. Gitelis S, Schajowicz F 1989 Osteoid osteoma and osteoblastoma. Orthoped Clin North Am 20: 313–325
9. Goldman A B, Schneider R, Pavlov H 1993 Osteoid osteoma of the femoral neck: report of four cases evaluated with isotopic bone scanning CT and MR imaging. Radiology 186: 227–231
10. Lucas D R, Unni K K, McLeod R A, O'Connor M I, Sim F H 1994 Osteoblastoma: clinicopathologic study of 306 cases. Human Pathol 25: 117–134
11. Mitchell M L, Ackerman L V 1986 Metastatic and pseudomalignant osteoblastoma: a report of two unusual cases. Skel Radiol 15: 213–218
12. Woods E R, Martel W, Mandel S H, Crabbe J P 1993 Reactive soft tissue mass associated with osteoid osteoma: correlation of MR imaging features with pathologic findings. Radiology 186: 221–225
13. Blau R A, Zwick D L, Westphal R A 1988 Multiple non ossifying fibroma. J Bone Joint Surg 70: 299–304
14. Ritsch P, Hajek P C, Pechman U 1989 Fibrous metaphyseal defects: magnetic resonance imaging appearance. Skel Radiol 18: 253–259
15. Jee W H, Choe B Y, Kang H S, Suh K J 1998 Non ossifying fibroma: characteristics at MR imaging with pathologic correlation. Radiology 209: 197–202
16. Pazzaglia U E, Pedrotti L, Beluffi G et al 1990 Radiographic findings in hereditary multiple exostoses and new theory of pathogenesis of exostoses. Pediatr Radiol 20: 594–597
17. Eich G F, Hoeffel J C, Tschappeler H, Gassner I, Willi U V 1998 Fibrous tumours in children: imaging features of a heterogeneous group of disorders. Pediatr Radiol 28: 500–509
18. Woertler K 2003 Benign bone tumors and tumor-like lesions: value of cross-sectional imaging. Eur Radiol 13: 1820–1835
19. Mahnken A H, Nolte-Ernsting C C, Wildberger J E et al 2003 Aneurysmal bone cyst: value of MR imaging and conventional radiography. Eur Radiol 13: 1118–1124
20. Jee W H, Choi K H, Choe B Y, Park J M, Shinn K S 1996 Fibrous dysplasia. MRI imaging characteristics with radiologic correlations. Am J Roentgenol 167: 1523–1527
21. Link M P, Eilber F 1997 Osteosarcoma. In: Pizzo P A, Poplack D G (eds) Principles and practice of pediatric oncology. Lippincott-Raven, Philadelphia, pp 889–920
22. Logan M P, Mitchell M J, Munk P L 1998 Imaging of variant osteosarcoma: with an emphasis on CT and MR imaging. Am J Roentgenol 171: 1531–1537
23. Meyer J S, Dormans J P 1998 Differential diagnosis of pediatric musculoskeletal masses. MRI Clin North Am 6: 561–577
24. Horovitz M E, Malawer M M, Woo S Y, Hicks M J 1997 Ewing's sarcoma family of tumors: Ewing's sarcoma of bone and soft tissue and the peripheral primitive neuroectodermal tumors. In: Pizzo P A, Poplack D G (eds) Principles and practice of pediatric oncology. Lippincott-Raven, Philadelphia, pp 831–863
25. Toma P, Lucigrai G, Marzoli A et al 1994 Prenatal diagnosis of metastatic adrenal neuroblastoma with sonography and MR imaging. Am J Roentgenol 162: 1183–1184
26. Siegel M J, Ishwaran H, Fletcher B D et al 2002 Staging of neuroblastoma at imaging: report of the radiology diagnostic oncology group. Radiology 223: 168–175
27. Brodeur G M, Pritchard J, Berthold F et al 1993 Revisions of the international criteria for neuroblastoma diagnosis, staging, and response to treatment. J Clin Oncol 11: 1466–1477
28. Abramson S J 1999 Neuroblastoma. In: Siegel M J (ed) Special course in pediatric radiology: current concepts in body imaging at the millenium. RSNA Inc, Oak Brook, pp 157–172
29. Couanet D, Geoffray A, Hartmann O et al 1988 Bone marrow metastases in children's neuroblastoma studied by magnetic resonance imaging: advances in neuroblastoma research. Prog Clin Biol Res 271: 547–555
30. Kushner B H 2004 Neuroblastoma: a disease requiring a multitude of imaging studies. J Nucl Med 45: 1172–1188

CHAPTER 70

Paediatric Neuroradiology

Roxana S. Gunny and W. K. 'Kling' Chong

NORMAL BRAIN MATURATION

Brain maturation is assessed by observing tissue characteristics related to myelination, as well as variations in morphology. Most of the changes associated with myelination occur in the first 2 years of life, but other changes in tissue characteristics occur as the brain matures. Gyral and sulcal development mainly occurs in utero or in the premature brain, but other morphological changes are observable later in life.

Normal myelination

The extent of myelination of the infant brain is assessed by magnetic resonance imaging (MRI) according to specific milestones analogous to the normal milestones of clinical development. As the brain matures there is progressive T1 and T2 shortening of the white matter due to changes in the lipid and water content of developing myelin and packing of white matter tracts[1]. This follows a centrifugal posterior-to-anterior and inferior-to-superior pattern and is virtually complete by the age of 2 years (Fig. 70.1). Advanced MRI techniques show progressive reduction in water diffusion, increased fractional anisotropy (assessed by diffusion tensor imaging), and increased magnetization transfer[2–4]. Brain myelination is detected in grey matter earlier on T2-weighted fast spin-echo (FSE) and in the white matter tracts earlier on T1-weighted spin-echo (SE) or inversion recovery (STIR) sequences. Most myelination occurs post-term in the first 8 months, although it may extend into adulthood. The brain should appear virtually fully myelinated on T2-weighted sequences by 2 years, with almost an adult appearance on T1-weighted sequences by 10 months (Fig. 70.2).

The newborn has limited motor function but a well-developed sensory system. Thus the myelination pattern seen at birth at full term is primarily in the sensory tracts. During the first 6 months of life the process of myelination is easiest to follow on T1-weighted images, where the myelinated areas appear bright. T2-weighted images are less sensitive and it takes much more myelin to produce a hypointense signal within the white matter. During this period T2-weighted images show only subtle myelination.

At full term, T1-weighted images should show high signal in the dorsal medulla and brain stem, the cerebellar peduncles, a small part of the cerebral peduncles, about a third of the posterior limb of the internal capsule, the central corona radiata, and the deep white matter in the region of the pre- and post-central gyrus[5]. Progression of myelination is seen in the optic radiations during the first months of life. The internal capsule will demonstrate T1 shortening within the anterior limb by 3 months, while on T2-weighted images the hypointensity due to myelin is not seen until about 8 months of age. The splenium of the corpus callosum on T2-weighted images becomes hypointense at 3 months of age. The hypointense signal extends anteriorly along the body and genu, and the complete corpus callosum is myelinated at 6 months[6].

After 6 months the signal pattern on T1-weighted images becomes less precise, and after 10 months the brain is fully myelinated by T1 criteria. T2-weighted images are then used to assess the myelination from 6 months to 24 months of age, when the signal pattern generally is fully mature and has a completely adult pattern, though the milestones of myelination are much more imprecise than during the first 6 months of life.

On T2 weighted images the first signs of mature subcortical white matter are found around the calcarine fissure at 4 months and in the pre- and post-central gyri at 8 months.

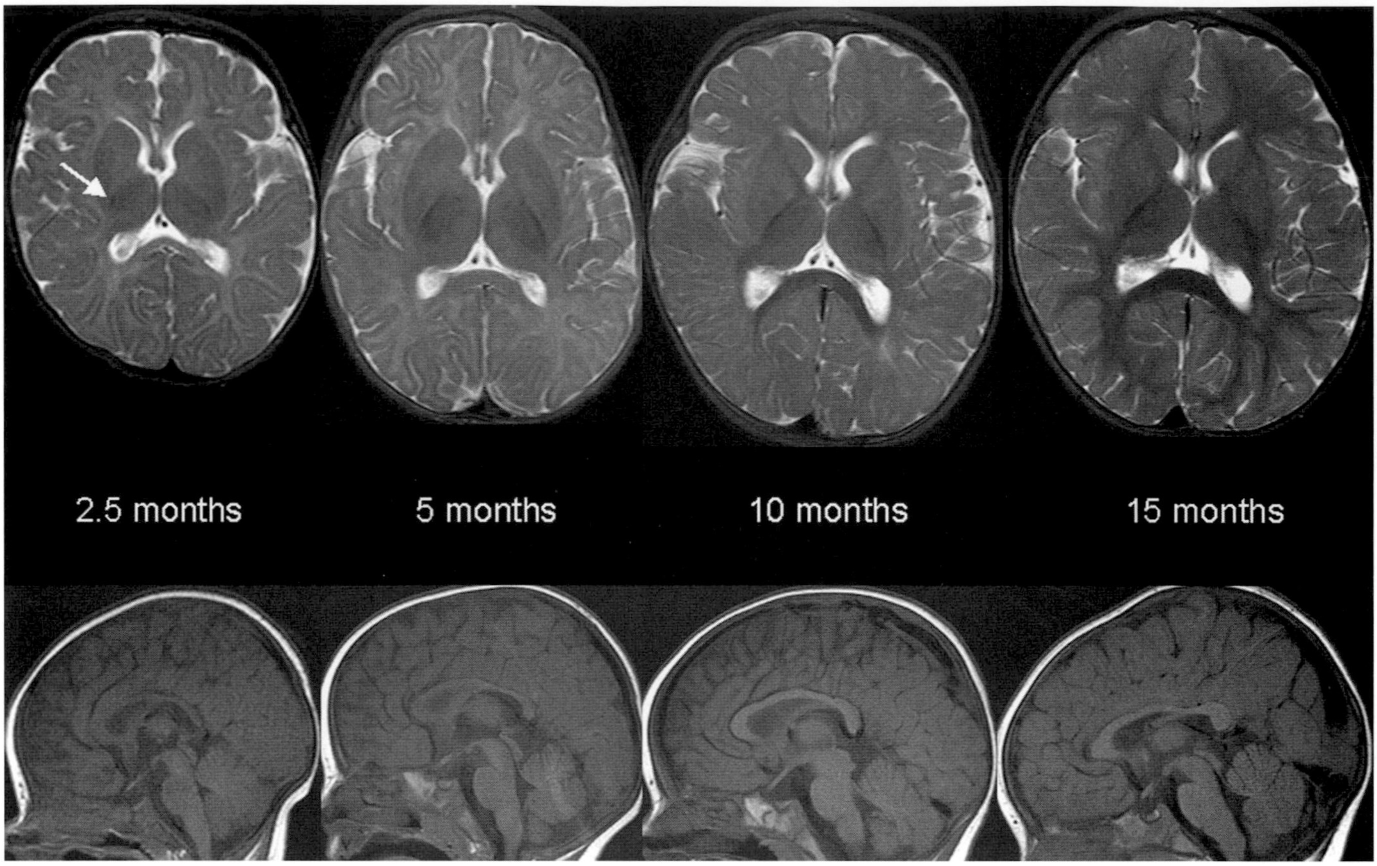

Figure 70.1 Normal brain development with age seen on T2- (top row) and T1-weighted (bottom row) MRI. On T2-weighted images myelination at term and at 2.5 months is seen centrally as signal hypointensity within the posterior limbs of the internal capsules. This progresses from posterior to anterior with age, as does myelination of the corpus callosum. Myelination also progresses centrally to peripherally. The sagittal T1-weighted image shows progressive bulking up of the corpus callosum. By 6 months the corpus callosum should reach approximately its normal childhood size. The splenium is slightly enlarged with respect to the genu.

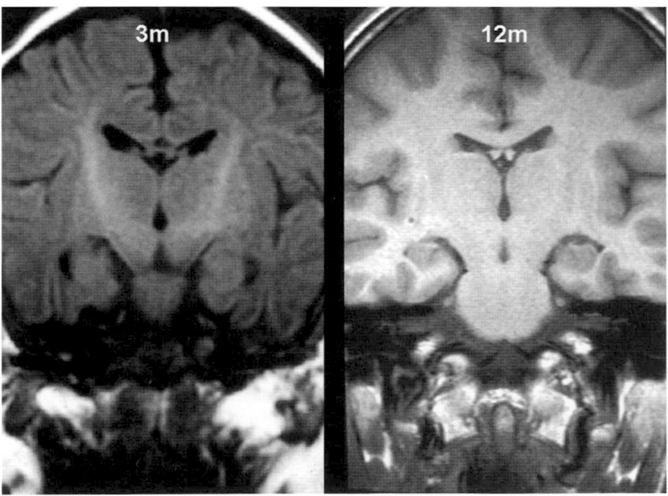

Figure 70.2 Normal brain myelination at 3 and 12 months. On T1-weighted MRI at term, T1 shortening is seen within the posterior limb of the internal capsule. This progresses posteriorly to anteriorly and centrally to peripherally until by 12 months the brain appears fully myelinated.

By 10 months the occipital subcortical white matter appears isointense with the overlying grey matter and finally shows mature hypointense signal around 1 year of age. This process proceeds anteriorly and by 18 months has finally reached the most frontal parts and the frontal poles of the temporal lobes.

Regions of persistent hyperintensity on T2-weighted sequences known as the 'terminal myelination zones'[7] may be seen within the peritrigonal areas well into adulthood, and can be distinguished from white matter disease by the presence of a rim of normal myelinated brain between these areas and the ventricular margin. Other areas may also persist as regions of signal hyperintensity beyond 2 years, e.g. in the fronto-temporal subcortical white matter, and should not be mistaken for disease (Fig. 70.3).

Normal gyration

Gyration is the process by which the individual gyri and sulci of the cerebral hemispheres form. The MRI appearances lag behind the extent of gyral formation seen at the same age at post-mortem. The surface of the cerebral hemispheres is initially smooth, with the interhemispheric fissure and Sylvian fissures having already formed by 16 weeks gestation. Other primary sulci, such as the callosal sulcus and parieto-occipital fissure, are recognizable at 22 weeks gestation, followed by the cingular and calcarine sulci. The central sulcus is seen in most infants by 27 weeks. Gyration then continues into the post-term period in a standardized and consistent sequence, beginning with the sensorimotor regions and visual pathways, areas that are also myelinating at the same time. The slowest regions of gyration are also those with the slowest myelination, such

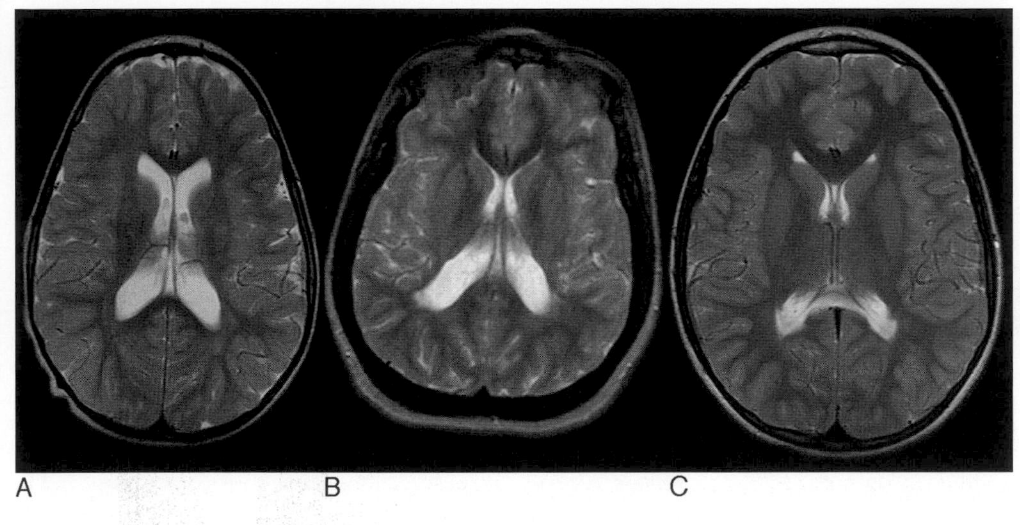

Figure 70.3 Normal terminal myelination zones compared to pathological states. (A) T2-weighted MRI shows signal hyperintensity adjacent to the trigones of the lateral ventricles but with a rim of darker signal between this and the ventricular margins. This is the normal appearance of the terminal myelination zones. (B) Periventricular signal hyperintensity extending down to the ventricular margin. The ventricles are dilated posteriorly and there is irregular scalloping of the ventricular margins in keeping with white matter volume loss. These are the typical features of periventricular leukomalacia due to hypoxic ischaemia. (C) Peritrigonal and splenial signal abnormality. The ventricles are not dilated. This is the typical pattern of adrenoleukodystrophy.

as the frontal and temporal poles. By term the gyral pattern is nearly the same as the appearance in adults with further deepening of the sulci occurring post-term. The Sylvian fissures are also wider and vertically oriented and these continue to mature post-term.[8,9]

Other post-natal maturational changes

Development of the corpus callosum begins with the posterior genu, body, and splenium, then the anterior genu and rostrum. All these components are present by 20 weeks gestation; however, it continues to grow in length and thickness through the rest of the fetal period and post-term. The adult appearance with full thickness of the corpus callosum is achieved by 8–10 months of age, and bulking up of the splenium as the visual pathways mature occurs by 4–6 months[10].

In the adult there are several regions where there is relative T2 hypointensity, considered to be due to the normal deposition of iron; these are the basal ganglia, particularly the globus pallidus, substantia nigra, and red nucleus. In the infant the basal ganglia begin to appear relatively T2 hypointense to cortex by about 6 months of age due to myelination, but the putamen and globus pallidus are isointense to each other and the internal capsule. They then become relatively bright with respect to white matter as this begins to myelinate. By 9 or 10 years there is a second stage of T2 shortening in the globus pallidus, substantia nigra and red nucleus, which reduces further during the second decade[11]. The dentate nuclei show similar though less marked changes by about age 15 years. This phase is due to iron deposition which continues throughout adult life.

In normal infants up to the age of 2 months the anterior pituitary gland has a convex upper border and is of relatively high T1-weighted signal[12]. From 2 months the pituitary gland has a flat surface and is isointense with grey matter. It slowly grows during childhood and ranges from 2 to 6 mm in vertical diameter until puberty when it enlarges again.

BRAIN STRUCTURAL MALFORMATIONS

Cerebellar malformations

Cerebellar hypoplasia

The cerebellum may be small due to lack of formation or cerebellar atrophy. Cerebellar hypoplasia an acquired insult, such as infection (especially congenital cytomegalovirus); an inborn error of metabolism, such as a glycosylation disorder; or unknown cause. Clinically the child may present with variable hypotonia or ataxia but these features may be very mild and there is no clear correlation between the severity of the imaging findings and the clinical presentation. Although the underlying aetiology is usually not elucidated, in around 10% of children the diagnosis includes carbohydrate-deficient glycoprotein syndrome, infantile neuroaxonal dystrophy (Fig. 70.4), pontocerebellar hypoplasia, spinocerebellar atrophies, Friedrich's ataxia and other rare syndromes[13]. The pons may also be small which may simply reflect the lack of synaptic connections from the hypoplastic cerebellum. The posterior fossa is of normal size and the cerebellum is of normal signal intensity.

Dandy–Walker complex

This encompasses a spectrum of cystic posterior fossa malformations from the complete Dandy–Walker malformation to persistent Blake's pouch and mega cisterna magna, all of which have in common an apparently focal extra-axial cerebrospinal fluid (CSF) collection which is continuous with the fourth ventricle and variable cerebellar hypoplasia[14]. Children with any of these developmental anomalies may present as incidental findings or with developmental delay, seizures and hydrocephalus. The Dandy–Walker malformation and its variants are associated with hydrocephalus and other midline anomalies, and can be an indicator for underlying clinical syndromes and chromosomal abnormalities. The classical Dandy–Walker malformation is characterized by cystic dilatation of the fourth ventricle, which almost fills the entire enlarged posterior fossa;

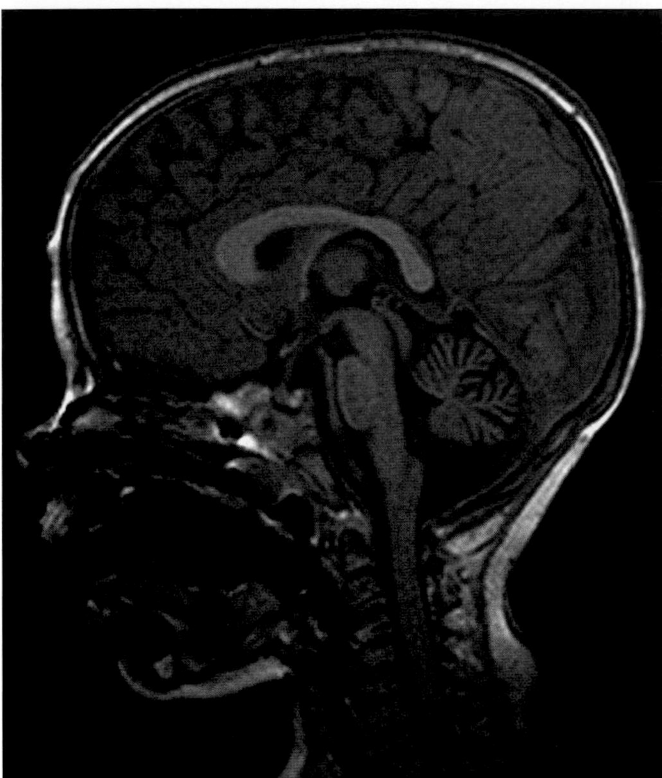

Figure 70.4 Child with infantile neuroaxonal dystrophy. The cerebellar folia are underformed and the fissures are widened. The brainstem is also small.

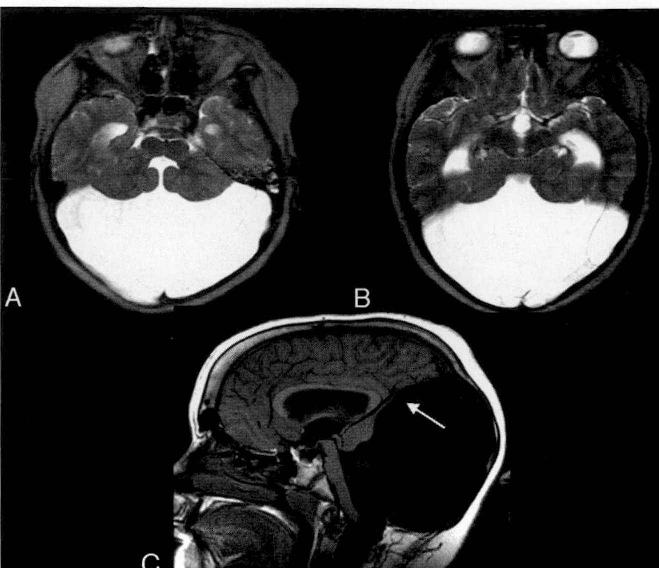

Figure 70.5 Dandy–Walker malformation. (A,B) The fourth ventricle opens into a large posterior fossa cyst. There is associated hydrocephalus. (C) The cerebellum is hypoplastic and a thin rim of cerebellar tissue is seen forming the wall of the posterior fossa cyst (arrow). The vein of Galen, straight sinus, and venous confluence are elevated above the level of the lambdoid suture.

the cerebellar vermis is hypoplastic and rotated or aplastic and the tentorium and venous confluence of the torcula are elevated (Fig. 70.5)[15]. Torcular–lambdoid inversion may be seen on plain radiography, computed tomography (CT) and MRI. At the mildest end of the spectrum, the mega cisterna magna is seen as an incidental finding of doubtful clinical significance and consists of an infracerebellar CSF collection (or normal cisternal space), occasionally with an enlarged posterior fossa but a normal cerebellum and fourth ventricle. These need to be distinguished from posterior fossa arachnoid cysts. Such arachnoid cysts do not communicate with the fourth ventricle. They may occasionally cause sufficient mass effect to warrant surgical intervention. The presence of crossing vessels and the falx cerebelli favours the mega cisterna magna over arachnoid cyst.

Joubert's syndrome and related disorders

The typical clinical syndrome is of hyperpnoea, abnormal eye movements and ataxia that is associated with a particular pattern of cerebellar dysgenesis[16]. The typical imaging findings may occasionally be seen in clinically normal children or in children without the full triad of clinical features, and there is some controversy as to the exact definition of this condition. In a few cases a specific genetic locus has been identified, and many syndromes with additional features such as renal cysts, ocular abnormalities, liver fibrosis, hypothalamic hamartoma and polymicrogyria have been classified with this anomaly, so that detection of the typical midbrain changes should prompt investigation for these. It is probably best to think of it as a generalized developmental disorder of the midbrain and hindbrain. The imaging findings reflect a failure of formation of the decussation of the superior cerebellar peduncles, lack of the pyramidal decussations and other anomalies of the midbrain crossing tracts and their nuclei. On cross-sectional imaging the fourth ventricle is enlarged with a 'batwing appearance' and there is a cleft in the vermis. The midbrain is small. The 'molar tooth' appearance seen on axial images arises from the lack of the superior cerebellar decussation and the superior peduncles also appear enlarged (Fig. 70.6)[17].

Rhombencephalosynapsis and other cerebellar malformations

Rhombencephalosynapsis is a very rare cerebellar malformation in which the cerebellar hemispheres are fused across the midline and there is hypoplasia or aplasia of the vermis[18]. Again, the clinical presentation is variable. It is associated with other midline supratentorial anomalies such as absence of the septum pellucidum and corpus callosum and holoprosencephaly.

L'Hermitte-Duclos or dysplastic cerebellar gangliocytoma is a developmental mass lesion with a distinctive radiological appearance in which there is enlargement of the cerebellar cortex usually affecting one hemisphere. On MRI there is a nonenhancing mass with diffusely enlarged cerebellar folia[19]. Pial enhancement may be demonstrated. There are many other forms of nonspecific cerebellar dysgenesis for which as yet there are no universally accepted classification systems. The Chiari malformations are discussed separately below as they represent separate entities.

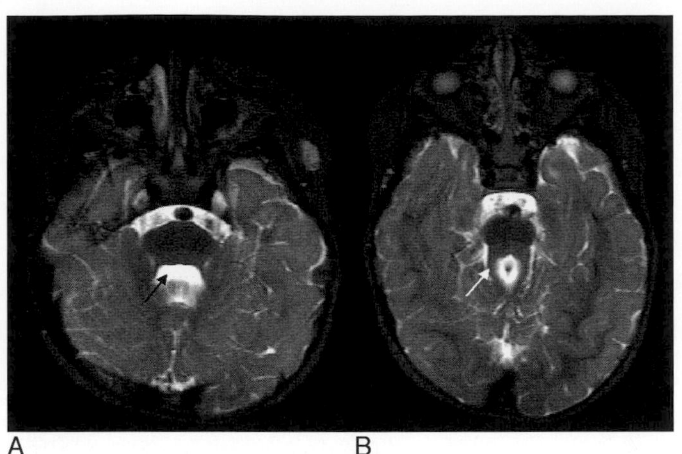

Figure 70.6 Child with Joubert's syndrome. (A) Typical batwing appearance to the fourth ventricle (arrow) and (B) prominent superior cerebellar peduncles with failure of the normal midline decussation (arrow). This gives the typical 'molar tooth' appearance. The midbrain is hypoplastic in this condition.

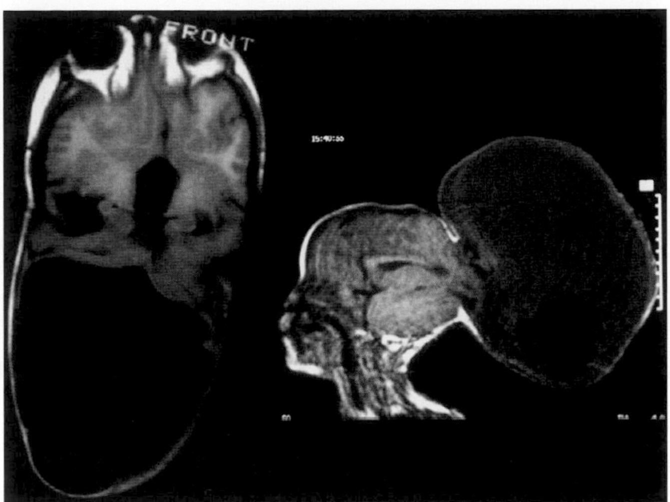

Figure 70.7 Parieto-occipital cephalocele with herniation of the brain and meninges through a calvarial defect. Most of the herniated component is in the form of a cerebrospinal fluid-containing meningocele.

Cerebral malformations[20–22]

The earliest malformations to appear relate to the formation of the neural tube, i.e. abnormalities of dorsal induction or cranial dysraphism (3–4 weeks gestation). Anencephaly, cephalocele and Chiari II (Arnold–Chiari) malformation are consequences of abnormalities of dorsal induction. The events following the formation of the neural tube are termed ventral induction, when the two separate cerebral hemispheres are formed (5–8 weeks). The holoprosencephalies are all abnormalities of ventral induction. The structures in the posterior fossa are also formed during this period. Neurones form and proliferate in the subependymal layer of the lateral ventricles known as the germinal matrix from around 7 weeks gestation. The neurones subsequently migrate peripherally along radially oriented microglia to form the layers of the cerebral cortex from 2 to 5 months' gestation, the deeper layers forming first.

Disorders of dorsal induction

Anencephaly is the most common cerebral malformation in the fetus and is incompatible with life. Most anencephalics are stillborn, but a few survive for a few days. Anencephaly in which there is no cerebral cortex should be distinguished from gross hydrocephalus in which there is a very thin, barely visible cerebral cortical mantle.

Cephalocele. A cephalocele is an extracranial protrusion of intracranial structures through a congenital defect of the skull and dura mater (Fig. 70.7). Unlike myelomeningoceles in the spine there is usually no skin defect. When the cephalocele contains only leptomeninges and CSF it is a meningocele, and when it also contains neural tissue, which is usually abnormal and nonfunctioning, it is an encephalocele. When this includes part of the ventricle it is called an encephalocystocele. The cephalocele may be palpable clinically and may be pulsatile. The majority of congenital cephaloceles occur in the occipital and frontal regions.

The primary role of imaging is to establish the presence of neural tissue, other intracranial malformations and hydrocephalus, preferably by MRI. Small meningoceles may not require surgery since their size may decrease with time, producing the appearance of an 'atretic meningocele'. The detection and localization of vascular structures is important before any neurosurgical intervention. Herniated neural tissue may have an obliterated blood supply and hence show signs of ischaemia.

Chiari II malformation (Arnold–Chiari). This is discussed here as a congenital malformation of the hindbrain that, for practical purposes, is always associated with myelomeningocele. Affected children usually present with hydrocephalus following repair of the myelomingocele after birth. Other symptoms of complications of the malformation include upper airway problems, such as apnoea and stridor, and feeding problems, such as dysphagia.

The Chiari II malformation consists of inferior displacement of the cerebellum, pons, medulla oblongata and cervical cord. Associated features include an inferiorly displaced and elongated fourth ventricle, beaking of the tectum, flattening of the ventral pons and low attachment of the tentorium[23,24]. The tentorial incisura is enlarged and the cerebellum herniates superiorly into the supratentorial space. The falx is partially absent or fenestrated with consequent interdigitation of gyri across the midline, and the massa intermedia of the thalami is enlarged. The foramen magnum is enlarged and 'shield-shaped' (Fig. 70.8).

Other malformations that may be associated with the Chiari II malformation include a lacunar skull dysraphism (lukenschadel), disorders of neuronal migration, malformation of the corpus callosum, a dorsal midline cyst and absence of the septum pellucidum.

The diagnosis can be readily made with CT by identifying the wide tentorial incisura, typical configuration of the foramen magnum and the small fourth ventricle and posterior fossa. Interdigitation of the cerebral hemispheres may be also identified. MRI is the best investigation to show complications, which include hydrocephalus, an isolated fourth ventricle, hydrosyringomyelia and compression of the craniocervical junction.

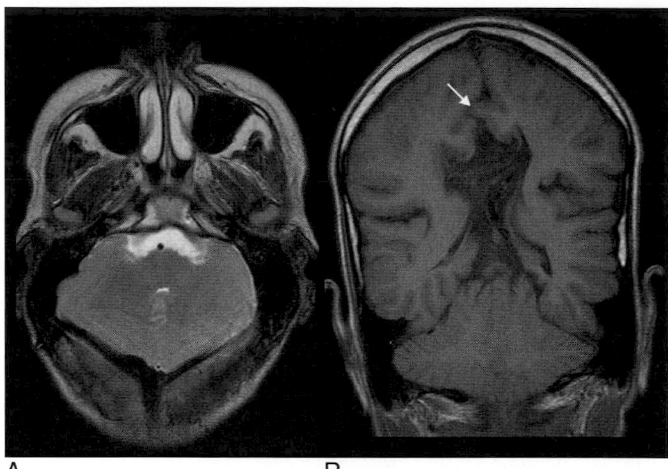

Figure 70.8 Chiari II malformation. (A) The posterior fossa is enlarged and 'shield shaped'. The fourth ventricle is small and slit-like. (B) The cerebellum towers superiorly through the tentorium and there is interdigitation of a cerebral gyrus through the fenestrated falx (arrow).

The fourth ventricle in Chiari II malformation should be slit-like: a normal or enlarged ventricle suggests hydrocephalus or that the ventricle may be isolated (Fig. 70.9).

Disorders of ventral induction

Holoprosencephaly is a midline malformation of ventral induction of the anterior brain, skull and face, resulting from the failure of the embryonic prosencephalon to undergo segmentation and cleavage into two separate cerebral hemispheres. Holoprosencephaly is associated with chromosomal abnormalities, facial clefting and various teratogenic factors including maternal diabetes.

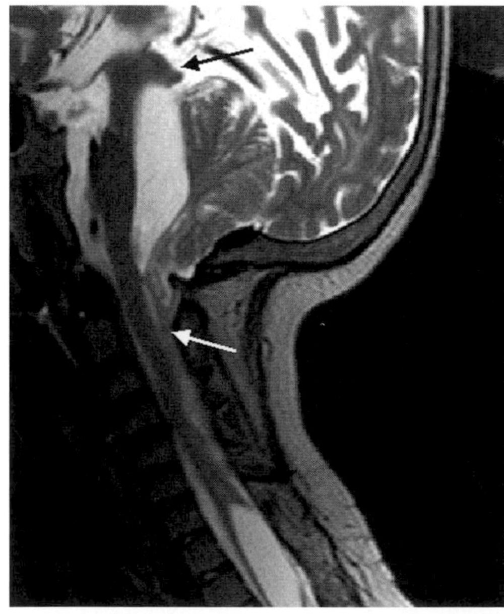

Figure 70.9 Chiari II malformation. The fourth ventricle, which should normally be small and slit-like in this condition, is enlarged, indicating hydrocephalus. There is cascading tonsillar tissue herniating through the foramen magnum (white arrow). Beaking of the tectal plate is also seen (black arrow), as well as a cervical spinal cord syringomyelic cavity.

Alobar holoprosencephaly is the severest form and affected fetuses are often spontaneously aborted. The ventricular system with a single cavity is in continuity with a large dorsal cyst (Fig. 70.10). Hydrocephalus prevails, causing macrocrania in spite of microcephaly.

Semilobar holoprosencephaly is less severe and there is less reduction in brain volume. Posteriorly the interhemispheric fissure is partially formed. The frontal lobes are fused, but the thalami are partially separated. There is still a single ventricle, but there is an indication of a third ventricle. The corpus callosum may be partially formed.

Lobar holoprosencephaly is associated with mild (or absent) facial malformations and intellectual abilities that range from mild impairment to normal. The brain is generally of normal volume and shows almost complete separation into two hemispheres, though in the depth of the frontal lobes there is continuous cerebral cortex between the two lobes.

Malformations of commissural and related structures

Agenesis of the septum pellucidum. Absence of the septum pellucidum is not a severe malformation, but should be recognized as an indicator of other cerebral malformations. Associated malformations are septo-optic dysplasia, agenesis of the corpus callosum, holoprosencephaly, Chiari II malformation, schizencephaly and other migration disorders. Septo-optic dysplasia or de Morsier's syndrome includes the triad of hypopituitarism, hypoplasia of the optic nerves and absence of the septum pellucidum (Fig. 70.11). The syndrome is not rare but the clinical manifestations are quite variable. On coronal T1-weighted MRI it is important to assess the size of the optic nerves and chiasm, as well as the pituitary gland.

Commissural agenesis or dysgenesis. The major interhemispheric commissural connections are the corpus callosum and anterior and posterior commissures. The corpus callosum may be partially formed (dysgenetic) or completely absent. The anterior part (posterior genu and anterior body) is formed before the posterior part (posterior body and splenium). Thus a small or absent genu or body, with an intact

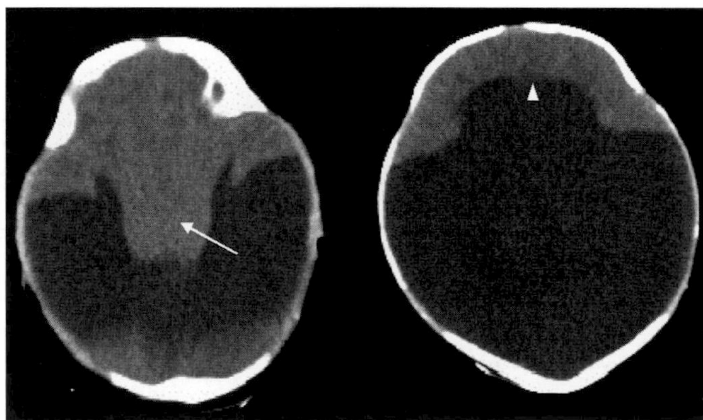

Figure 70.10 CT brain of this infant shows that the cerebral hemispheres have failed to form and there is no interhemispheric fissure or corpus callosum. Instead there is a thin pancake of cerebral tissue crossing the midline anteriorly (arrowhead) and a single holoventricle continuous with a large dorsal cyst. The midbrain and deep grey structures are fused into a single indiscriminate mass (arrow).

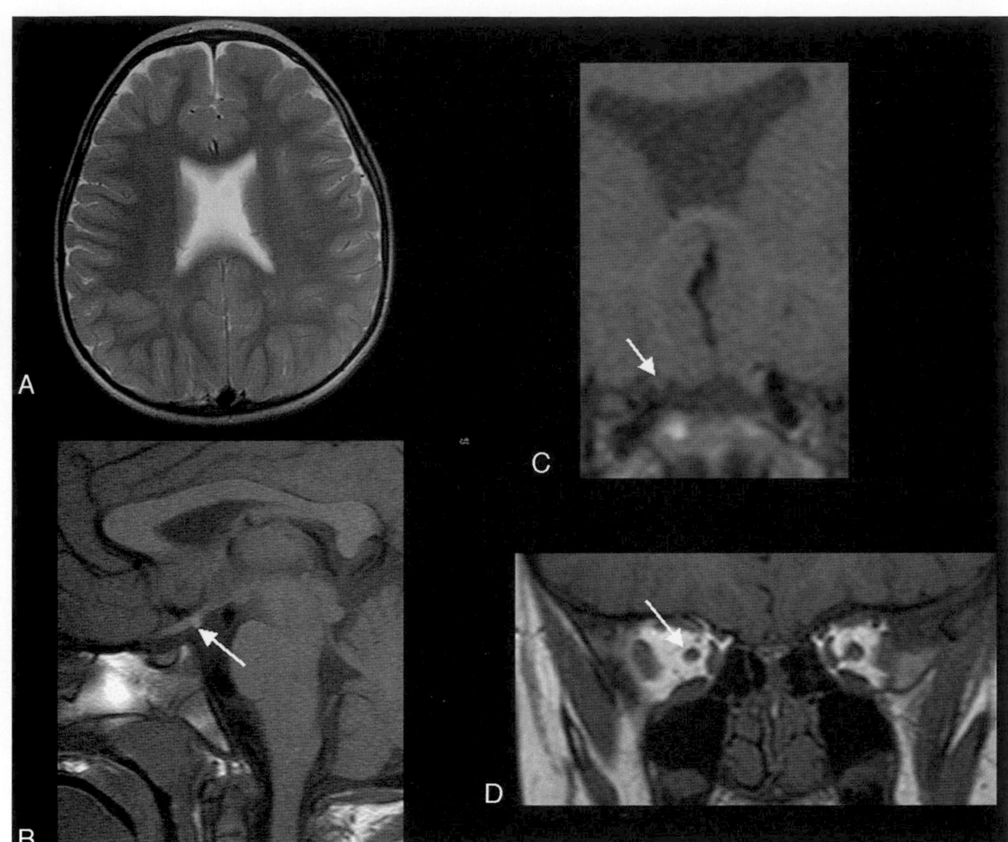

Figure 70.11 Septo-optic dysplasia in a child with HESX1 gene mutation. (A) The septum pellucidum is absent and the frontal horns have a typical box-like configuration. (B) The posterior pituitary gland is ectopic (arrow). (C,D) The right optic nerve is small (arrows).

splenium and rostrum, indicates secondary destruction rather than abnormal development. The structure develops between about 7 and 20 weeks gestation, which parallels the development of the rest of the cerebrum and the cerebellum; abnormalities of the corpus callosum are therefore commonly associated with other congenital malformations of the brain, such as the Chiari II malformation, the Dandy–Walker malformation, lipoma, abnormalities of neuronal migration and organization, dysraphic anomalies, encephaloceles, septo-optic dysplasia, ocular anomalies and other midline facial anomalies[25].

There are many well-defined syndromes in which callosal abnormalities feature, including Aicardi's syndrome characterized by seizures, intellectual impairment and brain abnormalities. Callosal agenesis is a feature of oculocerebrocutaneous syndrome or Delleman's syndrome (Fig. 70.12). Dysgenesis of the corpus callosum is also frequently seen in fetal alcohol syndrome.

The presence of parallel lateral ventricles with the third ventricle seen between them and without the normal convergence of the bodies of the ventricles indicates callosal agenesis and can be detected on axial imaging. It is thought that the interhemispheric cyst frequently seen with this malformation originates from the herniated third ventricle but has lost continuity with this structure. On sagittal MRI, partial

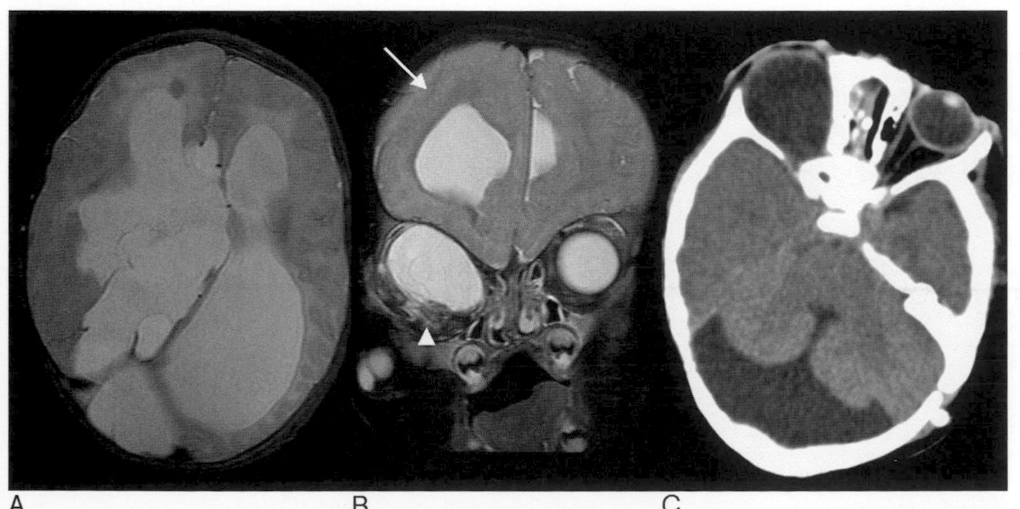

Figure 70.12 Child with skin lesions and right orbital cyst in oculocerebrocutaneous syndrome. (A) There is callosal agenesis with dorsal interhemispheric cysts. (B) The right cerebral hemisphere is dysplastic with thickening of the cortex and an indistinct grey–white matter junction (arrow). There is a cyst expanding the orbit with a small calcified globe seen inferiorly (arrowhead). (C) An associated Dandy–Walker posterior fossa malformation is also present.

or complete absence of the corpus callosum must be distinguished from a generally thinned one (which is more likely to be an acquired abnormality, e.g. ischaemia). In callosal agenesis the vertically oriented sulci extend right down to the ventricle and there is no horizontally running cingulate sulcus. Presence of one midline anomaly, such as callosal agenesis (Fig. 70.13), should prompt the reporting radiologist to look carefully for other midline anomalies that are frequently associated.

Malformations of neuronal migration and cortical organization

Abnormalities of the cerebral cortex are a common finding in children with developmental delay and children with partial epilepsy. The cortex is formed from neuroblasts that are generated in the germinal matrix, an ependymal layer of the ventricular wall. The neuroblasts migrate to the surface of the brain along radially oriented glia, passing neurones previously laid down to form the layers of cortex. Thus the six layers of the cortex are formed with the youngest neurones on the surface and the oldest ones adjacent to the subcortical white matter. The migration of the neuroblasts starts at about week 7 of gestation, is most intense during weeks 15–17 and is largely complete by weeks 23–24. When the process of neuronal migration is disturbed, there is a migration disorder resulting in morphologically abnormal cortex.

Schizencephaly

Schizencephaly is a defect that involves the complete cerebral mantle and connects the calvarium and the outer surface of the brain with the lateral ventricles. The defect is a cleft lined by grey matter and leptomeninges, which differentiates it from a transmantle infarction in which the defect is lined by white matter. The schizencephaly may have an 'open lip' with a wide open defect (Fig. 70.14), or a 'closed lip' when the cleft is closed but lined with grey matter entirely into the ventricle. The convolutional pattern of the cortex adjacent to the clefts is abnormal and consists of polymicrogyria.

The clinical features are variable, depending on the size and location of the lesion. Severe seizures are quite common, as is spasticity. Children with bilateral clefts have severe mental and psychomotor developmental delay. Wide clefts usually correlate with moderate to severe developmental delay, while children with narrow or closed-lipped lesions may only have hemiplegia and/or seizures. The location of the lesion is typically central, involving the pre- and post-central gyri. However, the clefts may also be found in parasagittal, frontal or occipital sites when the clinical manifestations are often mild.

In most cases the diagnosis is made with CT, but this may not detect all cases with closed lips, which are best detected using coronal T1-weighted MRI, preferably a three-dimensional (3D) volume acquisition. MRI also shows the abnormal appearance of the cortical mantle along the cleft and the cortex appearing thicker than normal owing to the presence of polymicrogyria. The contralateral hemisphere may also have developmental abnormalities, such as polymicrogyria and subependymal heterotopia. CT may show subependymal or parenchymal calcification in many cases, which suggests that one cause of schizencephaly may be intrauterine infection with cytomegalovirus.

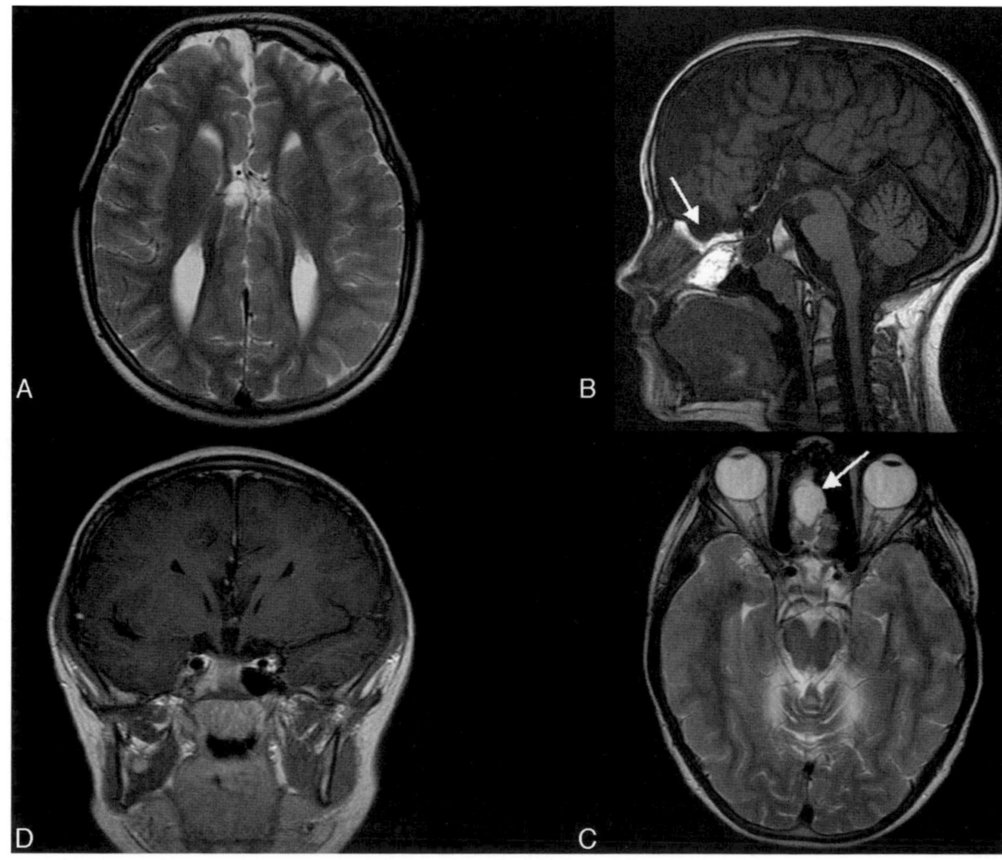

Figure 70.13 Callosal agenesis. (A) Axial T2-weighted MRI shows separated ventricles with parallel orientation. The superior part of the third ventricle is just seen. (B) Sagittal T1-weighted MRI through the midline confirms callosal agenesis. There is no cingulate sulcus and the vertically oriented cerebral sulci extend right down to the third ventricle. This finding is associated with other midline anomalies such as a fronto-ethmoidal cephalocele (arrow), seen also on the axial T2-weighted MRI (arrow, C). (D) The optic chiasm is absent.

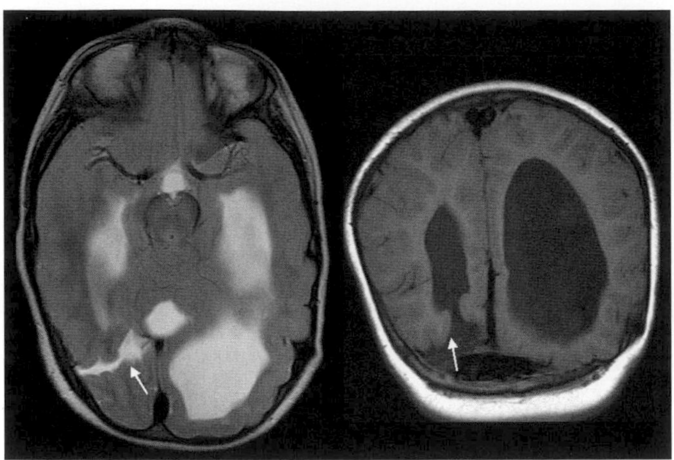

Figure 70.14 Schizencephaly with a grey matter-lined cleft (arrows) extending from the leptomeningeal surface through the brain parenchyma to the ventricular margin.

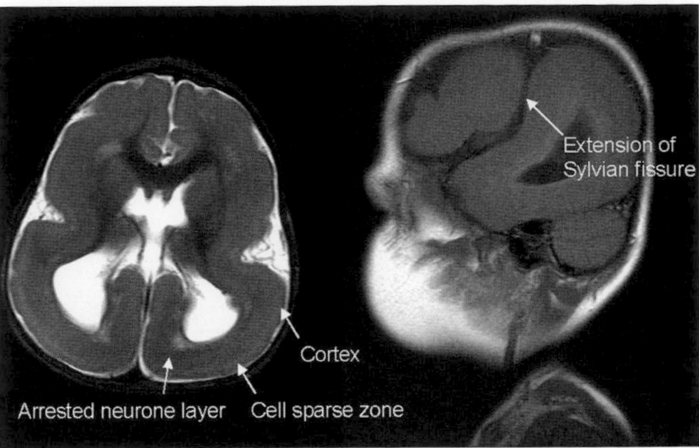

Figure 70.15 Classical with lissencephaly. This child was 'floppy' at birth and then had developmental delay, seizures, and strabismus. MRI shows a smooth gyral pattern which is slightly more developed frontally in keeping with classical lissencephaly (LIS1 mutation). The cerebral cortex is generally thin and there is a band of arrested neurones deep to the 'cell sparse zone'. The Sylvian fissures are vertically oriented and extend into a vertical cleft.

Lissencephaly–agyria–pachygyria

The lissencephaly–agyria–pachygyria group includes the severest forms of abnormal neuronal migration. Lissencephaly literally means 'smooth brain'. The brain has very few or no gyri, opercularization (development of the Sylvian fissures) is abnormal, and the Sylvian fissures are shallow. Other associated features are agenesis or hypoplasia of the corpus callosum or septum pellucidum. Agyria refers to the total absence of a convolutional pattern, i.e. there are no gyri or sulci, and is synonymous with 'complete lissencephaly'. In pachygyria, the gyri are relatively few and are unusually broad and flat. The entire brain is not affected and therefore it is also known as 'incomplete lissencephaly'. Macroscopically and on standard thick-slice MRI, pachygyria may be difficult to differentiate from polymicrogyria, but the latter may be distinguished more easily on higher resolution imaging, e.g. with volumetric T1-weighted imaging (e.g. MPRAGE, SPGR, FLASH).

In complete lissencephaly the brain surface is smooth and the Sylvian fissures are wide and vertically orientated. The cortex is thin; there is a 'cell-sparse zone' of white matter adjacent to it and a broad band of grey matter, the 'arrested neurones' that have failed to migrate to the cortex, deep to it (Fig. 70.15). The gyral pattern of the brain resembles the appearance of the 23–24-week normal fetal brain. The implication of this is that lissencephaly is unlikely to be reliably diagnosed on early fetal MRI, though there may be clues to the diagnosis before this, such as the immature appearance of the Sylvian fissures, cell-sparse zone and the broad band of arrested neurones.

With incomplete lissencephaly there is an antero-posterior (AP) gradation of gyral development. In the LIS1 mutation (chromosome 17) the fronto-temporal gyri are more developed than the parieto-occipital gyri and in the X-linked form the posterior gyri are more developed.

Cobblestone lissencephaly is the result of overmigration of neurones, and is characterized by thick meninges adherent to the smooth cortical surface. There is no recognizable lamination of the cortex. Large areas of heterotopia are prominent and delay in myelination is frequently present. The congenital muscular dystrophies (CMDs) are a heterogeneous group characterized clinically by hypotonia at birth, muscle weakness and joint contractures, developmental delay and seizures. They may demonstrate 'cobblestone lissencephaly', e.g. in Walker–Warburg syndrome with coexistent ocular abnormalities and Fukayama CMD with relatively normal eyes.

Grey matter heterotopia

Grey matter heterotopia refers to the occurrence of grey matter in an abnormal position anywhere from the subependymal layer to the cortical surface, but the term is usually reserved for ectopic neurones in locations other than the cortex. Its most common clinical presentation is as a seizure disorder.

Heterotopia can be subependymal, focal subcortical or band formed, or parallel to the ventricular wall (double cortex). They are isointense with cortical grey matter on all imaging sequences and do not enhance after the intravenous infusion of paramagnetic contrast agents.

Subependymal heterotopia are smooth and ovoid, with their long axis typically parallel to the ventricular wall, quite different from subependymal hamartomas in tuberous sclerosis which are irregular and have their long axis perpendicular to the ventricular wall (Fig. 70.16). Hamartomas are more heterogeneous depending on any calcification, gliois, etc., and do not have signal characteristics of grey matter. They may also enhance after the intravenous infusion of a paramagnetic contrast agent. Small isolated areas of heterotopia may be seen occasionally as incidental findings in normal patients.

Focal subcortical heterotopia produces variable motor and intellectual impairment, depending on the size and location of the lesions. The overlying cortex is thin with shallow sulci. The foci may be isolated or may coexist with other malformations such as schizencephaly, microcephaly, polymicrogyria, dysgenesis of the corpus callosum, or absence of the septum pellucidum.

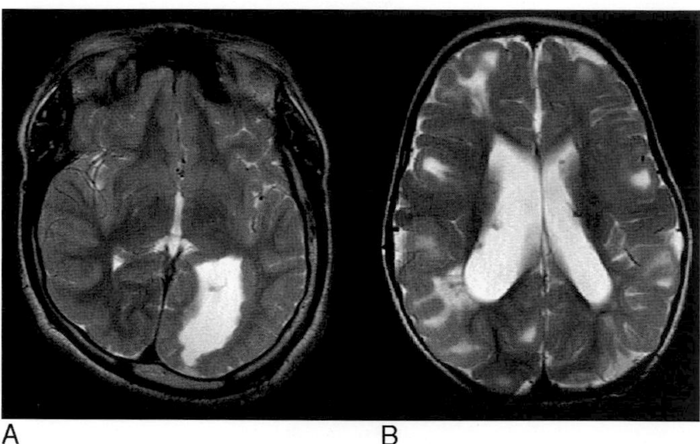

Figure 70.16 Subependymal grey matter heterotopia (A) and subependymal hamartomas of tuberous sclerosis (B). (A) Multiple subependymal continuous 'nodules' running along the ventricular margin with signal intensity isointense to grey matter. (B) Scattered nodules which project into the ventricles and with variable signal intensity. Some are markedly hypointense in keeping with calcification. Note also the multiple regions of cortical and subcortical white matter abnormality with slight mass effect in keeping with cortical tubers.

Band heterotopia or 'double cortex' is predominantly seen in girls (>90%). Although the imaging appearances are severe, the degree of developmental delay may be quite variable. Some children may even be normal except for a relatively mild seizure disorder. On imaging, band heterotopia appears as a homogeneous band of grey matter between the lateral ventricle and the cerebral cortex, separated from both by a layer of white matter. The overlying cortex is usually of normal thickness but has shallow sulci. Band heterotopia may be complete or partial, the latter predominantly involving the frontal lobes.

Polymicrogyria

This is considered to be a disorder of neuronal organization, occurring after neuronal migration. The extent of polymicrogyric cortex may vary from small, isolated, unilateral areas to larger areas of bilateral disease (Fig. 70.17). The appearances on imaging may also vary from apparently broad, thickened gyri mimicking pachygyria, to clearly overconvoluted multiple gyri, to subtle lesions that are difficult to detect even when using high-resolution 3D MRI sequences.

Transmantle cortical dysplasia

In transmantle cortical dysplasia, abnormal cells extend all the way from the wall of the ventricle to the cortex. The presenting signs and symptoms relate to the size and location of the lesion. Patients with involvement of just a small part of the cortex may have a normal neurological examination, though most patients with transmantle cortical dysplasia have complex partial epilepsy.

Large lesions are quite characteristic on neuroimaging but smaller ones may be very difficult to detect. Typical features include blurring of the junction between the cortex and the white matter, and hyperintensity (compared to the white matter on T2) extending from the lateral ventricular wall to the blurred cortex (Fig. 70.18). There is a correlation between abnormal venous drainage and dysplastic cortex so it can be useful to look for large cortical vessels on MRI in the search for the abnormal area of cortex. The lesion may sometimes be calcified and seen as a radially oriented band of T1 shortening extending down towards the ventricle. Occasionally the only clue to its presence may be a focus of calcification seen on CT.

Hemimegalencephaly

This is a structural malformation due to defective neuronal proliferation, migration and organization, leading to hamartomatous overgrowth of all or part of one hemisphere. It may occur in isolation or in association with syndromes such as proteus, epidermal naevus and Klippel–Trenaunay–Weber, syndromes neurofibromatosis type 1 (NF1) and tuberous sclerosis. The affected hemisphere contains regions of pachygyria, polymicrogyria, heterotopia, as well as dysmyelination and gliosis. Usually (but not always) the hemisphere is enlarged, there is diffuse cortical thickening, white matter signal abnormality and there may be calcification. The ipsilateral ventricle is enlarged and there is a very characteristic configuration of the frontal horn which is straight and pointed (Fig. 70.19). Occasionally this may be the only imaging clue to an underlying malformation.

Chiari I malformation

This may be considered a form of hindbrain deformation rather than a true malformation and is characterized by tonsillar descent. It may be an acquired condition and has occasionally been observed either to improve or worsen without interven-

Figure 70.17 Extensive bilateral cerebral hemisphere polymicrogyria. Virtually no normal cortex is seen. At first glance the cortex appears thickened but closer inspection reveals an overconvoluted gyral pattern and a 'lumpy bumpy' grey–white matter interface (including regions marked by white arrows). The Sylvian fissure is abnormally oriented with a parietal cleft that extends posteriorly (black arrow).

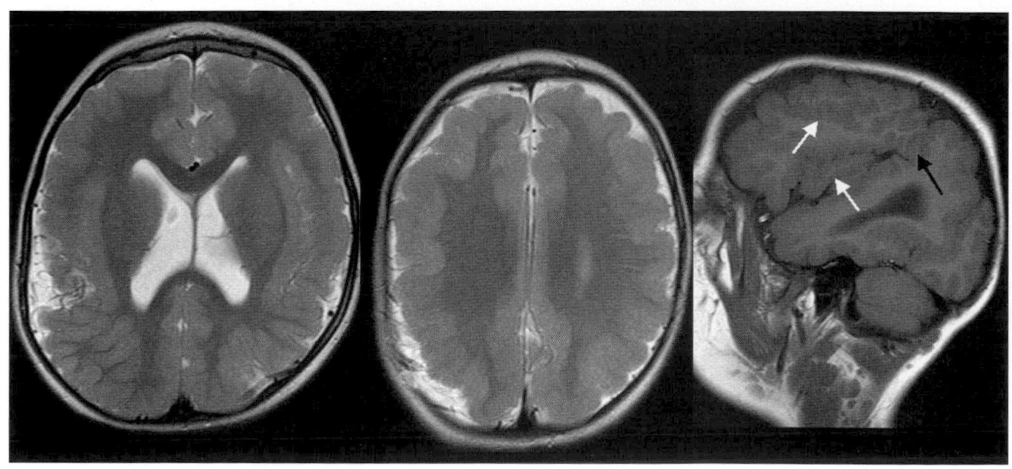

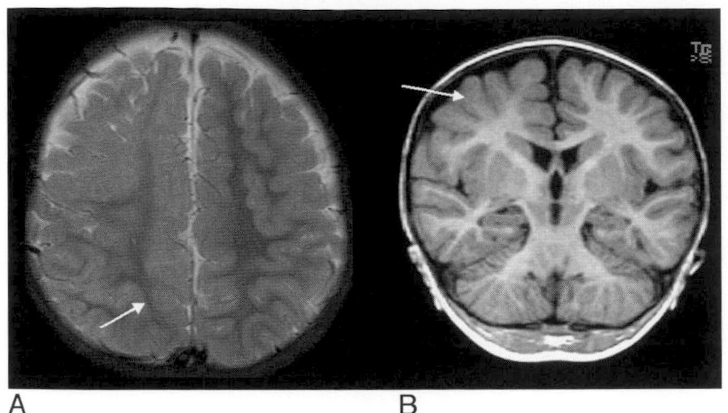

Figure 70.18 Child with focal seizures and right fronto-parietal lobe cortical dysplasia. (A) Axial T2-weighted MRI shows blurring of the right frontal grey–white matter junction and more extensive associated white matter signal hyperintensity involving most of the hemisphere, including the parietal lobe at this level (arrow). (B) Coronal T1 SPGR image (part of the volumetric dataset) also shows grey–white matter junction signal abnormality (arrow) and more subtle white matter change.

tion. Clinical symptoms are more likely when there is greater than 5 mm descent below the foramen magnum, and therefore descent below this level is considered to be clinically significant. However, MRI does not predict who is symptomatic. Children between 5 and 15 years have greater tonsillar descent up to 6 mm as a normal finding compared to children under 5 years or adults. There may be an associated syringomyelia. Symptoms include cough-induced headache, cranial nerve palsies and disassociated peripheral anaesthesia.

NEUROCUTANEOUS SYNDROMES

The neurocutaneous syndromes or phakomatoses are congenital malformations affecting particularly structures of ectodermal origin, i.e. the nervous system, skin and eye. The most frequently seen are NF1, tuberous sclerosis, neurofibromatosis type 2 (NF2), von Hippel–Lindau disease and Sturge–Weber syndrome[26,27].

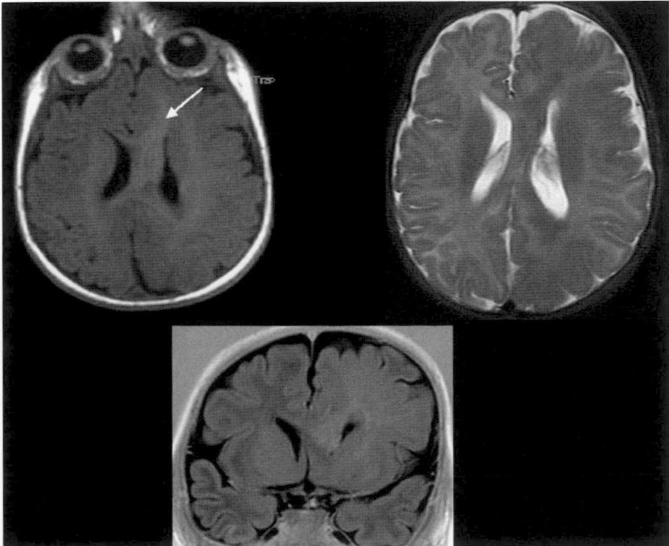

Figure 70.19 Hemimegalencephaly with overgrowth and enlargement of the left cerebral hemisphere. There is thickening of the cortex with broad, thickened gyri, underdeveloped sulci, and extensive white matter signal abnormality. Note the typical appearance of the frontal horn and genu of the corpus callosum, which is straight and points anteriorly (arrow).

Neurofibromatosis type 1

The most common neurocutaneous syndrome is NF1 with an incidence of 1 in 3000–4000 births. As well as being one of the most common inherited central nervous system (CNS) disorders, it is the most common autosomal dominant condition, due to a mutation on chromosome 17 which encodes for the tumour suppressor gene product neurofibromin, and the most common inherited tumour syndrome. Half are new mutations. The diagnosis is made on the basis of at least two major criteria (Table 70.1)[28]. Minor criteria are supportive of the diagnosis.

CNS tumours in NF1 include visual pathway gliomas, plexiform neurofibromas and cranial and peripheral nerve gliomas. These may be diagnosed radiologically without recourse to biopsy and the diagnostic criteria allow the diagnosis of NF1 to be made purely on neuroimaging or as an adjunct to clinical findings. Visual/optic pathway gliomas (OPGs) are usually WHO Grade I pilocytic astrocytomas and are the most common brain abnormality in NF1, occurring in up to 15% of patients. Most of these are diagnosed in childhood but only half are symptomatic. OPGs in NF1 are more likely to affect the optic nerves rather than the chiasm and post-chiasmatic pathways, as opposed to non-NF1 OPGs, and are also associated with a better prognosis. Once the tumour involves the chiasm and hypothalamus there is a risk of precocious puberty and a greater risk of visual deterioration[29]. They have a wide spectrum of biological behaviours ranging from static or minimal growth in most to rapidly increasing size in a minority.

Fusiform expansion of the nerve and widening of the optic foramen may be detected on CT, along with the very characteristic sphenoid wing dysplasia and plexiform neurofibroma. Although CT can detect the intra-orbital involvement of OPG, this involves irradiating the eye and is less sensitive than MRI for delineating tumour within the chiasm and intracranial extension. Other orbital features seen in NF1 include dilatation of the optic nerve sheaths due to dural ectasia and intra-orbital extension of plexiform neurofibroma. Variable

Table 70.1 DIAGNOSTIC CRITERIA FOR NEURO-FIBROMATOSIS TYPE 1

Major criteria	Minor criteria
Café-au-lait spots	Small stature
Freckling in the inguinal or axillary areas	Macrocephaly
One plexiform neurofibroma or two neurofibromas of any type*	Scoliosis*
Visual pathway glioma*	Pectus excavatus*
Two or more lisch nodules of iris	'Hamartomatous lesions' of NF1*
Distinctive osseous lesion, e.g. sphenoid dysplasia or thinning of cortex*	Neuropsychological abnormalities
First-degree relative with neurofibromatosis type 1 (NF1)	

*Radiologically detectable features.

extension into the chiasm, the lateral geniculate bodies or optic radiations is best detected on MRI. A suggested NF1 imaging protocol includes orbital MRI with axial and coronal dual-echo STIR, coronal and T1-weighted pre- and fat-saturation post-gadolinium images, all with a slice thickness of 3 mm or less. Images obtained with a fat-saturation pulse allow elimination of chemical shift artefact at the interface of the optic nerve sheath complex and intra-orbital fat, making assessment easier, and contrast medium improves visualization of the normal intra-orbital optic nerves.

The whole of the optic nerve may be expanded or there may be subarachnoid extension of tumour around a normal sized nerve. Tumour infiltration within the nerve causes variable enhancement of expanded nerve within the optic nerve sheath, whereas if the tumour is predominantly subarachnoid, a rim of enhancing tumour around a minimally enhancing nerve is detected. It is important to identify the expanded nerve within the optic nerve sheath in order to distinguish it from NF1-associated dural ectasia in which the optic nerve sheath is expanded by CSF rather than tumour. Generally these optic pathway tumours are kept under observation unless symptomatic or progressive (≤5%). Spontaneous involution of tumour is also well recognized.

There is an increased risk of other CNS tumours in NF1 with OPG. These are usually WHO Grade I pilocytic astrocyomas occurring in 1–3% of patients, particularly within the cerebellum and brainstem, although other low grade and higher grade tumours also occur. In the brainstem they are usually less aggressive than non-NF1 brainstem astrocytomas and are more likely to be seen in the medulla and midbrain (e.g. tectal plate gliomas) than the pons. A tectal plate tumour may cause aqueduct stenosis and hence hydrocephalus. These brainstem NF1 tumours are often biologically benign and may regress spontaneously, and therefore clinical management is generally not aggressive unless clinical/radiological tumour progression is seen.

Another characteristic lesion of NF1 is the so-called 'hamartomatous' changes of NF1, also known as 'unidentified bright objects (UBOs)', 'neurofibromatosis bright objects (NBOs)' or areas of myelin vacuolation. These are seen in 60–80% of NF1 cases, depending on the age at which the child is imaged, and in 95% of children with NF1 and OPG, and may have an impact on cognitive function[30]. They are few in number before the age of 4 years, increase in number and volume between 4 and 10 years and then decrease in the second decade, being rare over the age of 20. Therefore, they are rarely seen in the adult NF1 population. They appear as multiple T2 hyperintense lesions with minimal mass effect and no contrast enhancement in typical sites such as the pons, cerebellar white matter, internal capsules, basal ganglia, thalami and hippocampi. They have normal signal on T1-weighted images, apart from lesions in the basal ganglia which are often slightly T1 hyperintense (Fig. 70.20). Generally these features distinguish them from gliomas. Astrocytomas, however, may develop in the areas involved by UBOs and radiologically it is not always possible to distinguish them. Enhancement and increasing mass effect are suspicious for tumour development, in which case the involved areas should be kept under regular imaging review. Other non-CNS tumours recognized in NF1 include phaeochromocytoma, carcinoid, rhabdomyosarcoma and childhood chronic myeloid leukaemia.

Plexiform neurofibromas are one of the main diagnostic criteria of NF1. These are multinodular lesions formed when tumour involves either multiple trunks or multiple fascicles of a large nerve. Typical locations include the orbit growing along the ophthalmic division of the trigeminal nerve in association with progressive sphenoid wing dysplasia. They are hypodense on CT and generally do not enhance with contrast agents. On MRI they have a more heterogeneous appearance, of low T1-weighted signal intensity and T2-weighted hyperintensity, with variable contrast enhancement, although at least part of the tumour normally enhances. Extension occurs along the nerve pathways into the pterygomaxillary fissure, orbital apex/superior orbital fissure and cavernous sinus (Fig. 70.21). Other characteristic sites include the lumbosacral and brachial plexi. There is a malignant potential with transformation to fibrosarcoma quoted at between 2% and 12%. Neurofibromas are more homogeneous and well-defined lesions which cause diffuse expansion of nerves. It may be possible to distinguish plexiform from other types of neurofibroma radiologically. The former are more diffuse lesions. Neurofibromas appear on MRI as nodules seen along the spinal nerves of the cauda

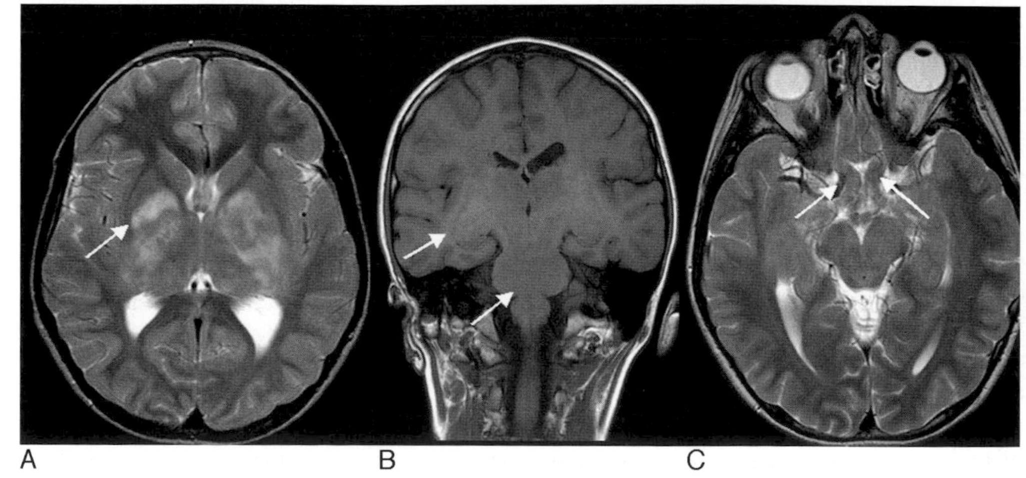

Figure 70.20 Child with neurofibromatosis type 1 (NF1). (A,B) There are very characteristic lesions within the lentiform nuclei, brainstem, and midbrain, the so-called 'hamartomatous' lesions or 'unidentified bright objects' of NF1 (arrows). They are hyperintense on T2-weighted imaging, with minimal mass effect. Basal ganglia lesions may demonstrate some T1 shortening, as in this case, or are hypointense on T1-weighted imaging. (C) There are also bilateral optic nerve gliomas extending into the optic chiasm (arrows).

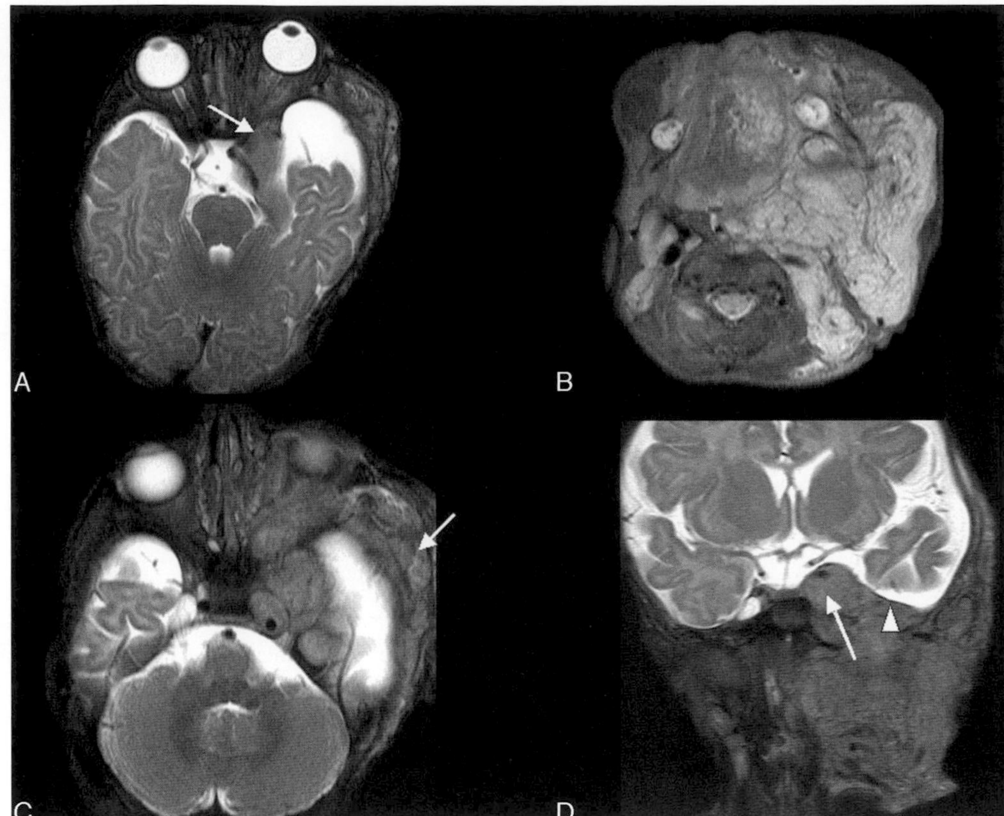

Figure 70.21 Infant with neurofibromatosis type 1. The diagnosis was made from these images. (A) There is sphenoid wing dysplasia causing expansion of the middle cranial fossa (arrow) and absence of the lateral orbital wall, which causes the 'bare orbit' sign (arrow) on AP plain radiographs. (B) There is an associated extensive plexiform neurofibroma involving the deep and superficial fascial spaces of the neck, tongue, and orbit. (C,D) This is almost indistinguishable on imaging from multiple cranial nerve fibromas involving the left cavernous sinus (arrows) and middle cranial fossa. Note the neurofibroma has extended through the foramen ovale and is elevating the dura, seen as a black line (arrowhead).

equina and, as they enlarge, they extend out through the neural exit foramina, enlarging them. They may have a central region of T2 hypointensity producing a target appearance. Malignant transformation in these is less common, and cannot be excluded radiologically, but suggestive features are local pain, rapid growth, large size, and internal heterogeneity.

NF1 is associated with some characteristic bone dysplasias, including lambdoid sutural dysplasia, thinning of long bone cortices and kyphoscoliosis with a high thoracic acute curve. One of the most common is sphenoid wing dysplasia marked by a bone defect which allows herniation of the temporal lobe through the orbit. On plain radiography this produces the 'empty' or 'bare' orbit (Fig. 70.21A). Clinically there may be pulsatile exophthalmos due to transmission of CSF pulsations. The globe may also be affected.

As well as kyphoscoliosis due to a primary skeletal dysostosis, there may be dural ectasia with vertebral scalloping and lateral meningoceles containing CSF. Scoliosis may be seen in association with an intrinsic spinal cord tumour or peripheral nerve neurofibroma.

Tuberous sclerosis

Tuberous sclerosis (TS) is a multisystem genetic neurocutaneous syndrome characterized by hamartomas, cortical tubers and benign neoplastic lesions (giant cell astrocytomas), with an incidence of around 1 in 5800 live births. The most frequently affected organs are the skin, brain, retina, lungs, heart, skeleton and kidneys, but the few manifestations that are associated with the reduced life expectancy seen in this condition are, in order of highest to lowest frequency, neurological disease (seizures and subependymal giant cell tumour), renal disease (angiomyolipoma and renal cell carcinoma), pulmonary disease (lymphangioleiomyomatosis and bronchopneumonia) and cardiovascular disease (rhabdomyosarcoma and aneurysm). TS is autosomal dominant with a high level of penetrance and variable phenotypic expression; 60–70% of cases are sporadic and two-gene mutations have been identified, TSC1 and TSC2, encoding protein products with a tumour suppressor function.

The classical clinical presentation of TS is the triad of intellectual impairment, epilepsy and adenoma sebaceum, but there is a wide phenotypic range. There are a large number of diagnostic primary, secondary and tertiary criteria for TS, some of which are radiological and which categorize TS as 'definite', 'probable' or 'possible'. Radiological primary criteria are the presence of calcified subependymal nodules while noncalcified subependymal nodules and tubers, cardiac rhabdomyoma and renal angiomyolipoma are secondary criteria[32,33]. In 80% of patients with TS, infantile spasms or myoclonic seizures are the presenting symptom. Conversely, 10% of children with infantile spasms will have evidence of TS, so structural MR neuroimaging is indicated in these children.

Ocular manifestations of TS include retinal hamartomas seen near the optic disc in 15% and are often bilateral and multiple. On CT they appear as nodular masses originating from the retina and when calcified may be difficult to distinguish from retinoblastomas unless there are also calcified subependymal nodules. Subretinal effusions may also be detected. Micro-ophthalmia and leukocoria are other features.

The intracranial manifestations include subependymal hamartomas or nodules (SENs), subependymal giant cell astrocytomas (GCAs), radially oriented linear bands and cortical tubers (Fig. 70.22). SENs are the most common lesion and are seen in 88–95% of individuals with TS. They may be calcified which is a useful diagnostic feature on CT or T2* MRI; calcification increases with age and is rarely detected under the age of 1 year[33]. Histologically they are indistinguishable from GCAs. The latter are determined by location in the caudothalamic groove adjacent to the foramen of Monro, progressive growth on serial imaging and the presence of hydrocephalus. Contrast enhancement may be seen in both SENs and GCAs. The lack of myelination in infants helps to identify white matter anomalies, which become less visible as myelination progresses[34]. SENs and linear parenchymal tuberous sclerosis lesions in infants under 3 months old are hyperintense on T1-weighted images and hypointense on T2-weighted images as opposed to the reverse pattern of signal intensity in older children and adults.

Sturge–Weber syndrome

Sturge–Weber syndrome is a congenital syndrome characterized by a port-wine naevus on the face and ipsilateral leptomeningeal angiomas with a primarily parieto-occipital distribution[35].

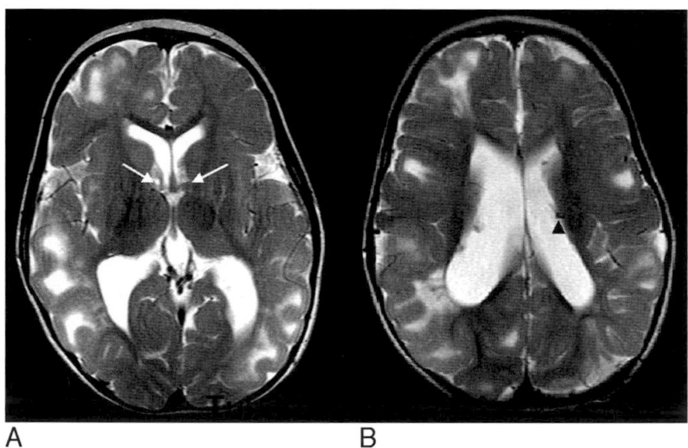

Figure 70.22 Intracranial manifestations of tuberous sclerosis. (A) Multiple tubers involving the cortex and subcortical white matter. Bilateral lesions are seen at the foramina of Monro, in keeping with giant cell astrocytomas (arrows). (B) Subependymal nodules project into the ventricles, some of which are markedly hypointense, in keeping with calcification (arrowhead).

Bilateral involvement may occasionally occur. The clinical manifestations include the onset of focal seizures, appearing during the first year of life, and developmental delay with progressive hemiparesis, hemianopsia and intellectual impairment. The seizures progressively become refractory to medication.

The leptomeningeal angiomas cause abnormal venous drainage with chronic ischaemia, leading ultimately to cortical atrophy and calcification, the latter feature being usually very prominent. By 2 years of age, skull radiographs may reveal 'tramline calcifications' within the cortices.

In early imaging the brain may look normal on CT as well as on MRI without intravenous contrast enhancement. The involved hemisphere progressively becomes atrophied and the pial angioma is seen as diffuse pial enhancement of variable thickness (Fig. 70.23)[36]. The ipsilateral white matter appears hypointense on T1-weighted images and hyperintense on T2-weighted images. Other findings include enlargement of the ipsilateral choroid plexus and dilatation of transparenchymal veins that communicate between the superficial and deep cerebral venous systems. In 'burnt out' cases the pial angioma may no longer be detected after contrast enhancement, leaving only a chronically shrunken and calcified hemisphere.

Neurofibromatosis type 2

This is located to an abnormality on chromosome 22 and occurs in 1 in 50 000 live births. Nearly all have bilateral vestibular schwannomas, other tumours such as meningiomas and other cranial and peripheral nerve schwannomas and ependymomas, including spinal tumours (Fig. 70.24). While in adults hearing loss is a common presentation, seizures and facial nerve palsy are more common in children.

Other neurocutaneous syndromes

These include hypomelanosis of Ito in which hypomelanotic skin lesions are associated with polymicrogyria, heterotopias and callosal dysgenesis, basal cell naevus syndrome and PHACES (posterior fossa malformations, facial haemangiomas, arterial anomalies, cardiac and eye anomalies and sternal cleft) syndromes. Neurocutaneous melanosis is a rare syndrome in which giant congenital melanocytic naevi on the skin are associated with intracranial melanosis (Fig. 70.25). Neuroimaging

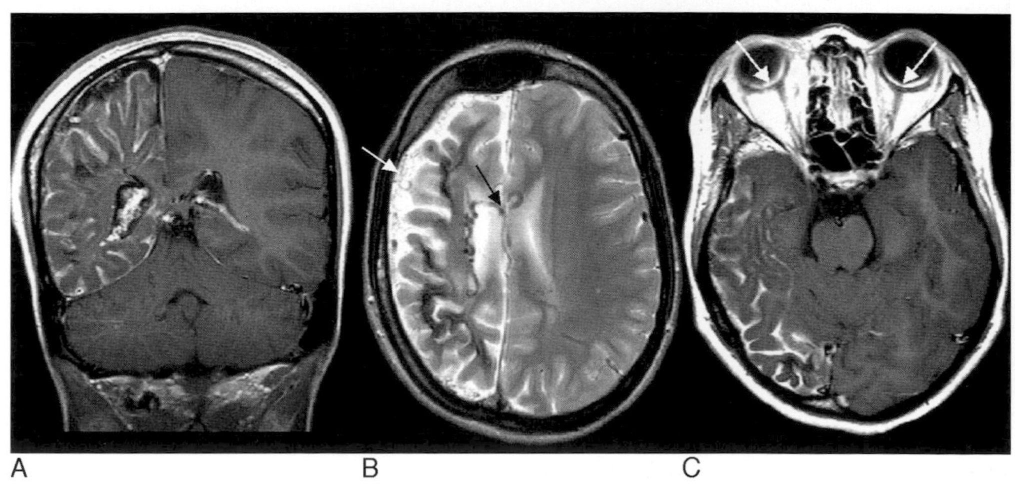

Figure 70.23 Sturge–Weber syndrome. (A) Coronal T1 post-contrast image shows an enhancing pial angioma overlying the right cerebral hemisphere which is atrophic. The right choroid plexus is enlarged. Foci of signal hypointensity within the gyri and adjacent white matter are due to calcification. (B) Axial T2-weighted image shows in addition prominent superficial cortical veins and ependymal veins (arrows). (C) Axial post-contrast T1-weighted image shows bilateral choroidal angiomas (arrows) in addition to the pial angioma.

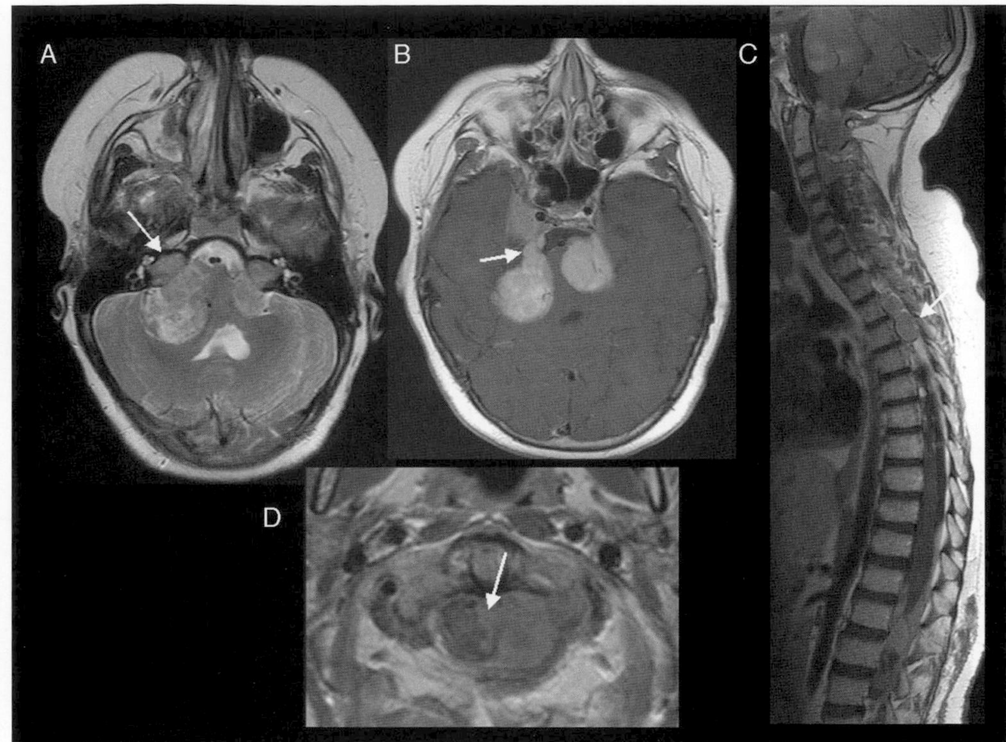

Figure 70.24 Neurofibromatosis type 2 (NF2). (A) Bilateral cerebellopontine angle masses extending into the internal auditory meati and causing expansion (arrow) in a child with NF2 and bilateral acoustic neuromas. (B) Trigeminal schwannomas extending into the cavernous sinus on the right. The arrow indicates the cisternal segment of the right trigeminal nerve. (C) Sagittal T1-weighted images show expansion of the neural exit foramina by enhancing nerve or nerve sheath tumours (arrow). (D) Axial image shows a mainly dural mass extending out through the neural foramen with a small intradural component (arrow).

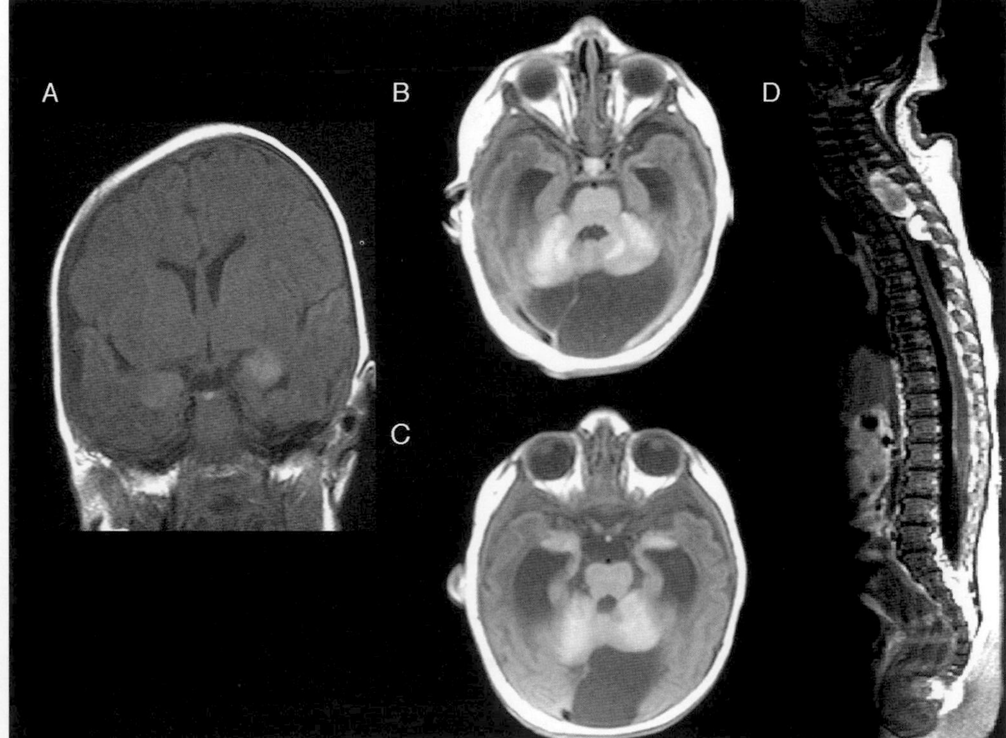

Figure 70.25 Child with giant pigmented naevus and neurocutaneous melanosis. (A) Initial coronal T1-weighted MRI shows the typical regions of T1 shortening within the amygdalae of the mesial temporal lobes. (B,C) Axial T1-weighted MRI obtained 2 years later shows hydrocephalus in addition to the regions of melanin deposition within the mesial temporal lobes and cerebellum. These do not show any enhancement. There is a posterior fossa arachnoid cyst, a described association. (D) Within the spine there is diffuse pial enhancement over the spinal cord in addition to focal haemorrhagic and partly enhancing extramedullary lesions, indicating malignant melanoma, which was subsequently confirmed histologically.

detects the clusters of melanocytes by the melanin that they are associated with, therefore appearing as regions of T1 shortening on MRI in characteristic locations: the anterior and mesial temporal lobe, cerebellum and pons. CT may detect areas of increased density but these are much more difficult to appreciate. Diffuse melanosis with intracranial and intraspinal leptomeningeal spread may occur and therefore hydrocephalus. Degeneration into malignant melanoma may occur.

SPINAL MALFORMATIONS

Normal development

The spinal cord forms during three embryological stages known as gastrulation (2–3 weeks), primary neurulation (3–4 weeks) and secondary neurulation (5–6 weeks). During gastrulation the embryonic bilaminar disc consisting of epiblast and hypoblast is converted to a trilaminar disc by migration of cells from the epiblast through Hensen's node, a focal region of thickening occurring at the cranial end of the midline 'primitive streak' of the disc. This results in the midline notochord and a layer that will form the future mesoderm. During primary neurulation the notochord induces the overlying ectoderm to become neurectoderm and form the neural plate. Subsequent folding and bending occurs until the margins unite to form the neural tube. The cranial end closes at day 25 while the caudal end closes a couple of days later. Finally the caudal cell mass arises from the primitive streak and undergoes retrogressive differentiation with cavitation. This is the origin of the fetal neural tissue and vertebrae distal to S2, and will become the conus medullaris. A focal expansion of the central canal known as the terminal ventricle occurs as a result of incomplete retrogressive differentiation. This may be seen as a normal asymptomatic finding in young children and may persist in a small minority into adulthood. It is seen on all post-mortem studies but is bigger in those detectable on MRI. Spinal dysraphisms can result from abnormalities occurring during any of these periods[37–39].

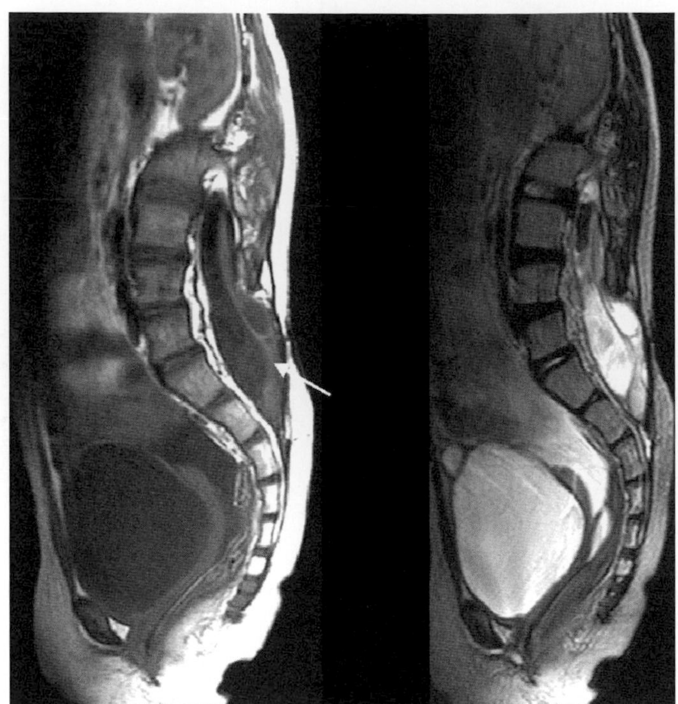

Figure 70.26 Repaired myelomeningocele in a child with Chiari II malformation. (A) The neural placode terminates inferiorly in the meningeal sac (arrow). The lumbosacral posterior vertebral elements have not formed. (B) Post-repair the skin is continuous over the defect.

Definitions

Spinal dysraphisms may be open, in which case nervous tissue is exposed, or closed, in which case the defect is covered by skin, although a cutaneous lesion such as a dimple, sinus, hairy naevus or haemangioma may be seen as a marker of an underlying defect in 50% of these cases[38,39]. Spina bifida refers to the failure of fusion of the posterior spinal bony elements. The neural placode is a flat segment of unneurulated nervous tissue that may be seen at the end of the spinal cord or at an intermediate position along its course. Tethered cord syndrome is a clinical diagnosis of progressive neurological deterioration (usually leg weakness, deformities such as scoliosis or foot abnormalities, loss of bladder and bowel function), presumed to be due to traction damage on the tethered cord. Although there may be some suggestive features such as an associated spinal cord syrinx, this is not a diagnosis made radiologically; the position of the conus or neural placode following successful surgical 'untethering' always remains unchanged. The level of the spinal cord termination has a Gaussian distribution. It is a popular misconception that the spinal cord lies lower in the neonate and continues to rise as the vertebral column grows during childhood. In fact most authors agree that it has reached its adult position by term, and in 98% lies above L2/3, the majority lying between T11/12 and L1/2[40,41]. The spinal cord termination should be considered convincingly abnormal if seen at or below L3.

Open spinal dysraphism

Most open spinal dysraphisms (OSDs) are myelomeningoceles and these are virtually always associated with Chiari II malformation (Fig. 70.26). The neural placode protrudes beyond the level of the skin and there is an expanded CSF-containing sac lined by meninges[38,39]. A small proportion of OSDs are myeloceles where the placode is flush with the surface and there is no meningocele component. Both disorders result from defective closure of the primary neural tube and persistence of unneurulated nervous tissue in the form of the neural placode, usually at the lumbosacral level at the spinal cord termination. Nerve roots arising from the everted ventral surface of the placode cross the widely dilated subarachnoid spaces of the meningocele to enter the neural exit foraminae. The posterior elements of the vertebral column and any other mesenchymal derivatives, such as the paravertebral muscles, remain everted. Hemimyelomeningoceles and hemimyeloceles may occur with diastematomyelia (split cord syndrome) and may be associated with an asymmetric skin abnormality. The clinical presentation is also very asymmetrical. These can be explained embryologically by failure of primary neurulation of one hemicord in addition to a gastrulation abnormality.

Myelomeningoceles are operated on soon after birth as if untreated the exposed neural tissue is prone to ulceration and infection. In some centres in utero repair has been correlated with subsequent failure to develop the typical hindbrain malformation of Chiari II, although other abnormalities such as the enlarged massa intermedia and falx fenestration persist. Hydrocephalus and the need for surgical drainage may also be delayed and even reduced. Hydrocephalus usually develops 2–3 days post-neonatal repair but may occur pre-operatively. Other causes of post-operative deterioration include re-tethering of the spinal cord and the development of a syrinx which may later cause scoliosis[42].

Closed spinal dysraphism

Closed spinal dysraphisms (CSDs) may be associated with cutaneous stigmata or a mass[43,44]. This may be a subcutaneous lipomatous mass overlying the spinal defect, as in lipomyeloceles and lipomyelomeningoceles, due to abnormal primary neurulation in which there is premature disjunction of the cutaneous ectoderm from the adjacent neuroectoderm, allowing mesenchymal elements to come into contact with the open neural tube. In a lipomyelocele the junction between the placode and the lipoma lies within the spinal canal (Fig. 70.27), while in lipomyelomeningoceles it lies outside. Typically the placode is rotated to one side while the meninges are herniated to the other.

A posterior meningocele consists of herniation of a CSF sac lined by dura and arachnoid through the spinal defect, resulting in a clinically apparent mass covered by skin. These are mainly lumbosacral but may be seen at any level. Anterior meningoceles are typically presacral, are seen with caudal agenesis and are present in older children and adults with low back pain and bladder/bowel disturbance. The terminal myelocystocele is a rare condition associated with syndromes such as VACTERL in which the central canal is dilated by a large hydromyelic cavity that herniates into a posterior meningocele through the posterior spinal bony defect. The cavity is usually discontinuous with the meningocele and lies inferiorly and posteriorly.

CSDs without a mass include simple intramedullary and intradural lipomas. These typically occur along the posterior midline in a subpial juxtamedullary location at the cervicothoracic level. Embryologically they are also the result of premature disjunction and the lipoma fills in the gap between the unopposed folds of the neural placode. On MRI they have the signal characteristics of fat, including signal suppression on STIR sequences.

The filum terminale lipoma is considered to arise from a disturbance of caudal regression. Fatty thickening of the filum terminale is detected on MRI, and may be more easily seen on axial T1-weighted sequences. This is estimated to occur in 1.5–5% of the normal adult population and may be considered a normal variant in the absence of the clinical tethered cord syndrome. The 'tight' filum terminale, also due to abnormal retrogressive differentiation, is a short, thick filum greater than 2 mm in diameter associated with clinical tethering and a low-lying spinal cord.

Dorsal dermal sinus

A dermal sinus is an epithelial-lined opening on the skin with variable fistulous extension to the dural surface, typically seen in the lumbosacral region and often associated with cutaneous stigmata, such as hairy naevus and capillary haemangioma[43,44]. Embryologically it arises from a failure of disjunction of neuroectoderm from cutaneous ectoderm. Dermal openings seen at the sacrococcygeal level are directed inferiorly below the thecal sac and are known as sacrococcygeal pits. They do not require further imaging. Those seen above the intergluteal cleft pass superiorly and may form a fistulous connection with the dural sac and warrant further investigation. On MRI they are seen as a thin linear strip of tissue hypointense to adjacent fat (Fig. 70.28). US may provide useful information about the intradural extension of the dermal sinus tract and the mobility of the conus[45].

Diastematomyelia

The split notochord syndromes are disorders of notochord midline integration. In diastematomyelia the spinal cord is split in two, with each hemicord having one anterior and one posterior grey matter horn[46,47]. In type I diastematomyelia there is a craniocaudal spectrum of abnormality ranging from partial clefting cranially to two complete dural sacs separated by an osteocartilaginous spur inferiorly. There may be plain radiographic features including scoliosis or hemivertebrae or bifid/fused vertebrae at the level of the bony spur. The bony spur in type I diastematomyelia is completely extradural, usually midline, though it may be seen coursing obliquely from the

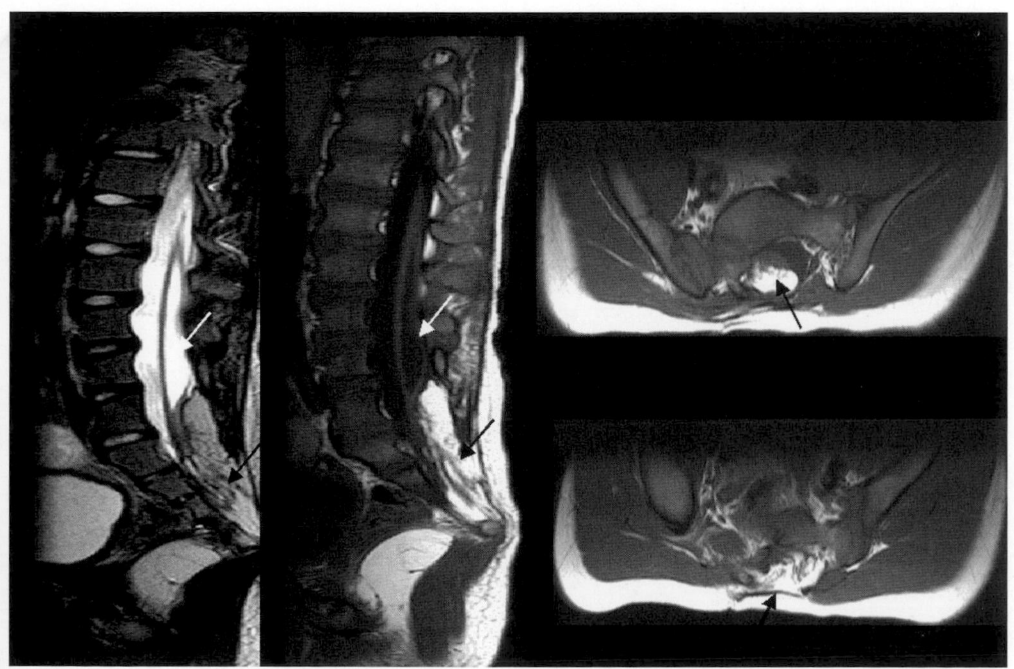

Figure 70.27 Closed spinal dysraphism. The spinal cord is too low and the neural placode terminates at the lumbosacral junction in a lipomyelocele (black arrows). There is an associated spinal cord syringomyelic cavity (white arrows). The posterior elements are deficient and everted.

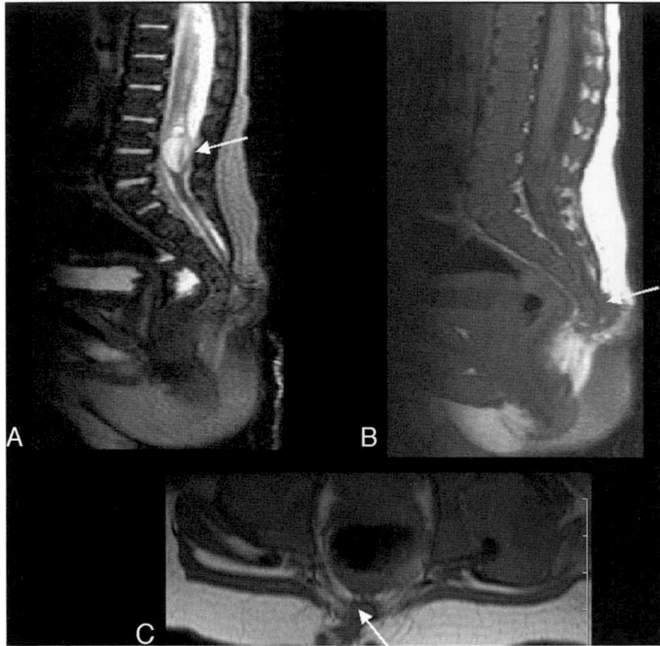

Figure 70.28 Dorsal dermal sinus. (A) The termination of the spinal cord is very low and there is a syringomyelic cavity with internal septations. In addition there is a more focal cyst within the conus confirmed at surgical untethering to be a dermoid cyst (arrow). (B,C) There is an associated dermal sinus track (arrows).

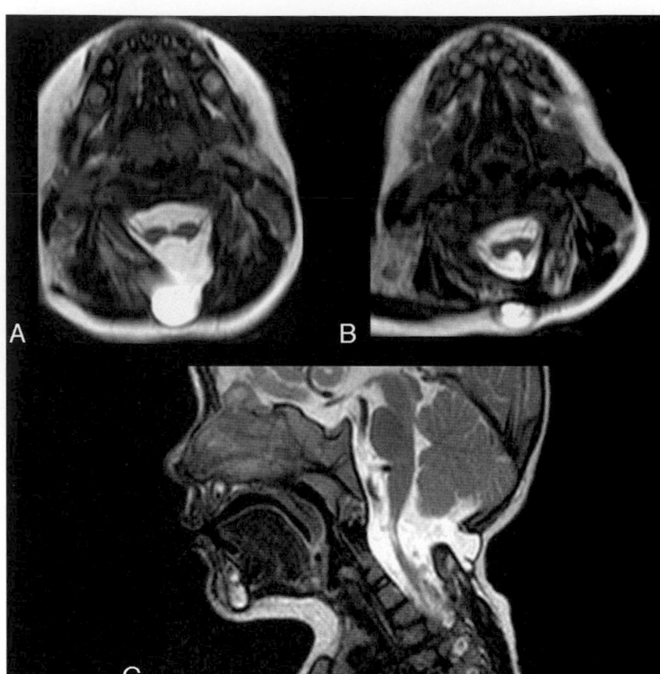

Figure 70.29 Cervical spinal cord diastematomyelia type II with associated craniocervical meningocele. (A) Sagittal T2-weighted MRI appears to show signal abnormality and thinning of the spinal cord, and is the clue to the diastematomyelia seen on the axial images. (B,C) Axial T2-weighted MRI shows that the cord has split into two hemicords. The apparent signal abnormality is in fact normal cerebrospinal fluid interspersed between the two hemicords. These re-unite inferiorly. The meningocele is seen herniating through a bony defect in the vertebral posterior elements.

posterior vertebrae to the laminae, and may be complete or incomplete. It is seen at the caudal end of the split and the hemicords fuse tightly just below it. On MRI marrow signal may be detected within it and distinguish it from a simple fibrous band. Above it the split is much longer. In rare cases, the separate dural sacs may terminate distally with different fates, one as a OSD and the other as a CSD. In diastematomyelia type II (Fig. 70.29) there is a single dural sac in which the two hemicords lie, and a fibrous septum, seen as a band of T2 hypointensity, may be seen passing intradurally between the two hemicords. There may be no septum or there may only be partial clefting of the cord. The conus is often low and there may be a tight or fatty filum. Both forms of diastematomyelia may be associated with hydromyelia.

Neurenteric cysts

The severest and rarest form of notochordal midline integration anomaly occurs with dorsal enteric fistulas and neurenteric cysts[48]. The cysts are usually seen intradurally anterior to the spinal cord and are derived from endodermal remnants trapped between a split notochord. They have signal characteristics of CSF or of proteinaceous fluid with T1 shortening (Fig. 70.30). The fistula connects the dorsal skin with bowel across a duplicated spine.

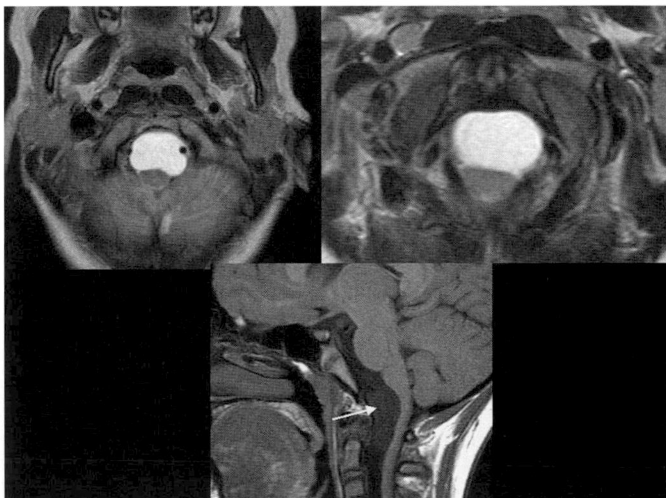

Figure 70.30 Neurenteric cyst ventral to the medulla and upper cervical spinal cord, displacing them posteriorly, and with the vertebral arteries displaced around it. The cyst is hyperintense on the T2-weighted images and there is also some mild T1 shortening (arrow).

Disorders of the caudal cell mass/caudal regression syndrome

The last group of developmental spinal abnormalities is those affecting development of the caudal cell mass[49]. Caudal agenesis and the rarer condition of segmental spinal dysgenesis are considered to occur as a result of apoptosis of notochordal cells which have not formed in their correct craniocaudal position. In caudal agenesis there is a severe abnormality which results in absence of the vertebral column at the affected level, as well as a truncated spinal cord, imperforate anus and genital anomalies. It may be seen with OEIS (omphalocele, exstrophy, imperforate anus, spinal defects), VACTERL and the Currarino triad in which there is partial sacral agenesis (or sometimes a 'scimitar'-shaped sacrum), anorectal malformation and a presacral mass which may be a teratoma or anterior meningocele[50–52]. In type I caudal agenesis, which affects secondary neurulation and formation of the caudal cell mass, but also primary neurulation of the distal true notochord, there is a high (often at T12) abrupt spinal cord termination with a characteristic wedge-shaped configuration and variable coccygeal to lower thoracic vertebral aplasia (Fig. 70.31). Clinically the neurological deficit due to absence of the distal spinal cord is stable. In type II caudal agenesis the true notochord is not affected and only the caudal cell mass is involved. The vertebral aplasia is less extensive with up to S4 present as the last vertebra. It may be difficult to detect partial agenesis of the conus because it is stretched and tethered to a fatty filum terminale, lipoma, lipomyelomeningocele, or anterior sacral meningocele. Finally, in segmental spinal dysgenesis there is a segmental abnormality affecting the spinal cord, segmental nerve roots and vertebrae, and associated with a congenital paraparesis and lower limb deformities. On imaging there is an acute angle kyphus, and the spine and spinal cord in the most severe cases may appear 'severed'. In less severe cases the cord is focally hypoplastic.

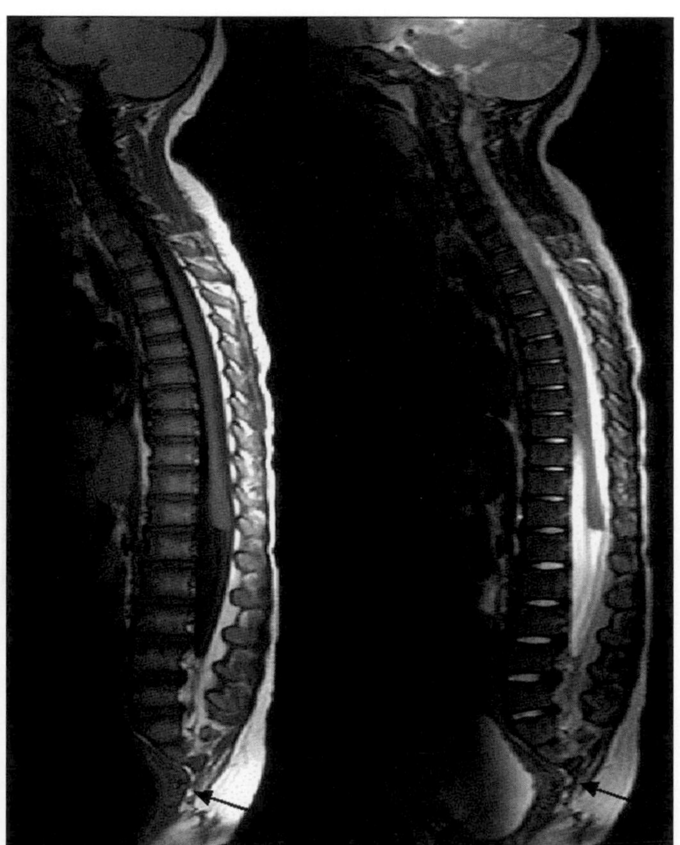

Figure 70.31 Caudal regression syndrome. The spinal cord is truncated with a typical blunt edge seen at the inferior margin of T12. The thecal sac terminates at the superior margin of L4. The sacrum distal to S2 is agenetic (arrows).

INBORN METABOLIC BRAIN DISORDERS

Metabolic disorders may be inborn or acquired. Inborn errors of metabolism may result from an enzyme deficiency leading to the build-up of a directly toxic metabolite, or have an indirect toxic effect by activation or inhibition of another metabolic pathway, leading to increased levels of a different toxic metabolite.

The inborn errors of metabolism may be subdivided according to a number of different classification systems, one of which is radiological. One system classifies them by cellular organelle involvement into mitochondrial (usually meaning disorders of mitochondrial energy metabolism), lysosomal and peroxisomal disorders. Another scheme classifies them by the biochemical enzyme pathway affected, e.g. the organic acidaemias, aminoacidopathies, or disorders of heavy metal metabolism. In the final classification scheme neuroimaging can be used to help classify them according to white or grey matter involvement, specifically by MRI. Interested readers can also refer to Van der Knaap and Valk[53] and Patay[54].

There are some general principles that may be helpful in detecting and characterizing the radiological features. The abnormalities of metabolic disease are characteristically bilateral and symmetrical. Assessment on MRI should include analysis of grey and white matter structures. When describing white matter abnormalities it is helpful to describe them in terms of general location (lobar involvement, centripetal/centrifugal distribution and AP gradient), juxtacortical U-fibre involvement, involvement of deep white matter structures such as the internal capsule, corpus callosum and white matter tracts such as the pyramidal tracts as they descend from the motor strip (precentral gyrus) through the posterior limbs of the internal capsules and cerebral peduncles to the decussation within the medulla and then into the spinal cord.

Assessment of the grey matter should include analysis of the cerebral and cerebellar cortex and basal ganglia and thalami for signal abnormality, swelling and volume loss. Signal changes include T2 and T1 prolongation, but faint T1 shortening within the basal ganglia may be seen also when there is calcification. Other deep grey structures include the red nuclei, and subthalamic and dentate nuclei. Calcification is much better assessed on CT. Macrocephaly is a useful clinical pointer to diseases such as megalencephalic leukodystrophy with subcortical cysts (MLC), Canavan's and Alexander's leukoencephalopathies, glutaric aciduria type I, GM2 gangliosidosis and L-2 hydroxyglutaric aciduria.

An assessment of the degree of myelination is useful as delay or hypomyelination is frequently seen in metabolic disorders. Although often nonspecific it is a helpful clue to an underlying neurometabolic condition. Myelination requires active energy-dependent metabolism and therefore may also be seen with cardiorespiratory illness. However, hypomyelination may also be seen as a general marker of developmental delay and correlates well with clinical developmental milestones. In premature infants the appropriate MRI markers for corrected age should be assessed before deciding that myelination is immature. There are also specific inherited hypomyelination disorders that may be detected on MRI as a myelination pattern which is immature for the child's age. These include Pelizaeus Merzbacher disease, in which T2-weighted imaging often shows more severe hypomyelination compared to T1-weighted imaging (Fig. 70.32).

Serial imaging should be assessed for progressive cerebral atrophy. This may involve white matter, shown as ventricular enlargement and thinning of the corpus callosum, cortical grey matter shown as sulcal widening, or deep grey matter with atrophy of the specific basal ganglia and thalamic structures.

Pathognomonic imaging patterns are seen in X-linked adrenoleukodystrophy (ALD), Alexander's disease, glutaric aciduria type I, Canavan's disease, L-2 hydroxyglutaricaciduria, neonatal maple syrup urine disease and MLCs, of which classic X-linked adrenoleukodystrophy is the most common leukodystrophy of children and affects 1 in 20 000 boys. It is due to a defect in a peroxisomal membrane protein leading to defective incorporation of fatty acids into myelin. Screening of family members of affected cases for the specific gene defect should be considered. Clinically boys present between the ages of 5 and 10 years with learning difficulties, behavioural problems, deteriorating gait and impaired visuospatial perception. Adrenal insufficiency may precede the CNS presentation or may be absent. Without bone marrow transplantation (which replaces the defective gene), the disease progresses to spastic paraparesis, blindness and deafness. Lorenzo's oil may also delay disease progression. Imaging features are of low attenuation on CT and T2-weighted hyperintensity on MRI in the posterior central white matter, specifically the splenium and peritrigonal white matter progressing to the corticospinal tracts and visual and auditory pathways. The regions of T2 signal abnormality show increased diffusion. The leading edge of the demyelination enhances, where there is active inflammation and disruption of the blood–brain barrier (Fig. 70.33). MR spectroscopy may detect early changes and may in the future guide early bone marrow transplantation before overt and irreversible changes in the white matter have occurred. Adrenomyeloneuropathy is a variation on ALD which presents in young adults or adolescents, usually boys, with progressive paraparesis and cerebellar signs. It has a less specific radiological pattern causing diffuse disease of the white matter, and it more commonly involves the cerebellum and less frequently the cerebral hemispheres.

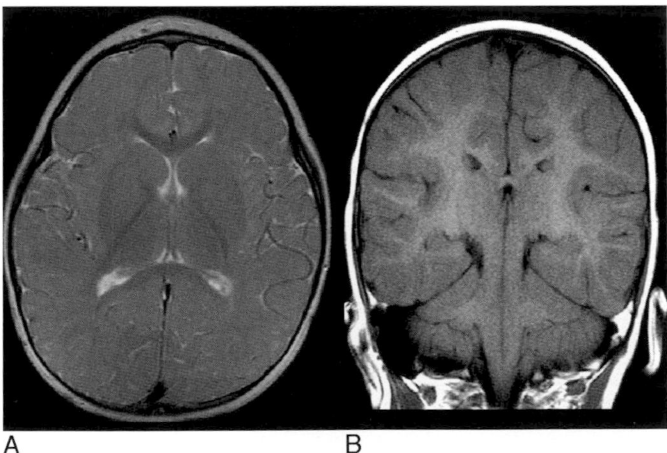

Figure 70.32 Pelizaeus Merzbacher disease in a 2 year old child with nystagmus and developmental delay. (A) Axial T2-weighted image shows dark regions of myelination in the posterior limbs of the internal capsules, splenium, and genu of the corpus callosum, and within the parieto-occipital lobe white matter. The rest of the cerebral hemispheres are not myelinated (the white matter is too bright). This pattern is severely delayed and equivalent approximately to an age of 6 months. (B) Paradoxically coronal T1-weighted MRI shows much more advanced myelination which appears virtually complete, with T1 shortening extending right out into the subcortical white matter.

In Alexander's disease, which has a neonatal, juvenile and adult form, imaging shows extensive white matter abnormality beginning in the frontal and periventricular white matter (Fig. 70.34). Large cystic cavities are seen within the frontal and temporal regions. The basal ganglia may also be involved. Contrast enhancement may be seen along the ventricular ependyma.

L-2 hydroxyglutaricaciduria is a slowly progressive disorder which is usually discovered in childhood or early adulthood, although it is likely to have started earlier than this. The clinical presentation is nonspecific with learning difficulties, epilepsy and pyramidal and cerebellar signs. The MRI findings show white matter involvement with peripheral involvement, particularly of the subcortical U fibres, internal, external and extreme capsules, sparing of the periventricular white matter and corpus callosum, and with a slight frontal predominance. There is macrocephaly. There is also grey matter involvement affecting the basal ganglia and sparing the thalami (Fig. 70.35).

Maple syrup urine disease (MSUD) is an autosomal recessive disorder in which an enzyme deficiency leads to an accumulation of amino acids (leucine, isoleucine and valine) and their metabolites.

MLC is a recently identified autosomal recessive leukodystrophy with macrocephaly.

Suggestive MRI patterns include methylmalonic acidaemia in which there is bilateral symmetrical involvement of the globus pallidus with sparing of the thalami and the rest of the basal ganglia (Fig. 70.36). The cerebral cortex is also normal. In the acute stage there is swelling and oedema of these structures while in the chronic phase there is imaging evidence of atrophy and gliosis. Bilateral pallidal involvement is also seen as T2 hyperintensity in other rarer inborn errors of metabolism, such as GAMT (guanidinoacetate methyltransferase deficiency), Kearns–Sayer syndrome and some acquired and toxic disorders, such as kernicterus and carbon monoxide poisoning (Fig. 70.36).

Disorders of heavy metal metabolism include Wilson's and Menke's diseases, both disorders of copper metabolism, molybdenum cofactor deficiency and disorders of magnesium and manganese metabolism. Wilson's disease results from defective extracellular copper transport and leads to multi-organ copper deposition. Hyperintensities on T2-weighted MRI are seen in the basal ganglia, midbrain and pons, thalami and claustra, and there is T1 shortening in the basal ganglia and thalami, as in other hepatic encepha-

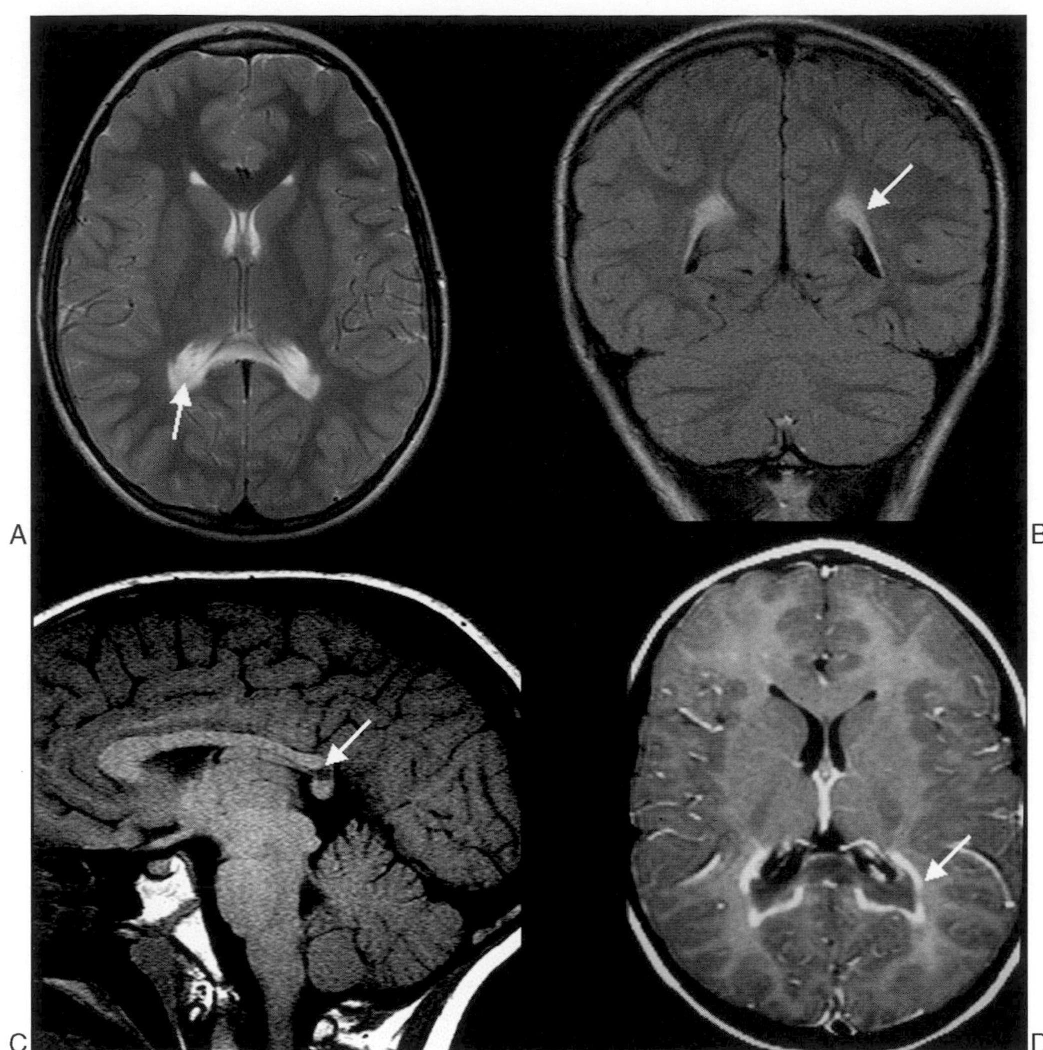

Figure 70.33 Adrenoleukodystrophy. MRI of a 6 year old boy with increasing gait disturbance and impaired vision demonstrates peritrigonal and splenial signal abnormality (increased signal on T2-weighted images and low signal on T1-weighted images), and (A,B,C, arrows) marginal enhancement at the leading edges where there is active inflammation, typical of adrenoleukodystrophy (D, arrow).

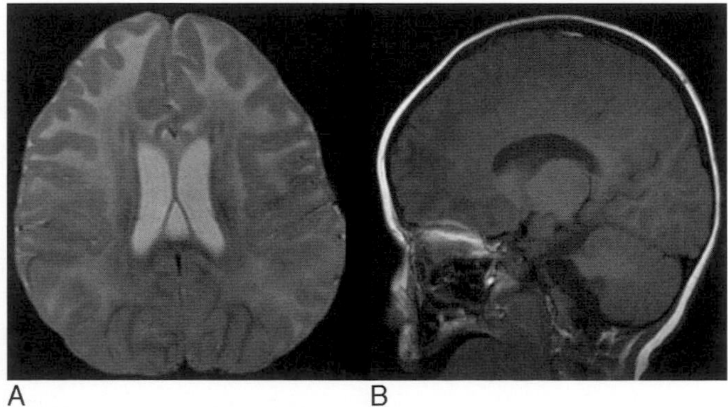

Figure 70.34 Child with Alexander's disease. Head circumference charts showed the child had macrocephaly. (A) Axial T2-weighted MRI shows extensive bilateral symmetrical deep and subcortical white matter signal hyperintensity with a frontal predominance and mild swelling. (B) Sagittal T1-weighted MRI shows corresponding low signal in the affected areas without evidence of cavitation but in keeping with oedema.

lopathies. Menke's disease is X-linked and affects transcellular copper metabolism at the level of the cell membrane. There is a systemic failure of copper-requiring enzymes, particularly those of the cytochrome c-oxidase system. They acquire connective tissue defects with 'kinky hair', inguinal herniae, hyperflexible joints and bladder diverticula. In the brain there is progressive cerebral atrophy which may allow subdural collections of CSF or subdural haematomas (and therefore mimics of nonaccidental head injury). The basal ganglia may also show T1 shortening. Children develop a severe cerebral vasculopathy in which vessels are tortuous and prone to dissection.

Disorders of cellular organelle function include mitochondrial, lysosomal and peroxisomal disorders. Mitochondria are involved in energy metabolism; lysosomes in the degradation of macromolecules, e.g. those involved in the maintenance of cell membrane integrity such as lipids and lipoproteins; and peroxisomes have a role in both catabolic and anabolic metabolism. Mitochondrial disorders include those of mitochondrial energy metabolism affecting oxidative phosphorylation, fatty acid oxidation and ketone metabolism. Respiratory chain disorders affect the respiratory chain, a multicomplex protein on the inner membrane of the mitochondria which has an integral role in oxidative phosphorylation and tend to be multisystem diseases. In the brain they may result in multiple cerebral infarcts in nonvascular territories. Leigh's disease can

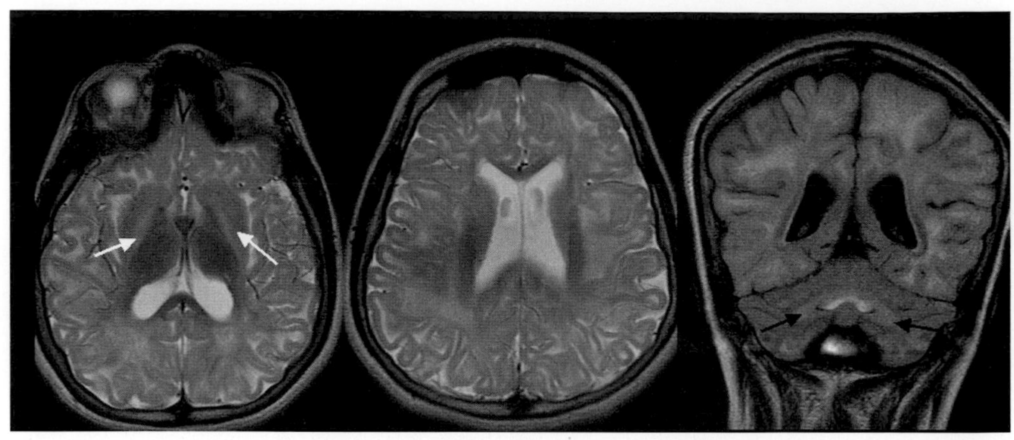

Figure 70.35 L-2 hydroxyglutaricaciduria axial T2-weighted MRI. Coronal FLAIR and show extensive white matter signal hyperintensity involving mainly deep and subcortical white matter but with relative sparing of the periventricular white matter, and bilateral pallidal involvement. The dentate nuclei are also abnormal.

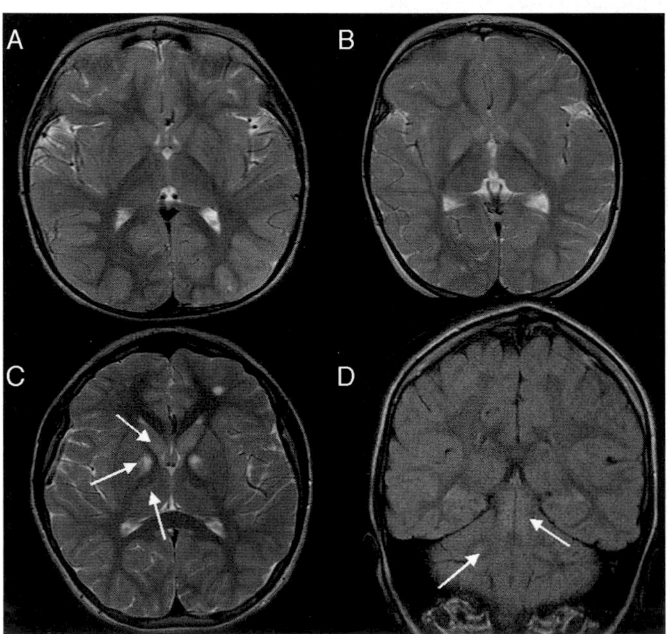

Figure 70.36 Examples of signal abnormality affecting both globus pallidi. (A) Kernicterus. (B) Methylmalonicacidaemia. (C) Kearns–Sayer syndrome. This child also has hyperintense signal in both caudate nuclei and thalami, left frontal white matter and (D) Dorsal midbrain and cerebellar dentate nuclei (arrows).

be caused not only by respiratory chain defects but also by enzyme disorders such as those of pyruvate and tricarboxylic acid metabolism. Bilateral typically symmetrical signal change is seen within the brainstem, deep cerebellar grey matter, subthalamic nuclei and basal ganglia (Fig. 70.37). The midbrain changes have been described as a 'panda face' with involvement of the substantia nigra and tegmentum, and the medulla is frequently involved and may account for the apneoic episodes often seen clinically. Cerebral grey matter infarction may also be seen. MELAS (mitochondrial encephalomyopathy with lactic acidosis and stroke-like episodes) is another mitochondrial disease, typically occurring between the ages of 4 and 15 years but which can occur at any age. Acute metabolic decompensation may be provoked by any insult which causes increased metabolic demand, e.g. febrile illness. Patients may also have a cardiomyopathy and endocrinopathies. Imaging features are those of cerebral infarcts in nonvascular territories and symmetrical basal ganglia calcification. Lysosomal disorders include Krabbe's disease and metachromatic leukodystrophy. Imaging features which might suggest Krabbe's disease are white matter changes, more severely posteriorly and centrally; basal ganglia and thalamic involvement, including T2 hypointensity; cerebellar white matter abnormality, sparing the dentate nuclei; and involvement of the pyramidal tracts within the brainstem. Peroxisomal disorders include Zellweger's syndrome and X-linked ALD. Imaging features of Zellweger's syndrome include severely delayed myelination, periventricular germinolytic cysts, peri-Sylvian polymicrogyria and grey matter heterotopias. When this combination is seen in the clinical context of severe hypotonia with visual and hearing deficits, seizures, hepatomegaly and jaundice, the pattern may be considered pathognomonic.

CRANIOSYNOSTOSIS[55]

Craniosynostosis is a disorder of growth, one of the manifestations of which is premature closure of one or more calvarial or skull base sutures. The three broad categories of craniosynostosis are the simple nonsyndromic type, usually involving one suture; complex syndromic forms involving many sutures; and secondary craniosynostosis due to disrupted growth caused by a wide range of insults such as drugs and metabolic bone disease or secondary to an underlying small brain, as in chronic, treated hydrocephalus or any other cause of microcephaly. The most common type of primary craniosynostosis is simple sagittal synostosis.

The diagnosis is made initially by clinical assessment of the skull shape. Imaging provides confirmatory evidence and information regarding the skull base and orbits, and is important in the assessment of intracranial complications of craniosynostosis, such as hydrocephalus and visual failure. Standard radiographs will allow assessment of the coronal, sagittal, lambdoid and metopic sutures on the AP view; lambdoid and sagittal sutures on the Towne's view; and coronal and lambdoid sutures

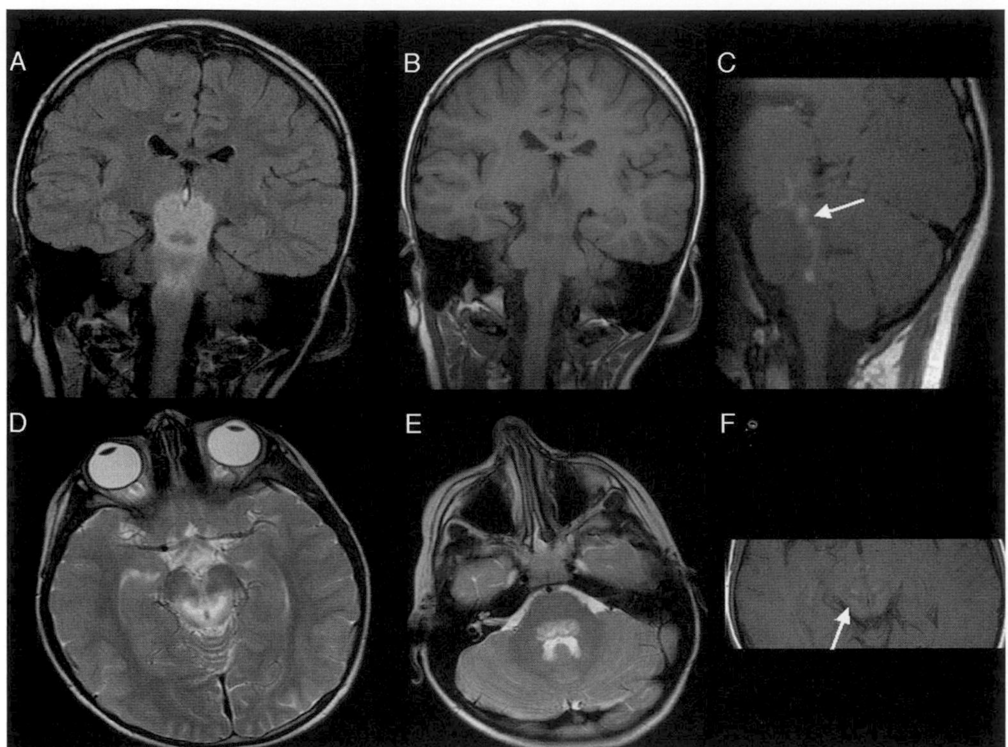

Figure 70.37 Leigh's disease. There is bilateral symmetrical signal hyperintensity on the coronal FLAIR (A) and axial T2 images (D), (E) matched by hypointensity on the coronal T1-weighted MRI (B) affecting the midbrain, pons, and medulla. Symmetrical contrast enhancement (C), (F) indicates breakdown of the blood–brain barrier in keeping with active disease.

on the lateral view in addition to assessment of the skull shape, foramen magnum and fontanelles. The affected suture may be absent, indistinct, show bridging sclerosis or a heaped up or beaked appearance, but also may appear normal if the synostosis is fibrotic not bony. Skull growth decreases perpendicular to the suture and increases parallel to it. Therefore, greater weight is given to the skull shape than the radiological evidence of direct sutural involvement. Conversely, if the sutures are not clearly visualized but the skull shape is normal, then craniosynostosis is unlikely.

Sagittal synostosis produces an elongated head shape called scaphocephaly (Fig. 70.38). Bicoronal synostosis causes brachycephaly or foreshortening in the AP direction which is accompanied by lateral elevation of the sphenoid wings producing the characteristic 'harlequin' deformity, upward slanting of the petrous apices and hypertelorism. Unicoronal synostosis causes anterior plagiocephaly or asymmetrical skull deformity and may be associated with compensatory growth on the unaffected side resulting in frontoparietal bossing (Fig. 70.39). Metopic synostosis causes trigonocephaly or 'keel deformity' and an AP view may show parallel, vertically oriented medial orbital walls. True unilateral lambdoid synostosis, the rarest form of monosutural synostosis, causes posterior plagiocephaly. This should be distinguished from the much more common positional or deformational plagiocephaly in which the suture is normal, and which is seen more often since the

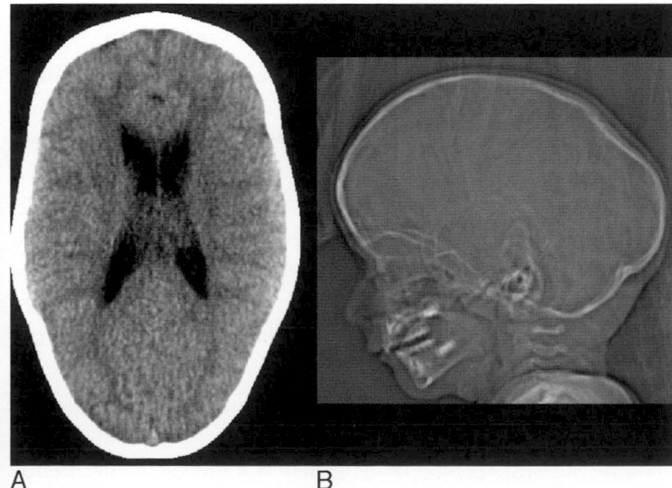

Figure 70.38 Sagittal synostosis. (A) Brain CT and (B) lateral scout view showing the typical 'boat-shaped' skull or scaphocephaly of sagittal synostosis.

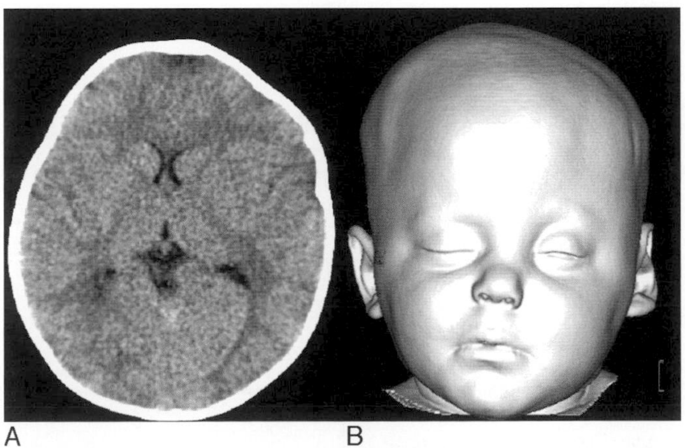

Figure 70.39 Unicoronal synostosis. (A) Axial CT and (B) 3D surface-shaded reformat show the asymmetrical head shape of left frontal plagiocephaly due to unicoronal craniosynostosis, with bossing seen on the right side.

1992 recommendation of the American Academy of Pediatrics to place newborns supine rather than prone in their cots to reduce the incidence of sudden infant death. In this case the skull deformity is caused by the child lying on one side in preference to the other, and may also be seen in torticollis or developmental delay. On plain radiographs and CT the lambdoid sutures appear open. Imaging of the spine may reveal segmentation anomalies, e.g. C5 and C6 in Apert's syndrome, and atlanto-occipital assimilation and basilar invagination in Apert's and Crouzon syndrome.

CT is more sensitive and specific than plain radiographs for detecting radiological evidence of craniosynostosis, such as sclerosis and bony bridging, and CT venography may be helpful to assess the jugular foramina, variations in venous anatomy and patency of the venous sinuses. 3D CT surface-shaded bone and soft tissue reconstructions or maximum intensity projections (MIPs) with a low milliampere technique may also be acquired, preferably in the craniofacial unit where treatment is being considered. The sutures should be assessed on both the axial 2D CT and 3D CT as either technique may miss relevant diagnostic features. There is also increasing prenatal diagnosis of craniosynostosis, particularly the syndromic forms, by ultrasound and fetal MRI.

In Apert's syndrome there are features of brachycephaly due to bicoronal synostosis, a wide open midline calvarial defect from the root of the nose to the posterior fontanelle in what would normally be the sagittal and metopic sutures and anterior fontanelle (Fig. 70.40). The sutures never form properly and instead bone islands appear within the defect, eventually coalescing to bony fusion by about 36 months. There is also hypertelorism with shallow anterior cranial fossae, depressed cribriform plate, as well as maxillary hypoplasia causing midface retrusion with exorbitism. Indeed the globe may actually sublux onto the cheek. The hand and feet deformities distinguish this condition from most other syndromic craniosynostoses and include syndactyly, phalangeal fusion and short radially deviated thumb producing the 'mitten' or more severe 'hoof' hand.

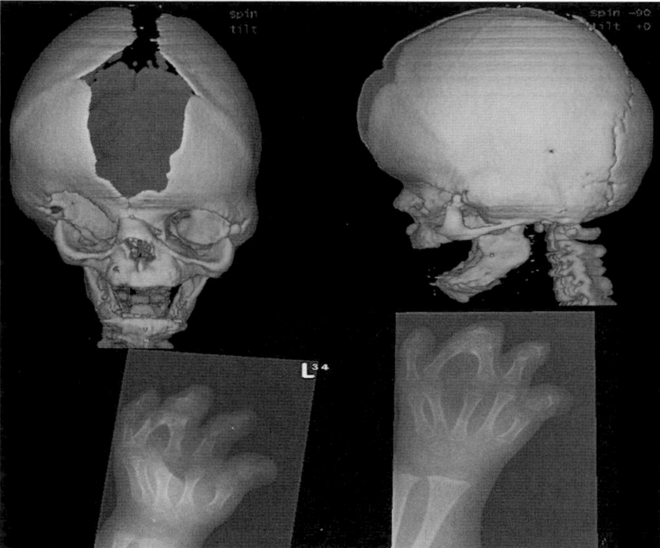

Figure 70.40 Apert's syndrome. (A,B) 3D CT surface-shaded display shows the wide open defect of the sagittal suture and brachycaphaly with bicoronal synostosis typical of Apert's syndrome. The coronal sutures appear fused and are ridged. (C,D) Plain radiographs of the hands show the 'mitten hand' appearance with syndactyly and shortened metacarpals.

Children with Crouzon's syndrome demonstrate a more complex syndromic synostosis involving the coronal, sagittal, metopic and squamosal sutures with early rather than late fontanelle closure. There is no midline calvarial defect but there is maxillary hypoplasia, hypertelorism, exorbitism and dental malocclusion. The limbs are usually clinically normal.

CT will detect any underlying structural brain abnormality. Although the brain usually appears structurally normal, midline anomalies such as callosal and septum pellucidum agenesis, limbic system abnormalities in Apert's, ventriculomegaly or distortion of the posterior fossa and skull base causing Chiari I malformations (tonsillar descent) may be detected. Tonsillar herniation is more frequently seen in Crouzon's syndrome, probably because there is more frequent skull base sutural synostosis in these conditions compared to Apert's.

Predicting raised intracranial pressure is known to be difficult by imaging, and correlation with clinical assessment is extremely important. Sometimes, however, direct invasive intracranial pressure (ICP) monitoring will be required. Hydrocephalus, seen in 4–25% of craniosynostosis and more commonly in the syndromic forms, may be multifactorial; possible aetiologies include tonsillar herniation and altered craniocervical junction CSF dynamics and venous hypertension due to venous foraminal narrowing, such as the jugular foramina, which ultimately may lead to venous occlusion and the development of venous collateral pathways such as enlargement of the stylomastoid emissary veins. Hydrocephalus is the most sensitive radiological indicator (see below) but only detects 40% of these children with raised ICP.

Finally CT may also be useful to assess the airway. Midface hypoplasia, small maxilla with dental overcrowding and basilar kyphosis may contribute to nasopharyngeal obstruction. Deviation of the nasal septum and choanal atresia may also be detected.

NEONATAL NASAL OBSTRUCTION: NASAL CAVITY STENOSIS/ATRESIA

The most common cause of neonatal nasal obstruction is mucosal oedema, followed by choanal atresia, skeletal dysplasias and congenital dacrocystocele due to distal nasolacrimal duct obstruction.

Choanal atresia

Choanal atresia/stenosis, a congenital malformation of the anterior skull base characterized by failure of canalization of the posterior choanae, is the most common form of nasal cavity stenosis. It may be bony and/or fibrous in nature, unilateral presenting in later childhood with chronic nasal discharge and bilateral presenting in newborns with respiratory distress, particularly during feeding and which is a surgical emergency. Bilateral forms are more likely to be syndromic (50%) than unilateral forms and common associations are Crouzon's, Treacher–Collins, CHARGE and Pierre–Robin syndromes.

The CHARGE syndrome describes the association of colobomas of the eye, heart defects, atresia of the choanae, retardation of growth and development, genitourinary anomalies and ear anomalies. The atresia is best evaluated on CT by direct axial and direct coronal imaging on a bone algorithm after administration of a nasal decongestant. The nasal cavity appears funnel shaped with a fluid level proximal to the obstruction. The posterior vomer is thickened and the nasal septum is deviated to the side of the stenosis. A bony, fibrous or membranous bridging bar across the posterior choana is seen (Fig. 70.41).

Skeletal dysplasias

Fibrous dysplasia is a benign congenital disorder in which bone is gradually replaced by fibrous tissue. McCune–Albright syndrome is a subtype of polyostotic fibrous dysplasia in which there is pituitary hypersecretion (hence precocious puberty but also Cushing's syndrome, etc.) and café-au-lait spots. Cherubism refers to fibrous dysplasia of the mandible and maxilla, and unlike the other forms of fibrous dysplasia is an inheritable condition. Typically the mandibular condyles are spared. The teeth may be displaced, impacted, resorbed, or appear to be floating.

Clinical symptoms other than cosmetic deformity relate to the site of bony involvement; hence cranial nerve impingement caused by narrowing of the skull base foramina, exophthalmos and optic foraminal narrowing caused by orbital involvement are all seen. On CT the typical lesion is a region of bony expansion with a 'ground-glass' appearance, but lesions may be lytic or sclerotic, or a combination of all three (Fig. 70.42).

BRAIN TUMOURS[56]

The United Kingdom Children's Cancer Study Group (UKCCSG) guidelines[57]

At initial presentation all paediatric brain tumours should have brain and whole spine MRI, including contrast-enhanced images. A suggested protocol includes T2-weighted FSE axial and coronal images of the brain, T1-weighted SE pre- and post-contrast imaging in at least two orthogonal planes, and post-contrast imaging of the whole spine. Ideally spine imaging should be performed at the outset; but if the need for surgery is immediate, then postoperative spinal imaging (pre- and post-contrast T1-weighted MRI to allow exclusion of T1 shortening due to post-surgical blood products) should be performed. The immediate postoperative MRI should be performed within 48 h (or 72 h maximum, according to the UKCCSG guidelines), the rationale being that post-surgical nodular enhancement which mimics tumour will not be seen before then. Post-surgical linear enhancement may be seen within this time period and indeed intra-operatively, and should therefore be interpreted with caution. The management strategy and frequency of subsequent surveillance imaging is determined by the tumour histology and presence of residual or recurrent tumour[58–60].

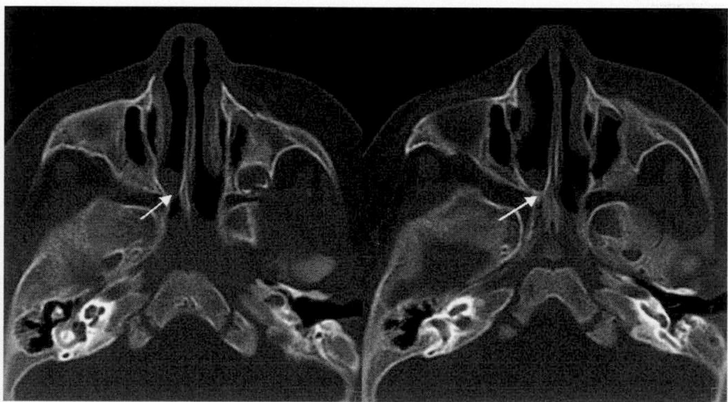

Figure 70.41 Choanal atresia. Axial skull base CT in a child with chronic nasal discharge shows right-sided choanal atresia. There is bony narrowing of the funnel-shaped posterior right choana down to a bony bridging bar (arrows) and pooling of secretions proximally.

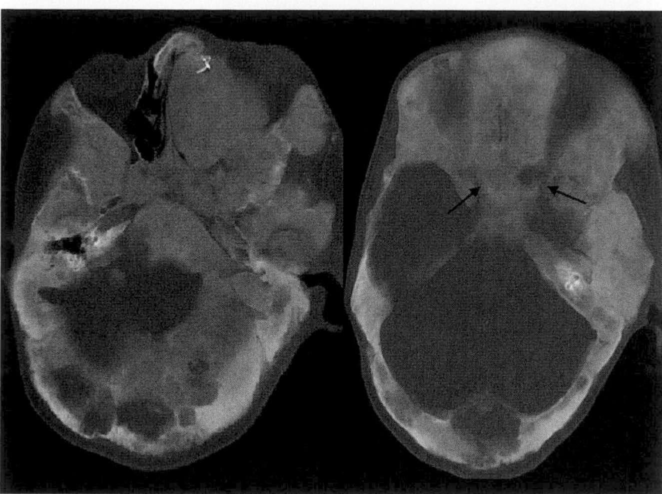

Figure 70.42 Polyostotic fibrous dysplasia with diffuse calvarial expansion, mixed lytic lesions, and sclerosis. The optic nerve canals are markedly narrowed (arrows).

Posterior fossa tumours

The most common intra-axial cerebellar tumours in children are medulloblastoma, pilocytic astrocytoma, ependymoma and atypical teratoid/rhabdoid tumour, of which medulloblastoma and astrocytoma are the most common. Cerebellar haemangioblastoma may be seen in the context of von Hippel–Lindau disease but otherwise is an unusual tumour in the paediatric age group. Other posterior fossa tumours include brainstem gliomas and extra-axial tumours, such as dermoid and epidermoid cysts, schwannoma, neurofibroma, meningioma and skull base lesions, such as Langerhans' cell histiocytosis, Ewing's sarcoma (Fig. 70.43) and glomus tumours.

Cerebellar tumours

Clinically all of these tumours may present as a 'posterior fossa' syndrome with lethargy, headache and vomiting due to hydrocephalus and/or direct involvement of the brainstem emetic centre. Before the fontanelles have closed infants may present with macrocephaly and sunsetting eyes. Truncal and gait ataxia is seen more often in older children and adults.

Medulloblastomas are highly malignant small, round cell tumours. They are slightly more common than pilocytic astrocytomas in most pathological series, are more common in boys, and account for 30–40% of posterior fossa tumours. They are

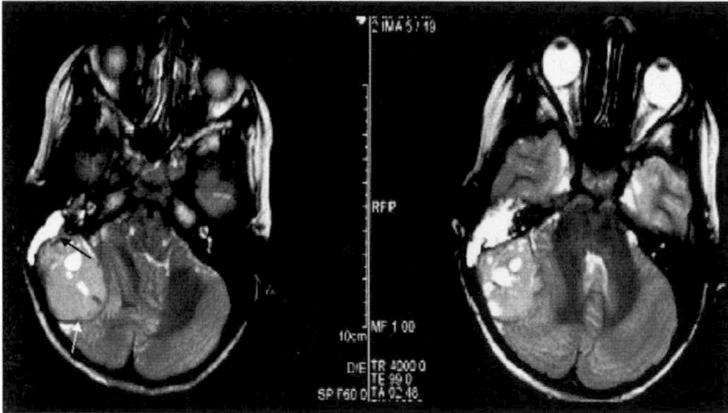

Figure 70.43 Ewing's sarcoma. This unusual posterior fossa tumour is also hypointense on the T2-weighted images but it is extradural. The dura is seen as a hypointense layer around the tumour and it erodes the right petrous bone. There are retained mastoid secretions. This was a Ewing's sarcoma of the skull base.

also associated with some rare oncogenetic disorders such as Li–Fraumeni syndrome, Gorlin's or basal cell naevus syndrome (with falcine calcification), Turcot and Cowden syndromes. They are aggressive, high-grade tumours (WHO Grade IV) and tend to have a shorter onset of symptoms, typically shorter than 1 month, compared to other cerebellar tumours. The peak age of presentation is 7 years but they have a wide range and may be seen from the neonatal period to late adulthood. There is a second peak in young adults presenting with the 'desmoplastic', less aggressive type of medulloblastoma, which is seen more frequently in the cerebellar hemisphere than the vermis. Occasionally there may be symptoms and signs or imaging evidence of intracranial or intraspinal leptomeningeal metastatic disease at presentation, a feature observed more commonly than with other posterior fossa tumours.

The typical appearance of the childhood medulloblastoma on CT is of a hyperdense midline vermian mass abutting the roof of the fourth ventricle, with perilesional oedema, variable patchy enhancement and hydrocephalus. The brainstem is usually displaced anteriorly rather than directly invaded. Cystic change, haemorrhage and calcification are frequently seen. On MRI, the mass is hypointense or isointense compared to grey matter. The CT finding of hyperdensity and MRI finding of T2 hypointensity, supported by the presence of restricted diffusion on diffusion-weighted imaging, are in our experience the most reliable observations in prospectively differentiating medulloblastoma (and atypical rhabdoid tumour which on imaging appears identical to medulloblastoma) from ependymoma or other posterior fossa tumours (Fig. 70.44, Table 70.2)[61]. Both the CT hyperdensity and MRI T2 signal hypointensity reflect the increased nuclear-to-cytoplasmic ratio and densely packed cells of the tumour, and are particularly useful in differentiating medulloblastomas with 'atypical' features, such as a lateral site involving the foramen of Luschka or extrusion through the foramen of Magendie, which are more commonly seen with ependymomas. Medulloblastomas demonstrate restricted diffusion and reduced N-acetyl asparatate (NAA) peak with an increased choline-to-creatine ratio, and occasionally lactate and lipid peaks on MR spectroscopy.

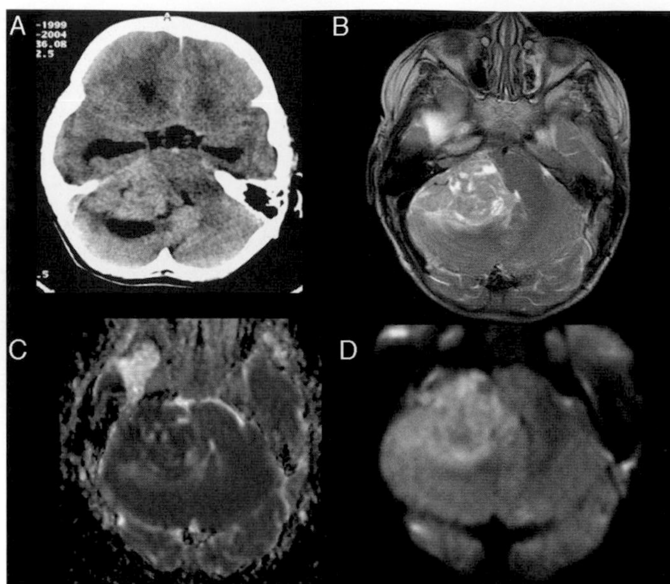

Figure 70.44 Medulloblastoma. (A) CT and (B–D) axial T2, ADC, and diffusion MRI show a mixed solid and cystic mass within the right cerebellopontine angle encroaching on the pons and fourth ventricle and causing hydrocephalus. The solid component is hyperdense on CT, hypointense on the T2-weighted sequence, and demonstrates restricted diffusion in keeping with a cellular tumour. Despite some less typical features, such as lateral site (more usually seen in older patients and associated with the desmoplastic variant) and cystic components, on the basis of the signal characteristics this was correctly diagnosed as a medulloblastoma.

Table 70.2 DIFFERENTIAL DIAGNOSIS OF POSTERIOR FOSSA TUMOUR WITH CT HYPERDENSITY AND T2 HYPOINTENSITY
Medulloblastoma/primitive neuroectodermal tumour /atypical teratoid/ rhabdoid tumour
Choroid plexus carcinoma
Ewings' sarcoma
Chondrosarcoma
Chordoma
Lymphoma
Langerhans' cell histiocytosis

In medulloblastoma, both intracranial and intraspinal subarachnoid dissemination should be actively looked for, and is seen in a third of cases at presentation, most often occurring as irregular, nodular leptomeningeal enhancement, (Fig. 70.45). Imaging is reported as being more sensitive than CSF cytology and false positives can be avoided by pre-operative imaging of the brain and spine. Occasionally, enhancement may not always be detected or may be very mild, making the detection of both disseminated disease and residual or recurrent tumour on surveillance imaging more difficult. Other features of leptomeningeal disease include sulcal and cisternal effacement and communicating hydrocephalus; thickening, nodularity and clumping of nerve roots; and pial 'drop' metastases along the surface of the spinal cord.

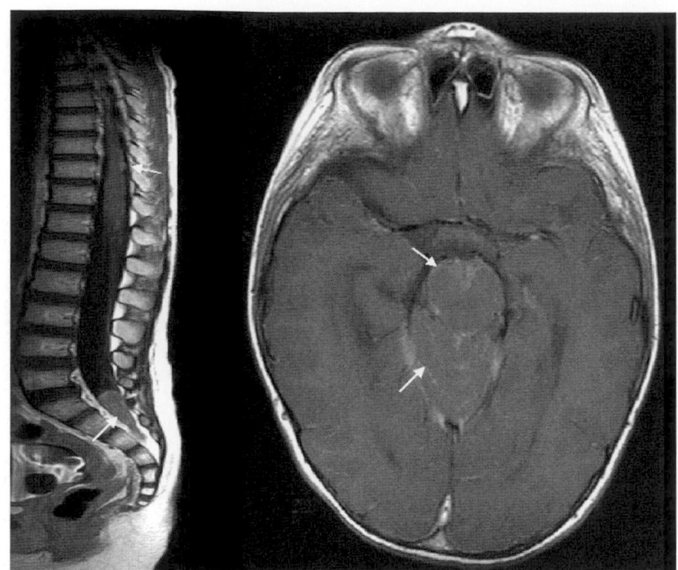

Figure 70.45 Medulloblastoma. Same patient as in Figure 70.44 with posterior fossa medulloblastoma has evidence of disseminated metastatic disease. There is nodular enhancement over the conus medullaris and a mass within the thecal sac in addition to pial enhancement over the midbrain and cerebellar folia (arrows).

Standard treatment for medulloblastoma is by surgical resection, with adjuvant craniospinal radiotherapy for those over 3 years of age (as the infant brain is more susceptible to radiation effects) and chemotherapy. The 5-year survival varies from 50% to 80%. Favourable prognostic factors include complete surgical resection, lack of CSF dissemination at presentation, onset in the second decade, female gender and lateral location within the cerebellar hemisphere. Surveillance imaging detects recurrences earlier than clinical presentation, allows earlier therapeutic intervention, and correlates with increased survival. There remain regional differences in outcome in the UK, emphasizing the importance of managing children with these tumours in a paediatric neuro-oncology centre with multidisciplinary support of neurosurgery, radiology and pathology.

Atypical teratoid/rhabdoid tumours are unusual malignant tumours with a poor prognosis. For practical purposes, the imaging features are indistinguishable from medulloblastoma/primitive neuroectodermal tumour (PNET). They are more aggressive tumours, are often large at the time of presentation and occur in slightly younger children, typically under the age of 2 years.

The next most common cerebellar tumour in children after medulloblastoma, and accounting for 30–40%, is the cerebellar low-grade astrocytoma (CLGA), which in most cases (85%) is a pilocytic tumour (WHO Grade I) and in up to 15% is a more diffuse fibrillary type with a higher histological grade. The 5-year survival for cerebellar pilocytic astrocytoma is in excess of 95% in most reported series, including the original description by Cushing in 1931. The CLGA is a well-circumscribed, slowly growing lesion of children and young adults, though it is occasionally seen in older people. There is an association with NF1 as there is for other neuro-axis pilocytic astrocytomas. The duration of symptom onset is more insidious than that of medulloblastomas, typically being intermittent over several months.

On CT and MRI the tumour is typically a cerebellar vermian or hemispheric tumour which is cystic with an enhancing mural nodule. The solid component is hypointense to isodense on CT, hyperintense on T2-weighted FSE and hypointense on T1-weighted sequences reflecting the hypocellular and loosely arranged tumoral architecture[62]. The solid component is highly vascular with a deficient blood–brain barrier and therefore enhances avidly and homogeneously (Fig. 70.46).

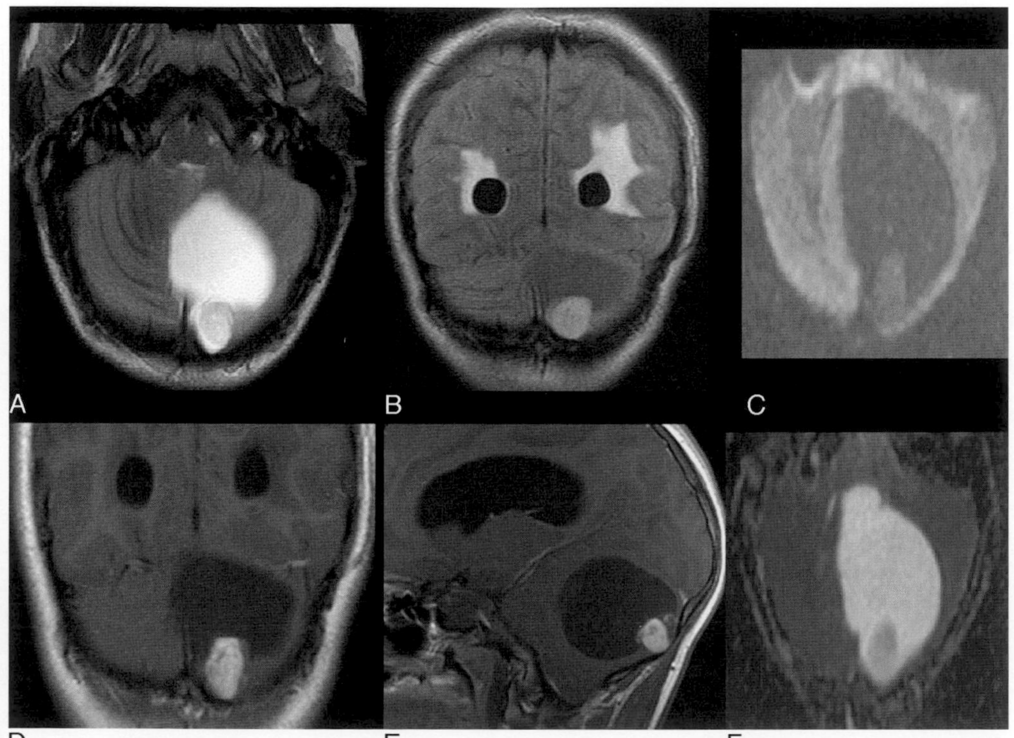

Figure 70.46 Cerebellar hemispheric tumour in a child with a history of ataxia, nausea, and vomiting over several months. (A,B,D,E) Axial T2, coronal FLAIR, coronal and sagittal T1 enhanced MRI show a left cerebellar hemispheric tumour with a large cystic component and solid homogeneously enhancing component which is bright on T2-weighted sequences (compare with the images of posterior fossa medulloblastoma, Figures 70.44 and 70.45). The solid component is not restricted on the diffusion-weighted image (C) and ADC map (F) compared to medulloblastoma and there is free diffusion in the cystic component.

Occasionally the pilocytic astrocytoma may present with diffuse nodular enhancement of the leptomeninges, indicating intracranial or intraspinal pial dissemination. This is typically seen with WHO Grade I tumours, does not imply a higher grade tumour and like the tumour primary tends to grow slowly.

Ependymomas (WHO Grade II) account for approximately 10% of paediatric posterior fossa tumours and the posterior fossa is the most common site for ependymomas in children. Their mean age at presentation is 6.4 years, with a range of 2 months to 16 years. They are well-defined tumours which typically originate from the floor or the roof of the fourth ventricle, extend into the cerebellopontine angle and extrude through the foramina of Luschka and Magendie (Fig. 70.47). Perivascular pseudorosettes and ependymal rosettes are the cardinal histopathological features. They are more cellular than CLGAs but usually demonstrate CT and MRI features consistent with a higher water content than medulloblastomas. Therefore they are still hypodense or isodense on CT, hypointense on T1 and isodense to hyperintense on MRI. Foci of microcystic change, haemorrhage and calcification are common features. They can also disseminate throughout the neuro-axis by leptomeningeal spread, although this is much less common then for medulloblastoma. Incomplete resection, age under 3 years and anaplastic histopathological features correlate with a worse prognosis. The 5-year progression-free survival is 50% but worse under the age of 2 years.

Children with von Hippel–Lindau disease may occasionally present with cerebellar haemangioblastoma (WHO Grade I), which in the sporadic form is usually a tumour of adults. It consists of a rich capillary network in addition to large vacuolated stromal cells. On imaging haemangioblastomas may mimic a CLGA with an intensely enhancing mural nodule and a cystic component. The tumour abuts the pial surface but unlike the CLGA it may be associated with prominent vascular flow voids. Haemorrhage and frank necrosis may occur but are less common.

Most brainstem tumours in children are astrocytomas. Medullary tumours may present with symptoms and signs of raised cranial pressure and cranial nerve dysfunction. The two major groups are diffuse tumours and focally exophytic tumours[63]. Diffuse tumours extend up and down the brainstem and are seen best as ill-defined signal hyperintensity on T2-weighted (including FLAIR) images in association with expansion of the brainstem. Their enhancement if present is usually minimal unless the tumour has been irradiated (Fig. 70.48). Focal exophytic tumours are usually dorsally exophytic, well-defined tumours, which do not extend along white matter tracts in the same ways as diffuse astrocytomas (hence their exophytic growth), but often enhance. They are usually Grade I pilocytic or Grade II astrocytomas and are associated with a better prognosis than diffuse astrocytomas, particularly focal tumours within the midbrain tectum[64]. Occasionally, however, anaplastic gangliogliomas or PNET tumours may appear like this.

Suprasellar tumours

Some knowledge of the typical clinical presentation of certain suprasellar tumours can be very helpful in differentiating them even before imaging. For example, hypopituitarism is more likely to be seen with craniopharyngioma, delayed puberty with hypothalamic astrocytoma or Langerhans' cell histiocytosis, and occasionally pituitary adenoma, precocious puberty due to hypothalamic infundibular lesions, such as Langerhans' cell histiocytosis, germinoma, craniopharyngioma, hamartoma and non-neoplastic granulomatous disease, such as sarcoidosis and tuberculosis. Large suprasellar mass lesions have the ability to produce hydrocephalus by obstruction at the foramen of Monro, and visual field defects by compression or involvement of the optic chiasm.

Craniopharyngioma

Although histologically benign (WHO Grade I), this tumour is associated with significant morbidity and mortality because of its site and often large size at presentation. It is the most common suprasellar tumour in children, accounting for 1–3% of intracranial tumours of all ages, but usually occurring from age 5 to 15 years. Most craniopharyngiomas have a suprasellar mass and a smaller intrasellar component. In 5% of cases it is purely intrasellar and may be difficult to distinguish from a Rathke's cleft cyst. Classically it appears as a calcified, mixed

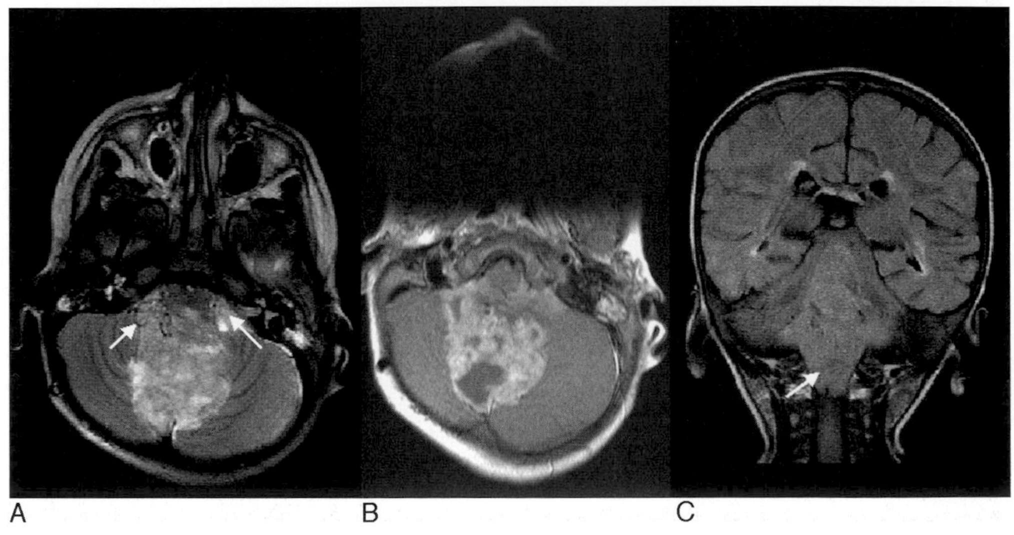

Figure 70.47 Ependymoma. (A–C) Axial T2, enhanced T1, and coronal FLAIR images showing a solid and microcystic fourth ventricular tumour extending out through the foramina of Luschka, Magendie, and the foramen magnum (arrows), the typical features of an ependymoma.

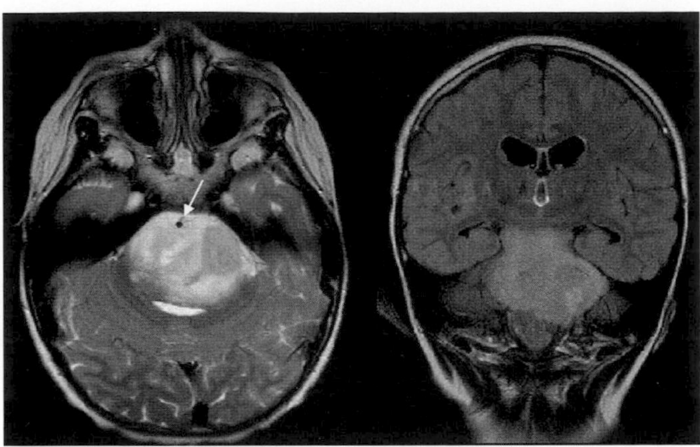

Figure 70.48 Diffuse brainstem astrocytoma. Note the mass effect within the pons distorting the fourth ventricle and the encasement of the basilar artery (arrow).

Table 70.3 DIFFERENTIAL OF ENHANCING INFUNDIBULAR LESIONS
Germinoma
Langerhans' cell histiocytosis
Lymphocytic hypophysitis
Granuloma (tuberculosis, sarcoid)

cystic and solid tumour with enhancement of the solid component and the cyst wall (Fig. 70.49). Large tumours may cause hydrocephalus and compression and distortion of the optic chiasm. The cystic components may extend behind the clivus and into any of the cranial fossae. On T1-weighted sequences the cyst may demonstrate T1 shortening due to proteinaceous components, which have been described macroscopically as appearing like 'machine oil'. The cystic components are of increased signal on T2-weighted FSE. MR spectroscopy demonstrates high lipid peaks. Surgical resection is often incomplete (in >20%) because of the close adherence of the tumour to the optic chiasm; despite this long-term survival is good (>90% in children).

Hypothalmic–optic pathway glioma

Astrocytomas of the optic chiasm and hypothalamus account for 10–15% of supratentorial tumours in children. Optic chiasm tumours often extend into the hypothalamus and vice versa; hence they are discussed here together. Optic nerve tumours are usually pilocytic astrocytomas with a very indolent course, while hypothalamic/chiasmatic tumours may be of higher histological grade and more aggressive biological behaviour.

CT and MRI both define involvement of the optic nerves. CT can detect expansion of the optic canal. However, MRI is the best modality for delineating expansion of the chiasm and hypothalamus and involvement of the posterior visual pathways (Fig. 70.50). Tumour appears isointense to hypointense on T1-weighted imaging and hyperintense on T2-weighted imaging. There may be diffuse fusiform expansion of the nerve from subarachnoid dissemination of tumour around the optic nerve. Enhancement is variable. The main differential diagnosis is from craniopharyngioma, which tends to present later, is usually calcified and is adherent to the chiasm rather than arising from it and causing expansion.

Infundibular tumours

These include germinomas and Langerhans' cell histiocytosis, both of which cause expansion and enhancement of the pituitary infundibulum (Fig. 70.51). Onset of diabetes insipidus appears to correlate with absence of high T1 signal in the posterior pituitary

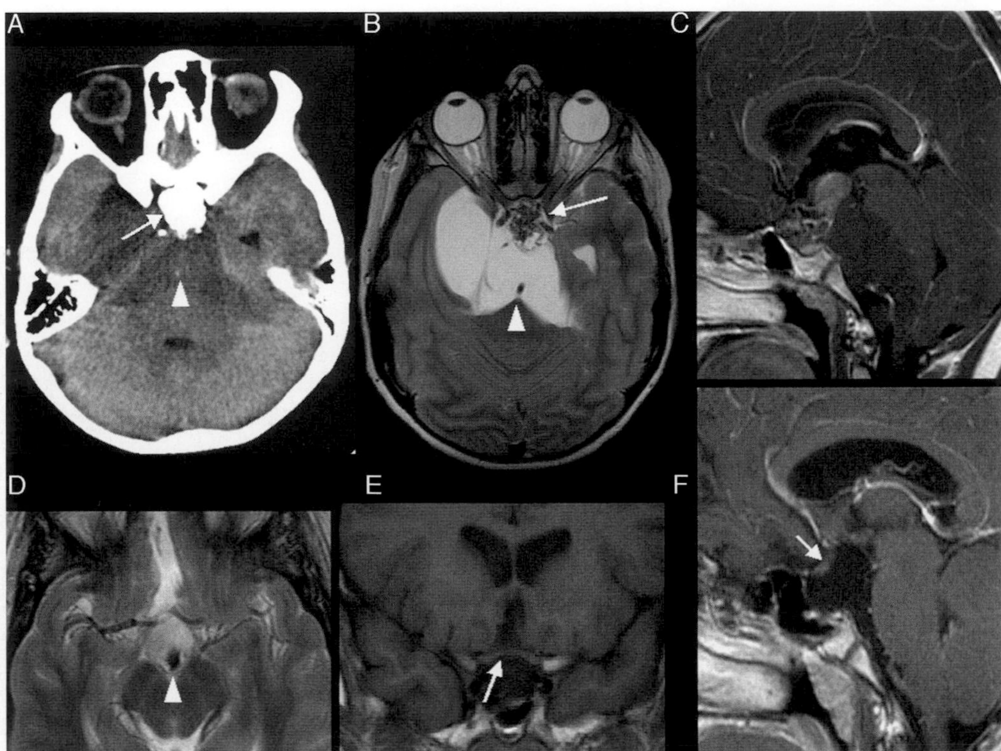

Figure 70.49 Craniopharyngiomas in two children. (A–C) The first child has a large suprasellar, pre-pontine and middle cranial fossa tumour which is causing considerable mass effect on the brainstem and is encasing the basilar artery (arrowheads). There are solid enhancing and calcified components (arrows). The cystic components are of higher density on CT and there is T1 shortening on MRI in keeping with proteinacous contents. (D–F) The second child has a smaller suprasellar lesion, which is also calcified (arrowhead). The optic chiasm is clearly separate from the lesion and is draped over the top (E,F).

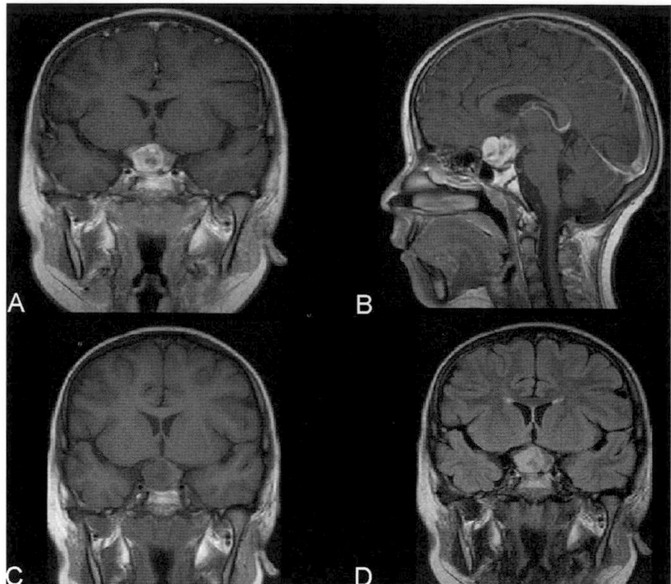

Figure 70.50 Hypothalmic–optic pathway glioma. (A) Coronal T1-weighted, (B) sagittal, and (C) coronal enhanced T1-weighted MRI, and (D) coronal FLAIR show an optic chiasm glioma. The chiasm is not identified separately from the tumour.

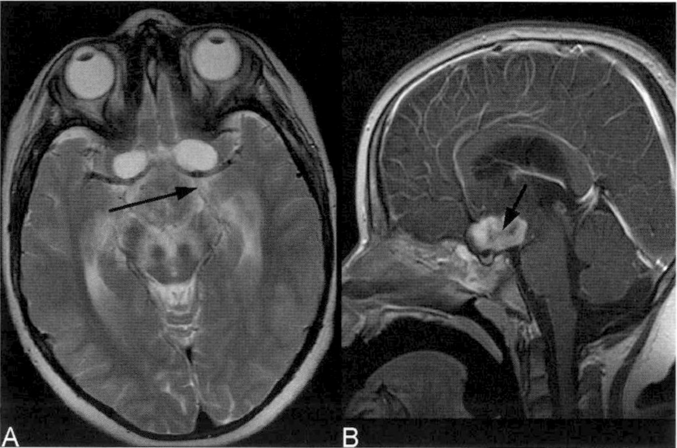

Figure 70.51 Langerhans' cell histiocytosis. (A) Axial T2-weighted image. (B) Sagittal T1-weighted post-contrast image. Suprasellar T2 hypointense and enhancing mass (arrows) with associated oedema extending superiorly along white matter tracts in a child with multisystem Langerhans' cell histiocytosis.

gland. The hypothalamic hamartoma (not a tumour by definition) presents either with precocious puberty or with gelastic seizures. These may be sessile or pedunculated and are well-defined lesions arising from the floor of the third ventricle and extending inferiorly into the suprasellar or interpeduncular cistern. They are typically isointense to grey matter on T1- and T2-weighted MRI and do not enhance (Fig. 70.52).

Pituitary tumours

Pituitary adenomas are uncommon in children but may present in adolescents, and account for 2% of all pituitary adenomas. The most common functional tumours are prolactinomas and corticotrophin- and growth hormone-secreting tumours. A quarter of paediatric pituitary tumours are nonfunctioning.

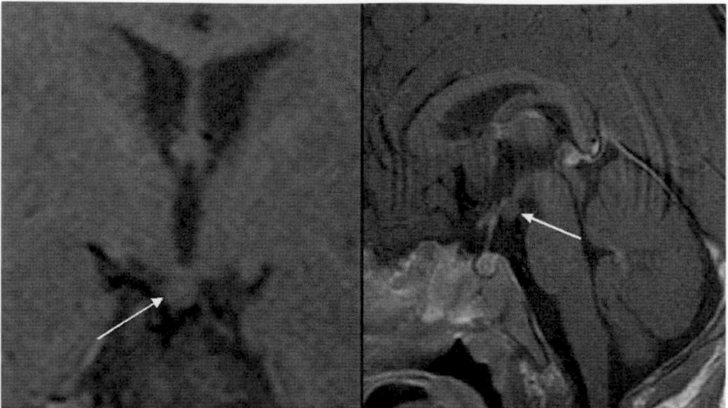

Figure 70.52 Hypothalamic hamartoma. Coronal T1 and sagittal T1-weighted post-contrast MRI shows a nonenhancing lesion arising from the floor of the third ventricle posterior to the pituitary infundibulum and projecting inferiorly into the suprasellar cistern (arrows).

The imaging appearances are the same as in adults. Rathke's cleft cysts are also rare in children.

Pineal region tumours

The pineal region is a descriptive term and encompasses the posterior third ventricle and its contents, including the pineal gland itself, the tectal plate and aqueduct, the posterior septum pellucidum, corpus callosum and thalami, internal cerebral veins in addition to the quadrigeminal cistern containing the posterior cerebral arteries, vein of Galen and straight sinus. Lesions may arise from any of these components and therefore the differential diagnosis of a pineal region tumour is wide. The most common lesions are germ cell tumours (GCTs), followed by primary pineal gland masses. Gliomas are also relatively common lesions at this site, usually derived from adjacent brain parenchyma. Pineal region tumours can cause hydrocephalus by obstruction of the cerebral aqueduct. Direct compression or invasion of the tectal plate, specifically the colliculi, may cause failure of upward gaze and convergence (Parinaud's syndrome). They may also cause precocious puberty.

Central nervous system germ cell tumours

CNS GCTs are primarily tumours of the young, over 90% occurring in the under 20 age group and with a peak incidence from age 10 to 12 years. They are more common in Asia but in the West account for 1% of intracranial neoplasms in children. Germinoma is the most common type of CNS GCT, followed by nonsecreting teratoma. Other GCTs include rarer secreting forms such as yolk sac, embryonal and choriocarcinoma, and may be of mixed cellular types, the latter associated with the worst prognosis.

Germinomas are characteristically found in the midline, in the pineal or suprasellar regions. A minority of lesions may be found in the basal ganglia, thalami, or cerebellum. Pineal and suprasellar lesions may be synchronous, and when so, are pathognomonic. Most pineal region GCTs occur in boys and suprasellar GCTs in girls. Pathologically the tumour is solid and consists of large, glycogen-rich germ line cells with variable desmoplastic stroma and lymphocytic infiltrate. Necrosis and haemorrhage are unusual with the exception of lesions seen in the basal ganglia.

Germinomas are classified as malignant tumours but respond extremely well to radiotherapy and may melt away over just a few days of treatment. Overall they are more common in young adolescent males. On CT they appear as a hyperdense, solid mass within the posterior third ventricle and enhance avidly and homogeneously. They tend to engulf the pineal gland which may be calcified. Occasionally this may be difficult to differentiate from intrinsic tumoral calcification more suggestive of a teratoma or primary pineal gland tumour, such as a pineoblastoma, although both of these lesions are typically more heterogeneous with haemorrhage and cyst formation. On MRI the cellularity of the tumour is reflected by T2 hypointensity relative to grey matter. The tumour may be less homogeneous than on CT and cystic change may be detected, although enhancement remains a marked feature. Germinomas demonstrate restricted diffusion. Synchronous germinomas in typical midline sites, such as the suprasellar region, and evidence of early CSF dissemination should be actively looked for.

Benign teratomas are very heterogeneous, mixed cystic, solid and well-defined masses characterized by calcification and fat. Enhancement is not usually seen unless there are areas of malignant degeneration. Other GCTs are also heterogeneous in appearance and do not contain fat, but the individual tumour types are not distinguishable radiologically.

Primary pineal tumours: pineoblastoma and pineocytoma

Pineoblastomas are malignant (WHO Grade IV), small, round cell tumours which histologically are similar to medulloblastomas and share similar imaging characteristics in terms of hyperdensity on CT and are hypointense to isointense signal on T2-weighted FSE relative to grey matter. They may contain areas of calcification and rarely haemorrhage. The solid parts of the tumour enhance intensely. They may be distinguished from Grade II pineocytomas by the age at presentation, as they occur most frequently in the first two decades of life compared to pineocytomas which are tumours of young adults; by their size (>3 cm); and by their relative T2-weighted hypointensity (Fig. 70.53).

Supratentorial hemisphere tumours

Overall supratentorial tumours occur as frequently as posterior fossa tumours in the paediatric age group but are more common under the age of 2 and over the age of 10, while posterior fossa tumours are more common from the ages of 2 to 10. The presenting symptoms are due to a large mass-occupying lesion and include headaches and vomiting. In the under 2 year old age group the tumour may be very large at the time of presentation; the fontanelles are open so that infants present with increasing head size as often as they do with hydrocephalus. Seizures are seen more particularly with temporal and frontal cortex lesions.

Astrocytomas

The most common paediatric cerebral hemispheric tumour is the astrocytoma, accounting for 30% of supratentorial brain tumours in children. In children under 2 years, other diagnoses should be considered; teratomas and desmoplastic infantile gangliogliomas are seen in neonates and PNET, atypical teratoid/rhabdoid tumours, and ependymomas are seen in slightly older infants. Some children who present with a longer history and refractory epilepsy may have low-grade, indolent glioneuronal tumours, including the dysembryoplastic neuroepithelial tumour.

As with cerebellar astrocytomas, hemispheric astrocytomas may be cystic with an enhancing mural nodule, entirely solid with variable enhancement or solid with a necrotic centre. On CT the solid part of the hemispheric astrocytoma is isodense or hypodense and on MRI T2-weighted sequences it is hyperintense, helping to distinguish these tumours from small, round cell tumours such as supratentorial PNET. They may rarely be multicentric. The histological grade cannot be reliably determined by the radiological features. Contrast enhancement can be seen in both low- and high-grade tumours. A simple cyst with nonenhancing walls, minimal surrounding oedema and a single enhancing mural nodule is more likely to be a pilocytic astrocytoma. Lesions containing haemorrhage and associated with marked adjacent oedema are more likely to be of higher grade. Glioblastoma is seen in children and in children is associated with a better prognosis than in adults. The pleomorphic

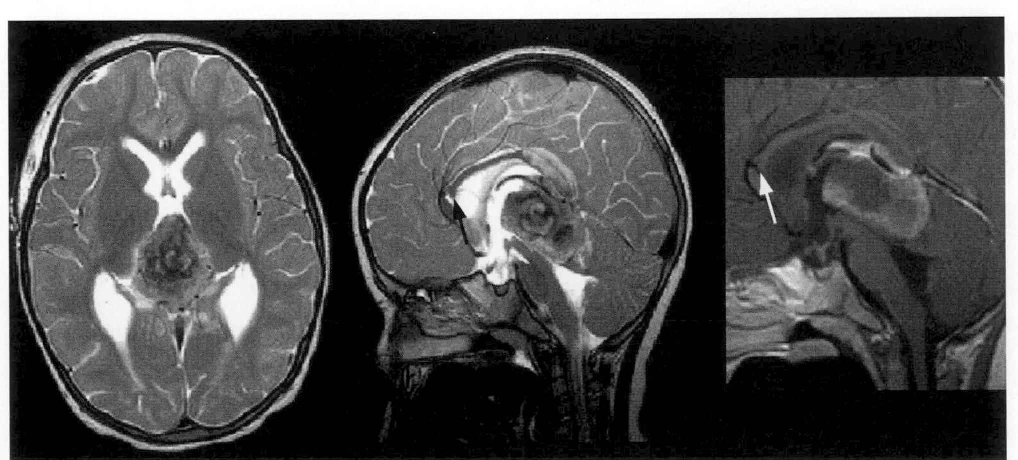

Figure 70.53 Pineoblastoma. (A) Axial, (B) sagittal T2-weighted fast spin-echo, and (C) enhanced sagittal T1-weighted MRI in a 2 year old girl show a pineal region tumour effacing the tectal plate. The hydrocephalus is treated by a frontal extraventricular drain (track through the genu of the corpus callosum marked by the arrows). The tumour is hypointense on the T2-weighted images with rings of lower signal consistent with calcification and haemorrhagic products, and peripheral rim enhancement, and was confirmed as a pineoblastoma.

xanthoastrocytoma is an uncommon astrocytoma of children and young adults. It is usually a WHO Grade II lesion, though may have anaplastic features. Typically it has a superficial location within the temporal lobe and consists of a cyst and enhancing mural nodule with minimal adjacent oedema. Radiologically it is often indistinguishable from ganglioglioma and some other glioneuronal tumour subtypes.

Ependymonas

Supratentorial ependymomas occur more commonly in boys with a peak incidence between the ages of 1 and 5 years, and again are similar to the posterior fossa ependymoma. However they are more usually extraventricular in site and therefore CSF dissemination is less common than with their posterior fossa equivalent. They are isodense to hyperdense, well-defined lesions on CT with variable enhancement of the solid component. Tumour heterogeneity with cystic areas and foci of calcification are common (Fig. 70.54). Haemorrhage may also be seen.

Primitive neuroectodermal tumours

PNET (WHO Grade IV) is a cellular tumour of primitive cell types and may be seen in children as young as 4 weeks to 10 years with a mean age of 5.5 years. A rare subtype that includes more neuronal cells is known as cerebral neuroblastoma. PNET is found more frequently in the posterior fossa than in the supratentorial compartment. Poor prognostic factors for PNET include age under 2 years and a supratentorial location. The 5-year survival drops from 85% for tumours in the posterior fossa to 34% for supratentorial tumours. They are frequently haemorrhagic, necrotic and have foci of calcification. The solid parts of the tumour are hyperdense on CT and hypointense on T2-weighted FSE. There is always some enhancement although the degree is variable. Although the tumour may appear well-defined radiologically, tumour cells are likely to extend beyond the apparent margins. Widespread dissemination of tumour both through the CSF space and to the lungs, liver and spleen, is not infrequent.

Medulloepithelioma is a rare, highly malignant tumour usually affecting children between the ages of 6 months and 5 years. Solid components are hypercellular; therefore, the density and signal characteristics may be similar to PNET. They are large at the time of presentation with extensive areas of haemorrhage and necrosis but may be distinguished from other tumours, including PNET, by their lack of contrast enhancement.

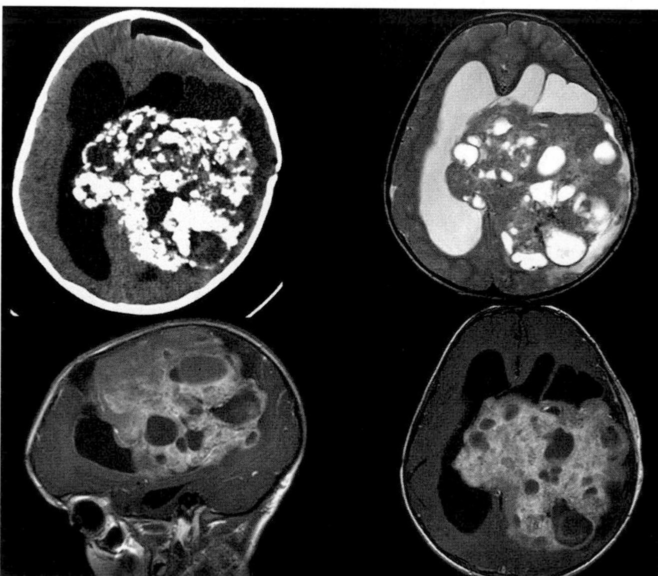

Figure 70.54 Supratentorial grade II ependymoma. The left cerebral hemisphere tumour extends across the midline into the right ventricle. (A) CT (post partial debulking) shows it is heavily calcified and (B–D) MRI (axial T2 enhanced, sagittal T1 and axial T1-weighted MRI) show a mixed cystic and solid heterogeneously enhancing tumour. There is associated hydrocephalus.

Desmoplastic infantile gangliomas

These typically present as a massive cyst with an enhancing cortically-based mural nodule in an infant with increased head size and bulging fontanelle. Adjacent dural enhancement may also be seen. The cyst, which is hypointense on T1, hyperintense on T2 and may contain septations, usually does not enhance.

Choroid plexus tumours

These are 'cauliflower-like' tumours arising from the epithelium of the choroid plexus and are more frequently benign (papilloma) than malignant (carcinoma). Both types may disseminate within the CSF space. They are the most common brain tumour in children under 1 year and present with hydrocephalus, possibly due to CSF hypersecretion or obstructive hydrocephalus due to haemorrhage, arachnoiditis or carcinomatosis in carcinomas. For papillomas the 5-year survival approaches 100% while for carcinomas it ranges from 25% to 40% with a higher survival if the tumour is completely resected.

On CT they are seen as hyperdense or isodense, lobulated 'frond-like', avidly and homogeneously enhancing masses with punctate calcifications, occasionally with haemorrhage and with hydrocephalus. The typical site is the trigone of the lateral ventricle, while in older children the cerebellopontine angle or fourth ventricle may be involved (Fig. 70.55). On MRI the papillary appearance is more readily appreciated: they are more mottled and isointense or hypointense on T1-weighted imaging with intense enhancement. Vascular flow voids, usually from choroidal arteries, are often seen in association, and arterial embolization may be considered before surgery in an attempt to reduce the vascularity of the tumour. Haemorrhage and localized vasogenic oedema are suggestive of carcinoma with invasion but the two histological types cannot be reliably distinguished on imaging.

Other intraventricular tumours include meningiomas, which are rare in children outside NF2 and ependymomas.

Dysembryoplastic neuroepithelial tumours

Dysembryoplastic neuroepithelial tumour (DNT) is a WHO Grade I benign tumour which classically presents with complex partial seizures in children and young adults under the age of 20. It is a cortically based lesion which may have associated foci of cortical dysplasia.

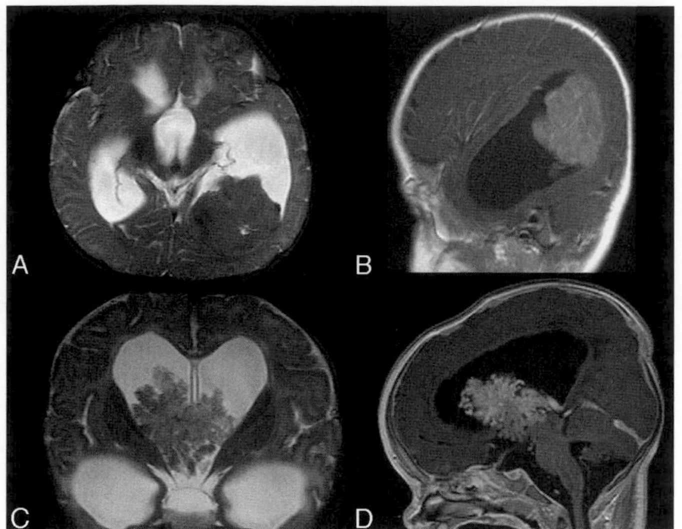

Figure 70.55 Choroid plexus tumours. (A,B) Axial T2, enhanced sagittal T1-weighted MRI in a boy aged 6 months demonstrate a lobulated homogeneously enhancing intraventricular tumour with relative T2 hypointensity, in keeping with a highly cellular tumour closely related to the choroid plexus. The ependyma is enhancing and the interface between tumour and adjacent brain is indistinct. Histology confirmed the tumour to be a choroid plexus carcinoma and this was subsequently embolized before surgery. There is a communicating hydrocephalus which may be due to increased cerebrospinal fluid production or to proteinaceous/haemorrhagic exudate. (C,D) A different child with choroid plexus papilloma. Choroid plexus tumours although commonly seen within the trigone of the lateral ventricle may arise from anywhere within the ventricular system. This child has a frondy choroid plexus papilloma arising within the third ventricle and extending superiorly through the foramina of Monro. In this case the hydrocephalus was obstructive.

On imaging it appears as a well-defined cortically based lesion with a characteristic 'bubbly' internal structure, minimal mass effect and no associated vasogenic oedema (Fig. 70.56). There may be some adjacent bony scalloping consistent with a long-standing lesion and a third of lesions demonstrate calcification. On MRI they are hypointense on T1 and have a hyperintense rim on FLAIR or proton density-weighted imaging. Most tumours do not enhance and if present, enhancement is faint and patchy.

CEREBROVASCULAR DISEASE AND STROKE

Stroke is an important paediatric illness with an incidence of around 2 cases per 100,000 children per annum. The aetiology of paediatric stroke is significantly different from adult stroke, as large artery atherosclerosis, cardio-embolic and small vessel disease combined account for only 10% of cases in children[65].

There have been several misconceptions regarding stroke in children. Paediatric stroke was said to be idiopathic, associated with a good prognosis with low recurrence rates and good recovery of motor function and school performance, and was minimally investigated on the assumption that this would not affect management. Recent work has shown that there are many different aetiologies associated with stroke in

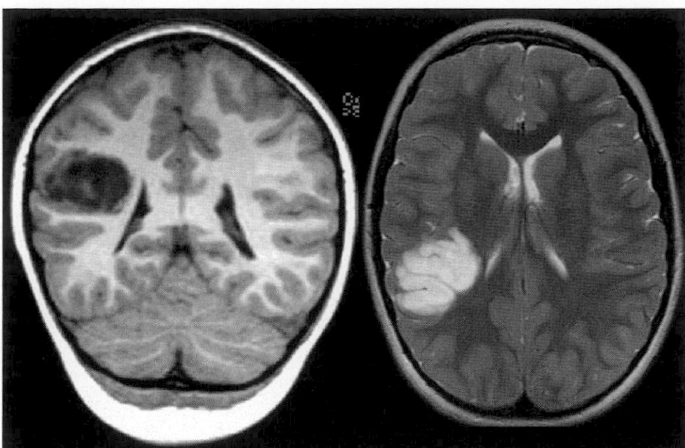

Figure 70.56 Dysembryoplastic neuroepithelial tumour (DNT) in a child with long-standing refractory focal epilepsy referred to the epilepsy surgical programme. Several MRI examinations over 3 years had shown no change in the appearances of this right inferior parietal lobe lesion. The lesion is well-defined, cortically based, extends towards the ventricular margin, and has the typical lobulated internal architecture of DNT.

children and a single episode may be multifactorial. Associated factors, some of which may be amenable to treatment, include congenital heart disease, anaemias, prothrombotic disorders such as protein C and S deficiencies, hyperhomocystinaemia, lipid abnormalities, recent infections and respiratory chain disorders (Fig. 70.57). Equally, long-term follow-up has shown a poor outcome with some degree of dependency in

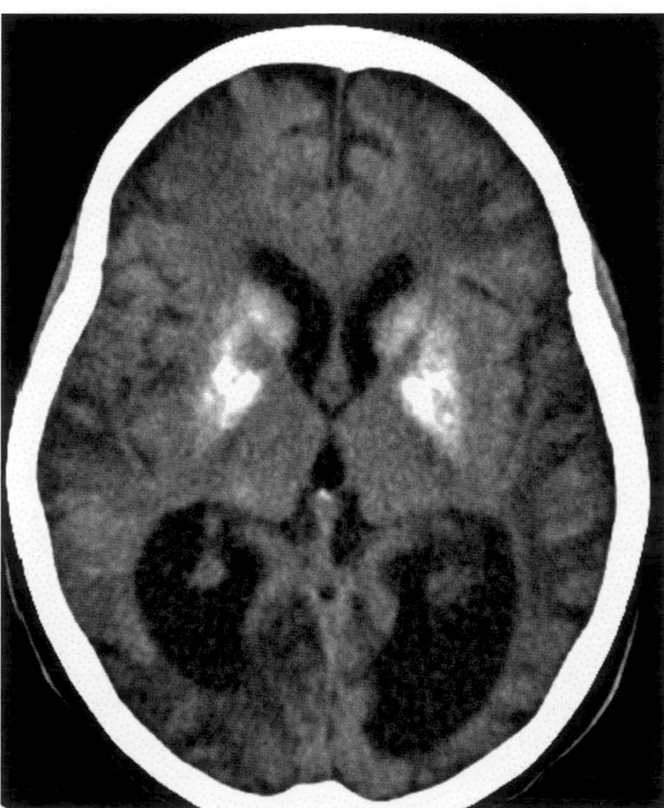

Figure 70.57 Strokes occurring in mitochondrial cytopathy. Bilateral symmetrical lentiform and caudate calcification and extensive cerebral infarction crossing arterial territories in a child with a mitochondrial disorder (MELAS).

60% of affected children. Although difficult to quantify due to selection bias, the risk of recurrence for ischaemic stroke ranges from 5% to 20%. Children who have a stroke at a young age have a worse physical and intellectual outcome and behavioural problems may be significant. Hence children with acute stroke should be referred to, or have their management discussed with a paediatric neurologist, and thoroughly investigated on each occasion to detect all potential risk factors. Cross-sectional brain imaging is mandatory in children presenting with clinical stroke. Brain MRI is recommended and should be performed as soon as possible after presentation. If MRI is not available within 48 h, CT is an acceptable initial alternative. Imaging should be undertaken urgently in those who have a depressed conscious level or whose clinical status is deteriorating[66].

The purpose of neuroimaging is to confirm the diagnosis and exclude alternative treatable lesions, as well as to help understand the underlying cause, guide treatment and monitor progression of the disease. The radiological findings of brain parenchymal involvement in stroke are not significantly different from findings in adults. There is however some evidence that restricted diffusion may occur for a shorter time in younger children and pseudonormalization may occur earlier than in adults. Vascular abnormalities in paediatric ischaemic stroke are common[67]. These are more frequently intracranial than extracranial, involve the anterior rather than posterior circulation and typically consist of occlusion of proximal large arteries, i.e. middle cerebral artery (MCA), anterior cerebral artery (ACA) and terminal internal carotid artery (ICA).

Sickle cell disease, a chronic haemolytic anaemia in which abnormal haemoglobin (HbS) forms with a tendency to cause red blood cells to distort and block small blood vessels, is the most common cause of ischaemic stroke in children worldwide. Even within this single disease entity there are several factors that contribute to stroke. These include a cerebral vasculopathy known as moya moya disease, an underlying predilection to infection, tissue hypoxia and precipitation of sickling vaso-occlusive crisis resulting from chronic anaemia, high white cell count, adenotonsillar hyperplasia causing obstructive sleep apnoea, cardiomegaly and a generalized procoagulant state.

Stroke in sickle cell disease is clinically apparent in 9% of children with sickle cell disease under the age of 20 years, but silent infarction occurs in as many as 25%. The imaging pattern of infarction is typically of arterial watershed infarction between the major cerebral arterial territories. A fifth of strokes in sickle cell disease may be haemorrhagic. The diploic space of the calvarium may be diffusely thickened due to increased haematopoiesis in order to compensate for the chronic haemolytic anaemia.

The brain MRI and circle of Willis MR angiogram (MRA) may show evidence of a cerebral vasculopathy known as moya moya syndrome. In this there is typically progressive stenosis of the terminal ICA and proximal segments of the major intracranial arteries (Fig. 70.58). There is a predilection for the anterior circulation. As the stenosis progresses, increased flow occurs through proximal collateral vessels, particularly the lenticulostriate and thalamoperforator arteries, resulting in the 'puff of smoke' appearance to which moya moya refers. These are seen as multiple small flow voids within the basal ganglia. Prominent transmedullary veins and pial enhancement may also be seen. Other acquired vascular abnormalities include aneurysms and small arteriovenous malformations.

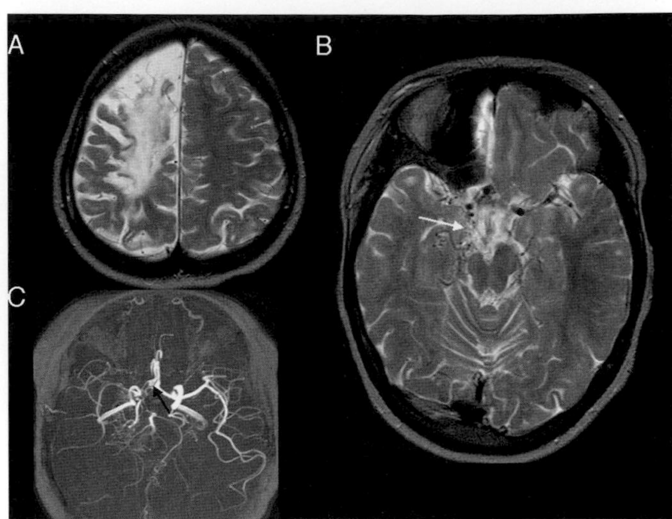

Figure 70.58 Sickle cell disease and moya moya syndrome. Child with extensive frontal, deep and posterior watershed infarction (A). (B) Shows extensive perimesencephalic 'moya moya' collaterals (arrow) and attenuated right middle cerebral artery (MCA) flow voids. (C) Compressed maximum intensity projection image shows narrowed terminal internal carotid artery (ICA), reduced filling of right MCA, and A1 segment of the anterior cerebral artery. There is an aneurysm at the A1/anterior communicating artery (ACOM) junction (arrow).

Referral to a neurosurgical paediatric centre for consideration of external-to-internal carotid (EC–IC) bypass may be indicated. At this point cerebral perfusion imaging to detect 'diffusion–perfusion mismatch' may be helpful in order to assess for critical ischaemia or to select which hemisphere should be revascularized first. This involves a bolus of intravenous contrast medium for MRI perfusion studies and it is important that the child with sickle cell disease is well hydrated for this. Surgical EC–IC bypass may be performed indirectly by mobilization of part of the temporalis muscle with its blood supply, the superficial temporal artery (STA) and laying it onto the pial surface of the brain, or by direct end-to-side anastomosis between the STA and distal MCA branch. Some centres use multiple calvarial burr holes alone to promote superficial angiogenesis and collateral revascularization. Post-operative MRA and perfusion imaging after successful EC–IC bypass should show flow through the STA and increased collateral flow within the distal MCA branches. Perfusion imaging will show increased cerebral blood volume and flow to the revascularized hemisphere.

Moya moya accounts for up to 30% of cerebral vasculopathy in paediatric stroke but it is not unique to sickle cell disease, being also idiopathic, secondary to NF1, cranial irradiation, Down's syndrome, human immunodeficiency virus (HIV) and even tuberculous meningitis. Postinfective angiitis associated with varicella zoster, in which the terminal ICA and proximal MCA are usually affected and there is infarction of the basal ganglia, is relatively common (Fig. 70.59). MRA in the majority (but not all) shows evidence of stabilization or remodelling and improvement of the angiographic appearances at 6-month follow-up.

Arterial dissection may occur intracranially but is also seen, as it is in young adults especially, not infrequently within the cervical arteries. Vertebral arterial dissection occurs most commonly as the vertebral artery exits the transverse foramen of C2 before passing posterolaterally over the lateral masses of C1 to enter the foramen magnum, and ICA dissection occurs above the bifurcation (Fig. 70.59C,D). Dissections may involve intracranial and extracranial arteries. There may be other rarer causes of cervical arterial disease with more diffuse involvement proximal to the bifurcation, e.g. that seen with the connective tissue disorders such as Marfan's, Ehlers–Danlos type IV, osteogenesis imperfecta type I, autosomal dominant polycystic kidney disease, fibromuscular dysplasia, or other causes of cystic medial necrosis and Menke's disease. Cervical arterial dissection may occur without an antecedent history of trauma. As this is a potentially treatable cause of stroke[68], we advocate in all paediatric stroke noninvasive imaging by MRA not only of the intracranial circle of Willis but also of the entire great arteries of the neck from their origins at the aortic arch to their intracranial terminations. Radiological criteria for the diagnosis of dissection are visualization of an intimal flap or a double lumen in the wall of the artery. These pathognomonic signs are detected in fewer than 10% of adult dissections by catheter angiography which remains the gold standard for diagnosis. However, tapering arterial occlusion, the 'string sign' or 'rat's tail' appearance (Fig. 70.59C,D), aneurysmal dilatation of the artery and eccentric mural thrombus are other less specific signs.

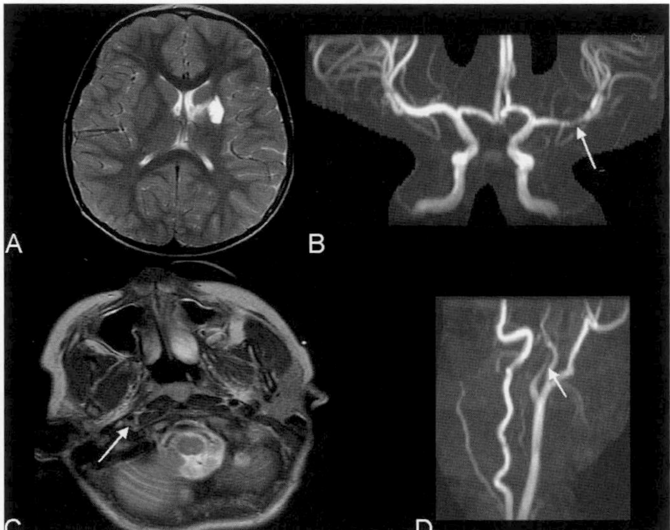

Figure 70.59 Vasculitis. (A,B) In a child with chicken pox vasculitis, axial T2 and maximum intensity projection (MIP) image of time of flight (TOF) circle of Willis MRA show a mature proximal left middle cerebral artery branch infarct with reduced and turbulent flow (arrow) and reduced distal filling. **Arterial dissection.** (C,D) In a 14 year old girl with acute onset left hemiplegia, large right middle cerebral artery territory infarct, and internal carotid artery (ICA) dissection is seen. On the axial T2-weighted image there is an eccentric filling defect within the lumen of the right internal carotid artery which is narrowed, confirming the presence of dissection (arrow). The MIP image of the TOF MRA shows a typical rat's tail appearance of a tapering stenosis distal to the right ICA bifurcation (arrow).

Vein of Galen aneurysmal malformations (VGAMs) are a rare cause of paediatric stroke but have a wide range of clinical presentations and account for 30% of vascular malformations in children. Their recognition is important as there is increasing evidence that appropriate endovascular treatment by neuroradiologists with specialist skill in dealing with paediatric high flow AV shunts in a multidisciplinary setting with access to neonatologists, anaesthetists and neurologists is associated with improved outcome. VGAMs are unique congenital malformations of the intracranial circulation characterized by an enlarged midline venous structure, a persistent embryological remnant, with multiple arteriovenous communications leading to aneurysmal dilatation, presumably secondary to high arteriovenous flow. Neonates may present with severe cardiac failure. In infants and children who present with VGAMs the degree of shunting is much smaller and they may have evidence of hydrocephalus with cerebral atrophy. Older children may have headaches and seizures, and also are more likely to develop intracerebral or subarachnoid haemorrhage.

MRI will demonstrate the dilated venous sac, location of fistulous connections and the arteries involved, venous drainage and any evidence of thrombus within the venous sac (Fig. 70.60). MRI can determine the extent of parenchymal damage, including focal infarctions and generalized cerebral atrophy, although CT is more sensitive for the parenchymal calcification which accompanies chronic venous hypertension. Angiography is the gold standard of diagnosis and ideally should be performed at the time of endovascular treatment. In imaging follow-up, evidence of significant arteriovenous shunting, progressive cerebral damage/atrophy and jugular vein occlusion as a chronic effect of venous hypertension should be sought.

HYPOXIC–ISCHAEMIC INJURY IN THE DEVELOPING BRAIN

Well-recognized patterns of brain injury have been attributed to hypoxic–ischaemic injury and are believed to vary according to the nature and severity of the insult and the degree of maturity of the developing brain[69–72]. The term *partial* hypoxic–ischaemic injury is used to describe an episode or episodes of hypoxia or hypoperfusion to the developing brain, whilst *profound* hypoxic–ischaemic injury is used to describe a briefer episode of anoxia or circulatory arrest. Injuries occurring in the first and early part of the second trimester of pregnancy are expected to result in brain malformations and will not be discussed further in this section. Injuries occurring later will be discussed below.

Preterm patterns

The so-called 'preterm' patterns of hypoxic–ischaemic injury tend to be seen in brains of about 20–35 weeks gestational age and are characterized clinically by a neonatal encephalopathy. Few survive a profound hypoxic–ischaemic injury, but if they do, the pattern of injury appears predominantly to affect

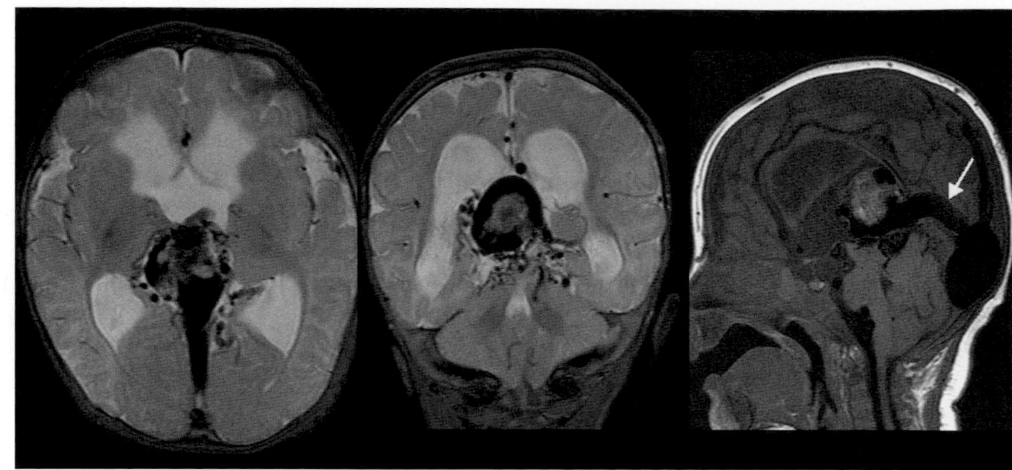

Figure 70.60 Vein of Galen malformation (partly occluded by embolization glue) showing residual flow through the promesencephalic vein, containing a combination of glue and thrombus, via the falcine sinus (arrow) towards the venous confluence. Arterial supply is via a number of choroidal vessels.

the thalami with relative sparing of the other deep grey matter structures. Partial hypoxic–ischaemic injury is believed to result in the most common pattern seen in this age group, which is that of periventricular leukomalacia (PVL), germinal matrix or periventricular haemorrhage and intraventricular haemorrhage (GM/IVH), also described as periventricular haemorrhagic infarction (PVHI)[71,72]. In extreme cases, cystic encephalomalacia may be seen. Outcome is determined by the degree of brain injury and is also influenced by any complications and the effectiveness of any intervention, such as CSF diversion procedures for hydrocephalus.

The physiological conditions necessary for the development of PVL are thought to be present from 25 to 34 weeks gestational age, the condition being most frequent in the older group, 30–33 weeks gestational age. The precise mechanisms responsible for these lesions are not fully understood, but this condition is usually considered to be a complication of prematurity and is probably multifactorial. The clinical picture is spastic diplegia or quadriplegia, often with visual impairment. Mental retardation is usually absent or mild, except in very severe cases, as are seizures[73].

The simplest theory suggests that there is cerebral hypoperfusion and hypoxia causing ischaemic infarction, which in 20% may be complicated by secondary haemorrhage following reperfusion of the damaged areas. The parts of the immature brain most sensitive to insufficient cerebral perfusion or hypoxia are found in the periventricular white matter, which is therefore the most common location of PVL. Factors such as respiratory problems, sepsis, necrotizing enterocolitis, feto-maternal haemorrhage, or hypoglycaemia are associated with PVL. PVL can also be seen in mature newborns but the early stages of damage are not seen as the lesion occurs in utero and is well into the sequence of pathological development by birth at term.

PVL results in infarction with oedema seen in the periventricular region. This may be seen as increased echogenicity on US. The damaged tissue undergoes cystic degeneration 10–20 d after the insult. Small, often confluent, cysts form in the periventricular white matter; these are usually transient and subsequently collapse. The detection of these cysts is the most reliable US finding of PVL in its early development (Fig. 70.61). As the cysts collapse, atrophy of the damaged brain tissue

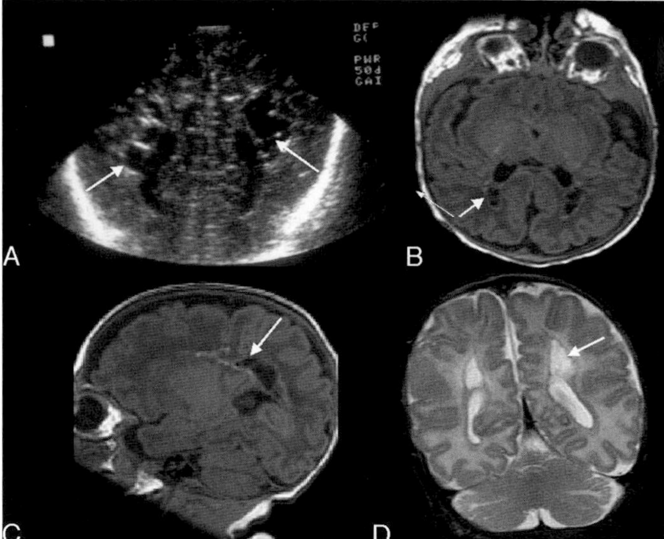

Figure 70.61 Early sign of periventricular leukomalacia. (A) US shows periventricular echolucencies (arrows), one of the earliest signs of periventricular leukomalacia. (B,C) On T1-weighted MRI sequences, these are seen posteriorly in the peritrigonal area and are lined by small focal regions of T1 shortening in keeping with haemorrhage (arrows).

follows and this process is first detected by the demonstration of secondary ventricular dilatation; in more severe cases there is a more generalized loss of brain tissue, particularly white matter. Ventricular dilatation beyond normal limits is usually detectable by US or CT 4–8 weeks after the injury, depending on the severity of the lesions, and persists throughout life as permanent tissue loss. The features of end-stage PVL result from the decreased amount of periventricular white matter adjacent to the trigones. There is ventricular dilatation with irregular ventricular margins and the distribution is characteristically worst in the parieto-occipital regions with sparing of the frontal and temporal regions. Injury to the remaining white matter is more difficult to detect and MRI is most reliable in demonstrating these end-stage changes of PVL, 1–2 years after the injury, when the myelination process is complete or almost complete. MRI then shows abnormal signal in the remaining periventricular white matter (Fig. 70.62).

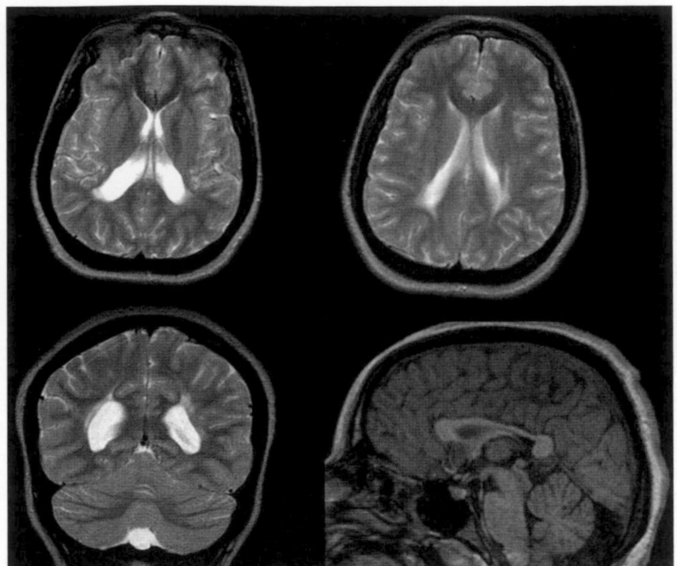

Figure 70.62 End-stage changes of periventricular leukomalacia. A child with spastic diplegia scanned much later in life (15 years) has the typical chronic changes of periventricular leukomalacia. There is posterior periventricular increased signal on T2-weighted images and enlargement of the ventricles posteriorly with irregular, scalloped margins, indicating white matter loss. The corpus callosum seen on the sagittal T1-weighted MRI is markedly thinned, particularly affecting the posterior body.

GM/IVH is also common in the immature brain but is possibly less significant in terms of subsequent handicap. The cause of IVH is also thought to be fluctuations in cerebral perfusion. The germinal matrix is in a process of involution after 24 weeks gestational age and its fragile vessels rupture easily. Its proximity to the lateral ventricle, from which it is separated only by ependyma, frequently results in rupture of haemorrhage into the ventricular system.

In some immature neonates with IVH, the amount of blood is excessive and it dilates the ventricle, causing congestion in the periventricular white matter, venous infarction and secondary haemorrhage. The lesions are often unilateral and anterior, and tend to occur in the group of neonates younger than 30 weeks gestational age. The findings are well seen on US which is used for grading the severity of disease. Later, resolution of the parenchymal haemorrhage results in either paraventricular cavities which may communicate with the ventricle or focal dilatations of the ventricles.

Term patterns

The 'term' patterns of hypoxic–ischaemic injury tend to be seen in brains of about 36–42 weeks gestational age at the time of the insult. The pattern that is attributed to profound hypoxic–ischaemic injury characteristically affects the brain regions that are most metabolically active and therefore most selectively vulnerable at the time of insult. These are the posterolateral putamina, ventrolateral thalami and adjacent capsular white matter. The hippocampi, peri-Rolandic (motor and sensory) cortex and visual cortex are also often affected, and the changes are typically bilateral and symmetrical. The cerebellar vermis is also recognized as selectively vulnerable in this context. This pattern is often matched with the clinical picture of dyskinetic or dystonic cerebral palsy[70,72].

The injuries attributed to partial hypoxic ischaemia are seen in a parasagittal distribution, typically involving a combination of cortex and subcortical white matter, and most often across the frontoparietal regions. Whilst usually bilateral, this pattern is not uncommonly asymmetric. A characteristic region of involvement is the posterior part of the Sylvian fissures. More characteristically, the greatest injury occurs at the base of the gyri, within the depths of the sulci, resulting in focal atrophy in these areas and a pattern recognized as ulegyria (Fig. 70.63). As with the preterm brain, more prolonged insults are thought to result in cystic encephalomalacia (Fig. 70.64). The predominant involvement of the cerebral hemipheres with relative sparing of the posterior fossa structures is a pattern that favours hypoxic–ischaemic injury over other causes of global brain injury at term, such as perinatal/neonatal infection.

The common clinical sequelae of this type of injury are microcephaly with severe mental retardation and spastic quadriplegia which may be asymmetric[74].

MISCELLANEOUS ACQUIRED TOXIC OR METABOLIC DISEASE

Kernicterus is the result of the toxic effect of neonatal unconjugated hyperbilirubinaemia on the brain. The brain regions

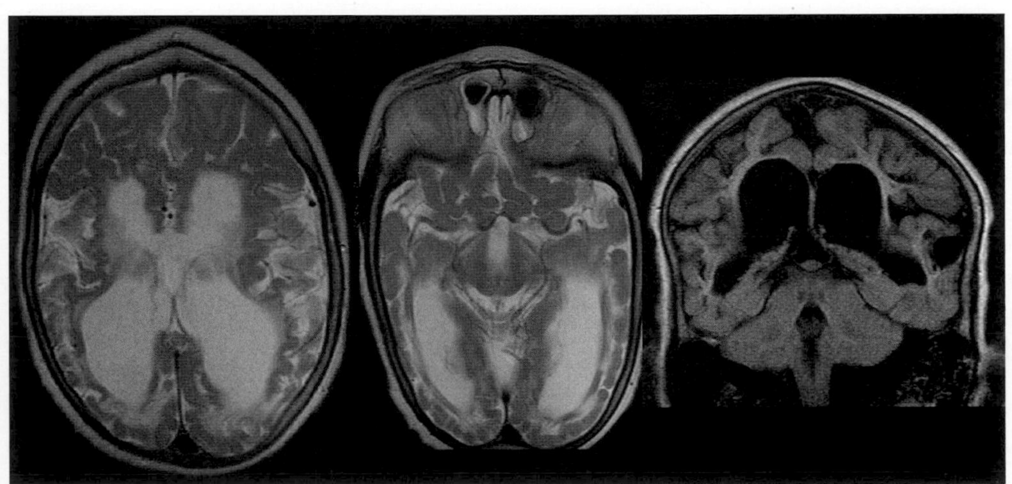

Figure 70.63 Hypoxic ischaemia at term, imaged in childhood. The gyri are thinner at their bases than at their apices. This is known as ulegyria and dates the hypoxic–ischaemic event to term. Note the relative preservation of the cerebellum and brainstem.

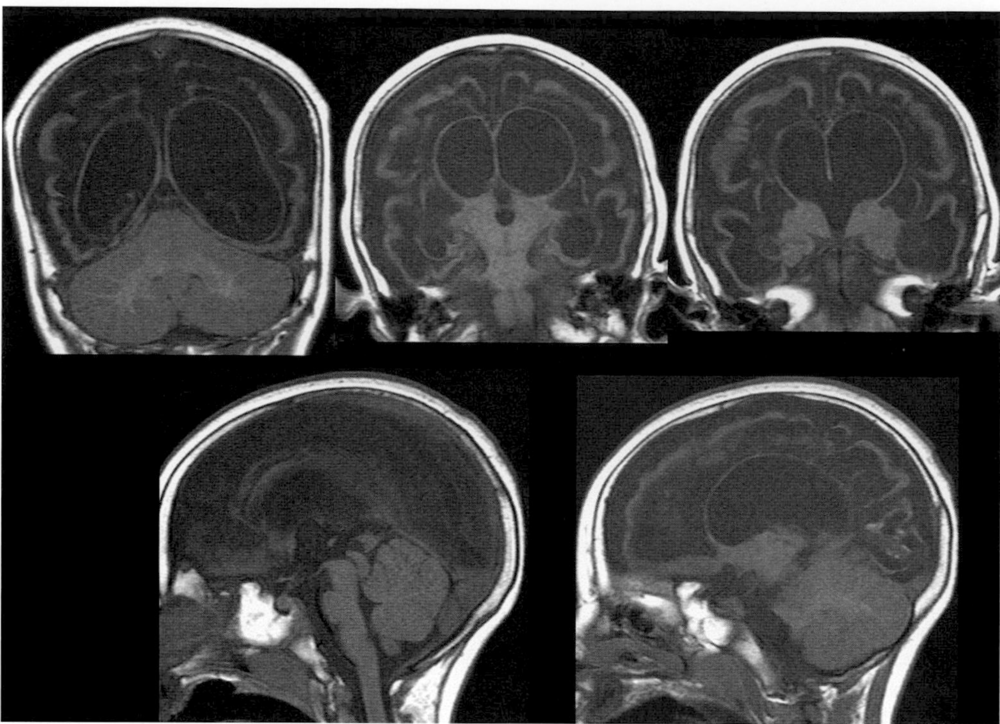

Figure 70.64 Prolonged hypoxic ischaemia resulting in multicystic encephalomalacia. There is cystic cavitation of most of the white matter with grossly thinned corpus callosum, leaving only a very thin rim of preserved cortical mantle.

that have selective susceptibility include the globus pallidi, subthalamic nuclei and hippocampi, as well as cranial nerves VIII, VII and III. Neonates with bilirubin encephalopathy have a depressed conscious level, hypotonia and seizures with opisthotonus. Delayed effects include extrapyramidal signs (athetosis), deafness, gaze palsies and developmental delay. In the acute stage there is signal abnormality with bilateral symmetrical T2 prolongation and swelling of the globus pallidi. There may be T1 shortening also. Eventually the pallidal changes will progress to atrophy with variable persistent gliotic change. US and CT are initially normal although later there may be evidence of calcification.

Hypoglycaemia may also present with a nonspecific encephalopathy subsequently leading to seizures. This is a problem particularly with neonates who have immature enzyme pathways and relatively poor glycogen reserves, particularly in the context of increased requirements due to sepsis or associated hypoxia–ischaemia but may also be the end result of some inborn errors of metabolism or hyperinsulinism. Imaging studies may show evidence of a diffuse encephalopathy but the findings are typically most severe in the parieto-occipital regions. There is T1 and T2 prolongation with swelling affecting the cortex and subcortical white matter with variable restricted diffusion (Fig. 70.65), progressing to the chronic sequelae of cerebral infarction with evidence of gliosis, cavitation and atrophy. Pallidal damage may also occur.

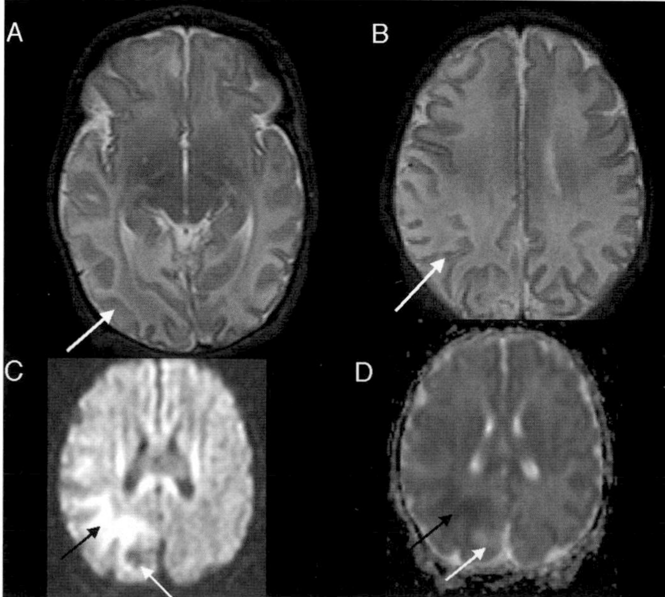

Figure 70.65 Neonate with seizures and hypoglycaemia shows (A,B) increased signal within the parieto-occipital cortex and white matter, with patchy loss of the normal cortical low signal (arrow). (C) Diffusion-weighted image and (D) ADC map show that the diffusion changes are a mixture of restricted (black arrows) and increased diffusion (white arrows). *All* of these changes, including the T2 and restricted areas of diffusion, completely resolved on follow-up.

Hypernatraemia is most commonly seen in premature infants, particularly if there is additional dehydration, e.g. due to diarrhoea. Affected infants have a depressed conscious level and irritability. There is an osmotic water shift from the intracellular to the extracellular space resulting in interstitial oedema, manifest by T1 and T2 prolongation with increased diffusion, but also in parenchymal haemorrhage as the brain shrinks and bridging dural veins are torn as they are pulled away from the calvarium.

Toxic exposure should be considered in children, particularly adolescents, with acute neurological symptoms and bilateral symmetrical grey matter involvement. Toxins include toluene or other organic solvents, cyanide and carbon monoxide poisoning.

INTRACRANIAL AND INTRASPINAL INFECTIONS

Congenital infections (TORCH)

These infections are acquired in utero or during passage through the birth canal; bacterial infections spread from the cervix to the amniotic fluid while toxoplasmosis, rubella, cytomegalovirus (CMV), syphilis and human immunodeficiency virus (HIV) spread via the transplacental route, and herpes simplex virus (HSV) is acquired from direct exposure to maternal type II herpetic genital lesions during delivery. The stage of brain development judged by the gestational age is more important than the actual organism in determining the pattern of CNS injury. Therefore in utero infections acquired before 16–18 weeks, when neurones are forming within the germinal matrix and migrating to form the cerebral cortex, produce lissencephaly and a small cerebellum. Spontaneous abortion is also a frequent outcome during this time. Between 18 and 24 weeks, when the cortical neurones are organizing but the immature brain is unable to mount an inflammatory response, the infective insult may produce localized dysplastic cortex and porencephaly. This is seen as a smooth-walled cavity isointense to CSF on all sequences in continuity with the ventricular system and without evidence of gliosis. From the third trimester onwards the insult results in asymmetrical cerebral damage with gliosis, cystic change and calcification.

CMV is the most common cause of serious viral infection in fetuses and neonates in the West, occurring in up to 1% of all births. It is acquired transplacentally and the vertical transmission rate is 30–40%. The classical manifestations of CMV disease at birth include hepatosplenomegaly, petechiae, thrombocytopenia, microcephaly, chorioretinitis and sensorineural deafness occurring in up to 10% of CMV infection, but there is also an increased risk of developing deafness and other neurological deficits up to 2 years after exposure. The mechanism of injury may be due to a direct insult to the germinal matrix cells leading to periventricular calcification, cortical malformations with microcephaly and cerebellar hypoplasia, or due to the virus causing a vascular insult.

Transfontanelle cranial US may demonstrate branching curvilinear hyperechogenicity in the basal ganglia, or 'lenticulostriate vasculopathy', which may also be seen with other congenital infections, hypoxic–ischaemia and trisomy 13 and 21. Infants affected in the second trimester have lissencephaly with a thin cortex, hypoplastic cerebellum, ventriculomegaly and periventricular calcification, which is more reliably detected on CT than MRI. Those injured later, probably during the period of cortical organization in the second trimester, have polymicrogyria, with less ventricular dilatation and cerebellar hypoplasia, and later infection produces parenchymal damage, large ventricles, calcification and haemorrhage without an underlying structural brain malformation. Temporal pole cysts are also a feature.

Toxoplasmosis is a protozoan infection caused by ingestion by the mother of *Toxoplasma gondii* oocytes in undercooked meat. The transmission rate is high and increases from 30% at 6 months' gestation to approaching 100% at term. The incidence of congenital infection is approximately 1 in 1000 to 1 in 3400 but it accounts for 1% of all stillbirths. When the CNS is involved the infection may cause a granulomatous meningitis or diffuse encephalitis. Most infants at birth are asymptomatic, although sequelae such as seizures, hydrocephalus and chorioretinitis may appear later. Imaging features of microcephaly and parenchymal calcification are similar to CMV infection although cerebellar hypoplasia and polymicrogyria are not seen, and the ventriculomegaly may be due to an active ependymitis causing obstructive hydrocephalus rather than diffuse cerebral damage (Fig. 70.66). The severity of brain involvement correlates with earlier maternal infection.

The CNS involvement in HSV is a rapidly disseminating diffuse encephalitis unlike the pattern of involvement in children or adults in which disease starts within the mesial temporal lobes and spreads within the limbic system. CT and MRI of neonatal infection show widespread asymmetrical regions of hypodensity or T2 hyperintensity mainly in the white matter. As the disease progresses there is increasing swelling and cortical involvement (CT cortical hyperdensity and T1/T2 shortening on MRI) and meningeal enhancement. Subsequent loss of brain parenchyma occurs early on, often as early as the second week, eventually resulting in profound cerebral atrophy, cystic encephalomalacia and calcification.

Congenital rubella is now very rare in the West following the introduction of mass immunization programmes, but immigrant populations remain at risk as do populations where uptake of the MMR vaccine is low. In the first 8 weeks, cataracts, glaucoma and cardiac malformations occur while in the third trimester infection may be asymptomatic. Brain imaging appearances demonstrate similar changes to other congenital infections depending on the timing of the insult.

It is estimated that over 60 million people worldwide are infected with HIV. Almost half are women and vertical transmission of HIV accounts for 90% of newly diagnosed cases. Children with congenitally acquired AIDS usually present between the ages of 2 months and 8 years with nonspecific signs such as hepatosplenomegaly and failure to thrive. Neonatal presentation is unusual. Affected children may develop a

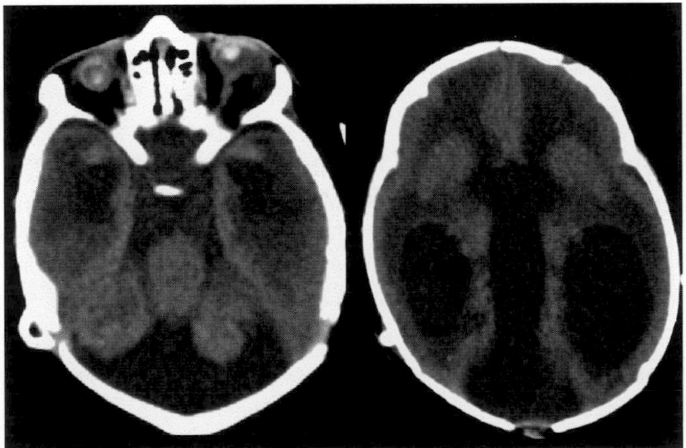

Figure 70.66 CT of a neonate with congenital TORCH infection. Both the globes are small and calcified (phthisis bulbi). There is a Dandy–Walker malformation and hydrocephalus with transependymal oedema.

progressive HIV encephalopathy in which dementia, spasticity and increasing head size occur. A more static form is also seen in which cognitive and motor developmental delay predominate. Global atrophy and bilateral basal ganglia calcification are the most common imaging findings. Diffuse symmetrical periventricular and deep white matter abnormalities are seen in almost half of children with HIV encephalopathy and are usually associated with mild atrophy. HIV may also cause corticospinal tract degeneration.

Meningitis

Meningitis is the most common infection in childhood. The diagnosis is made not on imaging but on the presence of clinical symptoms and signs and the results of lumbar puncture. Indeed in uncomplicated meningitis the imaging is usually normal, and the role of neuroimaging is to detect the complications of meningitis. Neuroimaging is indicated when the diagnosis is unclear, if the meningitis is associated with persistent seizures or focal neurological deficits, if symptoms or signs suggest raised intracranial pressure, or when recovery is unduly slow.

Pathophysiology

Organisms reach the meninges by five main routes: direct spread from an adjacent infection, especially otitis media and sinusitis; haematogenous spread; rupture of a superficial cortical abscess; passage through the choroid plexus; or from direct penetrating trauma. Cerebral infarction (venous and arterial) is seen in 30% of neonates with bacterial meningitis. Infection spreads along the adventitia of penetrating cortical vessels within the periventricular spaces. Arterial thrombosis may arise from the resulting arterial wall inflammation and necrosis, or from a similar process affecting the arteries that traverse basal meningitic exudates. Venous thrombosis and subsequent infarction is particularly common in the presence of subdural empyemas due to veins becoming thrombosed as they traverse the infected subdural space. Extension of the infection through thrombosed vessels into the brain parenchyma can result in cerebritis and abscess formation. Fibropurulent exudates in the basal cisterns, ventricular outlet foramina or over the brain convexity result in hydrocephalus due either to the obstruction of CSF flow or failure of resorption. Ventriculitis occurs in about 30% of children with meningitis and is particularly common in neonates with ependymal changes seen in severe or prolonged meningitis. Later on, ventricular enlargement may persist due to damage to the adjacent periventricular white matter and parenchymal loss.

Neonatal meningitis has two distinct clinical presentations. The first presents in the first few days of life with overwhelming generalized sepsis often in association with complicated labour, such as premature rupture of membranes. The second develops after the first week with milder systemic sepsis but with more meningitic features.

In older infants and children acute bacterial meningitis has a mortality of 5% in the developed world which rises to between 12% and 50% in developing countries where there is a high incidence of permanent neurological sequelae.

Uncomplicated meningitis

Although neuroimaging is not performed for this indication alone and is usually normal, occasionally meningeal enhancement may be seen on CT or MRI. MRI is more sensitive than CT but the sensitivity of either/both is insufficient to warrant imaging as a diagnostic test for meningitis. Imaging findings are more useful for chronic and granulomatous meningitides where dense enhancing basal exudates may be seen within the cisternal spaces. Recurrent meningitis is unusual and full neuro-axis imaging is often applied to identify underlying risk factors (see below).

Imaging of complications (Table 70.4)

Hydrocephalus may be detected on CT or MRI and may reflect a combination of obstructed CSF flow and impaired absorption. Ependymitis may cause debris/haemorrhage within the ventricular system resulting in obstructive hydrocephalus at the foramen of Monro, cerebral aqueduct and fourth ventricular outlet foramina. Purulent exudates may impair CSF absorption within the subarachnoid space resulting in communicating hydrocephalus.

Table 70.4 INTRACRANIAL COMPLICATIONS OF MENINGITIS IN INFANTS

Pathology	Imaging
Cerebritis	Diffuse hypodensity (CT), hyperintensity (T2-weighted MRI) involving cortex and white matter, gyral swelling, ill-defined enhancement
Abscess formation	Peripheral rim enhancement surrounding central necrotic cavity, adjacent oedema
Effusion	Cerebrospinal fluid density/signal subdural collection, no pathological enhancement
Empyema	Higher density (CT), restricted diffusion (MRI) subdural collection with pachymeningeal/dural enhancement
Deep venous thrombosis	Hyperdense expanded venous sinus (CT), lack of T2 flow void, expanded sinus (MRI), variable haemorrhagic venous infarction
Cavernous sinus thrombosis	Expanded cavernous sinus, filling defects on CTV, signal drop off MRV
Arterial thrombosis	Large arterial territory infarct, basal ganglia/thalamic small perforating arterial territory infarcts
Ventriculitis	Debris within ventricular system, hyperdense ependyma (pre-contrast), ependymal contrast enhancement, ventricular isolation
Hydrocephalus	Obstructive intraventricular (foramen of Monro, cerebral aqueduct), obstructive extraventricular, communicating
Deafness	CT/MRI evidence of labyrinthitis ossificans

Sterile subdural effusions are often seen as a complication of meningitis, particularly in neonates with *Streptococcus pneumoniae* or *Haemophilus influenzae*. They are not empyemas, do not need to be surgically treated and will regress as the meningitis is treated. On imaging, the subdural collections have density and signal characteristics similar to CSF on CT and MRI, though they may be slightly hyperintense to CSF on MRI.Enhancement is not usually seen; however, leptomeningeal (pial) enhancement, to be distinguished from pachymeningeal (dural) enhancement, may be seen as a result of underlying brain infarction or due to leptomeningeal inflammation.

Subdural empyemas may require urgent surgical drainage to prevent further cerebritis and cerebral infarction.These appear as more proteinaceous subdural collections (increased density on CT, intermediate T1 signal intensity relative to CSF, T2 hyperintensity) with pachymeningeal (dural) and leptomeningeal enhancement (Fig. 70.67).

Imaging evidence for ventriculitis, usually spread via the choroid plexus, comes from the finding of debris layered posteriorly within the ventricular system and ependyma which are hyperdense on CT. Hydrocephalus may be seen and there may be isolation of various components of the ventricular system resulting in some parts draining adequately while others remain dilated as debris obstructs the CSF outlet foramina. Infection may extend directly into the adjacent brain parenchyma causing cerebritis.

Thrombosis of deep venous sinuses and cortical veins may occur, particularly in children with dehydration (Fig. 70.68). The symptoms of deep venous sinus thrombosis, such as headache, impaired consciousness and prolonged fitting, cannot be distinguished from the symptoms of the underlying meningitis and neuroimaging is required for confirmation. Cavernous sinus thrombosis is uncommon, is more commonly seen with paranasal sinus, dental or orbital infection, and tends to present with ophthalmoplegia due to involvement of the cranial nerves II, IV, and VI as they pass through the cavernous sinus. Direct involvement of the cavernous carotid artery by infection may produce a mycotic aneurysm. In generalized sepsis, the sagittal and transverse sinuses are most commonly involved.

Deep venous sinus thrombosis may be seen as a hyperdense expanded sinus on unenhanced CT.As the thrombus becomes less dense, intravenous enhancement may demonstrate the 'empty delta' sign as a filling defect within the sinus lumen. A dense cortical vein may also be seen on CT but neither CT nor MRI can reliably detect cortical vein thrombosis.

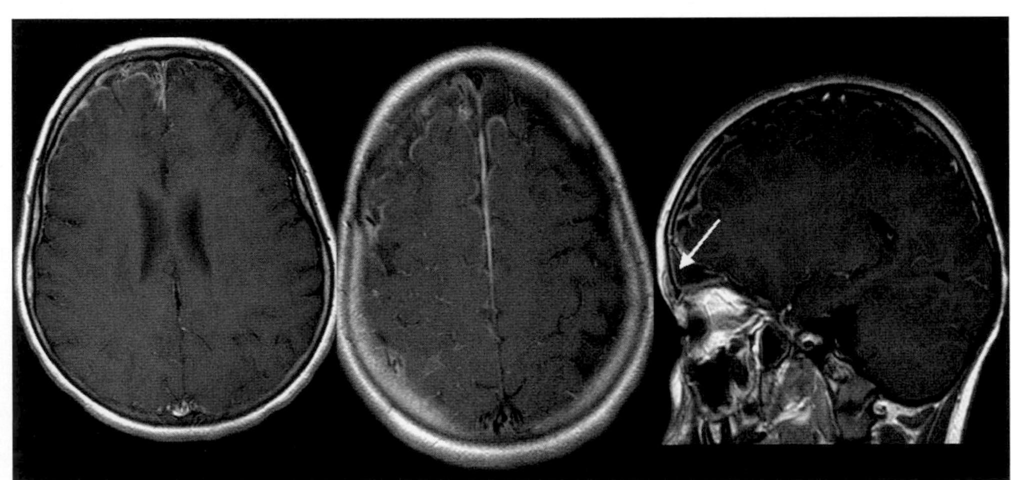

Figure 70.67 Bilateral subdural empyemas. There is leptomeningeal and pachymeningeal enhancement (arrows) most marked over the right cerebral convexity and extending back to the vertex (on the sagittal view). There is enhancing debris within the subdural space and the signal is slightly increased compared to cerebrospinal fluid. The source of infection was from the frontal sinus (arrow).

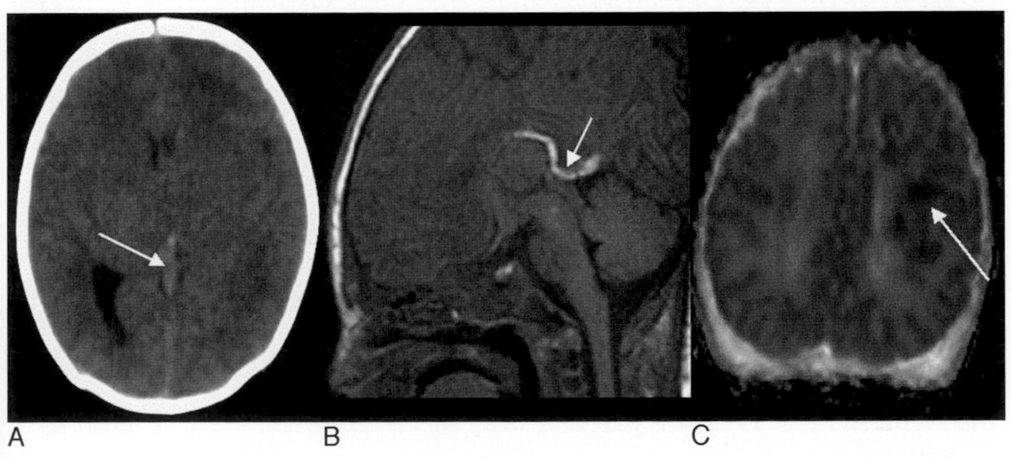

Figure 70.68 Venous sinus thrombosis in a child with recent history of nausea and vomiting. (A) CT shows hyperdense thrombus within the vein of Galen just reaching the internal cerebral veins (arrow). There is diffuse cerebral swelling with more hypodense change and swelling affecting the left hemisphere and thalami (B) Sagittal T1-weighted MRI confirms the diagnosis with T1 shortening in keeping with methaemoglobin in the internal cerebral veins and vein of Galen (arrow). (C) The ADC map shows patchy restricted diffusion (low signal) (arrow) within the deep white matter in keeping with infarction.

The diagnosis of deep venous sinus thrombosis may be missed in up to 40% of patients at CT; MRI with MR venography (MRV) is more sensitive. In the subacute phase thrombus is seen as T1 shortening within an expanded sinus and this finding may be sufficient to make the diagnosis. In the acute phase when the thrombus is isointense on T1-weighted imaging and hypointense on T2-weighted imaging it can be mistaken for flowing blood, although the sinus, in the latter, should not be expanded. MRV is useful to confirm absence of flow in the thrombosed sinus.

Venous infarction may occur in up to 40% of children with deep venous sinus thrombosis. Venous infarcts are often bilateral, do not conform to an arterial territory but to the territory of venous drainage, and are frequently haemorrhagic. They are parasagittal when the superior sagittal sinus is involved, thalamic when the internal cerebral veins or straight sinus/vein of Galen are involved, and temporal lobe when the transverse or sigmoid sinus or vein of Labbé (one of the deep superficial venous system anastomoses connecting the middle cerebral vein to the transverse sinus) are involved. On diffusion imaging there is a mixture of restricted and free diffusion even when nonhaemorrhagic.

Arterial infarction may be seen as wedge-shaped cortical and white matter hypodensity conforming to a major arterial territory on CT or as T2 hyperintensity and T1 hypointensity with cortical highlighting on MRI. The basal meningitis may occlude small perforating branches from the circle of Willis causing small infarcts in the region of the deep grey nuclei (basal ganglia and thalami).

Labyrinthitis ossificans, the most common cause of acquired deafness in childhood, is one of the sequelae of bacterial meningitis resulting from direct spread of infection from the meninges into the inner ear. Faint enhancement of the membranous labyrinth may be seen on enhanced T1-weighted images in acute infection. In some children inflammation persists; fibrosis and ossification subsequently develop and may be detected on high-resolution CT of the temporal bone, as increased density within the membranous labyrinth. High-resolution T2-weighted MRI (e.g. performed with 3DFT-CISS imaging) may be more sensitive than CT to the changes of labyrinthitis ossificans, and T2 signal drop-off may detect the fibrous stage before ossification when children are still suitable for cochlear implantation. Once the typical appearances of diffuse labyrinthitis ossificans develop, cochlear implantation is much more difficult (Fig. 70.69).

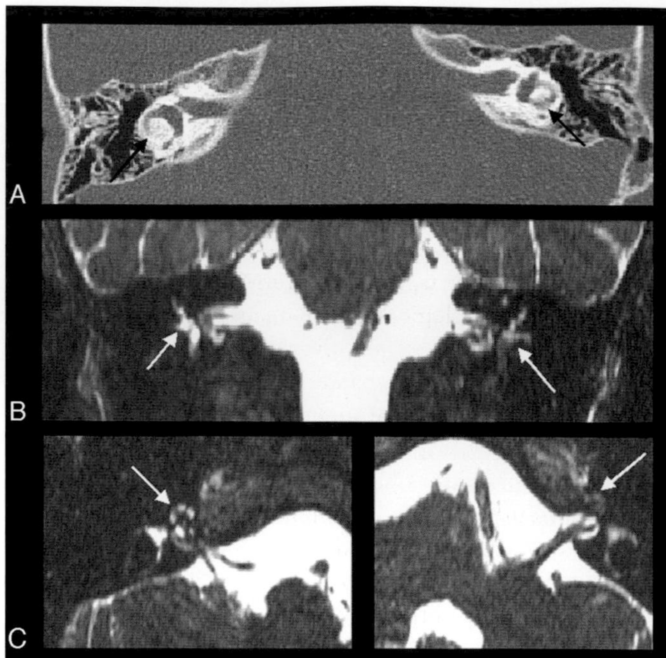

Figure 70.69 Child with recent meningitis and new sensorineural deafness. (A) High-resolution axial CT through the petrous bones shows increased density in keeping with calcification within the lateral semicircular canals (arrows). (B) Coronal and (C) axial CISS MRI shows reduced T2 signal within all the semicircular canals (arrows), particularly the left, confirmed on the oblique axial views (C). There is reduced signal within the cochlea, again worse on the left (arrows). These are typical features of labyrinthitis ossificans.

Tuberculous infection

Tuberculosis (TB) has risen in incidence recently, and while it remains a serious problem in children, there does not appear to have been an increase in tuberculous meningitis in children as yet, possibly due to targeted immunization of at-risk immigrant populations. TB may cause meningitis, cerebritis and abscess formation (tuberculomas). With leptomeningeal disease, which may be seen without evidence of miliary TB elsewhere, thick enhancing purulent soft tissue exudates may be seen in the subarachnoid space, particularly in the basal cisterns, and associated with hydrocephalus, basal ganglia and thalamic infarcts. Larger major arterial branch cortical infarcts are seen less frequently. Tuberculomas are seen as solid or ring-enhancing lesions, particularly at the grey–white matter junction.

Bacterial infection: cerebritis and abscess formation

Cerebritis is the earliest stage of purulent brain infection, may be focal or multifocal, and may resolve or evolve into frank abscess formation. Predisposing conditions include middle ear, dental and paranasal sinus infection, penetrating injury, postoperative complication or dermal sinus, immune deficiency, and any cause of arteriovenous shunting (e.g. cyanotic congenital heart disease). Fungal infection may also cause brain abscesses, particularly in immunocompromised children, but in this case the lesion may not be able to encapsulate because this requires the ability to mount an adequate immune response. Radiological differentiation between cerebritis and abscess formation is important because cerebritis may respond to antibiotics while an abscess may require surgical drainage as an adjunct. During the cerebritis stage CT and MRI show an ill-defined area of oedema with swelling with or without variable ill-defined enhancement and haemorrhagic transformation. As the infection becomes more established, focal areas may become walled-off and abscess formation occurs. On imaging this appears as a space-occupying lesion with a central region of pus manifest as low density on CT, or T2 hyperintensity on MRI, surrounded by an enhancing wall. The wall of the cavity may demonstrate T1/T2 shortening. Typically there is surrounding oedema. The central region of pus shows restricted diffusion and this may help to differentiate abscesses from necrotic or cystic tumours which usually demonstrate central areas of increased diffusion. Imaging can be used to monitor response to treatment although there may be a lag time between the resolution of imaging findings and clinical response.

Neurocysticercosis

Cysticercosis occurs from ingestion of the encysted form of *Taenia solium* (porcine tapeworm). Humans act as the intermediate host and neurological disease occurs as the host mounts an inflammatory response and the parasites die. In children a typical presentation is with parenchymal cysts associated with seizures, headache and focal neurological deficits. These may occur anywhere within the brain but typically at the grey–white matter interface. Calcification may occur and may be punctate within the solid component or may occur within the wall of the cyst. Perilesional oedema is the result of the inflammatory response to the dying larva. Lesions at various stages of development may be seen. Therefore active lesions seen as regions of oedema may coexist with ring or solid enhancing lesions with or without oedema, and with foci of calcification without oedema or enhancement which are burnt out lesions following the death of the parasite.

There are also leptomeningeal, intraventricular and racemose forms of neurocysticercosis. Leptomeningeal disease is demonstrated on CT or MRI by soft tissue filling the basal cisterns with marked contrast enhancement. Granulomata with variable calcification may be seen within the subarachnoid space. Hydrocephalus and brain infarcts are also complications. Intraventricular cysticerci are important to detect because of the risk of acute onset hydrocephalus and sudden death. MRI is more sensitive than CT at identifying the cysts with their scolex. In the racemose form there are multilobular cysts without a scolex within the subarachnoid space, typically in the cerebellopontine angles, suprasellar region and basal cisterns and Sylvian fissures. They may demonstrate enhancement and may coexist with leptomeningitis.

Viral encephalitis

The typical pattern of viral encephalitis is that of patchy and asymmetrical disease with a predeliction for grey matter. The anterior temporal and inferior frontal cortical regions are a classical location for herpes encephalitis. Another characteristic herpes virus pattern is the involvement of the hippocampi and cingulate gyrus as a limbic encephalitis. More widespread hemispheric involvement is seen with a variety of enteroviruses, echovirus and cocksackie virus in particular.

A more unusual pattern of deep grey matter and upper brainstem disease is seen with rare types of viral encephalitis. Patchy enhancement with oedema has been seen with Epstein–Barr virus infection and may also be mimicked by mycoplasma infection. Thalamic and upper brainstem involvement, occasionally with haemorrhagic change, is a feature of Japanese encephalitis and the related West Nile virus.

Acute cerebellitis presents infrequently in children with sudden onset of truncal ataxia, dysarthria, involuntary eye movements due to a swollen cerebellum, and nausea, headache and vomiting due to resulting hydrocephalus. Fever and meningism may also be present. The many causes of a swollen cerebellum include infectious (e.g. pertussis), post-infectious (e.g. acute disseminated encephalomyelitis [ADEM]), toxic, such as lead poisoning and vasculitis. Imaging shows effacement of the cerebellar fissures, enlarged cerebellum, signal abnormality affecting the cortex and white matter, and variable hydrocephalus. Although the cerebellar swelling may resolve spontaneously, surgical CSF diversion may be necessary as a temporary measure.

Infection in immunocompromised children

Children with primary, acquired or iatrogenic immunodeficiencies are vulnerable to opportunistic and unusual organisms. Examples include fungal infections such as aspergillosis, actinomyces and unusual bacterial infections such as atypical mycobacteria. The host's ability to develop an inflammatory response may be limited and the interpretation of images should be considered in this context. Contrast enhancement remains a useful hallmark. A diffuse pattern of nodular leptomeningeal and parenchymal disease may be seen. Conversely, focal large parenchymal abscesses or mycetomas may develop.

Spinal infections

The patterns of discitis and spondylitis in children are similar to those of young adults and do not need to be discussed in detail in this chapter. However, special mention should be made of congenital spinal abnormalities (see Chapter 51) that may harbour or increase the risk of spinal infection. These children may present with recurrent meningitis. Spinal imaging may reveal a dorsal dermal sinus tract or an intraspinal dermoid.

Brain and cord inflammation

Children may develop CNS disease known as acute disseminated encephalomyelitis (ADEM) following an infection, usually viral, or vaccination. This is assumed to be a post-infectious inflammatory immune-mediated phenomenon. Affected children present with focal neurological deficits, headache, fever and altered consciousness following a recent infection. Classically ADEM is a monophasic disease occurring at multiple sites within the brain and spinal cord. Most children recover completely, although 10–30% will have a permanent neurological deficit. Occasionally ADEM may present with relapses occurring within a few months of the original presentation, but these are still considered as part of a monophasic inflammatory process. When relapses occur that are more disseminated in time or place the diagnosis of multiple sclerosis (MS) may be made. On follow-up imaging, children with ADEM have no new lesions and complete or partial resolution of the majority of old lesions, while in MS there are new lesions which may or may not be symptomatic.

On MRI multiple asymmetrical areas of demyelination seen as increased signal intensity on T2-weighted imaging with swelling occur within the subcortical white matter of both hemispheres and may also involve the cerebellum and spinal cord. Cortical and deep grey matter may also be involved but to a lesser extent (Fig. 70.70). Diffusion-weighted imaging

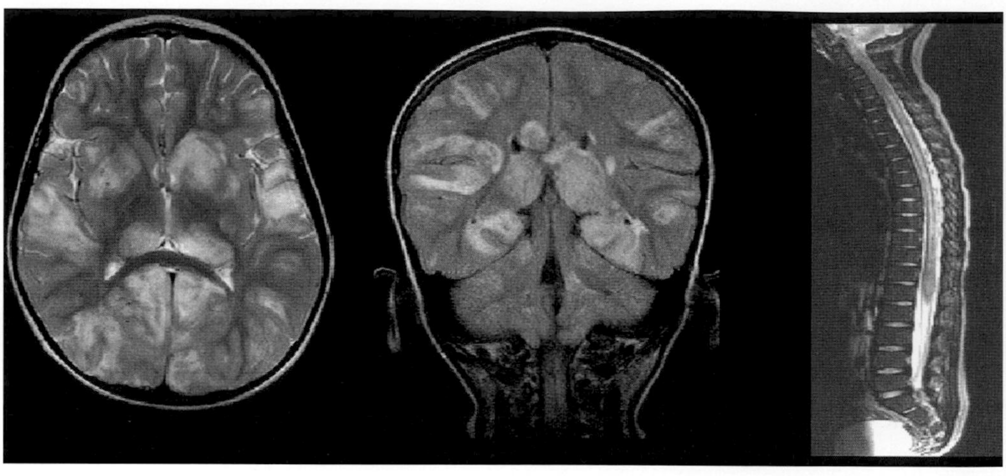

Figure 70.70 Acute disseminated encephalomyelitis in an 11 year old boy with recent viral illness and acute impaired consciousness. MRI shows bilateral, asymmetrical, mainly subcortical, cerebral hemisphere white matter lesions but also involving the cortex and deep grey matter. The cerebellum and spinal cord are also involved. There is focal swelling of the involved regions. The imaging features are typical of acute disseminated encephalomyelitis. The child made a full recovery.

shows increased free diffusion within the lesions. Occasionally, a fulminant haemorrhagic form may develop. Periventricular and callosal lesions (such as Dawson's fingers) are more in keeping with MS lesions while cortical abnormality is not seen with MS and deep grey matter involvement, though seen in both, is more frequent in ADEM. Other differentials include viral encephalitis, which typically is more cortically based, and vasculitis (the lesions should also show restricted diffusion).

TRAUMA

Birth trauma

Extracranial haemorrhage may be seen as a consequence of birth trauma and more often with instrumental delivery. It does not usually require imaging but may be detected on images done for intracranial assessment. Subgaleal haemorrhage may occur deep to the scalp aponeurosis. As there is a large potential space the extent of haemorrhage may occasionally be severe, requiring transfusion. Cephalhaematoma is a traumatic subperiosteal haemorrhage between the vault and the outer layer of periosteum and is therefore confined by the sutures. It may calcify peripherally where the periosteum calcifies. Very rarely forceps may cause skull fractures. These may be linear, depressed or 'ping pong' (depressed without a fracture line, but to be distinguished from an asymptomatic parietal depression which is a normal variant) with a cephalhaematoma overlying them. Caput succadaneum is due to diffuse oedema and bleeding under the scalp and is more commonly seen with prolonged vaginal or Ventouse delivery.

Birth trauma can result in a subdural haematoma, which may be seen even without instrumental delivery. Most are small, clinically silent and infratentorial, although they may extend above the tentorium cerebelli, and resolve spontaneously within 4 weeks. Occasionally they are large and associated with extensive intracranial haemorrhage and hydrocephalus. However, small posterior fossa subdural bleeds are common incidental findings on MRI when newborn infants are imaged for clinical CNS illness.

The spinal cord may be injured by distraction during a difficult delivery, usually a breech delivery, typically affecting the lower cervical and upper thoracic regions. The cord can be transected while the soft and compliant spine remains undamaged. A more common birth-related neurological injury is brachial plexus damage secondary to traction of the shoulder during a breech delivery of the head. Brachial plexus MRI may show CSF signal pseudomeningoceles around the avulsed nerve roots.

Growing skull fractures

Growing skull fractures are seen when there is a dural tear deep to the fracture and usually also when there is localized brain parenchymal damage, which may be associated with a focal neurological deficit or seizures (Fig. 70.71). CSF pulsation may keep the tear open, preventing healing of both the dura and the fracture. The fracture margins become progressively widened on serial radiographs and are bevelled and sclerotic. It usually occurs in children under 1 year with 90% occurring under the age of 3. A leptomeningeal cyst with arachnoid adhesions can cause further pressure erosion.

Spinal trauma

The investigation of spinal trauma in children requires knowledge of the normal appearances of the developing spine on plain radiographs. The distance between the anterior arch of

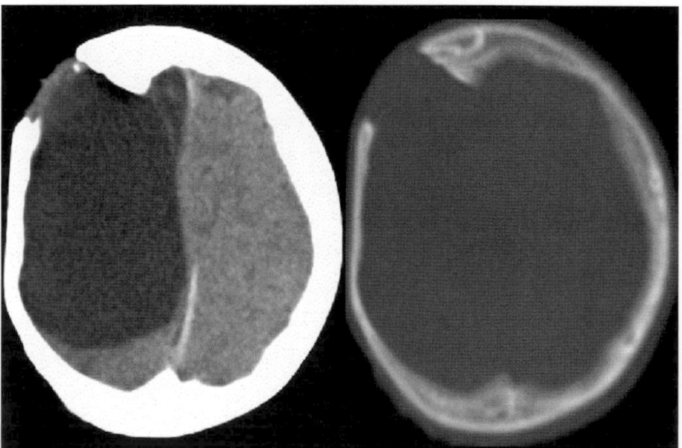

Figure 70.71 Large cerebral parenchymal defect in association with frontal bone defect which increased in size following a frontal bone linear fracture. Note the well corticated margins of the fracture.

C1 and the dens can be up to 5 mm in normal children, and there is increased mobility not only between C1 and C2 but also between C3 and C4. The prevertebral soft tissues should not exceed two-thirds of the width of the C2 vertebral body. Increased mobility in many children allows anterior 'pseudo-luxation' of C2 on C3 by up to 4 mm but the posterior elements should always remain correctly aligned and the distance should reduce in extension.

There is generalized ligamentous laxity of the immature spine. This may allow significant injury to the spinal cord in the absence of detectable bony injury causing SCIWORA (spinal cord injury without radiographic abnormality). In the appropriate clinical setting a proper evaluation may therefore require carefully performed flexion and extension views, and MRI to look for soft tissue and cord injury.

Atlanto-axial rotatory fixation

This entity is discussed in this section for convenience, although there is often little or no history of trauma in these cases. Torticollis is common in children. Most cases are acute and the symptoms disappear without treatment within a week. Rarely it may be caused by rotatory fixation between C1 and C2, and with variable degrees of subluxation, and may occur within a normal range of movement and without subluxation. Atlanto-axial rotatory fixation should be suspected if the symptoms of torticollis persist for more than 2 weeks. The diagnostic test (CT is best) must prove that there is a fixed relationship between C1 and C2 in all positions, and in particular, on turning the head to the opposite side of the clinical presentation. Atlanto-axial rotatory fixation is present if there is rotation between C1 and C2 which remains constant throughout all positions. The treatment is aggressive with traction; if it is unsuccessful, the atlanto-axial rotatory fixation will result in a permanent rotatory malalignment requiring surgery. Secondary degenerative changes and eventually fusion may occur.

Nonaccidental head injury

Imaging of the brain is particularly important for the diagnosis of the so-called 'shaken baby syndrome' (see also Chapter 68). The triad of retinal haemorrhages, subdural haemorrhages and encephalopathy is accepted as a useful marker for this condition. The mechanism for injury is thought to be that of vigorous or violent shaking or such shaking followed by an impact injury. The emphasis is on rapid and alternating forces of acceleration and deceleration acting on an unsupported head. The strength of force required to cause these injuries is unknown and not easy to study scientifically. However, experienced workers would agree that such injuries cannot occur from the normal handling of an infant or young child. Subarachnoid haemorrhage, cerebral contusions, lacerations or 'splits' in the brain parenchyma and diffuse cerebral oedema with little evidence of external impact injury are supportive hallmarks of the shaken baby syndrome.

During shaking, the brain also comes into contact with the inner surface of the skull, and there may also be a final impact, and cerebral contusions are seen. The mechanism behind the repeated trauma also causes shearing injuries in the brain, often located in the subcortical region at the junction of white and grey matter. MRI detects these injuries more frequently than CT. Brain oedema is a very important feature of the shaken baby syndrome, the mechanism of which is hypothesized to be due to hypoxic–ischaemic injury. The oedema is usually massive with reduced or absent grey–white matter differentiation, and is worst in the parieto-occipital regions. The basal ganglia, brainstem and cerebellum are, in turn, relatively preserved. The outcome of brain injury caused by shaking when severe brain oedema is present is usually grim. There is rapid destruction of brain tissue and significant atrophy becomes obvious after 2–3 weeks. In severe cases the end result is multicystic encephalomalacia, and microcephaly with marked mental and motor disability (Fig. 70.72).

HYDROCEPHALUS

The term 'hydrocephalus', literally 'water on the brain', is unfortunately a nonspecific term which refers to any condition in which the ventricles are enlarged, including cerebral atrophy. The clinical and radiological challenge is to identify those forms that are likely to benefit from intervention. Some qualifying terms have been used to distinguish some of these entities. The terms communicating and noncommunicating

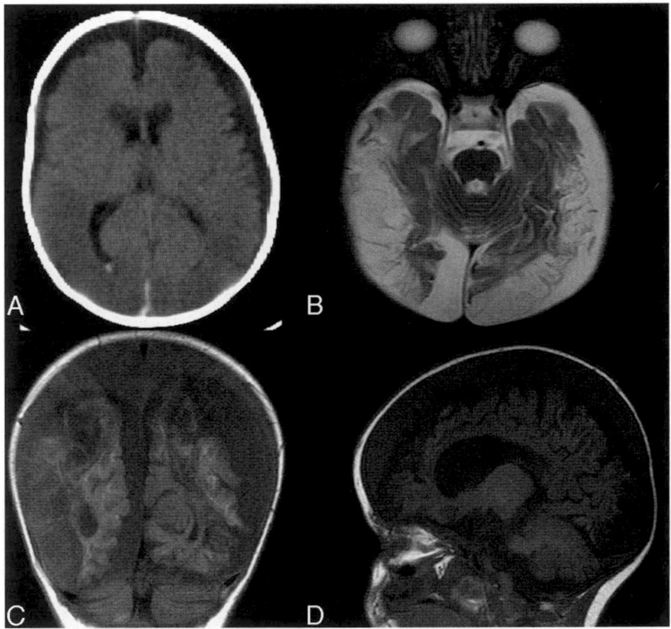

Figure 70.72 Brain injury in 'shaken baby syndrome'. (A) The initial CT shows posterior interhemispheric subdural and intraventricular blood. There are bilateral hypodense subdural collections overlying both hemispheres. Extensive bilateral hypodense parenchymal lesions consistent with contusions or infarction are seen. (B) Follow-up MRI shows evolution of the parenchymal damage with marked atrophy and large chronic subdural collections. (C) Coronal and (D) sagittal T1-weighted sequence shows the subdural collections have signal slightly greater than cerebrospinal fluid in keeping with proteinaceous contents from previous haemorrhage. There is cortical T1 shortening suggesting the parenchymal lesions are regions of cerebral infarction.

hydrocephalus are used to indicate extraventricular obstructive hydrocephalus and intraventricular obstructive hydrocephalus, respectively. These need to be distinguished from ventriculomegaly due to underlying lack of brain parenchyma, through atrophy or primary lack of brain development; some authors have suggested avoiding the use of the term hydrocephalus altogether for these cases. The concepts fail to hold true in a sizeable minority of cases, where the changes following intervention may not appear to follow expectations. For these, an appreciation of the complexities of CSF physiology may be helpful. Whilst it is generally accepted that those forms of hydrocephalus that are likely to benefit from interventions are caused by an imbalance between CSF production and absorption, the exact pathophysiology of these mechanisms remains poorly understood. CSF is produced by the choroid plexuses and is mostly absorbed through the brain and cord with a lesser contribution from the arachnoid granulations. There is a net flow of CSF through the ventricular system, from lateral to third to fourth ventricles, which is influenced by cerebrovascular pulsations.

Post-haemorrhagic and post-infective hydrocephalus account for a significant proportion of hydrocephalus presenting in neonates and infants. Apart from these, congenital causes include aqueductal stenosis/gliosis, Chiari II malformation (usually occurring after repair of the associated lumbosacral myelomeningocele) and other malformations such as the Dandy–Walker malformation. Rarer causes include congenital midline tumours and vascular (e.g. vein of Galen) malformations. Before closure of the fontanelles (i.e. up to 2 years), the most reliable clinical sign is progressive macrocephaly documented by serial head circumference measurements. Caution should be exercised in the case of an asymmetrical skull or preferential growth in one direction due to craniosynostosis, which may give a spuriously enlarged head circumference without hydrocephalus. Alongside an increasingly disproportionate head circumference which crosses centiles on growth charts, other features of hydrocephalus in this age group include frontal bossing, calvarial thinning, presence of a tense, bulging anterior fontanelle, sutural diastasis and enlargement of scalp veins. Sunsetting eyes with failure of upward gaze, lateral rectus palsies and leg spasticity due to stretching of the corticospinal tracts as they descend from the motor strip around the ventricles are also seen.

In older children posterior fossa neoplasms and aqueduct stenosis are the most common causes of hydrocephalus. Early morning headache, nausea, vomiting, papilloedema, leg spasticity, cranial palsies and alterations in conscious level are the dominant clinical features as the skull is rigid. The fontanelles have fused and the sutures are fusing, and therefore increasing head circumference, fontanelle bulging and sutural diastasis are not features.

Imaging indicators of intraventricular obstructive (non-communicating) hydrocephalus include dilatation of the temporal horns disproportionate to lateral ventricular dilatation, enlargement of the anterior and posterior recesses of the third ventricle with inferior convexity of the floor of the third ventricle, transependymal (periventricular interstitial) oedema and bulging of fontanelles (Fig. 70.73). The sulcal spaces, major fissures and basal cisterns are small or obliterated. A careful survey of the regional ventricular dilatation may reveal the location as well as the cause of obstruction. Other features, such as changes in the configuration of the frontal horns of the lateral ventricles, specifically widening of the radius of the frontal horn, and a decrease in the angle it makes with the midline plane, are less useful. Further features classically described in chronic hydrocephalus, such as erosion of the dorsum sellae and copper beaten skull, are even less reliable.

Extraventricular obstructive (communicating) hydrocephalus, however, may reveal a range of findings from ventricular and sulcal prominence to 'normal' CT/MRI appearances. It may have a variety of causes ranging from haemorrhage and proteinaceous cellular debris with infection and disseminated malignancy to venous hypertension from impaired venous drainage to impaired arterial compliance from diffuse arteriopathies. In some cases, a combination of both forms of obstructive hydrocephalus would be expected.

Assessment of the cortical sulci for effacement disproportionate to ventricular size in children can be difficult and it requires some knowledge of the normal appearances for age; in normal younger children, under two, the ventricles and subarachnoid spaces are more prominent, and should not be misinterpreted as 'atrophic' or due to hydrocephalus. Knowledge of the head size is important in making this distinction, being large in hydrocephalus and benign enlargement of the subarachnoid spaces, or small if there is cerebral atrophy. Again it may not be possible to be certain about the findings in the absence of serial measurements documenting trends. In benign enlargement of the subarachnoid spaces, there is believed to be a mismatch between the rate of skull growth and rate of growth of the developing brain. The child is neurologically normal. There is rapid skull growth, often to above the 95th centile by the time of presentation, but this then stabilizes and both the size of the subarachnoid spaces and head size have usually normalized by age 2 years. The extra space anterior to the cerebral convexities is distinguishable from subdural collections by lack of mass effect on the adjacent brain and the presence of crossing

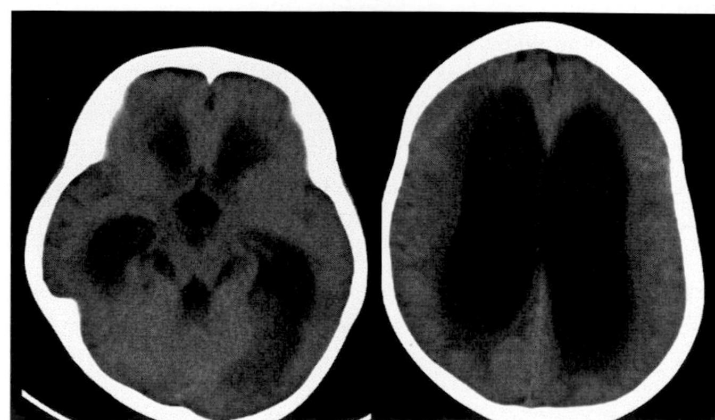

Figure 70.73 Child with mucopolysaccharidosis type I and hydrocephalus. The temporal horns and anterior recesses of the third ventricle are dilated. There is transependymal oedema and the cerebral sulci are effaced.

veins within the subarachnoid space. The importance of its recognition is to indicate that no intervention is required, with the expectation that the situation will normalize with age.

In the second decade the hemispheric cortical sulci become much less conspicuous and the ventricles less prominent, which should equally not be misinterpreted as due to cerebral oedema or the presence of a 'tight' brain. In this case in the normal child the basal cisterns should not be effaced.

An attempt should be made to identify a structural cause for the hydrocephalus. The narrowest parts of the ventricular system are the most susceptible to mechanical obstruction, i.e. the foramina of Monro, cerebral aqueduct and fourth ventricular outflow foramina. Masses causing obstructive hydrocephalus at the foramina of Monro include superior extension of suprasellar tumours and arachnoid cysts, colloid cysts, which may cause sudden acute and life-threatening hydrocephalus, and giant cell astrocytomas in tuberous sclerosis. Masses effacing the cerebral aqueduct include tectal plate gliomas, superior extension of midline posterior fossa tumours and brainstem diffuse astrocytomas and inferior extension of pineal region tumours. Atrial diverticula from dilated lateral ventricles may herniate into the quadrigeminal and supracerebellar cisterns and may also compress the tectum. These may be distinguished from large arachnoid cysts using multiplanar MRI to confirm continuity with the ventricular system.

More diffuse patterns of obstruction, including isolation of pockets of CSF, may be caused by haemorrhage, infection, disseminated tumour and reparative fibrosis. Clues to the underlying cause include evidence of haemosiderin staining or superficial siderosis in previous haemorrhage; focal atrophy or porencephaly from previous haematomas; the presence of hyperdense exudates in the basal cisterns, subarachnoid space and pial enhancement with infection or pial neoplastic dissemination.

Aqueduct stenosis is one of the most common causes of hydrocephalus in children but may present at any time from birth to adulthood. It may be developmental or acquired gliosis secondary to infection or intraventricular haemorrhage. Classically, the lateral and third ventricles are dilated and the fourth ventricle is of normal size, and there is no evidence of a tectal plate tumour. On sagittal MRI there is focal narrowing of the cerebral aqueduct, normally proximally at the level of the superior colliculi or at the intercollicular sulcus with posterior displacement of the tectal plate. Proximal to this the aqueduct is dilated (Fig. 70.74). Occasionally a congenital web may be seen as a very thin sheet of tissue across the distal aqueduct.

Overproduction of CSF is a very rare cause of hydrocephalus, most often seen with choroid plexus papillomas. These tumours may cause hydrocephalus by other mechanisms, e.g. obstructive hydrocephalus of the lateral ventricle due to mass effect at the body/trigone or foramen of Monro of the lateral ventricle, and haemorrhage within the ventricular system. A highly proteinaceous exudate produced by the tumour can cause communicating hydrocephalus due to impaired extraventricular drainage of CSF. Spinal cord tumours may be associated with hydrocephalus due to proteinaceous exudates or pial dissemination of disease, both causing impaired absorption of CSF. Indeed in the cases of unexplained hydrocephalus, spinal imaging is recommended to exclude a possible occult intraspinal lesion.

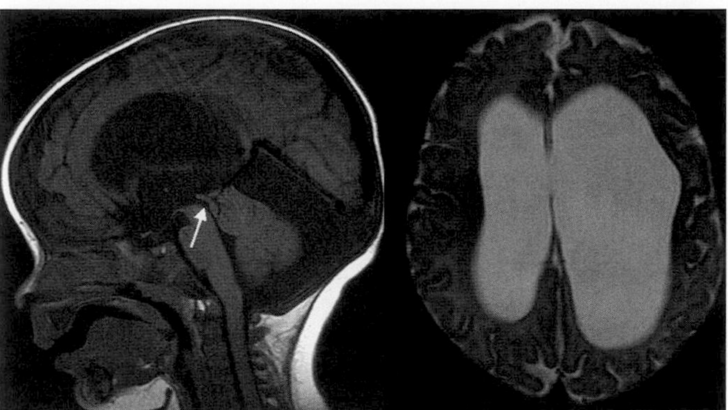

Figure 70.74 Child with aqueduct stenosis with a history of prematurity. There is dilatation of the lateral ventricles and proximal cerebral aqueduct (arrow). The hydrocephalus is long-standing as there is white matter volume loss and the anterior recesses of the third ventricle are not bulging. There is more focal damage in the left frontal lobe, probably due to previous germinal matrix haemorrhage. A posterior fossa arachnoid cyst is also noted.

Chiari II malformation is a common cause of hydrocephalus presenting early in life. The underlying aetiology is disputed; it may not be due to simple craniocervical junction obstruction but due to the displacement of the fourth ventricular outlet foramina within the spinal canal inferior to the foramen magnum, i.e. within the spinal canal, where the capacity for CSF absorption is reduced. Some specific features should be looked for when assessing these children for hydrocephalus or shunt malfunction. Children with occipital headaches at night probably have some degree of shunt malfunction which may present with potentially fatal signs of brainstem compression and apnoeic attacks. Also, the fourth ventricle should be slit-like, so the presence of a normal sized or enlarged fourth ventricle suggests a shunt malfunction or isolation of the fourth ventricle requiring diversion.

Finally, hydrocephalus may be seen as a consequence of raised intracranial venous pressure. Examples include syndromic skull base abnormalities in craniosynostosis(es) and leading to stenosis of the jugular outflow foramina. Vascular causes include venous thrombosis, the vein of Galen aneurysmal malformation and dural arteriovenous shunts. Persistent untreated raised intraventricular pressure may result in secondary parenchymal damage affecting adjacent white matter and resulting in impaired cognitive function, permanent spasticity and blindness.

As well as by removing the obstructive lesion, hydrocephalus can be treated by CSF diversion. This can be performed initially by external ventricular drainage, or more permanently by ventriculoperitoneal, ventriculoatrial shunting, or third ventriculostomy. Here a surgical defect is made in the floor of the third ventricle allowing CSF drainage into the suprasellar cistern.

Shunt malfunction from obstruction of the shunt by choroid plexus or glial tissue and subsequent ventricular dilatation is best assessed by comparison with baseline or previous imaging. In addition to a recurrence of the signs of hydrocephalus, there may be the appearance of fluid tracking along the length or the shunt tubing. Assessment of shunt tubing integrity may be made by plain radiograph imaging of the tube from the skull to the abdomen/pelvis. The scout view of a brain CT may also be useful to pick up disrupted shunt tubing or disconnection of the valve. As well as separation of the fragments, calcification may be seen at either end of the shunt disruption due to inflammation and fibrotic change where the shunt has become tethered and then distracted. Knowledge of the type of shunt inserted, or discussion with the neurosurgeon who inserted it, should allow distinction of the normal radiolucent components of the shunt (often as it exits the calvarium) from shunt distraction.

Patency of a third ventriculostomy can be inferred on MRI by visualizing the surgical defect and detecting rapid CSF flow through it into the suprasellar cistern, manifest as large hypointense flow voids on T2-weighted imaging. This may be aided by imaging without any flow compensation.

The incidence of shunt infection has declined over the years and in most neurosurgical centres runs at around 1–5%, being slightly higher in infants. Imaging may detect evidence of ventriculitis: enlarged ventricles with hyperdense ependyma on CT, ependymal enhancement and debris within the ventricular system. This may progress to cerebritis with devastating consequences for the developing brain parenchyma. Other shunt complications include the development of abdominal ascites, pseudocyst formation and perforated abdominal viscus. Rarely, shunted hydrocephalic patients may become symptomatic without ventricular dilatation and develop the 'slit ventricle' syndrome. This has a number of potential causes which include overdrainage of CSF, stiff, poorly compliant ventricles which allow raised intraventricular pressure without ventricular dilatation, intermittent shunt malfunction and headaches unrelated to the shunt.

SUMMARY

Paediatric neuroradiology is a subspecialist field drawing from knowledge and expertise in neuroimaging, paediatrics, embryology and genetics. Some skill is required in adapting neuroimaging techniques to suit the paediatric population, especially in terms of sedation/general anaesthesia. The range of conditions encountered is very different from that seen in adults. The management aims and options are also often different from adult cases.

REFERENCES

1. Barkovich A J 2000 Concepts of myelin and myelination in neuroradiology. Am J Neuroradiol 21: 1099–1109
2. Wimberger D M, Roberts T P, Barkovich A J et al 1995 Identification of 'premyelination' by diffusion weighted MRI. J Comput Assist Tomogr 19: 28–33
3. Huppi P S, Maier S E, Peded S et al 1998 Microstructural development of human newborn cerebral white matter assessed *in vivo* by diffusion tensor magnetic resonance imaging. Pediatr Res 44: 584–590
4. Engelbrecht V, Rassek M, Preiss S et al 1998 Age-dependent changes in magnetization transfer contrast of white matter in the pediatric brain. Am J Neuroradiol 19:1923–1929.
5. Barkovich A J 1998 MR of the normal neonatal brain: assessment of deep structures. Am J Neuroradiol 19: 1397–1403
6. Barkovich A J, Kjos B O, Jackson D E et al 1988 Normal maturation of the neonatal and infant brain: MR imaging at 1.5T. Radiology 166: 173–180
7. Yakovlev P I, Lecours A R 1967 The myelogenetic cycles of regional maturation of the brain. In: Minkowski A (ed) Regional development of the brain in early life. Oxford: Blackwell, pp 3–70
8. Van der Knaap M S, Van Wezel-Miejler G, Barth P G et al 1996 Normal gyration and sulcation in preterm and term neonates: appearance on MR images. Radiology 200: 389–396
9. Martin E, Kikinis R, Zuerrer M et al 1988 Developmental stages of human brain: an MR study. J Comput Assist Tomogr 12: 917–922
10. Barkovich A J, Kjos B O 1988 Normal postnatal development of the corpus callosum as demonstrated by MR imaging. Am J Neuroradiol 9: 487–491
11. Aoki S, Okada Y, Nishimura K et al 1989 Normal deposition of brain iron in childhood and adolescence: MR imaging at 1.5T. Radiology 172: 381–385
12. Cox T D, Elster A D 1991 Normal pituitary gland: changes in shape, size and signal intensity during the first year of life at MR imaging. Radiology 179: 721–724
13. Raemakaers V T, Heimann G, Reul J et al 1997 Genetic disorders and cerebellar structural abnormalities in childhood. Brain 120: 1739–1751
14. Tortori-Donati P, Fondelli M, Rossi A et al 1996 Cystic malformations of the posterior cranial fossa originating from a defect of the posterior membranous area: mega cisterna magna and persisting Blake's pouch: two separate entities. Childs Nerv Syst 12: 203–308
15. Hart M N, Malamud N, Ellis W G 1972 The Dandy–Walker syndrome. A clinicopathological study based on 28 cases. Neurology 22: 771–780
16. Joubert M, Eisenring J J, Robb J P et al 1969 Familial agenesis of the cerbellar vermis. A syndrome of episodic hyperpnea, abnormal eye movements, ataxia and retardation. Neurology 19: 813–825
17. Kendall B, Kingsley D, Lambert S R et al 1990 Joubert syndrome: a clinical–radiological study. Neuroradiology 31: 502–506
18. Toelle S P, Yalcinkaya C, Kocer N et al 2002 Rhombencephalosynapsis: clinical findings and neuroimaging in 9 children. Neuropediatrics 33: 209–214
19. Meltzer C C, Smirniotopoulos J G, Jones R V 1995 The striated cerebellum: an MR imaging sign in L'Hermitte-Duclos disease (dysplastic gangliocytoma). Radiology 194: 699–703
20. Barkovich A J 2002 Magnetic resonance imaging: role in the understanding of cerebral malformations. Brain Dev 24: 2–12
21. Wright L B, James C A, Glasier C M 2001 Congenital cerebral and cerebrovascular anomalies: magnetic resonance imaging. Top Magn Reson Imaging 12: 361–374.
22. Barkovich A J 2005 Congenital malformations of the brain and skull. In: Pediatric neuroradiology, 3rd edn. Philadelphia: Lippincott, Williams & Wilkins, ch 3
23. Naidich T P, McLone D G, Fulling K H 1983 The Chiari II malformation: Part IV. The hindbrain deformity. Neuroradiology 25: 179–197
24. Wolpert S M, Anderson M, Scott R M et al 1987 Chiari II malformation: MR imaging evaluation. Am J Roentgenol 149: 1033–1042
25. Hetts S W, Sherr E H, Chao S et al 2006 Anomalies of the corpus callosum: an MR analysis of the phenotypic spectrum of associated malformations. Am J Roentgenol 187: 1343–1348
26. Barkovich A J 2005 The phakomatoses. In: Paediatric neuroimaging, 3rd edn. Philadelphia: Lippincott, Williams & Wilkins, pp 440–504
27. Herron J, Darrah R, Quaghebeur G 2000 Intra-cranial manifestations of the neurocutaneous syndromes. Clin Radiol 55: 82–98
28. Neurofibromatosis. In: National Institutes of Health Consensus Development Conference. Arch Neurol 1988;575–578
29. Balcer L J, Liu G T, Heller G et al 2001 Visual loss in children with neurofibromatosis type 1 and optic pathway gliomas: relation to

tumor location by magnetic resonance imaging. Am J Ophthalmol 131: 442–445
30. Goh W H, Khong P L, Leung C S et al 2004 T2-weighted hyperintensities (unidentified bright objects) in children with neurofibromatosis 1: their impact on cognitive function. J Child Neurol 19: 853–858
31. Roach E S, Sparagana S P 2004 Diagnosis of tuberous sclerosis complex. J Child Neurol 19: 643–649.
32. Roach E S, Gomez M R, Northrup H 1998 Tuberous sclerosis complex consensus conference: revised clinical diagnostic criteria. J Child Neurol 13: 624–628
33. Kingsley D, Kendall B, Fitz C 1986 Tuberous sclerosis: a clinicoradiological evaluation of 110 cases with particular reference to atypical presentation. Neuroradiology 28: 171–190
34. Baron Y, Barkovich A J 1999 MR imaging of tuberous sclerosis in neonates and young infants. Am J Neuroradiol 20: 907–916
35. Braffman B, Naidich T P 1994 The phakomatoses: Part II. von Hippel–Lindau disease, Sturge–Weber syndrome, and less common conditions. Neuroimaging Clin N Am 4: 325–348
36. Marti -Bonmarti L, Menor F, Mulas F 1993 The Sturge–Weber syndrome: correlation between the clinical status and radiological CT and MRI findings. Childs Nerv Syst 9: 107–109
37. Naidich T P, Blaser S I, Delman B N et al 2002 Embryology of the spine and spinal cord, in Proceedings of the 40th Annual Meeting of the American Society of Neuroradiology, Vancouver, BC, May 13–17, pp 3–13
38. Barkovich A J 2005 Congenital anomalies of the spine. In: Barkovich A J (ed) Pediatric neuroimaging, 4th edn. Philadelphia: Lippincott Williams & Wilkins, 2005
39. Rossi A, Gandolfo C, Morana G, et al 2006 Current classification and imaging of congenital spinal abnormalities. Semin Roentgenol 41: 250–273
40. Rowland Hill C A, Gibson P J 1995 Ultrasound determination of the normal location of the conus medullaris in neonates. Am J Neonat Radiol 16: 469–472
41. Beek FJ, de Vries L S, Gerards L J, Mali W P 1996 Sonographic determination of the position of the conus medullaris in premature and term infants. Neuroradiology 38 (Suppl 1): S174–177
42. McLone D G, Dias M S 1991–1992 Complications of myelomeningocele closure. Pediatr Neurosurg 17: 267–273
43. Drolet B 1998 Birthmarks to worry about. Cutaneous markers of dysraphism. Dermatol Clin 16: 447–453
44. Thompson D 2000 Hairy backs, tails and dimples. Curr Paediatr 10: 177–183
45. Hughes J A, De Bruyn R, Patel K, Thompson D 2003 Evaluation of spinal ultrasound in spinal dysraphism. Clin Radiol 58: 227–233
46. Pang D, Dias M S, Ahab-Barmada M 1992 Split cord malformation. Part I: a unified theory of embryogenesis for double spinal cord malformations. Neurosurgery 31: 451–480
47. Pang D 1992 Split cord malformation. Part II: clinical syndrome. Neurosurgery 31: 481–500
48. Faris J C, Crowe J E 1975 The split notochord syndrome. J Pediatr Surg 10: 467–472
49. Duhamel B 1961 From the mermaid to anal imperforation: the syndrome of caudal regression. Arch Dis Child 36: 152–155
50. Carey J C, Greenbaum B, Hall B D 1978 The OEIS complex (omphalocele, exstrophy, imperforate anus, spinal defects). Birth Defects Orig Artic Ser 14: 253–263
51. Currarino G, Coln D, Votteler T 1981 Triad of anorectal, sacral, and presacral anomalies. Am J Roentgenol 137: 395–398
52. Pang D 1993 Sacral agenesis and caudal spinal cord malformations. Neurosurgery 32: 755–779
53. Van Der Knaap M S, Valk J 2005 Magnetic resonance imaging of myelination and myelination disorders, 3rd edn. Berlin: Springer Verlag
54. Patay Z 2005 Metabolic disorders. In: Carty H et al (eds) Imaging children, 2nd edn, vol 2. Edinburgh: Churchill Livingstone, pp 1899–1956
55. Hayward R, Jones B, Dunaway D, Evans R (eds) 2004 The clinical management of craniosynostosis. Clin Dev Med 163
56. World Health Organization 2000 Classification of tumours. Pathology and genetics. In: Kleihues P, Cavenee W (eds) Tumours of the nervous system. IARC Press Cambridge
57. Griffiths P D 1999 A protocol for imaging paediatric brain tumours. United Kingdom Children's Cancer Study Group (UKCCSG) and Societe Francaise D'Oncologie Pediatrique (SFOP) Panelists. Clin Oncol (R Coll Radiol) 11: 290–294
58. Saunders D E, Phipps K P, Wade A M et al 2005 Surveillance imaging strategies following surgery and/or radiotherapy for childhood cerebellar low-grade astrocytoma. J Neurosurg 102 (2 Suppl):172–178.
59. Saunders D E, Hayward R D, Phipps K P et al 2003 Surveillance neuroimaging of intracranial medulloblastoma in children: how effective, how often, and for how long? J Neurosurg 99: 280–286.
60. Good C D, Wade A M, Hayward R D et al 2001 Surveillance neuroimaging in childhood intracranial ependymoma: how effective, how often, and for how long? J Neurosurg 94: 27–32.
61. Rumboldt Z, Camacho D L, Lake D et al 2006 Apparent diffusion coefficients for differentiation of cerebellar tumors in children. Am J Neuroradiol 27: 1362–1369.
62. Arai K, Sato N, Aoki J et al 2006 MR signal of the solid portion of pilocytic astrocytoma on T2-weighted images: is it useful for differentiation from medulloblastoma? Neuroradiology 48: 233–237.
63. Fischbein N J, Prados M D, Wara W et al 1996 Radiologic classification of brain stem tumors: correlation of magnetic resonance imaging appearance with clinical outcome. Pediatr Neurosurg 24: 9–23.
64. Bowers D C, Georgiades C, Aronson L J 2000 Tectal gliomas: natural history of an indolent lesion in pediatric patients. Pediatr Neurosurg 32: 24–29.
65. Chong W K, Saunders D S, Ganesan V 2004 Stroke is an important paediatric illness. Pediatr Radiol 34: 2–4.
66. Paediatric Stroke Working Group 2004 Stroke in childhood. Clinical guidelines for diagnosis, management and rehabilitation. London: Clinical Effectiveness and Evaluation Unit, Royal College of Physicians.
67. Ganesan V, Prengler M, McShane M A, Wade A M, Kirkham F J 2003 Investigation of risk factors in children with arterial ischemic stroke. Ann Neurol 53: 167–173.
68. DeVeber G 2005 In pursuit of evidence-based treatments for paediatric stroke: the UK and Chest guidelines. Lancet Neurol 4: 432–436.
69. Barkovich A, Truwit C 1989 Brain damage from perinatal asphyxia: correlation of MR findings with gestational age. Am J Neuroradiol 11: 1087–1096
70. Barkovich A 1992 MR and CT evaluation of profound neonatal and infantile asphyxia. Am J Neuroradiol 13: 959–972
71. Barkovich A, Sargent S 1995 Profound asphyxia in the premature infant: Imaging findings. Am J Neuroradiol 16: 1837–1846
72. Krageloh-Mann I 2004 Imaging of early brain injury and cortical plasticity. Exp Neurol 190 (Suppl 1): S84–90
73. Krageloh-Mann I, Peterson D, Hagberg G, et al 1995 Bilateral spastic cerebral palsy – MRI pathology and origin. Analysis from a representative series of 56 cases. Dev Med Child Neurol 37: 379–397

SECTION 9

Miscellaneous Disorders

CHAPTER 71

Imaging of the Endocrine System

S. Aslam A. Sohaib, Andrea Rockall, Jamshed B. Bomanji, Jane Evanson and Rodney H. Reznek

- The hypothalamic–pituitary axis
- The thyroid gland
- The parathyroid glands
- Pancreatic and gastrointestinal endocrine disorders
- Carcinoid tumours
- The adrenal glands
- The female reproductive system
- The male reproductive system

Endocrine disorders result from excessive or deficient hormone production, which may be continuous or intermittent and may affect a single or multiple hormones. Hypofunction results from destruction or replacement of a gland by a tumour, infection, autoimmune processes, haemorrhage or infarction, or by compression from an adjacent mass lesion. Hyperfunction may be caused by hypertrophy, microadenoma, adenoma (single or multiple), or carcinoma of the endocrine gland. Over-production of a hormone may also arise from an 'ectopic' site. In most cases, this is due to a tumour that is usually, but not always, malignant (e.g., adrenocorticotropic hormone [ACTH] secretion by small-cell lung cancer).

The diagnosis of endocrine disease is usually based on clinical presentation and subsequent assay of the appropriate hormone. It is rare for radiological signs to suggest an unsuspected endocrine disease. There are few radiological signs that confirm the diagnosis when biochemical tests are equivocal. The challenge for imaging in endocrine disease lies in identifying the abnormality leading to the endocrine disorder. Although radiological investigations of endocrine disease now centre mostly on cross-sectional imaging techniques, a functional abnormality often needs to be corroborated by radionuclide imaging, venous sampling, or biochemistry. Cross-sectional imaging techniques are unable to distinguish between a functioning and a nonfunctioning tumour.

Imaging of the endocrine system differs in several ways from imaging in other body systems. Although a correlation between anatomical abnormality and functional abnormality is important, the degree of endocrine abnormality does not correlate with the size of the macroscopic lesion. Very small lesions can give rise to profound biochemical disturbance; attention to technique is therefore essential, as a small lesion may be missed. Furthermore, an endocrine disorder may arise from one of several sites within the endocrine system in addition to ectopic sites; for example, Cushing's syndrome may arise from anywhere within the hypothalamic–pituitary–adrenal axis or from an ectopic site. Detection of the source of Cushing's syndrome may require imaging of several different anatomical regions using multiple imaging techniques.

Due to the diversity of the endocrine system and its pathology, the imaging needs to be tailored to the endocrine gland or disease in question, as discussed in the sections below.

THE HYPOTHALAMIC–PITUITARY AXIS

ANATOMY AND PHYSIOLOGY

The hypothalamus is a thin layer of tissue that forms the floor and lower lateral walls of the third ventricle. It extends from the lamina terminalis and optic chiasm anteriorly to the mammillary bodies posteriorly (Fig. 71.1). The inferior surface of the hypothalamus between these structures is called the tuber cinereum. A swelling on its surface, the median eminence, is continuous with the infundibulum (pituitary stalk). The pituitary stalk tapers smoothly as it travels inferiorly from the hypothalamic origin to the pituitary insertion. The normal stalk is 3–3.5 mm wide at its origin and 2 mm wide near its insertion[1].

The hypothalamus controls pituitary function through direct neuronal links with the posterior lobe of the pituitary (neurohypophysis) and vascular links with the anterior lobe (adenohypophysis). Within the medial parts of the hypothalamus are a number of named hypothalamic nuclei (e.g., supraoptic and paraventricular nuclei), which manufacture hormones. Axons from the supraoptic and paraventricular nuclei transport

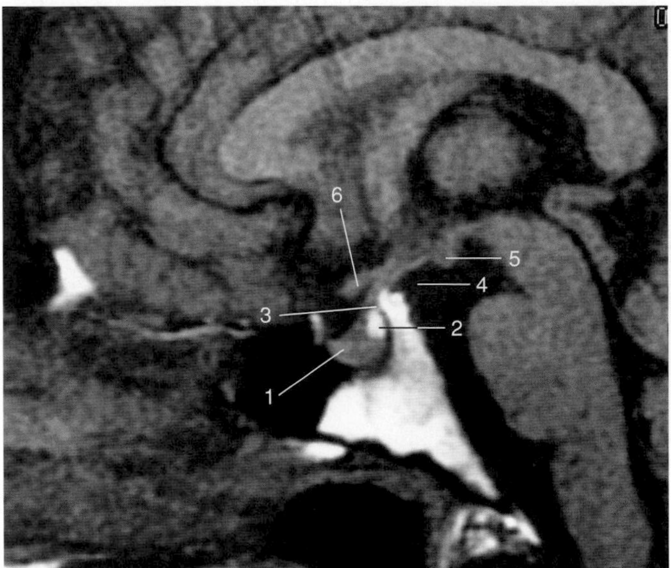

Figure 71.1 Normal pituitary gland. Unenhanced sagittal T1-weighted spin-echo images of a normal pituitary gland and hypothalamus. The anterior pituitary gland (1), posterior pituitary bright spot (2), pituitary stalk (3), tuber cinereum (4), mammillary bodies (5), sphenoid sinus (6) and optic chiasm (7) are identified.

vasopressin (antidiuretic hormone; ADH) and oxytocin down the stalk into the posterior lobe of the pituitary. Hypothalamic-releasing factors are delivered to the anterior lobe of the pituitary by a system of hypophyseal veins, which run from the hypothalamus to the vascular sinusoids of the anterior pituitary.

The pituitary gland is composed of two lobes that are physiologically, embryologically and anatomically distinct. The anterior lobe is the largest part and comprises 75% of the total volume. It arises from an invagination of Rathke's pouch from the fetal nasopharynx. It is composed of glandular cells that produce numerous hormones. Its predominant blood supply is from the hypophyseal-portal system, which also serves as the pathway by which hypothalamic-releasing hormones reach the pituitary. In adults, the anterior pituitary appears homogeneous and isointense to grey matter on T1- and T2-weighted MRI. The posterior lobe of the pituitary occupies the posterior third of the sella and arises embryologically from a down growth of the hypothalamus. It is characteristically of high signal on T1-weighted MRI sequences, i.e., 'posterior pituitary bright spot' (see Fig. 71.1). This high signal is ascribed to the vasopressin complex present within the axon terminals. Absence of this high signal is reported in patients with central diabetes insipidus[2]. However, the high signal may not be seen in all normal subjects[3]. An ectopic position of the posterior pituitary may be a normal variant, but can be associated with pituitary dwarfism (growth hormone [GH] deficiency)[4].

The pituitary gland occupies the sella turcica, which is a cup-shaped depression in the basisphenoid bone. The roof of the sella is formed by the diaphragma sella, a fold of dura, which is perforated to allow passage of the pituitary stalk. Above the diaphragma sella lies the suprasellar cistern the optic chiasm and the anterior cerebral arteries. The lateral walls of the pituitary fossa are formed by the cavernous sinuses containing the internal carotid arteries and cranial nerves III, IV, the first and second divisions of V and VI. Behind the sella is the pontine cistern containing the basilar artery. The cavernous sinus, pituitary gland and stalk lie outside the blood–brain barrier and, therefore, show significant enhancement after the administration of intravenous contrast medium.

The hypothalamus plays an important role in the regulation of the autonomic nervous system, temperature, appetite and sleep patterns. It also influences most endocrine glands through its effect on the pituitary gland (Table 71.1).

IMAGING TECHNIQUES

MRI and CT are the main techniques for evaluating the sella and juxtasellar region, with MRI being the technique of choice. Current imaging protocols for the hypothalamic–pituitary axis (HPA) typically utilize sagittal and coronal T1-weighted spin-echo sequences. In order to achieve high spatial resolution, thin slices (3 mm), and a small field of view (16–20 cm) is used. Alternatively a 3D-spoiled gradient-echo volume acquisition can be used. This results in thinner slices (1.5 mm) with good signal-to-noise ratio and can be reconstructed in all three planes. Susceptibility artefacts at air/bone interfaces may occur with these sequences. Dynamic T1-weighted spin-echo acquisition within 1–2 minutes after intravenous gadolinium slightly improves the sensitivity of MRI for the detection of small pituitary adenomas[5]. T2-weighted sequences are not as sensitive as contrast enhanced T1-weighted sequences for the detection of adenomas, but can occasionally prove useful.

There is still a role for CT in imaging the pituitary. There are a number of patients who cannot undergo MRI, and CT is also useful for detection of calcification, the presence of which

Table 71.1 PITUITARY HORMONES AND THEIR REGULATION

Pituitary lobe	Hormone	Releasing factor	Inhibitory factor	Target organ
Anterior	Corticotropin	CRH	ADH	Adrenal gland
	FSH, LH	GnRH	–	Gonads
	GH	GHRH	Somatotstatin	Liver, bone, fat
	Prolactin	VIP	Dopamine	Breast
	TSH	TRH	Somatotstatin	Thyroid
Posterior	ADH	–	–	Kidney
	Oxytocin	–	–	Breast, uterus

may influence the differential diagnosis. CT may contribute to preoperative planning particularly in regard to the pneumatization and anatomy of the sphenoid air sinus. Pituitary CT can be performed in the axial plane with thin (1 mm) contiguous sections following intravenous contrast medium. Images can then be reformatted in the coronal and sagittal planes.

The role of inferior petrosal venous sampling in pituitary tumour localization is discussed elsewhere.

DISORDERS OF THE HYPOTHALAMIC–PITUITARY AXIS

Dysfunction of the HPA typically results from intrinsic disorders of the HPA itself although lesions in adjacent structures (e.g., cavernous sinus) may involve the HPA. Hyperfunction of the HPA can give rise to a number of well-described syndromes depending on which hormone is being hypersecreted (Tables 71.2–71.7).

Pituitary hyperfunction is most commonly from a pituitary adenoma or occasionally from other pituitary lesions (e.g., hypophysitis).

Hypofunctioning states results from destruction of the HPA leading to the under production of hormone. Total or partial hypopituitarism may occur in patients with pituitary adenomas, with parasellar diseases, in those who have had pituitary surgery or radiation, or following head injury. The systemic radiological changes in adults with hypopituitarism are minimal (see Table 71.4).

The role of imaging in disorders of the HPA is to identify and characterize structural lesions, which may have caused the

Table 71.2 RADIOLOGICAL FEATURES OF ACROMEGALY

Skull	Vault thickened Paranasal and mastoid air cells enlarged Pituitary fossa enlarged Floor of the fossa asymmetrical or ballooned
Mandible	Prognathism with increased angle
Spine	Kyphosis Enlarged vertebral bodies Posterior scalloping of vertebral bodies
Chest	Increased antero-posterior diameter Ribs increased in calibre and length
Hands	General enlargement Enlarged bases of phalanges and terminal tufts, spade-like Enlarged muscle attachments
Feet	Thickening of 'heel pad': M > 23 mm, F > 21.5 mm
Long bones	Thickened by periosteal new bone formation
Joints	Widening of joint spaces due to thickened cartilage Premature degeneration (OA) changes (shoulders, hips, knees) Chondrocalcinosis
Soft tissues	Enlarged heart, kidneys, liver Calcification of pinna of ears

Table 71.3 RADIOLOGICAL FEATURES OF CUSHING'S SYNDROME

Skull	Pituitary fossa usually normal
Skeleton	Osteoporosis Vertebral collapse Kyphosis Concave vertebral margins Wedged vertebral bodies Rib fractures—multiple, painless with excess callus Necrosis of femoral heads Secondary osteoarthritis

Table 71.4 RADIOLOGICAL FEATURES OF HYPOPITUITARISM

Skull	Unfused sutures
Skeleton	Small but normal proportions (Lorain dwarf) Slender bones Small pituitary fossa Unfused epiphyses

Table 71.5 RADIOLOGICAL FEATURES OF HYPERTHYROIDISM (THYROTOXICOSIS)

Skull	Exophthalmos
Skeleton	Osteopenia Cortical striation—acropachy In childhood, early appearance and accelerated growth of ossification centres
Heart	Cardiac enlargement Cardiac failure
Thymus	Enlargement

Table 71.6 RADIOLOGICAL FEATURES OF HYPOTHYROIDISM (CRETINISM AND JUVENILE MYXOEDEMA)

Skull	Delayed closure of fontanelles Relatively large sella Poorly developed paranasal sinus Usually brachycephalic Dentition delayed: dental caries Wormian bones
Skeleton	Dwarfism Increased density
Ossification centres	Retarded growth Multicentric and irregular Bilateral and symmetrical
Epiphyses	Delayed fusion and appearance Inhomogeneous epiphyses Fine or coarse stippling Fragmentation
Spine	Kyphosis Flattening of bodies Increase in width of intervertebral space Bullet-shaped vertebral bodies, usually L1 and L2
Long bones	Short Dense transverse bands at metaphyseal ends
Pelvis	Narrow with coxa vara

Table 71.7 RADIOLOGICAL FEATURES OF MYXOEDEMA

Heart	Enlargement Pericardial effusion Heart failure
Body cavities	Pleural effusion Ascites
Gastrointestinal tract	Abnormalities of oesophageal peristalsis Decreased incidence of peristalsis Constipation 'Pseudo-obstruction'

endocrine abnormalities. It is important first to identify the primary anatomical site of the lesion. Lesions may be intrasellar, suprasellar, or combined intra- and suprasellar.

Intrasellar lesions

Normal variants: The normal pituitary size and shape varies with age and sex. The pituitary gland in neonates is rounder, brighter and relatively larger during the first 2 months of life than in later childhood. In adults, the average height of the pituitary is between 3.5 and 8 mm and is slightly larger in women than men. In pubertal girls and pregnant women the gland enlarges and often appears spherical or upwardly convex and may occasionally reach 10–11 mm in height. The anterior pituitary may also appear hyperintense in pregnant or postpartum women. Pubertal boys may have a slightly rounded, upward convex pituitary that measures up to 6–7 mm in height. The pituitary gland normally decreases in size with ageing, though there may be a slight increase in size in perimenopausal women[6].

In addition to the normal physiological changes in the pituitary with age and sex, the pituitary may enlarge during the administration of exogenous oestrogens, in central precocious puberty, with hypothalamic tumours, ectopic tumours secreting hypothalamic-releasing factors, and secondary to end organ failure, e.g., in hypothyroidism.

An empty sella is usually an incidental finding thought to be caused by a congenital defect in the diaphragm sellae, which allows pulsating cerebrospinal fluid (CSF) to expand the sella. This leads to compression and atrophy of the pituitary gland and expansion of the sella turcica. As the anterior pituitary has a large functional reserve, endocrine dysfunction only occurs if less than 10% of the gland remains active. On CT and MRI the pituitary gland is flattened to a thin rim along the floor of the sella turcica. The pituitary stalk remains in its normal position, a finding that differentiates an empty sella from a cystic tumour in which the stalk is displaced or obliterated. Occasionally intrasellar herniation of the optic nerve, chiasm, or tract into the empty sella is seen.

An acquired empty sella may occur with anterior pituitary haemorrhage secondary to pituitary gland necrosis following peripartum circulatory collapse (Sheehan syndrome) or from infarction of a pituitary adenoma.

Adenomas are the most common primary neoplasms of the pituitary. They are benign and slow growing. Those smaller than 10 mm in diameter are termed microadenomas (Fig. 71.2) and those larger than 10 mm termed macroadenomas (Figs 71.3, 71.4). Approximately 75% of patients with pituitary adenomas will have symptoms of hormone excess, while the remainder (those with nonfunctioning tumours) present with clinical findings related to tumour mass effect (e.g., headache, visual field defects, cranial nerve palsies). Pituitary adenomas are classified on the basis of electron microscopic and immunohistochemical criteria. On high-resolution CT, pituitary adenomas are typically hypodense compared with the normal gland on both unenhanced and contrast-enhanced images. Similarly, on MRI, 80–90% of microadenomas appear as a focal hypointense lesion compared with the normal gland

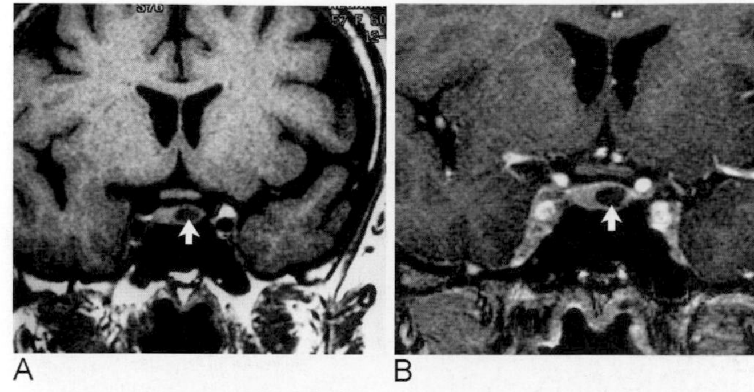

Figure 71.2 Pituitary microadenoma. Coronal T1-weighted spin echo images before (A) and after (B) gadolinium enhancement demonstrates a microadenoma (arrow) in the left side of the gland. The adenoma enhances less avidly than the rest of the gland.

on unenhanced T1-weighted images. After gadolinium, the adenoma enhances less avidly than the rest of the gland. The use of gadolinium increases the sensitivity of MRI for the detection of adenomas. Although up to 50% of microadenomas are hyperintense on T2-weighted sequences, overall T2-weighted sequences are less sensitive than T1-weighted sequences for detection of adenomas and are not used routinely. Other evidence of an adenoma includes focal erosion of the sella floor or focal convexity of the superior surface of the gland. Tilting of the pituitary stalk, which was once thought to be indirect evidence of an adenoma, is now considered to be unreliable as a diagnostic sign owing to the wide range of

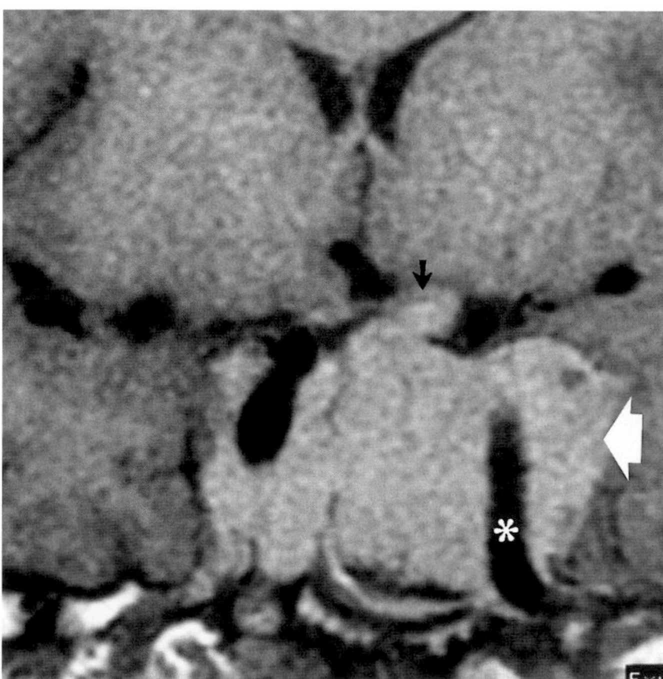

Figure 71.3 Pituitary macroadenoma. Unenhanced coronal T1-weighted spin-echo image demonstrates a pituitary macroadenoma. The presence of tumour tissue (white arrow) lateral to the black flow-void of the left carotid artery (*) indicates involvement of the cavernous sinus; the right cavernous sinus is also involved. A small suprasellar nodule of tumour deforms the left optic nerve (black arrow).

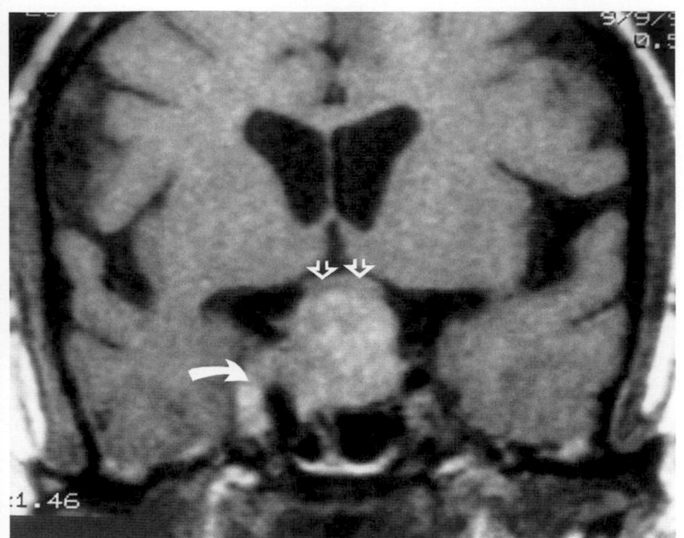

Figure 71.4 Pituitary macroadenoma with suprasellar extension. Unenhanced coronal T1-weighted spin-echo image demonstrates a pituitary macroadenoma extending into the right cavernous sinus (curved arrow) and extending upward into the suprasellar cistern to impinge on the optic chiasm (open arrows). The high signal from the tumour indicates the presence of recent haemorrhage.

normal variation[7]. Macroadenomas have similar signal characteristics to microadenomas, however, it is often not possible to identify any remaining normal pituitary tissue with larger lesions. Macroadenomas may grow upwards to compress the optic nerves and chiasm and/or may extend downward into the sphenoid sinus. It is important to diagnose cavernous sinus invasion by a pituitary adenoma, but unfortunately neither CT nor MRI has proved highly accurate in its preoperative detection. Encasement of the internal carotid artery is conclusive evidence. The identification of any tumour lying lateral to the lateral tangent of the intra and supracavernous internal carotid artery on coronal MRI is highly suggestive of cavernous sinus involvement. Cystic degeneration and haemorrhage are not uncommon in larger tumours but are also seen in microadenomas. Large pituitary adenomas are prone to develop infarction or haemorrhage owing to their tenuous blood supply. While this may present with fulminant and life-threatening pituitary apoplexy, it is far more frequently a subclinical phenomenon, being detected only at surgery or MRI. On MRI, over half of pituitary adenomas treated with bromocriptine will reveal evidence of haemorrhage that is clinically silent[8].

Postoperative imaging of the sella is difficult. Changes in its anatomy and that of its surroundings, the surgical technique used, inflammation and the quality and quantity of the implanted synthetic and organic materials are all factors that impede assessment of residual tumour. In practice, baseline imaging 3–4 months after pituitary surgery can give an accurate assessment of residual tumour.

Rathke's cleft cyst: Asymptomatic non-neoplastic pituitary cysts are found in approximately 11% of autopsies[9]. They arise from remnants of epithelium from Rathke's pouch. They are typically in the centre of the gland, although they can be laterally located or even suprasellar. Many of these cysts are isointense with CSF, however, if they contain proteinaceous fluid they may be hyperintense on T1- and T2-weighted sequences. The lack of contrast enhancement and absence of calcification usually allows distinction from craniopharyngiomas. Occasionally a Rathke's cleft cyst can enlarge and compress the chiasm.

Suprasellar lesions

The most common lesion in the suprasellar region is the pituitary macroadenoma with suprasellar extension (see intrasellar adenomas above). Other common lesions include craniopharyngiomas, meningioma, hypothalamic/chiasmatic glioma and aneurysm. Uncommon lesions include metastases, meningitis and granulomatous disease.

Craniopharyngiomas are encapsulated cystic tumours of the sella or suprasellar region (Fig. 71.5), which originate from epithelial remnants of Rathke's pouch. There is a bimodal age distribution; one peak between 5 and 10 years and the second smaller peak between 50 and 60 years. Typical presentation in childhood is with headache and raised intracranial pressure. Visual impairment and hypopituitarism may be present. MRI reveals a predominantly suprasellar mass that has both cystic and solid elements. The cystic portions of the tumour are characteristically hyperintense on T1- and T2-weighted sequences. The signal characteristics are due to the cholesterol crystals present in the cyst fluid, at surgery this fluid appears like 'engine-oil'. The solid portions of the tumour enhance with gadolinium. These tumours are locally invasive, hard to resect and have a tendency to recur. Calcification is typical and is easier to identify on CT, appearing as an area of hypointensity on MRI. Less typical appearances of craniopharyngioma include purely solid masses and entirely intrasellar lesions. Craniopharyngiomas in the older age group are more likely to be solid, less likely to be calcified and have a better prognosis.

Parasellar meningiomas can arise from any dural surface in the sellar region, This includes the anterior clinoid processes, the diaphragma sella, tuberculum or dorsum sellae, or

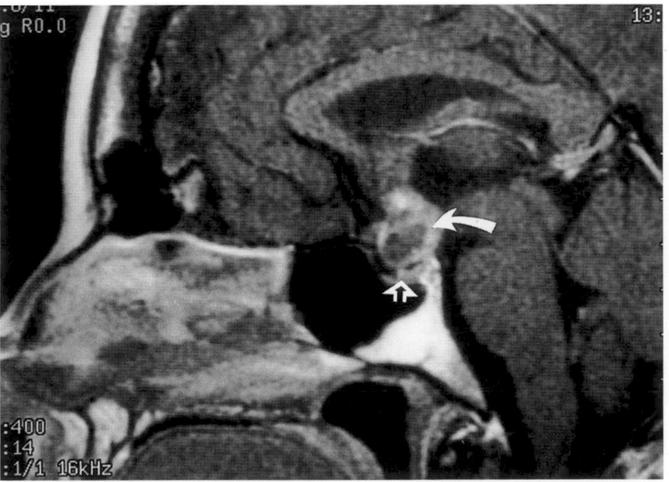

Figure 71.5 Craniopharyngioma. Enhanced sagittal T1-weighted spin echo images demonstrates a recurrent craniopharyngioma (curved arrow). The mass is suprasellar and clearly separate from the normal pituitary gland (open arrow). There is patchy enhancement but no cystic component is visible.

the cavernous sinuses. Their appearances on CT and MRI are similar to those of meningiomas elsewhere. A clear plane separating the tumour from the pituitary gland is often visible at high-resolution MRI. Meningiomas of the cavernous sinuses may cause constriction of the internal carotid artery, a feature not seen in pituitary adenomas.

Primary hypothalamic tumours, such as gliomas, are uncommon. It is often difficult to identify whether a tumour in this site has arisen from the optic chiasm or the hypothalamus, particularly if it is a large mass. Chiasmatic gliomas are found mainly in children and may be associated with neurofibromatosis type 1. These tumours have a tendency to spread along the optic pathways, and T2-weighted sequences should be used to assess signal change along the optic radiation. These tumours are usually low grade, may be cystic, may or may not enhance and do not calcify.

Germinomas are solid tumours arising from germ cells and typically occurring between the ages of 5 and 25 years. Although the pineal is the most common location for these lesions, they can also occur primarily in the suprasellar region and may be multicentric (Fig. 71.6). Diabetes insipidus and visual impairment are often the presenting feature. On MRI they appear as homogeneous solid masses often involving the pituitary stalk and optic chiasm. They are slightly hypointense on T1-weighted sequences and slightly hyperintense on T2-weighted sequences. Enhancement is prominent and homogeneous.

Metastases to the sellar region account for approximately 1% of sellar masses and they most commonly arise from lung, breast, kidney, gastrointestinal tract, or nasopharyngeal tumours. There is usually clinical evidence of widespread metastatic disease. Metastases are usually suprasellar or combined intra- and suprasellar in position. They show varying degrees of enhancement and calcification is extremely rare.

Vascular lesions: Aneurysms of the supraclinoid internal carotid artery are important to recognize. MRI shows a typical area of black flow void (on spin-echo sequences). Partially thrombosed aneurysms may have more complex signal characteristics. Aneurysms of the cavernous portion of the internal carotid artery can expand the cavernous sinus and extend into the pituitary fossa.

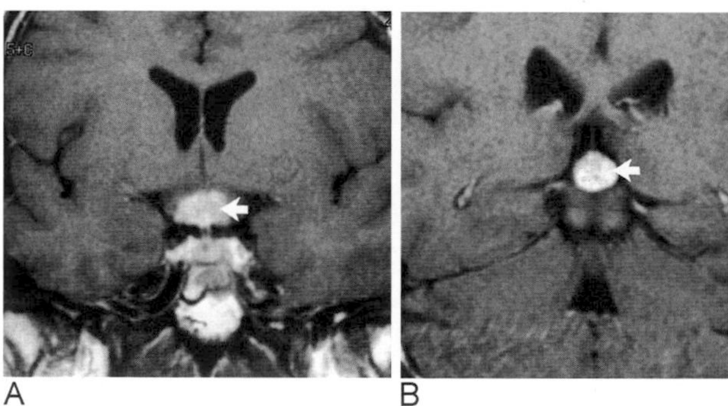

Figure 71.6 Germinoma. Coronal T1-weighted spin echo image after intravenous injection of gadolinium demonstrates homogeneously enhancing masses (arrow) in the (A) suprasellar and (B) pineal regions. The masses were isointense prior to contrast (not shown)

Suprasellar arachnoid cysts show smooth margins and have CSF signal intensity. They do not calcify or enhance. They may enlarge displace and compress the third ventricle. On fluid attenuation inversion recovery (FLAIR) and diffusion-weighted sequences they are identical to CSF within the ventricles.

Hypothalamic (tuber cinerum) hamartoma is a congenital non-neoplastic heterotopia. The clinical presentation is usually that of precocious puberty although gelastic (laughing) seizures may occur. On MRI the hamartoma is seen as a sessile or pedunculated well-defined lesion arising from the tuber cinereum (Fig. 71.7). This is isointense to grey matter on T1-weighted images and isointense (or slightly hyperintense) to grey matter on T2-weighted images[10]. There is no calcification or enhancement.

Other causes of infundibular masses include Langerhans cell histiocytosis, sarcoid lymphoma and metastases. Involvement of the infundibulum with one of these processes usually enlarges it to a diameter greater than 4.5 mm or greater than that of the basilar artery[1]. CT or MRI shows an enhancing, usually homogeneous mass.

THE THYROID GLAND

ANATOMY AND PHYSIOLOGY

The thyroid gland is located in the anterior part of the neck with the lateral lobes lying on either side of the trachea joined across the midline by the isthmus. Each lobe measures approximately 40 × 20 × 20 mm. The pretracheal fascia binds the thyroid to the trachea, and it moves with the trachea on swallowing. An accessory lobe, the pyramidal lobe may be present in up to 50% of the population and usually arises from the thyroid isthmus[11].

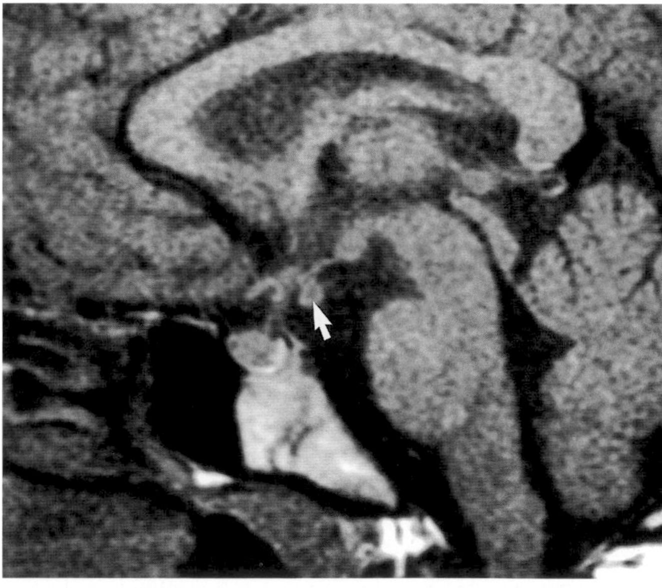

Figure 71.7 Hypothalamic hamartoma. Unenhanced sagittal T1-weighted spin echo image demonstrates a hypothalamic hamartoma (arrow). This arises from the inferior surface of the tuber cinereum and is isointense with other grey matter.

The thyroid produces two major hormones, thyroxine (T4) and tri-iodothyronine (T3). The production of these hormones from the thyroid is regulated via thyroid-stimulating hormone (TSH) secreted by the anterior pituitary, which in turn is regulated by TSH-releasing hormone (TRH) released from the hypothalamus.

IMAGING TECHNIQUES

Ultrasound

Ultrasound (US) provides the best anatomical representation of the thyroid gland. Using high-resolution (7.5–10 MHz) probes, modern machines provide excellent spatial resolution and allow nodules as small as 2–3 mm to be detected.

Radionuclides

Radionuclide imaging of the thyroid provides functional information that complements the anatomical information obtained from US. Several radionuclide-labelled agents are currently used to image the thyroid.

Technetium-99m (^{99m}Tc) pertechnetate is the most widely used thyroid-imaging agent and is used as a first-line diagnostic tool in the evaluation of the thyroid. The pertechnetate anion is actively concentrated across the epithelium of a number of tissues via the same ion channel as the iodide anion. In addition to the thyroid gland, this includes the choroid plexus, salivary glands and gastric mucosa. Although pertechnetate is concentrated within the thyroid, unlike iodide it is not incorporated into thyroglobulin. Pertechnetate is excreted unchanged by the kidneys, salivary glands and gut. Before imaging, markers are placed on any palpable abnormalities, the cricoid and suprasternal notch. Imaging begins 20 minutes after the intravenous injection of sodium pertechnetate. Anterior, left and right oblique views are obtained and uptake of the injected activity is measured (normal 0.4–4.0%). The uptake of pertechnetate provides a map of the trapping function of thyroid tissue. Usually, uniform uptake of pertechnetate is seen throughout both lobes, but sometimes it concentrates in the isthmus or in the pyramidal lobe.

Radioisotopes of iodine permit tracer studies of the entire metabolic pathway of iodine within the thyroid. This includes trapping, organification, coupling, hormone storage and secretion. Oral iodides, radiographic contrast media and iodine-containing drugs compete with these radioisotopes and should be avoided before studies with radioisotopes of iodine. Iodine-123 (^{123}I) decays by electron capture with a single gamma-ray photon of 159 keV (which is ideal for imaging) and releases no beta particles. Its low radiation dose and short half-life (13 h) makes it an excellent radiotracer for functional evaluation of the thyroid. The disadvantages of ^{123}I are its limited availability and high cost of production, as it requires a cyclotron. ^{123}I is given intravenously and imaging is performed 2–6 hours and 18–24 hours after administration, at which time most of the iodine within the thyroid is present as radio-iodotyrosine residues on thyroglobulin, reflecting hormonogenesis.

[F-18]-2-fluoro-2-deoxyglucose ([F-18]FDG) has recently become the most commonly used radiopharmaceutical for clinical positron emission tomography (PET) studies in cancer patients. FDG is transported into cancer cells like glucose. The more aggressive thyroid cancers, which often do not accumulate radio-iodine, do accumulate [F-18]FDG. The main clinical indication is in patients with residual or recurrent thyroid cancer with raised thyroglobulin and a negative radio-iodine whole-body survey. [F-18]FDG-PET imaging may also be helpful in anaplastic and some medullary carcinomas of the thyroid.

Other radiotracers used in thyroid imaging: Thallium-201 (^{201}Tl) uptake is seen in various thyroid disorders, including cancers, subacute and chronic thyroiditis and Graves' disease. Its main clinical application is in patients with residual or recurrent thyroid cancer with raised thyroglobulin and a negative radio-iodine whole-body survey. In 29% of such patients, ^{201}Tl can detect residual disease. ^{99m}Tc-methoxy-isobutylisonitrile (^{99m}Tc-MIBI) is also concentrated by thyroid tissue, and its role in thyroid imaging is similar to that of ^{201}Tl. ^{99m}Tc-MIBI images have better resolution and are easier to interpret than ^{201}Tl-scintigrams. However, because of considerable hepatic and abdominal activity with ^{99m}Tc-MIBI, ^{201}Tl is preferred if these areas are suspected sites of disease. ^{99m}Tc-tetrofosmin has similar imaging properties to ^{99m}Tc-MIBI. ^{201}Tl, ^{99m}Tc-MIBI and ^{99m}Tc-tetrofosmin do not require the withdrawal of thyroid-suppressive treatment unlike radio-iodine. In the investigation of medullary thyroid cancer ^{123}I-metaiodobenzylguanidine (^{123}I-MIBG), pentavalent ^{99m}Tc DMSA and indium-111-diethylenetriaminepentaacetic acid-octreotide (^{111}In-DTPA-octreotide) may be used[12]. However, with rising calcitonin levels and negative ^{123}I-MIBG, pentavalent ^{99m}Tc-DMSA and ^{111}In-DTPA-octreotide imaging, [F-18]FDG-PET is useful.

Computed tomography and magnetic resonance imaging

MRI and CT have a limited role in the evaluation of thyroid disease. They may occasionally be used to demonstrate the extent of local invasion or local recurrence of thyroid malignancy and to detect the presence of retrosternal and retrotracheal extension of thyroid enlargement.

THYROID DISORDERS

Thyroid nodules

One of the most common clinical problems is in patients presenting with a solitary palpable thyroid nodule. Its importance is due to the fact that thyroid cancer most often presents as a solitary thyroid nodule. However, thyroid nodules are extremely common: 4–7% of adults have palpable nodules[13]. The majority are benign, due to cysts, thyroiditis, adenomas, or colloid nodules. Investigation is directed towards detecting the 5–10% of palpable thyroid nodules that are malignant[12].

US, often the first imaging investigation, is of value in establishing whether a palpable nodule is solitary, cystic or part of a multinodular process such as multinodular goitres. In approximately 25% of patients, clinically solitary palpable nodules are shown by US to be multiple. Multinodular goitres have a lower incidence of malignancy (1–6%) than is associated with a single 'cold' nodule that is malignant (15–25% of cases).

US cannot reliably distinguish between benign and malignant thyroid nodules, but is however extremely effective in distinguishing between solid and cystic lesions. Purely cystic lesions with no soft tissue component are very rarely cancers, and in most institutions are managed with fine-needle aspiration. Certain US features increase the likelihood of malignancy of a thyroid nodule; notably, invasion into surrounding tissues, which results in loss of clear definition of the tissue planes. US is more sensitive than clinical examination in the detection of enlarged cervical nodes. Cervical lymph nodes, infiltrated by papillary carcinoma of the thyroid, may be entirely cystic and mimic other cystic masses of the neck, such as a branchial cyst, while calcification may be seen within nodes invaded by medullary carcinoma. Microcalcification smaller than 2 mm in diameter with acoustic shadowing suggests malignancy, as it is observed in about 60% of carcinomas but only 2% of benign nodules[14].

Ultrasound-guided fine-needle aspiration for cytology (FNAC) is the most reliable nonoperative method for obtaining a definitive diagnosis and is important in the selection of patients for surgery. Overall, the sensitivity of FNAC for the detection of malignancy in both cystic and solid lesions ranged from 90 to 100%. However, false-positives occur quite frequently, so the specificity is only 55% for solid nodules and 52% for cystic lesions[15]. Other drawbacks of FNAC are that it may be less sensitive for cystic papillary carcinomas[15] and that it is not possible to differentiate between follicular adenoma and adenocarcinoma, as histologically the distinction relies on documenting capsular or venous invasion. Many centres now perform US-guided core biopsy for these reasons.

Radionuclide thyroid scintigraphy is used to determine the functional status of nodules. Nodules may be 'cold', 'warm', or 'hot', depending on the uptake of tracer compared with normal thyroid. Pitfalls inherent in the use of these terms are well recognized: a superficial cold nodule may appear to be functioning because normal thyroid tissue behind it is visualized; or a superficial functioning nodule may appear hot because of photons emanating from the deeper, normal tissue.

Thyroid cancers concentrate less radio-iodine (only 1%) than normal thyroid tissue and hence appear 'cold' in the presence of normal thyroid tissue (Fig. 71.8). Rarely, well-differentiated thyroid cancers have preserved trapping function, but virtually no capacity for iodine organification, therefore giving the appearance of function on early imaging (trapping phase) but becoming 'cold' on delayed images. This drawback can be overcome by acquiring delayed images of functioning nodules. Most 'cold' nodules are adenomas, colloid nodules, or foci of thyroiditis or rarely intrathyroid lymph nodes, lymphomas, or metastases. Approximately 10–25% of nonfunctioning ('cold') solitary nodules are malignant. 'Cold' nodules always require further assessment, usually by fine-needle aspiration cytology, core biopsy and/or excision biopsy. This combined imaging approach reduces significantly the rate of unnecessary surgery for benign nonfunctioning nodes.

Functioning nodules account for approximately 30% of solitary nodules, and one third to one half are autonomous. In euthyroid individuals, the autonomous and nonautonomous nodules can be differentiated by the administration of T3, which uniformly suppresses the uptake of iodide by both the TSH-dependent nodule and the extranodular normal tissue, but not by the autonomous nodule. The diagnosis of autonomous function can also be made by the demonstration of suppressed extranodular tissue on repeating the data acquisition following the administration of TSH. Approximately 10–20% of euthyroid subjects with autonomous nodules become hyperthyroid within 6 years, of whom half show an elevation in T3 only ('T3 toxicosis'). Scintigraphic progression of the disorder (progressive suppression of extranodular uptake) parallels the decline in serum TSH concentration, but hyperthyroidism rarely occurs until a nodule reaches 30 mm in diameter. Malignant autonomous nodules usually produce hyperthyroidism.

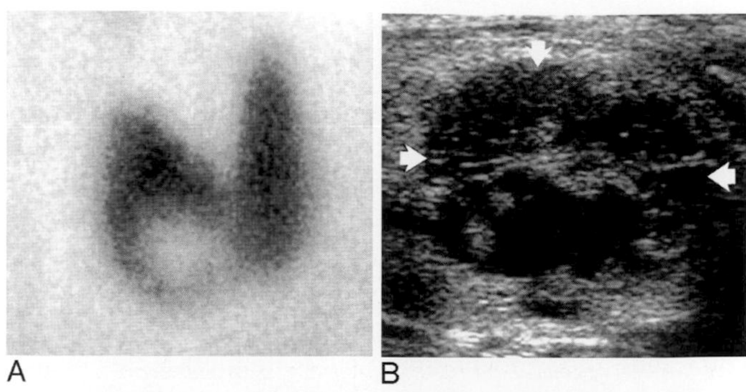

Figure 71.8 Thyroid carcinoma presenting as a cold nodule. (A) ^{99m}Tc-pertechnetate scintigram shows a 'cold' nodule in the lower pole of the right lobe of the thyroid gland. (B) Transverse ultrasound corresponding to the lesion in (A) shows an inhomogeneous nodule (arrows).

The 'hot' appearance of a nodule is not synonymous with autonomy; indeed, it often represents a spared focus of normal thyroid tissue (or a TSH-dependent nodule) in a gland otherwise involved in a destructive process (typically Hashimoto's thyroiditis). Diagnosis can be made by the T3-suppression test.

Multinodular goitre is generally, but not always, a benign disorder, and dominant cold nodules, especially enlarging ones, require further evaluation by aspiration biopsy. Autonomous foci are common and, when extensive, ultimately result in hyperthyroidism (toxic multinodular goitre, Plummer's disease), one of the nodules often being dominant.

Thyroid cancer

Thyroid cancer is uncommon and accounts for only 0.5% of all cancer deaths[12]. All forms of thyroid cancer occur more frequently in women than men and the peak incidence is seen in young women aged 25–35 years. Radiation exposure is the most important aetiological factor, but other risk factors include iodine excess, genetic predisposition and alcohol excess. The main histological subtypes of thyroid cancers are papillary, follicular, medullary and anaplastic cancers.

Papillary cancers are the most common type and account for 50–80% of all thyroid malignancy. They are characteristically low-grade tumours with good prognosis. These tumours are usually multicentric histologically and spread to lymph nodes early, but distant metastases are rare. Metastatic lymph nodes may be normal in size, cystic, calcified, haemorrhagic, or may contain colloid. Papillary carcinomas concentrate radio-iodine.

Follicular cancers account for 10–40% of thyroid cancers. They are slow-growing but have a tendency to spread via the bloodstream and disseminate to bone, liver, or lung and only rarely metastasize to regional lymph nodes. Hurthle cell tumours comprise 20% of follicular carcinomas; these are more common in women, they usually do not take up radio-iodine and metastases are frequently undetected. In such cases, ^{201}Tl, ^{99m}Tc-MIBI or ^{99m}Tc-tetrofosmin may be useful.

Anaplastic thyroid cancers are undifferentiated tumours and are the most malignant. They have a poor prognosis and are usually treated with radiotherapy rather than surgery. Lymphatic metastases occur in the majority of patients and are often necrotic. These neoplasms do not concentrate radio-iodine. On US they are often hypoechoic, and on CT punctate calcification and necrosis are frequently present.

Medullary carcinomas originate from the parafollicular C cells. Medullary carcinomas are usually solitary lesions that may invade locally, spread to regional nodes, or undergo haematogenous spread to lung, bone, or liver and may be sporadic or familial. The familial form occurs with multiple endocrine neoplasia (MEN) type II syndrome (Table 71.8) or with other endocrine neoplasms. Patients may present with ectopic hormone production, and calcitonin is normally elevated. Unlike papillary and follicular tumours, medullary tumours do not concentrate radio-iodine but radionuclides specific for neuroendocrine tissue such as ^{123}I-MIBG and somatostatin analogues may be used to evaluate patients with medullary cancer (Fig. 71.9).

Lymphomas account for 10% of thyroid malignancies and are mostly non-Hodgkin type. They occur in one third of patients with Hashimoto's thyroiditis. Imaging cannot distinguish between lymphoma and thyroiditis[16]. Patients usually present with a rapidly enlarging thyroid mass. They tend to involve the nodes and spread to the gastrointestinal tract.

Table 71.8 MULTIPLE ENDOCRINE NEOPLASIA (MEN)

MEN Type I
Parathyroid adenoma or hyperplasia (hyperthyroidism)
Pancreatic islet cell tumours
Pituitary adenoma
MEN Type IIA
Parathyroid hyperplasia
Adrenal medullary tumour
Medullary thyroid cancer
MEN Type IIB
Medullary thyroid cancer
Adrenal medullary tumour
Marfanoid features, multiple cutaneous and mucosal neuromas, neurofibromas and gastrointestinal ganglioneuroma

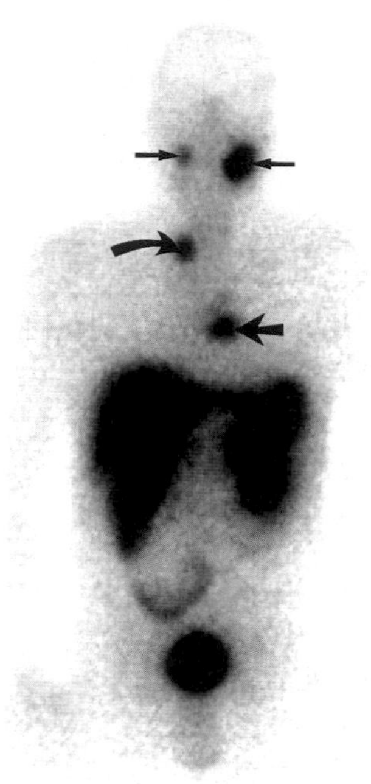

Figure 71.9 MEN Type IIB. ^{111}In-pentetreotide image shows a patient with medullary carcinoma of the thyroid (curved arrow) and bilateral glomus tumours (small arrows) and a paraganglioma (large arrow) in lower mediastinum.

Thyroid lymphoma presents most commonly as a solitary nodule (80%) or as multiple nodules. The nodule is hypoechoic on US[17], hypodense on CT, and of high signal intensity on T2-weighted MRI[18]. Necrosis and calcification is uncommon.

Metastatic tumour presenting on the thyroid is uncommon. Clinically, the most commonly detected primary is renal cancer[19].

The diagnosis of thyroid malignancy is confirmed by cytology or histology from a thyroid nodule or after the removal of a cervical lymph node. Imaging is useful to delineate the extent of the tumour, detect metastatic disease and for follow-up of treated patients to detect local recurrence and distant spread. The main factors determining the prognosis include the patient's age, size of the tumour, degree of differentiation, invasion and nodal and distant metastases.

Treatment and follow-up of thyroid cancer

Patients with thyroid cancer are usually treated with a total thyroidectomy. This enables subsequent follow-up with ^{131}I-scintigraphy and serum thyroglobulin measurement. Subtotal operations are followed by ^{131}I-ablation therapy. Clinical evaluation, repeat scintigraphy and serum thyroglobulin measurement are performed 6–12 months later to assess the adequacy of ablation and to detect and treat metastatic disease under elevated TSH drive. Whole-body iodine imaging is performed after discontinuing thyroid hormone (for 4 weeks for T4 or for 2 weeks for T3) and establishing that TSH concentrations are $>30\,\mu mol\ L^{-1}$ [20]. It is also possible to image these patients without discontinuing thyroid medication using recombinant TSH, although slightly better results are achieved by suspending conventional thyroid medication.^{131}I-whole-body imaging can identify most functioning metastases (Fig. 71.10), which are usually in the neck, lungs, or bone[20]. Lung metastases are clearly seen on ^{131}I-imaging. The scintigraphic detection of metastases is increased when the patient is imaged about 7 days after a therapeutic dose of ^{131}I. The sensitivity and specificity of ^{131}I-scintigraphy for detecting metastatic disease due to differentiated thyroid cancers is 42–62% and 99–100%, respectively[21,22]. Both the sensitivity and specificity of serum thyroglobulin are in the range 55–78%, depending on the presence or absence of anti-thyroglobulin antibody[23]. In patients with raised thyroglobulin concentrations and a negative ^{131}I-whole-body survey, the sensitivity of ^{201}Tl, ^{99m}Tc-MIBI, ^{99m}Tc-tetrofosmin and [F-18]FDG-PET is 49%, 88%, 89% and 94% respectively[23–25]. High specificity has also been reported with [F-18]FDG-PET.

In patients with medullary carcinoma, following removal serum calcitonin concentrations are used to diagnose recurrence. When elevated, pentavalent ^{99m}Tc-DMSA or ^{111}In-DTPA-octreotide or ^{123}I-MIBG have been used for the detection and documentation of recurrent or residual disease[12]. In cases of ^{123}I-MIBG-positive disease, therapy with ^{131}I-MIBG can be instituted.

In the detection of recurrent disease, MRI has a positive predictive value of 82% and a negative predictive value of 86% in the neck[26]. Like CT, false-positive results can be caused by inflammatory lymphatic hyperplasia and granulation tissue. Nevertheless, there is a distinct advantage to using MRI rather than US or CT in the detection of recurrent disease[26]. US is useful during follow-up to detect neck masses or lymph nodes.

Screening for thyroid cancer

Following radiation therapy to the neck, there is an increased risk of papillary and follicular thyroid carcinoma. For example, in patients who have received radiotherapy for Hodgkin's disease, the risk of developing thyroid cancer is about 15%[27]. The carcinoma is unlikely to develop within 5 years of exposure to radiation; therefore, beyond 5 years, US provides a useful, sensitive and relatively inexpensive means of screening a population at risk for thyroid cancer[27].

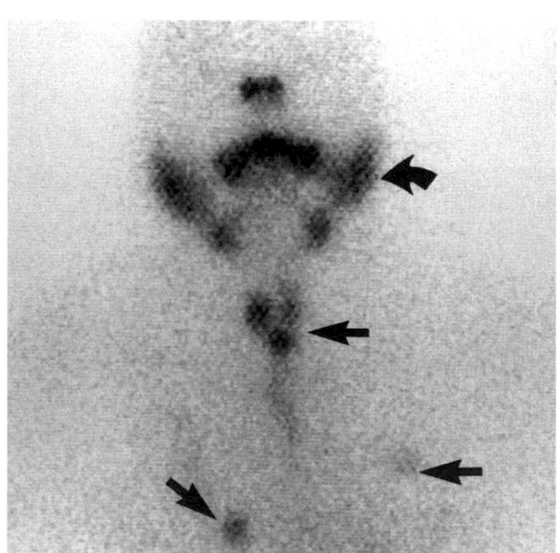

Figure 71.10 Well-differentiated thyroid carcinoma imaged 3 days after ^{131}Iodine (150 mCi, 5.55 GBq). Imaging shows increased uptake in thyroid bed, right hilar region and left upper chest (arrows). Salivary activity is also noted which is a normal feature (curved arrow).

Hyperthyroidism

Hyperthyroidism is most commonly due to Graves' disease or autonomous toxic nodules (Plummer's disease). Other causes of hyperthyroidism include iodide-induced hyperthyroidism, thyroiditis and rarely hyperthyroidism secondary to a pituitary, hypothalamic, or ectopic source such as struma ovarii. Hyperthyroidism is diagnosed clinically and biochemically. Imaging may be helpful in identifying the cause and in the follow-up of patients managed with radio-iodine.

Graves' disease is an autoimmune disorder in which a circulating immunoglobulin, produced largely by intrathyroidal lymphocytes, stimulates the thyroid gland by binding to TSH receptors. If this sequence of events occurs in a thyroid that is normal to begin with, the result is diffuse toxic goitre. Scintigraphy reveals high and uniform uptake of tracer in the enlarged gland (Fig. 71.11). At US the gland is often diffusely hyperechoic without discrete nodules. There is a characteristic increase in thyroid vasculature on colour Doppler (see Fig. 71.11) especially in patients with active hyperthyroidism. Approximately 5–10% of the population have underlying thyroid disease to start with, and Graves' disease may be superimposed upon solitary thyroid nodules, multinodular goitre, or Hashimoto's thyroiditis, and the imaging will reflect this. The combination of Graves' disease and a functioning nodule is called Marine–Lenhart syndrome. This entity is important as 50% of the nodules are radioresistant: this gives rise to unusual scintigraphic findings following ^{131}I-therapy.

Toxic multinodular goitre (Plummer's disease) may present either as a toxic goitre with hyperfunctioning nodules and suppressed stroma or as diffuse toxicity of the thyroid stroma with intervening nodules. A single toxic nodule shows high uptake of tracer and the remaining normal thyroid tissue may show poor or virtually no activity on the images. Toxic multinodular goitre that is not associated with any of the autoimmune manifestations of Graves' disease is the most common cause of toxicosis in elderly patients.

Hypothyroidism

Hypothyroidism may be primary (endogenous thyroid disorder), secondary (decreased TSH production due to pituitary disease) or tertiary (decreased TRH secretion from hypothalamic disorders). The most common causes of primary hypothyroidism include surgery or radiation ablation for Graves' disease or thyroid cancer, primary idiopathic hypothyroidism, Hashimoto's thyroiditis (see below), iodine deficiency and congenital hypothyroidism. In neonates with suspected primary congenital hypothyroidism based on screening (heel-stick blood levels of T4 and TSH), the ^{99m}Tc-pertechnetate scan is a useful adjunct procedure. The ^{99m}Tc-pertechnetate helps to confirm the presence of a normal gland in patients with a false-positive screening test and to differentiate between the three sub-groups of primary congenital hypothyroidism: (A) nonvisualization of functioning thyroid tissue; (B) hypoplastic and ectopic glands; and (C) dyshormonogenesis[28].

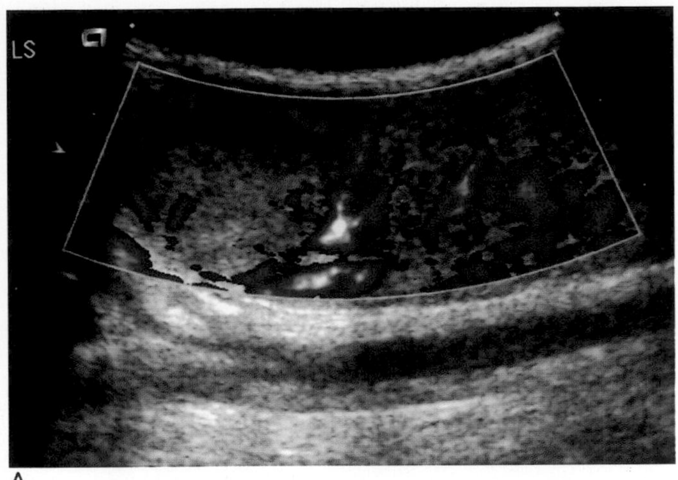

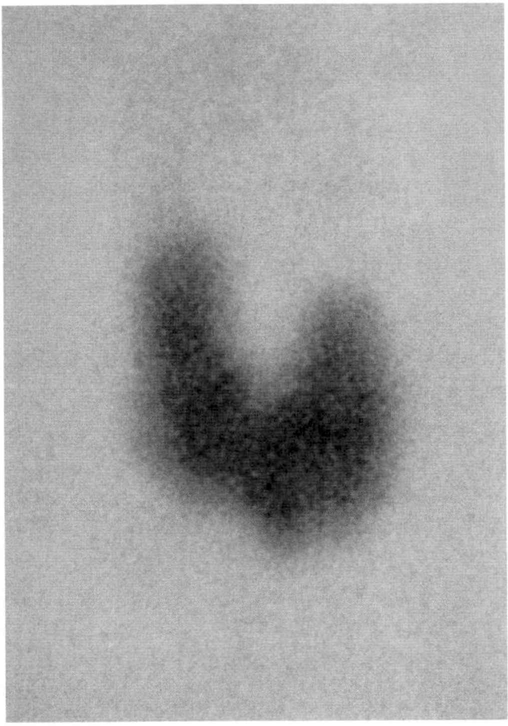

Figure 71.11 Graves' disease. (A) Longitudinal ultrasound with colour Doppler shows diffusely increased vascularity of the thyroid gland. (B) ^{99m}Tc-pertechnetate imaging shows a diffusely increased tracer uptake.

Thyroiditis

Hashimoto's thyroiditis (chronic lymphocystic thyroiditis) is an autoimmune destructive disorder. On scintigraphy, there is no typical pattern. Uptake is most commonly heterogeneous and patchy, but may be uniformly increased or decreased. At US the gland shows a variety of patterns. The thyroid may be normal or enlarged in size and is diffusely abnormal with a heterogeneous echo texture. There may be numerous poorly defined hypoechoic regions separated by fibrous strands. Discrete nodules and adjacent adenopathy are less commonly seen. End-stage disease may show a fibrotic gland that is small, ill defined and heterogeneous. US is performed to follow up Hashimoto's disease to check for malignancy and the development of large nodules within the gland increase the possibility of superimposed non-Hodgkin lymphoma.

Silent or painless thyroiditis is another autoimmune disorder in which radio-iodine uptake is initially very low, but in the recovery (hypothyroid) phase it may be normal to elevated. The scintigram in mild, subacute (viral) thyroiditis generally shows patchy uptake in an enlarged and tender thyroid gland. With extensive disease, the uptake is markedly suppressed by both the disruptive effect of inflammation and the ensuing hyperthyroidism. Riedel's thyroiditis is characterized by a fibrosing reaction that destroys the thyroid. The thyroid is hypoechoic on US and hypodense on CT[29]. On MRI, the thyroid is of low signal intensity on T1- and T2-weighted images[29]. In acute suppurative thyroiditis the affected portion of the gland is enlarged and heterogeneous on cross-sectional imaging. Focal abscess may develop with disease progression, and there may be associated myositis and cellulitis in the adjacent neck. Imaging is used to exclude a fistula (from the pyriform sinus) as a cause of the thyroiditis.

Congenital disorders

During fetal development, the thyroid descends from the base of the tongue (foramen caecum) to the low anterior neck. The thyroid is attached to the tongue base by the thyroglossal duct. During the caudal descent, the duct elongates and then degenerates and abnormal development or aberrant descent results in a spectrum of congenital lesions.

Ectopic thyroid tissue may occur anywhere from the foramen caecum, along the thyroglossal tract to the pretracheal, mediastinal, pericardiac area. Residual tissue at the foramen caecum is called a 'lingual thyroid'. A lingual thyroid is rarely associated with the presence of a normally positioned thyroid gland. Following total thyroidectomy, an ectopic focus within the thyroglossal tract near the centre of the hyoid bone is commonly seen, and must not be mistaken for a metastasis of thyroid cancer.

Hypoplasia or agenesis of a lobe almost always involves the left side[30]; conversely, a small right lobe is usually the result of disease rather than anatomical variation.

Incomplete degeneration of a thyroglossal cyst may result in a persistent fistulous tract or thyroglossal duct cyst. More than half of these cysts have normal thyroid tissue in their walls[11]. Thyroglossal cysts are infrahyoid in 65%, suprahyoid in 20% and in the hyoid region in 15%[11]. Uncomplicated cysts have the appearances of a typical cyst on cross-sectional imaging. Occasionally, if the cyst is infected, haemorrhagic, or has a high protein content, it may appear as hyperdense on CT, of high signal intensity on T1- and T2-weighted MRI (Fig. 71.12), and have internal echo at US. Rarely, thyroglossal cyst may undergo malignant change usually into a papillary carcinoma, which may be suspected if a soft tissue component exists within or around the cyst.

THE PARATHYROID GLANDS

ANATOMY AND PHYSIOLOGY

The parathyroid glands are derived from the endoderm of the third and fourth pharyngeal pouches. There are usually four

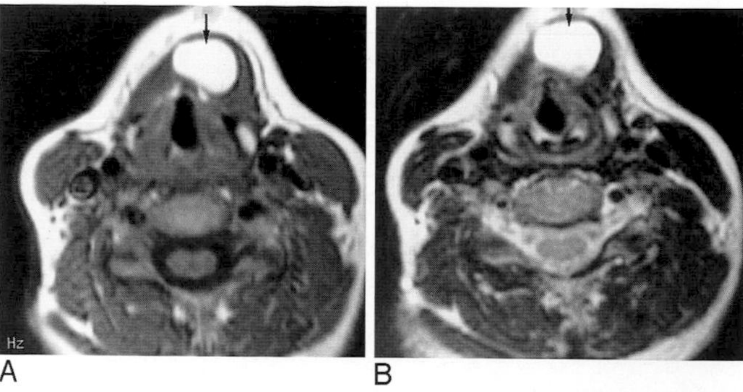

Figure 71.12 Thyroglossal duct cyst. (A) Axial T1-weighted spin-echo and (B) T2-weighted fast spin-echo images show a well-defined high signal intensity thyroglossal duct cyst just anterior to the hyoid bone.

glands, which lie behind the thyroid, but there may be as few as two or as many as six. Approximately 2.5% of the population have five glands. Each parathyroid gland measures approximately 5 × 3 × 1 mm and weighs 35 mg. Compared with the thyroid, the parathyroid glands are hypoechoic on US and have lower attenuation on CT than the thyroid. Approximately 80% of abnormal parathyroid glands are situated in and immediately adjacent to the thyroid. Ectopic glands may be found anywhere from the level of the third pharyngeal pouch, just behind the angle of the mandible at the level of the hyoid bone, down to the aortic root. Up to 5% may be in the posterior mediastinum.

Parathormone (PTH), together with vitamin D and calcitonin, maintains normal serum calcium levels by acting on bone, kidney and intestine.

PARATHYROID DISORDERS

Hypoparathyroidism

Hypoparathyroidism is most commonly due to accidental removal of the parathyroid glands or their ablation by radio-iodine therapy. Less frequently, hypoparathyroidism occurs in association with autoimmune disorders, including Addison's disease, pernicious anaemia and chronic thyroiditis. Rarely, aplasia or hypoplasia of the parathyroids occurs. Congenital causes of hypoparathyroidism include di George syndrome, which is associated with agenesis of the thymus.

The skeleton is usually normal in patients with hypoparathyroidism and the principal radiological manifestation of the disease is calcification of the basal ganglia and areas of the cerebrum and cerebellum. Ectopic calcification may also occur in periarticular or subcutaneous tissue.

Pseudohypoparathyroidism is an inherited disorder in which the biochemical finding of hypocalcaemia and hyperphosphataemia are similar to that found in hypoparathyroidism but do not respond to treatment with parathormone. Affected individuals are short in stature with short metacarpals, metatarsals and phalanges. The fourth and fifth metacarpals in particular are affected. The teeth are hypoplastic with defective enamel, and calcification may be present in the basal ganglia, cerebellum and skin. Children are moon-faced and may have deformities due to chronic tetany.

Pseudo-pseudohypoparathyroidism is a rare disorder exhibiting the same skeletal syndrome as pseudohypoparathyroidism but with normal blood chemistry.

Hyperparathyroidism

In hyperparathyroidism, increased concentrations of parathyroid hormones cause hypercalcaemia and increased urinary calcium excretion. This may result in nephrocalcinosis, renal calculi and bone disease.

The causes of primary hyperparathyroidism are, in order of frequency: single adenoma (80%), hyperplasia (15%), carcinoma (4%) and multiple adenoma (1%). Very rarely, ectopic excretion occurs, particularly with bronchial carcinoma. Secondary hyperparathyroidism results from parathyroid hyperplasia in response to hypocalcaemia. Tertiary hyperparathyroidism follows prolonged hypocalcaemia (as in chronic renal failure) and an autonomous adenoma forms.

The diagnosis of hyperparathyroidism is based on biochemical findings. Imaging is performed purely to localize parathyroid tumours and abnormal glands before surgery. The effects of hyperparathyroidism on the skeleton are discussed elsewhere.

Localization of abnormal parathyroid gland

The need for preoperative localization depends on the approach of individual surgeons. An experienced surgeon can achieve a cure rate of approximately 95% in primary hyperparathyroidism following initial exploration of the neck. Under these circumstances, preoperative localization is unlikely to add significantly to these results, or to reduce the operation time[31]. Other authors recommend unilateral neck dissection if one abnormal gland is demonstrated on preoperative images, only proceeding to bilateral exploration if the second ipsilateral gland appears abnormal at the time of operation[32]. A unilateral neck dissection allows a considerable reduction in operating time. It is advocated that a localization study should be performed in those patients who require reoperation, when the surgical cure rate without preoperative localization is 30–40% lower than in patients being operated on for the first time. Even though an increased proportion of abnormal glands will lie in an ectopic site, the pathological gland is still most likely to be located in the neck. In these patients, imaging before surgery improves the results by identifying the location of a parathyroid tumour[33,34].

On US, parathyroid adenomas typically appear as oval, well-defined anechoic or hypoechoic masses posterior to the thyroid gland. They tend to be of the order of 10 mm in diameter but can grow to a very large size (4–5 cm). As glands become larger, they are more likely to be multilobulated and to contain echogenic areas, cysts and calcifications.

There are several problems in the localization of parathyroid adenomas by US. Retropharyngeal, retro-oesophageal and mediastinal parathyroid glands, which account for 5–15% of all glands, are not easily accessible by US. Occasionally, in primary hyperplasia, one gland may predominate; simulating a solitary parathyroid adenoma. An exophytic thyroid nodule can be indistinguishable from a parathyroid nodule and a

PTH assay on fine-needle aspiration of the nodule will often resolve this problem. Other false-positive US diagnoses can result when hyperplastic lymph nodes, prominent longus colli muscles and sympathetic ganglia are misinterpreted as parathyroid adenomas. Intraoperative US has been shown to be of value during reoperation for primary hyperparathyroidism, assisting the surgeon in localizing the abnormal glands and reducing the operating time.

Computed tomography does not have any advantage over ultrasound in detecting an adenoma located in a normal parathyroid site, but is very useful for detecting abnormalities lying in sites inaccessible to ultrasound, such as behind the trachea, in the mediastinum, or in an undescended inferior parathyroid gland in the carotid sheath. These are all sites where adenomas are missed at initial neck exploration. CT is, therefore, a very useful localization procedure when performed before reoperation for persistent hyperparathyroidism. It is usually successful at identifying low cervical adenomas, but only 50% of mediastinal adenomas are detected.

Magnetic resonance imaging is increasingly being used for localizing abnormal parathyroid glands. Parathyroid adenomas typically are isointense to muscle on T1-weighted images, and of high signal intensity on T2-weighted images. However, approximately 30–40% of abnormal parathyroid glands do not have conventional signal characteristic[35] and must be identified on the basis of abnormal size and location.

Radionuclide imaging with ^{201}Tl or ^{99m}Tc-MIBI, using a subtraction technique whereby the image of the thyroid gland as shown by ^{99m}Tc or ^{123}I is removed, is a noninvasive technique for tumour localization (Fig. 71.13). ^{99m}Tc-MIBI can also be used on its own to detect adenomas (Fig. 71.14); early (15 min post injection) and delayed (90 min post injection) images are acquired for this purpose. ^{99m}Tc-MIBI is more sensitive than ^{201}Tl in preoperative data acquisition and in patients undergoing reoperation. Cumulative analysis of ^{99m}Tc-MIBI scintigraphy in patients with hyperparathyroidism demonstrates a sensitivity of 90% for single adenomas, 55% for abnormal glands in patients with multiglandular disease and 75% for recurrent hyperparathyroidism; the specificity for primary adenomas has been shown to be 98%[36]. The availability of ^{99m}Tc-MIBI single photon emission tomography (SPET)/CT and intra-operative detection of adenomas using hand-held gamma probes is becoming more popular, especially in patients who have undergone previous neck exploration. Autografted normal parathyroid glands can also be imaged with ^{99m}Tc-MIBI[37]. In patients where surgical re-exploration is being planned, but with negative conventional scintigraphy, ^{11}C-methionine PET/CT should also be considered.

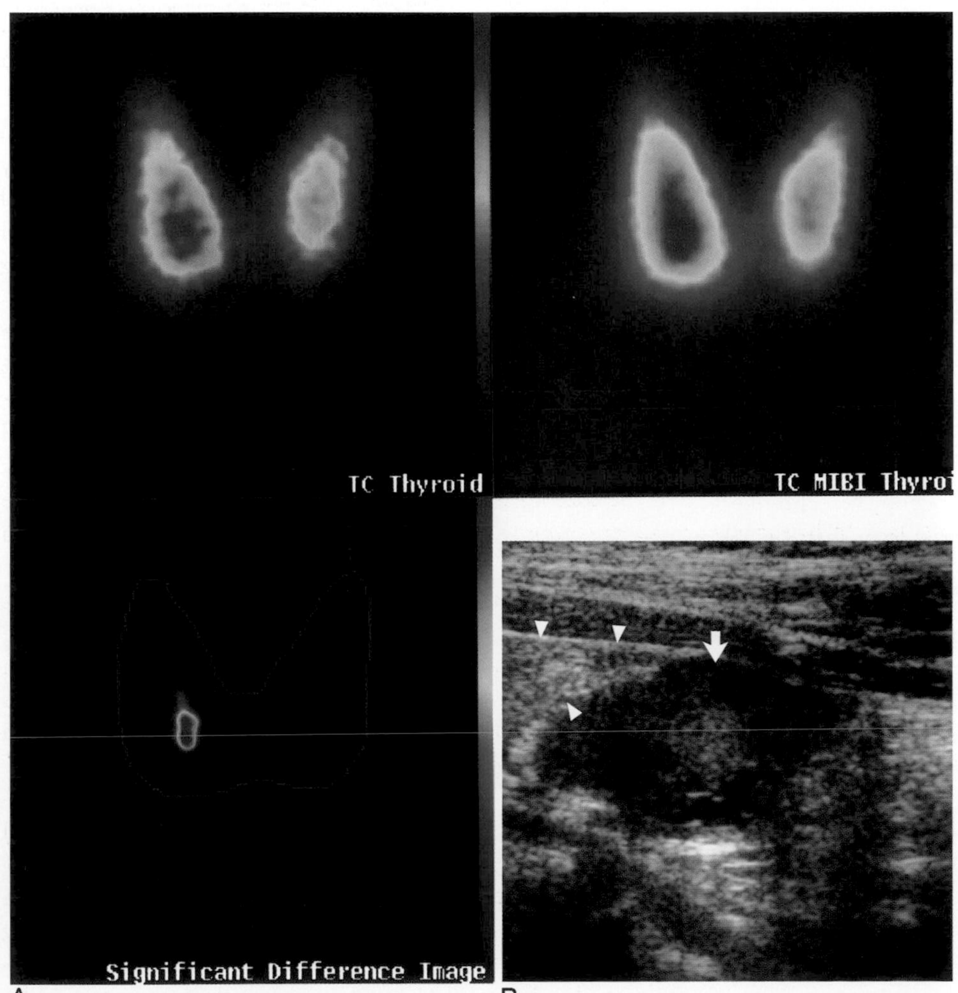

Figure 71.13 Parathyroid adenoma. (A) Left top figure shows ^{99m}Tc-pertechnetate scintigram, which shows uptake by thyroid tissue only. Right top figure shows ^{99m}Tc-MIBI with uptake in both thyroid and parathyroid tissue. Left bottom figure shows the subtraction image locating the parathyroid adenoma behind the lower pole of the right lobe of the thyroid gland. (B) Longitudinal ultrasound confirms the parathyroid adenoma (arrow) posterior to the lower pole of the right lobe of the thyroid gland (arrowheads).

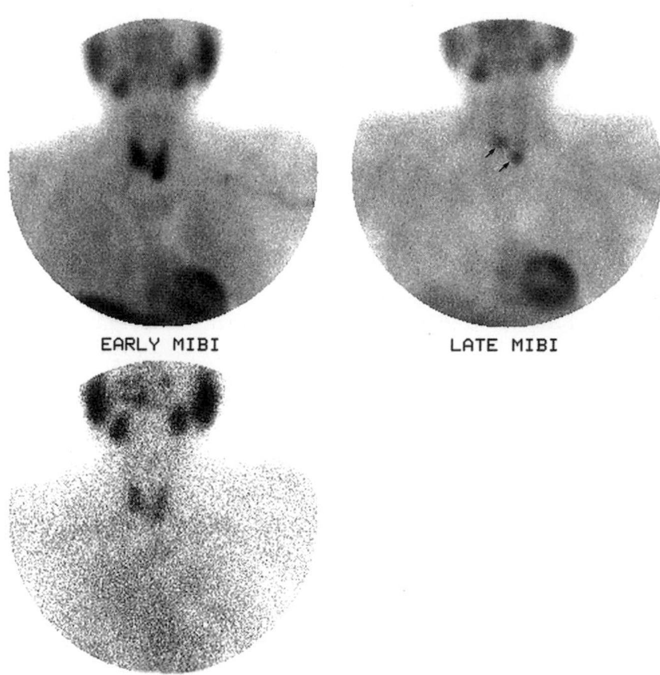

Figure 71.14 Multiple parathyroid adenoma. Left top figure shows the early ^{99m}Tc-MIBI scintigram, which shows uptake by thyroid and parathyroid tissue. The retention of tracer in parathyroid is significantly longer than normal thyroid tissue and the right top figure shows retention of ^{99m}Tc-MIBI in two parathyroid adenomas (arrows) near the lower pole of the thyroid gland. Left bottom figure shows conventionally obtained ^{99m}Tc-pertechnetate scintigram 20 minutes after injection for comparison.

Angiography and venous sampling are usually used as a last resort in difficult cases. The ablation of parathyroid adenomas has been reported following successful selective angiography.

The accuracy of imaging techniques in localizing parathyroid disease

There is great variation in the reported accuracy of imaging techniques in the localization of parathyroid disease. The overall sensitivity for identifying parathyroid adenomas with ^{99m}Tc-sestamibi ranges from 80 to 95%, which is significantly higher than that of ^{201}Tl[34,36,38,39]. The specificity is high at 91–98%. The sensitivity of radiopharmaceutical techniques to demonstrate hyperplasia is lower (55%) than that for the detection of parathyroid adenomas[36,40], and the sensitivity for the detection of pathology at reoperation is 75%[36]. Modern US using high-resolution (7.5–10 MHz) probes is only slightly less sensitive than nuclear medicine; the highest reported sensitivity for identifying an adenoma is 82%[26,41]. The specificity, however, is high, ranging from 78 to 100% [40]. As with all imaging techniques, the sensitivity of US falls to around 60% in identifying hyperplastic glands and to about 50% when localizing parathyroid pathology following a previous operation[34,41]. The sensitivity of CT in identifying parathyroid adenomas is similar to that of US, with specificities ranging from 92 to 95%[34,38]. After failed exploration of the neck, sensitivity of 44–50% has been reported. The results for MRI are similar to those for CT[34,38,40]. CT appears to be less sensitive than MRI in localizing mediastinal parathyroid adenomas in most studies.

PANCREATIC AND GASTROINTESTINAL ENDOCRINE DISORDERS

DIABETES MELLITUS

Diabetes mellitus is by far the most common endocrine disorder. It is characterized by chronic elevation of blood glucose level, for which a cause is not usually identified. Occasionally, diabetes mellitus is secondary to damage to the pancreas such as chronic pancreatitis and haemochromatosis. The diagnosis of diabetes is made on fasting blood-glucose measurement. Patients with diabetes have many radiological features (Table 71.9). These are attributable to complications from diabetes.

Table 71.9 RADIOLOGICAL FEATURES OF DIABETES MELLITUS

Cardiovascular system	Arterial calcification: aortic, iliac, femoral, carotid
	Myocardial infarction
	Heart failure
	Atheromatous plaques, stenosis
	Obstruction
Respiratory system	Infections
Genitourinary system	Pyelonephritis
	Papillary necrosis
	Emphysematous interstitial nephritis
	Perirenal abscess
	Nephrosclerosis—small contracted kidneys
	Cystitis, cystitis emphysematosa
	Neuropathic bladder
	Ureteric reflux
	Gas in pelviureteric systems
	Vas deferens calcification
Skeletal system	Osteomyelitis, secondary to overlying skin necrosis
	May have gas in soft tissues
	Charcot's or neuropathic foot
	Periarticular bone fragmentation with soft tissue calcification
	Resorption of terminal tufts of terminal phalanges
	Localized osteoporosis, especially feet
	Subluxations
	Fragmentation of femoral heads
	Generalized retarded maturation of bones
Gastrointestional system	Gastroparesis
	Acute gastric dilatation
	Colonic pseudo-obstruction
	Small bowel malabsorption pattern
Gall bladder	Emphysematous cholecystitis
Neonates	Large infants
	Hyaline membrane disease

Many are related to the duration of the disease and are the result of degenerative cardiovascular lesions in the eyes, heart, brain, kidneys, bladder, peripheral nervous system and musculoskeletal system. Other radiological abnormalities are due to infective, neuropathic, or metabolic changes. The role for radiology in patients with diabetes depends on the medical problems of the individual patients.

ISLET-CELL TUMOURS

Islet-cell tumours are a range of rare neoplasms of neuroendocrine origin arising in or near the pancreas. The normal islets cells of Langerhans in the pancreas contain B cells (which secrete insulin), A cells (glucagon), D cells (somatostatin), D1 cells (pancreatic polypeptide, PP) and D2 cells (vasoactive intestinal peptide, VIP). The majority (85%) of islet-cell tumours secrete one or more of these hormones, or other substances not normally found in the adult pancreas (although often present in the fetal pancreas), notably gastrin.

Functioning tumours

Functioning tumours are named according to the main hormone produced, and patients usually present with the clinical features of this excessive hormone secretion. These tumours may be either benign or malignant, solitary or multiple, or form part of the multiple endocrine neoplasia syndrome (MEN). The diagnosis is almost always made biochemically and the role of imaging is to localize the tumour prior to surgery and to look for evidence of malignancy or metastases.

Insulinomas are the most frequent functioning pancreatic tumours and account for 50% of all islet-cell tumours[42]. They produce spontaneous hypoglycaemia, which is relieved by glucose and associated with high levels of plasma insulin and C peptide. Insulinomas are usually solitary and benign: 10% are malignant, 10% are multiple and 4% are associated with MEN I, in which case multiple tumours are usually present. Insulinomas are usually very small: 90% are less than 2 cm and 50% less than 1.3 cm in diameter[43]. When multiple, the individual lesions are smaller (mean diameter 9 mm versus 13 mm)[44]. Malignant insulinomas tend to be larger than benign ones (2.5–12 cm diameter)[43].

Gastrinomas are the second most common functioning islet-cell tumour of the pancreas accounting for 20% of all islet-cell tumours[42]. They give rise to Zollinger–Ellison syndrome, which comprises increased gastric acid secretion, diarrhoea and peptic ulceration. The diagnosis is established by the demonstration of a raised fasting serum-gastrin level with high basal gastric acid output. Over 90% of gastrinomas are found in the 'gastrinoma triangle' bounded by the third part of the duodenum, the neck of the pancreas and the porta hepatis[45]. Gastrinomas are multiple in 20–40% of patients and often extrapancreatic, with 20% found in the duodenum. Gastrinomas are frequently malignant with metastatic spread occurring to the liver and local lymph nodes. They tend to be small: 38% of pancreatic and all duodenal tumours are less than 1 cm in diameter at diagnosis. One third of cases are associated with MEN I in which multiplicity is the rule and there is a tendency to recurrence.

Glucagonomas are rare, cause nonketogenic diabetes mellitus and a characteristic migrating, necrolytic rash, as well as stomatitis, diarrhoea and venous thrombosis. The tumours have an average diameter of 4–7 cm at diagnosis and are malignant in approximately 60% of cases.

VIPomas produce watery diarrhoea, hypokalaemia and achlorhydria (Verner–Morrison syndrome). The tumours range in diameter from 2 to 7 cm at diagnosis. The site of the tumour is intrapancreatic in 90% of cases, with the remainder (mainly gangliomas or ganglioneuroblastomas) originating in the sympathetic chain or adrenal medulla. Most extrapancreatic tumours are benign but 50% of pancreatic VIPomas are malignant.

Somatostatinomas are very rare, slow growing tumours, which produce the clinical triad of gallstones, diabetes mellitus and steatorrhoea. These tumours arise either from the pancreas or duodenum. Duodenal somatostatinomas occur in association with neurofibromatosis and are usually periampullary in position.

Nonfunctioning tumours

Nonfunctioning tumours account for 15% of pancreatic neuroendocrine tumours. They do not usually present until the tumour is large enough to cause symptoms from mass effect. The tumours tend to be large, solid and malignant but are usually slow growing.

Imaging islet-cell tumours

Transabdominal ultrasound usually demonstrates an islet-cell tumour as a well-circumscribed mass of lower echogenicity and finer echo texture than normal pancreas (Fig. 71.15). There may be a hyperechoic rim and larger tumours may show evidence of necrosis or calcification. Occasionally masses, especially gastrinomas, may be hyperechoic. Some lesions are isoechoic and are seen due to a hypoechoic halo around the lesion or due to the distortion of the gland. Liver

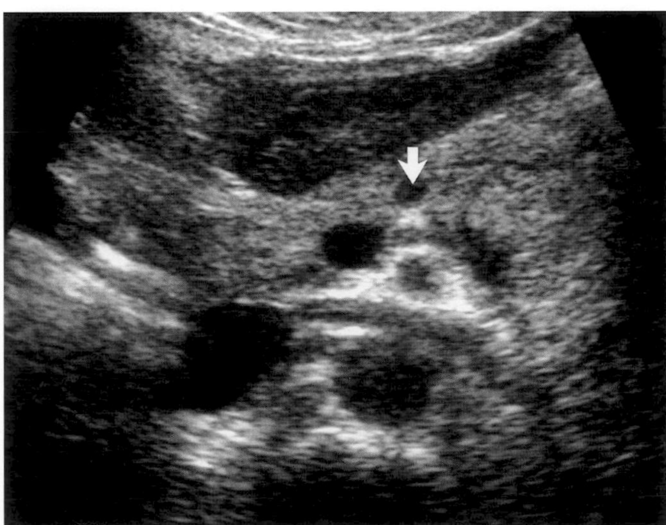

Figure 71.15 Insulinoma. Transverse ultrasound through the upper abdomen shows a small hypoechoic insulinoma (arrow) in the neck of the pancreas.

metastases are mostly hyperechoic or heterogeneous, and larger lesions may show evidence of cystic degeneration[43]. The overall detection rate for insulinomas is approximately 25–63% but can be up to 70% if the pancreas is adequately visualized. The reported detection rate for gastrinomas is worse, with only 30% of lesions identified[46]. The sensitivity is better for the detection of intrapancreatic gastrinomas than extrapancreatic lesions. The low sensitivity of transabdominal US is due to overlying bowel gas, deep location of the pancreas and limited resolution of with 3.5–5 MHz probes.

Endoscopic ultrasound (EUS) is superior to transabdominal US due to the use of high-frequency probes (7.5–12 MHz) placed in close proximity to the pancreas and duodenum (Fig. 71.16). In experienced hands, it has a high sensitivity in detecting tumours of the pancreatic head but has been less successful for lesions of the pancreatic tail and duodenum wall. Sensitivities as high as 79–100% have been reported for intrapancreatic lesions[47]. The procedure is relatively invasive and the equipment and expertise not widely available. However, in many centres, it is now considered a first-line investigation in patients with biochemical evidence of insulinoma.

Intraoperative ultrasound (IOUS), like EUS, is highly operator-dependent, but in experienced hands it is extremely effective for the identification of insulinomas at surgery. It is much less effective, however, for the identification of gastrinomas, since it is unable to identify extrapancreatic tumours of this type. Intraoperative US does not replace preoperative localization of islet-cell tumours but is used as an adjunct to palpation.

Computed tomography is the most widely used method for localizing islet-cell tumours. Most islet-cell tumours are isodense on unenhanced CT and will not be seen without intravenous administration of contrast medium unless they are large enough to deform the pancreatic outline. Occasional small tumours may be apparent as a hyperdense mass. Calcification may occur in up to 20% and is more common in malignant than benign tumours. Larger lesions may show central necrosis and are also more likely to calcify. On contrast-enhanced CT, islet-cell tumours are generally seen as a rounded area that enhances more than the surrounding pancreas (Fig. 71.17), although hypodense lesions do occur[48]. Hepatic metastases are seen as low-attenuation areas

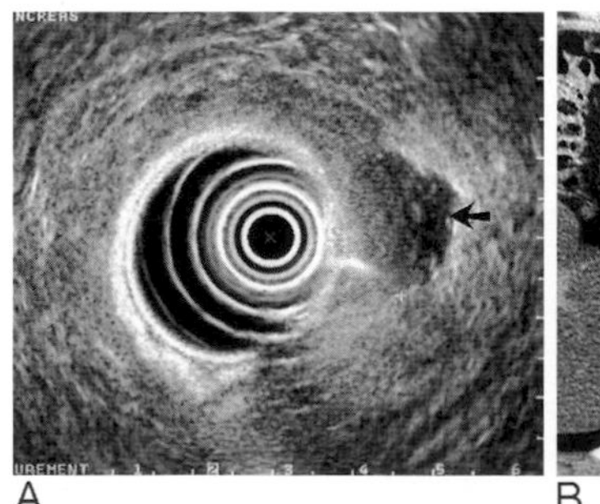
A

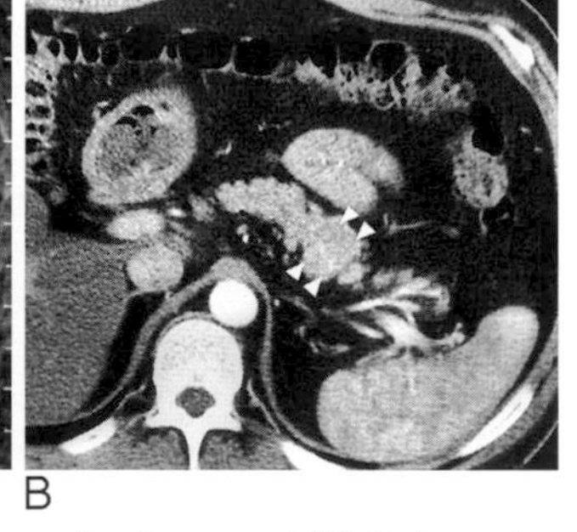
B

Figure 71.16 Insulinoma on endoscopic ultrasound. (A) Endoscopic ultrasound shows a hypoechoic tumour (arrow) in the tail of the pancreas, which is seen on the (B) contrast-enhanced CT as a bulge in the tail of the pancreas (arrowheads).

on unenhanced CT. Central necrosis is common in larger lesions and calcification may occur. Following intravenous contrast medium injection, the lesions, which are highly vascular, enhance. Solitary lesion may be indistinguishable from a haemangioma.

Biphasic enhanced CT, with thin primary collimation in the arterial phase followed by parenchymal phase imaging has a very high sensitivity (94%) for the detection of small pancreatic islet-cell tumours when compared with multiphasic CT without thin sections (57%) or conventional CT imaging (29%)[42,49]. Combining biphasic thin collimation CT with EUS has been reported to have a sensitivity of 100%[42].

Magnetic resonance imaging is increasingly being used in the localization of islet-cell tumours. Studies comparing MRI and CT have shown that MRI has greater sensitivity than CT, particularly for smaller islet-cell tumours. In general, islet-cell tumours are of lower signal intensity on T1-weighted images and higher signal intensity on T2-weighted images than normal pancreas (Fig. 71.18)[50].

Arteriography With the development of cross-sectional imaging, arteriography has decreased in importance in localizing pancreatic neuroendocrine tumour. Meticulous arteriographic technique should include selective arteriography of the superior mesenteric artery, the splenic artery, the gastroduodenal artery, the dorsal pancreatic artery, the common hepatic artery and any accessory hepatic arteries. Hepatic arteriography is performed both to demonstrate the arterial anatomy for the surgeon and to identify any liver metastases. Islet-cell tumours typically appear as a well-circumscribed blush in the arterial and early venous phase (Fig. 71.18). Abnormal feeding vessels may be seen in large tumours. Vascular liver lesions may be seen in the case of a malignant tumour. This technique is very operator-dependent. This may partly account for the widely varying reported sensitivities of selective angiography, which for insulinoma is between 43% and 94%[51] and for gastrinomas between 64% and 100%. In patients with multiple tumours, the sensitivity for individual lesions is lower. Lesions may be missed on angiography because they are too small or hypovascular or are obscured by the blush of adjacent bowel or spleen. False positives result from misinterpretation of blush of adjacent bowel, splenunculus, or angioma.

Venous sampling allows functional radiological localization of insulinomas and gastrinomas. In arterial stimulation and venous sampling (ASVS), selective pancreatic arterial injections of a secretagogue (calcium for insulinoma and secretin for gastrinoma) are made and hepatic venous effluent is sampled. When arteries supplying the tumour are injected, there is a rise in the hepatic venous hormone concentration. ASVS detects lesions not seen on cross-sectional studies[52]. Arteriography is usually combined with ASVS to give a high sensitivity for the detection and localization of functioning tumours. In cases where arteriography is negative, ASVS will localize the tumour to a region of the pancreas. ASVS is less reliant on operator expertise and consequently has a high reported sensitivity of 80–90%[51].

Transhepatic portal venous sampling (TPVS) is performed by transhepatic catheterization of the right portal vein. Samples for hormonal analysis are obtained from the splenic

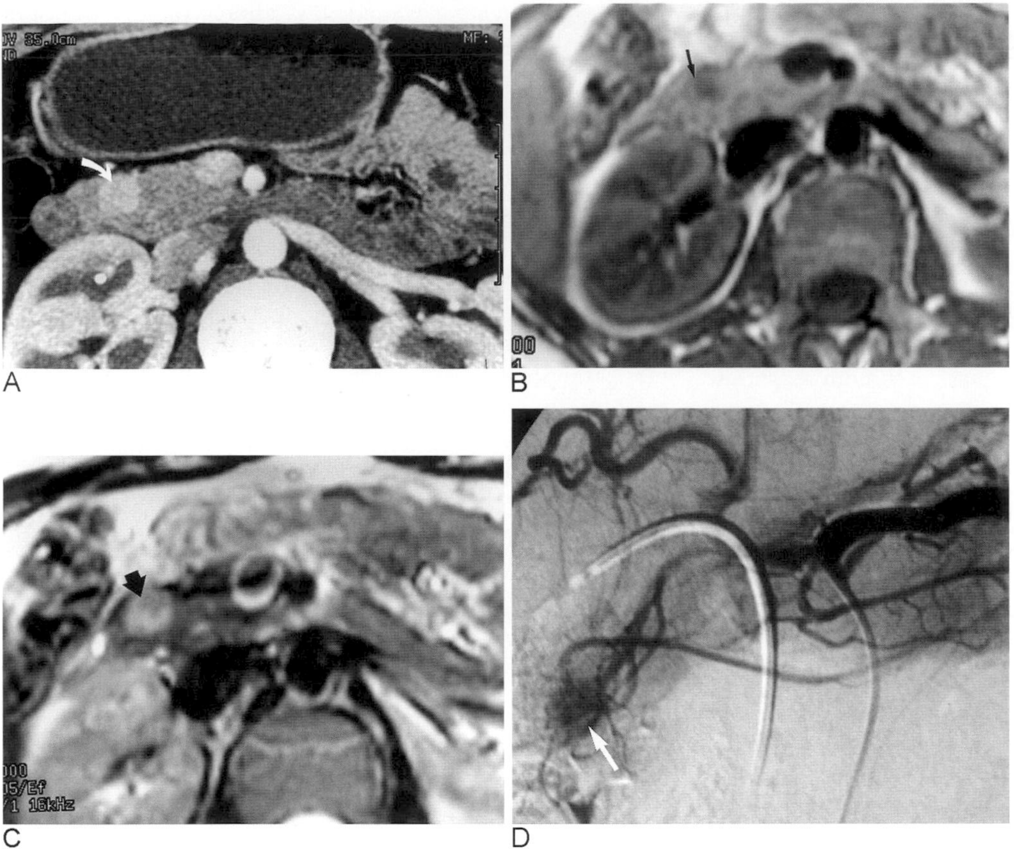

Figure 71.17 Insulinoma. (A) Contrast enhanced spiral CT demonstrating a small brightly enhancing insulinoma (curved arrow) in the head of the pancreas. (B) Axial T1-weighted spin echo MR image and (C) T2-weighted fast spin echo image show the corresponding lesion (arrow) on MRI of low signal intensity on the T1- and high signal intensity on the T2-weighted images. (D) A coeliac arteriogram in the same patient shows the vascular blush of the insulinoma (arrow).

vein, superior and inferior mesenteric veins, portal trunk and pancreatic veins. TPVS only localizes the tumour to a region of the pancreas. TPVS is an invasive procedure with a risk of hepatic arteriovenous fistulae, haemobilia and superior mesenteric artery occlusion and significant mortality. It is reserved for patients with suspected insulinoma if all other preoperative tests are negative[51] and is seldom used nowadays.

Scintigraphy for neuroendocrine tumours of the pancreas and bowel can be performed using radiolabelled somatostatin analogues and vasoactive intestinal peptide (^{123}I-VIP). The

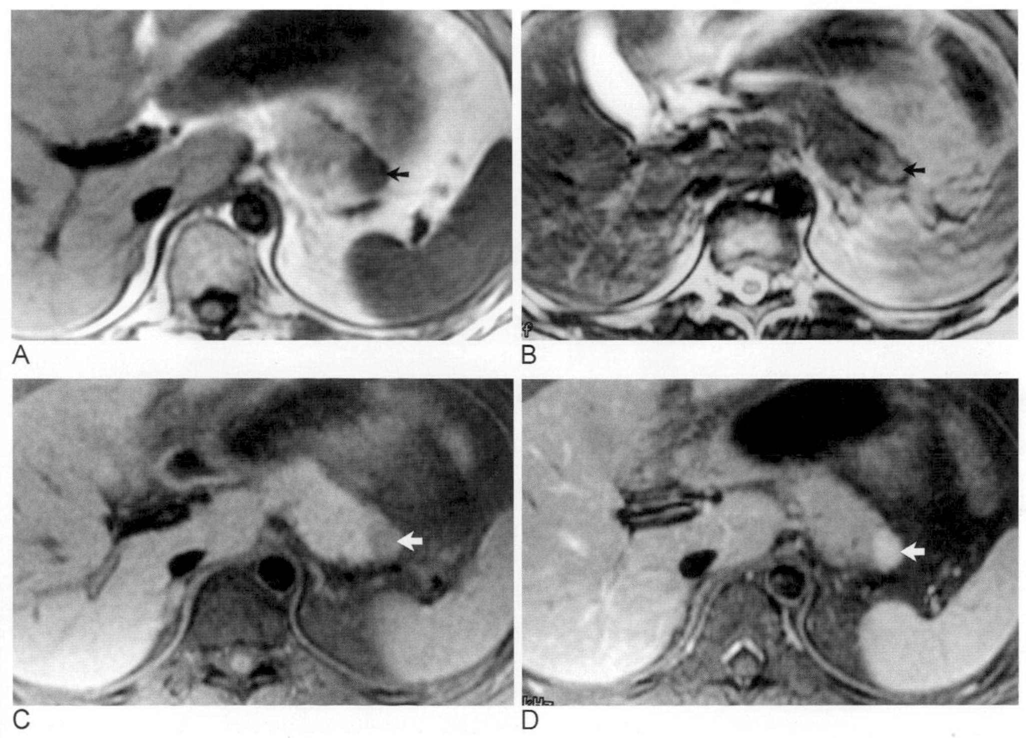

Figure 71.18 A small non-functioning islet-cell tumour in a patient with MEN type 1 syndrome. Axial T1-weighted spin-echo (A), T2-weighted fast spin-echo (B), and fat-suppressed T1-weighted spin echo image before (C) and after (D) intravenous gadolinium administration show the typical signal intensity pattern for islet-cell tumour on the various sequences in addition to the marked enhancement following intravenous gadolinium.

radiolabelled somatostatin analogue ^{111}In-pentetreotide is used to image a variety of somatostatin receptor-positive tumours. The main advantages of scintigraphy are its ability to image the whole body and to detect tumours or their metastases as small as 1 cm in diameter, especially in areas not under clinical suspicion. These imaging techniques can also be used to monitor the effects of therapy[53]. These small tumours can also be located at surgery using hand-held gamma probes. Table 71.10 summarizes the proportions of tumours that show uptake on scintigraphy. More recently ^{68}Ga-octreotate, ^{11}C-5-hydroxytryptophan and ^{11}C-L-dihydroxyphenylalanine PET/CT have been introduced to improve tumour diagnosis and localization.

Localization of islet-cell tumours

The localization of islet-cell tumour presents a challenge to the radiologist as several imaging techniques are capable of demonstrating the tumour and no one technique is superior to the others. A rational approach to the localization of these tumours requires careful consideration of cost, sensitivities and availability of the imaging techniques. In most cases, initial imaging with a combination of US and CT or MRI will demonstrate the tumour and hepatic metastases. If these tests are negative or equivocal arteriography (with ASVS) is the next line of investigation. If the tumour remains undetected, further investigation depends on local expertise. EUS has emerged as a highly sensitive test for the detection of small pancreatic tumours and may also demonstrate extrapancreatic gastrinomas. IOUS is a useful adjunct to palpation at the time of surgery. Somatostatin-receptor imaging is useful in somatostatin receptor positive tumour not detected on other imaging techniques.

CARCINOID TUMOURS

Carcinoid tumours are neuroendocrine neoplasms occurring most commonly within the gastrointestinal system, less frequently in the respiratory tract and thymus and very rarely at other sites. Hormonal products can be demonstrated within cellular neurosecretory granules in all carcinoid tumours, but systemic manifestations of hormonal secretion are rare. A small number of patients may present with symptoms, related to the release of 5-hydroxytryptamine (5-HT) and other vasoactive metabolites, which include skin flushing, intestinal hypermotility bronchoconstriction, cardiac valvular fibrosis and liver enlargement. Carcinoid syndrome is present in cases with hepatic metastases. Carcinoid tumours may also produce ACTH resulting in Cushing's syndrome, most commonly due to lung carcinoid. The resulting occult ectopic ACTH can often be extremely difficult to localize as sampling of the systemic veins is usually negative[54].

Carcinoid tumours often have a relatively indolent course and prolonged survival is not uncommon even in the presence of distant metastases with reported survival rates of more than 80% at 5 years.

Gastrointestinal carcinoids are found in the appendix (45%), the small bowel (25%) and colorectum (25%). Symptoms result from local fibrosis with obstruction or from endocrine effects; the latter usually from an ileal carcinoid after it has metastasized to the liver. Gastrointestinal tumours are sometimes diagnosed on barium examinations as intramural tumours or constrictive lesions. On CT, although the primary tumour may not be seen, mesenteric infiltration and fibrosis produce a characteristic appearance of a soft tissue mass in the mesentery with a radiating stellate pattern of linear densities.

Carcinoid liver metastases can be shown by US or CT or MRI, angiography being reserved for patients in whom hepatic arterial embolization is planned. Hepatic metastases are typically hypervascular and are optimally depicted during the arterial phase of a contrast-enhanced CT or MRI (Fig. 71.19) and may calcify. These tumours may appear isoattenuating when compared with adjacent hepatic parenchyma during the portal venous phase of enhancement. In our experience, MRI following administration of MnDPDP, a liver-specific contrast agent, increases the ability to detect neuroendocrine liver metastases with a high level of interobserver reproducibility.

Bronchial carcinoids represent 1% of pulmonary neoplasms and appear as well-circumscribed nodules or masses on chest radiographs. Patients with bronchial carcinoid present with chest symptoms such as cough, recurrent infection, or haemoptysis. Approximately 2% of bronchial carcinoid tumours present with an endocrine disturbance, and approximately 1%

Table 71.10 PROPORTIONS OF TUMOURS THAT SHOW UPTAKE ON SCINTIGRAPHY

Type of tumour	^{111}In-pentetreotide (%)	^{123}I-VIP (%)
Gastrinomas	80	–
Glucagonomas	95	–
Carcinoid	86	85
Insulinomas	61	82
Somatostatinomas	100	–
VIPomas	80	100

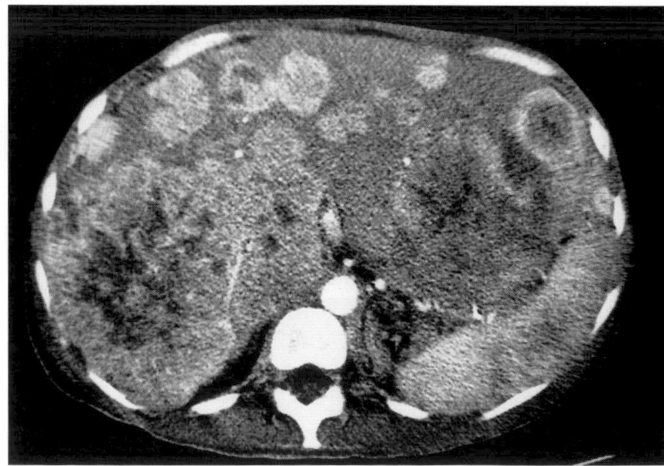

Figure 71.19 Carcinoid liver metastases. 'Arterial' phase contrast enhanced CT shows multiple highly vascular lesions typical of metastases from a primary neuroendocrine tumour.

of cases of Cushing's syndrome are secondary to bronchial carcinoid through the ectopic production of ACTH or corticotropin-releasing hormone (CRH). Bronchial carcinoids represent the most common source of ectopic ACTH production in patients presenting with Cushing's syndrome[54]. The causative bronchial carcinoid is usually very small and is often difficult to identify. Biochemically, the syndrome is often difficult to distinguish from a pituitary cause of excess ACTH, hence the term occult ectopic ACTH production[54].

Thymic carcinoids usually manifest as an anterior mediastinal mass in adults. The majority of patients present with symptoms related to compression or invasion of the mediastinal structures. Approximately 50% of thymic carcinoids are functionally active resulting most commonly in Cushing's syndrome. CT and MRI may be helpful in the evaluation of patients with occult, hormonally active lesions[55].

Radionuclide imaging plays an important role in the localization and management of these tumours. The ability of these tumours to concentrate ^{123}I- or ^{131}I-MIBG allows scintigraphy to be performed with a cumulative sensitivity of 71%[56]. The most common midgut carcinoids (appendix and distal ileum) probably concentrate the radiolabelled MIBG more readily than those in the foregut and hindgut. The main use for ^{123}I-MIBG scintigraphy is as a prelude to ^{131}I-MIBG therapy, for which good palliative results are obtained. ^{111}In-pentetreotide has also been used to image these tumours, which has a higher sensitivity (86%) than MIBG. Recently, lutetium-177-octreotate (a somatostatin analogue) has been used for targeted radionuclide therapy of these tumours.

THE ADRENAL GLANDS

ANATOMY AND PHYSIOLOGY

The right adrenal gland lies posterior to the inferior vena cava and the left adrenal gland anteromedial to the upper pole of the left kidney (Fig. 71.20). The adrenal glands have an arrowhead configuration, with a body and medial and lateral limbs.

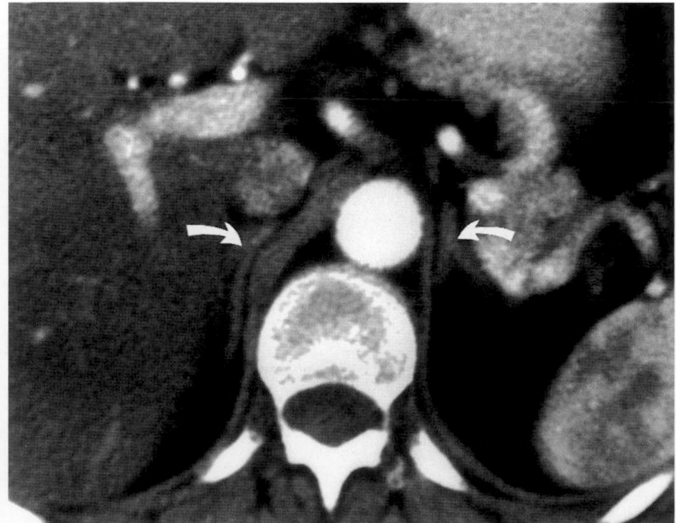

Figure 71.20 Normal adrenal glands. Contrast enhanced CT of normal adrenal glands (arrows).

The normal adrenals extend 2–4 cm in the craniocaudal direction, and the thickness of the adrenal body and limbs does not exceed 9–10 mm and 4–5 mm, respectively[57].

The adrenal glands have an inner medulla and outer cortex. The outer zone of the cortex, the zona glomerulosa, secretes mineralocorticoids (largely aldosterone), which controls salt and water metabolism. The inner cortical zones, the zona fasciculata and zona reticularis, secrete glucocorticoids and androgens responding to ACTH from the hypothalamic-pituitary axis, which is in turn inhibited by the cortisol.

The medulla, derived from the primitive neuroectoderm, consists of chromaffin cells, which produce catecholamines, adrenaline (epinephrine) and noradrenaline (norepinephrine). Their metabolites (excreted in urine) include vanillyl mandelic acid (VMA). The medulla is almost entirely localized within the body of the adrenal gland.

TECHNIQUES FOR INVESTIGATING THE ADRENAL GLANDS

Ultrasound is seldom used in the detection of adrenal mass lesions in adults as the normal adrenal glands and small adrenal lesions remain difficult to visualize, especially in obese patients.

Computed tomography is currently the technique of choice in detecting and evaluating adrenal lesions. Thin collimation allows accurate density measurements of adrenal lesions. Intravenous administration of contrast medium helps to distinguish the adrenal glands from adjacent vessels and to assess the vascularity of an adrenal mass, and to characterize individually detected masses.

Magnetic resonance imaging offers an alternative method for imaging the adrenal gland. Imaging protocols usually consists of axial T1- and T2-weighted sequences. Imaging in the coronal and sagittal planes helps to identify invasion into adjacent structures by large mass lesions. Chemical-shift imaging sequences are performed to differentiate between benign and malignant adrenal masses. Intravenous contrast media are administered to differentiate between solid and cystic masses and to assess the vascularity of a lesion.

Radionuclide imaging: Radiopharmaceuticals can be grouped into two categories—adrenocortical and adrenomedullary imaging agents. Radiolabelled analogues of cholesterol, such as ^{131}I-6β-iodomethyl-19-norcholesterol (NP-59), are used to identify and localize masses that result in adrenal cortical dysfunction. MIBG, an analogue of guanethidine, is concentrated in sympathoadrenal tissue, and is thus used to image adrenomedullary disorders. ^{131}I- and ^{123}I-MIBG have the advantage of being able to screen the whole body for sympathomedullary tissue.

Venous sampling is extremely accurate in the preoperative localization of the source of abnormal hormone secretion. It is, however, an invasive procedure, requiring long fluoroscopy times and high radiation exposures. Even in experienced hands, failure to catheterize the adrenal veins occurs in 10–30% of cases. Complications are frequently seen and include adrenal infarction, adrenal vein thrombosis, adrenal haemorrhage, hypotensive crises and adrenal insufficiency. Venous sampling is best reserved for patients in whom findings are equivocal on cross-sectional imaging.

Percutaneous adrenal biopsy has an accuracy of 80–90%[58]. Minor complications include abdominal pain, haematuria, nausea and small pneumothoraces. Major complications that necessitate treatment occur in 3–5% of cases and include pneumothoraces that require intervention and haemorrhage. Biopsy of an unsuspected phaeochromocytoma can be life-threatening due to a catecholamine 'storm'. The complication rate varies with the approach used, but does not appear to be related to the size of the needle used[58].

IMAGING OF ADRENAL LESIONS

Adrenocortical hyperfunction[59]

Endogenous Cushing's syndrome

Endogenous Cushing's syndrome is the result of an excess of ACTH production in 75% of cases and excess cortisol from an adrenal neoplasm in 25% of cases. The diagnosis of Cushing's syndrome depends predominantly on the clinical and biochemical findings. The aims of imaging are to identify the source of excess ACTH production either from a pituitary tumour or an ectopic ACTH source, and to localize or exclude a unilateral adrenal mass. The appearance of the adrenal gland in Cushing's syndrome will depend on the aetiology of the syndrome[60,61].

ACTH-dependent Cushing's syndrome A pituitary cause (i.e., Cushing's disease) is responsible in approximately 85% of cases and the remainder are due to ectopic ACTH secretion, which may be overt or occult. Overt ectopic ACTH production is usually clinically apparent and presents with a short history, lacks the clinical features of Cushing's syndrome, and is most commonly from a small-cell lung cancer. Occult ectopic ACTH-secreting tumours present with a more chronic clinical picture, often indistinguishable from Cushing's syndrome due to pituitary or adrenal adenoma. The source of occult ectopic ACTH is most commonly a bronchial carcinoid tumour; less frequently an islet-cell tumour of the pancreas, phaeochromocytoma, medullary thyroid carcinoma, or thymic carcinoid tumours are the source. In ACTH-dependent Cushing's syndrome, the adrenals show hyperplastic changes (Fig. 71.21) in 71% of cases, with the glands largest in patients with ectopic ACTH production[60].

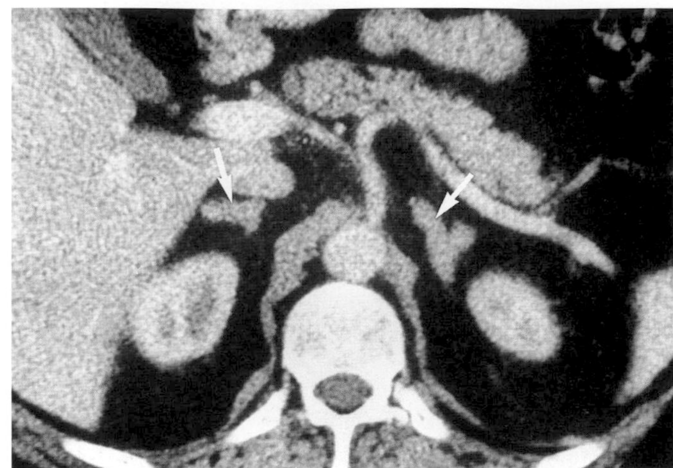

Figure 71.21 Bilateral adrenal hyperplasia (arrows) in a patient with Cushing's disease.

Adrenocortical adenomas account for 10–20% of cases of Cushing's syndrome. Functioning adrenal cortical adenomas responsible for Cushing's syndrome are usually larger than 2 cm in diameter (Fig. 71.22). The contralateral gland is usually normal, but occasionally is atrophic because of reduced ACTH secretion. On cross-sectional imaging, most adenomas are homogeneous, although some may be heterogeneous because of focal areas of necrosis or haemorrhage, which is seen in larger masses.

Adrenal carcinomas account for 10–15% of cases of Cushing's syndrome. Most of these tumours exceed 6 cm in diameter at the time of presentation and are readily detected on US, CT, or MRI (Figs 71.23, 71.24). On CT, these tumours are heterogeneous, with areas of necrosis and calcification. Approximately 15% of carcinomas are less than 6 cm in diameter and may resemble adenomas. Adrenal carcinomas may invade adjacent organs, extend into the inferior vena cava, and involve lymph nodes and metastases to the liver, lung and bone. Functional imaging using [F-18]FDG-PET/CT can be used to map the full extent of spread.

Rare adrenal causes of Cushing's syndrome[61] include primary pigmented nodular adrenocortical disease (which may be associated with cardiac myxomas, skin pigmentation and testicular tumours in Carney complex) and primary macronodular hyperplasia.

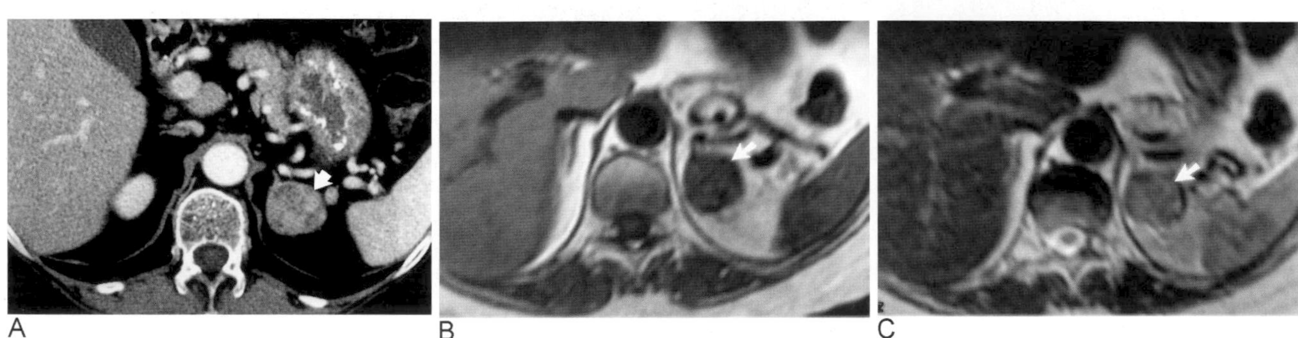

Figure 71.22 Cushing's syndrome due to adrenocortical adenoma. (A) Contrast enhanced CT, (B) T1-weighted spin-echo and (C) T2-weighted fast spin-echo images all showing a 3 cm adenoma (arrows) in the left adrenal gland.

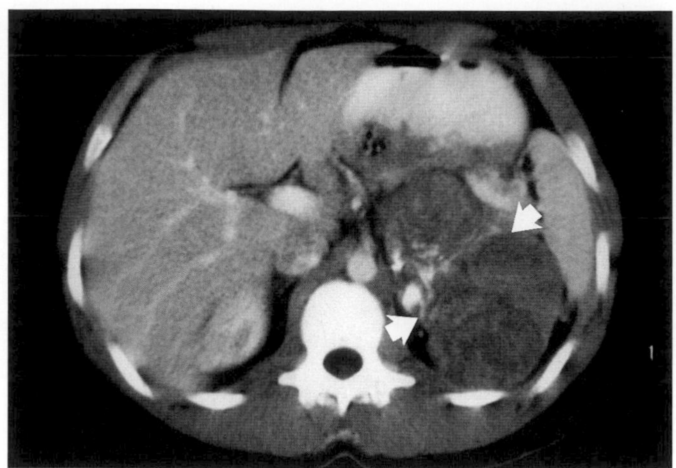

Figure 71.23 Adrenal carcinoma. Contrast-enhanced CT demonstrating a large partly calcified, inhomogeneously enhancing left adrenal cancer (arrows).

Primary hyperaldosteronism

Primary hyperaldosteronism (Conn's syndrome) results from a benign cortical adenoma (Fig. 71.25) in 79% of cases, bilateral adrenal hyperplasia (Fig. 71.26) in 20% of cases, and is rarely due to an adrenocortical carcinoma. Imaging plays an important role in distinguishing between the causes of primary hyperaldosteronism, as surgery should be considered for adenomas and bilateral hyperplasia is best treated medically.

Adrenocortical adenomas (Conn's tumour) tend to be small, with an average size of approximately 1.6–1.8 cm. These adenomas are of low density on CT (less than 10 HU) because of high cytoplasmic lipid content. They do not enhance significantly after intravenous injection of contrast medium and rarely calcify. On MRI, most adenomas appear slightly hypointense or isointense relative to the liver on T1-weighted images and slightly hyperintense or isointense relative to hepatic parenchyma on T2-weighted images (see Fig. 71.25)[62]. The sensitivity of CT in detecting these adenomas is 70–90%; its specificity exceeds 90%[63]. MRI is probably as sensitive and as specific as CT[62,64]. When successful, venous sampling is the most accurate means of localizing aldosteronomas, with a sensitivity approaching 100% and a positive predictive value of 90%[65].

Adrenal scintigraphy with a cholesterol-based radiopharmaceutical such as ^{131}I-6β-iodomethyl-19-norcholesterol (NP-59) and dexamethasone suppression can distinguish between a unilateral adenoma and bilateral hyperplasia. As with CT, the sensitivity of the technique is dependent in part on the size of the adenoma and its accuracy compares unfavourably with that of CT. Because of this, and also because the procedure is time-consuming and expensive, it is seldom used.

In practice, when CT or MRI identifies a solitary adenoma, further imaging before surgery is unnecessary. Venous sampling is reserved for cases in whom both adrenal glands appear normal (as a micronodule may be undetected), where there are bilateral nodules that may be due to nodular hyperplasia or multiple adenomata, and where there is disagreement between the imaging and biochemistry findings.

Adrenogenital syndrome

Androgen-producing tumours of the adrenals are usually carcinomas, less commonly adenomas. They usually exceed 2 cm in diameter and have the same characteristics described elsewhere for adenomas and carcinomas[66]. In patients with virilism, imaging is used to detect a tumour in the adrenals, ovaries, or testes.

The most common adrenal cause of excess androgens in childhood is congenital adrenocortical hyperplasia. This usually results from an inborn enzyme deficiency, which causes a partial block to the synthesis of adrenocortical steroids and an increase in the production of androgens. The compensatory elevation of ACTH results in gross enlargement of the adrenals, easily recognizable on CT or MRI. Long-term stimulation can result in transformation of a hyperplastic nodule into an adenoma or even a carcinoma[58].

Adrenal medullary tumours

Phaeochromocytomas are catecholamine-producing tumours that arise from the paraganglion cells anywhere in the

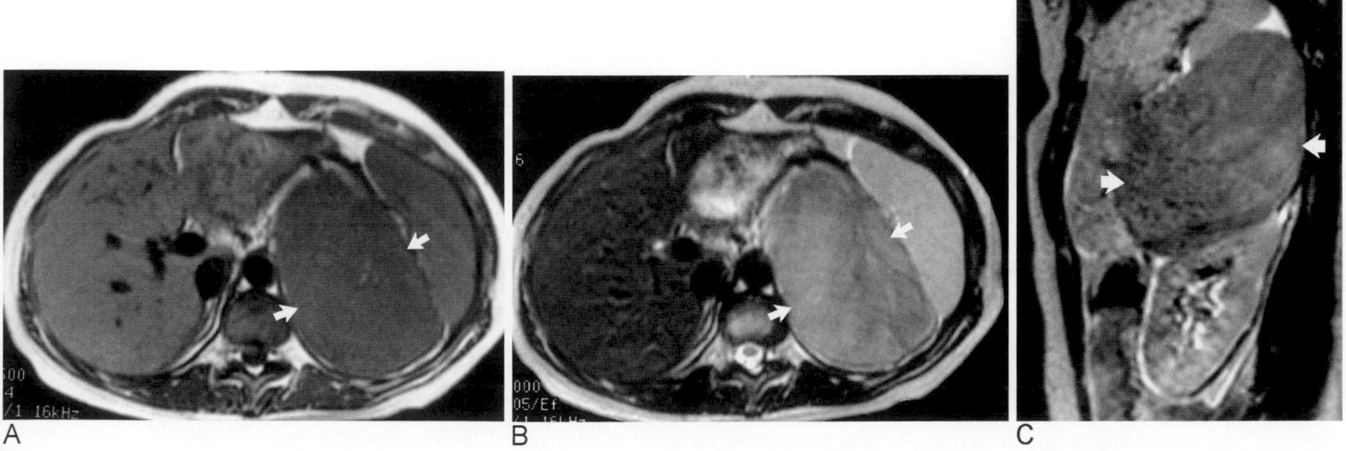

Figure 71.24 Adrenal carcinoma on MRI. (A) Axial T1-weighted spin-echo, (B) axial and (C) sagittal T2-weighted fast spin-echo images show a large left adrenal cancer (arrows). The size of the lesion and the high signal intensity on the T2-weighted images are typical of an adrenal carcinoma.

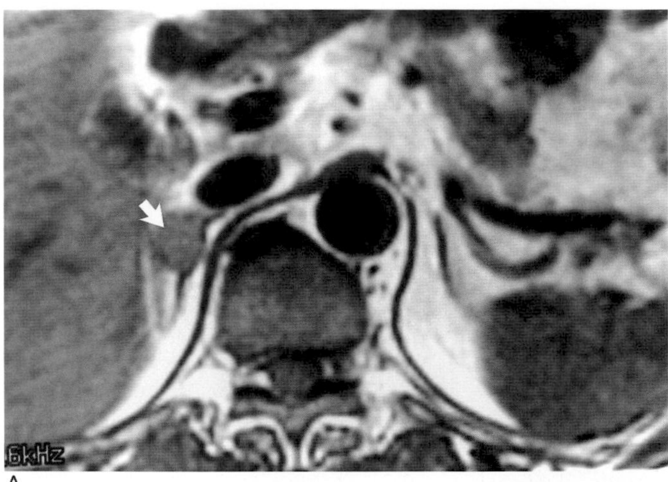
A

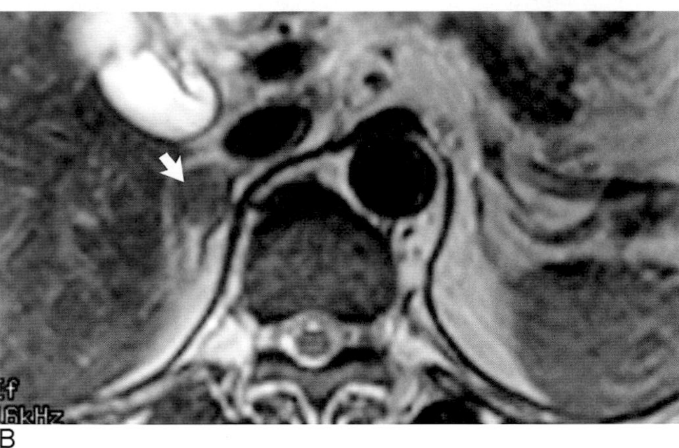
B

Figure 71.25 Conn's syndrome due to an adrenocortical adenoma. (A) T1-weighted spin-echo and (B) T2-weighted fast spin-echo images showing the typical appearance of a small aldosterone-producing adenoma (arrow) in the right adrenal gland.

autonomic nervous system. Phaeochromocytomas originate in the adrenal medulla in 90% of cases; most extra-adrenal phaeochromocytomas arise in the paravertebral sympathetic ganglia, in the organ of Zuckerkandl or, rarely, in the bladder[67]. About 90% of adrenal medullary phaeochromocytomas are functional, but only 50% of sympathetic and 1% of parasympathetic tumours produce excess catecholamines. Ninety per cent of phaeochromocytomas are sporadic, the remaining 10% being associated with neuroectodermal disorders such as neurofibromatosis, tuberous sclerosis, von Hippel–Lindau syndrome, or multiple endocrine neoplastic syndrome. Multiple phaeochromocytomas occur in up to 10% of sporadic cases, but in as many as 30% when associated with a neuroectodermal syndrome. Approximately 10% of phaeochromocytomas are malignant.

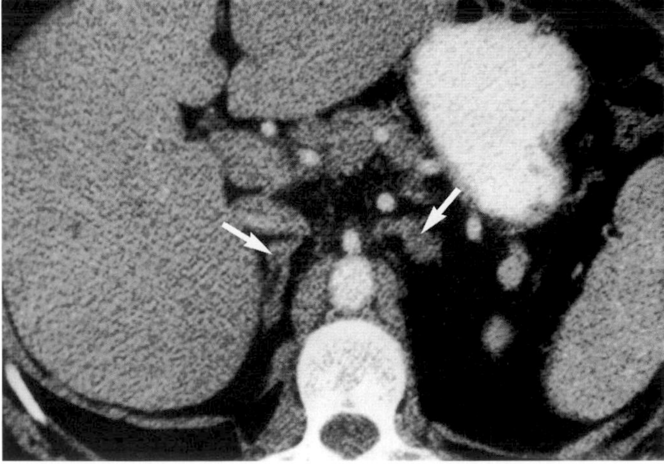

Figure 71.26 Conn's syndrome due to bilateral nodular adrenal hyperplasia. Contrast-enhanced CT shows small nodules in the adrenal glands (arrows).

On unenhanced CT, phaeochromocytomas appear as round masses of similar density to surrounding soft tissue structures. Phaeochromocytomas frequently undergo marked necrosis, so that the mass may have a fluid-filled centre (Fig. 71.27). Calcification occurs occasionally and is usually speckled. In sporadic cases of phaeochromocytoma, the tumour tends to be large with an average size of 5 cm[58]. The lesions are often smaller when detected in patients with multiple endocrine abnormalities as they are often specifically sought. Phaeochromocytomas show intense enhancement following intravenous injection of contrast medium. Unlike ionic contrast media, adrenergic blockade to prevent hypertensive crisis is not required with non-ionic contrast media[68]. The overall accuracy of CT in detecting adrenal phaeochromocytomas is very high, with a sensitivity of 93–100% and a positive predictive value greater than 90%.

On MRI, phaeochromocytomas are hypointense on T1-weighted images and usually markedly hyperintense on T2-weighted images (Fig. 71.28). Although their appearance on T2-weighted images is typical it is not specific, as there is some similarity in appearance with adrenal metastasis. Atypical signal intensity on T2-weighted images is seen in 35% of phaeochromocytomas[58]. CT and MRI are equally accurate for identifying adrenal phaeochromocytomas.

On US, phaeochromocytomas are well-defined, round or ovoid masses with uniform reflectivity. Large tumours frequently undergo haemorrhage or necrosis with loss of homogeneity (see Fig. 71.27). The accuracy of US in detecting phaeochromocytomas is less than CT, MRI, or MIBG scintigraphy, particularly for small or ectopic tumours.

MIBG scintigraphy is especially useful for the detection of ectopic phaeochromocytomas and also for the identification of metastatic or locally recurrent disease, because, unlike US, CT, or MRI, it is inherently a whole-body imaging technique. Phaeochromocytomas are seen as an abnormal focal area of increased activity. The sensitivity of MIBG scintigraphy in detecting functioning phaeochromocytomas is slightly less than 90%, and its specificity exceeds 90%. However, a positive MIBG study always requires correlation with CT or MRI. In metastatic disease, ^{131}I-MIBG therapy provides an important palliative therapeutic option.

Neuroblastoma—See paediatric chapter (Chapter 69).

Hypoadrenalism

Hypoadrenalism is usually due to primary idiopathic atrophy, in western countries, and imaging of the adrenals is seldom undertaken. However, imaging can be useful in identifying a potentially treatable cause. In patients with idiopathic atrophy, the glands are extremely small and may be difficult

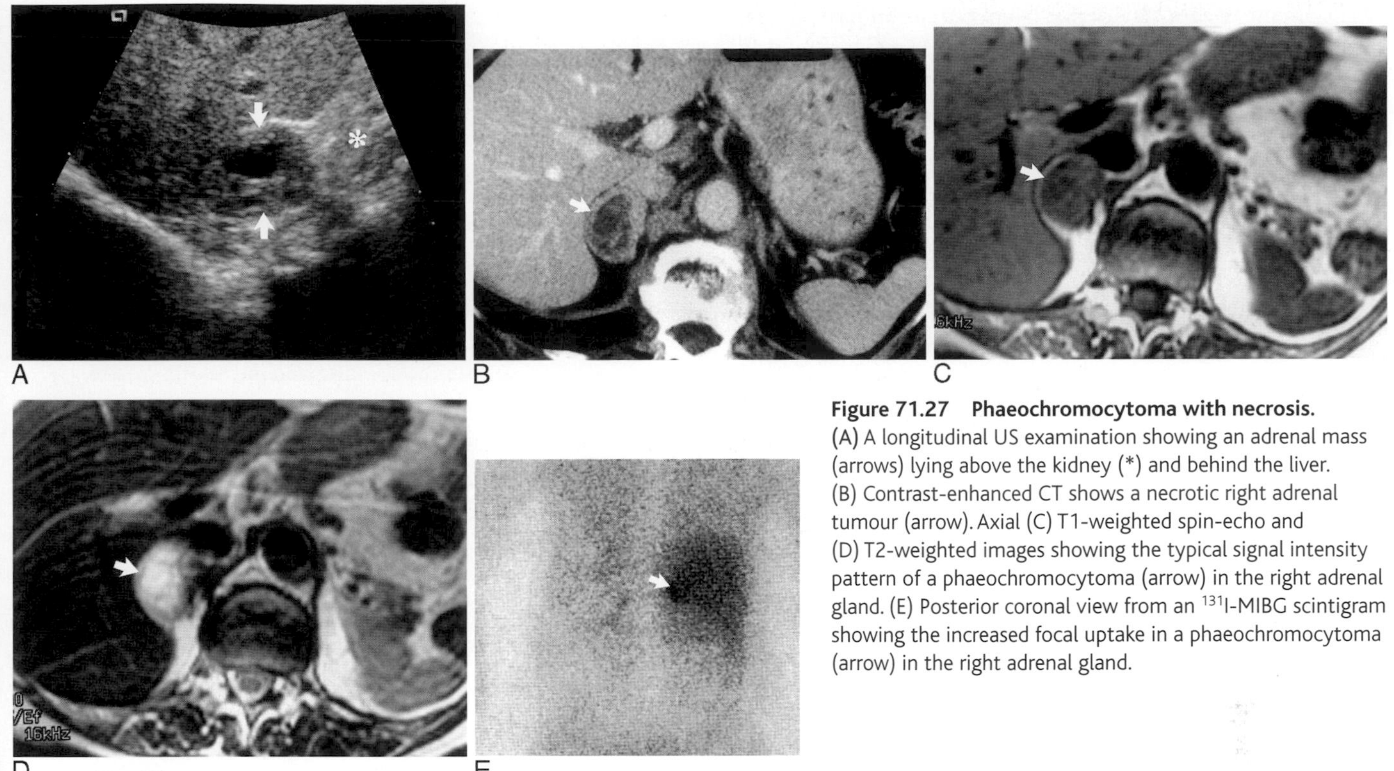

Figure 71.27 Phaeochromocytoma with necrosis. (A) A longitudinal US examination showing an adrenal mass (arrows) lying above the kidney (*) and behind the liver. (B) Contrast-enhanced CT shows a necrotic right adrenal tumour (arrow). Axial (C) T1-weighted spin-echo and (D) T2-weighted images showing the typical signal intensity pattern of a phaeochromocytoma (arrow) in the right adrenal gland. (E) Posterior coronal view from an ^{131}I-MIBG scintigram showing the increased focal uptake in a phaeochromocytoma (arrow) in the right adrenal gland.

to identify. Small adrenal glands may also be seen in chronic tuberculosis (see below). Enlarged glands are most commonly due to tuberculosis, but occasionally may be due to amyloid, sarcoidosis, metastatic disease, haemochromatosis, fungal infection, or adrenal haemorrhage. If Addison's disease develops suddenly then imaging techniques may be useful to confirm the presence of bilateral haemorrhage.

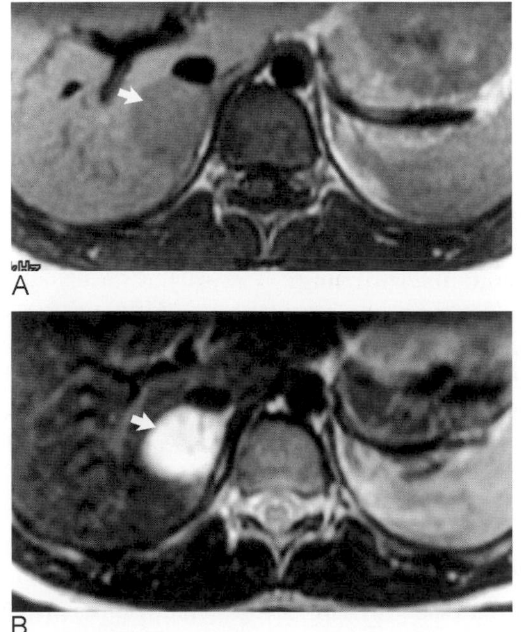

Figure 71.28 Phaeochromocytoma on MRI. Axial (A) T1-weighted spin-echo and (B) T2-weighted fast spin-echo images showing a right adrenal phaeochromocytoma (arrow). The very high signal intensity is typical of a phaeochromocytoma.

Adrenal disorders not resulting in altered hormonal activity

Non-hyperfunctioning adrenal adenomas are detected incidentally in up to 5% of CT examinations[58]. The number and size of these nodules increase with age and are most common in obese diabetics and elderly women. These 'silent' adenomas are thought to represent non-neoplastic overgrowth of adrenocortical cells of the zona fasciculata. The appearance of non-hyperfunctioning and hyperfunctioning adenomas on cross-sectional imaging is similar[61].

Primary adrenocortical carcinomas are rare and highly malignant. Ninety per cent produce steroids but only half cause symptoms related to excess hormone production. Functioning carcinomas most commonly result in Cushing's syndrome, but virilization or feminization and hyperaldosteronism may also occur. Most carcinomas are usually large (> 6 cm in diameter) at the time of diagnosis and are more commonly seen on the left; only about 10% are bilateral. The imaging characteristics of carcinomas are described above.

Adrenal metastases are most commonly from tumours of the lung, kidney, melanoma, breast, digestive tract and ovary. Adrenal metastases very rarely result in hypoadrenalism. The presence of an adrenal mass in a patient with known malignancy does not necessarily indicate metastatic disease, because 40–50% are nonmetastatic and represent adenomas. Metastases tend to be larger than adenomas, less well-defined, inhomogeneous and have a thick, irregular enhancing rim after injection of intravenous contrast medium. They are more commonly unilateral than bilateral. On MRI, they are typically hypointense compared with the liver on T1-weighted images and relatively hyperintense on T2-weighted images. The adrenal glands may show diffuse enlargement without evidence of metastases in patients with known malignancy[69,70].

Primary adrenal lymphoma is very rare, tends to be extranodal and has a poor prognosis. The adrenal glands are enlarged but maintain their adreniform shape. The adrenal glands are more commonly involved in widespread lymphoma, being detected on imaging in about 4% of cases of non-Hodgkin lymphoma, but at autopsy in up to 25% of cases. On CT, secondary adrenal lymphoma usually appears as solid homogeneous masses of soft tissue density, which enhance slightly after intravenous injection of contrast medium. Calcification is unusual without previous radiotherapy.

Adrenal cysts are uncommon, usually unilateral and occur more often in women than men. Adrenal cysts are usually endothelial or epithelial in origin but may also be parasitic or pseudocysts. Pseudocysts are thought to represent the result of previous haemorrhage. Adrenal cysts have the same characteristics on imaging as cysts seen elsewhere in the body (Fig. 71.29), i.e., they are well-defined, thin-walled fluid-filled structures that show no enhancement after intravenous injection of contrast medium. Calcification is seen in 15% of adrenal cysts, which is often peripheral and curvilinear. On MRI, adrenal cysts are usually markedly hypointense on T1-weighted images and markedly hyperintense on T2-weighted images. However, the presence of proteinaceous material, infectious debris, or haemorrhage within the cyst can cause increased signal intensity on T1-weighted images.

Adrenal myelolipomas are rare, benign neoplasms composed of fat and bone-marrow tissue in varying proportions. Most are asymptomatic and nonfunctioning and identified incidentally on imaging. However, there are isolated reports of endocrine abnormalities associated with myelolipomas[71]. Haemorrhage or necrosis within the tumour may cause pain and also lead to discovery of these lesions. The diagnosis of these lesions is based on the demonstration of fat within an adrenal mass (Fig. 71.30). However, the proportion of fat within the lesion may vary and those with only a small proportion of fat may be difficult to differentiate from other adrenal masses[72]. Nevertheless, the use of narrow collimation on CT will usually allow the demonstration of any fat that is present. The fat component of these lesions can also be readily shown on MRI, with signal intensity similar to fat on all pulse sequences.

Infection: In granulomatous infections (tuberculosis, histoplasmosis, or blastomycosis), there is usually bilateral but asymmetric involvement of the adrenal glands. In active infection the adrenals are enlarged and inhomogeneous in density on CT particularly after contrast medium enhancement, when numerous small nonenhancing areas, of caseous necrosis, can often be seen (Fig. 71.31). Calcification may be seen in the acute phase or during healing and long-standing infection results in atrophic glands. Percutaneous biopsy is often required to confirm the diagnosis of granulomatous disease and to identify the organism. In AIDS patients with extrapulmonary *Pneumocystis carinii* infection, there may be punctuate or coarse calcification in the adrenal gland as well as in the spleen, liver, kidney and lymph nodes. Adrenal abscesses are rare, most being found in neonates with pre-existing adrenal haemorrhage. The abscess appears as a thick-walled cystic lesion.

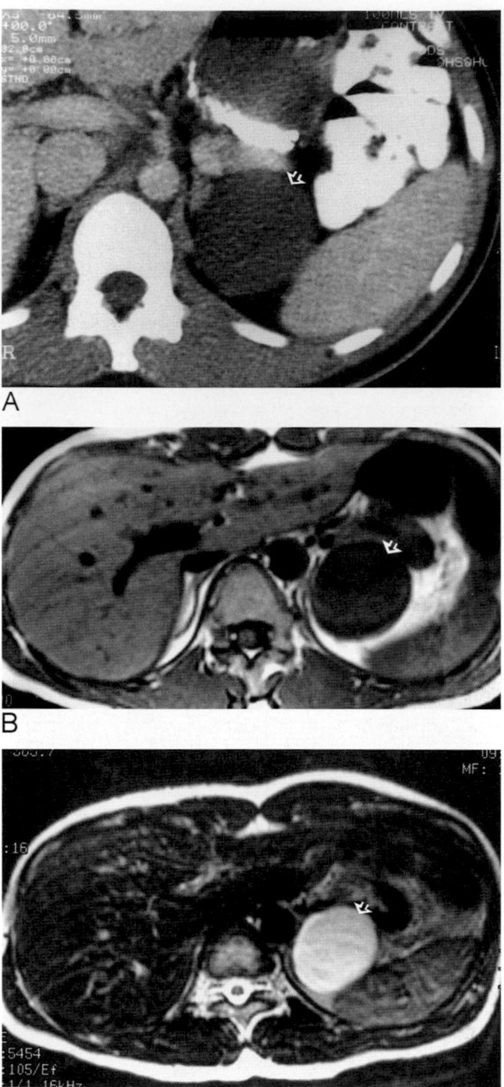

Figure 71.29 Adrenal cyst. (A) Contrast-enhanced CT showing the typical appearance of a cyst (arrow) within the left adrenal gland. (B) T1-weighted spin-echo image shows the low signal intensity of a simple cyst (arrow). (C) T2-weighted fast spin-echo image shows the uniformly high signal intensity of a fluid filled lesion (arrow).

Adrenal haemorrhage is usually clinically silent. It is seen on CT in 2% of patients who sustain severe trauma. The most common CT feature of adrenal injury is a round or oval adrenal haematoma (83%), followed by uniform adrenal enlargement (9%) or diffuse irregular haemorrhage obliterating the gland (9%). Non-traumatic adrenal haemorrhage is usually associated with anticoagulants (or other bleeding disorders), stress caused by surgery, sepsis (in particular meningococcal) and hypotension. Approximately 80% of adrenal haemorrhages are unilateral and most commonly on the right side (Fig. 71.32). Adrenal haemorrhage usually resolves but occasionally the haematoma liquefies and persists as a pseudocyst. The size and appearance of an adrenal haematoma varies with its age. On CT, in the acute or subacute phase, the enlarged adrenals are of increased density

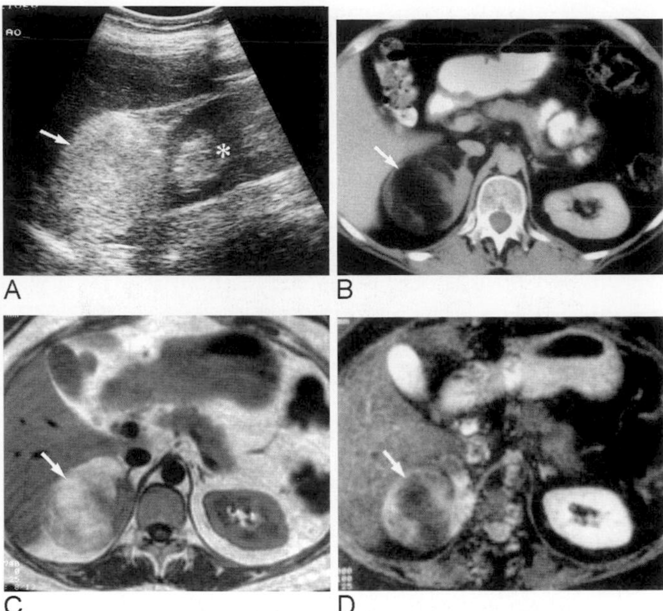

Figure 71.30 Myelolipoma. (A) A longitudinal ultrasound showing a hyperechoic mass (arrow) lying above the right kidney (*) and behind the liver. (B) Contrast-enhanced CT showing large right adrenal mass (arrow) consisting predominantly of fat. (C) Corresponding T1-weighted MRI showing a mass consists predominantly of fat of similar intensity to the surrounding perirenal fat. (D) STIR sequence showing suppression of the signal from fat within the mass (arrow). (After Peppercorn P D, Reznek R H 1997 State-of-the-art CT and MRI of the adrenal gland. Eur Radiol 7: 822–836, with permission).

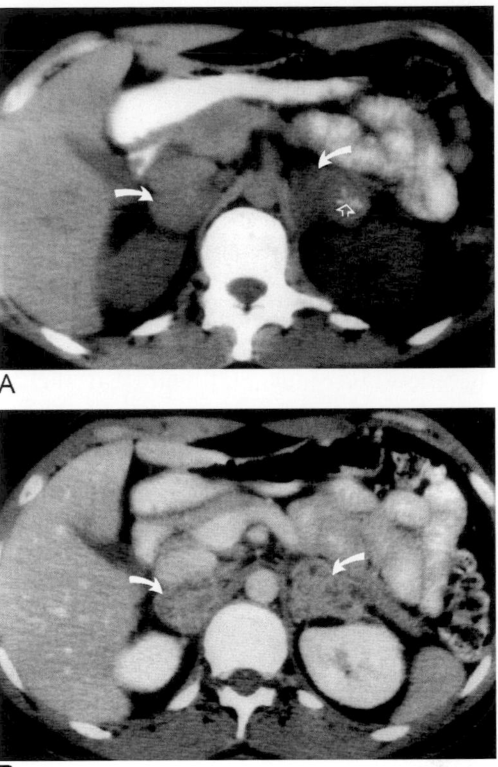

Figure 71.31 Adrenal gland tuberculosis. (A) Nonenhanced CT showing bilateral adrenal masses (curved arrows) with punctuate calcification in the left adrenal gland (open arrow). (B) Following intravenous injection of contrast media there are the typical nonenhancing areas within the gland (curved arrows) corresponding to multiple small caseating granulomata. (After Peppercorn P D, Reznek R H 1997 State-of-the-art CT and MRI of the adrenal gland. Eur Radiol 7: 822–836, with permission).

(50–70 HU) and follow-up studies show reductions in the density and size of the lesion. Calcification may develop a few months after the adrenal haemorrhage. On MRI, intracellular deoxyhaemoglobin in the acute phase causes signal loss on T1- and T2-weighted images. Subacutely, methaemoglobin causes bright signal intensity on T1-weighted images. Chronic adrenal haemorrhage often has low signal intensity on T1- and T2-weighted images because of calcification and haemosiderin deposition.

The 'incidentally' discovered adrenal mass

Adrenal masses are found incidentally in up to 5% of abdominal CT examinations. In the assessment of an incidentally discovered adrenal mass, the initial step is biochemical evaluation. The type of biochemical abnormality then dictates further management. It is important to note that if there is no history of malignancy, a unilateral non-hyperfunctioning adrenal mass rarely, if ever, represents a metastasis unless there is a known underlying malignancy, and the differential diagnosis rests usually between adenoma and carcinoma.

Though small adrenal masses are more likely to be benign, it has been shown that size alone is poor at discriminating between adenomas and non-adenomas[73]. The measurement of the CT attenuation value of the mass can be helpful. Unlike malignant lesions, benign adenomas generally contain intracellular lipid and thus have a lower CT attenuation value. An attenuation value of less than 10 HU on non-contrast-enhanced CT has an extremely high specificity and acceptable sensitivity for a benign cortical adenoma. Much greater overlap is seen after enhancement. However, malignant masses tend to have a rapid loss of attenuation value following intravenous contrast material injection. The percentage absolute and relative enhancements on the delayed imaging at 10 and 15 minutes have been shown to be useful in discriminating benign from malignant adrenal mass. Absolute percentage loss of enhancement of greater than 60% at 10 minutes has 100% specificity for the diagnosis benign adenoma[74].

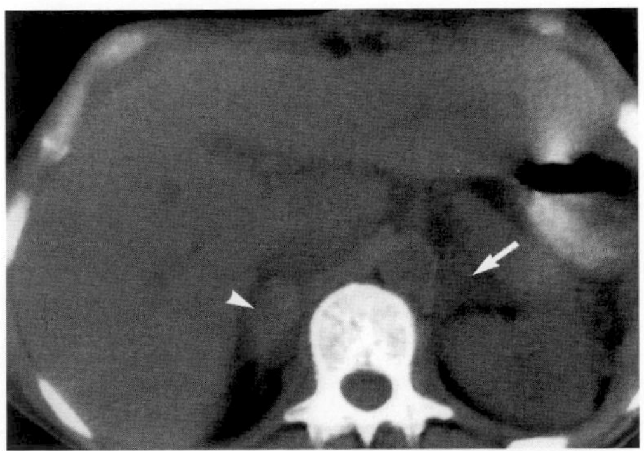

Figure 71.32 Adrenal haemorrhage. Non-enhanced CT showing bilateral enlargement due to adrenal haemorrhage (arrow). An area of high attenuation due to bleeding is demonstrated within the right adrenal gland (arrowhead).

Chemical shift imaging on MRI may also be used to characterize adrenal masses (Fig. 71.33). As with CT, the characterization is based on the detection of intracellular lipid in benign adenomas. When sufficient loss of signal has been demonstrated in adrenal masses on chemical shift imaging, a specificity of 100% has been reported for benign adenomas[58].

Cholesterol-based radiopharmaceutical imaging can also be used in evaluating an incidental adrenal mass. Cholesterol-based scintigraphy may show increased uptake in a non-functioning adenoma, whereas distorted, absent or reduced uptake suggests pathology such as carcinoma or other space-occupying lesions. Recently, PET with [F-18]FDG has also been reported to be able to differentiate between benign adenomas and metastases.

THE FEMALE REPRODUCTIVE SYSTEM

The ovaries have both germinal and hormonal functions, which are modulated by hypothalamic and pituitary hormones. The adult ovaries function cyclically with changes in hormone levels. Ovarian endocrine dysfunction may present with failure to develop secondary sex characteristics, amenorrhoea, galactorrhoea, or infertility.

Amenorrhoea, failure of ovulation, may be either primary (i.e., where no menstruation has previously occurred) or secondary (i.e., when there is loss of menstruation following previous periods). In the investigation of amenorrhoea, pregnancy must be excluded before recourse to other biochemical or imaging investigations. In primary amenorrhoea, imaging plays an important role in the exclusion of gross urogenital anatomical defects before proceeding to more complex biochemical assessment.

Turner's syndrome is the classical form of ovarian dysgenesis. These patients have a 45-XO karyotype and elevated follicle-stimulating hormone (FSH) concentrations. They have 'streak ovaries' and a small uterus. Patients with Turner's syndrome may also have a high arched palate, a webbed neck, widely-spaced nipples, poorly developed breasts, cubitus valgus, short fourth metacarpals, beaked vertebral bodies and osteoporosis. Pelvic gonadal dysgenesis may occur with a normal karyotype; in Swyer syndrome, an XY karyotype is associated with gonadal dysgenesis. The importance of recognizing this condition lies in the 25% incidence of associated ovarian tumours, such as dysgerminomas, which occur up to the age of 20 years. Annual pelvic US is recommended in these patients to detect any such ovarian tumour.

FUNCTIONING OVARIAN TUMOURS

Ovarian tumours that cause virilization include Sertoli–Leydig cell tumours, Brenner tumours and the rare lipoid cell tumours. Granulosa-theca cell tumours are the most common oestrogen-producing tumours but may also release testosterone. Cross-sectional imaging techniques show these tumours are predominantly solid or solid and cystic[75]. There are no specific features to help distinguish between functioning ovarian tumours or with other ovarian neoplasm.

THE MALE REPRODUCTIVE SYSTEM

Like the ovaries, the testes have both germinal and hormonal functions, which are modulated by the hypothalamic and pituitary hormones. Gonadotropin-releasing hormone (GnRH) from the hypothalamus controls FSH and luteinizing hormone (LH) secretion. In men FSH is responsible for initiating

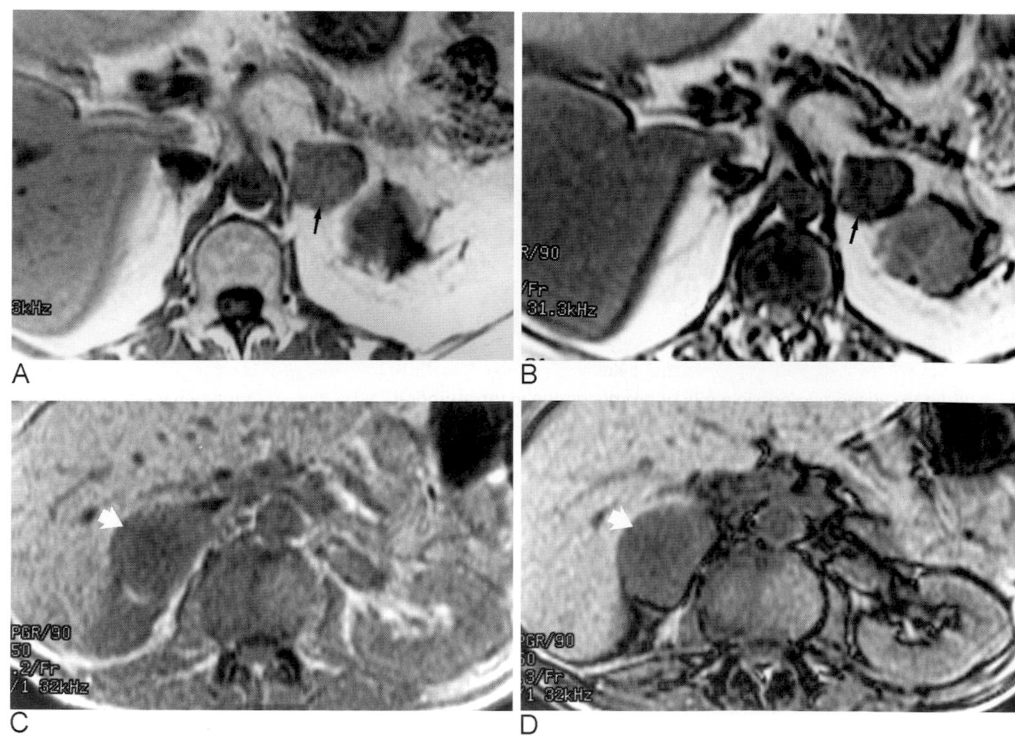

Figure 71.33 Chemical shift imaging to evaluate incidentally discovered adrenal masses. In-phase (A) and out-of-phase (B) images in a benign adrenal adenoma (arrow). The out-of-phase image shows marked loss of signal intensity within the adenoma indicating presence of intracellular lipid in keeping with a benign adenoma. In-phase (C) and out-of-phase (D) images in an adrenal metastasis from a colon cancer (arrow). The out-of-phase images show that there has been no loss of signal intensity and, therefore, the presence of intracellular fat has not been demonstrated.

spermatogenesis and LH stimulates Leydig cells to produce androgens.

Primary abnormalities of the testes are best imaged using US and MRI may be of benefit where US is inconclusive. Abnormalities of testicular function have different consequences depending on the phase of life in which they first become manifest, i.e., in fetal development, puberty, or adult life.

ANDROGEN EXCESS

Primary tumours of either adrenal glands or testes, or congenital adrenal hyperplasia may give rise to excessive androgen production in childhood, resulting in precocious puberty. Primary germ cell tumour (seminoma or teratoma) or nongerminal (interstitial or Sertoli cell) tumour may also cause androgen excess.

ANDROGEN DEFICIENCY

Androgen deficiency may result either from primary testicular failure or secondary to abnormality in the hypothalamic–pituitary axis (see above). In primary testicular disorders, serum testosterone levels are decreased and gonadotropin levels are elevated. The diagnosis is made on clinical grounds, biochemical assay, and the demonstration of chromosomal abnormality. Imaging has a minimal role in the diagnosis and management of these patients.

REFERENCES

1. Tien R D, Newton T H, McDermott M W, Dillon W P, Kucharczyk J 1990 Thickened pituitary stalk on MR images in patients with diabetes insipidus and Langerhans cell histiocytosis. Am J Neuroradiol 11: 703–708
2. Sato N, Ishizaka H, Yagi H, Matsumoto M, Endo K 1993 Posterior lobe of the pituitary in diabetes insipidus: dynamic MR imaging. Radiology 186: 357–360
3. Brooks B S, el Gammal T, Allison J D, Hoffman W H 1989 Frequency and variation of the posterior pituitary bright signal on MR images. Am J Roentgenol 153: 1033–1038
4. Kelly W M, Kucharczyk W, Kucharczyk J et al 1988 Posterior pituitary ectopia: an MR feature of pituitary dwarfism. Am J Neuroradiol 9: 453–460
5. Bartynski W S, Lin L 1997 Dynamic and conventional spin-echo MR of pituitary microlesions. Am J Neuroradiol 18: 965–972
6. Tsunoda A, Okuda O, Sato K 1997 MR height of the pituitary gland as a function of age and sex: especially physiological hypertrophy in adolescence and in climacterium. Am J Neuroradiol 18: 551–554
7. Ahmadi H, Larsson E M, Jinkins J R 1990 Normal pituitary gland: coronal MR imaging of infundibular tilt. Radiology 177: 389–392
8. Yousem D M, Arrington J A, Zinreich S J, Kumar A J, Bryan R N 1989 Pituitary adenomas: possible role of bromocriptine in intratumoral hemorrhage. Radiology 170: 239–243
9. Teramoto A, Hirakawa K, Sanno N, Osamura Y 1994 Incidental pituitary lesions in 1,000 unselected autopsy specimens. Radiology 193: 161–164
10. Hahn F J, Leibrock L G, Huseman C A, Makos M M 1988 The MR appearance of hypothalamic hamartoma. Neuroradiology 30: 65–68
11. Loevner L A 1996 Imaging of the thyroid gland. Semin Ultrasound CT MR 17: 539–562
12. Hussain H K, Britton K E, Grossman A B, Reznek R H 2004 Thyroid cancer. In: Husband J E, Reznek R H (eds) Imaging in Oncology. Taylor and Francis, London, pp 669–710
13. Hegedus L 2004 Clinical practice. The thyroid nodule. N Engl J Med 351: 1764–1771
14. Clark O H, Duh Q Y 1991 Thyroid cancer. Med Clin North Am 75: 211–234
15. de los Santos E T, Keyhani-Rofagha S, Cunningham J J, Mazzaferri E L 1990 Cystic thyroid nodules. The dilemma of malignant lesions. Arch Intern Med 150: 1422–1427
16. Shibata T, Noma S, Nakano Y, Konishi J 1991 Primary thyroid lymphoma: MR appearance. J Comput Assist Tomogr 15: 629–633
17. Hopkins C R, Reading C C 1995 Thyroid and parathyroid imaging. Semin Ultrasound CT MR 16: 279–295
18. Takashima S, Ikezoe J, Morimoto S H et al 1988 Primary thyroid lymphoma: evaluation with CT. Radiology 168: 765–768
19. Haugen B R, Nawaz S, Cohn A et al 1994 Secondary malignancy of the thyroid gland: a case report and review of the literature. Thyroid 4: 297–300
20. Maisey M N 1998 Thyroid imaging. In: Grossman A B (ed) Clinical Endocrinology. Blackwell Science Ltd, London, pp 298–314
21. Grunwald F, Schomburg A, Bender H et al 1996 Fluorine-18 fluorodeoxyglucose positron emission tomography in the follow-up of differentiated thyroid cancer. Eur J Nucl Med 23: 312–319
22. Dietlein M, Scheidhauer K, Voth E, Theissen P, Schicha H 1997 Fluorine-18 fluorodeoxyglucose positron emission tomography and iodine-131 whole-body scintigraphy in the follow-up of differentiated thyroid cancer. Eur J Nucl Med 24: 1342–1348
23. Chung J K, So Y, Lee J S et al 1999 Value of FDG PET in papillary thyroid carcinoma with negative ^{131}I whole-body scan. J Nucl Med 40: 986–992
24. Alam M S, Kasagi K, Misaki T et al 1998 Diagnostic value of technetium-99m methoxyisobutyl isonitrile (99mTc-MIBI) scintigraphy in detecting thyroid cancer metastases: a critical evaluation. Thyroid 8: 1091–1100
25. Gallowitsch H J, Mikosch P, Kresnik E, Unterweger O, Gomez I, Lind P 1998 Thyroglobulin and low-dose iodine-131 and technetium-99m-tetrofosmin whole-body scintigraphy in differentiated thyroid carcinoma. J Nucl Med 39: 870–875
26. Auffermann W, Clark O H, Thurnher S, Galante M, Higgins C B 1988 Recurrent thyroid carcinoma: characteristics on MR images. Radiology 168: 753–757
27. Healy J C, Shafford E A, Reznek R H et al 1996 Sonographic abnormalities of the thyroid gland following radiotherapy in survivors of childhood Hodgkin's disease. Br J Radiol 69: 617–623
28. Sfakianakis G N, Ezuddin S H, Sanchez J E, Eidson M, Cleveland W 1999 Pertechnetate scintigraphy in primary congenital hypothyroidism. J Nucl Med 40: 799–804
29. Perez F F, Cordido C F, Pombo F F, Mosquera O J, Villalba M C 1993 Riedel thyroiditis: US, CT, and MR evaluation. J Comput Assist Tomogr 17: 324–325
30. Melnick J C, Stemkowski P E 1981 Thyroid hemiagenesis (hockey stick sign): a review of the world literature and a report of four cases. J Clin Endocrinol Metab 52: 247–251
31. Krubsack A J, Wilson S D, Lawson T L et al 1989 Prospective comparison of radionuclide, computed tomographic, sonographic, and magnetic resonance localization of parathyroid tumors. Surgery 106: 639–644; discussion 644–646
32. Lucas R J, Welsh R J, Glover J L 1990 Unilateral neck exploration for primary hyperparathyroidism. Arch Surg 125: 982–984; discussion 984–985
33. Al-Sayer H M, Krukowski Z H, Williams V M, Matheson N A 1985 Fine needle aspiration cytology in isolated thyroid swellings: a prospective two year evaluation. Br Med J (Clin Res Ed) 290: 1490–1492
34. Levin K E, Gooding G A, Okerlund M et al 1987 Localizing studies in patients with persistent or recurrent hyperparathyroidism. Surgery 102: 917–925
35. Lee V S, Spritzer C E 1998 MR imaging of abnormal parathyroid glands. Am J Roentgenol 170: 1097–1103
36. Pattou F, Huglo D, Proye C 1998 Radionuclide scanning in parathyroid diseases. Br J Surg 85: 1605–1616

37. Sierra M, Herrera M F, Herrero B et al 1998 Prospective biochemical and scintigraphic evaluation of autografted normal parathyroid glands in patients undergoing thyroid operations. Surgery 124: 1005–1010
38. Kohri K, Ishikawa Y, Kodama M et al 1992 Comparison of imaging methods for localization of parathyroid tumors. Am J Surg 164: 140–145
39. Denham D W, Norman J 1998 Cost-effectiveness of preoperative sestamibi scan for primary hyperparathyroidism is dependent solely upon the surgeon's choice of operative procedure. J Am Coll Surg 186: 293–305
40. Price D C 1993 Radioisotopic evaluation of the thyroid and the parathyroids. Radiol Clin North Am 31: 991–1015
41. Miller D L, Doppman J L, Shawker T H et al 1987 Localization of parathyroid adenomas in patients who have undergone surgery. Part I. Noninvasive imaging methods. Radiology 162: 133–137
42. Noone T C, Hosey J, Firat Z, Semelka R C 2005 Imaging and localization of islet-cell tumours of the pancreas on CT and MRI. Best Pract Res Clin Endocrinol Metab 19: 195–211
43. King C M, Reznek R H, Dacie J E, Wass J A 1994 Imaging islet cell tumours. Clin Radiol 49: 295–303
44. Gorman B, Charboneau J W, James E M et al 1986 Benign pancreatic insulinoma: preoperative and intraoperative sonographic localization. Am J Roentgenol 147: 929–934
45. Power N, Reznek R H 2002 Imaging pancreatic islet cell tumours. Imaging 14: 147–159
46. London J F, Shawker T H, Doppman J L et al 1991 Zollinger-Ellison syndrome: prospective assessment of abdominal US in the localization of gastrinomas. Radiology 178: 763–767
47. McLean A M, Fairclough P D 2005 Endoscopic ultrasound in the localisation of pancreatic islet cell tumours. Best Pract Res Clin Endocrinol Metab 19: 177–193
48. Smith T R, Koenigsberg M 1990 Low-density insulinoma on dynamic CT. Am J Roentgenol 155: 995–996
49. King A D, Ko G T, Yeung V T, Chow C C, Griffith J, Cockram C S 1998 Dual phase spiral CT in the detection of small insulinomas of the pancreas. Br J Radiol 71: 20–23
50. Owen N J, Sohaib S A, Peppercorn P D et al 2001 MRI of pancreatic neuroendocrine tumours. Br J Radiol 74: 968–973
51. Jackson J E 2005 Angiography and arterial stimulation venous sampling in the localization of pancreatic neuroendocrine tumours. Best Pract Res Clin Endocrinol Metab 19: 229–239
52. Pereira P L, Roche A J, Maier G W et al 1998 Insulinoma and islet cell hyperplasia: value of the calcium intraarterial stimulation test when findings of other preoperative studies are negative. Radiology 206: 703–709
53. Sandler M P, Delbeke D 1993 Radionuclides in endocrine imaging. Radiol Clin North Am 31: 909–921
54. Vincent J M, Trainer P J, Reznek R H et al 1993 The radiological investigation of occult ectopic ACTH-dependent Cushing's syndrome. Clin Radiol 48: 11–17
55. Hanson J A, Sohaib S A, Newell-Price J et al 1999 Computed tomography appearance of the thymus and anterior mediastinum in active Cushing's syndrome. J Clin Endocrinol Metab 84: 602–605
56. Bomanji J, Conry B G, Britton K E, Reznek R H 1988 Imaging neural crest tumours with ^{123}I-metaiodobenzylguanidine and X-ray computed tomography: a comparative study. Clin Radiol 39: 502–506
57. Vincent J M, Morrison I D, Armstrong P, Reznek R H 1994 The size of normal adrenal glands on computed tomography. Clin Radiol 49: 453–455
58. Sohaib S A, Reznek R H 2000 Adrenal imaging. BJU Int ; 86 (suppl 1): 95–110
59. Sohaib SA, Rockall AG, Reznek RH. Imaging functional adrenal disorders. Best Pract Res Clin Endocrinol Metab 2005; 19: 293–310
60. Sohaib S A, Hanson J A, Newell-Price J et al 1999 The CT appearance of the adrenal glands in adrenocorticotrophic hormone (ACTH)-dependent Cushings syndrome. Am J Roentgenol 172: 997–1002
61. Rockall A G, Babar S A, Sohaib S A et al 2004 CT and MR imaging of the adrenal glands in ACTH-independent Cushing syndrome. Radiographics 24: 435–452
62. Sohaib S A, Peppercorn P D, Allan C et al 2000 MRI in primary hyperaldosteronism (Conn's syndrome). Radiology 214: 527–531
63. Lingam R K, Sohaib S A, Vlahos I et al 2003 CT of primary hyperaldosteronism (Conn's syndrome): the value of measuring the adrenal gland. Am J Roentgenol 181: 843–849
64. Lingam R K, Sohaib S A, Rockall A G et al 2004 Diagnostic performance of CT versus MR in detecting aldosterone-producing adenoma in primary hyperaldosteronism (Conn's syndrome). Eur Radiol 14: 1787–1792
65. Sheaves R, Goldin J, Reznek R H et al 1996 Relative value of computed tomography scanning and venous sampling in establishing the cause of primary hyperaldosteronism. Eur J Endocrinol 134: 308–313
66. Hanson J A, Weber A, Reznek R H et al 1996 Magnetic resonance imaging of adrenocortical adenomas in childhood: correlation with computed tomography and ultrasound. Pediatr Radiol 26: 794–799
67. Sahdev A, Sohaib A, Monson J P, Grossman A B, Chew S L, Reznek R H 2005 CT and MR imaging of unusual locations of extra-adrenal paragangliomas (pheochromocytomas). Eur Radiol 15: 85–92
68. Mukherjee J J, Peppercorn P D, Reznek R H et al 1997 Pheochromocytoma: effect of nonionic contrast medium in CT on circulating catecholamine levels. Radiology 202: 227–231
69. Vincent J M, Morrison I D, Armstrong P, Reznek R H 1994 Computed tomography of diffuse, non-metastatic enlargement of the adrenal glands in patients with malignant disease. Clin Radiol 49: 456–460
70. Jenkins P J, Sohaib S A, Trainer P J, Lister T A, Besser G M, Reznek R 1999 Adrenal enlargement and failure of suppression of circulating cortisol by dexamethasone in patients with malignancy. Br J Cancer 80: 1815–1819
71. Jenkins P J, Chew S L, Lowe D G, Reznek R H, Wass J A 1994 Adrenocorticotrophin-independent unilateral macronodular adrenal hyperplasia occurring with myelolipoma: an unusual cause of Cushing's syndrome. Clin Endocrinol (Oxf) 41: 827–830
72. Musante F, Derchi L E, Zappasodi F et al 1988 Myelolipoma of the adrenal gland: sonographic and CT features. Am J Roentgenol 151: 961–964
73. Korobkin M, Brodeur F J, Yutzy G G et al 1996 Differentiation of adrenal adenomas from nonadenomas using CT attenuation values. Am J Roentgenol 166: 531–536
74. Al Hawary M M, Francis I R, Korobkin M 2005 Non-invasive evaluation of the incidentally detected indeterminate adrenal mass. Best Pract Res Clin Endocrinol Metab 19: 277–292
75. Sohaib S A, Husband J E, Reznek R H 2004 Ovarian cancer. In: Reznek RH, Husband JE, editors. Imaging in Oncology. Taylor and Francis, London, 429–466
76. Peppercorn P D, Reznek R H 1997 State-of-the-art CT and MRI of the adrenal gland. Eur Radiol 7: 822–836

CHAPTER 72

Reticuloendothelial Disorders: Lymphoma

Sarah J. Vinnicombe and Rodney H. Reznek

- Epidemiology
- Histopathological classification
- Staging, investigation and management
- Lymph node disease in lymphoma
- Extranodal manifestations of lymphoma
- Burkitt lymphoma
- Lymphoma in the immunocompromised
- Monitoring response to therapy
- Surveillance and detection of relapse
- Conclusion

The lymphomas are a complex group of diseases divided into two broad groups: Hodgkin's disease (HD), or Hodgkin's lymphoma (HL) and lymphomas other than Hodgkin's disease, the non-Hodgkin's lymphoma (NHL). The overall incidence of NHL is increasing globally, with age-adjusted incidence rates for NHL being highest in more developed countries. Recent figures from the USA give an incidence of 15.5 per 100 000 persons per year, representing a 73% increase since the early 1970s[1]. This is due in part to secondary lymphoma arising in the setting of AIDS, but a steady increase had been noted before the AIDS epidemic. In the corresponding period, the incidence of HD has remained relatively steady at around 3.7 per 100 000.

EPIDEMIOLOGY

Age

Hodgkin's disease has a peak incidence in the 20–30 year age group, with a second, smaller peak in the elderly population that is becoming less evident, partly because of a refinement of the classification of NHL. The incidence of NHL increases exponentially with age after 20 years. The subtypes of lymphoma encountered differ in frequency between the adult and paediatric groups, with a strong bias towards precursor B- and T-lymphoblastic lymphoma and Burkitt lymphoma in childhood. Lymphomas with less typical age distribution include mediastinal large B-cell lymphoma, which has a peak incidence between 25 and 35 years and mantle cell lymphoma, which is more common in those over 60 years.

Infectious agents

Oncogenic lymphotrophic DNA and RNA viruses have been implicated in many NHL types. The single most important agent in this regard is the herpes virus, Epstein–Barr virus (EBV). The EBV genome was first detected in cultured African Burkitt lymphoma cells and is known to be present in over 90% of such cases. EBV is important as a trigger for lymphoproliferations/lymphomas occurring in congenital immunodeficiencies, iatrogenically immunosuppressed organ transplant recipients, patients receiving maintenance chemotherapy and patients receiving combined immunosuppressive therapy for collagen disorders. EBV is also found in HD (mostly the mixed cellularity type) and patients who have had infectious mononucleosis are at increased risk of HD. The retrovirus human lymphotropic virus type 1 (HTLV-1) is implicated in the causation of adult T-cell lymphoma, which is endemic in certain areas of the globe, particularly in East Africa, the Caribbean, southwest Japan and New Guinea. Human herpesvirus 8 (HHV-8) has been implicated as a cause of primary effusion lymphoma, a rare type of large cell lymphoma confined to serous-lined body cavities, which occurs with highest frequency in the HIV-positive population.

Bacterial overgrowth can also promote lymphomagenesis. In gastric lymphoma of mucosa-associated lymphoid tissue (MALT) type, *Helicobacter pylori* infection has been shown to be necessary for the development and early proliferation of the lymphoma.

Immunosuppression

A variety of lymphomas are associated with pre-existing immunosuppression. The degree of immunosuppression is important in determining the lymphoma type that may emerge. In organ-specific autoimmune diseases, such as Hashimoto's thyroiditis and Sjögren's syndrome, extranodal marginal zone lymphomas of MALT type can arise within the affected organ. In severe immunodeficiency states, such as the congenital immunodeficiencies, AIDS and after organ transplantation, the lymphomas are very often EBV-driven large B-cell lymphomas.

In the setting of systemic collagen diseases, there is an increase in haematological malignancy and patients receiving immunosuppressive therapy for these conditions are at still greater risk. The types of haematological malignancy that arise are quite varied, but there is a slight excess of myeloma and small B-lymphocytic lymphoma.

Genetic factors

It is known that the risk of developing haematological malignancy is greater in patients with a family history of disease. This increased risk does not extend to the histological type or lineage of the tumours in question, such that one family member may have HD whereas a relative may have NHL or myeloid leukaemia.

Gender and race

It has long been recognized that there is a slight predominance of NHL and HD in men (1.1–1.4 to 1). The incidence of NHL and HD varies by race, with a higher frequency in whites than blacks or Asians. Certain NHL types cluster according to race, for example the natural killer (NK) T-cell lymphomas are most frequently encountered in oriental populations.

HISTOPATHOLOGICAL CLASSIFICATION

Non-Hodgkin's lymphoma

Many of the difficulties that beset early taxonomists in the classification of NHL have been overcome with improved immunological and molecular methods of diagnosis, resulting in a new classification scheme, the Revised European–American Lymphoma (REAL) classification. This depended on a triad of morphology, immunophenotype and molecular methods for defining disease entities, as well as clinical features[2], differentiating it from earlier morphologically based classifications. The scheme forms the backbone of the second WHO classification of tumours of haematopoietic and lymphoid tissues[3]. A summary of the WHO classification is given in Table 72.1. The WHO classification stratifies neoplasms by lineage into distinct disease entities and is a real advance in the ability to identify disease accurately and consistently.

Hodgkin's disease

Biological studies have shown that Hodgkin's disease is a true lymphoma, many pathologists preferring the term Hodgkin's lymphoma (HL). The defining cell of HD is the Reed–Sternberg cell, a large, binucleated blast cell. Mononuclear counterparts are called Hodgkin cells. The Reed–Sternberg cells and their variants are a minority population accounting for less than 5% of the volume of any involved lymph node. The balance is made up of reactive non-neoplastic T cells, histiocytes, plasma cells, eosinophils and fibroblasts, varying in proportion according to the histological subtype. Since the 1960s, so-called classical HD has been subclassified into four histological types, indicated below along with their relative frequencies in western populations:

Table 72.1 WHO CLASSIFICATION OF LYMPHOID NEOPLASMS

Neoplasm	Percentage of NHL*
B-CELL NEOPLASMS	85.0
Precursor B-cell neoplasms	
Precursor B-lymphoblastic leukaemia/lymphoma	
Mature B-cell neoplasms	
CLL/small lymphocytic lymphoma	6.7
B-cell prolymphocytic leukaemia	
Lymphoplasmacytic (lymphoplasmacytoid) lymphoma	1.2
Splenic marginal zone lymphoma	< 1.0
Hairy cell leukaemia	
Plasma cell myeloma	
Solitary plasmacytoma of bone	
Extraosseous plasmacytoma	
Extranodal marginal zone B-cell lymphoma of mucosa associated lymphoid tissue (MALT)	7.6
Nodal marginal zone lymphoma	1.8
Follicular lymphoma	22.0
Mantle cell lymphoma	6.0
Diffuse large B-cell lymphoma (BCL)	32.0
Mediastinal (thymic)	2.4
Intravascular	
Primary effusion lymphoma	
Burkitt lymphoma/leukaemia	1.0
B-CELL PROLIFERATIONS OF UNCERTAIN MALIGNANT POTENTIAL	
Lymphomatoid granulomatosis	
Post-transplant lymphoproliferative disorder, polymorphic	
T-CELL AND NK-CELL NEOPLASMS	14.0
Precursor T-cell neoplasms	
Precursor T-lymphoblastic lymphoma/leukaemia	1.7
Blastic NK-cell lymphoma	
Mature T-cell and NK-cell neoplasms	
T-cell prolymphocytic leukaemia	
T-cell large granular lymphocytic leukaemia	
Aggressive NK-cell leukaemia	
Adult T-cell leukaemia/lymphoma	2.4
Extranodal NK-/T-cell lymphoma, nasal type	< 1.0
Enteropathy-type T-cell lymphoma	
Hepatosplenic T-cell lymphoma	<0.001
Subcutaneous panniculitis-like T-cell lymphoma	1.0
Mycosis fungoides	
Sézary syndrome	1.2
Primary cutaneous anaplastic large cell lymphoma	
Peripheral T-cell lymphoma, unspecified	
Angioimmunoblastic T-cell lymphoma	7.0
Anaplastic large cell lymphoma	

Neoplasm	Percentage of NHL*
T-CELL PROLIFERATIONS OF UNCERTAIN MALIGNANT POTENTIAL	
Lymphoid papulosis	
HODGKIN'S LYMPHOMA	
Nodular lymphocyte-predominant HL	
Classical HL	
Nodular sclerosis classical HL	
Lymphocyte-rich classical HL	
Mixed cellularity classical HL	
Lymphocyte-depleted classical HL	

*Approximate frequency – refers to lymph node biopsies in adults, with 1% accounting for the very rare entities.

- lymphocyte-rich classical HD—5%
- mixed cellularity (MC) classical HD—20–25%
- nodular sclerosing (NS) classical HD—70%
- lymphocyte-depleted (LD) classical HD—<5%.

In the nodular sclerosing type, substantial fibroblastic activity results in segmentation of involved nodes into cellular nodules separated by thick bands of collagen. It typically presents as a bulky mediastinal mass. In mixed cellularity HD, classical Reed–Sternberg cells are mixed with sheets of inflammatory elements. It is commoner in developing countries and in patients with HIV infection, as is the rare lymphocyte-depleted HL. Both have an aggressive clinical course.

All four classical subtypes share the same immunophenotype and together constitute 95% of all cases of HD. A second distinct entity is nodular lymphocyte predominant HD, which was probably misdiagnosed as lymphocyte-rich classical HD in the past. It has a different morphology, immunophenotype and clinical course from classical HD and latent EBV infection is not a feature.

STAGING, INVESTIGATION AND MANAGEMENT

Hodgkin's disease

Staging

The so-called Cotswold's modification[4] of the original Ann Arbor staging classification was designed to take into account prognostic factors such as the volume of lymph node masses and modern imaging techniques such as CT may be used in staging. This classification is shown in Table 72.2.

Most patients present with lymph node enlargement, most often in the cervical chains. Up to 40% have B symptoms (fever, drenching night sweats and weight loss of more than 10% of the person's bodyweight). Patients may also complain of other constitutional symptoms, such as pruritus, fatigue, anorexia and rarely alcohol-induced pain at the site of enlarged lymph nodes. Clinical examination usually reveals peripheral lymphadenopathy, most commonly in the neck. Axillary nodal enlargement occurs in up to 20% and inguinal disease in up to 15%, although exclusive infradiaphragmatic nodal disease is seen in under 10% at presentation. Splenomegaly may be evident on clinical examination in up to 30% of patients.

Tissue biopsy (often image guided) is essential to make the diagnosis. Investigations will comprise a blood count and erythrocyte sedimentation rate (ESR), together with liver biochemistry, renal function and serum urate. A chest radiograph is mandatory because mediastinal involvement is common. CT may show involvement of intrathoracic, abdominal or pelvic lymph nodes. A bone marrow aspirate and trephine biopsy should be performed in all patients except those with stage I disease, in whom the likelihood of bone marrow infiltration is negligible.

Prognosis and treatment

The prognosis of HD depends on:

- age (poorer prognosis in older patients)
- tumour subtype (see above)
- raised ESR
- mutiple sites of disease
- bulky mediastinal disease (see Table 72.2)
- B symptoms.

Treatment is almost invariably given with curative intent. The choice of treatment will depend predominantly on stage and the presence or absence of adverse prognostic factors.

Localized disease (Stages IA and IIA) The majority of patients with early stage favourable disease are treated with radiotherapy, provided that all of the involved sites can safely be encompassed within the radiation field. Patients presenting with a

Table 72.2 COTSWOLD'S MODIFICATION OF THE ANN ARBOR STAGING CLASSIFICATION OF HODGKIN'S DISEASE

Stage	Classification
I	Involvement of a single lymph node region (I) or a single extralymphatic organ or site (IE)
II	Involvement of two or more lymph node regions on the same side of the diaphragm (II) or one or more lymph node regions plus an extralymphatic site (IIE)
III	Involvement of lymph node regions on both sides of the diaphragm (III) (the spleen is included in stage III) subdivided into: III(1): involvement of spleen and/or splenic hilar, coeliac and portal nodes III(2): with para-aortic, iliac, or mesenteric nodes
IV	Involvement of one or more extralymphatic organs, e.g. lung, liver, bone, bone marrow, with or without lymph node involvement
Additional qualifiers denote the following:	A: asymptomatic B: fever, night sweats and weight loss of >10% body weight X: bulky disease (defined as a lymph node mass >10 cm in diameter or, if involving the mediastinum, a mass greater than one third of the intrathoracic diameter at the level of T5 E: involvement of a single extranodal site, contiguous with a known nodal site

large mediastinal mass (i.e. a mass greater than one-third of the intrathoracic diameter at the level of T5) are generally treated with a moderate amount of chemotherapy initially, so as to shrink the mass before radiotherapy and avoid excessive irradiation of lung parenchyma and subsequent radiation fibrosis.

Advanced disease (Stages IIB, IIIA/B and IVA/B) Treatment comprises extensive combination chemotherapy in the first instance, with or without subsequent consolidatory radiotherapy to sites of 'bulky' disease, to reduce the risk of local recurrence.

Though HD is highly radiosensitive, in recent years there has been a trend towards the avoidance of radiotherapy in young patients because of the significant increase in secondary cancers, notably of the thyroid and breast, both areas included in the classical mantle radiotherapy field.

Failure to achieve an initial complete, or almost complete, response to first line treatment and recurrence in the first year are both associated with a very poor prognosis. Similarly, patients who develop recurrent HD more than once will almost certainly eventually die as a consequence of the disease. By comparison, patients who develop recurrent HD some years after receiving treatment for localized disease can be given further combination chemotherapy and still be cured.

Non-Hodgkin's lymphoma

Local diagnosis of NHL requires an adequate tissue biopsy and an experienced histopathologist. Some lesions, for example, retroperitoneal, mediastinal and mesenteric masses, may be amenable to ultrasound or CT-guided core-needle biopsy, which may safely yield adequate tissue for histological diagnosis and immunophenotyping[5].

Staging

By comparison to HD, the histological subtype of NHL has a major bearing on treatment. As in HD, the clinical stage of the disease carries strong prognostic significance, a more advanced stage being associated with a significantly worse prognosis[6]. Staging investigations are essential. The Cotswold's modification of the Ann Arbor staging system has been largely adopted for clinical usage in NHL. Since the majority of patients present with widespread disease, all newly diagnosed patients should undergo detailed physical examination, including examination of the fauces and testes. CT of the neck, chest, abdomen and pelvis is mandatory, together with a bone marrow aspirate and trephine biopsy, owing to the propensity of many NHL to infiltrate the bone marrow. Depending on the pattern of symptoms, other radiological investigations such as plain radiographs, skeletal scintigraphy or MRI may be indicated. However many of these tests may be replaced by PET-CT once this technique becomes more widely available.

Prognosis and treatment

The prognosis of NHL varies tremendously, depending upon the histological subtype. In order to evaluate therapies better and to choose the most appropriate treatment for a given patient, the International Prognostic Index (IPI) was developed[6]. Five factors were statistically associated with significantly inferior overall survival:

- age >60 years
- elevated serum lactate dehydrogenase (LDH)
- performance status >1 (i.e. nonambulatory)
- advanced stage III or IV
- presence of >1 extranodal site of disease.

The IPI is strictly speaking only applicable to diffuse large B-cell lymphoma (DLBCL) and more recently a similar prognostic index has been developed for lower grade follicular lymphomas, where the important factors are considered to be:

- age >60 years
- elevated serum LDH
- haemoglobin <12 g/dl
- advanced stage III or IV
- more than four nodal sites of disease.

Treatment is nearly always with combination chemotherapy, since around 80% of patients will have advanced disease (stage III or IV) at presentation. Radiotherapy alone is considered for the small proportion of patients with stage I disease and no adverse factors, in whom surgical excision alone is considered inappropriate.

LYMPH NODE DISEASE IN LYMPHOMA

In HD, lymph node involvement is usually the only manifestation of disease, whereas in NHL nodal disease is frequently associated with extranodal sites of tumour. At presentation, differences exist between the patterns of lymph node involvement in HD and NHL. Lymph nodes tend to be larger in NHL than HD; indeed in nodular sclerosing and lymphocyte-depleted HD, nodal enlargement may be minimal. Typically, involved nodes tend to displace adjacent structures rather than invade them, except in the case of diffuse large B-cell lymphoma, which is often locally aggressive.

Imaging nodal disease

At present, size is the only criterion by which lymph nodes demonstrated on CT or MRI are considered to be involved, though clustering of multiple small nodes, for example within the anterior mediastinum or the mesentery, is suggestive. A maximum short-axis diameter of 10 mm is taken to be the upper limit of normal, depending upon the exact site within the neck, thorax, abdomen, or pelvis. Thus within the neck, the jugulodigastric node can measure up to 13 mm short axis diameter, whereas those in the gastrohepatic ligament and porta hepatis are considered abnormal if they measure more than 8 mm in diameter. Retrocrural nodes greater than 6 mm are taken as enlarged[7] and in the pelvis the upper limit of normal is regarded as 8 mm[8]. Lymph nodes at some sites, such as the splenic hilum, presacral and perirectal areas, are not usually visualized on cross-sectional imaging and, when demonstrated, are likely to be abnormal whatever the size.

Enlarged lymph nodes in both HD and in NHL are usually homogeneous and of soft-tissue density on CT. They may show mild or moderate uniform enhancement after intravenous injection of contrast medium. Calcification is uncommon but may be seen on post-treatment scans. Necrosis is rarely seen in large nodal masses in both HD (particularly nodular sclerosing HD) and aggressive NHL, more frequently after treatment. On MRI, lymph nodes are easily identified as relatively low to intermediate signal intensity masses on T1-weighted images, of intermediate to high signal on T2-weighted images and which may have very high signal intensity on short-tau inversion recovery (STIR) sequences. Though the signal intensity of involved nodes and the presence of necrosis do not appear to have much prognostic significance, there is some evidence that within large lymphomatous masses, heterogeneous T2 signal at MRI or heterogeneous enhancement at CT are associated with a worse outcome.

Choice of imaging technique

The ability of CT to demonstrate enlarged lymph nodes throughout the body and detect associated lesions in soft-tissue structures, together with a high level of reproducibility, have all contributed to CT becoming the treatment of choice for the staging and follow-up of lymphoma. Ultrasound will readily show lymph node enlargement in the coeliac regions, splenic hilum and porta hepatis[9]. Frequently, however, the entire retroperitoneum cannot be shown, limiting its value in staging. Typically on ultrasound, lymphomatous nodal involvement produces uniform hypoechoic lobulated masses. The pattern of vascular perfusion as demonstrated by power Doppler interrogation may suggest the diagnosis, lymphomatous nodes having rich central and peripheral perfusion. The main value of ultrasound in lymphoma lies not in routine staging but in confirming that a palpable mass is in fact nodal, or in solving specific problems related to detection of involvement of tumour in the liver, spleen, or kidney. Although the accuracy of MRI in detecting lymph node involvement is equal to that of CT (and indeed better in some areas such as the supraclavicular fossa and within the pelvis), it has no particular advantage over CT in this respect and its role is essentially adjunctive, to solve problems in the identification of lymph node pathology or in monitoring response to treatment[10–12].

Although lymphangiography was shown to be equal, or slightly superior, to CT for detecting nodal lymphoma in the 1980s, it had many disadvantages, which have led to the almost universal abandonment of the technique. Radioisotope studies using gallium-67 (Ga-67) and the positron emitter, 2[F-18]fluoro-2-deoxy-D-glucose ([F-18]FDG), can demonstrate viable tumour cells within nodes with high sensitivity. However, the accuracy of gallium-67 is dependent upon several factors including cell type, location and the size of the lesion. Its accuracy is greater for HD and high-grade NHL than for other forms and decreases for lesions measuring less than 2 cm, even with optimal technique. It performs poorly below the diaphragm because of normal splenic and bowel activity and a significant number of lymphomas are non-gallium-avid. For these reasons, it has no role as an isolated tool in the staging of lymphoma.

Numerous studies have shown that positron emission tomography (PET) using [F-18]FDG (FDG-PET) is at least as accurate as CT in the depiction of nodal and extranodal disease[13,14] and more sensitive than Ga-67. It results in clinically significant upstaging in up to 10–20% of patients and as a result, changes in therapy, particularly in HD[15,16]. In NHL, it indicates tumour burden as well as the presence or absence of extranodal disease, though occasional false negative studies occur with very low grade lymphomas such as MALT types. Despite the proven advantages of FDG-PET, until recently few authorities would have recommended its use as an isolated staging tool. However, the advent of combined PET-CT will potentially revolutionize staging, since for the first time it is possible to assess both morphological and functional abnormalities accurately.

Neck

Between 60 and 80% of patients with HD present with cervical lymphadenopathy. The spread of the disease is most frequently to contiguous nodal groups, with involvement of the internal jugular chain first and spread to other deep lymphatic chains in the neck, supraclavicular fossae and axillae. Patients with supraclavicular or bilateral neck adenopathy are at increased risk of infradiaphragmatic disease.

Cervical adenopathy is less common in NHL, although involved nodes may be much larger. Extranodal disease with or without associated adenopathy is common, Waldeyer's ring being the site most frequently involved. Approximately 40–60% of patients who present with head and neck involvement will have disseminated NHL. Involved nodal groups tend to be noncontiguous. Lymph nodes greater than 10 mm in diameter are generally considered enlarged. Minimally enlarged discrete lymph nodes seen in the neck in patients with lymphoma usually have a well-defined contour, but once tumour has broken beyond the confines of the node, the fat planes between the nodal mass and adjacent structures are lost. Central necrosis within a lymph node is rarely seen. Imaging with CT or MRI has a useful role in evaluating the neck in patients with lymphoma, as it may identify enlarged nodes which are impalpable. It is useful to assess treatment response, particularly in patients treated with radiotherapy, where post-treatment fibrosis renders clinical assessment difficult and it may identify recurrence in such patients.

Thorax

Nodes within the thorax are involved at the time of presentation in 60–85% of patients with HD and 25–40% of patients with NHL[17,18]. Nodes larger than 1 cm short axis diameter at CT or MRI are considered enlarged. Any intrathoracic group of nodes may be affected, but all the mediastinal sites other than paracardiac and posterior mediastinal nodes are more frequently involved in HD than NHL. The frequency of nodal involvement in HD is as follows[18]:

- prevascular and paratracheal—84% (Figs 72.1, 72.2)
- hilar—28% (Fig. 72.2)
- subcarinal—22% (Fig. 72.2).

Other sites, which account for about 5% of all involved nodal groups, include the aortopulmonary window, the anterior diaphragmatic group, the internal mammary (Fig. 72.1) and the posterior mediastinal group (Fig. 72.2). In NHL involvement of the hilar and subcarinal groups is rarer, occurring in 9%

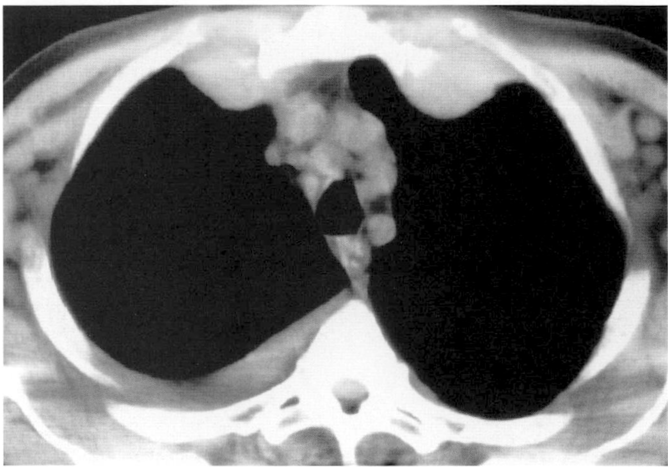

Figure 72.1 Internal mammary lymphadenopathy. Unenhanced CT showing marked enlargement of the internal mammary lymph nodes bilaterally. Note the minimal bilateral axillary and paratracheal lymph node enlargement and small right pleural effusion.

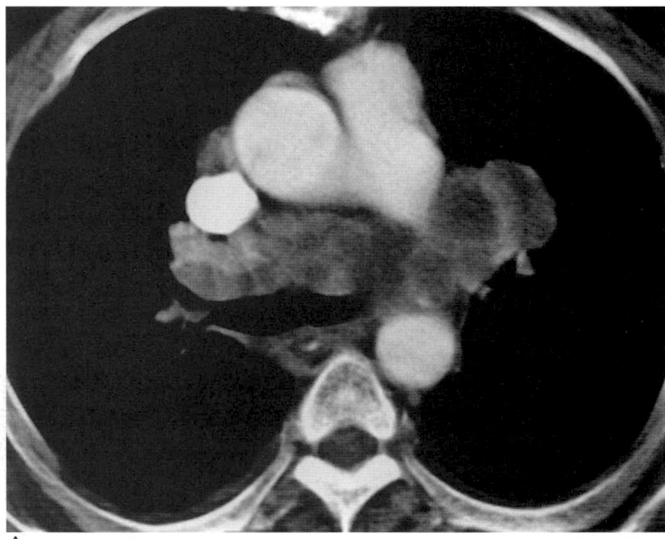

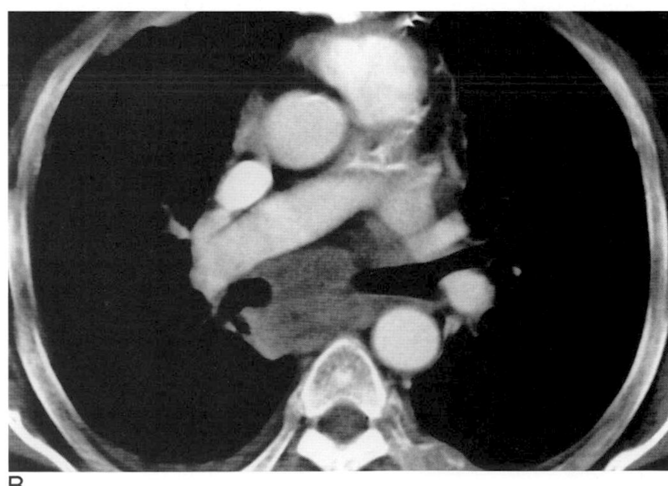

Figure 72.2 Middle mediastinal nodal disease. (A) Contrast-enhanced CT showing marked enlargement of the paratracheal and precarinal group of nodes, extending laterally into the left aortopulmonary nodes and continuing inferiorly into the subcarinal group (B) in the same patient.

and 13% respectively, whereas superior mediastinal nodes are involved in 35%[19].

The great majority of cases of HD show enlargement of two or more nodal groups, whereas only one nodal group is involved in up to half of the cases of NHL. Almost all patients with nodular sclerosing HD have disease in the anterior mediastinum. Hilar nodal enlargement is rare without associated mediastinal involvement, particularly in HD. The posterior mediastinum is infrequently involved, but if disease is present in the lower part of the mediastinum, contiguous retrocrural disease is likely. Although paracardiac nodes are rarely involved at presentation in HD, they may become important as sites of recurrence, as they are not included in the classical 'mantle' radiation field. In most cases lymphadenopathy is bilateral but asymmetrical and nodes may be discrete or matted together.

In HD and NHL, large anterior mediastinal masses usually represent thymic infiltration as well as a nodal mass (Fig. 72.3). Cystic change can be recognized at CT and MRI with large anterior mediastinal masses, especially in mediastinal large B-cell lymphoma (previously called sclerosing large B-cell lymphoma). A large anterior mediastinal mass in HD is recognized as an adverse prognostic feature. As indicated above, such a feature alters management strategy and defines the need for more aggressive initial therapy.

In 10% of patients with HD, CT will demonstrate unsuspected mediastinal nodal enlargement despite a normal chest radiograph and these patients have a poorer prognosis. As a result, CT of the chest will change stage and alter management in up to 25% of patients with HD. The therapeutic impact is less in patientswith NHL.

Abdomen and pelvis

The pattern of the disease below the diaphragm is markedly different in HD and NHL. At presentation the retroperitoneal nodes are involved in 25–35% of patients with HD and 45–55% of patients with NHL[20]. Mesenteric lymph nodes are involved in more than half the patients with NHL and less than 5% of patients with HD[20,21]. Other sites, as in the porta hepatis and around the splenic hilum, are also less frequently involved in HD than NHL (Fig. 72.4).

In HD, nodal spread is predictably from one lymph node group to another through directly connected lymphatic pathways[22]. Nodes are frequently of normal size or only minimally enlarged[23]. Spread from the mediastinum occurs through the lymphatic vessels to the retrocrural nodes, coeliac axis and so on. Around the coeliac axis, multiple normal-sized nodes may be seen, which can be difficult to evaluate because involved, normal-sized nodes are frequent in HD[23]. The coeliac axis, splenic hilar and porta hepatis nodes are involved in about 30% of patients and splenic hilar nodal involvement is almost always associated with diffuse splenic infiltration (Fig. 72.4). In the porta hepatis (Fig. 72.4), the node of the foramen of Winslow (porta caval node), lying between the portal vein and the inferior vena cava, is important, as it is often overlooked and may be the only site of disease relapse. This node has a triangular or lozenge shape; its normal transverse diameter is up to 3 cm and in the anteroposterior plane is approximately 1 cm.

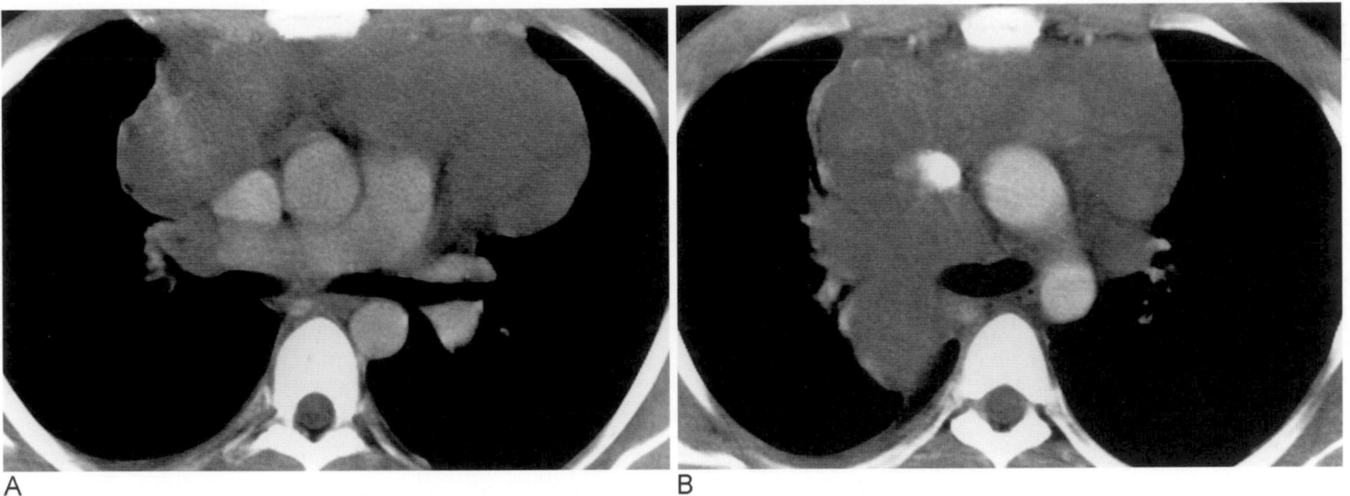

Figure 72.3 Mediastinal masses in lymphoma. (A) Contrast-enhanced CT showing a large anterior mass in a young patient with Hodgkin's disease. No other disease was demonstrated. (B) Contrast-enhanced CT in a patient with mediastinal diffuse large B-cell lymphoma (non-Hodgkin's). The mass is involving the anterior and middle mediastinum. This subtype of non-Hodgkin's lymphoma carries a poor prognosis and, as in this patient, often involves the abdominal viscera.

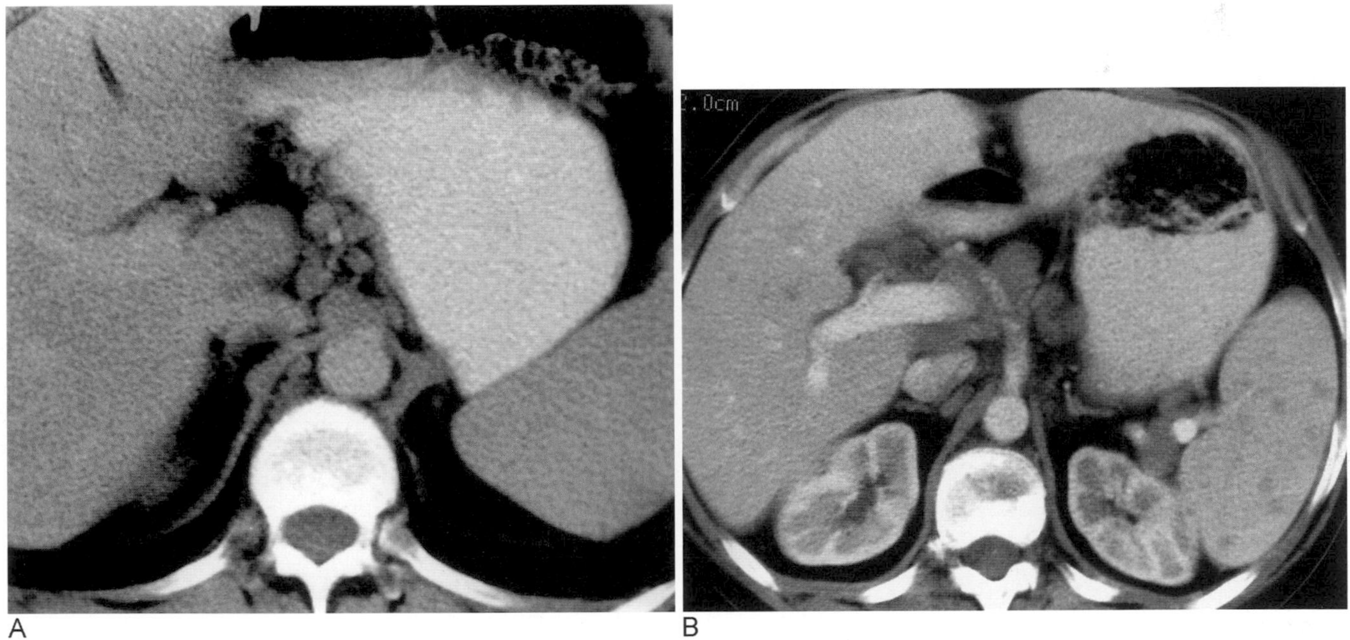

Figure 72.4 Upper abdominal lymph node enlargement. (A) Contrast-enhanced CT showing enlarged lymph nodes in the gastrohepatic ligament. Minimal lymph node enlargement (exceeding 6 mm) is also seen in the right retrocrural region. (B) Contrast-enhanced CT showing lymph node enlargement in the region of the splenic hilum around the coeliac axis and in the porta hepatis. Multiple small, nonenhancing foci are demonstrated within the spleen, typical of splenic involvement.

In NHL, nodal involvement is frequently noncontiguous and bulky and is more frequently associated with extranodal disease. Discrete mesenteric nodal enlargement or masses may be seen with or without retroperitoneal nodal enlargement. Large volume nodal disease in both mesentery and retroperitoneum may give rise to the so-called 'hamburger' sign, in which a loop of bowel is compressed between two large nodal masses. In NHL, regional nodal involvement is frequently seen in patients with primary extranodal lymphoma involving an abdominal viscus. Involved nodes tend to enhance uniformly and the presence of central necrosis or multilocular enhancement should suggest an alternative diagnosis such as tuberculosis or atypical infection.

In the pelvis, all nodal groups may be involved in both HD and NHL. Presentation with enlarged inguinal or femoral lymphadenopathy is seen in less than 20% of HD, but when it does occur, careful attention must be paid to the pelvic nodes on imaging, as these will be the next contiguous site of spread. In patients with massive pelvic disease, MRI is helpful for delineating the full extent of tumour and the effect on the adjacent organs.

EXTRANODAL MANIFESTATIONS OF LYMPHOMA

Involvement of extranodal sites by lymphoma usually occurs in the presence of widespread advanced disease elsewhere. Such secondary involvement occurs in both HD and NHL and it is a recognized adverse prognostic feature. However, in approximately 30–40% of cases, primary involvement of an extranodal site occurs, with lymph node involvement limited to the regional group of nodes—stages I–IIE. Both primary and secondary extranodal involvement is more common in NHL than HD. As primary extranodal HD is extremely rare, rigorous exclusion of disease elsewhere is essential before this diagnosis can be made. The incidence of extranodal involvement in NHL depends on a number of factors, including the age of the patient, the presence of pre-existing immunodeficiency and the pathological subtype of lymphoma. There is an increased incidence of extranodal disease in children, especially in the gastrointestinal tract, the major abdominal viscera and extranodal locations in the head and neck,[24] and in the immunocompromised host. In both these patient groups, the high incidence of extranodal involvement is a reflection of the fact that such lymphomas are usually of the more aggressive histological subtypes. As the frequency of NHL is increasing (both in the general population and in the immunocompromised), the incidence of extranodal disease is rising faster than that of nodal disease[25]. For example, primary lymphomas of the CNS and orbit are increasing in frequency at a rate of 10% and 6%, respectively, per annum.

Of the various pathological forms of NHL, mantle cell (a diffuse low-grade B-cell lymphoma), lymphoblastic lymphomas (80% of which are T-cell), Burkitt (small cell noncleaved) and MALT lymphomas demonstrate a propensity to arise in extrandal sites.

CT generally performs well in the depiction of extranodal disease, though there are certain instances where ultrasound or MRI are preferred. FDG-PET is more sensitive than CT because of its ability to identify splenic and bone marrow infiltration[14], though limited availability has precluded its use in this regard.

Thorax

Pulmonary parenchymal involvement

Several categories of lymphomatous lung involvement can be identified:

- that associated with existing or previously treated intrathoracic nodal disease
- that associated with widespread extrathoracic disease
- primary pulmonary HD
- primary pulmonary NHL.

Some authors also separate out AIDS-related lymphomas (ARL), which commonly affect the lungs and the post-transplant lymphoproliferative disorders (PTLDs)[26].

There is lung involvement at presentation in just under 4% of patients with NHL, but in approximately 12% of patients with HD. It usually occurs by direct extension of nodal disease, which is generally evident radiographically, into the adjacent parenchyma, hence its paramediastinal or perihilar location. In this circumstance there is no effect on stage; the 'E' lesion. Patients with HD presenting with an intrapulmonary lesion in the absence of demonstrable mediastinal disease are unlikely to have lymphomatous disease of the lung, unless there has been previous mediastinal or hilar irradiation, when recurrence may be confined to the lungs. Conversely, in NHL, nodal disease is absent in 50% of those patients with pulmonary or pleural involvement.

As nodal disease progresses or relapses, lung involvement becomes commoner in HD and NHL, such that 30–40% of patients with HD have pulmonary involvement at some stage during the course of the disease[27].

Radiographic appearances The radiographic appearances are extremely variable, but the commonest pattern is that of one or more discrete nodules, with or without cavitation, which tend to be less well defined and less dense than those of primary or metastatic carcinoma, which they otherwise resemble (Figs 72.5, 72.6)[28]. The disease tends to spread along lymphatic channels and involves lymphoid follicles around bronchovascular divisions, resulting in peribronchial nodula-

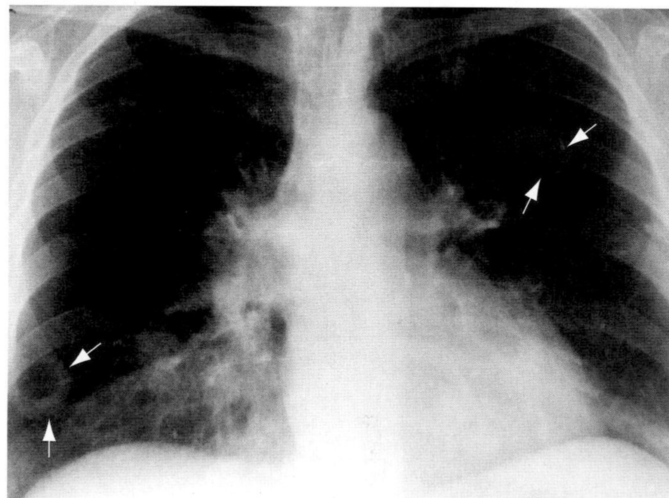

Figure 72.5 Hodgkin's disease with cavitating lung lesions. Chest radiograph showing bilateral hilar lymph node enlargement and multiple cavitating lung nodules (arrows).

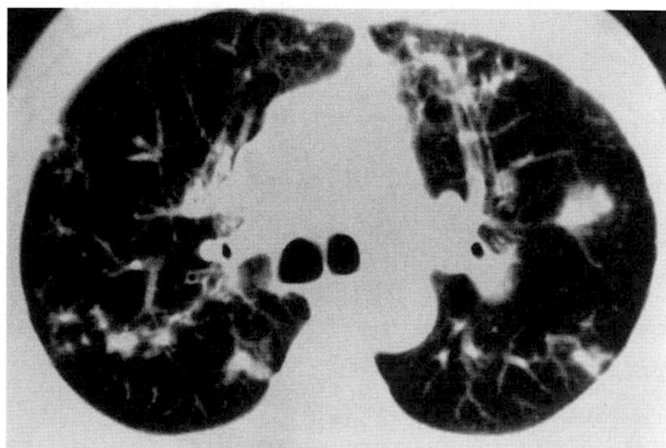

Figure 72.6 Pulmonary involvement in a patient with Hodgkin's disease. CT performed at the time of presentation, showing widespread ill-defined intrapulmonary nodular shadowing scattered throughout both lungs. Early cavitation can be seen in a peripheral nodule in the left lung.

tion spreading out from the hila, which can result in streaky shadowing visible on chest radiographs and at CT.

A more unusual pattern is for the lymphoma to fill the pulmonary acini, producing rounded or segmental areas of consolidation with air bronchograms (Fig. 72.7). Small nodulations along the bronchial wall may enable differentiation from infective consolidation. A rare pattern of disease is widespread interstitial reticulonodular shadowing, producing a lymphangitic picture. Another rare manifestation is atelectasis, which results from endobronchial lymphoma rather than extrinsic compression by nodal disease.

Several problems exist in the differential diagnosis of pulmonary involvement in lymphoma, which includes drug-induced changes, the effect of radiotherapy and opportunistic infection during or following chemotherapy, particularly in patients with antecedent immunosuppression.

Primary pulmonary lymphoma

Primary pulmonary lymphoma accounts for less than 1% of all lymphomas and is usually low-grade B-cell NHL, arising from MALT or bronchus-associated lymphoid tissue (BALT). BALT lymphomas are low-grade lymphomas of small lymphocytic type which tend to occur in the fifth to sixth decades, have an indolent course with 5-year survivals of over 60% and tend to remain extranodal, although lymph node involvement can occur with advanced disease[29]. Many patients will have a prior history of inflammatory or autoimmune disease, such as Sjögren's syndrome, collagen vascular disease and dysgammaglobulinaemia[30]. The imaging findings are nonspecific with the single commonest manifestation being a solitary nodule. Multiple nodules, or one or more rounded or segmental areas of consolidation[31], are also seen. These can persist unchanged for long periods. Pleural effusions are seen in up to 20% of cases[30].

In the remaining 15–20% of patients, primary lung lymphoma is due to high-grade NHL. The most common finding on a chest radiograph is of a solitary or multiple pulmonary nodules, which characteristically grow rapidly. Primary pulmonary HD is extremely rare. The most frequently described finding is single or multiple nodules with upper zone predominance and a relatively high incidence of cavitation.

Pleural disease

Pleural effusions, usually accompanied by mediastinal lymphadenopathy, occur at presentation in 10% of patients with NHL and 7% of patients with HD (Fig. 72.8)[32], though they may be detected on CT in 50% of patients with mediastinal nodal disease. They are usually exudates secondary to central lymphatic or venous obstruction, rather than direct malignant involvement and therefore clear promptly with treatment of the mediastinal disease. Pulmonary involvement need not be present. Focal pleural masses do occur at presentation but are more commonly seen in recurrent disease, when they are generally accompanied by an effusion[32].

Pericardium and heart

Direct pericardial and cardiac involvement can occur with high-grade peripheral T-cell and large B-cell lymphomas. Such direct spread to involve the heart is rare, except in patients with AIDS related lymphoma (ARL) and post-transplant lymphoproliferative disorders (PTLD) who may present with acute onset of heart block, tamponade, or congestive cardiac failure. Pericardial effusions occur in 6% of patients with HD at the time of presentation and are associated with large masses adjacent to the heart. For staging, effusions are regarded as evidence of pericardial involvement. Small pericardial effusions are often seen at CT during treatment, the aetiology of which is unclear. They usually resolve with time, although some pericardial thickening may remain.

Thymus

It is rare for HD to arise primarily in the thymus, but involvement of the thymus by HD in association with enlarged mediastinal nodes occurs in 30–50% of patients at presentation. Mediastinal large B-cell lymphoma characteristically involves the thymus, occurring typically in young women

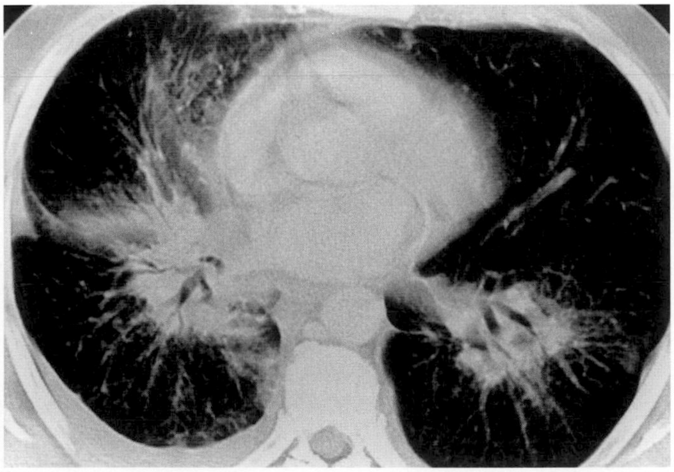

Figure 72.7 Lung involvement in Hodgkin's disease. CT showing peribronchial streaking and consolidation radiating from both hila. This pattern reflects spread along the peribronchial lymphatics.

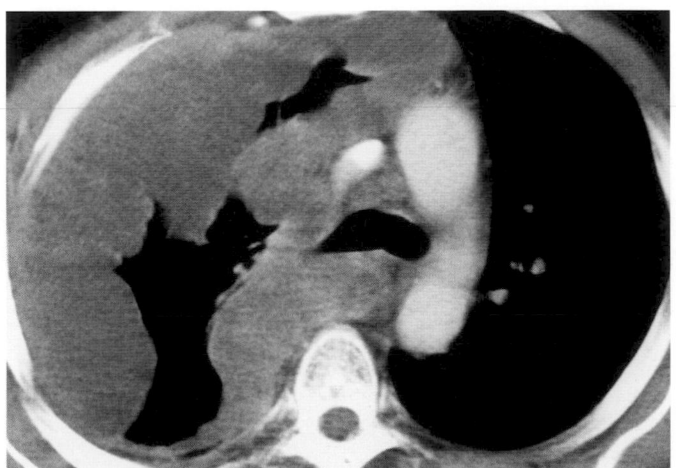

Figure 72.8 Pleural disease in lymphoma. CT showing a typical appearance of pleural involvement in a patient with NHL. There is a lobulated mass encasing the right hemithorax involving all the pleural surfaces, encasing and narrowing the superior vena cava.

between the ages of 25 and 40 years (Fig. 72.3B). Rapidly growing bulky disease is typical and up to 40% have superior vena caval obstruction, which is rare with other lymphomas.

On CT, differentiation of enlarged mediastinal lymph nodes from thymic involvement is often difficult as the thymus involved by lymphoma usually has a homogeneous soft-tissue density or a heterogeneous nodular appearance. On MRI as well, the gland is often of mixed signal intensity similar to that of involved nodes. Nevertheless, thymic involvement usually retains the shape of the normal thymus and has a smooth contour, whereas nodal masses are usually lobulated. CT or MRI may occasionally demonstrate cysts up to 3 cm in diameter, which can persist or even increase in size following regression of the rest of the involved gland with successful treatment. Calcification may be present at the outset or may develop during treatment[33,34].

Benign thymic rebound hyperplasia can develop after completion of chemotherapy, which can be difficult to differentiate from recurrent disease. Unfortunately, functional imaging with gallium-67 or FDG-PET may not always differentiate between the two and clinical correlation combined with follow-up studies may be necessary.

Chest wall

In HD, spread into the chest wall usually occurs by direct infiltration from an anterior mediastinal mass, especially from an internal mammary chain. In HD or NHL, chest wall masses can also spread from axillary or supraclavicular nodes, or arise de novo within the chest wall. Bony destruction is rare and should suggest a diagnosis of carcinoma or infection rather than lymphoma. Thoracic wall disease is better shown by MRI than CT, particularly on T2-weighted or STIR sequences, where there is excellent contrast between the mass and normal low signal intensity muscle. This facilitates more accurate planning of radiotherapy portals[35].

Breast

Lymphoma of the breast is usually associated with widespread disease elsewhere. Primary NHL of the breast is rare, accounting for approximately 2% of all lymphomas and under 0.5% of all malignant breast neoplasms. The age distribution is bimodal, with the first peak occurring during pregnancy and lactation, often high-grade or Burkitt and affecting both breasts diffusely with an inflammatory picture. Mammography shows thickening of the skin and trabeculae[36]. There is a second peak at around 50 years when patients present with discrete masses, solitary in 66% of cases. Bilateral disease occurs in up to 13%. The masses are usually fairly well defined and there is little accompanying architectural distortion or skin thickening. Secondary involvement is characterized by multiple nodules, with associated large-volume adenopathy. Calcification has not been described in primary or secondary disease.

Hepatobiliary system and spleen

Liver

Liver involvement is present in up to 15% of adult patients with NHL at presentation, though this figure is higher in the paediatric population and with recurrent disease. In HD, liver involvement occurs in about 5% of patients at presentation, almost invariably in association with splenic HD. True primary hepatic lymphoma is rare but the incidence is rising, up to 25% of affected patients being hepatitis B or C positive.

Pathologically, diffuse microscopic infiltration around the portal tracts is the most common form of involvement. CT and MRI are therefore insensitive in the detection of liver involvement. However, hepatomegaly strongly suggests the presence of diffuse infiltration (in contradistinction to the significance of splenomegaly). Larger focal areas of infiltration are only present in 5–10% of patients with hepatic lymphoma. Cross-sectional imaging may demonstrate miliary nodules or larger solitary or multiple masses, resembling metastases (Fig. 72.9).

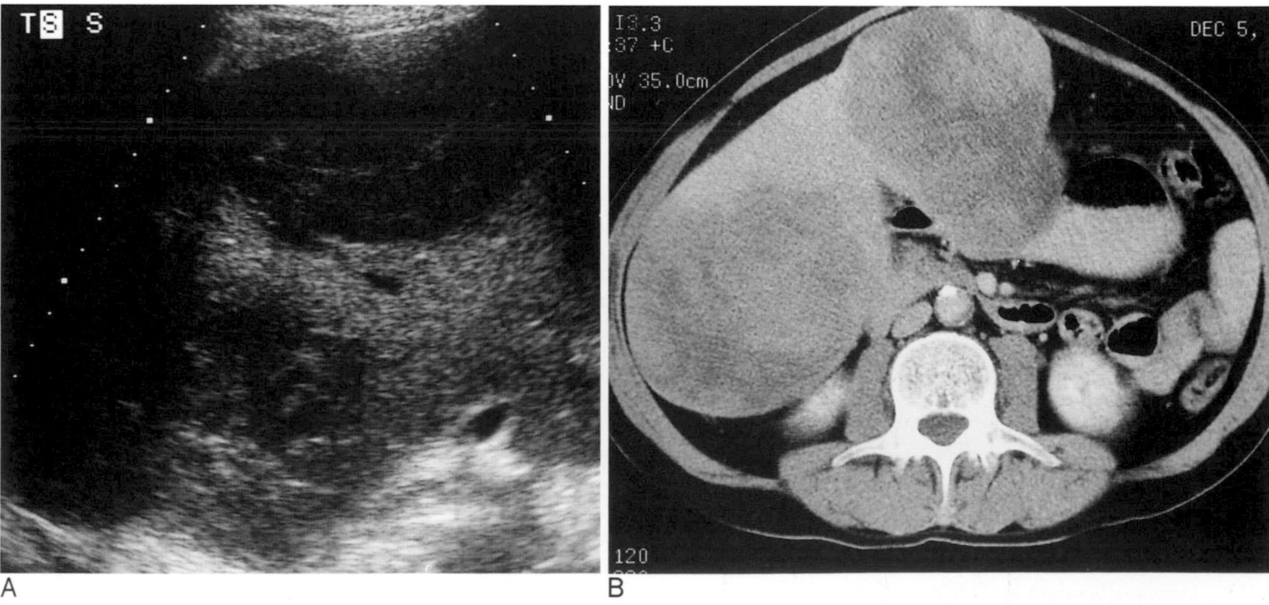

Figure 72.9 Lymphomatous infiltration of the liver. (A) Transverse ultrasound of the liver, showing multiple large hypoechoic lesions corresponding to the large focal masses demonstrated on contrast-enhanced CT (B).

On ultrasound they are usually well defined and hypoechoic; on CT they are hypodense before and after intravenous injection of contrast medium; and on MRI they are of higher signal intensity than the surrounding parenchyma on T2-weighted sequences. Superparamagnetic iron oxide particles can increase the conspicuity of such focal deposits. Occasionally, especially in children, periportal infiltration is manifest as periportal low attenuation tissue at CT (Fig. 72.10).

Non-Hodgkin's lymphoma of the bile ducts and gallbladder is rare but occurs with relatively high frequency in patients with ARL.

Spleen

The spleen is involved in 30–40% of patients with HD at the time of presentation, usually in the presence of nodal disease above and below the diaphragm (stage III), but in a small proportion it is the sole focus of intra-abdominal disease. In the majority of patients, the involvement is microscopic and diffuse and thus particularly difficult to identify on cross-sectional imaging, as splenomegaly does not necessarily indicate involvement; 33% of patients have splenomegaly without infiltration and, conversely, 33% of normal-sized spleens are found to contain tumour following splenectomy. Measurements of splenic volume and splenic indices are not generally utilized.

Focal splenic deposits occur in only about 10–25% of cases which, when they are more than 1 cm in diameter, can be demonstrated on any form of cross-sectional imaging (Fig. 72.4B). Up to 40% of patients with NHL have splenic involvement at some stage. Imaging findings include a solitary mass, military nodules, or multiple masses, all of which tend to have a nonspecific appearance. The differential diagnosis of multiple masses includes opportunistic infection and granulomatous disease.

In early studies, the sensitivity of ultrasound and CT for the detection of splenic involvement was extremely low (about 35%), although in a more recent study ultrasound was more sensitive than CT in detecting nodules down to 3 mm in size (63 vs. 37%)[37]. Detection of small focal nodules has improved with the advent of multidetector CT (MDCT) and powered contrast medium injection, with optimal splenic parenchymal opacification. MRI with superparamagnetic iron oxide may improve the diagnostic accuracy but is seldom undertaken to assess splenic status. However, FDG-PET can detect splenic disease more accurately than CT or gallium scintigraphy. In the past, the poor sensitivity of imaging for the detection of splenic involvement in HD necessitated staging laparotomy with splenectomy but the development of effective combination chemotherapy with good salvage regimens has led to this practice being abandoned.

Primary splenic NHL is rare, accounting for 1% of all patients with NHL. Patients present with splenomegaly, often marked and focal masses are usual. Splenic involvement is also a particular feature of certain other pathological subtypes of NHL, such as mantle cell lymphoma and splenic marginal zone lymphoma. Infarction is a well-recognized complication.

Gastrointestinal tract

The gastrointestinal tract is the commonest site of primary extranodal NHL, accounting for 30–45% of all extranodal presentations. It is the initial site of lymphomatous involvement in up to 10% of all adult patients and up to 30% of children[24]. As elsewhere, primary HD of the gastrointestinal tract is most unusual. Secondary involvement of the gastrointestinal tract is extremely common, usually from direct extension from involved mesenteric or retroperitoneal lymph nodes and consequently multiple sites of involvement occur.

Primary lymphomas arise from lymphoid tissue of the lamina propria and the submucosa of the bowel wall and occur most frequently below the age of 10 years (usually Burkitt lymphoma, BL) and in the sixth decade (MALT type and enteropathy-associated T-cell type). Primary gastrointestinal lymphoma is usually unifocal; accepted criteria for the diagnosis of primary disease include:

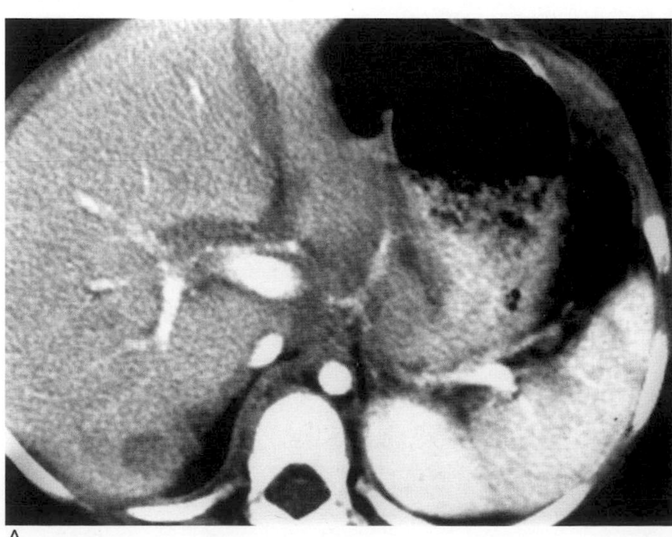
A

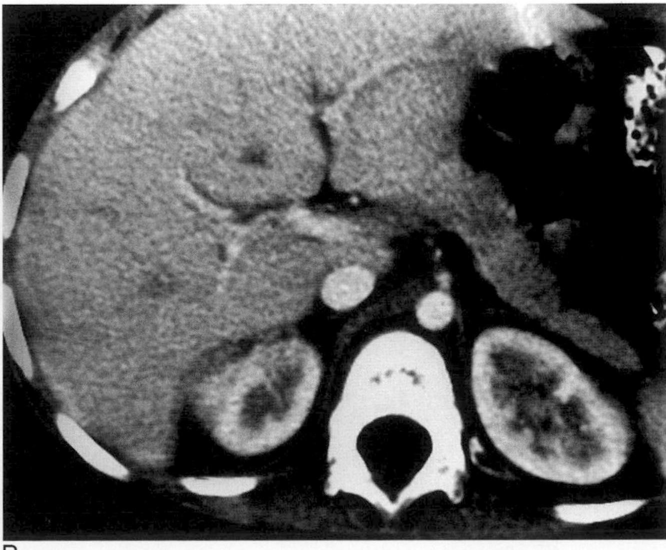
B

Figure 72.10 Periportal lymphoma. (A) Contrast-enhanced CT in a child with NHL, showing infiltration of low-density lymphomatous tissue from the porta hepatis, encasing the main portal vein, extending alongside the right portal vein. A solitary focal abnormality is seen posteriorly within the liver. (B) A follow-up after chemotherapy shows complete resolution of the disease.

- an absence of superficial or intrathoracic lymph node enlargement
- no involvement of the liver or spleen
- a normal white cell count
- no more than local regional lymph node enlargement.

In both primary and secondary cases, the stomach is most frequently involved (50%), followed by the small bowel (35%) and large bowel (15%).

Stomach

Primary lymphoma accounts for about 2–5% of all gastric tumours[38]. It originates in the submucosa, affecting the antrum more commonly than the body and the cardia. Radiologically the appearances reflect the gross pathological findings; common appearances are multiple nodules, some with central ulceration, or a large, fungating lesion with or without ulceration. About a third of patients have diffuse infiltration with marked thickening of the wall and narrowing of the lumen, sometimes with extension into the duodenum indistinguishable from linitis plastica. Only about 10% are characterized by diffuse enlargement of the gastric folds, similar to the pattern seen in hypertrophic gastritis (Fig. 72.11).

As the disease originates in the submucosa, the signs described above are best demonstrated on barium studies or endoscopically, but these investigations do not reflect the true extent of gastric wall thickening and accompanying nodal involvement, which is well shown on CT. Typically, infiltration of adjacent organs is unusual, unlike in gastric carcinoma[39], though it may occur in DLBCL in Table 72.1. In gastric MALT lymphomas, mural thickening may be minimal; CT is then of limited value and endoscopic ultrasound is more useful in staging, prognostication and assessment of response (Fig. 72.12). Low-grade MALT lymphoma is more likely to cause shallow ulceration and nodulation, whereas high-grade lymphoma can produce more massive gastric infiltration and polypoid masses.

Small bowel

Lymphoma accounts for up to 50% of all primary tumours of the small bowel, occurring most frequently in the terminal ileum and becoming progressively less frequent proximally, such that duodenal lymphomas are rare (Fig. 72.13). In children the disease is almost exclusively ileocaecal. Most are of B-cell lineage. The disease is multifocal in up to 50% of cases and because the disease originates in the lymphoid follicles, mural thickening with constriction of segments of bowel is typical. Patients commonly present with obstructive symptoms. Bowel wall thickening is well demonstrated on CT (Fig. 72.14). With progressive tumour spread through the submucosa and muscularis mucosa, long tube-like segments result. Aneurysmal dilatation of long segments of bowel also develop, presumably due to infiltration of the autonomic plexus. Such alternating areas of dilatation and constriction are a common manifestation of small bowel infiltration.

Occasionally the lymphomatous infiltration is predominantly submucosal, which results in multiple nodules or polyps of varying size scattered throughout the small bowel, but predominantly in the terminal ileum. It is this form of lymphoma that typically results in intussusception, usually in the ileocaecal region. This is the commonest cause of intussusception in children older than 6 years. Barium studies typically

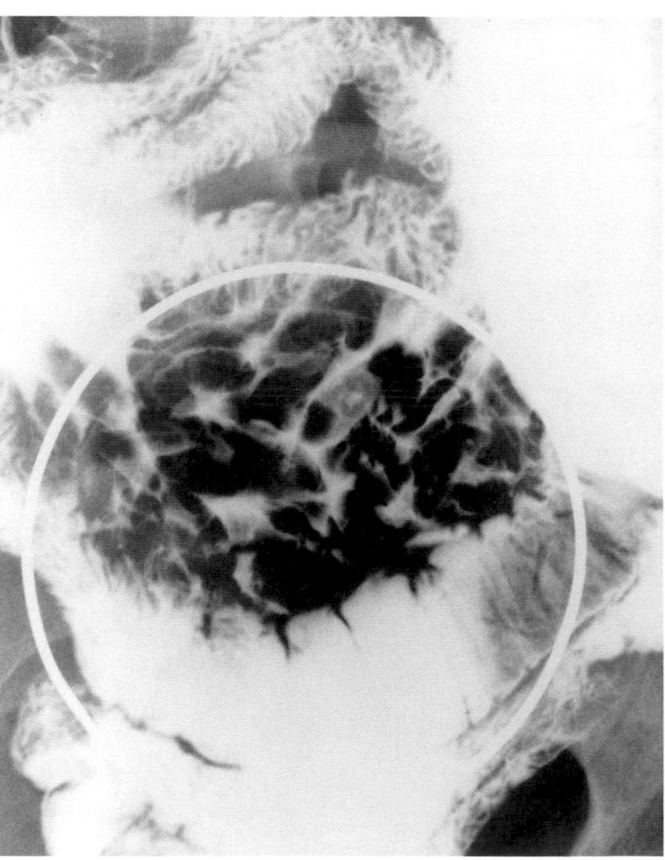

Figure 72.11 Gastric lymphoma. Double-contrast barium meal study (with compression) showing marked rugal hypertrophy. Note areas of ulceration.

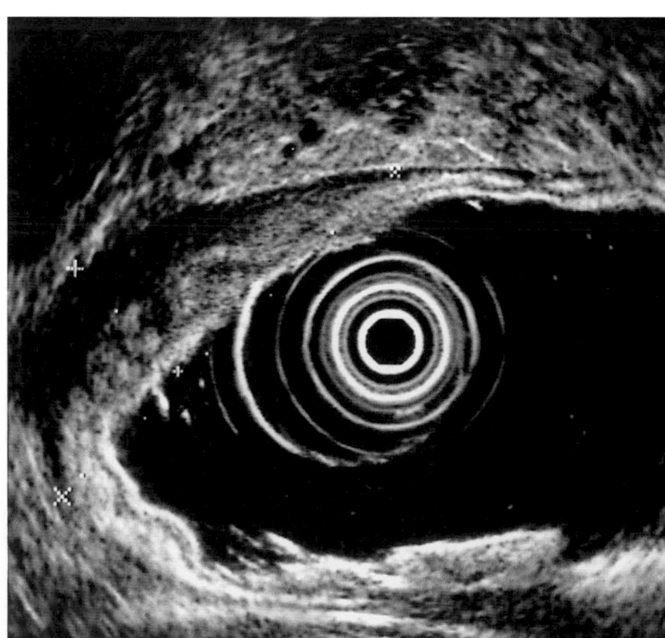

Figure 72.12 MALT lymphoma. Endoscopic ultrasound showing a narrow sheet of low echogenic tissue in the submucosa (arrowed). (Image courtesy of Dr A. McLean, Department of Diagnostic Imaging, St Bartholomew's Hospital, London.)

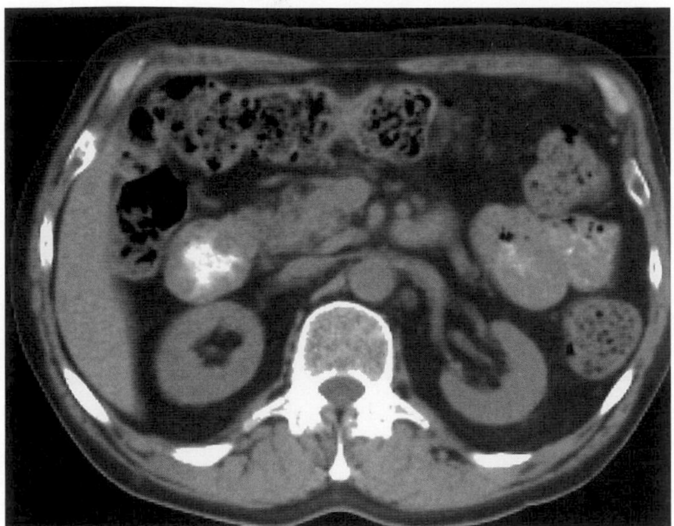

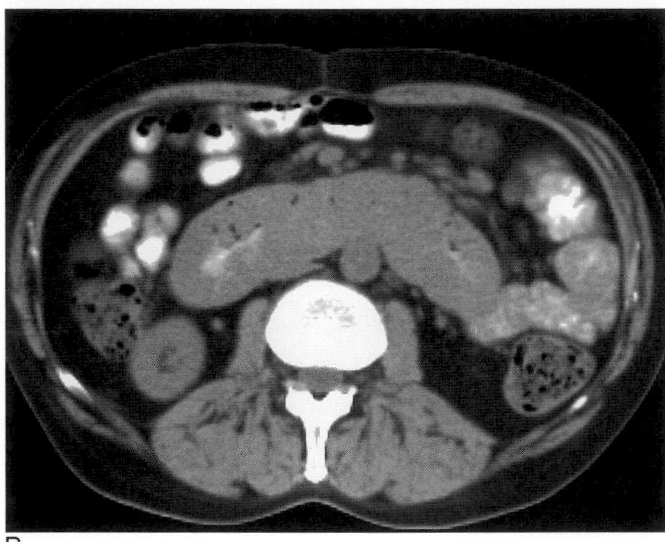

Figure 72.13 Non-Hodgkin's lymphoma involving the duodenum. (A, B) Diffuse concentric gross thickening of the duodenal wall due to lymphomatous infiltration. Note multiple prominent lymph nodes in the mesentery and retroperitoneum.

show multiple polypoid filling defects, with or without central ulceration and irregular thickening of the valvulae.

Enteropathy associated T-cell lymphoma and immunoproliferative small intestinal disease (alpha-chain disease) commonly present with clinical and imaging features of malabsorption, but acute presentations with perforation are common. Often the whole small intestine is affected, especially the duodenum and jejunum. In the small bowel (and colon), MALT lymphoma is manifest as mucosal nodularity, which can be appreciated in barium studies.

Secondary invasion of the small bowel is commonly seen when large mesenteric lymph node masses cause displacement, encasement or compression of the bowel. Peritoneal disease identical to that seen with ovarian carcinoma generally occurs late in advanced disease, though it may be seen at presentation in BL.

Colon and rectum

Primary colonic lymphomas are usually of Burkitt or MALT subtypes, but account for under 0.1% of all colonic neoplasms,

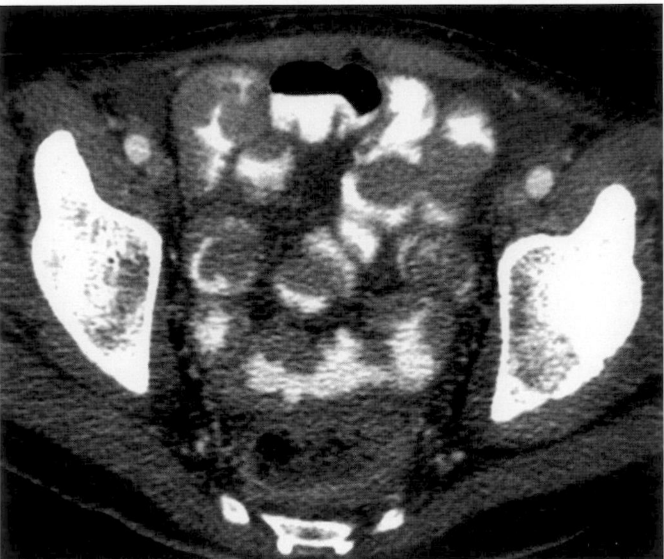

Figure 72.14 Small bowel involvement in lymphoma. CT showing marked nodular thickening of multiple loops of ileum secondary to infiltration by low-density lymphomatous material.

most arising in the caecum and rectum. The most common pattern of the disease is a diffuse or segmental distribution of small nodules 0.2–2.0 cm in diameter, typically with intact mucosa (Fig. 72.15). A less common form of the disease is a solitary polypoid mass, often in the caecum, indistinguishable from carcinoma on imaging unless there is concomitant involvement of the terminal ileum, which is more suggestive of lymphoma.

In advanced disease, there may be marked thickening of the colonic or rectal folds resulting in focal strictures, fissures or ulcerative masses with fistula formation. In the rectosigmoid, lymphomatous strictures are generally longer than carcinomatous strictures and irregular excavation of the mass strongly suggests lymphoma. Involvement of the anorectum is a feature of ARL. Patients usually present with obstruction and rectal bleeding.

Oesophagus

Involvement of the oesophagus is extremely unusual and begins as a submucosal lesion, usually in the distal third of the oesophagus, resulting in smooth luminal narrowing with intact

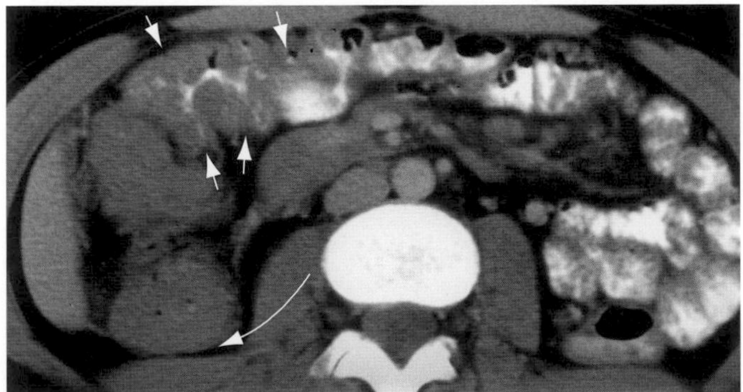

Figure 72.15 Involvement of large bowel in non-Hodgkin's lymphoma. CT showing marked and extensive diffuse, uniform thickening of the wall of the transverse colon (arrow). Mesenteric nodes can also be identified. There is also very marked thickening of the wall of the ascending colon (curved arrow) and caecum.

overlying mucosa. Later, ulceration can develop. Secondary involvement by contiguous spread from adjacent nodal disease is more common but rarely results in dysphagia.

Pancreas

Primary pancreatic lymphoma accounts for only 1.3% of all pancreatic malignancies and 2% of patients with NHL. Intrinsic involvement of the pancreas usually results in a solitary mass lesion, usually in the head of the pancreas, indistinguishable from primary adenocarcinoma on US, CT, or MRI[40]. Biliary or pancreatic ductal obstruction can occur. Calcification and necrosis are rare. Less commonly, diffuse uniform enlargement of the pancreas is seen. As elsewhere, involvement is far more common in NHL than in HD.

Secondary pancreatic involvement is seen in association with disease elsewhere and usually results from direct infiltration from adjacent nodal masses, either focal or massive.

Genitourinary tract

Although the genitourinary tract is not commonly involved at the time of presentation (<5%), more than 50% of patients will have involvement of some part of the genitourinary tract at autopsy. The testicle is the most commonly involved organ, followed by the kidney and the perirenal space; only rarely are the bladder, prostate, uterus, vagina, or ovaries involved. True primary genitourinary lymphoma is rare, as there is normally very little lymphoid tissue within the genitourinary tract.

Kidneys

Despite the sensitivity of CT in detecting lymphomatous renal masses, a discrepancy exists between the frequency of involvement diagnosed antemortem and postmortem, probably explained by the fact that renal involvement is a late phenomenon. Renal involvement is identified in around 3% of patients undergoing staging CT. Detection of renal involvement rarely alters the stage of the disease; close to 90% of cases are in association with high-grade NHL; in more than 40% of patients the disease occurs at the time of recurrence only and renal function is usually normal[41].

On imaging, the commonest disease pattern, seen in 60%, is multiple masses (Fig. 72.16). On ultrasound these masses are hypoechoic with little posterior acoustic enhancement. On CT, the masses may show typical 'density reversal pattern' before and after administration of contrast medium, with the lesion being more dense than the surrounding parenchyma before contrast medium administration and less dense after. A solitary renal mass is seen in only 5–15% of cases and may be indistinguishable from renal cell carcinoma (Fig. 72.17)[41,42]. An important feature of renal masses occurring in NHL is that in over 50% of cases there is no evidence of retroperitoneal lymph node enlargement detectable on CT.

Direct infiltration of the kidney by contiguous retroperitoneal nodal masses is the second most common type of renal involvement, accounting for about 25% of cases. There is often associated encasement of the renal vessels and extension into the renal hilum and sinus. Radiologically the appearance can closely resemble transitional cell carcinoma of the renal pelvis. In a further 10%, soft-tissue mass(es) are seen in the perirenal

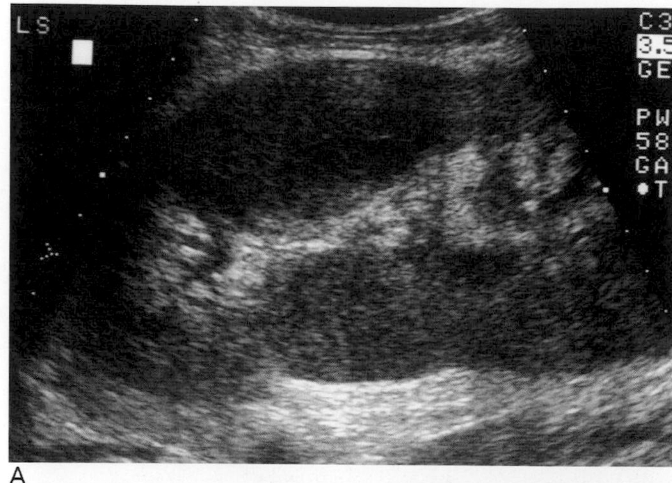

A

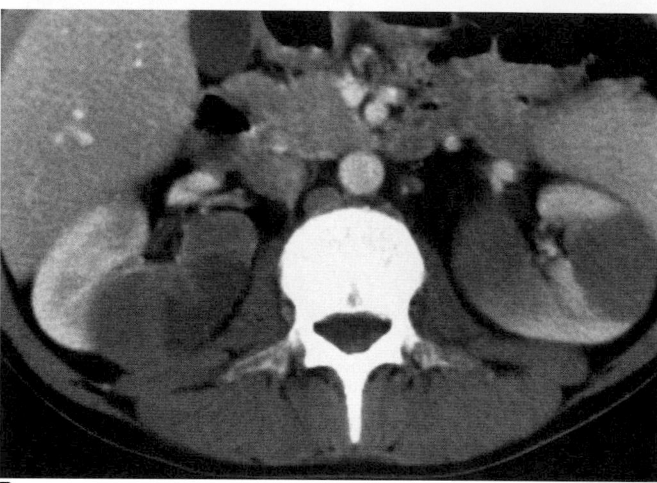

B

Figure 72.16 Multiple lymphomatous renal masses. (A) Longitudinal ultrasound of the left kidney showing multiple hypoechoic masses. (B) CT in the same patient showing multiple masses, well defined from the normally enhancing adjacent renal parenchyma. Note the absence of retroperitoneal lymph node enlargement.

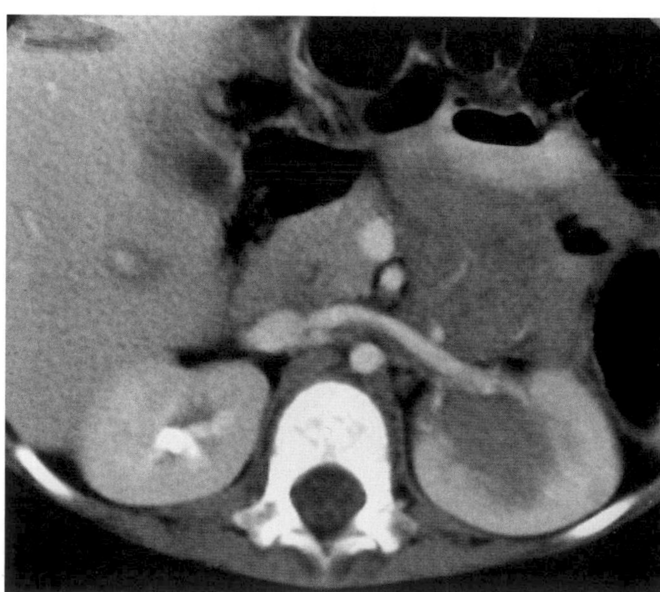

Figure 72.17 Renal lymphomatous mass. A left renal mass is seen within the renal pelvis on contrast-enhanced CT in a patient with non-Hodgkin's lymphoma. The inferior aspect of a large pancreatic mass is also seen, extending anteriorly from the left renal vein.

space, occasionally encasing the kidney without any evidence of invasion of the parenchyma (Fig. 72.18).

Diffuse intrinsic infiltration of the kidney resulting in global enlargement is the least common manifestation of renal lymphomatous involvement. On ultrasound, the kidneys are diffusely enlarged and uniformly hypoechoic. On CT, the appearance following intravenous injection of contrast medium is variable, but usually the normal parenchymal enhancement is replaced by homogeneous nonenhancing tissue.

Bladder

The urinary bladder is a rare site of primary extranodal involvement, accounting for less than 1% of all bladder tumours[43]. It occurs more frequently in women in the sixth decade, often with a history of recurrent cystitis. Small cell and MALT types are seen, both characteristically producing large multilobular submucosal masses with minimal or no mucosal ulceration. Transmural spread into adjacent pelvic organs can occur, well demonstrated on cross-sectional imaging (Fig. 72.19). The prognosis is generally good.

Secondary lymphoma of the bladder is found in 10–15% of patients with lymphoma at autopsy. It is manifest either as intrinsic bladder disease or as contiguous spread from adjacent involved nodes. Microscopic involvement is far more common than gross infiltration, but both can be associated with haematuria. On CT the appearances are usually nonspecific and indistinguishable from transitional cell carcinoma, producing either diffuse widespread thickening of the bladder wall or a large nodular mass.

Prostate

Primary prostatic lymphoma is also extremely rare, but in contradistinction to primary bladder NHL it carries a very poor prognosis. It is generally intermediate to high grade and produces irritative obstructive symptoms. Histological examination usually shows diffuse infiltration with spread into the peri-prostatic tissues. Solitary nodules are uncommon. More frequently, prostatic involvement is secondary to spread from the adjacent nodes in the setting of advanced disease.

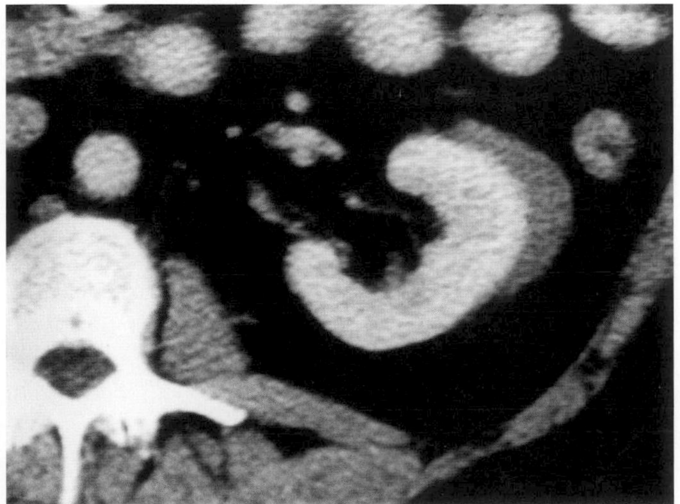

Figure 72.18 Perirenal lymphoma. Postcontrast CT showing a mass in the perirenal space.

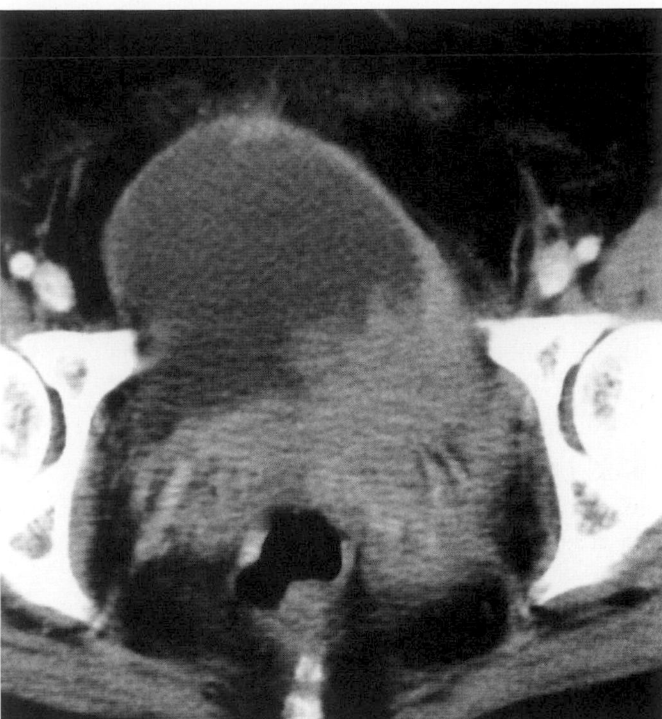

Figure 72.19 Bladder lymphoma. Contrast-enhanced CT of the pelvis in a female patient showing an irregular soft-tissue mass of lymphomatous tissue infiltrating the lumen at the base of the bladder and resulting in asymmetrical thickening of the left bladder wall.

Testis

Testicular lymphoma accounts for about 5% of primary testicular tumours overall and 25–50% of those in patients over 50 years; it is the commonest primary tumour over the age of 60 years. It is vanishingly rare in HD but is seen at presentation in approximately 1% of all patients of NHL, usually with DLBCL or BL. There is an association with lymphoma of Waldeyer's ring, the skin and central nervous system. Patients usually present with a painless testicular swelling and in up to 25% of cases the involvement is bilateral. Relapse can occur in the contralateral testis.

Ultrasonically, the lesions usually have a nonspecific appearance, with focal areas of decreased echogenicity, or a more diffuse decrease in reflectivity of the testicle (without any focal abnormality). At present, MRI does not appear to have advantage over ultrasound in the detection of testicular involvement[44].

Because of the association with disease elsewhere, staging must always include ultrasonic evaluation of the contralateral testis and whole body CT. Cranial CT or MRI and CSF examination should also be considered.

Female genital tract

Isolated lymphomatous involvement of the female genital organs is rare, accounting for approximately 1% of extranodal NHL. Nearly 75% of women affected are postmenopausal and present with vaginal bleeding. It affects the cervix more frequently than the uterus and vagina. Involvement of these gynaecological organs is best demonstrated by MRI, where primary lymphoma of the cervix and/or vagina is characterized by a large soft-tissue mass with high signal intensity on

T2-weighting and clearly distinguished from the surrounding normal tissues (Fig. 72.20)[45]. Involvement of the uterine body usually produces diffuse enlargement, often with a lobular contour similar to a fibroid. Characteristically the mucosa and underlying junctional zone are intact. Primary uterine lymphoma has a good prognosis and MRI can demonstrate complete resolution.

Primary ovarian lymphoma, by contrast, has a very poor prognosis as it often presents late and disease is frequently bilateral. It is less common than uterine lymphoma. The usual pathological subtypes are DLBCL or BL. Imaging appearances are identical to those of ovarian carcinoma, although haemorrhage, necrosis and calcification are relatively rare.

Adrenal glands

Primary adrenal lymphoma is extremely rare, usually occurring in men over the age of 60.

Secondary involvement of the adrenals is detected in about 6% of patients undergoing routine abdominal staging CT, usually in the presence of widespread retroperitoneal disease. Adrenal insufficiency is most unusual, even with bilateral disease. The appearance on cross-sectional imaging is indistinguishable from that of metastases (Fig. 72.21). Bilateral adrenal hyperplasia in the absence of metastatic involvement has also been described[46].

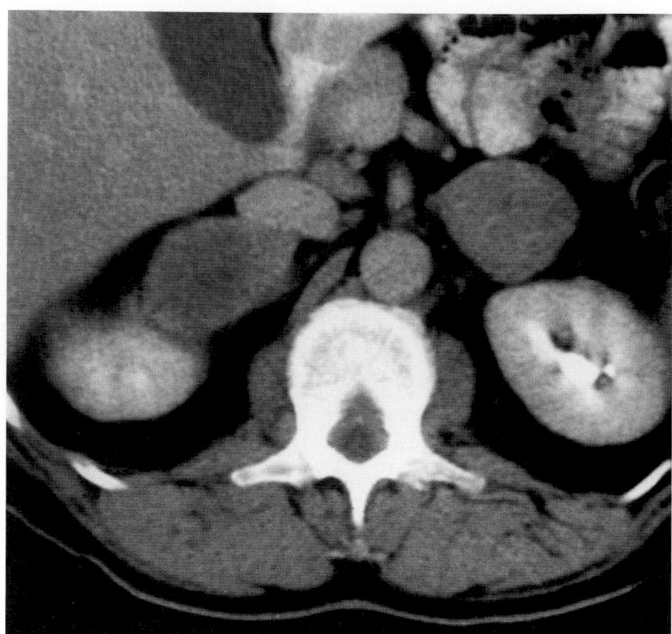

Figure 72.21 Adrenal lymphoma. Contrast-enhanced CT showing bilateral large inhomogeneous soft-tissue masses. No other evidence of disease could be detected elsewhere and a core biopsy showed the presence of non-Hodgkin's lymphoma.

Musculoskeletal system

Involvement of the bone, bone marrow and skeletal muscles can occur in both HD and NHL. Bone and bone marrow are particularly important sites of disease relapse and any skeletal symptoms following previous treatment for lymphoma should always raise the suspicion of bone disease. It should be borne in mind that involvement of osseous bone does not necessarily imply bone marrow involvement (unless it is particularly widespread); skeletal radiography has no predictive value in determining marrow involvement.

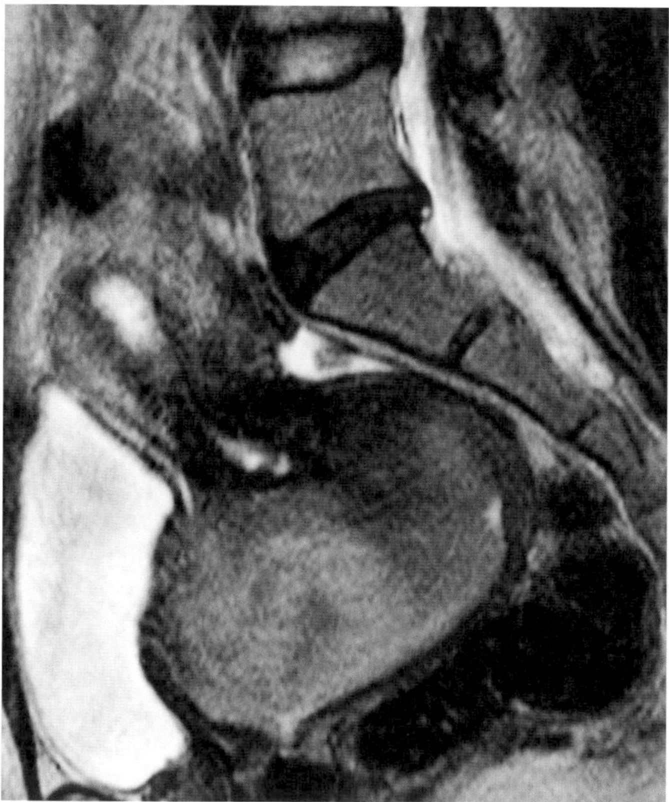

Figure 72.20 Lymphoma of the cervix. Sagittal T2-weighted MRI showing a large mass of intermediate to high signal intensity. The mass is substantially larger than is usually seen in a squamous carcinoma of the cervix. Biopsy showed an aggressive B-cell lymphoma.

Bone marrow

Since the bone marrow is an integral part of the reticuloendothelial system, lymphoma may arise within the marrow as true primary disease. It is then categorized as stage IE disease. More often, however, the marrow is involved as part of a disseminated process, when it is categorized as stage IV disease.

In NHL, marrow involvement is present in 20–40% of patients at presentation and is associated with a poorer prognosis than liver or lung involvement. Bone marrow biopsy is therefore included in the staging of NHL. Such routine staging bone marrow biopsy increases the stage in up to 30% of cases, usually from stage III to stage IV[47]. In low-grade NHL, involvement tends to be diffuse, whereas in high-grade NHL the marrow is more likely to be affected focally; hence the increased incidence of marrow positivity with bilateral iliac crest biopsies in this situation. In HD, marrow involvement at presentation is rare but will develop during the course of the disease in 5–15% of patients. Bone marrow biopsy, therefore, is not considered necessary as part of the initial staging of patients with clinical early stage HD.

Magnetic resonance imaging is extremely sensitive in detecting bone marrow involvement, with involved areas having low signal intensity on T1-weighted images and high signal on STIR sequences[48,49]. It can upstage as many as 30% of patients with negative iliac crest biopsies. A positive MRI study appears to confer a poorer prognosis regardless of bone marrow biopsy status. However, given the obvious need to examine the cytology of bone marrow, the precise role of MRI in the initial staging of patients with lymphoma is unclear.

FDG-PET is also very sensitive for bone marrow involvement at presentation, upstaging a similar proportion of patients as MRI when compared to bone marrow biopsy. Occasional false negative studies occur with both techniques, especially with microscopic infiltration (under 5%) and low-grade lymphoma. Both modalities can be used to monitor the effects of treatment, especially where other imaging modalities have failed to demonstrate the disease. A particular problem after treatment is the presence of myeloid hyperplasia, which can produce false positive studies, especially if granulocyte colony-stimulating factor has been administered.

Bone

True primary lymphoma of bone is nearly all NHL and accounts for almost 1% of all NHL. The criteria for the diagnosis of primary lymphoma of bone require that:

- only a single bone is involved
- there is unequivocal histological evidence of lymphoma
- other disease is limited to regional areas at the time of presentation
- the primary tumour precedes metastases by at least 6 months.

The diagnosis of true primary bone lymphoma is made less often than in the past, probably because better imaging has allowed detection of synchronous disease elsewhere, indicating that the apparent 'primary' osseous involvement is in fact secondary. This is particularly the case in children. Infiltration of bone can also occur secondarily by direct invasion from adjacent soft-tissue masses. The average age at presentation is 24 years; 50% of cases occur in patients between 10 and 30 years old; it affects males more frequently than females; and usually occurs in the appendicular skeleton, involving the femur, tibia and humerus in descending order of frequency.

Radiographic evidence of secondary bone involvement is present during the course of the disease in 20% of patients with HD, appearing in 4% at initial presentation. Secondary involvement of bone is present in 5–6% of patients with NHL, although it is more frequent in children with NHL[24]. The axial skeleton is much more commonly affected than the appendicular skeleton.

Whether primary or secondary, bone lesions in NHL are permeative and osteolytic in just under 80% of cases, sclerotic in only 4% and mixed in 16% (Fig. 72.22)[50]. By comparison, HD typically gives sclerotic or mixed sclerotic and lytic lesions (86%) and is far less frequently lytic (14% of cases). In HD, most lesions are found in the skull, the spine and the femora. The classic finding is the sclerotic 'ivory' vertebra. Nevertheless, radiographically, primary and secondary NHL, HD and other bone tumours (such as Ewing's sarcoma and other small round cell tumours) may be indistinguishable.

Soft-tissue disease typically may involve adjacent bones; anterior mediastinal and paravertebral masses not infrequently involve the sternum and vertebrae, respectively, resulting in scalloping or destruction.

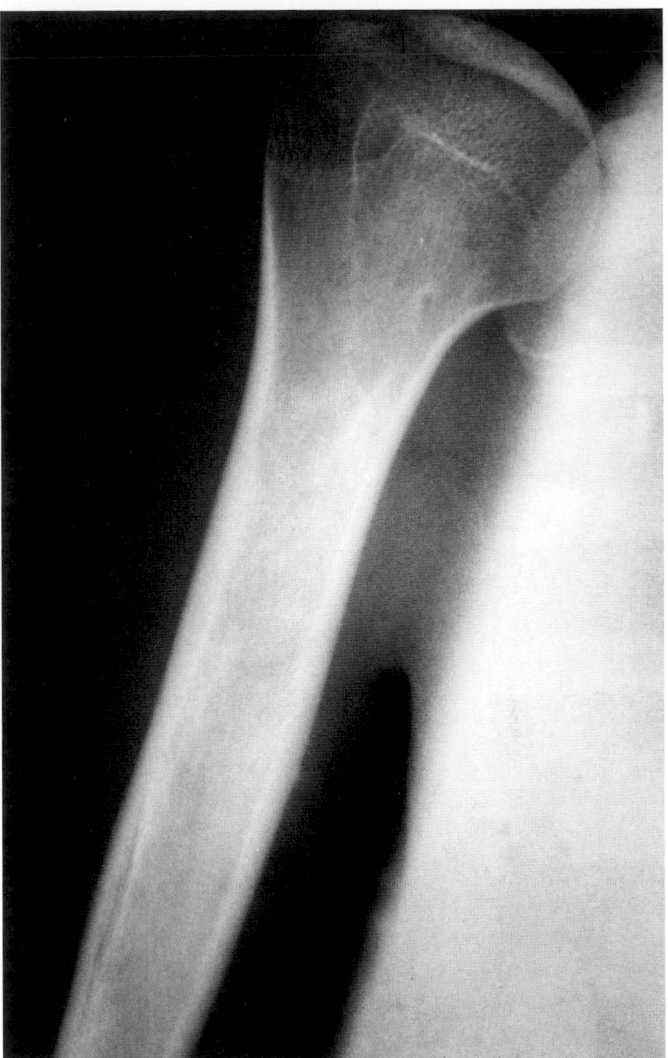

Figure 72.22 Primary non-Hodgkin's lymphoma of bone. Plain radiograph of the humerus of a 14-year-old child showing a poorly defined sclerotic lesion in the proximal humerus. Further investigation revealed no other sites of lymphomatous disease.

Screening for bone involvement at the time of presentation is not routine but is reserved for patients with specific complaints. Radionuclide radiology has a sensitivity of close to 95% in the detection of bone involvement, far greater than plain radiography. MRI depicts the disease in much more detail, often demonstrating a greater extent of associated extraosseous involvement and degree of marrow infiltration and is the method of choice in local staging of primary bone lymphoma[51]. It is also of value in the assessment of response to treatment. FDG-PET is yet more accurate than radionuclide radiology and has a high positive predictive value in the detection of osseous involvement (Fig. 72.23).

Central nervous system

Primary

Primary CNS lymphoma (PCNSL) is restricted to the craniospinal axis, with no evidence of systemic disease and is nearly always intracranial. It is increasing in incidence, accounting for over 3% of all primary brain tumours and up to nearly 30% of cases of NHL in some series. This is in part due to an

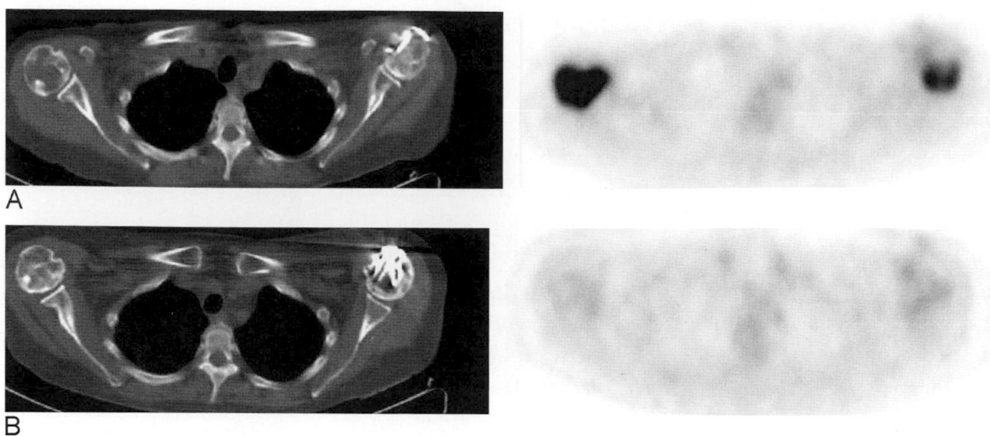

Figure 72.23 Non-Hodgkin's lymphoma of bone. (A) Axial CT on bone settings at the level of the humeri with corresponding axial PET image. Lymphomatous deposits in both humeral heads are intensely metabolically active. Note pathological fracture on the right. (B) After successful treatment, there has been complete metabolic resolution. (By kind permission of Dr Gary Cook, Department of Radiology, The Royal Marsden Hospital, London.)

association with immunosuppressive therapy after cardiac and renal transplant and with immunodeficiency states, as up to 6% of patients with AIDS can be expected to develop PCNSL during the course of the disease. It can occur at any age but peaks between the ages of 40 and 60 years. A second, smaller peak occurs in the first decade of life. Presentation is that of an intracranial space-occupying lesion or personality changes, as the lesions are often frontal. Fits are rare.

More than 50% of tumours occur within the cerebral white matter, close to or within the corpus callosum[52]. Most touch the ependymal lining of the ventricles or the leptomeningeal surfaces. A butterfly distribution with spread across the corpus callosum is a typical finding. In about 15% of cases, the lesions affect the deep grey matter of the thalamus and basal ganglia and only about 10% arise in the posterior fossa, usually near the midline. In about 15% of cases the disease is multifocal.

The tumour mass is typically isodense or of increased density on unenhanced CT and in 90% of cases it enhances homogeneously. Calcification virtually never occurs and there is relatively little surrounding vasogenic oedema or mass effect[53]. On MRI, the masses are typically isointense on T1- and T2-weighted sequences. As at CT, there is homogeneous enhancement after the administration of gadolinium-DTPA (Fig. 72.24), though atypical forms with rim enhancement can occur with AIDS-related PCNSL.

Secondary

Secondary CNS involvement occurs during the course of lymphoma in 15% of patients with NHL. Certain groups are known to be at risk: those with stage IV disease, testicular or ovarian presentation; those with high-grade histology (lymphoblastic and immunoblastic histologies) and also BL. Secondary CNS involvement is so rare in HD that a space-occupying lesion in the brain of a patient with known HD should prompt consideration of a second diagnosis. Although intra-axial masses do occur, with imaging features similar to primary lymphoma, secondary involvement has a much greater tendency to involve the extracerebral spaces (epidural, subdural and subarachnoid) and the spinal epidural and subarachnoid spaces.[53] In the basal meninges, such encasement results in presentation with cranial nerve palsies. MRI with intravenous injection of gadolinium-DTPA is superior to CT in the detection of such subdural and leptomeningeal disease, which is seen as enhancing plaques over the cerebral convexities and around the basal meninges[54].

Contrast-enhanced MRI can also demonstrate spinal leptomeningeal disease (Fig. 72.25), but there is a significant false negative rate, higher than that for leptomeningeal carcinomatosis[55].

Disease in the spinal epidural space can cause spinal cord compression and cauda equina syndromes. This is a late manifestation of HD, but can be the presenting feature of NHL (Fig. 72.26). Epidural extension of tumour into the spinal canal from a paravertebral mass is the commonest cause, resulting in a so-called 'dumb-bell' tumour. The dura itself usually acts as an effective barrier to the intrathecal spread of tumour and on occasion the disease is limited to the neural foramen. A small number of patients with high-grade NHL have vertebral involvement that results in epidural spread and extrinsic compression of the theca.

Though all these patterns of epidural spread can occasionally be depicted at CT, subtle disease is readily missed unless actively sought and is much better demonstrated by MRI.

Orbit

Primary orbital lymphomas occur most commonly in patients between 40 and 70 years of age and typically present as a slow-growing, diffusely infiltrative tumour for which the main differential diagnosis is from the nonmalignant condition, orbital pseudotumour. It is almost always due to NHL and is the most common primary orbital malignancy in adults, accounting for 10–15% of orbital masses[53] and 4% of all primary extranodal NHL. Secondary orbital involvement occurs in approximately 3.5–5.0% of both HD and NHL. In both the primary and secondary forms, the clinical manifestations will depend on the site of involvement. Retrobulbar lymphoma infiltrates around and through the extraocular muscles, causing proptosis and ophthalmoplegia, but rarely disturbing visual acuity. The conjunctiva, lacrimal glands and eyelids can all be involved. Lacrimal gland involvement displaces the globe downwards and is often bilateral. Bilaterality does not appear to alter prognosis, which is generally good in all the primary forms. In patients with an orbital lymphomatous mass, about half will be found to have an extracentral nervous system primary site of origin. CT and MRI can both demonstrate the

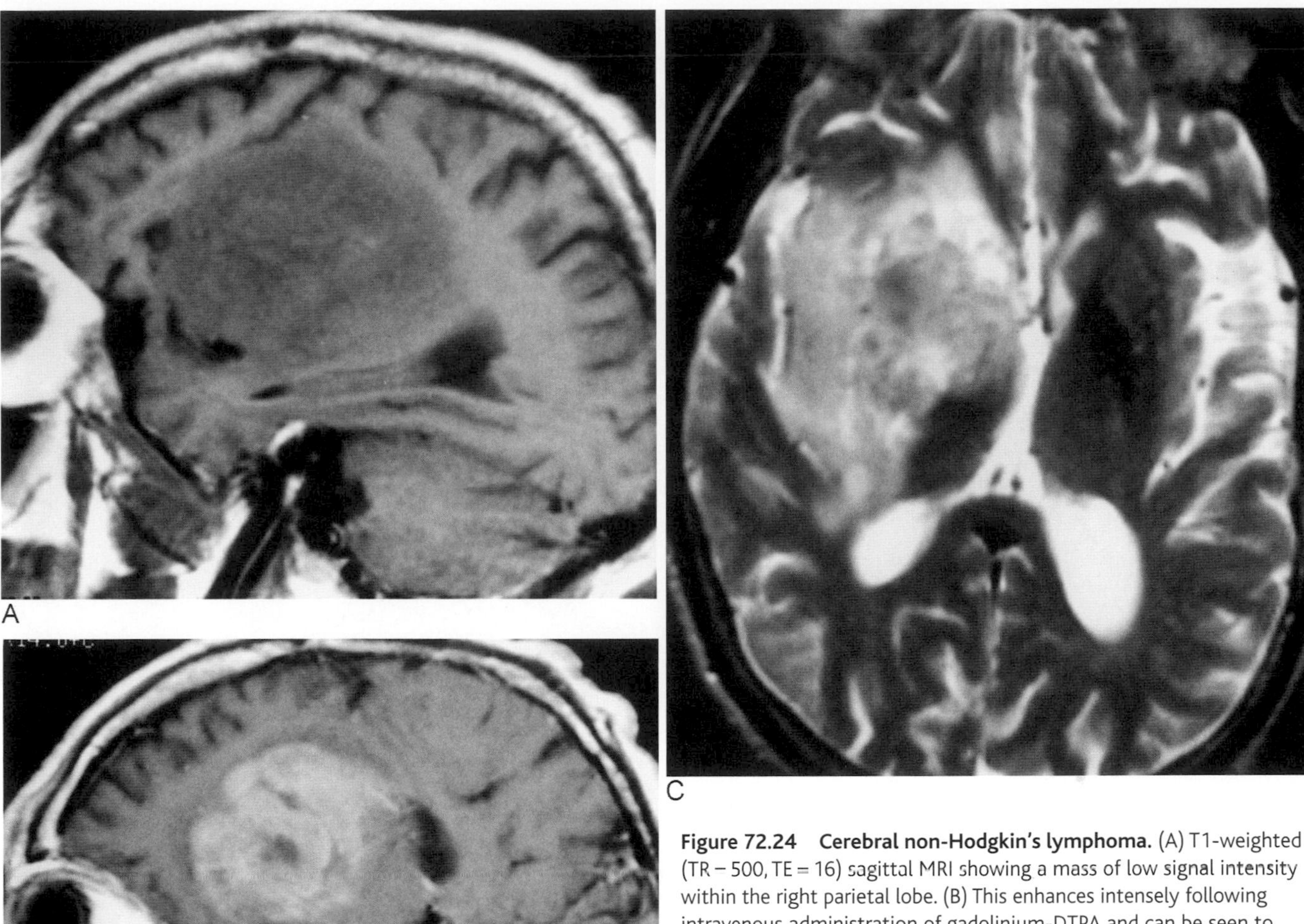

Figure 72.24 Cerebral non-Hodgkin's lymphoma. (A) T1-weighted (TR – 500, TE = 16) sagittal MRI showing a mass of low signal intensity within the right parietal lobe. (B) This enhances intensely following intravenous administration of gadolinium-DTPA and can be seen to be causing marked mass effect with compression of the right lateral ventricle on (C), an axial T2-weighted (TR = 3800, TE = 95) image.

site of a mass, but the latter is best for the assessment of the presence, if any, of intracranial extension (Fig. 72.27).

Head and neck lymphoma

Although HD typically involves the cervical lymph nodes as the presenting feature, true extranodal involvement of sites in the head and neck region is rare. By comparison, in NHL, 10% of patients present with extranodal head and neck involvement. About half of these will prove to have disseminated lymphoma. Extranodal NHL accounts for approximately 5% of head and neck cancers.

Waldeyer's ring

Waldeyer's ring is the commonest site of head and neck lymphoma and there is a close link with involvement of the gastrointestinal tract, which may be synchronous or metachronous. This is probably a reflection of the fact that many are of the MALT type. Hence some centres include abdominal CT and/or endoscopy as part of staging, since up to 30% of patients will have advanced disease at presentation. Waldeyer's ring comprises lymphoid tissue in the nasopharynx, oropharynx, the faucial and palatine tonsil and the lingual tonsil. A diagnosis of NHL is suggested by circumferential involvement or multifocality. Secondary invasion from adjacent nodal masses is also a common occurrence.

NHL comprises 8% of tumours of the paranasal sinuses. In the West, the disease affects middle-aged men and the maxillary sinus is most commonly involved, whereas the aggressive diffuse T-cell type (that forms part of the 'lethal midline granuloma' syndrome) typically affects younger Asians. Whilst paranasal sinus involvement often presents with acute facial swelling and pain and disease often spreads from one sinus to the other in a contiguous fashion, bony destruction is considerably less marked than in squamous cell carcinomas.

MRI is the preferred imaging technique for evaluating head and neck lymphoma due to high tissue contrast between tumour adjacent to normal structures. Its multiplanar capability

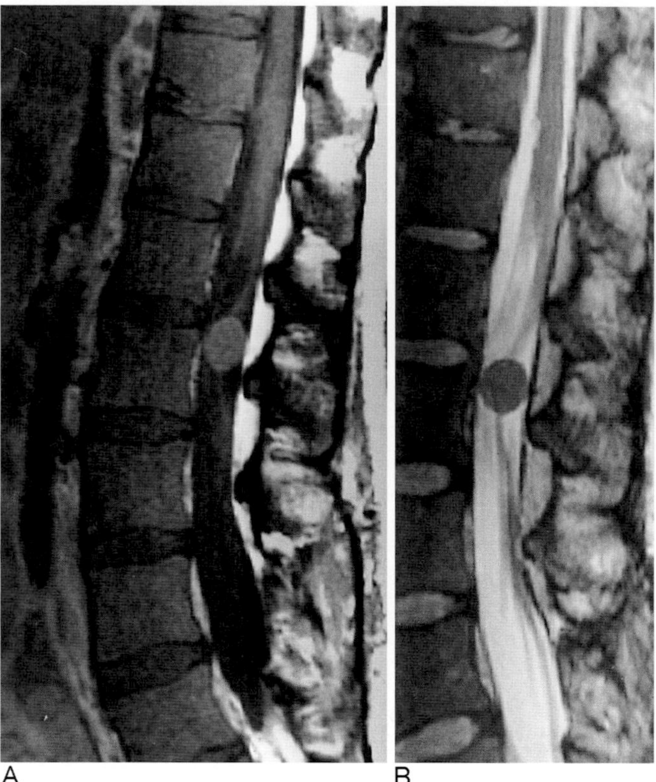

Figure 72.25 Meningeal deposits in lymphoma. (A) Sagittal T1-weighted MRI (TR = 500, TE = 14) showing a well-defined lesion within the dura due to a lymphomatous deposit within the meninges. (B) The lesion is also clearly seen on a fast spin-echo T2-weighted image (TR = 6000, TE = 95/Ef).

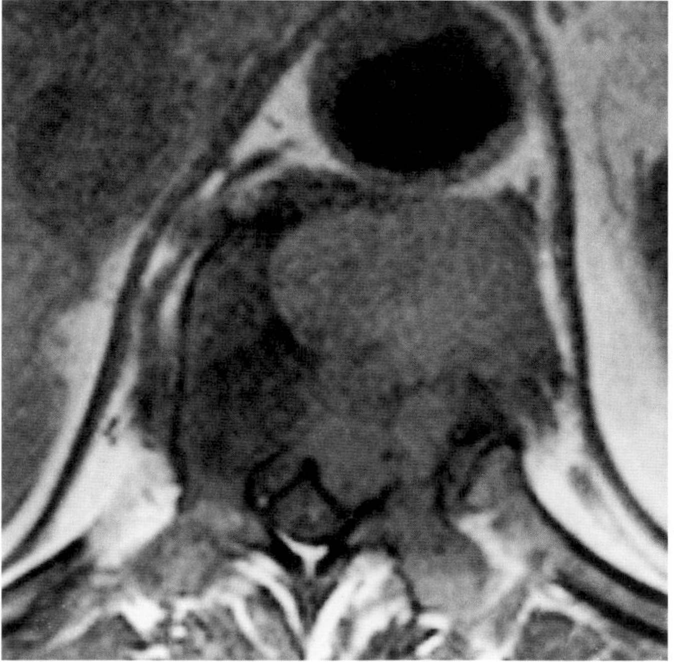

Figure 72.26 Lymphomatous infiltration of the spinal canal. T1-weighted (TR = 800, TE = 12) MRI showing a mass of intermediate to high signal intensity in the paravertebral soft tissues, extending into the vertebral body and into the spinal canal. The mass is displacing the theca.

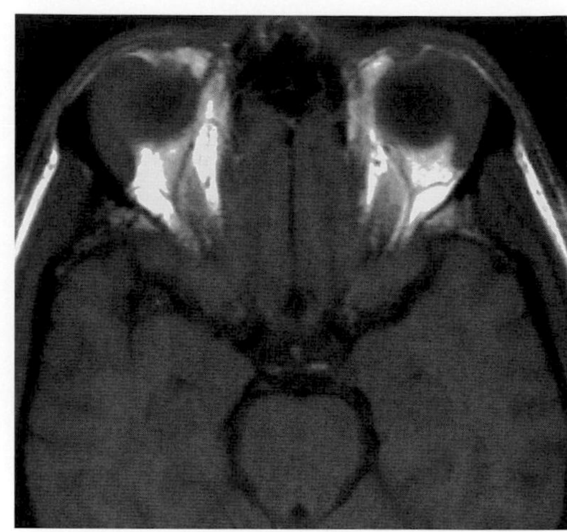

Figure 72.27 Bilateral orbital lymphoma. T1-weighted MRI in the axial plane demonstrating bilateral orbital masses arising in the region of the lacrimal glands.

allows clear demonstration of the full extent of disease and permits detection of tumour spread into the cranial cavity from the infratemporal fossa and orbit.

Salivary glands

All the salivary glands may be involved in lymphoma but the parotid gland is most frequently affected. Single or multiple well-defined masses are seen, which are of higher density than the surrounding gland on CT, hypoechoic on ultrasound and of intermediate signal intensity on T1- and T2-weighted MRI sequences. Many of the patients are middle-aged women and a history of Sjögren's disease is common.

Thyroid

Non-Hodgkin's lymphoma accounts for 2% of malignant tumours of the thyroid. MALT type lymphomas arise in women in association with Hashimoto's disease. However, DLBCL also occurs, such patients presenting with a rapidly growing mass and obstructive symptoms. Direct spread of tumour beyond the gland and involvement of adjacent lymph nodes is common. At ultrasound these masses are relatively hypoechoic and at CT they usually have a lower attenuation than the normal gland and may show peripheral enhancement following injection of intravenous contrast medium.

MUCOSA ASSOCIATED LYMPHOID TISSUE (MALT) LYMPHOMAS

The MALT lymphomas arise from mucosal sites that normally have no organized lymphoid tissue, but within which acquired lymphoid tissue has arisen as a result of chronic inflammation or autoimmunity. Examples include Hashimoto's thyroiditis, Sjögren's syndrome and *Helicobacter*-induced chronic follicular gastritis. Patients with Sjögren's syndrome (lymphoepithelial sialadenitis) are at 44 times the risk of developing lymphoma, of which over 80% are MALT type and patients with Hashimoto's thyroiditis have a 70-fold increased risk of thyroid lymphoma.

The histological hallmark of MALT lymphoma is the presence of lymphomatous cells in a marginal zone around reactive follicles, which can spread into the epithelium of glandular tissues to produce the characteristic lymphoepithelial lesion. In up to 30%, transformation to large cell lymphoma occurs.

Adults with a median age of 60 are most often affected, with a slight female preponderance. Most patients present with stage IE or IIE disease, which tends to be indolent. Bone marrow involvement is seen in only 20%, but the frequency varies depending on the primary site. Multiple extranodal sites are involved in up to 10%, but this does not appear to have the same poor prognostic import as in other forms of NHL. Nonetheless, extensive staging investigations may be necessary[56].

The commonest site of involvement is the gastrointestinal (GI) tract (50%) and within the GI tract, the stomach is most often affected (around 85% of cases). The small bowel and colon are involved in immunoproliferative small intestinal disease (IPSID), previously known as *alpha-chain disease*. Other sites commonly affected include the lung, head, neck, ocular adnexae, skin, thyroid and breast. In the thyroid, MALT lymphomas can present as diffuse enlargement or as large nodules. MALT lymphomas of the lacrimal glands present as a mass or periorbital swelling. CT and MRI depict uni- or bilateral enhancing masses with a nonspecific appearance. Up to 20% of lymphomas involving Waldeyer's ring are of MALT type. The tonsils are most commonly affected, the commonest pattern being asymmetrical thickening of the pharyngeal mucosa. This is well shown by CT and MRI.

BURKITT LYMPHOMA (BL)

Burkitt lymphoma is a highly aggressive B-cell variant of NHL, associated with Epstein–Barr virus (EBV) in a variable proportion of cases.

Three clinical variants are recognized:

- endemic (African) type
- sporadic (nonendemic)
- immunodeficiency associated.

Though these tumours are extremely aggressive and rapidly growing, they are potentially curable. They account for only 2–3% of NHL in immunocompetent adults, but 30–50% of all childhood lymphoma is BL. Immunodeficiency associated BL is seen chiefly in association with HIV infection and may be the initial manifestation of AIDS. EBV is identified in up to 40% of cases. Extranodal disease is common and all three variants are at risk for CNS disease.

In the endemic form, the jaws and orbit are involved in 50% of cases, producing the 'floating tooth sign' on plain radiography. The ovaries, kidneys and breast may be involved. The sporadic forms have a predilection for the ileocaecal region and patients can present with acute abdominal emergencies such as intussusception. Again, ovaries, kidneys and breasts are commonly involved. Retroperitoneal and paraspinal disease can cause paraplegia, the presenting feature in up to 15%. Thoracic disease is rare; in a recent series, 50% had disease confined to the abdomen[57]. Leptomeningeal disease can be seen at presentation and is a site of relapse.

LYMPHOMA IN THE IMMUNOCOMPROMISED

The WHO classification recognizes four broad groupings associated with an increased incidence of lymphoma and lymphoproliferative disorders[3]:

- primary immunodeficiency syndromes
- infection with the human immunodeficiency virus (HIV)
- iatrogenic immunosuppression after solid organ or bone marrow allografts
- iatrogenic immunosuppression from methotrexate (usually for autoimmune disorders).

The development of lymphoma in these settings is multifactorial, but mostly related to defective immune surveillance, with or without chronic antigenic stimulation.

Lymphomas associated with HIV

Lymphoma is the first AIDS-defining illness in up to 5% of HIV patients. The incidence of all subtypes of NHL is increased 60–200 fold. Various types are seen, including those seen in immunocompetent patients, such as BL and DLBCL, but some occur much more frequently in the HIV population (e.g. primary effusion lymphoma and plasmablastic lymphoma of the oral cavity). The incidence of HD is also increased up to eightfold. DLBCL tends to occur later, when CD4 counts are under $100 \times 10^{6-} L^{-1}$, whereas BL occurs in less immunodeficient patients. EBV positivity occurs in up to 70%; PCNSL is associated with EBV in over 90% of cases and EBV positivity is seen in nearly all cases of HD associated with HIV.

Most tumours are aggressive, with advanced stage, bulky disease and a high serum LDH at presentation. Most have a marked propensity to involve extranodal sites, especially the GI tract, CNS (less frequent with the advent of highly active antiretroviral therapy), liver and bone marrow. Multiple sites of extranodal involvement are seen in over 75% of cases[58]. Peripheral lymph node enlargement is relatively uncommon.

In the chest, NHL is usually extranodal; pleural effusions and lung disease are common, with nodules, acinar and interstitial opacity being described. Hilar and mediastinal nodal enlargement is generally mild. There is a wide differential diagnosis and in one study the presence of cavitation, small nodules under 1 cm in diameter and nodal necrosis predicted for mycobacterial infection rather than lymphoma.

Within the abdomen, the GI tract, liver, kidneys, adrenal glands and lower genitourinary tract are commonly involved. Mesenteric and retroperitoneal nodal enlargement is less common than in immunocompetent patients, but there are no real differences in the CT features of patients with or without AIDS.

Regarding PCNSL, certain features such as rim enhancement and multifocality are seen more often than in the immunocompetent population. This can cause confusion with cerebral toxoplasmosis, though the location of PCNSL in the deep white matter is suggestive. Quantitative FDG-PET uptake can help in the differentiation of these conditions.

Post-transplant lymphoproliferative disorders (PTLD)

These occur in 2–4% of solid organ transplant recipients, depending on the type of transplant, the lowest frequency being seen in renal transplant recipients (1%) and the highest in heart–lung or liver–bowel allografts (5%). Marrow allograft recipients in general have a low risk (1%). Most are associated with EBV infection and appear to represent EBV-induced monoclonal or, more rarely, polyclonal B-cell or T-cell proliferation as a consequence of immune suppression[3]. The clinical features are variable, correlating with the type of allograft and type of immunosuppression. PTLD develops earlier in patients receiving cyclosporine rather than azathioprine (mean interval 48 months). EBV positive cases occur earlier than EBV negative cases, the latter occurring 4–5 years after transplantation. In all cases, extranodal disease is disproportionately commoner. In patients receiving azathioprine, the allograft itself and the CNS are often involved, whereas in patients who have received cyclosporine, the GI tract is affected more than the CNS. The bone marrow, liver and lung are often affected, with multiple intrapulmonary masses, pleural effusions, involvement of multiple segments of bowel and the transplanted organ all being reported[59].

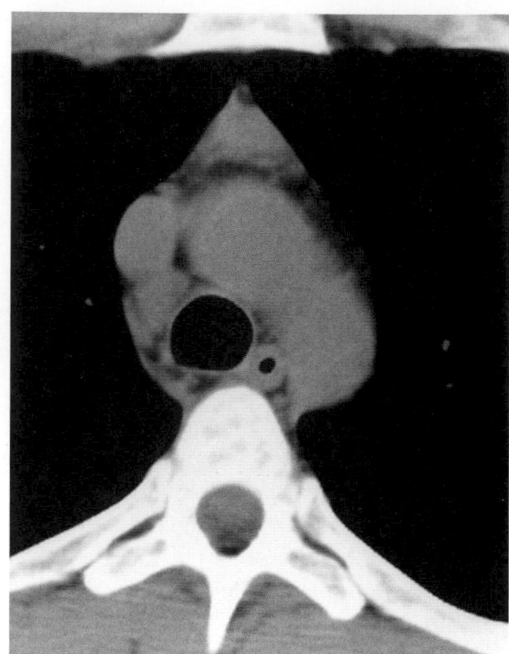

Figure 72.28 Thoracic residual mass in a patient with Hodgkin's disease. After treatment, follow-up CT at 6 months shows a residual right paratracheal mass. Surveillance CTs done several years later have demonstrated the stability of this small mass, consistent with inactive residual disease.

MONITORING RESPONSE TO THERAPY

Achievement of complete response after treatment is the most important factor for predicting prolonged survival in both HD and NHL. Imaging plays a critical role in monitoring response to treatment and in assessing the degree of response. The chest radiograph is useful in assessing response when there is intrathoracic disease; it is repeated at each monthly visit. Although the chest radiograph will show a response early in the treatment course, changes due to radiotherapy, thymic cyst formation or rebound thymic hyperplasia often make the mediastinum difficult to assess on a chest radiograph, particularly in children. Therefore, response cannot be monitored reliably and CT is necessary for the evaluation of response (Fig. 72.28). In patients with intra-abdominal disease, serial CT is of course essential (Fig. 72.29). Assessment of response requires the measurement of a number of marker lesions before, during and after therapy, especially in the setting of clinical trials and here the reproducibility and reliability of MDCT is a great advantage. Nonetheless, there is significant interobserver variation in the measurement of masses and, wherever possible, well-defined regular masses above and below the diaphragm should be assessed[60].

The optimal timing of such reassessment has not been widely investigated. In many centres the practice is to assess patients fully 1 month after completion of therapy. Others favour an interim CT study after two cycles of chemotherapy, especially for patients enrolled in clinical trials. The timing will often depend on local clinical practice and on the availability of resources. The speed of modern CT systems has largely removed the need for limited studies advocated in the past. Contrast medium is routinely administered in most centres, since without it assessment of extranodal and visceral disease is difficult.

Response criteria

Standardized response criteria are essential for clinical research and comparison of different therapies and these now exist for both HD and NHL. In HD, a complete response is designated when there is no clinical or radiological evidence of disease after treatment. A separate category of complete remission—unconfirmed/uncertain—exists for cases in which there is no clinical evidence of disease, but there is a radiological abnormality that is not consistent with previous therapy. Residual masses should be investigated with imaging and highly suspicious lesions may require biopsy. Criteria for response in NHL are similar[61]. Here, complete remission requires:

- Complete disappearance of all detectable clinical and radiological evidence of disease.
- All nodal masses to have decreased to normal (<1.5 cm in greatest transverse diameter for nodes that were >1.5 cm pretherapy). Nodes initially between 1 and 1.5 cm must have decreased to 1 cm or less.
- The spleen, if previously enlarged on CT, must be normal in size and any focal deposits should have resolved.
- If the marrow was involved, it must be clear. Marrow biopsy is used for this criterion.

As with HD, a category exists for complete remission—unconfirmed. This allows for a residual mass of more than 1.5 cm short axis diameter (SAD) but which must have regressed by more than 75% of the sum of the products of the greatest diameters (SPD) of the original mass.

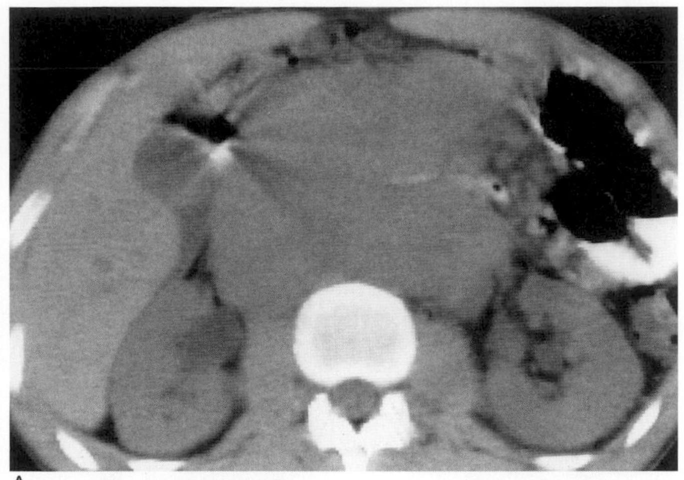

A

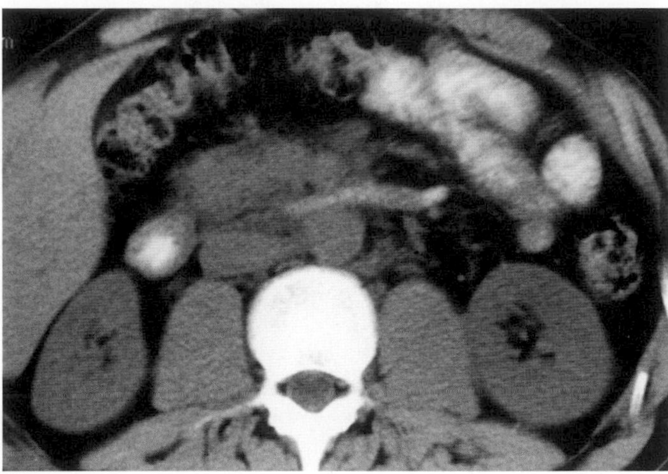

B

Figure 72.29 Abdominal residual mass (A) Unenhanced CT in a patient with non-Hodgkin's lymphoma presenting with a large **mesenteric nodal mass.** (B) Follow-up CT performed 1 year after treatment shows a marked reduction in the size of the mass but persistent low-density soft tissue within the mesentery encasing the mesenteric vessels, which was stable 3 years later.

A partial response (PR) is defined as a greater than 50% decrease in the SPD of masses, with a similar decrease in the size of any splenic or hepatic nodules and no evidence of progressive disease. Progressive disease (PD) is defined as a 50% or greater increase from nadir in the SPD of an established mass or the appearance of a new lesion.

FDG-PET in monitoring of response

Recently, there has been considerable interest in the use of functional imaging (gallium-67 SPECT and, notably, FDG-PET) after a few cycles of chemotherapy for the purposes of prognostication. The value of gallium imaging is limited by its lower sensitivity and by the significant proportion of non-gallium-avid tumours. FDG-PET performed after one to three cycles of chemotherapy appear to predict eventual outcome in NHL more accurately than PET at the end of treatment and more accurately than conventional imaging, especially with diffuse histologies[62,63]. Such early FDG-PET imaging allows a change in therapy and may avoid potential toxicity from ineffective therapy[64].

Residual masses

Successfully treated, enlarged nodes often return to normal size in both HD and NHL. However, a 'sterilized' mass of fibrous tissue can persist (Figs 72.28,72.29). This phenomenon occurs in up to 85% of patients treated for HD (usually within the mediastinum) and 40% of patients with NHL[34,65,66]. Such residual masses occur more frequently in patients with bulky disease, at least in HD. Whether such residual masses predispose to relapse is uncertain. Determination of the nature of such residual masses and exclusion of active disease with imaging is a major challenges in oncological radiology.

Computed tomography

On CT, residual masses are those that are greater than 1.5 cm SAD, which have nonetheless reduced by more than 75% of the SPD of the pre-treatment mass. CT cannot distinguish between fibrotic tissue and residual active disease on the basis of density alone, hence the very low positive predictive value of CT in determining the likelihood of relapse after treatment. Nevertheless, up until very recently, serial CT performed every 2–3 months was the most widely used method of determining the nature of a residual mass. Masses that remain static after 1 year are considered inactive, whereas any increase in size is highly suggestive of relapse.

MRI

MRI may help to differentiate active tumour and necrosis[67]. Most tumours have high T2 signal intensity and with response this decreases, possibly reflecting the development of fibrosis. Persistent heterogeneous high T2 signal or recurrent high signal in a residual mass suggest residual or recurrent disease respectively. However, small foci of tumour can remain within a low signal area[12], hence the fairly low sensitivity of MRI. In addition, false positive studies are common especially early on after treatment because of nonspecific inflammation and necrosis.

Radionuclide imaging

Gallium-67 is still sometimes used to monitor the effects of treatment, since it is taken up by viable tumour cells but not by fibrous or necrotic tissue. If no uptake is shown in a residual mass that was previously gallium-avid, it can be inferred that the mass is fibrotic in nature. It has been shown that persistent uptake of gallium-67 in a residual mass after treatment is a bad prognostic sign[68–70]. It is a far better predictor of disease relapse than CT in both HD and NHL. The limitations of gallium scanning have been discussed above, but in addition, it is a difficult isotope to use. Furthermore, nonspecific treatment related inflammation, rebound thymic hyperplasia and benign hilar uptake can all cause false positive studies.

Positron emission tomography

With the development of whole body and PET-CT systems FDG-PET has become a realistic alternative to other anatomical and functional imaging. Other PET tracers such as [C-11] methionine have also been described but remain in the research arena. The great advantage of FDG-PET lies in its ability to detect and quantify changes in functional/metabolic activity long before structural changes have taken place, hence its value in prognostication early after commencement of treatment as described above. At the end of treatment, FDG-PET has a very high positive predictive value for early relapse, with or without a residual mass at CT[71–73]. The specificity, overall accuracy and positive predictive value of FDG-PET are much higher than those of CT[74,75]. There are only a few studies directly comparing FDG-PET and gallium-67 but these do suggest that FDG-PET is more sensitive and has a greater overall accuracy[76]. It is likely therefore that it will have an increasingly important role in identifying relapse before conventional imaging can do so (Fig. 72.30). The greater sensitivity means that false positive studies can be a problem and it is essential that studies are interpreted in the light of the clinical findings and other imaging studies[77]. Pneumonitis and thymic hyperplasia are recognized causes of false positive studies. It should be recognized that FDG-PET predicts for early relapse and false negative studies do occur with late relapse.

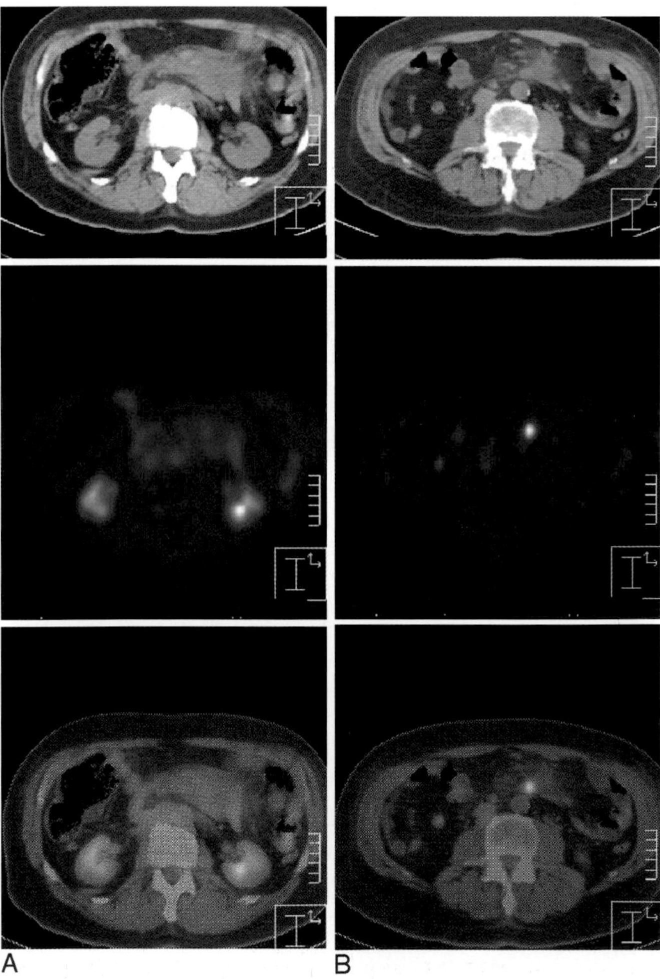

Figure 72.30 PET in monitoring disease progress. (A) CT, PET and fused PET-CT images demonstrating a large residual mass that is PET negative. (B) At a lower level, there is a small nodule in the inferior part of the mass that is metabolically active, indicating residual disease. (By kind permission of Dr Gary Cook, Department of Radiology, The Royal Marsden Hospital, London.)

SURVEILLANCE AND DETECTION OF RELAPSE

Relapse after satisfactory response to initial treatment occurs in 10–40% of patients with HD and over 50% of patients with NHL. In HD, relapse usually occurs within the first 2 years after treatment and patients are followed up closely during this period, although CT is not usually required unless clinical features suggest the possibility of recurrence. Strategies for follow-up with imaging vary between institutions. In patients with residual masses in HD and NHL, follow-up depends on the size of the mass, the site of involvement and the extent of disease; it is therefore impossible to define strict guidelines for each clinical situation.

For patients who attain CR or CR_u (i.e. in whom there is a Ga-67 or FDG-PET negative residual mass), it has been argued that routine imaging is desirable to detect asymptomatic early relapse, so that salvage therapy can be offered. In this situation, CT may be of limited value, since it may take some time before there is an appreciable increase in the size of the residual mass. Indeed, a number of studies have shown that relapse is rarely identified by conventional imaging before patients become symptomatic[78–80]. However, functional imaging can identify early relapse before CT and indeed, before the development of clinical signs[81].

Given the wealth of comparative data consistently showing a higher sensitivity for FDG-PET in the detection of disease compared to CT, especially at extranodal sites and the lower radiation dose (9 mSv vs. 30 mSv), there are theoretical reasons why PET might be adopted as a routine surveillance procedure[82]. However there is as yet little in the literature on the efficacy of PET in this role. In cases of suspected relapse, the development of a positive PET scan is highly suggestive and it is in this situation that PET-CT is likely to have a significant therapeutic impact, allowing percutaneous guided biopsies which can then direct therapy by establishing relapse and identifying transformation.[5]

CONCLUSION

Management of patients with lymphoma depends heavily on the imaging findings, which are vital in initial staging of the disease, prognostication and monitoring response to treatment. The radiologist needs to understand the fundamental aspects of tumour biology and behaviour and must appreciate the factors that will influence therapy. When reporting a study, it is no longer sufficient for the radiologist to document the presence of nodal enlargement above and below the diaphragm and to make imprecise comments upon the volume of disease. It is necessary to record the number of sites of nodal disease; the presence and sites of bulky disease; the presence of any extranodal disease; and factors which may influence delivery of therapy, such as central venous thrombosis or hydronephrosis. As indicated above, pitfalls still exist in monitoring response, particularly in evaluating the true nature of residual masses and this is one area where the increased availability of PET and the advent of PET-CT can be expected to have a huge impact. However, further research is needed in this exciting area before the precise roles of PET and PET-CT can be defined and their place in the investigative algorithm established. For all of these reasons, the radiologist has become a pivotal member of the multidisciplinary team managing patients with lymphoma.

REFERENCES

1. Lin A Y, Tucker M A 1998 Epidemiology of Hodgkin's disease and non-Hodgkin's lymphoma. In: Canellos G, Lister T A, Sklar J L (eds) The Lymphomas. London,W B Saunders, pp 43–61
2. Harris N L, Jaffe E S, Stein H, et al 1994 A revised European–American classification of lymphoid neoplasms: a proposal from the International Lymphoma Study Group. Blood 84: 1361–1392
3. World Health Organization Classification of Tumours 2001 Pathology & Genetics. Tumours of Haematopoietic and Lymphoid Tissues. Lyon, IARC Press
4. Lister T A, Crowther D, Sutcliffe S B, et al 1989 Report of a committee convened to discuss the evaluation and staging of patients with Hodgkin's disease. J Clin Oncol 7: 1630–1636
5. Pappa V I, Hussain H K, Reznek R H, et al 1996 The role of image-guided core needle biopsy in the management of patients with lymphoma. J Clin Oncol 14: 2427–2430
6. Shipp M, Harrington D, Anderson J, et al 1993 Development of a predictive model for aggressive lymphoma: the international NHL prognostic factors project. N Engl J Med 329: 987–994
7. Callen P W, Korobkin M, Isherwood I 1997 Computed tomography evaluation of the retrocrural prevertebral space. Am J Roentegenol 129: 907–910
8. Vinnicombe S, Norman A, Husband J, Nicolson V 1995 Normal pelvic lymph nodes: documentation by CT scanning after bipedal lymphangiography. Radiology 194: 349–355
9. Carroll B A 1982 Ultrasound of lymphoma. Semin Ultrasound 3(2): 114–122
10. Dooms G C, Hricak H, Crooks L, et al 1984 Magnetic resonance imaging of the lymph nodes. Comparison with CT. Radiology 153: 719–728
11. Greco A, Jeliffe A M, Maher J E, et al 1988 MR imaging of lymphomas: impact on therapy. J Comput Assist Tomogr 19: 785–791
12. Hill M, Cunningham D, MacVicar D, et al 1993 Role of magnetic resonance imaging in predicting relapse in residual masses after treatment of lymphoma. J Clin Oncol 11: 2273–2278
13. Moog F, Bangerter M, Diederichs C G, et al 1997 Lymphoma: role of whole-body 2-deoxy-2-[F-18]fluoro-D-glucose (FDG) PET in nodal staging. Radiology 203: 795–800
14. Moog F, Bangerter M, Diederichs C G, et al 1998 Extranodal malignant lymphoma: detection with FDG-PET versus CT. Radiology 206: 475–481
15. Bangerter M, Moog F, Buchmann I, et al 1998 Whole-body 2-[^{18}F]-fluoro-2-deoxy-D-glucose positron emission tomography (FDG-PET) for accurate staging of Hodgkin's disease. Ann Oncol 9: 1117–1122.
16. Jerusalem G, Warland V, Najjar F, et al 1999 Whole-body ^{18}F-FDG-PET for the evaluation of patients with Hodgkin's disease and non-Hodgkin's lymphoma. Nucl Med Commun 20: 13–20
17. Filly R, Blank N, Castellino R A 1976 Radiographic distribution of intrathoracic disease in previously untreated patients with Hodgkin's disease and non-Hodgkin's lymphoma. Radiology 120: 277–281
18. Castellino R A, Blank N, Hoppe R T, et al 1986 Hodgkin's disease: contribution of chest CT in the initial staging evaluation. Radiology 160: 603–605
19. Castellino R A, Hilton S, O'Brien J P, et al 1996 Non-Hodgkin's lymphoma: contribution of chest CT in the initial staging evaluation. Radiology 199: 129–131
20. Castellino R A, Marglin S, Blank N 1980 Hodgkin's disease, the non-Hodgkin's lymphomas and the leukaemias in the retroperitoneum. Semin Roentgenol 15: 288–301
21. Goffinet D R, Warnke R, Dunnick N R, et al 1977 Clinical and surgical (laparotomy) evaluation of patients with non-Hodgkin's lymphomas. Cancer Treat Rep 61: 981–992
22. Rosenberg S A, Kaplan H S 1966 Evidence for an orderly progression in the spread of Hodgkin's disease. Cancer Res 26: 1225–1231
23. Stomper P C, Cholewinski S P, Park J, et al 1993 Abdominal staging of thoracic Hodgkin disease: CT-lymphangiography-Ga-67 scanning correlation. Radiology 187: 381–386
24. Ng Y Y, Healy J C, Vincent J M et al 1994 The radiology of non-Hodgkin's lymphoma in childhood: a review of 80 cases. Clin Radiol 49: 594–600
25. Devesa S S, Fears T 1992 Non-Hodgkin's lymphoma time trends: United States and international data. Cancer Res 52: 5432s
26. Lee K S, Kim Y, Primack S L 1997 Imaging of pulmonary lymphomas. Am J Roentgenol 168: 339–345
27. Cobby M, Whipp E, Bullimore J, et al 1990 CT appearances of relapse of lymphoma in the lung. Clin Radiol 41: 232–238
28. Lewis E R, Caskey C I, Fishman E K 1991 Lymphoma of the lung: CT findings in 31 patients. Am J Roentgenol 156: 711–714
29. Sutcliffe S B, Gospodarowicz M K 1998 Primary extranodal lymphomas. In: Canellos G, Lister T A, Sklar J L (eds) The lymphomas. Philadelphia, W B Saunders, pp 449–479
30. O'Donnell P G, Jackson S A, Tung K T, et al 1998 Radiological appearances of lymphoma arising from mucosa associated lymphoid tissue (MALT) in the lung. Clin Radiol 53: 258–263
31. Murray K A, Chor P J, Turner J F 1996 Intrathoracic lymphoproliferative disorders and lymphoma. Curr Probl Diagn Radiol 25: 77–108
32. Celikoglu F, Teirstein A S, Krellenstein D J, et al 1992 Pleural effusion in non-Hodgkin's lymphoma. Chest 101: 1357–1360
33. Wernecke K, Vassalo P, Rutsch F, et al 1991 Thymic involvement in Hodgkin's disease: CT and sonographic findings. Radiology 181: 375–383
34. Spiers A S, Husband J E, MacVicar A D 1997 Treated thymic lymphoma: comparison of MR imaging with CT. Radiology 203: 369–376
35. Carlsen S E, Bergin C J, Hoppe R T 1993 MR imaging to detect chest wall and pleural involvement in patients with lymphoma: effect on radiation therapy planning. Am J Roentgenol 160: 1191–1195
36. Liberman L, Giess C S, Dershaw D D, et al 1994 Non-Hodgkin lymphoma of the breast: imaging characteristics and correlation with histopathologic findings. Radiology 192: 157–160
37. Munker R, Stengel A, Stabler A, et al 1995 Diagnostic accuracy of ultrasound and computed tomography in the staging of Hodgkin's disease. Verification by laparotomy in 100 cases. Cancer 76: 1460–1466
38. Brady L W, Asbell S O 1980 Malignant lymphoma of the gastrointestinal tract. Radiology 137: 291–298
39. Megibow A J, Balthazar E J, Naidich D P, et al 1983 Computed tomography of gastrointestinal lymphoma. Am J Roentgenol 141: 541–543
40. Shirkhoda A, Ros P R, Farah J, et al 1990 Lymphoma of the solid abdominal viscera. Radiol Clin North Am 28: 785–799
41. Reznek R H, Mootoosamy I, Webb J A, et al 1990 CT in renal and perirenal lymphoma: a further look. Clin Radiol 42: 233–238
42. Bailey J E, Roubidoux M A, Dunnick N R 1998 Secondary renal neoplasms. Abdom Imaging 23: 266–274
43. Aigen A B, Phillips M 1986 Primary malignant lymphoma of the urinary bladder. Urology 28: 235–237
44. Thurnher S, Hricak H, Carroll P R, et al 1988 Imaging the testis: comparison between MR imaging and US. Radiology 167: 631–636
45. Kim Y S, Koh B H, Cho O K, et al 1997 MR imaging of primary uterine lymphoma. Abdom Imaging 22: 441–444
46. Vincent J M, Morrison I D, Armstrong P, et al 1994 Non-metastatic enlargement of the adrenal glands in patients with malignant disease. Clin Radiol 49: 456–460
47. Pond G D, Castellino R A, Horning S, et al 1989 Non-Hodgkin's lymphoma: influence of lymphography, CT and bone marrow biopsy on staging and management. Radiology 170: 159–164
48. Döhner H, Gückel F, Knauf W, et al 1989 Magnetic resonance imaging of bone marrow in lymphoproliferative disorders: correlation with bone marrow biopsy. Br J Haematol 73:12–17
49. Hoane B R, Shields A F, Porter B A, et al 1991 Detection of lymphomatous bone marrow involvement with magnetic resonance imaging. Blood 78: 728–738

50. Ngan H, Preston B J 1975 Non-Hodgkin's lymphoma presenting with osseous lesions. Clin Radiol 26: 351–356

51. Stroszczynski C, Oellinger J, Hosten N, et al 1999 Staging and monitoring of malignant lymphoma of the bone: comparison of ^{67}Ga scintigraphy and MRI. J Nucl Med 40: 387–393

52. Hobson D E, Anderson B A, Carr I, et al 1986 Primary lymphoma of the central nervous system: Manitoba experience and review of literature. Can J Neurol Sci 13: 55–61

53. Zimmerman R A 1990 Central nervous system lymphoma. Radiol Clin North Am 28: 697–721

54. Chamberlain M C, Sandy A D, Press G A 1990 Leptomeningeal metastasis: a comparison of gadolinium-enhanced MR and contrast-enhanced CT of the brain. Neurology 40: 435–438

55. Yousem D M, Patrone P M, Grossman R I 1990 Leptomeningeal metastases: MR evaluation. J Comput Assist Tomogr 14: 255–261

56. Raderer M, Vorbeck F, Formanek M, et al 2000 Importance of extensive staging in patients with mucosa-associated lymphoid tissue (MALT)-type lymphoma. Br J Cancer 83: 454–457

57. Johnson K A, Tung K, Mead G, et al 1998 The imaging of Burkitt's and Burkitt-like lymphoma. Clin Radiol 53: 835–841

58. Radin D R, Esplin J A, Levine A M, et al 1993 AIDS-related non-Hodgkin's lymphoma: abdominal CT findings in 112 patients. Am J Roentgenol 160: 1133–1139

59. Pickhardt P J, Siegel M J 1998 Abdominal manifestations of posttransplantation lymphoproliferative disorder. Am J Roentgenol 171: 1007–1013

60. Hopper K D, Kasales C J, Van Slyke M A, et al 1996 Analysis of interobserver and intraobserver variability in CT tumor measurements. Am J Roentgenol 167: 851–854

61. Cheson B D, Horning S J, Coiffier B, et al. 1999 Report of an international workshop to standardize response criteria in non-Hodgkin's lymphoma. J Clin Oncol 1999;17:1244–12**53.**

62. Mikhaeel N G, Timothy A R, O'Doherty M J, et al 2000 18-FDG-PET as a prognostic indicator in the treatment of aggressive non-Hodgkin's lymphoma—comparison with CT. Leuk Lymphoma 39: 543–553

63. Spaepen K, Stroobants S, Dupont P, et al 2001 Prognostic value of positron emission tomography (PET) with fluorine-18 fluorodeoxyglucose ([^{18}F]FDG) after first-line chemotherapy in non-Hodgkin's lymphoma: is [^{18}F]FDG-PET a valid alternative to conventional diagnostic methods? J Clin Oncol 19: 414–419

64. Kostakoglu L, Coleman M, Leonard J P, et al 2002 PET predicts prognosis after 1 cycle of chemotherapy in aggressive lymphoma and Hodgkin's disease. J Nucl Med 43: 1018–1027

65. Surbone A, Lango D L, de Vitra V T, et al 1988 Residual abdominal masses in aggressive non-Hodgkin's lymphoma after combination chemotherapy: significance and management. J Clin Oncol 6: 1832–1837

66. Jochelson M, Mauch P, Balikian J, et al 1985 The significance of the residual mediastinal mass in treated Hodgkin disease. J Clin Oncol 3: 637–640

67. Rahmouni A, Tempany C, Jones R, et al 1993 Lymphoma. Monitoring tumor size and signal intensity with MR imaging. Radiology 188: 445–451

68. Front D, Israel O 1995 The role of Ga-67 scintigraphy in evaluating the results of therapy of lymphoma patients. Semin Nucl Med 26: 60–71

69. Israel O, Front D, Epelbaum R, et al 1990 Residual mass and negative gallium scintigraphy in treated lymphoma. J Nucl Med 31: 365–368

70. Kaplan W D, Jochelson M S, Herman T S, et al 1990 Gallium-67 imaging: a predictor of residual tumour viability and clinical outcome in patients with diffuse large-cell lymphoma. J Clin Oncol 8: 1966–1970

71. Jerusalem G, Beguin Y, Fassotte M F, et al 1999 Whole-body positron emission tomography using ^{18}F-fluorodeoxyglucose for posttreatment evaluation in Hodgkin's disease and non-Hodgkin's lymphoma has higher diagnostic and prognostic value than classical computed tomography scan imaging. Blood 94: 429–433

72. Naumann R, Vaic A, Beuthien-Baumann B, et al 2001 Prognostic value of positron emission tomography in the evaluation of post-treatment residual mass in patients with Hodgkin's disease and non-Hodgkin's lymphoma. Br J Haematol 115: 793–800

73. Weihrauch M R, Re D, Scheidhauer K, et al 2001 Thoracic positron emission tomography using ^{18}F-fluorodeoxyglucose for the evaluation of residual mediastinal Hodgkin disease. Blood 98: 2930–2934

74. Cremerius U, Fabry U, Neuerburg J, et al 1998 Positron emission tomography with ^{18}F-FDG to detect residual disease after therapy for malignant lymphoma. Nucl Med Commun 19: 1055–1063

75. Stumpe K D, Urbimelli M, Steinert H C, et al 1998 Whole body positron emission tomography using FDG for staging of lymphoma: effectiveness and comparison with computed tomography. Eur J Nucl Med 25: 721–728

76. Van Den Bosche B, Lambert B, De Winter F, et al 2002 ^{18}FDG-PET versus high-dose ^{67}Ga scintigraphy for restaging and treatment follow-up of lymphoma patients. Nucl Med Commun 23:1079–1083

77. Bakheet S M, Powe J 1998 Benign causes of 18-FDG uptake on whole body imaging. Semin Nucl Med 28: 352–358

78. Weeks J C, Yeap B Y, Canellos G P, et al 1991 Value of follow-up procedures in patients with large-cell lymphoma who achieve a complete remission. J Clin Oncol 9: 1196–1203

79. Radford J A, Eardley A, Woodman C, et al 1997 Follow up policy after treatment for Hodgkin's disease: too many clinic visits and routine tests? A review of hospital records. Br Med J 314: 343–346

80. Elis A, Blickstein D, Klein O, et al 2002 Detection of relapse in non-Hodgkin's lymphoma: role of routine follow-up studies. Am J Hematol 69: 41–44

81. Front D, Bar-Shalom R, Epelbaum R, et al 1993 Early detection of lymphoma recurrence with gallium-67 scintigraphy. J Nucl Med 34: 2101–2104

82. Jerusalem G, Beguin Y, Fassotte M, et al 2003 Early detection of relapse by whole-body positron emission tomography in the follow-up of patients with Hodgkin's disease. Ann Oncol 14: 123–130

CHAPTER 73

Reticuloendothelial Disorders: The Spleen

S. Aslam A. Sohaib and Rodney H. Reznek

- Imaging techniques
- Normal anatomy
- Splenomegaly
- Malignant mass lesions
- Splenic infection
- Splenic trauma
- Other splenic disorders

IMAGING TECHNIQUES

Plain radiography is not routinely used in the evaluation of the spleen. The splenic outline may be seen on a plain radiograph especially if it is enlarged (Fig. 73.1).

On ultrasound (US) the spleen is readily visualized. The normal splenic parenchyma shows a homogenous low-level echo pattern, which is generally of slightly lower reflectivity than hepatic parenchyma. Ultrasound is useful for detecting and characterizing focal lesions within the spleen as cystic or solid. Colour Doppler US is useful for differentiating vascular structures such as normal vessels from nonvascular structures such as pancreatic pseudocysts.

The use of microbubble US contrast media may aid in identifying and characterizing splenic abnormalities[1].

On non-enhanced computed tomography (CT) the normal spleen is homogeneous and has an attenuation of 35–55 HU, that is 5–10 HU less than that of liver. The spleen is optimally evaluated following intravenous injection of contrast medium. The spleen normally enhances heterogeneously immediately after injection of a bolus of contrast material. Only after a minute or more does the splenic parenchyma achieve uniform homogeneous enhancement (Fig. 73.2). This is thought to reflect the variable blood flow within different compartments of the spleen and should not be misinterpreted for disease.

On magnetic resonance imaging (MRI) the splenic parenchyma is of lower signal intensity than the liver and slightly greater signal than muscle on T1-weighted images. On T2-weighted sequences, the spleen shows higher signal intensity than the liver (Fig. 73.3). The signal intensity of normal splenic parenchyma and many pathological processes are similar. Consequently, the use of contrast enhanced MRI is important for evaluating the spleen. Intravenous gadolinium-based contrast agents are most commonly used. Images are acquired using a dynamic breath-hold T1-weighted spoiled gradient echo sequence after injection of a bolus of gadolinium intravenously. As on CT, the spleen shows heterogeneous enhancement on the dynamic contrast enhanced MRI (Fig. 73.4). Superparamagnetic iron oxide particles injected intravenously have been used to evaluate the spleen. These particles are taken up by the reticuloendothelial system and lower the signal intensity of the normal spleen, thereby increasing the conspicuousness of focal abnormalities in the spleen.

Radionuclide imaging with technetium-99m (^{99m}Tc) labelled sulphur or tin colloid imaging of the spleen for the detection of focal abnormalities has been replaced by cross-sectional imaging. For specific imaging of the spleen, ^{99m}Tc-labelled denatured autologous red blood cells are used.

Angiography with selective catheterization of the coeliac axis or splenic artery provides excellent visualization of the splenic and portal veins. In many patients it is possible to show the main splenic artery and normal splenic and portal veins using intravenous subtraction angiography.

Percutaneous biopsy of splenic lesions may be performed for cytological or histological diagnosis. This results in a high diagnostic rate (55–90%) and the complication rate is low[2]. Splenic abscess may be treated successfully with aspiration or percutaneous drainage.

NORMAL ANATOMY

The spleen forms from multiple foci of mesenchymal cells in the dorsal mesogastrium. During embryological development, the dorsal mesentery moves to the left with the development of the stomach. As it grows to the left the spleen becomes covered with peritoneum of the greater sac. The anterior portion of the dorsal mesogastrium that extends from the greater

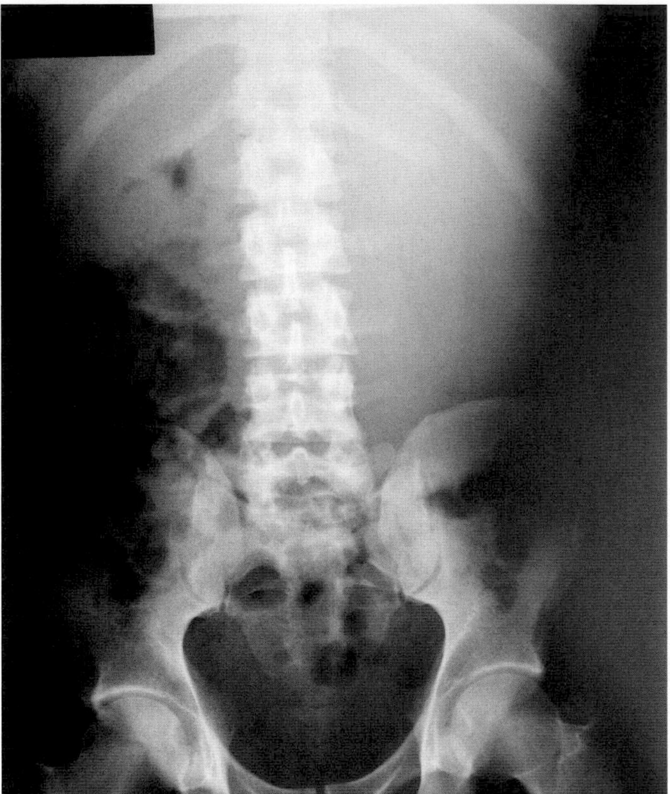

Figure 73.1 Splenomegaly. Plain radiograph showing the splenic outline in a patient with splenomegaly due to chronic myeloid leukaemia.

curvature of the stomach to the spleen becomes the gastrosplenic ligament. The posterior portion of the dorsal mesogastrium extending from the spleen to the left kidney becomes the splenorenal ligament, which transmits the tip of the pancreatic tail and splenic vessels towards the splenic hilum. Both ligaments carry veins, which are potential anastomotic channels between the portal and systemic venous system.

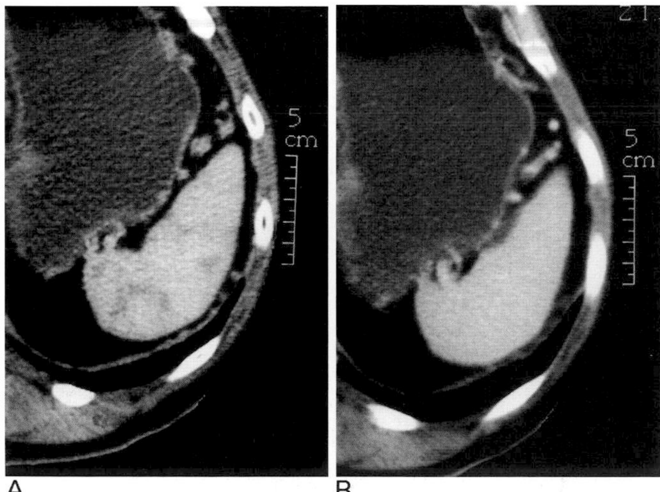

Figure 73.2 Normal splenic enhancement on CT. (A) Dynamic contrast-enhanced CT obtained 30 s after bolus injection of contrast media showing the heterogeneous enhancement pattern. (B) A delayed image shows uniform opacification of the spleen.

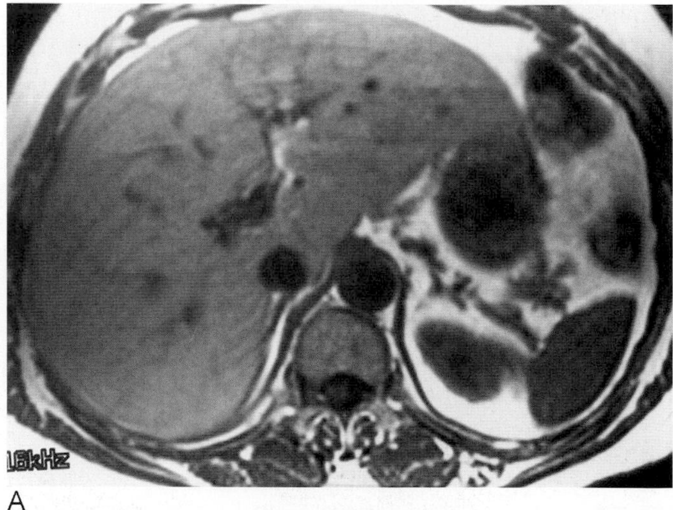

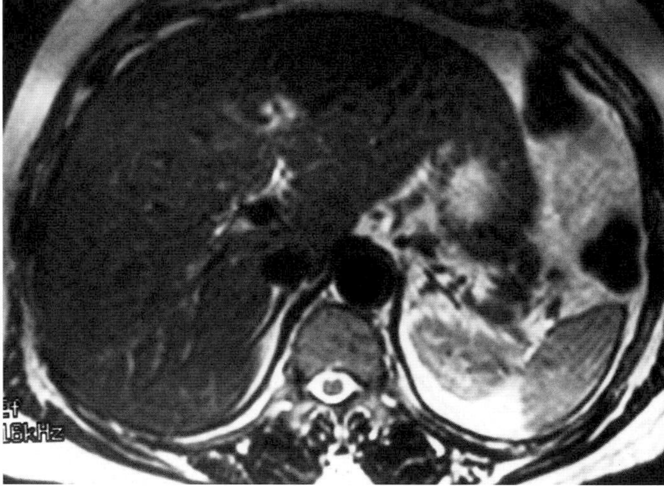

Figure 73.3 Normal spleen on MRI. Axial (A) T1-weighted spin-echo and (B) T2-weighted fast-spin-echo images showing the normal signal intensity of the spleen.

The adult spleen lies in the left hypochondrium at the level of the 10th rib in the mid axillary line. The spleen has diaphragmatic and visceral surfaces. The visceral surface is related to the stomach and left kidney. The spleen has a superior and inferior border and is notched on its inferior border. The vessels and nerve enter the spleen at the hilum on the visceral surface.

The spleen is composed of a supporting connective tissue framework comprising its capsule and trabeculae, and a unique functional parenchyma made up of red and white pulp. The spleen has important haematological and immunological functions.

Spleen size

The normal adult spleen measures approximately 12–15 cm length, 4–8 cm in antero-posterior diameter and 3–4 cm in thickness[3]. However, the irregular shape and oblique orientation of spleen mean that these linear measurements are of limited use. Furthermore, splenic volume varies greatly from one individual to another, and the normal spleen decreases in size

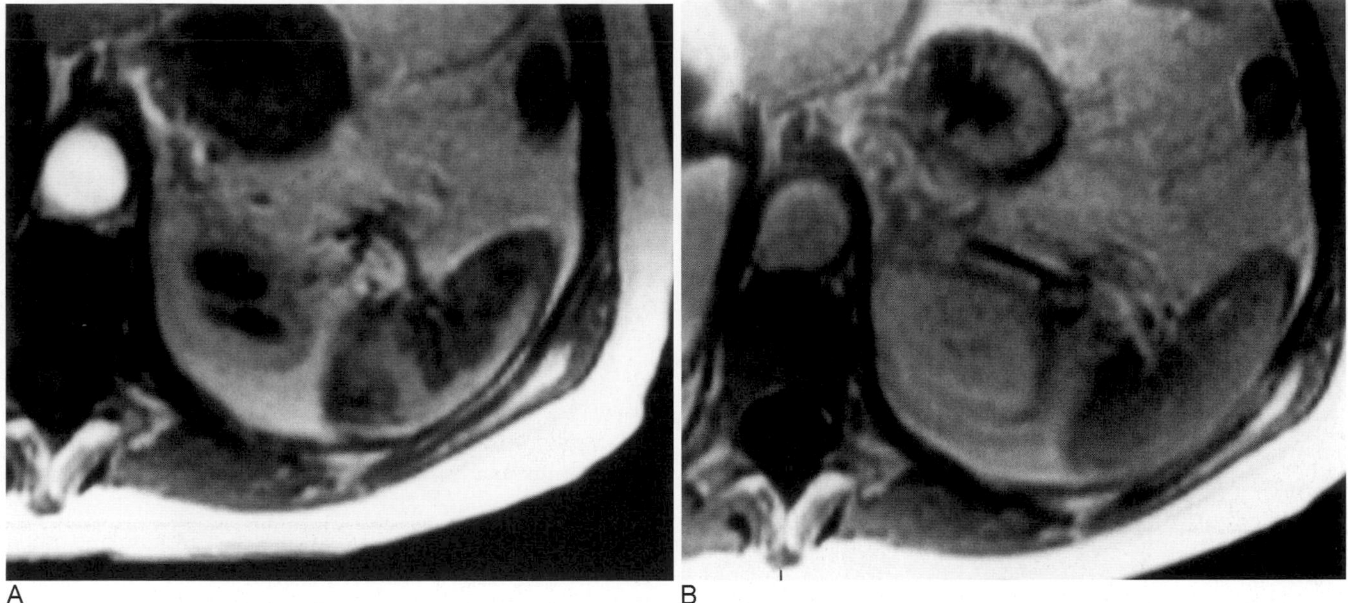

Figure 73.4 Normal splenic enhancement on MRI. (A) A dynamic breath-hold axial T1-weighted spoiled gradient-echo image obtained 30 s after bolus injection of gadolinium shows inhomogeneous enhancement. (B) The delayed image shows uniform enhancement of the spleen.

with age. Normal in vivo adult splenic volume ranges from 107 to 314 cm^3[3,4]. Splenic size can be assessed on imaging. On plain radiography vertical length measurement is the single best indicator of splenic size. A length greater than 11 cm is associated with a 70% probability of splenomegaly[5]. Ultrasound can be used to determine changes in spleen size with serial measurement and the long axis of the spleen is less than 12 cm in 95% of the population[6]. Ultrasound assessment of splenic size correlates well with CT splenic volume[7]. Determination of splenic volume on CT using summation of cross-sectional areas is very accurate with errors in the range of 3–5%[7]. However, this technique is cumbersome and, in practice, on CT or MRI most observers judge splenic volume by subjective evaluation. Rounding of the normally crescentic shape, extension of the spleen anterior to the aorta or below the right hepatic lobe or rib cage are further clues to splenomegaly. On cross-sectional imaging a more accurate method for the assessment of the splenic volume is the splenic index, i.e., the product of the length, width and thickness. The normal splenic index is between 120 and 480 cm^3[3,8].

Normal variants and congenital anomalies

The shape and position of the normal spleen can vary considerably. Commonly, a bulge from the posterior margin of the spleen may extend medially and simulate a mass on urography. In 15–20% of individuals the posterolateral border of the spleen lies posterior to the left kidney. This is known as a retrorenal spleen. Residual clefts between adjacent lobulations may mimic lacerations. The upside down spleen is a variant in which the splenic hilum is directed superiorly towards the hemidiaphragm.

Accessory spleen (splenunculus) refers to ectopic splenic tissue of congenital origin, unlike splenosis, which refers to ectopic splenic tissue that results from trauma (see below). Accessory spleens are present in 10–30% of the population, and can be single or multiple. They usually occur near the splenic hilum (75%), but may be found in its suspensory ligaments or in the tail of the pancreas and, rarely, elsewhere in the abdomen. The blood supply to an accessory spleen is usually derived from the splenic artery with drainage into the splenic vein. Accessory spleens vary in size from a few millimetres to several centimetres in diameter. After splenectomy, an accessory spleen can hypertrophy dramatically causing recurrence of problems in patients who have undergone splenectomy for hypersplenism. The typical accessory spleen has a smooth, round or ovoid shape (Figs 73.5, 73.6). Its imaging appearance (i.e., echo-texture, or attenuation, or signal intensity) is similar to that of the parent spleen.

The **wandering spleen** is a congenital variant in which laxity of the suspensory ligament permits the spleen to move about in the abdomen. It affects children and women of childbearing age and is usually asymptomatic unless torsion occurs. The imaging findings are of an abdominal mass with a size appropriate for the spleen with the absence of the spleen in the normal location. It may be possible to recognise the characteristic shape of the spleen and to trace the splenic vasculature back to its origin. The density and pattern of enhancement may also suggest the diagnosis. However, if there is uncertainty as to whether the mass is truly an ectopically located spleen, radionuclide scintigraphy with ^{99m}Tc-labelled denatured autologous red blood cells usually resolves the issue.

Polysplenia is a rare complex congenital syndrome characterized by partial visceral heterotaxia (situs ambiguous) and concomitant levo-isomerism (bilateral left-sidedness). It is associated with multiple, highly variable cardiovascular and

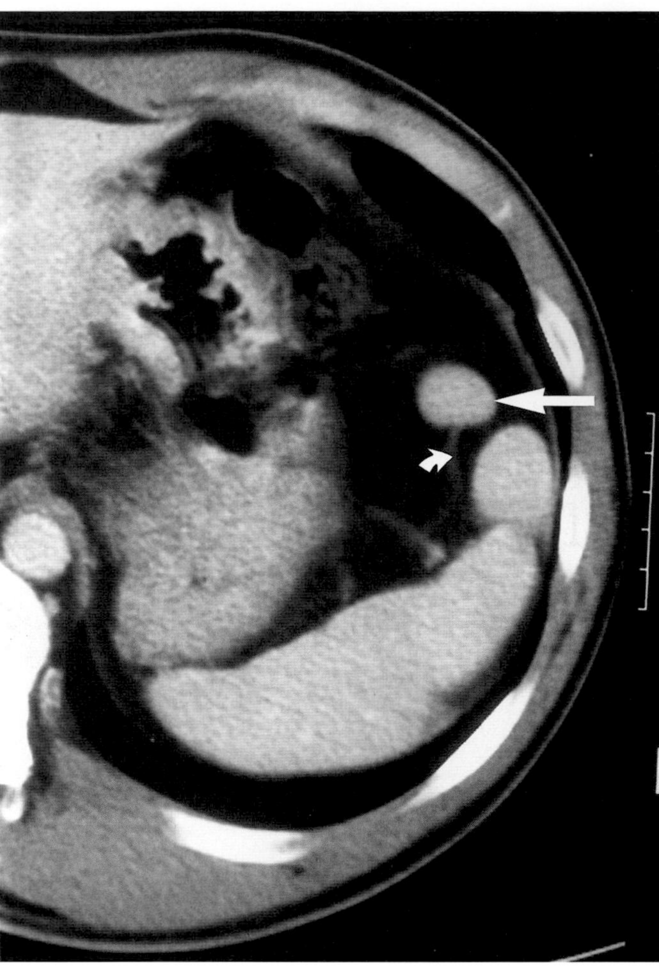

Figure 73.5 Accessory spleen. Contrast-enhanced CT shows a small accessory spleen (arrow) anterior to the spleen. Note the draining vein (curved arrow) from the accessory spleen can be seen to join the other veins draining the main spleen.

visceral anomalies. The abdominal anomalies include a right-sided stomach, midline or left-sided liver, malrotation of the intestine, a short pancreas and inferior vena cava anomalies. The spleen is divided into 2–16 masses, which are located in either the right or left upper quadrant along the greater curve of the stomach. Less commonly, there are one or two large spleens along with several smaller splenunculi.

The congenital asplenia syndrome (right isomerism) is characterized by an absent spleen and multiple anomalies in both the abdomen and thorax. Many of its features are those of right isomerism, e.g., situs ambiguous with bilateral right sidedness.

Splenogonadal fusion is a rare congenital anomaly characterized by fusion of splenic tissue and gonad[9]. It is thought that this anomaly is due to an adhesion between the gonadal primordia and developing spleen prior to gonadal descent. The functioning splenic tissue is located in close proximity to gonadal tissue. Splenogonadal fusion occurs predominantly in male patients and the left gonad is nearly always affected. It is usually asymptomatic but may cause confusion with testicular malignancy.

SPLENOMEGALY

There are many causes of splenomegaly (Table 73.1). The imaging appearances are usually non-specific and only occasionally can imaging provide a clue to the underlying cause, e.g., abdominal lymph node enlargement may suggest lymphoma or sarcoidosis.

Benign mass lesions

Splenic cyst

Non-neoplastic splenic cysts can be divided into true (primary) cysts, which possess a cellular lining, and false (secondary) cysts, which have no cellular lining. True cysts are either parasitic (echinococcal) or nonparasitic (epithelial). True, nonparasitic, i.e., epithelial (also called epidermoid, mesothelial, or primary) cysts are congenital in origin. They are more common in women than in men and usually occur in childhood or adolescence[10]. In 80% of cases congenital splenic cysts are unilocular and solitary. A false cyst, i.e., pseudocyst, is post-traumatic in origin and is thought to represent the final stage in the evolution of a splenic haematoma.

On CT/MRI, splenic cysts are well defined, of water density or signal intensity, and show no enhancement after intravenous injection of contrast medium (Figs 73.7, 73.8). It is usually difficult to distinguish between true and false cysts on imaging, but certain characteristics may be useful in differentiating between them. On US, false cysts may contain internal echoes from debris and show echogenic foci with distal shadowing due to calcification in the wall. On CT, cyst wall calcification can be seen in 14% of true cysts and 50% of false cysts[11]. Cyst wall trabeculation or peripheral septation occurs in 86% of true cysts and 17% of false cysts. High attenuation cysts may occur in up to one third of false cysts. On MRI, false cysts may have variable signal intensity on T1-weighted images, depending on the degree of proteinaceous material or haemorrhage present.

Splenic hydatid cysts occur in less than 5% of cases of echinococcosis, and in approximately 75% of patients with echinoccoccal involvement of the spleen other structures are involved, the liver being the most common. The appearance on imaging of splenic hydatidosis depends on the age of the cyst and any associated complication. On US, a hydatid cyst may be anechoic or have mixed echogenicity due to intracystic components, e.g., scolices. Separation of the membrane produces the 'water-lily' sign—an undulating, linear collection of echoes within the cyst. Daughter cysts give the characteristic appearance of a cyst enclosed within a cyst. On CT, hydatid cysts are well-defined low-density lesions that do not enhance after intravenous injection of contrast medium, except for possible ring-like enhancement of the external cyst wall. The cyst wall may calcify, and the presence of a complete ring of calcification suggests an inactive lesion. On MRI, hydatid cysts are well-defined, rounded spaces occupying lesions with signal intensity similar to water. However, depending on the protein content or haemorrhage in the cyst, the signal intensity on T1-weighted sequences may vary. Daughter cysts have slightly

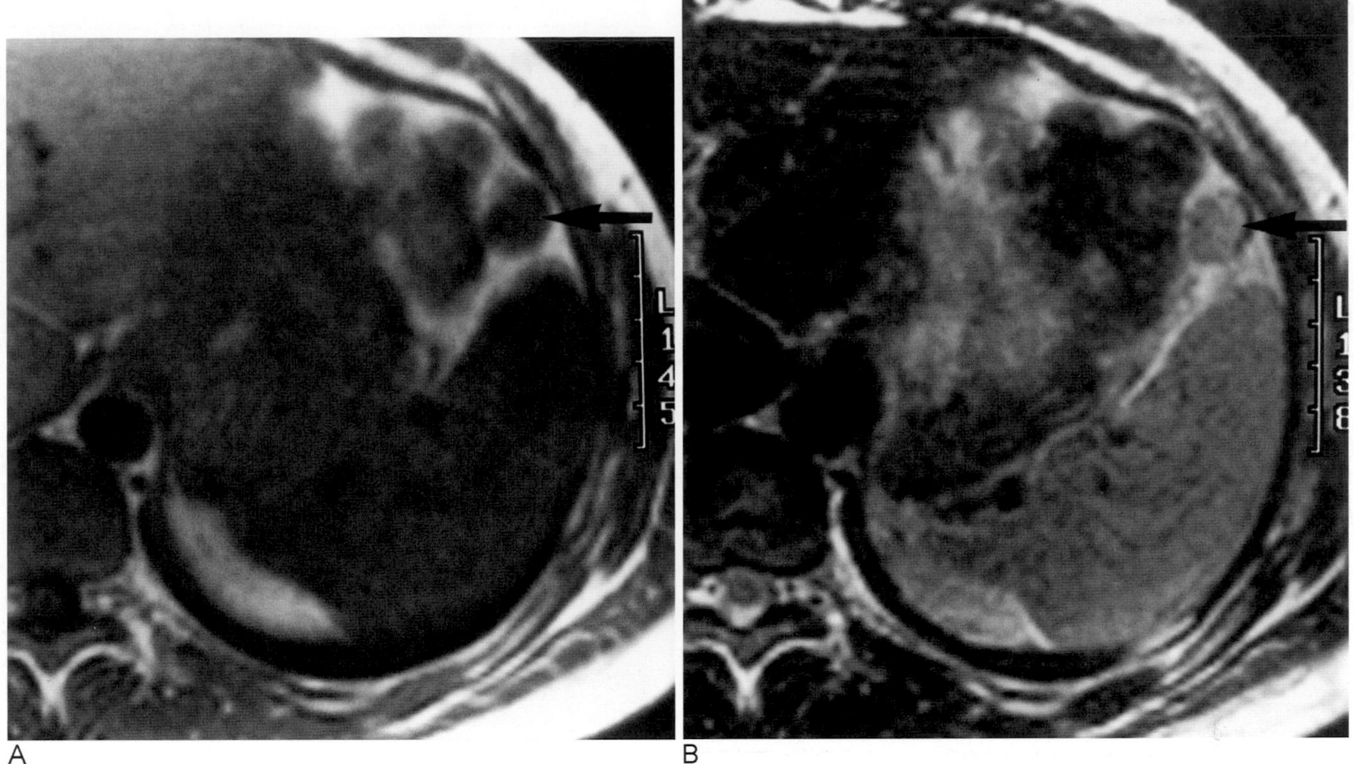

Figure 73.6 Accessory spleen on MRI. Axial (A) T1-weighted spin-echo and (B) T2-weighted fast-spin-echo images shows a small accessory spleen (arrow) anterior to the spleen. The signal intensity of the accessory spleen corresponds to that of the spleen on all sequences.

lower signal than the main cyst on T1-weighted images. A thick, low-intensity rim surrounding the cyst is usually present. This rim corresponds to a dense fibrous capsule encasing the parasitic membrane. As the appearance of a hydatid cyst is non-specific, differentiating hydatid cysts from other cystic lesions can be difficult. The presence of daughter cyst, hepatic involvement and positive serology may be helpful in the differential diagnosis.

The differential diagnosis of a splenic cyst includes abscess, acute haematoma, intrasplenic pancreatic pseudocyst, cystic neoplasm (lymphangioma or haemangioma) and cystic metastasis.

Haemangioma

Haemangioma is the most common primary benign neoplasm of the spleen, occurring in 0.03–14% of cases at autopsy[12]. Splenic haemangiomas can be multiple (Fig. 73.9) and part of a generalised angiomatosis as in Klippel–Trénaunay–Weber syndrome. Most lesions are detected incidentally but large haemangiomas can lead to splenic rupture and anaemia, thrombocytopenia and coagulopathy (Kasabach–Merritt syndrome).

The imaging characteristics of splenic haemangiomas range from solid to mixed to purely cystic lesions[13]. The US appearance is non-specific, and may show cystic areas. On CT, haemangiomas may appear either solid or cystic and may enhance in a similar pattern to hepatic haemangioma[14]. Some lesions are relatively avascular or show slow filling of contrast material. The MRI appearance is also similar to hepatic haemangioma. The lesion is of lower signal intensity than, or isointense to, the spleen on T1-weighted images, and of high signal intensity on T2-weighted images. T2-weighted images may show heterogeneous signal intensity representing mixed solid and cystic component of the haemangioma. T1-weighted images may shows areas of high signal due to subacute haemorrhage or proteinaceous fluid.

Lymphangioma

Lymphangioma may occur as single or multiple lesions, are usually asymptomatic, and are categorized as capillary, cavernous, or cystic depending on the size of the abnormal lymphatic channels. In the spleen the cystic type is most common. On US they appear as hypoechoic masses occasionally containing septation and debris[15]. CT shows multiple thin-walled, well-marginated cysts, often subcapsular in location. No enhancement is seen and the attenuation measurements vary from 15–35 HU[16].

Hamartoma

Splenic hamartomas (also called splenomas, or nodular hyperplasia of the spleen) are rare benign lesions composed of an anomalous mixture of normal splenic elements with red pulp predominating[17]. The hamartoma occurs singly or less commonly as multiple nodules. On US, hamartomas are hyperechoic relative to the spleen and sometimes have a cystic component[18]. On CT, they appear iso- or hypodense on unenhanced images with occasional lesions showing cystic components. On MRI, they are isointense on T1-weighted and hyperintense on T2-weighted sequences[15]. On CT and MRI, following intravenous contrast material, they usually show slow enhancement with late 'filling in'[19].

Table 73.1 CAUSES OF SPLENOMEGALY
Congestive
Portal hypertension
Cirrhosis
Cystic fibrosis
Splenic vein obstruction
Neoplasms
Leukaemia / lymphoma
Storage disease
Gaucher's disease
Niemann–Pick disease
Amyloidosis
Histiocytosis
Collagen vascular
Systemic lupus erythematosus
Rheumatoid / Felty syndrome
Haemolytic anaemias
Haemoglobinopathies
Hereditary spherocytosis
Infections
Hepatitis
Malaria
Infectious mononucleosis
Tuberculosis
Typhoid
Extramedullary haematopoiesis
Myelofibrosis
Miscellaneous
Sarcoidosis
Porphyria

MALIGNANT MASS LESIONS

Lymphoma (see Chapter 72)

Splenic lymphoma is usually a manifestation of generalized lymphoma and is the most common splenic malignancy. Primary splenic lymphoma, which is usually of the non-Hodgkin type, is rare and comprises 1–2% of all lymphomas[20]. It is estimated that, at the time of diagnosis, splenic involvement is present in 25–35% of patients with Hodgkin's or non-Hodgkin lymphoma (NHL)[21]. In patients with NHL splenic involvement is associated with infiltrated para-aortic nodes in approximately 70% of patients. On imaging, splenic involvement in lymphoma can take several forms: (A) homogeneous enlargement, (B) miliary nodules, (C) multifocal, 1–10 cm lesions (Figs 73.10, 73.11), or (D) single solitary mass. Necrosis of a large lesion can give rise to an irregular cystic lesion[22]. Radiologically visible calcification has been reported in aggressive lesions and after chemotherapy[23].

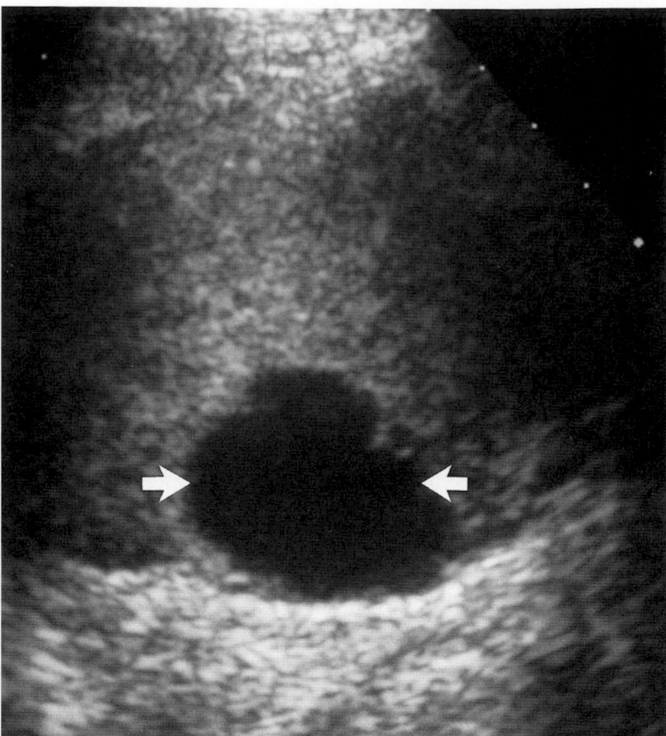
A

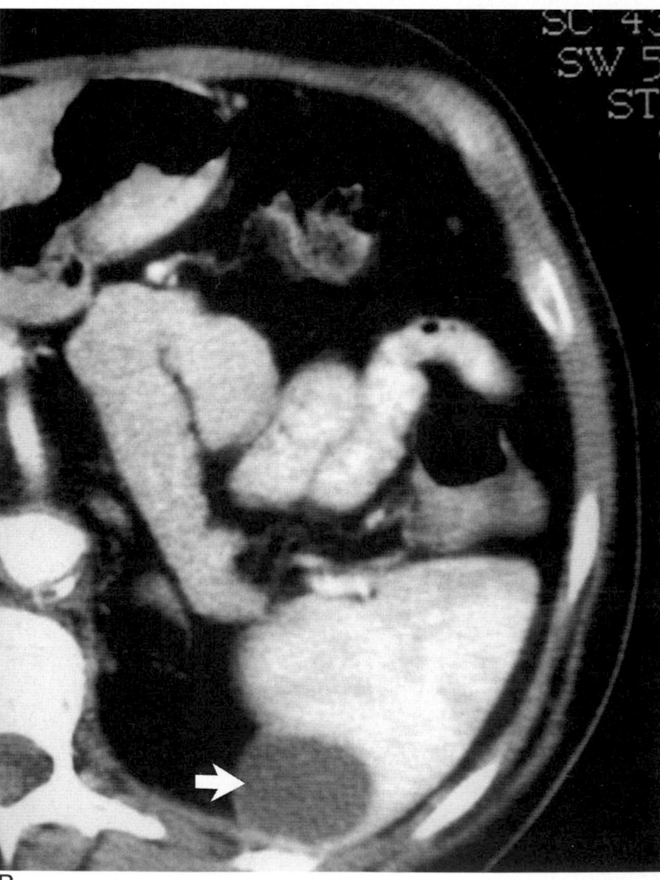

B

Figure 73.7 Splenic cyst. (A) Ultrasound and (B) contrast-enhanced CT showing the typical appearances of a splenic cyst (arrow).

Other primary malignant tumours

Splenic angiosarcoma is very rare but is the most common non-lymphoid primary malignant tumour of the spleen. The prognosis is very poor as only 20% of patients survive lon-

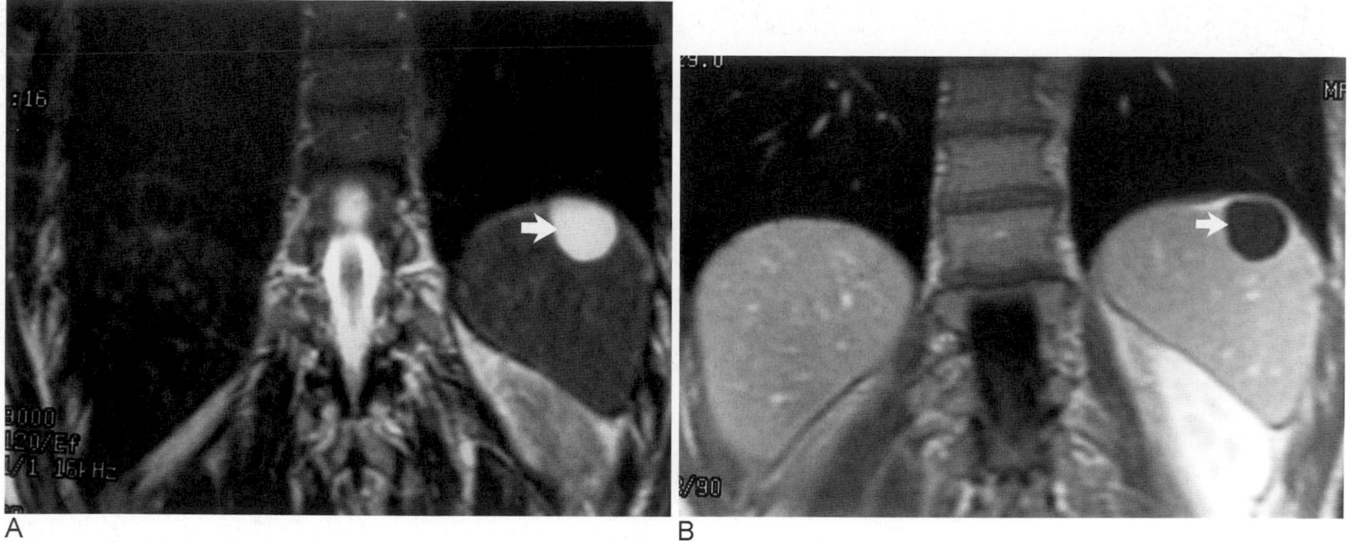

Figure 73.8 Splenic cyst on MRI. (A) Coronal T2-weighted fast-spin-echo and (B) a dynamic breath-hold coronal T1-weighted spoiled gradient-echo image obtained 2 minutes after gadolinium injection shows the typical appearance of splenic cyst (arrow) on MRI.

ger than 6 months. Approximately 70% of all angiosarcoma metastasize to the liver and approximately 30% undergo spontaneous rupture[24]. Imaging reveals an enlarged spleen with a poorly defined mass, and there may be areas of haemorrhage.

Other primary tumours of the spleen are very rare and include fibrosarcoma, leiomyosarcoma, malignant teratoma and malignant fibrous histocytoma.

Metastatic disease

Metastatic deposits in the spleen are unusual, occurring in only 0.3–10.3% of patients with malignancy where metastases have occurred in multiple organs[25]. Splenic metastases are usually asymptomatic and are usually found at autopsy or at imaging. The most common primary site for splenic metastases are the breast, lung, colorectal, ovary and skin (melanoma).

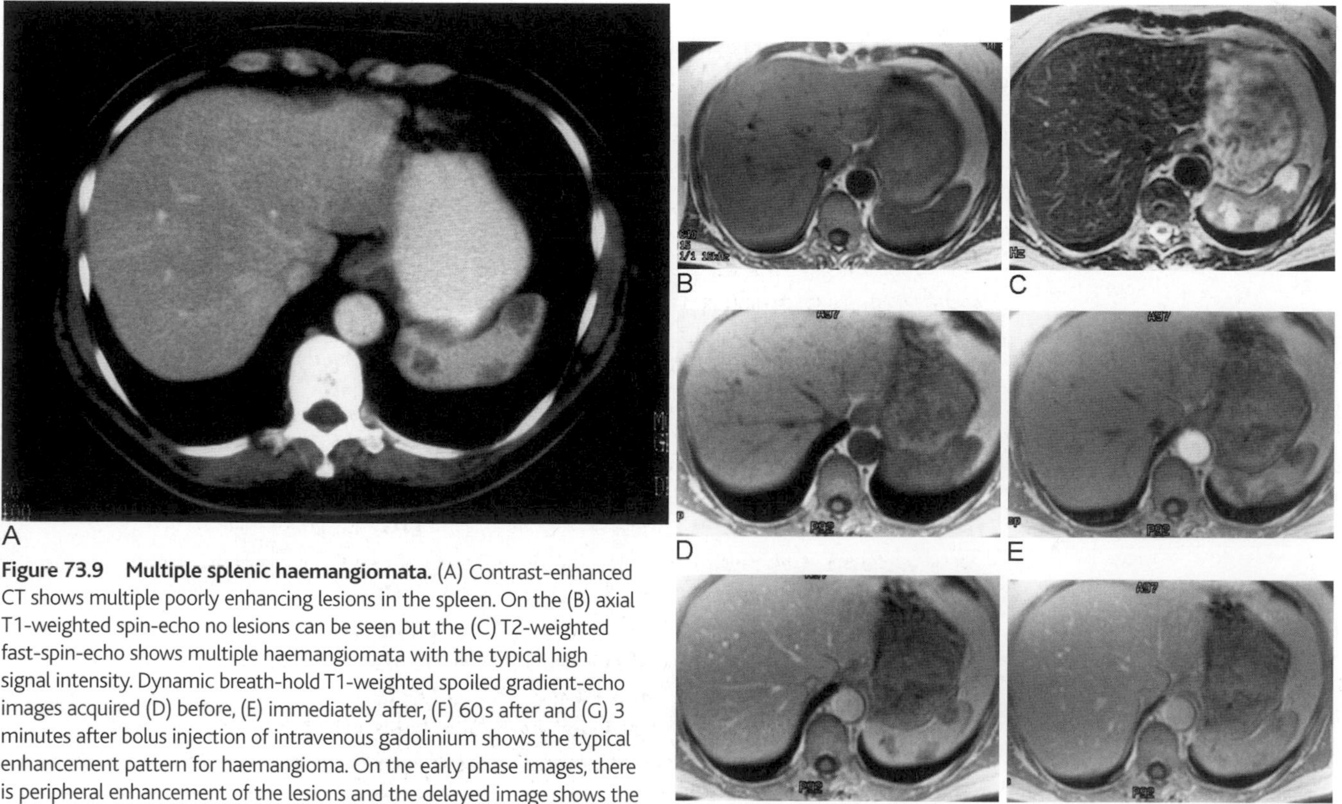

Figure 73.9 Multiple splenic haemangiomata. (A) Contrast-enhanced CT shows multiple poorly enhancing lesions in the spleen. On the (B) axial T1-weighted spin-echo no lesions can be seen but the (C) T2-weighted fast-spin-echo shows multiple haemangiomata with the typical high signal intensity. Dynamic breath-hold T1-weighted spoiled gradient-echo images acquired (D) before, (E) immediately after, (F) 60 s after and (G) 3 minutes after bolus injection of intravenous gadolinium shows the typical enhancement pattern for haemangioma. On the early phase images, there is peripheral enhancement of the lesions and the delayed image shows the haemangioma to be isointense to the rest of the spleen.

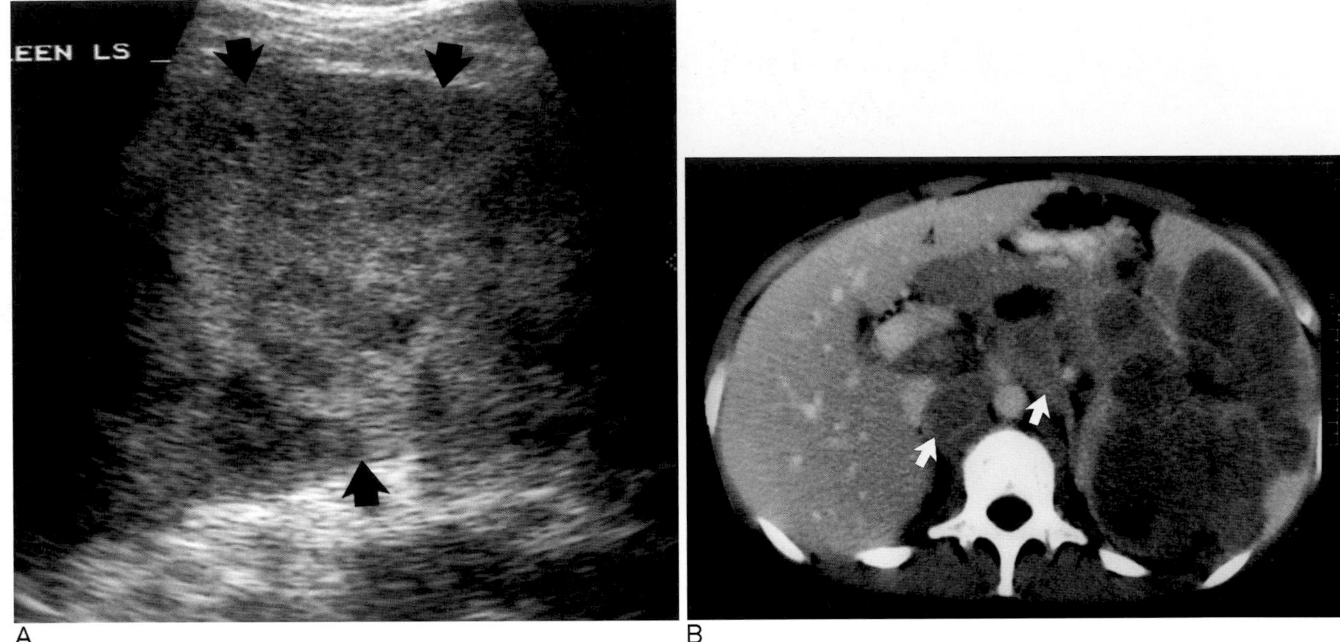

Figure 73.10 Lymphoma. (A) Ultrasound and (B) contrast-enhanced CT in a patient with non-Hodgkin's lymphoma involving the spleen. The ultrasound shows a large spleen (arrows) with multiple, poorly defined hypoechoic lesions. On the CT, enlarged intra-abdominal lymph nodes (arrows) can also be seen.

Splenic involvement may either be due to surface disease from peritoneal spread of cancer or parenchymal disease from haematogenous spread.

Parenchymal splenic metastases most frequently appear as multiple nodules. On CT, nodular metastases appear as rounded hypodense lesions (Fig. 73.12). Cystic lesions may occur with metastases from ovary (Fig. 73.13), breast, endometrium and skin (melanoma). Calcification is uncommon but occurs typically in patients with a mucinous adenocarcinoma primary. Peritoneal implants in patients with ovarian, gastrointestinal, or pancreatic cancer can cause scalloping of the splenic capsular surface.

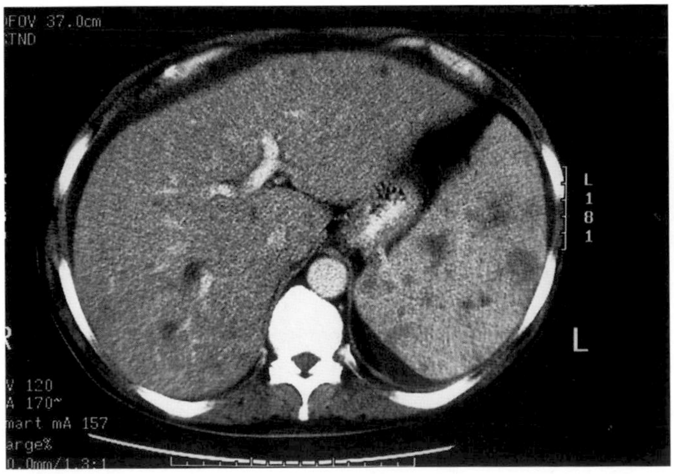

Figure 73.11 Lymphoma. Contrast-enhanced CT in a patient with non-Hodgkin's lymphoma involving the liver and spleen. Multiple small poorly defined nodules can be seen in both liver and spleen. A trace of ascites can also be seen anterior to the liver.

SPLENIC INFECTION

Splenic infection is uncommon and in 70% of cases is the result of haematogenous spread from primary infection elsewhere. Endocarditis is the most common cause; others include urinary tract infection, wound infection, appendicitis and pneumonia. Abscesses are present in other organs in 15–20% of patients with splenic abscess[26]. Direct spread of infection from adjacent organs may also occur. Noninfectious predisposing factors include diabetes, immunosuppression, sickle-cell disease, splenic injury and infarction.

Bacterial splenic abscess is most commonly due to staphylococci, streptococci, or salmonella. On US, splenic abscesses have a variable appearance: they may be hypoechoic

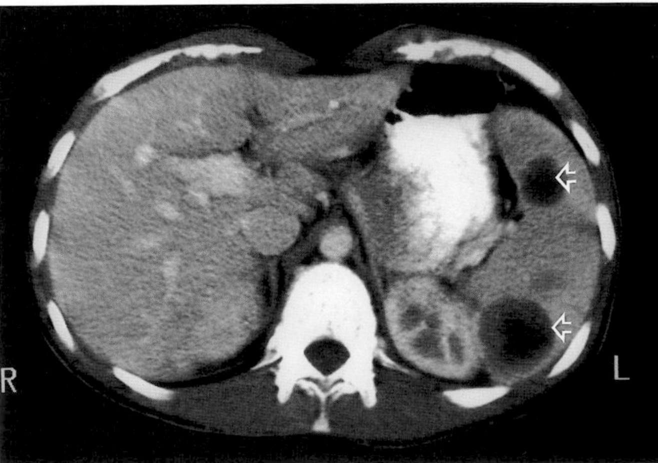

Figure 73.12 Splenic metastases. Contrast-enhanced CT showing multiple deposits (arrows) from malignant melanoma.

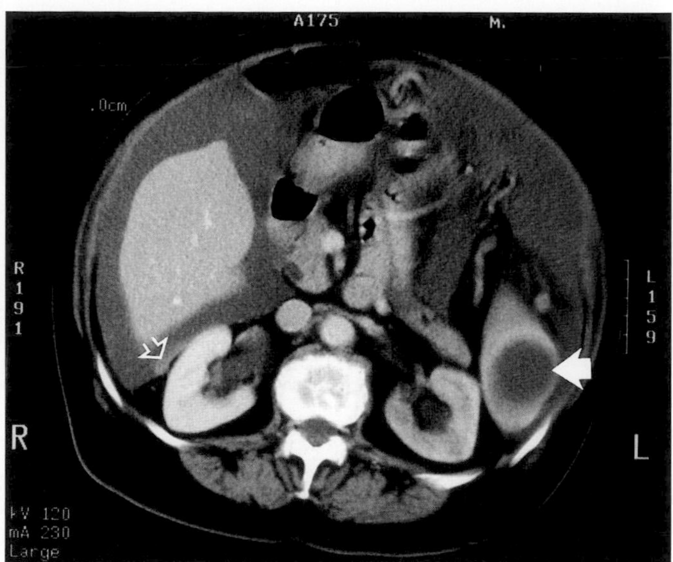

Figure 73.13 Cystic splenic metastasis. Contrast-enhanced CT shows a cystic splenic metastasis (arrow) in a patient with advanced ovarian cancer. There are also peritoneal deposits (open arrow) and malignant ascites present.

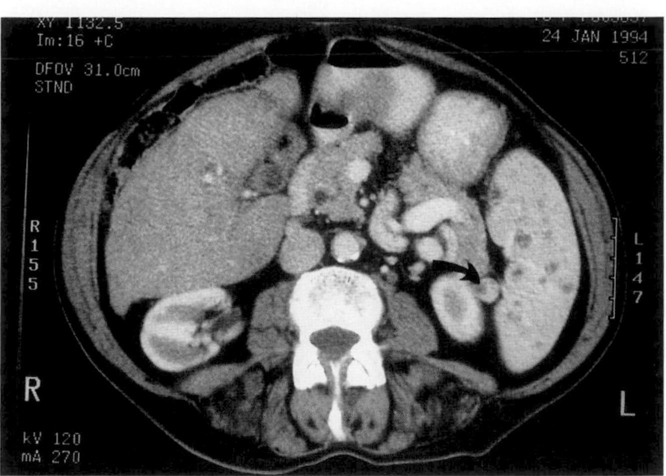

Figure 73.14 Splenic candidiasis. Contrast-enhanced CT shows multiple tiny hypodense lesions in the spleen from candidal microabscess. A small accessory spleen (curved arrow) at the splenic hilum is also involved.

or cystic with an irregular wall containing debris, septation and air bubbles. On CT, splenic abscesses appear as spherical or slightly lobulated non-enhancing areas of low attenuation. The rim is often of equal attenuation to the surrounding spleen but an enhancing capsule may be seen. Gas is present in only a small number of splenic abscesses. The use of CT or US-guided drainage is becoming an acceptable alternative to splenectomy[27].

Infection of the spleen with *Mycobacterium tuberculosis* usually occurs in a miliary form by haematogenous dissemination. Miliary tuberculosis may appear as irregular areas of low attenuation. Often there is mild splenomegaly, and infarcts from septic emboli may be present. Other evidence of intra-abdominal tuberculosis may be present, such as lymphadenopathy, high attenuation ascites on CT, peritoneal thickening, or hepatomegaly. Evolution of the splenic lesions ultimately gives rise to healed calcified granuloma often incidentally noted on CT.

With increasing prevalence of immunosuppression, fungal infection is becoming more common. The most common pathogens are candida, aspergillus and cryptococcus[28]. Fungal infection in the spleen is most likely to appear as a miliary or multifocal process. On CT, hepatosplenic candidiasis (Fig. 73.14) may appear as multiple rounded areas of decreased attenuation producing a "bull's-eye" lesion with hypoattenuating foci and a central core of higher attenuation; or as tiny 2–5 mm lesions of increased attenuation due to calcification. Calcification is seen in treated candida microabscesses and lesions caused by other fungi, especially histoplasma, mycobacteria and *Pneumocystis carinii*. Fungal abscesses in neutropenic patients are often small and not always detectable with any imaging technique.

Patients with acquired immune deficiency syndrome (AIDS) infrequently have fungal microabscesses seen in other immunocompromised patients. More often, several small hypoattenuating foci seen in the spleen are due to granulomas or abscesses caused by mycobacteria or *P. carinii*. On CT, this appears as splenomegaly with focal lesion and several scattered punctuate calcification. Calcification may occur before or after treatment.

SPLENIC TRAUMA

Splenic trauma may follow blunt or penetrating injuries and may be spontaneous or iatrogenic. The spleen is the most commonly injured organ in cases of blunt abdominal trauma. Ultrasound may be used to evaluate the abdomen and may show splenic injury (Fig. 73.15). However, CT is the investigation of choice for the evaluation and delineation of the extent of splenic injury. Intravenous administration of contrast material is needed for adequate evaluation of splenic trauma as areas of haematoma and laceration may be isodense to splenic parenchyma on non-contrast-enhanced CT. Injury to the spleen can take the form of laceration, intrasplenic haematoma, subcapsular haematoma, or infarction. Splenic laceration appears as an irregular linear area of hypodensity on contrast-enhanced CT (Fig. 73.16); intrasplenic haematoma as a hypodense area of nonperfused spleen on the contrast-enhanced CT; a subcapsular haematoma as a crescentic collection of fluid that distorts the underlying spleen. A congenital splenic cleft may mimic laceration, but typically these are smooth and there is no perisplenic blood. A decrease in the overall splenic enhancement to less than that of the liver has been noted in traumatized hypotensive patients and should not be misinterpreted as representing splenic vascular injury. Haemoperitoneum almost always accompanies significant splenic injury. If there is significant intra-abdominal fluid, the presence of local perisplenic clot (i.e., a 'sentinel clot') suggests splenic injury as the site of bleeding. This sentinel clot has a homogeneous appearance with an attenuation coefficient greater than 60 HU[29]. Perisplenic haematoma may have

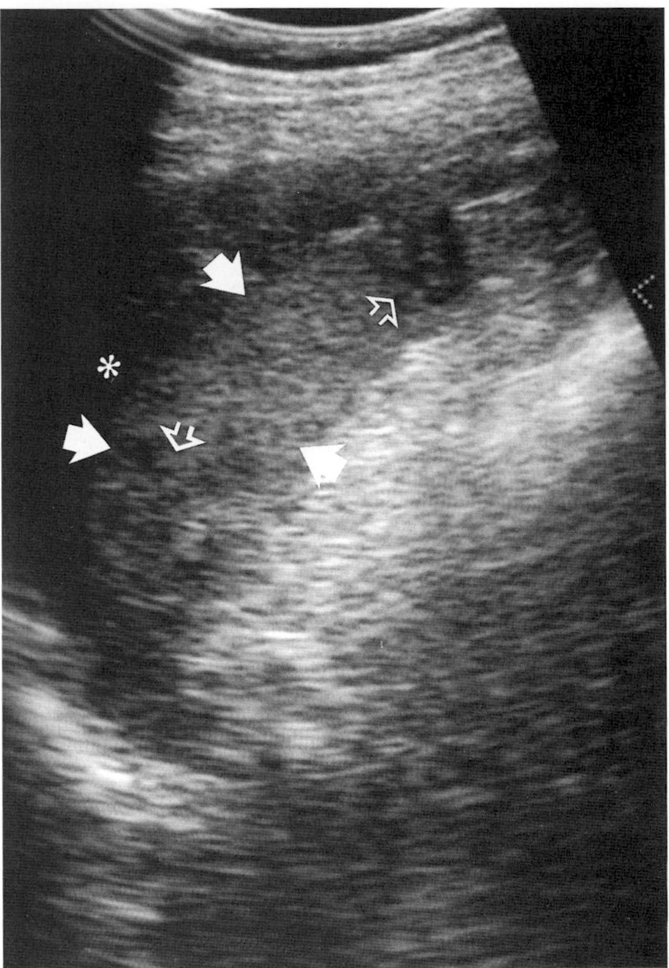

Figure 73.15 Splenic injury. A longitudinal ultrasound showing splenic lacerations (open arrows) and perisplenic fluid/haematoma (asterisks) around the spleen (arrows). (Courtesy of Dr J.A.W. Webb.)

a multilayered or 'onion skin' appearance if there are repeated episodes of bleeding. Pseudoaneurysm formation can occur following trauma, which appears as a focal well-circumscribed area of vascular enhancement within the splenic parenchyma.

Several CT grading systems have been devised in an attempt to identify patients with splenic trauma who may undergo successful nonsurgical treatment[30,31]. Recent studies have shown that although CT is an accurate means of evaluating splenic injury it cannot be used to reliably determine the need for surgical intervention or to predict clinical outcome[31,32].

Delayed splenic rupture—i.e., haemorrhage from splenic rupture occurring more than 48 hours after trauma—may occur in a few patients in whom the initial CT was normal[32]. This may be genuinely delayed and secondary to a splenic fracture in which there is little initial haemorrhage. Alternatively, poor contrast opacification of the spleen, rendering the haematoma isodense with splenic parenchyma on images acquired soon after trauma, may result in splenic trauma being unidentified if unenhanced images were not obtained[32].

CT may be used to monitor healing of splenic injury, as documented by progressive diminution of perisplenic and intrasplenic haematoma or laceration. Progressive enlargement on serial CT is not an indicator of clinical deterioration. It is likely that, in acutely injured patients, the spleen contracts secondary to intravascular volume depletion and sympathetic drive. With time and volume replacement the spleen returns to normal size.

Splenosis

Splenosis represents the heterotopic autotransplantation of splenic tissue that usually follows traumatic rupture of the splenic capsule. The splenic remnant implants on the serosal surfaces of the abdomen and chest, derives its blood supply from surrounding tissues, and is indistinguishable from normal spleen histologically. The radiological diagnosis of splenosis requires awareness of the condition and a history of splenic trauma. Imaging may show one or several homogeneous, solid, well-circumscribed, noncalcified soft tissue nodules. The splenules have a variable shape, are poorly marginated and are closely related to the tissue from which they receive their blood supply. ^{99m}Tc-sulphur colloid or ^{99m}Tc-labelled heat denatured erythrocytes show uptake in splenic tissue and may be used to diagnose splenosis[33]. MRI

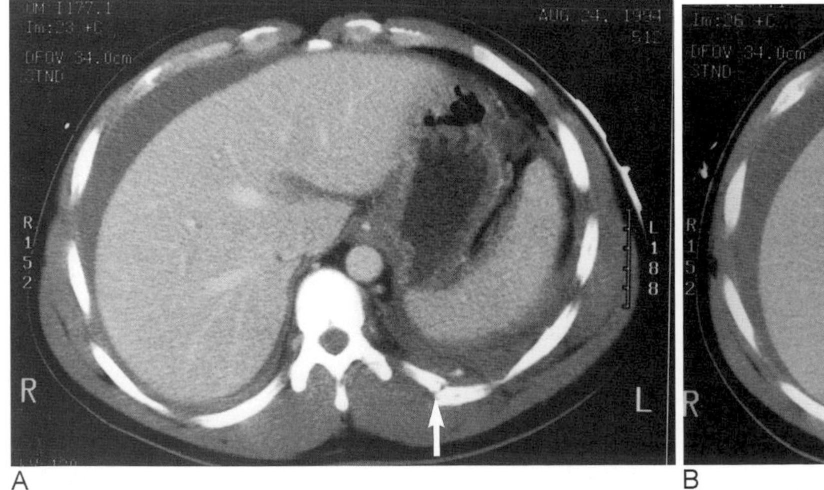

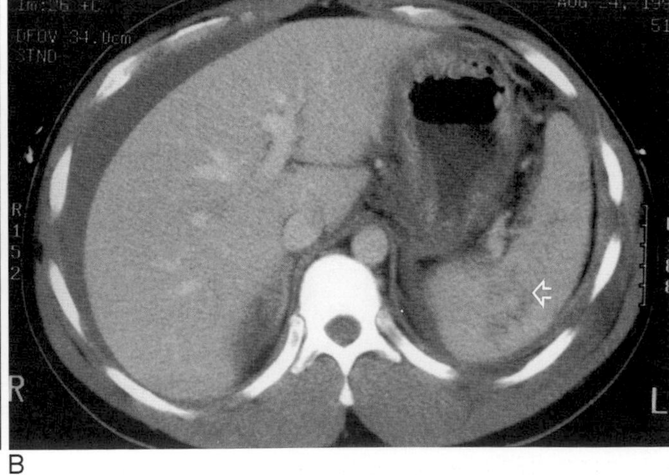

Figure 73.16 Splenic injury. Contrast-enhanced CT in a man who fell from a ladder. (A)There is fracture of the left 10th rib (arrow) with perisplenic fluid and ascites. (B) Splenic laceration (open arrow) was also identified on CT.

with supramagnetic iron-oxide particles has also been used to diagnose splenosis[34]

OTHER SPLENIC DISORDERS

Splenic infarcts may occur from embolic disease, atherosclerosis, arteritis, splenic artery aneurysm, sickle-cell disease, or mass lesion compressing splenic vasculature, e.g., pancreatic masses. Splenic infarction may be diffuse or focal. On CT, infarcts typically appear as sharply marginated, low-density wedge-shaped areas (Fig. 73.17). Occasionally infarcts may be multiple, resulting in poorly defined hypodense lesions. When the entire spleen is infarcted, only rim enhancement of the capsule occurs from capsular vessels[3]. Splenic infarction can also been seen on MRI, and haemorrhagic infarcts have a high signal on T1- and T2-weighted images.

Splenic sarcoidosis is usually asymptomatic, and the spleen may be involved in up to 60% of patients. The presentation and appearance of the spleen may mimic lymphoma. Imaging findings include splenomegaly, hypodense nodules in the spleen on CT, and coexistent lymphadenopathy. The chest radiograph may be normal in 25% of patients with splenomegaly or discrete nodules in the spleen[35].

Iron deposition in the reticuloendothelial system, haemosiderosis, may occur in patients receiving multiple blood transfusions and can sometimes be identified on CT by its increased attenuation. MRI is more sensitive than CT for demonstrating iron deposition. The paramagnetic properties of deposited iron results in diffuse diminished signal intensity of the spleen relative to the musculature on T1- and T2-weighted images (Fig. 73.18).

Splenic involvement in amyloidosis may be nodular or diffuse[36]. The nodular form involves the lymphoid follicle, and appears on CT as discrete low-attenuation masses within an enlarged spleen. In the diffuse form, with infiltration of the red pulp, the spleen is of low attenuation with poor contrast enhancement. Spontaneous splenic rupture may occur due to vascular fragility and acquired coagulopathy associated with amyloidosis. On MRI, low signal intensity in the spleen has been noted on T2-weighted images[37].

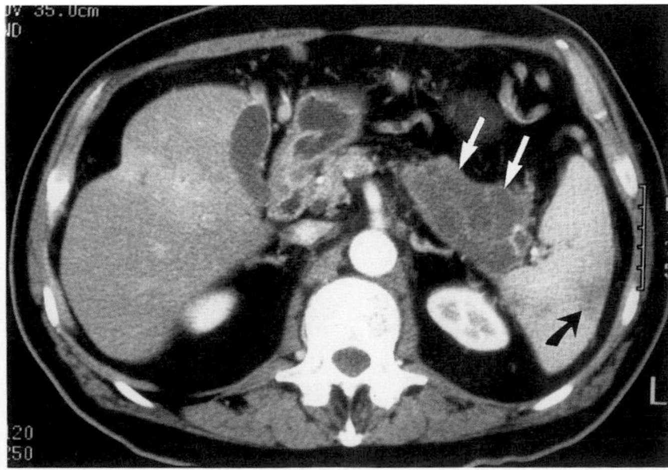

Figure 73.17 Splenic infarct. Contrast-enhanced CT shows a tumour mass (arrows) in the tail of the pancreas is causing occlusion to the splenic vein and a splenic infarct (black arrow)

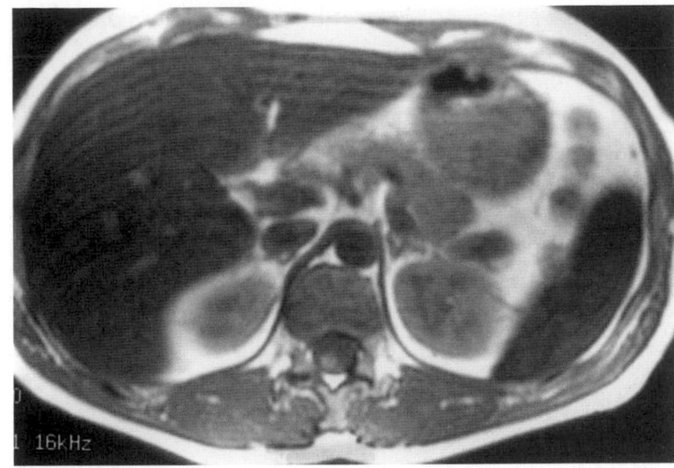
A

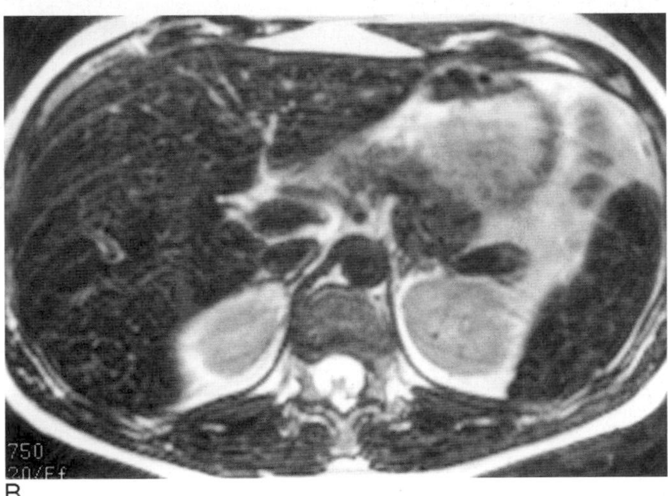
B

Figure 73.18 Haemosiderosis. Axial (A) T1-weighted spin-echo and (B) T2-weighted fast-spin-echo images show the very low signal intensity of the liver and spleen with respect to the skeletal muscle due to iron deposition in a patient with leukaemia who has had multiple blood transfusions.

In sickle-cell anaemia the appearance of the spleen depends on the duration of the disease and whether the patient has the homozygous (sickle-cell disease) or the heterozygous (sickle-cell trait) form of the condition. Disease complications will also alter the appearance of the spleen. Splenic infarction is common in both forms of sickle-cell anaemia. Repeated infarction in sickle-cell anaemia eventually results in a shrunken spleen containing diffuse microscopic deposits of calcium and iron. Acute splenic sequestration is a common complication of sickle-cell disease during childhood and may occur in the heterozygous form of the condition at any age. It results from sudden trapping of a large amount of blood in the spleen, resulting in splenic enlargement and a rapid decrease in haematocrit. On CT, the spleen is enlarged with peripheral low-attenuation regions from infarcts interspersed with higher attenuation areas from haemorrhage and pooling of blood. MRI shows the corresponding changes due to infarction and haemorrhage. Functional asplenia occurs in sickle-cell anaemia and may be indicated by the absence of tracer uptake on a ^{99m}Tc-sulphur colloid scintigraphy. Deposition of iron (haemosiderois) and calcium in sickle-cell anaemia results in an echogenic spleen on US, high attenuation on CT and low signal intensity on T1- and T2-weighted MRI.

ACKNOWLEDGEMENTS

We would like to thanks Mrs Julie Jessop for help with the manuscript preparations.

REFERENCES

1. Peddu P, Shah M, Sidhu P S 2004 Splenic abnormalities: a comparative review of ultrasound, microbubble-enhanced ultrasound and computed tomography. Clin Radiol 59: 777–792
2. Lucey B C, Boland G W, Maher M M, Hahn P F, Gervais D A, Mueller P R 2002 Percutaneous nonvascular splenic intervention: a 10-year review. Am J Roentgenol 179: 1591–1596.
3. Warshauer D M, Koehler R E 1998 Spleen. In: Lee J K, Sagel S S, Stanley R J, Heiken J P (eds) CT with MRI Correlation. Lippencott-Raven, Philadelphia, 845–872
4. Prassopoulos P, Daskalogiannaki M, Raissaki M, Hatjidakis A, Gourtsoyiannis N 1997 Determination of normal splenic volume on computed tomography in relation to age, gender and body habitus. Eur Radiol 7: 246–248
5. Whitley J E, Maynard C D, Rhyne A L 1966 A computer approach to the prediction of spleen weight from routine films. Radiology 86: 73–76
6. Dardenne A N 1993 The Spleen. In: Cosgrove D O, Meire H B, Dewbury K C D (eds) Clinical Ultrasound. Churchill Livingstone, Edinburgh, 353–365
7. Lamb P M, Lund A, Kanagasabay R R, Martin A, Webb J A, Reznek R H 2002 Spleen size: how well do linear ultrasound measurements correlate with three-dimensional CT volume assessments? Br J Radiol 75: 573–577
8. Strijk S P, Wagener D J, Bogman M J, de Pauw B E, Wobbes T 1985 The spleen in Hodgkin disease: diagnostic value of CT. Radiology 154: 753–757
9. Carragher A M 1990 One hundred years of splenogonadal fusion. Urology 35: 47175.
10. Younger K A, Hall C M 1990 Epidermoid cyst of the spleen: a case report and review of the literature. Br J Radiol 63:652–653
11. Dawes L G, Malangoni M A 1986 Cystic masses of the spleen. Am Surg 52: 333–336
12. Rabushka L S, Kawashima A, Fishman E K 1994 Imaging of the spleen: CT with supplemental MR examination. Radiographics 14:307–332
13. Duddy M J, Calder C J 1989 Cystic haemangioma of the spleen: findings on ultrasound and computed tomography. Br J Radiol 62:180–182
14. Ros P R, Moser R P J, Dachman A H, Murari P J, Olmsted W W 1987 Hemangioma of the spleen: radiologic-pathologic correlation in ten cases. Radiology 162: 73–77
15. Mortelé K J, Merjo P J, Kunnen M 2000 Tumoral pathology of the spleen. In: DeSchepper A M, Vanhoenacker F (eds) Medical Imaging of the Spleen. Spinger-Verlag, Berlin, pp 101–123
16. Pistoia F, Markowitz S K 1988 Splenic lymphangiomatosis: CT diagnosis. Am J Roentgenol 150: 121–122
17. Dachman A H, Friedman A C 1993 Radiology of the Spleen. Mosby-Year Book Inc, St Louis
18. Norowitz D G, Morehouse H T 1989 Isodense splenic mass: hamartoma, a case report. Comput Med Imaging Graph 13:347–350
19. Ohtomo K, Fukuda H, Mori K, Minami M, Itai Y, Inoue Y 1992 CT and MR appearances of splenic hamartoma. J Comput Assist Tomogr 16: 425–428
20. Long J C, Aisenberg A C 1974 Malignant lymphoma diagnosed at splenectomy and idiopathic splenomegaly. A clinicopathologic comparison. Cancer 33: 1054–1061
21. Castellino R A 1986 Hodgkin disease: practical concepts for the diagnostic radiologist. Radiology 159: 305–310
22. Harris N L, Aisenberg A C, Meyer J E, Ellman L, Elman A 1984 Diffuse large cell (histiocytic) lymphoma of the spleen. Clinical and pathologic characteristics of ten cases. Cancer 54: 2460–2467
23. Marti-Bonmati L, Ballesta A, Chirivella M 1989 Unusual presentation of non-Hodgkin lymphoma of the spleen. Can Assoc Radiol J 40: 49–50
24. Mahony B, Jeffrey R B, Federle M P 1982 Spontaneous rupture of hepatic and splenic angiosarcoma demonstrated by CT. Am J Roentgenol 138: 965–966
25. Lam K Y, Tang V 2000 Metastatic tumors to the spleen: a 25-year clinicopathologic study. Arch Pathol Lab Med 124: 526–530
26. Tikkakoski T, Siniluoto T, Paivansalo M, et al 1992 Splenic abscess. Imaging and intervention. Acta Radiol 33: 561–565
27. Thanos L, Dailiana T, Papaioannou G, Nikita A, Koutrouvelis H, Kelekis D A 2002 Percutaneous CT-guided drainage of splenic abscess. Am J Roentgenol 179: 629–632
28. Chew F S, Smith P L, Barboriak D 1991 Candidal splenic abscesses. AJR Am J Roentgenol 156: 474
29. Orwig D, Federle M P 1989 Localized clotted blood as evidence of visceral trauma on CT: the sentinel clot sign. Am J Roentgenol 153: 747–749
30. Buntain W L, Gould H R, Maull K I 1988 Predictability of splenic salvage by computed tomography. J Trauma 28: 24–34
31. Mirvis S E, Whitley N O, Gens D R 1989 Blunt splenic trauma in adults: CT-based classification and correlation with prognosis and treatment. Radiology 171: 33–39
32. Umlas S L, Cronan J J 1991 Splenic trauma: can CT grading systems enable prediction of successful nonsurgical treatment? Radiology 178: 481–487
33. Gunes I, Yilmazlar T, Sarikaya I, Akbunar T, Irgil C 1994 Scintigraphic detection of splenosis: superiority of tomographic selective spleen scintigraphy. Clin Radiol 49: 115–117
34. Storm B L, Abbitt P L, Allen D A, Ros P R 1992 Splenosis: superparamagnetic iron oxide-enhanced MR imaging. Am J Roentgenol 159: 333–335
35. Warshauer D M, Dumbleton S A, Molina P L, Yankaskas B C, Parker L A, Woosley J T 1994 Abdominal CT findings in sarcoidosis: radiologic and clinical correlation. Radiology 192: 93–98
36. Kozicky O J, Brandt L J, Lederman M, Milcu M 1987 Splenic amyloidosis: a case report of spontaneous splenic rupture with a review of the pertinent literature. Am J Gastroenterol 82: 582–587
37. Rafal R B, Jennis R, Kosovsky P A, Markisz J A 1990 MRI of primary amyloidosis. Gastrointest Radiol 15: 199–201

FURTHER READING

Dachman A H, Friedman A C 1993 Radiology of the Spleen. St Louis, Mosby-Year Book Inc

DeSchepper A M, Vanhoenacker F 2000 Medical Imaging of the Spleen. Berlin, Spinger-Verlag

CHAPTER 74

Myeloproliferative and Similar Disorders

Dennis J. Stoker and Asif Saifuddin

- Red cell disorders
- White cell disorders
- Plasma cell dyscrasias
- Reticuloendothelial disorders
- Haemophilia and other disorders of blood coagulation; bleeding disorders

This chapter deals with disorders of proliferation of the bone marrow and allied conditions. In many respects these disorders are dissimilar, but they do not fit conveniently under any other heading or classification. Magnetic resonance imaging (MRI) is now the primary technique for imaging bone marrow disorders[1].

The cells of the bone marrow consist mainly of:

1 red cell precursors
2 white cell precursors
3 cells of the reticuloendothelial system
4 plasma cells
5 megakaryocytes.

Many of these cells are also found in other parts of the body.

The word 'reticuloses' has been avoided as an omnibus term for these disorders. The only disorder designated a 'reticulosis' (reticuloendotheliosis) is histiocytosis, a disease of unknown aetiology.

RED CELL DISORDERS

In late fetal life and infancy, the entire bone marrow is utilized for red blood cell (RBC) formation, supplemented by extramedullary erythropoiesis in the liver and spleen. As the child becomes older and RBC lifespan increases, erythropoiesis is withdrawn from the liver and spleen, then gradually from the diaphyses of the long bones, so that, by the age of 18–20 years, active bone marrow is confined to the axial skeleton, the flat bones and the proximal ends of the femora and humeri. This explains why metastases to bone preferentially involve these sites[2]. The process of withdrawal will not occur with a need for extra erythropoiesis and the process reverses in the presence of increased RBC destruction. Many of the features of normal marrow erythropoiesis have been categorized using MRI.

The anaemias

Only chronic anaemias affect the radiographic appearances of bone. Anaemias that do not produce reactive erythropoiesis (e.g., aplastic anaemia) do not affect the skeletal radiograph.

The more severe and prolonged the anaemia, the greater the bony change. The haemolytic anaemias are the most severe anaemias.

CHRONIC HAEMOLYTIC ANAEMIAS—THE HAEMOGLOBINOPATHIES

The haemoglobin molecule consists of a protein (globin) and four haem groups, each with four pyrole rings surrounding an iron atom. The protein moiety consists of 574 amino acids arranged in four spiral polypeptide chains. The different chains are designated by letters of the Greek alphabet (α, β) and the three normal haemoglobins (Hbs) A, A_2 and F each contain two α chains, differing only in their second pairs.

Three types of haemoglobinopathy are found:

1 Thalassaemias—inherited defects of Hb A synthesis with inadequate manufacture of α- or β-chains.
2 Haemoglobin variants—inherited defects of Hb A synthesis producing abnormal α- or β-chains. All the variants differ from Hb A by the substitution of only one amino acid in the chain, e.g. Hb S (sickle-cell anaemia) where valine is substituted for glutamine at residue 6 in the β-chain.
3 Combination of thalassaemia and abnormal haemoglobin, e.g. Hb S-thalassaemia.

Thalassaemia

Beta-thalassaemia is prevalent in Europe and the Near East, while α-thalassaemia is encountered in the Far East. Alpha-thalassaemia is less easily detected haematologically and its incidence may be higher than generally accepted. Varieties unique to Southeast Asians include haemoglobin H disease (a severe form of α-thalassaemia) and Hb E/β-thalassaemia. In African-Americans, both the thalassaemia traits are common but symptomatic thalassaemia is rare.

Thalassaemia is transmitted by an autosomal dominant gene and exists in two forms—homozygous (thalassaemia major) and heterozygous (thalassaemia minor and thalassaemia minima). In β-thalassaemia, the low level of Hb A is partially supplemented by fetal haemoglobin (Hb F) and Hb A_2, whilst in α-thalassaemia, Hb H is formed of four β chains. None of these substitute haemoglobins is as effective an oxygen carrier as Hb A and neither are the cells containing them as long-lived; hence the need for erythroid hyperplasia.

Clinical features

Thalassaemia major causes a severe anaemia in infants and young children, with a high mortality. Bone changes produce a rodent-like facies and hepatosplenomegaly is the rule. In later childhood, cardiac enlargement mirrors the degree of anaemia. Physical retardation is present in severe cases, with severely affected children dying in infancy.

Homozygous α-thalassaemia, due to both parents transmitting the abnormal gene, is a major cause of hydrops fetalis in the Far East[3].

Radiological features[4]

In children, the medulla enlarges relative to the cortex, leading to bony expansion and cortical thinning. In long bones, this results in the characteristic Erlenmeyer flask appearance, also found in conditions such as Gaucher's disease. Within the medulla, trabecular thinning initially occurs, followed by trabecular coarsening due to new bone formation, the changes being most marked in the metacarpals and phalanges (Fig. 74.1), which become cylindrical or even biconvex. The ribs are similarly affected with club-like anterior ends. A 'rib-within-a-rib' appearance may also be seen due to subperiosteal extension of haemopoietic tissue through the rib cortex. This typically occurs in the mid and anterior portions of the ribs (Figure 74.2A).

Extramedullary erythropoiesis occurs in severe cases surviving to adulthood, the most common sites being the thoracic paravertebral region by extension from the adjacent ribs (Figure 74.2B), the mediastinum and presacral region. Epidural extension from paraspinal extramedullary erythropoiesis may result in spinal cord compression. These features are optimally demonstrated by MRI, which also demonstrates diffuse reduction in marrow signal intensity (SI) on T1-weighted (T1W) images due to marrow reconversion (Fig.74.3).

With severe childhood disease, the paranasal sinuses develop poorly and often contain red marrow, accounting for the facial abnormalities and dental malocclusion. The ethmoid cells are spared since they contain no red marrow. The

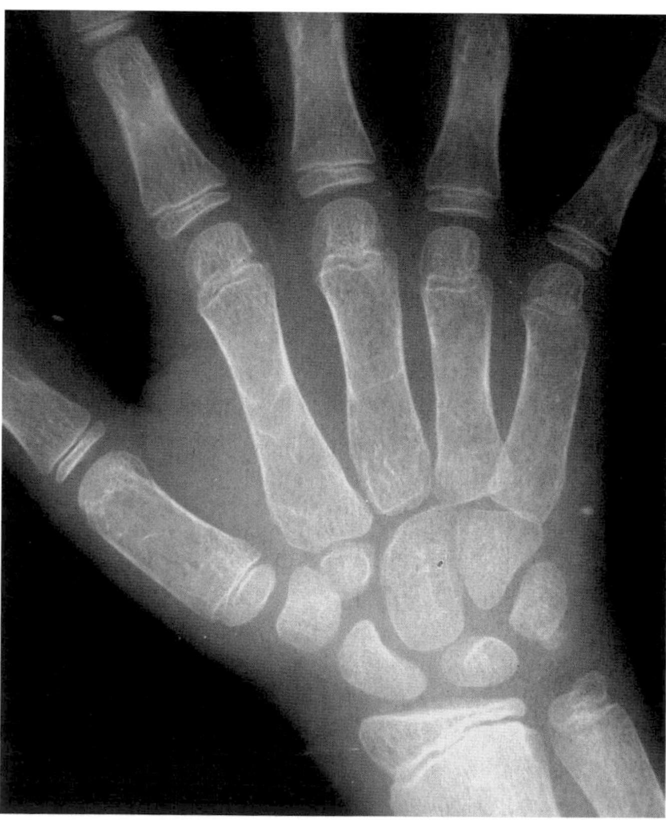

Figure 74.1 Thalassaemia. Hand showing osteopenia with thinning of the cortices, loss of tubulation and a coarsened medullary pattern.

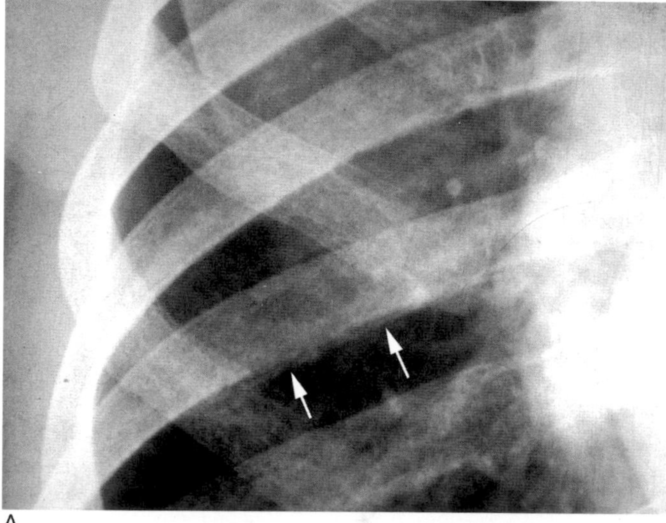

A

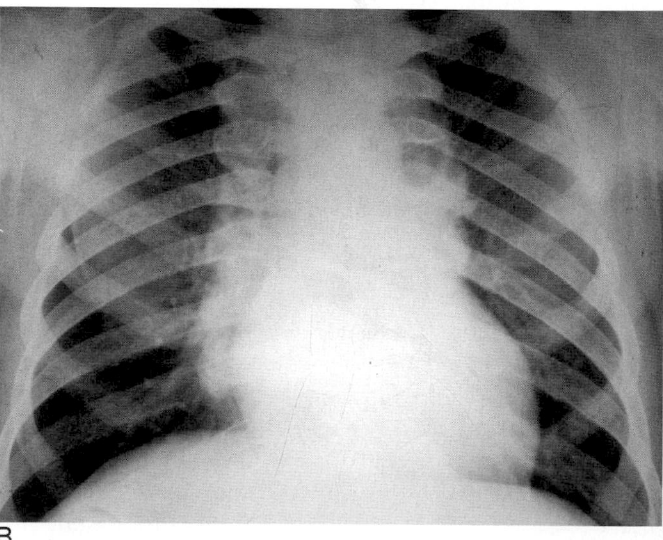

B

Figure 74.2 Thalassaemia. (A) The ribs appear mildly expanded with periostitis producing a bone-within-a-bone appearance (arrows). (B) Chest radiograph showing generalized osteopenia and massive paraspinal widening due to extramedullary erythropoiesis.

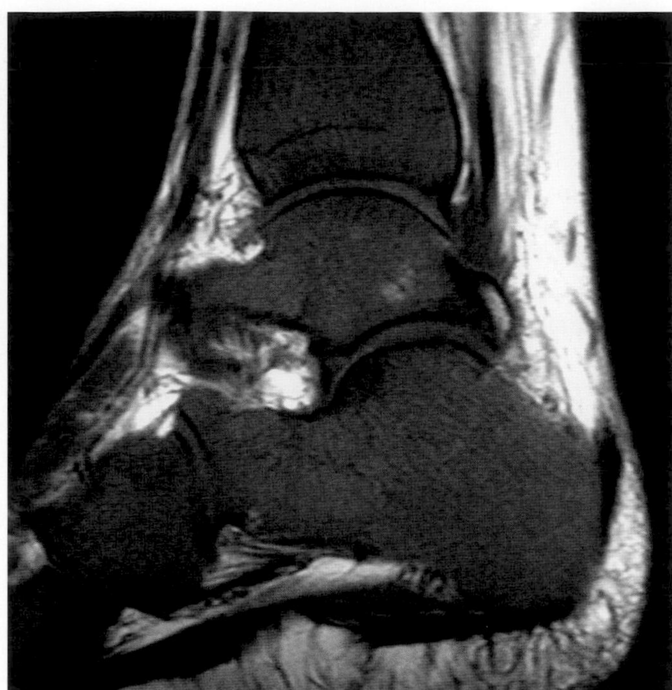

Figure 74.3 Thalassaemia. Sagittal T1-weighted spin-echo MRI of the ankle showing diffuse reduction of marrow signal intensity due to reconversion.

diploë of the skull vault are widened except in the occiput. These changes occur earliest and most severely in the frontal bone producing the classical 'hair-on-end' appearance (Figure 74.4). Spinal changes consist of generalized osteopenia, resulting in compression fractures and biconcavity of the vertebral bodies. Scoliosis occurs in over 50% of children with thalassaemia major, while platyspondyly is reported as a side effect of hypertransfusion.

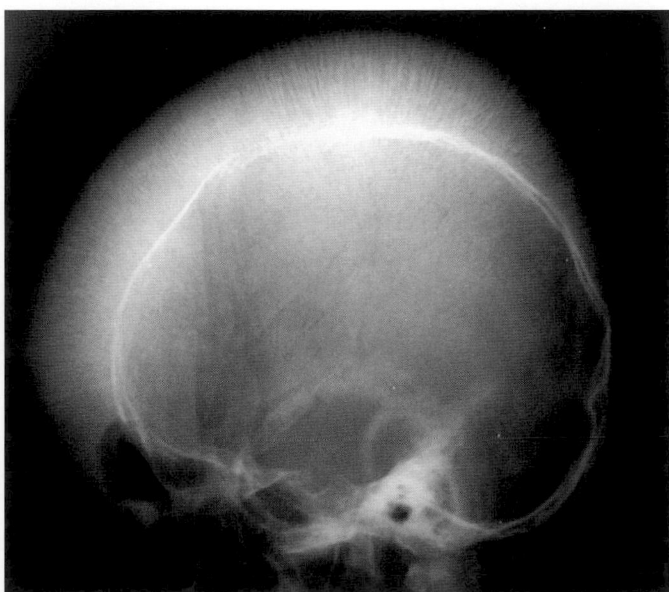

Figure 74.4 Thalassaemia. Lateral radiograph of the skull showing gross expansion of the diploë and loss of definition of the outer table with sparing of the occipital bone. A gross 'hair-on-end' appearance is shown.

Premature fusion of the growth plates may contribute to short stature. These radiological changes are reported in 10–15% of patients, generally occur after 10 years of age and most commonly affect the proximal humerus and distal femur. Desferoxamine therapy may also result in morphological changes in the long bone metaphyses.

In thalassaemia minor and thalassaemic variants, only widespread osteopenia is seen. Transfusion therapy may prevent most of these skeletal changes if instituted in early childhood but may result in iron overload. Quantitative MRI is an accurate noninvasive method for assessing hepatic iron concentration, reducing the need for liver biopsy.

Problems in older age include cardiomegaly, rickets, spinal deformities, neural compression, fractures and severe osteopenia.

Sickle-cell disease[5]

The clinical findings in sickle-cell disease (SCD) are explained by the physical properties of the abnormal haemoglobin. When oxygen tension falls and Hb S is converted to its reduced form, its low solubility produces semicrystalline tactoids, which distort the cell membrane into a sickle shape. Sickle cells are mechanically fragile and show an abnormal metabolism. They are removed from the circulation by the reticuloendothelial system and hence have a short circulating life. Sickle cells obstruct small blood vessels, leading to stasis and tissue hypoxia/anoxia.

The full clinical and radiological picture occurs in the homozygous sickle-cell subject (Hb S-S). When only one parent carries the abnormal gene, the sickle-cell trait (Hb S-A) occurs, without anaemia but with sickling to a lesser degree.

Clinical features

Sickle-cell disease affects people of African racial origin and approximately 8–10% of black Americans have sickle cell trait but only 0.2% have sickle cell anaemia. The anaemia of SCD is not as marked as in thalassaemia major. Cardiomegaly is present in 80% of homozygous cases and heart failure may occur due to the anaemia, obliterative pulmonary vascular disease, or ischaemic heart disease. Hepatomegaly and pigment gallstones are common, although splenomegaly is infrequent after the age of 10 years due to repeated splenic infarction. Most patients with homozygous SCD die by the age of 50 years.

The most striking clinical features are due to vaso-occlusive sickle crises, which result in infarctions. Rib or sternal infarcts may simulate heart or lung disease. Abdominal crises mimic an acute abdomen. Soft tissue involvement results in ulcers and muscle infarction, which are well demonstrated by MRI.

Sickle variants show less anaemia with fewer crises. However, bone infarction, especially of the femoral head, affects patients with Hb S-C disease five times more often than those with Hb S-S, although the overall prevalence of Hb S-C is only one third that of the homozygous disease. This may reflect the longer survival in Hb S-C disease.

In sickle-cell trait (Hb S-A), significant anaemia and bone infarction are rare. However, infarction of the spleen and renal papillary necrosis do occur.

Radiological features[6]

The changes in SCD and its variants are similar, varying only in degree. Changes can be divided into those due to marrow hyperplasia, bone infarction and secondary osteomyelitis.

Marrow hyperplasia This is more severe in the homozygous disease. As in thalassaemia major, osteopenia occurs with initial cortical and trabecular thinning, although bony modelling defects are less common. In two thirds of patients with SCD, the vertebrae become biconcave as the intervertebral discs compress the vertebral end plates.

The diploic space of the skull is widened and, although development of the paranasal sinuses is usually normal, maxillary enlargement with dental protrusion has been reported. The outer table of the skull is thinned, but a 'hair-on-end' appearance is infrequent. Marrow reconversion is well demonstrated by MRI, with replacement of normal fatty marrow by intermediate SI on T1W images.

Bone infarction This is estimated to be at least 50 times more common than osteomyelitis in SCD. In children, bone infarction occurs most frequently in the hands and feet resulting in destructive lesions with associated periostitis and soft tissue swelling (Figure 74.5). The resulting dactylitis is termed 'hand–foot syndrome' and typically occurs before the age of 4 years and rarely after the age of 7 years. In adolescents and adults, infarction occurs more in the metaphyses and epiphyses. The earliest radiological evidence of bone infarction is laminar periosteal reaction followed by patchy medullary destruction. Healing leads to reactive sclerosis. MRI shows medullary oedema on T2-weighted (T2W) and short tau inversion recovery (STIR) sequences with associated periostitis and adjacent soft tissue inflammation, making differentiation from osteomyelitis difficult. With healing, these areas assume a low SI due to fibrosis and medullary sclerosis.

Infarction of the vertebral body occurs in approximately 10% of patients and is usually due to venous thromboembolism in the central part of the vertebral end plate, with collapse producing a stepped depression (Figure 74.6). The floor of the depression forms a flat sclerotic margin during healing. This appearance is almost pathognomonic of SCD but has also been reported in Gaucher's disease. Overgrowth of an adjacent vertebral body producing a so-called 'tower' vertebra is also reported.

Diaphyseal infarctions are also common, with localized metadiaphyseal osteolysis and periosteal reaction in the older child and young adult. Infarction of the metaphyses on either side of the knee is common and may lead to premature fusion

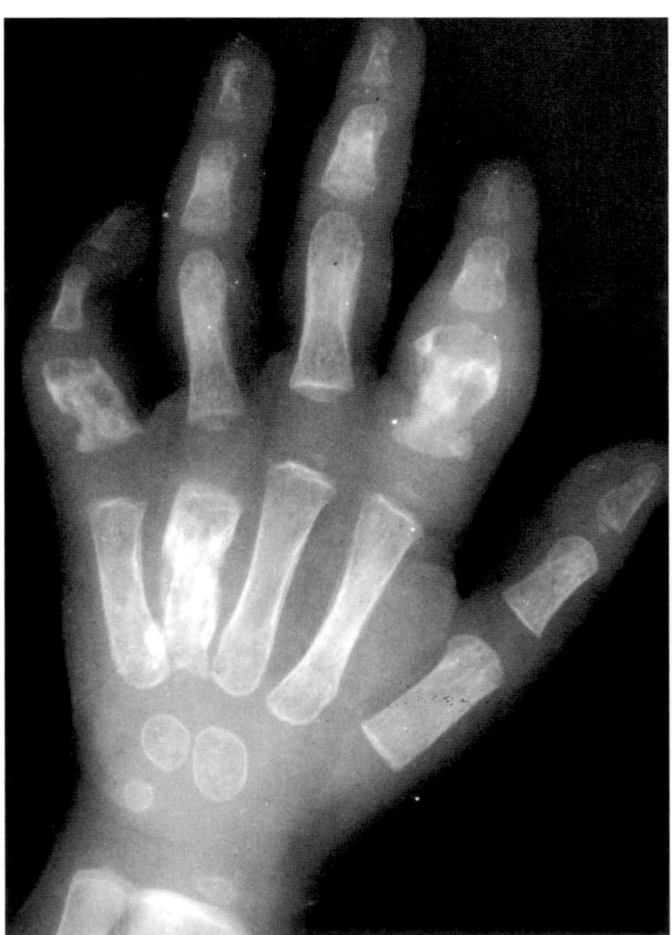

Figure 74.5 Sickle-cell disease. Infarction in several of the metacarpals and proximal phalanges has resulted in bone destruction and swelling of the soft tissues.

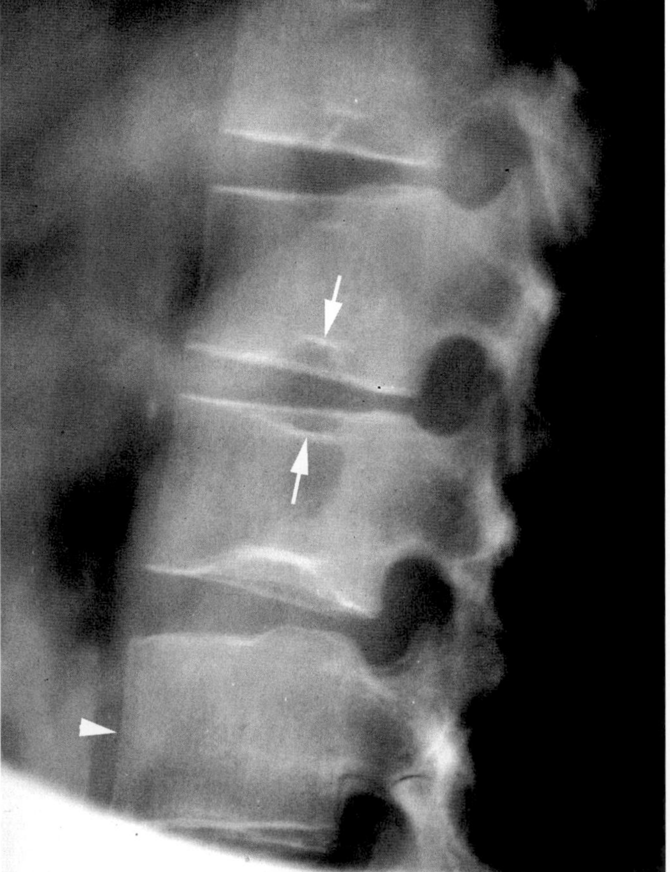

Figure 74.6 Sickle-cell disease. The classical 'stepped depression' of the vertebral end plates is seen (arrows). Note increased height of the adjacent 'tower' vertebra (arrowhead).

of the growth plates. Asymmetrical shortening of tubular bones (e.g., hands or feet) is a common sequel to childhood sickling crises. Pathological fracture occurs in some patients.

Osteonecrosis is common, particularly in the proximal femur and proximal humerus. SCD is the most common cause of osteonecrosis of the femoral head in children, while approximately 50% of all patients will develop osteonecrosis by the age of 35 years. MRI will initially demonstrate infarction as epiphyseal oedema. Radiographic abnormalities include mixed lysis and sclerosis with a sub-chondral fracture being typical (Figure 74.7). Eventually, secondary osteoarthritis will supervene.

Chronic ischaemia or multiple small infarctions in SCD may produce cortical thickening which is both endosteal and periosteal, with narrowing of the marrow cavity (Figure 74.8). Splitting of the cortex may give rise to a bone-within-a-bone

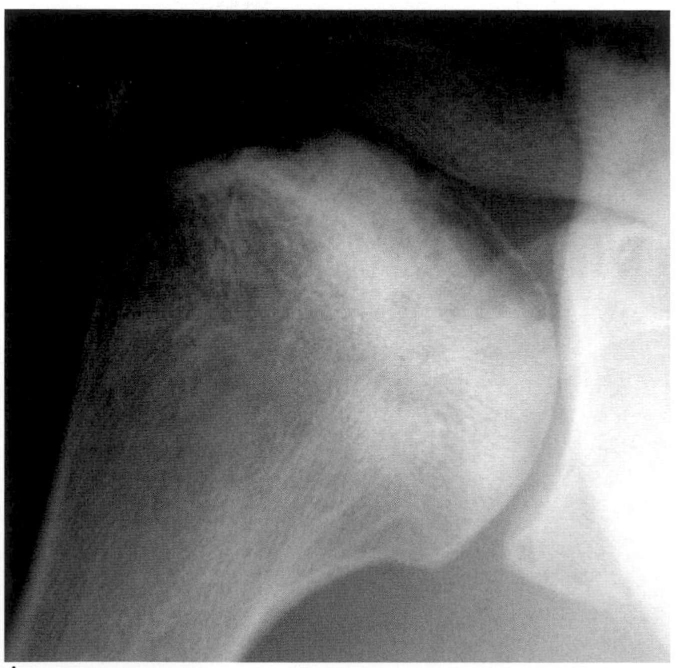
A

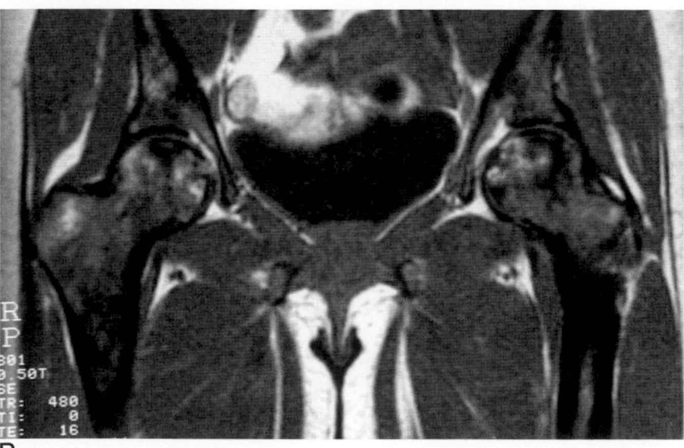

B

Figure 74.7 Sickle-cell disease. (A) Infarction of the humeral head has led to the separation of an osteochondral fragment of the subarticular bone with adjacent reactive medullary sclerosis. (B) Coronal T1-weighted spin-echo MRI of the proximal femora showing patchy hypointensity within the marrow due to marrow hyperplasia and bilateral femoral head osteonecrosis.

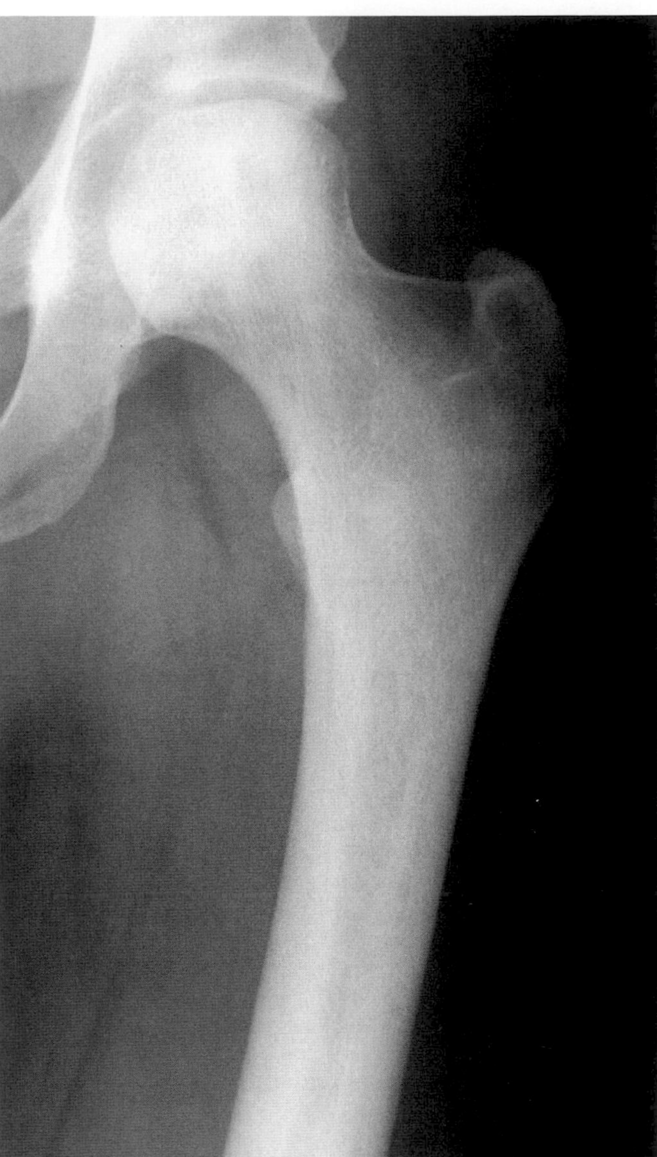

Figure 74.8 Sickle-cell disease. Chronic changes with generalized sclerosis, thickening of the cortex and narrowing of the marrow cavity.

appearance, while secondary myelofibrosis causes medullary sclerosis.

Secondary osteomyelitis

This usually complicates bone infarction and it may be difficult to distinguish clinically or radiologically between an infarct with infection and one without. Salmonella osteomyelitis is common in African children.

Osteomyelitis causes increased bone destruction with multilaminar periostitis and eventual sequestration and involucrum formation (Figure 74.9). Any infection potentiates local sickling of red cells due to stasis and reduced oxygen tension. Lung infection causes hypoxia and provokes major sickling crises. Early diagnosis of bone infection by MRI[7] is important. MRI typically demonstrates poorly defined marrow oedema and the presence of regions of marrow enhancement on fat-suppressed post-contrast T1W images is strongly associated with infection. Ultrasound (US) may differentiate infection

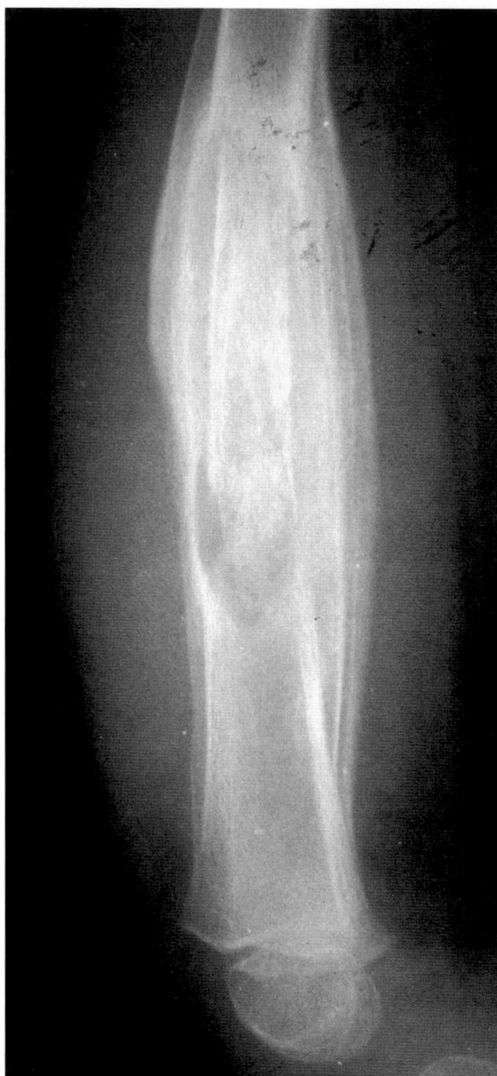

Figure 74.9 Sickle-cell disease. Lateral radiograph of the femur showing features of chronic salmonella osteomyelitis with gross cortical thickening and a central sequestrum.

from infarction by the thickness of subperiosteal fluid collections and guide aspiration, both for symptomatic relief and obtaining material for culture[8].

OTHER ANAEMIAS AND BONE MARROW DYSCRASIAS

Iron-deficiency anaemia

Although this is a common disease, radiographic evidence of bone change is apparent only in infancy.

Polycythaemia vera

This disorder results in excess erythroid, myeloid and megakaryocytic elements with elevation of the haemoglobin level to above 17.5 g L^{-1} and an RBC count persistently greater than $6.0 \times 10^{11} L^{-1}$. Any skeletal change results from occasional bone infarction due to increased viscosity of the blood. The superimposition of leukaemia and myeloid metaplasia is relatively common and MRI can readily depict conversion of cellular marrow to fatty marrow and vice versa in polycythaemia vera and myeloid metaplasia[9].

Myelofibrosis[10] (agnogenic myeloid metaplasia, myeloid metaplasia, myelosclerosis)

Primary myelofibrosis is a slowly progressive marrow disorder of unknown aetiology. It affects men and women equally, with an age range of 20–80 years (median age 60 years). It should only be diagnosed once causes of secondary myelofibrosis have been excluded. The disorder presents insidiously with weakness, dyspnoea and weight loss. Antecedent polycythaemia is common, but obliteration of the marrow by fibrosis or bony sclerosis soon leads to a moderate normochromic normocytic anaemia. Leukocytosis is usually present with some immature white cell forms. Haemopoiesis takes place in the liver and spleen, which become enlarged in 72% and 94% of cases, respectively. Extramedullary haemopoiesis is also reported in lymph nodes, lung, choroid plexus, kidney, etc. The natural history is one of slow deterioration, with death typically occurring 2–3 years after diagnosis.

Radiological features

Bone sclerosis is the major radiological finding, being evident in approximately 30–70% of cases. Typically, this is diffuse (Figure 74.10A) or occasionally patchy, occurring most often in the axial skeleton and metaphyses of the femur, humerus and tibia. Sclerosis is due to trabecular and endosteal new bone formation, resulting in reduced marrow diameter. In the established disease, lucent areas are due to fibrous tissue reaction. Periosteal reaction occurs in one third of cases, most often in the medial aspects of the distal femur and proximal tibia. The skull may show a mixed sclerotic and lytic pattern.

MRI appearances vary depending upon the tissue contained in the marrow. Knowledge of the age-related distribution of fatty and cellular marrow is important. Generally, the high SI of marrow fat is replaced on both T1W and T2W sequences by low SI (Figure 74.10B). Additional features include arthropathy due to haemarthrosis and secondary gout, occurring in 5–20% of cases. Also, infiltration of the synovium by bone marrow elements may result in polyarthralgia and polyarthritis.

Secondary myelofibrosis is the end stage of the myeloproliferative syndrome and occurs to a greater or lesser degree in leukaemia, lymphoma, Gaucher's disease, toxic exposure, carcinomatosis and even infection.

Radiological differentiation between other causes of increased bone density may be difficult, but the presence of anaemia and splenomegaly should suggest the diagnosis in this age group. Radiological differential diagnosis includes osteopetrosis, fluorosis, mastocytosis, carcinomatosis and adult SCD.

WHITE CELL DISORDERS

Leukaemia[11,12]

Acute lymphocytic leukaemia (ALL) accounts for 80%, acute myeloblastic leukaemia (AML) for 10% and other types for 10% of cases. Acute leukaemia is the most common malignancy of childhood, while chronic leukaemias predominate in adults but sometimes terminate in an acute blastic form. Radiographic demonstration of bone lesions in children is relatively

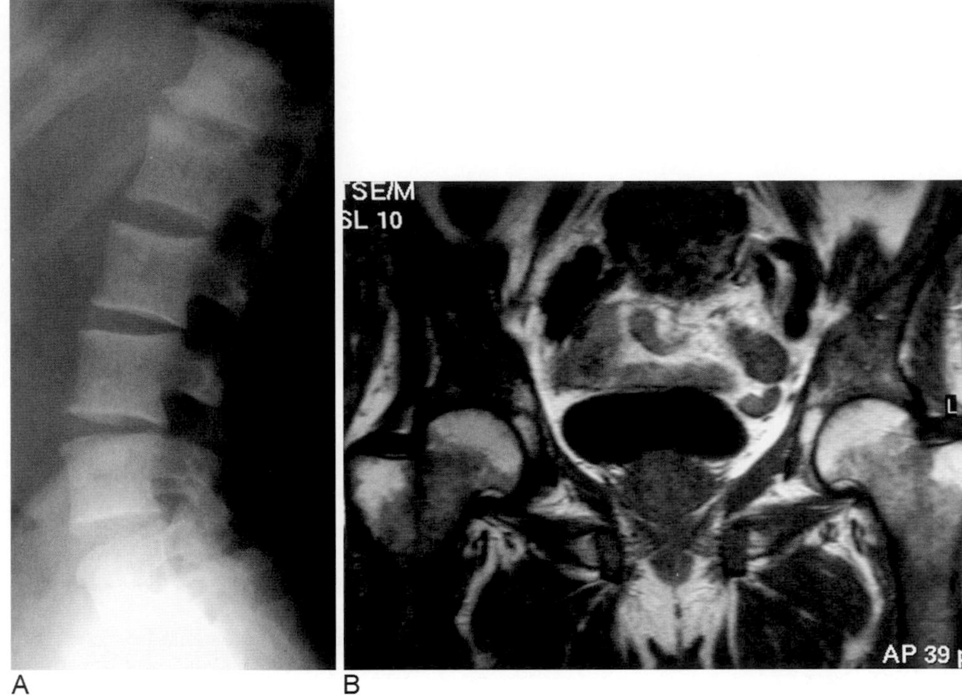

Figure 74.10 Myelofibrosis. (A) Lateral radiograph of the lumbar spine showing diffuse vertebral body sclerosis. (B) Coronal T1-weighted spin-echo MRI showing patchy reduction of marrow signal intensity in the pelvic bones and proximal femora.

common. Skeletal lesions in adults tend to be uncommon and focal, often simulating metastases.

Clinical features

The acute disease is often insidious, with non-specific malaise, anorexia and weight loss. Limb pain and pathological fracture are common. Bone pain at presentation is five times more common in children than adults, being reported in 21–59% of cases.

Adults are most commonly affected by ALL and chronic myeloid leukaemia (CML). Most skeletal lesions in adults affect sites of residual red marrow—axial skeleton and proximal ends of the femora and humeri. Chronic lymphatic leukaemia (CLL) is a disease of the elderly, characterized by enlargement of the spleen and lymph nodes with skeletal involvement being rare except as a terminal event.

Radiological features

Approximately 75% of children with leukaemia develop radiographic evidence of skeletal involvement during the course of their disease, while radiological evidence of bone involvement is reported in 41–75% at time of presentation. Overproduction of leukaemic cells causes trabecular and endosteal cortical destruction and eventually extraosseous extension. The bone changes in children include diffuse osteopenia, metaphyseal lucencies, diffuse bone destruction, osteolytic or osteoblastic lesions and periosteal reaction. Pathological fractures occur in association with osteopenia of the spine (Fig.74.11A), while approximately 1% of children treated for leukaemia develop osteonecrosis.

Diffuse osteopenia is reported in 16–41% of cases and may be either metabolic in aetiology, due to protein and mineral deficiencies, or may be related to diffuse marrow infiltration with leukaemic cells. The effects of corticosteroids and chemotherapy also contribute to osteoporosis.

Metaphyseal lucent bands are identified at time of presentation in up to 80% of cases and are commonly the earliest radiographic finding. They primarily affect sites of maximum growth, such as the distal femur, proximal tibia and distal radius, but other metaphyses and the vertebral bodies are affected later. They are typically 2–15 mm in width (Fig.74.11B). These changes are non-specific, with the differential diagnosis including generalized infection, although this is more common in infancy. In children over the age of 2 years, leukaemia is more likely.

More extensive involvement results in diffuse, permeative bone destruction (Fig.74.11C) similar to the spread of highly malignant tumours such as Ewing sarcoma. The cortex becomes eroded on its endosteal surface and may ultimately be destroyed. The permeative pattern is reported in 18% of leukaemic children and may indicate a poor prognosis.

Osteolytic lesions secondary to bone destruction typically have a moth-eaten appearance and most commonly affect the metaphyses of long bones (Figure 74.11D). Such lesions are reported in 10–40% of patients and predispose to pathological fracture. A particular focal lesion in AML is granulocytic sarcoma (chloroma), which is usually located in the skull, spine, ribs, or sternum of children. This is an expanding geographical tumour caused by a collection of leukaemic cells and reported to occur in 4.7% of patients.

Osteosclerosis is rare, being reported in 6% of cases. Sclerotic changes in the metaphyses of long bones may occur spontaneously or as a result of therapy. Mixed lytic/sclerotic lesions are identified in around 18% of children. Periosteal reaction is reported in 2–50% of cases and may occur in isolation or in association with destructive cortical lesions. It is due to haemorrhage or proliferation of leukaemic deposits deep to the periosteum. Non-specific cortical destruction may involve

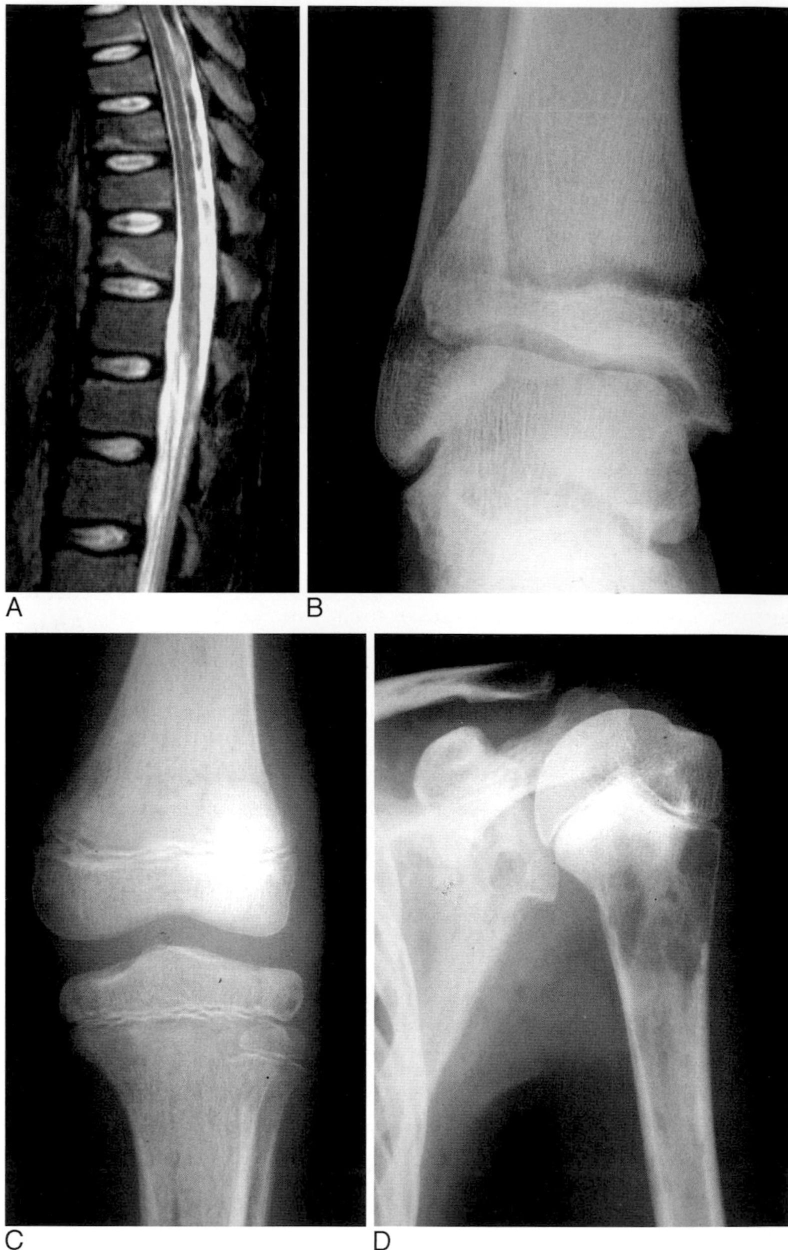

Figure 74.11 Acute leukaemia. (A) Sagittal fat-suppressed T2-weighted fast spin-echo MRI of the thoracic spine showing multilevel wedge compression fractures due to osteopenia as the presenting feature of acute myeloblastic leukaemia (AML). (B) Metaphyseal lucent bands in the distal tibia in a patient with acute lymphocytic leukaemia (ALL). (C) Permeative pattern of bone destruction in the distal femoral and proximal tibial metaphyses. (D) Multiple lytic areas of bone destruction in the proximal humeral metaphysis and scapula.

the medial aspect of the proximal humerus, tibia and sometimes femur.

In adults, skeletal lesions are less common and have to be differentiated from metastases or a primary malignant bone neoplasm.

MRI typically demonstrates diffuse marrow infiltration with reduction of T1W SI in affected areas[13,14]. A change from normal to nodular to diffuse low SI can be seen with disease progression, together with an increase in the extent of SI abnormality. Response to therapy is also demonstrable. However, a potential problem is the difficulty in differentiating areas of fibrosis from active disease and in the identification of bone marrow abnormalities in children successfully treated for ALL[15]. MRI can identify complications of treatment such as osteonecrosis[16] and may also have a part to play in monitoring marrow transplantation.

Mastocytosis[17,18] (mast cell reticulosis, urticaria pigmentosa)

Mastocytosis is a disorder of mast cell proliferation within different body tissues that can result in a variety of clinical syndromes, including urticaria pigmentosa, systemic mastocytosis and mast cell leukaemia. Urticaria pigmentosa accounts for 80–90% of cases and is a self-limiting condition that typically affects children. Systemic mastocytosis accounts for less than 10% of cases and usually occurs in adults. Clinical symptoms resemble lymphoma or leukaemia and the condition can be fatal. The liver, spleen, lymph nodes, skin and bone marrow can all be affected.

Radiological features

Skeletal changes are usually evident in early adult life and affect 10% of patients with urticaria pigmentosa alone, but

70% of patients with systemic mastocytosis. Radiography is insensitive to marrow infiltration, but two patterns may be observed. The first is the presence of small osteolytic or osteoblastic lesions (Figure 74.12), which may disappear spontaneously. The second is diffuse involvement, often sclerotic or mixed in type, where trabecular thickening accounts for the generalized osteosclerosis. Superimposed on this may be a fine reticular or nodular sclerosis. These changes are demonstrated most often in the vertebrae, skull, ribs and pelvis. Differential diagnoses include myelofibrosis, fluorosis, carcinomatosis and lymphoma. MRI may be normal or show a variety of marrow infiltration patterns, including homogeneous and heterogeneous areas of reduced SI on T1W images[17,18]. The spine is always affected and spinal compression fracture is a recognized complication.

Lymphoma[19,20]

The lymphomas are diseases of the lymphatic and reticuloendothelial system. Skeletal involvement usually indicates extensive or late disease (Stage IV). Primary osseous non-Hodgkin's lymphoma (NHL) is rare, while primary osseous Hodgkin's lymphoma even rarer.

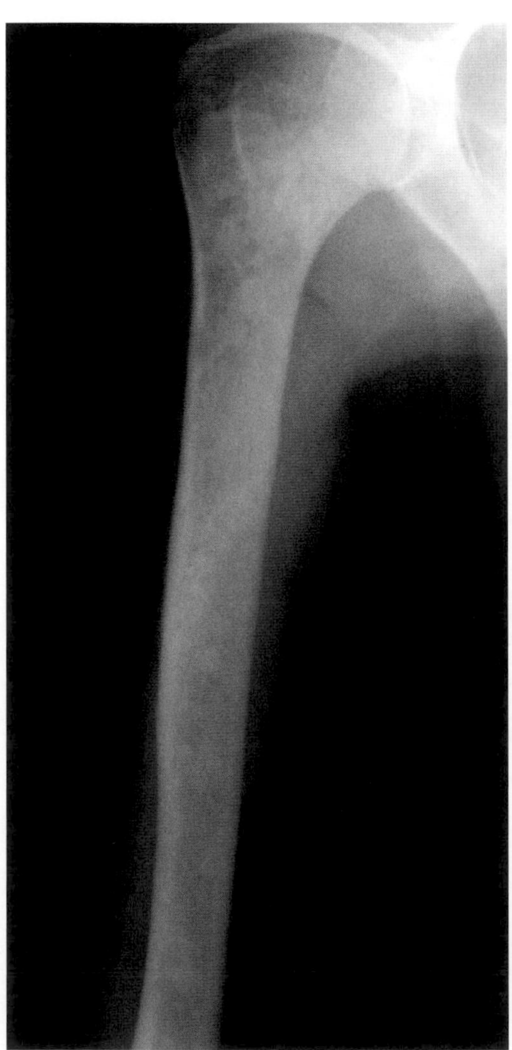

Figure 74.12 Mastocytosis. Radiograph of the humerus demonstrating multiple small osteoblastic lesions.

Hodgkin's disease

The incidence of Hodgkin's disease (HD) has decreased over the past 30 years. Approximately 2% of patients with HD present initially with a skeletal lesion. The prevalence of bone involvement at autopsy is almost 75%. However, at clinical assessment, bone involvement is reported in 15–20% of cases, especially in the more aggressive histological sub-types (mixed cellularity, lymphocyte depletion). Secondary malignancies complicate treated HD in 5–10% of cases.

Clinical features

Three quarters of patients present between 20 and 30 years of age, with a second peak over the age of 60 years. A slight male predominance (1.4:1) is found. Sites of bony involvement are predominantly those containing red marrow, with the majority (75%) in the axial skeleton. Identification of a solitary bony lesion necessitates full staging.

Radiological features

Approximately one third of skeletal lesions are solitary and scintigraphy is mandatory to identify further lesions. Osteolytic lesions or mixed lesions account for almost 90% of cases, the remainder being purely sclerotic.

In the spine, HD most commonly causes sclerosis, although it is an uncommon cause of 'ivory' vertebra. Vertebral collapse takes place early with lytic lesions. The disc spaces are usually preserved but when reduced, it may be difficult to exclude infection. Preservation of the vertebral end plate favours HD. Erosion of the anterior border of one or more vertebral bodies is also found occasionally (Figure 74.13), possibly by direct spread from affected prevertebral lymph nodes. Such features are best shown with MRI. In the thoracic region, paravertebral masses may precede radiographic or scintigraphic evidence of bony involvement.

Rib involvement is common, with multiple lytic lesions associated with soft tissue masses predominating. Occasionally the ribs appear expanded. In the pelvis, involved nodes may invade the bone directly, usually in the posterior half of the ilium. Mixed lesions are relatively common and the ischium and pubic rami may show expansion. Direct haematogenous involvement of the sternum is common. The typical lesion is lytic and expanding, associated with a soft tissue mass.

The differential diagnosis includes metastases, leukaemia and NHL. Individual lesions may appear benign, particularly when showing a well-defined sclerotic margin. Biopsy is always required to establish the diagnosis, although non-skeletal lesions may be more accessible.

Non-Hodgkin's lymphoma

The term non-Hodgkin's lymphoma embraces a variety of follicular and diffuse lymphocytic lymphomas. NHL represents a monoclonal proliferation of B cells, T cells, or histiocytes. They represent only 2% of malignant tumours (excluding skin cancers) in Britain. Recently, AIDS[21] and transplant-related NHL have increased in prevalence, usually as high-grade B-cell disease. Such tumours primarily affect the central nervous system, chest and abdomen, although involvement of the skeleton is probably

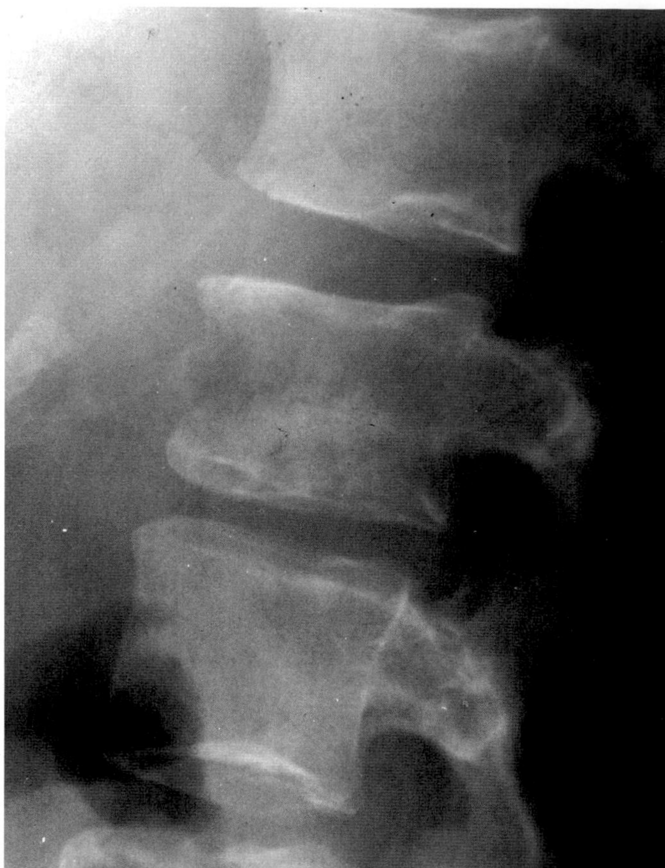

Figure 74.13 Hodgkin's disease. Coned lateral radiograph shows erosion of the anterior cortex of the second lumbar vertebra.

increasing. Primary lymphoma of bone is described with the primary malignant tumours of bone in Chapter 48.

Secondary skeletal involvement occurs in 15–25% and is probably more common in children. Detection of an osseous lesion at initial presentation is uncommon. Children with generalized NHL tend to have widespread skeletal involvement manifest as osteopenia. MRI tends to show foci before the diffuse infiltration of the established disease. MRI may also be used to stage disease and will occasionally demonstrate marrow disease despite negative iliac crest biopsy. Although the MRI appearances are non-specific, the presence of a paravertebral soft tissue mass with maintenance of the cortical outline of the vertebral body is highly suggestive of lymphoma[22].

Burkitt's lymphoma[23]

Burkitt's lymphoma is a high-grade NHL with distinctive clinical and histological features. A causative relationship to the Epstein–Barr virus and more recently HIV, is probable. A 74% 4-year survival rate is reported.

The disease shows a male to female ratio of 2:1, affecting mainly African children. Large tumours affect the jawbones and abdominal viscera. The mean age is 7 years, with a range of 2–16 years. Added to this endemic (African) group are the nonendemic cases, mainly in white children. The jaw is the initial focus in about 50% of patients, although less so in nonendemic cases. Other sites of involvement include the pelvis, long bones and bones of the hands and feet.

Radiological features

The jaw lesion is generally destructive, starting in the medulla and later affecting the cortex. Bone destruction and dental displacement in the enlarging soft tissue mass give the appearance of 'floating' teeth (Figure 74.14). Lesions in other bones show similar appearances and periosteal reaction may be present in all locations.

Full assessment and staging is required for this multicentric neoplasm. Treatment is primarily with chemotherapy.

PLASMA CELL DYSCRASIAS[24]

Plasmacytoma (solitary myeloma)

Plasmacytoma is apparently solitary at presentation and accounts for approximately 2% of patients with plasma cell dyscrasias. It may remain localized for many years but more than 30% progress quite rapidly to generalized myelomatosis.

Presentation with pain is common, but uncomplicated plasmacytoma may be asymptomatic. Although presentation below 40 years of age is uncommon, the age of presentation tends to be earlier and the age range wider than in multiple myeloma (MM). As plasma protein changes are related to the total tumour mass, protein electrophoresis is often normal and the erythrocyte sedimentation rate (ESR) normal or only slightly elevated.

Radiological features

Plasmacytoma is typically lytic and destructive with sclerosis being rare. The lesion arises in the medulla and the radiological features suggest a relatively slow growth rate.

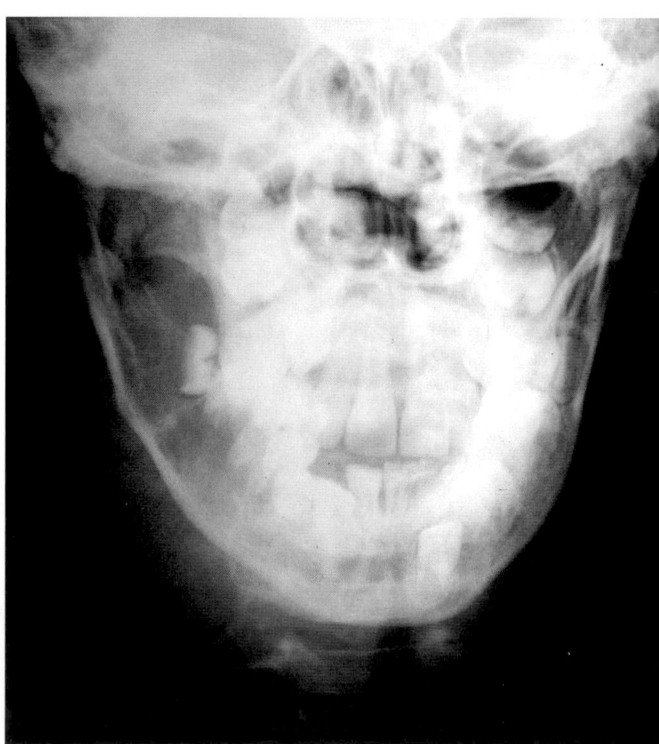

Figure 74.14 Burkitt's lymphoma. Destruction of the right side of the mandible has resulted in 'floating teeth' and an associated large soft tissue mass.

The margin is often well defined and cortical thinning with expansion is usually present. Apparent trabeculation or a 'soap bubble' appearance is common (Figure 74.15) and an associated soft tissue mass is frequently seen. Affected sites usually contain persistent red marrow and include the axial skeleton, pelvis, proximal femur, proximal humerus and ribs. Peripheral lesions are rare. Following the diagnosis of plasmacytoma, MRI of the spine and pelvis is indicated to identify additional lesions, which may be seen in up to 80% of cases. Occult lesions may also be demonstrated by [F-18]-fluoro-deoxyglucose positron emission tomography ([F-18]FDG-PET).

Involvement of a vertebral body is common, sometimes leading to early collapse. Extension across the disc space is a rare feature (Figure 74.16). The differential diagnosis includes metastatic carcinoma, which rarely destroys two or three bodies in continuity and infection. A solitary plasmacytoma in the spine may show characteristic MRI features, particularly the presence of peripheral thickened trabeculae[25].

In long and flat bones, plasmacytoma may resemble an aneurysmal bone cyst or an expanding metastasis.

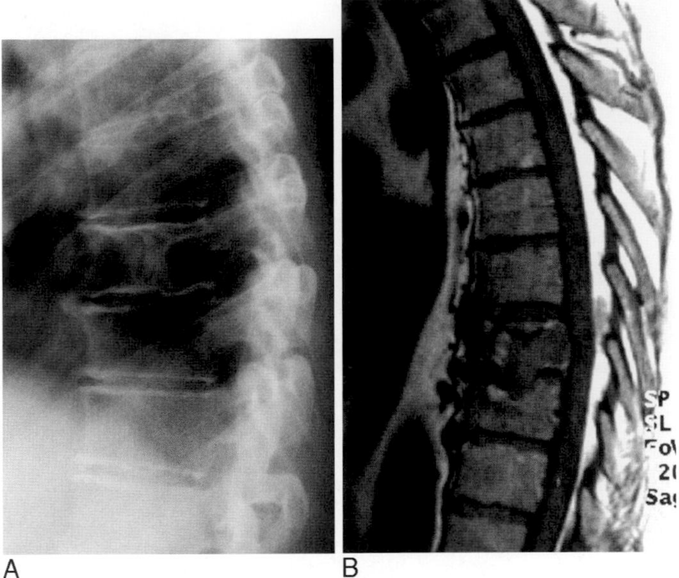

Figure 74.16 Plasmacytoma of the spine. (A) Lateral radiograph shows a lytic destructive lesion showing minor collapse. (B) Sagittal T1-weighted spin-echo MRI demonstrates extension across the disc space.

Multiple myeloma

Multiple myeloma is the most common primary malignant neoplasm of bone and is the predominant plasma cell dyscrasia, accounting for approximately 1% of all malignant disease and 10% of haematological malignancies. The incidence of newly diagnosed cases in the USA is 3–4/100 000 population per year.

Clinical features

Three-quarters of affected patients are over 50 years of age with a median age of 65 years and approximately 3% of patients presenting before the age of 40 years. There is a male predominance of up to 2:1. Widespread involvement of the skeleton is present in 80%, the axial skeleton and proximal ends of the limb bones being particularly involved. Fever, pain, backache and weakness are common symptoms.

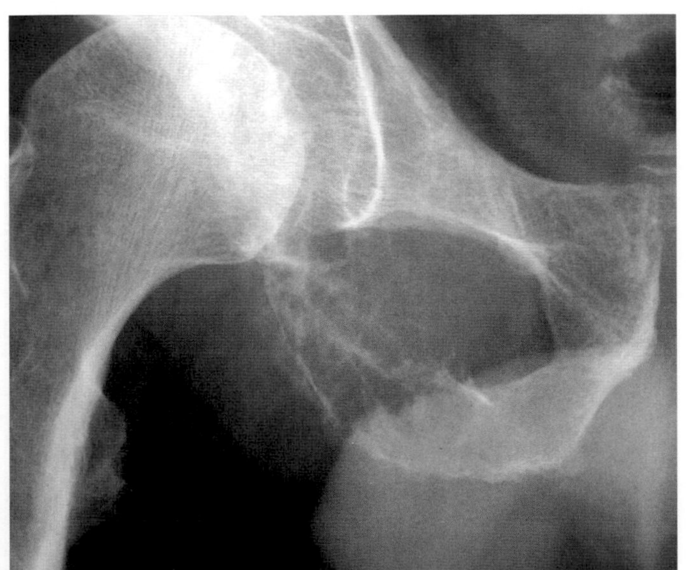

Figure 74.15 Plasmacytoma. Antero-posterior radiograph shows a slightly expanded lytic lesion with apparent trabeculation in the inferior pubic ramus.

With generalized skeletal involvement, production of an abnormal paraprotein leads to a wide m-band on plasma electrophoresis. This paraprotein elevates the ESR, which is frequently over 100 mm h^{-1}. Production of light-chain immunoglobulins results in Bence Jones proteinuria in over 50% of patients. Chronic renal failure is a major cause of death in MM, while risk factors for acute renal failure include hypercalcaemia, dehydration, infection and Bence Jones proteinuria. In MM, the administration of intravenous contrast media is not totally free from risk and caution has to be exercised in performing excretion urography. Particularly, the patient *must* be well hydrated. Amyloidosis is reported in approximately 20% of patients with MM.

Radiological features[26,27]

The classical appearance of MM consists of well-defined 'punched-out' lesions throughout the skeleton, most characteristic in the skull. The only common differential diagnosis in this age group is metastatic disease. The presence of multiple small (up to 20 mm), well-defined, round or oval lesions is more suggestive of MM.

Diffuse osteopenia usually involves the spine and may result in multiple compression fractures (Fig.74.17). Pathological fracture of the vertebrae affects approximately 50% of patients at some stage. Fractures of the tubular bones heal readily with normal amounts of callus.

Osteoblastic or mixed lesions are rare in untreated patients. Following radiotherapy, marginal sclerosis may be observed. Examples of purely sclerotic myeloma are recognized and may be associated with polyneuropathy, organomegaly, endocrinopathy, monoclonal gammopathy and skin changes (POEMS syndrome).

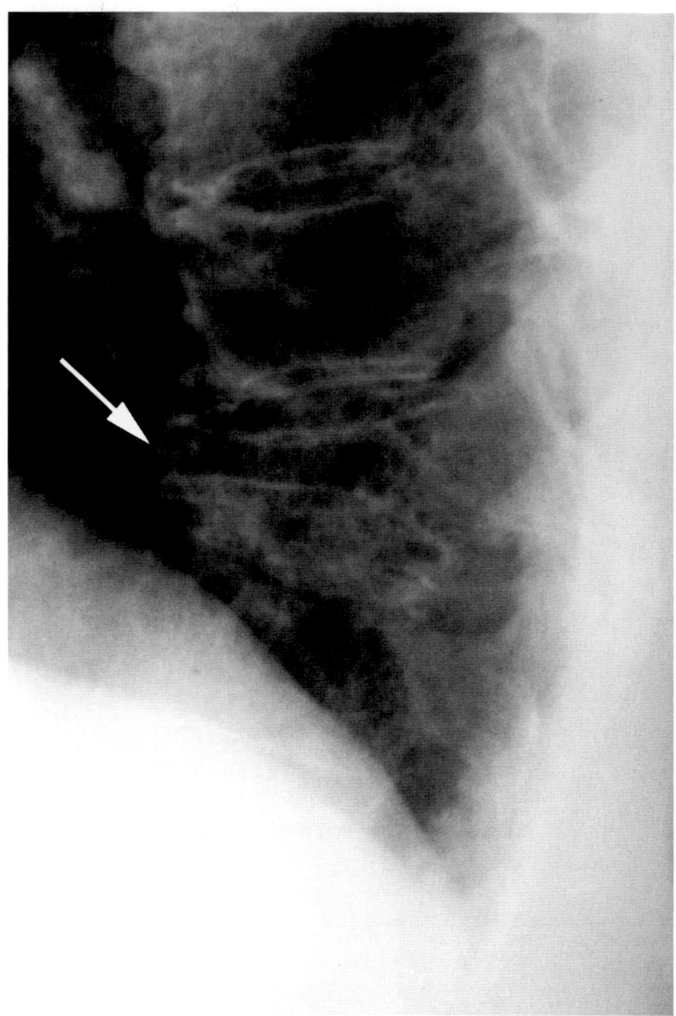

Figure 74.17 Multiple myeloma. Lateral radiograph of the lower thoracic spine showing diffuse osteopenia and pathological collapse of T11 (arrow).

Scintigraphy remains an important method of demonstrating the extent of skeletal involvement. However, MM may be underestimated by this technique, many lesions showing normal uptake or photopenia, probably because of their nonosteoblastic nature. Thus the skeletal survey is still widely employed; whole-body MR and CT may become more widely used in the future. Scintigraphy may pick up lesions in bones such as the ribs where radiography is less sensitive. Symptomatic lesions are more likely to be detected by a combination of radiography and scintigraphy. Fluorine-18 FDG PET, however, has been shown to be more sensitive than skeletal survey in demonstrating MM lesions[28].

The MRI appearances in MM are variable. A normal marrow pattern may be seen at presentation in 50–75% of patients with early untreated (Stage 1) MM and in 20% of patients with advanced (Stage 3) MM. A focal pattern consists of localized areas of decreased SI on T1W images with corresponding increased SI on T2W and STIR images (Fig.74.18A,B). Occasionally, focal lesions may be relatively hyperintense on T1W and be identified only on T2W images. The diffuse pattern manifests as generalized reduction of marrow SI on T1W, such that the intervertebral discs appear hyperintense compared with the vertebral bodies. The marrow appears hyperintense on T2W and STIR images and shows diffuse enhancement following gadolinium. Finally, a 'variegated' pattern is described, which consists of multiple tiny foci of reduced SI on T1W and hyperintensity on T2W/STIR on a background of normal marrow (Fig.74.18C). This pattern is seen almost always in early disease. These patterns have some prognostic value, in that patients with diffuse marrow abnormality on MRI will have a poorer outcome than those with a normal MRI pattern.

Vertebral fractures in MM occur in 55–70% of cases and may be either benign due to diffuse osteopenia or pathological due to tumour infiltration. The majority occur in the thoracolumbar region. MRI is valuable in the differentiation of benign versus malignant collapse[29]: benign collapse is suggested by the presence of normal marrow SI in the chronic stage or band-like marrow oedema in the acute stage, with some preservation of normal fatty marrow, normal SI within the pedicles (Fig.74.19), homogeneous contrast enhancement and retropulsion of the posterosuperior corner of the vertebral body into the canal; conversely, pathological collapse is suggested by diffuse reduced T1W SI throughout the vertebral body, involvement of the neural arch, soft tissue extension and posterior bulging of the vertebral body cortex (see Fig.74.18A). Application of these criteria suggests that one third of vertebral fractures in MM are pathological while two thirds are benign.

Other plasma cell dyscrasias

Plasma cell disorders cover a wide range of severity, with most symptomatic types occurring at the malignant end of the spectrum. Three types of heavy-chain disease are described (*a*, *t*, *m*). All produce a lymphoma-like illness and may show skeletal lesions indistinguishable from MM.

Waldenström's macroglobulinaemia resembles MM but produces a high-molecular-weight IgM. Skeletal changes are present in about 50% of cases[30]. Correlation of abdominal CT and spinal MRI findings is advantageous as abdominal lymphadenopathy and diffuse marrow involvement are common in the more advanced disease[31].

Light-chain deposition disease is a variant of myeloma. The MRI appearances in the spine show multiple small hypointense foci on T1W, T2W and STIR sequences[32].

RETICULOENDOTHELIAL DISORDERS

LANGERHANS CELL HISTIOCYTOSIS[33,34]

Langerhans cell histiocytosis (LCH) is an extremely heterogeneous clinical disorder, which embraces Letterer–Siwe disease (LSD), Hand–Schüller–Christian disease (HSCD) and eosinophilic granuloma (EG). LCH is a non-neoplastic proliferation of Langerhans cells of unknown aetiology.

Letterer–Siwe disease (disseminated histiocytosis)

Letterer–Siwe disease is a rare acute form of the disease. Visceral lesions predominate and, as most cases are fatal, bone

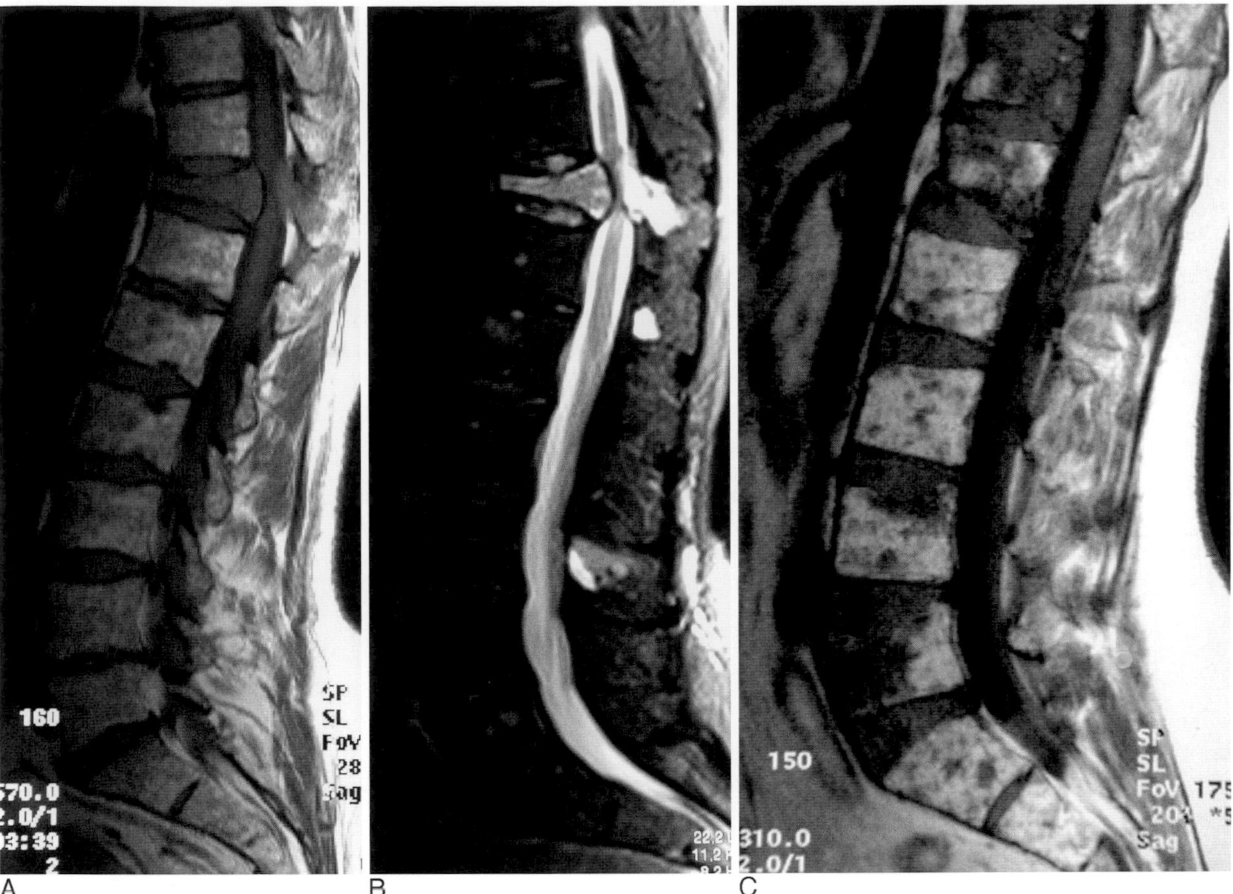

Figure 74.18 Multiple myeloma. (A) Sagittal T1-weighted spin-echo and (B) fat-suppressed T2-weighted fast spin-echo MRI showing pathological collapse of T11 with cord compression and multiple smaller areas of focal marrow involvement. (C) Sagittal T1-weighted spin-echo MRI showing the variegated pattern of marrow involvement.

lesions may never be identified in life. LSD affects infants and children under 2 years of age and has been reported as early as 1 month of age. Splenomegaly, hepatomegaly and lymphadenopathy with anaemia predominate. Patients present with fever and failure to thrive, and the disease is usually fatal if untreated.

Radiological features

Bone lesions resemble those of the other histiocytoses but are often widespread. Destructive medullary lesions affect flat bones and the metaphyses of long bones. Infants with skeletal lesions seem to have a better prognosis than those without, but this may be because they have survived the acute visceral stage. Diagnosis is established by biopsy of material from lymph nodes or bone. Differential diagnosis includes acute lymphoma, leukaemia and metastatic neuroblastoma.

Hand–Schüller–Christian disease (multifocal histiocytosis)

Hand–Schüller–Christian disease is almost as rare as LSD, being a disorder of childhood with a more chronic course. Approximately 70% of patients present before the age of 5 years. The classical triad of calvarial lesions, exophthalmos and diabetes insipidus is found in only 10% of cases. Approximately 75% of these patients go on to disease-free survival but require hormone replacement. About 50% of patients develop diabetes insipidus early in the disease. One quarter develop unilateral or bilateral exophthalmos due to histiocytosis of the bony orbit.

Radiological features

Skeletal lesions are similar to, but more numerous than those of eosinophilic granuloma. Large geographic areas of destruction are observed in the calvaria (Figure 74.20). Lesions of the jaw are present in approximately 40%, with destruction mainly of the alveolar margins, leading to 'floating' teeth in the radiolucent matrix. In long bones, metaphyseal and diaphyseal lesions are initially lytic, but later heal with periosteal reaction and medullary sclerosis. Pelvic and vertebral body lesions are common. At presentation, most skeletal lesions are at the same stage of development. Although morbidity is severe, the overall mortality is only 10%, predominantly from infection.

Eosinophilic granuloma (solitary or pauciostotic histiocytosis)

Although rare, this benign type of histiocytosis is more common than both the others put together. Lesions are mainly confined to bone. Approximately 80% present before the age of 10 years, although the disease is also seen in adolescents, young adults and occasionally as late as 60 years. A male to female ratio of 2:1 is reported. Presentation is usually with pain and local tenderness, while pathological fracture is rare. The

Figure 74.19 MRI features of benign collapse. Sagittal T1-weighted spin-echo MRI in the midsagittal (A) and parasagittal (B) planes showing marrow oedema, which is not filling the vertebral body or extending into the pedicles. Note also the absence of extraosseous tissue.

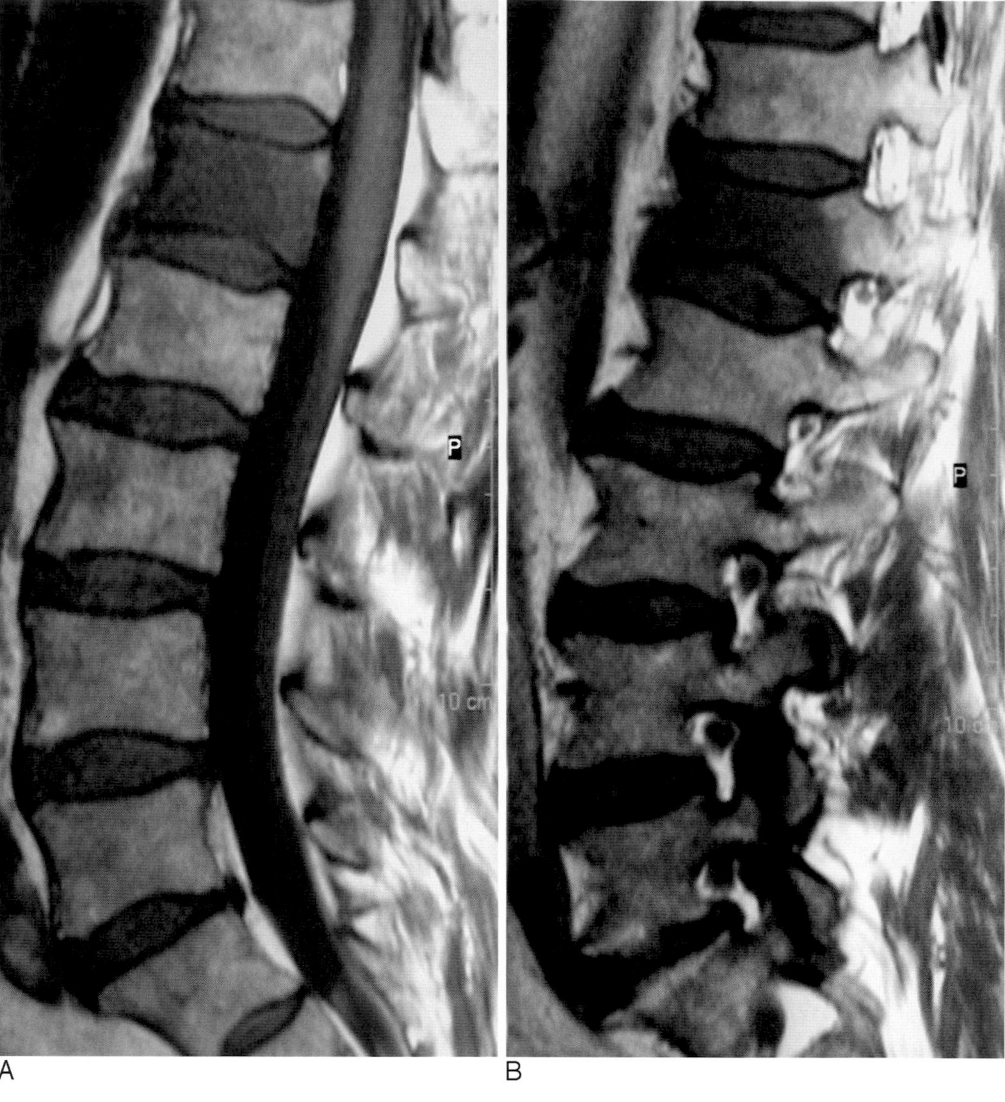

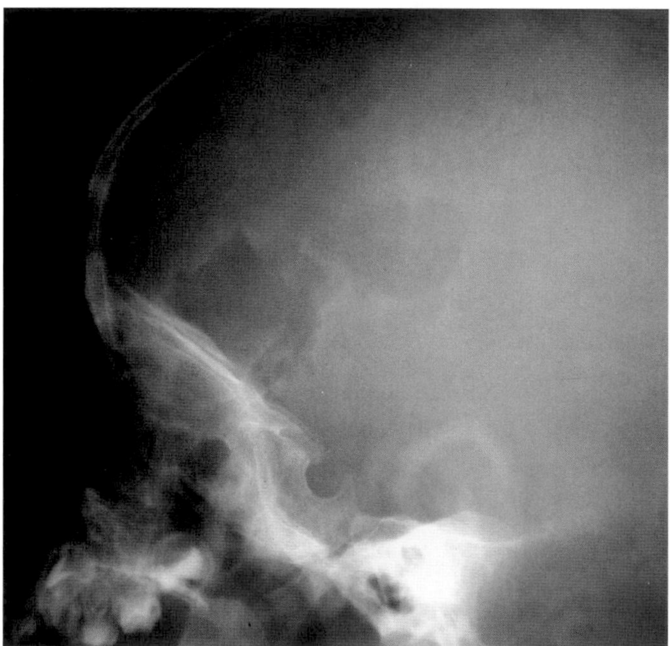

Figure 74.20 Langerhans cell histiocytosis. Geographic lytic lesions of the skull vault in Hand–Schüller–Christian disease.

ESR is either normal (in under half the patients) or shows a moderate elevation (<60 mm h^{-1}).

More than 50% of cases involve the skull, spine, pelvis, ribs and mandible. Long bone involvement is typically in the diaphyses of the femur, tibia and humerus. Lesions of the hands and feet are rare. Multiple lesions are demonstrated in approximately 10% of cases at presentation. This probably underestimates the incidence, as many lesions are not synchronous. Scintigraphy may demonstrate lesions as either focal 'hot' or 'cold' spots but is not as sensitive as skeletal survey. Whilst multiple skeletal lesions tend to suggest a more severe form of histiocytosis, as many as eight bony lesions have been found in a patient without extraskeletal involvement.

Radiological features

Geographic destruction of bone is characteristic, particularly in the skull where tangential views show a bevelled edge to the defect, indicating destruction of the two tables to a differing degree. In the paediatric spine, the thoracic region is most commonly involved (54%), followed by the lumbar (35%) and cervical (11%) regions. The classical spinal lesion, termed vertebra plana (Figure 74.21), where the vertebral body becomes

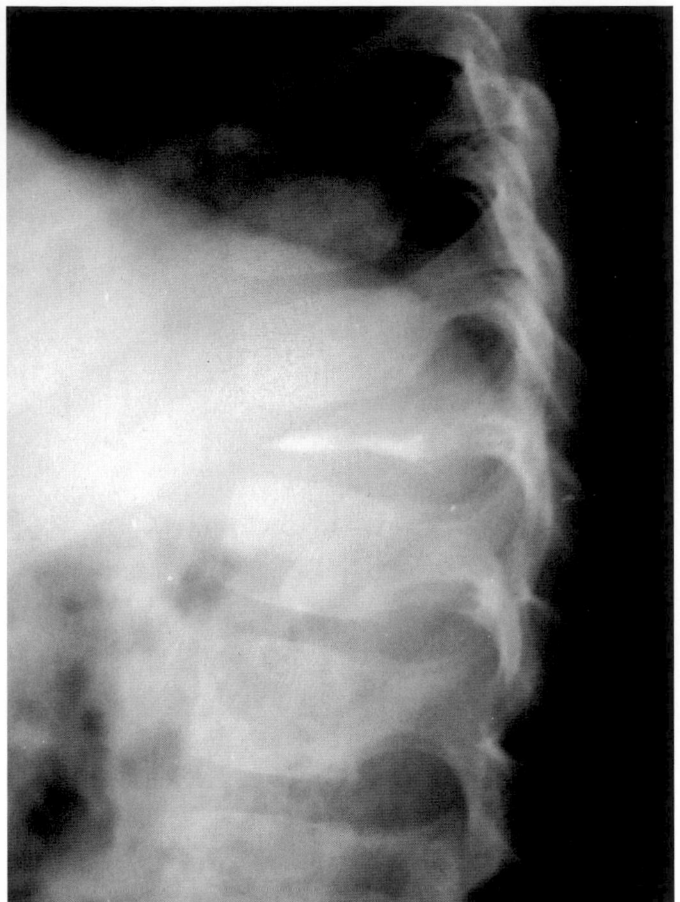

Figure 74.21 Langerhans cell histiocytosis. Vertebra plana of T11 is demonstrated.

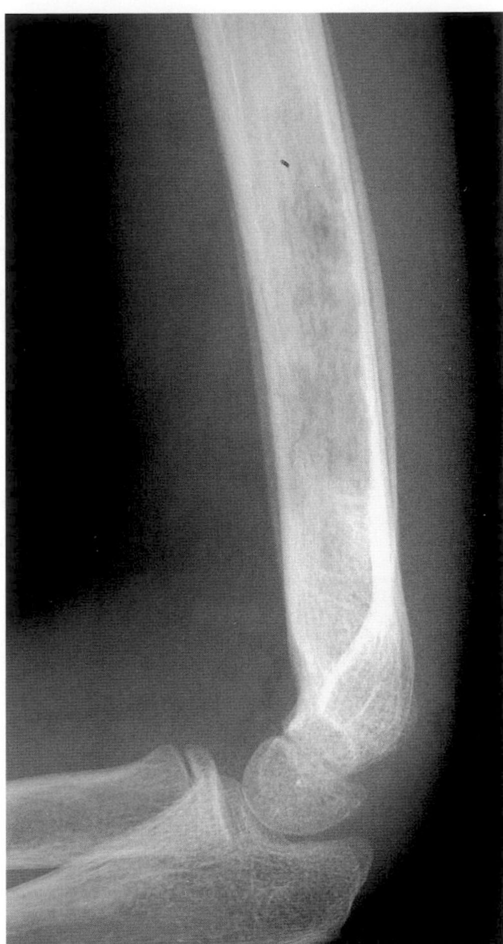

Figure 74.22 Langerhans cell histiocytosis of the humerus. Distal metadiaphyseal lesion showing permeative destruction and periosteal reaction.

flattened and often wafer-thin, is not one of the most common findings. LCH is the most common cause of paediatric vertebral collapse and restoration of about two thirds of vertebral height may be expected with healing. A small paravertebral mass is occasionally present and probably represents associated haemorrhage. Infection (particularly tuberculosis), primary Ewing sarcoma and metastatic tumours can also produce vertebra plana, but are uncommon at this site in the typical age group.

EG in flat or long bones produces a less well-defined medullary lesion. Endosteal erosion is common, as is a linear periosteal reaction (Figure 74.22). Such lesions may simulate infection or low-grade neoplasms and early biopsy is advisable, as the diagnostic histological features are often obscured by healing. Unusual radiographic features include epiphyseal lesions, transphyseal lesions, extracranial 'button' sequestra, posterior vertebral arch lesions and lesions arising in rare sites such as the clavicle and small bones of the hands and feet[35].

The MRI findings are non-specific and most commonly consist of a focal lesion with extensive marrow and soft tissue oedema, which is of low SI on T1W sequences and high SI on T2W or STIR images (Figure 74.23)[36]. Rarer features include fluid–fluid levels and dural extension of spinal lesions. Extraosseous involvement is reported in 30% of cases and may be due to extension from bone disease or may be isolated to the soft tissues[37]. In patients with multilevel spinal disease, MRI is able to differentiate active from healing lesions and thus guide needle biopsy[38] (Figure 74.24).

Healing usually takes a matter of months and it is unusual for new lesions to appear more than 6 months after the original focus. EG is a benign and self-limiting condition and radiotherapy is best avoided.

GAUCHER'S DISEASE[39]

Gaucher's disease is the most common lipid storage disorder and is due to a genetic enzyme (glucocerebrosidase) deficiency, which results in the accumulation of the lipid glucocerebroside in the lysosomes of monocytes and macrophages. These engorged cells are called Gaucher cells and the accumulation of Gaucher cells within a variety of organ systems accounts for the symptoms of the disorder. Many of those affected are Ashkenazi Jews (approximately 1 of every 400–600), but all races are vulnerable. Three types are recognized: the common Type 1, which is non-neuronopathic and the rare neuronopathic Types 2 (acute) and 3 (subacute).

An infantile form may occur as early as 2 weeks of age, mainly in non-Jewish patients. It is characterized by hepatosplenomegaly, lymphadenopathy and neurological complications. Anaemia and haemorrhage are common. Death is usual before the age of 2 years, mainly due to involvement of the central nervous system.

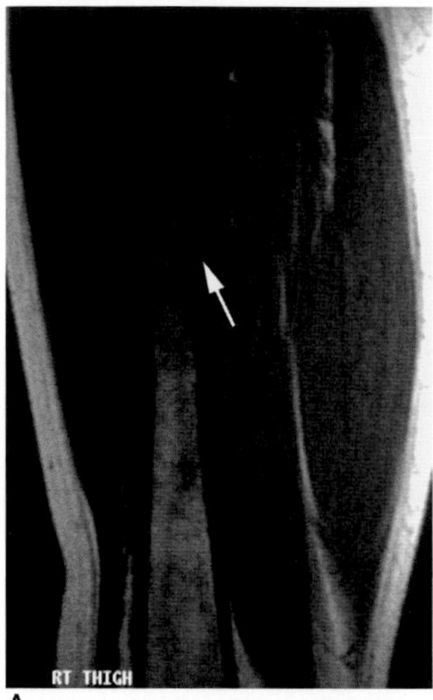

A

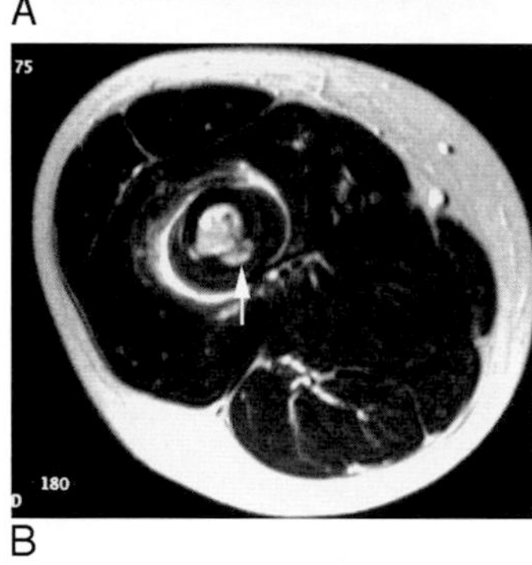
B

Figure 74.23 Langerhans cell histiocytosis of the femur. (A) Coronal T1-weighted spin-echo and (B) axial T2-weighted fast spin-echo MRI showing a focal lesion causing endosteal scalloping (arrow), with associated periostitis and reactive marrow and soft tissue oedema.

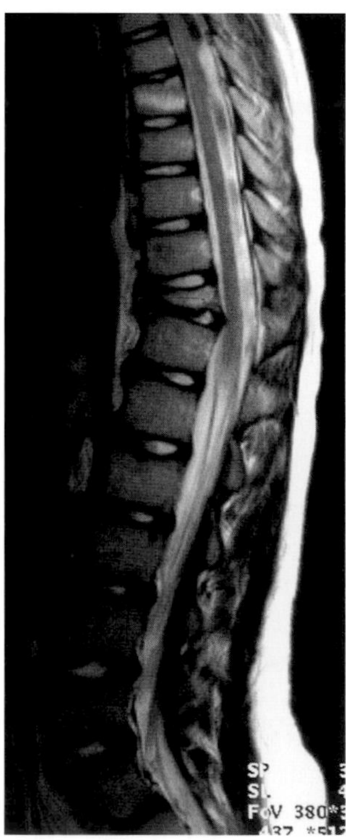

Figure 74.24 Langerhans cell histiocytosis of the spine. Sagittal T2-weighted fast spin-echo MRI of the thoracolumbar spine showing collapse of T11 with oedema also in T7, indicating an active lesion.

The adult form mainly affects older children and young adults, but older adults are not exempt. The adult disease may also present with hepatosplenomegaly, abdominal pain and ascites. Both dull bone pain and acute painful crises occur. Bone crises are characterized by acute episodes of severe skeletal pain, fever, leukocytosis and raised ESR.

Radiological features[40,41]

Acute bone crises may show periosteal reaction on radiography, focal photopenic areas on scintigraphy and marrow oedema on MRI. The condition must be differentiated from osteomyelitis, which also complicates Gaucher's disease.

Radiological features relate to lipid storage effects and bone necrosis. The large amounts of lipid in the marrow spaces cause osteopenia (Figure 74.25A). Loss of normal modelling of the long bones in childhood results in the Erlenmeyer flask appearance of their ends (Figure 74.25B). However, this appearance is common to other marrow-expanding disorders. Lytic areas of various size and a 'soap bubble' appearance may be seen. The cortex is scalloped on its endosteal surface and becomes thinned. Osteopenia is associated with an increased risk of pathological fracture. Osteosclerosis may also occur as a healing response following bone infarction. Metaphyseal notching of the humerus is also a characteristic feature and is thought to be secondary to increased bone turnover.

Bone infarction is common and either due to interference of blood supply by lipid-laden cells or to fat embolism. Episodes of bone pain, fever and elevation of ESR may indicate osteonecrosis. Bone infarction involves particularly the subarticular bone of the femoral and humeral heads, the metaphyseal regions of long bones and the vertebral bodies, in which case vertebral collapse with or without cord compression may occur.

MRI is most useful in evaluating the extent of marrow infiltration (Figure 74.26), being manifest as either homogeneous or heterogeneous reduced SI on T1W images and increased SI on T2W images. Such changes are always present in the spine. Complications such as bone infarction, osteomyelitis and fracture can also be assessed, as can response to enzyme replacement therapy (ERT).

The prevalence of bone changes depends upon whether ERT has been administered. In the absence of ERT, 94% of patients will demonstrate some form of osseous radiological abnormality, including Erlenmeyer flask deformity (61%), osteopenia (50%), bone infarction and osteonecrosis (35%), fractures (26%) and lytic lesions (18%). All of these features are less common in patients receiving ERT.

NIEMANN-PICK DISEASE

Niemann-Pick disease is a rare autosomal recessive disorder of phospholipid metabolism affecting mainly Jewish infants, with death being common in the first 2 years. It resembles Gaucher's disease but with the deposition of sphingomyelin in foam cells. The radiographic changes resemble Gaucher's disease, but are less common. Four phenotypes have been described. The MRI findings in Type B disease include low SI within the femoral marrow on T1W and T2W sequences together with hypodense splenic nodules on CT[42].

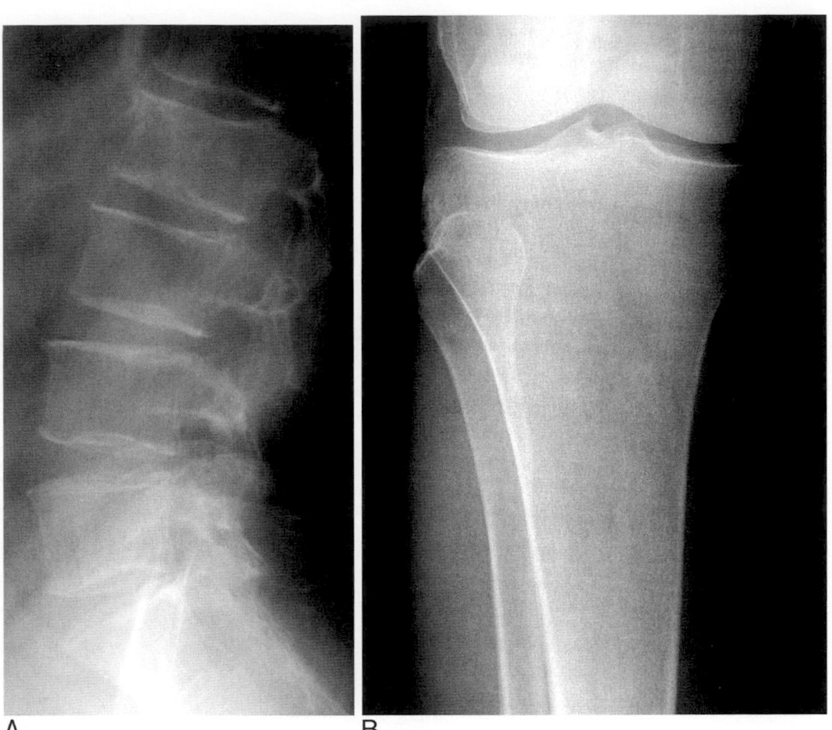

Figure 74.25 Gaucher's disease. (A) Lateral radiograph of the lumbar spine shows diffuse osteopenia and partial collapse of L2. (B) The tibia shows mild expansion, the Erlenmeyer-flask deformity, with associated cortical thinning and osteopenia.

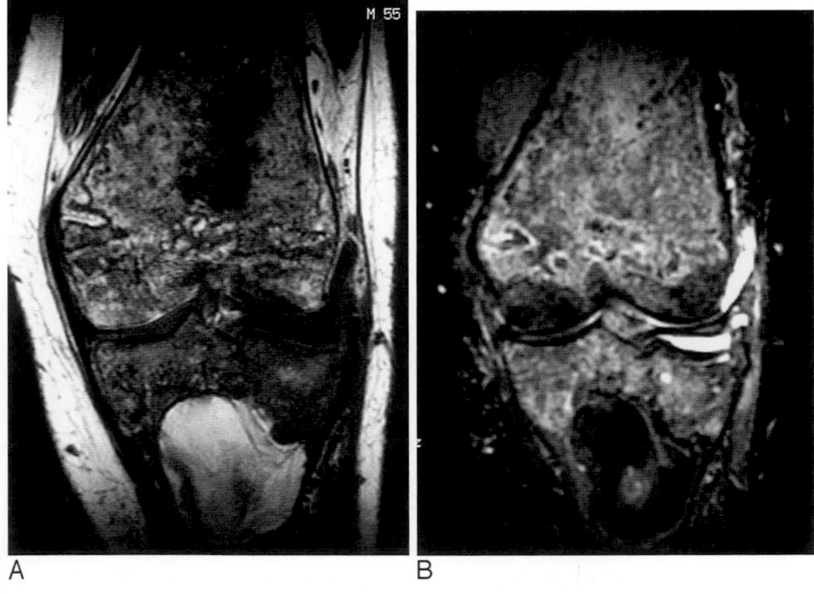

Figure 74.26 Gaucher's disease. Coronal T1-weighted spin-echo (A) and short tau inversion recovery (STIR). (B) MRI of the proximal tibia showing inhomogeneous marrow signal intensity changes due to a combination of infiltration and marrow fibrosis.

HAEMOPHILIA AND OTHER DISORDERS OF BLOOD COAGULATION; BLEEDING DISORDERS

Three major inherited disorders are considered:

1 classic haemophilia (haemophilia A)
2 Christmas disease (haemophilia B)
3 von Willebrand's disease.

All produce the same radiological appearances, the diseases differing only in the frequency and severity of the observed changes. Very occasionally, a patient of either sex may develop antibodies to antihaemophilic globulin and develop an acquired form of haemophilia. The prevalence of haemophilia and Christmas disease is approximately 1 in 10 000, with haemophilia A being more common.

Haemophilia[43] (haemophilia A)

Haemophilia A is an X-linked recessive disorder resulting from deficiency of Factor VIII. Bleeding, which usually follows minor trauma, may occur in the first year of life and 70% of haemophiliacs have experienced haemarthrosis by the age of 2 years. Repeated haemarthroses result in chronic arthropathy and eventually premature osteoarthritis. Soft tissue haemorrhage, often close to muscle attachments, produces another lesion characteristic of the disease, the haemophilic pseudotumour.

Christmas disease (haemophilia B)

Named after the first patient studied, this disorder is due to deficiency of Factor IX and is also an X-linked recessive disease. It is less severe than haemophilia and about one fifth as common.

Von Willebrand's disease

Inherited as a dominant character and affecting both sexes, von Willebrand's disease is due to both a capillary defect and a deficiency in Factor VIII. The coagulation defect is mild and only occasionally causes significant skeletal abnormality. The severity of the disease relates to the level of Factor VIII in the blood, which is variable.

Radiological features

In patients with severe haemophilia, 85% of all bleeding events involve the joints. Acute haemarthrosis simulates a tense joint effusion of any cause, although periarticular osteoporosis may indicate previous episodes. MRI is more accurate than clinical examination at identifying haemarthrosis and US may also have a role in early detection. The most common joints involved are the knee, elbow, ankle, hip and shoulder. Repeated episodes of haemorrhage result in progressive joint damage referred to as haemophilic arthropathy.

Haemorrhage initially occurs into the synovium and eventually extends into the joint space. Recurrent haemarthrosis results in a chronic haemorrhagic synovitis and articular cartilage damage. Hyperaemia results in periarticular osteopenia, epiphyseal overgrowth and premature closure of the growth plates. Pannus similar to that occurring in rheumatoid arthritis causes marginal erosions. Loss of secondary trabeculae leads to a permanent coarsening of the trabecular pattern, while growth arrest lines indicate the episodic nature of the disorder. Fibrosis results in joint contracture and intraosseous haemorrhage produces subarticular cysts, which predispose to sub-chondral collapse. Synovial thickening together with osteopenia make the soft tissues appear radiographically denser. An absolute increase in the soft tissue density may also occur due to concentration of haemosiderin by macrophages in the periarticular regions (Figure 74.27).

The knee is the most common joint involved. Radiological features include enlargement of the distal femoral and proximal tibial epiphyses, varus or valgus deformity, squaring of the inferior pole of the patella with patellar overgrowth and widening of the intercondylar notch (Figure 74.28A). Eventually, advanced secondary OA develops.

In the elbow, chronic hyperaemia causes accelerated appearance of the ossification centres and overgrowth of the radial head. Pressure erosion of the radial notch of the ulna, large lytic lesions of the proximal ulna and erosion of the trochlear notch are also seen (Figure 74.28B).

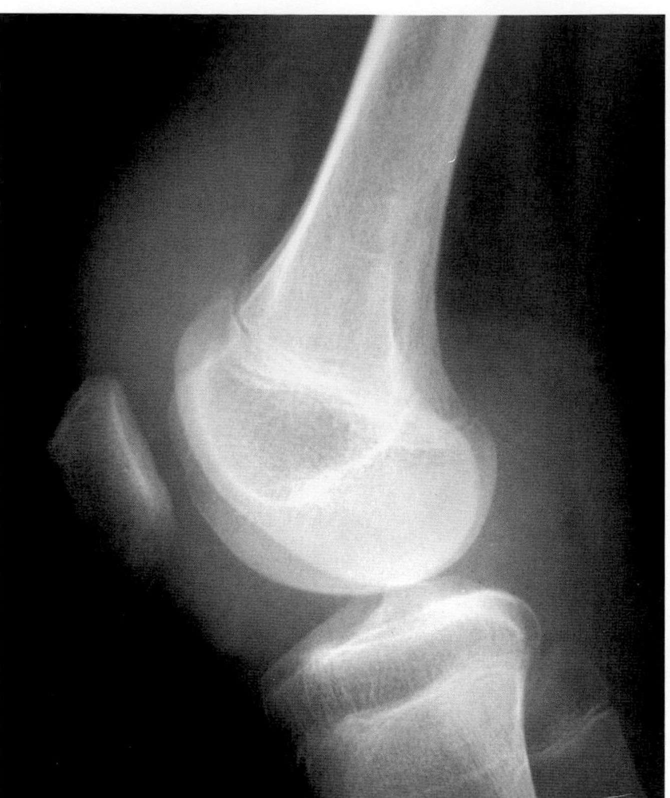

Figure 74.27 Haemophilia. Lateral radiograph of the knee shows extensive, hyperdense synovitis.

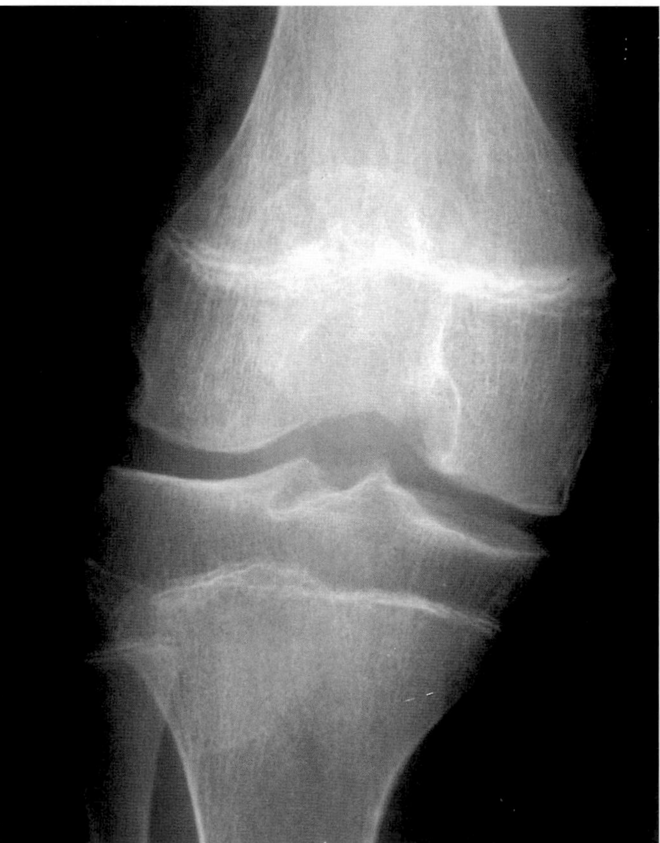

A

Figure 74.28 Haemophilia. (A) Antero-posterior radiograph of the knee showing epiphyseal overgrowth and enlargement of the intercondylar notch.

Continued

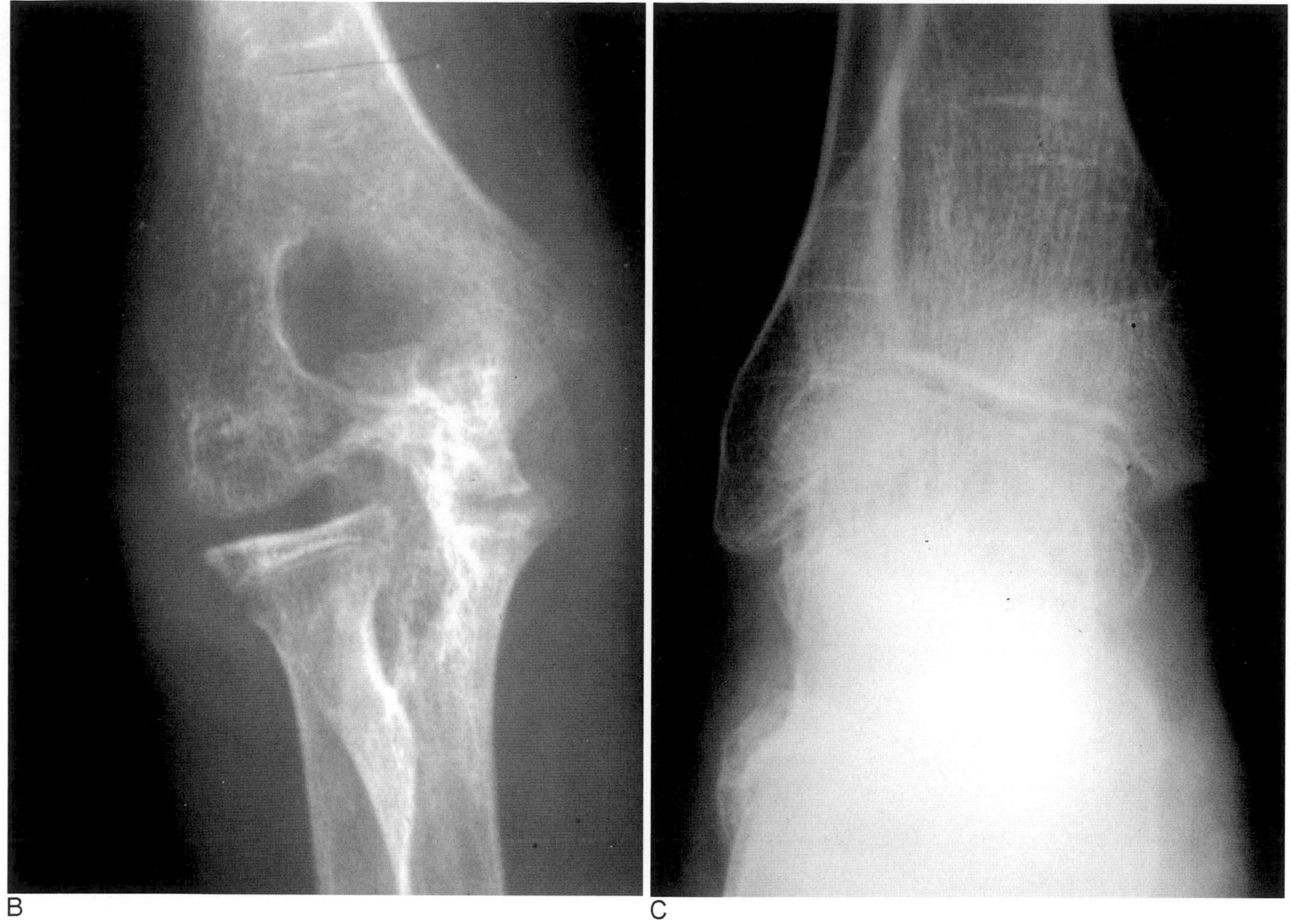

Figure 74.28, Cont'd (B) Antero-posterior radiograph of the elbow showing erosion of the radial notch of the ulna. (C) Antero-posterior radiograph of the ankle showing medial tibiotalar slant and secondary osteoarthritis.

In the ankle, asymmetric growth of the distal tibial epiphysis results in medial tibiotalar slant (Figure 74.28C). Marked flattening of the talar dome, a variety of ankle and foot deformities and rarely ankylosis of the ankle or subtalar joints may be seen.

Typical radiographic features of osteonecrosis may be evident in the hip and may simulate Perthes' disease, eventually resulting in coxa magna. Protrusio acetabuli and secondary OA are also seen, while haemorrhage into the growth plate may result in slipped epiphysis. Coxa valga may result from delayed weight-bearing.

MRI shows the earliest evidence of haemarthrosis, manifest as a low SI intra-articular blood clot within a hyperintense joint effusion. Fluid–fluid levels may also be seen. In chronic cases, the haemosiderin-laden synovium appears irregularly thickened and markedly hypointense on T2W images, particularly gradient echo sequences. Other features include focal cartilage defects and sub-chondral cysts.

Small soft tissue haematomas are common and, when repetitive, may lead to contractures. Of more importance is the infrequent progressive haemorrhage close to muscle attachments, usually with no history of injury resulting in the haemophilic pseudotumour. This is more common in adults, with a reported incidence of 1.56%. Most are reported in the pelvis, thigh, or calf. Subperiosteal or intraosseous haemorrhage causes pressure erosion of the bone, particularly the iliac blade in relation to the extensive origin of the iliacus muscle (Figure 74.29) and the femur. Pathological fracture may be the first manifestation of a haemophilic pseudotumour of bone.

Radiographically, a haemophilic pseudotumour appears as a soft tissue mass, which may be calcified. Bone lesions may show geographic lytic destruction with cortical thickening. CT identifies the thick, relatively hyperdense pseudocapsule with a hypodense centre. The MRI SI varies with the age of the contained blood, progressing from being isointense with muscle in the first week on T1W and subsequently becoming hyperintense on both T1W and T2W images. The wall tends to be hypointense because of its contained haemosiderin. Mural nodules provide a highly characteristic appearance. Treatment is by management of the haemophilia and exploratory operation is to be avoided.

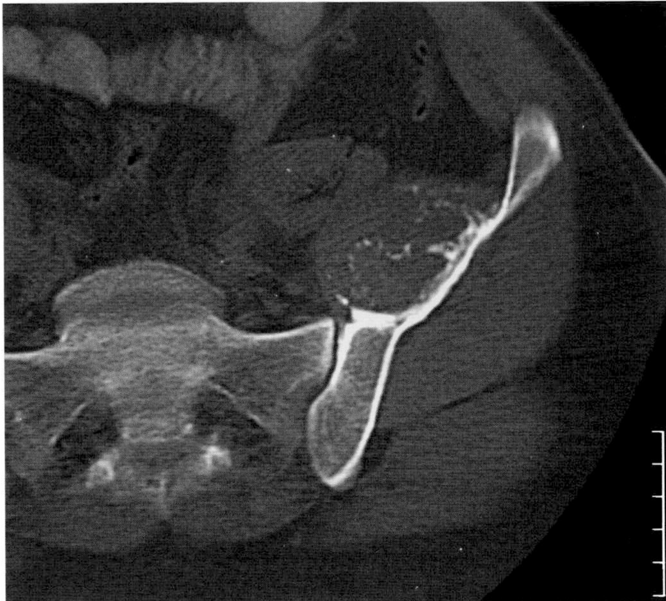

Figure 74.29 Haemophilic pseudotumour. CT study shows scalloping of the ilium, with an adjacent calcified soft tissue mass within the iliacus muscle. (Courtesy of Dr Sajid Butt, Consultant Radiologist, Royal National Orthopaedic Hospital Trust.)

REFERENCES

1. Vanel D, Dromain C, Tardivon A 2000 MRI of bone marrow disorders. Eur Radiol 10: 224–229
2. Kricun M E 1985 Red-yellow marrow conversion: its effect on the location of some solitary bone lesions. Skeletal Radiol 14: 10–19
3. Chui D H, Waye J S 1998 Hydrops fetalis caused by alpha-thalassaemia: an emerging health care problem. Blood 91: 2213–2222
4. Tunaci M, Tunaci A, Engin G et al 1999 Imaging features of thalassaemia. Eur Radiol 9: 1804–1809
5. Fixler J, Styles L 2002 Sickle cell disease. Pediatr Clin North Am 49: 1193–1210
6. Lonergen G J, Cline D B, Abbondanzo S L 2001 Sickle cell anemia. Radiographics 21: 971–994
7. Umans H, Haramati N, Flusser G 2000 The diagnostic role of gadolinium enhanced MRI in distinguishing between acute medullary bone infarct and osteomyelitis. Magn Reson Imaging 18: 255–262
8. Booz M M Y, Hariharan V, Aradi A J, Malki A A 1999 The value of ultrasound and aspiration in differentiating vaso-occlusive crisis and osteomyelitis in sickle-cell disease patients. Clin Radiol 54: 636–639
9. Kaplan K R, Mitchell D G, Steiner R M et al 1992 Polycythemia vera and myelofibrosis: correlation of MR imaging, clinical and laboratory findings. Radiology 183: 329–334
10. Guermazi A, de Kerviler E, Cazals-Hatem D, Zagdanski A M, Frija J 1999 Imaging findings in patients with myelofibrosis. Eur Radiol 9: 1366–1375
11. Gallagher D J, Phillips D J, Heinrich S D 1996 Orthopaedic manifestations of acute paediatric leukemia. Orthop Clin North Am 27: 635–644
12. Parker B R 1997 Leukemia and lymphoma in childhood. Radiol Clin North Am 35: 1495–1516
13. Moulopoulos L A, Dimopoulos M A 1997 Magnetic resonance imaging of the bone marrow in hematologic malignancies. Blood 90: 2127–2147
14. Vande Berg B C, Lecouvet F E, Michaux L, Ferrant A, Maldague B, Malghem J 1998 Magnetic resonance imaging of the bone marrow in hematological malignancies. Eur Radiol 8: 1335–1344
15. Ojala A E, Paakko E, Lanning F P, Harila-Saari A H, Lanning B M 1998 Bone marrow changes on MRI in children with acute lymphoblastic leukaemia 5 years after treatment. Clin Radiol 53: 131–136
16. Ojala A E, Paakko E, Lanning F P, Lanning M 1999 Osteonecrosis during the treatment of childhood acute lymphoblastic leukemia: a prospective MRI study. Med Pediatr Oncol 32: 11–17
17. Avila N A, Ling A, Metcalfe D D, Worobec A S 1998 Mastocytosis: magnetic resonance imaging patterns of marrow disease. Skeletal Radiol 27: 119–126
18. Roca M, Mota J, Giraldo P, Garcia Erce J A 1999 Systemic mastocytosis: MRI of bone marrow involvement. Eur Radiol 9: 1094–1097
19. Ruzek K A, Wenger, D E 2004 The multiple faces of lymphoma of the musculoskeletal system. Skeletal Radiol 33: 1–8
20. Mengiardi B, Honegger H, Hodler J et al 2005 Primary lymphoma of bone: MRI and CT characteristics during and after successful treatment Am J Roentgenol 184: 185–192
21. Aboulafia A J, Khan F, Pankowsky D, Aboulaia D M 1998 AIDS-associated secondary lymphoma of bone: a case report with review of the literature. Am J Orthopedics 27: 128–134
22. Moulopoulos L A, Dimopoulos M A, Vourtsi A, Gouliamos A, Vlahos L 1999 Bone lesions with soft-tissue mass: magnetic resonance imaging diagnosis of lymphomatous involvement of the bone marrow versus multiple myeloma and bone metastases. Leuk Lymphoma 34: 179–184
23. Spina M, Tirelli U, Zagonel V et al 1998 Burkitt's lymphoma in adults with and without human immunodeficiency virus infection: a single-institution clinicopathologic study of 75 patients. Cancer 82: 766–774
24. Wilson C S 2004 The plasma cell dyscrasias. Cancer Treat Res 121: 113–144
25. Shah B K, Saifuddin A, Price G J 2000 Magnetic resonance imaging of spinal plasmacytoma. Clin Radiol 55: 439–445
26. Lecouvet F E, Vande Berg B C, Malghem J, Maldague B E 2001 Magnetic resonance and computed tomography imaging in multiple myeloma. Seminars in Musculoskeletal Radiol 5: 43–55
27. Angtuaco E J, Fassas A B, Walker R, Sethi R, Barlogie B 2004 Multiple myeloma: clinical review and diagnostic imaging. Radiology 231:11–23
28. Schirrmeister H, Bommer M, Buck A K et al 2002 Initial results in the assessment of multiple myeloma using F-18 FDG PET. Eur J Nucl Med Mol Imaging 29: 361–366
29. Uetani M, Hashmi R, Hayashi K 2004 Malignant and benign compression fractures: differentiation and diagnostic pitfalls on MRI. Clin Radiol 59: 124–131
30. Venness M, Pearson K D, Einstein A B, Fahey J L 1972 Osseous manifestations of Waldenstrom's macroglobulinaemia. Radiology 102: 497–504
31. Moulopoulos L A, Dimopoulos M A, Varuna D G K et al 1993 Waldenstrom macroglobulinaemia: MR imaging of the spine and CT of the abdomen and pelvis. Radiology 188: 669–673
32. Baur A, Stabler A, Lamerz R, Bartl R, Reiser M 1998 Light chain deposition disease in multiple myeloma: MR imaging features correlated with histopathological findings. Skeletal Radiol 27: 173–176
33. Kilborn T N, Teh J, Goodman T R 2003 Paediatric manifestations of Langerhans cell histiocytosis: a review of the clinical and radiological findings. Clin Radiol 58: 269–278
34. Azouz E M, Saigal G, Rodriguez M M, Podda A 2005 Langerhans' cell histiocytosis: pathology, imaging and treatment of skeletal involvement. Pediatr Ra diol 35: 103–115
35. Hindman B W, Thomas R D, Young L W, Yu L 1998 Langerhans cell histiocytosis: unusual skeletal manifestations observed in thirty-four cases. Skeletal Radiol 27: 177–181
36. Beltran J, Aparisi F, Bonmati L M, Rosenberg Z S, Present D, Steiner G C 1993 Eosinophilic granuloma: MRI manifestations. Skeletal Radiol 22: 157–161
37. Schmidt S, Eich G, Hanquinet S, Tschappeler H, Waibel P, Gudinchet F 2004 Extra-osseous involvement of Langerhans' cell histiocytosis in children. Pediatr Radiol 34: 313–321

38. Kaplan G R, Saifuddin A, Pringle J A, Noordeen M H, Mehta M H 1998 Langerhans' cell histiocytosis of the spine: use of MRI in guiding biopsy. Skeletal Radiol 27: 673–676
39. Wenstrup R J, Roca-Espiau M, Weinreb N J, Bembi B 2002 Skeletal aspects of Gaucher disease: a review. Br J Radiol 75 (suppl 1): A2–A12
40. Maas M, Poll L W, Terk M R 2002 Imaging and quantifying skeletal involvement in Gaucher disease. Br J Radiol 75 (suppl 1): A13–A24
41. McHugh K, Olsen E O E, Vellodi A 2004 Gaucher disease in children: radiology of non-central nervous system manifestations. Clin Radiol 59: 117–123
42. Muntaner L, Galmes A, Chabas A, Herrera M 1997 Imaging features of type-B Niemann-Pick disease. Eur Radiol 7: 361–364
43. Kerr R 2003 Imaging of musculoskeletal complications of hemophilia. Semin Musculoskelet Radiol 7; 127–136

CHAPTER 75

Principles of Oncological Radiology

David MacVicar

DIAGNOSIS OF PRIMARY NEOPLASMS

Until the second half of the 20th century, surgery was the principal method for attempting to cure solid tumours and until computers revolutionized radiological imaging, open surgical biopsy was the usual method of making a pathological diagnosis of cancer. Plain film radiography could detect pulmonary masses and bony lesions, and the radiologists of the past were highly skilled at detecting displacement of mediastinal lines and other radiological signs, which might escape the scrutiny of today's practitioners who have been trained in the era of cross-sectional imaging. However, a detailed understanding of normal imaging anatomy remains fundamental to all attempts at diagnosis. Put simply, if something is present that is not an identifiable normal structure, it could be a tumour. There are many potential pitfalls, such as retroperitoneal vascular structures that can mimic lumps and lymph nodes. However, thorough knowledge of variations will allow an abnormal mass to be identified with confidence.

In the majority of cases, a cancer patient presents with symptoms and signs, and appropriate investigations are arranged, including imaging. On plain radiography or cross-sectional imaging, a potentially abnormal structure is then detected and the issue is raised of how best to make a diagnosis. If a lesion is detected radiologically, it is often the radiologist who is approached first to confirm the suspected diagnosis. There are only a few diagnoses that can be made with confidence from imaging characteristics, for example, ovarian dermoid and other fat-containing tumours, and lesions that are obviously cystic. In most cases there is a differential diagnosis. However, a variety of techniques may yield a pathological diagnosis including cytological examination of fine needle aspiration samples, specimens from automatic cutting needles and surgical biopsies. In some circumstances needle techniques should be avoided. If lymphoma is suspected, the pathologist would much prefer a complete and intact superficial lymph node, which allows characterization of nodal architecture, to a fine needle aspiration or cutting needle biopsy.

Certain principles should be followed when needle aspiration or percutaneous core biopsy is being planned:

1. The technique chosen should enable sufficient tissue to be obtained for adequate diagnosis.
2. The coagulation parameters should be checked and appropriate measures taken to minimize the risk of haemorrhage.
3. When biopsying multiple lesions, the same instrument should not be used for different lesions.

A variety of fine needles are available for obtaining cytological samples. Fig. 75.1 shows the Westcott-type needle. Ideally a cytologist would be present while the specimen is being obtained to stain and interpret cytology samples immediately. However, it is often necessary for the radiologist to assess the suitability of the sample and prepare slides, which are interpreted later. It is important for radiologists undertaking such procedures to be familiar with the preferred preparation technique, which may involve air-drying or application of alcohol or other fixatives.

There are several types of cutting needles used for core biopsy. The Tru-Cut needle has a central trocar that makes the initial movement forward, exposing a slot. The sheath is then advanced over the slot, cutting a piece of tissue into the slot, and the entire apparatus is withdrawn, with a core specimen contained in the slot.

Coaxial systems offer a method of increasing the amount of tissue available for histological examination through a single

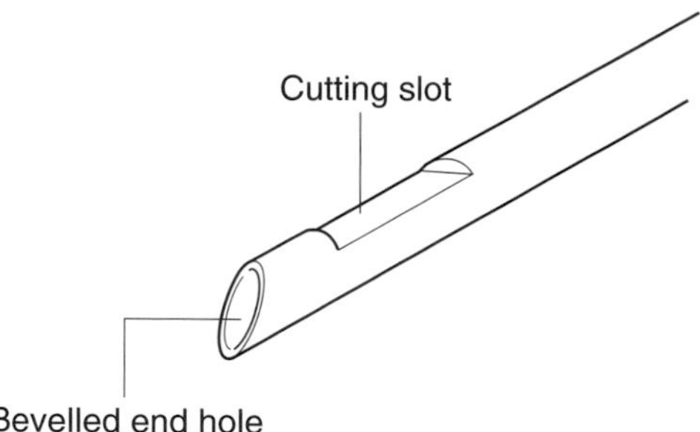

Figure 75.1 Diagram of Westcott-type needle. This is used for aspiration of cytology samples. There is an end hole and a cutting side hole. Vacuum is applied when a central trocar is withdrawn following satisfactory placement of needle.

puncture site. The principle involves placement of a needle from which the sharpened trocar is removed to leave a hollow unsharpened cannula in the mass for biopsy (Fig. 75.2). An automatic cutting needle can then be placed down the cannula. Several cores can then be obtained, and different parts of the lesion may be sampled by angling the cannula slightly in a variety of directions. Since only one puncture is made of the skin and intervening tissue planes, more tissue is obtained without increasing the risk of track seeding.

Preparation of core biopsies should also be discussed with the examining pathologist. Most specimens can be placed in formalin but others require preparation for special staining techniques. If the first attempt at image-assisted tissue diagnosis is inconclusive, a decision will then need to be made whether further attempts are made or open surgical biopsy should be carried out. There are no strict rules as to how many attempts should be made, but the reason for diagnostic failure is of importance. Some tumours such as pancreatic carcinoma frequently have relatively few malignant cells and may require repeat percutaneous biopsy or laparoscopic investigation. The degree of risk involved in repeat biopsy, the technical ease with which the specimen was obtained, and the likelihood of achieving positive tissue diagnosis on the second attempt should all be taken into account.

STAGING SYSTEMS

Since attempts to treat cancer in a systematic way began, staging systems have been devised which provide a description of the anatomical extent of tumour, an early example being Dukes' staging classification of colorectal cancer. Over the years, many staging systems have borne the name of eminent doctors (e.g., the Robson staging classification of renal tumours), organizations (e.g., the Fédération Internationale de Gynécologie et d'Obstétrique classification systems for cervical, uterine and other gynaecological neoplasms), or institutions (e.g., the Royal Marsden Hospital staging classification for testicular germ cell tumours). A path of convergent evolution has been followed towards the tumour–node–metastasis (TNM system), which is espoused by the American Joint Committee on Cancer (AJCC) and the Union Internationale Contre le Cancer (UICC). The aims of a staging system are:

1 To allow rational selection of primary therapy and assessment of the necessity for adjuvant treatment.
2 To give some indication of likely prognosis.
3 To assist in evaluation of results of treatment.
4 To enable exchange of information between cancer treatment centres.
5 To contribute to the continuing investigation of human cancer.

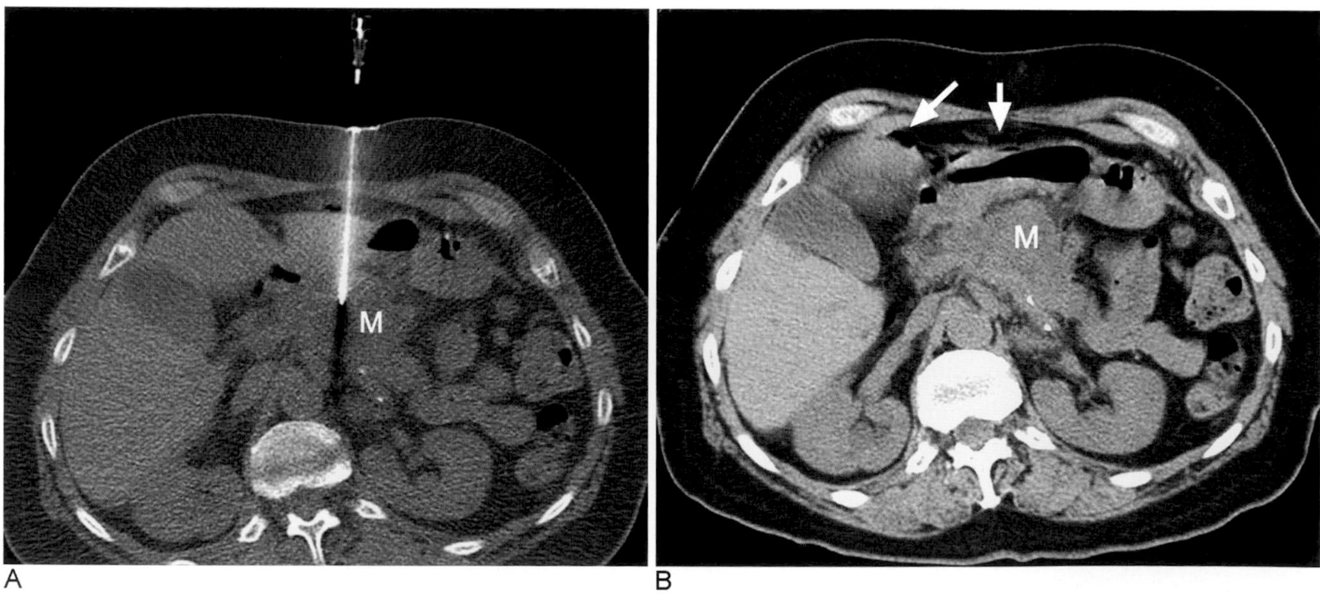

Figure 75.2 Coaxial system for biopsy. (A) A coaxial needle has been introduced into a pancreatic mass (M) through the gastric antrum. Dense artefact is present at the tip of the trocar. Once the trocar is withdrawn, an automatic cutting needle of appropriate length is introduced through the cannula left in situ, and multiple biopsies can be obtained by angling in a variety of directions. (B) Once the system is withdrawn, limited free gas is present outside the stomach (arrows). No clinical symptoms developed and the patient was discharged 6 hours after the procedure.

An ideal staging system should be internationally agreed and acknowledged, and applicable to all clinical circumstances in oncology. It should also be simple, precise and consistent and convey some prognostic information to facilitate best practice. The TNM system comes close to fulfilling these criteria, and is growing in influence. The TNM classification of malignant tumours and the AJCC cancer staging handbook are now in their sixth editions[1,2]. The system was originally devised by Pierre Denoix in the 1940s and, over the subsequent decades, it has been modified. Since the 1970s, imaging has become increasingly important in defining the anatomical extent of disease. The way in which imaging is used depends on the primary tumour and also the category being investigated.

'T' category entails evaluation of local tumour extent. 'N' category entails evaluation of nodal involvement. 'M' category entails evaluation of disease at distant sites. The 'T' category, which may have the prefix 'c' to indicate 'clinical' staging, although this is frequently omitted, has several standard forms of notation:

Tx indicates that primary tumour cannot be assessed.
Tis indicates in situ disease with no evidence of invasion.
T0 indicates no visible evidence of primary tumour.
T1–T4 indicates increasing degrees of local tumour extent.

These divisions may be adapted with the addition of subdivisions indicated by letters for greater flexibility in different tumour types. Although staging of the primary from T1 to T4 follows broad principles and there are some similarities between tumour types, refinements and adaptations for individual tumours are common, and the oncological radiologist would be unwise to try and remember all of the details. For this reason, the TNM classification of malignant tumours or similar publication should be an ever-present bench book.

The 'N' category has similar notation. Direct spread of primary tumour into an adjacent lymph node is classified as nodal spread. Nx is where regional lymph nodes cannot be assessed, N0 is where no regional lymph node metastases are present and N1, N2 and N3 indicate increasing involvement of regional lymph nodes. 'M' category assesses distant metastasis where Mx indicates that distant metastasis cannot be assessed, M0 indicates there are no distant metastases and M1 indicates the presence of distant metastasis. The category M1 may be further specified indicating which organs are involved. For example, PUL indicates pulmonary metastases, OSS indicates osseous metastases and HEP indicates hepatic metastases.

A number of general rules apply when using the clinical TNM staging system. Firstly, all tumours must be confirmed by microscopy. Clinical stage is assigned by physical examination, imaging and other relevant investigations, but may be amended as pathological information becomes available. If there is doubt what stage should be assigned, the lower category should be used. Therefore, an imaging investigation that is suspicious but not diagnostic of (for example) spread to the pelvic sidewall will be disregarded unless supplemented by further imaging or confirmation by histopathology. Once assigned, the pre-treatment TNM stage is recorded in the patient's records and remains unchanged through subsequent treatment. For multiple synchronous primary tumours, the tumour with the highest 'T' category is used for staging purposes. For synchronous primary tumours arising in paired organs, each tumour should be assigned a separate TNM stage.

In modern usage the TNM system has many advantages of clarity of communication, but it also has some disadvantages. Inconsistencies within the staging of certain tumours, such as Stage T1 carcinoma of the cervix, may be small but significant.

Some common tumours are still not routinely staged using the TNM system. Examples include Hodgkin's disease, which remains within the Cotswold modification of the Ann Arbor staging system; cutaneous melanomas are still staged using Clarke levels, although the TNM system has attempted to mimic Clarke levels with T-stage equivalents, and brain tumours are not staged within the TNM system. The complexity of the TNM system has led to a system of stage grouping, which is published within the AJCC system. Stage groups of 0–4 are assigned as tumour becomes more extensive and widespread.

It should also be remembered that the clinical TNM stage is modified in the light of pathological findings and given the prefix pTNM stage where microscopic extent of disease is known. The anatomical extent of disease on imaging is only one of the important pieces of information, and decision making at diagnosis is influenced by factors such as the histological grade of the tumour and its expected biological behaviour and the age and general fitness of the patient[3].

STAGING PRIMARY TUMOURS AT THE TIME OF DIAGNOSIS

Organizational aspects of cancer management

Health care provision in more economically developed countries has been a politically sensitive topic for many years. Following the Calman–Hine Report of 1995[4], the UK government published the NHS Cancer Plan in 2000[5]. Both publications are broad in their scope and draw attention to reduction of risk of cancer by discouraging smoking and improving diet. It is also suggested that screening programmes for colorectal, prostatic and ovarian cancer might be added to the existing screening programmes for breast and cervical cancer. A further aim is to reduce inequalities in cancer care on the basis of geography and social class. The NHS Cancer Plan, being a political document primarily, sets targets such as a maximum one-month interval between diagnosis and treatment for all cancers by the year 2005. An important organizational development suggested initially in the Calman–Hine Report is of the setting up of networks intended to deliver a uniform standard of high-quality care to all patients. Three levels at which care is delivered are proposed:

1 Primary Care Trusts are seen as the initial focus and are encouraged to plan strategic commissioning and provision of cancer services not just at the time of diagnosis but through to palliative care.

2 Designated cancer units should be created in district hospitals across the nation. These should be of a size to support clinical teams with sufficient expertise and facilities to manage common cancers.
3 Designated cancer centres should provide expertise in the management of all cancers including common cancers within their immediate locality and less common cancers by referral from cancer units. They will provide specialist diagnostic and therapeutic techniques including radiotherapy.

There are several aims implicit in the setting up of these networks. They should ensure that patients referred for management of their cancer will see specialists with experience in that disease. Multidisciplinary consultation and management are essential, and each cancer unit will have links to a cancer centre. Service delivery plans are prepared and conceived by the cancer networks as a whole. Peer reviews of cancer services are arranged to ensure uniformity of practice and service delivery. Although there will be some variations in patterns of practice, cancer units or cancer centres that use different methods of treatment should be expected to justify them on scientific or logistical grounds. Collection of cancer data by local and national registries has been formalized so that incidence, survival and mortality data can be compared. Over the past 10 years, networks were developed by the Cancer Services Collaborative and at the time of writing there are 41 established cancer networks in England and Wales.

One of the effects of the development of multidisciplinary teams is to place the radiologist at the heart of decision-making. There are few specialties that rely more heavily on imaging than oncology, and assessment of the anatomical extent of tumour at diagnosis forms the basis of many therapeutic decisions. For rational decision-making, all new presentations of cancer should be assessed at a multidisciplinary meeting and in busy cancer networks these can become large and prolonged. The time needed for preparation is considerable, and organizational aspects such as the ability to preview electronic or hard-copy images require investment in equipment as well as protected time. In the NHS Cancer Plan, it was acknowledged that there is a relative shortage of expertise in diagnostic specialties such as radiology and pathology, but these problems have yet to be fully addressed in the UK. However, the forum of the multidisciplinary meeting (MDM) gives the radiologist the opportunity to direct colleagues to using the most suitable investigation in a timely fashion at diagnosis and in follow-up.

Choice of staging investigations

To function optimally within the multidisciplinary team (MDT), the radiologist would benefit from in-depth knowledge of the biological behaviour of an individual tumour type. The interaction with clinical colleagues in decision-making can be an extremely useful way of furthering knowledge and understanding of disease processes and the time-honoured teaching maxim 'you see what you look for and you look for what you know' remains valid. A second facet of the radiologist's role is to understand available technology with which to investigate and detect tumour spread. However, it is not clear to what extent technology directly affects patient health, and a strategy has been devised for evaluating the chain of events that leads from an observer making an imaging report using data from a technique which may be innovative or unproven, through to its effect on patient care. Effectiveness of diagnostic imaging may be assessed at five levels[6]:

1 technical performance
2 diagnostic performance
3 diagnostic impact
4 therapeutic impact
5 impact on health.

Technical performance describes the facility to obtain high-quality images that will allow correct diagnostic interpretation.

Diagnostic performance assesses the ability of a technique to diagnose or stage tumour correctly. In the radiological literature, diagnostic performance is routinely measured in terms of sensitivity, specificity, positive predictive value (PPV) and negative predictive value (NPV), and accuracy of the technique summarizes the overall diagnostic performance. The decision to use one imaging technique for staging cancer is frequently based on information provided on diagnostic performance.

Diagnostic impact is determined by the influence of imaging on the physician's or surgeon's diagnostic confidence and whether a new technology will replace a previously established method. It may be easy to demonstrate diagnostic impact when a technique such as lymphangiography disappears altogether from oncological practice to be replaced by cross-sectional imaging.

Therapeutic impact reflects the alteration in management of a patient based on imaging results. This may also be easy to demonstrate, for example, when the demonstration of disseminated metastatic disease renders a surgical approach to the primary tumour inappropriate.

Impact on health may be more difficult to evaluate, and it can be argued that in some tumour types early diagnosis of metastatic disease has no positive impact on health as the diagnostic information is in advance of the ability to treat the disease effectively.

The way in which these levels interact informs the radiologist within the MDT and there are frequently complex factors to evaluate before imaging protocols are embedded in the framework for patient management for a specific tumour type. It is useful to illustrate principles of staging investigations with some examples of primary tumours.

Staging of rectal cancer

Rectal cancer is a good example of a tumour in which a staging system has evolved and changed over a period of more than 70 years, and technical refinement of surgery over the past 20 years has gone hand-in-hand with increasingly sophisticated imaging of the primary tumour such that imaging is now central to decision-making. It remains true that the vast majority of patients with rectal cancer should be offered surgery, as local symptoms due to growth within the pelvis are associated with severe pain that can be difficult to palliate. However, the timing of surgery and the role of neoadjuvant chemotherapy and radiotherapy depend on local tumour stage at the time of diagnosis. In 1932, Dukes highlighted the importance of extramural spread in the prediction of local recurrence and survival. He also observed that lymph node invasion was present in 14% of patients with tumours confined to the bowel wall and 43% of patients with tumours extending beyond the serosa[7]. A number of other prognostic indicators have subsequently been identified including the pattern of local spread (a well-circumscribed margin implies a better prognosis than a widely infiltrated tumour with ill-defined borders). Spread beyond the peritoneal membrane results in a high incidence of both local recurrence and transcoelomic dissemination; invasion of extramural veins by tumour and extent and number of tumour involved lymph nodes are all independent predictors of a poor prognosis. For many years the preferred operation for rectal cancer was synchronous combined abdominoperineal excision of rectum (known as AP resection). However, total mesorectal excision has become the gold standard since its introduction in the 1970s[8]. In this technique, the surgeon dissects from above and finds the mesorectal plane. As the lymphatic vessels and nodes draining the tumour are located throughout the mesorectum, if this is divided or disrupted during surgical excision, spillage of malignant cells may occur and involved nodes may be left in situ. This increases the likelihood of local recurrence, and excision of the rectum is best achieved by dissection down the mesorectal fascia allowing the mesorectum and rectum to be removed en bloc without disruption of the presacral fascia and the underlying venous plexus. The surgically excised specimen may then be sectioned transversely and the circumferential resection margin (CRM) examined for tumour involvement. The presence of tumour at the extremity of the resection margin is a major prognostic factor[9]. In recent years, MRI has been shown to be the investigation of choice in demonstrating spread of tumour within the mesorectum and the mesorectal plane itself (Figs 75.3, 75.4). It is possible to demonstrate the relationship of the tumour to the anal canal, indicating the potential for sphincter-preserving surgery (Fig. 75.5). Criteria have been developed in pathologically correlated series for staging of the primary tumour and nodes within the mesorectum. Effectively, MRI can provide a 'road map' for the surgeon and recent studies have shown that the pathological status of the CRM can be predicted[10,11]. Other prognostic factors such as extramural venous invasion and peritoneal penetration can be demonstrated. If locally advanced disease with mural penetration is demonstrated, chemotherapy and radiation therapy may be employed to downstage the primary prior to an attempt at surgery, allowing a more tailored preoperative strategy.

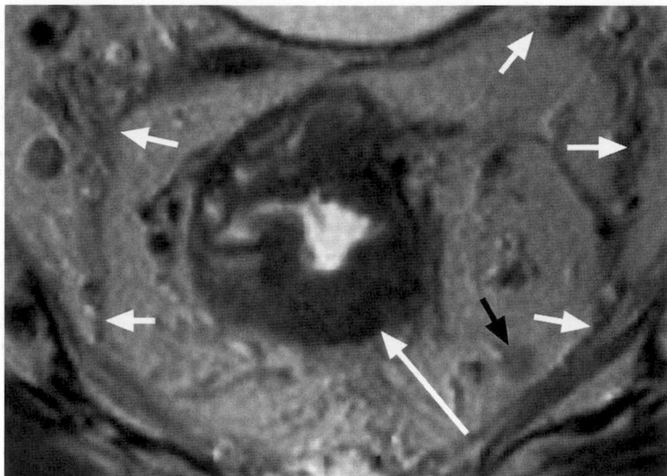

Figure 75.3 T2-weighted MRI through rectum. There is diffuse low-signal tumour in the rectal wall predominantly to the left of the midline with a well-circumscribed margin (long arrow). The mesorectal fascia is clearly demonstrated (short arrows). A small nodule of intermediate signal is demonstrated within the mesorectum (black arrow). However, there is no evidence of spread to the mesorectum. Subsequent total mesorectal excision demonstrated clear circumferential resection margin (CRM) with tumour confined to the rectal wall and reactive nodes only within the mesorectum.

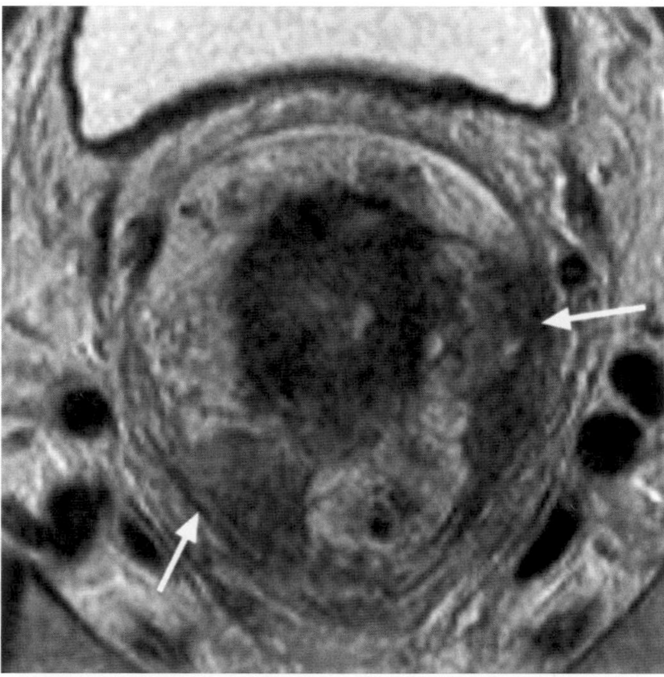

Figure 75.4 T2-weighted MRI of rectum in paraxial plane. There is an irregular tumour of the rectum obliterating normal mural anatomy. Further tumour is present within the mesorectum, extending up to the mesorectal fascia (arrows). The circumferential resection margin (CRM) would be tumour-involved, and neoadjuvant treatment with chemotherapy and radiotherapy may help to downstage the tumour prior to consideration of surgery.

Recent studies at our own institution have demonstrated that the incidence of tumour at the circumferential resection margin was 2% in patients diagnosed by MRI as likely to have a safe resection margin for immediate surgery. Overall incidence of positive resection margins in those patients seen by the MDT, including those who had undergone preoperative chemotherapy and radiotherapy for disease diagnosed by MRI to be locally advanced at initial presentation, was 8.5%. In a group of patients not assessed by the MDT, positive resection margins were present in 24%[12]. The implication is clear: all

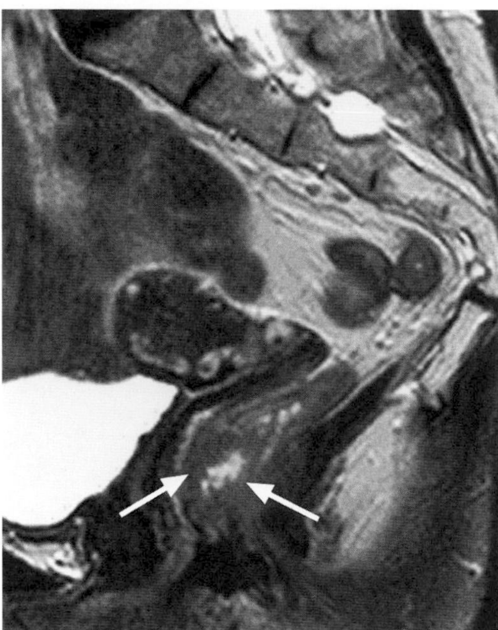

Figure 75.5 Sagittal MRI of a low rectal tumour. This demonstrates the tumour extending inferiorly into the anal sphincter (arrows). Sphincter preserving surgery and re-anastomosis will not be technically possible.

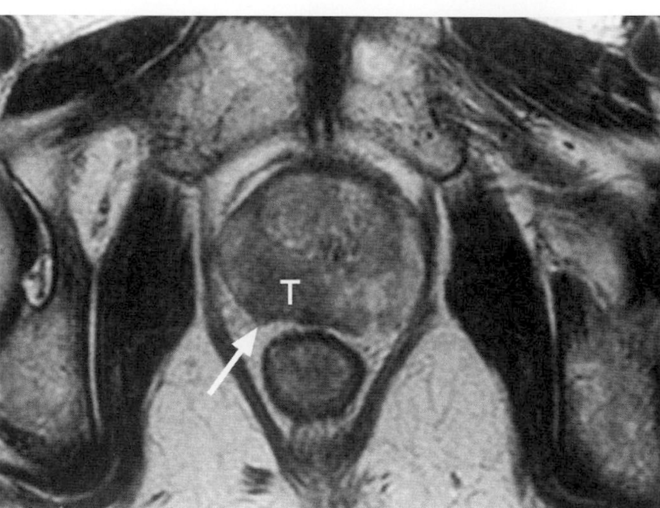

Figure 75.6 T2-weighted MRI of prostate. There is low-signal tumour (T) in the peripheral zone of the prostate. Tumour extends to the capsular margin (arrow) but there is no confirmatory evidence of extracapsular spread. Local staging by MRI criteria is T2.

patients newly diagnosed with rectal cancer should be assessed within the framework of a cancer network by a multidisciplinary team to ensure that up-to-date investigation and treatment is available.

Preoperative staging for distant disease is another facet that may be considered by the MDT. CT is usually employed to assess for retroperitoneal nodal disease and hepatic and pulmonary metastatic disease. However, CT is demonstrably less accurate for the staging of the primary rectal tumour. The presence of metastatic disease does not contraindicate surgery to the primary tumour, as local control is necessary for symptomatic relief. Small-volume metastatic disease in liver and lungs may also be amenable to surgery.

Staging of other pelvic cancers

MRI is particularly well-suited to staging pelvic neoplasms. The studies of the Radiologic Diagnostic Oncology Group (RDOG) demonstrated that for detection of extracapsular spread of prostate cancer, values of sensitivity and specificity were highest with MRI (Fig. 75.6). Endorectal ultrasound gave slightly lower sensitivity, specificity and overall accuracy than MRI, but both imaging techniques were an improvement on clinical staging[13,14]. There has also been considerable interest in the effect of endorectal coil imaging on staging accuracy. Two studies have been published of meta-analyses of the literature on staging prostate cancer and the effect of changing technology, including the use of endorectal MRI coils, and the results indicate a wide range of reported sensitivity and specificity. In prostate cancer, it is difficult to demonstrate a clear impact of high-technology imaging on patient health. One of the reasons for this is that the optimal treatment of prostate cancer remains controversial and the natural history of the disease is heterogeneous[15,16].

In the case of cervical cancer, imaging is not a formal part of the FIGO staging system, which is still widely employed, especially in Africa where the disease is extremely common. However, in the UK and USA cross-sectional techniques including CT and MRI are widely used, and MRI is recognized as a very valuable technique in the assessment of parametrial spread (Fig. 75.7)[17].

Staging of head and neck cancer

Tumours of the paranasal sinuses, nasopharynx and oral cavity present unique challenges to the radiologist and surgeon. Staging classifications of primary tumours are complex, with differences in the definition of T stages depending on which sinus or which part of the oral cavity is involved. It is an area of practice probably best left to experts, and one of the types of imaging where long, exhaustively detailed reports are justified. MRI and CT both have a role in staging these tumours. It is important to identify tumour margins and differentiate tumour from secretions, and to identify intracranial extension and bony and nodal involvement to help plan surgery or radiotherapy. The advantages of CT are that acquisition is fast and CT is more sensitive in the detection of bony destruction. However, CT is not as good as MRI in differentiating tumour from secretions and may, therefore, be limited in determining the full extent of tumour. It is also less effective than MRI in demonstrating perineural tumour and intracranial extension (Fig. 75.8). However, MRI may be degraded by movement artefact, particularly as patients with bulky pharyngeal or oral tumours may find it difficult not to swallow during the procedure. There has been considerable recent interest in positron emission tomography (PET) and PET/CT in the assessment of head and neck tumours, particularly for detecting nodal involvement (Fig. 75.9). The head and neck region contains numerous lymph nodes, and in patients without head and neck tumours these nodes are frequently visible. It would be a significant advantage if PET were able to discriminate reliably which nodes are likely to be tumour-involved[18].

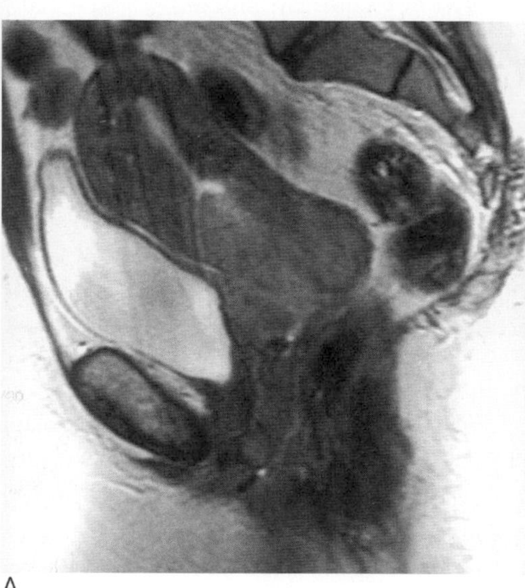
A

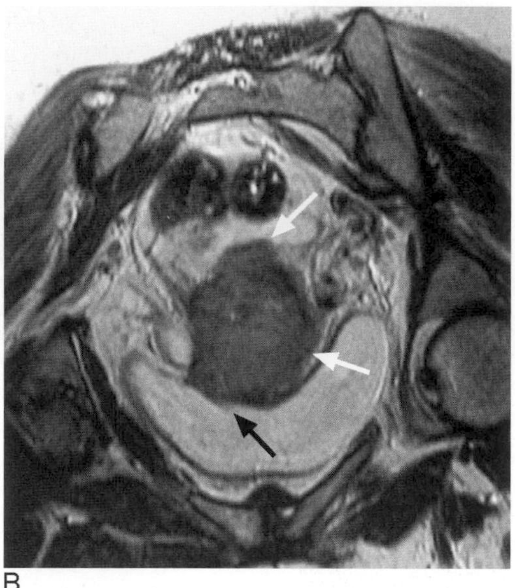
B

Figure 75.7 MRI of the pelvis. (A) T2-weighted sagittal image of the pelvis demonstrating a tumour of the cervix, disrupting the zonal anatomy of the cervix and extending cranially into the uterine cavity. (B) Paraxial T2-weighted MRI perpendicular to the long axis of the cervix. There is parametrial spread (arrows) with involvement of the posterior wall of the urinary bladder (black arrow).

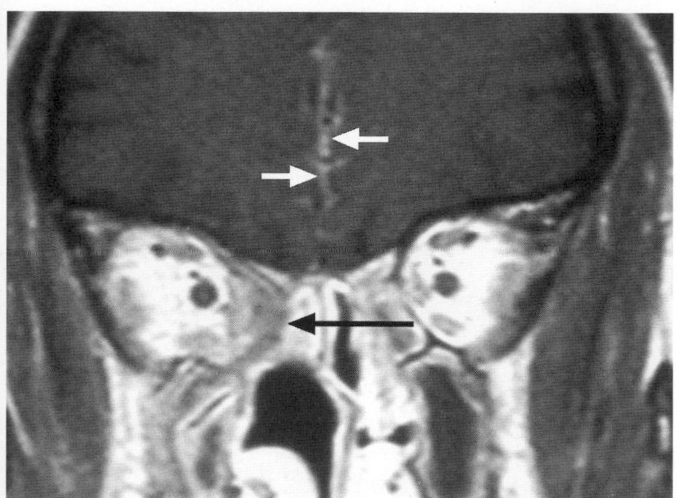

Figure 75.8 Coronal gadolinium-enhanced T1-weighted MRI of paranasal sinuses. Following surgery for rhabdomyosarcoma of the right maxillary antrum, tumour has recurred in the ethmoid region, invading the medial aspect of the right orbit (long arrow). There is also abnormal enhancement of the leptomeninges between the frontal lobes (short arrows) indicating parameningeal spread, most likely through the cribriform plate. This pattern of spread is relatively common in the clinical context of head and neck rhabdomyosarcoma.

Staging of breast cancer

Breast cancer is another disease where surgical techniques have undergone frequent revision, from the days of very radical surgery in the 1950s, to lumpectomy favoured in the 1970s and more recent regimens involving wide local excision or quadrantectomy followed by radiotherapy. Although many primary breast tumours can be staged by clinical examination, planning of local management may benefit from imaging. When multifocal disease is suspected or tumour is diffuse, contrast-enhanced MRI has very high sensitivity for lesion detection. However, specificity is lower as areas of gadolinium enhancement within the breast do not necessarily represent cancer. Ultrasound has the advantage of staging the primary tumour, detecting abnormal lymph nodes in the axilla and facilitating fine-needle aspiration for cytology if abnormal nodes are detected. The concept of sentinel-node detection prior to surgery also involves imaging. The principle is that the first lymph node in a nodal bed draining from a tumour will show metastatic disease if lymphatic spread has occurred. Absence of metastatic disease in a sentinel node in patients with breast cancer has been reported to have a negative predictive value for axillary nodal disease of 98%[19]. A combined technique using injected blue dye and an isotope, which is then localized by gamma camera imaging before surgery and with an intraoperative gamma probe during surgery, is usually recommended. However, the exact technique that should be used, and also the validity of the concept remain controversial. Once again, the MDT is a useful forum in which to debate the correct approach for an individual patient[20,21].

GUIDELINES ON STAGING INVESTIGATIONS

The brief examples above highlight the complexities of choosing the most appropriate imaging investigations. National

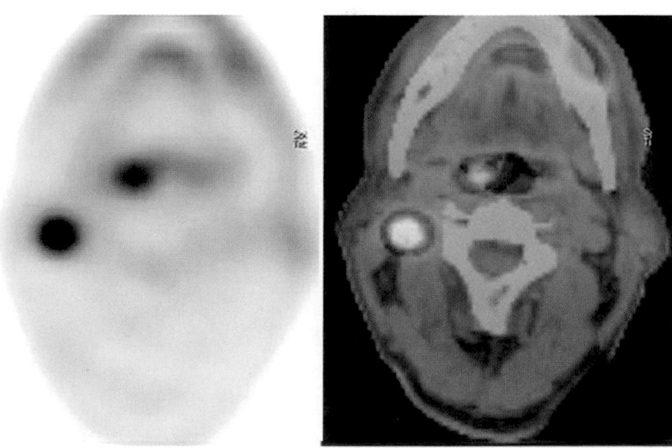

Figure 75.9 Computed tomography/positron emission tomography (PET/CT) of a patient presenting with an enlarged node in the right side of the neck showing increased uptake of ^{18}F-fluoro-deoxyglucose (^{18}F-FDG). There is also an area of increased uptake in the right side of the pharynx representing a primary squamous carcinoma, which was clinically occult.

bodies such as the Royal College of Radiologists have provided guidelines to assist in the choice of investigation. *'Making the Best Use of a Radiology Department'* has wide-ranging guidelines covering all aspects of radiology and has a section on oncological imaging. The 6th edition is in preparation at the time of writing, and the 5th edition (MBUR 5) makes recommendations for choices in common solid tumours[22]. The guidelines frequently give a choice of cross-sectional imaging techniques, recognizing that local availability and the preference and experience of individual radiologists is an important consideration. MBUR 5 has become a basis of guidelines adopted throughout Europe and the Royal College of Radiologists has also recently published recommendations on the use of CT, MRI and PET/CT in the imaging of malignancies[22–24].

STAGING FOR DISTANT DISEASE

Surveillance of asymptomatic patients

Following the diagnosis of a primary tumour decisions need to be made on how extensive the search for metastases should be, how it should be carried out and for how long imaging surveillance should continue. The approach differs between tumour types, and depends on the initial local (T) staging and tumour biology. Another factor to consider is whether there is a biochemical marker for the tumour, a rise in which would indicate the likelihood of a relapse that could subsequently be anatomically demonstrated by imaging. A good example of a tumour in which surveillance programmes are appropriate is nonseminomatous germ-cell tumours (NSGCT) of the testis. Following orchidectomy, CT staging of chest, abdomen and pelvis is usually undertaken. Seventy per cent of patients will be demonstrated to have no lymph node, pulmonary, or other metastatic spread and will subsequently not relapse. However, 30% of patients with a normal CT study at the time of orchidectomy will relapse: 80% of this group will relapse within 1 year and 95% will relapse within 2 years. Two thirds of these have a rise in tumour markers, but the remainder are marker-negative. Cytotoxic chemotherapy for relapse is effective with cure rates in excess of 90%. It is, therefore, justifiable to continue CT surveillance for 2 years, and at our Institution the follow-up examinations are performed at 3, 6, 9, 12, 18 and 24 months, although there is no definite evidence that follow-up imaging at six-monthly or even yearly intervals worsens prognosis. However, if large volume disease is allowed to develop, this has an adverse prognostic significance, so shortening the inter-examination interval empirically makes sense[25].

A further example where imaging is used to detect asymptomatic disease is colorectal carcinoma. Surgery in patients with resectable hepatic metastatic disease gives a 40% 5-year survival, compared with survival rates close to zero in untreated patients[26]. Current strategies now aim to reduce the volume of hepatic metastatic disease so that previously nonresectable disease may undergo surgery with curative intent[27]. There is growing evidence that intensive follow-up that incorporates monitoring of carcinoembryonic antigen (CEA) and CT of chest, abdomen and pelvis contributes to detection of metastatic disease in patients who subsequently proceed to potentially curative resection[28,29]. CT has adequate sensitivity for detection of hepatic and pulmonary metastases, but ultrasound and MRI have a role in characterizing liver lesions (Fig. 75.10). ^{18}F-fluoro-deoxyglucose positron emission tomography (^{18}F-FDG-PET) and PET/CT may prove to be valuable in early detection of metastatic disease, particularly in areas where CT alone lacks sensitivity such as the peritoneal cavity (Fig. 75.11). PET/CT is a valuable problem-solving technique when CEA is rising, and other imaging techniques fail to demonstrate the site of recurrence.

The frequency and duration of imaging follow-up is controversial, but is influenced by factors such as the T stage of the colorectal primary, histology and factors that help to predict relapse, such as positive CRM and vascular invasion. These principles may be applied to any tumour type, and should be influenced by the likelihood of detection of metastatic disease.

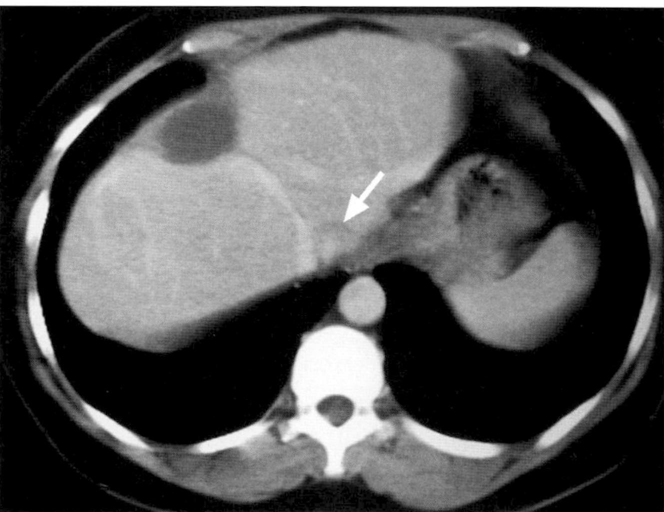

A

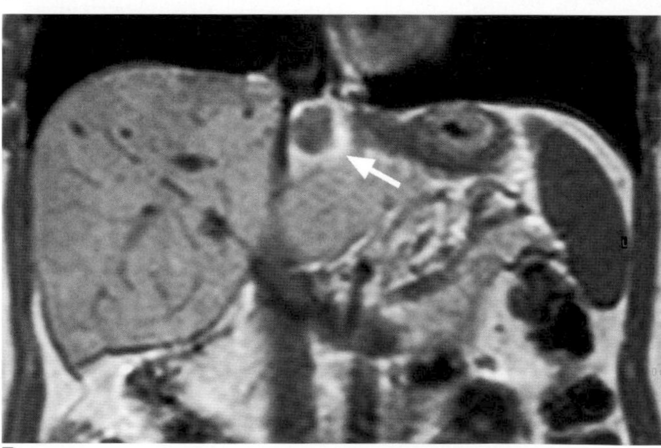

B

Figure 75.10 CT and MRI of a patient following hepatic metastasectomy. (A) Follow-up CT in a patient after hepatic metastasectomy (low-attenuation post-surgical defect shown anteriorly). There is an intermediate attenuation abnormality in the upper liver close to the diaphragmatic surface (arrow). (B) Further investigation with mangafodipir trisodium (Mn-DPDP)-enhanced liver imaging shows perilesional enhancement on T1-weighted MRI 24 hours after administration of the contrast agent. This appearance is typical of a metastasis (arrow).

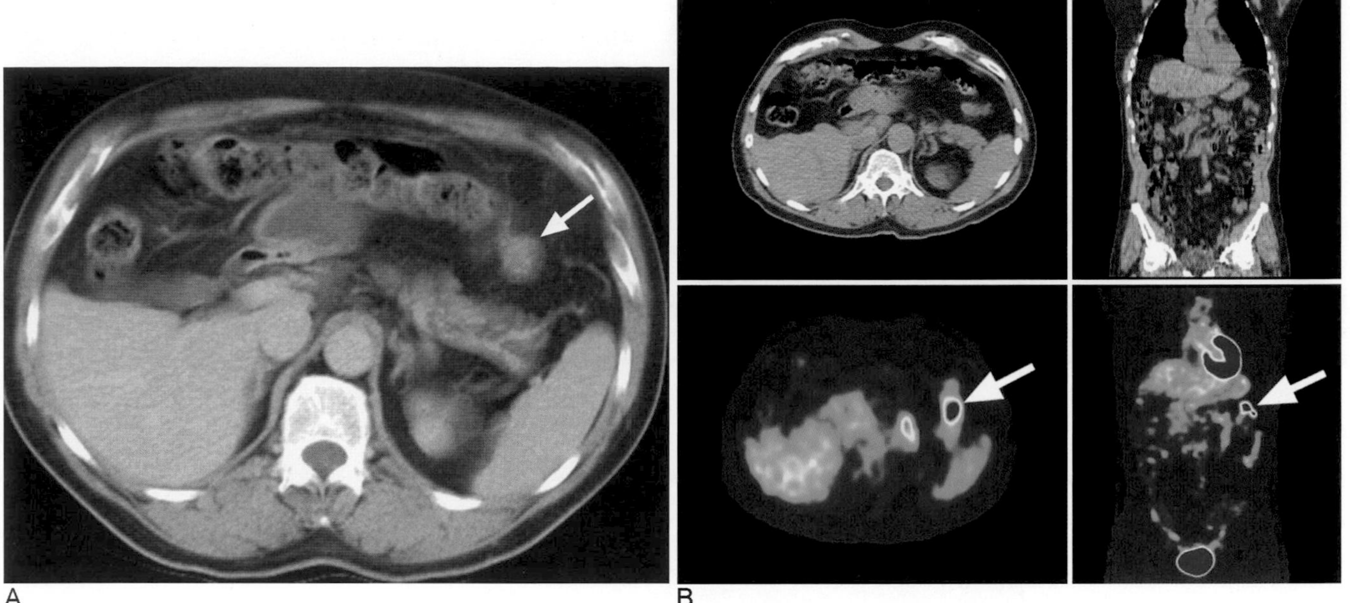

Figure 75.11 CT and PET/CT following resection of colonic carcinoma. (A) A year after resection of a colonic carcinoma, CT shows evidence of nodularity in the peritoneal surfaces of the left upper quadrant (arrow). (B) PET/CT demonstrates increased uptake in the left upper quadrant (arrow) confirming peritoneal recurrence.

Following treatment of primary breast cancer, there is considerable variation in practice. Some surgeons request chest radiography, liver ultrasound examination and radionuclide bone examination whereas others request whole body CT. In T1 and T2 primary tumours (less than 5 cm) the incidence of metastatic disease at the time of diagnosis is extremely low. In a series of almost 500 consecutive patients who were imaged at diagnosis with chest radiograph, liver ultrasound examination and radionuclide bone examination, no metastases were found in patients with T1 tumours. In patients with T4 tumours, the rate of detection of metastases was 8%. Overall, distant metastases were found at the time of primary diagnosis in 3.9% of patients[30]. However, there is limited evidence that detection of metastatic breast cancer in asymptomatic patients improves 5-year survival[31,32]. In testicular NSGCT, relapse is eminently treatable with cytotoxic chemotherapy. In colorectal cancer, surgery for metastatic disease is beneficial, but in breast cancer surveillance protocols are less useful, owing to the natural history of the disease. Such factors need to be considered for each individual tumour type before embarking on prolonged and costly investigation.

RESTAGING OF SYMPTOMATIC PATIENTS

Once a patient has been diagnosed with a malignant tumour it becomes the most important element of their medical history. Any prolonged or persistent complaint will usually precipitate a search for recurrence. Lethargy, fatigue and weight loss are frequent symptoms, but imaging investigation is easier to direct when there are localizing symptoms such as abdominal pain or distension, dyspnoea, bone pain, or a neurological event. The choice of investigation should be directed appropriately, for example, patients with abdominal pain should first be investigated with an ultrasound examination of the abdomen. A knowledge of the pattern of disease spread will assist choice and interpretation of investigations. With a history of colorectal cancer, hepatic pain from metastatic disease is likely, whereas ovarian tumours are more likely to disseminate through the peritoneal cavity, causing poorly localized abdominal pain and ascites.

Acute bone pain can be investigated with plain radiography, but more frequently radionuclide bone examinations are used. Most tumours can metastasize to bone, but breast, prostate, lung, kidney and thyroid do so particularly frequently. However, some metastases are not detectable by radionuclide bone examination, because of their failure to excite sufficient osteoblastic response. For example, in breast cancer 7% of patients with a normal skeletal scintigram have metastatic bone disease on MRI (Fig. 75.12)[33].

A neurological presentation, such as a convulsion in a patient with a previous diagnosis of cancer, is best investigated with CT or MRI of the brain. The cause of dyspnoea may be diagnosed using chest radiography. There is a trend towards whole-body imaging to search for metastases, and CT of the thorax, abdomen and pelvis is often requested without any real attempt to investigate the presenting symptom. Whole-body CT is a widely available test, but some authors have suggested whole-body PET or whole-body MRI using the short tau inversion recovery (STIR) sequence[34-35]. Potentially, the greatest disadvantage of whole-body imaging techniques is that they will generate false-positive findings, or diagnose recurrence for which treatment is not possible or not necessary. It should always be borne in mind when investigating symptoms in a patient with a history of cancer that the diagnosis of metastatic disease is a major blow for the patient, and the diagnosis should only be made when there is a high degree of certainty. The imaging findings should be consistent with the known patterns of metastatic spread for

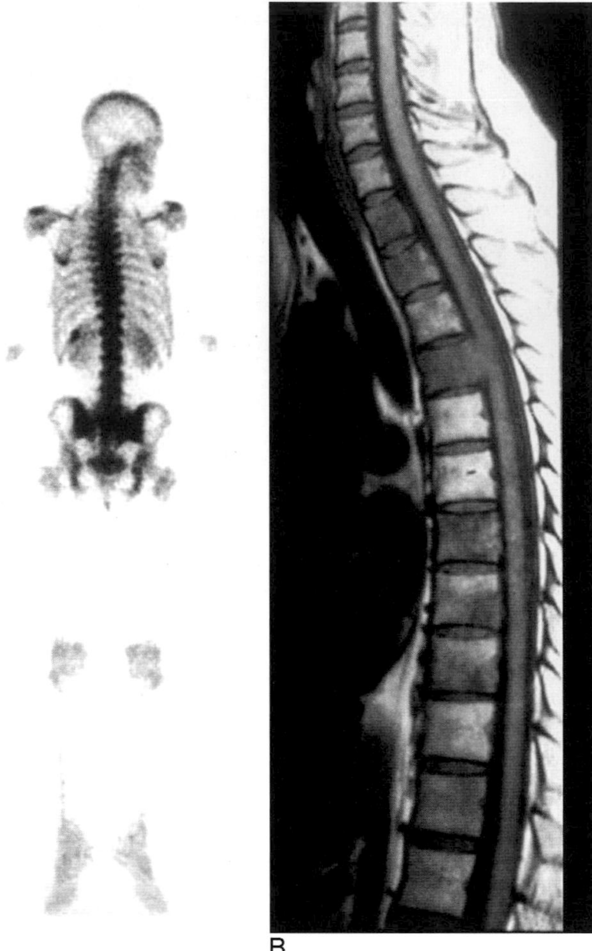

Figure 75.12 Patient previously diagnosed with breast cancer presenting with back pain. (A) Skeletal Scintigram. There are no focal areas of abnormal uptake in the skeleton. (B) T1-weighted sagittal MRI study of spine demonstrating multiple areas of low signal in the vertebral bodies consistent with bony metastases. Mechanical cord compression is threatened in the upper thoracic area. MRI was performed a week after scintigraphy.

the relevant tumour. If the imaging features are unconvincing or atypical, it is preferable to delay a positive finding of metastatic disease rather than to overdiagnose.

FOLLOW-UP IMAGING ON TREATMENT

General strategies for imaging

When disseminated disease is diagnosed according to the principles outlined above, it is likely that the patient will have systemic cytotoxic chemotherapy. It is important to have an evaluative framework, of which imaging forms an important part. Imaging investigations can demonstrate a reduction in tumour size, but this should be seen within the context of the patient's clinical well-being on toxic therapy and other factors such as biochemical tumour markers. In specialist cancer centres, the majority of patients are on clinical trials, which may stipulate the timing and technique of follow-up investigations. Even if the patient is not on a clinical trial, it is important to have some reproducible and objective technique that will allow directly comparable measurements to be made. For these reasons, CT is the most frequently used follow-up technique. Ultrasound and MRI can be used but, if MRI is employed, it is important to ensure that the same imaging protocol and sequences are used at each attendance. The frequency of follow-up investigations depends on the toxicity of treatment and the perceived likelihood of response. Physician preference is also a consideration, and it is noticeable that some clinicians adopt shorter follow-up intervals for similar treatment regimens. There is also some pressure from the pharmaceutical industry to document reduction in tumour bulk. Overall survival rate remains the best objective parameter of efficacy of treatment, but demonstration of some form of objective response earlier in the course of disease encourages development of certain medications.

Measurements

Effective systemic chemotherapy and cross-sectional imaging developed side by side during the 1970s, and it became clear that a common language and definition of guidelines for the assessment of objective tumour response was necessary. The World Health Organization (WHO) proposed the system that remains in widespread use today[36-37]. Miller et al[37] recommended that a partial response should be designated when bi-dimensional measurement of a single lesion shows greater than 50% reduction in cross-sectional area (perpendicular diameters should be measured). Separate categories are available where one-dimensional measurements only are obtainable, but no consideration is given to calculation of tumour volumes. It also states that objective response can be determined clinically, radiologically, biochemically or by surgical/pathological re-staging. The WHO criteria remain useful but more recently an attempt has been made to simplify and standardize methods. The response evaluation criteria in solid tumours (RECIST) were proposed by the European Organization for Research and Treatment of Cancer (EORTC) in collaboration with the National Cancer Institute (NCI) in the USA and the National Cancer Institute of Canada Clinical Trials Group[38].

The RECIST criteria allow one-dimensional measurement of target lesions and the sum of these is used rather than the product of two perpendicular linear measurements. A partial response is defined of at least a 30% decrease in the sum of the longest diameter of target lesions, taking as a reference the baseline sum of longest diameters (Table 75.1). The aim of the RECIST criteria was to simplify the way in which information is gathered and recorded, and not necessarily to increase precision. The fundamental problem of observer variability and subjectivity remains. It is still the responsibility of an investigator to select lesions for measurement, but one of the important recommendations of the RECIST Group was that results of trials claiming response by measurement should be validated by an independent review committee. Having participated in such committees, it is the opinion of the author that it is the experience and objectivity of the observer/investigator that remains the main source of variation in reporting trials rather than the response evaluation criteria used.

Table 75.1 DEFINITION OF OBJECTIVE RESPONSE ACCORDING TO THE WHO* AND RECIST* CRITERIA

	WHO	RECIST
Response	Change in the sum of the products of the two longest perpendicular diameters	Modification of the sum of the longest diameter of each target
Complete response	Disappearance of all target lesions with no residual lesion, confirmed at 4 weeks	Disappearance of all target lesions, confirmed at 4 weeks
Partial response	50% or more decrease in tumour load (single or multiple lesions) without a 25% increase in the size of any measurable lesion, confirmed at 4 weeks	30% or more decrease in the sum of the longest diameter(s) of target lesions, taking as reference the baseline sum of the longest diameter(s), confirmed at 4 weeks
Stable disease	Absence of criteria of partial response or progressive disease	Absence of criteria of partial response or progressive disease
Progressive disease	At least a 25% increase in size of measurable lesions or appearance of new lesions	At least a 20% increase in the sum of the longest diameter of target lesions, taking as reference the smallest sum of the longest diameter(s) recorded since the treatment started, or the appearance of one or more new lesions

*RECIST = Response evaluation criteria in solid tumours; WHO = World Health Organization.

Anatomical measurement criteria fail to take account of functional changes within tumour. Likewise cyst formation and necrosis within tumours cannot be assessed by size criteria alone. It remains important to assess size alterations within the context of the clinical state of the patient and the natural history of the disease.

Imaging residual masses

A post-treatment residuum is frequently seen in several solid tumours, such as lung cancer, lymphoma and metastatic NSGCT. A wide variety of imaging techniques have been used in an attempt to predict the likelihood of recurrence in these residual masses. Investigation has been most intensive in lymphoma. Enlargement of a residual mass on CT is strong evidence of disease recurrence, but it is hoped that it will be possible to identify residual or recurrent disease earlier using functional techniques. Radionuclide imaging with Gallium-67 has been used, and there is good evidence of a high sensitivity for ^{18}FDG-PET in detection of residual disease. There are theoretical reasons for using PET as a routine surveillance procedure following treatment. However, at the time of writing, there is no clear evidence to support this strategy.

MRI has also been evaluated in the investigation of residual lymphoma masses. Reduction in signal intensity on T2-weighted images during treatment is taken as a sign of successful treatment, leaving a fibrotic residuum. However, MRI has not become a routine investigation because of high false-negative and false-positive rates. Patient populations can be classified into groups at low- or high-risk for relapse[39]. Imaging features suggestive of residual disease may help to select patients for repeat biopsy or further treatment, for example, with adjuvant radiotherapy. However, as treated cancer can leave abnormal tissue detectable by imaging, imaging alone is unreliable in predicting the pathological nature of the residuum.

IMAGING OF TREATMENT TOXICITY

Radiotherapy and/or chemotherapy can affect all tissues of the body. Imaging features and the timing of their appearance vary from organ to organ. Radiotherapy causes acute change by a direct physical inflammatory process and later effects as a result of an ischaemic insult. Anticancer drugs have direct cytotoxic effects, but may also cause hypersensitivity reactions. Some organs are more susceptible to tissue damage than others, although observed imaging changes are not always of clinical importance. Interpretation is facilitated by a knowledge of the type and timing of treatment.

Lung

A radiological diagnosis of radiation pneumonitis is made when there is evidence of acute radiotherapy change in the lungs, but this is always accompanied by clinical symptoms. Radiation pneumonitis usually appears 6–8 weeks after completion of treatment with 35–40 Gy, but is not generally seen at radiation doses below 30 Gy. It is almost always seen at doses over 40 Gy and will appear earlier than 6 weeks. It becomes most extensive 3–4 months after completion of radiotherapy. The histological appearance is of diffuse alveolar damage. At a later stage, an organizing fibrosis develops, which becomes complete 9–12 months after termination of therapy. The histological appearances are non-specific, but the distinguishing feature on plain film radiography and CT is a straight edge corresponding to a radiation field. When there is significant volume loss, traction effects occur and there may be bronchiectatic changes.

Neoadjuvant cytotoxic chemotherapy enhances the effect of radiation causing earlier radiation pneumonitis and more severe fibrosis. Drugs most commonly implicated include dactinomycin, doxorubicin, bleomycin, cyclophosphamide, mitomycin and vincristine. There is a growing list of cytotoxic drugs that are recognized to cause pulmonary parenchymal damage independent of radiation therapy. Bleomycin is used in the treatment of NSGCT, lymphoma and squamous cell carcinoma. The toxic effect is dose-dependent and exacerbated by the use of other agents in combination chemotherapy, adjuvant radiation therapy and oxygen therapy. Early radiographic abnormality is typically a reticular nodular pattern of interstitial disease, which is most severe in the basal segments. Lung damage may be progressive, leading to pulmonary fibrosis, which may be severe and cause traction pneumothorax and pneumomediastinum (Fig. 75.13).

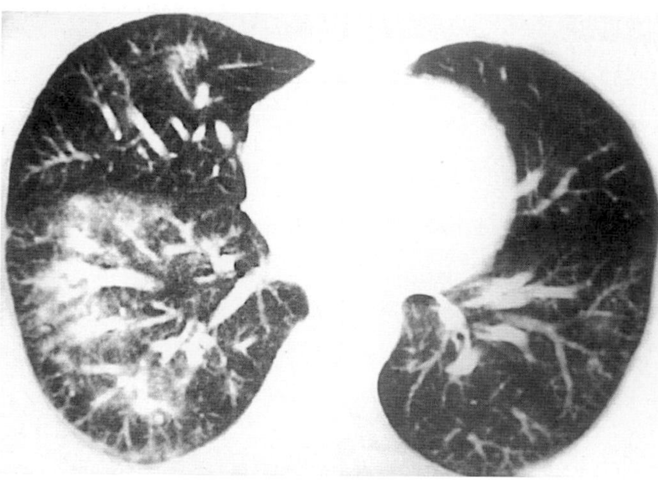

Figure 75.13 CT of acute bleomycin toxicity. This shows widespread predominantly basal interstitial change.

Busulfan, which is used in haematological malignancy, causes interstitial lung damage. Methotrexate is responsible for a hypersensitivity reaction, which results in alveolar shadowing and sometimes in mediastinal adenopathy. If methotrexate therapy is prolonged, the lung damage may progress to fibrosis. Treatment related lung toxicity can usually be seen on plain radiography, but CT is more sensitive[40-41].

Bone and bone marrow

Osseous changes in response to radiation were first described by Ewing as long ago as the 1920s. Local demineralization and osteopenia are the earliest and often the only post-radiation changes noted on plain radiography. Later changes include mixed lytic and sclerotic areas and trabecular coarsening, which may develop 2 or more years after radiotherapy. Spontaneous fractures and aseptic necrosis can occur, but, in general, radiation damage to bone is becoming less common as a result of high-energy mega-voltage radiotherapy and more accurate dose distribution. However, the effect on bone marrow is frequently seen on MRI at relatively low doses, from 15–20 Gy. Haemopoietic bone marrow converts to fatty marrow, resulting in a high signal on T1-weighted sequences. Following treatment of metastatic bone disease or primary bone tumour with radiotherapy or chemotherapy, the marrow can take on a bizarre appearance on MRI that is virtually uninterpretable. For example, following treatment of lymphoma or neuroblastoma diffusely involving the bone marrow, the latter will usually alter its appearance, sometimes reverting to normal, but often leaving an array of mixed residual signal changes (Fig. 75.14).

Neurotoxicity

Therapeutic radiation to the brain induces an ischaemic insult, which is manifested as abnormality within the deep cerebral white matter. This is best demonstrated by MRI, where diffuse high signal is present on T2-weighted images or using the fluid attenuation inversion recovery (FLAIR) sequence. Similar changes may be seen within the spinal cord as a result of radiation myelitis. White matter changes may also be identified with cytotoxic medications (Fig. 75.15) including fluorouracil,

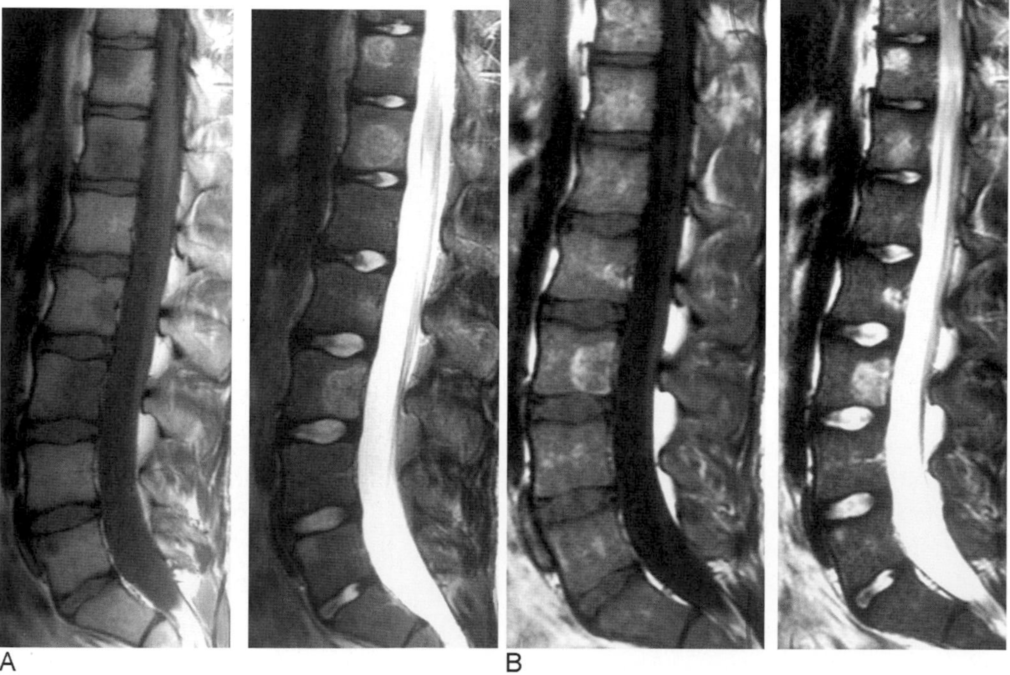

Figure 75.14 Lymphoma of lumbar spine pre- and post-treatment. (A) Sagittal MRI of lumbar spine showing lymphoma in bone marrow. On T1-weighted sequence (left) low signal is returned from the marrow cavity of T11/12 and L2, 3 and 5. Corresponding focal areas of high signal are identified on the T2-weighted sequence (right). Uptake of ^{18}F-fluoro-deoxyglucose (^{18}F-FDG) on PET was increased in these vertebrae. (B) Following chemotherapy, the T1-weighted sequence (left) shows a generalized increase of signal in the marrow cavities and focal high signal corresponding to previous tumour involved areas. The signal is also increased on T2-weighted imaging (right) at these sites, although uptake of ^{18}F-FDG was normal. Although clearly abnormal, this MRI appearance was interpreted as successful treatment of lymphoma, and the patient remains disease-free 12 months after completion of therapy.

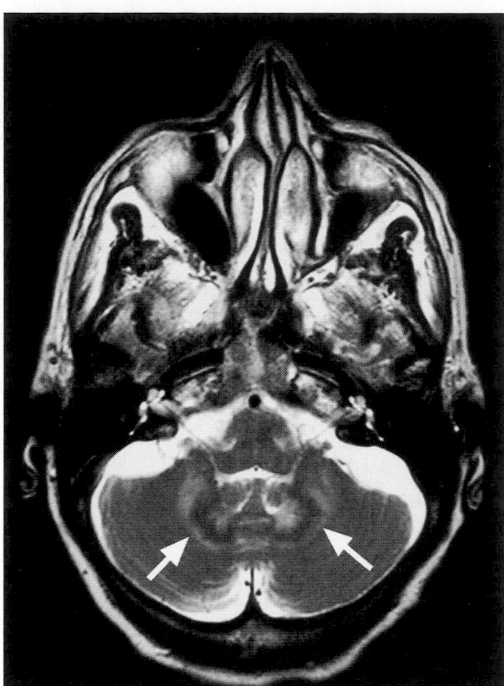

Figure 75.15 T2-weighted MRI of posterior fossa. This shows diffuse high signal in cerebellum (arrows) following treatment with fluorouracil.

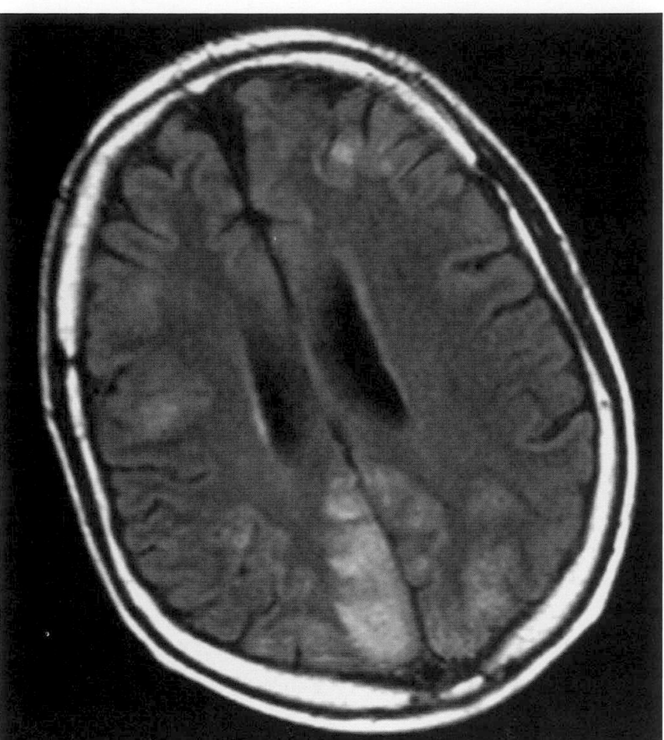

Figure 75.16 MRI axial fluid attenuation inversion recovery sequence. This shows high signal in the parafalcine posterior grey and white matter with isolated areas of abnormal signal in both frontal lobes. This appearance is typical of the reversible posterior leukoencephalopathy syndrome seen following bone marrow transplantation, frequently attributed to toxicity from cyclosporine.

levamisole and intrathecal methotrexate. As with lung toxicity, a growing number of cytotoxic agents has been implicated in central neurotoxic events. Following bone marrow transplantation, immunosuppressive drugs, including cyclosporine, cause a reversible posterior leukoencephalopathy syndrome (RPLS), which has a characteristic distribution of grey and white matter change (Fig. 75.16).

Peripheral neuropathy is common with cytotoxic agents such as vincristine, but has no imaging features. However, radiation damage to the brachial plexus is occasionally encountered following treatment for breast cancer. This is due to an ischaemic insult to the vasa nervorum of the brachial plexus. Thickening of the elements of the brachial plexus within the radiation field is seen on MRI (Fig. 75.17). This is difficult to distinguish from the infiltrative forms of recurrent breast cancer. However, if there is no mass lesion, and if appropriate symptoms and clinical signs are present, MRI is an accurate way of diagnosing radiation induced brachial plexopathy[42].

Hepatic toxicity

Many cytotoxic chemotherapy regimens induce abnormality of liver function. The change most frequently observed on imaging is hepatic steatosis. This may be reversible even if treatment is continued, which can be a source of confusion as contrast parameters within the liver in the presence of metastases can alter radically between examinations interval. It is, therefore, important to continue using the same imaging protocols throughout the treatment regimen.

Cardiotoxicity

Radiation to the thorax may cause acute and chronic pericarditis, cardiomyopathy and, in the long term, coronary artery

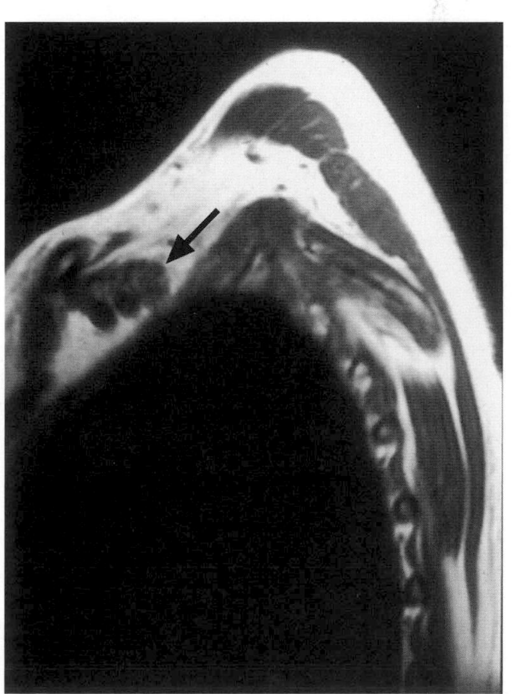

Figure 75.17 T1-weighted sagittal MRI. This shows thickening of the cords of the brachial plexus (arrow) as a result of radiation therapy. The patient had symptomatic brachial plexopathy, which has remained stable over several years.

disease and valvular dysfunction. A more frequent problem for the cancer patient is cardiotoxicity from cytotoxic agents; for example, doxorubicin is known to cause some degree of myocardial dysfunction in 50% of asymptomatic patients. In extreme cases, life-threatening congestive cardiac failure can develop. Circulatory problems may also develop due to fluid overload during hyper-hydration, which is necessary in a number of treatment regimens. Agents such as asparaginase can precipitate abnormalities of coagulation, resulting in venous thrombosis.

CONCLUSION

Oncological radiology demands a sound knowledge of anatomy and understanding of patterns of spread and biological behaviour of individual tumour types. In these respects it is similar to other imaging specialities, but there are also many toxic effects of treatment and associated conditions, which must be discriminated from manifestations of the underlying malignancy. An accurate clinical history and a high level of multidisciplinary cooperation greatly enhance the practice of oncological radiology.

ACKNOWLEDGEMENTS

I would like to acknowledge my colleagues Dr Dow-Mu Koh, Dr Bhuey Sharma and Dr Aslam Sohaib for supplying some figures, and Mrs Janet Macdonald and Mrs Maureen Watts for their help in the preparation of the images and manuscript.

REFERENCES

1. Sobin L, Wittekind C (eds) 2002 UICC: TNM Classification of Malignant Tumours, 6th edn. John Wiley & Sons, New York
2. Greene F L, Page D L, Balch C M et al (eds) 2002 AJCC: Cancer Staging Manual, 6th edn. Springer-Verlag, New York
3. Gospodarowicz M K, Henson D E, Hutter R V P, O'Sullivan B, Sobin L H, Wittekind C H (eds) 2001 Union Internationale Contre le Cancer (UICC): Prognostic factors in cancer, 2nd edn. Wiley New York
4. Calman K, Hine D 1999 Calman-Hine Report. A Policy Framework for Commissioning Cancer Services: A Report by the Expert Advisory Group on Cancer to the Chief Medical Officers of England and Wales. April 1995. Available: www.dh.gov.uk
5. Dept of Health 2000 The NHS Cancer Plan: a plan for investment, a plan for reform. Available: www.dh.gov.uk
6. Mackenzie R, Dixon A K 1995 Measuring the effects of imaging: an evaluative framework. Clin Radiol 50: 513–518
7. Dukes C E 1932 The classification of cancer of the rectum. J Path Bact 35: 323
8. Heald R J 1995 Total mesorectal excision is optimal surgery for rectal cancer: A Scandinavian consensus. Br J Surg 82: 1297–1299
9. Quirke P, Durdey P, Dixon M F et al 1986 Local recurrence of rectal adenocarcinoma due to inadequate surgical resection. Histopathological study of lateral tumour spread and surgical excision. Lancet 2: 996–999
10. Beets-Tan R G, Beets G L, Vliegen R F et al 2001 Accuracy of magnetic resonance imaging in prediction of tumour-free resection margin in rectal cancer surgery. Lancet 357: 497–504
11. Brown G, Radcliffe A G, Newcombe R G et al 2003 Preoperative assessment of prognostic factors in rectal cancer using high-resolution magnetic resonance imaging. Br J Surg 90: 355–364
12. Burton S, Brown G, Daniels I R 2006 MRI directed multidisciplinary team preoperative treatment strategy: the way to eliminate positive circumferential margins? Br J Cancer 94: 351–357
13. Rifkin M D, Zerhouni E A, Gatsonis C A et al 1990 Comparison of magnetic resonance imaging and ultrasonography in staging of early prostate cancer. Results of a multi-institutional cooperative trial. N Engl J Med 323: 621–626
14. Tempany C M, Zhou X, Zerhouni E A et al 1994 Staging of prostate cancer: results of Radiology Diagnostic Oncology Group project comparison of three MR imaging techniques. Radiology 192: 47–54
15. Sonnad S S, Langlotz C P, Schwartz J S 2001 Accuracy of MR imaging for staging prostate cancer: a meta-analysis to examine the effect of technologic change. Acad Radiol 8: 149–157
16. Engelbrecht M R, Jager G J, Laheij R J 2002 Local staging of prostate cancer using magnetic resonance imaging: a meta-analysis. Eur Radiol 12: 2294–2302
17. Hawnaur J M, Johnson R J, Buckley C H et al 1994 Staging, volume estimation and assessment of nodal status in carcinoma of the cervix: comparison of magnetic resonance imaging with surgical findings. Clin Radiol 49: 443–452
18. Halfpenny W, Hain S F, Biassoni L et al 2002 FDG-PET. A possible prognostic factor in head and neck cancer. Br J Cancer 86: 512–516
19. Turner R R, Ollila D W, Krasne D L et al 1997 Histopathologic validation of sentinel lymph node hypothesis for breast carcinoma. Ann Surg 226: 271–278
20. Albertini J J, Lyman G H, Cox C et al 1996 Lymphatic mapping and sentinel node biopsy in the patient with breast cancer. J Am Med Assoc 276: 1818–1822
21. Querci della Rovere G, Bird P A 1998 Sentinel-lymph-node biopsy in breast cancer. Lancet 352: 421–422
22. Royal College of Radiologists 2003 Making the Best Use of a Department of Clinical Radiology. Guidelines for Doctors, 5th edn. Ref: BFCR(03)3. Royal College of Radiologists, London
23. European Guidelines for Radiological Investigations. Online: http://ec.europa.eu/energy/nuclear/radioprotection/publication/118_en.pdf
24. The Royal College of Radiologists 2006 Recommendations for Cross-Sectional Imaging in Cancer Management. Ref:RCR(06)1, The Royal College of Radiologists, London
25. MacVicar D 1993 Staging of testicular germ cell tumours. Clin Radiol 47: 149–158
26. Choti M A, Sitzmann J V, Tiburi M F et al 2002 Trends in long-term survival following liver resection for hepatic colorectal metastases. Ann Surg 235: 759–766
27. Shankar A, Leonard P, Renaut A J et al 2001 Neo-adjuvant therapy improves resectability rates for colorectal liver metastases. Ann R Coll Surg Engl 83: 85–88
28. Renehan A G, Egger M, Saunders M P et al 2002 Impact on survival of intensive follow up after curative resection for colorectal cancer: systematic review and meta-analysis of randomised trials. BMJ 324: 813
29. Chau I, Allen M J, Cunningham D et al 2004 The value of routine serum carcino-embryonic antigen measurement and computed tomography in the surveillance of patients after adjuvant chemotherapy for colorectal cancer. J Clin Oncol 22: 1420–1429
30. Schneider C, Fehr M K, Steiner R A et al 2003 Frequency and distribution pattern of distant metastases in breast cancer patients at the time of primary presentation. Arch Gynecol Obstet 269: 9–12
31. Yeh K A, Fortunato L, Ridge J A et al 1995 Routine bone scanning in patients with T1 and T2 breast cancer: a waste of money. Ann Surg Oncol 2: 319–324
32. Miller K D, Weathers T, Haney L G et al 2003 Occult central nervous system involvement in patients with metastatic breast cancer: prevalence, predictive factors and impact on overall survival. Ann Oncol 14: 1072–1077

33. Jones A L, Williams M P, Powles T J et al 1990 Magnetic resonance imaging in the detection of skeletal metastases in patients with breast cancer. Br J Cancer 62: 296–298
34. Rostom A Y, Powe J, Kandil A et al 1999 Positron emission tomography in breast cancer: a clinicopathological correlation of results. Br J Radiol 72: 1064–1068
35. Walker R, Kessar P, Blanchard R et al 2000 Turbo STIR magnetic resonance imaging as a whole-body screening tool for metastases in patients with breast carcinoma: preliminary clinical experience. J Magn Reson Imaging 11: 343–350.
36. World Health Organization 1979 WHO Handbook for Reporting Results of Cancer Treatment. World Health Organization, Geneva, Switzerland, 48
37. Miller A B, Hoogstraten B, Staquet M et al 1981 Reporting results of cancer treatment. Cancer 47: 207–214
38. Therasse P, Arbuck S G, Eisenhauer E A et al 2000 New guidelines to evaluate the response to treatment in solid tumors. European Organization for Research and Treatment of Cancer, National Cancer Institute of the United States, National Cancer Institute of Canada. Natl Cancer Inst 92: 205–216
39. Hill M, Cunningham D, MacVicar D et al 1993 Role of magnetic resonance imaging in predicting relapse in residual masses after treatment of lymphoma. J Clin Oncol 11: 2273–2278
40. Morrison D A, Goldman A L 1979 Radiographic patterns of drug-induced lung diseases. Radiology 131: 299–304
41. Libshitz H I, Shuman L S 1984 Radiation-induced pulmonary change: CT findings. J Comput Assist Tomogr 8: 15–19
42. Qayyum A, MacVicar A D, Padhani A R et al 2000 Symptomatic brachial plexopathy following treatment for breast cancer: utility of MR imaging with surface-coil techniques. Radiology 214: 837–842

Index

Alphabetization is word-by-word.
Page numbers followed by 't' refer to tables.
Page numbers in italic refer to figures.